MW01204098

Principles and Practice of
Palliative Care *and*
Supportive Oncology

FIFTH EDITION

EDITORS

Ann M. Berger, MSN, MD

Pain and Palliative Care
Bethesda, Maryland

Joseph F. O'Neill, MD, MS, MPH

Pain and Palliative Care
Bethesda, Maryland

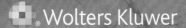 Wolters Kluwer

Philadelphia • Baltimore • New York • London
Buenos Aires • Hong Kong • Sydney • Tokyo

Acquisitions Editor: Nicole Dernoski
Development Editor: Sean McGuire
Editorial Coordinator: Linda Christina
Marketing Manager: Julie Sikora
Production Project Manager: Bridgett Dougherty
Design Coordinator: Larry Pezzato
Manufacturing Coordinator: Beth Welsh
Prepress Vendor: SPi Global

Fifth Edition

Copyright © 2022 Wolters Kluwer

4th Edition Copyright © Lippincott Williams & Wilkins, a Wolters Kluwer business, 2013; 3rd Edition Copyright © Lippincott Williams & Wilkins, 2007; 2nd Edition Copyright © 2002 by Lippincott Williams & Wilkins; 1st Edition Copyright © 1998 by Lippincott-Raven Publishers. All rights reserved. This book is protected by copyright. No part of this book may be reproduced or transmitted in any form or by any means, including as photocopies or scanned-in or other electronic copies, or utilized by any information storage and retrieval system without written permission from the copyright owner, except for brief quotations embodied in critical articles and reviews. Materials appearing in this book prepared by individuals as part of their official duties as U.S. government employees are not covered by the above-mentioned copyright. To request permission, please contact Wolters Kluwer at Two Commerce Square, 2001 Market Street, Philadelphia, PA 19103, via email at permissions@lww.com, or via our website at shop.lww.com (products and services).

9 8 7 6 5 4 3 2 1

Printed in China

Cataloging-in-Publication Data available on request from the Publisher

ISBN: 978-1-9751-4368-8

This work is provided "as is," and the publisher disclaims any and all warranties, express or implied, including any warranties as to accuracy, comprehensiveness, or currency of the content of this work.

This work is no substitute for individual patient assessment based upon healthcare professionals' examination of each patient and consideration of, among other things, age, weight, gender, current or prior medical conditions, medication history, laboratory data and other factors unique to the patient. The publisher does not provide medical advice or guidance and this work is merely a reference tool. Healthcare professionals, and not the publisher, are solely responsible for the use of this work including all medical judgments and for any resulting diagnosis and treatments.

Given continuous, rapid advances in medical science and health information, independent professional verification of medical diagnoses, indications, appropriate pharmaceutical selections and dosages, and treatment options should be made and healthcare professionals should consult a variety of sources. When prescribing medication, healthcare professionals are advised to consult the product information sheet (the manufacturer's package insert) accompanying each drug to verify, among other things, conditions of use, warnings and side effects and identify any changes in dosage schedule or contraindications, particularly if the medication to be administered is new, infrequently used or has a narrow therapeutic range. To the maximum extent permitted under applicable law, no responsibility is assumed by the publisher for any injury and/or damage to persons or property, as a matter of products liability, negligence law or otherwise, or from any reference to or use by any person of this work.

shop.lww.com

To our spouses and children, whose love and support make our work possible:

Carl, Stephen, and Rebecca Berger
Walter Atha

CONTRIBUTING AUTHORS

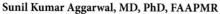

Sunil Kumar Aggarwal, MD, PhD, FAAPMR
Codirector
AIMS Institute
Affiliate Assistant Professor of Medicine and
    Geography
University of Washington
Seattle, Washington

Alyx Rosen Aigen, MD
Assistant Professor
Dr. Phillip Frost Department of Dermatology and
    Cutaneous Surgery
University of Miami Miller School of
    Medicine
Director of Dermatologic Surgery
Jackson Memorial Hospital
Miami, Florida

Christopher Ahern, DO
Section of General Internal Medicine
Palliative Care Program
Yale University
New Haven, Connecticut

Tim A. Ahles, PhD
Director, Neurocognitive Research Laboratory
Department of Psychiatry and Behavioral
    Sciences
Memorial Sloan Kettering Cancer Center
New York, New York

Ivy Akid, MD
Palliative Faculty
Department of Internal Medicine
Johns Hopkins University School of Medicine
Baltimore, Madison

Karine A. Al Feghali, MD, MSc
Clinical Fellow
Department of Radiation Oncology
The University of Texas MD Anderson Cancer
    Center
Houston, Texas

Sara R. Alcorn, MD, MPH, PhD
Director of Clinical Operations and Assistant
    Professor
Department of Radiation Oncology and Molecular
    Radiation Sciences
The Sidney Kimmel Comprehensive Cancer Center
    at the Johns Hopkins University School of
    Medicine
Baltimore, Maryland

Terry Altilio, LCSW, ACSW, APHSW-C
Palliative Social Work Consultant
Mt. Kisco, New York

Victoria Anderson, MSN, CRNP
Senior Nurse Practitioner
Laboratory of Clinical Immunology and
    Microbiology
National Institute of Allergy and Infectious Diseases
National Institutes of Health
Bethesda, Maryland

John R. Bach, MD
Professor of Physical Medicine and Rehabilitation
Department of Physical Medicine and Rehabilitation
Professor of Neurology
Department of Neurology
Director of the Center for Ventilation Management
    Alternatives and Pulmonary Rehabilitation
University Hospital
New Jersey Medical School
Rutgers University
Newark, New Jersey

Karen Baker, CRNP
Pain and Palliative Care Service
Bethesda, Maryland

Yevgeniy Balagula, MD
Department of Medicine
Albert Einstein College of Medicine
The Bronx, New York

Lauren A. Baldassarre, MD, FACC, FSCMR, FSCCT
Associate Professor of Cardiovascular Medicine and
    Radiology & Biomedical Imaging
Cardio-oncology Director
Cardiac MR/CT Cardiology Director
Department of Internal Medicine
Yale School of Medicine
New Haven, Connecticut

Terry L. Barrett, MD
Fellow Physician, Hospice and Palliative
    Medicine
Department of Internal Medicine
University of California, Los Angeles and West Los
    Angeles VA Medical Center
Los Angeles, California

Lynda Kwon Beaupin, MD
Cancer and Blood Disorders Institute
Johns Hopkins All Children's Hospital
St. Petersburg, Florida

Ann M. Berger, MSN, MD
Pain and Palliative Care
Bethesda, Maryland

Rebecca Berger, ARNP, CPNP-AC
Cancer and Blood Disorders Institute
Johns Hopkins All Children's Hospital
St. Petersburg, Florida

Karen Blackstone, MD, FAAHPM
Director, Palliative Care Services
Department of Geriatrics and Extended Care
Washington DC Veterans Affairs Medical Center
Washington, District of Columbia

Joann N. Bodurtha, MD, MPH, FAAP, FACMG
Professor of Genetic Medicine, Oncology,
    and Pediatrics
Departments of Genetic Medicine, Oncology, and
    Pediatrics
Johns Hopkins University School of Medicine
Johns Hopkins University School of Nursing
Department of Health, Behavior and Society
Johns Hopkins University Bloomberg School of
    Public Health
Baltimore, Madison

Nina L. Bray, MD
Palliative Care Specialist
Hospice Taranaki
New Plymouth, New Zealand

Mary Brown, MA Ed
Founder, Cannabinoid Therapy Educator
SMJ Consulting
Chief Clinic Officer
Canvas Therapeutics
Seattle, Washington

Eduardo Bruera, MD
FT McGraw Chair in the Treatment of Cancer
Chair, Department of Palliative, Rehabilitation, &
    Integrative Medicine
The University of Texas MD Anderson Cancer Center
Houston, Texas

Gary T. Buckholz, MD, HMDC, FAAHPM
Clinical Professor
Department of Medicine
University of California, San Diego Health
San Diego, California

M. Jennifer Cheng, MD
Staff Clinician
Pain and Palliative Care Service
Clinical Center
National Institutes of Health
Bethesda, Maryland

Hae Lin Cho, BA
Fellow
Department of Bioethics
Clinical Center
National Institutes of Health
Bethesda, Maryland

Caroline Chung, MD, MSc, FRCPC, CIP
Associate Professor
Department of Radiation Oncology
The University of Texas MD Anderson Cancer Center
Houston, Texas

Elizabeth L. Cobbs, MD, FACP, AGSF
Chief of Geriatrics and Extended Care at the Wash-
    ington DC VA Medical Center
GWU Geriatrics Fellowship Program Director
Founding Program Director of the GWU Hospice
    and Palliative Medicine Fellowship
Department of Geriatrics and Hospice and Palliative
    Medicine
George Washington University School of Medicine
    and Health Sciences
Washington, District of Columbia

Stephen Connor, PhD
Executive Director
Worldwide Hospice Palliative Care Alliance
London, United Kingdom

Sebastian Cousins, MD
Fellow, Pulmonary Disease and Critical Care Medicine
Department of Medicine
MedStar Washington Hospital Center
Washington, District of Columbia

Jennifer M. Cuellar-Rodriguez, MD
Senior Associate Physician
Director, Transplant Infectious Diseases Consult
    Service
Laboratory of Clinical Immunology and Microbiology
Division of Intramural Research
National Institute of Allergy and Infectious
    Diseases
Bethesda, Maryland

**Schuyler C. Cunningham, MSW, LICSW, LCSW-C,
OSW-C, BCD**
Director
The Center for Neurocognitive Excellence
Washington, District of Columbia

Pierce DiMauro, BA
Graduate MSN/DNP Student
Department of Acute Care
School of Nursing
Columbia University Irving Medical Center
New York, New York

Pallavi Doddakashi, MD
Clinical Assistant Professor of Medicine
Department of Internal Medicine
George Washington University School of Medicine
    and Health Sciences
Washington, District of Columbia

Laura Drach, DO
Palliative Medicine
Johns Hopkins All Children's Hospital
St. Petersburg, Florida

Donato G. Dumlao, MD, FACP
Supportive Cancer Care Program
Banner MD Anderson Cancer Center
Gilbert, Arizona

Christen R. Elledge, MD
Department of Radiation Oncology and Molecular
    Radiation Sciences
Johns Hopkins University School of Medicine
Baltimore, Maryland

Egidio Del Fabbro, MD
Professor
Palliative Care Endowed Chair and Program Director
Division of Hematology, Oncology and Palliative Care
Department of Internal Medicine
Richmond, Virginia

Jane M. Fall-Dickson, PhD, RN
Associate Professor, and Assistant Chair, Research
Department of Professional Nursing Practice
School of Nursing & Health Studies, Georgetown
    University
Washington, District of Columbia

Betty Ferrell, RN, PhD, MA, FAAN, FPCN, CHPN
Professor and Director
Division of Nursing Research and Education
City of Hope National Medical Center
Duarte, California

Valerie A. Cruz Flores, MD, FAAP
Attending Physician, Pediatric Hematology–
    Oncology, Neuro-Oncology
Cancer & Blood Disorders Institute
Johns Hopkins All Children's Hospital
St. Petersburg, Florida

Alexandra M. Gaynor, PhD
Postdoctoral Research Fellow
Department of Psychiatry and Behavioral
    Sciences
Memorial Sloan Kettering Cancer Center
New York, New York

Juan C. Gea-Banacloche, MD
Senior Associate Consultant
Division of Infectious Diseases
Mayo Clinic Arizona
Phoenix, Arizona

Ruthann M. Giusti, MS, MD
Attending Physician
Pain and Palliative Care Service
Warren G Magnuson Clinical Center
National Institutes of Health
Bethesda, Maryland

Clara Van Gerven, MSW
Hospice Social Worker
Casey House
Montgomery Hospice
Rockville, Maryland

Christine Grady, RN, PhD
Bethesda, Maryland

Hunter Groninger, MD
Associate Professor
Department of Medicine
Georgetown University
Washington, District of Columbia

Mariana Henry, MPH
Research Assistant
Section of Cardiovascular Medicine
Yale University School of Medicine
New Haven, Connecticut

Mary K. Hughes, APRN, CNS, CT
Clinical Nurse Specialist
Department of Psychiatry
The University of Texas MD Anderson Cancer
    Center
Houston, Texas

Sarah C. Hull, MD, MBE
Assistant Professor of Clinical Medicine
Section of Cardiovascular Medicine
Associate Director
Program for Biomedical Ethics
Yale University School of Medicine
New Haven, Connecticut

Jessica Israel, MD
Senior Vice President, Geriatrics and Palliative Care
RWJ Barnabas Health
West Orange, New Jersey

Laura D. Johnson, MDiv
Palliative Care Chaplain
Section of Palliative Care
MedStar Washington Hospital Center
Washington, District of Columbia

Mohana B. Karlekar, MD, FAAHPM
Assistant Professor
Section of Palliative Medicine
Vanderbilt University Medical Center
Nashville, Tennessee

Vaughan L. Keeley, PhD, FRCP
Consultant Physician in Lymphedema and Honorary
    Professor (University of Nottingham)
Lymphedema Department
Royal Derby Hospital
Derby, United Kingdom

Anne M. Kelemen, LICSW, APHSW-C
Social Work Supervisor
Section of Palliative Care
Department of Medicine
MedStar Washington Hospital Center
Assistant Professor of Medicine
Georgetown University Medical Center
Washington, District of Columbia

Teresa Khoo, MD
Assistant Clinical Professor
Department of Medicine
David Geffen School of Medicine of the University of
    California at Los Angeles
Los Angeles, California

Philip S. Kim, MD
Center for Interventional Pain Spine
Bryn Mawr, Pennsylvania
LLC Newark
Newark, Delaware

Monique C. King, MA, CCC-SLP
Speech Language Pathologist
Rehabilitation Medicine Department
Mark O. Hatfield Clinical Research
    Center
National Institutes of Health
Bethesda, Maryland

Madeline R. Kozak
Nursing Student
Department of Professional Nursing
School of Nursing & Health Studies
Georgetown University
Washington, District of Columbia

Carol Kummet, MSW, LICSW, MTS
Palliative Care Social Worker
Social Work and Care Coordination
University of Washington Medical Center
Seattle, Washington

Elizabeth Kvale, MD, MSPH
Program Leader of Survivorship & Supportive
    Care
Livestrong Cancer Institutes
Associate Professor
Department of Internal Medicine
University of Texas at Austin Dell Medical
    School
Austin, Texas

Han Le, DO
Hospice and Palliative Medicine Fellow
Department of Pain and Palliative Care
National Institutes of Health Clinical Center
Bethesda, Maryland

Tanya J. Lehky, MD
Chief
EMG Section
National Institute of Neurological Disorders and
    Stroke
National Institutes of Health
Bethesda, Maryland

Jonathan Scott Leventhal, MD
Department of Dermatology
Yale School of Medicine
New Haven, Connecticut

Ben A. Lin, MD, PhD
Director of Echocardiography
Assistant Professor of Clinical Medicine
Division of Cardiovascular Medicine
Keck School of Medicine
University of Southern California
Los Angeles, California

Angela K. M. Lipshutz, MD, MPH
Attending Physician
Pain and Palliative Care Service
National Institutes of Health Clinical Center
Bethesda, Maryland

Russell R. Lonser, MD
Chair
Department of Neurological Surgery
Cochair
Neurological Institute
Ohio State University Wexner Medical Center
Columbus, Ohio

Charles L. Loprinzi, MD
Regis Professor of Breast Cancer Research
Division of Medical Oncology
Mayo Clinic
Rochester, Minnesota

Matthew J. Loscalzo, LCSW, APOS Fellow
Liliane Elkins Professor in Supportive Care Programs
Administrative Director, Sheri & Les Biller Patient
    and Family Resource Center
Executive Director, Department of Supportive Care
    Medicine
Professor, Department of Population Sciences
City of Hope–National Medical Center
Duarte, California

Fade Mahmoud, MD, FACP
Medical Oncologist
T. W. Lewis Melanoma Center of Excellence
Banner MD Anderson Cancer Center
Gilbert, Arizona

Margaret M. Mahon, PhD, CRNP, FAAN, FPCN
Nurse Practitioner
Pain and Palliative Care
Clinical Center
National Institutes of Health
Bethesda, Maryland

Sonia Malani, ND
Resident Physician
AIMS Institute
Seattle, Washington

Andrew Mannes, MD, MBA, ME
Chief
Department of Perioperative Medicine
Clinical Center at the National Institutes
    of Health
Bethesda, Maryland

Emily J. Martin, MD
Assistant Clinical Professor
Department of Medicine
David Geffen School of Medicine at the University of
    California, Los Angeles
Los Angeles, California

Katrazyna McNeal
Department of Psychiatry and Behavioral Sciences
Memorial Sloan Kettering Cancer Center
New York, New York

Alexandra L. McPherson, PharmD, MPH
Palliative Care Clinical Pharmacy Specialist
Department of Medicine
MedStar Washington Hospital Center
Washington, District of Columbia

Mary Lynn McPherson, PharmD, MA, MDE, BCPS
Professor and Executive Director,
    Advanced Post-Graduate Education
    in Palliative Care
Executive Program Director, Online Master of
    Science and Graduate Certificate Program in
    Palliative Care
Department of Pharmacy Practice
    and Science
University of Maryland School of Pharmacy
Baltimore, Maryland

Ambereen K. Mehta, MD, MPH
Assistant Professor
Palliative Care Program
Department of Medicine
Johns Hopkins Bayview Medical Center
Baltimore, Maryland

Susan E. Merel, MD, FACP
Associate Professor, General Internal
    Medicine
Associate Clerkship Director, Medicine Student
    Programs
Communication Training Project Lead,
    Cambia Palliative Care Center of
    Excellence
University of Washington School of
    Medicine
Seattle, Washington

Adam R. Metwalli, MD
Professor of Surgery and Chief of Urology
Howard University College of Medicine and Howard
    University Hospital
Washington, District of Columbia

Sumi K. Misra, MD, MPH, FAAHPM
Associate Professor
Section of Palliative Medicine
Nashville Veterans Administration Hospital
Vanderbilt University Medical Center
Nashville, Tennessee

Maria Pia Morelli, MD, PhD
Assistant Professor
Gastrointestinal Medical Oncology Department
The University of Texas MD Anderson Cancer Center
Houston, Texas

R. Sean Morrison, MD
Icahn School of Medicine at Mount Sinai
New York, New York

Ryan R. Nash, MD, MA, FACP, FAAHPM
Hagop S. Mekhjian, MD, Chair in Medical Ethics
    and Professionalism
Director, The Ohio State University Center for
    Bioethics and Medical Humanities
Director and Associate Professor with Tenure,
    Division of Bioethics
Department of Biomedical Education and Anatomy
The Ohio State University College of Medicine
Columbus, Ohio

Paul Noufi, MD
General Adult Psychiatrist, Consultation–Liaison
    Psychiatrist, Pain and Palliative Care Fellow
Department of Palliative Medicine
MedStar Washington Hospital Center
Washington, District of Columbia

Joseph F. O'Neill, MD, MS, MPH
Pain and Palliative Care
Bethesda, Maryland

Brianna Olamiju, MD
Department of Dermatology
Yale School of Medicine
New Haven, Connecticut

Rachel Ombres, MD
Fellow
Department of General Internal Medicine
The University of Texas MD Anderson Cancer
    Center
Houston, Texas

Judith A. Paice, PhD, RN
Director, Cancer Pain Program
Division of Hematology and Oncology
Feinberg School of Medicine
Northwestern University
Chicago, Illinois

Sonika Pandey, MD
Assistant Professor
Department of Medicine
The George Washington University
Director–Outpatient and Palliative Care, Geriatrics
    and Extended Care
VA Medical Center
Washington, District of Columbia

Maryland Pao, MD, FAACAP, FACLP, FAPA
Clinical and Deputy Scientific Director
National Institute of Mental Health
National Institutes of Health
Bethesda, Maryland

Gregory Pappas, MD, PhD
Washington, District of Columbia

Hiren V. Patel, MD, PhD
Section of Urologic Oncology
Rutgers Cancer Institute of New Jersey
Rutgers Robert Wood Johnson Medical School
New Brunswick, New Jersey

Laura Patel, MD, FAAHPM
Chief Medical Officer
Transitions LifeCare
Raleigh, North Carolina

Xiao P. Peng, MD, PhD
Pediatrics–Medical Genetics Combined Resident
   (Postgraduate Year 4)
Departments of Pediatrics and Genetic Medicine
Johns Hopkins University School of Medicine
Baltimore, Maryland

Jacob W. Phillips, DO
Hospice and Palliative Medicine Fellow
Department of Hospice and Palliative
   Medicine
George Washington University School of Medicine
   and Health Sciences
Washington, District of Columbia

Christopher J. Pietras, MD
Associate Clinical Professor
Palliative Care Program Director
Geriatrics–Palliative Medicine Fellowship Program
   Director
Department of Medicine
David Geffen School of Medicine of the University of
   California at Los Angeles
Los Angeles, California

Peter A. Pinto, MD
Head, Prostate Cancer Section
Urologic Oncology Branch
Center for Cancer Research
National Cancer Institute
Bethesda, Maryland

Elizabeth Prsic, MD
Director, Adult Inpatient Palliative Care
Director, Supportive Care Unit
Firm Chief for Operations and QualityMedical
   Oncology
Assistant Professor
Department of Internal Medicine
Yale School of Medicine
Yale New Haven Hospital/Yale Cancer Center
New Haven, Connecticut

Christina M. Puchalski, MD, MS, FACP, FAAHPM
Founder and Director
George Washington Institute for Spirituality and
   Health
Professor, Medicine and Health Sciences
George Washington University School of Medicine
   and Health Sciences
Washington, District of Columbia

Jason G. Ramirez, MD
Staff Physician
Anesthesiology
George E. Wahlen VA Salt Lake City Health Care
   System
Salt Lake City, Utah

Haniya Raza, DO, MPH
Chief, Psychiatry Consultation Liaison Service
Office of the Clinical Director
National Institute of Mental Health
National Institutes of Health
Bethesda, Maryland

Alvin L. Reaves III, MD, FACP, FAAHPM
Medical Director for Palliative and Supportive
   Care
US Acute Care Solutions
Shady Grove Medical Center Adventist
   HealthCare
Rockville, Maryland

Christine S. Ritchie, MD, MSPH
Director of Research
Division of Palliative Care and Geriatric Medicine
Director
Morgan Institute Center for Aging and Serious
   Illness
Massachusetts General Hospital
Center for Palliative Care
Harvard Medical School
Cambridge, Massachusetts

Jaydira Del Rivero, MD
Assistant Research Physician
Developmental Therapeutics Branch
Center for Cancer Research
National Cancer Institute
National Institutes of Health
Bethesda, Maryland

James C. Root, PhD
Associate Attending Neuropsychologist
Neurocognitive Research Laboratory
Memorial Sloan Kettering Cancer Center
New York, New York

Maleeha Ruhi, MD
Hospice and Palliative Medicine
   Physician
Capital Caring Health
Arlington, Virginia

Elizabeth Ryan, PhD, ABPP-Cn
Associate Professor
Neurocognitive Research Lab
Associate Attending Neuropsychologist, Psychiatry
    Service
Department of Psychiatry and Behavioral Sciences
Memorial Sloan Kettering Cancer Center
New York, New York

Biren Saraiya, MD
Assistant Professor of Medicine
Division of Medical Oncology
Section of Solid Tumor Oncology
Rutgers Cancer Institute of New Jersey
Rutgers Robert Wood Johnson Medical School
New Brunswick, New Jersey

Nabeel Sarhill, MD
Assistant Professor
Medical Oncology and Hematology
UT RGV School of Medicine
Harlingen, Texas

Erica Schockett, MD
Director, Inpatient Palliative Medicine
Assistant Professor of Medicine
Department of Internal Medicine
George Washington University School of Medicine
    and Health Sciences
Washington, District of Columbia

Lee Schwartzberg MD, FACP
Chief Medical Officer
OneOncology
Medical Director
West Cancer Center and Research Institute
Clinical Professor of Medicine
University of Tennessee Health Science Center
Memphis, Tennessee

Anna Sedney, MD
Palliative Medicine
Johns Hopkins All Children's Hospital
St. Petersburg, Florida

Brian Shinder, MD
Section of Urologic Oncology
Rutgers Cancer Institute of New Jersey
Rutgers Robert Wood Johnson Medical
    School
New Brunswick, New Jersey

Nicole Shirilla, MD, MEd, MA
Assistant Professor
Division of Bioethics
Department of Biomedical Education and Anatomy
Division of Palliative Medicine
Department of Internal Medicine
The Ohio State University College of Medicine
Columbus, Ohio

Eric A. Singer, MD, MA, MS, FACS
Associate Chief of Urology and Urologic
    Oncology
Associate Professor of Surgery and Radiology
Rutgers Cancer Institute of New Jersey
Rutgers Robert Wood Johnson Medical School
New Brunswick, New Jersey

Beth I. Solomon, MS, CCC-SLP
Senior Lead, Speech Language Pathologist
Rehabilitation Medicine Department
Mark O. Hatfield Clinical Research Center
National Institutes of Health
Bethesda, Maryland

Stacie Stapleton, MD
Chief of Oncology Division
Cancer and Blood Disorders Institute
Johns Hopkins All Children's Hospital
St. Petersburg, Florida

Katelyn Stepanyan, MD
Associate Program Director, Hospice & Palliative
    Medicine Fellowship
Assistant Clinical Professor
Department of Medicine
UCLA David Geffen School of Medicine
Los Angeles, California

Ryan D. Stephenson, DO
Assistant Professor of Medicine
Division of Medical Oncology
Section of Solid Tumor Oncology
Rutgers Cancer Institute of New Jersey
Rutgers Robert Wood Johnson Medical
    School
New Brunswick, New Jersey

Jessica Streufert, RRT
Cannabinoid Therapy Educator
SMJ Consulting
Seattle, Washington

Linda J. Stricker, MSN, RN, CWOCN
Program Director, WOC Nursing Education
R.B. Turnbull, Jr. MD School of WOC Nursing
    Education
Cleveland Clinic
Cleveland, Ohio

Thomas Strouse, MD, DLFAPA, FACLP, FAAHPM
Maddie Katz Professor
Palliative Care Research and Education
Medical Director
UCLA Resnick Neuropsychiatric Hospital
Department of Psychiatry
Semel Institute
UCLA David Geffen School of Medicine
Los Angeles, California

Joan M. Teno, MD, MS
Professor of Medicine
Division of General Internal Medicine and
    Geriatrics
Oregon Health & Science University
Portland, Oregon

Cindy S. Tofthagen, PhD, APRN, AOCNP, FAANP, FAAN
Associate Professor of Nursing   .
Division of Nursing Research
Mayo Clinic
Jacksonville, Florida

Ryan Tourtellot, DO
Clinical Fellow
Pain and Palliative Care Service
National Institutes of Health Clinical Center
Bethesda, Maryland

Martha L. Twaddle, MD, FACP, FAAHPM, HMDC
The Waud Family Medical Directorship
Palliative Medicine & Supportive Care
Clinical Professor of Medicine
Northwestern Feinberg School of Medicine
Chicago, Illinois

Krishna Upadhyaya, MD
Cardiologist with Ascension Medical Group
Department of Cardiology
Columbia St. Mary's Hospital Milwaukee
Milwaukee, Wisconsin

Lakshmi Vaidyanathan, MD, MBA
Medical Director
Palliative Medicine & Population Health
University of Maryland Shore Regional Health
Easton, Maryland

Jaya Vijayan, MD, FAAFP, FAAHPM
Medical Director, Palliative Care
Holy Cross Health
Silver Spring, Maryland

Charles F. von Gunten, MD, PhD
Vice President
Medical Affairs
Hospice and Palliative Medicine
OhioHealth
Columbus, Ohio

Liping Wang, MD
Deputy Chief Physician
Department of Neurology
Peking University Third Hospital
Beijing, China

Xiao-Min Wang, MD, PhD
Department of Anaesthesiology
The University of Hong Kong
Hong Kong, SAR, China

Xin Shelley Wang, MD, MPH
Professor
Department of Symptom Research
The University of Texas MD Anderson Cancer
    Center
Houston, Texas

Sharon M. Weinstein, MD, FAAHPM
Associate Professor of Anesthesiology
Adjunct Professor of Pediatrics
School of Medicine
University of Utah
Salt Lake City, Utah

Jasmine Williams, MD, MBA
PACT (Pediatric Advance Care Team)
    Physician
Children's Healthcare of Atlanta
Assistant Professor
Emory University School of Medicine
Atlanta, Georgia

Vanessa Wookey, MD
Hematology Oncology Fellow
Division of Hematology and Oncology
Department of Internal Medicine
University of Tennessee Health Science
    Center
Memphis, Tennessee

Sara Yumeen
Department of Dermatology
Yale School of Medicine
New Haven, Connecticut

James R. Zabora, ScD, MSW, FAPOS, FAOSW
Assistant Director for Community Outreach &
    Engagement
Sidney Kimmel Comprehensive Cancer Center at
    Johns Hopkins
The Johns Hopkins School of Medicine
Baltimore, Maryland

Shali Zhang, MD
Department of Dermatology
Hawaii Pacific Health Straub Medical
    Center

Zhang-Jin Zhang, MD, PhD
School of Chinese Medicine
The University of Hong Kong
Hong Kong, SAR, China

PREFACE

The term "palliative care" is derived from the Latin *pallium:* meaning to cloak or cover. The editors of this textbook like the Canadian Palliative Care Association's expansion upon the WHO definition of palliative care:

Palliative care, as a philosophy of care, is the combination of active and compassionate therapies intended to comfort and support individuals and families who are living with a life-threatening illness. During periods of illness and bereavement, palliative care strives to meet physical, psychological, social, and spiritual expectations and needs, while remaining sensitive to personal, cultural, and religious values, beliefs, and practices. Palliative care may be combined with therapies aimed at reducing or curing the illness, or it may be the total focus of care.

At its core, then palliative care makes it its business to provide maximum quality of life and minimize (cover) suffering. In oncology, the related term "supportive care" refers to those aspects of medical care concerned with physical, psychosocial, practical, and spiritual issues experienced by the patient who has cancer and those (families, loved ones, communities, and professionals) who care for and about them. Supportive oncology encompasses the patient's needs arising from the cancer itself as well as those stemming from antineoplastic therapies and other medical interventions.

In 1990, the World Health Organization (WHO) published a landmark document entitled Cancer Pain Relief and Palliative Care,[1] which clearly defined, on a global scale, barriers and needs for improved pain and symptom control for cancer patients. In 2014, the World Health Assembly built upon this by adopting a resolution that called upon the WHO and all member states to improve access to palliative care as a core component of their health systems.[2] Closer to home, in 2016, the American Society of Clinical Oncology (ASCO) promulgated practice guidelines stating that all patients with advanced cancer (defined as those with distant metastases, late-stage disease, cancer that is life limiting, and/or with prognosis of 6 to 24 months) should receive dedicated palliative care services, early in the disease course, concurrent with active treatment.[3]

In developing this textbook, the editors have brought together those elements of palliative care that are most helpful to the health care professional and have provided detailed and in-depth guidance on their use in supporting patients receiving active cancer treatment as well for those for whom disease-directed therapy is not warranted or wanted. Consistent with ASCO guidance, the editors view these interventions as a necessary and vital aspect of medical care for all cancer patients, from the time of diagnosis until death.

Most patients will have a significant physical symptom requiring treatment at the time of their cancer diagnosis. Even when cancer can be effectively treated and a cure or life prolongation is achieved, there are always physical, psychosocial, or spiritual concerns that must be addressed to maintain function and optimize the quality of life. For patients whose cancer cannot be effectively treated, palliative care must be the dominant mode—focusing intensely on the control of distressing symptoms and the psychosocial, practical, and spiritual impact of impending disability and death. Planning for the end of life and ensuring that death occurs with a minimum of suffering and in a manner consistent with the values and desires of the patient and family are fundamental elements of this care. Palliative care, as a desired approach to comprehensive cancer care, is appropriate for all health care settings, including the clinic, acute care hospital, long-term care facility, or home hospice.

Palliative care and the related concept of supportive care involve the collaborative efforts of an interdisciplinary team. This team must include the cancer patient and his or her family, care givers, and involved health care providers. Integral to effective palliative care is the opportunity and support necessary for both care givers and health care providers to work through their own emotions related to the care they are providing.

In organizing this textbook, the editors have recognized the important contributions of medical research and clinical care that have emerged from the disciplines of hospice and palliative medicine; medical, radiation, and surgical oncology; nursing; neurology and neuro-oncology; anesthesiology; psychiatry and psychology; pharmacology; and many others. The text includes chapters focusing on the common physical symptoms experienced by the cancer patient; a review of specific supportive treatment modalities, such as nutritional support, hydration, palliative chemotherapy, radiotherapy, and surgery; and finally, a review of more specialized topics, including survivorship issues, medical ethics, spiritual care, quality of life, and supportive care in the elderly and pediatric patients.

---

[1]https://apps.who.int/iris/handle/10665/39524
[2]www.who.int/news-room/fact-sheets/detail/palliative-care
[3]https://ascopubs.org/doi/full/10.1200/JCO.2016.70.1474

The fifth edition of *Principles and Practice of Palliative Care and Supportive Oncology* is the product of months of work by a large number of contributors, all aimed at helping those who care for patients with cancer. As with previous editions, the editors and authors have endeavored to create authoritative and up-to-date reviews of research and clinical care best practices in palliative care and supportive oncology, presented with a focus on practical, clinical application. We continue to emphasize integrated interdisciplinary care, collaborating with the patient and family to shape care that respects and prioritizes the patient's goals, values, and preferences. It is our hope that this effort will be a source of both help and inspiration to all who practice palliative care and supportive oncology.

The fifth edition contains updated and revised chapters throughout. There are new chapters including cannabinoids in palliative care, survivorship issues in pediatrics, cancer genetics, noninvasive ventilation, global issues, and physician-assisted suicide. There are many promising new cancer treatments on the horizon. No matter what these new treatments will offer in terms of curing the disease or prolonging life, cancer will remain a devastating illness, not only for the affected patients but also for their families, community, and health care providers. Providing excellent, supportive care will continue to be a goal for all health care providers.

Ann M. Berger, MSN, MD
Joseph F. O'Neill, MD, MS, MPH

ACKNOWLEDGMENTS

We would like to thank all of the contributors to this volume for their tireless effort and superb work. Without their dedication, wisdom, experience, and generosity, this book would not be possible. We are grateful to our families, friends, and colleagues who support us in body, mind, and spirit through the joys and challenges of life and of publishing. Most importantly, we are grateful to our patients—the true heroes of all medical education—who teach us. We lost one of the great palliative medicine leaders, Richard Payne, MD, since the last edition of this book and we honor his life and work with every page of this edition. We thank our publisher, Wolters Kluwer, and their staff especially Sean McGuire whose oversight, gentle prodding, and years of experience were essential to the success of the book and Linda Christina for her efforts in helping us get the book completed.

CONTENTS

Symptoms and Syndromes

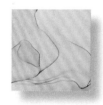 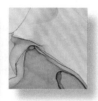 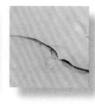 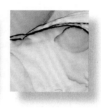 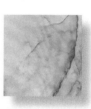

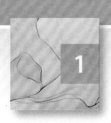

1 Neuropathic, Bone, and Visceral Pain Syndromes

Terry L. Barrett and Emily J. Martin

Nociception is the physiologic process by which tissue nociceptors, also known as A-delta and C-nerve fibers, are activated and sensitized. Pain corresponds to our awareness of nociception and has been defined by the International Study for Pain as "an unpleasant sensory and emotional experience associated with tissue damage or described in terms of such damage" (1).

In the clinical setting, pain may occur as a response to a noxious event in the tissue, such as tissue inflammation due to a burn injury, or as a response to activation of the nervous system pain pathways. In the first case, the pain signal presumably originates from "healthy" tissue nociceptors activated or sensitized by the local release of algogenic substances (e.g., protons, prostaglandins, bradykinin, adenosine, and cytokines). This type of pain is referred to as *nociceptive* and is often characterized by a gnawing or aching sensation. In the second case, the pain signal is generated ectopically by abnormal peripheral nerve fibers involved in pain transmission and/or by abnormal pain circuits in the central nervous system (CNS). This type of pain has been called *neuropathic*; it is characterized by sharp, burning, or lancinating pain.

Notably, the distinction between nociceptive and neuropathic pain is often blurred. Indeed, as discussed in the subsequent text, neuropathic pain may arise from inflammation (i.e., inflammatory neuropathic pain) (2). Further, inflammatory and neuropathic mechanisms may be present concurrently or sequentially. Visceral pain represents another common pain syndrome and, while it shares similarities to both nociceptive and neuropathic pain, is associated with its own unique pain pathways.

DIFFICULT PAIN SYNDROMES: PERIPHERAL AND CENTRAL MECHANISMS

The nociceptive pain signal is transmitted from the peripheral nociceptors through the dorsal horn of the spinal cord and the thalamus to the cortex. In the periphery, nociceptors can be activated by chemical products of tissue damage and inflammation, which include prostanoids, serotonin, bradykinin, cytokines, adenosine, adenosine-5′-triphosphate, histamine, protons, free radicals, and growth factors. These agents can activate afferent fibers or sensitize them to a range of mechanical, thermal, and chemical stimuli. Notably, a proportion of the afferent fibers that are normally unresponsive to noxious stimuli ("silent" or "sleeping" nociceptors) can be "awakened" by inflammatory chemicals and be stimulated to contribute to pain and hyperalgesia. The products of tissue damage and inflammation interact with receptors located on the A-delta fibers and C-nerve fibers to initiate membrane excitability and intracellular transcriptional changes.

Most neuropathic pain conditions develop after partial injuries to the peripheral nervous system (PNS). For example, as observed in animal models of partial nerve injury, both injured and uninjured primary sensory neurons acquire the ability to express genes de novo and, therefore, change their phenotype (phenotypic shift). Nerve endings develop sensitivity to a number of factors, such as prostanoids and cytokines (e.g., tumor necrosis factor-α [TNF-α]) (3–6). One example is the upregulation or induction of catecholamine receptors in undamaged nociceptors; in this condition, nociceptors are activated by noradrenaline and the resulting neuropathic pain has been called *sympathetically maintained pain* (*SMP*) (7,8). Reversal of the phenotypic shift is associated with the reduction of neuropathic pain (9).

Recent findings suggest that during cancer (and other pathologic inflammatory conditions), a number of diffusible factors might be involved in causing a "neuropathic spin" in the pain state (10). Tissue-related growth factors (e.g., nerve growth factor [NGF]) in combination with specific proinflammatory cytokines (e.g., TNF-α and interleukin [IL]-1β (11)) might sensitize nociceptors and generate ectopic and spontaneous activity in tissue receptors. In these instances, the pain syndrome could be classified as inflammatory neuropathic pain. There is considerable hope that the identification of the diffusible factors causing altered gene expression in the dorsal root ganglia sensory neurons will direct research to discover more effective treatments. In the PNS, several elements of the cellular "machinery" that are thought to be relevant to the development of pathologic pain have been identified as potential targets for analgesic drugs. In the CNS, in particular within the spinal cord, a variety of neurobiology events can occur during the course of an ongoing peripheral tissue damage and inflammation (12). Early and aggressive pain interventions and the use of specific therapies that disengage gene expression might be sufficient to uncouple the phenotypic shift and reverse a difficult pain syndrome into an easy-to-treat condition.

NEUROPATHIC PAIN

Clinical Findings and Diagnosis

The clinical interview of a patient with pain should focus on questions about onset, duration, progression, character, and nature of complaints suggestive of neurologic deficits (e.g., persistent numbness in a body area and focal weakness), as well as complaints suggestive of sensory dysfunction (e.g., touch-evoked pain, intermittent abnormal sensations, spontaneous burning, and shooting pains). Notably, patients may report only sensory symptoms and have no neurologic deficits. The assessment should also include a discussion of any alleviating factors that the patient has identified.

Patients with neuropathic pain may present with some or all of the following abnormal sensory symptoms and signs:

- *Paresthesias*: spontaneous, intermittent, painless, and abnormal sensations
- *Dysesthesias*: spontaneous or evoked unpleasant sensations, such as annoying sensations elicited by cold stimuli or pinprick testing
- *Allodynia*: pain elicited by nonnoxious stimuli (i.e., clothing, air movement, and tactile stimuli) when applied to the symptomatic cutaneous area; allodynia may be mechanical (static, e.g., induced by application of a light pressure, or dynamic, e.g., induced by moving a soft brush) or thermal (e.g., induced by a nonpainful cold or warm stimulus)
- *Hyperalgesia*: an exaggerated pain response to a mildly noxious (mechanical or thermal) stimulus applied to the symptomatic area
- *Hyperpathia*: a delayed and explosive pain response to a stimulus applied to the symptomatic area

Allodynia, hyperalgesia, and hyperpathia represent positive abnormal findings, as opposed to hypesthesia and anesthesia, which represent negative findings of the neurologic sensory examination. Heat hyperalgesia and deep mechanical allodynia (i.e., tenderness on soft tissue palpation) are findings that are commonly present in the cutaneous epicenter of an inflammatory pain generator, also known as the *zone of primary hyperalgesia*. These findings are indicative of PNS sensitization and are related to a local inflammatory state. On the other hand, the skin surrounding the site of inflammation, also known as the *zone of secondary hyperalgesia*, may present the finding of mechanical allodynia, which can be elicited, for example, by stroking the area with a soft brush. Secondary hyperalgesia is indicative of CNS sensitization. Patients affected by SMP typically complain of cold allodynia or hyperalgesia. This is assessed by providing a cold stimulus, such as a cold metallic tuning fork, to the painful region for a few seconds.

Clinical and research tools to assess and measure the intensity and quality of neuropathic pain include the Brief Pain Inventory (BPI), the Neuropathic Pain Scale (NPS), and the McGill Pain Questionnaire (MPQ), among others (13). The BPI is a questionnaire that consists of 15 items asking the patient about average pain and worst pain in the past week, whether the patient has received relief from pain treatment, and whether the pain has interfered with daily activities (14). It is well validated for both cancer and non-cancer pain (15). Its major disadvantage is the time it takes to complete (5 to 15 minutes), which makes it challenging to repeatedly administer in the setting of acute pain (16). The NPS is a self-report scale for measuring neuropathic pain. It consists of 12 distinct questions, which ask about intensity and quality of the patient's pain. In validation studies, it has been found to have a good predictive power in discriminating between major subgroups of patients with neuropathic pain (13). The NPS was not designed to diagnose neuropathic pain, rather it is a tool that helps measure intensity of neuropathic pain and may be useful in assessing a patient's response to therapeutic interventions (16). The MPQ is a 20-item questionnaire designed for adult patients with a variety of pain syndromes. It aims to evaluate not only the intensity of pain but also the emotional impact and cognitive evaluation of pain (17).

Cancer-Related Neuropathic Pain Syndromes

Table 1.1 (18) lists common neuropathic pain syndromes that have been reported in association with cancer. Neuropathy may result from one or more cancer-related mechanisms (19), for example, compression, mechanical traction, inflammation, or infiltration of nerve trunks or plexi caused by the progression of the primary cancer or by metastatic disease affecting bone or soft tissues. Head and neck cancer and skull-based tumors can cause painful cranial neuropathies by direct nerve compression. Salivary gland cancers may cause painful facial neuropathies. Breast or lung cancer

TABLE 1.1 NEUROPATHIC PAIN SYNDROMES RELATED TO CANCER

Neuropathic pain syndromes	Clinical examples
Cranial nerve neuralgias	Base of skull or leptomeningeal metastases and head and neck cancers
Mononeuropathy and other neuralgias	Rib metastases with intercostal nerve injury
Radiculopathy	Epidural mass and leptomeningeal metastases
Cervical plexopathy	Head and neck cancer with local extension and cervical lymph node metastases
Brachial plexopathy	Lymph node metastases from breast cancer or lymphoma and direct extension of Pancoast tumor
Lumbosacral plexopathy	Extension of colorectal cancer, cervical cancer, sarcoma, or lymphoma and breast cancer metastases
Paraneoplastic peripheral neuropathy	Small cell lung cancer and antineuronal nuclear antibodies type 1
Central pain	Spinal cord compression
Cachexia	Compression or entrapment neuropathies

Adapted from Martin LA, Hagen NA. Neuropathic pain in cancer patients: mechanisms, syndromes, and clinical controversies. *J Pain Symptom Manage.* 1997;14:99-117.

can infiltrate the brachial plexus and cause painful plexitis. Pelvic or retroperitoneal cancer may invade the lumbosacral plexus. If the meninges are affected (meningeal carcinomatosis), the involvement of adjacent roots, spinal nerves, and plexi can occur. Metastatic disease or lymphoma can cause meningeal carcinomatosis and affect multiple spinal roots. Peripheral neuropathies with pain and dysesthesia may also be observed in the presence of lymphomas. Acute inflammatory demyelinating polyneuropathy of the Guillain-Barré syndrome type may occur with lymphomas, particularly Hodgkin's disease.

Antineoplastic therapeutic agents such as platinum-based agents, taxoids, and vincristine may cause painful neuropathies; these are usually distal symmetrical polyneuropathies, but can manifest as a mononeuropathy. For additional information on chemotherapy-induced neuropathy, please see Chapter 6. Postradiation plexopathies may arise when >60 Gy (6,000 rad) of irradiation is given to the patient as a radiation dose. Surgical resection of cancers may result in traumatic injuries to peripheral nerves with the subsequent development of painful neuromas. For example, postthoracotomy pain can be caused by injury to the intercostal nerves and postmastectomy pain may arise through injury to the intercostobrachial nerve. Compression or entrapment neuropathies occur in the presence of cachexia; for example, patients with cancer who have lost substantial fat and muscle body weight are prone to develop peroneal neuropathies.

While rare, paraneoplastic autoimmune syndromes due to antineuronal antibodies may present as painful neuropathies. Patients who complain of burning dysesthesias in their feet, hands, and face in the setting of diagnosed or undiagnosed carcinoma may have antineuronal nuclear antibodies type 1 (ANNA-1), also known as *anti-Hu*. Painful dysesthesias develop first in one limb and then progress to involve other limbs, face, scalp, and trunk over weeks or months. In these patients, deep tendon reflexes are reduced or absent and muscle strength is preserved (20).

Therapeutic Interventions for Neuropathic Pain

Management of severe neuropathic pain can be a challenge, often requires a combination of therapies. Treatment includes a wide range of modalities, ranging from opioid and nonopioid analgesics, neuropathic adjuvant medication, interventional pain procedures, implantable devices, and surgery. Table 1.2 tabulates the pharmacotherapy used in neuropathic pain.

Antiepileptic Drugs

Antiepileptic drugs (AEDs) are important agents in the management of neuropathic pain. In particular, the gabapentinoid anticonvulsants, gabapentin and pregabalin, have both established efficacy in treating neuropathic pain. Gabapentin is FDA approved for the treatment of postherpetic neuralgia (PHN), and there is good evidence available that supports its efficacy across other neuropathic pain states, particularly diabetic neuropathy (21,22). The gabapentin analog pregabalin is FDA approved for the treatment of PHN and painful diabetic neuropathy. The

TABLE 1.2 PHARMACOTHERAPY OF NEUROPATHIC PAIN

Class	Medication	Typical dosing	Comments
First line			
Gabapentinoids	Gabapentin	Slow titration to 600 mg t.i.d. Maximum daily dose: 3,600 mg	Dose reduce for renal insufficiency
	Pregabalin	Start with 150 mg b.i.d. or t.i.d. Maximum daily dose: 600 mg	
Serotonin norepinephrine reuptake inhibitors (SNRIs)	Duloxetine	Start with 30 mg daily Maximum daily dose: 60 mg	Caution in renal or liver disease
	Venlafaxine	Start at 37.5 mg daily Maximum daily dose: 225 mg	
Tricyclic antidepressants (TCAs)	Nortriptyline	Start with 25 mg qhs Maximum daily dose: 150 mg	Risk of anticholinergic side effects and serotonin syndrome
	Amitriptyline	Start with 10–25 mg qhs Maximum daily dose: 150 mg (75 mg in older adults)	
Second line			
Topical agents	Capsaicin 8% patch	1–4 patches applied to the painful area for 30–60 min every 3 mo PRN	Avoid eyes or mucosa; avoid in diabetic peripheral neuropathy
	Lidocaine 5% patch	1–3 patches to the painful area for up to 12 h	Avoid more than three patches at one time
Combinations	Gabapentinoid + TCA		Avoid in older adults
	Gabapentinoid + SNRI		
Opioids	Tramadol	Start with 50 mg b.i.d. to q.i.d. PRN Maximum daily dose: 400 mg	Risk of serotonin syndrome and seizures; dose reduce in renal insufficiency

Adapted from Finnerup NB, Attal N, Haroutounian S, et al. Pharmacotherapy for neuropathic pain in adults: a systematic review and meta-analysis. *Lancet Neurol.* 2015;14(2):162-173.

gabapentinoids were originally created to mimic the action of the neurotransmitter GABA; however, their mechanism of action does not involve the GABA receptor. Instead, it acts on the $\alpha2\delta$-1 subunit of voltage-gate calcium channels in dorsal root ganglion neurons and dorsal horn neurons, inhibiting nerve injury-induced trafficking of $\alpha1$ pore-forming units (23). More recently, concerns have been raised about the potential for abuse of gabapentin and pregabalin, particularly in patients with a history of substance use disorder (24).

Trigeminal neuralgia, a neuropathic condition characterized by a brief excruciating, lancinating pain in the distribution of the trigeminal nerve, responds extremely well to carbamazepine or oxcarbazepine. Lamotrigine has shown some efficacy in treating carbamazepine-resistant trigeminal neuralgia (25). Topiramate has been anecdotally used in the treatment of complex regional pain syndrome (CRPS) type 1 (26). A recent randomized controlled trial (RCT) compared topiramate to gabapentin in the treatment

of diabetic polyneuropathy and found that they were similarly effective (27). Several other AEDs (e.g., levetiracetam, zonisamide, oxcarbazepine, and tiagabine) have become available for medical use, and some of these, along with topiramate, may have analgesic effect in primary headache and perhaps in neuropathic pain (28,29). However, a recent Cochrane review noted that, while there was evidence to support the use of gabapentin and pregabalin in some neuropathic pain conditions, there was insufficient evidence to make a recommendation regarding the use of clonazepam, phenytoin, or valproic acid and there was low-quality evidence for the use of carbamazepine. Further, lamotrigine, oxcarbazepine, and topiramate all had reasonable quality evidence to suggest little or no effect in neuropathic pain (30,31). There is also evidence to suggest that the combination of gabapentin and morphine may result in superior analgesic effect at lower doses, compared with either agent alone. This has been demonstrated in both neuropathic pain and postoperative pain (32–34).

Opioids

Opioids are currently the most potent and effective analgesics used to treat acute pain. Long considered to be ineffective for neuropathic pain, opioids have demonstrated efficacy in several recent clinical trials (35–38). A recent Cochrane review which analyzed 31 total RCTs regarding efficacy of opioids in neuropathic pain found equivocal evidence for short-term (<24 hours) use of opioids for neuropathic pain, but found that intermediate term (<12 weeks) demonstrated significant efficacy of opioids over placebo, suggesting a possible role for opioids in the management of neuropathic pain (39).

The analgesic action of the pure opioid agonists (e.g., morphine, fentanyl, oxycodone, hydromorphone, and oxymorphone) is well established. Among all the analgesic medications currently available, the most powerful and effective drugs are still the agents acting on the μ-, κ-, and Δ-opioid receptors. Opioid receptors are located not only in the CNS (primarily in the dorsal horn) but also on peripheral nociceptors. Opioids may also have a relevant peripheral analgesic effect during painful inflammatory states (40). Interestingly, animal studies suggest that the addition of an extremely low dose of an opioid receptor antagonist (e.g., naltrexone) to morphine in a ratio of 1:1,000 may enhance the analgesic efficacy of the opioid agonists (41).

Tramadol is an analgesic agent with a weak μ-opioid agonistic effect. Its potency is comparable to that of a codeine-acetaminophen preparation. Although some trials showed potential benefit of tramadol in neuropathic pain (40–43), a recent Cochrane review of the available evidence concludes that the evidence for use of tramadol for this indication is modest, and generally of low or very low quality (44).

Methadone is an opioid agonist with unique properties. Methadone consists of a racemic mixture of the D and L isomers—the D isomer has more N-methyl-D-aspartate (NMDA) properties and the L isomer has more opioid properties. Methadone has an intrinsic NMDA receptor antagonistic effect, which adds adjuvant analgesic effect in the setting of neuropathic pain (discussed in more detail in subsequent text).

Common side effects of opioids include constipation, sedation, pruritus, and nausea/vomiting. Except for constipation, tolerance occurs within a few days for most of these side effects. Respiratory depression, although rare, is the most feared complication. Also, rare, opioid-induced neurotoxicity may occur, especially in the setting of rapid dose titration. Side effects can often be managed with additional pharmacotherapy or with rotation to another opioid. When converting opioids, it is wise to refer to an opioid conversion table, such as the one included in Table 1.3, and to dose reduce to account for incomplete cross-tolerance.

Opioid titration and opioid rotation are essential concepts in the management of neuropathic pain. To determine adequate opioid responsiveness, a careful titration of the opioid dose is necessary. Pure opioid agonists have no true "ceiling

TABLE 1.3 EQUIANALGESIC POTENCY CONVERSION FOR CANCER PAIN

Drug	Equianalgesic dose (mg)	
	Intramuscular[a,b]	Oral
Morphine	10	60[c]
Codeine	130	200
Heroin	5	60
Hydromorphone	1.5	7.5
Levorphanol	2	4
Meperidine	75	300
Methadone	10	20
Oxycodone	15	30
Oxymorphone	1	10 (rectal)

[a]Based on single-dose studies in which an intramuscular dose of each drug listed was compared with morphine to establish relative potency. Oral doses are those recommended when changing from a parenteral to an oral route.
[b]Although no controlled studies are available, in clinical practice it is customary to consider the doses of opioid given intramuscularly, intravenously, or subcutaneously to be equivalent.
[c]The conversion ratio of 10 mg of parenteral morphine to 60 mg of oral morphine is based on a potency study in patients with acute pain.
Note: All intramuscular and oral doses listed are considered to be equivalent in analgesic effect to 10 mg of intramuscular morphine.

dose" for analgesia and do not cause direct organ damage. The maximum daily dose of opioid-acetaminophen combination medications, however, is limited by acetaminophen.

Antidepressants

Antidepressants also play an important role in the treatment of chronic pain. Tricyclic antidepressants (TCAs), such as amitriptyline, nortriptyline, and desipramine (45), have established efficacy in the treatment of neuropathic pain. They have been used successfully for the treatment of painful diabetic neuropathy and PHN and provided pain relief in nondepressed patients affected by neuropathic pain. Notably, TCAs such as amitriptyline, doxepin, and imipramine have been found to have potent local anesthetic properties. TCAs frequently have poorly tolerated adverse effects, including cardiotoxicity, confusion, urinary retention, orthostatic hypotension, nightmares, weight gain, drowsiness, dry mouth, and constipation. These medications are difficult to titrate, and at times, patients may need to stop the medication because of side effects.

Duloxetine and venlafaxine are antidepressants with analgesic properties similar to that of TCAs but without the anticholinergic and antihistamine effects of the TCAs (46–48). Duloxetine is a serotonin-norepinephrine reuptake inhibitor that is approved by the FDA for the treatment of pain secondary to diabetic neuropathy (48,49). It is also recommended by the American Society of Clinical Oncology for the treatment of chemotherapy-induced peripheral neuropathy (CIPN) (50). A slow-release preparation of bupropion, a dopamine, and norepinephrine, serotonin reuptake inhibitor, has also been shown to effectively treat neuropathic pain, although the data are limited (51). Selective serotonin reuptake inhibitors (SSRIs), such as paroxetine and fluoxetine, are effective antidepressants, but lack analgesic properties. While being used for the management of comorbidities such as anxiety, depression, and insomnia, which frequently affect patients with chronic neuropathic pain, SSRIs have not shown the same efficacy as TCAs in the treatment of neuropathic pain (45).

Local Anesthetics

The data supporting the use of transdermal lidocaine in the treatment of pain due to localized peripheral neuropathy are mixed. A 2014 Cochrane review found insufficient evidence from randomized trials to recommend the use of transdermal lidocaine for neuropathic pain (52); however, there are randomized studies that have found transdermal lidocaine to be effective

at addressing neuropathic pain (53,54) The FDA has approved transdermal lidocaine for the treatment of postherpetic pain (55), and there is early evidence to suggest that the 5% lidocaine patch provides benefit for other neuropathic pain states (56), including diabetic neuropathy (57), CRPS, postmastectomy pain, and HIV-related neuropathy (58).

Intravenous lidocaine and oral mexiletine have been shown to be effective in the management of refractory neuropathic pain (59,60). Lidocaine and mexiletine are local anesthetic and anti-arrhythmic agents. They function as nonspecific sodium channel blockers and, notably, have analgesic properties similar to some AEDs (e.g., lamotrigine and carbamazepine). When used at analgesic concentrations, they function to inhibit the abnormal, spontaneous firing of sodium channels that develop along injured nerves and their dorsal root ganglia without suppressing normal nerve or cardiac conduction. Through their action on sodium channels, these agents inhibit both central and peripheral pain pathways. Systemic lidocaine is also noted to have anti-inflammatory properties. Lidocaine tends to be better tolerated, as mexiletine is commonly associated with gastrointestinal side effects (e.g., nausea and diarrhea). Both medications are contraindicated in the presence of second-degree and third-degree atrial-ventricular conduction blocks. While the evidence is limited, these medications can be considered for patients with neuropathic pain that is refractory to first- or second-line agents (61–63).

Interestingly, sodium channel-blocking properties are also found in several AEDs, such as carbamazepine, oxcarbazepine, and lamotrigine, and in the TCAs, such as amitriptyline, doxepin, and imipramine (63–65).

Adjuvants and Nonopioid Analgesics for Neuropathic Pain

In addition to the agents discussed in the preceding text, many medications from a variety of pharmacologic classes can be classified as adjuvant analgesics and used "off label" in the management of patients with chronic intractable pain. In many cases, the mechanisms supporting this analgesic enhancement are still unknown. At present, the evidence that these medications may possess analgesic properties for the treatment of neuropathic pain has mostly been derived from preliminary clinical investigations and observations.

α_2-Adrenergic Agonists

Medications acting on the α_2-adrenergic spinal receptors (e.g., clonidine and tizanidine) have been clinically recognized as analgesics (9,66).

α_2-Adrenergic agonists are known to have a spinal antinociceptive effect. Controlled trials have shown the effectiveness of intraspinal clonidine for controlling pain (66,67). Clonidine has been found to potentiate intrathecal opioid analgesia. Moreover, transdermal clonidine has a local antiallodynic effect in patients with SMP (68). Topical clonidine, an α_2-adrenergic agonist, has an analgesic effect in SMP. Clonidine causes local inhibition of noradrenaline release by acting on the adrenergic α_2-autoreceptors of the sympathetic endings (68). In one recent study, application of topical clonidine gel significantly reduced the level of pain in subjects with diabetic neuropathy (69). Tizanidine is a relatively short-acting, oral α_2-adrenergic agonist with a much lower hypotensive effect than clonidine. Tizanidine has been used for the management of spasticity. However, animal studies and clinical experience indicate the usefulness of tizanidine for a variety of painful states, including neuropathic pain disorders (70–72). The most common side effects of the α_2-adrenergic agonists are somnolence and dizziness (to which tolerance usually develops).

Capsaicin

Capsaicin is the natural substance present in hot chili peppers. Capsaicin activates the recently cloned vanilloid neuronal membrane receptor (73). A single administration of a large dose of capsaicin, after an initial depolarization, appears to produce a prolonged deactivation of capsaicin-sensitive nociceptors. The analgesic effect is dose dependent and may last for several weeks. Capsaicin must be compounded topically at high concentrations (>1%) and administered under local or regional anesthesia (74). Over-the-counter creams must be applied several times a day for many weeks. Controlled studies at low capsaicin concentrations (0.075% or less) have shown mixed results, possibly because of noncompliance. A recent study found that capsaicin 8% patch provides significant pain relief in CIPN and may lead to regeneration and restoration of sensory nerve fibers (75).

NMDA Antagonists

Evidence gleaned from animal experiments shows that NMDA receptors play an important role in the central mechanisms of hyperalgesia and chronic pain (76). There is evidence to suggest that NMDA antagonists may prevent or counteract opioid analgesic tolerance (77,78). Dextromethorphan, memantine, and ketamine are NMDA antagonists that may be considered as adjuvants in the management of hyperalgesic neuropathic states poorly responsive to opioid analgesics (79–82).

Ketamine. At sub-anesthetic doses (infusions <1 mg/kg/h and oral solution doses of <0.5 mg/kg), ketamine has analgesic properties. Ketamine is increasingly being used as an adjuvant to opioids for refractory neuropathic pain. When added as an adjuvant to opioids, ketamine increases pain relief by 20% to 30% and allows opioid dose reduction by 25% to 50% and can be used in both adult and pediatric patients (79,80). Ketamine is able to alter the nociceptive input at the spinal level; because of the potential neurotoxicity of intrathecal racemic ketamine, the administration of the active compound $S(+)$-ketamine may be a valuable alternative (82). When taken orally, ketamine undergoes extensive first pass metabolism to norketamine, which is an active metabolite. While ketamine has a plasma half-life of 2.5 to 3 hours, the plasma half-life of norketamine is 12 hours. The onset of intravenous ketamine is approximately 5 minutes, while the onset of action is 30 minutes when taken orally. Topical ketamine can provide effective palliation of mucositis pain induced by radiation therapy (81).

Methadone. As mentioned previously, methadone is a racemic mixture of the isomers D-methadone and L-methadone. D-Methadone has been shown to possess NMDA receptor antagonist activity (83). A recent Cochrane review concluded that there was insufficient evidence regarding the use of methadone in the treatment of neuropathic pain (84), although it is noted to be effective clinically (85,86). Of interest is the possibility that NMDA antagonists may prevent or counteract opioid analgesic tolerance (77). Given its long half-life and unpredictable interindividual pharmacokinetic variation, it should be prescribed by experienced clinicians.

In addition to the above limitations, methadone has been associated with QTc prolongation, which may predispose patients to potentially fatal arrhythmias. The American Pain Society issued a clinical practice guideline regarding methadone safety in 2014, which included guidance regarding cardiac testing prior to initiating methadone. Prior to initiation of oral methadone, in patients with risk factors with QTc prolongation, a baseline ECG is recommended. If the QTc interval is >500 milliseconds, methadone initiation is not recommended.

Cannabinoids

Evidence from preclinical and clinical studies indicates that cannabinoids have analgesic properties (78,83,87) that are chiefly mediated via the endocannabinoid signaling system. Cannabinoids are a class of drugs that take their name from the cannabinoid botanical *Cannabis sativa* from which they were first isolated and include herbal preparations of cannabis as well as synthetic, semisynthetic, and extracted cannabinoid preparations (78,87). Public interest in the use of cannabis for a variety of medical purposes has increased in recent years. Thirty-three states have implemented laws legalizing the use of medical marijuana. However, marijuana remains classified as a schedule I drug under federal legal status, and as such, it has not gone through the FDA approval process. This leaves regulations regarding cultivation, product testing and packaging/labeling requirements up to individual states and has resulted in wide regulatory variations across the country (88). Historically, in oncology, the main approved therapeutic use of cannabinoids has been in the prevention of nausea and vomiting caused by chemotherapy. In patients with cancer or acquired immunodeficiency syndrome, Δ-9-*trans*-tetrahydrocannabinol (Δ-9-THC) can be used to increase the appetite and treat weight loss. Several studies have now been carried out to assess the therapeutic effectiveness of cannabinoids as analgesics. Cannabis and the major active constituent of cannabis, Δ-9-THC, have been shown to have antinociceptive effects. Cannabinoids appear to have a predominant antiallodynic/antihyperalgesic effect (78,83,87). Interestingly, the addition of inactive doses of cannabinoids to low doses of μ-opioid agonists appears to potentiate opioid antinociception (89,90).

The results of a series of randomized, placebo-controlled clinical trials performed by regional branches of the University of California have demonstrated that inhaled cannabis holds therapeutic value in the treatment of neuropathic pain. Two studies examined neuropathic pain resulting from painful HIV sensory neuropathy (91,92). One examined neuropathic pain of varying causes, including HIV neuropathy, diabetic neuropathy, brachial plexus avulsion, and CRPS (93), while the other used an experimental model of neuropathic pain with heat and capsaicin tested in healthy volunteers (94). The largest study involved 55 patients with HIV-associated neuropathic pain who were randomized in a double-blind fashion to inhaled cannabis of up to three cannabis (3.56% THC) cigarettes daily for 5 days or placebo (91). Results showed that smoked cannabis relieved chronic neuropathic pain (34% reduction, $p = 0.03$), and more than 50% of patients experienced at least a 30% reduction in pain intensity ($p = 0.04$). Anxiety, sedation, disorientation, confusion, and dizziness occurred more often in cannabis recipients, but these effects were rated as between "none" and mild.

The three separate University of California clinical trials of inhaled cannabis for chronic neuropathic pain involved a total of 127 patients. The results from these studies have been convergent, with all demonstrating a significant decrease in pain after cannabis administration. The magnitude of effect in these studies, expressed as the number of patients needed to treat to produce one positive outcome, was comparable to current therapies. A recent outpatient RCT of patients with chronic post-traumatic or postsurgical refractory neuropathic pain using inhaled cannabis conducted by researchers at McGill showed favorable results in concordance with the University of California studies (95). A recent systematic review and meta-analysis of 42 RCTs reviewed the efficacy of cannabis-based medications for pain management. It concluded that moderate- to high-quality evidence supporting the use of cannabis-based medications for treatment of chronic pain patients, especially for neuropathic pain. This review was limited by heterogeneity of the data available to review. There was wide variability in the cannabinoid derivatives used, the treatment indications, dosages, route, and in the study designs themselves (96).

Synthetic cannabinoids have also been studied in clinical trials. For example, in chronic neuropathic pain, 1′,1′-dimethylheptyl-Δ8-tetrahydrocannabinol-11-oic acid (CT-3) was shown to be more effective than placebo and without major unfavorable side effects. Twenty-one patients with chronic neuropathic pain were randomized to a double-blind, placebo-controlled, crossover trial. Three hours after the administration, the visual analog scale values of those in the treatment group differed significantly from those of the placebo group ($p < 0.02$), whereas after 8 hours, the differences between the two groups were less marked. Dry mouth and fatigue were the most common side effects ($p < 0.02$) (78).

In summary, neuropathic pain is an indication for which cannabinoids may be of benefit; however, most studies are of short trial duration with small sample sizes. High-quality head-to-head trials focused on pain relief and functional outcomes are needed to further characterize safety issues and efficacy with this class of medications.

Anti-inflammatory and Immunomodulatory Agents

A short course of corticosteroids may be considered for severe inflammatory neuropathic pain such as that seen with malignant infiltration of the brachial or lumbosacral plexus, roots, or nerve trunks. Nonsteroidal anti-inflammatory drugs (NSAIDs), for example, cyclooxygenase (COX) type-1 and type-2 inhibitors, and acetaminophen have been of little benefit in the treatment of severe neuropathic pain. Several lines of evidence indicate that TNF-α, as well as other proinflammatory interleukins, may play a key role in the mechanism of pathologic intractable pain. Thalidomide has been shown to prevent hyperalgesia caused by nerve constriction injury in rats (97,98) and is known to inhibit TNF-α production. TNF-α antagonists or newly developed thalidomide analogs with a better safety profile may play a relevant role in the prevention and treatment of otherwise intractable painful disorders (99).

Bisphosphonates (e.g., pamidronate and clodronate) have been reported to be efficacious in the treatment of not only bone cancer pain but also CRPS, a neuropathic inflammatory pain syndrome (77,78). The analgesic effect of bisphosphonate is poorly understood. It may be related to the inhibition and apoptosis of activated cells such as osteoclasts and macrophages. This leads to a decreased release of proinflammatory cytokines in the area of inflammation. In animal models of neuropathic pain (sciatic nerve ligature), bisphosphonates reduced the number of activated macrophages infiltrating the injured nerve, reduced Wallerian nerve fiber degeneration, and decreased experimental hyperalgesia (100). A more recent study has shown that bisphosphonates attenuate spinal microglia activation and p38 MAPK signaling pathway (101).

GABA Agonists

Baclofen is an analog of the inhibitory neurotransmitter GABA and has a specific action on the GABA-B receptors. It has been used for many years as an effective spasmolytic agent. Baclofen also has shown effectiveness in the treatment of trigeminal neuralgia (38). Clinical experience supports the use of low-dose baclofen to potentiate the antineuralgic effect of carbamazepine in trigeminal neuralgia. Baclofen has also been used intrathecally to relieve intractable spasticity and may have a role as an adjuvant when added to spinal opioids for the treatment of intractable neuropathic pain and spasticity. The most common side effects of baclofen are drowsiness, weakness, hypotension, and confusion. It is important to note that discontinuation of baclofen always requires a slow tapering to avoid the occurrence of seizures and other severe neurologic manifestations.

Benzodiazepines (e.g., alprazolam, lorazepam, and diazepam) are GABA-A agonists. Their clinical use in patients with chronic pain is controversial. In a controlled trial, patients with PHN did worse when treated with lorazepam than with placebo or amitriptyline (102). Benzodiazepine-related side effects include depression and disruption of physiologic sleep. In combination with opioids, benzodiazepines cause significant cognitive impairment (103).

Invasive Interventions

Implantable devices, such as spinal cord stimulators (SCSs) intrathecal pumps (IPs), are additional options for the management of intractable neuropathic pain. SCSs work by sending mild electric pulses to the spinal cord, thereby masking and modifying the pain signal. IPs are used to deliver a variety of agents, such as opioids, clonidine, local anesthetics, ziconotide, and baclofen into the cerebrospinal fluid. At this time, only two intrathecally administered medications have been FDA approved for pain: morphine and ziconotide (104). IPs can improve pain and increase functioning in patients whose pain is not adequately controlled after a reasonable trial of systemic opioid therapy or in those who cannot tolerate systemic opioid therapy due to side effects (105,106). Before implantation of an intrathecal morphine pump, treatment trials must show that the patient's pain is somewhat opioid responsive. The combination of intrathecal opioids and bupivacaine enhances the effectiveness of the analgesic regimen and reduces the need for ablative or neurolytic techniques. IPs can be implanted permanently once trials are successful. Ziconotide is a synthetic conopeptide that antagonizes N-type voltage-gated calcium channels and has been shown in multiple studies to improve pain scores. Its use is limited, however, by its narrow therapeutic window and possible side effect, which include dizziness, postural hypotension, nystagmus, and confusion (107).

Many studies suggest that motor cortex stimulation may relieve neuropathic pain, although the mechanism of action is not well understood. For certain intractable neuropathic pain disorders, neuroablative procedures might be considered. For example, the dorsal root entry zone (DREZ) lesion has been recommended for the treatment of intractable pain from painful brachial plexopathy. DREZ can also be useful for relieving pain from head and neck cancer. The decision to perform neuroablative surgery should be made only after a thorough comprehensive assessment has been carried out by a multidisciplinary team of pain medicine specialists and after conservative management has failed to produce any improvement in the patient's quality of life. Cordotomy can be an effective treatment for pathologic unilateral pelvic and leg pain. By sectioning the anterolateral quadrant of the spinal cord, interruption occurs in the spinothalamic tract with subsequent loss of contralateral pain and temperature sensation. The procedure can be done as a percutaneous radiofrequency ablation at C1-C2 or through laminectomy. Cordotomy appears to be more effective in addressing intermittent shooting pain than steady burning pain. Unfortunately, the benefit tends to subside with time, and, therefore, its use in treating chronic pain receives little attention. Dorsal root rhizotomies may be beneficial for patients with chest wall pain. It has been hypothesized that malignancies may induce pain through somatic and visceral mechanisms. Midline myelotomy has been proposed as a way of treating visceral pain associated with cancer. Discrete midline myelotomies have also been performed in patients with abdominal/pelvic pain due to cancer with encouraging results (108). A recent case series suggests that use of an IP in combination with neurosurgical ablation (myelotomy or cordotomy) may allow for more effective control of severe, refractory cancer pain (109).

MALIGNANT BONE PAIN

Incidence and Pathophysiology

Metastasis to bone is the most common cause of pain in patients with cancer (110). Bone pain is usually associated with direct tumor invasion and is often severe and debilitating. Tumors that metastasize to bone most commonly originate in the breast, lung, prostate, thyroid, and kidney; these lesions may be either blastic or lytic. Multiple myeloma, by contrast, is known for causing painful lytic lesions. More than two-thirds of patients with radiographically detectable lesions will experience bone pain, although many patients experience pain even before skeletal metastases become radiographically apparent (110,111).

Immunohistochemical studies have revealed an extensive network of nerve fibers both within and in the vicinity of skeletal structures, including the periosteum, cortical and trabecular bone, and bone marrow. Thinly myelinated and unmyelinated sensory fibers, as well as sympathetic fibers, occur throughout these tissues. Although the periosteum is the most densely innervated tissue, when the total volume of each tissue is considered, the bone marrow receives the greatest total number of sensory nerve fibers (112). These sensory fibers express multiple signaling molecules, including neuropeptides and neurotrophins. Recently, studies have shown that cancer cells in the bone induce sprouting and reorganization of sensory and sympathetic fibers in the periosteum, creating an increase in nerve fiber density and formation of neuroma-like structures, which may contribute to breakthrough or movement-induced pain (113).

The presence of receptors for some neuropeptides (e.g., calcitonin gene-related peptide and substance P) on osteoclasts and osteoblasts and the capacity of these receptors to regulate osteoclast formation and bone formation and resorption have recently been described. Because NGF has been shown to modulate inflammatory neuropathic pain states, in most recent animal models of cancer bone pain, NGF antibody antagonist therapy has also been shown to produce significant reduction in both ongoing and movement-related pain behavior (114). This treatment was more effective than morphine (115).

It is believed that skeletal lesions result, at least in part, from a disruption of the normal balance between bone formation and bone resorption. In the process, bone nociceptors respond to changes in the bone marrow, as well as cortical, trabecular, and periosteum microenvironments. Inflammatory, immunologic, and neuropathic mechanisms develop in the bone in response to the cancer insult and the patient experiences pain. As osteolysis continues, the bone integrity declines and patients become vulnerable to other complications, including pathologic fractures, nerve compression syndromes, spinal instability, and hypercalcemia. A full review of the pathophysiology of bone metastasis can be found in Chapter 5.

Clinical Findings and Diagnosis

Pain is commonly the presenting symptom of bone metastases, and the presence of focal pain in a patient with cancer should trigger an investigation. Patients may experience a deep throbbing pain punctuated by sharper intense pain, often triggered by movement (incident or breakthrough pain). On examination, there may also be focal tenderness and swelling at the affected sites. Range of motion may be severely limited, especially if the joint space is involved. In many patients, normal activities such as deep breathing, coughing, or moving an affected limb can cause intense, often unbearable, pain. Pain may be localized or referred to various sites. For example, involvement of the hip may cause referred pain to the knee or groin. Bone pain due to metastases should be differentiated from other bone pain syndromes that are caused by non-neoplastic conditions such as osteoarthritis, osteoporotic fractures, and osteomalacia.

Bone pain may be focal, multifocal, or generalized. Multifocal pain is commonly experienced by patients with multiple sites of bony metastases, although approximately 25% of patients with bone metastases do not complain of pain and a patient with multiple sites of osseous metastases may only have a few painful sites. There is a well-described generalized bone pain syndrome that occurs when there is replacement of bone marrow by tumor. This is observed with myeloproliferative malignancies and less commonly with solid tumors (116).

Plain film radiography, CT, MRI, and bone scintigraphy can be used to image osseous metastases. MRI is the most accurate diagnostic tool and is more sensitive than the other modalities at detecting early osseous lesions. Since MRI is not always clinically feasible, CT imaging can also be diagnostic and is more sensitive than plain film radiography. In the setting of lytic bone lesions, plain films characteristically reveal a "moth-eaten" appearance. Bone scintigraphy should be regarded as an adjunct to the former tests but can be useful when identifying the extent of bone lesions throughout the body.

The location of the lesion and the extent of cortical involvement influence the risk of pathologic fracture. For example, the incidence of fracture is cited to be 3.7% when 25% to 50% of the cortex was involved, 61% when the degree of cortical involvement ranged between 50% and 75%, and 79% when >75% of the cortex was involved (117). Although any tumor can metastasize to the bone and result in a pathologic fracture, mammary carcinoma is responsible for 50% of such fractures. Multiple myeloma is the second most common cancer to cause pathologic fractures.

Vertebral Lesions

The vertebral bodies are the most common sites of osseous metastases; more than two-thirds of vertebral metastases are found in the thoracic spine. This is attributed to the presence of a valveless plexus of epidural veins called the *Batson's plexus* in which blood flows rostrally or caudally. This may serve as a route for the metastatic spread of some cancers. The lumbosacral and cervical spine account for approximately 20% and 10% of bone metastases, respectively. Additionally, 85% of patients have multiple-level involvement (118). Early recognition of pain syndromes of the vertebral bodies is critical because the pain can indicate impending compression of adjacent neural structures.

Occipital pain can indicate the destruction of the atlas or fracture of the odontoid process and may be a sign of impending spinal cord compression at the cervicomedullary junction (119). Metastasis at this spinal level is uncommon, occurring in just 0.5% of all cases of spinal metastasis; however, these cases often require surgical intervention for both pain control and appropriate stabilization (120).

Bone metastases at the level of C7-T1 vertebral bodies can cause a pain referral pattern at the infrascapular area, with upper back pain and muscle spasm (121). When T12 or L1 is affected by bone metastases, the referral pattern can often be at the iliac crest or sacroiliac joint; imaging could miss the metastases if directed at the pelvis. Sacral

syndrome can develop from bone metastases, and referred and/or radiating pain can arise in the buttock, posterior thigh, or perineum (122,123). In addition to this skeletal component, involvement of adjacent structures, such as nerves or muscles, may produce other types of pain. Involvement of adjacent nerve tissue of the peripheral system, such as the lumbar plexus, or central system, such as the spinal cord, can produce both neuropathic pain syndromes and neurologic deficits. Severe back pain is the initial symptom in many patients who present with epidural compression and warrants prompt evaluation. Back pain typically precedes epidural compression. Clinically, there is a rapid, crescendo type of pain with epidural disease. There may or may not be a lancinating quality to the pain or a band-like tightness that wraps around the chest or abdomen. If epidural disease is not diagnosed and treated in a timely manner, paraplegia or quadriplegia secondary to spinal cord compression may occur.

Therapeutic Interventions for Malignant Bone Pain

There are numerous options for the treatment of pain related to bone metastases, including opioid therapy, specific pharmacotherapy, radiotherapy, systemic radionuclide therapy, and surgery (Table 1.4). With appropriate use of these measures, even patients with severe pain can expect to achieve relief.

Anti-inflammatory Drugs

Corticosteroids. Steroid therapy may be considered for severe inflammatory pain, especially when bone cancer infiltrates or compresses adjacent nerve tissue, such as the spinal cord or brachial or lumbosacral plexi. High-dose steroids are used in epidural disease for pain control and for decompression while definitive treatment is planned (124,125). High-dose steroids are also indicated for patients with increased intracranial pressure secondary to a mass effect of intracranial tumors.

Nonsteroidal Anti-inflammatory Drugs (NSAIDs). NSAIDs are commonly used in the treatment of mild to moderate bone pain. NSAIDs share a common mechanism of action, which is the inhibition of COX and, therefore, prostaglandin (PG) production. PGs function to generate pain by stimulating peripheral sensory neurons in the setting of inflammation. The mechanism of action of NSAIDs has been further elucidated by the discovery of two distinct isoforms of COX (COX-1 and COX-2). COX-1 is the constitutive isoform present in, for example, the stomach, kidney, and platelets. Conversely, the inducible isoform, COX-2, usually

TABLE 1.4 THERAPEUTIC INTERVENTIONS FOR BONE PAIN

	Denosumab	Zoledronic acid	Pamidronate
Agent class	• Fully human monoclonal antibody to RANKL	• Nitrogen-containing bisphosphonate	• Nitrogen-containing bisphosphonate
Indications	• Prevention of SREs from bone metastases due to solid tumors	• Bone metastases from solid tumors, MM, and HCM • For prostate cancer with progression after ≥1 previous hormonal therapy	• Bone metastases in solid tumors, MM, and HCM
Dosing and administration	• 120 mg s.c. every 4 wk	• 4 mg i.v. every 3–4 wk • HCM 4 mg, potential for retreatment if inadequate response (allow minimum of 7 d between treatments)	• Bone metastases, 90 mg i.v. over 4 h every 4 wk • HCM, 60–90 mg i.v. as single dose over 2–24 h
Adverse events	• Fatigue/asthenia, hypophosphatemia, nausea, dyspnea, hypocalcemia, and ONJ	• Fatigue, nausea, bone pain and myalgias, fever, hypocalcemia, subtrochanteric fracture, ONJ, and renal toxicity	• Monitor serum calcium, phosphate, magnesium, and potassium levels in patients with HCM; transient fever; renal toxicity; ONJ; and musculoskeletal symptoms
Safety information	• Can cause severe hypocalcemia; calcium levels lower if CrCl < 30 mL/min • Calcium and vitamin D supplementation recommended • ONJ rate 2.2% in clinical trials; oral exam recommended before starting therapy; avoid invasive dental procedures during therapy	• Due to potential renal toxicity, must obtain baseline CrCl; ZA dose based on CrCl and serum creatinine • Measure serum creatinine level before each dose; withhold treatment for renal deterioration • Calcium and vitamin D supplementation recommended • ONJ rate 1.3% in clinical trials; oral exam recommended before starting therapy; avoid invasive dental procedures during therapy	• Due to potential renal toxicity, assess baseline and subsequent serum creatinine levels before treatment • Oral exam recommended before starting therapy; avoid invasive dental procedures during therapy • Calcium and vitamin D supplementation recommended • Closely monitor patients with preexisting anemia, leukopenia, or thrombocytopenia for first 2 wk after treatment
FDA approval date	• 2010: bone metastases • Not approved for HCM or MM	• 2001: HCM • 2002: broad bone metastases including MM	• 1991: HCM • 1995: MM and breast cancer

MM, multiple myeloma; ONJ, osteonecrosis of the jaw; HCM, hypercalcemia of malignancy; SRE, skeletal-related events; RANKL, Rank ligand.

becomes expressed in cells after being activated by proinflammatory cytokines. COX-1 and COX-2 inhibition results in both the adverse and beneficial effects of NSAIDs. The anti-inflammatory and analgesic effects of different NSAIDs are generally considered equal; however, the frequency with which they produce side effects varies. Caution must be exercised when using NSAIDs in patients with hypertension, impaired renal function, or heart failure. COX-2 inhibitors have fewer gastrointestinal side effects; however, they are noted to have vascular prothrombotic effects. Given the different COX inhibitors available, one must consider the patient's history of response and the efficacy, safety, and cost-effectiveness of the specific agent to be prescribed.

Bone-Modifying Agents

Bisphosphonates. Some of the most important drugs that have emerged in the battle against bone pain are the bisphosphonates, the synthetic analogs of pyrophosphate that bind hydroxyapatite crystals of the bone with a high affinity. They reduce resorption of bone by inhibiting osteoclastic activity and osteolysis. Bisphosphonate therapy has proved to be highly valuable in the management of numerous bone-related conditions, including hypercalcemia, osteoporosis, multiple myeloma, and Paget's disease of bone. First-generation bisphosphonates, such as etidronate, have been largely replaced by second-generation bisphosphonates, including pamidronate, as well as third-generation bisphosphonates, including zoledronic acid and ibandronate. Multiple studies have demonstrated the efficacy of second- and third-generation bisphosphonates in reducing pain in bone metastases (126,127). Zoledronic acid significantly reduces the overall risk of developing a skeletal-related event, such as pathologic fracture, spinal cord compression, hypercalcemia of malignancy, and the need for surgery or radiation to bone in patients with bone metastasis by an additional 20% in comparison with pamidronate and significantly improves pain and quality of life (128). Ibandronate has been shown to provide significant and sustained relief from metastatic bone pain, improving patient functioning and quality of life. The oral and intravenous formulations of ibandronate appear to have comparable efficacy and treatment with a loading dose of ibandronate has been shown to produce pain reduction within days (129). With a favorable long-term safety profile and the added convenience and flexibility offered by its efficacious oral formulation, ibandronate represents a good therapeutic option for metastatic bone disease management.

Rank Ligand Inhibition. Rank ligand is a protein that stimulates osteoclasts in patients with metastatic bone disease. Increased Rank ligand helps drive a vicious cycle of bone destruction, which can lead to devastating skeletal-related events and severe bone pain (130). Denosumab is a Rank ligand inhibitor used for solid tumor bone metastases, with the exclusion of multiple myeloma. Recent studies have shown denosumab to be superior to zoledronic acid in preventing skeletal-related events (131). One large study of 1,432 subjects with hormone-resistant prostate cancer who were randomized to receive placebo or denosumab found that treatment with denosumab was associated with delayed symptoms of metastases, extended the time to the first bone metastases, and increased bone metastasis-free survival by an average of more than 4 months, although there was no survival difference between the two groups (132).

Calcitonin. Calcitonin may have several pain-related indications in patients who have bone pain, including osseous metastases. The most frequent routes of absorption are intranasal and subcutaneous injection. Calcitonin reduces resorption of bone by inhibiting osteoclastic activity and osteolysis.

Radiotherapy

Radiation therapy is an effective, well-tolerated modality in the management of painful bone metastases. Between 60% and 85% of patients experience clinically significant pain relief following treatment, with complete pain relief achieved in 15% to 58% of patients (133). The extent and duration of pain relief following irradiation can vary based on the type and location of the lesion. While the onset of pain relief may occur as early as 1 to 2 weeks after treatment, full palliative effect is typically experienced at 4 to 6 weeks. It is estimated that 30% to 40% of patients may experience a "pain flare" or transient worsening of pain typically lasting 1 to 2 days at the irradiated site. A short course of dexamethasone has been shown to reduce the frequency of these events.

Most patients are treated with external beam radiation therapy, in which a high-energy X-rays are generated outside the body (typically by a linear accelerator) and are directed at the tumor site. While these X-rays preferentially damage cancer cells, healthy cells can be injured if they receive high enough doses of radiation. In the setting of curative intent radiation therapy, a high total dose of radiation is desired. To reduce the risk of delayed, long-term side effects in adjacent healthy tissues, this total dose of radiation is divided into smaller doses, called fractions, which are delivered over multiple daily sessions, thereby allowing healthy tissues time to repair. In comparison, when radiation is delivered with palliative intent, a much lower total dose of radiation is required and therefore conventional dose fractionation is not necessary.

Over 30 randomized trials have compared outcomes associated with different dose fractionation schemes commonly utilized in the management of painful bone metastases, including 30 Gy in 10 fractions, 24 Gy in 6 fractions, 20 Gy in 5 fractions, and 8 Gy in 1 fraction. The data overwhelmingly support the use of single fraction radiation therapy for uncomplicated, painful bone metastases. Single fraction treatment is just as effective as multi-fractionated regimens while also reducing treatment burden and cost (134–136). While in some studies, the rate of retreatment was significantly higher in the single fraction group, it is thought that this is largely due to increased willingness on the part of the provider to re-irradiate after a lower total dose delivered among those treated with single fraction therapy and increased reluctance to re-irradiate after a higher total dose delivered among those receiving multi fractionated treatment (134,137).

While a single fraction of 8 Gy is almost always appropriate in the setting of uncomplicated, painful bone metastases, multifractionated regimens that allow for a higher total dose of may be indicated in certain clinical situations. These include patients with lytic lesions and an impending pathologic fracture, patients with a symptomatic pathologic fracture, and patients with lesions associated with substantial extraosseous involvement (138).

Radiopharmaceuticals

Bone-targeting radiopharmaceuticals are systemically administered radioactive compounds that localize to areas of osteoblastic activity to deliver radiation to the sites of osteoblastic or mixed osteoblastic/osteolytic bone metastases. Radiopharmaceuticals can be an effective method for alleviating metastatic bone pain, especially in the setting of scattered painful bone metastases, for which external beam radiotherapy is impossible because of the large field of irradiation (139,140). Due to the latency of therapeutic effect, these agents are most appropriate for use in patients with a life expectancy of at least 3 months (141). The most common and major safety concern related to the adverse effects from radiopharmaceuticals is bone marrow toxicity. Although this side effect is typically reversible, their use is relatively contraindicated in patients with severe myelotoxicity. Severe renal dysfunction (glomerular filtration rate [GFR] <30 mL/min) is also a relative contraindication to the use of radiopharmaceuticals, as the agents are really cleared and the longer they remain in circulation, the greater the risk of myelotoxicity.

Strontium 89 (^{89}Sr). The radioisotope ^{89}Sr is a divalent ion, similar to calcium. It is incorporated into bone with a 10-fold higher uptake seen at the site of metastatic bone lesions compared to normal bone (142). Approximately 80% of patients experience at least partial pain relief and a reduction in analgesic use is seen in 71% to 81% of treated patients. The onset of pain relief is typically between 1 and 4 weeks after treatment with a duration of relief ranging from 3 to 15 months (143). Patients who responded well to initial treatment tend to benefit from retreatment, although those who did not experience sufficient relief with the first dose are unlikely to achieve relief with subsequent treatment.

Samarium-153 Ethylene Diamine Tetramethylene Phosphonate. ^{153}Sm-ethylene diamine tetramethylene phosphonate (^{153}Sm-EDTMP) is a widely available and extensively tested radiopharmaceutical for systemic therapy in patients with multiple skeletal metastases. Its use is approved for any secondary bone lesion that has been shown to accumulate the traditional marker in bone scans, that is, technetium Tc 99m-methylene diphosphonate (Tc 99m-MDP). The short half-life, the relatively low-energy β-emissions, and the γ-emissions make the ^{153}Sm an attractive radionuclide, allowing therapeutic delivery of short-range electrons at relatively high dose (144).

Rhenium-186 Hydroxyethylidene Diphosphonate. Rhenium-186 hydroxyethylidene diphosphonate (^{186}Re-HEDP) is a potentially useful radiopharmaceutical agent for the palliation of bone pain, having numerous advantageous characteristics. Bone marrow toxicity is limited and reversible, which makes repetitive treatment safer. Studies using ^{186}Re-HEDP have shown encouraging clinical results of palliative therapy, with an overall response rate of about 70% in painful bone metastases (145). It is effective for fast palliation of painful bone metastases from various tumors and the effect tends to last longer if patients are treated early in the course of their disease. It is preferred to radiopharmaceuticals with a long half-life in patients who have been pretreated with bone marrow-suppressive chemotherapy.

Surgery

When weighing the risks and benefits of surgery in the management of painful bone metastases, it is critical to assess the patient's ability to tolerate the procedure. In patients for whom the prognosis is less than a month, surgery is rarely indicated. Patients with cardiopulmonary disease should have a thorough operative assessment. Orthopedic stabilization of the affected skeletal segment can be helpful for patients with large lytic lesions who are at risk for fracture and can improve the overall quality of life for many patients. Vertebroplasty and kyphoplasty may be efficacious in treating painful vertebral metastasis. Vertebroplasty is the injection of bone cement, generally poly (methyl methacrylate), into a vertebral body. Kyphoplasty is the placement of a balloon into the vertebral body, followed by an inflation/deflation sequence to create a cavity before the cement injection. These procedures are most often performed in a percutaneous manner on an outpatient or short-stay basis. The risks associated with the procedures are low, but serious complications, such as spinal cord compression, nerve root compression, venous embolism, and pulmonary embolism, including cardiovascular collapse, may occur (146).

VISCERAL PAIN

Visceral pain represents a pain phenotype distinct from that of somatic or neuropathic pain. Mediated by unique peripheral and central pathways, visceral pain results from the activation of visceral nociceptors, often in the setting of inflammation, compression, distention, infiltration, or stretching, or contraction of the thoracic, abdominal, or pelvic viscera. Visceral pain can also occur in the absence of clear underlying pathology, as seen in functional disorders.

Clinical Findings and Diagnosis

Visceral pain is typically described as dull, squeezing, colicky, gnawing, or aching. It can be intermittent or continuous and is generally poorly localized due to the low density of visceral innervation and degree of divergence of visceral input in the CNS. Visceral pain is frequently referred to somatic sites; this is due to the convergence of visceral and somatic afferent inputs to the CNS. Since the referred pain is generally localized, it may be challenging to differentiate from pain of true somatic origin. Viscero-visceral convergence, which leads to referred pain from one visceral organ to another, can also occur. Visceral pain is frequently associated with autonomic changes such as pallor, diaphoresis, nausea, gastrointestinal disturbances, and changes in blood pressure, heart rate, and body temperature (147). Further, emotional states and stress are known to influence the perception of visceral pain through supra-spinal modulation (148).

Hepatic capsular stretch or diaphragmatic irritation is commonly seen with primary hepatocellular carcinoma or hepatic metastases. The pain tends to be dull and aching located in the right subcostal region or referred to the right shoulder, and exacerbated by movement or deep inspiration. The treatment for this syndrome is analgesic doses of corticosteroids given in divided dose and opioid analgesics (149).

Back pain is common in pancreatic cancer, endometrial cancer, or in the setting of retroperitoneal lymphadenopathy. The pain is exacerbated on recumbency and alleviated with forward flexion. The pain is typically dull, diffuse, and poorly localized. This type of pain should be differentiated from epidural metastasis, and a careful examination and appropriate imaging can confirm the diagnosis.

Intestinal distention resulting from intraluminal obstruction due to a gastrointestinal tumor, adhesions, and intra-abdominal or pelvic masses causes a pain syndrome characterized by colicky pain. It is often associated with nausea and/or vomiting, anorexia, and bloating. This pain syndrome can also result from atonic bowel due to ischemia, autonomic denervation, or primary cancer therapies including radiotherapy.

Visceral carcinomatosis is frequently associated with visceral abdominal pain in the setting of peritoneal inflammation, malignant adhesions, and ascites. Tense ascites produce discomfort from abdominal wall stretching and can also manifest as low back pain. Pelvic and perineal pain can occur in malignancies that arise in the pelvis, including colorectal and genitourinary tumors. This pain syndrome is often characterized by both nociceptive and neuropathic components. Occasionally, patients experience painful spasms in the rectum, bladder, or urethra. The visceral component of this pain syndrome can be marked by tenesmus.

Therapeutic Interventions for Visceral Pain

While it is understood that visceral pain can be modulated at the peripheral, spinal, and supraspinal levels, our understanding of the specific mechanisms is limited, as is the availability of targeted pharmacologic agents. We do know that certain receptors are involved in the downregulation of visceral pain; these include gamma aminobutyric acid-B (GABA-B) channels, kappa and mu opioid receptors, and somatostatin receptors. Ion channels and inflammatory processes are also established targets for treatment. In general, it is thought that combinations of analgesics may be more effective than the use of single agents and that visceral pain is best managed using a multimodal approach (150).

Opioid analgesics can be effective in the management of acute visceral pain although common opioid side effects, such as constipation and nausea, may exacerbate symptoms. Interestingly, opioids have also been shown to cause a paradoxical visceral hypersensitivity in some settings (151). Kappa and mu opioid receptors are located along the gastrointestinal tract and on visceral afferents, and it is thought that differential activation of these receptors might be responsible for this visceral hyperalgesia (152,153). For example, oxycodone, which is a kappa and mu opioid receptor agonist has been shown to reduce visceral pain more effectively than morphine, which is primarily a mu opioid receptor agonist (153). Opioid-induced visceral hyperalgesia is best managed by rotating to a different opioid, lowering the opioid dose, or adding a gabapentinoid, which may reduce visceral hypersensitivity caused by morphine (154).

There is evidence to suggest that adjuvant analgesics should be considered early in the management of visceral pain, although there are few clinical trials and the data are largely based on animal models. Gabapentinoids exert an effect on visceral nociception both centrally and peripherally. NMDA receptor antagonists have been shown to reduce visceral pain and can act synergistically with opioids (155). TCAs and serotonin norepinephrine reuptake inhibitors are thought to improve visceral pain through increased norepinephrine activity. Gamma aminobutyric acid receptor-B (GABA-B) agonists, such as baclofen, have been shown to modulate visceromotor signals due to colorectal distention in animal models (156). Acetaminophen and NSAIDS may also provide relief in some patients with mild symptoms. Octreotide should be considered in the setting of intestinal obstruction and has also been noted to reduce visceral hyperalgesia (157). Anticholinergic medications may provide relief of visceral spasms. For example, hyoscyamine is commonly used for gastrointestinal spasms and oxybutynin is used for painful bladder spasms due to overactive bladder pathology. Given the side effect profile of most anticholinergic agents, in certain clinical situations, symptoms may be exacerbated with their use. Corticosteroids are often used in the management of visceral pain syndromes including capsular stretch or organ distention.

The use of tunneled intraspinal catheter systems, neurolytic blockades, neuroablative procedures, radiotherapy, or palliative surgeries may be options if pharmacologic management is insufficient. For more information regarding bowel obstruction and treatment options, please see Chapter 15.

Neurolytic Blockade for Visceral Pain

Neurolytic blockade can be efficacious for visceral-related pain in cancer; however, it is usually reserved for patients with a limited prognosis and well-localized pain syndromes. Nerve blocks that are specifically for visceral pain lack durability and have an analgesic benefit of 6 months or less in some cases. Neurolytic blocks are primarily viewed as adjuvant therapy and not as a replacement for systemic pharmacotherapy for cancer pain. Alcohol and phenol are the most widely used agents (158).

Intrapleural phenol block has been reported to be helpful in managing visceral pain associated with esophageal cancer (159). Certain types of thoracic pain from invasion of the chest wall secondary to a pleural tumor may respond to intercostal neurolytic blocks or paravertebral blockade.

Neurolytic block of the celiac plexus is well described in the literature and has proven efficacy in patients with pancreatic cancer and epigastric and/or back pain. Celiac plexus block has also been used successfully in treating visceral pain from upper abdominal malignancies. In one prospective randomized trial of patients with pancreatic cancer, the pain relief provided by a neurolytic celiac plexus block was equal to that provided by systemic opioids with fewer side effects (160). Data also support the use of intraoperative neurolytic blockade of the celiac plexus for unresectable pancreatic tumor (161). Neurolysis of the superior hypogastric plexus has been used for the treatment of visceral pain from cancer of the lower abdomen and pelvis, including gynecologic, colorectal, and genitourinary malignancies. However, some of these cancers may have a significant retroperitoneal pain component, which may lead to poor results with this type of neurolysis. Reportedly, the procedure seems to carry minimal risks in terms of complications (162). Neurolysis of the ganglion

impar is used for intractable rectal and perineal pain in patients who often suffer from urgency. The ganglion is located at the sacrococcygeal junction. There are limited published data on this procedure. Intrathecal neurolytic blockade might be indicated for patients with advanced or terminal malignancy, with intractable, unilateral pain affecting only a few dermatomes (preferably of the thoracic region). The most common complications of intrathecal neurolysis are persistent pain, limb weakness, and urinary and rectal dysfunction.

Epidural neurolytic blockade can be performed by the insertion of a catheter, so that multiple repeated injections can be administered. Epidural neurolysis has been used successfully for unilateral or bilateral pain of thoracic and abdominal visceral origin. It has been described as a procedure safer than intrathecal neurolysis. The duration of analgesia may vary from 1 to 3 months (163).

CONCLUSION

Neuropathic, bone, and visceral pain syndromes can be difficult to treat and are best addressed using a comprehensive, multimodal approach. The number and variety of management options can be confusing and intimidating, even for physicians specializing in the treatment of pain. Dose titration is an important principle to be familiar with when using analgesics, in particular, opioids, antiepileptics, and antidepressants. The treating physician should be sure to (a) know how to conduct a comprehensive pain assessment, (b) determine the predominant mechanism(s) underlying the pain syndrome, (c) understand the pharmacology of the analgesics and the indications for the procedures under consideration, (d) know how to appropriate titrate the dose of medications used, and (e) recognize and manage side effects of medications and procedure-related adverse events.

REFERENCES

1. Merskey H, Bogduk N, eds. *Classification of Chronic Pain. IASP Task Force on Taxonomy.* 2nd ed. Seattle, WA: IASP Press; 1994:209-214.
2. Pappagallo M. Peripheral neuropathic pain. In: Pappagallo M, ed. *The Neurological Basis of Pain.* New York, NY: McGraw-Hill; 2005:321-341.
3. Allan SM, Tyrrell PJ, Rothwell NJ. Interleukin-1 and neuronal injury. *Nat Rev Immunol.* 2005;5:629-640.
4. Empl M, Renaud S, Erne B, et al. TNF-alpha expression in painful and nonpainful neuropathies. *Neurology.* 2001;56:1371-1377.
5. Lindenlaub T, Sommer C. Cytokines in sural nerve biopsies from inflammatory and non-inflammatory neuropathies. *Acta Neuropathol.* 2003;105:593-602.
6. Schafers M, Lee DH, Brors D, et al. Increased sensitivity of injured and adjacent uninjured rat primary sensory neurons to exogenous tumor necrosis factor-alpha after spinal nerve ligation. *J Neurosci.* 2003;23:3028-3038.

7. Raja SN, Turnquist JL, Meleka S, et al. Monitoring adequacy of alpha-adrenoceptor blockade following systemic phentolamine administration. *Pain.* 1996;64(1):197-204.

8. Ali Z, Raja SN, Wesselmann U, et al. Intradermal injection of norepinephrine evokes pain in patients with sympathetically maintained pain. *Pain.* 2000;88:161-168.

9. Scholz J, Woolf CJ. Mechanisms of neuropathic pain. In: Pappagallo M, ed. *The Neurological Basis of Pain.* New York, NY: McGraw-Hill; 2005:71-94.

10. Kim HK, Park SK, Zhou JL, et al. Reactive oxygen species play an important role in a rat model of neuropathic pain. *Pain.* 2004;111(1-2):116-124.

11. Schafers M, Brinkhoff J, Neukirchen S, et al. Combined epineurial therapy with neutralizing antibodies to tumor necrosis factor-alpha and interleukin-1 receptor has an additive effect in reducing neuropathic pain in mice. *Neurosci Lett.* 2001;310:113-116.

12. Watkins LR, Milligan ED, Maier SF. Glial activation: a driving force for pathological pain. *Trends Neurosci.* 2001;24(8):450-455.

13. Galer BS, Jensen MP. Development and preliminary validation of a pain measure specific to neuropathic pain: the Neuropathic Pain Scale. *Neurology.* 1997;48:332-338.

14. Cleeland CS, Ryan KM. Pain assessment: global use of the Brief Pain Inventory. *Ann Acad Med Singapore.* 1994;23:129-138.

15. Keller S, Bann CM, Dodd SL, Schein J, Mendoza TR, Cleeland CS. Validity of the brief pain inventory for use in documenting the outcomes of patients with noncancer pain. *Clin J Pain.* 2004;20(5):309-318.

16. Correll DJ. The measurement of pain: objectifying the subjective. *Pain Manage.* 2007;1:197-211.

17. Katz J, Melzack R. The McGill Pain Questionnaire: development, psychometric properties, and usefulness of the long-form, short-form, and short-form-2. In: Turk DC, Melzack R, eds. *Handbook of Pain Assessment.* New York, NY: The Guilford Press; 2011:45-66.

18. Martin LA, Hagen NA. Neuropathic pain in cancer patients: mechanisms, syndromes, and clinical controversies. *J Pain Symptom Manage.* 1997;14:99-117.

19. Amato AA, Collins MP. Neuropathies associated with malignancy. *Semin Neurol.* 1998;18:125-144.

20. Zis P, Varrassi G. Painful peripheral neuropathy and cancer. *Pain Ther.* 2017;6:115-116.

21. Backonja M, Glanzman RL. Gabapentin dosing for neuropathic pain: evidence from randomized, placebo-controlled clinical trials. *Clin Ther.* 2003;25:81-104.

22. Backonja M, Beydoun A, Edwards KR, et al. Gabapentin for the symptomatic treatment of painful neuropathy in patients with diabetes mellitus: a randomized controlled trial. *JAMA.* 1998;280:1831-1836.

23. Kukkar A, Bali A, Singh N, et al. Implications and mechanism of action of gabapentin in neuropathic pain. *Arch Pharm Res.* 2013;36:237-251.

24. Bonnet U, Scherbaum N. How addictive are gabapentin and pregabalin? A systematic review. *Eur Neuropsychopharmacol.* 2017;27(12):1185-1215. doi:10.1016/j.euroneuro.2017.08.430.

25. Zakrzewska JM, Chaudhry Z, Nurmikko TJ, et al. Lamotrigine (lamictal) in refractory trigeminal neuralgia: results from a double-blind, placebo controlled, crossover trial. *Pain.* 1997;73:223-230.

26. Pappagallo M. Preliminary experience with topiramate in the treatment of chronic pain syndromes. Poster presented at: The 17th annual meeting, American Pain Society, 1998, San Diego, CA.

27. Nazarbaghi S, Amiri-Nikpour MR, Eghbal AF, et al. Comparison of the effect of topiramate versus gabapentin on neuropathic pain in patients with polyneuropathy: a randomized clinical trial. *Electron Physician.* 2017;9(10):5617-5622.

28. Shi W, Liu H, Zhang Y, et al. Design, synthesis, and preliminary evaluation of gabapentin-pregabalin mutual prodrugs in relieving neuropathic pain. *Arch Pharm (Weinheim).* 2005;338:358-364.

29. Pappagallo M. Newer antiepileptic drugs: possible uses in the treatment of neuropathic pain and migraine. *Clin Ther.* 2003;25:2506-2538.

30. Wiffen PJ, Derry S, Moore RA, et al. Antiepileptic drugs for neuropathic pain and fibromyalgia—an overview of Cochrane reviews. *Cochrane Database Syst Rev.* 2013;2013(11):CD010567.

31. Finnerup NB, Attal N, Haroutounian S, et al. Pharmacotherapy for neuropathic pain in adults: a systematic review and meta-analysis. *Lancet Neurol.* 2015;14(2):162-173.

32. Gilron I, Bailey JM, Tu D, et al. Morphine, gabapentin, or their combination for neuropathic pain. *N Engl J Med.* 2005;352:1324-1334.

33. Arumugam S, Lau CS, Chamberlain RS. Use of preoperative gabapentin significantly reduces postoperative opioid consumption: a meta-analysis. *J Pain Res.* 2016;9:631-640.

34. Jiang Y, Li J, Lin H, et al. The efficacy of gabapentin in reducing pain intensity and morphine consumption after breast cancer surgery: a meta-analysis. *Medicine (Baltimore).* 2018;97(38):e11581.

35. Gimbel JS, Richards P, Portenoy RK. Controlled-release oxycodone for pain in diabetic neuropathy: a randomized controlled trial. *Neurology.* 2003;60:927-934.

36. Raja SN, Haythornthwaite JA, Pappagallo M, et al. Opioids versus antidepressants in postherpetic neuralgia: a randomized, placebo-controlled trial. *Neurology.* 2002;59:1015-1021.

37. Rowbotham MC, Twilling L, Davies PS, et al. Oral opioid therapy for chronic peripheral and central neuropathic pain. *N Engl J Med.* 2003;348:1223-1232.

38. Suzuki R, Chapman V, Dickenson AH. The effectiveness of spinal and systemic morphine on rat dorsal horn neuronal responses in the spinal nerve ligation model of neuropathic pain. *Pain.* 1999;80:215-228.

39. McNicol ED, Midbari A, Eisenberg E. Opioids for neuropathic pain. *Cochrane Database Syst Rev.* 2013;(8): CD006146.

40. Pappagallo M. Aggressive pharmacologic treatment of pain. In: Pisetsky DS, Bradley L, eds. *Pain Management in the Rheumatic Diseases. Rheumatic Disease Clinics of North America.* Philadelphia, PA: WB Saunders; 1999:193.

41. Crain SM, Shen KF. Antagonists of excitatory opioid receptor functions enhance morphine's analgesic potency and attenuate opioid tolerance/dependence liability. *Pain.* 2000;84:121-131.

42. Harati Y, Gooch C, Swenson M, et al. Double-blind randomized trial of tramadol for the treatment of the pain of diabetic neuropathy. *Neurology.* 1998;50:1842-1846.

43. Sindrup SH, Madsen C, Brosen K, et al. The effect of tramadol in painful polyneuropathy in relation to serum drug and metabolite levels. *Clin Pharmacol Ther.* 1999;66:636-641.

44. Duehmke RM, Derry S, Wiffen PJ, Bell RF, Aldington D, Moore RA. Tramadol for neuropathic pain in adults. *Cochrane Database Syst Rev.* 2017;6(6):CD003726.

45. Max MB, Lynch SA, Muir J, et al. Effects of desipramine, amitriptyline, and fluoxetine on pain in diabetic neuropathy. *N Engl J Med.* 1992;326:1250-1256.

46. Grothe DR, Scheckner B, Albano D. Treatment of pain syndromes with venlafaxine. *Pharmacotherapy.* 2004;24:621-629.

47. Marchand F, Alloui A, Pelissier T, et al. Evidence for an antihyperalgesic effect of venlafaxine in vincristine-induced neuropathy in rat. *Brain Res.* 2003;980:117-120.

48. Rowbotham MC, Goli V, Kunz NR, et al. Venlafaxine extended release in the treatment of painful diabetic neuropathy: a double-blind, placebo-controlled study. *Pain.* 2004;110:697-706.

49. Goldstein DJ, Lu Y, Detke MJ, et al. Duloxetine vs. placebo in patients with painful diabetic neuropathy. *Pain.* 2005;116:109-118.

50. Hershman DL, Prevention and management of chemotherapy-induced peripheral neuropathy in survivors of adult cancers. *J Clin Oncol.* 2014;32(18):1941-1967.

51. Semenchuk MR, Sherman S, Davis B. Double-blind, randomized trial of bupropion SR for the treatment of neuropathic pain. *Neurology.* 2001;57:1583-1588.

52. Derry S, et al. Topical lidocaine for neuropathic pain in adults. *Cochrane Database Syst Rev.* 2014;(7):CD010958.

53. Rowbotham MC, Davies PS, Verkempinck C, et al. Lidocaine patch: double-blind controlled study of a new treatment method for post-herpetic neuralgia. *Pain.* 1996;65:39-44.

54. Demant DT, et al. Pain relief with lidocaine 5% patch in localized peripheral neuropathic pain in relation to pain phenotype. *Pain.* 2015;156:11:2234-2244.

55. Galer BS, Rowbotham MC, Perander J, et al. Topical lidocaine patch relieves postherpetic neuralgia more effectively than a vehicle topical patch: results of an enriched enrollment study. *Pain.* 1999;80:533-538.

56. Devers A, Galer BS. Topical lidocaine patch relieves a variety of neuropathic pain conditions: an open-label study. *Clin J Pain.* 2000;16:205-208.

57. Hart-Gouleau S, Gammaitoni A, Galer B, et al. Open label study of the effectiveness and safety of lidocaine patch 5% (Lidoderm) in patients with painful diabetic neuropathy [abstract]. Program and abstracts of the IASP 10th World Congress of Pain. Seattle, WA: IASP; 2002.

58. Berman SM, Justis JV, Ho M, et al. Lidocaine patch 5% (Lidoderm) significantly improves quality of life (QOL) in HIV-associated painful peripheral neuropathy [abstract]. Program and abstracts of the IASP 10th World Congress of Pain. Seattle, WA: IASP; 2002.

59. Wallace MS. Calcium and sodium channel antagonists for the treatment of pain. *Clin J Pain.* 2000;16: S80-S85.

60. Challapalli V, Tremont-Lukats IW, McNicol ED, et al. Systemic administration of local anesthetic agents to relieve neuropathic pain. *Cochrane Database Syst Rev.* 2005;2005(4):CD003345.

61. Lee JT, Sanderson CR, Xuan W, et al. Lidocaine for cancer pain in adults: a systematic review and meta-analysis. *J Palliat Med.* 2019;22:3.

62. Kandil E, Melikman E, Adinoff B. Lidocaine infusion: a promising therapeutic approach for chronic pain. *J Anesth Clin Res.* 2017;8(1):697.

63. Lai J, Hunter JC, Porreca F. The role of voltage-gated sodium channels in neuropathic pain. *Curr Opin Neurobiol.* 2003;13:291-297.

64. Hains BC, Klein JP, Saab CY, et al. Upregulation of sodium channel Na(v)1.3 and functional involvement in neuronal hyperexcitability associated with central neuropathic pain after spinal cord injury. *J Neurosci.* 2003;23:8881-8892.

65. Roza C, Laird JM, Souslova V, et al. The tetrodotoxin-resistant Na+ channel Na(v)1.8 is essential for the expression of spontaneous activity in damaged sensory axons of mice. *J Physiol.* 2003;550:921-926.

66. Khan ZP, Ferguson CN, Jones RM. Alpha-2 and imidazoline receptor agonists. Their pharmacology and therapeutic role. *Anaesthesia.* 1999;54:146-165.

67. Eisenach JC, Rauck RL, Buzzanell C, et al. Epidural clonidine analgesia for intractable cancer pain: phase I. *Anesthesiology.* 1989;71:647-652.

68. Davis KD, Treede RD, Raja SN, et al. Topical application of clonidine relieves hyperalgesia in patients with sympathetically maintained pain. *Pain.* 1991;47:309-317.

69. Campbell CM, Kipnes MS, Stouch BC, et al. Randomized control trial of topical clonidine for treatment of painful diabetic neuropathy. *Pain.* 2012;153(9):1815-1823.

70. Fogelholm R, Murros K. Tizanidine in chronic tension-type headache: a placebo controlled double-blind cross-over study. *Headache.* 1992;32:509-513.

71. Fromm GH, Aumentado D, Terrence CF. A clinical and experimental investigation of the effects of tizanidine in trigeminal neuralgia. *Pain.* 1993;53:265-271.

72. McCarthy RJ, Kroin JS, Lubenow TR, et al. Effect of intrathecal tizanidine on antinociception and blood pressure in the rat. *Pain.* 1990;40:333-338.

73. Caterina MJ, Schumacher MA, Tominaga M, et al. The capsaicin receptor: a heat-activated ion channel in the pain pathway. *Nature.* 1997;389:816-824.

74. Robbins WR, Staats PS, Levine J, et al. Treatment of intractable pain with topical large-dose capsaicin: preliminary report. *Anesth Analg.* 1998;86:579-583.

75. Anand P, Elsafa E, Privitera R, et al. Rational treatment of chemotherapy-induced peripheral neuropathy with capsaicin 8% patch: from pain relief towards disease modification. *J Pain Res.* 2019;12:2039-2052.

76. Bennett GJ. Update on the neurophysiology of pain transmission and modulation: focus on the NMDA-receptor. *J Pain Symptom Manage.* 2000;9:S2-S6.

77. Price DD, Mayer DJ, Mao J, et al. NMDA-receptor antagonists and opioid receptor interactions as related to analgesia and tolerance. *J Pain Symptom Manage.* 2000;19:S7.

78. Russo EB. The role of cannabis and cannabinoids in pain management. In: Weiner RS, ed. *Pain Management: A Practical Guide for Clinicians.* 6th ed. Boca Raton, FL: CRC Press; 2002:357-375.

79. Fitzgibbon EJ, Viola R. Parenteral ketamine as an analgesic adjuvant for severe pain: development and retrospective audit of a protocol for a palliative care unit. *J Palliat Med.* 2005;8:49-57.

80. Lossignol DA, Obiols-Portis M, Body JJ. Successful use of ketamine for intractable cancer pain. *Support Care Cancer.* 2005;13:188-193.

81. Slatkin NE, Rhiner M. Topical ketamine in the treatment of mucositis pain. *Pain Med.* 2003;4:298-303.

82. Vranken JH, van der Vegt MH, Kal JE, et al. Treatment of neuropathic cancer pain with continuous intrathecal administration of S(+)-ketamine. *Acta Anaesthesiol Scand.* 2004;48:249-252.

83. Davis AM, Inturrisi CE. D-Methadone blocks morphine tolerance and N-methyl-D-aspartate-induced hyperalgesia. *J Pharmacol Exp Ther.* 1999;289:1048-1053.

84. McNicol ED, Ferguson MC, Schumann R. Methadone for neuropathic pain in adults. *Cochrane Database Syst Rev.* 2017;5(5):CD012499.

85. Altier N, Dion D, Boulanger A, Choiniere M. Management of chronic neuropathic pain with methadone: a review of 13 cases. *Clin J Pain.* 2005;21:364-369.

86. Madden K, Bruera E. Very-low-dose methadone to treat refractory neuropathic pain in children with cancer. *J Palliat Med.* 2017;20(11):1280-1283.

87. Aggarwal SK, Carter GT, Sullivan MD, ZumBrunnen C, Morrill R, Mayer JD. Medicinal use of cannabis in the United States: historical perspectives, current trends, and future directions. *J Opioid Manag.* 2009;5:153-168.

88. Klieger SB, Gutman A, Allen L, et al. Mapping medical marijuana: state laws regulating patients, product safety, supply chains and dispensaries, 2017. *Addiction.* 2017;112(12):2206-2216.

89. Cichewicz DL. Synergistic interactions between cannabinoid and opioid analgesics. *Life Sci.* 2004;74(11):1317-1324.

90. Narang S, Gibson D, Wasan AD, et al. Efficacy of dronabinol as an adjuvant treatment for chronic pain patients on opioid therapy. *J Pain.* 2008;9(3):254-264.

91. Abrams DI, Jay CA, Shade SB, et al. Cannabis in painful HIV-associated sensory neuropathy: a randomized placebo-controlled trial. *Neurology.* 2007;68:515-521.

92. Ellis R, Toperoff W, Vaida F, et al. Smoked medicinal cannabis for neuropathic pain in HIV: a randomized, crossover clinical trial. *Neuropsychopharmacology.* 2008;34(3):672-680.

93. Wilsey B, Marcotte T, Tsodikov A, et al. A randomized, placebo-controlled, crossover trial of cannabis cigarettes in neuropathic pain. *J Pain.* 2008;9(6):506-521.

94. Wallace M, Schulteis G, Atkinson JH, et al. Dose-dependent effects of smoked cannabis on capsaicin-induced pain and hyperalgesia in healthy volunteers. *Anesthesiology.* 2007;107(5):785-796.

95. Ware MA, Wang T, Shapiro S, et al. Smoked cannabis for chronic neuropathic pain. *CMAJ.* 2010;182(14):E694-E701.

96. Aviram J, Samuelly-Leichtag G. Efficacy of cannabis-based medicines for pain management: a systematic review and meta-analysis of randomized controlled trials. *Pain Physician.* 2017;20;E755-E796.

97. Sommer C, Marziniak M, Myers RR. The effect of thalidomide treatment on vascular pathology and hyperalgesia caused by chronic constriction injury of rat nerve. *Pain.* 1998;74:83-91.

98. Ribeiro RA, Vale ML, Ferreira SH, et al. Analgesic effect of thalidomide on inflammatory pain. *Eur J Pharmacol.* 2000;391:97-103.

99. George A, Marziniak M, Schafers M, et al. Thalidomide treatment in chronic constrictive neuropathy decreases endoneurial tumor necrosis factor-alpha, increases interleukin-10 and has long-term effects on spinal cord dorsal horn met-enkephalin. *Pain.* 2000;88:267-275.

100. Liu T, van Rooijen N, Tracey DJ. Depletion of macrophages reduces axonal degeneration and hyperalgesia following nerve injury. *Pain.* 2000;86:25-32.

101. Yao Y, et al. Alendronate attenuates spinal microglial activation and neuropathic pain. *J Pain.* 2016;17:8:7889-7903.

102. Max MB, Schafer SC, Culnane M, et al. Amitriptyline, but not lorazepam, relieves postherpetic neuralgia. *Neurology.* 1988;38:1427-1432.

103. Haythornthwaite JA, Menefee LA, Quatrano-Piacentini AL, et al. Outcome of chronic opioid therapy for non-cancer pain. *J Pain Symptom Manage.* 1998;15:185-194.

104. Deer TR, et al. Polyanalgesic Consensus Conference 2012: recommendations for the management of pain by intrathecal (intraspinal) drug delivery: report of an interdisciplinary expert panel. *Neuromodulation.* 2012;15(5):436-464.

105. Pope JE, Deer TR. Guide to implantable devices for intrathecal therapy. *Pract Pain Manage.* 2013;3(8): 1-11.

106. Brogan S, Junkins S. Interventional therapies for the management of cancer pain. *J Support Oncol.* 2010;8(2):52-59.

107. Bruel BM, Burton AW. Intrathecal therapy for cancer-related pain. *Pain Med.* 2016;17(12):2404-2421.

108. Nauta HJ, Soukup VM, Fabian RH, et al. Punctate midline myelotomy for the relief of visceral cancer pain. *J Neurosurg.* 2000;92:125-130.

109. Bentley JN, Viswanathan A, Rosenberg WS, et al. Treatment of medically refractory cancer pain with a combination of intrathecal neuromodulation and neurosurgical ablation: case series and literature review. *Pain Med.* 2014;15:1488-1495.

110. Banning A, Sjogren P, Henriksen H. Pain causes in 200 patients referred to a multidisciplinary cancer pain clinic. *Pain.* 1991;45:45-48.

111. Heindal W, et al. The diagnostic imaging of bone metastases. *Dtsch Arztebl Int.* 2014;111(44):741-747.

112. Mach DB, Rogers SD, Sabino MC, et al. Origins of skeletal pain: sensory and sympathetic innervation of the mouse femur. *Neuroscience.* 2002;113:155-166.

113. Falk S, Bannister K, Dickenson AH. Cancer pain physiology. *Br J Pain.* 2014;8(4):154-162.

114. Jimenez-Andrade M, Ghilardi JR, Castañeda-Corral G, et al. Preventive or late administration of anti-NGF therapy attenuates tumor-induced nerve sprouting, neuroma formation, and cancer pain. *Pain.* 2011;152:2564-2574.

115. Sevcik MA, Ghilardi JR, Peters CM, et al. Anti-NGF therapy profoundly reduces bone cancer pain and the accompanying increase in markers of peripheral and central sensitization. *Pain.* 2005;115:128-141.

116. Jonsson OG, Sartain P, Ducore JM, et al. Bone pain as an initial symptom of childhood acute lymphoblastic leukemia: association with nearly normal hematologic indexes. *J Pediatr.* 1990;117:233-237.

117. Fidler M. Incidence of fracture through metastases in long bones. *Acta Orthop Scand.* 1981;52:623-627.

118. Wong DA, Fornasier VL, MacNab I. Spinal metástasis; the obvious, the occult, and the impostors. *Spine.* 1990;15:1-4.

119. Sundaresan N, Galicich JH, Lane JM, et al. Treatment of odontoid fractures in cancer patients. *J Neurosurg.* 1981;54:187-192.

120. Rustagi T, Mashaly H, Mendel E. Posterior occiput-cervical fixation for metastasis to upper cervical spine. *J Craniovertebr Junction Spine.* 2019;10(2):119-126.

121. Stark RJ, Henson RA, Evans SJ. Spinal metastases. A retrospective survey from a general hospital. *Brain.* 1982;105:189-213.

122. Portenoy RK, Galer BS, Salamon O, et al. Identification of epidural neoplasm. Radiography and bone scintigraphy in the symptomatic and asymptomatic spine. *Cancer.* 1989;64:2207-2213.

123. Ruff RL, Lanska DJ. Epidural metastases in prospectively evaluated veterans with cancer and back pain. *Cancer.* 1989;63:2234-2241.

124. Ettinger AB, Portenoy RK. The use of corticosteroids in the treatment of symptoms associated with cancer. *J Pain Symptom Manage.* 1988;3:99-103.

125. Vecht CJ, Haaxma-Reiche H, van Putten WL, et al. Initial bolus of conventional versus high-dose dexamethasone in metastatic spinal cord compression. *Neurology.* 1989;39:1255-1257.

126. Mystakidou K, Katsouda E, Stathopoulou E, et al. Approaches to managing bone metastases from breast cancer: the role of bisphosphonates. *Cancer Treat Rev.* 2005;31:303-311.

127. Smith MR. Osteoclast-targeted therapy for prostate cancer. *Curr Treat Options Oncol.* 2004;5:367-375.

128. Wardley A, Davidson N, Barrett-Lee P, et al. Zoledronic acid significantly improves pain scores and quality of life in breast cancer patients with bone metastases: a randomised, crossover study of community vs

hospital bisphosphonate administration. *Br J Cancer.* 2005;92:1869-1876.

129. Gordon DH. Efficacy and safety of intravenous bisphosphonates for patients with breast cancer metastatic to bone: a review of randomized, double-blind, phase III trials. *Clin Breast Cancer.* 2005;6:125-131.

130. Ogawa K, Mukai T, Arano Y, et al. Development of a rhenium-186-labeled MAG3-conjugated bisphosphonate for the palliation of metastatic bone pain based on the concept of bifunctional radiopharmaceuticals. *Bioconjug Chem.* 2005;16:751-757.

131. Gül G, Sendur MA, Aksoy, S, et al. A comprehensive review of denosumab for bone metastasis in patients with solid tumors. *Curr Med Res Opin.* 2016;31(1): 133-145.

132. Smith MR, Saad F, Coleman R, et al. Denosumab and bone metastasis-free survival in men with castration-resistant prostate cancer: results of a phase 3, randomised, placebo controlled trial. *Lancet.* 2012; 379(9810):39-46.

133. Johnstone C, Lutz ST. External beam radiotherapy and bone metastases. *Ann Palliat Med.* 2014;3(2): 114-122.

134. Steenland E, Leer JW, van Houwelingen H, et al. The effect of a single fraction compared to multiple fractions on painful bone metastases: a global analysis of the Dutch Bone Metastases Study. *Radiother Oncol.* 1999;52: 101-109.

135. Hartsell WF, Scott CB, Bruner DW, et al. Randomized trial of short- versus long-course radiotherapy for palliation of painful bone metastases. *J Natl Cancer Inst.* 2005;97:798-804.

136. Konski A, DeSilvio M, Harsell W, et al. Continuing evidence for poorer treatment outcomes for single male patients: retreatment data from RTOG 97 14. *Int J Radiat Oncol Biol Phys.* 2006;66:229-233.

137. Rich SE, Chow R, Raman S, et al. Update of the systematic review of palliative radiation therapy fractionation for bone metastases. *Radiother Oncol.* 2018;126(3): 547-557.

138. Van der Linden YM, Dijkstra PD, Kroon HM, et al. Comparative analysis of risk factors for pathological fracture with femoral metastases. *J Bone Joint Surg Br.* 2004;86:566-573.

139. Mundy GR. Metastasis to bone: causes, consequences and therapeutic opportunities. *Nat Rev Cancer.* 2002;2: 584-593.

140. Kantoff PW, Higano CS, Shore ND, et al. Sipuleucel-T immunotherapy for castration-resistant prostate cancer. *N Engl J Med.* 2010;363:411-422.

141. Handkiewicz-Junak D, Poeppel TD, Bodei L, et al. EANM guidelines for radionuclide therapy of bone metastases with beta-emitting radionuclides. *Eur J Nucl Med Mol Imaging.* 2018;45(5):846-859. doi:10.1007/s00259-018-3947-x.

142. Robinson RG, Blake GM, Preston DF, et al. Strontium-89: treatment results and kinetics in patients with painful metastatic prostate and breast cancer in bone. *Radiographics.* 1989;9(2):271-281.

143. Finlay IG, Mason MD, Shelley M. Radioisotopes for the palliation of metastatic bone cancer: a systematic review. *Lancet Oncol.* 2005;6(6):392-400.

144. Maini CL, Bergomi S, Romano L, et al. 153Sm-EDTMP for bone pain palliation in skeletal metastases. *Eur J Nucl Med Mol Imaging.* 2004;31(suppl 1):S171-S178.

145. Lam MG, de Klerk JM, van Rijk PP. 186Re-HEDP for metastatic bone pain in breast cancer patients. *Eur J Nucl Med Mol Imaging.* 2004;31(suppl 1):S162-S170.

146. Burton AW, Rhines LD, Mendel E. Vertebroplasty and kyphoplasty: a comprehensive review. *Neurosurg Focus.* 2005;18(3):e1.

147. Sikandar S, Dickenson AH. Visceral pain: the ins and outs, the ups and downs. *Curr Opin Support Palliat Care.* 2012;(1):17-26.

148. Grundy L, Erickson A, Brierly SM. Visceral pain. *Annu Rev Physiol.* 2019;81:261-284.

149. Farr WC. The use of corticosteroids for symptom management in terminally ill patients. *Am J Hosp Care.* 1990;7:41-46.

150. Davis MP. Drug management of visceral pain: concepts from basic research. *Pain Res Treat.* 2012;2012:265605.

151. Okada-Ogawa A, Porreca F, Meng ID. Sustained morphine-induced sensitization and loss of diffuse noxious inhibitory controls in dura-sensitive medullary dorsal horn neurons. *J Neurosci.* 2009;29(50):15828-15835.

152. Lian B, Vera-Portocarrero L, King T, et al. Opioid-induced latent sensitization in a model of non-inflammatory viscerosomatic hypersensitivity. *Brain Res.* 2010;1358:64-70.

153. Staahl C, Christrup LL, Andersen SD, et al. A comparative study of oxycodone and morphine in a multimodal, tissue-differentiated experimental pain model. *Pain.* 2006;123(1-2):28-36.

154. Bannister K, Sikandar S, Bauer CS, et al. Pregabalin suppresses spinal neuronal hyperexcitability and visceral hypersensitivity in the absence of peripheral pathophysiology. *Anesthesiology.* 2011;115(1):144-152.

155. McRoberts JA, Coutinho SV, Marvizón JC, et al. Role of peripheral N-methyl-D-aspartate (NMDA) receptors in visceral nociception in rats. *Gastroenterology.* 2001;120(7):1737-1748.

156. Lindström E, Brusberg M, Ravnefjord A, et al. Oral baclofen reduces visceral pain-related pseudo-affective responses to colorectal distension in rats: relation between plasma exposure and efficacy. *Scand J Gastroenterol.* 2011;46(6):652-662.

157. Ripamonti C, Mercadante S, Groff L, et al. Role of octreotide, scopolamine butylbromide, and hydration in symptom control of patients with inoperable bowel obstruction and nasogastric tubes: a prospective randomized trial. *J Pain Symptom Manage.* 2000;19:23-34.

158. Cousins MJ. Techniques for neurolytic neural blockade. In: Cousins MJ, Bridenbaugh PO, eds. *Neural Blockade in Clinical Anesthesia and Management of Pain.* 3rd ed. Philadelphia, PA: Lippincott Williams & Wilkins; 1998:1007-1061.

159. Lema MJ, Myers DP, Leon-Casasola O, et al. Pleural phenol therapy for the treatment of chronic esophageal cancer pain. *Reg Anesth.* 1992;17:166-170.

160. Mercadante S. Celiac plexus block versus analgesics in pancreatic cancer pain. *Pain.* 1993;52:187-192.

161. Mercadante S, Nicosia F. Celiac plexus block: a reappraisal. *Reg Anesth Pain Med.* 1998;23:37-48.

162. Plancarte R, Leon-Casasola OA, El Helaly M, et al. Neurolytic superior hypogastric plexus block for chronic pelvic pain associated with cancer. *Reg Anesth.* 1997;22:562-568.

163. Korevaar WC. Transcatheter thoracic epidural neurolysis using ethyl alcohol. *Anesthesiology.* 1988;69:989-993.

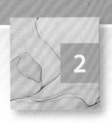

2 Opioid Pharmacotherapy

Alexandra L. McPherson, Mary Lynn McPherson, and Judith A. Paice

Opioids and their derivatives have been used for centuries to relieve pain. Their contribution to relief of suffering is well established. Earliest records of opioid use are centuries old, extending back to the ancient Egyptians. In the 1600s, Thomas Sydenham promoted the use of laudanum, a mixture of opium, saffron, cinnamon, and cloves in wine (1). Two centuries later, the pharmacist Wilhelm Sertürner extracted morphine from poppy juice, calling this substance morphium after Morpheus, the Greek god of sleep (1). Since that time, many new opioids have been developed, and medicine's understanding of the pharmacodynamics, pharmacokinetics, and pharmacogenomics of these compounds has increased greatly. This, in turn, has led to improvements in their clinical application, for relief not only of pain but of dyspnea, cough, and intractable diarrhea as well.

Despite these advances, opioids continue to generate fear, misunderstanding, and controversy. The evolving opioid crisis in which we are currently embroiled has certainly not helped the situation (2). In order to provide optimal pain and symptom relief for patients, misconceptions about opioids must be addressed. This must start with a strong knowledge base regarding the pharmacology and clinical application of opioids.

PHARMACOLOGY OF OPIOIDS

To fully appreciate the optimal clinical use of opioids, the clinician must understand the pharmacodynamics (the mechanism of opioid analgesia) and the pharmacokinetics (the process by which opioids are absorbed, distributed, metabolized, and excreted) of this class of drugs. The pharmacogenomics of opioids helps explain the variability in response seen in the clinical setting.

Pharmacodynamics

Opioids act through three major types of opioid receptors, including μ (MOR for μ-opioid receptor), δ (DOR for δ-opioid receptor), and κ (KOR for κ-opioid receptor). These receptors are distributed widely throughout the nervous system, including the peripheral nerves, spinal cord, and brain (3). The highest density of opioid receptors

appears in laminae I and II of the dorsal horn of the spinal cord (4). Opioid receptors are also found in the brainstem, including the periaqueductal gray, nucleus raphe magnus, and locus caeruleus, areas known to be involved in the mediation of opioid analgesia (5). Opioid receptors have also been found on immune cells.

Opioid receptors are G protein coupled, activating a complex cascade of events. These include increased conduction through potassium channels, which hyperpolarizes the sensory neuron. Opioid receptor binding results in diminished conduction through calcium channels, resulting in decreased release of neurotransmitters involved in nociception. Finally, opioid receptor binding leads to inhibition of adenylate cyclase. Together, these actions contribute to the analgesia that results when an opioid agonist binds to the above receptors.

Pharmacokinetics

As with all other compounds, the absorption, distribution, metabolism, and elimination of an opioid influence the efficacy of the drug. Alterations are of particular concern when caring for patients with advanced malignancy or other life-threatening illnesses because any of these phases of opioid pharmacokinetics may be altered by extensive disease.

Absorption

Absorption is influenced by the lipophilicity of an agent. Morphine and hydromorphone have a partition coefficient (octanol/water) of 1 compared with 115 for methadone and 820 for fentanyl (6,7). Therefore, fentanyl can cross biologic membranes more avidly when compared with morphine, making it the more appropriate agent for transdermal and transmucosal delivery. The lipophilicity affects the time to maximal serum concentration (C_{max}). The C_{max} for a hydrophilic drug, such as morphine, is approximately 60 minutes after oral administration, 30 minutes after subcutaneous (sub.q.) delivery, and 6 minutes or more after intravenous (i.v.) delivery. The half-life of oral morphine is approximately 4 hours. Because steady state is reached in approximately 4 to 5 half-lives, it will be reached within approximately 16 to 20 hours of regular immediate-release oral morphine administration. Little is known about the alterations in absorption of opioids that occur when patients have extensive disease. For example, factors such as shortened transit time may delay the absorption of oral opioids, particularly long-acting or sustained-release compounds.

Distribution

Plasma proteins and lipid solubility of a particular opioid affect the distribution of the drug throughout the vasculature (8). Other mediating factors include body fat stores and total body water. All of these factors listed above can be significantly altered in older adults or in persons with cachexia and dehydration, the common sequelae of advanced disease.

Metabolism

Most opioids are metabolized through glucuronidation, dealkylation, or other processes and are then excreted by the kidneys. Although some metabolites produce analgesia (e.g., morphine-6-glucuronide [M6G]), they may also contribute to neurotoxicity (9). Myoclonus has been associated with both morphine-3-glucuronide (M3G) and hydromorphone-3-glucuronide (H3G), metabolites that appear to pose a risk for accumulating in patients receiving high doses of opioid for extended periods or in those with renal disease (9,10). Metabolism is known to be affected by advanced age, liver disease, genetics, and other factors that are prominent in palliative care.

Elimination

Most opioids are excreted renally, with only methadone being eliminated fecally. Experience suggests that patients with renal failure or those receiving dialysis might benefit from the use of agents that are more readily dialyzable, such as fentanyl, as opposed to morphine or codeine (11). However, even in patients who have undergone a successful renal transplantation, the large variability in the kinetics of fentanyl after surgery supports the axiom that all opioid therapy must be individualized (12). Much more research is needed on the interaction between advanced disease and the pharmacokinetics of opioids.

Pharmacogenomics

Numerous factors are responsible for the interpatient variability seen in the response to medications such as the patient's age, organ function (renal, hepatic), body habitus, comorbidities, and concomitant medication therapy (13). In recent years, the significant impact of genetic polymorphisms has been recognized as a major influence on medication responsiveness. The field of pharmacogenomics is rapidly growing, and much evidence for the variability in response to opioids seen in the clinical setting is related to inborn properties caused by genetic variability (14). The MOR was cloned in 1993 and was called *MOR-1*. Additional work has identified splice variants of the MOR-1 receptor, with different localization of the splice variants within the nervous system (15). The efficacy of morphine varies among the variants, and this may explain, in part, the variability in response to opioids seen in the clinical setting, including efficacy and adverse effects. The translation of this information to the clinical experience includes the practice of opioid rotation when a particular opioid agonist either is ineffective or produces unmanageable adverse effects.

Another clear clinical example of the contribution of pharmacogenomics to the variability of opioid responsiveness is variations in the CYP2D6 gene (16). Opioids such as codeine, oxycodone, hydrocodone, and tramadol possess limited analgesic effect as administered, and require metabolism to new pharmacologically active moieties to realize their full analgesic potential. There are over 80 unique alleles of CYP2D6 and variations in expression influence the metabolic fate and pharmacodynamic potential of opioids (both therapeutic and toxic effects) (17). Based on allele expression, individuals can be categorized as "extensive metabolizers" (normal enzyme activity; most individuals fall in this category), "poor metabolizers" (no enzyme activity), "intermediate metabolizers" (low enzyme activity) or "ultrarapid metabolizers" (high enzyme activity). Up to 10% of the populations are considered poor metabolizers, over half of Asians are intermediate metabolizers, and some populations have a substantial number of individuals considered to be ultrarapid metabolizers (approximately one-third of Ethiopian/Nigerian individuals, 20% of Saudis) (17). With opioids such as codeine and tramadol that require biotransformation to their pharmacologically active opioid analgesic, a poor or intermediate metabolizer may not achieve pain relief. Conversely, an ultrarapid metabolizer at the CYP2D6 enzyme may experience a toxic reaction to codeine or tramadol, potentially including respiratory depression and death (18,19). For this reason, the US Food and Drug Administration (FDA) has restricted the use of codeine and tramadol in children and recommends against use in breast-feeding women (20).

One example of the role of pharmacogenomics in cancer pain control is related to the catechol-*O*-methyltransferase (*COMT*) gene, which inactivates dopamine, epinephrine, and norepinephrine in the nervous system. A study of 207 white patients with cancer found that polymorphism of the *COMT* gene contributes to variability in response to morphine in pain control (21). A common functional polymorphism (Val158Met) leads to a significant variation in the COMT enzyme activity, with the Met form displaying lower enzymatic activity. Patients with the Val/Val genotype needed more morphine when compared with the Val/Met and Met/Met genotype groups. The investigators could not explain these differences by other factors such as duration of opioid treatment, performance status, time since diagnosis, perceived pain intensity, adverse symptoms, or time until death. Much more research is needed to fully understand the pharmacogenetics of opioids and their implications for those with cancer or other life-threatening illnesses.

CLINICAL APPLICATION

Opioids are a critical component of the armamentarium used to control pain in palliative care. They are indicated in moderate to severe pain, as well as in the management of cough, dyspnea, and severe diarrhea. Because opioids alter pain signal transmission and perception throughout the nervous system, they have an analgesic effect despite the underlying pathophysiology of pain. In fact, despite earlier beliefs, opioids have been shown to be effective in providing relief of neuropathic pain.

Specific Opioids

Opioids are generally categorized as agonists, partial agonists, and mixed agonist–antagonists. Additionally, antagonists to opioids may be used to counteract adverse effects of opioids.

Agonists

Numerous opioid agonists are available for clinical use. These agents can be subcategorized as alkaloids and synthetic opioids (Table 2.1). Attributes associated with the more commonly used opioids are described in the following text and in Table 2.2.

Codeine. Codeine is a relatively weak opioid that is frequently administered in combination with acetaminophen. Codeine is a prodrug that is metabolized by glucuronidation primarily to codeine-6-glucuronide and to a much lesser degree to norcodeine and morphine, which is subsequently metabolized to M3G, morphine-6-glucuronide, and normorphine (22). As described earlier in the section Pharmacogenomics, codeine is converted to morphine by CYP2D6. The polymorphism seen in this enzyme between various ethnic groups, and between individuals, leads to significant variability in the therapeutic response. Of greatest concern are the ultrarapid metabolizers

TABLE 2.1 OPIOIDS BY CLASSIFICATION

Agonists
Alkaloids
  Morphine
  Codeine
Semisynthetic opioids—hydrocodone, hydromorphone, oxycodone, and oxymorphone
Synthetic opioids
  Phenylpiperidine derivatives—fentanyl, sufentanil, alfentanil, remifentanil, and meperidine
  Diphenylheptane derivatives—methadone
  Morphinan derivatives—levorphanol
  Novel formulations—tramadol and tapentadol

Partial Agonists
Semisynthetic—buprenorphine

Mixed Agonist–Antagonists
Semisynthetic alkaloid—nalbuphine
Synthetic benzomorphan derivative—pentazocine
Synthetic morphinan derivative—butorphanol

Antagonists
Naloxone
Naltrexone
Methylnaltrexone

who metabolize codeine to its active form much faster than usual, resulting in dangerously high serum concentrations, potentially leading to respiratory depression that could result in death. This is more common in the pediatric patient population and has led to changes in drug labeling per the FDA, restricting the use of codeine-containing products in children and breast-feeding mothers as discussed above (20).

Fentanyl. Fentanyl is a highly lipid-soluble synthetic opioid that may be administered by parenteral (i.v., i.m., sub.q [off-label]), epidural, transdermal, and transmucosal routes of administration. Case reports have also been published demonstrating the use of nebulized fentanyl for pain and dyspnea (23,24). Fentanyl is highly potent (approximately 75 to 100 times more potent than morphine on an mg-to-mg basis) and is typically dosed in micrograms (25). Fentanyl is extensively metabolized by CYP3A4 (to nonactive metabolite, norfentanyl), and therefore may be subject to drug interactions (26). Questions arise about the efficacy of fentanyl and related compounds, alfentanil, remifentanil, and sufentanil, in the face of extremes in body weight. A study of i.v. fentanyl for acute postoperative pain in lean and obese patients found no relationship between plasma levels required for analgesia and total body weight. Therefore, using weight-based i.v. dosing (or milligram per kilogram dosing) in patients with cachexia could lead to underdosing, whereas the same practice in the obese patient could lead to overdosing (27). A small study of cancer patients receiving fentanyl patches revealed that cachectic

TABLE 2.2 PROPERTIES OF COMMONLY USED OPIOIDS

Agent	Routes	Formulations	Starting dose for adults[a]	Other
Codeine	Oral	Codeine sulfate 15, 30, or 60 mg tablets Tylenol No. 2 (15 mg codeine/300 mg acetaminophen) Tylenol No. 3 (30 mg codeine/300 mg acetaminophen) Tylenol No. 4 (60 mg codeine/300 mg acetaminophen) Codeine/acetaminophen liquid (5 mL = 12 mg codeine/120 mg acetaminophen)	Oral: 30–60 mg	Converted to morphine by CYP2D6; poor metabolizers obtain little pain relief
Fentanyl	Intraspinal Parenteral Transdermal Transmucosal Sublingual	Fentanyl solution for i.v. Fentanyl patch (Duragesic, generics) 12, 25, 37.5, 50, 62.5, 75, 87.5, or 100 μg/h Fentanyl oral transmucosal lozenge (Actiq, generics) 200, 400, 600, 800, 1,200, or 1,600 μg Fentanyl transmucosal buccal tablets (Fentora, generics) 100, 200, 400, 600, 800 μg Fentanyl transmucosal sublingual tablets (Abstral) 100, 200, 300, 400, 600, 800 μg Fentanyl nasal (Lazanda) 100, 300, 400 μg/actuation Fentanyl sublingual liquid (Subsys) 100, 200, 400, 600, 800, 1,200, 1,600 μg	NA	Transdermal fentanyl 25 μg/h approximately equal to 50 mg oral morphine
Hydrocodone	Oral	Hydrocodone bitartrate extended-release capsule (Zohydro ER, generics) 10, 15, 20, 30, 40, 50 mg Hydrocodone bitartrate extended-release tablet (Hysingla ER) 20, 30, 40, 60, 80, 100, 120 mg Hydrocodone/acetaminophen oral tablet (2.5, 5, 7.5, or 10 mg hydrocodone/325 mg acetaminophen) Hydrocodone/acetaminophen oral tablet (5, 7.5, or 10 mg hydrocodone/300 mg acetaminophen) Hydrocodone/acetaminophen oral elixir (15 mL = 10 mg hydrocodone/300 mg acetaminophen) Hydrocodone/acetaminophen oral solution (15 mL = 7.5 or 10 mg hydrocodone/325 mg acetaminophen) Hydrocodone/ibuprofen oral tablet (2.5, 5, 7.5, or 10 mg hydrocodone/200 mg ibuprofen)	Oral: 5–10 mg	Role of CYP2D6 unclear
Hydromorphone	Oral Parenteral Rectal	Hydromorphone solution for i.v. Hydromorphone oral tablet (Dilaudid, generics) 2, 4, or 8 mg Hydromorphone 24-h extended release tablet (Exalgo, generics) 8, 12, 16, 32 mg Hydromorphone suppository, 3 mg	Oral: 4–8 mg	Toxicity may be due in part to hydromorphone-3-glucuronide

(Continued)

TABLE 2.2 PROPERTIES OF COMMONLY USED OPIOIDS (*Continued*)

Agent	Routes	Formulations	Starting dose for adults[a]	Other
Levorphanol	Oral	Levorphanol oral tablet, 2 or 3 mg	Oral: 2–3 mg	Long half-life; repeated dosing may lead to accumulation Increased incidence of psychotomimetic effects
Meperidine	Oral Parenteral	Meperidine oral tablet 50, 100 mg Meperidine oral syrup 50 mg/5 mL Meperidine solution for injection (Demerol, generics)	Not recommended	Not recommended because of toxic metabolite, normeperidine; mainly used in the management of rigors
Methadone	Oral Parenteral	Methadone oral concentrate 10 mg/mL Methadone oral solution 5 mg or 10 mg/5 mL Methadone oral tablet 5, 10 mg Methadone oral soluble tablet 40 mg Methadone solution for injection, 10 mg/mL	See text	See text and Tables 3.3 and 3.4
Morphine	Intraspinal Oral Parenteral Rectal	Morphine immediate release (15, 30 mg) Morphine extended release, 12-h (MS Contin, Oramorph SR, Arymo ER, MorphaBond ER, generics) 15, 30, 50, 60, 100, 200 mg Morphine extended release, 24-h (Kadian, generics) 10, 20, 30, 40, 50, 60, 75, 80, 90, 100, 120, 200 mg Morphine oral solution 20 mg/5 mL, 10 mg/5 mL Morphine oral concentrate 100 mg/5 mL, 20 mg/mL (listed as two separate products) Morphine suppository 5, 10, 20, 30 mg	Oral: 15–30 mg	Kadian may be used as sprinkles Toxicity may be due in part to morphine-3-glucuronide
Oxycodone	Oral	Oxycodone immediate-release tablet (Roxicodone, generics) 5, 10, 15, 20, 30 mg Oxycodone immediate-release tablet (abuse deterrent) (Oxaydo) 5, 7.5 mg Oxycodone extended-release tablet (OxyContin, generics) 10, 15, 20, 30, 40, 60, 80 mg Oxycodone extended-release capsule (Xtampza ER) 9, 13.5, 18, 27, 36 mg Oxycodone oral solution 5 mg/5 mL Oxycodone oral concentrate 100 mg/5 mL Oxycodone/acetaminophen oral tablet (2.5, 5, 7.5, or 10 mg oxycodone/300 mg acetaminophen) Oxycodone/acetaminophen oral tablet (2.5, 5, 7.5, or 10 mg oxycodone/325 mg acetaminophen)	Oral: 5–10 mg	Xtampza ER may be used as sprinkles

Drug	Route	Formulations	Starting Dose	Comments
Oxymorphone	Oral	Oxymorphone immediate release (Opana, generics) 5, 10 mg Oxymorphone extended release (Opana ER, generics) 5, 7.5, 10, 15, 20, 30, 40 mg	Oral: 5–10 mg	
Tapentadol	Oral	Tapentadol immediate release (Nucynta) 50, 75, 100 mg Tapentadol extended release (Nucynta ER) 50, 100, 150, 200, 250 mg	Oral: 50 mg	
Tramadol	Oral	Tramadol immediate release (Ultram, generics) 50, 100 mg Tramadol extended release (Ultram ER, ConZip, generics) 100, 150, 200, 300 mg Tramadol oral reconstituted suspension (Synapryn FusePaq) 10 mg/mL	Oral: 50 mg	C-IV controlled substance Maximum recommended total daily dose: 400 mg/d Avoid taking in combination with other serotonergic medications (e.g., SSRIs, SNRIs, TCAs, triptans)

[a]Starting doses are approximations for opioid-naive adult patients.

patients had lower plasma concentrations when compared with normal weight patients (28). This does not preclude the use of fentanyl patches in cachectic patients, but it reinforces the need for individualized dosing and frequent reassessment.

Hydrocodone. Hydrocodone is a semisynthetic opioid that is more potent than codeine and is found in combination products containing acetaminophen and ibuprofen. It is also found in several antitussive combination products. These additives limit the use of hydrocodone in palliative care when higher opioid doses are required. Hydrocodone is a prodrug that is metabolized by CYP2D6 to its active metabolite, hydromorphone, and by CYP3A4 to the inactive metabolite, norhydrocodone. Laboratory evidence suggests that CYP2D6 polymorphism may alter the analgesic response to hydrocodone (29).

Hydromorphone. Hydromorphone is a derivative of morphine, with similar properties, and is available as oral tablets (both immediate- and extended-release), as parenteral formulations, and as a rectal suppository (30). Because it is highly soluble and approximately 5 times more potent than morphine, hydromorphone is used frequently in palliative care when small volumes are needed for sub.q. infusions. Hydromorphone undergoes glucuronidation and the primary metabolite is H3G (22). Recent experience suggests that this metabolite may lead to opioid neurotoxicity, similar to that seen with morphine metabolites, including myoclonus, hyperalgesia, and seizures (10,31,32). This appears to be of particular risk with high doses, with prolonged use, or in persons with renal dysfunction (33).

Methadone. Methadone has been gaining renewed popularity in the management of severe, persistent pain, yet it has several characteristics that complicate its use. Methadone is a synthetic MOR and DOR agonist and *N*-methyl-D-aspartate (NMDA) receptor antagonist, with affinity similar to that of ketamine (34). This activity at the NMDA receptor is believed to be of particular benefit in neuropathic pain and in the management of hyperalgesia. Methadone also blocks the reuptake of serotonin and norepinephrine, another potentially favorable attribute to its use in treating neuropathic pain. Methadone has been shown to be noninferior to fentanyl in treating radiation-induced nociceptive pain with head and neck cancer, and superior to fentanyl in treating neuropathic pain in the same cancer population (35,36). Methadone has also been shown to be effective when used in a low dose, used adjunctively to more traditional regularly scheduled opioids (37). A Cochrane review concluded there was limited evidence of the efficacy and safety of methadone in chronic neuropathic pain; however, a second Cochrane review concluded that methadone has similar analgesic benefits to morphine, and a role in the management of cancer pain in adults (38,39).

The prolonged plasma half-life of methadone (ranging from 15 to 60+ hours; average is 24 hours) allows for a relatively convenient dosing schedule of every 8 to 12 hours. Furthermore, methadone is much less expensive than comparable doses of commercially available prolonged-release formulations.

Another advantage of methadone is the availability of multiple dosage formulations (tablets, oral solution, highly concentrated oral solution, and parenteral) and routes of administration (oral, transmucosal, rectal, intravenous, and neuraxial) (40). Nasal administration has also been reported to be effective, but preparations are not commercially available. The ratio of oral to parenteral methadone is 2:1 (when transitioning from oral to parenteral; conversion in the opposite direction is more conservative) and that of oral to rectal is 1:1 (41,42). Subcutaneous methadone infusions may produce local irritation, although using a more dilute solution or changing the needle more frequently can mediate this. Intramuscular administration may be unpredictable, and local tissue reactions may occur.

The pharmacokinetics of methadone varies greatly between individuals, and causes for the variability include protein binding, CYP3A4 activity, urinary pH, and other factors. Methadone binds avidly to α_1-glycoprotein, the level of which is increased in advanced cancer, leading to decreasing amounts of unbound methadone and initially delaying the onset of effect. As a result, the interindividual variability of the pharmacokinetics of methadone is more pronounced in patients with cancer (34).

Methadone is metabolized primarily by CYP3A4, but also by CYP2D6 and CYP1A2 (34,43,44). Drugs that induce CYP3A4 enzymes accelerate the metabolism of methadone, resulting in reduced serum levels of the drug. Patients report shortened analgesic periods or reduced overall pain relief (45). Drugs that inhibit CYP3A4 enzymes slow down methadone metabolism, potentially leading to sedation and respiratory depression. Table 2.3 lists many agents commonly used in palliative care that are CYP3A4 inducers and inhibitors. While there are numerous medications that may interact with methadone, an easy way to remember potential interacting medications is "the three A's"—amiodarone, anti-infectives, and antidepressants (25). We must also consider drug interactions that can result in additive pharmacodynamic effects, such

TABLE 2.3 AGENTS USED IN PALLIATIVE CARE THAT MAY INTERACT WITH METHADONE

Inhibitors of CYP3A4 (may increase serum methadone levels)	Inducers of CYP3A4 (may lower serum methadone levels)
Amiodarone	Carbamazepine
Aprepitant	Dexamethasone
Clarithromycin	Efavirenz
Cimetidine	Ethanol (acute use)
Ciprofloxacin	Isoniazid
Delavirdine	Lopinavir
Diazepam	Nevirapine
Dihydroergotamine	Oxcarbazepine
Diltiazem	Pentobarbital
Disulfiram	Phenobarbital
Erythromycin	Phenytoin
Ethanol (chronic use)	Rifampin
Fluconazole	Risperidone
Fluoxetine	Spironolactone
Haloperidol	St. John's wort
Ketoconazole	Topiramate
Nicardipine	
Norfloxacin	
Omeprazole	
Paroxetine	
Thioridazine	
Venlafaxine	
Verapamil	

as "increased risk of sedation and sleep-disordered breathing when using lorazepam (and other benzodiazepines) and methadone together" (40).

Urinary pH can account for a significant amount of the variability seen in methadone plasma levels. Clearance of methadone is greater when the pH is more acidic (46). As a result, urinary alkalizers, such as sodium bicarbonate, will decrease methadone excretion. Other factors that alter methadone kinetics include drug interactions. In addition to the CYP3A4 interactions listed previously, others have been described. For example, the proton pump inhibitor omeprazole increases gastric pH, thereby increasing the rate of absorption.

Although the extended half-life of methadone allows for longer dosing intervals, it also increases the potential of drug accumulation, leading to delayed sedation and respiratory depression. This may occur 2 to 5 days after initiating the drug or increasing the dose, which is why close monitoring is essential. Another consequence of prolonged or high-dose opioid administration, myoclonus, has been reported with methadone use (47). Finally, controversy exists about the role of methadone in QTc interval prolongation, which increases the risk of developing torsade de pointes (TdP), a potentially fatal arrhythmia. While methadone "does not have a direct adverse effect on the myocardium," it delays cardiac repolarization, which can result in QT prolongation (40). This is of particular significance in patients with positive risk factors for

QT prolongation at baseline, including electrolyte abnormalities (hypokalemia, hypomagnesemia), hepatic impairment, structural heart disease, and genetic predisposition (40). We must also consider other medications with the potential for causing QT prolongation, including haloperidol, olanzapine, ondansetron, and tricyclic antidepressants, all of which are commonly used in the palliative care patient population (40).

Some question whether this is due to preservatives in the parenteral formulation, although the syndrome has been reported with oral administration of methadone as well (48). A study of 100 patients taking methadone found that one-third had prolonged QT-wave intervals on electrocardiogram, occurring more frequently in men, yet there did not appear to be a risk of serious prolongation (49,50). This was confirmed in a prospective study of cancer patients receiving methadone that revealed elevated QTc to be common at baseline and that elevations beyond 500 ms after initiating therapy were rare (51).

Patients currently receiving methadone maintenance treatment (MMT) for substance use disorder will have developed cross-tolerance to opioids and, as a result, will require higher doses than opioid-naïve patients (52). Prescribing methadone for substance use disorders requires a special registration in the United States. As a result, prescriptions provided for methadone to manage pain in palliative care should include the statement "for pain."

Methadone is a very potent opioid; in opioid-naïve patients dosing should generally begin between 2 and 5 mg/d, not to exceed 7.5 mg/d and given in two divided doses (40). Per the American Pain Society, and an expert consensus white paper on safe and appropriate use of methadone in hospice and palliative care, patients receiving up to 60 mg a day of oral morphine equivalent would begin methadone using a similar dosing strategy (40). Because methadone has an average elimination half-life of 24 hours, it takes approximately 5 days to achieve steady state; therefore the methadone dose should not be increased before 5 days. It is also important that the total daily dose of methadone not be increased by >5 mg/d; once a patient reaches 30 to 40 mg of methadone a day or more, the total daily methadone dose may be increased by 10 mg/d (40).

When converting to methadone from a different opioid, calculate the oral morphine equivalent total daily dose, if the patient was not already taking oral morphine. There are numerous suggested conversion ratios from oral morphine to oral methadone ranging from 2:1 to >40:1. The recommendation from the expert consensus white paper for patients under 65 years of age and receiving >60

TABLE 2.4 METHADONE DOSE RATIOS

Oral morphine equivalent (OME) (mg/d)	
0–60	2–5 mg/d (not to exceed 7.5 mg/d) in two divided doses
	Conversion ratio to oral methadone
>60–199 OME and <65 years of age	10 mg OME:1 mg oral methadone
>200 OME and/or >65 years of age	20 mg OME:1 mg oral methadone

Note: These ratios are generally accepted in clinical practice, although these serve only as a guide to converting an opioid to methadone. Many factors can increase or decrease serum methadone levels, and caution is advised. Frequent assessment of pain and sedation are warranted when converting to methadone or when increasing the dose.

but <199 mg oral morphine equivalents per day is a 10:1 conversion (morphine:methadone). For patients who are over 65 years of age, OR receiving 200 mg or more oral morphine equivalents per day, it is recommended to use a 20:1 conversion ratio (morphine:methadone). These recommendations are summarized in Table 2.4.

There are a variety of protocols recommended for converting from other opioids to methadone beyond the equianalgesic conversion factor. For example, there is the "rapid stop" method (stop the original opioid, start the calculated methadone dose), the "ad libitum" method (stop the original opioid and select a dose of methadone to be taken "as needed"; patient self-titrates to the dose necessary to control pain), and a method that uses a 3- to 5-day crossover titration (titrating original opioid dose down while titrating methadone dose up) (25). No single method has proven to be superior to the other methods, and the precaution that methadone is best dosed by experienced practitioners is wise advice. For both opioid-naïve and opioid-tolerant patients beginning methadone therapy, consider other medications the patient is receiving and make dosage adjustments as appropriate (e.g., reduce calculated dose in the presence of an enzyme inhibitor).

Morphine. In the past, morphine was considered the "gold standard." We now recognize that because of the wide variability in response, the most appropriate opioid is the agent that works best for a given patient. Morphine is a useful compound for many patients, in that there is a wide range of formulations and routes available for its use (53,54). Initial adverse effects are similar to those of all other opioids, including sedation and

nausea that should be anticipated and treated appropriately. These generally resolve within a few days (55). Long-term effects, such as constipation, should be prevented. An active metabolite of morphine, M3G, may contribute to myoclonus, seizures, and hyperalgesia (increasing pain), particularly when clearance is impaired because of renal impairment (22,46,56). In differentiating adverse effects and metabolic effects, the time course of onset should be determined. Adverse effects generally occur soon after the drug has been absorbed, whereas metabolite-induced effects are generally delayed by several days. When adverse effects do not respond to appropriate management, conversion to an equianalgesic dose of a different opioid is recommended.

Oxycodone. Oxycodone is a semisynthetic opioid available as both immediate- and extended-release tablets and liquid formulations. A recent systematic review found the equianalgesic ratio between morphine and oxycodone to be 1.5:1 (57). Metabolites of oxycodone include noroxycodone (inactive) and oxymorphone (active). In addition to binding to the MOR, oxycodone binds to the KOR and DOR. Side effects appear to be similar to those experienced with morphine. One study comparing these two long-acting formulations in persons with advanced cancer found that oxycodone produced less nausea and vomiting; however, a recent systematic review found no difference between these agents (58,59).

Oxymorphone. Oxymorphone is a semisynthetic derivative of morphine that is available in the United States as both immediate- and extended-release oral formulations, as well as a parenteral solution (60). Oxymorphone is thought to be twice as potent as morphine, and it does not appear to induce or inhibit the CYP2D6 or CYP3A4 enzyme pathways (61,62). The prevalence of adverse effects appears to be similar to other opioids (53).

Tapentadol. Tapentadol is a relatively new synthetic opioid that has a dual mechanism of action—it binds to the MOR and inhibits the reuptake of norepinephrine—making it useful in both nociceptive and neuropathic pain. It is an active compound (as opposed to a prodrug) with no active metabolites and therefore is less prone to enzyme-related drug interactions (63). In clinical trials, there appear to be fewer gastrointestinal adverse effects when compared with oxycodone (64,65). Despite being a dual mechanism drug, tapentadol is scheduled as a C-II controlled substance similar to other strong opioids.

Tramadol. Tramadol is a synthetic analog of codeine that binds to the MOR and blocks the reuptake of serotonin and norepinephrine. Because of the inhibited reuptake of monoamines, the use of tramadol should be avoided in patients on selective serotonin reuptake inhibitors or tricyclic antidepressants due to the increased risk of seizure and serotonin syndrome. Tramadol is extensively metabolized by CYP2D6 to its active metabolite, O-desmethyl tramadol, and therefore analgesia may be reduced in poor metabolizers of CYP2D6 (66). Tramadol is thought to be approximately one-tenth as potent as morphine in patients with cancer (66). Individuals on higher doses of tramadol or who have a history of seizures may be at increased risk for seizures. The ceiling dose of tramadol is 400 mg/d and is dose adjusted in renal impairment. Both immediate- and extended-release oral formulations are available. In a double-blind study of tramadol in cancer patients, adverse effects, including vomiting, dizziness, and weakness, were more likely when compared with hydrocodone and codeine (67). A large cohort study from the United Kingdom found an increased risk of hospitalization due to hypoglycemia in patients receiving tramadol compared with codeine (68). Due to its dual mechanism of action, naloxone is only partially effective in reversing tramadol toxicity. While naloxone will reverse respiratory depression, it does not reverse the monoamine effects (e.g., tachycardia, hypertension, seizure) if present. Tramadol is a C-IV controlled substance.

Other Opioids. Meperidine is not recommended in palliative care or cancer pain management because of the neurotoxic effects of its metabolite, normeperidine. Levorphanol is an analog of morphine that binds to MOR, KOR, and DOR; is an antagonist at NMDA receptors; and is a monoamine reuptake inhibitor. It is not widely used, in part because of limited availability and expense.

Partial Agonists

Buprenorphine is a highly lipophilic, semisynthetic thebaine derivative with a unique pharmacological profile that provides several advantages over traditional MOR agonists (69). It is a partial MOR agonist and weak KOR antagonist with a prolonged terminal half-life, which allows for less frequent dosing. Buprenorphine undergoes extensive first-pass metabolism and has very low oral bioavailability, which is why it is not typically administered orally but it is available in numerous other formulations (intravenous, subcutaneous [Sublocade], sublingual [Subutex, and in combination with naloxone (Suboxone)], buccal [Belbuca], and transdermal [Butrans]). The buccal and transdermal formulations are indicated for pain management in the United States; these may be of particular benefit when patients are no longer able to swallow. Buprenorphine is metabolized to its active metabolite, norbuprenorphine,

by CYP3A4 and therefore may be subject to drug–drug interactions. A recent study examined the potential interaction between buprenorphine and cannabis (CYP3A4 inhibitor) and found higher concentrations of both buprenorphine and norbuprenorphine in cannabis users (70). Despite the common misconception, there is no ceiling effect on analgesia and development of tolerance is less likely to occur due to KOR antagonism. Buprenorphine is approximately 75 to 115 times as potent as morphine and has been shown to be efficacious in various pain subtypes, including cancer pain and neuropathic pain (71–73). There is, however, a dose-ceiling effect on respiratory depression and euphoriant effect at doses up to 32 mg/d (74,75). It is important to note that there is still a risk of respiratory depression and overdose if buprenorphine is taken concomitantly with benzodiazepines, alcohol, and/or other CNS depressants. Buprenorphine is a Schedule III controlled substance that may help mitigate some of the barriers patients are currently facing in obtaining opioids in the midst of the opioid epidemic.

Case reports and clinical trials suggest that transdermal buprenorphine, a partial agonist, is useful in cancer pain (76–78). Additionally, a randomized placebo-controlled study in patients with cancer pain revealed an analysis effect of this therapy (79). However, breakthrough medication consisted of sublingual buprenorphine, a product not commercially available in the United States. A recent consensus panel endorsed its use for cancer pain (80), and a small open-label study's suggestion of using i.v. morphine for breakthrough pain did not alter the analgesic effects of the transdermal buprenorphine (81). The interaction of pure and partial opioid agonists may lead to reduced analgesia.

Mixed Agonist–Antagonists

Mixed agonist–antagonist opioid analgesics, including butorphanol, nalbuphine, and pentazocine, exhibit a ceiling effect for analgesia, are more likely to cause psychotomimetic effects, and can precipitate withdrawal if given to a patient physically dependent on a pure opioid agonist (82). As a result, these agents are not recommended in cancer pain management.

Antagonists

Opioid antagonists, such as parenteral and intranasal naloxone, have been used to reverse acute adverse effects, primarily respiratory depression, caused by opioids. Oral naloxone has been shown to be effective in relieving opioid-induced constipation (OIC), although one must use bad-tasting solutions intended for parenteral administration

(83). Furthermore, higher doses, up to 8 to 12 mg, can reverse analgesia. Agents such as methylnaltrexone, naloxegol, and alvimopan (among others) act peripherally to block opioid receptor binding within the gastrointestinal tract and will be discussed in *Constipation* (84).

Definitions

Misconceptions about terms such as tolerance, physical dependence, and addiction contribute to inadequate management of pain (Table 2.5). Education of professionals, patients, family members, and the public is needed to overcome the many misconceptions and biases that limit the effective use of this class of analgesics. See Chapter 44 for specific information on substance-abuse issues in palliative care.

Routes of Opioid Administration

Numerous routes of opioid administration that are of particular benefit in palliative care are available. In a study of patients with cancer at 4 weeks, 1 week, and 24 hours before death, the oral route of opioid administration was continued in 62%, 43%, and 20% of patients, respectively (90). When

TABLE 2.5 DEFINITIONS ASSOCIATED WITH OPIOIDS

Addiction
Addiction is a treatable, chronic medical disease involving complex interactions among brain circuits, genetics, the environment, and an individual's life experiences. People with addiction use substances or engage in behaviors that become compulsive and often continue despite harmful consequences (85).

Physical Dependence
Physical dependence is a state of adaptation that is manifested by a drug class–specific withdrawal syndrome that can be produced by abrupt cessation, rapid dose reduction, decreased blood level of the drug, and/or administration of an antagonist (86).

Tolerance
Tolerance is a state of adaptation in which repeated exposure to a drug induces changes that result in a diminishment of one or more of the drug's effects over time (87).

Pseudoaddiction
Pseudoaddiction is the mistaken assumption of addiction in a patient who is receiving inadequate analgesia. Patients with pseudoaddiction may display aberrant drug-related behaviors; however, they cease after their pain has been adequately treated (88).

Pseudotolerance
Pseudotolerance is the misconception that the need for increasing doses of drug is due to tolerance rather than disease progression or other factors (89).

oral delivery is no longer useful, many alternative routes exist. Sublingual, buccal, rectal, transdermal, sub.q., intramuscular (i.m.), i.v., pulmonary, nasal, spinal, and peripheral (topical) routes of administration have all been described (91). However, the fact that a drug can be administered by a particular route does not imply that it is effective. Lipid solubility and the size of the molecule influence the transport of the opioid across biological membranes, affecting the pharmacokinetics of the agent. The unique clinical challenge of caring for a person unable to swallow because of anatomic abnormalities or loss of consciousness at the end of life leads to the desire to find alternative routes. Yet, the attributes of the compound must first be considered.

Oral, Sublingual, and Buccal

Numerous options are available when patients are able to swallow tablets or capsules, including immediate-release and long-acting solid dosage formulations, as well as liquids. Morphine's bitter taste may be prohibitive, especially if immediate-release tablets are left in the mouth to dissolve if the patient cannot normally swallow. For patients with dysphagia, several options are available. The 24-hour, long-acting morphine capsule can be broken open and the "sprinkles" placed in applesauce or other soft foods. Oral morphine or oxycodone solution can be swallowed or small volumes (0.5 to 1 mL) of a concentrated solution (e.g., 20 mg/mL) can be placed sublingually or buccally in patients whose voluntary swallowing capabilities are more significantly limited (92–95). However, buccal or sublingual uptake of morphine is slow and not very predictable because of its hydrophilic chemical nature (96). In fact, most of the analgesic effect of morphine administered in this manner is due to the drug trickling down the throat and the resultant absorption through the gastrointestinal tract. Methadone oral solution has been shown to be well tolerated and effective when instilled in the buccal cavity as compared to oral administration (97). When administering an oral solution in the buccal cavity, particularly in patients with an impaired level of consciousness, it is important to prop the upper body up about 30 degrees to minimize the risk of aspiration (25). Topical morphine mouthwash has been studied to treat chemotherapy-induced oral mucositis (98).

Fentanyl is commercially available in six different transmucosal (sublingual or buccal) formulations (99,100). These include a compressed lozenge of fentanyl citrate (Actiq), fentanyl effervescent buccal tablet (Fentora), buccal soluble film (Onsolis), sublingual oral disintegrating fentanyl citrate (Abstral), intranasal fentanyl spray (Lazanda), and sublingual fentanyl spray (Subsys) (25). These products are indicated for cancer patients over age 18, who are considered to be "opioid tolerant." Prescribers must enroll in the Transmucosal Immediate Release Fentanyl (TIRF) Risk Evaluation Mitigation (REMS) program to prescribe, dispense, or distribute these medications (inpatient and hospice providers are exempt).

Enteral and Rectal

If already in place, enteral feeding tubes can be used to access the gut when patients can no longer swallow opioids. The size of the tube should be considered when placing long-acting morphine "sprinkles" to avoid obstruction of the tube. The rectal, stomal, or vaginal route can be used to administer medication when oral delivery is unreasonable. Commercially prepared suppositories, compounded suppositories, or microenemas can be used to deliver the drug into the rectum or stoma. Sustained-release morphine tablets have been used rectally, with resultant delayed time to peak plasma level and approximately 90% of the bioavailability being achieved by oral administration (101). Rectal methadone has a bioavailability approximately equal to that of oral methadone (102). The "Macy Catheter" is a novel device that allows for crushing appropriate tablets, or opening capsules as permitted, and administering by the rectal route of administration (103). Thrombocytopenia, neutropenia, or painful lesions preclude the use of these routes. Additionally, delivering medications through these routes can be difficult for family members, especially when the patient is obtunded or unable to assist in turning.

Nasal

Nasal fentanyl, hydromorphone, and morphine have been investigated (31,104,105). A fentanyl nasal spray is available for breakthrough cancer pain, as described above (106).

Parenteral

Parenteral administration includes both sub.q. and i.v. delivery, routes that are frequently used in palliative care when other methods are ineffective (53). Intramuscular opioid delivery is inappropriate in the palliative care setting because of the pain associated with this route and the variability in systemic uptake of the drug (82). The i.v. route provides rapid drug delivery, but it requires vascular access. Subcutaneous boluses have a slower onset and a lower peak effect when compared with i.v. boluses (107), although continuous infusions are equianalgesic (108,109). Subcutaneous infusions may include rates of up to 10 mL/h (110) (although most patients absorb 2 to 3 mL/h with

least difficulty). Volumes of sub.q. drug delivery greater than these are poorly absorbed.

Neuraxial (Epidural/Intrathecal)

Neuraxial, or intraspinal routes, including epidural and intrathecal delivery, may allow administration of drugs, such as opioids, local anesthetics, and/or α-adrenergic agonists, in palliative care settings (111). Reviews have concluded that neuraxial opioid therapy in patients with pain due to cancer is often effective when other interventions have not been successful (112,113). One must consider the complexity of the equipment used to deliver these medications and the potential caregiver burden. Additionally, not all centers have health care professionals on staff with the specialized knowledge to provide these therapies. Finally, cost is a significant concern related to high-tech procedures.

Intraspinal delivery should be considered when patients experience intolerable adverse effects to opioids and other analgesics, despite aggressive management. Additionally, patients who do not obtain adequate relief from aggressive titration of systemic opioids and other analgesics should be considered for intraspinal drug administration. When systemic opioids are relatively ineffective, this suggests the need for the addition of a local anesthetic, such as bupivacaine, to the infusion. Additionally, pain that is bilateral or midline and is not responsive to systemic analgesics might best be treated with intraspinal drug administration because nerve blocks or other ablative procedures are generally not indicated in these circumstances.

Spinal Delivery Systems. Percutaneous catheters attached to an external infusion device can be used to deliver medications through the epidural or intrathecal space. Patients with a longer life span would likely benefit from a more permanent catheter that is tunneled to reduce the risk of infection. Dislodgement and infection are the most common complications. Subcutaneous ports, similar to those used to access the venous system, can be implanted and are approved for epidural delivery. Although technically an implanted system, the port must be constantly accessed with a deflected tip needle to allow continuous infusions by an external pump. Implanted pumps are battery driven and programmable, allowing more precise delivery of the drug. There is a potential for reduced risk of infection because the pump is entirely implanted. However, they are more expensive and require specially trained staff to refill the device as well as equipment to make programming changes that allow changes in the rate of drug delivery.

Agents Administered Spinally. Opioids given intraspinally typically include morphine, hydromorphone, fentanyl, remifentanil, and sufentanil. The more lipophilic compounds, such as fentanyl, remifentanil, and sufentanil, are likely to be administered epidurally, whereas more hydrophilic agents, including morphine and hydromorphone, are delivered intrathecally. Adverse effects include those seen with systemic administration of an opioid, with a greater prevalence of pruritus and urinary retention. Local anesthetics are beneficial when treating neuropathic pain, particularly in the pelvis and lower extremities. Clonidine, an α_2-adrenergic agonist, has been shown to be of benefit in providing relief of postoperative, cancer, and labor pain. Hypotension is a potentially dose-limiting adverse effect. The N-specific calcium channel blocker, ziconotide, has been shown to produce analgesia when delivered intrathecally, although the therapeutic window is narrow and adverse effects can be significant.

The Polyanalgesic Consensus Conference (PACC) by Deer et al. have provided a series of three articles that provide extensive guidance on intrathecal drug delivery, including candidate and drug selection, trialing therapies, dosing and monitoring (114–116).

Topical

Because of the hydrophilic nature of morphine, creams and patches that contain morphine are unlikely to provide analgesia when applied to intact skin. An analysis of the bioavailability of topical morphine gel applied to the intact skin of the wrist, identical to the formulation used in some hospices, revealed no measurable serum levels (117). Controversy exists about whether topical morphine or other opioids might be useful in providing pain relief when applied to open areas, such as burns, pressure ulcers, or skin lesions due to venous stasis or sickle cell disease. Several case reports and open-label trials indicate that this might be an effective route (118–120). However, a randomized controlled trial of topical morphine used to treat painful skin ulcers found no benefit when compared with placebo (121). An analysis of the bioavailability of morphine when delivered to open ulcers found little systemic uptake, a possible explanation for the lack of efficacy (122).

Various recipes of compounded topical pain creams have been trialed to treat localized chronic pain. Brutcher et al. evaluated the efficacy of three different multi-ingredient topical pain creams to treat localized pain classified as neuropathic, nociceptive, or mixed (123). After 3 months of therapy, the compounded creams were shown to be no better than placebo creams.

Topical lidocaine 5% patches are approved for the treatment of postherpetic neuralgia, and case reports and open-label studies have shown some efficacy in cancer pain (124). Additionally, topical nonsteroidal anti-inflammatory agents (e.g., diclofenac) and topical capsaicin may be beneficial to treat pain, particularly localized pain from a comorbid condition.

Transdermal

Transdermal fentanyl has been used extensively, and a wide range of dosing options (12, 25, 37.5, 50, 62.5, 75, 87.5, and 100 µg/h patches) makes this route particularly useful in palliative care (93). Fever, diaphoresis, cachexia, morbid obesity, and ascites may have a significant impact on the absorption, predictability of blood levels, and clinical effects of transdermal fentanyl, although studies are lacking. There is some suggestion that transdermal fentanyl may produce less constipation when compared with long-acting morphine; yet, the studies demonstrating this effect are small and not sufficiently powered to evaluate this effect (125). A small subset of patients will develop skin irritation because of the adhesive in any patch. Most topical antihistamines have an oil base and would preclude adherence by the patch. Spraying an aqueous steroid inhaler (intended to treat asthma) on the skin and allowing it to dry before applying the patch will often prevent rashes.

A small proportion of patients will experience decreased analgesic effects after only 48 hours of applying a new patch; this should be accommodated by determining whether a higher dose is tolerated with increased duration of the effect or a more frequent (q48h) patch change should be scheduled. As with all long-acting preparations, breakthrough pain medications should be made available to patients using immediate-release opioids.

Transdermal buprenorphine is another transdermal opioid option, indicated for pain severe enough to require daily, around-the-clock, long-term opioid treatment and for which alternative treatment options are inadequate. Available as a 5-, 7.5-, 10-, 15-, and 20-µg/h transdermal patch, transdermal buprenorphine may be administered to opioid-naïve patients and those routinely receiving <30 mg oral morphine equivalents per day, with the 5 µg/h patch. Patients receiving between 30 and 80 mg oral morphine equivalents per day should be tapered down to no more than 30 mg oral morphine equivalent per day; after 7 days the patient may begin transdermal buprenorphine 10 µg/h. The prescribing information recommends that transdermal buprenorphine is not an appropriate therapeutic option for patients requiring >80 mg of oral morphine equivalents per day (126). While there are data supporting the efficacy of transdermal buprenorphine in cancer pain as discussed above, a Cochrane review concluded that as an opioid, buprenorphine should likely be considered more of a fourth-line opioid, and the role of transdermal buprenorphine is not clear (127).

Adverse Effects

The adverse effects associated with opioids are generally well known, although the underlying mechanism for each of these effects might not be fully articulated. More common adverse effects include constipation, cognitive impairment, nausea and vomiting, and sedation. Less common effects include myoclonus, pruritus, urinary retention, and respiratory depression. These may be dose limiting or result in discontinuation of therapy, but there are strategies that can help prevent or mitigate these adverse effects while maintaining adequate pain management.

Constipation

Patients receiving palliative care frequently experience constipation, in part because of opioid therapy. OIC, which is defined by the Rome IV criteria, affects between 40% and 60% of cancer patients and significantly impacts quality of life (128). Opioids cause constipation through several mechanisms—reducing peristalsis and fluid secretion, increasing fluid reabsorption, and increasing sphincter tone—and tolerance does not occur over time. Symptoms or complications that can accompany constipation include abdominal pain, bloating, nausea, vomiting, early satiety, reflux, anal fissure, hemorrhoids, and/or bowel obstruction. The American Gastroenterological Association (AGA), the European Society for Medical Oncology (ESMO), and the Multinational Association of Supportive Care in Cancer (MASCC) recently updated their clinical practice guidelines on the management of OIC and constipation in advanced cancer (128–130). A prophylactic bowel regimen should be started when commencing opioid analgesic therapy (131). A daily stimulant laxative (e.g., senna) titrated upward is generally warranted. In a study of hospitalized patients with cancer, many of whom were taking opioids, those in the senna-only group had more bowel movements than did those in the senna-docusate group (132). Bulking or high-fiber agents (e.g., psyllium) are rarely effective and may contribute to worsening constipation, particularly in patients with insufficient fluid intake. Oil-based products, such as mineral oil, are not indicated because they prevent the absorption of fat-soluble vitamins, cause incontinence, and may lead to aspiration in bedbound

patients. Peripherally acting μ-opioid receptor antagonists (PAMORAs), such as methylnaltrexone, block opioid receptors within the gastrointestinal tract without affecting analgesia and are typically reserved for refractory OIC (133). See Table 2.6 for a list of agents used to prevent and treat OIC. See Chapter 14 for a complete discussion on the management of constipation.

Cognitive Impairment

Anecdotally, patients taking opioids for pain control often report "fuzzy" thinking and an inability to concentrate or perform simple cognitive tasks (such as balancing a checkbook). Few studies have been conducted to explore this phenomenon. A double-blind, crossover, controlled trial of patients on sustained-release opioids for pain control examined cognitive performance and memory after administration of oral immediate-release morphine or placebo. There were significant differences in pain reduction, but little effect on sedation. Interestingly, both transient anterograde and retrograde memory impairment and reduced performance on a complex tracking task were observed in those receiving morphine (134). A recent systematic review including older patients with cancer and chronic noncancer pain found mixed results, with cognitive changes occurring more commonly at higher mean opioid doses (approximately 120 to 190 mg oral morphine equivalent daily dose) (135). More studies are needed to fully understand the effects of opioids on cognitive functioning, and a brief screening tool to aid in clinical assessment would be beneficial.

Nausea and Vomiting

Nausea and vomiting as a result of initial opioid administration are relatively common because of the activation of the chemoreceptor trigger zone in the medulla, enhanced vestibular sensitivity, and delayed gastric emptying. Habituation occurs in most cases within days to weeks. Around-the-clock antiemetic therapy can be effective during this initial period. If persistent, assess for other causes. Table 2.7 provides recommendations for the management of opioid-induced nausea and vomiting. See Chapter 13 for a thorough discussion on the assessment and treatment of persistent nausea and vomiting.

Sedation

Excessive sedation may occur with initial dosing of opioids. It is important to distinguish accumulating, opioid-induced sedation from "catch-up" sleep that may occur once pain is better controlled. Regardless, it is important to ensure that the patient remains easily arousable.

TABLE 2.6 OPIOID-INDUCED CONSTIPATION

Prevention

Stimulant laxatives

Senna

Recommended starting dose: 17.2 mg/d (2 tabs)

Onset of laxative effect: 6–12 h

Bisacodyl

Recommended starting dose: 5 mg/d (oral) or 10 mg/d (rectal suppository)

Onset of laxative effect: 6–12 h

Management of preexisting or intermittent constipation

Category	Agent and dose
Osmotic agents	Polyethylene glycol 17–34 g (1–2 heaping tablespoons or 1–2 packets) mixed in 4–8 ounces of water, juice, soda, coffee, or tea
	Lactulose 15–30 mL orally/day
	Milk of magnesia 15–60 mL/day
	Glycerin 1 rectal suppository/day
Peripherally acting mu opioid receptor antagonists (PAMORAs)	Methylnaltrexone (Relistor) <38 kg: 0.15 mg/kg sub.q. every other day PRN 38 to < 62 kg: 8 mg sub.q. every other day PRN 62–114 kg: 12 mg sub.q. every other day PRN >114 kg: 0.15 mg/kg sub.q. every other day PRN
	Naldemedine (Symproic) 0.2 mg orally once daily
	Naloxegol (Movantik) 25 mg orally once daily in the morning; if not tolerated, reduce dose to 12.5 mg (indicated for chronic noncancer pain)
Other	Linaclotide (Linzess) 72 or 145 µg orally once daily at least 30 minutes prior to the first meal of the day (indicated for chronic idiopathic constipation)
	Lubiprostone (Amitiza) 24 µg orally twice daily (indicated for chronic noncancer pain)
Saline laxatives	Magnesium citrate 1–2 bottles/day

- If patients are unable to swallow or too weak to assist in evacuation of the stool, laxative suppositories (such as bisacodyl) are indicated; sub.q. methylnaltrexone may be useful when opioids are implicated
- Glycerin suppositories coat the rectal mucosa, providing some pain relief when stools are hard and painful to evacuate and helping to prevent tissue damage
- For patients with neuromuscular dysfunction affecting the bowel (e.g., spinal cord compression), bowel training may be helpful; this includes preventive agents, along with the use of bisacodyl at the same time each day
- Saline-type enemas (e.g., Fleet) may be indicated if suppositories are ineffective; however, these can be associated with electrolyte disturbances and they should be used with caution.

Tolerance to this effect generally develops; however, if sedation persists, one can first try lowering the opioid dose. If dose reduction is ineffective or simply not feasible due to pain severity, the use of psychostimulants may be beneficial. Starting doses include dextroamphetamine 2.5 to 5 mg p.o. every morning and midday or methylphenidate 5 to 10 mg p.o. every morning and 2.5 to 5 mg midday (134). Adjust both the dose and the timing to prevent nocturnal insomnia and monitor for undesirable psychotomimetic effects (such as agitation, hallucinations, and irritability). A study conducted in patients with cancer allowed "as-needed" dosing of methylphenidate to manage opioid-induced sedation. Doses up to 20 mg/d did not result in sleep disturbances or agitation, although most subjects took doses in the afternoon and evening (136). Modafinil, an agent approved to manage narcolepsy, has been reported to relieve opioid-induced sedation with once-daily dosing (137). The usual starting dose of modafinil is 100 to 200 mg p.o. once daily in the morning.

Myoclonus

Myoclonus, which is defined as "sudden, brief, involuntary muscle jerks either irregular or rhythmic," occurs more commonly with high-dose opioid therapy and has been reported following

TABLE 2.7 MANAGEMENT OF OPIOID-INDUCED NAUSEA AND VOMITING

- Rule out other causes of nausea and vomiting and treat accordingly
  - A. Other medications (antibiotics, anticonvulsants, antidepressants, antiparkinsonian medications, NSAIDs, vitamins)
  - B. Tumor (increased intracranial pressure)
  - C. Treatment (radiation to thorax or upper abdomen; chemotherapy)
  - D. Bowel obstruction or constipation
  - E. Metabolic abnormalities
  - F. Anxiety

- Treat with centrally acting antiemetics
  - A. Butyrophenones
    - i. Haloperidol 0.5–5 mg every 6 h orally or 0.5–2 mg every 6 h i.v.; fewer adverse effects at lower doses; as effective as phenothiazines
  - B. Atypical antipsychotics
    - i. Olanzapine 2.5–5 mg orally q12–24h
  - C. Phenothiazines
    - i. Trimethobenzamide 300 mg orally every 6–8 h or 200 mg per rectum every 6–8 h
    - ii. Prochlorperazine 10 mg orally every 6 h or 25 mg per rectum every 12 h; side effects may limit routine use, more sedating than haloperidol
  - D. Prokinetic agents
    - i. Metoclopramide 5–10 mg orally or i.v. every 6 h; administer prior to meals +/− bedtime
  - E. Serotonin antagonists

- Ondansetron 4 mg orally or i.v. every 8 h

- Consider dexamethasone 4–8 mg every day (although optimal dose is unknown); effective in nausea/vomiting due to raised intracranial pressure

- If vestibular component to the nausea is present, add meclizine 25 mg every 6 h orally

- If nausea and/or vomiting occur upon opioid initiation, consider administering scheduled antiemetics for the first 2–3 days of opioid therapy, then slowly withdraw to determine whether the patient has developed tolerance to this effect

- If these interventions are inadequate, consider opioid rotation

---

various routes of administration (intrathecal, intravenous, and oral) (138,139). Dose reduction or opioid rotation may be useful because metabolite accumulation may be implicated, particularly in the case of renal dysfunction (46,47,56,140). A lower relative dose of the substituted drug may be possible because of incomplete cross-tolerance. Benzodiazepines, such as clonazepam at a starting dose of 0.5 to 1 mg p.o. q6–8h, and increased as needed and tolerated, may be useful in patients who are able to take oral preparations. Lorazepam can be given sublingually if the patient is unable to swallow. Parenteral administration of lorazepam or midazolam may be indicated if symptoms progress. If rapid opioid dose reduction is warranted, there may be a role for ketamine (141). Grand mal seizures associated with high-dose parenteral opioid infusions have been reported, requiring aggressive interventions that include benzodiazepines, barbiturates, and propofol (32).

Pruritus

Pruritus is a less common adverse effect, occurring in 2% to 10% of patients on chronic opioid therapy; however, the risk increases with epidural or intrathecal administration (142). When pruritus occurs in the palliative care patient, other etiologies should also be explored. Opioid rotation may be indicated because there appears to be variability in the prevalence of pruritus associated with various opioids (108). Antihistamines (such as diphenhydramine) are the most common first-line approach when treatment is indicated, although these agents produce sedation and are rarely totally effective as they do not address the centrally mediated component of opioid-induced pruritus. Several studies have reported that prophylactic 5-HT$_3$ receptor antagonists, including ondansetron, have resulted in decreased incidence, severity, and need for treatment of pruritus following opioid administration (143–145). There may also be a role for nalbuphine and low-dose naloxone, but available data are somewhat limited. Switching to a different opioid may also be a useful strategy. Chapter 19 provides a thorough review of pruritus.

Respiratory Depression

Respiratory depression is greatly feared, although in palliative care, this occurs rarely because most patients are opioid tolerant. Clinicians and family members often fear "giving the last dose" of an opioid. Existing data suggest a lack of correlation between opioid dose, timing of opioid administration, and patient death (146,147). There are, however, patient- and treatment-specific risk factors for opioid-induced sedation and respiratory depression, some of which include known or suspected sleep-disordered breathing, various comorbidities (e.g., history of cardiac and/or pulmonary disease, impaired renal function, impaired hepatic function, obesity, and substance use disorder), requirement for aggressive titration and dosing of opioids to manage pain, continuous opioid infusion in opioid-naïve patients, concomitant administration of sedating agents (e.g., benzodiazepines, antihistamines), and history of naloxone administration (148,149). When respiratory depression (rate <8/min and/or hypoxemia [O_2 saturation <90%]) occurs and the cause is clearly associated with opioid use, cautious and slow titration of naloxone should be instituted. Standard doses of naloxone may cause abrupt opioid reversal with pain and autonomic crisis. Dilute one ampule of naloxone (0.4 mg/mL) in 10 mL of injectable saline (final concentration 40 μg/mL) and inject 1 mL every 2 to 3 minutes while closely monitoring the level of consciousness and respiratory rate. Because the duration of effect of naloxone is approximately 30 minutes, the depressant effects of the opioid will recur at 30 minutes and persist until the plasma levels decline (often 4 or more hours) or until the next dose of naloxone is administered (108). If the patient has been on methadone, a continuous infusion of naloxone may be warranted because of the long half-life of this opioid.

Principles of Opioid Use

Effective pain control requires interdisciplinary care that incorporates a thorough assessment, which informs the development of a multimodal treatment plan. Optimally, the plan includes pharmacologic and nonpharmacologic therapies. Because opioids are the mainstay of this treatment plan, clinicians caring for patients must understand the basic principles of opioid use that build on the information previously presented in this chapter (Table 2.8).

Prevent and Treat Pain

As much as possible, pain should always be prevented and managed aggressively once it occurs. Prevention includes adequate premedication before invasive procedures and also incorporates patient education to take an immediate-release opioid before a painful activity (e.g., bathing, riding in car, wound care).

When in the hospital setting, opioids may be ordered around the clock rather than p.r.n. As-needed dosing of an opioid requires the patient to determine when the pain is sufficiently intense to call the nurse. Furthermore, there is great reluctance to "bother" the nurse coupled with a fear of appearing to be "addicted" to the medication. In a study conducted on an inpatient medicine unit, around-the-clock dosing provided significantly lower pain intensity with no increased risk of adverse effects (150).

Use of Long-Acting and Breakthrough Opioids

Long-acting or sustained-release oral opioid preparations allow convenience and are believed to enhance adherence to the treatment. There are a number of formulations currently available in the United States, including once-daily morphine, twice-daily morphine, twice-daily oxycodone, twice-daily oxymorphone, once-daily hydromorphone, and transdermal fentanyl and buprenorphine. Methadone is often included in this list because it can be given every 8 or 12 hours. Selection is based on the patient's ability to obtain relief with a particular opioid; the need for an oral, enteral, or transdermal delivery method; support in the home to adhere to a particular regimen; and preference. When using these sustained-release oral formulations, as well as transdermal agents, several principles should be considered:

1. First, titrate with a short-acting product, such as immediate-release morphine, oxycodone, or hydromorphone; then determine the dose that provides relief during a 24-hour period and convert this dose to an equivalent sustained-release opioid.
2. Immediate-release opioids should be available for breakthrough pain, with each dose calculated as approximately 10% to 15% of the 24-hour total sustained-release opioid and offered every 2, 3, or 4 hours, or even as frequently as every hour.
3. If the patient consistently requires more than two or three doses of breakthrough medication in a 24-hour period, the total breakthrough dose needed during that time should be added to the sustained-release dose (63).

There is great variability in opioid requirements, so the dose of the opioid necessary to relieve pain is the correct dose for that individual.

Opioid Rotation

When the treatment of opioid-induced adverse effects is not successful, changing to an alternative opioid, also called *opioid rotation* or *switching*, can be useful. Convert the daily dose of the current opioid, such as morphine, to the equivalent dose of an alternate opioid, such as hydromorphone, using equianalgesic tables as a guide. The 24-hour equianalgesic dose is usually reduced by approximately 25% to 50% because of incomplete cross-tolerance

TABLE 2.8 PRINCIPLES OF OPIOID ADMINISTRATION IN PALLIATIVE CARE

- Screen for pain frequently; conduct a thorough assessment when the patient reports experiencing pain.

- Consider symptoms that frequently occur with pain, including fatigue, depression, and others.

- Use opioids as part of a multimodal treatment plan that incorporates nonopioids, adjuvant analgesics, cancer therapies when appropriate, nerve blocks, and other ablative procedures as warranted, as well as nonpharmacologic strategies.

- Because pain includes physical, emotional, social, spiritual, and other factors, multidisciplinary care is required.

- Prevent pain whenever possible.

- Prevent and manage opioid-related adverse effects.

- Use sustained-release opioids combined with short-acting opioids for rescue doses.
  A. Rescue doses are generally 10%–15% of the 24-h sustained-release dose.
  B. Rescue doses for parenteral administration are 50%–100% of the hourly i.v. or sub.q. rate.

- Rotate opioids when unmanageable adverse events occur or when relief is inadequate despite aggressive titration.
  A. Calculate the appropriate dose using an equianalgesic chart.
  B. Reduce the dose by ~25%–50% to account for cross-tolerance.

- Consider patient-related factors when selecting the route of administration.
  A. If the patient has dysphagia, choose transdermal or parenteral delivery.
  B. Determine whether equipment and cost of parenteral or spinal administration will place a hardship on family caregivers.

- Educate patients and families about the most effective strategies for using pharmacologic and nonpharmacologic management.
  A. Diaries, flow sheets, and pill boxes will help promote adherence.
  B. Knowing how and when to use p.r.n. medications is particularly difficult for many patients and family members; reinforce this information repeatedly.
  C. Differentiate p.r.n. medications for pain, nausea and vomiting, and anxiety through color-coding or copying pictures of the pills onto a small poster that explains their use.
  D. Consider the patient and family's literacy level when providing any instructional material.

- When financial barriers to obtaining opioids exist, explore patient assistance programs.
  A. www.needymeds.com
  B. www.togetherrxaccess.com
  C. www.cancer.org/Treatment/index

- Never abruptly discontinue an opioid.
  A. Gradually reduce the dose by ~25%–50% to prevent distressing symptoms associated with the abstinence syndrome: agitation, sleeplessness, abdominal cramping, diarrhea, lacrimation, yawning, and piloerection.

and is titrated as needed (25). Ongoing evaluation of the efficacy of any analgesic regimen is essential, and doses of drug must be titrated on the basis of the patient's self-report of pain.

Multimodal Therapy

For the complicated pain syndromes often seen in advanced disease, opioids alone are rarely sufficient. Adjuvant analgesics, nonsteroidal anti-inflammatory drugs, and interventional approaches, along with cognitive–behavioral and physical approaches, are warranted (82). See Chapters 2 to 4 for information on other pharmacologic therapies, nonpharmacologic approaches, and interventional procedures for pain control.

CONCLUSION

For most patients with pain associated with cancer or advanced disease, relief is possible through the use of opioids and other therapies. An understanding of opioid pharmacotherapy is a critical component of pain management in those with cancer or other life-threatening illnesses. The evolving field of pharmacogenomics reinforces and informs the clinical observation that all regimens must be individualized to the patient's needs and responses. One envisions a time when screening to determine the optimal response to a particular opioid will be widely available, preventing the trial and error approach currently required.

Although the science of pain mechanisms and opioid pharmacotherapy is advancing rapidly, myths and misperceptions about addiction persist. In fact, there appears to be an even greater fear of addiction as media attention to celebrity addictive disease increases. To address these misunderstandings, patients, family members, and, often, other clinicians need extensive education. Pain in people with life-threatening illness is a serious problem in health care that can be addressed only through the combined efforts of scientists, clinicians, regulators, and the public to ensure the availability of opioids to provide relief.

REFERENCES

1. Zimmerman M. The history of pain concepts and treatment before IASP. In: Mersky H, Loeser J, Dubner R, eds. *The Paths of Pain 1975-2005*. Seattle, WA: International Association for the Study of Pain; 2005:1-21.
2. Volkow ND, Blanco C. The changing opioid crisis: development, challenges and opportunities. *Mol Psychiatry*. 2020. doi: 10.1038/s41380-020-0661-4. [Epub ahead of print].
3. Stein C. Opioid receptors. *Annu Rev Med*. 2016;67:433-451.
4. Yaksh TL, Rudy TA. Analgesia mediated by a direct spinal action of narcotics. *Science*. 1976;192(4246):1357-1358.
5. Pasternak GW. Mu opioid pharmacology: 40 years to the promised land. *Adv Pharmacol*. 2018;82:261-291.
6. Jackson KC II. Opioid pharmacokinetics. In: Davis M, Glare P, Hardy J, eds. *Opioids in Cancer Pain*. New York, NY: Oxford University Press; 2005:43-52.
7. Mazak K, Noszal B, Hosztafi S. Advanced in physicochemical profiling of opioid compounds of therapeutic interest. *ChemistryOpen*. 2019;8:879-887.
8. Jensen TS, Yaksh TL. Comparison of antinociceptive action of morphine in the periaqueductal gray, medial and paramedial medulla in rat. *Brain Res*. 1986;363(1):99-113.
9. Klimas R, Mikus G. Morphine-6-glucuronide is responsible for the analgesic effect after morphine administration: a quantitative review of morphine, morphine-6-glucuronide, and morphine-3-glucuronide. *Br J Anaesth*. 2014;113(6):935-944.
10. Thwaites D, McCann S, Broderick P. Hydromorphone neuroexcitation. *J Palliat Med*. 2004;7(4):545-550.
11. Dean M. Opioids in renal failure and dialysis patients. *J Pain Symptom Manage*. 2004;28(5):497-504.
12. Koehntop DE, Rodman JH. Fentanyl pharmacokinetics in patients undergoing renal transplantation. *Pharmacotherapy*. 1997;17(4):746-752.
13. Obeng AO, Hamadeh I, Smith M. Review of opioid pharmacogenetics and considerations for pain management. *Pharmacotherapy*. 2017;37(9):1105-1121.
14. Klepstad P, Dale O, Skorpen F, et al. Genetic variability and clinical efficacy of morphine. *Acta Anaesthesiol Scand*. 2005;49(7):902-908.
15. Pasternak GW. Molecular biology of opioid analgesia. *J Pain Symptom Manage*. 2005;29(suppl 5):S2-S9.
16. Gualberto R, Kost JA. Fundamental considerations for genetically-guided pain management with opioids based on CYP2D6 and OPRM1 polymorphisms. *Pain Physician*. 2017;21:E611-E621.
17. Kaye AD, Garcia AJ, Hall OD, et al. Update on the pharmacogenomics of pain management. *Pharmacogenomics Pers Med*. 2019;12:125-143.
18. Fulton CR, Zang Y, Desta Z, et al. Drug-gene and drug-drug interactions associated with tramadol and codeine therapy in the INGENIOUS trial. *Pharmacogenomics*. 2019;20(6):397-408.
19. Miotto K, Cho AK, Khalil MA, et al. Trends in tramadol: pharmacology, metabolism, and misuse. *Anesth Clin Pharmacol*. 2017;124(1):44-51.
20. US Food and Drug Administration. FDA restricts use of prescription codeine pain and cough medicines and tramadol pain medicines in children; recommends against use in breastfeeding women. Drug Safety Communications; 2017. https://www.fda.gov/media/104268/download. Accessed April 25, 2020.
21. Rakvag TT, Klepstad P, Baar C, et al. The Val158Met polymorphism of the human catechol-O-methyltransferase (*COMT*) gene may influence morphine requirements in cancer pain patients. *Pain*. 2005;116(1-2):73-78.
22. Lotsch J. Opioid metabolites. *J Pain Symptom Manage*. 2005;29(suppl 5):S10-S24.
23. Sathyan G, Jaskowiak J, Evashenk M, et al. Characterization of the pharmacokinetics of the fentanyl HCl patient-controlled transdermal system (PCTS): effect of current magnitude and multiple-day dosing and comparison with IV fentanyl administration. *Clin Pharmacokinet*. 2005;44(suppl 1):7-15.
24. Mystakidou K, Katsouda E, Tsilika E, et al. Transdermal therapeutic fentanyl-system (TTS-F). *In Vivo*. 2004;18(5):633-642.
25. McPherson ML. *Demystifying Opioid Conversion Calculations: A Guide to Effective Dosing*. Bethesda, MD: American Society of Health-System Pharmacists; 2018.
26. Smith HS. Opioid metabolism. *Mayo Clin Proc*. 2009; 84(7):613-624.
27. Shibutani K, Inchiosa MA Jr, Sawada K, et al. Pharmacokinetic mass of fentanyl for postoperative analgesia in lean and obese patients. *Br J Anaesth*. 2005;95(3): 377-383.
28. Heiskanen T, Matzke S, Haakana S, Gergov M, Vuori E, Kalso E. Transdermal fentanyl in cachectic cancer patients. *Pain*. 2009;144:218-222.
29. Hutchinson MR, Menelaou A, Foster DJR, et al. CYP2D6 and CYP3A4 involvement in the primary oxidative metabolism of hydrocodone by human liver microsomes. *Br J Clin Pharmacol*. 2004;57(3):287-297.
30. Murray A, Hagen NA. Hydromorphone. *J Pain Symptom Manage*. 2005;29(suppl 5):S57-S66.
31. Finn J, Wright J, Fong J, et al. A randomised crossover trial of patient controlled intranasal fentanyl and oral morphine for procedural wound care in adult patients with burns. *Burns*. 2004;30(3):262-268.
32. Golf M, Paice JA, Feulner E, et al. Refractory status epilepticus. *J Palliat Med*. 2004;7(1):85-88.
33. Lee M, Leng M, Cooper R. Measurements of plasma oxycodone, noroxycodone and oxymorphone levels in a patient with bilateral nephrectomy who is undergoing haemodialysis. *Palliat Med*. 2005;19(3):259-260.
34. Benmebarek M, Devaud C, Gex-Fabry M, et al. Effects of grapefruit juice on the pharmacokinetics of the enantiomers of methadone. *Clin Pharmacol Ther*. 2004;76(1):55-63.
35. Haumann J, van Kuijk SMJ, Geurts JW, et al. Methadone versus fentanyl in patients with radiation-induced neuropathic pain with head and neck cancer: a randomized controlled noninferiority trial. *Pain Pract*. 2018;18(3):331-340.
36. Haumann J, Geurts JW, van Kuijk SM, et al. Methadone is superior to fentanyl in treating neuropathic pain in patients with head-and-neck cancer. *Eur J Cancer*. 2016;65:121-129.

37. Furst P, Lundstrom S, Klepstad P, et al. Improved pain control in terminally ill cancer patients by introducing low-dose oral methadone in addition to ongoing opioid treatment. *J Palliat Med.* 2018;21(2):177-181.
38. McNicol ED, Ferguson MC, Schumann R. Methadone for neuropathic pain in adults. *Cochrane Database Syst Rev.* 2017;(5):5-7. Art. No.: CD012499. doi: 10.1002/14651858.CD012499.pub2.
39. Nicholson AB, Watson GR, Derry S, et al. Methadone for cancer pain. *Cochrane Database Syst Rev.* 2017;(2). Art. No.: CD003971. doi: 10.1002/14651858.CD003971.pub4.
40. McPherson ML, Walker KA, Davis MP, et al. Safe and appropriate use of methadone in hospice and palliative care: Expert consensus white paper. *J Pain Symptom Manage.* 2019;57(3):635-645.
41. Gagnon C. The use of methadone in the care of the dying. *Eur J Palliat Care.* 1997;4:152-158.
42. Gonzalez-Barboteo J, Porta-Sales J, Sanchez D, et al. Conversion from parenteral to oral methadone. *J Pain Palliat Care Pharmacother.* 2008;22:200-205.
43. Kharasch ED, Hoffer C, Whittington D, et al. Role of hepatic and intestinal cytochrome P450 3A and 2B6 in the metabolism, disposition, and miotic effects of methadone. *Clin Pharmacol Ther.* 2004;76(3):250-269.
44. Wang J-S, DeVane CL. Involvement of CYP3A4, CYP2C8, and CYP2D6 in the metabolism of (R)- and (S)-methadone in vitro. *Drug Metab Dispos.* 2003;31(6):742-747.
45. Ferrari A, Coccia CPR, Bertolini A, et al. Methadone—metabolism, pharmacokinetics and interactions. *Pharmacol Res.* 2004;50(6):551-559.
46. Smith MT. Neuroexcitatory effects of morphine and hydromorphone: evidence implicating the 3-glucuronide metabolites. *Clin Exp Pharmacol Physiol.* 2000;27(7):524-528.
47. Sarhill N, Davis MP, Walsh D, et al. Methadone-induced myoclonus in advanced cancer. *Am J Hosp Palliat Care.* 2001;18(1):51-53.
48. Krantz MJ, Kutinsky IB, Robertson AD, et al. Dose-related effects of methadone on QT prolongation in a series of patients with torsade de pointes. *Pharmacotherapy.* 2003;23(6):802-805.
49. Cruciani RA, Sekine R, Homel P, et al. Measurement of QTc in patients receiving chronic methadone therapy. *J Pain Symptom Manage.* 2005;29(4):385-391.
50. Reddy S, Fisch M, Bruera E. Oral methadone for cancer pain: no indication of Q-T interval prolongation or torsades de pointes. *J Pain Symptom Manage.* 2004;28(4):301-303.
51. Reddy S, Hui D, El Osta B, et al. The effect of oral methadone on the QTc interval in advanced cancer patients: a prospective pilot study. *J Palliat Med.* 2010;13:33-38.
52. Peles E, Schreiber S, Gordon J, et al. Significantly higher methadone dose for methadone maintenance treatment (MMT) patients with chronic pain. *Pain.* 2005;113(3):340-346.
53. Mercadante S. Intravenous morphine for management of cancer pain. *Lancet Oncol.* 2010;11:484-489.
54. Swarm R, Abernethy AP, Anghelescu KL, et al. Adult cancer pain. *J Natl Compr Canc Netw.* 2010;8:1046-1086.
55. Hanks GW, Conno F, Cherny N, et al. Morphine and alternative opioids in cancer pain: the EAPC recommendations. *Br J Cancer.* 2001;84(5):587-593.
56. Andersen G, Jensen NH, Christrup L, et al. Pain, sedation and morphine metabolism in cancer patients during long-term treatment with sustained-release morphine. *Palliat Med.* 2002;16(2):107-114.
57. Mercadante S, Caraceni A. Conversion ratios for opioid switching in the treatment of cancer pain: a systematic review. *Palliat Med.* 2011;5:504-515.
58. Lauretti GR, Oliveira GM, Pereira NL. Comparison of sustained-release morphine with sustained-release oxycodone in advanced cancer patients. [see comment]. *Br J Cancer.* 2003;89(11):2027-2030.
59. King SJ, Reid C, Forbes K, Hanks G. A systematic review of oxycodone in the management of cancer pain. *Palliat Med.* 2011;5:454-470.
60. Gabrail NY, Dvergsten C, Ahdieh H. Establishing the dosage equivalency of oxymorphone extended release and oxycodone controlled release in patients with cancer pain: a randomized controlled study. *Curr Med Res Opin.* 2004;20(6):911-918.
61. Sloan P. Review of oral oxymorphone in the management of pain. *Ther Clin Risk Manage.* 2008;4:777-787.
62. Adams M, Pieniaszek HJ Jr, Gammaitoni AR, Ahdieh H. Oxymorphone extended release does not affect CYP2C9 or CYP3A4 metabolic pathways. *J Clin Pharmacol.* 2005;45:337-345.
63. Langford RM, Knaggs R, Farguhar-Smith P, Dickenson AH. Is tapentadol different from classical opioids? A review of the evidence. *Br J Pain.* 2016;10(4):217-221.
64. Prommer EE. Tapentadol: an initial analysis. *J Opioid Manage.* 2010;6:223-226.
65. Wade WE, Spruill WJ. Tapentadol hydrochloride: a centrally acting oral analgesic. *Clin Ther.* 2009;31:2804-2818.
66. Grond S, Sablotzki A. Clinical pharmacology of tramadol. *Clin Pharmacokinet.* 2004;43(13):879-923.
67. Rodriguez RF, Bravo LE, Castro F, et al. Incidence of weak opioids adverse events in the management of cancer pain: a double blind comparative trial. *J Palliat Med.* 2007;10:56-60.
68. Fournier J, Azoulay L, Yin H, Montastruc J, Suissa S. Tramadol use and the risk of hospitalization for hypoglycemia in patients with noncancer pain. *JAMA Intern Med.* 2015;175(2):186-193. doi: 10.1001/jamainternmed.2014.6512.
69. Davis MP. Twelve reasons for considering buprenorphine as a frontline analgesic in the management of pain. *J Support Oncol.* 2012;10(6):209-219.
70. Vierke C, Marxen B, Boettcher M, et al. Buprenorphine-cannabis interaction in patients undergoing opioid maintenance therapy. *Eur Arch Psychiatry Clin Neurosci.* 2020. doi: 10.1007/s00406-019-01091-0. [Epub ahead of print].
71. Sittl R, Likar R, Poulsen-Nautrup B. Equipotent doses of transdermal fentanyl and transdermal buprenorphine in patients with cancer and noncancer pain: results of a retrospective cohort study. *Clin Ther.* 2005;27:225-237.
72. Przeklasa-Muszynska A, Dobrogowski J. Transdermal buprenorphine in the treatment of cancer and noncancer pain-the results of multicenter studies in Poland. *Pharmacol Rep.* 2011;63(4):935-948.
73. Penza P, Campanella A, Martini A, et al. Short- and intermediate-term efficacy of buprenorphine TDS in chronic painful neuropathies. *J Peripher Nerv Syst.* 2008;13(4):283-288.
74. Dahan A, Yassen A, Romberg R, et al. Buprenorphine induces ceiling in respiratory depression but not in analgesia. *Br J Anaesth.* 2006;96(5):627-632.
75. Dahan A, Yassen A, Bijl H, et al. Comparison of the respiratory effects of intravenous buprenorphine and fentanyl in humans and rats. *Br J Anaesth.* 2005;94(6):825-834.
76. Ahn JS, Lin J, Ogawa S, et al. Transdermal buprenorphine and fentanyl patches in cancer pain: a network systematic review. *J Pain Res.* 2017;10:1963-1972.

77. Pergolizzi JV, Taylor R, LeQuang JA, et al. Pain control in Latin America: the optimized role of buprenorphine in the treatment of cancer and noncancer pain. *Pain Ther.* 2019;8:187-201.

78. O'Brien T, Ahn JS, Chye R, et al. Understanding transdermal buprenorphine and a practical guide to its use for chronic cancer and non-cancer pain management. *J Opioid Manage.* 2019;15(2):147-158.

79. Sittl R, Griessinger N, Likar R. Analgesic efficacy and tolerability of transdermal buprenorphine in patients with inadequately controlled chronic pain related to cancer and other disorders: a multicenter, randomized, double-blind, placebo-controlled trial. *Clin Ther.* 2003;25(1):150-168.

80. Pergolizzi JV Jr, Mercandante S, Echaburu AV, et al. The role of transdermal buprenorphine in the treatment of cancer pain: an expert panel consensus. *Curr Med Res Opin.* 2009;25:1517-1528.

81. Mercadante S, Villari P, Ferrera P, et al. Safety and effectiveness of intravenous morphine for episodic breakthrough pain in patients receiving transdermal buprenorphine. *J Pain Symptom Manage.* 2006;32:175-179.

82. Miaskowski C, Cleary J, Burney R, et al. *Guideline for the Management of Cancer Pain in Adults and Children. APS Clinical Practice Guidelines Series No. 3.* Glenview, IL: American Pain Society; 2005.

83. Meissner W, Schmidt U, Hartmann M, et al. Oral naloxone reverses opioid-associated constipation. *Pain.* 2000;84(1):105-109.

84. Yuan C-S. Clinical status of methylnaltrexone, a new agent to prevent and manage opioid-induced side effects. *J Support Oncol.* 2004;2(2):111-117; discussion 119-122.

85. American Society of Addiction Medicine. Definition of addiction. https://www.asam.org/Quality-Science/definition-of-addiction. Accessed May 10, 2020.

86. American Society of Addiction Medicine. The ASAM national practice guideline for the use of medications in the treatment of addiction involving opioid use; 2015. https://www.asam.org/docs/default-source/practice-support/guidelines-and-consensus-docs/asam-national-practice-guideline-supplement.pdf. Accessed May 10, 2020.

87. Jage J. Opioid tolerance and dependence—do they matter? *Eur J Pain.* 2005;9(2):157-162.

88. Greene MS, Chambers RA. Pseudoaddiction: fact or fiction? An investigation of the medical literature. *Curr Addict Rep.* 2015;2(4):310-317.

89. Weissman DE, Haddox JD. Opioid pseudoaddiction—an iatrogenic syndrome. *Pain.* 1989;36(3):363-366.

90. Coyle N, Adelhardt J, Foley KM, et al. Character of terminal illness in the advanced cancer patient: pain and other symptoms during the last four weeks of life. [comment]. *J Pain Symptom Manage.* 1990;5(2):83-93.

91. Kestenbaum MG, Vilches AU, Messersmith S, et al. Alternative routes to oral opioid administration in palliative care: a review and clinical summary. *Pain Med.* 2014;15:1129-1153.

92. Zeppetella G. Sublingual fentanyl citrate for cancer-related breakthrough pain: a pilot study. *Palliat Med.* 2001;15(4):323-328.

93. Jandhyala R, Fullarton JR, Bennett MI. Efficacy of rapid-onset oral fentanyl formulations vs. oral morphine for cancer-related breakthrough pain: a meta-analysis of comparative trials. *J Pain Symptom Manage.* 2013;46(4):573-580.

94. Hoskin PJ, Hanks GW, Aherne GW, et al. The bioavailability and pharmacokinetics of morphine after intravenous, oral and buccal administration in healthy volunteers. *Br J Clin Pharmacol.* 1989;27:499-505.

95. Norman C, Maynard L. Buccal opioids for breakthrough pain in children with life-limiting conditions receiving end-of-life care. *Int J Palliat Nurs.* 2019;25(10):472-479.

96. Weinberg DS, Inturrisi CE, Reidenberg B, et al. Sublingual absorption of selected opioid analgesics. *Clin Pharmacol Ther.* 1988;44(3):335-342.

97. Spaner D. Effectiveness of the buccal mucosa route for methadone administration at the end of life. *J Palliat Med.* 2014;17(11):1252-1265.

98. Cerchietti LCA, Navigante AH, Korte MW, et al. Potential utility of the peripheral analgesic properties of morphine in stomatitis-related pain: a pilot study. *Pain.* 2003;105(1-2):265-273.

99. Schug SA, Ting S. Fentanyl formulations in the management of pain: an update. *Drugs.* 2017;77:747-763.

100. Zeppetella G. Evidence-based treatment of cancer-related breakthrough pain with opioids. *JNCCN.* 2013;11(suppl 1):S37-S43.

101. Gourlay GK. Sustained relief of chronic pain. Pharmacokinetics of sustained release morphine. *Clin Pharmacokinet.* 1998;35(3):173-190.

102. Dale O, Sheffels P, Kharasch ED. Bioavailabilities of rectal and oral methadone in healthy subjects. *Br J Clin Pharmacol.* 2004;58(2):156-162.

103. Macygin KMC, Kulstad E, Mokszycki R, et al. Evaluation of the Macy Catheter®: a rectal catheter for rapid medication and fluid administration. *Expert Rev Med Devices.* 2018;6:407-414.

104. Rudy AC, Coda BA, Archer SM, et al. A multiple-dose phase I study of intranasal hydromorphone hydrochloride in healthy volunteers. *Anesth Analg.* 2004;99(5):1379-1386 (table of contents).

105. Fitzgibbon D, Morgan D, Dockter D, et al. Initial pharmacokinetic, safety and efficacy evaluation of nasal morphine gluconate for breakthrough pain in cancer patients. *Pain.* 2003;106(3):309-315.

106. Mercadante S, Radbruch L, Davies A, et al. A comparison of intranasal fentanyl spray with oral transmucosal fentanyl citrate for the treatment of breakthrough cancer pain: an open-label, randomized, crossover trial. *Curr Med Res Opin.* 2009;25:2805-2815.

107. Parsons HA, Shukkoor A, Quan H, et al. Intermittent subcutaneous opioids for the management of cancer pain. *J Palliat Med.* 2008;11:1319-1324.

108. Miaskowski C, Blair M, Chou R, et al. *Principles of Analgesic Use in the Treatment of Acute Pain and Cancer Pain.* 6th ed. Glenwood, IL: American Pain Society; 2008.

109. Nelson KA, Glare PA, Walsh D, et al. A prospective, within-patient, crossover study of continuous intravenous and subcutaneous morphine for chronic cancer pain. *J Pain Symptom Manage.* 1997;13(5):262-267.

110. Anderson SL, Shreve ST. Continuous subcutaneous infusion of opiates at end-of-life. *Ann Pharmacother.* 2004;38:1015-1023.

111. Baker L, Lee M, Regnard C, et al. Evolving spinal analgesia practice in palliative care. *Palliat Med.* 2004;18(6):507-515.

112. Ballantyne JC, Carwood C, Gupta A, et al. Comparative efficacy of epidural, subarachnoid, and intracerebroventricular opioids in patients with pain due to cancer. *Cochrane Database Syst Rev.* 2005;(2). Art. No.:CD005178. doi: 10.1002/14651858.CD005178.

113. Farquhar-Smith P, Chapman S. Neuraxial (epidural and intrathecal) opioids for intractable pain. *Br J Pain.* 2012;6(1):25-35.

114. Deer TR, Pope JE, Hayek SM, et al. The Polyanalgesic Consensus Conference (PACC): recommendations on intrathecal drug infusion systems best practices and guidelines. *Neuromodulation.* 2017;20:96-132.

115. Deer TR, Hayek SM, Pope JE, et al. The Polyanalgesic Consensus Conference (PACC): recommendations for trialing of intrathecal drug delivery infusion therapy. *Neuromodulation.* 2017;20:133-154.

116. Deer TR, Pope JE, Hayek SM, et al. The Polyanalgesic Consensus Conference (PACC): recommendations for intrathecal drug delivery: guidance for improving safety and mitigating risks. *Neuromodulation.* 2017;20:155-176.

117. Paice JA, Von Roenn JH, Hudgins JC, et al. Morphine bioavailability from a topical gel formulation in volunteers. *J Pain Symptom Manage.* 2008;35:314-320.

118. Zeppetella G, Paul J, Ribeiro MDC. Analgesic efficacy of morphine applied topically to painful ulcers. *J Pain Symptom Manage.* 2003;25(6):555-558.

119. Ballas SK. Treatment of painful sickle cell leg ulcers with topical opioids. *Blood.* 2002;99(3):1096.

120. Long TD, Cathers TA, Twillman R, et al. Morphine-infused silver sulfadiazine (MISS) cream for burn analgesia: a pilot study. *J Burn Care Rehabil.* 2001;22(2):118-123.

121. Vernassiere C, Cornet C, Trechot P, et al. Study to determine the efficacy of topical morphine on painful chronic skin ulcers. *J Wound Care.* 2005;14(6):289-293.

122. Ribeiro MDC, Joel SP, Zeppetella G. The bioavailability of morphine applied topically to cutaneous ulcers. *J Pain Symptom Manage.* 2004;27(5):434-439.

123. Brutcher RE, Kurihara C, Bicket MC, et al. Compounded topical pain creams to treat localized chronic pain: a randomized controlled trial. *Ann Intern Med.* 2019;170:309-318.

124. Garzon-Rodriguez C, Casals MM, Calsina-Berna A, et al. Lidocaine 5% patches as an effective short-term co-analgesic in cancer pain. Preliminary results. *Support Care Cancer.* 2013;21(11):153-158.

125. Muijsers RB, Wagstaff AJ. Transdermal fentanyl: an updated review of its pharmacological properties and therapeutic efficacy in chronic cancer pain control. *Drugs.* 2001;61(15):2289-2307.

126. *Butrans Prescribing Information.* Purdue Pharma LP. http://app.purduepharma.com/xmlpublishing/pi.aspx?id=b. Accessed May 10, 2020.

127. Schmidt-Hansen M, Bromham N, Taubert M, et al. Buprenorphine for treating cancer pain. *Cochrane Database Syst Rev.* 2015;(3):CD009596. doi: 10.1002/14651858.CD009596.pub4.

128. Larkin PJ, Cherny NI, La Carpia D, et al. Diagnosis, assessment and management of constipation in advanced cancer: ESMO Clinical Practice Guidelines. *Ann Oncol.* 2018;29:iv111-iv125.

129. Crockett SD, Greer KB, Heidelbaugh JJ, Falck-Ytter Y, Hanson BJ, Sultan S. American Gastroenterological Association Institute Guideline on the Medical Management of opioid-induced constipation. *Gastroenterology.* 2019;156(1):218-226.

130. Davies A, Leach C, Caponero R, et al. MASCC recommendations on the management of constipation in patients with advanced cancer. *Support Care Cancer.* 2020;28:23-33.

131. Ishihrara M, Iihara H, Okayasu S, et al. Pharmaceutical interventions facilitate premedication and prevent opioid-induced constipation and emesis in cancer patients. *Support Care Cancer.* 2010;12:1531-1538.

132. Hawley PH, Byeon JJ. A comparison of sennosides-based bowel protocols with and without docusate in hospitalized patients with cancer. *J Palliat Med.* 2008;11(4):575-581.

133. Thomas J, Karver S, Cooney GA, et al. Methylnaltrexone for opioid-induced constipation in advanced illness. *N Engl J Med.* 2008;358:2332-2343.

134. Rozans M, Dreisbach A, Lertora JJL, et al. Palliative uses of methylphenidate in patients with cancer: a review. *J Clin Oncol.* 2002;20(1):335-339.

135. Pask S, Dell-Olio M, Murtagh FEM, Boland JW. The effects of opioids on cognition in older adults with cancer and chronic noncancer pain: a systematic review. *J Pain Symptom Manage.* 2020;59(4):871-893.

136. Bruera E, Driver L, Barnes EA, et al. Patient-controlled methylphenidate for the management of fatigue in patients with advanced cancer: a preliminary report. *J Clin Oncol.* 2003;21(23):4439-4443.

137. Webster L, Andrews M, Stoddard G. Modafinil treatment of opioid-induced sedation. *Pain Med.* 2003;4(2):135-140.

138. Sedighinejad A, Nationwide BN, Haghighi M, et al. Comparison of the effects of low-dose midazolam, magnesium sulfate, remifentanil and low-dose etomidate on prevention of etomidate-induced myoclonus in orthopedic surgeries. *Anesth Pain Med.* 2016;6(2):e35333.

139. Woodward OB, Naraen S, Naraen A. Opioid-induced myoclonus and hyperalgesia following a short course of low-dose oral morphine. *Br J Pain.* 2017;11(1):32-35.

140. Mercadante S. Pathophysiology and treatment of opioid-related myoclonus in cancer patients. *Pain.* 1998;74(1):5-9.

141. Winegarden J, Carr DB, Bradshaw S. Intravenous ketamine for rapid opioid dose reduction, reversal of opioid-induced neurotoxicity, and pain control in terminal care: case report and literature review. *Pain Med.* 2016;17(4):644-649.

142. Reich A, Szepietowski JC. Opioid-induced pruritus: an update. *Clin Exp Dermatol.* 2009;35:2-6.

143. Iatrou CA, Dragoumanis CK, Vogiatzaki TD, et al. Prophylactic intravenous ondansetron and dolasetron in intrathecal morphine-induced pruritus: a randomized, double-blinded, placebo-controlled study. *Anesth Analg.* 2005;101(5):1516-1520.

144. Wang W, Zhou L, Sun L. Ondansetron for neuraxial morphine-induced pruritus: a meta-analysis of randomized controlled trials. *J Clin Pharm Ther.* 2017;42(4):383-393.

145. Bonnet MP, Marret E, Josserand J, et al. Effect of prophylactic 5-HT3 receptor antagonists on pruritus induced by neuraxial opioids: a quantitative systematic review. *Br J Anaesth.* 2008;101(3):311-319.

146. Sykes N, Thorns A. The use of opioids and sedatives at the end of life. *Lancet Oncol.* 2003;4(5):312-318.

147. Thorns A, Sykes N. Opioid use in last week of life and implications for end-of-life decision-making. *Lancet.* 2000;356(9227):398-399.

148. Pawasauskas J, Stevens B, Youssef R, et al. Predictors of naloxone use for respiratory depression and oversedation in hospitalized adults. *Am J Health Syst Pharm.* 2014;71(9):746-750.

149. Rosenfield WW, Betcher JA, Shah R, et al. Findings of a naloxone database and its utilization to improve safety and education in a tertiary care medical center. *Pain Pract.* 2016;16(3):327-333.

150. Paice JA, Noskin GA, Vanagunas A, et al. Efficacy and safety of scheduled dosing of opioid analgesics: a quality improvement study. *J Pain.* 2005;6(10):639-643.

3 Nonpharmacologic Management of Pain

Ryan Tourtellot and Angela K. M. Lipshutz

Pain is one of the most common and most feared symptoms associated with cancer. In a systematic review of the prevalence of pain in patients with cancer, pain was reported by 59% of patients undergoing treatment for cancer, 64% of patients with advanced disease, and 33% of patients after curative treatment (1). Unfortunately, undertreatment of cancer pain is not uncommon; in fact, a third of patients with cancer pain may be undertreated (2). Unrelieved pain can have profound effects on overall quality of life (3). Patients with uncontrolled pain suffer from anxiety and depression and often fear pain more than death (4).

Medications remain the mainstay of treatment for cancer pain. The most well-known and widely-accepted algorithm for the pharmacologic treatment of cancer pain is that put forward by the World Health Organization (WHO) (5). The WHO algorithm recommends immediate administration of medications and consideration for around the clock rather than as needed dosing, as well as the use of nonopioid medications, opioid medications, and adjuvants (6). The algorithm contains the well-known three-step ladder, which specifically recommends escalating the intensity of treatment from non-opioid analgesics to weak opioids and finally to strong opioids until the patient's pain is controlled.

However, since pain encompasses not only physical, but also psychosocial–spiritual dimensions, the treatment of cancer pain requires more than just pharmacologic interventions. Nonpharmacologic modalities play an integral role in the treatment of cancer pain, and, as such, are widely used among cancer patients (7–9). In 2019, the National Comprehensive Cancer Network published guidelines for the treatment of adult cancer pain that recommend nonpharmacologic modalities for cancer pain as an adjunct to medications (10). Likewise, the American Society of Clinical Oncologists (11,12) and the American Society of Anesthesiologists (13) support the combination of pharmacologic and nonpharmacologic modalities in the treatment of cancer pain.

Numerous nonpharmacologic modalities are employed for the treatment of cancer pain, more than could be adequately described in the context of this chapter. Further, many of these modalities lack a rigorous evidence base for their efficacy (14). This chapter focuses on the most widely used and accepted nonpharmacologic interventions for cancer pain, with particular attention paid to those modalities for which there is evidence of efficacy.

RATIONALE FOR NONPHARMACOLOGIC INTERVENTIONS

In his *Treatise of Man* published in 1664, French philosopher René Descartes described the "pain pathway" as a simple matter of a single neural thread relaying information about a stimulus in the body to the brain (15). Cancer pain specialists now know the experience of pain to be far more complex. Melzack's neuromatrix theory broadens the concept of a single neural thread to include a neural network that integrates input from the somatosensory, limbic, and thalamocortical systems (16,17). The complex experience of pain reflects the activity of numerous brain inputs, not only from peripheral nociception but also from other aspects of sensorimotor, cognitive, and emotional processing (18).

In the 1960s, Dame Cicely Saunders, founder of the modern hospice movement, defined the concept of total pain as suffering encompassing physical, psychological, social, emotional, and spiritual elements (Fig. 3.1) (19,20). Indeed, there is a broad and expanding volume of literature on the psychosocial-spiritual factors that may cause or influence the experience of pain. Psychological distress is known to directly impact the experience of pain (21). Depression, anxiety, anger, and mood disturbances are correlated with higher levels of perceived cancer-related pain (21,22). Conversely, patients with higher levels of social support report lower levels of cancer pain intensity (23,24). Patients' coping styles also influence the experience of pain, with maladaptive methods of coping increasing the experience of cancer-related pain, and allowing other areas of life to be adversely affected by pain (25–27).

Clearly, the experience of pain is affected not only by direct injury to tissue but also by cognitive, emotional, and psychosocial–spiritual contributions. It

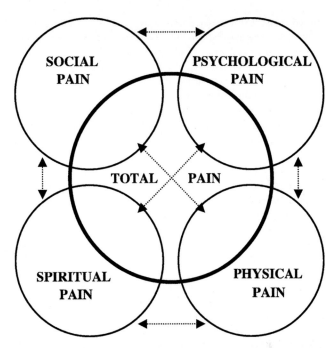

Figure 3.1 The experience of total pain. (Reprinted with permission from LWW/ Wolters Kluwer Health. Mehta A, Chan LS. Understanding of the concept of "total pain": a prerequisite for pain control. *J Hospice Palliat Nurs*. 2008;10(1):26-32. Ref (19).)

stands to reason, therefore, that a pain management approach that includes therapies to address these various dimensions of suffering will more effectively treat the whole patient with cancer who is experiencing pain.

PSYCHOSOCIAL–SPIRITUAL INTERVENTIONS FOR CANCER PAIN

Psychosocial–spiritual interventions have been shown to lead to improved pain control in patients with cancer-related pain (28). There are several psychosocial–spiritual approaches that have strong or promising empirical evidence to support their efficacy in treating such patients. These approaches can be grouped into three broad categories: self-regulatory approaches, cognitive-behavioral therapy (CBT), and spiritual care. All of these modalities can be used safely and effectively in combination with pharmacologic approaches to treat cancer-related pain.

Self-regulatory Approaches

Relaxation

Relaxation is the central theme running through many self-regulatory techniques employed for pain management in patients with cancer. Relaxation therapies, techniques, and training will be referenced frequently in subsequent sections of this chapter as important components of most self-regulatory approaches, including biofeedback, hypnosis, and mindfulness. Relaxation focuses on the identification of sources of tension within the mind and body, followed by the practice of

systematic methods such as diaphragmatic breathing, progressive muscle relaxation (29–31), or guided imagery to reduce tension and alter the perception of physical pain (32). It may improve pain symptoms by reducing the physical tension and emotional stressors and by facilitating the ability to become comfortable, rest, and fall asleep (33). Relaxation has been shown to be effective for chronic pain management related to a variety of noncancer illnesses, including migraine headaches (34), musculoskeletal pain (35), and low back pain (36). Studies have repeatedly found relaxation to be one of the most frequently used complementary therapies by cancer survivors (37). A controlled study in hospitalized oncology patients performed in the 1990s examined the efficacy of relaxation techniques involving deep breathing, muscle relaxation, and imagery compared with no relaxation (38). Results showed a significant reduction in subjective pain ratings and in the use of nonopioid analgesics. Another study randomized 58 women with breast cancer to progressive muscle relaxation or massage therapy for 30-minute sessions, 3 times a week for 5 weeks (39). The control group received usual care. Both the progressive muscle relaxation group and the massage group had significantly lower pain scores as compared with the standard treatment group.

Relaxation via guided imagery and progressive muscle relaxation also helps alleviate pain and improve quality of life in hospice patients with advanced cancer. In a study done by De Paolis et al., 91 hospice patients with cancer of various etiologies were randomized to receive combination guided imagery/progressive muscle relaxation for 20 minutes versus usual care and assessed regarding pain before and 2 hours after the intervention (29). Patients in the intervention group reported a greater decrease in pain intensity after the intervention as compared to the control group. In addition, patients who received guided imagery/progressive muscle relaxation reported less anxiety and depressive symptoms.

Biofeedback

Biofeedback is a noninvasive process for monitoring physiologic functions such as breathing, heart rate, and blood pressure and then altering that function, most commonly through relaxation therapy. Instrumentation is used to measure and relay information to the patient regarding their vital signs, electroencephalography (EEG) or brain waves, electromyography or muscle tension, and peripheral skin temperature. Over time and with the guidance of a trained practitioner, the patient learns to control these physiologic functions without the need for instrumentation in order to improve symptoms including pain (40). Biofeedback is commonly used in epilepsy, autism, and psychotic disorders and has also been well-studied in the setting of chronic noncancer pain, low back pain, joint pain, headache, and procedural pain (41). However, the use of biofeedback has not been extensively studied in cancer patients or cancer survivors. Hetkamp et al. evaluated four studies and two cases of biofeedback in cancer patients and noted that EEG feedback shows promise in alleviating pain and other symptoms, including chemotherapy-induced peripheral neuropathy, fatigue, mood, and cognitive impairment (40). Of note, all of the included studies were specific to the breast cancer population, with the exception of one pediatric study. A randomized controlled trial (RCT) of electromyography biofeedback-assisted relaxation in cancer-related pain in patients with advanced cancer showed significantly lower pain intensity scores in the treatment arm (42). Two-thirds of patients in the intervention groups reported a reduction of at least 30% in pain intensity from baseline and half obtained a reduction of at least 50% in pain intensity from baseline. In contrast, patients in the control arm, who received usual care, reported an average increase of 14% in pain intensity from baseline.

An earlier analysis of the literature suggested that the improvement in pain with biofeedback is confounded by the use of relaxation techniques in order to achieve the desired alterations of physiologic functions (43). In fact, relaxation techniques are an integral component of biofeedback training, and whether biofeedback can independently improve pain without relaxation may be difficult to examine.

Hypnosis

Hypnosis is the guided induction of a deeply relaxed state in which patients are directed to focus their awareness and imagine improvement in symptoms or changes in behavioral response (44). Once in this state of heightened and focused concentration, known as a hypnotic trance, patients can be given therapeutic suggestions to change their perception of pain (22,45). The efficacy of hypnosis has been well established for procedural pain (45–47), anticipatory nausea and vomiting (48), and various types of chronic pain (49–51). In the oncology population specifically, hypnosis is beneficial in the setting of pain related to breast biopsy (52,53), lumbar puncture (54), and bone marrow aspirates and biopsies (55,56). Additionally, the National Institutes of Health Technology Assessment Panel on Integration of Behavioral and Relaxation Approaches Into the Treatment of Chronic Pain and Insomnia found strong evidence for hypnosis in alleviating cancer-related pain (57). Likewise, Syrjala et al., in a review of meta-analyses and RCTs, found strong evidence for the use of hypnosis in treating cancer-related pain, including pain from the disease itself as well as associated treatments, procedures, and surgeries (44). Hypnosis is also useful in the pediatric oncology population. Pediatric and adolescent patients may more easily and quickly reach therapeutic trance states, with less direction compared to adults, and are more suggestive to therapeutic goals (58). Liossi et al. examined venipuncture-induced pain in children with cancer in the age group of 6 to 16 (54). Forty-five pediatric patients were randomized to receive local anesthetic, local anesthetic plus hypnosis, or local anesthetic plus attention. Patients receiving local anesthetic plus hypnosis reported significantly less procedure-related pain and demonstrated less behavioral distress during the procedure than patients in the other two groups. The same group of researchers performed two trials examining hypnosis in pediatric cancer patients undergoing lumbar puncture for hematologic malignancies and obtained similar results (59,60). Integrating hypnosis with acupuncture and yoga in pediatric patients has also shown promising results (61).

The role of hypnosis in end of life cancer patients is less clear, however. A review done by Rajasekaran et al. regarding the use of hypnotherapy to treat symptoms of terminally ill adult cancer patients concluded that the quality of the available evidence is inadequate to make a recommendation, and further research is required to understand the role of hypnotherapy in cancer patients at the end of life (62).

Mindfulness/Meditation

Mindfulness is the nonjudgmental, intentional, and conscious awareness of the present moment (63), which can be used to facilitate reduction in stress, anxiety, and depression (64). Various mindfulness practices exist; among the more common are focused attention, where the patient focuses on in-the-moment variation quality and the characteristics of sensory, emotional, and cognitive events, and open monitoring which is more inclusive of perceived thoughts and emotions without evaluation or judgment (65). Similarly, meditation is defined as "a practice of harmonizing mental states and consciousness." (66)

Mindfulness and meditation are often integrated into other mind–body modalities of nonpharmacologic pain management such as hypnosis, guided imagery, relaxation, and CBT. A recent systematic review and meta-analysis of 60 studies involving 6,404 patients with chronic pain of diverse etiologies undergoing mind body therapies revealed a moderate to large improvement in pain outcomes associated with meditation, as well as a small decrease in opioid requirement, opioid craving, and opioid misuse (67). In a review of two systematic reviews and three RCTs of mindfulness in noncancer patients, Lachance et al. suggest that mindfulness may be more clinically effective than pharmacology depending on the outcome measured and the population involved, and no study found mindfulness to be significantly less effective than traditional pharmacologic interventions (63). Furthermore, the benefit of mindfulness-based interventions persists in long-term; in a systematic review of 16 mindfulness-based interventions in chronic pain patients, benefit persisted at long-term follow-up ranging from 3 months to 3 years, regardless of the initial assessment period (68).

Ngamkham et al. performed a systematic review of mindfulness interventions for cancer-related pain (64). They found that mindfulness interventions, including meditation, can influence both physical pain and psychological variables, such as anxiety, stress, and depression. However, given the paucity of studies and the risk of bias, they call for future research in to determine the role of mindfulness in the treatment of cancer pain.

One potential benefit of mindfulness and meditation is that they can be practiced easily, for brief periods of time, in a variety of settings. Indeed, meditation instruction and practice can be performed in novel ways, such as via an integrative medicine self-care app, which, in a waiting room setting for oncology patients, reduced stress and anxiety (69).

Cognitive-Behavioral Therapy

CBT is the psychotherapeutic approach that emphasizes how our thought processes, framing, and behaviors can affect how we feel (70,71). CBT theorizes that what an individual thinks and believes about his or her symptoms, including thoughts about a symptom's meaning, controllability, and consequences, influences how that symptom is experienced (33). By helping individuals improve or resolve their maladaptive emotions, thoughts, and behaviors through a goal-oriented, systematic procedure (32,70,71), it has been used as an adjuvant to treat a variety of noncancer pain and is becoming increasing more popular as a modality to assist in cancer pain as well. Through systematic counseling, patients learn cognitive strategies and coping skills to change their thoughts and behaviors. Treatment sessions are interactive and use a combination of instruction, review of home practice, positive reinforcement, guided practice, behavioral rehearsal, and problem solving (Table. 3.1) (27,70).

Numerous studies support the efficacy of CBT for chronic pain both in patients with and without cancer. A 2012 *Cochrane Review* examined the effect of CBT on all types of chronic noncancer pain (72). Forty-two RCTs encompassing 4,788 patients examined the effects of CBT and behavioral therapy on chronic pain reduction immediately following treatment and at 6 or greater months posttreatment. CBT had a small to

TABLE 3.1 COGNITIVE-BEHAVIORAL PAIN MANAGEMENT PROTOCOL

Session	Topics	Pain Management Goals
1	Rationale for CBT	
2	Progressive relaxation training	Diverting attention away from pain
3	Guided imagery	
4	Using focal points	Altering activity patterns
5	Activity pacing	
6	Pleasant activity scheduling	Reducing negative pain-related emotions
7	Identifying negative thoughts	
8	Challenging negative thoughts	
9	Goal setting	Applying and maintaining skills in everyday situations
10	Skills maintenance	

CBT, cognitive-behavioral therapy.
Adapted from Keefe FJ, Abernethy AP, Campbell LC Psychosocial approaches to understanding and treating disease-related pain. *Annu Rev Psychol.* 2005;56:601-630.

moderate effect on pain as compared to usual care; interestingly, this effect was mostly noted immediately after treatment and dissipated at follow-up. CBT also had a small positive effect on disability and reduction in catastrophizing.

Randomized studies of the effect of CBT focusing on cancer-related pain have also shown benefit. Syrjala et al. conducted some of the first RCTs comparing CBT with treatment as usual for mucositis pain in patients receiving bone marrow transplantation for hematologic cancers (56,73). Only in the second study did CBT result in lower reported pain as compared to those who did not receive CBT (56). In this study, 94 patients with oral mucositis were randomized to 5 weeks of training in a "package" of cognitive-behavioral coping skills, which included relaxation and imagery, training solely in relaxation and imagery, therapist support, or treatment as usual. Patients who received either relaxation and imagery or the package of cognitive-behavioral coping skills reported significantly less pain than patients who received therapist support or treatment as usual.

Another study of 131 patients with cancer-related pain evaluated the efficacy of a profile-tailored CBT program compared with either standard CBT or usual care (74). CBT patients received five 50-minute treatment sessions. Compared with standard CBT and usual care patients, profile-tailored CBT patients reported significant improvements in worst pain, least pain, and interference of pain with sleep immediately after intervention. And, the results seemed to persist long-term; 6 months after the intervention, both CBT groups reported significantly less average pain and current pain as compared to patients who received usual care. In contrast, Anderson et al. randomized 57 patients taking opioids for chronic cancer-related pain to one of three cognitive behavioral interventions or wait-list control (75). Patients in the three intervention groups were given audiotapes describing the cognitive-behavioral techniques and written instructions on practicing regularly at home. Patients who practiced relaxation and distraction reported significantly lower pain intensity immediately after listening to the cognitive-behavioral tapes as compared with the control group. However, the pain reduction was not long-lasting, with no significant difference in pain intensity or pain interference found between groups 2 weeks after the intervention.

Spiritual Care

Spirituality has been described as "the aspect of humanity that refers to the way individuals seek and express meaning and purpose and the way they experience their connectedness to the moment, to self, to others, to nature, and to the significant or sacred" (76). It plays an important part in patients' derivation of hope and how they cope with a serious illness like cancer. And, spiritual distress can contribute to total pain. Patients who report greater levels of spiritual well-being report better quality of life, decreased rates of depression, and less anxiety and distress (77). Unfortunately, spiritual distress is common, reported by about 20% of cancer patients. Unmet spiritual needs include such things as a need to find inner peace, finding hope and connection to the world, finding meaning or purpose in life, giving and receiving love, talking to other people about their fears and worries, and being seen as a person up until the point of their death (78).

In a joint guidance statement, the American Society of Clinical Oncology (ASCO) and the American Academy of Hospice and Palliative Medicine (AAHPM) include spiritual/cultural assessment and management as one of the core domains of high-quality palliative care in oncology practices (79). ASCO, in their guidelines on global care in resource constrained settings, recommends that spiritual care should be provided by trained providers and should be culturally appropriate (80). They cite the growing body of research noting the impact of spirituality and religion on aspects of care such as quality of life, coping, depression, anxiety, and social health and functioning. Given the impact of these domains on total pain, spiritual assessment and spiritual care is an important modality in the nonpharmacologic management of pain.

PHYSIATRIC AND BODY-BASED INTERVENTIONS

Physiatry, or physical medicine and rehabilitation, is a field of medicine that traditionally treats patients with anatomic injuries or deformities with the goal of returning the patient to function. However, the physiatric model can also be employed effectively as a nonpharmacologic means of enhancing pain control in patients with cancer-related pain. Several of these modalities have been shown to be effective in cancer-related pain. One category of physiatric intervention that this chapter addresses is nociceptive modulation, which includes the practice of massage, transcutaneous electrical nerve stimulation (TENS), acupuncture, and touch therapy. Other physical or body-based modalities that may be helpful in treating cancer-related pain include restoration or preservation of normal biomechanics, such as therapeutic exercise and the use of adaptive orthotics to allow pain-free mobility and self-care.

Nociceptive Modulation

Massage Therapy

Massage therapy involves manipulation of the body's soft tissues using a variety of manual techniques through the application of pressure and traction. The most commonly used techniques include traditional Swedish massage, Thai massage, shiatsu, reflexology, myofascial release, and manual lymphatic drainage. Experts recommend consulting with a licensed professional massage therapist to determine the best method to utilize for individual patients (81). Evaluating the effectiveness of massage can be difficult given the wide variety of techniques and variability in practitioner ability, as well as difficulty identifying the appropriate control group.

The National Comprehensive Cancer Network recommends the use of massage in its treatment guidelines for refractory cancer pain (10), and major cancer centers such as Memorial Sloan-Kettering have been using and studying the use of massage for cancer-related pain for several decades (82). Massage has been shown in systematic reviews and meta-analyses to be beneficial for cancer-related pain as compared to active comparators or usual care; in addition, massage is effective for pain in pediatric cancer patients, patients undergoing stem cell transplantation, and patients with metastatic bone pain (83).

Although widely considered to be safe, certain considerations and precautions must be taken for the cancer patient. Deep tissue massage should be avoided in cancer patients with coagulopathy or thrombocytopenia due to the risk of bleeding or bruising (84). Therapists should perform only light massage in the area of bony metastasis to avoid fracture. An open wound, rashes, and radiation dermatitis should not be massaged due to the risk of increased pain and infection (81).

Reflexology. Reflexology is a type of massage in which physical pressure is applied to specific reflex points located on parts of the body—typically the feet, but sometimes the hands or ears—that are believed to correspond to different body organs and systems. By using or adjusting how pressure is applied, the massage therapist aims to alter or improve the perception of pain at distal sites. Although interest in the use of reflexology in the treatment of pain has increased recently, there remains a paucity of data on the effects of reflexology on cancer pain, and the existing literature shows mixed results. In a systematic review of five studies of reflexology in cancer patients, the authors concluded that data were limited and no firm conclusions could be made; however, they admit that reflexology may confer benefits over foot massage or no intervention for pain, as well as shortness of breath and anxiety (85). Indeed, reflexology may confer benefits beyond pain symptoms, with studies also suggesting benefit in nausea and fatigue (86). Further research is needed to determine the potential role for reflexology in the treatment of cancer pain.

Myofascial Release. Myofascial release is a commonly used subtype of massage therapy that focuses on the restoration of normal length–tension relationships of muscles and fascia. Fascial release techniques are used to release contracted fascia. Practitioners use vigorous "hands-on" compression and stretching to alter the mobility of affected tissues. Multiple sessions with a skilled practitioner are generally required. Release of fascial contractures may be required before patients can tolerate therapeutic exercise or aerobic conditioning. Trigger point release is a type of myofascial release that involves the strategic application of pressure to discrete foci of increased muscle tone called trigger points (87). Sustained pressure is applied to a circumscribed, symptomatic area in conjunction with passive range of motion.

Myofascial release is most commonly used in the treatment of myofascial pain syndrome, a regional pain syndrome characterized by the presence of myofascial trigger points—tight, hypertonic, palpable bands of skeletal muscle fibers—that can cause distal referred pain, motor, and autonomic effects (87–91). Hypertonic muscles, which function as pain generators, are common in cancer patients, occurring in 45% of post mastectomy patients within 1 year (88), and 15% to 40% of head and neck cancer patients (91). Indeed, many conditions that are associated with cancer can produce fascial contractures, including radiation fibrosis, immobility, postsurgical scarring, and pain-engendered muscle spasms.

Among cancer patients, myofascial release is most frequently studied in breast cancer. It has been shown in several RCTs to improve localized chronic pain and mobility in breast cancer patients who underwent surgery, as compared to traditional massage, usual care, or manual lymphatic drainage (92–94) as well as a decrease in the number of active trigger points (94).

Transcutaneous Electrical Nerve Stimulation

TENS is the application of an electrical current to the skin to stimulate nerve fibers in an effort to inhibit the transmission of pain (95–98). A recent *Cochrane Review* determined that while there may be some benefit for cancer patients with bone pain associated with movement, the overall evidence for TENS in treating pain cancer patients remains inconclusive due to lack of suitable RCTs

(99). Nonetheless, TENS is generally well tolerated without serious side effects, and a trial can be considered when pharmacologic and/or procedural approaches fail to control pain.

Acupuncture

The practice of acupuncture has its roots in ancient Chinese traditional medicine. It involves the insertion of very fine sterile needles into the skin at precise locations—acupuncture points—to treat various diseases and symptoms (100). Figure 3.2 depicts acupuncture points along meridian lines, as illustrated by noted Chinese physician Hua Shou circa 1341 (101). Although the mechanism is not fully understood, acupuncture has been shown to increase the release of calcitonin gene-related peptide, neuropeptide Y, and vasoactive intestinal peptide during and after treatment (102). MRI studies have shown that acupuncture can induce brain activation in the hypothalamus and nucleus accumbens while also inducing deactivation of the amygdalae and hippocampus (103). There is substantial evidence supporting the use of acupuncture for low back pain (104), dental pain (105), headache (106), and chemotherapy-induced nausea and vomiting (107). Acupuncture should be

avoided in patients with severe thrombocytopenia, coagulopathy, or neutropenia due to the risk of bleeding or infection.

Several systematic reviews have been conducted to evaluate the efficacy of acupuncture, specifically for cancer-related pain (100,108–110). In a recent systematic review of 17 RCTs and meta-analysis of 14 trials encompassing 2,031 patients, He et al. found that acupuncture, as compared to sham acupuncture, was associated with decreased pain in cancer patients (109). Additionally, patients who received acupuncture or acupressure in addition to pharmacological analgesics had decreased opioid use. These findings are consistent with prior findings that acupuncture was beneficial in the treatment of malignancy-associated and oncological surgery pain (110,111). Indeed, Chen et al. randomized 66 patients with late-stage cancer to receive acupuncture at three to five of their most severe tender points or to receive medication according to the World Health Organization three-step analgesic ladder (111). Acupuncture and medication patients were divided and matched into groups of mild, moderate, and severe pain. Patients in the medication group with mild pain took aspirin, moderate pain took codeine,

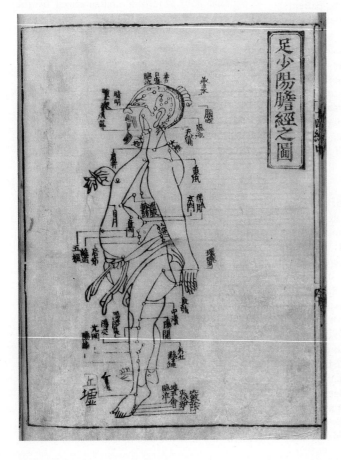

Figure 3.2 Traditional rendering of Chinese acupuncture meridians. Hua S. Jūshikei hakki. Edo, Japan: Suharaya Heisuke kankō, Kyōhō gan; 1716. https://collections.nlm.nih.gov/catalog/nlm:nlmuid-8105422-bk. Accessed January 28, 2020. Courtesy of the National Library of Medicine (101).

and severe pain took morphine. While each group achieved significant pain relief, those receiving acupuncture and medication had significantly greater pain relief than those receiving medication alone (94% vs. 87.5%).

Acupuncture has also been shown to be beneficial specifically in cancer patients with neuropathic pain. Alimi et al. randomized 90 patients with cancer and neuropathic pain to true auricular acupuncture, auricular acupuncture at placebo sites, or auricular seeds implanted at placebo sites (112). After 2 months of treatment, patients receiving true auricular acupuncture reported a decrease in pain intensity of 36% from baseline compared with 2% in the placebo groups. While the two acupuncture groups were blinded to the intervention, neither the acupuncturist nor the auricular seed groups could be blinded.

Importantly, acupuncture may not be beneficial in all cancer-related pain. Several studies have found no benefit for acupuncture in pain related to hormone therapy, radiation therapy, or chemotherapy (110,113). Nonetheless, the American Society of Clinical Oncology Clinical Practice Guidelines note that the use of acupuncture in cancer-related pain is evidence based, and the benefits of acupuncture outweigh the risk in select patients (11).

Touch Therapies

Touch therapies consist of healing touch, therapeutic touch, and Reiki, which are closely related touch-mediated therapies that have considerable overlap in theory and application (114,115). All of these therapies are based on the principle that the body is a complex energy system that can be affected by another to promote well-being, healing, and symptomatic relief (116,117). These therapies involve use of a practitioner's hands on or above a patient's body with the intention of promoting physical healing and emotional, mental, and spiritual balance (117,118).

A *Cochrane Review* found that all three types of touch therapies have a modest effect in pain relief (119). While the lack of sufficient data made the results inconclusive, the authors assert that the existing evidence supports the use of touch therapies in pain relief. Post-White et al. assessed healing touch as an intervention for pain in patients receiving chemotherapy (118). Two hundred and thirty patients were randomized to healing touch, massage therapy, or caring presence. Results showed that after four weekly sessions, patients receiving either healing touch or massage therapy had significantly lower pain ratings than those receiving caring presence alone. In a more recent RCT, Tabatabaee et al. randomized 90 male patients with cancer to seven sessions of therapeutic touch, placebo,

or usual care over a 4-week period. The intervention group received therapeutic touch via a variety of purposeful movements with the hands close to the patient, performed by a trained touch therapist who continuously examined and adjusted the various perceived energy fields and auras. For the placebo group, the therapist placed his/her hands near the patient, but roved about with no particular order and at greater distance. The control group received routine care. Patients who received therapeutic touch reported a significant decrease in pain levels as compared to the placebo and control groups (120).

A small study by Olson et al. randomized 24 patients with cancer pain to either standard opioid management plus rest or opioids plus Reiki (121). Participants either rested for 1.5 hours or received two Reiki treatments on days 1 and 4, 1 hour after their first afternoon analgesic dose. Participants receiving Reiki experienced significantly improved pain control following treatment compared with standard opioid management alone. However, there was no overall reduction in opioid use in either group.

Restoration and Preservation of Normal Biomechanics

Therapeutic Exercise

Therapeutic exercise encompasses a range of interventions, including general physical fitness, aerobic exercise, muscle strengthening, and flexibility and stretching exercises. There are several studies suggesting the effectiveness of therapeutic exercise in treating some of the nonpain symptoms of cancer, such as fatigue and nausea in breast cancer patients undergoing chemotherapy (122), or radiotherapy-induced trismus in patients with head and neck cancer (123). Recently, there has been more interest in the role of exercise therapy specifically for the treatment of pain in cancer patients and survivors.

Cantarero-Villanueva et al. evaluated the effects of a water physical therapy program versus usual care on cervical and shoulder pain in 66 breast cancer survivors (124). The intervention consisted of 24 one-hour sessions over 8 weeks. Patients in the intervention group reported improvement in neck and shoulder/axillary pain, but no significant changes in pain hyperalgesia. Likewise, a RCT of an Internet-based tailored exercise program versus usual care in 81 breast cancer survivors found that telerehabilitation significantly improved both pain severity and pain interference (125). In addition, progressive resistance exercise training was superior to standardized therapeutic exercise in ameliorating pain and disability in a RCT of 52 head and neck cancer survivors with postsurgical pain secondary to spinal accessory nerve damage (126). Cheville et al. performed a RCT of a home-based exercise program versus usual care in 66 adults with stage IV lung or colorectal cancer (127). The exercise group was instructed during a single physiotherapy visit and then exercised for 4 or more days per week for 8 weeks. At week 8, the intervention group reported improvement in mobility, fatigue, and sleep quality, but no difference in pain.

Yoga and tai chi can also be considered forms of therapeutic exercise. Although both have been shown to have positive effects on the treatment of chronic noncancer pain (83), as well as a positive impact on depression, fatigue, and overall quality of life in cancer patients, convincing evidence of the beneficial effect of these modalities on cancer pain is lacking (128,129).

Notably, in their clinical practice guidelines, the Society for Integrative Oncology states that regular exercise can have many positive roles in cancer pain and recommends having patients evaluated by a qualified exercise specialist (130).

Orthotics

Orthotics are braces designed to alter articular mechanics when the integrity of such mechanics is compromised. They may be used therapeutically to provide support, restore normal alignment, protect vulnerable structures, address soft tissue contractures, substitute for weak muscles, or maintain joints in positions of least pain. This last application can be very helpful as an adjunct in cancer pain, particularly in the case of bone metastases. The use of orthotics for patients with cancer-related pain must always be considered within the framework of patient comfort. It is important to refer patients to orthotists or physical medicine and rehabilitative specialists to ensure that they are provided with appropriate orthoses. Since rehabilitative specialists may not have extensive experience in dealing with patients with cancer-related pain, it is important to communicate the patients' symptom burdens, prognoses, goals of care, and financial constraints to help ensure that patients receive the orthoses that best meet their unique needs and pain symptoms.

THERAPEUTIC RECREATION AND CREATIVE ARTS THERAPY

Therapeutic recreation is the systematic utilization of recreation and other activity-based interventions to improve psychological and physical health, recovery, and well-being and facilitate full participation in life (131). In this chapter, we focus on animal-assisted therapy, one of the many therapeutic recreation interventions. Creative arts therapy, including music therapy, dance/movement therapy, and various forms of art therapy aims to generate creative energy as a healing force. Such therapies are becoming more common in noncancer and cancer patients alike and may be helpful in decreasing symptom burden and improving well-being among patients with serious, chronic, and/or terminal illnesses.

Art Therapy

According to the American Association of Art Therapists, the goal of art therapy is to "enrich the lives of individuals, families, and communities through active art-making, creative process, applied psychological theory, and human experience." (132) This goal is achieved through integrative methods and visual and symbolic expression that circumvents the limitations of language.

Studies have suggested that clinical art therapy may be beneficial for patients with cancer. Lefevre et al. assessed 28 cancer patients taking part in 63 art therapy sessions. These sessions reduced global distress by 47% and were also associated with a significant reduction in pain, anxiety, fatigue, and depression (133). Likewise, of 177 patients with terminal cancer in a hospice unit in Taiwan who engaged in image appreciation and hands-on painting, nearly three-quarters reported feeling much or very much more relaxed after the art therapy session, and over half reported feeling much or very much better physically (134). In a review of 27 RCTs of 1,576 cancer patients randomized to receive clinical art therapy, Puetz et al. note that art therapy yielded a reduction in anxiety, depression, and pain. These effects were more pronounced in hospitalized patients compared to those seen in an outpatient setting (135). Conversely, a systematic review and meta-analysis of 13 trials consisting of 606 patients with breast cancer showed an improvement in anxiety, but no significant effect on depression, quality of life, or pain (136).

Music Therapy

The American Association of Music Therapy defines music therapy as the use of music to address the physical, emotional, cognitive, and social needs of individuals (137). Music therapy is administered in a number of ways as part of the patient–therapist relationship (138), including listening and reflecting on music and producing or creating music (139).

Music therapy has been reported to provide improvements in physical, emotional, spiritual, and social well-being. A meta-analysis of 91 RCTs by Lee et al. revealed that music interventions may provide pain relief across various settings, including acute pain, procedural pain, chronic pain, and cancer-specific pain (140). A meta-analysis of music therapy in patients with cancer suggests that music therapy significantly ameliorates pain, with the greatest effectiveness in adults and patients who select their own music (141). Music interventions were also associated with improvements in anxiety, depression, and fatigue. In a more recent study in terminally ill cancer patients, music therapy was associated with improvements with regard to life closure, well-being, relaxation, worry, and pain (142).

Animal-Assisted Therapy

Animal-assisted therapy is the increasingly popular use of animals, most commonly dogs, who are trained to be calm, obedient, and comforting to patients suffering from a variety of medical illnesses including cancer (143–145). It has been shown to reduce physiologic markers of stress, increase endorphins, reduce loneliness, and improve patient mood, cognitive function, anxiety, and pain (145,146). In a study of patients undergoing chemotherapy, when given the option of having treatment with or without a therapy dog present, 86% elected to have the therapy dog present (147). Those accompanied by a therapy dog reported less anxiety and depression as compared to those who did not have a therapy dog; however, no improvement in pain was observed. In a study of 42 patients with head and neck cancer undergoing combined chemotherapy and radiation, animal-assisted therapy was associated with increases in social and emotional well-being (148), both of which can effect a patient's perception of pain.

Animal-assisted therapy is also quite common in pediatric oncology; in a survey of the top 20 pediatric oncology hospitals, 18 reported having an animal-assisted therapy program (146). In a study of 24 children with leukemia and solid tumors receiving outpatient treatment for cancer, animal-assisted therapy with dogs was associated with a significant decrease in pain, irritation, and stress by self-report, as well as improvement in anxiety, confusion, and tension as reported by caregivers (149).

CONCLUSION

Patients with cancer-related pain are increasingly turning to nonpharmacologic methods as adjuncts to traditional medication-based treatments. Recent theory and research suggest that psychosocial–spiritual factors play an important role in the experience of pain. Although evidence is limited, literature suggests that interventions designed to address psychosocial–spiritual factors may benefit many patients with cancer-related pain. Additionally, physiatric and body-based approaches, as well as recreational and creative arts interventions have been shown to be an effective means of nonpharmacologic management for many patients with cancer who suffer from pain. Larger studies are needed to further explore the full potential of this field of cancer pain management. Nevertheless, the available evidence for nonpharmacologic cancer pain management should enhance clinicians' confidence in recommending these interventions to their patients.

REFERENCES

1. van den Beuken-van Everdingen MH, de Rijke JM, Kessels AG, Schouten HC, van Kleef M, Patijn J. Prevalence of pain in patients with cancer: a systematic review of the past 40 years. *Ann Oncol.* 2007;18(9):1437-1449.
2. Greco MT, Roberto A, Corli O, et al. Quality of cancer pain management: an update of a systematic review of undertreatment of patients with cancer. *J Clin Oncol.* 2014;32(36):4149-4154.
3. Te Boveldt N, Vernooij-Dassen M, Burger N, Ijsseldijk M, Vissers K, Engels Y. Pain and its interference with daily activities in medical oncology outpatients. *Pain Physician.* 2013;16(4):379-389.
4. Singh P, Chaturvedi A. Complementary and alternative medicine in cancer pain management: a systematic review. *Indian J Palliat Care.* 2015;21(1):105-115.
5. Stjernsward J. WHO cancer pain relief programme. *Cancer Surv.* 1988;7(1):195-208.
6. Stjernsward J, Colleau SM, Ventafridda V. The World Health Organization Cancer Pain and Palliative Care Program. Past, present, and future. *J Pain Symptom Manage.* 1996;12(2):65-72.
7. Ernst E, Cassileth BR. The prevalence of complementary/alternative medicine in cancer: a systematic review. *Cancer.* 1998;83(4):777-782.
8. Eisenberg DM, Davis RB, Ettner SL, et al. Trends in alternative medicine use in the United States, 1990-1997: results of a follow-up national survey. *JAMA.* 1998;280(18):1569-1575.
9. Richardson MA, Sanders T, Palmer JL, Greisinger A, Singletary SE. Complementary/alternative medicine use in a comprehensive cancer center and the implications for oncology. *J Clin Oncol.* 2000;18(13):2505-2514.
10. Swarm RA, Paice JA, Anghelescu DL, et al. Adult Cancer Pain, Version 3.2019, NCCN Clinical Practice Guidelines in Oncology. *J Natl Compr Canc Netw.* 2019;17(8):977-1007.
11. Paice JA, Portenoy R, Lacchetti C, et al. Management of chronic pain in survivors of adult cancers: American Society of Clinical Oncology Clinical Practice Guideline. *J Clin Oncol.* 2016;34(27):3325-3345.
12. Lyman GH, Greenlee H, Bohlke K, et al. Integrative therapies during and after breast cancer treatment: ASCO Endorsement of the SIO Clinical Practice Guideline. *J Clin Oncol.* 2018;36(25):2647-2655.
13. Practice guidelines for cancer pain management. A report by the American Society of Anesthesiologists Task Force on Pain Management, Cancer Pain Section. *Anesthesiology.* 1996;84(5):1243-1257.
14. Bardia A, Barton DL, Prokop LJ, Bauer BA, Moynihan TJ. Efficacy of complementary and alternative medicine therapies in relieving cancer pain: a systematic review. *J Clin Oncol.* 2006;24(34):5457-5464.

15. Descartes R, Clerselier C, de La Forge L, Schuyl F. *L'homme... et un traitté De la formation du foetus du mesme autheur.* Charles Angot.

16. Melzack R. From the gate to the neuromatrix. *Pain.* 1999;(suppl 6):S121-S126.

17. Melzack R, Wall PD. Pain mechanisms: a new theory. *Science.* 1965;150(3699):971-979.

18. Cassileth BR, Keefe FJ. Integrative and behavioral approaches to the treatment of cancer-related neuropathic pain. *Oncologist.* 2010;15(suppl 2):19-23.

19. Mehta A, Chan LS. Understanding of the concept of "total pain": a prerequisite for pain control. *J Hospice Palliat Nurs.* 2008;10(1):26-32.

20. Ong CK, Forbes D. Embracing Cicely Saunders's concept of total pain. *BMJ.* 2005;331(7516):576.

21. Zaza C, Baine N. Cancer pain and psychosocial factors: a critical review of the literature. *J Pain Symptom Manage.* 2002;24(5):526-542.

22. Breitbart W, Gibson CA. Psychiatric aspects of cancer pain management. *Primary Psychiatry.* 2007;14(9):81-91.

23. Ferrell BR, Grant MM, Funk BM, Otis-Green SA, Garcia NJ. Quality of life in breast cancer survivors: implications for developing support services. *Oncol Nurs Forum.* 1998;25(5):887-895.

24. Koopman C, Hermanson K, Diamond S, Angell K, Spiegel D. Social support, life stress, pain and emotional adjustment to advanced breast cancer. *Psychooncology.* 1998;7(2):101-111.

25. Snow-Turek AL, Norris MP, Tan G. Active and passive coping strategies in chronic pain patients. *Pain.* 1996;64(3):455-462.

26. Utne I, Miaskowski C, Bjordal K, Paul SM, Jakobsen G, Rustoen T. Differences in the use of pain coping strategies between oncology inpatients with mild vs. moderate to severe pain. *J Pain Symptom Manage.* 2009;38(5):717-726.

27. Keefe FJ, Abernethy AP, Campbell LC. Psychological approaches to understanding and treating disease-related pain. *Annu Rev Psychol.* 2005;56:601-630.

28. Abernethy A, Keefe F, McCrory D, Scipio C, Matchar DJD. *Technology Assessment on the Use of Behavioral Therapies for Treatment of Medical Disorders: Part 2—Impact on Management of Patients with Cancer Pain.* North Carolina: Duke Center for Clinical Health Policy Research; 2005.

29. De Paolis G, Naccarato A, Cibelli F, et al. The effectiveness of progressive muscle relaxation and interactive guided imagery as a pain-reducing intervention in advanced cancer patients: a multicentre randomised controlled non-pharmacological trial. *Complement Ther Clin Pract.* 2019;34:280-287.

30. Kapogiannis A, Tsoli S, Chrousos G. Investigating the effects of the progressive muscle relaxation-guided imagery combination on patients with cancer receiving chemotherapy treatment: a systematic review of randomized controlled trials. *Explore (NY).* 2018;14(2):137-143.

31. Charalambous A, Giannakopoulou M, Bozas E, Marcou Y, Kitsios P, Paikousis L. Guided imagery and progressive muscle relaxation as a cluster of symptoms management intervention in patients receiving chemotherapy: a randomized control trial. *PLoS One.* 2016;11(6):e0156911.

32. Kerns RD, Sellinger J, Goodin BR. Psychological treatment of chronic pain. *Annu Rev Clin Psychol.* 2011;7:411-434.

33. Kwekkeboom KL, Cherwin CH, Lee JW, Wanta B. Mind-body treatments for the pain-fatigue-sleep disturbance symptom cluster in persons with cancer. *J Pain Symptom Manage.* 2010;39(1):126-138.

34. Kaushik R, Kaushik RM, Mahajan SK, Rajesh V. Biofeedback assisted diaphragmatic breathing and systematic relaxation versus propranolol in long term prophylaxis of migraine. *Complement Ther Med.* 2005;13(3):165-174.

35. Middaugh SJ, Woods SE, Kee WG, Harden RN, Peters JR. Biofeedback-assisted relaxation training for the aging chronic pain patient. *Biofeedback Self Regul.* 1991;16(4):361-377.

36. McCauley JD, Thelen MH, Frank RG, Willard RR, Callen KE. Hypnosis compared to relaxation in the outpatient management of chronic low back pain. *Arch Phys Med Rehabil.* 1983;64(11):548-552.

37. Bell RM. A review of complementary and alternative medicine practices among cancer survivors. *Clin J Oncol Nurs.* 2010;14(3):365-370.

38. Sloman R, Brown P, Aldana E, Chee EJCN. The use of relaxation for the promotion of comfort and pain relief in persons with advanced cancer. *Contemp Nurse.* 1994;3(1):6-12.

39. Hernandez-Reif M, Field T, Ironson G, et al. Natural killer cells and lymphocytes increase in women with breast cancer following massage therapy. *Int J Neurosci.* 2005;115(4):495-510.

40. Hetkamp M, Bender J, Rheindorf N, et al. A systematic review of the effect of neurofeedback in cancer patients. *Integr Cancer Ther.* 2019;18:1534735419832361.

41. Astin JA. Mind-body therapies for the management of pain. *Clin J Pain.* 2004;20(1):27-32.

42. Tsai PS, Chen PL, Lai YL, Lee MB, Lin CC. Effects of electromyography biofeedback-assisted relaxation on pain in patients with advanced cancer in a palliative care unit. *Cancer Nurs.* 2007;30(5):347-353.

43. Burish TG, Jenkins RA. Effectiveness of biofeedback and relaxation training in reducing the side effects of cancer chemotherapy. *Health Psychol.* 1992;11(1):17-23.

44. Syrjala KL, Jensen MP, Mendoza ME, Yi JC, Fisher HM, Keefe FJ. Psychological and behavioral approaches to cancer pain management. *J Clin Oncol.* 2014;32(16):1703-1711.

45. Montgomery GH, Schnur JB, Kravits K. Hypnosis for cancer care: over 200 years young. *CA Cancer J Clin.* 2013;63(1):31-44.

46. Lang EV, Berbaum KS, Faintuch S, et al. Adjunctive self-hypnotic relaxation for outpatient medical procedures: a prospective randomized trial with women undergoing large core breast biopsy. *Pain.* 2006;126(1-3):155-164.

47. Lang EV, Berbaum KS, Pauker SG, et al. Beneficial effects of hypnosis and adverse effects of empathic attention during percutaneous tumor treatment: when being nice does not suffice. *J Vasc Interv Radiol.* 2008;19(6):897-905.

48. Richardson J, Smith JE, McCall G, Richardson A, Pilkington K, Kirsch I. Hypnosis for nausea and vomiting in cancer chemotherapy: a systematic review of the research evidence. *Eur J Cancer Care (Engl).* 2007;16(5):402-412.

49. Elkins G, Jensen MP, Patterson DR. Hypnotherapy for the management of chronic pain. *Int J Clin Exp Hypn.* 2007;55(3):275-287.

50. Jensen M, Patterson DR. Hypnotic treatment of chronic pain. *J Behav Med.* 2006;29(1):95-124.

51. Patterson DR, Jensen MP. Hypnosis and clinical pain. *Psychol Bull.* 2003;129(4):495-521.

52. Schnur JB, Bovbjerg DH, David D, et al. Hypnosis decreases presurgical distress in excisional breast biopsy patients. *Anesth Analg.* 2008;106(2):440-444.

53. Spiegel D, Bloom JR. Group therapy and hypnosis reduce metastatic breast carcinoma pain. *Psychosom Med*. 1983;45(4):333-339.

54. Liossi C, White P, Hatira P. A randomized clinical trial of a brief hypnosis intervention to control venipuncture-related pain of paediatric cancer patients. *Pain*. 2009;142(3):255-263.

55. Snow A, Dorfman D, Warbet R, et al. A randomized trial of hypnosis for relief of pain and anxiety in adult cancer patients undergoing bone marrow procedures. *J Psychosoc Oncol*. 2012;30(3):281-293.

56. Syrjala KL, Donaldson GW, Davis MW, Kippes ME, Carr JE. Relaxation and imagery and cognitive-behavioral training reduce pain during cancer treatment: a controlled clinical trial. *Pain*. 1995;63(2):189-198.

57. Integration of behavioral and relaxation approaches into the treatment of chronic pain and insomnia. NIH Technology Assessment Panel on Integration of Behavioral and Relaxation Approaches into the Treatment of Chronic Pain and Insomnia. *JAMA*. 1996;276(4): 313-318.

58. Sawni A, Breuner CC. Clinical hypnosis, an effective mind-body modality for adolescents with behavioral and physical complaints. *Children (Basel)*. 2017;4(4):19.

59. Liossi C, Hatira P. Clinical hypnosis in the alleviation of procedure-related pain in pediatric oncology patients. *Int J Clin Exp Hypn*. 2003;51(1):4-28.

60. Liossi C, White P, Hatira P. Randomized clinical trial of local anesthetic versus a combination of local anesthetic with self-hypnosis in the management of pediatric procedure-related pain. *Health Psychol*. 2006;25(3): 307-315.

61. Kaiser P, Kohen DP, Brown ML, Kajander RL, Barnes AJ. Integrating pediatric hypnosis with complementary modalities: clinical perspectives on personalized treatment. *Children (Basel)*. 2018;5(8):108.

62. Rajasekaran M, Edmonds PM, Higginson IL. Systematic review of hypnotherapy for treating symptoms in terminally ill adult cancer patients. *Palliat Med*. 2005;19(5):418-426.

63. Lachance CC, McCormack S. CADTH rapid response reports. In: *Mindfulness Training for Chronic Nonmalignant Pain Management: A Review of the Clinical Effectiveness, Cost-effectiveness and Guidelines*. Ottawa, ON: Canadian Agency for Drugs and Technologies in Health; 2019.

64. Ngamkham S, Holden JE, Smith EL. A systematic review: mindfulness intervention for cancer-related pain. *Asia Pac J Oncol Nurs*. 2019;6(2):161-169.

65. Zeidan F, Vago DR. Mindfulness meditation-based pain relief: a mechanistic account. *Ann N Y Acad Sci*. 2016;1373(1):114-127.

66. Araujo RV, Fernandes AFC, Nery IS, Andrade E, Nogueira LT, Azevedo FHC. Meditation effect on psychological stress level in women with breast cancer: a systematic review. *Rev Esc Enferm USP*. 2019;53:e03529.

67. Garland EL, Brintz CE, Hanley AW, et al. Mind-body therapies for opioid-treated pain: a systematic review and meta-analysis. *JAMA Intern Med*. 2019;180(1): 91-105.

68. Reiner K, Tibi L, Lipsitz JD. Do mindfulness-based interventions reduce pain intensity? A critical review of the literature. *Pain Med*. 2013;14(2):230-242.

69. Bao T, Deng G, DeMarzo LA, et al. A technology-assisted, brief mind-body intervention to improve the waiting room experience for chemotherapy patients: randomized quality improvement study. *JMIR Cancer*. 2019;5(2):e13217.

70. Daniels S. Cognitive behavior therapy for patients with cancer. *J Adv Pract Oncol*. 2015;6(1):54-56.

71. Hofmann SG, Asnaani A, Vonk IJJ, Sawyer AT, Fang A. The efficacy of cognitive behavioral therapy: a review of meta-analyses. *Cognit Ther Res*. 2012;36(5):427-440.

72. Williams ACdC, Eccleston C, Morley S. Psychological therapies for the management of chronic pain (excluding headache) in adults. *Cochrane Database Syst Rev*. 2012;11(11):CD007407.

73. Syrjala KL, Cummings C, Donaldson GW. Hypnosis or cognitive behavioral training for the reduction of pain and nausea during cancer treatment: a controlled clinical trial. *Pain*. 1992;48(2):137-146.

74. Dalton JA, Keefe FJ, Carlson J, Youngblood R. Tailoring cognitive-behavioral treatment for cancer pain. *Pain Manag Nurs*. 2004;5(1):3-18.

75. Anderson KO, Cohen MZ, Mendoza TR, Guo H, Harle MT, Cleeland CS. Brief cognitive-behavioral audiotape interventions for cancer-related pain: immediate but not long-term effectiveness. *Cancer*. 2006;107(1):207-214.

76. Puchalski CM, Vitillo R, Hull SK, Reller N. Improving the spiritual dimension of whole person care: reaching national and international consensus. *J Palliat Med*. 2014;17(6):642-656.

77. Lee Y-H. Spiritual care for cancer patients. *Asia Pac J Oncol Nurs*. 2019;6(2):101-103.

78. Ripamonti CI, Giuntoli F, Gonella S, Miccinesi G. Spiritual care in cancer patients: a need or an option? *Curr Opin Oncol*. 2018;30(4):212-218.

79. Bickel KE, McNiff K, Buss MK, et al. Defining high-quality palliative care in oncology practice: an American Society of Clinical Oncology/American Academy of Hospice and Palliative Medicine Guidance Statement. *J Oncol Pract*. 2016;12(9):e828-e838.

80. Osman H, Shrestha S, Temin S, et al. Palliative care in the global setting: ASCO Resource-Stratified Practice Guideline. *J Glob Oncol*. 2018;4:1-24.

81. Corbin L. Safety and efficacy of massage therapy for patients with cancer. *Cancer Control*. 2005;12(3):158-164.

82. Cassileth BR, Vickers AJ. Massage therapy for symptom control: outcome study at a major cancer center. *J Pain Symptom Manage*. 2004;28(3):244-249.

83. Tick H, Nielsen A, Pelletier KR, et al. Evidence-based nonpharmacologic strategies for comprehensive pain care: the Consortium Pain Task Force White Paper. *Explore (NY)*. 2018;14(3):177-211.

84. Cassileth BR, Deng GE, Gomez JE, Johnstone PA, Kumar N, Vickers AJ. Complementary therapies and integrative oncology in lung cancer: ACCP evidence-based clinical practice guidelines (2nd edition). *Chest*. 2007;132(3 suppl):340s-354s.

85. Wilkinson S, Lockhart K, Gambles M, Storey L. Reflexology for symptom relief in patients with cancer. *Cancer Nurs*. 2008;31(5):354-360; quiz 361-352.

86. Özdelikara A, Tan M. The effect of reflexology on chemotherapy-induced nausea, vomiting, and fatigue in breast cancer patients. *Asia Pac J Oncol Nurs*. 2017;4(3):241-249.

87. Hasuo H, Ishihara T, Kanbara K, Fukunaga M. Myofascial trigger points in advanced cancer patients. *Indian J Palliat Care*. 2016;22(1):80-84.

88. Torres Lacomba M, Mayoral del Moral O, Coperias Zazo JL, Gerwin RD, Goni AZ. Incidence of myofascial pain syndrome in breast cancer surgery: a prospective study. *Clin J Pain*. 2010;26(4):320-325.

89. Saxena A, Chansoria M, Tomar G, Kumar A. Myofascial pain syndrome: an overview. *J Pain Palliat Care Pharmacother*. 2015;29(1):16-21.

90. Sagar SM, Dryden T, Wong RK. Massage therapy for cancer patients: a reciprocal relationship between body and mind. *Curr Oncol*. 2007;14(2):45-56.

91. Kalichman L, Menahem I, Treger I. Myofascial component of cancer pain review. *J Bodyw Mov Ther.* 2019;23(2):311-315.

92. Massingill J, Jorgensen C, Dolata J, Sehgal AR. Myofascial massage for chronic pain and decreased upper extremity mobility after breast cancer surgery. *Int J Ther Massage Bodywork.* 2018;11(3):4-9.

93. Serra-Ano P, Ingles M, Bou-Catala C, Iraola-Lliso A, Espi-Lopez GV. Effectiveness of myofascial release after breast cancer surgery in women undergoing conservative surgery and radiotherapy: a randomized controlled trial. *Support Care Cancer.* 2019;27(7): 2633-2641.

94. Fernandez-Lao C, Cantarero-Villanueva I, Fernandez-de-Las-Penas C, del Moral-Avila R, Castro-Sanchez AM, Arroyo-Morales M. Effectiveness of a multidimensional physical therapy program on pain, pressure hypersensitivity, and trigger points in breast cancer survivors: a randomized controlled clinical trial. *Clin J Pain.* 2012;28(2):113-121.

95. Claydon LS, Chesterton LS, Barlas P, Sim J. Dose-specific effects of transcutaneous electrical nerve stimulation (TENS) on experimental pain: a systematic review. *Clin J Pain.* 2011;27(7):635-647.

96. Wu PI, Meleger A, Witkower A, Mondale T, Borg-Stein J. Nonpharmacologic options for treating acute and chronic pain. *PM R.* 2015;7(11 suppl):S278-S294.

97. Lee JE, Anderson CM, Perkhounkova Y, Sleeuwenhoek BM, Louison RR. Transcutaneous electrical nerve stimulation reduces resting pain in head and neck cancer patients: a randomized and placebo-controlled double-blind pilot study. *Cancer Nurs.* 2019;42(3):218-228.

98. Vance CGT, Dailey DL, Rakel BA, Sluka KA. Using TENS for pain control: the state of the evidence. *Pain Manag.* 2014;4(3):197-209.

99. Hurlow A, Bennett MI, Robb KA, Johnson MI, Simpson KH, Oxberry SG. Transcutaneous electric nerve stimulation (TENS) for cancer pain in adults. *Cochrane Database Syst Rev.* 2012;(3):CD006276.

100. Lee H, Schmidt K, Ernst E. Acupuncture for the relief of cancer-related pain—a systematic review. *Eur J Pain.* 2005;9(4):437-444.

101. Hua S. Jūshikei hakki. Edo, Japan: Suharaya Heisuke kankō, Kyōhō gan; 1716. https://collections.nlm.nih.gov/catalog/nlm:nlmuid-8105422-bk. Accessed January 28, 2020.

102. Dawidson I, Angmar-Mansson B, Blom M, Theodorsson E, Lundeberg T. Sensory stimulation (acupuncture) increases the release of vasoactive intestinal polypeptide in the saliva of xerostomia sufferers. *Neuropeptides.* 1998;32(6):543-548.

103. Wu MT, Hsieh JC, Xiong J, et al. Central nervous pathway for acupuncture stimulation: localization of processing with functional MR imaging of the brain—preliminary experience. *Radiology.* 1999;212(1): 133-141.

104. Berman BM, Langevin HM, Witt CM, Dubner R. Acupuncture for chronic low back pain. *N Engl J Med.* 2010;363(5):454-461.

105. Ernst E, Pittler MH. The effectiveness of acupuncture in treating acute dental pain: a systematic review. *Br Dent J.* 1998;184(9):443-447.

106. Melchart D, Linde K, Fischer P, et al. Acupuncture for recurrent headaches: a systematic review of randomized controlled trials. *Cephalalgia.* 1999;19(9):779-786; discussion 765.

107. Lee A, Done ML. The use of nonpharmacologic techniques to prevent postoperative nausea and vomiting: a meta-analysis. *Anesth Analg.* 1999;88(6):1362-1369.

108. Paley CA, Johnson MI, Tashani OA, Bagnall AM. Acupuncture for cancer pain in adults. *Cochrane Database Syst Rev* 2011(1):CD007753.

109. He Y, Guo X, May BH, et al. Clinical evidence for association of acupuncture and acupressure with improved cancer pain: a systematic review and meta-analysis. *JAMA Oncol.* 2019;6(2):271-278.

110. Chiu HY, Hsieh YJ, Tsai PS. Systematic review and meta-analysis of acupuncture to reduce cancer-related pain. *Eur J Cancer Care (Engl).* 2017;26(2).

111. Chen ZJ, Guo YP, Wu ZC. [Observation on the therapeutic effect of acupuncture at pain points on cancer pain]. *Zhongguo Zhen Jiu.* 2008;28(4):251-253.

112. Alimi D, Rubino C, Pichard-Leandri E, Fermand-Brule S, Dubreuil-Lemaire ML, Hill C. Analgesic effect of auricular acupuncture for cancer pain: a randomized, blinded, controlled trial. *J Clin Oncol.* 2003;21(22):4120-4126.

113. Chien T-J, Liu C-Y, Chang Y-F, Fang C-J, Hsu C-H. Acupuncture for treating aromatase inhibitor-related arthralgia in breast cancer: a systematic review and meta-analysis. *J Altern Complement Med.* 2015;21(5):251-260.

114. Jackson E, Kelley M, McNeil P, Meyer E, Schlegel L, Eaton M. Does therapeutic touch help reduce pain and anxiety in patients with cancer? *Clin J Oncol Nurs.* 2008;12(1):113-120.

115. Potter PJ. Energy therapies in advanced practice oncology: an evidence-informed practice approach. *J Adv Pract Oncol.* 2013;4(3):139-151.

116. Wardell DW, Weymouth KF. Review of studies of healing touch. *J Nurs Scholarsh.* 2004;36(2):147-154.

117. Tabatabaee A, Tafreshi MZ, Rassouli M, Aledavood SA, AlaviMajd H, Farahmand SK. Effect of therapeutic touch in patients with cancer: a literature review. *Med Arch.* 2016;70(2):142-147.

118. Post-White J, Kinney ME, Savik K, Gau JB, Wilcox C, Lerner I. Therapeutic massage and healing touch improve symptoms in cancer. *Integr Cancer Ther.* 2003; 2(4):332-344.

119. So PS, Jiang Y, Qin Y. Touch therapies for pain relief in adults. *Cochrane Database Syst Rev.* 2008(4):CD006535.

120. Tabatabaee A, Tafreshi MZ, Rassouli M, Aledavood SA, AlaviMajd H, Farahmand SK. Effect of therapeutic touch on pain related parameters in patients with cancer: a randomized clinical trial. *Mater Sociomed.* 2016;28(3):220-223.

121. Olson K, Hanson J, Michaud M. A phase II trial of Reiki for the management of pain in advanced cancer patients. *J Pain Symptom Manage.* 2003;26(5):990-997.

122. Johnsson A, Demmelmaier I, Sjovall K, Wagner P, Olsson H, Tornberg AB. A single exercise session improves side-effects of chemotherapy in women with breast cancer: an observational study. *BMC Cancer.* 2019;19(1):1073.

123. Scherpenhuizen A, van Waes AM, Janssen LM, Van Cann EM, Stegeman I. The effect of exercise therapy in head and neck cancer patients in the treatment of radiotherapy-induced trismus: a systematic review. *Oral Oncol.* 2015;51(8):745-750.

124. Cantarero-Villanueva I, Fernandez-Lao C, Fernandez-de-Las-Penas C, et al. Effectiveness of water physical therapy on pain, pressure pain sensitivity, and myofascial trigger points in breast cancer survivors: a randomized, controlled clinical trial. *Pain Med.* 2012;13(11):1509-1519.

125. Galiano-Castillo N, Cantarero-Villanueva I, Fernandez-Lao C, et al. Telehealth system: a randomized controlled trial evaluating the impact of an internet-based exercise intervention on quality of life, pain, muscle

strength, and fatigue in breast cancer survivors. *Cancer*. 2016;122(20):3166-3174.

126. McNeely ML, Parliament MB, Seikaly H, et al. Effect of exercise on upper extremity pain and dysfunction in head and neck cancer survivors: a randomized controlled trial. *Cancer*. 2008;113(1):214-222.

127. Cheville AL, Kollasch J, Vandenberg J, et al. A home-based exercise program to improve function, fatigue, and sleep quality in patients with Stage IV lung and colorectal cancer: a randomized controlled trial. *J Pain Symptom Manage*. 2013;45(5):811-821.

128. Buffart LM, van Uffelen JG, Riphagen, II, et al. Physical and psychosocial benefits of yoga in cancer patients and survivors, a systematic review and meta-analysis of randomized controlled trials. *BMC Cancer*. 2012;12:559.

129. Wayne PM, Lee MS, Novakowski J, et al. Tai Chi and Qigong for cancer-related symptoms and quality of life: a systematic review and meta-analysis. *J Cancer Surviv*. 2018;12(2):256-267.

130. Deng GE, Frenkel M, Cohen L, et al. Evidence-based clinical practice guidelines for integrative oncology: complementary therapies and botanicals. *J Soc Integr Oncol*. 2009;7(3):85-120.

131. About Recreational Therapy. National Council for Therapeutic Recreation Certification. 2020. https://www.nctrc.org/about-ncrtc/about-recreational-therapy/. Accessed January 21, 2020.

132. About Art Therapy. American Art Therapy Association. 2020. https://www.arttherapy.org/upload/2017_DefinitionofProfession.pdf. Accessed January 21, 2020.

133. Lefèvre C, Ledoux M, Filbet M. Art therapy among palliative cancer patients: aesthetic dimensions and impacts on symptoms. *Palliat Support Care*. 2016;14(4):376-380.

134. Lin MH, Moh SL, Kuo YC, et al. Art therapy for terminal cancer patients in a hospice palliative care unit in Taiwan. *Palliat Support Care*. 2012;10(1):51-57.

135. Puetz TW, Morley CA, Herring MP. Effects of creative arts therapies on psychological symptoms and quality of life in patients with cancer. *JAMA Intern Med*. 2013;173(11):960-969.

136. Boehm K, Cramer H, Staroszynski T, Ostermann T. Arts therapies for anxiety, depression, and quality of life in breast cancer patients: a systematic review and meta-analysis. *Evid Based Complement Alternat Med*. 2014;2014:103297.

137. What is Music Therapy? American Music Therapy Association. 2020. https://www.musictherapy.org/about/musictherapy/. Accessed January 21, 2020.

138. Bradt J, Shim M, Goodill SW. Dance/movement therapy for improving psychological and physical outcomes in cancer patients. *Cochrane Database Syst Rev*. 2015;1(1):CD007103.

139. Atiwannapat P, Thaipisuttikul P, Poopityastaporn P, Katekaew W. Active versus receptive group music therapy for major depressive disorder—a pilot study. *Complement Ther Med*. 2016;26:141-145.

140. Lee JH. The effects of music on pain: a meta-analysis. *J Music Ther*. 2016;53(4):430-477.

141. Tsai HF, Chen YR, Chung MH, et al. Effectiveness of music intervention in ameliorating cancer patients' anxiety, depression, pain, and fatigue: a meta-analysis. *Cancer Nurs*. 2014;37(6):E35-E50.

142. Warth M, Kessler J, van Kampen J, Ditzen B, Bardenheuer HJ. 'Song of Life': music therapy in terminally ill patients with cancer. *BMJ Support Palliat Care*. 2018;8(2):167-170.

143. Marcus DA. Complementary medicine in cancer care: adding a therapy dog to the team. *Curr Pain Headache Rep*. 2012;16(4):289-291.

144. Harper CM, Dong Y, Thornhill TS, et al. Can therapy dogs improve pain and satisfaction after total joint arthroplasty? A randomized controlled trial. *Clin Orthop Relat Res*. 2015;473(1):372-379.

145. Petranek S, Pencek J, Dey M. The effect of pet therapy and artist interactions on quality of life in brain tumor patients: a cross-section of art and medicine in dialog. *Behav Sci (Basel)*. 2018;8(5):43.

146. Chubak J, Hawkes R. Animal-assisted activities: results from a survey of top-ranked pediatric oncology hospitals. *J Pediatr Oncol Nurs*. 2016;33(4):289-296.

147. Orlandi M, Trangeled K, Mambrini A, et al. Pet therapy effects on oncological day hospital patients undergoing chemotherapy treatment. *Anticancer Res*. 2007;27(6c):4301-4303.

148. Fleishman SB, Homel P, Chen MR, et al. Beneficial effects of animal-assisted visits on quality of life during multimodal radiation-chemotherapy regimens. *J Community Support Oncol*. 2015;13(1):22-26.

149. Silva NB, Osório FL. Impact of an animal-assisted therapy programme on physiological and psychosocial variables of paediatric oncology patients. *PLoS One*. 2018;13(4):e0194731.

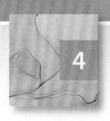

4 Interventional Approach to Pain

Philip S. Kim, Andrew Mannes, and Russell R. Lonser

Interventional and neurosurgical procedures can be utilized to supplement pharmacologic and complementary approaches to treat pain. Pharmacologic therapies are described elsewhere in this text and include principles of analgesic management using opioid agents and adjuvant medications. The primary indications for interventional techniques are either for patients whose pain is poorly responsive to systemic analgesic therapies or for those who suffer from intolerable side effects, in whom efforts to manage adverse effects are unsuccessful. Patients can experience severe dose-limiting side effects that prevent optimal titration to therapeutic levels. For example, systemic opioids can produce constipation, nausea, vomiting, or sedation.

Patient's response to analgesic medicinal therapies has been best described in the cancer population. The oral administration of analgesics based on recommendations, including those outlined by the World Health Organization, has provided satisfactory relief to most patients. However, the poorly relieved pain experienced by 5% to 15% of the approximately 500,000 patients who die each year from cancer represents a significant need for additional methods, including interventional and neurosurgical procedures, that can offer symptom relief (1).

Aside from optimizing pain control while minimizing side effects, interventional pain therapies can also enhance functional abilities and physical and psychological well-being, enhancing the patient's quality of life (2). It has also been reported that better pain management utilizing interventional techniques may result in increased life. Further, reducing patient visits for symptom management could potentially reduce costs (3). Recent econometric analysis suggests that interventional techniques using intrathecal pump therapy compared to conventional medical therapy are associated with lower health care cost and utilization.

INITIAL EVALUATION

For the interventionalist, it is important to understand the patient's prognosis, associated comorbidities, and patient's and family's expectations. An initial evaluation for interventional pain therapies should ascertain the patient's general medical condition along with the primary disease. A complete history is required, including a general medical, disease-specific (e.g., patients with oncologic disorders need to be thoroughly evaluated for possible local recurrence or new metastases), and pain histories. Specific pain history would include the following: quality of pain, pain intensity, alleviating and exacerbating factors, temporal characteristics, duration, and associated features (e.g., numbness, weakness, vasomotor changes). Psychosocial evaluation should assess the presence of psychological symptoms (e.g., anxiety, depression), and psychiatric disorders (e.g., major depression, delirium) should be similarly addressed. The nature and meaning of the presenting pain needs to be distinguished from anxiety and suffering affecting all aspects of one's life. The ability to cope and the availability of psychosocial support systems need to be assessed and reinforced with proper health and social professionals. A final assessment should determine the patient's expectation of therapeutic interventional options.

The physical examination includes a general medical examination, with emphasis on neurologic findings. Specific examination of the site of pain and surrounding anatomic regions are important. For example, if a patient has profound motor and sensory deficits in a particular region, neurolysis techniques become a more acceptable therapeutic option.

Appropriate selection of an intervention is based on therapeutic goals. If the presenting pain is expected to be transient (pain that will be alleviated by primary radiation therapy or chemotherapy, pain that is associated with the treatment of the primary disease, or pain that is), then the intervention should likewise be reversible. However, if the pain is expected to be chronic, a technique that results in more permanent effects is indicated. Life expectancy must be considered when selecting an appropriate intervention. If the patient's life expectancy is short, treatment strategies should strive to minimize the frequency and level of interventions and recovery time and should focus on optimizing a patient's quality of life. A patient with a longer life expectancy may warrant more extensive

TABLE 4.1 COMPARISON OF INTERVENTIONAL PAIN PROCEDURES

	Nerve blocks	Neurolytic procedures	Neurostimulation	Neuraxial infusion
Advantages	Ease of performance Useful for diagnostic and therapeutic relief	Ease of performance Provides long-term relief	Nondestructive Reversible	Nondestructive Reversible
Disadvantages	Provides short-term relief	Risk of associated sensory and motor deficits	Requires costly equipment and surgical implantation	Requires costly equipment and possible surgical implantation Requires pharmaceutical and ancillary support

and expensive interventions (i.e., implantable devices). Certain procedures may not be indicated for patients with longer life expectancy such as neuroablative procedures that are associated with permanent loss of function or a theoretical risk of developing deafferentation pain syndromes.

Therefore, once a definitive diagnosis has been made, a treatment plan should characterize the expected outcome, define contingencies, and plan for reassessment. Longitudinal monitoring of pain and response to interventional therapies is essential and allows implementation of additional options (e.g., complementary therapies, pharmacologic strategies, and behavioral and psychological approaches).

This chapter includes some of the frequently utilized procedures in the palliative care pain population (Table 4.1). Not all indications and contraindications are included, and consultation with a pain practitioner should be considered before referring the patient for evaluation and treatment.

APPROACHES TO INTERVENTIONS

Pharmacologic management of pain can be viewed as a continuum of indirect and direct drug delivery paradigms. Indirect drug delivery (i.e., systemic analgesia) refers to the administration of an analgesic into the bloodstream, which is then transported to the receptor site in neural tissue:

1. By systemic absorption
2. By formulation of depot for sustained and continuous release
3. Through the bloodstream

Direct drug delivery is the administration of an agent to the targeted neural tissue involved in nociception. By delivering directly to the nociceptive pathways, one can achieve a pronounced analgesic effect at a lower dose with fewer side effects. An example of this is comparing equianalgesic morphine doses in the intrathecal, epidural, and intravenous spaces (Table 4.2) (4,5).

Interventional pain therapies are usually minimally invasive techniques that can be divided into direct drug delivery, neuroablation, neural blockade, and neurostimulation. Direct drug delivery involves the administration of analgesics, usually opioids and local anesthetics, directly into nociceptive pathways. Other potential agents such as α_2-agonists and calcium channel blockers can be administered. Neuroablation refers to direct chemical, thermal, or surgical destruction of nociceptive pathways. Neurostimulation or neuroaugmentation refers to the application of direct electrical stimulation to inhibit nociceptive transmission. Not all pain, however, can be adequately addressed using these techniques. In such cases, one can consider consultation with a neurosurgeon and interventional pain specialist about surgical intervention.

Direct Drug Delivery

Neuraxial direct drug delivery involves accessing the epidural or subarachnoid (intrathecal) space by a needle or the placement of a continuous infusion system. In general, neuraxial infusion should be considered when severe pain cannot be controlled with systemic drugs and/or because of dose-limiting toxicities. Neuraxial infusions

TABLE 4.2 EQUIANALGESIC MORPHINE CONVERSIONS AMONG ROUTES OF ADMINISTRATION

Oral	Parenteral	Epidural	Subarachnoid
300 mg =	100 mg =	10 mg =	1 mg

can also be considered when there is an immediate need for using various nonopioid analgesics. Specifically, local anesthetics can have a profound analgesic effect on many intractable opioid-unresponsive pain conditions. Although it is possible to give local anesthetic systemically, higher local concentrations can be achieved, resulting in profound neural blockade through direct drug delivery.

Neuraxial delivery systems have two components: an intraspinal or epidural catheter and a delivery mode (e.g., bolus dosing, syringe pump, internal port, or internal or external pump). There are basically five types of neuraxial drug delivery systems, and familiarization with these systems allows the clinician to understand the respective advantages and disadvantages of each (4,6).

The simplest, least expensive, and least invasive option, a percutaneous catheter, is typically made of nylon, polyurethane, or polyamide and can be wire reinforced. These catheters are routinely placed in surgical and obstetric patients to manage operative and postoperative pain and are designed for short-term use (<1 week). But a catheter may be maintained for longer periods without problems and may suffice for the duration of the patient's life. If there is a complication, these catheters can be discontinued by removing the dressing and withdrawing the catheter (7,8). However, these catheters can cause localized tissue reaction at the site of insertion, can migrate, and are susceptible to accidental displacement.

The next type of drug delivery system uses the same type of catheter as that mentioned in the preceding text, but it is tunneled subcutaneously to decrease the incidence of migration. Placement can be performed in a clinic and requires a small incision with multiple needle insertions. Tunneling the catheter is better suited for the outpatient or the home-bound patient.

Implanted catheters with subcutaneous injection site are technologically more advanced and require a minor surgical procedure, resulting in higher costs (for placement). Sterile preparation and the use of fluoroscopy are essential. These systems can be placed in the epidural or intrathecal space. There are two basic designs: exteriorized and completely internalized injection port. In the first design, the proximal catheter is tunneled from the exit site in the back and exteriorized usually along the midaxillary line. This catheter can include an antimicrobial cuff that reduces both infection and catheter migration. In the second design, the port is supported by bone, usually a rib, so as to facilitate needle insertion. It can be used for intermittent bolus dosing or accessed for continuous infusions.

A totally implanted catheter with implanted infusion pump is available in two basic designs.

The simpler design is a constant fixed infusion pump in which the dose can be adjusted by a clinician changing the concentration. The second type includes a programmable, infusion pump with a drug reservoir, an electronic module, and an antenna allowing reprogramming of drug flow rates (Flowonics). The clinician controls the pump through an external programmer head (such as a pacemaker) to alter the dose, give single doses, or change the continuous infusion rate. Pump system like Medtronic and Flowonics will allow the patient to receive a medical direct bolus of medication when the device is activated.

Typically, a percutaneous test catheterization of the epidural or intrathecal space would be performed to assess the efficacy and starting doses of medication before implanting a permanent delivery system. Some practitioners have advocated eliminating pump trial to reduce health cost and utilization on patient and family (9,10). There are several approaches to trial the drugs, including bolus dosing, by accessing the intrathecal space with a spinal needle or by placement of a catheter and continuous infusion—either in the epidural or intrathecal space. Ideally, the method utilized for clinical assessment would best emulate the intended route (e.g., a trial with a continuous intrathecal catheter for evaluating future implantable pump placement). Although the complication rate is low, implantable devices can have problems with catheter failure, infection, seroma, wound dehiscence, and catheter tip fibroma formation (reported with high-concentration morphine) (5,11,12). They also require health care provider visits for routine refills and adjustment of dosing.

The selection of the appropriate neuraxial drug(s) and delivery system for an individual patient is based on several considerations (5,13).

1. Patient life expectancy
2. Economics and cost-effectiveness
3. Choice of epidural versus subarachnoid route of administration

Patient life expectancy and duration of need are difficult to predict. The more sophisticated implantable systems are expensive devices that require a trial catheter, adjustments of medications, and a surgical procedure for placement. One study by Bedder et al. suggest that an implanted pump system is a more viable financial alternative compared to other drug delivery systems for a period over 3 months (14). The less sophisticated percutaneous and tunneled catheters are best suited for patients with a limited life expectancy of <1 month. Both epidural and subarachnoid drug delivery can be equally effective. The duration of therapy will usually predict the type of infusion system selected. Catheter obstruction, fibrosis, and loss of analgesic efficacy are well described in long-term epidural drug systems (4). Therefore, intrathecal drug delivery systems are best suited for a protracted duration of therapy (>3 months). A decision-making algorithm for using neuraxial analgesia is shown in Figure 4.1 (9).

Multiple pharmacologic preparations have been administered through the neuraxial drug delivery systems. The gold standard is morphine, which is widely used and successful. When intrathecal morphine provides inadequate relief, other opioids, such as hydromorphone, meperidine, methadone, fentanyl, and sufentanil, have been used. As tolerance develops, one might switch opioids and/or use them in combination with coanalgesics, which include local anesthetics (e.g., tetracaine, bupivacaine), α_2-agonists (e.g., clonidine), and GABA B agonists (baclofen). Ziconotide, a calcium channel blocker that is the synthetic equivalent of a peptide produced by a snail, has been approved for use in intrathecal pumps (15). Drug selection is based on the patient's pain symptoms using clinical strategies that have been developed (e.g., Comprehensive consensus based guidelines on intrathecal drug delivery systems in the treatment of pain caused by cancer pain, updated 2017) (5,16). The guidelines and algorithms were developed by an expert panel, evaluating existing literature and algorithms for various intrathecal drugs (8). The optimal drug dosage, concentration, and issues related to compounding of drugs have been reviewed (8).

Complications from neuraxial catheter and pump placement may result from anatomic changes, infection, fluid collection, catheter migration, or device failure. Patients with suspected block of the subarachnoid circulation due to tumor extension or subarachnoid hemorrhage/arachnoiditis may have a poor response to the delivery of intrathecal analgesia. Evidence of an obstruction should be sought using magnetic resonance imaging (MRI) or myelography to determine the level of obstruction. Retesting the efficacy of analgesia by placing the injectant proximal to the obstruction may yield improved analgesic response. Migration or fracture of the catheter should be suspected if the patient reports sudden changes in pain relief or if a fluid collection is seen at the insertion site. Percutaneously placed catheters can be bolused with a test dose of a local anesthetic to assess function. Myelography should be performed with implantable catheters or pumps (through a side port) to determine catheter placement and function when displacement or catheter rupture is suspected.

An infection of the site does not always necessitate immediate removal of a catheter. Superficial infections may only require a course of antibiotics. However, persistent or progressive tissue infection or central nervous system (CNS) involvement necessitates immediate removal of the catheter and/or pump (17).

A growing body of case reports and studies supports the benefits of direct drug (intrathecal) delivery systems in cancer pain patients (5,9). In a study of 202 patients experiencing refractory cancer pain who were randomized to receive either an implantable drug delivery system or comprehensive medical

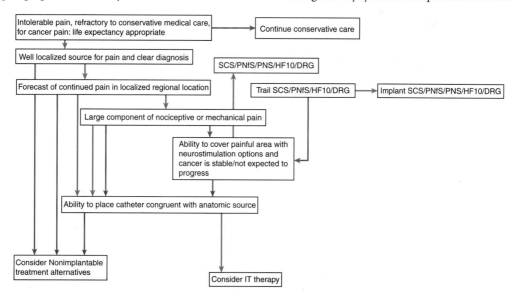

Figure 4.1 A decision-making algorithm for patients with refractory cancer-related pain. IT-PCA, intrathecal patient-controlled analgesia; DRG, dorsal root stimulation; HF10, high frequency; PNfS, peripheral field stimulation; PNS, peripheral nerve stimulation; SCS, spinal cord stimulation; *green arrows* indicate affirmation or positive response; *red arrows* signify negative response. (From Deer TR, Pope JE, Hayek SM, et al. The Polyanalgesic Consensus Conference (PACC): recommendations on intrathecal drug infusion systems best practices and guidelines. *Neuromodulation.* 2017;20(2):96-132. doi:10.1111/ner.12538.)

management, the patients receiving implantable intrathecal pump had reported successful pain control with a reduction in common drug toxicities such as fatigue and diminished level of consciousness (3). Overall, there was an improvement in the quality-of-life measures and survival over the 6 months in the patients receiving implantable intrathecal pump. A systematic review with identification of six randomized controlled studies has shown improved outcomes with intrathecal therapies for cancer pain patients (18). A recent study has shown significant benefit using bupivacaine in external pump system for cancer pain patients (19). Recent econometric analysis suggests that intrathecal drug delivery care compared to conventional medication is more cost-effective (20).

Peripheral Nerve/Plexus Drug Delivery

Blockade of peripheral nerves and neural plexuses is commonly performed to provide regional anesthesia and analgesia to patients undergoing surgical procedures (21,22). Modified constant infusion systems typically deliver local anesthetics directly to peripheral nerves and neural plexuses in patients with inadequate analgesia or intolerable toxicities from systemic medications. Specific localized pain syndromes related to a mononeuropathy, plexopathy, and peripheral neuropathy may benefit from peripheral nerve infusion.

Continuous neural blockade of the brachial plexus is common for postoperative pain. A technique of placing a catheter along the brachial plexus and self-contained infusion system has been described (23). A case report describes the successful 2-week management of pain from Pancoast's syndrome with a brachial plexus infusion system using local anesthetics (24). Other potential areas where neural infusion could be performed include the lumbosacral plexus, paravertebral and selected peripheral nerves, and sympathetic chain.

The current self-contained peripheral nerves/plexuses infusion system is a modification of neuraxial infusion systems (22,25). The advantages of this system are the simplicity and the minimal invasiveness of the placement of the system. However, the patient can experience a localized tissue reaction or catheter migration and has a risk of infection for implantations of >1-month duration. Implantable technology must be improved to provide a completely implanted infusion system for long-term continuous nerve/plexuses analgesic infusion.

Neural blockade with longer-acting local anesthetics such bupivacaine can provide hours of relief until a more long-term solution can be offered. A liposomal bupivacaine has been used for interscalene blocks, delivering 72 hours of analgesia (26). Potential use of long-acting bupivacaine formulation for other sites has yet to investigate. This window of analgesia can also provide time to titrate systemic medications such as steroids, antidepressants, and anticonvulsants. Many times, diagnostic neural blockade will predict the response to neuroablative techniques.

Neuroablation

Neuroablation should be initiated in the following conditions (2,27):

1. If systemic therapies fail to provide adequate relief and quality of life
2. If neuraxial drug administration fails
3. To accommodate patient preference
4. Early in the natural history of disease (e.g., cancer) in the presence of discrete well-defined pain generators

Contemporary minimally invasive neurolytic techniques can be divided into chemical lysis, cryoneurolysis, and radiofrequency and surgical ablation (28). Chemical neurolysis involves the injection of a destructive chemical such as alcohol or phenol. Historically, other chemicals such as chlorocresol, ammonium salts, and iced and hypertonic saline have been used. Ethyl alcohol dehydrates and precipitates neural tissue. Phenol (carbonic acid) denatures neural tissue as well, with an apparently lower incidence of neuritis. Radiofrequency neurolysis has numerous advantages compared to chemical neurolysis. Radiofrequency neurolysis involves the placement of insulated needles to localize nociceptive pathways and then pinpoint a heat lesion. The extent of the lesion can be controlled by the size of the probe, duration of application, and the temperature at the tip of the needle. Because a more precise controlled lesion can be performed, radiofrequency lesioning is preferred for cordotomy, rhizotomy, and gangliolysis. The use of pulsed radiofrequency as an alternative to conventional radiofrequency ablation (RFA) techniques is being explored. This technique uses a narrow pulsed current, allowing for cooling time, and a lower tissue temperature (42°C in pulsed radiofrequency vs. 80°C in RFA) with no histologic signs of tissue damage (29). Several studies have reported reversible antinociceptive effects; therefore, pulsed radiofrequency may be better suited for treating patients with reversible disease or treatment related pain (29).

Like radiofrequency neurolysis, cryoneurolysis has an advantage in producing a controlled lesion. Cryoneurolysis is produced by disrupting neuronal transmission by allowing rapid expansion of compressed gas, causing the formation of an "ice ball" at the tip of the needle (30,31). Nerves encompassed in the frozen tissue develop ice crystals that result in degeneration. However, the architecture of the perineurium and epineurium is not affected, thereby allowing resprouting of the axons without subsequent neuroma formation. The clinical effects are variable and are a function of precise needle tip localization (duration of freezing and lowest temperature achieved). The longevity of the effects needs to be considered when utilizing this technique. If the pain is expected to resolve, the recovery of nerve function would be desirable. However, if the targeted pain is expected to be chronic, relief from symptoms may be short lived. Rarely, peripheral and central nerves can be surgically interrupted. Neurosurgical techniques are included in greater detail in this chapter.

Neurolytic procedures, by definition, often cause irreversible damage to the neurons, but other structures in proximity to the intended site can be damaged because of extension of the therapy or accidental needle migration. Therefore, the resulting effects may include not only the neurons responsible for conveying pain but also lesion neurons that convey touch, proprioception, bladder and bowel control, and motor function. Therefore, these procedures are best performed by trained and experienced practitioners. Although not essential, using local anesthetic blocks is a good trial before implementing an irreversible blockade. It will emulate the level of pain relief that can be provided by the neurolytic procedure while allowing the patient to experience other side effects associated with deafferentation. This includes evaluating the untoward effects such as "numbness" in the affected region that some patients find less desirable than the original pain.

The efferent neuronal pathway can also be a target for interventional therapies. Botulism toxin, a neurotoxin produced by *Clostridium botulinum*, blocks acetylcholine release from nerve terminals, resulting in muscle relaxation (32). Therapeutic benefit can be achieved by carefully injecting botulinum toxin A into various muscle groups in patients with myofascial pain, migraines, and spastic conditions (33).

Neurolytic Procedures

Head and Neck Pain

Peripheral neurolysis can be done at various neural structures throughout the body (28). The head and neck region is richly innervated, and disease resulting in pain in this region (e.g., cancer) is difficult to manage. Pain is often aggravated by simple movements related to coughing, swallowing, talking, and eating. The cranial nerves typically affected by neoplastic growth and surgical and radiation therapy are V, VII, IX, and X. Potential problems exist for the pain interventionalist in understanding anatomic distortion due to cancer

and cancer therapies. The avoidance of damage to cranial nerves IX and X is critical for ventilatory and swallowing control.

The cell bodies of the sensory neurons innervating the face, forehead, and upper neck are localized to the trigeminal ganglia (cranial nerve V). The ganglia or branches of the afferent fibers can be selectively targeted by several approaches. Surgical rhizotomies have been supplanted by percutaneous approaches and open surgical microvascular decompression. Radiofrequency thermogangliolysis is the most popularly utilized technique, with >14,000 cases reported in 33 publications (28). Technically similar to chemical neurolysis, a radiofrequency probe is placed along the divisions of the trigeminal ganglion through the foramen ovale, and a brief thermal lesion is performed. In one large series, at 2-year follow-up, 28.3% of patients had recurrence of symptoms after one treatment and 8.3% has recurrence after multiple treatments (34). Trigeminal balloon compression is a surgical approach in which a Fogarty balloon catheter is placed and inflated to perform neurolysis, with reported results being similar to those of radiofrequency neurolysis (35). Microvascular decompression is discussed in the section other Neurosurgical Procedures. Eye pain can also be conveyed along the fifth cranial nerve. Pain symptoms may arise from localized pathology or may be referred (e.g., migraine), and patient referral to an ophthalmologist is warranted.

Intractable hiccups (singultus) can be treated with phrenic nerve blocks (28). This is done with fluoroscopic guidance to determine whether one hemidiaphragm is predominant in spasm and should be blocked. If the local anesthetic block is successful, a neurolytic phrenic technique can be done surgically or with RFA (36).

Upper and Lower Extremity

Upper and lower extremity pain can be difficult to treat with interventional neurolytic approaches. The nerves of the brachial and lumbosacral plexuses are mainly mixed nerves with motor and sensory components. Difficulties exist in selectively blocking only the sensory components of the nerves and plexuses. Subarachnoid and dorsal root neurolysis can be performed with a limited incidence of motor deficits (28). The injection of phenol in the brachial plexus provided four patients with cancer with good to excellent pain relief for 12 weeks (28). Intractable shoulder pain was managed effectively with suprascapular neurolysis using phenol or absolute alcohol (28). A recent case report used 5% phenol in a transforaminal approach for cancer-related pain in the upper extremity with excellent results (37).

Thorax and Abdomen

Thoracic and abdominal wall pain can be treated with multiple intercostal or paravertebral nerve blocks. If adequate relief is obtained, a percutaneous neurolysis can be performed. Subarachnoid neurolysis can also be performed if the dermatome(s) involved in the pain generator can be identified. Doyle reported a series of 46 hospice patients treated with multiple phenol intercostal blocks (38). The patients received a range of total relief from 1 to 6 weeks (mean: 3 weeks). Peripheral neurolysis of various branches of the lumbosacral plexus (iliohypogastric, ilioinguinal) has been similarly performed for pain in the lower abdomen/pelvic region (39). A recent review of sacroiliac pain related to tumor showed significant relief using lateral branch denervation of multiple lumbar and sacral levels (40).

Sympathetic Ganglion Neurolytic Blocks

Neuropathic, intra-abdominal, pelvic, and perineal pain can be treated with various sympathetic ganglion neurolytic approaches (41). Unlike the somatic nerves, selective blockade of the sympathetic nervous system will not result in altered motor or sensory function (although other sympathetic mediated function may be lost).

Celiac plexus and splanchnic blocks are among the frequently utilized neurolytic blocks for neuropathic or cancer pain (42,43). Sympathetic blocks are indicated for treating abdominal and referred back pain secondary to abdominal pathology, especially pancreatic cancer. Pancreatic cancer involving the head of the pancreas is more responsive than that of the tail of the pancreas (44). In addition to providing pain relief, celiac plexus blocks can reduce sympathetic tone, leaving unopposed parasympathetic activity, thereby enhancing gastrointestinal motility—a major benefit for patients with cancer requiring systemic opioids. Serious complications involving the kidney, lung, aorta, and vena cava have been minimized with fluoroscopic or computed tomographic (CT) guidance and modification of the original techniques. A randomized study of early intervention of alcohol versus placebo celiac blocks demonstrated statistically significant pain relief and prolonged survival ranging from 3 to 9 months in alcohol-treated patients (45). A preemptive interventional approach may lead to improved survival rates, but more studies are needed. Another comparison study revealed that patients who underwent celiac plexus neurolysis had improvement in pain and elevated mood with associated increase in life expectancy (46).

An alternative therapy to the celiac axis neurolysis targets the nerves that condense to form the plexus, specifically the greater, lesser, and least splanchnic nerves (derived from the thoracic chain) (27). Neuroablative therapy applied to the splanchnic nerves can achieve the same therapeutic result as celiac plexus neurolysis, although some practitioners think the technique is safer. The lesions must be applied bilaterally, but there is less likelihood for intraperitoneal, bowel, or arterial injections or trauma to these structures. Retrospective study reveals significant relief with bilateral thoracic splanchnic thermocoagulation (47). A novel approach to celiac plexus is endoscopic ultrasound in a series of patient with success (48).

Interventional pain therapies for intractable perineal pain are predisposed to the potential risk of rectal and urinary incontinence. In cases of preexisting incontinence with surgical diversion, a neurolytic subarachnoid saddle block is simple and effective. Other target structures for pelvic and perineal pain include the superior hypogastric plexus and ganglion impar. The superior hypogastric plexus consists of sympathetic and parasympathetic fibers that innervate the pelvis including the vagina, uterus, cervix, testis, ovaries, and bladder (49). Patients with advanced disease experiencing refractory pain in this region could obtain significant pain relief with a neuroablative procedure.

Sympathetic innervation to the head, neck, and upper extremities can be interrupted with a stellate ganglion block and the lower extremities with a lumbar sympathetic block. An initial injection or series of injections with local anesthetics are useful for diagnosis and possibly for treatment. A successful injection will reduce the patient's pain symptoms and produce evidence of sympathetic blockade (e.g., temperature chance in affected limb) without somatic motor or sensory loss. If symptom relief is reproducible but transient, a trial using a dorsal column stimulator or a neurodestructive procedure using RFA, chemical neurolysis, or surgical procedure can be considered. Early initiation of treatment after an injury or the appearance of symptoms may elicit a better response than that seen with patients who have experienced chronic symptoms.

Other neurolytic approaches may involve interruption of various CNS pathways. Subarachnoid and epidural neurolysis have been reported in various case reports and series (28,50). The disadvantage is the potential spread of these chemicals on other central structures, leading to potential myelopathies. Painful conditions may require multiple-level neurolysis, greatly compounding the probability of serious complications. The use of implantable intrathecal drug therapy has reduced the need for this procedure.

Neurostimulation

Neurostimulation is the application of precisely targeted electrical stimulation on nociceptive pathways. Electric stimulation has a long history in medicine in treating various ailments. Beyond the application of electrodes on the skin such as a transcutaneous electrical nerve stimulation (TENS), electrodes have been applied directly to nociceptive pathways.

Spinal cord stimulation (SCS) uses epidural electrodes placed along the dorsal columns to block nociception (51,52). The system entails the surgical placement of epidural electrodes, cables, and radiofrequency transmitter or battery. Minimal discomfort is encountered in the placement of the system and in the postoperative period.

The mechanism of SCS is based on the gate control theory (51). It postulates that stimulating large nerve fibers (A-beta fibers) can inhibit or modulate smaller nerve fibers (A delta or C fibers) transmitting nociceptive input, possibly at the dorsal root or horn of the spinal cord. Strategically placed epidural electrodes stimulate the dorsal columns (A-beta fibers) to inhibit or modulate nociceptive input (A delta or C fibers). Ongoing research suggests that SCS may inhibit transmission in the spinothalamic tract, activate central inhibitory mechanisms influencing sympathetic efferent neurons, and release various inhibitory neurotransmitters. New waveforms, closed loop systems, high frequency, and multiplex programming are the advanced technology that may provide better outcomes for chronic pain patients (53). Dorsal root stimulation has emerged as novel approach for complex regional pain syndromes (54).

SCS can be applied to treat neuropathic pain conditions including arachnoiditis, complex regional pain syndrome (formerly, reflex sympathetic dystrophy), neuropathies, brachial and lumbosacral plexopathies, radiculopathies, deafferentation syndromes, phantom limb pain, and postherpetic neuralgia (deer, tasker). Visceral syndromes such as interstitial cystitis, chronic abdominal pain, and chronic pancreatitis have been treated with limited success. SCS for cancer pain is limited to the dynamic nature and progression of neoplasms. SCS may have a role in stable neuropathic cancer pain related to cancer treatments and stable neoplasms. Specifically for cancer pain, a Cochrane review identified four case series, which showed improved pain relief and reduced analgesic consumption (55).

Peripheral nerve stimulation (PNS) has developed for specific localized neuropathic conditions that follows the same concept of SCS with electrical stimulation of specific nerve fibers and pathways (56). Modification and miniaturization of electrodes and battery allow placement of systems throughout the body. As with SCS, a gate control therapy is proposed as the initial mechanism with ongoing studies elucidating complex array of pathway and mechanisms of nociception. Specific targets of PNS include almost all plexuses and peripheral nerves.

PERCUTANEOUS VERTEBRAL AUGMENTATION

Percutaneous vertebral augmentation are image-guided, outpatient procedures, which may be used to treat pain associated with vertebral compression fractures caused by metastatic tumors or osteoporosis (57,58). Kyphoplasty is vertebroplasty with the creation of cavity prior placement of the cement. Most vertebroplasties and kyphoplasty are performed for osteoporotic compression fractures, but patients with cancer pain can experience significant symptom relief with this procedure. Patients with anterior osteolytic lesions that are not amenable to surgical interventions may be candidates for this less invasive intervention. Contraindications for vertebroplasty and kyphoplasty include >70% vertebral collapse, epidural disease, asymptomatic stable fractures, or infection (57). However, there is growing evidence that these guidelines may not be absolute contraindications (58).

During vertebroplasty and kyphoplasty, one or two bone biopsy needles are inserted into the collapsed vertebral body through a small incision in the patient's back and acrylic bone cement is injected through the cannula to stabilize the fracture. The procedure typically requires a local anesthetic; conscious sedation is sometimes helpful, depending on the patient's condition and tolerance for medications that can compound hypotension. For many patients, however, vertebroplasty and kyphoplasty provide immediate (within 72 hours) and lasting relief from pain. Many patients are able to increase their level of activities within only a few days of the procedure.

Some clinical studies have reported conflicting success with vertebroplasty (59,60). A meta-analysis of 59 studies show kyphoplasty was superior to vertebroplasty in providing pain relief in cancer-related vertebral compression fractures and associated with a lower rate of complications (61). Both procedures have an extremely low complication rates including infection, an allergic reaction to methacrylates, pulmonary embolism from intravascular injection, and weakness from displacement of fracture or extravasation of the injection into the intrathecal space.

NEUROSURGICAL PROCEDURES FOR PAIN

Despite optimized medical therapy and the use of interventions, some patients will still not achieve a satisfactory level of symptom control and may require neurosurgical procedures for pain relief. Although these procedures can be quite effective in treating specific cancer pain syndromes, careful patient selection is critical to maximize potential benefit. Neurosurgical treatment of medically refractory cancer pain usually involves the interruption of the specific involved pain-sensory pathways. These interventions most often include cordotomy, myelotomy, and other nervous system ablative procedures.

Cordotomy

Cordotomy is used for patients with unilateral medically intractable cancer pain below the level of C5 (62,63). Cordotomy involves lesioning of the anterior spinothalamic tract of the spinal cord that transmits nociceptive impulses from the contralateral half of the body. Interruption of this tract can be performed by an open operation or percutaneously. Because percutaneous cordotomies can be performed under local anesthesia with minimal morbidity, it has become the preferred technique. Percutaneous cordotomies are performed by placing a needle through the neck contralateral to the pain (because the spinothalamic tract fibers have crossed the spinal cord by this point) at the C1-C2 level under CT scan guidance (63). Once the placement of the needle tip in the anterior spinothalamic tracts is confirmed, a permanent thermal lesion is made.

Cordotomy can provide excellent pain relief immediately after the procedure in >90% of patients (63). The effectiveness of this operation diminishes with time, and at 1 year after cordotomy, 50% to 60% of patients will continue to have adequate pain control. Beyond 1 year, 40% of patients will continue to have adequate analgesia. Complications are rare (usually <5%) and frequently transient. Complications include ataxia, ipsilateral paresis, bowel/bladder dysfunction, ipsilateral Horner's syndrome, sexual dysfunction, respiratory problems (sleep apnea or respiratory failure), and dysesthesias. Because there is a possibility of loss of ipsilateral diaphragmatic function with cordotomy, preoperative pulmonary function studies and dynamic radiographic studies should be performed to assess respiratory and diaphragmatic function. Patients with any pain ipsilateral to cordotomy will often see an exacerbation of this pain (*mirror-image pain*) and may require a second, staged cordotomy on the contralateral side.

Myelotomy

Myelotomy is primarily used for bilateral or midline pain in the lower half of the body (64). Patients with medically intractable pelvic, lower extremity, visceral, and perineal pain are potential candidates.

Classically, myelotomy has been described as incising through the posterior midline of the spinal cord to ventral pia. It is hypothesized that this interrupts the second-order crossing spinothalamic pain fibers and has been designed to create a level of analgesia corresponding to the level and extent of interruption. This procedure is typically performed in the thoracolumbar region, and a number of open and closed techniques have been described (64).

Because of the variability in reported techniques, the region treated for relief from pain, and follow-up, it is difficult to draw definitive conclusions about the effectiveness of this technique. Nevertheless, some studies have shown that myelotomy provides pain relief in 80% to 90% of patients immediately after the procedure. Similar to other neurosurgical procedures for pain, the effectiveness of this operation diminishes with time, with reports of variable pain relief at distant time points (approximately 25% to 70% of patients with continued adequate relief). Myelotomy is generally well tolerated with a low rate of morbidity. Complications (approximately 10%) include temporary weakness of the lower extremities, transient loss of pain and temperature sensation, bowel/bladder incontinence, and dysesthesias. Reported mortality rates are generally in the range of 1% to 2%.

OTHER NEUROSURGICAL PROCEDURES

Mesencephalotomy

Candidates for mesencephalotomy include patients with cancer pain of the head and neck or cancer pain of the proximal upper extremity, or in those with diaphragmatic paralysis in whom cordotomy may be dangerous (65). Mesencephalotomy involves stereotactically creating a lesion in the rostral midbrain in structures lying just medial to the lateral spinothalamic tract (65). The results of several small, uncontrolled, retrospective studies suggest that 50% to 75% of patients may have significant pain relief, over both the short term (months) to several years (up to 5-year follow-up in some studies). Lesions at the level of the superior colliculus are more likely to be successful but also more commonly lead to problems such as difficulty with extraocular movements and binocular vision (up to 10%) than do lesions that are placed slightly lower in the midbrain, at the level of the inferior colliculus.

Hypophysectomy

Candidates for hypophysectomy include patients with severe bone pain as a result of metastatic disease (breast or prostate carcinomas) (66). Although both animal studies and clinical work has shown a connection between the pituitary gland and hypothalamus and pain and pain relief, the exact mechanisms remain poorly understood. Several groups in the 1960s and 1970s reported satisfying results with respect to both pain relief and tumor regression in up to 60% of patients treated with total hypophysectomy through a transsphenoidal approach. Other methods of hypophysectomy, such as direct transsphenoidal injection of absolute ethanol and Gamma knife radiation, have also been shown to provide moderate or even complete pain relief in most selected patients (67,68). These results can be difficult to predict, however, and may result from a variety of factors, including endocrine effects due to loss of cortisol, thyroid-stimulating hormone, or growth hormone, or due to stimulation of endorphin pathways; activation of stress-analgesic responses; or even a direct neurolytic effect. The natural consequence of the removal of the pituitary is panhypopituitarism, which carries with it significant morbidity. In addition, the need to perform these procedures under general anesthesia in patients who have been medically compromised potentially has led to waning interest in these approaches, except in carefully selected situations.

Microvascular Decompression

Microvascular decompression, an open neurosurgical approach, is based on the theory that aberrant torturous vessels compress the trigeminal nerve root entry zone at the brainstem, causing pain. By surgically placing an Ivalon or Teflon sponge between the artery and nerve, one can alleviate the facial pain. In one study, 90% of patients had sustained pain relief over 5 years and 46% recurrence of pain in 8.5 years (34,35,69).

SUMMARY

Whether treating a patient's pain resulting from a life-treating disease or from a nonmalignant source (chronic low back pain), interventional or surgical procedures may dramatically improve a patient's quality of life. Although they provide additional valuable tools when a medicinal or complementary approach fails to provide satisfactory symptom relief, the variability of patient presentation, including progression of disease, results in tremendous unpredictability of the outcome results. Pain may be alleviated in the treated site(s) while other pain elsewhere will not be affected. The distribution of locally administered drug(s) can also be variable, leading to a lessening rather than the complete resolution of the pain symptoms. The duration of the therapeutic

effects may be only transient because of incompleteness of the procedure's effects. In rare cases, the intervention may further transiently aggravate or even permanently worsen pain symptoms, or other adverse events may further deteriorate the patient's quality of life. Therefore, the risks and benefits must be carefully weighed. Several texts on interventional pain that provide additional information on the indications, procedure, and risks are included in the references (70,71).

Despite the above cautions, advances in pain interventional techniques continue to improve the therapeutic benefit while reducing the risks. Imaging techniques allow greater visualization and, therefore, facilitate greater ease and precision in needle placement. This provides greater specificity in targeting pain pathways and reduces untoward effects. Further, new therapies that target novel sites are in various stages of clinical development. For example, neurolytic drugs that delete only pain-specific fibers (sparing other afferent and efferent pathways) have demonstrated safety and efficacy in preclinical testing (72,73).

Finally, more work is needed to validate the use of some of the many current pain interventions. Although interventional techniques are frequently utilized, many therapies have not undergone rigorous blinded controlled studies to determine efficacy. This is by no means an easy task and represents an ethical dilemma because of the necessity of withholding therapies that could increase suffering in this patient group.

REFERENCES

1. Meuser T, Pietruck C, Radbruch L, Stute P, Lehmann KA, Grond S. Symptoms during cancer pain treatment following WHO-guidelines: a longitudinal follow-up study of symptom prevalence, severity and etiology. *Pain.* 2001;93(3):247-257. doi:10.1016/S0304-3959(01)00324-4.
2. Tay W, Ho K-Y. The role of interventional therapies in cancer pain management. *Ann Acad Med Singapore.* 2009;8(11):989-997. doi:10.1161/JAHA.115.002867.
3. Smith TJ, Staats PS, Deer T, et al. Randomized clinical trial of an implantable drug delivery system compared with comprehensive medical management for refractory cancer pain: impact on pain, drug-related toxicity, and survival. *J Clin Oncol.* 2002;20(19):4040-4049. doi:10.1200/JCO.2002.02.118.
4. Ferrante FM. Neuraxial infusion in the management of cancer pain. *Oncol (willist Park).* 1999;13(5 suppl 2):30-36.
5. Upadhyay SP, Mallick PN. Intrathecal drug delivery system (IDDS) for cancer pain management: a review and updates. *Am J Hosp Palliat Med.* 2012;29(5):388-398. doi:10.1177/1049909111426134.
6. Coffey RJ, Owens ML, Broste SK, et al. Mortality associated with implantation and management of intrathecal opioid drug infusion systems to treat noncancer pain. *Anesthesiology.* 2009;111(4):881-891. doi:10.1097/ALN.0b013e3181b64ab8.
7. Smitt PS, Tsafka A, Teng-Van De Zande F, et al. Outcome and complications of epidural analgesia in patients

with chronic cancer pain. *Cancer.* 1998;83(9):2015-2022. doi:10.1002/(SICI)1097-0142(19981101)83:9<2015::AID-CNCR19>3.0.CO;2-R.

8. Deer TR, Pope JE, Hayek SM, et al. The Polyanalgesic Consensus Conference (PACC): recommendations for intrathecal drug delivery: guidance for improving safety and mitigating risks. *Neuromodulation.* 2017;20(2):155-176. doi:10.1111/ner.12579.

9. Deer TR, Pope JE, Hayek SM, et al. The Polyanalgesic Consensus Conference (PACC): recommendations on intrathecal drug infusion systems best practices and guidelines. *Neuromodulation.* 2017;20(2):96-132. doi:10.1111/ner.12538.

10. Deer TR, Prager J, Levy R, et al. Polyanalgesic Consensus Conference-2012: recommendations on trialing for intrathecal (intraspinal) drug delivery: report of an interdisciplinary expert panel. *Neuromodulation.* 2012;15(5):420-435. doi:10.1111/j.1525-1403.2012.00450.x.

11. Yaksh TL, Hassenbusch S, Burchiel K, Hildebrand KR, Page LM, Coffey RJ. Inflammatory masses associated with intrathecal drug infusion: a review of preclinical evidence and human data. *Pain Med.* 2002;3(4):300-312. doi:10.1046/j.1526-4637.2002.02048.x.

12. Deer, T. Pharmacology of intrathecal drug delivery in the spinal cord. *Reg Anesth Pain Med.* 2014;39(5):E33-#34. doi:10.1097/AAP.0000000000000142.

13. Mercadante S. Neuraxial techniques for cancer pain. *Reg Anesth Pain Med.* 1999;24(1):74-83. doi:10.1097/00115550-199924010-00014.

14. Bedder MD, Burchiel K, Larson A. Cost analysis of two implantable narcotic delivery systems. *J Pain Symptom Manage.* 1991;6(6):368-373. doi:10.1016/0885-3924(91)90028-3.

15. Staats PS, Yearwood T, Charapata SG, et al. Intrathecal ziconotide in the treatment of refractory pain in patients with cancer or AIDS: a randomized controlled trial. *J Am Med Assoc.* 2004;291(1):63-70. doi:10.1001/jama.291.1.63.

16. Deer TR, Pope JE, Hayek SM, et al. The Polyanalgesic Consensus Conference (PACC): recommendations on intrathecal drug infusion systems best practices and guidelines. *Neuromodulation.* 2017;2016:96-132. doi:10.1111/ner.12538.

17. Deer TR, Levy R, Prager J, et al. Polyanalgesic Consensus Conference-2012: recommendations to reduce morbidity and mortality in intrathecal drug delivery in the treatment of chronic pain. *Neuromodulation.* 2012;15(5):467-482. doi:10.1111/j.1525-1403.2012.00486.x.

18. Myers J, Chan V, Jarvis V, Walker-dilks C. Intraspinal techniques for pain management in cancer patients: a systematic review. *Support Care Cancer.* 2010;18(2);137-149. doi:10.1007/s00520-009-0784-2.

19. Reif I, Wincent A, Stiller C-O. Intrathecal analgesia by bupivacaine is not enhanced by coadministration of morphine in patients with severe cancer-related pain: a randomized double-blind cross-over study. *Int J Clin Pharmacol Ther.* 2017;55(6):525-532. doi:10.5414/cp202955.

20. Stearns LJ, Hinnenthal J, Hammond B, Berryman E, Janjan NA. Health services utilization and payments in patients with cancer pain: a comparison of intrathecal drug delivery vs. conventional medical management. *Neuromodulation.* 2016;19(2):204-205. doi:10.1111/ner.12384.

21. Ripamonti CI, Bandieri E, Roila F. Management of cancer pain: ESMO clinical practice guidelines. *Ann Oncol.* 2011;22(Supplement 6):69-77. doi:10.1093/annonc/mdr390.

22. Ilfeld BM. Continuous peripheral nerve blocks in the hospital and at home. *Anesthesiol Clin.* 2011;29(2):193-211. doi:10.1016/j.anclin.2011.04.003.

23. Ilfeld BM, Morey TE, Wright TW, Chidgey LK, Enneking FK. Continuous interscalene brachial plexus block for postoperative pain control at home: a randomized, double-blinded, placebo-controlled study. *Anesth Analg.* 2003;96(4):1089-1095. doi:10.1213/01.ANE.0000049824.51036.EF.

24. Swerdlow M. Spinal and peripheral neurolysis for managing Pancoast syndrome. *Adv Pain Res Ther.* 1982;4:135-143.

25. Klein SM, Greengrass RA, Grant SA, Higgins LD, Nielsen KC, Steele SM. Ambulatory surgery for multiligament knee reconstruction with continuous dual catheter peripheral nerve blockade. *Can J Anesth.* 2001;48(4):375-378. doi:10.1007/BF03014966.

26. Abildgaard JT, Lonergan KT, Tolan SJ, et al. Liposomal bupivacaine versus indwelling interscalene nerve block for postoperative pain control in shoulder arthroplasty: a prospective randomized controlled trial. *J Shoulder Elb Surg.* 2017;26(7):1175-1181. doi:10.1016/j.jse.2017.03.012.

27. De Leon-Casasola OA. Neurolysis of the sympathetic axis for cancer pain management. *Tech Reg Anesth Pain Manage.* 2005;9(3):161-166. doi:10.1053/j.trap.2005.06.009.

28. Patt RB, Millard R. A role for peripheral neurolysis in the management of intractable cancer pain. *Pain.* 1990;5(suppl):S358. doi:10.1016/0304-3959(90)92832-b.

29. Cohen SP, Van Zundert J. Pulsed Radiofrequency. *Reg Anesth Pain Med.* 2010;35(1):8-10. doi:10.1097/aap.0b013e3181c7705f.

30. Kim PS, Ferrante FM. Cryoanalgesia: a novel treatment for hip adductor spasticity and obturator neuralgia. *Anesthesiology.* 1998;6(3):345-360. doi:10.1097/00000542-199808000-00036.

31. Trescot AM. Cryoanalgesia in interventional pain management. *Pain Physician.* 2003;6(3):345-360.

32. Lavelle ED, Lavelle W, Smith HS. Myofascial trigger points. *Anesthesiol Clin.* 2007;25:841-851. doi:10.1016/j.anclin.2007.07.003.

33. Zhou JY, Wang D. An update on botulinum toxin a injections of trigger points for myofascial pain. *Curr Pain Headache Rep.* 2014;18(1):386. doi:10.1007/s11916-013-0386-z.

34. Meglio M, Cioni B, Moles A, Visocchi M. Microvascular decompression versus percutaneous procedures for typical trigeminal neuralgia: personal experience. *Stereotact Funct Neurosurg.* 1990;54-55:76-79. doi:10.1159/000100194.

35. Mullan S, Lichtor T. percutaneous microcompression of the trigeminal ganglion. *J Neurosurg.* 1983;23(2):270. doi:10.3171/jns.1983.59.6.1007.

36. Twycross RG, Fairfield S. Pain in far-advanced cancer. *Pain.* 1982;14(3):303-310. doi:10.1016/0304-3959(82)90137-3.

37. Candido KD, Philip CN, Ghaly RF, Knezevic NN. Transforaminal 5% phenol neurolysis for the treatment of intractable cancer pain. *Anesth Analg.* 2010;110(1):216-219. doi:10.1213/ANE.0b013e3181c0ecd5.

38. Doyle D. Nerve blocks in advanced cancer. *Practitioner.* 1982;226(1365):539, 541-544.

39. Kawaguchi M, Hashizume K, Iwata T, Furuya H. Percutaneous radiofrequency lesioning of sensory branches of the obturator and femoral nerves for the treatment of hip joint pain. *Reg Anesth Pain Med.* 2001;26(6):576-581. doi:10.1053/rapm.2001.26679.

40. Hutson N, Hung JC, Puttanniah V, Lis E. Interventional pain management for sacroiliac tumors in the oncologic population: a case series and paradigm approach. 2017;18(5):959-968. doi:10.1093/pm/pnw211.

41. Mercadante S, Klepstad P, Kurita GP, Sjøgren P, Giarratano A. Sympathetic blocks for visceral cancer pain management: a systematic review and EAPC recommendations. *Crit Rev Oncol Hematol.* 2015;96(3):577-583. doi:10.1016/j.critrevonc.2015.07.014.

42. Black A, Dwyer B. Coeliac plexus block. *Anaesth Intensive Care.* 1973;1(4):315-318.

43. Kress HG. Interventional techniques for cancer patients. *Eur J Pain.* 2009;13(1):S3-S4. doi:http://dx.doi.org/10.1016/S1090-3801%2809%2960011-2.

44. Rykowski JJ, Hilgier M. Efficacy of neurolytic celiac plexus block in varying locations of pancreatic cancer: influence on pain relief. *Anesthesiology.* 2000;92(2):347-354. doi:10.1097/00000542-200002000-00014.

45. Lillemoe KD, Cameron JL, Kaufman HS, Yeo CJ, Pitt HA, Sauter PK. Chemical splanchnicectomy in patients with unresectable pancreatic cancer: a prospective randomized trial. *Ann Surg.* 1993;217(5):447-455. doi:10.1097/00000658-199305010-00004.

46. Staats PS, Hekmat H, Sauter P, Lillemore K. The effects of alcohol celiac plexus block, pain, and mood on longevity in patients with unresectable pancreatic cancer: a double-blinded, randomized, placebo-controlled study. *Pain Med.* 2001;2(1):28-34.

47. Papadopoulos D, Kostopanagiotou G, Batistaki C. Bilateral thoracic splanchnic nerve radiofrequency thermocoagulation for the management of end-stage pancreatic abdominal cancer pain. *Pain Physician.* 2013;16(2):125-133.

48. Sharma V, Rana SS, Bhasin DK. Endoscopic ultrasound guided interventional procedures. *World J Gastrointest Endosc.* 2015;7(6):628-642. doi:10.4253/wjge.v7.i6.628.

49. Cariati M, De Martini G, Pretolesi F, Roy MT. CT-guided superior hypogastric plexus block. *J Comput Assist Tomogr.* 2002;26(3):428-431. doi:10.1097/00004728-200205000-00019.

50. Wagner KJ, Sprenger T, Pecho C, et al. [Risks and complications of epidural neurolysis—a review with case report]. *Anasthesiol Intensivmed Notfallmed Schmerzther.* 2006;41(4):213-222. doi:10.1055/s-2006-925232.

51. Melzack R, Wall PD. Pain mechanisms: a new theory. *Science.* 1965;150(3699):971-979.

52. Tsuda T, Tasker RR. [Percutaneous epidural electrical stimulation of the spinal cord for intractable pain—with special reference to deafferentation pain]. *No Shinkei Geka.* 1985;13(4):409-415.

53. Deer TR, Mekhail N, Provenzano D, et al. The appropriate use of neurostimulation of the spinal cord and peripheral nervous system for the treatment of chronic pain and ischemic diseases: the neuromodulation appropriateness consensus committee. *Neuromodulation.* 2014;17(6):515-550. doi:10.1111/ner.12208.

54. Pope JE, Deer TR, Kramer J. A systematic review: current and future directions of dorsal root ganglion therapeutics to treat chronic pain. *Pain Med (United States).* 2013;14(10):1477-1496. doi:10.1111/pme.12171.

55. Peng L, Min S, Zejun Z, Wei K, Bennett MI. Spinal cord stimulation for cancer-related pain in adults [systematic review]. *Cochrane Database Syst Rev.* 2015;2015(6):CD009389.

56. Slavin KV. Peripheral nerve stimulation for neuropathic pain. *Eur Neurol Rev.* 2012;7(4):244-248.

57. Jensen ME, Kallmes DF. Percutaneous vertebroplasty in the treatment of malignant spine disease. *Cancer J.* 2002;8(2):194-206. doi:10.1097/00130404-200203000-00013.

58. Hentschel SJ, Burton AW, Fourney DR, Rhines LD, Mendel E. Percutaneous vertebroplasty and kyphoplasty performed at a cancer center: refuting proposed contraindications. *J Neurosurg Spine.* 2005;2(4):436-440.

59. Buchbinder R, Osborne RH, Ebeling PR, et al. A randomized trial of vertebroplasty for painful osteoporotic vertebral fractures. *N Engl J Med.* 2009;361:557-568. doi:10.1056/NEJMoa0900429.

60. Kallmes DF, Comstock BA, Heagerty PJ, et al. A randomized trial of vertebroplasty for osteoporotic spinal fractures. *N Engl J Med.* 2009;361:569-579. doi:10.1056/NEJMoa0900563.

61. Bhargava A, Trivedi D, Kalva L, Tumas M, Hooks M, Speth J. Management of cancer-related vertebral compression fracture: comparison of treatment options: a literature meta-analysis. *J Clin Oncol.* 2009;27(15 suppl).

62. White JC, Sweet WH, Hawkins R, Nilges RG. Anterolateral cordotomy: results, complications and causes of failure. *Brain.* 1950;73(3):346-367. doi:10.1093/brain/73.3.346.

63. Kanpolat Y, Ugur HC, Ayten M, Elhan AH. Computed tomography-guided percutaneous cordotomy for intractable pain in malignancy. *Neurosurgery.* 2009;64(3 Suppl):ons187-ons193.

64. Hong D, Andrén-Sandberg Å. Punctate midline myelotomy: a minimally invasive procedure for the treatment of pain in inextirpable abdominal and pelvic cancer. *J Pain Symptom Manage.* 2007;33(1):99-109. doi:10.1016/j.jpainsymman.2006.06.012.

65. Bosch DA. Stereotactic rostral mesencephalotomy in cancer pain and deafferentation pain. *J Neurosurg.* 2009;75(5):747-751. doi:10.3171/jns.1991.75.5.0747.

66. Laws ER. Transsphenoidal hypophysectomy. *J Neurosurg.* 2007;107(2):458-471. doi:10.3171/JNS-07/08/0458.

67. Niranjan A, Bowden G, Flickinger JC, Lunsford LD. Gamma knife radiosurgery. In: *Principles and Practice of Stereotactic Radiosurgery.* New York, NY: Springer; 2015. doi:10.1007/978-1-4614-8363-2_8.

68. Lippitz B, Lindquist C, Paddick I, Peterson D, O'Neill K, Beaney R. Stereotactic radiosurgery in the treatment of brain metastases: the current evidence. *Cancer Treat Rev.* 2014;40(1):48-59. doi:10.1016/j.ctrv.2013.05.002.

69. Montano N, Conforti G, Di Bonaventura R, Meglio M, Fernandez E, Papacci F. Advances in diagnosis and treatment of trigeminal neuralgia. *Ther Clin Risk Manag.* 2015;11:289-299. doi:10.2147/TCRM.S37592.

70. Lamacraft G, Cousins MJ. Neural blockade in chronic and cancer pain. *Int Anesthesiol Clin.* 1997;35(2):131-153.

71. Manchikanti L, Kaye AD, Falco FJE, Hirsch JA. *Essentials of Interventional Techniques in Managing Chronic Pain.* International Association for the Study of Pain: Springer; 2018. doi:10.1007/978-3-319-60361-2.

72. Fink DJ, Wechuck J, Mata M, et al. Gene therapy for pain: results of a phase I clinical trial. *Ann Neurol.* 2011;70(2):207-212. doi:10.1002/ana.22446.

73. Karai L, Brown DC, Mannes AJ, et al. Deletion of vanilloid receptor 1-expressing primary afferent neurons for pain control. *J Clin Invest.* 2004;113(9):1344-1352. doi:10.1172/JCI20449.

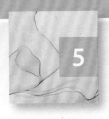

5 Treatment Planning in Palliative Radiotherapy

Christen R. Elledge and Sara R. Alcorn

INTRODUCTION

Up to 50% of radiotherapy treatments are delivered with palliative intent (1–5), and approximately 40% of patients with advanced cancers will receive palliative radiation therapy (RT) at some point in their disease course (6). However, due to factors such as the high degree of variability in the presentation of patients receiving palliative RT, urgency related to treatment planning for palliative cases, and minimal research on the breadth of treatments delivered with palliative intent, there is little guidance on treatment planning for palliative RT. This chapter aims to guide radiation oncologists through the treatment planning process and to provide information about a broad range of techniques available for use in order to provide appropriate, effective, and safe palliative RT.

SIMULATION

General Approach

The treatment simulation is a critical first step of the RT planning process, and further treatment planning and delivery depend on the adequacy and quality of the simulation. Treatment simulation is performed to determine (a) an appropriate and reproducible treatment position with immobilization devices, (b) the location of targets as well as nearby critical structures at risk, and (c) placement of isocenter and proper beam arrangements. Three commonly used simulation techniques, conventional simulation, clinical setup, and computed tomography (CT) simulation, are described below. Table 5.1 summarizes the advantages and disadvantages of each simulation technique.

Conventional Simulation

In cases requiring urgent or emergent delivery of palliative RT, a conventional simulation may be used. A conventional simulation is performed on a radiographic simulator that is capable of diagnostic kilovoltage (kV) imaging and fluoroscopy. The other components of the conventional simulator, such as the couch and gantry head, resemble a linear accelerator.

During a conventional simulation, the patient is placed on the couch in the desired treatment position. Immobilization devices are constructed to facilitate the reproducibility of patient setup for each fraction and to restrict interfraction (between radiation fractions) and intrafraction (within one fraction) movement. The radiation oncologist delineates the treatment field borders on the patient's skin using radiopaque markers, and orthogonal fluoroscopic imaging is obtained to determine isocenter. Once isocenter has been selected, orthogonal kV images (typically anteroposterior [AP] and lateral) are obtained for setup documentation and verification via comparison to megavoltage (MV) portal images (7). At this point, different beam positions (gantry angles, collimator angles), field sizes, and couch positions can be simulated in order to geographically optimize the delivery of radiation to the treatment area delineated by the physician. Finally, the laser coordinate system in the simulator room is used to mark the location of the isocenter on the patient. Simultaneously, other treatment planning information can be obtained such as the source-to-surface distance (SSD) and patient thickness.

The primary advantage of a conventional simulation is that it can be performed quickly for urgent or emergent palliative cases. Secondly, there are fewer limitations to patient positioning and to the size and shape of immobilization devices. For patients who cannot be placed in a supine position, some facilities have a special treatment chair in which the patient can be simulated while sitting in an upright position (8). Additionally, for some treatments such as of the distal upper extremity, it may be more comfortable for the patient to be seated next to the treatment couch with the affected extremity placed on the couch. Such positioning cannot be accommodated with CT simulators due to the restrictive size of the bore and the requirement for the patient to be positioned supine or prone on the couch during scanning. An additional advantage to conventional simulation is that the field visualization is directly on the patient's skin, which can be helpful for bulky disease that is externally visible (such as large, painful adenopathy). Finally, the fluoroscopic imaging capability

TABLE 5.1 SUMMARY OF THE ADVANTAGES AND DISADVANTAGES OF TREATMENT SIMULATION TECHNIQUES

Technique	Advantages	Disadvantages
Conventional simulation	• Fast • Permits use of a wide range of immobilization devices • Allows for unique treatment positions (including sitting) • Fluoroscopy can be used for a limited assessment of tumor motion • Allows for comparison of simulation images (kV) to MV portal images for treatment setup verification	• Limited tumor visualization • Conformal treatment planning is impossible • Limited ability to perform dose calculations to targets or OARs • Other imaging studies cannot be fused • Limited motion management options (abdominal compression may still be performed)
Clinical setup	• Fast • Permits use of a wide range of immobilization devices • Allows for unique treatment positions (including sitting) • Requires only one setup for simulation and delivery of the first fraction	• Limited tumor visualization • Conformal treatment planning is not possible • No shaped fields beyond the secondary collimator • Other imaging studies cannot be fused • Not possible to calculate dose to specific volumes or OARs • Limited motion management options (abdominal compression may still be performed)
CT simulation	• Provides 3-D anatomical information allowing for superior delineation of targets and critical structures • Allows for conformal RT planning and, thus, safer dose escalation when needed • Allows for volumetric radiation dose calculation • Simulation CT images may be fused with other 3-D imaging modalities (PET, MRI) to improve target delineation • Generation of a DRR allows for a virtual simulation and visualization of targets from a beam's eye view • DRR may be compared to MV portal images for setup verification or cone-beam CT may be directly compared to the simulation CT images • Multiple motion management strategies available	• Immobilization devices and patient positioning are limited by the CT bore size • Patient must be simulated either supine or prone on the couch; although some devices provide a minimal incline, the patient cannot be sitting up • Requires a CT technologist or radiation therapist with CT simulation training

allows for a limited assessment of tumor motion, which can be helpful for designing treatment margins (9). The primary disadvantage of a conventional simulation is the lack of 3-dimensional (3-D) visualization of patient anatomy; this makes identification and delineation of disease extent more difficult. In addition, due to the lack of 3-D visualization, conformal planning is not possible, which may increase treatment toxicity due to excess dose to nearby organs at risks (OARs) (10–15).

Clinical Setup

Given technical improvements in CT imaging and increased popularity of 3-D-based treatment planning, the use of conventional simulators has decreased dramatically across the United States, and many departments no longer have a conventional simulator (8). In some institutions, for patients with significant discomfort who cannot tolerate a CT scan, a "clinical setup" can serve as an alternative, quick approach to conventional simulation.

To perform a clinical setup, the patient is brought into the linear accelerator vault and placed on the treatment couch in the desired treatment position with appropriate immobilization. The radiation oncologist and radiation therapist set the treatment couch so the laser is at midplane and midline on the patient within the desired treatment field to determine source-to-axis distance (SAD). The radiation oncologist then specifies the location of the isocenter, gantry angles, and collimator angles. Using the specified parameters, double exposure (open field and planned field) portal

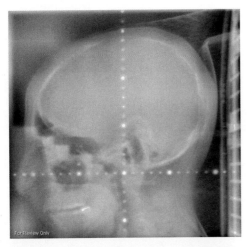

Figure 5.1 Port film obtained during a clinical setup of a patient treated urgently to the brain and upper cervical spine for symptomatic leptomeningeal disease.

images are acquired. Once the radiation oncologist has approved the treatment field, the final location of the isocenter is marked on the patient, calipers are used to measure the patient separation at isocenter, and the SSD is measured. Dosimetric verification software is used to perform a monitor unit (MU) calculation based on the jaw settings, beam energy, SSD, and machine calibration parameters. At most institutions, a secondhand calculation is performed by a medical physicist to verify the MU calculation obtained from the dosimetric software. Figure 5.1 shows an example of a patient treated to the brain and upper cervical spine for leptomeningeal disease using a clinical setup.

The advantages of a clinical setup are that (a) it is relatively quick, (b) it does not require a CT simulation procedure, (c) the patient does not have to be transferred from the simulator to the treatment couch, which may be critical to consider for patients with limited mobility or significant pain, and (d) there are fewer limitations on immobilization devices or patient positioning than with CT simulation. The primary disadvantage to this approach is that MV portal images have very poor soft tissue resolution, and there may be little to no ability to localize tumor volumes. RT fields are based on anatomic landmarks, and dose to specific OARs cannot be calculated. At our institution, multifraction palliative RT cases that initially require a clinical setup are generally resimulated with a CT simulation once the patient is able to tolerate a CT scan. This provides a means for potentially minimizing treatment-related toxicity and for documenting estimated cumulative doses to OARs for past and future treatments.

CT Simulation

The CT simulation has become the most common simulation technique used in the United States and, to date, is the only 3-D imaging modality employed for RT dose calculations (16). The CT simulation allows for virtual representation of both the patient and the linear accelerator; as such, it is sometimes referred to as a "virtual simulation" (17). First, the patient is positioned in the desired treatment position on a flat table-top couch that closely resembles the linear accelerator treatment couch. All immobilization devices required for treatment are used to position the patient prior to scanning. Additional treatment devices such as tissue-equivalent bolus can be placed on the patient prior to scanning. There is an indexing system on the couch surface that is similar to the indexing system used on the treatment couch. Devices such as head rests and breast boards can be indexed on both the CT couch and treatment couch to improve the reproducibility of patient setup. The CT scanner has a wide bore—usually >75 cm—to accommodate immobilization devices (18). Figure 5.2 shows an image of a modern CT simulator.

An AP, 2-dimensional (2-D) topogram or "scout view" is obtained prior to performing the CT scan. Reviewing the topogram allows the physician and

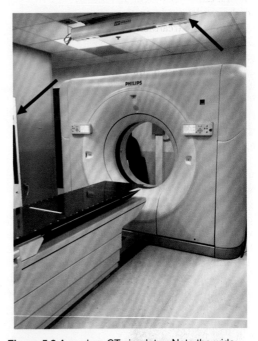

Figure 5.2 A modern CT simulator. Note the wide-bore to accommodate immobilization devices and the flat-top couch. The indexing system can also be seen along the vertical edges of the couch. The laser coordinate system is mounted on the ceiling and to each side of the CT scanner (*black arrows*).

radiation therapists to check patient alignment and positioning and to make final adjustments to the patient prior to full scan acquisition. The desired superior, inferior, and lateral scan limits are also selected based on the topogram and physician order. The CT scan is then acquired using preset protocols depending on treatment site. Intravenous (IV) or oral contrast may be administered to improve visualization of targets or OARs. After the CT images have been acquired, the radiation oncologist can review the scan and set the isocenter for treatment.

The isocenter is generally placed in the geometric center of the treatment field but can also be strategically positioned near bony landmarks or implanted fiducials if useful for future setup verification. Computer software is used to align the laser coordinate system in the room so the position of the isocenter can be marked on the patient at the time of simulation. Usually one anterior and two lateral marks are permanently tattooed on the patient. Alternatively, "pre-marks" or "reference marks" can be marked on the patient by therapists at the time of simulation to designate a "virtual" isocenter. Then, the physician or dosimetrist can set the isocenter at the time of treatment planning and shifts will be applied from the "pre-marks" (virtual isocenter) to the treatment isocenter on the first day of treatment. At that time, permanent marks can be made on the patient to denote the location of the treatment isocenter. An illustration of this approach is shown in Figure 5.3. After the patient has been marked, the patient may leave the clinic and the rest of the treatment planning can be performed using treatment planning software.

The simulation software will then generate a digitally reconstructed radiograph (DRR) to replace the simulation film. DRRs are generated by averaging CT values along a line from a digital "source"

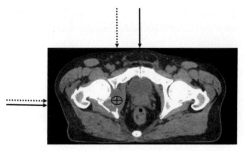

Figure 5.3 A CT simulation was performed and "pre-marks" were placed by radiation therapists at a midline, midplane location (*solid arrows*). Later, the physician sets the treatment isocenter (*circle with crosshairs/dashed arrows*). The distance between the *solid arrows* and the *dashed arrows* represents the necessary shifts to be made from "pre-marks" to isocenter prior to treatment.

to a digital "film." A computer uses these CT values to construct a "digital" simulator film that would traditionally be obtained using kV imaging on a conventional simulator (18). The DRR allows the radiation oncologist to view the treatment field from the "beam's eye view" (BEV) and to select the most appropriate gantry angle, collimator angle, couch angle, field size, and blocks when 3-D conformal radiotherapy (3-D CRT) is planned (see Treatment Volume Delineation). Additionally, at the time of treatment, MV portal images can be compared to the DRR for setup and isocenter verification. Alternatively, if 3-D image guidance is used, the cone beam CT (CBCT) can be compared to the simulation CT for setup and isocenter verification. Figure 5.4 provides an example of these different image types from a patient treated to a painful, sacroiliac joint metastasis.

A CT simulation provides several advantages over 2-D approaches. The first is that a simulation

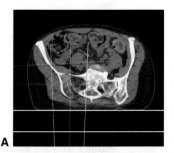 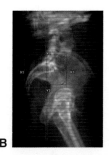 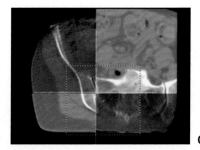

A   **B**   **C**

Figure 5.4 Representative images of a patient treated to a painful sacroiliac joint metastasis. CT simulation showing desired treatment region (*red*), posteroanterior (PA) treatment beam, and right lateral treatment beam **(A)**. DRR as viewed from the right lateral treatment beam **(B)**. Fusion of simulation CT scan (*upper right* and *lower left* panels) and CBCT (*upper left* and *lower right* panels) used for isocenter and setup verification **(C)**.

CT scan allows for 3-D visualization of patient anatomy. CT images are generally acquired in the axial dimension and then reconstructed and reformatted so they may be viewed in axial, coronal, and sagittal planes (19). This allows the radiation oncologist to view images of patient anatomy in multiple dimensions and to accurately identify and delineate radiation targets as well as nearby OARs. IV or oral contrast administration may further improve visualization and delineation of targets as well as OARs. In addition, other 3-D diagnostic imaging studies such as positron emission tomography (PET) scans or magnetic resonance imaging (MRI) scans may be fused with the simulation CT to further improve identification and delineation of radiation targets and OARs.

Once volumes have been delineated, radiation oncologists can prescribe dose to specific volumes while sparing nearby OARs. This volume-based planning approach allows for the shaping of conformal dose distributions with the potential for relative sparing of nearby OARs. This may allow for dose escalation strategies when appropriate. Secondly, a simulation CT allows for accurate radiation dose calculations to targets and OARs. This may be of critical importance for palliative radiation treatments, as many cases involve reirradiation of targets or significant overlap with prior curative- or palliative-intent RT fields. Finally, the use of a CT simulation allows for several motion management strategies for targets affected by respiratory motion.

The disadvantages of a CT simulation are as follows: (a) patient positioning and immobilization devices are limited by the bore size, (b) they require a radiation therapist trained in operating the CT simulator, thus limiting the availability of use for urgent/emergent treatments when the radiation oncology department may not be fully staffed, (c) it is more time consuming than a clinical setup, and (d) it requires the patient to be positioned in the treatment position at two different locations, which may be difficult for patients with severe discomfort or limited mobility.

CT Simulation: Motion Management

Modern CT simulators are capable of obtaining helical or axial multislice scans with fast acquisition times to provide a high-resolution, volumetric, 3-D reconstruction of patient anatomy (18). However, if there is movement during CT scan acquisition due to swallowing, respiration, cardiac movement, peristalsis, rectal or bladder filling, or physical patient movement, the resulting CT scan may be blurred due to "motion artifact." Notably, respiratory motion can lead to significant motion artifact and distortion of the anatomy during CT

imaging of the thorax and upper abdomen. Such respiratory motion can result in inaccurate contouring of targets and OARs, incorrect radiation dose calculations, and even "geographic misses," where there is displacement of the target out of the radiation field during treatment (18,20). Historically, very large margins, up to 2.5 cm, were required when treating thoracic or upper abdominal tumors to account for respiratory motion (21). These large margins led to increased normal tissue toxicity and prohibited dose escalation to targets. As such, several techniques including abdominal compression, breath hold techniques, 4D-CT, and gating have been developed to help reduce respiratory motion or to track the motion of targets and OARs during the respiratory cycle. The primary advantages and disadvantages of each technique are summarized in Table 5.2.

Abdominal compression uses pressure applied to the abdomen to reduce diaphragmatic excursion during inspiration, limiting motion of targets and OARs in the chest and upper abdomen (22–25). The advantages of abdominal compression are that it is a simple technique that does not require sophisticated imaging or treatment technology. The disadvantages of this approach are that abdominal compression (a) may cause significant pain, discomfort or anxiety in some patients, which may have the paradoxical effect of increasing respiratory motion (26,27); (b) cannot be used in significantly overweight and obese patients (28); (c) increases the time required for daily patient setup (27); and (d) may push abdominal OARs in closer proximity to the target (29).

A second approach utilizes breath hold techniques for both simulation and treatment. One such popular approach, active breathing control (ABC), was first described by Wong et al. in 1999 (21). ABC uses an apparatus that is placed in the patient's mouth to continuously monitor breathing (Fig. 5.5). At a preset lung volume during either inspiration or expiration, airflow to the patient is blocked, thereby immobilizing respiration at a consistent lung volume and ensuring reproducibility (21). The patient is asked to hold the breath for as long as comfortably possible, and the patient's maximum breath hold duration is recorded. During treatment, the radiation beam will be turned on for the length of the breath hold and then turned off during free breathing. The patient is given a nose clip to prevent breathing through the nares and a push button to place in the hand that the patient is instructed to push during the breath hold and to release if he or she needs to come out of the breath hold sooner than anticipated. Early feasibility studies of this approach found that patients preferred breath hold during inspiration

TABLE 5.2 SUMMARY OF ADVANTAGES AND DISADVANTAGES OF SEVERAL RESPIRATORY MOTION MITIGATION TECHNIQUES

Technique	Advantages	Disadvantages
Abdominal compression	• Simple, easy to use • Inexpensive	• May cause significant pain, discomfort, or anxiety in some patients • Cannot be used in overweight/obese patients • Increases daily setup time • May push abdominal OARs closer to RT target
ABC	• Helpful for tumors with significant excursion (>1 cm) with respiration to reduce treatment margins • Limits motion artifacts on CT imaging • Reproducible	• Not all patients are able to perform breath holds • Requires additional technology • Increased time for simulation because patients often need coaching • Increased treatment time
4D-CT	• Patients are not required to perform breath holds • Provides an accurate spatial map of the shape and trajectory of tumor movement (decreasing the risk of a geographic miss) • Limits motion artifacts on CT	• Increased simulation time • Increase radiation dose due to CT simulation • Requires additional technology • Not reproducible if the patient's breathing pattern changes during treatment
Gating	• Patients are not required to perform breath holds • Limits motion artifact on CT • Reproducible	• Increased simulation time • Increased treatment times • Requires additional technology

as opposed to expiration, and thus most centers use ABC to immobilize respiration near the peak of inspiration (21). Another option is to use voluntary deep-inspiration breath hold (DIBH), which can be performed with verbal instructions to the patient to "take a deep breath, and hold it." The treatment beam is turned on during breath hold, and the patient is instructed to resume normal breathing once the beams have been turned off. With the latter approach, no additional equipment is required, and it is less invasive than ABC. However, the breath hold may be less reproducible without the measurements and respiratory immobilization afforded by the ABC device. The greatest disadvantage of both breath hold techniques is that patients have to be fit enough to hold their breath, usually up to a minimum of 15 to 20 seconds. This is not feasible for many patients requiring palliative RT.

A third approach to motion management is the use of a 4-D CT, where the fourth dimension is time. A full discussion of 4-D CT technology is beyond the scope of this chapter, but the basic principle is that a 4-D CT provides information

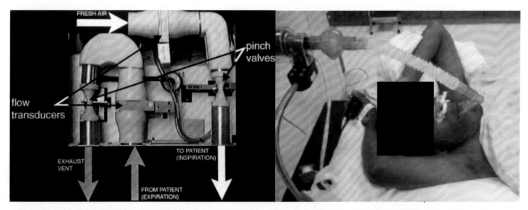

Figure 5.5 Adapted ventilator used for ABC (*left*). (Adapted from Wong JW, Sharpe MB, Jaffray DA, et al. The use of active breathing control (ABC) to reduce margin for breathing motion. *Int J Radiat Oncol Biol Phys*. 1999;44:911-919, with permission.) Patient with ABC device in place (*right*). Note the nose clip to prevent breathing through the nares and control button placed in the patient's right hand.

about how a structure varies in its 3-D location across time (i.e., across the respiratory cycle). 4-D CT scan acquisition is obtained by oversampling at each couch position so that organ motion is captured at different phases of the respiratory cycle. Simultaneously, the breathing cycle is monitored and recorded, and CT data are separated into bins based on the phase of the respiratory cycle in which the image was obtained (30). Thus, the 4-D CT minimizes image distortion due to motion and also provides a visual map of how the target and OARs move with respiration (18). Depending on the CT density of the target, the maximum intensity projection (MIP) or minimum intensity projection (MinIP), along with the scan images showing the minimum and maximum excursion, is used to contour an internal target volume (ITV). The MIP is a single image set reflecting the highest density value encountered in each voxel throughout the respiratory cycle. It is particularly helpful in delineation of lung tumors where the tumor is hyperdense compared to surrounding aerated lung (31). Similarly, the MinIP may be used for hypodense targets such as liver tumors (32,33). The advantages of a 4D-CT are that (a) there is a reduction in motion artifact and distortion, allowing for more accurate contouring of targets and OARs, (b) the radiation oncologist is provided with a spatial map of the shape and trajectory of tumor motion due to respiration, thereby reducing the chance of a geographic miss, and (c) the patient is not required to perform a breath hold. The primary disadvantages of this approach are the increased scan acquisition time, increased radiation dose to the patient, and costs of software and respiratory tracking technology.

A fourth approach to motion management is the use of gating for simulation and treatment. To use this approach, patients are positioned on the CT couch in the desired treatment position, and an external infrared reflector is placed on the patient's lower chest or upper abdomen. As the patient breathes, the reflector's movement is tracked by an infrared camera located at the foot of the CT couch (34). This motion is analyzed by software that allows the CT scanner to acquire images during specific "windows" of the respiratory cycle. In one commercially available system, there are two gating options: phase or amplitude (35). In the phase mode, images are acquired during a certain phase of the respiratory cycle (usually end-expiration or end-inspiration). Alternatively, images may be acquired based on the amplitude of the patient's breathing (35). The physician then contours the volumes based on the CT images obtained during the specified window of the CT simulation. The same technique used for simulation is subsequently employed during treatment. For instance, if a phase mode is used to capture end-inspiration during CT simulation, the linear accelerator beam will turn on during this same phase window for treatment. Ultimately, this allows for synchronization of radiation delivery with the respiratory cycle within specific windows based on phase or amplitude. The primary advantages of this approach are that (a) there is decreased motion artifact, resulting in more accurate contouring of targets and OARs and (b) the patient is not required to perform any breath holds. The primary disadvantages are that special gating software and hardware are required and simulation scan acquisition and treatment times are longer (33,36).

Simulations for Stereotactic Treatments

Advances in patient immobilization, diagnostic imaging, daily pretreatment imaging, and treatment planning techniques have allowed radiation oncologists to deliver stereotactic, highly conformal ablative radiation while sparing surrounding normal structures. Stereotactic radiation therapy such as stereotactic radiosurgery (SRS) or stereotactic body radiation therapy (SBRT) is increasingly being used for palliative radiotherapy treatments, particularly for the treatment of brain metastases or reirradiation of spinal metastases. There are a few additional considerations when performing a simulation for a planned stereotactic treatment. First, due to the narrow margins used with stereotactic treatments, the immobilization devices designed at the time of simulation should provide precise immobilization that is comfortable and reproducible. For brain metastases, rigid immobilization can be achieved through the use of a stereotactic head frame such as those used for Gamma Knife radiosurgery or with the use of a customized, thermoplastic head mask that is secured to the treatment table. For extracranial sites, thermoplastic molds and vacuum-locking bags should be considered for patient immobilization. For treatment areas where rigid immobilization is not possible, the use of a HexaPOD (Elekta) or other similar devices that use an infrared camera to enable submillimeter patient positioning accuracy with six degrees of freedom (translation and rotation) should be considered (37). When designing stereotactic treatments for tumors located in the abdomen or thorax, motion mitigation strategies such as abdominal compression, ABC, 4D-CT, or gating should be used. Finally, due to the small targets and narrow margins used for stereotactic treatments, a thin slice simulation CT is required for contouring and treatment planning, and a slice thickness of 1 to 2 mm is recommended, particularly for small targets (33,38).

Illustrative Palliative RT Case #1

Palliative RT cases often require creativity with patient setup, simulation, and treatment planning due to the wide variety of anatomic disease sites requiring treatment in patients who often have significant discomfort and pain, have been heavily pretreated, and may have markedly advanced disease presentations. One such case has been selected to demonstrate the ingenuity required for some palliative radiation treatments.

A 69-year-old female patient presented with refractory mycosis fungoides with painful lesions on the plantar aspects of both feet (Fig. 5.6). The lesions were too superficial to be treated with high-energy MV photons and the contour irregularity of her feet presented dosimetric challenges for electron treatment. The use of tissue-equivalent bolus wrapped around the feet would cause significant air gaps due to the contour irregularity of her feet and reproducibility of daily setup would be limited, particularly given the painful nature of the lesions. The decision was made to treat both feet in a water bath to provide adequate dose build up to allow for photon irradiation. Six layers of 1 cm tissue-equivalent bolus was added under her feet to allow for adequate dose buildup to the plantar surface. She was treated with 15 MV opposed lateral beams to a dose of 2,160 cGy in 12 fractions (180 cGy/fraction) with an excellent clinical response and resolution of pain. During treatment, she experienced minor skin breakdown, and was managed with supportive wound care and small doses of oral opioid analgesics.

TREATMENT VOLUME DELINEATION

General Approach

After deciding to treat a patient with RT, the radiation oncologist must then select the target volume to be irradiated. For definitive, curative-intent RT, the entirety of the gross tumor volume (GTV) and surrounding subclinical, microscopic disease is treated to curative doses. However, in the context of palliative radiotherapy, the goal of treatment is to alleviate symptoms due to tumor burden. As such, treatment volumes often do not encompass microscopic disease, and in many cases, do not cover all gross disease. The radiation oncologist must weigh the benefits of treating larger volumes with the costs of increased normal tissue toxicity. The decision to proceed with 2-D or 3-D treatment planning may be based on patient factors (e.g., inability to lie flat, urgency of the case), clinic factors (e.g., availability of CT simulation equipment, availability of a CT technologist or radiation therapist to operate the CT simulator), or other factors (e.g., cost-effectiveness, insurance approval).

2-D Approach

For 2-D treatments, anatomical landmarks are used to determine treatment fields. If bulky disease can be visualized by the radiation oncologist on or

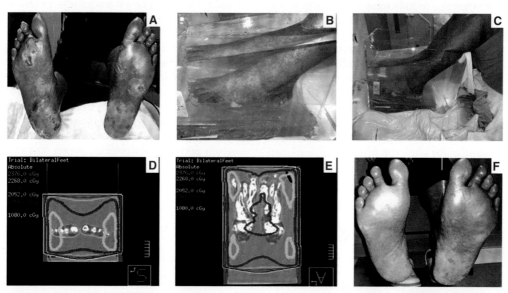

Figure 5.6 Pretreatment images of a patient with refractory, painful mycosis fungoides lesions with involvement of the plantar surfaces of both feet **(A)**. She was treated with her feet in a water bath with 6 cm of tissue-equivalent bolus underneath her feet to allow for adequate dose buildup to the plantar aspect of her feet **(B and C)**. Axial **(D)** and coronal **(E)** views of the dose distribution are shown. Six months post-RT, she had complete resolution of the lesions and pain **(F)**.

through the skin, this disease may be marked with radiopaque markers prior to imaging. Additionally, if the patient has significant pain in a certain location, a radiopaque marker can be placed over the site of pain to localize the treatment target. The location of critical organs, such as the spinal cord, can also be blocked based on knowledge of anatomical landmarks.

3-D Approach

With the use of 3-D treatment planning, the radiation oncologist uses the simulation CT to define target volumes as well as nearby OARs. A common nomenclature for radiation targets has been developed by the International Commission on Radiation Units and Measurements (ICRU) (39). As per this report, visible tumor seen on imaging is contoured as the GTV (Fig. 5.7). Other diagnostic imaging studies such as diagnostic-quality CT scans, MRIs, or PET scans may be fused with the simulation CT scan to aid in GTV delineation. If treatment of occult, microscopic disease extension is deemed clinically appropriate, the radiation oncologist may contour this additional volume or isotropically expand the GTV to cover it. The combined GTV and surrounding area at risk for occult, microscopic disease is called the clinical target volume (CTV). However, in general, a CTV is not created for palliative RT cases, as the goal of treatment is alleviation of symptoms and not eradication of disease. An additional margin is added to the GTV or CTV to account for motion of the target due to daily setup uncertainty, physiologic motion due to internal organs (e.g., peristalsis, bladder filling), respiratory motion (if an ITV is not made), and patient movement while on the treatment couch. The combined GTV or CTV with this additional margin is referred to as the planning target volume (PTV). The size of PTV margins depend on the type and frequency of image guidance used for setup verification, the susceptibility of the target to physiologic organ motion, the use and type of respiratory motion management, and the type of immobilization

device. Ideally, treatment would be delivered only to the PTV, but due to the physical limitations of radiation delivery and fall-off, the treated volume is the "volume described by an isodose surface, selected and specified by the radiation oncologist" (39). Finally, all nearby OARs should be contoured at least 5 cm superior and inferior to the target for accurate dose calculations when coplanar beams are used. More generous superior and inferior extent may be required when non-coplanar beams are employed (see Advanced Techniques: Intensity Modulated Radiation Therapy and Stereotactic Treatment Planning.)

Beam Selection, Arrangement, and Blocking

Using the radiographs obtained from the conventional simulator or the DRR obtained from a CT simulator, the radiation oncologist can select beam angles, collimator angles, and couch angles that provide adequate coverage of the treatment volume based on anatomic landmarks or a 3-D constructed PTV. Beam arrangements should also be selected to prevent unnecessary irradiation of OARs. For example, palliative radiotherapy used to treat the upper cervical spine should be delivered using opposed laterals instead of an anteroposterior (AP)/posteroanterior (PA) beam arrangement to avoid treating through the oral cavity. Beam energies are selected based on target depth and geometry. For 3-D CRT treatments, low-energy beams (4 to 6 MV) can be used for moderately deep tumors. If using parallel opposed low-energy beams, the patient thickness in the beam pathway should not exceed 17 cm (40). Higher energy beams (10 MV or greater) can be used for the treatment of deep-seated targets. In addition, the beam weighting can be modified to improve target coverage or decrease dose to OARs. For instance, when treating the lumbar spine with an AP/PA beam arrangement, the radiation oncologist may increase the weighting of the posterior beam to decrease dose in the anterior portion of the patient, sparing dose to the small bowel.

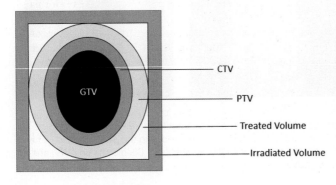

Figure 5.7 Schematic representation of various volumes defined by the ICRU. (Adapted from ICRU Report 50: Prescribing, Recording, and Reporting Photon Beam Therapy.)

Common beam arrangements used for palliative RT include single beam fields, parallel opposed fields, three field techniques, and four field box techniques. A single beam can be used for relatively superficial targets such as bulky supraclavicular adenopathy, or moderately deep targets, such as the spine in thin patients. However, for deeper targets, a single beam may deliver excessive dose to superficial tissues and can lead to very inhomogeneous dose distributions (41). For deeper targets, multiple beams intersecting at the target are required to deliver adequate dose to the target while sparing surrounding OARs. The most simple multiple beam approach uses parallel opposed fields. Parallel opposed fields produce a fairly uniform dose distribution with the highest dose near the skin surface and a minimum dose at mid-depth (41). If using an AP/PA beam arrangement for a target volume located more anteriorly, the anterior beam is given a greater weight such that more dose is delivered from the anterior beam than the posterior beam. Three-field and four-field approaches build on these same principles with the use of additional beams.

The initial field size is set by moving the secondary collimator jaws. The field size should encompass the entirety of the PTV (or desired treatment field based on anatomic landmarks) with an additional margin to account for dose fall-off at the edge of the treatment beams. This additional margin is sometimes referred to as an "aperture margin," and it is generally recommended to be a minimum of 7 to 8 mm to ensure adequate coverage of the PTV (39,42,43). The penumbra of a beam from a modern linear accelerator is predominantly determined by the range of secondary electrons generated in tissue. The range of these secondary electrons increases with increasing beam energy and decreasing tissue density, leading to a loss of electronic equilibrium and a subsequent decrease in radiation dose deposition at the periphery of the beam (44,45). As such, the aperture margin should be increased for higher energy beams and targets located near low density tissue such as the lungs (42,45). At our institution, the total margin used for palliative cases that encompasses concepts of CTV, PTV, and aperture margin is generally the GTV plus 1 to 2 cm. Specifically for spinal lesions treated with 2-D or 3-D plans, our margins typically extend to one vertebral body above and one vertebral body below the target level in superior–inferior extent. A 1 to 2 cm radial margin is generally applied around the entire individual vertebra at the involved level.

When designing radiotherapy with a 2-D approach, once the physician has set the gantry angle, collimator angle, and couch angle, simulation radiographs are performed from the desired beam angles. The initial size of the treatment field can be set by adjusting the secondary collimator jaws. The physician can then draw treatment blocks on the simulation images, and Cerrobend blocks can be fabricated to shield nearby critical structures or uninvolved tissues (46). These blocks are loaded onto block trays, which are placed in the gantry head at the time of treatment. With 3-D treatment planning, the physician first defines the PTV and OARs. Then, beam angles are selected to provide adequate coverage to the target volume while avoiding OARs. The treatment field is set by adjusting the secondary collimator jaws. If additional blocking is required, the multileaf collimator (MLC) can be used. In both approaches, adequate aperture margins should be used to ensure sufficient coverage of the desired treatment volume.

Palliative Radiation Therapy Doses

Before dosimetry is able to design an RT plan, the radiation oncologist must prescribe a dose and fractionation regimen. A full discussion of dose and fractionation selection is beyond the scope of this chapter, but Table 5.3 provides a short summary of common fractionation regimens used in palliative radiotherapy. When deciding on the dose and fractionation, the radiation oncologist should consider the histology of the tumor, the location of the tumor and nearby OARs, the anticipated life span of the patient, prior history of RT, and risk of acute and late effects of RT. In general, if there is evidence that shorter fractionation regimens are noninferior to longer treatment schedules, shorter regimens should be used to reduce treatment costs and improve convenience for patients (69).

TREATMENT PLANNING AND DOSIMETRY

2-D Approach

Once the physician has used the conventional simulator to specify gantry angles, collimator angles, couch angles, field sizes, and block placement, the dose is generally prescribed to midplane for parallel opposed fields or to isocenter if using a multiple-field technique. No further dose optimization can be performed, which is generally reasonable for palliative RT cases in which low doses are used for symptom relief.

3-D-CRT Approach

Once the physician has drawn the PTV and OARs, placed the beams, and designed the blocks, the plan then goes to dosimetry for further optimization and dose calculations. The dosimetrist can alter

TABLE 5.3 COMMON DOSE AND FRACTIONATION SCHEDULES USED FOR PALLIATIVE RADIATION THERAPY

Clinical scenario	Commonly used dose and fractionation regimens[a]
Painful bone metastases (47–53)	8 Gy in 1 fx 20 Gy in 5 fx 24 Gy in 6 fx 30 Gy in 10 fx
Spinal cord compression/cauda equina syndrome (54–56)	8 Gy in 1 fx 20 Gy in 5 fx 30 Gy in 10 fx 37.5 Gy in 15 fx 40 Gy in 20 fx
Bleeding or pain in pelvic sites (bladder, rectum, gynecologic sites, etc.) (57–65)	8 Gy in 1 fx 10 Gy in 1 fx (can be repeated monthly up to two more times if needed) 14.8 Gy in 4 fx delivered b.i.d. over 2 d (can be repeated up to 2 times every 3–4 wk) 20–25 Gy in 5 fx 30 Gy in 10 fx
Cough, hemoptysis, airway obstruction, SVC syndrome (62,66–68)	8 Gy in 1 fx 10 Gy in 1 fx 17 Gy in 2 fx given 1 week apart 20 Gy in 5 fx 30 Gy in 10 fx
Brain metastases (whole-brain RT) (69–71)	20 Gy in 5 fx 30 Gy in 10 fx 37.5 Gy in 15 fx 40 Gy in 20 fx
Esophageal obstruction/bleeding (72,73)	8 Gy in 1 fx 20–25 Gy in 5 fx 30 Gy in 10 fx 39 Gy in 13 fx
Pain, airway obstruction, or bleeding from locally advanced head and neck cancers (62,74,75)	8 Gy in 1 fx 14.8 Gy in 4 fx delivered b.i.d. over 2 d (can be repeated up to 2 times every 3–4 wk) 20 Gy in 5 fx 30 Gy in 10 fx

[a]Stereotactic body radiation therapy (SBRT) and stereotactic radiosurgery (SRS) dose and fractionation regimens have not been included in this table.
Fx, fraction; Gy, Gray; RT, radiation therapy.

the beam energies and beam weighting to improve target volume coverage and decrease radiation dose to nearby OARs. Additional beam modifiers such as compensators, segments, or wedges can be introduced into the beam to increase conformality and homogeneity of the dose distribution. Wedges are wedge-shaped pieces of steel or lead that are placed in front of the beam to increase the homogeneity of the dose distribution. Wedges may be (a) "internal" and moved into the field by a motor within the gantry head, (b) "external" and require physical placement by a radiation therapist onto a tray within the gantry head, or (c) "dynamic." A dynamic wedge is produced by moving one of the jaws from the secondary collimator across the beam during treatment leading to a wedge-shaped dose distribution (34). Segmented fields (or "field in field technique") use one or more (but usually <7 for 3-D-CRT planning) segments, or smaller fields than the primary field, to improve dose coverage and homogeneity (76–78). The use of segmented fields became possible after the development of the MLC and computerized treatment planning systems. Finally, the dosimetrist may add an additional beam to improve PTV coverage and/or dose homogeneity. This approach to treatment planning where beam angles, beam weights, field segments, and other parameters are selected first and then further optimized to produce the desired dose distribution is known as forward planning.

Illustrative Palliative RT Case #2

A 58-year-old gentleman presented with a large metastatic lesion in the C5 vertebral body compressing the nerve root and resulting in severe pain. The initial plan used opposed lateral beams, but the dose to the larynx and oral cavity were felt to be excessively high. The dosimetrist created an alternative plan with a wedge pair of opposed oblique beams and an additional posterior beam. The alternative plan improved target coverage while allowing for greater sparing of the oral cavity and larynx. He was treated to a dose of 3,000 cGy in 10 fractions with a good clinical response (Fig. 5.8).

Advanced Techniques: Intensity Modulated Radiation Therapy and Stereotactic Treatment Planning

It is beyond the scope of this chapter to discuss the complexities of intensity-modulated radiation therapy (IMRT) or stereotactic treatment planning in detail. As a vast oversimplification, IMRT divides the radiation beams up into discrete "beamlets," and MLCs are used to modify the intensity of the radiation across beamlets allowing for the delivery of highly conformal RT. As a first step in IMRT planning, the physician uses the simulation CT scan to delineate target volumes and OARs. The physician also then provides the dosimetrist with a list of objectives and constraints to be used for treatment planning. Objectives are metrics that measure the quality of the plan, and constraints are conditions that must always be satisfied or else the plan is considered unacceptable (79). The dosimetrist then selects couch and gantry angles and assigns different priorities, or "weights," to the constraints and objectives, thus

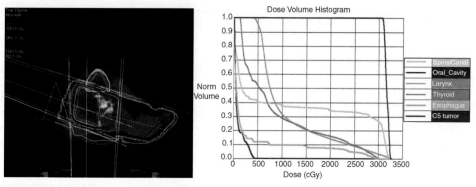

Figure 5.8 A C5 lesion (*red*) treated with a wedge pair of opposed oblique beams and an additional posterior beam (*left*) with the associated plan dose–volume histogram (DVH, *right*).

specifying a desired radiation dose distribution. Subsequently, the treatment planning system uses an inverse planning approach to calculate an intensity map for each beam segment. This process can be repeated many times during optimization before arriving at a satisfactory plan.

There are three broad delivery modes of IMRT, (a) step-and-shoot, (b) sliding window, and (c) volumetric modulated arc therapy (VMAT). Step-and-shoot and sliding window are considered "static modes" as they only deliver radiation from specific beam angles. Step-and-shoot sets the MLCs at planned positions to modulate the intensity of the beam; then, the beam shuts off, and the leaves move to the next position. In this mode, the beam is only on when the leaves and gantry head are both static (80). In sliding window mode, the leaves move across the beam while the beam is on in order to paint the desired intensity map. However, as the gantry head rotates to the next position, the beam is off (80). In VMAT mode, the MLC leaves continuously move, and the gantry rotates through an arc across the patient while the beam remains on. The dose rate is continuously varied to provide different beam weighting for various incident angles (80). The advantage of IMRT is that it provides a highly conformal dose distribution allowing for further dose escalation while minimizing treatment toxicity. The disadvantages are that (a) the treatment planning is complex and time and labor intensive, (b) there is an increase in low dose irradiation to the whole body, (c) dose distributions are more inhomogeneous than with 3-D CRT, and (d) treatment duration is longer. These disadvantages generally limit the use of IMRT for palliation to cases of reirradiation. In addition, IMRT may be considered for patients with long anticipated life expectancies for whom "aggressive palliation" to curative or near-curative doses may be appropriate, or for patients who may significantly benefit from the highly conformal nature of the treatments (e.g., major salivary glands may only be spared if IMRT is used).

Stereotactic treatment planning begins with the radiation oncologist contouring the target volume and surrounding OARs. Critical structures within 10 cm of the target should be contoured due to the use of noncoplanar beam arrangements. The GTV should be contoured and, if 4-D CT is used, an ITV should be created based on the 4-D CT to account for respiratory motion. PTV expansion margins are disease site and institution specific, but are generally much smaller than 3-D CRT or IMRT margins. For instance, at our institution, a 1-mm isotropic expansion from GTV to PTV is used for SRS treatments for intact brain metastases while a 5-mm isotropic expansion from ITV to PTV is used for lung SBRT. Once the contours have been completed, they are sent to the dosimetrist along with the planning objectives and constraints. Stereotactic treatments are characterized by a highly conformal high dose region with steep dose gradients outside of the high-dose volume (33). This is often achieved through the use of many noncoplanar, nonoverlapping beams. In addition, stereotactic plans are normalized to around the 80% isodose line resulting in a heterogeneous dose distribution with a high hot spot within the target. Beam energies should be selected with a consideration of penumbral effects, which are increased with higher energy beams and lower density tissue (42). For this reason, 6-MV beams are usually used for lung SBRT, but higher energy beams may be used in the liver or spine (33). Beams are generally weighted so that dose fall-off is isotropic, but if there is a nearby critical structure beam weighting can be changed to "push" fall-off dose away from the critical structure. Heterogeneity corrections are critically important for accurate dose calculations when delivering stereotactic RT as dose variations up to 10% have been reported when heterogeneity corrections were not applied (81).

Electron Treatments

Electron treatments can be particularly useful for palliative RT in which the desired treatment target is located on the surface of the patient or at a shallow depth. For example, electrons are often used to palliate cutaneous lesions, rib metastases, and sternal metastases. Electron treatments may use a clinical setup if the lesion is visible on the skin surface and can be outlined by the radiation oncologist at the time of setup. For deeper targets or targets that may be affected by surface heterogeneity or surrounding tissue heterogeneity (bone, lung, nose, etc.), a CT simulation is often performed. Tissue equivalent bolus may be placed at the time of simulation to improve dose homogeneity by flattening out surface irregularities and/or reducing the electron penetration in certain regions (82). Tissue equivalent or brass bolus may also be used to increase the surface dose to very superficial targets.

If using a clinical setup technique, the radiation oncologist may use the light field from the gantry head to determine the secondary collimator jaw settings. If further field shaping is desired, lead blocks may be manufactured or lead strips may be used. When CT simulation is performed, the radiation oncologists contours the GTV, CTV, and PTV similar to photon planning. Most palliative cases treated with electrons can be treated with a single field. The physician then chooses the beam energy, beam angle, and field size. The beam energy is selected based on the depth of the target at the deepest point of the tumor. A close approximation of the necessary beam energy can be calculated by multiplying the depth of the target by 3 (therapeutic electron range) (83). The beam direction should be selected such that the beam is perpendicular to the skin at the level of the target (en-face) in order to maximize the penetration of the electrons (82). Finally, to ensure adequate dose coverage of the PTV, the beam aperture should be designed so there is at least a 1-cm margin between the aperture and PTV due to decreased radiation dose deposition at the beam penumbra (82). Once the dose is calculated, the beam weighting can be changed to further improve dose coverage and homogeneity.

CONFORMAL PLAN EVALUATION

Once the dosimetrist has created a plan, the radiation oncologist should systematically review and evaluate the plan to determine if it is a satisfactory plan or if further modification and/or optimization is required. The first step is to review the isodose distributions superimposed on the patient's simulation CT while scrolling through the CT image set. This initial inspection provides 3-D visual-ization of the target coverage, dose homogeneity, and conformality of the radiation dose to the target volume. The value (dose) and location of "hot spots" and "cold spots" can be reviewed. Ideally, hot spots should be located within the GTV (or at least the PTV), but if it is not the case, the radiation oncologist should ensure hot spots are not within a critical structure such as the spinal cord. The value and location of hot spots can be modified by altering the number of beams, beam angles, beam energies, beam weighting, beam modifiers (segments, wedges, etc.), or by creating "avoidance structures" to reduce hot spots in a particular location (84). During plan evaluation, the physician should examine the path of the beams to ensure they are not unnecessarily traversing uninvolved tissues (such as the arms) or other OAR. Next, as a further check of the safety, coverage, and quality of the plan, the DVH is reviewed to assess if volumetric dose objectives and constraints are satisfied. The most common source of dose objectives and constraints for normal tissue toxicity is provided by reports published by the "QUANTEC" (Quantitative Analysis of Normal Tissue Effects in the Clinic) group. These reports are available to members of the American Association of Physicists in Medicine (AAPM) and in a special edition published in 2010 in the International Journal of Radiation Oncology, Biology and Physics (IJROBP) (85–108). Other sources of dose objectives and constraints come from prospective trials and retrospective reviews.

Finally, if treating with a stereotactic plan, an evaluation of the dose conformality to the target should be performed. The conformality of the prescription dose is evaluated by the conformity index, which is a ratio of the 95% isodose volume to the target volume. Ideally this ratio should be close to 1. To evaluate the steepness of the dose gradient, the maximum dose at a 2-cm radius outside the PTV (D_{2cm}) and a ratio of the 50% isodose volume to the PTV ($R_{50\%}$) may also be assessed (33). Specific guidelines on these metrics for different disease sites are provided online (www.rtog.org). If further modification and/or optimization is required to improve the quality of the plan, the entire plan evaluation process should be repeated after any modification. If the radiation oncologist feels the plan is satisfactory, the plan goes on to the next stage of the treatment planning process (quality assurance [QA] checks) and then on to treatment delivery.

For palliative radiation in the setting of retreatment, an attempt can be made to fuse past and present RT plans in order to create a composite plan. This provides an estimate of the cumulative dose to OARs over all courses of RT. Of note, care should be taken to account for different fractional doses used in separate plans by calculating the biologically effective dose (BED) received by a particular OAR for each plan. BED from each plan can then be summed and converted to more interpretable units, such as the equivalent dose in 2-Gy fractions (EQD2). When composite doses to OARs exceed thresholds commonly employed, the radiation oncologist may elect to (a) lower the dose of the present plan to stay under a specified constraint, (b) switch to a more conformal planning modality if feasible, (c) recommend non-RT alternatives for palliation, or (d) treat to a dose in excess of the constraint after careful discussion of the pros and cons of this approach with the patient. If the exceeded constraint is associated with a late effect that may evolve months to years after radiotherapy, such an effect may not be meaningful for a patient with an anticipated short life expectancy.

QUALITY ASSURANCE

Radiation therapy uses sophisticated and increasingly complex technology to deliver high doses of radiation to specific targets. Throughout the process of treatment planning from the CT simulation to the delivery of the treatment beam, there are QA checks that must be performed along every step of the process. Comprehensive reviews of all of the different QA checks performed in each stage of the treatment planning and treatment delivery processes are available through the AAPM (109) and International Atomic Energy Agency (IAEA) (110–112). In addition, the final step prior to treatment delivery is a QA check performed by medical physicists to ensure the accuracy, quality, and safety of the treatment plan prior to treatment delivery. For 3-D conformal RT, this consists primarily of confirming the site, a check to ensure the prescription dose matches what is being delivered, and a second dose calculation. For IMRT plans, the site and prescription dose are verified and patient-specific IMRT QA is performed. IMRT QA is performed by (a) designing a QA phantom (often a diode array), (b) calculating the expected dose along the diode array, (c) delivering the RT plan to the phantom, and (d) comparing the expected dose distribution to the delivered dose distribution (113). To pass IMRT QA, the delivered dose should be within 3% of the expected dose at each point. If the dose is not within 3%, the software searches the dose distribution to find a nearby point that is within 3% of the expected dose. This distance is referred to as the "distance to agreement" and should be within 3 mm. If such a point is found within 3 mm, the point is considered to pass. In general, 95% of the diodes should pass (114). IMRT QA may also be used for some stereotactic treatments that use standard linear accelerators for delivery.

TREATMENT DELIVERY: IMAGE GUIDANCE

General Approach

Image guidance may be used to verify setup accuracy prior to treatment delivery (to reduce interfractional error) and to monitor for target movement during treatment delivery (to reduce intrafractional error). Although image guidance is not used until treatment delivery, the radiation oncologists must consider what type of image guidance they wish to use at an earlier point in the treatment process as this information is used to design PTV margins. In general, image guidance strategies can largely be divided into 2-D and 3-D approaches. For the purposes of palliative radiotherapy, MV portal imaging, kV imaging, and CBCT are the most commonly used approaches for image guidance and are discussed in further detail below. All pretreatment imaging increases time on the treatment table, and thus, care should be taken to select the minimum level of appropriate image guidance when managing patients with significant discomfort or unstable conditions.

2-D Image Guidance

MV portal imaging and kilovoltage x-ray imaging are the two most commonly used modalities for 2-D image guidance. Portal imaging uses the gantry head along with an electronic portal imaging device (EPID), which consists of a flat-panel imager composed of amorphous silicon (115). The portal images produced using the MV beam have low soft tissue resolution but can be used to align skeletal anatomy or implanted fiducials prior to treatment delivery. The frequency of pretreatment portal imaging is determined by the radiation oncologist, but common schedules include once at the beginning of treatment, weekly, or daily. Double exposure portal images can be taken with the open field (to verify anatomic landmarks used for setup) and through the beam aperture to verify the size, shape, and position of the treatment field. The disadvantages of portal imaging for setup verification are (a) higher dose of radiation delivered to the patient than kV plain films and (b) poor image quality with particularly low soft tissue resolution.

X-rays produced by kV imaging are an additional option for 2-D image guidance. These kV imagers can be mounted on the gantry head orthogonal to the MV therapy beam or mounted on the ceiling with film detectors located on the floor (providing oblique orthogonal image pairs) (116). Most kV imaging systems are also capable of fluoroscopy to monitor motion of targets and OARs. Kilovoltage imaging provides superior imaging quality and exposes the patient to a lower radiation dose than does portal imaging. However, because the patient is not imaged from the gantry through the field aperture, kV images cannot be used to verify the size or shape of the treatment field.

3-D Image Guidance

Many modern linear accelerators are equipped with kV imaging sources with flat panel detectors orthogonal to the MV treatment beam. These kV imaging sources are often capable of plain radiography, fluoroscopy, and CBCT providing multiple pretreatment imaging verification techniques. CBCT images are acquired by rotating the kV imaging source around the patient and obtaining multiple projection radiographs, which are then reconstructed with a filtered back-projection algorithm to obtain a 3-D volumetric image (117,118). A CBCT image can be acquired in 40 to 120 seconds. The greatest advantage of the use of CBCT is that it provides a 3-D visualization of patient anatomy at the time of treatment and allows for direct comparison with simulation CT images. In addition, respiration-correlated 4D-CT has been developed, which allows the physician to review the motion of the tumor as an additional aspect of setup verification (119). The disadvantages of CBCT are (a) scan acquisition times can be long (up to 2 minutes) due to regulations on gantry rotation speed to 1 revolution per minute, (b) images being susceptible to motion artifact due to long acquisition times, (c) increased time required for patient setup (scan acquisition, registration, patient shifts, etc.), and (d) increased dose of radiation received by the patient.

SUMMARY

Palliative RT is a highly effective modality used for symptom alleviation in patients with locally advanced or metastatic cancer. Each portion of the treatment planning process from simulation, target delineation, design of the radiation plan, and delivery of the RT can be tailored depending on the goals of treatment as well as patient-specific factors such as anticipated life expectancy, ability to tolerate treatment positions, disease location and extent, and risk of acute and late effects of radiation therapy.

REFERENCES

1. van Oorschot B, Rades D, Schulze W, Beckmann G, Feyer P. Palliative radiotherapy—new approaches. *Semin Oncol.* 2011;38:443-449.
2. Murphy JD, Nelson LM, Chang DT, Mell LK, Le QT. Patterns of care in palliative radiotherapy: a population-based study. *J Oncol Pract.* 2013;9:e220-e227.
3. Janjan NA. An emerging respect for palliative care in radiation oncology. *J Palliat Med.* 1998;1:83-88.
4. Wei RL, Mattes MD, Yu J, et al. Attitudes of radiation oncologists toward palliative and supportive care in the United States: Report on national membership survey by the American Society for Radiation Oncology (ASTRO). *Pract Radiat Oncol.* 2017;7:113-119.
5. Wu SY, Singer L, Boreta L, Garcia MA, Fogh SE, Braunstein SE. Palliative radiotherapy near the end of life. *BMC Palliat Care.* 2019;18:29.
6. Lam TC, Tseng Y. Defining the radiation oncologist's role in palliative care and radiotherapy. *Ann Palliat Med.* 2019;8:246-263.
7. Galvin JM. The CT-simulator and the Simulator-CT: advantages, disadvantages, and future developments. In: Smith AR, ed. *Radiation Therapy Physics.* Berlin, Heidelberg: Springer Berlin Heidelberg; 1995:19-32.
8. Mutic S, Purdy J, Michalski J, Perez C, Vijayakumar S. The simulation process in the determination and definition of the treatment volume and treatment planning. In: Levitt SH, Purdy JA, Perez CA, Vijayakumar S, eds. *Technical Basis of Radiation Therapy: Practical Clinical Applications.* 4th ed. Heidelberg, Germany: Springer; 2006:107-133.
9. Baker GR. Localization: conventional and CT simulation. *Br J Radiol.* 2006;79:S36-S49.
10. McJury M, Fisher PM, Pledge S, et al. The impact of virtual simulation in palliative radiotherapy for non-small-cell lung cancer. *Radiother Oncol.* 2001;59:311-318.
11. Tomé WA, Steeves RA, Paliwal BP. On the use of virtual simulation in radiotherapy of the intact breast. *J Appl Clin Med Phys.* 2000;1:58-67.
12. Nagata Y, Okajima K, Murata R, et al. Three-dimensional treatment planning for maxillary cancer using a CT simulator. *Int J Radiat Oncol Biol Phys.* 1994;30:979-983.
13. Nishioka T, Shirato H, Arimoto T, et al. Reduction of radiation-induced xerostomia in nasopharyngeal carcinoma using CT simulation with laser patient marking and three-field irradiation technique. *Int J Radiat Oncol Biol Phys.* 1997;38:705-712.
14. Gripp S, Doeker R, Glag M, et al. The role of CT simulation in whole-brain irradiation. *Int J Radiat Oncol Biol Phys.* 1999;45:1081-1088.
15. Chao M, Gibbs P, Tjandra J, Darben P, Lim-Joon D, Jones IT. Evaluation of the use of computed tomography versus conventional orthogonal X-ray simulation in the treatment of rectal cancer. *Australas Radiol.* 2005;49:122-126.
16. Pereira GC, Traughber M, Muzic RF Jr. The role of imaging in radiation therapy planning: past, present, and future. *Biomed Res Int.* 2014;2014:231090.
17. Karangelis G, Zamboglou N. CT-based virtual simulation for external beam radiation therapy. *Int Congr Ser.* 2001;1230:492-499.
18. Mihailidis DN, Papanikolaou N. Treatment simulation. In: Khan FM Gibbons JP, Sperduto PW, eds. *Khan's Treatment Planning in Radiation Oncology.* 4th ed. Philadelphia, PA: Wolters Kluwer; 2016:29-45.
19. Pelc NJ. Recent and future directions in CT imaging. *Ann Biomed Eng.* 2014;42:260-268.
20. Li XA, Stepaniak C, Gore E. Technical and dosimetric aspects of respiratory gating using a pressure-sensor motion monitoring system. *Med Phys.* 2006;33:145-154.

21. Wong JW, Sharpe MB, Jaffray DA, et al. The use of active breathing control (ABC) to reduce margin for breathing motion. *Int J Radiat Oncol Biol Phys*. 1999;44:911-919.

22. Han K, Cheung P, Basran PS, Poon I, Yeung L, Lochray F. A comparison of two immobilization systems for stereotactic body radiation therapy of lung tumors. *Radiother Oncol*. 2010;95:103-108.

23. Baba F, Shibamoto Y, Tomita N, et al. Stereotactic body radiotherapy for stage I lung cancer and small lung metastasis: evaluation of an immobilization system for suppression of respiratory tumor movement and preliminary results. *Radiat Oncol*. 2009;4:15.

24. Negoro Y, Nagata Y, Aoki T, et al. The effectiveness of an immobilization device in conformal radiotherapy for lung tumor: reduction of respiratory tumor movement and evaluation of the daily setup accuracy. *Int J Radiat Oncol Biol Phys*. 2001;50:889-898.

25. Heinzerling JH, Anderson JF, Papiez L, et al. Four-dimensional computed tomography scan analysis of tumor and organ motion at varying levels of abdominal compression during stereotactic treatment of lung and liver. *Int J Radiat Oncol Biol Phys*. 2008;70:1571-1578.

26. Bouilhol G, Ayadi M, Rit S, et al. Is abdominal compression useful in lung stereotactic body radiotherapy? A 4DCT and dosimetric lobe-dependent study. *Phys Med*. 2013;29:333-340.

27. Bissonnette JP, Franks KN, Purdie TG, et al. Quantifying interfraction and intrafraction tumor motion in lung stereotactic body radiotherapy using respiration-correlated cone beam computed tomography. *Int J Radiat Oncol Biol Phys*. 2009;75:688-695.

28. Hu Y, Zhou YK, Chen YX, Zeng ZC. Magnitude and influencing factors of respiration-induced liver motion during abdominal compression in patients with intrahepatic tumors. *Radiat Oncol*. 2017;12:9.

29. Campbell WG, Jones BL, Schefter T, Goodman KA, Miften M. An evaluation of motion mitigation techniques for pancreatic SBRT. *Radiother Oncol*. 2017;124:168-173.

30. Chen GTY, Rietzel ERM. 4D CT simulation. In: Bortfeld T, Schmidt-Ullrich R, De Neve W, Wazer DE, eds. *Image-Guided IMRT*. 1st ed. Berlin, Germany: Springer; 2006:247-257.

31. Muirhead R, McNee SG, Featherstone C, Moore K, Muscat S. Use of maximum intensity projections (MIPs) for target outlining in 4DCT radiotherapy planning. *J Thorac Oncol*. 2008;3:1433-1438.

32. Liu J, Wang JZ, Zhao JD, Xu ZY, Jiang GL. Use of combined maximum and minimum intensity projections to determine internal target volume in 4-dimensional CT scans for hepatic malignancies. *Radiat Oncol*. 2012;7:11.

33. Foster RD, Ramirez E, Timmerman RD. Stereotactic ablative radiotherapy. In: Khan FM, Gibbons JP, Sperduto PW, eds. *Khan's Treatment Planning in Radiation Oncology*. 4th ed. Philadelphia, PA: Wolters Kluwer; 2016:227-243.

34. Mageras GS, Yorke E. Deep inspiration breath hold and respiratory gating strategies for reducing organ motion in radiation treatment. *Semin Radiat Oncol*. 2004;14:65-75.

35. Morin RL, Serago C, Vallow L. Respiratory gating for radiotherapy. *J Am Coll Radiol*. 2006;3:372-374.

36. Pan T, Lee TY, Rietzel E, Chen GT. 4D-CT imaging of a volume influenced by respiratory motion on multi-slice CT. *Med Phys*. 2004;31:333-340.

37. Jiang P, Zhang X, Wei S, Zhao T, Wang J. Set-up error and dosimetric analysis of HexaPOD evo RT 6D couch combined with cone beam CT image-guided intensity-modulated radiotherapy for primary malignant

38. Srivastava SP, Cheng CW, Das IJ. The effect of slice thickness on target and organs at risk volumes, dosimetric coverage and radiobiological impact in IMRT planning. *Clin Transl Oncol*. 2016;18:469-479.

39. Landberg T, Chavaudra J, Dobbs J, et al. Report 50. *J Int Comm Radiat Units Meas*. 2016;os26:NP-NP.

40. Khan FM. Introduction: process, equipment, and personell. In: Khan FM, Gibbons JP, Sperduto PW, eds. *Treatment Planning in Radiation Oncology*. 4th ed. Philadelphia, PA: Wolters Kluwer; 2016:3-11.

41. McDermott PN, Orton CG. *Dose Distributions in Two and Three Dimensions. The Physics and Technology of Radiation Therapy*. Madison, WI: Medical Physics Publishing; 2010.

42. Sharpe MB, Miller BM, Wong JW. Compensation of x-ray beam penumbra in conformal radiotherapy. *Med Phys*. 2000;27:1739-1745.

43. INTERNATIONAL ATOMIC ENERGY AGENCY. Transition from 2-D Radiotherapy to 3-D Conformal and Intensity Modulated Radiotherapy. IAEA-TEC-DOC-1588, IAEA, Vienna, Austria. 2008.

44. Ekstrand KE, Barnes WH. Pitfalls in the use of high energy X rays to treat tumors in the lung. *Int J Radiat Oncol Biol Phys*. 1990;18:249-252.

45. Hunt MA, Desobry GE, Fowble B, Coia LR. Effect of low-density lateral interfaces on soft-tissue doses. *Int J Radiat Oncol Biol Phys*. 1997;37:475-482.

46. Chen GTY, Sharp GC, Wolfgang JA, Pelizzari CA. Imaging in radiotherapy. In: Khan FM, Gibbons JP, Sperduto PW, eds. *Khan's Treatment Planning in Radiation Oncology*. 4th ed. Philadelphia, PA: Wolter Kluwer; 2016:12-28.

47. Steenland E, Leer JW, van Houwelingen H, et al. The effect of a single fraction compared to multiple fractions on painful bone metastases: a global analysis of the Dutch Bone Metastasis Study. *Radiother Oncol*. 1999;52:101-109.

48. Hartsell WF, Scott CB, Bruner DW, et al. Randomized trial of short- versus long-course radiotherapy for palliation of painful bone metastases. *J Natl Cancer Inst*. 2005;97:798-804.

49. Lutz S, Balboni T, Jones J, et al. Palliative radiation therapy for bone metastases: update of an ASTRO evidence-based guideline. *Pract Radiat Oncol*. 2017;7:4-12.

50. Chow E, Harris K, Fan G, Tsao M, Sze WM. Palliative radiotherapy trials for bone metastases: a systematic review. *J Clin Oncol*. 2007;25:1423-1436.

51. Chow E, Zeng L, Salvo N, Dennis K, Tsao M, Lutz S. Update on the systematic review of palliative radiotherapy trials for bone metastases. *Clin Oncol (R Coll Radiol)*. 2012;24:112-124.

52. van der Linden YM, Steenland E, van Houwelingen HC, et al. Patients with a favourable prognosis are equally palliated with single and multiple fraction radiotherapy: results on survival in the Dutch Bone Metastasis Study. *Radiother Oncol*. 2006;78:245-253.

53. Meeuse JJ, van der Linden YM, van Tienhoven G, Gans RO, Leer JW, Reyners AK. Efficacy of radiotherapy for painful bone metastases during the last 12 weeks of life: results from the Dutch Bone Metastasis Study. *Cancer*. 2010;116:2716-2725.

54. Rades D, Stalpers LJ, Veninga T, et al. Evaluation of five radiation schedules and prognostic factors for metastatic spinal cord compression. *J Clin Oncol*. 2005;23:3366-3375.

55. Maranzano E, Trippa F, Casale M, et al. 8Gy single-dose radiotherapy is effective in metastatic spinal cord compression: results of a phase III randomized multicentre Italian trial. *Radiother Oncol*. 2009;93:174-179.

tumor of the cervical spine. *J Appl Clin Med Phys*. 2020;21(4):22-30.

56. Rades D, Lange M, Veninga T, et al. Final results of a prospective study comparing the local control of short-course and long-course radiotherapy for metastatic spinal cord compression. *Int J Radiat Oncol Biol Phys.* 2011;79:524-530.

57. Onsrud M, Hagen B, Strickert T. 10-Gy single-fraction pelvic irradiation for palliation and life prolongation in patients with cancer of the cervix and corpus uteri. *Gynecol Oncol.* 2001;82:167-171.

58. Hodson DI, Krepart GV. Once-monthly radiotherapy for the palliation of pelvic gynecological malignancy. *Gynecol Oncol.* 1983;16:112-116.

59. Halle JS, Rosenman JG, Varia MA, Fowler WC, Walton LA, Currie JL. 1000 cGy single dose palliation for advanced carcinoma of the cervix or endometrium. *Int J Radiat Oncol Biol Phys.* 1986;12:1947-1950.

60. Spanos W Jr, Guse C, Perez C, Grigsby P, Doggett RL, Poulter C. Phase II study of multiple daily fractionations in the palliation of advanced pelvic malignancies: preliminary report of RTOG 8502. *Int J Radiat Oncol Biol Phys.* 1989;17:659-661.

61. Kim DH, Lee JH, Ki YK, et al. Short-course palliative radiotherapy for uterine cervical cancer. *Radiat Oncol J.* 2013;31:216-221.

62. Sapienza LG, Ning MS, Jhingran A, et al. Short-course palliative radiation therapy leads to excellent bleeding control: a single centre retrospective study. *Clin Transl Radiat Oncol.* 2019;14:40-46.

63. Lacarriere E, Smaali C, Benyoucef A, Pfister C, Grise P. The efficacy of hemostatic radiotherapy for bladder cancer-related hematuria in patients unfit for surgery. *Int Braz J Urol.* 2013;39:808-816.

64. Jereczek-Fossa BA, Marvaso G. Palliative radiation therapy in bladder cancer: a matter of dose, techniques and patients' selection. *Ann Palliat Med.* 2019;8:786-789.

65. Johnstone C, Rich SE. Bleeding in cancer patients and its treatment: a review. *Ann Palliat Med.* 2017;7:265-273.

66. Fairchild A, Harris K, Barnes E, et al. Palliative thoracic radiotherapy for lung cancer: a systematic review. *J Clin Oncol.* 2008;26:4001-4011.

67. Rodrigues G, Videtic GM, Sur R, et al. Palliative thoracic radiotherapy in lung cancer: an American Society for Radiation Oncology evidence-based clinical practice guideline. *Pract Radiat Oncol.* 2011;1:60-71.

68. Sundstrom S, Bremnes R, Aasebo U, et al. Hypofractionated palliative radiotherapy (17 Gy per two fractions) in advanced non-small-cell lung carcinoma is comparable to standard fractionation for symptom control and survival: a national phase III trial. *J Clin Oncol.* 2004;22:801-810.

69. Jones JA, Lutz ST, Chow E, Johnstone PA. Palliative radiotherapy at the end of life: a critical review. *CA Cancer J Clin.* 2014;64:296-310.

70. Tsao MN, Rades D, Wirth A, et al. Radiotherapeutic and surgical management for newly diagnosed brain metastasis(es): An American Society for Radiation Oncology evidence-based guideline. *Pract Radiat Oncol.* 2012;2:210-225.

71. Rades D, Bohlen G, Dunst J, et al. Comparison of short-course versus long-course whole-brain radiotherapy in the treatment of brain metastases. *Strahlenther Onkol.* 2008;184:30-35.

72. Murray LJ, Din OS, Kumar VS, Dixon LM, Wadsley JC. Palliative radiotherapy in patients with esophageal carcinoma: a retrospective review. *Pract Radiat Oncol.* 2012;2:257-264.

73. Walterbos NR, Fiocco M, Neelis KJ, et al. Effectiveness of several external beam radiotherapy schedules for palliation of esophageal cancer. *Clin Transl Radiat Oncol.* 2019;17:24-31.

74. Grewal AS, Jones J, Lin A. Palliative radiation therapy for head and neck cancers. *Int J Radiat Oncol Biol Phys.* 2019;105:254-266.

75. Corry J, Peters LJ, Costa ID, et al. The 'QUAD SHOT'—a phase II study of palliative radiotherapy for incurable head and neck cancer. *Radiother Oncol.* 2005;77:137-142.

76. Stefanovski Z, Smichkoska S, Petrova D, Lazarova E. Advantages of the technique with segmented fields for tangential breast irradiation. Conference on medical physics and biomedical engineering; 2013; Macedonia, The Former Yugoslav Republic of: Association for Medical Physics and Biomedical Engineering of R. Macedonia. p. 80.

77. Ludwig V, Schwab F, Guckenberger M, Krieger T, Flentje M. Comparison of wedge versus segmented techniques in whole breast irradiation: effects on dose exposure outside the treatment volume. *Strahlenther Onkol.* 2008;184:307-312.

78. Gulyban A, Kovacs P, Sebestyen Z, et al. Multisegmented tangential breast fields: a rational way to treat breast cancer. *Strahlenther Onkol.* 2008;184:262-269.

79. J. U. Intensity modulated radiation therapy: photons. In: Khan FM, Gibbons JP, Sperduto PW, eds. *Treatment Planning in Radiation Oncology.* Philadelphia, PA: Wolters Kluwer; 2016:122-149.

80. Herman TDLF, Schnell E, Young J, et al. Dosimetric comparison between IMRT delivery modes: Step-and-shoot, sliding window, and volumetric modulated arc therapy—for whole pelvis radiation therapy of intermediate-to-high risk prostate adenocarcinoma. *J Med Phys.* 2013;38:165-172.

81. Xiao Y, Papiez L, Paulus R, et al. Dosimetric evaluation of heterogeneity corrections for RTOG 0236: stereotactic body radiotherapy of inoperable stage I-II non-small-cell lung cancer. *Int J Radiat Oncol Biol Phys.* 2009;73:1235-1242.

82. Antolak JA. Electron beam treatment planning. In: Khan FM, Gibbons JP, Sperduto PW, eds. *Khan's Treatment Planning in Radiation Oncology.* 4th ed. Philadelphia, PA: Wolters Kluwer; 2016:288-312.

83. McDermott PN, Orton CG. *Electron beam dosimetry. The Physics and Technology of Radiation Therapy.* Madison, WI: Medical Physics Publishing; 2010.

84. Yorke ED, Jackson A, Kutcher GJ. Treatment plan evaluation. In: Khan FM, Gibbons JP, Sperduto PW, eds. *Khan's Treatment Planning in Radiation Oncology.* 4th ed. Philadelpha, PA: Wolters Kluwer; 2016:377-394.

85. Bentzen SM, Constine LS, Deasy JO, et al. Quantitative analyses of normal tissue effects in the clinic (QUANTEC): an introduction to the scientific issues. *Int J Radiat Oncol Biol Phys.* 2010;76:S3-S9.

86. Bentzen SM, Parliament M, Deasy JO, et al. Biomarkers and surrogate endpoints for normal-tissue effects of radiation therapy: the importance of dose—volume effects. *Int J Radiat Oncol Biol Phys.* 2010;76:S145-S150.

87. Bhandare N, Jackson A, Eisbruch A, et al. Radiation therapy and hearing loss. *Int J Radiat Oncol Biol Phys.* 2010;76:S50-S57.

88. Dawson LA, Kavanagh BD, Paulino AC, et al. Radiation-associated kidney injury. *Int J Radiat Oncol Biol Phys.* 2010;76:S108-S115.

89. Deasy JO, Bentzen SM, Jackson A, et al. Improving normal tissue complication probability models: the need to adopt a "data-pooling" culture. *Int J Radiat Oncol Biol Phys.* 2010;76:S151-S154.

90. Deasy JO, Moiseenko V, Marks L, Chao KSC, Nam J, Eisbruch A. Radiotherapy dose-volume effects on salivary gland function. *Int J Radiat Oncol Biol Phys.* 2010;76:S58-S63.

91. Gagliardi G, Constine LS, Moiseenko V, et al. Radiation dose-volume effects in the heart. *Int J Radiat Oncol Biol Phys*. 2010;76:S77-S85.

92. Jackson A, Marks LB, Bentzen SM, et al. The lessons of QUANTEC: recommendations for reporting and gathering data on dose-volume dependencies of treatment outcome. *Int J Radiat Oncol Biol Phys*. 2010;76:S155-S160.

93. Jaffray DA, Lindsay PE, Brock KK, Deasy JO, Tomé WA. Accurate accumulation of dose for improved understanding of radiation effects in normal tissue. *Int J Radiat Oncol Biol Phys*. 2010;76:S135-S139.

94. Jeraj R, Cao Y, Ten Haken RK, Hahn C, Marks L. Imaging for assessment of radiation-induced normal tissue effects. *Int J Radiat Oncol Biol Phys*. 2010;76:S140-S144.

95. Kavanagh BD, Pan CC, Dawson LA, et al. Radiation dose-volume effects in the stomach and small bowel. *Int J Radiat Oncol Biol Phys*. 2010;76:S101-S107.

96. Kirkpatrick JP, van der Kogel AJ, Schultheiss TE. Radiation dose-volume effects in the spinal cord. *Int J Radiat Oncol Biol Phys*. 2010;76:S42-S49.

97. Lawrence YR, Li XA, el Naqa I, et al. Radiation dose-volume effects in the brain. *Int J Radiat Oncol Biol Phys*. 2010;76:S20-S27.

98. Marks LB, Bentzen SM, Deasy JO, et al. Radiation dose-volume effects in the lung. *Int J Radiat Oncol Biol Phys*. 2010;76:S70-S76.

99. Marks LB, Ten Haken RK, Martel MK. Guest editor's introduction to QUANTEC: a users guide. *Int J Radiat Oncol Biol Phys*. 2010;76:S1-S2.

100. Marks LB, Yorke ED, Jackson A, et al. Use of normal tissue complication probability models in the clinic. *Int J Radiat Oncol Biol Phys*. 2010;76:S10-S19.

101. Mayo C, Martel MK, Marks LB, Flickinger J, Nam J, Kirkpatrick J. Radiation dose-volume effects of optic nerves and chiasm. *Int J Radiat Oncol Biol Phys*. 2010;76:S28-S35.

102. Mayo C, Yorke E, Merchant TE. Radiation associated brainstem injury. *Int J Radiat Oncol Biol Phys*. 2010;76:S36-S41.

103. Michalski JM, Gay H, Jackson A, Tucker SL, Deasy JO. Radiation dose-volume effects in radiation-induced rectal injury. *Int J Radiat Oncol Biol Phys*. 2010;76:S123-S129.

104. Pan CC, Kavanagh BD, Dawson LA, et al. Radiation-associated liver injury. *Int J Radiat Oncol Biol Phys*. 2010;76:S94-S100.

105. Rancati T, Schwarz M, Allen AM, et al. Radiation dose-volume effects in the larynx and pharynx. *Int J Radiat Oncol Biol Phys*. 2010;76:S64-S69.

106. Roach M III, Nam J, Gagliardi G, El Naqa I, Deasy JO, Marks LB. Radiation dose-volume effects and the penile bulb. *Int J Radiat Oncol Biol Phys*. 2010;76:S130-S134.

107. Viswanathan AN, Yorke ED, Marks LB, Eifel PJ, Shipley WU. Radiation dose-volume effects of the urinary bladder. *Int J Radiat Oncol Biol Phys*. 2010;76:S116-S122.

108. Werner-Wasik M, Yorke E, Deasy J, Nam J, Marks LB. Radiation dose-volume effects in the esophagus. *Int J Radiat Oncol Biol Phys*. 2010;76:S86-S93.

109. Fraass B, Doppke K, Hunt M, et al. American Association of Physicists in Medicine Radiation Therapy Committee Task Group 53: quality assurance for clinical radiotherapy treatment planning. *Med Phys*. 1998;25:1773-1829.

110. INTERNATIONAL ATOMIC ENERGY AGENCY, Commissioning and Quality Assurance of Computerized Planning Systems for Radiation Treatment of Cancer, Technical Reports Series No. 430, IAEA, Vienna, Austria; 2004.

111. INTERNATIONAL ATOMIC ENERGY AGENCY, Specification and Acceptance Testing of Radiotherapy Treatment Planning Systems, IAEA-TECDOC-1540, IAEA, Vienna, Austria; 2007.

112. INTERNATIONAL ATOMIC ENERGY AGENCY, Commissioning of Radiotherapy Treatment Planning Systems: Testing for Typical External Beam Treatment Techniques, IAEA-TECDOC-1583, IAEA, Vienna, Austria; 2008.

113. Kavanaugh JA, Klein EE, Mutic S, Van Dyk J. Commissioning and quality assurance. In: Khan FM, Gibbons JP, Sperduto PW, eds. *Khan's Treatment Planning in Radiation Oncology*. 4th ed. Philadelphia, PA: Wolters Kluwer; 2016:98-121.

114. McDermott PN, Orton CG. *Special Modalities in Radiation Therapy. The Physics and Technology of Radiation Therapy*. Madison, WI: Medical Physics Publishing; 2010.

115. Baker SJ, Budgell GJ, MacKay RI. Use of an amorphous silicon electronic portal imaging device for multileaf collimator quality control and calibration. *Phys Med Biol*. 2005;50:1377-1392.

116. Li G, Mageras, GS, Dong L, Mohan R. Image-guided radiation therapy. In: Khan FM, Gibbons JP, Sperduto PW, eds. *Khan's Treatment Planning in Radiation Oncology*. 4th ed. Philadelphia, PA: Wolters Kluwer; 2016:177-202.

117. Boda-Heggemann J, Lohr F, Wenz F, Flentje M, Guckenberger M. kV cone-beam CT-based IGRT: a clinical review. *Strahlenther Onkol*. 2011;187:284-291.

118. Jaffray DA, Siewerdsen JH, Wong JW, Martinez AA. Flat-panel cone-beam computed tomography for image-guided radiation therapy. *Int J Radiat Oncol Biol Phys*. 2002;53:1337-1349.

119. Sonke JJ, Zijp L, Remeijer P, van Herk M. Respiratory correlated cone beam CT. *Med Phys*. 2005;32:1176-1186.

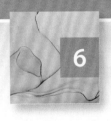

6 Pathophysiology of Chemotherapy-Induced Peripheral Neuropathy

Xiao-Min Wang, Jane M. Fall-Dickson, Zhang-Jin Zhang, and Tanya J. Lehky

INTRODUCTION

Chemotherapy-induced peripheral neuropathy (CIPN) is a common dose-limiting side effect of taxanes, platinum compounds, vinca alkaloids, epothilones, bortezomib, thalidomide, lenalidomide, and more recently, checkpoint inhibitors (1,2). CIPN commonly occurs in 30% to 40% of patients undergoing chemotherapy treatment, ranging from 10% to 90% of patients (3). The incidence is dependent on type of chemotherapy, CIPN assessment used, and timing of the assessment (4). CIPN is one of the main reasons that patients decide to stop chemotherapy treatment before completion. Early termination of chemotherapy limits the ability of oncologists to administer the optimal and aggressive regimens that improve cancer survival (3,5–7). Thus, CIPN remains a challenging treatment sequela for both patients and clinicians. For patients, CIPN can be a life-long burden, particularly for younger cancer survivors. Health-related quality of life is impaired in patients with CIPN because of associated fatigue, psychological distress, inability to work, and increased health care utilization. Although a variety of neuroprotective approaches have been investigated in both experimental studies and clinical trials, there is no available preventive strategy or effective treatment for CIPN because its etiology has not been fully elucidated. Therefore, defining the mechanisms of CIPN is critical to develop preventive and treatment strategies and to enhance health-related quality of life.

Most chemotherapeutic drugs penetrate the blood–brain barrier poorly but readily penetrate the blood–nerve barrier (BNB) and preferentially accumulate within the dorsal root ganglia (DRG) and peripheral nerves (8). This mechanism of action may be related in part to the relative deficiency and higher permeability of the BNB at the areas of the dorsal root ganglion (DRG) and nerve terminals (9). Additionally, endoneurial compartments have no lymphatic system to remove toxins (10). These factors increase peripheral nerve vulnerabilities to toxicity when compared with the central nervous system (CNS). Thus, chemotherapy-induced neurotoxicity mainly targets the peripheral nervous system (PNS) and manifests as peripheral neuropathies. Although there are cases of CNS toxicity manifesting as encephalopathy, these cases are rare and mostly unpredictable (11). For this reason, this chapter focuses mainly on chemotherapy-induced neuropathophysiology in the PNS, focusing on the localized lesions, followed by description of the known mechanisms underlying CIPN.

WHAT IS CIPN?

CIPN is primarily a polyneuropathy, with simultaneous malfunction of many peripheral nerves. The symptoms most commonly associated with CIPN are related to sensory neuropathy with mild limb weakness frequently noted on examination. Numbness, burning, tingling, pain, and weakness in the limbs are the most common symptoms reported to oncologists. The onset of symptoms can be subacute, such as paclitaxel acute pain syndrome (P-APS) (12), or may gradually progress over time. Initially, patients frequently feel abnormal positive symptoms including tingling, burning pain, or negative symptoms of numbness. These symptoms often start symmetrically in the toes and fingers and spread proximally in a "stocking and glove" distribution. Many patients complain of difficulty in walking due to loss of sensation in the feet and not able to pick up small items because of numbness in the fingertips. Chemotherapy may also affect the autonomic nervous system with anhidrosis in the limbs. Dysfunction of the autonomic nervous system can affect gastrointestinal (GI) motility and cause orthostatic intolerance. The incidence and severity of CIPN is influenced by multiple factors, including chemotherapy dose intensity, cumulative chemotherapy dose, duration of infusion, and combination regimen, as well as, age and preexisting conditions, such as diabetes, vitamin B_{12} deficiency, alcohol abuse, and prior chemotherapy exposure. Additionally, it is well-known that people with Charcot-Marie-Tooth (CMT) disease have severe worsening of their inherited neuropathy following treatment with vincristine. Advancing genetics research has led to preliminary evidence that additional genetic factors may also play a role in the incidence and severity of CIPN (13,14).

CIPN presents with unique clinical characteristics that are different from those seen with peripheral nerve injury in diabetes, metabolic neuropathy, or trauma. Table 6.1 summarizes the

TABLE 6.1 CHARACTERISTICS OF PERIPHERAL NEUROPATHY INDUCED BY COMMON CHEMOTHERAPEUTIC AGENTS

	Taxanes (Paclitaxel, Docetaxel)	Platinum (Cisplatin, Carboplatin, Oxaliplatin)	Vinca Alkaloids (Vincristine, Vinblastine, Vinorelbine, Vindesine)	Bortezomib	Thalidomide
Anticancer drugs					
Treatment	Breast, ovarian, non-small cell lung cancer	Testicular, ovarian, lung, bladder, colorectal cancers	Hematological cancers Pediatric sarcomas	Multiple myeloma	Multiple myeloma
Incidence	30%–60% (overall)	30%–100% (overall) Early (90%),[a] late (60%)[b]	30%–50% (overall)	30%–55% (overall) 10%–20% (severe)	25%–80% (overall) 28% (severe)
Symptoms	Symmetrical painful paresthesias or numbness in a stocking-glove distribution, sensory loss Motor symptoms at high dose	Symmetrical painful paresthesias or numbness in a stocking-glove distribution Early: cold allodynia and hyperalgesia Later: loss of motor function Long-term chronic sensory neuropathy	Symmetrical sensorimotor painful neuropathy: tingling paresthesias, proprioceptive loss, areflexia, and ataxia Constipation Muscle weakness Gait dysfunction	Hallmark: sensory painful neuropathy, resistant to treatment	Symmetrical distal paresthesias, dysesthesias Sensory painful neuropathy Muscle cramps
Main toxic targets	Axons and Schwann cells	Dorsal root ganglia	Axons	Axons	Axon Dorsal root ganglia
Possible mechanisms	Microtubule disruption Mitochondrial dysfunction Neurofilament accumulation DRG damage Damage blood supply to PNS	Bind to DNA adducts → apoptosis Anterograde axonal neuropathy Myelin sheath damage Channelopathy (Na^+, Ca^{2+}, K^+) Damage blood supply to PNS	Dysfunctions of mitochondria and endoplasmic reticulum Microtubule disruption Autoimmune Inflammation	Binds to the proteasome complex, leading to cell cycle interruption and apoptosis Mitochondrial disturbance Microtubule disruption	Antiangiogenesis Direct toxic effects on the DRG Neurotrophin dysregulation
Molecular genetic profiles	Matrix metalloproteinase-3 and CD163 IL-1, TNF, and CD11b Voltage-dependent calcium channel $\alpha_2\delta$-1 (**dorsal spinal cord**) ITGBL1	TRPM8 Voltage-dependent calcium channel $\alpha_2\delta$-1 (DRG)	TRPM8 ITGBL1, AURKA, MK167	RHOBTB2, CPCT1C ITGBL1, SOX8	
Single-nucleotide polymorphisms	ABCB1	ERCC1, GSTP1, C118T, GSTP1	PARP1, LTA, GLI1 ABCC1, DPYD, *ADRB2*, *CAMKK1*, *CYP2C9*, *NFATC2*, *ID3*, *SLC10A2*, *CYP2C8*	ALOX12, IGF1R, SOD2, MYO5A, MBL2, PPARD, ERCC4, ERCC3	ABCA1, ICAM, PPARD, *SLC12A6*, SERPINB2, SLC12A6, *LIG4*

aEarly onset—after first cycle of induction of treatment.
bLate onset—after two to three cycles of induction treatment.
DRG, dorsal root ganglia; PNS, peripheral nervous system; IL-1, interleukin 1; TNF, tumor necrosis factor.

characteristics of peripheral neuropathy induced by the most commonly used chemotherapeutic agents. These features include the following:

1. Chemotherapy-related neuropathic pain can often simultaneously begin in the hands and feet because of toxicity to the DRG. This is different from typical neuropathic pain associated with diabetes, which causes a length-dependent painful neuropathy that initially affects the feet.

2. The most common clinical presentation is sensory symptoms of pain, tingling, and numbness, rather than motor symptoms. The severity of symptoms is dose-dependent, with higher doses of a chemotherapeutic agent leading to worsening of symptoms. The neuropathic symptoms can progress after chemotherapy is stopped, in a phenomenon called "coasting" observed with platinum-based drugs.

3. Chemotherapeutic drugs are associated with different types of neuropathy depending on their mechanism of action; cisplatin causes sensory neuropathies because of DRG toxicity, while vincristine causes sensory and motor neuropathies due to diffuse damage of microtubules in the axons. Histological findings have indicated that, unlike painful peripheral neuropathies due to trauma and diabetes, CIPN-related pain can occur in the absence of axonal degeneration in peripheral nerves. This may be an effect of inflammatory cytokines, ion-channel perturbations, and effect on pain receptors.

4. Known onset and extent of neuronal or nerve injury induced by chemotherapeutic drugs provides an opportunity for translational work through both basic and clinical research to test prevention clinical trials for CIPN.

PATHOPHYSIOLOGY OF CIPN

Various CIPN mechanisms have been proposed based on the findings of in vitro and in vivo animal models. However, the pathophysiology of CIPN has not yet been fully established and can vary with different classifications of chemotherapeutic agents. An elucidation of the underlying mechanisms of peripheral neuropathy is imperative to identify potential targets for the prevention and treatment of CIPN. At the histological level, it has been generally accepted that chemotherapeutic drugs commonly induce (a) axonopathy or distal axonal neuropathy, causing a "dying back" axonal degeneration; (b) ganglionopathy, affecting cell bodies in the DRG; and (c) myelinopathy with primary segmental demyelination (15). At the cellular level, chemotherapeutic agents damage microtubules and interfere with microtubule-based axonal transport; interrupt mitochondrial function;

or directly target DNA (16). Peripheral nerve degeneration or small fiber neuropathy occurs that leads to sensitization and spontaneous activity of these fibers through an increase in voltage-gated sodium and calcium channels, which then facilitates the release of substance P and glutamate and leads to hyperexcitability of these fibers. Figure 6.1 illustrates the proposed targets of chemotherapy-induced neurotoxicity in the PNS.

Taxane compounds, including paclitaxel and docetaxel, bind to β-tubulin subunits, stabilize polymerization, and interfere with microtubule dynamics. Tubulin is a primary component of microtubules and the basis of cellular cytoskeletal structure. Microtubules are fundamental to axonal transport processes, providing trophic factors and energy for the long axons of peripheral nerves. In vitro, paclitaxel exposure induces marked microtubule aggregation in large myelinated axons (17) and DRG (18), and correspondingly, paclitaxel interferes with anterograde axonal transport (19). It has been postulated that taxanes elicit neurotoxic action through interaction with microtubules in the long axons of peripheral nerves, perhaps because microtubules are the key components in axonal transport. Thus, microtubule damage and subsequent dysfunction of axonal transport have long been associated with taxane-induced axonopathy (20).

Vinca alkaloid compounds include vincristine, vinblastine, vinorelbine, vindesine, and vinflunine. Axonal sensorimotor neuropathy induced by vincristine often occurs early during treatment and manifests itself by paresthesias followed by motor weakness. Histological studies show that vincristine causes lesions of axonal degeneration in both small and large fibers by disorientation of microtubules and disruption of the myelin sheath, leading to a decrease in nerve conduction velocity (21). Vincristine-induced neuropathic pain is characterized by abnormal spontaneous discharges in the A-fiber and C-fiber primary afferent neurons (22), but pain is not always a prominent feature of vincristine-induced peripheral neuropathy (23).

Similar to taxanes, vinca alkaloids bind to tubulin and inhibit microtubule dynamics (24). The affinity for tubulin differs among vinca alkaloid compounds (vincristine, vinblastine, vinorelbine, and vinflunine in descending order). As a result, vincristine produces significant alterations in axonal cytoskeletal structure, including microtubule disorientation and neurofilament accumulation (25,26), which contribute to interruption of axonal transport (27) and result in Wallerian-like axonal degeneration and axonopathy (25,26,28). In addition, these compounds have also been reported to produce direct axonal toxicity in vitro (29). Both taxanes and vinca alkaloids affect the stability of

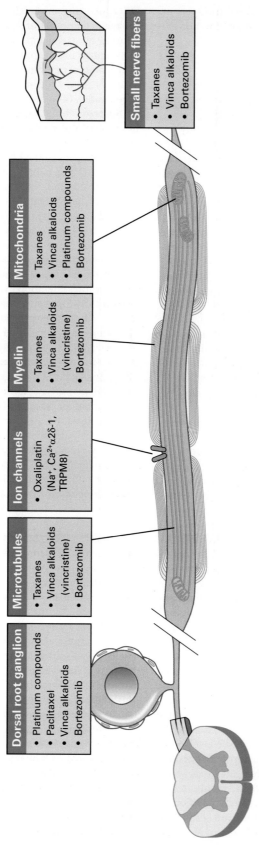

Dorsal root ganglion
- Platinum compounds
- Paclitaxel
- Vinca alkaloids
- Bortezomib

Microtubules
- Taxanes
- Vinca alkaloids (vincristine)
- Bortezomib

Ion channels
- Oxaliplatin (Na$^+$, Ca^{2+}α2δ-1, TRPM8)

Myelin
- Taxanes
- Vinca alkaloids (vincristine)
- Bortezomib

Mitochondria
- Taxanes
- Vinca alkaloids
- Platinum compounds
- Bortezomib

Small nerve fibers
- Taxanes
- Vinca alkaloids
- Bortezomib

Figure 6.1 A proposed diagram illustrating the targets of most commonly used chemotherapy-induced neurotoxicity in the peripheral nervous system.

microtubules and disrupt the axonal transport of growth factors and molecules essential to normal nerve function.

Platinum compounds, including cisplatin, carboplatin, and oxaliplatin, predominantly target and accumulate in the DRG. This preferential accumulation might be partially due to the relative deficiency of the BNB in peripheral nerves, especially in the DRG area, and their high affinity for the DRG cells (30). These compounds form DNA intrastrand adducts and interstrand cross-links that lead to DNA derangement, morphologic changes, and subsequent apoptosis (31,32). Platinum compounds exert direct damage on neurons and non-neuronal cells in the DRG, and the levels of platinum in DRG of treated patients correlate with the severity of CIPN (16,33–35). Histological study reveals axonal loss associated with a secondary DRG atrophy. Therefore, platinum compound-associated symptoms, such as cisplatin-induced peripheral neuropathy, are described as a primary sensory neuronopathy rather than an axonopathy (36). Other effects of platinum compounds include oxidative stress and mitochondria dysfunction triggering neuronal apoptosis (37). Cisplatin can also disrupt axonal microtubule growth that may also contribute to the cisplatin-induced peripheral neuropathy (38).

The platinum compounds, specifically cisplatin, share the "coasting" phenomenon in which symptoms and clinical signs often do not start until the end of treatment or continually worsen even after the cessation of treatment (39). This particularly troublesome aspect of cisplatin neurotoxicity prevents timely discontinuation of treatment in most patients with chemotherapy-induced neurotoxicity. Oxaliplatin-induced peripheral neuropathy has a distinctive spectrum of symptoms in addition to chronic presentations. Oxaliplatin also provokes an acute, cold-induced, and transient syndrome characterized by paresthesias in the distal extremities and perioral region that usually appear during infusion or within hours after infusion, and last 1 to 2 days. This acute transient neurotoxicity occurs in nearly all patients (82% to 92% of all neurotoxicity grades) (33). It is thought that the acute form of oxaliplatin toxicity may be associated with transit dysfunction of nodal axonal sodium or potassium channels leading to the neurophysiological finding of neuromyotonia (40). More precisely, oxalate, an oxaliplatin metabolite, is thought to be involved in the cold hyperalgesia, due to calcium or magnesium chelation by oxalate released from the drug, which adversely affects ion channels and synaptic transmission (41,42). Additionally, gene expression of transient receptor potential melastatin 8 (TRPM8, a cold thermal sensor channel) is increased in mouse DRG following oxaliplatin treatment, suggesting the mediating effect of TRPM8 on cold allodynia induced by oxaliplatin (43). Alteration of axonal ion channels may be responsible for the immediate neuropathic symptoms following oxaliplatin treatment and, over time, may result in chronic axonal degeneration (44).

Bortezomib, a novel proteasome inhibitor, induces painful sensory neuropathy with moderate or severe neurotoxicity reported in up to 30% of patients. The clinical hallmark of bortezomib-induced CIPN is painful sensory neuropathy that can be severe and resistant to treatment. Similar to other chemotherapeutic agents, bortezomib-induced motor impairment occurs occasionally. Neurophysiologic evaluation reveals a deficit of three major nerve fibers, A-β, A-δ, and C fibers, in patients with bortezomib-induced pain (45). In animal models, short-term treatment with bortezomib causes alteration in both DRG and peripheral nerves (46), whereas long-term treatment with bortezomib induces peripheral nerve axonopathy characterized by small fiber neuropathy (47).

Bortezomib is an inhibitor of proteasomes. The proteasome pathway facilitates the destruction of ubiquitinated protein and is critical for normal cellular activity (48). Bortezomib binds to the proteasome complex, leading to cell cycle interruption and apoptosis. Because of the importance of the proteasome pathway, bortezomib may exert neurotoxicity via multiple mechanisms, such as protein aggregation and cytoskeletal damage in DRG neurons (49), disruption in tubulin polymerization leading to axonal loss (50,51), and mitochondrial disturbance and injury in Schwann cells that lead to demyelination (46). In a preclinical animal model, exposure to bortezomib caused pathological lesions in Schwann cells and myelin with intracytoplasmic vacuolization (46). A more severe demyelination neuropathy has been described with a combination therapy of bortezomib and thalidomide (52). In addition, recent studies also suggest that bortezomib inhibits some cytokines and transcription factors, including nuclear factor-kappa B (NF-κB) (53). The NF-κB cell signaling pathway is involved in the promotion of neuronal survival (54). Thus, bortezomib, interfering with this pathway, leads to cell cycle arrest, apoptosis, and angiogenesis inhibition (55).

There are several examples of the basic mechanisms in which specific chemotherapeutic agents can cause axonal damage and peripheral neuropathy. Although these mechanisms of chemotherapy-induced neurotoxicity differ among classes of chemotherapeutic agents, all neurotoxic chemotherapeutic agents cause a common sensory disruption leading to painful paresthesias. These mechanisms alone do not explain the development of acutely painful neuropathies that occur even prior to the pathological loss of axons or alterations in the diagnostic testing for neuropathy. Thus, the common sensory disruption induced by these chemotherapeutic agents may result from a shared mechanism that is most probably not specifically associated with their antineoplastic mechanisms. Mitochondrial dysfunction and inflammatory cytokines may be additional critical factors in the induction of CIPN.

Thalidomide, a glutamic acid derivative, is generally associated with a length-dependent predominantly sensory neuropathy (56–58). It may also be associated with motor and autonomic neuropathies. Thalidomide-related CIPN is very dose-dependent, with cumulative doses of 20 g having high rates of CIPN, which limits its use. The newer analogues, lenalidomide and pomalidomide, have less neurotoxicity. The mechanism of action in CIPN is not well-understood though it is known to inhibit tumor necrosis factor-alpha (TNF-α) and block NF-κB. Inhibition of NF-κB has a negative effect on sensory neuron survival (59) and may be a potential cause of the thalidomide-related CIPN.

Check-point inhibitors include ipilimumab, nivolumab, and pembrolizumab. They are designed to inhibit the association of the program death ligand 1 (PDL-1) protein on the tumor cell with the receptor, programmed cell death protein (PD-1) on T-cells. This inhibition enhances the body's ability to mount an immune response to the tumor and induce apoptosis. Checkpoint inhibitors can induce a wide-range of autoimmune disorders including peripheral neuropathies (1). The most common neuropathy is a demyelinating neuropathy, either Guillain-Barré syndrome or chronic inflammatory demyelinating polyneuropathy. Acute painful axonal neuropathies have also been observed (1). Immune-mediated demyelination and cellular infiltration is the proposed mechanism for checkpoint inhibitor–related neuropathies (60).

MITOCHONDRIAL DYSFUNCTION CONTRIBUTION TO CIPN

Recent data from clinical and experimental studies indicate that interference with the energy mechanisms of axons through damage to mitochondria may play an important role in chemotherapy-induced neurotoxicity, particularly in the painful sensory disruption. Mitochondrial dysfunction and dysregulation of Ca^{2+} homeostasis have been implicated in chemotherapy-induced neurotoxicity because intracellular Ca^{2+} level plays an essential role in axonal degeneration via initiation of a cascade of damaging cellular processes. Paclitaxel,

vincristine, and oxaliplatin cause prominent abnormalities in axonal mitochondria, including swelling (61) and microtubule–mitochondrial aggregation (62). Bortezomib influences mitochondrial and endoplasmic reticulum integrity in animal models, particularly in myelin-producing Schwann cells, which leads to myelin sheath degeneration and myelinopathy (46,50). Recent research has confirmed the presence of defects in mitochondrial respiratory complexes I and II in peripheral nerves taken from rats with painful peripheral neuropathy after treatment with paclitaxel and oxaliplatin-induced peripheral neuropathy (63).

Energy depletion and deficiency leads to oxygen consumption and adenosine triphosphate (ATP) product decrease in axons that result in dysfunction of the energy-dependent Na/K-ATP pump. The energy-dependent Na/K-ATP pump is the key component in maintaining the normal membrane resting/action potential. Impaired mitochondrial function causes energy deficit and subsequently results in the abnormal spontaneous discharge of A-fiber and C-fiber that accounts for the sensation of pain and dysesthesia. In animal models, treatment with acetyl-L-carnitine (ALC), an agent synthesized in the mitochondria and known to improve mitochondrial function (64), decreases the spontaneous discharges of A-fiber and C-fiber and also prevents and reverses painful CIPN (22,61,65). In clinical trials, the efficacy of ALC has been demonstrated through reduction in the severity of existing sensory peripheral neuropathy in patients treated with paclitaxel or cisplatin (66). There have been randomized, placebo-controlled trials that investigated the intervention effects of ALC on painful peripheral neuropathy induced by paclitaxel or sagopilone in breast or prostate cancer patients that showed reduced severity of neuropathic symptoms (67,68).

INFLAMMATORY CYTOKINES: A TARGET FOR CIPN

Emerging data in clinical and experimental studies strongly support the critical role of pro-inflammatory cytokines in the development and persistence of peripheral neuropathic pain (69–72). This mechanism is probably initiated with infiltration of immune cells into the PNS and subsequent interactions of macrophages and T lymphocytes with neurons and their satellite cells in DRG, as well as Schwann cells. The end result is release of cytokines and chemokines into the peripheral nerve milieu. As an example, administration of paclitaxel and oxaliplatin shows notable changes in the neurons and surrounding satellite cells in the DRG and peripheral nerves accompanied by behavioral changes such as allodynia and hyperalgesia. Both drugs up-regulate the CD4+ and CD8+ T-cells though more notable increase in chemokines with paclitaxel (73). These pathological changes also include increased expression of activating transcription factor 3 (ATF3) in both neuronal and nonneuronal cells in DRG, peripheral nerves, and Schwann cells. ATF3 is a marker of nerve injury and was observed in neuronal nuclei in DRG of paclitaxel-treated rats (18,74–76). In animal models, the increased ATF3 expression occurred as early as 1 day after paclitaxel infusion, which is the time point patients first report pain in the course of P-APS. Interestingly, it appears that the initial intensity of acute pain in P-APS predicts the severity of symptoms associated with sensory peripheral neuropathy, specifically, the severity of burning and shooting pain at the later phase (12).

Macrophage infiltration in response to chemotherapy-induced injury leads to a subsequent production and secretion of various cytokines (TNF-α, interleukin [IL]-1β, IL-6, and IL-8), chemokine C-C motif ligand 2 (CCL2) and characteristically heparin-binding proteins (CXC family), growth factors, and inflammatory mediators such as bradykinin, prostaglandins, serotonin, and nitric oxide (NO), which are the potential mediators for the development of peripheral neuropathy (77). These molecules promote continued neuroinflammation through recruitment of macrophages (78). TNF-α and IL-1β can directly sensitize nociceptors and increase axonal spontaneous discharges by directly stimulating A-fiber and C-fiber (79). Intrathecal injection of IL-1ra and IL-10 gene therapy suppresses the expression of TNF-α and IL-1β in DRGs and attenuates paclitaxel-induced neuropathic pain in animal experiments (80,81). The antinociceptive effect of IL-10 may be associated with its inhibitory effect on the expression of TNF-α and IL-1β, as well as, through inducible nitric oxide (NO) synthase (82,83). These findings provide evidence that proinflammatory cytokines, chemokines, and their receptors and signaling pathways are involved in the development of chemotherapy-induced neuropathic pain. Therefore, characterization of cytokine and chemokine expression after chemotherapy might yield a new insight into the development of CIPN and elucidate targets for the development of effective prevention or treatment strategies for CIPN.

In summary, the release of proinflammatory cytokines/chemokines by activated macrophages, satellite cells in the DRG, and Schwann cells may be the primary cause of pain in CIPN, which is an early sign of initial peripheral neuropathy in most cancer patients undergoing chemotherapy treatment. Therefore, targeting the production

of proinflammatory cytokines may be a promising therapeutic strategy for prevention or relief of CIPN, especially for pain. Extracellular matrix metalloproteinases (MMPs) control the integrity of the BNB, myelin protein turnover, and phenotypic remodeling of glia and neurons. The specific role of MMPs in the pathogenesis of painful peripheral neuropathy is believed to relate to their control of cytokine release. Pharmacologic inhibition of MMPs or administration of small interfering RNA for MMPs produced immediate and sustained attenuation of mechanical allodynia (84,85). Treatment with the MMP inhibitor GM6001 or minocycline significantly reduced the mechanical allodynia after nerve injury (85,86). Minocycline, a broad-spectrum tetracycline antibiotic, has been reported to attenuate neuropathic pain (87) by inhibition of MMP3 up-regulation, macrophage accumulation, and proinflammatory cytokine release in the paclitaxel-treated rats. Treatment with minocycline effectively prevents both taxol-induced mechanical hyperalgesia and intraepidermal nerve fiber (IENF) loss in rats (86). Its inhibitory effect on cytokine release has been reported to be associated with its suppression of the NF-κ pathway (88). Therefore, minocycline protects against cytokine-related damage to axons and Schwann cells (89). However, its inhibitory effect seems most effective when treatment begins prior to nerve injury (90) because that minocycline does not reverse existing hypersensitivity after nerve injury (91). Pretreatment with minocycline inhibits macrophage infiltration and activation, suppresses ATF3 expression in DRGs, and partially blocks the loss of IENFs (86,92). Therefore, it is not difficult to understand its preventive effect on the mechanical allodynia and hyperalgesia induced by chemotherapeutic drugs (92,93) and the potential promising role for minocycline in CIPN.

EPIGENETIC REGULATION OF CIPN

A recent study reported that the incidence of developing CIPN is significantly decreased in patients concurrently treated with chemotherapy and valproic acid (VPA), a nonselective histone deacetylase (HDAC) inhibitor (94). Emerging evidence suggests that the development of neuropathic pain involves epigenetic modulation, and up-regulation of HDACs has been linked to impaired synaptic plasticity (95) and neuropathic pain (96).

It is worth noting that only 1% to 7% of all genes are found to be regulated by HDACs and that all excitatory amino acid transporters (EAATs) that have been studied to date are regulated by HDACs (97,98). In the spinal dorsal horn, glutamate is the dominant excitatory neurotransmitter released synaptically by primary afferent terminals, excitatory neurons, and descending terminals from supraspinal regions (99). The synaptically released glutamate is rapidly taken up by EAATs, to ensure high-fidelity sensory transmission, preventing nonsynaptic neuronal excitation, and hyperactivity. Excessive glutamate in synaptic clefts results in neuronal excitotoxicity that contributes to synaptic plasticity and central sensitization leading to neuropathic pain (97,100). EAATs serve to terminate the excitatory signal by clearance of excessive glutamate and maintain optimal glutamatergic homeostasis. Preclinical studies have shown that both excitatory amino acid transporter 2 (EAAT2/GLT-1) and vesicular-glutamate transporter 2 (VGLUT2) in the spinal dorsal horn are involved in the development and maintenance of CIPN. EAAT2 is the most abundant type expressed in the spinal dorsal and accounts for over 80% of synaptic glutamate clearance (100). Whereas VGLUT2, highly expressed in axon terminals of unmyelinated primary afferent fibers in lamina I-II (101,102), is responsible for active release and transport of glutamate into synaptic clefts. Dysregulation of EAAT2 and VGLUT2 have been reported to play the essential role in the initiation and maintenance of CIPN. HDACs have been shown to down-regulate EAAT2 and VPA reversed HDAC-induced down-regulation of EAAT2. Therefore, HDAC inhibitors might be a potential new class of drugs to be used as analgesics to target the development of CIPN (103). Furthermore, considering the significances of HDAC inhibitors in suppressing cancer cells, increasing the sensitivity of cancer cells to chemotherapeutic drugs, and attenuating cancer-associated chronic pain, developing HDAC inhibitors to treat CIPN will benefit cancer management in multiple dimensions.

DIAGNOSTIC TESTING FOR CIPN

Different methodologies can be used to diagnose and evaluate severity of CIPN. Oncologic clinical trials frequently rely on patient-reported outcomes such as the Common Terminology Criteria for Adverse Events (CTCAE) to determine the presence of CIPN although it may not be the most sensitive measure of CIPN (4). Other patient reported outcomes include the Total Neuropathy Scale (TNS), Patient Neurotoxicity Questionnaire (PNQ), fatigue scales, and quality of life measures such as the SF-36 questionnaire (4). Although these are important outcome measures, they are not designed to quantify the degree on nerve injury. Clinical evaluation of motor strength, sensory examination, and deep tendon reflexes provide

some objective measures of nerve function. Nerve conduction studies are the most frequent neurophysiologic test performed for CIPN. Although very reproducible, nerve conduction studies have a slight delay in detecting nerve injury (104) and are limited to evaluation of large diameter nerve fibers. Thus, they are not sensitive to small-fiber neuropathies and may correlate poorly with patient reported paresthesias and pain (105). Several other methodologies have been assessed for evaluating CIPN (106). Quantitative sensory testing (QST) is a psychobiometric technique that measures vibration, and cool and heat-pain thresholds and has been used to assess CIPN in clinical trials. Skin biopsies for intraepidermal nerve fiber density (IENFD) is sensitive to detecting small fiber neuropathies but is limited by the number of times a biopsy can be obtained. Autonomic testing, including QSART, which is a test of sympathetic sweat function in the limbs and another test for small fiber neuropathy, has not been found to be sensitive in the diagnosis of CIPN. There are newer techniques of laser-evoked potentials and corneal confocal microscopy that may be useful in the diagnosis of CIPN. Also, nerve imaging, either with MRI neurography or high-resolution ultrasound, could be used in the future to evaluate neuropathies.

In addition to diagnostic techniques, biomarkers can be used in clinical practice as diagnostic and prognostic tools to identify diseases and to monitor disease activity and treatment response. Cytokines and proinflammatory proteins could be potential biomarkers to predict the onset of CIPN and identify the early damage of axons (107), but more research is needed before these biomarkers are clinically useful.

POTENTIAL TREATMENT MODALITIES OF CIPN

CIPN results from the cumulative effect of chemotherapy on mitochondrial function, oxidative stress, ion channel activation, and up-regulation of proinflammatory cytokines resulting in nerve injury (108). It is reasonable to target these mechanisms for treatment of CIPN. Antioxidants such as glutathione prevent the accumulation of platinum adducts with DNA although it has not been shown to reduce platinum-based neurotoxicity. Ion channel targeted therapies including lidocaine and mexiletine reduce allodynia in rat models, but there is lesser evidence in human studies. Calcium and magnesium infusions inhibit Na channels but also have limited effect in preventing CIPN and may affect efficacy of chemotherapeutic agents. Anti-inflammatory agents, metformin and minocycline, and antioxidants, amifostine and mangafodipir have limited efficacy and can have dose-limiting side effects. Neurotransmitter-based therapy includes the commonly used antidepressants and epileptic medication used in the treatment of symptoms of painful neuropathy. Of all these targeted therapies, duloxetine, a combined serotonin and norepinephrine inhibitor, is the only drug that has been clinically proven to be effective in alleviating symptoms of CIPN although other agents, such as venlafaxine in this category may have some degree of efficacy. None of these agents have shown any efficacy in preventing CIPN (109).

Alternative therapies have been explored for treating CIPN though there are limited controlled studies. Vitamin E, L-glutamine, goshajinkigan, and omega-3 fatty acids have shown some benefit in small clinical trials (110). One nutraceutical, ALC, appears to be detrimental to CIPN when administered during chemotherapy treatment. Two studies showed a positive effect of acupuncture in alleviating pain symptoms (111). Massage, mind–body practice, and exercise may have beneficial effects on CIPN but lack controlled studies.

APPROACH TO THE PATIENT WITH CIPN

Common approaches to treating the CIPN would be an initial trial of duloxetine, which is a combined serotoninergic and norepinephrine inhibitor and with a known clinical efficacy in CIPN (112). Venlafaxine, which also is a combined serotonergic and norepinephrine inhibitor, may be another consideration. Other antidepressants such as amitriptyline, desipramine, and nortriptyline could also be considered although the anticholinergic side effects may be intolerable. Another frequent treatment of CIPN is the use of gabapentin, or pregabalin. Clinical studies show these two agents have modest effects in CIPN (113), and thus, this class of drugs is considered if duloxetine is not tolerated or is not providing relief of symptoms. Topical salves containing lidocaine, salicylates, or capsaicin could be used to complement oral medication or when oral medications are not tolerated (114). Complementary therapy such as acupuncture (115) shows some benefit in CIPN and could be used in addition to other treatment modalities. Other complementary practices such as massage, yoga, meditation, and prescribed exercise may also be incorporated into CIPN treatment (110). Most of the complementary therapy modalities lack valid controlled clinical trials to demonstrate efficacy but are generally safe and easy to administer to patients as adjuncts to more traditional medications. If the neuropathy is related to a checkpoint-inhibitor and likely immune-mediated, then immunomodulation with steroids or intravenous immunoglobulin (IVIG) should be considered (1).

CONCLUSION

CIPN presents a unique manifestation of the precise time and extent of neuronal or nerve injury induced by chemotherapeutic agents and provides opportunities to conduct preemptive trials in the preclinical and clinical setting. If CIPN can be blocked or attenuated by a preventative therapy, it is more likely that a full and more aggressive chemotherapy regimen can be administered and completed. The combined effect will be to increase the survival rate of patients with cancer treated with these agents and enhance these patients' HR-QOL because of less residual CIPN.

REFERENCES

1. Gu Y, Menzies AM, Long GV, Fernando SL, Herkes G. Immune mediated neuropathy following checkpoint immunotherapy. *J Clin Neurosci.* 2017;45:14-17.
2. Zajaczkowska R, Kocot-Kepska M, Leppert W, Wrzosek A, Mika J, Wordliczek J. Mechanisms of chemotherapy-induced peripheral neuropathy. *Int J Mol Sci.* 2019;20(6):1451.
3. Wolf S, Barton D, Kottschade L, Grothey A, Loprinzi C. Chemotherapy-induced peripheral neuropathy: prevention and treatment strategies. *Eur J Cancer.* 2008;44(11):1507-1515.
4. Molassiotis A, Cheng HL, Lopez V, et al. Are we misestimating chemotherapy-induced peripheral neuropathy? Analysis of assessment methodologies from a prospective, multinational, longitudinal cohort study of patients receiving neurotoxic chemotherapy. *BMC Cancer.* 2019;19(1):132.
5. Mielke S, Sparreboom A, Mross K. Peripheral neuropathy: a persisting challenge in paclitaxel-based regimes. *Eur J Cancer.* 2006;42(1):24-30.
6. Pasini F, Durante E, De Manzoni D, Rosti G, Pelosi G. High-dose chemotherapy in small-cell lung cancer. *Anticancer Res.* 2002;22(6B):3465-3472.
7. Cocconi G, Bisagni G, Ceci G, et al. Three new active cisplatin-containing combinations in the neoadjuvant treatment of locally advanced and locally recurrent breast carcinoma: a randomized phase II trial. *Breast Cancer Res Treat.* 1999;56(2):125-132.
8. Cavaletti G, Cavalletti E, Oggioni N, et al. Distribution of paclitaxel within the nervous system of the rat after repeated intravenous administration. *Neurotoxicology.* 2000;21(3):389-393.
9. Alessandri-Haber N, Dina OA, Yeh JJ, Parada CA, Reichling DB, Levine JD. Transient receptor potential vanilloid 4 is essential in chemotherapy-induced neuropathic pain in the rat. *J Neurosci.* 2004;24(18):4444-4452.
10. Weimer LH. Medication-induced peripheral neuropathy. *Curr Neurol Neurosci Rep.* 2003;3(1):86-92.
11. Sioka C, Kyritsis AP. Central and peripheral nervous system toxicity of common chemotherapeutic agents. *Cancer Chemother Pharmacol.* 2009;63(5):761-767.
12. Loprinzi CL, Reeves BN, Dakhil SR, et al. Natural history of paclitaxel-associated acute pain syndrome: prospective cohort study NCCTG N08C1. *J Clin Oncol.* 2011;29(11):1472-1478.
13. Cliff J, Jorgensen AL, Lord R, Azam F, Cossar L, Carr DF, et al. The molecular genetics of chemotherapy-induced peripheral neuropathy: a systematic review and meta-analysis. *Crit Rev Oncol Hematol.* 2017;120:127-140.

14. Fukuda Y, Li Y, Segal RA. A mechanistic understanding of axon degeneration in chemotherapy-induced peripheral neuropathy. *Front Neurosci.* 2017;11:481.

15. Argyriou AA, Koltzenburg M, Polychronopoulos P, Papapetropoulos S, Kalofonos HP. Peripheral nerve damage associated with administration of taxanes in patients with cancer. *Crit Rev Oncol Hematol.* 2008;66(3):218-228.

16. Windebank AJ, Grisold W. Chemotherapy-induced neuropathy. *J Peripher Nerv Syst.* 2008;13(1):27-46.

17. Cavaletti G, Tredici G, Braga M, Tazzari S. Experimental peripheral neuropathy induced in adult rats by repeated intraperitoneal administration of taxol. *Exp Neurol.* 1995;133(1):64-72.

18. Jimenez-Andrade JM, Peters CM, Mejia NA, Ghilardi JR, Kuskowski MA, Mantyh PW. Sensory neurons and their supporting cells located in the trigeminal, thoracic and lumbar ganglia differentially express markers of injury following intravenous administration of paclitaxel in the rat. *Neurosci Lett.* 2006;405(1-2):62-67.

19. Theiss C, Mazur A, Meller K, Mannherz HG. Changes in gap junction organization and decreased coupling during induced apoptosis in lens epithelial and NIH-3T3 cells. *Exp Cell Res.* 2007;313(1):38-52.

20. Scuteri A, Nicolini G, Miloso M, et al. Paclitaxel toxicity in post-mitotic dorsal root ganglion (DRG) cells. *Anticancer Res.* 2006;26(2A):1065-1070.

21. Rosenthal S, Kaufman S. Vincristine neurotoxicity. *Ann Intern Med.* 1974;80(6):733-737.

22. Xiao WH, Bennett GJ. Chemotherapy-evoked neuropathic pain: abnormal spontaneous discharge in A-fiber and C-fiber primary afferent neurons and its suppression by acetyl-L-carnitine. *Pain.* 2008;135(3):262-270.

23. Casey EB, Jellife AM, Le Quesne PM, Millett YL. Vincristine neuropathy. Clinical and electrophysiological observations. *Brain.* 1973;96(1):69-86.

24. Leveque D, Jehl F. Molecular pharmacokinetics of catharanthus (vinca) alkaloids. *J Clin Pharmacol.* 2007;47(5):579-588.

25. Sahenk Z, Brady ST, Mendell JR. Studies on the pathogenesis of vincristine-induced neuropathy. *Muscle Nerve.* 1987;10(1):80-84.

26. Topp KS, Tanner KD, Levine JD. Damage to the cytoskeleton of large diameter sensory neurons and myelinated axons in vincristine-induced painful peripheral neuropathy in the rat. *J Comp Neurol.* 2000;424(4):563-576.

27. Macfarlane BV, Wright A, Benson HA. Reversible blockade of retrograde axonal transport in the rat sciatic nerve by vincristine. *J Pharm Pharmacol.* 1997;49(1):97-101.

28. Tanner KD, Levine JD, Topp KS. Microtubule disorientation and axonal swelling in unmyelinated sensory axons during vincristine-induced painful neuropathy in rat. *J Comp Neurol.* 1998;395(4):481-492.

29. Silva A, Wang Q, Wang M, Ravula SK, Glass JD. Evidence for direct axonal toxicity in vincristine neuropathy. *J Peripher Nerv Syst.* 2006;11(3):211-216.

30. Holmes J, Stanko J, Varchenko M, et al. Comparative neurotoxicity of oxaliplatin, cisplatin, and ormaplatin in a Wistar rat model. *Toxicol Sci.* 1998;46(2):342-351.

31. Cavaletti G, Fabbrica D, Minoia C, Frattola L, Tredici G. Carboplatin toxic effects on the peripheral nervous system of the rat. *Ann Oncol.* 1998;9(4):443-447.

32. McDonald ES, Windebank AJ. Cisplatin-induced apoptosis of DRG neurons involves bax redistribution and cytochrome c release but not fas receptor signaling. *Neurobiol Dis.* 2002;9(2):220-233.

33. Wilkes G. Peripheral neuropathy related to chemotherapy. *Semin Oncol Nurs.* 2007;23(3):162-173.

34. Chaudhry V, Rowinsky EK, Sartorius SE, Donehower RC, Cornblath DR. Peripheral neuropathy from taxol and cisplatin combination chemotherapy: clinical and electrophysiological studies. *Ann Neurol.* 1994;35(3):304-311.

35. Legha SS. Vincristine neurotoxicity. Pathophysiology and management. *Med Toxicol.* 1986;1(6):421-427.

36. Walsh TJ, Clark AW, Parhad IM, Green WR. Neurotoxic effects of cisplatin therapy. *Arch Neurol.* 1982;39(11):719-720.

37. Huff LM, Sackett DL, Poruchynsky MS, Fojo T. Microtubule-disrupting chemotherapeutics result in enhanced proteasome-mediated degradation and disappearance of tubulin in neural cells. *Cancer Res.* 2010;70(14):5870-5879.

38. Tulub AA, Stefanov VE. Cisplatin stops tubulin assembly into microtubules. A new insight into the mechanism of antitumor activity of platinum complexes. *Int J Biol Macromol.* 2001;28(3):191-198.

39. Hilkens PH, Planting AS, van der Burg ME, et al. Clinical course and risk factors of neurotoxicity following cisplatin in an intensive dosing schedule. *Eur J Neurol.* 1994;1(1):45-50.

40. Lehky TJ, Leonard GD, Wilson RH, Grem JL, Floeter MK. Oxaliplatin-induced neurotoxicity: acute hyperexcitability and chronic neuropathy. *Muscle Nerve.* 2004;29(3):387-392.

41. Benoit E, Brienza S, Dubois JM. Oxaliplatin, an anticancer agent that affects both Na+ and K+ channels in frog peripheral myelinated axons. *Gen Physiol Biophys.* 2006;25(3):263-276.

42. Grolleau F, Gamelin L, Boisdron-Celle M, Lapied B, Pelhate M, Gamelin E. A possible explanation for a neurotoxic effect of the anticancer agent oxaliplatin on neuronal voltage-gated sodium channels. *J Neurophysiol.* 2001;85(5):2293-2297.

43. Gauchan P, Andoh T, Kato A, Kuraishi Y. Involvement of increased expression of transient receptor potential melastatin 8 in oxaliplatin-induced cold allodynia in mice. *Neurosci Lett.* 2009;458(2):93-95.

44. Krishnan AV, Goldstein D, Friedlander M, Kiernan MC. Oxaliplatin-induced neurotoxicity and the development of neuropathy. *Muscle Nerve.* 2005;32(1):51-60.

45. Cata JP, Weng HR, Burton AW, Villareal H, Giralt S, Dougherty PM. Quantitative sensory findings in·patients with bortezomib-induced pain. *J Pain.* 2007;8(4):296-306.

46. Cavaletti G, Gilardini A, Canta A, et al. Bortezomib-induced peripheral neurotoxicity: a neurophysiological and pathological study in the rat. *Exp Neurol.* 2007;204(1):317-325.

47. Meregalli C, Canta A, Carozzi VA, et al. Bortezomib-induced painful neuropathy in rats: a behavioral, neurophysiological and pathological study in rats. *Eur J Pain.* 2010;14(4):343-350.

48. Rajkumar SV, Richardson PG, Hideshima T, Anderson KC. Proteasome inhibition as a novel therapeutic target in human cancer. *J Clin Oncol.* 2005;23(3):630-639.

49. Csizmadia V, Raczynski A, Csizmadia E, Fedyk ER, Rottman J, Alden CL. Effect of an experimental proteasome inhibitor on the cytoskeleton, cytosolic protein turnover, and induction in the neuronal cells in vitro. *Neurotoxicology.* 2008;29(2):232-243.

50. Filosto M, Rossi G, Pelizzari AM, et al. A high-dose bortezomib neuropathy with sensory ataxia and myelin involvement. *J Neurol Sci.* 2007;263(1–2):40-43.

51. Poruchynsky MS, Sackett DL, Robey RW, Ward Y, Annunziata C, Fojo T. Proteasome inhibitors increase tubulin polymerization and stabilization in tissue culture cells: a possible mechanism contributing to

peripheral neuropathy and cellular toxicity following proteasome inhibition. *Cell Cycle*. 2008;7(7):940-949.

52. Chaudhry V, Cornblath DR, Ferguson A, Borrello I. Characteristics of bortezomib- and thalidomide-induced peripheral neuropathy. *J Peripher Nerv Syst*. 2008;13(4):275-282.

53. An J, Sun YP, Adams J, Fisher M, Belldegrun A, Rettig MB. Drug interactions between the proteasome inhibitor bortezomib and cytotoxic chemotherapy, tumor necrosis factor (TNF) alpha, and TNF-related apoptosis-inducing ligand in prostate cancer. *Clin Cancer Res*. 2003;9(12):4537-4545.

54. Maggirwar SB, Sarmiere PD, Dewhurst S, Freeman RS. Nerve growth factor-dependent activation of NF-kappaB contributes to survival of sympathetic neurons. *J Neurosci*. 1998;18(24):10356-10365.

55. Balayssac D, Ferrier J, Descoeur J, et al. Chemotherapy-induced peripheral neuropathies: from clinical relevance to preclinical evidence. *Expert Opin Drug Saf*. 2011;10(3):407-417.

56. Koeppen S. Treatment of multiple myeloma: thalidomide-, bortezomib-, and lenalidomide-induced peripheral neuropathy. *Oncol Res Treat*. 2014;37(9):506-513.

57. Cundari S, Cavaletti G. Thalidomide chemotherapy-induced peripheral neuropathy: actual status and new perspectives with thalidomide analogues derivatives. *Mini Rev Med Chem*. 2009;9(7):760-768.

58. Zara G, Ermani M, Rondinone R, Arienti S, Doria A. Thalidomide and sensory neurotoxicity: a neurophysiological study. *J Neurol Neurosurg Psychiatry*. 2008;79(11):1258-1261.

59. Fernyhough P, Smith DR, Schapansky J, et al. Activation of nuclear factor-kappaB via endogenous tumor necrosis factor alpha regulates survival of axotomized adult sensory neurons. *J Neurosci*. 2005;25(7):1682-1690.

60. Zhu J, Zou L, Zhu S, et al. Cytotoxic T lymphocyte-associated antigen 4 (CTLA-4) blockade enhances incidence and severity of experimental autoimmune neuritis in resistant mice. *J Neuroimmunol*. 2001;115(1-2):111-117.

61. Flatters SJ, Bennett GJ. Studies of peripheral sensory nerves in paclitaxel-induced painful peripheral neuropathy: evidence for mitochondrial dysfunction. *Pain*. 2006;122(3):245-257.

62. Raine CS, Roytta M, Dolich M. Microtubule-mitochondrial associations in regenerating axons after taxol intoxication. *J Neurocytol*. 1987;16(4):461-468.

63. Zheng H, Xiao WH, Bennett GJ. Functional deficits in peripheral nerve mitochondria in rats with paclitaxel- and oxaliplatin-evoked painful peripheral neuropathy. *Exp Neurol*. 2011;232(2):154-161.

64. Virmani A, Gaetani F, Binienda Z. Effects of metabolic modifiers such as carnitines, coenzyme Q10, and PUFAs against different forms of neurotoxic insults: metabolic inhibitors, MPTP, and methamphetamine. *Ann N Y Acad Sci*. 2005;1053:183-191.

65. Jin HW, Flatters SJ, Xiao WH, Mulhern HL, Bennett GJ. Prevention of paclitaxel-evoked painful peripheral neuropathy by acetyl-L-carnitine: effects on axonal mitochondria, sensory nerve fiber terminal arbors, and cutaneous Langerhans cells. *Exp Neurol*. 2008;210(1):229-237.

66. Bianchi G, Vitali G, Caraceni A, et al. Symptomatic and neurophysiological responses of paclitaxel- or cisplatin-induced neuropathy to oral acetyl-L-carnitine. *Eur J Cancer*. 2005;41(12):1746-1750.

67. Pachman DR, Barton DL, Watson JC, Loprinzi CL. Chemotherapy-induced peripheral neuropathy: prevention and treatment. *Clin Pharmacol Ther*. 2011;90(3): 377-387.

68. Campone M, Berton-Rigaud D, Joly-Lobbedez F, et al. A double-blind, randomized phase II study to evaluate the safety and efficacy of acetyl-L-carnitine in the prevention of sagopilone-induced peripheral neuropathy. *Oncologist*. 2013;18(11):1190-1191.

69. Uceyler N, Kafke W, Riediger N, et al. Elevated proinflammatory cytokine expression in affected skin in small fiber neuropathy. *Neurology*. 2010;74(22):1806-1813.

70. Scholz J, Woolf CJ. The neuropathic pain triad: neurons, immune cells and glia. *Nat Neurosci*. 2007;10(11):1361-1368.

71. Watkins LR, Maier SF. Beyond neurons: evidence that immune and glial cells contribute to pathological pain states. *Physiol Rev*. 2002;82(4):981-1011.

72. Mantyh PW. Cancer pain and its impact on diagnosis, survival and quality of life. *Nat Rev Neurosci*. 2006;7(10):797-809.

73. Makker PG, Duffy SS, Lees JG, et al. Characterisation of immune and neuroinflammatory changes associated with chemotherapy-induced peripheral neuropathy. *PLoS One*. 2017;12(1):e0170814.

74. Peters CM, Jimenez-Andrade JM, Jonas BM, et al. Intravenous paclitaxel administration in the rat induces a peripheral sensory neuropathy characterized by macrophage infiltration and injury to sensory neurons and their supporting cells. *Exp Neurol*. 2007;203(1):42-54.

75. Peters CM, Jimenez-Andrade JM, Kuskowski MA, Ghilardi JR, Mantyh PW. An evolving cellular pathology occurs in dorsal root ganglia, peripheral nerve and spinal cord following intravenous administration of paclitaxel in the rat. *Brain Res*. 2007;1168:46-59.

76. Nishida K, Kuchiiwa S, Oiso S, et al. Up-regulation of matrix metalloproteinase-3 in the dorsal root ganglion of rats with paclitaxel-induced neuropathy. *Cancer Sci*. 2008;99(8):1618-1625.

77. Sommer C, Kress M. Recent findings on how proinflammatory cytokines cause pain: peripheral mechanisms in inflammatory and neuropathic hyperalgesia. *Neurosci Lett*. 2004;361(1-3):184-187.

78. Tofaris GK, Patterson PH, Jessen KR, Mirsky R. Denervated Schwann cells attract macrophages by secretion of leukemia inhibitory factor (LIF) and monocyte chemoattractant protein-1 in a process regulated by interleukin-6 and LIF. *J Neurosci*. 2002;22(15):6696-6703.

79. Schafers M, Sorkin L. Effect of cytokines on neuronal excitability. *Neurosci Lett*. 2008;437(3):188-193.

80. Bethea JR, Nagashima H, Acosta MC, et al. Systemically administered interleukin-10 reduces tumor necrosis factor-alpha production and significantly improves functional recovery following traumatic spinal cord injury in rats. *J Neurotrauma*. 1999;16(10):851-863.

81. Ledeboer A, Jekich BM, Sloane EM, et al. Intrathecal interleukin-10 gene therapy attenuates paclitaxel-induced mechanical allodynia and proinflammatory cytokine expression in dorsal root ganglia in rats. *Brain Behav Immun*. 2007;21(5):686-698.

82. Plunkett JA, Yu CG, Easton JM, Bethea JR, Yezierski RP. Effects of interleukin-10 (IL-10) on pain behavior and gene expression following excitotoxic spinal cord injury in the rat. *Exp Neurol*. 2001;168(1):144-154.

83. Abraham KE, McMillen D, Brewer KL. The effects of endogenous interleukin-10 on gray matter damage and the development of pain behaviors following excitotoxic spinal cord injury in the mouse. *Neuroscience*. 2004;124(4):945-952.

84. Kawasaki Y, Xu ZZ, Wang X, et al. Distinct roles of matrix metalloproteases in the early- and late-phase development of neuropathic pain. *Nat Med*. 2008;14(3): 331-336.

85. Kobayashi H, Chattopadhyay S, Kato K, et al. MMPs initiate Schwann cell-mediated MBP degradation and mechanical nociception after nerve damage. *Mol Cell Neurosci*. 2008;39(4):619-627.

86. Boyette-Davis J, Xin W, Zhang H, Dougherty PM. Intraepidermal nerve fiber loss corresponds to the development of taxol-induced hyperalgesia and can be prevented by treatment with minocycline. *Pain*. 2011;152(2): 308-313.

87. Mika J, Osikowicz M, Makuch W, Przewlocka B. Minocycline and pentoxifylline attenuate allodynia and hyperalgesia and potentiate the effects of morphine in rat and mouse models of neuropathic pain. *Eur J Pharmacol*. 2007;560(2-3):142-149.

88. Nikodemova M, Watters JJ, Jackson SJ, Yang SK, Duncan ID. Minocycline down-regulates MHC II expression in microglia and macrophages through inhibition of IRF-1 and protein kinase C (PKC)alpha/betaII. *J Biol Chem*. 2007;282(20):15208-15216.

89. Keilhoff G, Schild L, Fansa H. Minocycline protects Schwann cells from ischemia-like injury and promotes axonal outgrowth in bioartificial nerve grafts lacking Wallerian degeneration. *Exp Neurol*. 2008;212(1): 189-200.

90. Mika J. Modulation of microglia can attenuate neuropathic pain symptoms and enhance morphine effectiveness. *Pharmacol Rep*. 2008;60(3):297-307.

91. Raghavendra V, Tanga F, DeLeo JA. Inhibition of microglial activation attenuates the development but not existing hypersensitivity in a rat model of neuropathy. *J Pharmacol Exp Ther*. 2003;306(2):624-630.

92. Liu CC, Lu N, Cui Y, et al. Prevention of paclitaxel-induced allodynia by minocycline: effect on loss of peripheral nerve fibers and infiltration of macrophages in rats. *Mol Pain*. 2010;6:76.

93. Cata JP, Weng HR, Dougherty PM. The effects of thalidomide and minocycline on taxol-induced hyperalgesia in rats. *Brain Res*. 2008;1229:100-110.

94. Wadia RJ, Stolar M, Grens C, Ehrlich BE, Chao HH. The prevention of chemotherapy induced peripheral neuropathy by concurrent treatment with drugs used for bipolar disease: a retrospective chart analysis in human cancer patients. *Oncotarget*. 2018;9(7):7322-7331.

95. Yamakawa H, Cheng J, Penney J, et al. The transcription factor Sp3 cooperates with HDAC2 to regulate synaptic function and plasticity in neurons. *Cell Rep*. 2017;20(6):1319-1334.

96. Descalzi G, Ikegami D, Ushijima T, Nestler EJ, Zachariou V, Narita M. Epigenetic mechanisms of chronic pain. *Trends Neurosci*. 2015;38(4):237-246.

97. Martinez-Lozada Z, Guillem AM, Robinson MB. Transcriptional regulation of glutamate transporters: from extracellular signals to transcription factors. *Adv Pharmacol*. 2016;76:103-145.

98. Butler R, Bates GP. Histone deacetylase inhibitors as therapeutics for polyglutamine disorders. *Nat Rev Neurosci*. 2006;7(10):784-796.

99. Mahmoud S, Gharagozloo M, Simard C, Gris D. Astrocytes maintain glutamate homeostasis in the CNS by controlling the balance between glutamate uptake and release. *Cells*. 2019;8(2):184.

100. Osikowicz M, Mika J, Przewlocka B. The glutamatergic system as a target for neuropathic pain relief. *Exp Physiol*. 2013;98(2):372-384.

101. Wang ZT, Yu G, Wang HS, Yi SP, Su RB, Gong ZH. Changes in VGLUT2 expression and function in pain-related supraspinal regions correlate with the pathogenesis of neuropathic pain in a mouse spared nerve injury model. *Brain Res*. 2015;1624:515-524.

102. Li JL, Fujiyama F, Kaneko T, Mizuno N. Expression of vesicular glutamate transporters, VGluT1 and VGluT2, in axon terminals of nociceptive primary afferent fibers in the superficial layers of the medullary and spinal dorsal horns of the rat. *J Comp Neurol*. 2003;457(3):236-249.

103. Krukowski K, Ma J, Golonzhka O, et al. HDAC6 inhibition effectively reverses chemotherapy-induced peripheral neuropathy. *Pain*. 2017;158(6):1126-1137.

104. du Bois A, Schlaich M, Luck HJ, et al. Evaluation of neurotoxicity induced by paclitaxel second-line chemotherapy. *Support Care Cancer*. 1999;7(5):354-361.

105. Cavaletti G, Nicolini G, Marmiroli P. Neurotoxic effects of antineoplastic drugs: the lesson of pre-clinical studies. *Front Biosci*. 2008;13:3506-3524.

106. Argyriou AA, Park SB, Islam B, et al. Neurophysiological, nerve imaging and other techniques to assess chemotherapy-induced peripheral neurotoxicity in the clinical and research settings. *J Neurol Neurosurg Psychiatry*. 2019;90:1361-1369.

107. Vincenzetti S, Pucciarelli S, Huang Y, et al. Biomarkers mapping of neuropathic pain in a nerve chronic constriction injury mice model. *Biochimie*. 2019;158:172-179.

108. Hu S, Huang KM, Adams EJ, Loprinzi CL, Lustberg MB. Recent developments of novel pharmacologic therapeutics for prevention of chemotherapy-induced peripheral neuropathy. *Clin Cancer Res*. 2019;25(21):6295-6301.

109. Hou S, Huh B, Kim HK, Kim KH, Abdi S. Treatment of chemotherapy-induced peripheral neuropathy: systematic review and recommendations. *Pain Physician*. 2018;21(6):571-592.

110. Brami C, Bao T, Deng G. Natural products and complementary therapies for chemotherapy-induced peripheral neuropathy: a systematic review. *Crit Rev Oncol Hematol*. 2016;98:325-334.

111. Li K, Giustini D, Seely D. A systematic review of acupuncture for chemotherapy-induced peripheral neuropathy. *Curr Oncol*. 2019;26(2):e147-e154.

112. Hu LY, Mi WL, Wu GC, Wang YQ, Mao-Ying QL. Prevention and treatment for chemotherapy-induced peripheral neuropathy: therapies based on CIPN mechanisms. *Curr Neuropharmacol*. 2019;17(2):184-196.

113. de Andrade DC, Jacobsen Teixeira M, Galhardoni R, et al. Pregabalin for the prevention of oxaliplatin-induced painful neuropathy: a randomized, double-blind trial. *Oncologist*. 2017;22(10):1154-e105.

114. Coderre TJ. Topical drug therapeutics for neuropathic pain. *Expert Opin Pharmacother*. 2018;19(11): 1211-1220.

115. Akhand O, Galetta MS, Cobbs L, et al. The new Mobile Universal Lexicon Evaluation System (MULES): a test of rapid picture naming for concussion sized for the sidelines. *J Neurol Sci*. 2018;387:199-204.

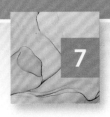

7 Cancer-Related Fatigue

Xin Shelley Wang

INTRODUCTION

Cancer-related fatigue (CRF) is one of the most prevalent symptoms reported by cancer patients and survivors—and one that presents many challenges. Most epidemiological studies of fatigue indicate that it occurs more frequently and more severely than do other symptoms in patients with cancer during the course of their disease and its treatment, regardless of the type of cancer or type of therapy; an early study described the CRF as "both pervasive and profound" (1). In another study, a significantly greater percentage of cancer patients than healthy individuals reported severe fatigue (rated 7 or higher on a 0 to 10 scale) (2). CRF often persists even among cancer survivors who have no evidence of active disease (3,4).

Such findings underline the importance of establishing a standardized method for assessing and managing fatigue in routine clinical oncology care (5,6). Efforts to develop educational and research initiatives that would help patients and health care providers better understand and treat fatigue began in the late 1990s (1), and since then, knowledge of CRF has progressed, allowing new hypotheses to be generated for further study. Nonetheless, knowledge about the pathophysiological mechanisms of CRF is still limited, and an effective intervention for fatigue in oncology patient care has yet to be established.

In this chapter, we define CRF, summarize the available research on clinical factors and underlying mechanisms of CRF, discuss methodological issues in measuring CRF and interpreting fatigue assessment results, and review innovations in CRF management.

DEFINING CRF

Characteristics of CRF: Many definitions of CRF share similar features. For example, seven characteristics of CRF in Table 7.1 that have been defined by the working group Assessing the Symptoms of Cancer Using Patient-Reported Outcomes (ASCPRO) (7) describe CRF as physical, subjective, temporal, emotional, cognitive, unusual, and affecting the patient's ability to function. Similarly, the

well-known and accepted National Comprehensive Cancer Network (NCCN) guidelines on fatigue define CRF as "a distressing, persistent, subjective sense of physical, emotional, and/or cognitive tiredness or exhaustion related to cancer or cancer treatment that is not proportional to recent activity and interferes with usual functioning" (8–10).

Fatigue could be described clinically with a range of terms, such as weariness, exhaustion, lassitude, weakness, malaise, discomfort, impatience, or the inability to perform aspects of normal functioning. Although patients with CRF use a variety of phrases to describe their fatigue, more often than not they characterize themselves as "suffering" from fatigue. However, the distinction between patient perception of CRF and that of "typical" fatigue remains somewhat vague. CRF may be ever-present or transient (a "fatigue attack," in which its onset is more rapid than that of typical fatigue). CRF can last longer, can drain more energy, and is more severe and unrelenting than typical fatigue. Because CRF overlaps with multifactorial physical and psychological disorders, it has been recognized as falling into "muddy water" conceptually. The European Association for Palliative Care has recognized both a physical and a cognitive dimension to fatigue and recommends that screening for fatigue include both a question about weakness to cover the physical dimension and a question about tiredness to cover the cognitive dimension (11).

Qualitatively define CRF: Data from qualitative studies could help to create a simplified approach to understanding CRF. For example, a qualitative study compared the key domains of adaptation for "tired," "fatigued," and "exhausted" in patients with cancer, suggesting that behavioral changes in sleep quality, stamina, cognition, and emotional reactivity may serve as early markers of impending fatigue and that decreased control over body processes and reduced social interaction may be signs that an individual has entered a state of fatigue (12). Qualitative research on CRF suggested that the word "tiredness" does not adequately capture the multidimensional nature of the CRF experience (13).

Impact on functioning: CRF negatively affects a patient's daily functioning and can diminish

TABLE 7.1 CHARACTERISTICS OF FATIGUE

Characteristic	Terms indicative of the characteristic	% Definitions including characteristic
Subjective	Self-report, self-perception	58
Physical sensation	Severity of sensations, including exhaustion, decreased energy, weakness, malaise, tiredness, lassitude	92
Unusual	Unrelieved by rest, unusual, abnormal, not proportional to activity, unusual need for rest, unpredictable	42
Impact on functioning	Decreased function, decreased capacity for work, decreased quality of life, difficulty completing tasks, poor sleep quality, withdrawal from activities, debilitation	66
Unpleasant emotions	Helplessness, vulnerability, distress, reactivity, impatience, anxiety, emotional numbness, unpleasant experience, emotional lability	54
Decreased cognitive ability	Decreased attention, decreased concentration, decreased motivation, memory deficits, decreased mental capacity, decreased capacity for mental work	46
Temporal variability	Pervasive, chronic, acute, persistent, episodic	58

Reprinted from Barsevick AM, Cleeland CS, Manning DC, et al. ASCPRO recommendations for the assessment of fatigue as an outcome in clinical trials. *J Pain Symptom Manage.* 2010;39(6):1086-1099, © 2010, with permission from Elsevier.

quality of life. It can be so overwhelming that patients elect to discontinue treatment, or oncologists may give patients a "treatment holiday" to recover from severe symptom burden. A quantitative study found that CRF-related interference with functioning, as measured by the Brief Fatigue Inventory, helped differentiate fatigue severity levels (2). An increase in a patient's worst-fatigue rating was associated with an increase in interference with patient function (12,14).

CLINICAL FACTORS AND OTHER CONDITIONS ASSOCIATED WITH CRF

The NCCN guidelines for managing fatigue attribute the causes of CRF to both the cancer and cancer therapy (8). CRF can occur during any phase of the disease, and it often results from a combination of cancer progression and the body's acute or late response to cancer therapy, plus the impact from other medical and psychological conditions and chronic illness.

Disease-related CRF: This is often observed in patients newly diagnosed with cancer. Unusual tiredness is frequently the first indicator that something is amiss (15). In a study of elderly patients newly diagnosed with various cancers, higher levels of fatigue were found in patients with late-stage disease than in patients with early-stage lung cancer (14,16). In patients with advanced cancer, tumor progression affects multiple organ systems and causes neurological and physiological changes in skeletal muscle that are potentially relevant to CRF.

Cancer therapy–related CRF: Cancer treatment can induce CRF and exacerbate existing CRF (5,17–20). A history of chemotherapy was independently associated with severe CRF in patients with various types of advanced cancer (21). Chemotherapy-related toxicities, such as hematological, gastrointestinal-tract, and neural toxicities, may also increase CRF severity. For some chemotherapy regimens, CRF is an expected adverse event, and patients receiving such regimens as standard care during acute treatment often accept CRF as the price they must pay to achieve a cure. For patients undergoing maintenance therapy (such as patients with chronic myeloid leukemia receiving long-term imatinib therapy), CRF is often a critical factor in deciding whether or not to withdraw from treatment.

Other cancer therapies, such as definitive surgery, radiotherapy, stem cell transplantation, targeted therapy, cellular therapy, and immunotherapy, can also induce or exacerbate CRF. Patients with cancer often experience postoperative fatigue immediately after a curative surgical procedure, although increased analgesia has been shown to attenuate immediate postsurgical fatigue (22). Gradual increases in fatigue severity have been observed during radiotherapy or concurrent chemoradiation following accumulated dose received (5,17–20). Radiotherapy or chemoradiation therapy can induce anemia, diarrhea, anorexia, weight loss, and chronic pain, any of which may be associated with an increase in CRF. When high-dose chemotherapy is paired with stem-cell transplantation, patients experience a dip in white blood cell count after the transplant, which has been found to be associated with a peak in fatigue levels (23,24). In patients with breast cancer, hormone treatment has been associated with lethargy and lack of energy equivalent in severity to the postradiotherapy fatigue experienced by patients with prostate cancer during hormone treatment (25). In addition, fatigue is one of the most common side effects of many tyrosine kinase inhibitors (26). Even though fatigue is a well-known issue for cancer patients and survivors, CRF was not noted among a list of adverse drug reactions that occurred after initial labels for targeted anticancer agents were approved on the basis of randomized phase III clinical trials (27), and there are few existing data on the impact of CRF-related drug discontinuation on disease control.

CRF in cancer survivorship: Even for cancer survivors who have completed therapy and have no evidence of active disease, CRF can be a persistent and functionally bothersome symptom. A population-based survey of 1-year cancer survivors revealed that fatigue was 1 of 3 most negative symptoms (along with depression and pain) among 67 symptoms affecting health-related quality of life (28). Fatigue is also perceived to be a significant problem in child and young-adult cancer survivors. Meeske et al. found that 30% of 161 long-term survivors of acute lymphoblastic leukemia whose cancer was diagnosed before the age of 18 years reported having fatigue, and that fatigue was highly associated with depression (29). In a multicenter study of 1,897 adult long-term survivors of childhood cancer (those who had a cancer diagnosis before age 21 and survived at least 5 years after the diagnosis), the overall prevalence of CRF was 19% among all survivors and 15% among the acute lymphoblastic leukemia survivors, after adjustment for medical and socioeconomic factors, including depression (30). Survivors were significantly more fatigued than their siblings. Survivors with fatigue were also more likely to experience depression than were survivors who did not have fatigue. These findings indicate that long-term follow-up care should include psychological assessments and interventions for childhood cancer survivors at highest risk (31).

Comorbidities and CRF: Research has revealed that chronic medical conditions and their treatments (e.g., pain, disturbed sleep, decreased activity levels, infections, anemia, nutritional deficiencies, dehydration, electrolyte disturbances, cardiac deconditioning, pulmonary disorders, neuromuscular disorders, thyroid dysfunction, liver failure, renal insufficiency, and diabetes), psychosocial stress and emotional distress (e.g., anxiety, depression, and environmental reinforcers), and concurrent exposure to sedating medications

(e.g., opioids, anxiolytics) can also contribute to CRF in patients with cancer, although the exact nature of these multiple influences cannot be determined. In addition, most patients with cancer are of advanced age, increasing the likelihood that they suffer from comorbidities that are also risk factors for CRF. The association of fatigue and cognitive impairment has not been well studied in the general population (32), whereas a strong association has been reported among patients under chemotherapy for early breast cancer (33).

POTENTIAL UNDERLYING MECHANISMS OF CRF

Increasing research has carefully documented the development of fatigue and how it interacts with potential biological-mechanism targets in specific cohorts. While numerous challenges exist in the translational area of biomedical sciences for narrowing down host factors related to CRF, some progress has been made in identifying a biomarker that could serve as an objective measure of fatigue. Few neuroimaging studies have examined CRF expression in the human brain, and animal models representing CRF have not been established. Translational work is needed to find a mechanism-driven intervention for fatigue.

Genomic variants on etiology studies: CRF does not develop in all patients at risk for it. Increasing research demonstrated that most genomic variants on the inflammatory and immune response pathways, including the neuro-proinflammatory cytokine pathway, have statistically significant associations with CRF (34). It is believed that the susceptibility to fatigue may be influenced by genetic factors, including single nucleotide polymorphisms (SNPs), especially in the regulatory regions of relevant genes. SNPs in regulatory pathways of immune and neurotransmitter systems were found to play important roles in the etiologies of chronic fatigue syndrome, CRF, and other disease-related fatigue, given that elevated fatigue and specific polymorphisms in tumor necrosis factor (TNF)-α, IL-1β, IL-4, and IL-6 genes were revealed for all three subgroups of fatigue (35). The review supports the continued use of genetic and epigenetic perspectives in assessing the role neurotransmitters play in persistent fatigue among cancer survivors (31,32).

Constellation of mechanisms causes CRF: Patients with cancer—especially those undergoing aggressive therapy, those with advanced disease, and those who have accompanying medical comorbidities or psychological disorders—rarely experience just one severe symptom. CRF often accompanies a cluster of other moderate to severe symptoms, such as pain, distress, poor appetite, drowsiness, and

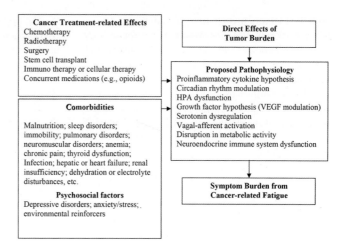

Figure 7.1 Proposed potential etiologies of cancer-related fatigue.

disturbed sleep. In a large case-controlled study of survivors with breast cancer, depression and pain were the strongest predictors of fatigue (3). This suggests that a complex interplay exists between the etiological agent (e.g., cancer treatment, infections, use of centrally acting drugs) and the patient's susceptibility to fatigue.

However, lack of clear pathophysiological explanations hampers our ability to determine whether a constellation of mechanisms causes CRF or whether a centrally mediated disorder characterized by CRF exists. Although the underlying etiology of fatigue is not yet fully understood, several working hypotheses to explain the mechanisms of this complex phenomenon have been suggested. Figure 7.1 presents the proposed etiologies of CRF.

The Proinflammatory Cytokine Hypothesis

The proinflammatory cytokine hypothesis, one of the primary proposed explanations of CRF, suggests that dysregulated inflammation and its toxic downstream effects constitute a significant biological basis for CRF and other cancer-related symptoms (15,23,36–40). As a typical nonspecific symptom in patients with cancer, fatigue is similar to certain sickness behaviors observed in animal models in studies of the behavioral effects of cytokine administration (41). Basic research on activation of immune-to-brain communication pathways in response to continued activation of the peripheral immune system indicates that proinflammatory cytokine (mainly IL-1β and TNF-α) signaling to the brain leads to an exacerbation of sickness behavior in vulnerable individuals, who develop a constellation of behavioral changes that include fatigue, disturbed sleep, and symptoms of depression (41). Increased expression of positive acute phase proteins such as C-reactive protein

and decreased expression of negative acute phase proteins such as albumin are also highly correlated with persistent CRF (42). Certain inflammatory biomarkers (IL-6 and TNF-α) were identified in vivo and in vitro (43); these biomarkers are associated with activation of innate immune cells and T cells (44).

The role of activation of the proinflammatory cytokine network in fatigue and other symptoms has been under investigation since the 1990s, although the relevance of these findings is limited by few translational studies confirming the results. In a quantitative review and meta-analysis of 18 studies, Schubert et al. found that CRF was associated with increased circulating levels of IL-6, IL-1 receptor antagonist, and neopterin (45). Reductions in fatigue were observed in patients given antagonists of TNF-α as an intervention for improving the tolerability of chemotherapy (46). More recently, clinical studies have indicated that TNF-α signaling plays a role in postchemotherapy fatigue in patients with early-stage breast cancer (47). A temporal association was also found between serum or plasma inflammatory markers induced by aggressive cancer therapy and the development of fatigue and a cluster of other sickness symptoms (pain, disturbed sleep, drowsiness, and poor appetite) that affect physical functioning in patients with cancer (23,48,49). Inflammatory process associated with tumor growth can cause abnormalities in energy metabolism and inhibit muscle function: Inagaki et al. found that elevated levels of plasma IL-6 were associated with increased levels of fatigue in terminally ill patients with cancer (50).

A deeper understanding of the relationship between fatigue and pain syndrome with the activation of proinflammatory microglia may bring new information on factors involved in CRF (51). These potential factors involve multiple effects on neurotransmission, neuroendocrinology, neuroplasticity, and the autonomic nervous system. In this model, fatigue can be understood as an evolutionary, meaningful symptom protective of the organism.

The development of the whole spectrum of symptoms of depression in response to cytokines is well established in both animal models and humans, especially in the context of cytokine immunotherapy (52–55). Current research indicates that activation of the tryptophan-degrading enzyme indoleamine 2,3-dioxygenase generates neurotoxic metabolites (56). A recent study indicated that, independent of its potential effect on tumor clearance, inhibition of IDO does not improve cancer-related symptoms (57). In cancer patients treated with IFN-α, hypermetabolism in the left putamen and nucleus accumbens probably related to reduced dopaminergic neurotransmission was associated with fatigue and lack of energy (58).

Fatigue from chronic neurological disease: Studies of the chronic physical and mental fatigue seen in many neurological diseases could also help improve understanding of CRF. Such fatigue is not accompanied by the profound weakness and persistent or progressive cognitive decline or failure of peripheral neuromuscular function seen in multiple sclerosis, chronic HIV infection, or Parkinson's disease. The neuroanatomy of cytokine-induced depression is focused on the brain circuits, with evidence of decreased baseline activity in the frontal and temporal cortex and the insula and increased activity in the cerebellum and subcortical and limbic regions (59). In patients with neurological disorders including multiple sclerosis, fatigue appears to result from a failure in the integration of limbic input and motor functions within the basal ganglia, affecting the striatal–thalamic–frontal cortical system (60). The origin of fatigue in patients with multiple sclerosis supports the idea that a specific dysfunction or involvement of the basal ganglia might contribute to fatigue (61). To understand the anatomical pathway of fatigue, further investigation into the potential shared mechanisms of and interventions for neurological disease–associated fatigue and CRF is thus warranted.

Other Hypotheses

Proinflammatory cytokines may act independently to produce CRF or may overlap or work synergistically with such mechanisms as vagal-afferent activation, hypothalamic–pituitary–adrenal (HPA) axis disruption, serotonin dysregulation, growth-factor activation, and circadian rhythm modulation. These mechanisms may act either directly or indirectly on the brain.

The vagal-afferent activation hypothesis posits that cancer and its treatment activate vagal-afferent nerves through the peripheral release of neuroactive molecules, resulting in decreased somatic motor output and sustained changes in brain regions associated with fatigue (15,36).

The HPA-disruption hypothesis is based on the theory that tumor-related or treatment-related dysregulation of HPA function can lead to endocrine changes that cause or contribute to fatigue (15,36). Reduced levels of cortisol and/or cortisol resistance may allow for increased levels of proinflammatory cytokines.

The serotonin dysregulation hypothesis suggests that cancer or its treatment induces increases in brain serotonin that alter HPA-axis functioning and reduces the patient's ability to perform physical activities (36). However, most of these studies have been carried out in the context of endurance training, so that their relevance to CRF is doubtful (62).

The growth-factor hypothesis associates treatment-induced fatigue with elevated levels of vascular endothelial growth factor, which stimulates the formation of new blood vessels necessary for tumor growth and metastasis, thereby decreasing the blood supply and energy of other organs including muscles and brain (63).

The circadian rhythm modulation hypothesis focuses on secretion rhythms of the stress hormone cortisol and their relation to rest–activity patterns. Elevated transforming growth factor-α levels have been associated with fatigue (64), flattened circadian rhythms, and loss of appetite in patients with metastatic colorectal cancer. Fatigue has also been associated with alterations in rest–activity cycles, which produce the sleep disruptions commonly seen in patients with cancer. A sleep disorder could cause disturbed arousal mechanisms or, equally plausibly, be an indicator of a disorder of arousal. These disorders could be primary or related to metabolic disturbances or the use of centrally acting drugs. However, findings on this topic remain inconclusive; one reason is that the methods for measuring circadian rhythms were inconsistent and that further research with larger sample sizes and more heterogeneous populations (most were focused on patients with breast cancer) is needed (65).

Fundamental disruption in metabolic activity has also been hypothesized as a potential cause of CRF. Cancer and its treatment may disrupt the metabolism of adenosine triphosphate, a major source of energy for skeletal-muscle contraction (15,36). Abnormalities in energy metabolism may be related to increased energy need (the hypermetabolic state that can accompany tumor growth, infection, fever, or surgery), decreased substrates (e.g., anemia, hypoxemia of any cause, poor nutrition), or abnormal accumulation of muscle metabolites (e.g., lactate) that impair intermediate metabolism or the normal functioning of muscles. Nutritional status as a mediator of CRF in older people has been discussed recently (66). Immobility and lack of exercise may also lead to reduced efficiency of neuromuscular functioning.

Risk factors beyond those involving the neuroendocrine immune system have also been proposed as mechanisms underlying CRF. For example, anemia leads to hypoxia, which can compromise organ function and induce fatigue (67). Longitudinal studies have promoted a better understanding of how CRF fluctuates according to various triggers and critical moderating factors, which should ultimately advance efforts to develop methods of mechanism-driven symptom intervention and prevention.

MEASURING CRF

Even though CRF can cause observable behavioral manifestations and is often accompanied by an objective decrement in performance and by other symptoms, CRF itself is a subjective experience and cannot be directly measured by an observer. Subjective patient reports (patient-reported outcomes [PROs]) have become the standard method for assessing dimensions of fatigue, as well as its severity and interference with daily activities. The United States Food and Drug Administration (FDA) encourages investigators to use standardized, psychometrically validated PROs measures in clinical research for symptom intervention (68). Validated measurement tools are essential for evaluating the treatment and management of CRF and for conducting translational mechanism studies and epidemiological studies with fatigue as a primary outcome. Even so, patient-reported measures of CRF provide little specific diagnostic information, while objective measures of CRF that are based on physiological or behavioral markers are frustratingly lacking.

The multifactorial nature of fatigue makes it especially difficult to measure. Even so, although initial efforts to develop a patient-reported measure of fatigue after World War I were ineffective, it is now widely accepted that a validated fatigue-assessment process is possible. Existing validated fatigue measures typically assess severity and the degree to which fatigue interferes with daily life, yet these results should be integrated, on a patient-by-patient basis, with assessments of other factors, such as the quality, temporal pattern, and history of the fatigue and expectations associated with the specific patient's disease phase or treatment status. To be clinically meaningful, a fatigue assessment should also examine the impact of fatigue on physical function, social function, cognition, mood, and other facets of quality of life. The assessment process must give clinical consideration to potential etiologies, such as cancer treatment and current systemic disorders, which should help identify any treatable causes of fatigue.

Selecting an Assessment Tool

Although the FDA has encouraged investigators to use PRO measures in their research (68), most fatigue data from clinical studies come from clinician ratings using the National Cancer Institute's Common Terminology Criteria for Adverse Events (NCI CTCAE). Further, no single standardized patient-report instrument for CRF or other forms of chronic fatigue has been adopted broadly, either in clinical practice or in research. In 2007, Hjollund et al. noted that between 1975 and 2004, more than 250 fatigue-assessment tools were developed for use in patients with either cancer or neurological or systemic disorders (69); some tools have "crossed over" to be used in additional patient populations. Of these, 150 were used only once. These tools vary in their construction (coverage, structure), frequency of use, recommended frequency of administration, scoring, and psychometric properties. These tools also vary by the type of response collected. For example, with verbal descriptor scales, patients select a category to describe their fatigue, such as "none," "mild," "moderate," or "severe." In visual analog scales (VAS), patients mark their fatigue severity along a line. In numerical rating scales (NRS), patients rate their fatigue severity on a numbered scale with a verbal anchor at each end (e.g., "no fatigue" and "fatigue as bad as you can imagine").

Tools for measuring persistent fatigue should be both practical and psychometrically sound, require the rating to occur within a reasonable recall period, present the instructions in easily understood terms, incorporate easy-to-use scales and standardized rules for administration and scoring, and be sensitive enough to detect changes in patient experience. To facilitate cross-cultural validation and comparison, the tool should also be easily translatable into other languages. Most importantly, a good fatigue assessment tool should allow for consistent interpretation of the data.

Although no consensus on the dimensional structure of fatigue has been reached (70), the fatigue assessment tools currently available may be categorized as unidimensional or multidimensional. Quick and easy unidimensional measures used for screening purposes provide such basic information as whether fatigue is present or absent and, if present, its intensity, severity, or impact. Unidimensional measures can be used to determine whether more-comprehensive clinical examination is needed and, when used in research or clinical trials, can provide enough data to track changes in fatigue both over time and in response to treatment. Examination of the various facets of fatigue—the mental–cognitive, physical, and emotional domains—requires a multidimensional measure. Because the experience of CRF is subjective and the impact of fatigue on everyday life varies from patient to patient, the information provided by a multidimensional measure can be valuable.

Unidimensional measures: Using theory-driven exploratory factor analysis to examine a 72-item data bank from a sample of 555 patients with cancer, Lai et al. reported that CRF is sufficiently unidimensional for measurement approaches that require or assume unidimensionality (71).

Unidimensional measures for CRF can be single-item tools like the widely used NCCN patient-reported fatigue intensity rating (8), which has a 0 to 10 numeric scale, or the NCI CTCAE (version 3.0) (72), which uses a 5-point Likert scale rated by medical staff. Another example is the single-item score given for "fatigue at its worst" on the Brief Fatigue Inventory, which asks patients to rate their level of worst fatigue/tiredness on a 0 to 10 scale during the past 24 hours (2). This item can be used as a rapid screening tool or a continual-monitoring variable in clinical practice (73).

Unidimensional measures for CRF may have multiple items, as do the Brief Fatigue Inventory (2) and the Fatigue Severity Scale (74). Multiple-item unidimensional measures with good reliability can generate usable results even when a small percentage of responses are missing. A unidimensional measure of CRF may also be a validated subscale of a larger quality-of-life measurement tool, such as the 13-item fatigue subscale of the Functional Assessment of Cancer Therapy (75), or three items on the European Organization for Research and Treatment of Cancer QLQ-C30 (76).

Multidimensional measures: Although the psychometric accuracy of unidimensional measures may be satisfactory, unidimensional measures fall short of assessing the full spectrum of CRF (5). Unlike unidimensional measures, multidimensional measures can distinguish physical from mental fatigue and measure responses in dimensions relating to affective functioning and activity. The relatively short and simple Multidimensional Fatigue Inventory (MFI-20) is a commonly used measure of fatigue, and its General Fatigue subscale can serve as a global index of fatigue severity (77). PROMIS-Fatigue CAT as a screening tool has been developed (78), and international psychometric validation of an EORTC quality of life module measuring cancer related fatigue (EORTC QLQ-FA12) has also been reported (79). Some multidimensional scales are too long for very ill patients to complete, however, and many of these measures use original phrases or idiomatic expressions that can hinder translation into other languages or cultural settings.

Interpreting Fatigue-Assessment Results

As an outcome measure, CRF can be an important component of drug trials and clinical practice. A reduction in CRF could represent reduced treatment toxicity, improved palliation for advanced disease, increased quality assurance and patient satisfaction with medical care, or improved functional and health status for cancer survivors. Thus, accurate interpretation of CRF assessment data is very important, whereas inadequate assessment can be a substantial barrier to good fatigue management in the clinic. Standardized fatigue assessment may expand the attention and resources provided to address this common and debilitating symptom.

Threshold to trigger an intervention in screening: One way to begin interpreting fatigue severity is to define levels at which symptoms interfere with physical and affective functioning and to analyze differences between cancer patients and healthy individuals. Functional impairment or interference was found to increase as fatigue worsened (80), which is consistent with pain-research findings (81–83). The severity of fatigue may be the most informative indicator of the need for intervention. The boundary between mild–moderate and severe fatigue may be a clinically meaningful indicator for determining whether a fatigue intervention is effective. The best example of fatigue severity delineated by mild–moderate versus severe ratings is the NCCN practice guideline for clinical management of CRF (10). A population-based study provided evidence to support the NCCN Guideline consensus that cutpoints for differentiating between mild and moderate fatigue are 3/4 on a 0 to 10 rating scale, and cutpoints for differentiating between moderate and severe fatigue are 6/7 (14). In clinical implementation, such research becomes more important to increase the utility of PRO measures in real-world patient care.

Prevalence: After defining the boundary of severity of fatigue for a given scale, another application is to draw a picture of symptom prevalence. Due to the differences in CRF scales, mapping the result has been challenging. Although mostly reported in breast cancer patients or survivors, CRF is more severe in lung cancer patients during active treatment and in a similar severity among other cancer patients during and after treatment.

Response shift: Tracking changes in self-report over time can introduce response shift, a phenomenon that occurs when patients judge their level of fatigue differently after having experiences that alter their own internal standards, values, or conceptualizations. The possibility of response shift raises methodological concerns, because it can lead to underreporting of fatigue as patients adapt to more severe "normal" levels of fatigue after therapy. For example, response shift occurred in a group of patients receiving radiotherapy who retrospectively minimized their pretreatment fatigue severity compared with their current fatigue levels (84). A meta-analysis of 19 quality-of-life studies revealed response shifts for several measures, with the largest mean effect size of response shift for fatigue (0.32), followed by global quality of life, physical role limitation, psychological well-being, and pain (85). Importantly, the patient's illness perception, coping skills, and mood may have long-lasting effects on his or her eventual adaptation to chronic fatigue and must be considered in any interpretation of fatigue results.

INTERVENTIONS FOR CRF

Although a standard intervention for CRF has not yet been established, more evidence-based recommendations are emerging for management. Current treatments for CRF include individual interventions for various treatable secondary conditions as causes of fatigue (see Fig. 7.1). Guidelines for the general supportive care of CRF have been developed by NCCN (10) and the Oncology Nursing Society (ONS) (86), with general strategies for the management of fatigue for active treatment, posttreatment, and end of life. National clinical practice guidelines (87) and product labeling from the United States FDA should direct individualized management of patients with cancer-related or treatment-associated anemia. Open communication between the patient, family, and caregiving team can facilitate better management of CRF and enhance understanding of its effects on daily life (8,11).

A growing number of clinical trials aimed at developing and testing pharmacological and non-pharmacological treatments for fatigue have been reported in the past decade. Systematic reviews and meta-analyses have analyzed the efficacy of some of the most-reported interventions, discussed below. Mitchell and Berger have created a list of interventions for which there is evidence of efficacy in treating CRF, along with interventions whose efficacy has not been established or is supported only by expert opinion (88). Nonetheless, the generalizability of the CRF intervention studies analyzed remains limited. Improvements in methodological quality and documentation can be gained through more-careful study design and adherence to better reporting standards, such as the Consolidated Standard of Reporting Trials (CONSORT) (89,90), both of which would provide more accurate data on the efficacy of psychosocial therapy for CRF.

Pharmacological Treatments

For purposes of supportive/palliative care, a 2015 executive summary provided no evidence-based recommendations for use of a specific drug to treat CRF (91). However, there was a very high degree of statistical and clinical heterogeneity in the trials.

Psychostimulants

In an early meta-analysis of five placebo-controlled trials, psychostimulants showed a small but significant improvement in fatigue (91,92). The most-studied psychostimulant used to treat CRF is methylphenidate, which works by directly stimulating adrenergic receptors and indirectly causing the release of dopamine and norepinephrine from presynaptic terminals (93). Methylphenidate is generally well tolerated in cancer patients; the data support prescribing 10 to 20 mg daily. Insomnia and agitation are the most common side effects, but these are mostly reversible with discontinuation of the treatment. Close monitoring is recommended, especially for the first few days of treatment. A large placebo effect has been reported in most trials with stimulants; therefore, a clinical trial with a larger sample size would be helpful for making conclusive recommendations for the use of methylphenidate to treat CRF.

Modafinil, another central nervous system stimulant, is used to treat narcolepsy. Fava et al. reported that modafinil is a well-tolerated and potentially effective augmenting agent for patients with fatigue and sleepiness who are partial responders to selective serotonin reuptake inhibitors (94). In a phase III, randomized, placebo-controlled, double-blind trial, modafinil significantly benefited 631 patients undergoing chemotherapy who had severe fatigue at baseline (95). It significantly improved daytime sleepiness but had no effect on depression.

Antidepressants

It is not known whether fatigue and depression share pathophysiological characteristics; however, efforts have been made to treat fatigue with antidepressants in depressed cancer patients. Morrow et al. reported that in a multicenter, double-blind, randomized, placebo-controlled study of paroxetine administered to fatigued cancer patients undergoing chemotherapy, paroxetine produced a significant reduction in depressive symptoms but not in fatigue (96). Roscoe et al. reported a more favorable outcome from a double-blind placebo-controlled trial (97).

Bupropion may benefit patients with CRF because its ability to increase dopaminergic neurotransmission (9,98). Further study is needed to determine whether fatigue can be treated effectively with other classes of antidepressants in patients undergoing various modes of cancer therapy.

Anti-inflammatory Agents

The use of steroids to treat persistent CRF does not appear to be warranted, in part because of concerns about long-term use of steroids, and in part because steroids appear to have no effect or increased fatigue. An analysis of four randomized, placebo-controlled trials indicated that a mean of 8 weeks of progestational steroid therapy did not reduce fatigue in a group of patients receiving palliative care without chemotherapy (overall z score, 1.06; $p = 0.29$) (99). In men with castration-resistant prostate cancer (100), grade 3 to 4 fatigue was approximately double in patients who received daily corticosteroids as part of their antineoplastic treatment (5.58; 95% CI = 4.33 to 6.98) versus those who did not (2.67%; 95% CI = 1.53 to 4.11).

Minocycline is a readily available, low-cost, low-toxicity antibiotic with anti-inflammatory properties. Several mechanism-driven phase II randomized, double-blind, placebo-controlled trials investigated the effect of minocycline in reducing radiotherapy-related symptom burden in patients with non-small cell lung cancer or head and neck cancer, including fatigue, with positive outcomes (101,102). However, negative results were found in similarly designed studies in patients treated with chemotherapy for advanced pancreatic cancer or colorectal cancer (103,104).

Traditional Chinese Medicine and Guarana

Ginseng is a widely used tonic agent with a potent smell and aftertaste that are difficult to mask—a challenging impediment to its use in blinded randomized trials (105). Because ginseng is easily acquired at health food stores, patients may not think of it as medication. Research into American ginseng in patients with CRF has indicated that patients receiving the highest study dose showed the most improvement in overall energy levels and overall mental, physical, spiritual, and emotional well-being (106,107).

Based on the traditional Chinese medicine (TCM) theory and a long history of well-adopted practice of fatigue management in China, Renshen Yangrong Tang (RSYRT) therapy elicits a statistical and clinical improvement of fatigue severity and functioning through a 6-week phase II randomized, active controlled trial in Chinese cancer survivors (108). No grade 3 to 4 toxicities were observed, and effectiveness started from 4 weeks. Patients using herbal treatments should exercise caution because of possible profound drug interactions with active cancer treatments.

Guarana (*Paullinia cupana*) is a plant native to the Amazon basin with energy-enhancing and tonic properties known to the local people. Dry extract of guarana, at a dose of 75 mg once per day, has been reported to reduce fatigue associated with therapy in breast cancer patients, with no significant side effects and at a relatively low cost (109). These effects are thought to be mainly due to the methylxanthine present in the plant's seeds.

Study participants with unexplained chronic fatigue of unknown etiology lasting for at least 6 months reported that the alternative treatments coenzyme Q10 and dehydroepiandrosterone were the most helpful (110).

Placebo Effect

The efficacy of placebo was never the main objective of any serious investigation until a recent report included 29 studies with 3,758 participants in a meta-analysis (111). It concluded that placebo treatments had a significant effect on CRF: 29% (95% CI = 25% to 32%) of patients taking a placebo reported a significant improvement in CRF compared with 36% of patients treated with other interventions ($p = 0.030$). The magnitude of placebo effect in RCTs of drugs to relieve CRF was further reviewed in a recent study with 30 RCTs, which also concluded as "nontrivial in size and statistically significant" (112). The established knowledge for placebo effect needs to be accounted in fatigue intervention trials and in patient care strategies.

NONPSYCHOLOGICAL AND ACTIVITY-BASED INTERVENTIONS

By current guidelines, nonpharmacological interventions are the first recommendation for CRF. A recent Bayesian network meta-analysis evaluating the comparative effects and ranks of all major nonpharmacological interventions reported that different interventions have their own sets of advantages for addressing CRF, based on various fatigue assessment tools (113). Interest has been growing in the role of cognitive factors (e.g., tendency to perceive catastrophe) and behavioral factors (e.g., physical activity) in exacerbating and prolonging fatigue. A 2017 meta-analysis of randomized clinical trials in adults with cancer, using CRF severity as an outcome and testing of exercise, psychological, exercise plus psychological, or pharmaceutical interventions (114) recommended behavioral intervention, exercise, and psychological interventions to be used as frontline treatment for CRF, due to their effectiveness for reducing CRF during and after cancer treatment that is not attributable to time, attention, and education, and specific intervention modes, and they were found to be significantly better than available pharmaceutical options.

Exercise: A meta-analysis conducted by Schmitz et al. suggested that exercise is an effective way to manage CRF both during and after treatment, although the effect sizes were small (115). The Cochrane collaboration published a meta-analysis of 9 studies of the effects of aerobic or resistance exercise on CRF for 452 women receiving adjuvant therapy for breast cancer (116). Although the difference in improvement in patient-reported fatigue between the intervention and control groups was not statistically significant in these patients, exercise appeared to result in improved physical fitness and, as a result, in improved capacity for performing activities of daily life. These studies involved a range of exercise types (walking, cycling, swimming, resistive exercise, combined exercise), intensity (with most programs at 50% to 90% of the estimated VO_2 maximum heart rate, from twice a day to two times per week), degree of supervision, and duration (from 2 weeks to 1 year).

Psychosocial interventions: These may include cognitive–behavioral therapy, coping skills training, motivational therapy, mindfulness-based stress reduction, and psychoeducational or educational therapies, which may be combined with mind–body elements such as yoga, relaxation breathing, or progressive muscle relaxation. In 2017, a systematic review and meta-analysis of nonpharmacological therapy published by Cochrane collaboration (117) summarized 14 studies ($N = 535$) of the effects of psychosocial intervention for fatigue in cancer patients. There was insufficient and very low-quality evidence to support their use for fatigue reduction, with most studies having small samples, leading to uncertainty of conclusion. Previously, Jacobsen et al. reported a small effect size for 18 psychosocial intervention studies (support-group therapy and individual psychotherapy, both of which provided education, coping strategy programs, tailored behavioral interventions, and professionally or self-administered stress-management training) for significantly improved CRF (118).

Educational interventions: From a 2016 review (119), a low quality of evidence from 12 of 14 randomized studies demonstrated a small effect on reducing fatigue intensity, fatigue's interference with daily life, and general fatigue, and could have a moderate effect on reducing fatigue distress.

Structured rehabilitation programs: Rehabilitation programs have reported significant and sustained improvement in persistent fatigue, especially in cancer survivors. Tailoring the program based on the patient's current level of energy and stage along the treatment trajectory is necessary (120).

Acupuncture: A recent review with meta-analysis reported of acupuncture (121) with a marked effect in patients with CRF from 10 randomized clinical trials, regardless of concurrent anticancer treatment, particularly among breast cancer patients. Regarding the dose of acupuncture used to treat CRF, 20 to 30 minutes/session three times/week for 2 or 3 weeks, twice weekly for 2 weeks and weekly for 6 weeks, and weekly for 6 weeks had substantial effects on CRF. It suggests that the procedure may be an effective way of controlling CRF and other symptoms (122,123).

IMPLEMENTING GUIDELINES FOR OPTIMAL FATIGUE MANAGEMENT

Evidence-based guidelines for managing CRF are increasingly available. The 2015 Canadian Association of Psychosocial Oncology (CAPO) CRF guidelines, along with the American Society of Clinical Oncology (ASCO) (124), the NCCN (10), and the ONS (125) present the strongest evidence for use of screening and surveillance for fatigue and recommendations for interventions based on the stage of treatment to assist primary care and other clinicians (126).

Yet there are barriers and enablers for efforts to implement practice guidelines. Studies reported that it is feasible to adopt the guidelines, if refined for ease of use and if CRF management is integrated into policy and practice (126,127). To enhance implementation, a better plan for guideline dissemination and application is needed, including patient-level education, professional education on symptom assessment and management, and finally health care system enhancements for better access to and reimbursement of integrated supportive care service (128).

CONCLUSION

CRF is a common and distressing symptom because it interferes with multiple aspects of daily life. Debilitating fatigue can be produced by cancer or its treatment, especially in patients undergoing active cancer treatment, and it can be a persistent symptom for some survivors who have otherwise been cured of their cancer. The mechanism underlying CRF is poorly understood, and although awareness and study of this symptom have grown in recent years, consistent assessment and effective management of CRF have not been priorities in routine medical practice.

A 2003 National Institutes of Health State-of-the-Science Statement (129) called for additional adequately funded prospective studies of pain, depression, and fatigue—both alone and in combination—which has stimulated tremendous growth in clinical investigations of the effectiveness of interventions for CRF. Improving understanding of fatigue will require epidemiological studies and increased reporting of effective therapies. Well-designed clinical trials are needed to evaluate both pharmacological and nonpharmacological methods for treating CRF. Education about CRF should be made available to all patients and their caregivers: accurate and age-appropriate information about conditions like CRF alleviates much of the stress and anxiety brought on by poor communication about of the likelihood of CRF during treatments.

Advancing fatigue research and clinical management will also require the measurement of fatigue in a reliable and valid manner that examines widely accepted dimensions, both for screening and for use in clinical trials. Numerous subscales, unidimensional measures, and multidimensional measures exist, and the establishment of a single, standard tool for measuring symptoms was not recommended in the FDA's PROs guidance (68). Rather, clinicians and researchers should consider individual circumstances, good clinical practice, and research goals as guides for choosing the most appropriate fatigue measurement tool.

Effective treatment of the root causes of CRF will require a much better understanding of the underlying pathophysiological mechanisms of CRF, which remain largely unknown. The development of mechanism-driven fatigue interventions from physiological–behavioral fatigue research, implementation of guidelines for experimental designs, and discovery of biomarkers to identify high-risk individuals would provide patients with greater symptom control.

REFERENCES

1. Vogelzang NJ, Breitbart W, Cella D, et al. Patient, caregiver, and oncologist perceptions of cancer-related fatigue: results of a tripart assessment survey. The Fatigue Coalition. *Semin Hematol.* 1997;34(3 suppl 2):4-12.
2. Mendoza TR, Wang XS, Cleeland CS, et al. The rapid assessment of fatigue severity in cancer patients: use of the Brief Fatigue Inventory. *Cancer.* 1999;85(5):1186-1196.
3. Bower JE, Ganz PA, Desmond KA, Rowland JH, Meyerowitz BE, Belin TR. Fatigue in breast cancer survivors: occurrence, correlates, and impact on quality of life. *J Clin Oncol.* 2000;18(4):743-753.
4. Servaes P, Gielissen MF, Verhagen S, Bleijenberg G. The course of severe fatigue in disease-free breast cancer patients: a longitudinal study. *Psychooncology.* 2007;16(9):787-795.
5. Prue G, Rankin J, Allen J, Gracey J, Cramp F. Cancer-related fatigue: a critical appraisal. *Eur J Cancer.* 2006; 42(7):846-863.
6. Cleeland CS, Mendoza TR, Wang XS, et al. Assessing symptom distress in cancer patients: the M.D. Anderson Symptom Inventory. *Cancer.* 2000;89(7):1634-1646.
7. Barsevick AM, Cleeland CS, Manning DC, et al. ASCPRO recommendations for the assessment of fatigue as an outcome in clinical trials. *J Pain Symptom Manage.* 2010;39(6):1086-1099.
8. Mock V, Atkinson A, Barsevick AM, et al. Cancer-related fatigue. Clinical Practice Guidelines in Oncology. *J Natl Compr Canc Netw.* 2007;5(10):1054-1078.
9. Berger AM, Mooney K, Alvarez-Perez A, et al. Cancer-related fatigue, version 2.2015. *J Natl Compr Canc Netw.* 2015;13(8):1012-1039.
10. NCCN. Cancer-related fatigue 2020. https://www.nccn.org/professionals/physician_gls/pdf/fatigue.pdf
11. Radbruch L, Strasser F, Elsner F, et al. Fatigue in palliative care patients—an EAPC approach. *Palliat Med.* 2008;22(1):13-32.
12. Olson K. A new way of thinking about fatigue: a reconceptualization. *Oncol Nurs Forum.* 2007;34(1):93-99.
13. Scott JA, Lasch KE, Barsevick AM, Piault-Louis E. Patients' experiences with cancer-related fatigue: a review and synthesis of qualitative research. *Oncol Nurs Forum.* 2011;38(3):E191-E203.
14. Wang XS, Zhao F, Fisch MJ, et al. Prevalence and characteristics of moderate to severe fatigue: a multicenter study in cancer patients and survivors. *Cancer.* 2014;120(3):425-432.
15. Wang XS. Pathophysiology of cancer-related fatigue. *Clin J Oncol Nurs.* 2008;12(5 suppl):11-20.
16. Given CW, Given B, Azzouz F, Kozachik S, Stommel M. Predictors of pain and fatigue in the year following diagnosis among elderly cancer patients. *J Pain Symptom Manage.* 2001;21(6):456-466.
17. Wang XS, Fairclough DL, Liao Z, et al. Longitudinal study of the relationship between chemoradiation therapy for non-small-cell lung cancer and patient symptoms. *J Clin Oncol.* 2006;24(27):4485-4491.
18. Hickok JT, Morrow GR, Roscoe JA, Mustian K, Okunieff P. Occurrence, severity, and longitudinal course of twelve common symptoms in 1129 consecutive patients during radiotherapy for cancer. *J Pain Symptom Manage.* 2005;30(5):433-442.
19. Knobel H, Loge JH, Nordøy T, et al. High level of fatigue in lymphoma patients treated with high dose therapy. *J Pain Symptom Manage.* 2000;19(6):446-456.
20. Jacobsen PB, Hann DM, Azzarello LM, Horton J, Balducci L, Lyman GH. Fatigue in women receiving adjuvant chemotherapy for breast cancer: characteristics, course, and correlates. *J Pain Symptom Manage.* 1999;18(4):233-242.
21. Minton O, Strasser F, Radbruch L, Stone P. Identification of factors associated with fatigue in advanced cancer: a subset analysis of the European palliative care research collaborative computerized symptom assessment data set. *J Pain Symptom Manage.* 2012;43(2):226-235.
22. Rubin GJ, Hotopf M. Systematic review and meta-analysis of interventions for postoperative fatigue. *Br J Surg.* 2002;89(8):971-984.

23. Wang XS, Shi Q, Williams LA, et al. Serum interleukin-6 predicts the development of multiple symptoms at nadir of allogeneic hematopoietic stem cell transplantation. *Cancer.* 2008;113(8):2102-2109.

24. Anderson KO, Giralt SA, Mendoza TR, et al. Symptom burden in patients undergoing autologous stem-cell transplantation. *Bone Marrow Transplant.* 2007;39(12): 759-766.

25. Stone P, Hardy J, Huddart R, A'Hern R, Richards M. Fatigue in patients with prostate cancer receiving hormone therapy. *Eur J Cancer.* 2000;36(9):1134-1141.

26. Guevremont C, Alasker A, Karakiewicz PI. Management of sorafenib, sunitinib, and temsirolimus toxicity in metastatic renal cell carcinoma. *Curr Opin Support Palliat Care.* 2009;3(3):170-179.

27. Seruga B, Sterling L, Wang L, Tannock IF. Reporting of serious adverse drug reactions of targeted anticancer agents in pivotal phase III clinical trials. *J Clin Oncol.* 2011;29(2):174-185.

28. Shi Q, Smith TG, Michonski JD, Stein KD, Kaw C, Cleeland CS. Symptom burden in cancer survivors 1 year after diagnosis: a report from the American Cancer Society's Studies of Cancer Survivors. *Cancer.* 2011;117(12):2779-2790.

29. Meeske KA, Siegel SE, Globe DR, Mack WJ, Bernstein L. Prevalence and correlates of fatigue in long-term survivors of childhood leukemia. *J Clin Oncol.* 2005;23(24):5501-5510.

30. Mulrooney DA, Ness KK, Neglia JP, et al. Fatigue and sleep disturbance in adult survivors of childhood cancer: a report from the childhood cancer survivor study (CCSS). *Sleep.* 2008;31(2):271-281.

31. Zeltzer LK, Recklitis C, Buchbinder D, et al. Psychological status in childhood cancer survivors: a report from the Childhood Cancer Survivor Study. *J Clin Oncol.* 2009;27(14):2396-2404.

32. Menzies V, Kelly DL, Yang GS, Starkweather A, Lyon DE. A systematic review of the association between fatigue and cognition in chronic noncommunicable diseases. *Chronic Illn.* 2019:1742395319836472.

33. Gullett JM, Cohen RA, Yang GS, et al. Relationship of fatigue with cognitive performance in women with early-stage breast cancer over 2 years. *Psychooncology.* 2019;28(5):997-1003.

34. Tariman JD, Dhorajiwala S. Genomic variants associated with cancer-related fatigue: a systematic review. *Clin J Oncol Nurs.* 2016;20(5):537-546.

35. Wang T, Yin J, Miller AH, Xiao C. A systematic review of the association between fatigue and genetic polymorphisms. *Brain Behav Immun.* 2017;62:230-244.

36. Ryan JL, Carroll JK, Ryan EP, Mustian KM, Fiscella K, Morrow GR. Mechanisms of cancer-related fatigue. *Oncologist.* 2007;12(suppl 1):22-34.

37. Cleeland CS, Bennett GJ, Dantzer R, et al. Are the symptoms of cancer and cancer treatment due to a shared biologic mechanism? A cytokine-immunologic model of cancer symptoms. *Cancer.* 2003;97(11):2919-2925.

38. Kurzrock R. The role of cytokines in cancer-related fatigue. *Cancer.* 2001;92(6 suppl):1684-1688.

39. Lee BN, Dantzer R, Langley KE, et al. A cytokine-based neuroimmunologic mechanism of cancer-related symptoms. *Neuroimmunomodulation.* 2004;11(5):279-292.

40. Dantzer R, O'Connor JC, Freund GG, Johnson RW, Kelley KW. From inflammation to sickness and depression: when the immune system subjugates the brain. *Nat Rev Neurosci.* 2008;9(1):46-56.

41. Dantzer R, Kelley KW. Twenty years of research on cytokine-induced sickness behavior. *Brain Behav Immun.* 2007;21(2):153-160.

42. Orre IJ, Murison R, Dahl AA, Ueland T, Aukrust P, Fossa SD. Levels of circulating interleukin-1 receptor antagonist and C-reactive protein in long-term survivors of testicular cancer with chronic cancer-related fatigue. *Brain Behav Immun.* 2009;23(6):868-874.

43. Collado-Hidalgo A, Bower JE, Ganz PA, Cole SW, Irwin MR. Inflammatory biomarkers for persistent fatigue in breast cancer survivors. *Clin Cancer Res.* 2006;12(9):2759-2766.

44. Bower JE, Ganz PA, Aziz N, Fahey JL. Fatigue and proinflammatory cytokine activity in breast cancer survivors. *Psychosom Med.* 2002;64(4):604-611.

45. Schubert C, Hong S, Natarajan L, Mills PJ, Dimsdale JE. The association between fatigue and inflammatory marker levels in cancer patients: a quantitative review. *Brain Behav Immun.* 2007;21(4):413-427.

46. Monk JP, Phillips G, Waite R, et al. Assessment of tumor necrosis factor alpha blockade as an intervention to improve tolerability of dose-intensive chemotherapy in cancer patients. *J Clin Oncol.* 2006;24(12):1852-1859.

47. Bower JE, Ganz PA, Irwin MR, Kwan L, Breen EC, Cole SW. Inflammation and behavioral symptoms after breast cancer treatment: do fatigue, depression, and sleep disturbance share a common underlying mechanism? *J Clin Oncol.* 2011;29(26):3517-3522.

48. Wang XS, Shi Q, Williams LA, et al. Inflammatory cytokines are associated with the development of symptom burden in patients with NSCLC undergoing concurrent chemoradiation therapy. *Brain Behav Immun.* 2010;24(6):968-974.

49. Bower JE, Ganz PA, Tao ML, et al. Inflammatory biomarkers and fatigue during radiation therapy for breast and prostate cancer. *Clin Cancer Res.* 2009;15(17):5534-5540.

50. Inagaki M, Isono M, Okuyama T, et al. Plasma interleukin-6 and fatigue in terminally ill cancer patients. *J Pain Symptom Manage.* 2008;35(2):153-161.

51. Conrad R, Geiser F, Mucke M. [Pain and fatigue—a systematic review]. *Z Psychosom Med Psychother.* 2018;64(4):365-379.

52. Payne J, Piper B, Rabinowitz I, Zimmerman B. Biomarkers, fatigue, sleep, and depressive symptoms in women with breast cancer: a pilot study. *Oncol Nurs Forum.* 2006;33(4):775-783.

53. Raison CL, Capuron L, Miller AH. Cytokines sing the blues: inflammation and the pathogenesis of depression. *Trends Immunol.* 2006;27(1):24-31.

54. Dantzer R, Capuron L, Irwin MR, et al. Identification and treatment of symptoms associated with inflammation in medically ill patients. *Psychoneuroendocrinology.* 2008;33(1):18-29.

55. Miller AH, Ancoli-Israel S, Bower JE, Capuron L, Irwin MR. Neuroendocrine-immune mechanisms of behavioral comorbidities in patients with cancer. *J Clin Oncol.* 2008;26(6):971-982.

56. Irwin MR, Miller AH. Depressive disorders and immunity: 20 years of progress and discovery. *Brain Behav Immun.* 2007;21(4):374-383.

57. Vichaya EG, Vermeer DW, Budac D, et al. Inhibition of Indoleamine 2,3 dioxygenase does not improve cancer-related symptoms in a murine model of human papilloma virus-related head and neck cancer. *Int J Tryptophan Res.* 2019;12:1178646919872508.

58. Capuron L, Pagnoni G, Demetrashvili MF, et al. Basal ganglia hypermetabolism and symptoms of fatigue during interferon-alpha therapy. *Neuropsychopharmacology.* 2007;32(11):2384-2392.

59. Fitzgerald PB, Laird AR, Maller J, Daskalakis ZJ. A meta-analytic study of changes in brain activation in depression. *Hum Brain Mapp.* 2008;29(6):683-695.

60. Chaudhuri A, Behan PO. Fatigue in neurological disorders. *Lancet.* 2004;363(9413):978-988.

61. Tellez N, Alonso J, Rio J, et al. The basal ganglia: a substrate for fatigue in multiple sclerosis. *Neuroradiology.* 2008;50(1):17-23.

62. Davis JM, Bailey SP. Possible mechanisms of central nervous system fatigue during exercise. *Med Sci Sports Exerc.* 1997;29(1):45-57.

63. Mills PJ, Parker B, Dimsdale JE, Sadler GR, Ancoli-Israel S. The relationship between fatigue and quality of life and inflammation during anthracycline-based chemotherapy in breast cancer. *Biol Psychol.* 2005;69(1):85-96.

64. Rich T, Innominato PF, Boerner J, et al. Elevated serum cytokines correlated with altered behavior, serum cortisol rhythm, and dampened 24-hour rest-activity patterns in patients with metastatic colorectal cancer. *Clin Cancer Res.* 2005;11(5):1757-1764.

65. Payne JK. Altered circadian rhythms and cancer-related fatigue outcomes. *Integr Cancer Ther.* 2011;10(3):221-233.

66. Azzolino D, Arosio B, Marzetti E, Calvani R, Cesari M. Nutritional status as a mediator of fatigue and its underlying mechanisms in older people. *Nutrients.* 2020;12(2):444.

67. Hurter B, Bush NJ. Cancer-related anemia: clinical review and management update. *Clin J Oncol Nurs.* 2007;11(3):349-359.

68. US Department of Health and Human Services, Food and Drug Administration (FDA), Center for Drug Evaluation and Research (CDER), Center for Biologics Evaluation and Research (CBER), Center for Devices and Radiological Health (CDRH). *Guidance for Industry Patient-Reported Outcome Measures: Use in Medical Product Development to Support Labeling Claims.* Silver Spring, MD. 2009. https://www.fda.gov/media/77832/download

69. Hjollund NH, Andersen JH, Bech P. Assessment of fatigue in chronic disease: a bibliographic study of fatigue measurement scales. *Health Qual Life Outcomes.* 2007;5:12.

70. Jacobsen PB. Assessment of fatigue in cancer patients. *J Natl Cancer Inst Monogr.* 2004;(32):93-97.

71. Lai JS, Crane PK, Cella D. Factor analysis techniques for assessing sufficient unidimensionality of cancer related fatigue. *Qual Life Res.* 2006;15(7):1179-1190.

72. Basch E, Iasonos A, McDonough T, et al. Patient versus clinician symptom reporting using the National Cancer Institute Common Terminology Criteria for Adverse Events: results of a questionnaire-based study. *Lancet Oncol.* 2006;7(11):903-909.

73. Escalante CP, Manzullo EF, Lam TP, Ensor JE, Valdres RU, Wang XS. Fatigue and its risk factors in cancer patients who seek emergency care. *J Pain Symptom Manage.* 2008;36(4):358-366.

74. Krupp LB, LaRocca NG, Muir-Nash J, Steinberg AD. The fatigue severity scale. Application to patients with multiple sclerosis and systemic lupus erythematosus. *Arch Neurol.* 1989;46(10):1121-1123.

75. Yellen SB, Cella DF, Webster K, Blendowski C, Kaplan E. Measuring fatigue and other anemia-related symptoms with the Functional Assessment of Cancer Therapy (FACT) measurement system. *J Pain Symptom Manage.* 1997;13(2):63-74.

76. Aaronson NK, Ahmedzai S, Bergman B, et al. The European Organization for Research and Treatment of Cancer QLQ-C30: a quality-of-life instrument for use in international clinical trials in oncology. *J Natl Cancer Inst.* 1993;85(5):365-376.

77. Smets EMA, Garssen B, Bonke B, De Haes JCJM. The multidimensional Fatigue Inventory (MFI) psychometric qualities of an instrument to assess fatigue. *J Psychosom Res.* 1995;39(3):315-325.

78. Leung YW, Brown C, Cosio AP, et al. Feasibility and diagnostic accuracy of the Patient-Reported Outcomes Measurement Information System (PROMIS) item banks for routine surveillance of sleep and fatigue problems in ambulatory cancer care. *Cancer.* 2016;122(18):2906-2917.

79. Weis J, Tomaszewski KA, Hammerlid E, et al. International psychometric validation of an EORTC quality of life module measuring cancer related fatigue (EORTC QLQ-FA12). *J Natl Cancer Inst.* 2017;109(5). doi: 10.1093/jnci/djw273.

80. Cleeland CS, Wang XS. Measuring and understanding fatigue. *Oncology.* 1999;13(11 A):91-97.

81. Serlin RC, Mendoza TR, Nakamura Y, Edwards KR, Cleeland CS. When is cancer pain mild, moderate or severe? Grading pain severity by its interference with function. *Pain.* 1995;61(2):277-284.

82. Cleeland CS, Ryan KM. Pain assessment: global use of the Brief Pain Inventory. *Ann Acad Med Singapore.* 1994;23(2):129-138.

83. Cleeland CS, Gonin R, Hatfield AK, et al. Pain and its treatment in outpatients with metastatic cancer. *N Engl J Med.* 1994;330(9):592-596.

84. Visser MR, Smets EM, Sprangers MA, de Haes HJ. How response shift may affect the measurement of change in fatigue. *J Pain Symptom Manage.* 2000;20(1):12-18.

85. Schwartz CE, Bode R, Repucci N, Becker J, Sprangers MA, Fayers PM. The clinical significance of adaptation to changing health: a meta-analysis of response shift. *Qual Life Res.* 2006;15(9):1533-1550.

86. Mitchell SA Beck SL, Eaton LH. Putting evidence into practice (PEP): fatigue. In: Eaton LH, Tipton JM, eds. *Putting Evidence Into Practice: Improving Oncology Patient Outcomes.* 1st ed. Pittsburgh PA: Oncology Nursing Society; 2009:149-174.

87. National Comprehensive Cancer Network (NCCN). NCCN clinical practice guidelines in oncology: cancer- and chemotherapy-induced anemia. *Oncology (Williston Park).* 2006;20(8 suppl 6):12-15.

88. Mitchell SA, Lawrence TS, Rosenberg SA, eds. *Cancer: Principles & Practice of Oncology: Primer of the Molecular Biology of Cancer.* Philadelphia, PA: Wolters Kluwer Health/Lippincott Williams & Wilkins; 2011:2387-2392.

89. Moher D, Jones A, Lepage L. Use of the CONSORT statement and quality of reports of randomized trials: a comparative before-and-after evaluation. *JAMA.* 2001;285(15):1992-1995.

90. Moher D, Schulz KF, Altman DG. The CONSORT statement: revised recommendations for improving the quality of reports of parallel-group randomised trials. *Lancet.* 2001;357(9263):1191-1194.

91. Mucke M, Cuhls H, Peuckmann-Post V, Minton O, Stone P, Radbruch L. Pharmacological treatments for fatigue associated with palliative care. *Cochrane Database Syst Rev.* 2015;(5):CD006788.

92. Minton O, Richardson A, Sharpe M, Hotopf M, Stone PC. Psychostimulants for the management of cancer-related fatigue: a systematic review and meta-analysis. *J Pain Symptom Manage.* 2011;41(4):761-767.

93. Breitbart W, Alici Y. Psychostimulants for cancer-related fatigue. *J Natl Compr Canc Netw.* 2010;8(8):933-942.

94. Fava M, Thase ME, DeBattista C, Doghramji K, Arora S, Hughes RJ. Modafinil augmentation of selective serotonin reuptake inhibitor therapy in MDD partial responders with persistent fatigue and sleepiness. *Ann Clin Psychiatry.* 2007;19(3):153-159.

95. Morrow GR, Jean-Pierre P, Roscoe JA, et al. A phase III randomized, placebo-controlled, double-blind trial of a eugeroic agent in 642 cancer patients reporting fatigue during chemotherapy: a URCC CCOP Study. *J Clin Oncol.* 2008;26(15_suppl):9512.

96. Morrow GR, Hickok JT, Roscoe JA, et al. Differential effects of paroxetine on fatigue and depression: a randomized, double-blind trial from the University of Rochester Cancer Center Community Clinical Oncology Program. *J Clin Oncol.* 2003;21(24):4635-4641.

97. Roscoe JA, Morrow GR, Hickok JT, et al. Effect of paroxetine hydrochloride (Paxil) on fatigue and depression in breast cancer patients receiving chemotherapy. *Breast Cancer Res Treat.* 2005;89(3):243-249.

98. Moss EL, Simpson JS, Pelletier G, Forsyth P. An open-label study of the effects of bupropion SR on fatigue, depression and quality of life of mixed-site cancer patients and their partners. *Psychooncology.* 2006;15(3):259-267.

99. Minton O, Richardson A, Sharpe M, Hotopf M, Stone P. A systematic review and meta-analysis of the pharmacological treatment of cancer-related fatigue. *J Natl Cancer Inst.* 2008;100(16):1155-1166.

100. Ferro M, Di Lorenzo G, de Cobelli O, et al. Incidence of fatigue and low-dose corticosteroid use in prostate cancer patients receiving systemic treatment: a meta-analysis of randomized controlled trials. *World J Urol.* 2019;37(6):1049-1059.

101. Wang XS, Shi Q, Mendoza T, et al. Minocycline reduces chemoradiation-related symptom burden in patients with non-small cell lung cancer: a phase 2 randomized trial. *Int J Radiat Oncol Biol Phys.* 2020;106(1):100-107.

102. Gunn GB, Mendoza TR, Garden AS, et al. Minocycline for symptom reduction during radiation therapy for head and neck cancer: a randomized clinical trial. *Support Care Cancer.* 2020;28(1):261-269.

103. Wang XS, Shi Q, Bhadkamkar NA, et al. Minocycline for symptom reduction during oxaliplatin-based chemotherapy for colorectal cancer: a phase II randomized clinical trial. *J Pain Symptom Manage.* 2019;58(4):662-671.

104. Kamal M, Wang XS, Shi Q, et al. A randomized, placebo-controlled, double-blind study of minocycline for reducing the symptom burden experienced by patients with advanced pancreatic cancer. *J Pain Symptom Manage.* 2020;59(5):1052.e1-1058.e1.

105. Elam JL, Carpenter JS, Shu XO, Boyapati S, Friedmann-Gilchrist J. Methodological issues in the investigation of ginseng as an intervention for fatigue. *Clin Nurse Spec.* 2006;20(4):183-189.

106. Laino, C. Ginseng may relieve cancer treatment fatigue. *Mayo Clin Health Lett.* 2007;25:4. https://www.webmd.com/cancer/news/20070604/ginseng-may-relieve-cancer-fatigue#1

107. Barton DL, Soori GS, Bauer B, et al. A pilot, multi-dose, placebo-controlled evaluation of american ginseng (panax quinquefolius) to improve cancer-related fatigue: NCCTG trial N03CA. *J Clin Oncol.* 2007;25(18_suppl):9001.

108. Xu Y, Wang XS, Chen Y, Shi Q, Chen TH, Li P. A phase II randomized controlled trial of Renshen Yangrong Tang herbal extract granules for fatigue reduction in cancer survivors. *J Pain Symptom Manage.* 2020;59(5):966-973.

109. Campos MP, Hassan BJ, Riechelmann R, Del Giglio A. Cancer-related fatigue: a review. *Rev Assoc Med Bras (1992).* 2011;57(2):211-219.

110. Bentler SE, Hartz AJ, Kuhn EM. Prospective observational study of treatments for unexplained chronic fatigue. *J Clin Psychiatry.* 2005;66(5):625-632.

111. Junior PNA, Barreto CMN, de Iracema Gomes Cubero D, Del Giglio A. The efficacy of placebo for the treatment of cancer-related fatigue: a systematic review and meta-analysis. *Support Care Cancer.* 2020;28(4):1755-1764.

112. Roji R, Stone P, Ricciardi F, Candy B. Placebo response in trials of drug treatments for cancer-related fatigue: a systematic review, meta-analysis and meta-regression.

BMJ Support Palliat Care. 2020. doi:10.1136/bmjspcare-2019-002163.

113. Wu C, Zheng Y, Duan Y, et al. Nonpharmacological interventions for cancer-related fatigue: a systematic review and Bayesian network meta-analysis. *Worldviews Evid Based Nurs.* 2019;16(2):102-110.

114. Mustian KM, Alfano CM, Heckler C, et al. Comparison of pharmaceutical, psychological, and exercise treatments for cancer-related fatigue: a meta-analysis. *JAMA Oncol.* 2017;3(7):961-968.

115. Schmitz KH, Holtzman J, Courneya KS, Masse LC, Duval S, Kane R. Controlled physical activity trials in cancer survivors: a systematic review and meta-analysis. *Cancer Epidemiol Biomarkers Prev.* 2005;14(7):1588-1595.

116. Furmaniak AC, Menig M, Markes MH. Exercise for women receiving adjuvant therapy for breast cancer. *Cochrane Database Syst Rev.* 2016;(9):CD005001.

117. Poort H, Peters M, Bleijenberg G, et al. Psychosocial interventions for fatigue during cancer treatment with palliative intent. *Cochrane Database Syst Rev.* 2017;(7):CD012030.

118. Jacobsen PB, Donovan KA, Vadaparampil ST, Small BJ. Systematic review and meta-analysis of psychological and activity-based interventions for cancer-related fatigue. *Health Psychol.* 2007;26(6):660-667.

119. Bennett S, Pigott A, Beller EM, Haines T, Meredith P, Delaney C. Educational interventions for the management of cancer-related fatigue in adults. *Cochrane Database Syst Rev* 2016;(11):CD008144.

120. van Weert E, Hoekstra-Weebers JEHM, May AM, Korstjens I, Ros WJG, van der Schans CP. The development of an evidence-based physical self-management rehabilitation programme for cancer survivors. *Patient Educ Couns.* 2008;71(2):169-190.

121. Zhang Y, Lin L, Li H, Hu Y, Tian L. Effects of acupuncture on cancer-related fatigue: a meta-analysis. *Support Care Cancer.* 2018;26(2):415-425.

122. Balk J, Day R, Rosenzweig M, Beriwal S. Pilot, randomized, modified, double-blind, placebo-controlled trial of acupuncture for cancer-related fatigue. *J Soc Integr Oncol.* 2009;7(1):4-11.

123. Molassiotis A, Sylt P, Diggins H. The management of cancer-related fatigue after chemotherapy with acupuncture and acupressure: a randomised controlled trial. *Complement Ther Med.* 2007;15(4):228-237.

124. Bower JE, Bak K, Berger A, et al. Screening, assessment, and management of fatigue in adult survivors of cancer: an American Society of Clinical oncology clinical practice guideline adaptation. *J Clin Oncol.* 2014;32(17):1840-1850.

125. Mitchell SA, Hoffman AJ, Clark JC, et al. Putting evidence into practice: an update of evidence-based interventions for cancer-related fatigue during and following treatment. *Clin J Oncol Nurs.* 2014;18(suppl):38-58.

126. Pearson EJ, Morris ME, McKinstry CE. Cancer-related fatigue: appraising evidence-based guidelines for screening, assessment and management. *Support Care Cancer.* 2016;24(9):3935-3942.

127. Pearson EJM, Morris ME, McKinstry CE. Cancer related fatigue: implementing guidelines for optimal management. *BMC Health Serv Res.* 2017;17(1):496.

128. Berger AM, Mooney K. Dissemination and implementation of guidelines for cancer-related fatigue. *J Natl Compr Canc Netw.* 2016;14(11):1336-1338.

129. Patrick DL, Ferketich SL, Frame PS, et al. National Institutes of Health state-of-the-science conference statement: symptom management in cancer: pain, depression, and fatigue, July 15-17, 2002. *J Natl Cancer Inst.* 2003;95(15):1110-1117.

8 Fever and Sweats

Christopher Ahern and Elizabeth Prsic

TEMPERATURE AND ASSOCIATED SYMPTOMS

Temperature has long been recognized as an integral clinical indicator in medicine and was included in the cardinal signs of inflammation described as "calor, dolor, tumor, rubor" by Celsus in the first century (1). The measurement of temperature may be taken either centrally (rectally) or peripherally (orally, axillary, temporally, or by tympanic membrane). Normal body temperature is maintained at 37°C and is tightly controlled within a narrow range through diverse heat conservation and dissipation mechanisms (2).

Fever is defined as any elevation in the core body temperature above the normal range. More commonly, a temperature >38°C is considered a clinically significant fever. According to American Society of Clinical Oncology and the Infectious Disease Society of America, a fever in neutropenic patients is defined as a single temperature reading >38.3°C or a temperature >38°C sustained over an hour (3). The term fever of unknown origin (FUO) is used commonly, and often incorrectly, in the daily practice of medicine. A true FUO is defined as an illness lasting at least 3 weeks with a fever higher than 38.3°C on more than one occasion and which lacks a definitive diagnosis after 1 week of hospital evaluation (4).

Fever is often accompanied by other symptoms, including sweating and rigors. Sweating, when it accompanies fever, is a cooling response by the body wherein heat is released from the body as it evaporates water on the skin's surface. Rigors and shivering also contribute to temperature control (2). Nonshivering thermogenesis, a process involving heat production in brown adipose tissue, is important in the temperature control of infants.

CONTROL OF TEMPERATURE

Core body temperature is controlled by neurologic mechanisms centered in the hypothalamus. Fever is the result of up-regulation of the hypothalamic temperature set point by endogenous pyrogens, inflammatory cytokines, or drugs (2). Fever is initiated by the increased production of interleukins IL-1, IL-6, tumor necrosis factor, interferon-alpha, and other pyrogenic cytokines by phagocytic cells in tissue and blood. These cytokines stimulate the increased production of prostaglandin (especially PGE2) in the anterior hypothalamus, which in turn leads to an increase in the hypothalamic set-point temperature (2,5).

As a result of the reset hypothalamic temperature, the body increases the core body temperature to this new level (Fig. 8.1). Shivering and rigors, initiated by mechanisms within the anterior hypothalamus, contribute to temperature control through thermogenesis (2). Cold temperatures activate centers in the posterior hypothalamus, which initiate rhythmic contraction of skeletal muscle to promote heat production (2). Rapid muscle spasms increase endogenous heat production, contributing to temperature elevation, and appear more commonly with rapid rises in temperature (6). The sympathetic nervous system is involved in heat generation and retention, in particular through increased sympathetic tone and vasoconstriction (2). Nonshivering thermogenesis, a process involving heat production in brown adipose tissue, is important in the temperature control of infants. For adult humans, warming behaviors (putting on additional layers of clothing, increasing temperature of external environment) contribute significantly to physiologic heat retention.

The continued presence of pyrogen at the hypothalamus results in the maintenance of this higher temperature. Eventually, as a result of either a decrease in the quantity of pyrogen or the administration of an antipyretic, the hypothalamic temperature is reset to a lower or normal level. The core body temperature is therefore lowered through various mechanisms for cooling including vasodilation of skin blood vessels through decreased sympathetic tone, and increased sweating through sympathetic cholinergic response (2). These control mechanisms may be suppressed in patients administered steroids or anti-inflammatory agents, in children, or in the elderly. Although fever appears to be associated with enhanced function of the immune system, it must nonetheless be noted that a direct connection between such

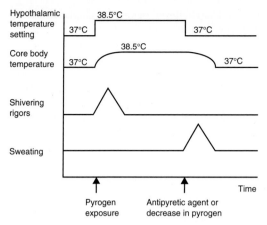

Figure 8.1 Physiologic mechanisms associated with fever and accompanying symptoms. (Adapted from Boulant JA. Thermoregulation. In: Mackowiak P, ed. *Fever: Basic Mechanisms and Management*. New York, NY: Raven Press; 1991:1-22, with permission.)

phenomena and a beneficial effect of fever on outcome of infections has not been established. Fever, in fact, may be deleterious in the setting of autoimmune disorders or infections (7).

Fever is pathophysiologically distinct from hyperthermia and hyperpyrexia. In hyperthermia, thermoregulation of the hypothalamus remains intact, but exogenous factors such as excessive heat, or endogenous heat production override the physiologic drive for normothermia. Heat-dissipating mechanisms are unable to keep up with heat production, which can lead to acute or fatal events if not treated (2). Malignant hyperthermia, characterized by substantial increases in metabolic rate, oxygen consumption, and increased heat production, can be caused by inhalational anesthetics in susceptible individuals (2).

Hyperpyrexia is body temperature >41.5°C, which can be seen in the setting of sepsis or more commonly associated with central nervous system hemorrhage. Hyperpyrexia should be managed with cooling measures, as well as antipyretics (6).

FEVER IN SPECIAL POPULATIONS

Elderly

With increased age and frailty, elderly patients may mount a less robust febrile response, even in the presence of serious infection, due to impaired functioning in one of more of the body's thermoregulatory systems (e.g., hypothalamic activation, vasoconstriction, shivering, brown adipose tissue thermogenesis). Indeed, a fever may be absent or markedly blunted in 20% to 30% of geriatric cases of infection (8). Though recorded temperatures may not be markedly elevated, these patients are

recognized to be at high risk for poor clinical outcomes. Thus, a lower threshold for diagnosis of fever in frail, older patients is commonly utilized. In such cases, diagnostic criteria for a fever are a single oral temperature >37.8°C or persistent oral or tympanic membrane temperature >37.2°C or a rise in temperature of ≥ 1.1°C above a patient's baseline temperature (8).

Children

The parameters for diagnosis of fever in infants and young children vary from that of the adult population, due in part to the higher metabolic rate and greater surface-area-to-body-weight ratio in pediatric patients. For children up to 3 months of age, the consensus definition for fever of concern is a rectal temperature >100.4°F (38.0°C). For children 3 to 36 months of age, fever is defined as a rectal temperature of 100.4°F to 102.2°F (38°C to 39°C), and "fever of concern" is defined as a rectal temperature above 102.2°F (>39°C).

Pediatric febrile seizures occur in 3% to 4% of children between 6 months and 5 years of age. Febrile seizures occur in the presence of a body temperature of 100.4°F or higher, most commonly on the first day of illness. Febrile seizures are by definition not associated with intracranial infection or defined cause, and, despite frequent parental concern to the contrary, these brief benign convulsive episodes are not associated with brain damage. Most notable in the context of this chapter is the fact that treatment of fever with antipyretics is not associated with decreased incidence of febrile seizure occurrence.

ETIOLOGY OF FEVER IN CANCER PATIENTS

Fever is common in patients with cancer, even in the absence of infection. Febrile etiologies in patients with cancer will be considered in relation to the pathophysiology of fever.

Tumor

Tumor fever, while common, is a diagnosis of exclusion. Fever associated with oncologic or hematologic malignancy is believed to be associated with the release of pyrogens, either directly from a tumor or from tumor stimulation of immunologic mechanisms that cause an elevation in temperature through action on the hypothalamus. Cytokines specifically involved in fever production include tumor necrosis factor α, IL-1 and IL-6, and interferon, although they are involved in fever related to both malignancy and infection (9). Differentiating between fevers related to tumor and infection is challenging. A recent study identified

TABLE 8.1 TUMORS CLASSICALLY ASSOCIATED WITH FEVER

Hodgkin's disease
Lymphoma
Leukemia
Renal cell carcinoma
Myxoma
Osteogenic sarcoma

shaking chills, decline in baseline performance status, and change in baseline neutrophil:lymphocyte ratio to be statistically significant factors indicative of infection rather than tumor fever (10).

Fever is commonly associated with both hematologic malignancies and solid tumors. The most common malignancies associated with fever include Hodgkin's and non-Hodgkin's lymphoma, acute and chronic leukemia, soft tissue sarcoma, renal cell carcinoma, and atrial myxoma (9) (Table 8.1). Tumor fever is important in the differential diagnosis of FUO. Between 15% and 20% of fevers of unknown origin in adults are eventually attributed to malignancy (11). In children, under 10% of FUO are attributed to malignancy (12). In patients with neutropenia, secondary to either malignancy or cancer treatment, timely fever assessment and management are critical.

Pel-Ebstein fever pattern is characterized by febrile episodes that present daily over many weeks, with alternating afebrile periods (13,14) (Fig. 8.2). The Pel-Ebstein fever is historically associated with Hodgkin's lymphoma. Overall, this presentation is rare in the modern clinical setting (13). While B-symptoms are certainly important clinically, the eponymous Pel-Ebstein fever is largely relegated to historical interest and is of limited diagnostic or prognostic value.

Febrile Neutropenia

Although infection and fever can be a common presentation in patients with cancer, it is of particular concern in patients with neutropenia. Neutropenia, defined as peripheral blood absolute neutrophil count ≤1,500/μL, results from either decreased production or increased destruction of white blood cells. Severe neutropenia is defined as a peripheral blood absolute neutrophil count <500/μL or anticipated decrease to <500/μL within 48 hours. Clinically significant infection risk rises with severity of neutropenia. Risk factors for the development of fever in the setting of neutropenia have been identified and include a rapid decrease in the neutrophil count and prolonged, severe neutropenia >10 days (15). Decreased

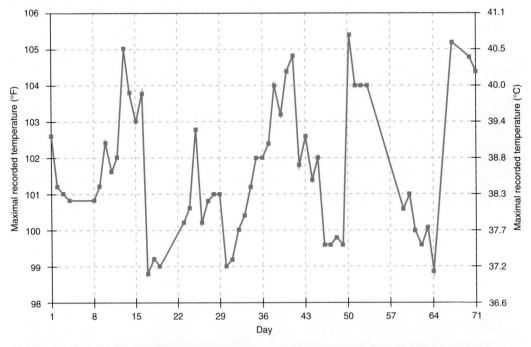

Figure 8.2 A 50-year-old man had fever, night sweats, and nonproductive cough for 10 weeks. He took antipyretic medications during the febrile periods. His wife recorded his temperatures, shown in the preceding text, on 56 of the 71 days. Biopsy of a rapidly enlarging cervical lymph node revealed nodular sclerosing Hodgkin's lymphoma. The patient's fevers and other symptoms promptly disappeared after the first cycle of doxorubicin, bleomycin, vinblastine, and dacarbazine. (From Good GR, Dinubile MJ. Images in clinical medicine. Cyclic fever in Hodgkin's disease (Pel-Ebstein fever). *N Engl J Med.* 1995;332:436, with permission.)

production by the bone marrow may result either from disease involving the marrow or from myelosuppression due to chemotherapy. Other factors that may alter infectious risk in the patient with neutropenia include phagocyte function, the status of the patient's immune system, alterations in the physical defense barriers of the patient's immune system, and alterations in the physical defense barriers of the body (e.g., mucositis). Given immunosuppression inherent in patients with febrile neutropenia, temperature should not be measured rectally to avoid possible introduction of infection through mucosal trauma.

In addition to malignancy and chemotherapy, other causes of neutropenia include drug-induced, hypersplenism, and infections, most commonly HIV, EBV, cytomegalovirus, hepatitis A and B, measles, varicella, *Rickettsia*, and anaplasmosis (16). Finally, increased destruction of neutrophils may occur through autoimmune mechanisms.

Chemotherapy regimens confer varying risks of severe neutropenia. If risk of febrile neutropenia following chemotherapy is ≥20%, guidelines recommend prophylaxis with myeloid colony-stimulating factors (17).

Management of Febrile Neutropenia

Current guidelines recommend prompt assessment, and initiation of empiric antibiotics within 1 hour of triage for patients presenting with febrile neutropenia (3). Patients should receive monotherapy with an antipseudomonal beta-lactam agent or piperacillin–tazobactam. Other agents may be considered for initial regimen if antibiotic resistance is suspected or proven, or in the setting of complications (e.g., hypotension, pneumonia). Aerobic gram-positive cocci coverage is not recommended as initial empiric therapy, except in specific clinical settings such as catheter-related infections, skin or soft tissue infections, pneumonia, or hemodynamic instability (17). Antifungal coverage should be considered in high-risk patients with persistent fever after 4 to 7 days of broad-spectrum antibiotics and no identified fever source. The duration of therapy is dependent upon the underlying infection, if identified, and the duration of severe neutropenia (17).

Infections in Febrile Neutropenia

A microbiological source of infection is identified in only 10% to 20% of patients presenting with febrile neutropenia. Only 20% to 30% of patients with febrile neutropenia present with a clinically documented infection (e.g., cellulitis without isolated pathogen). The majority of documented infections are thought to be caused by translocation of endogenous bacterial flora (Palmore 2018).

Despite thorough inpatient assessment, roughly half of patients presenting with febrile neutropenia have a FUO (18,19). Prior to the 1980s, gram-negative bacilli were the most commonly identified source of infection in patients with febrile neutropenia. More recently, gram-positive bacteria have become the predominant infectious etiology of fever among patients with cancer (20). However, trends towards multidrug-resistant gram-negative organisms as well as vancomycin-resistant *Enterococcus faecium* among patients with hematologic malignancies have been documented (21). The etiology of febrile neutropenia differs between hematologic and oncologic malignancies, as well as between patient populations (e.g., elderly vs. children) (22).

The risk of invasive fungal infection in patients for whom duration of severe neutropenia is expected to be ≤7 days is very low. For these patients, prophylaxis is not recommended. For high-risk patients especially, invasive fungal infections should be considered in the evaluation of febrile neutropenia. In high-risk patients who have persistent fever after 4 to 7 days of broad-spectrum antibiotics and no identified source of fever, empiric antifungal coverage should be added to therapy (17). Invasive fungal infections are associated with prolonged duration and severity of neutropenia, longer duration of chemotherapy, and extended antibiotic exposure. The fungal species most commonly associated with febrile neutropenia are *Candida* spp and *Aspergillus* spp. Both prophylactic and empiric antifungal regimens must include coverage of these pathogens.

Febrile neutropenia in patients with cancer is associated with a substantial risk of morbidity and mortality. Several evidence-based tools including the MASCC (Multinational Association for Supportive Care in Cancer) Score may be used to identify patients with febrile neutropenia who are at lower risk of complications and may be managed outpatient (3). The MASCC score was developed through a multinational study, which identified a risk index score to stratify patients with febrile neutropenia (23). Predictive factors included blood pressure, presence of chronic obstructive pulmonary disease or solid tumor, previous fungal infection in patients with hematologic malignancies, outpatient status, status of hydration, and age in relation to 60 years (Table 8.2). A MASCC risk index score ≥21 identified low-risk patients with positive predictive value of 91%, specificity of 68%, and sensitivity of 71%. Patients at low risk of complications in the setting of febrile neutropenia may be managed with oral antibiotics in the outpatient setting after initial evaluation (24).

TABLE 8.2 MULTINATIONAL ASSOCIATION FOR SUPPORTIVE CARE IN CANCER SCORING INDEX

Characteristic	Score
Burden of illness: no or mild symptoms	5
Burden of illness: moderate symptoms	3
Burden of illness: severe symptoms	0
No hypotension (systolic BP > 90 mm Hg)	5
No chronic obstructive pulmonary disease	4
Solid tumor/lymphoma with no previous fungal infection	4
No dehydration	3
Outpatient status (at onset of fever)	3
Age <60 years	2

Scores ≥21 are at low risk of complications.
Points attributed to the variable "burden of illness" are not cumulative. The maximum theoretical score is therefore 26.

Febrile Neutropenia in Pediatric Population

There are currently six validated pediatric risk stratification strategies for low-risk patients, all of which rely on a single assessment at presentation (Table 8.3). According to the American Society of Clinical Oncology, no schema has been proven superior but each of them is validated in the proper setting. Thus, it is recommended that the chosen schema be locally validated and applied to all pediatric cancer patients presenting with febrile neutropenia in order to identify low-risk patients (25).

In order to guide treatment course, ASCO recommends obtaining blood cultures at onset from all lumens of any central venous catheters and to consider peripheral blood culture collected concurrent with central lines. Clean-catch midstream urinalysis and culture should be considered if readily available, and chest radiography only in patients with signs of respiratory involvement.

In those pediatric patients assessed to have features of high-risk febrile neutropenia, current recommendations are for empirical monotherapy with either an antipseudomonal beta-lactam, a fourth generation cephalosporin, or a carbapenem. Addition of a second gram-negative agent or a glycopeptide is recommended only for patients who are clinically unstable, when resistance is suspected, or if local antibiograms demonstrate a high rate of pathogen resistance.

In pediatric patients with low-risk febrile neutropenia, initial outpatient management or step-down oral antibiotic management can be considered if the infrastructure exists to ensure close monitoring and follow-up. Indeed, four studies demonstrated no difference in outcomes between those low-risk patients randomized to inpatient and outpatient management (27–30).

Per ASCO, pediatric patients at high risk for invasive fungal disease (IFD) include those with diagnoses of acute myeloid leukemia, high-risk acute lymphoblastic leukemia (ALL) or relapsed acute leukemia, children undergoing allogeneic hematopoietic stem cell transplant, children with prolonged neutropenia, and children receiving high-dose corticosteroids. All other patients with febrile neutropenia should be categorized as low risk for IFD.

It is recommended to initiate empirical antifungal therapy with either caspofungin or liposomal amphotericin B in high-risk patients with prolonged (>96 hours) febrile neutropenia not responsive to initial broad-spectrum antibiotics. For patients with persistent febrile neutropenia beyond 96 hours who are low risk for IFD, there is a weak recommendation against empirical therapy for IFD in low-risk patients (25).

Location

A detailed history and physical examination is critical in determining the location of infection in a febrile patient. Patients undergoing chemotherapy are at higher risk of infection at any site related to immune suppression, invasive procedures, radiation, and drug-specific toxicities. Among patients with cancer, there are particularly broad potential sites of infection.

Immunosuppressed patients are at increased risk of infection throughout the gastrointestinal tract. Mucositis is of particular concern in certain therapeutic settings (5-fluorouracil, high-dose methotrexate, mucosal radiation exposure) as it impairs physiologic defenses and increases risk of infection further in vulnerable patients. Oral candidiasis is frequently observed in immunosuppressed patients. Dental problems whether related to mucositis, gingivitis, xerostomia, radiation, or bisphosphonates also figure prominently for infection risk among patients undergoing cancer therapy, or in the survivorship setting. *Clostridium difficile* infection may present with fever and diarrhea and is common in patients in both hospital- and community-acquired settings. Cancer chemotherapy and *C. difficile* infection may be related to both the antimicrobial effect of chemotherapy agents as well as associated immunosuppression (31). In the gastrointestinal tract, spontaneous bacterial peritonitis should be considered in patients with ascites, fever, and abdominal pain. Cholangitis is also common, particularly among patients who have had recent instrumentation or

TABLE 8.3 VALIDATED PEDIATRIC RISK STRATIFICATION STRATEGIES FOR LOW-RISK PATIENTS

Schema-related factors	Rackoff (4)	Alexander (5)	Rondinelli (6)	Santolaya (7)	Ammann (8)	Ammann (9)
Patient- and disease-related factors	None	AML, Burkitt's lymphoma, induction ALL, progressive disease, relapsed with marrow involvement	2 points for central venous catheter, 1 point for age ≤5 years	Relapsed leukemia, chemotherapy within 7 days of episode	Bone marrow involvement, central venous catheter, pre–B-cell leukemia	4 points for chemotherapy more intensive than ALL maintenance
Episode-specific factors	Absolute monocyte count	Hypotension; tachypnea or hypoxia <94%; new CXR changes; altered mental status; severe mucositis, vomiting, or abdominal pain; focal infection; other clinical reason for inpatient treatment	4.5 points for clinical site of infection, 2.5 points for no URTI, 1 point each for fever > 38.5°C, hemoglobin ≤70 g/L	CRP ≥ 90 mg/L, hypotension, platelets ≤50 g/L	Absence of clinical signs of viral infection, CRP > 50 mg/L, white blood cell count ≤500/µL, hemoglobin >100 g/L	5 points for hemoglobin ≥90 g/L, 3 points each for white blood cell count <300/µL, platelet <50 g/L
Rule formulation	Absolute monocyte count ≥100/µL = low risk of bacteremia; HSCT = high risk	Absence of any risk factor = low risk of serious medical complication; HSCT = high risk	Total score <6 = low risk of serious infectious complication; HSCT = high risk	Zero risk factors or only low platelets or only <7 days from chemotherapy = low risk of invasive bacterial infection	Three or fewer risk factors = low risk of significant infection; HSCT = high risk	Total score < 9 = low risk of adverse FN outcome; HSCT = high risk
Demonstrated to be valid[a]	United States, Madsen (10)	United Kingdom, Dommett (11), Arif (12)	Brazil, Rondinelli (6)	South America, Santolaya (13)	Europe, Ammann (9), Macher (14), Arif (12)	Europe, Miedema (15)

[a]Valid refers to clinically adequate discrimination of a group at low risk of complications.

ALL, acute lymphoblastic leukemia; AML, acute myeloid leukemia; CRP, C-reactive protein; CXR, chest radiography; HSCT, hematopoietic stem cell transplantation; URTI, upper respiratory tract infection.

From Lehrnbecher T, Phillips R, Alexander S, et al. Guideline for the management of fever and neutropenia in children with cancer and/or undergoing hematopoietic stem-cell transplantation. *J Clin Oncol.* 2012;30(35):4427-4438. Ref. (26).

malignant obstruction in the bile duct. Typhlitis is highly morbid and more common in patients with hematologic malignancy and prolonged, severe neutropenia.

Patients with pulmonary tumors, either primary or metastatic, may be at risk of postobstructive pneumonia or fever related to atelectasis. Dysphagia and aspiration events increase risk of aspiration pneumonia and pneumonitis. Ventilator-associated pneumonia also figures prominently in the intensive care setting.

Urinary catheter placement increases the risk of urinary tract infection as does the presence of urinary obstruction, or instrumentation. The presence of asymptomatic bacteriuria in a catheterized patient without neutropenia is not usually an indication for antibiotic treatment.

Central nervous system infections can be difficult to diagnose and typically require lumbar puncture to confirm. Infection is a relatively common complication of Ommaya reservoirs, used to administer intraventricular chemotherapy. Infections occur in 1 of every 20 patients with the device (32). Ommaya reservoir infections are more likely to occur in those with previous radiotherapy or in whom repeated surgical procedures have been necessary (33). Most infections are due to coagulase-negative staphylococcus (32,34). The majority (70%) of patients in a retrospective analysis at Memorial Sloan-Kettering Cancer Center presented with fever and/or headache, and half had the reservoir removed during treatment of the infection (32).

The skin is also a common site of infection that may range from infected decubitus ulcers to cellulitis or herpes zoster. Particular attention to sites of recent surgery or instrumentation is essential in assessing infection. Fistulae wherever present, abolish physiological barriers, promoting bacterial translocation and infection, and often mucosal injury. Finally, the use of percutaneous catheters in oncology creates another portal for the introduction of infection in patients with cancer. Overall, totally implantable venous access ports are associated with a lower risk of central line–associated bloodstream infections (CLABSI) than external central venous catheters. A meta-analysis and systemic review found a significantly lower risk (relative risk [RR], 0.44; 95% confidence interval [CI], 0.31 to 0.62; $p < 0.00001$) of CLABSI with totally implantable venous access ports compared to external central venous catheters, with subgroup analyses demonstrating infection reduction greatest in adult patients (35).

Transfusion Related

Blood products, administered extensively to patients with cancer, may be associated with febrile reactions. Febrile nonhemolytic transfusion reactions occur in up to 1.0% of blood transfusions but are less common in leukocyte-reduced products. These reactions are caused by preformed anti-WBC antibodies in the recipient. If recurrent, acetaminophen premedication is administered. Delayed hemolytic transfusion reactions may also present with fever, jaundice, or anemia. These reactions occur 1 to 2 weeks following transfusions, and result from an anamnestic immune response to incompatible red cell antigens (36).

More serious and rare are acute hemolytic transfusion reactions. These are related to preformed antibodies to incompatible blood product (1:76,000) or ABO incompatibility (1:40,000). Patients may present with fever, chills, hypotension, renal failure, back pain, or hemoglobinuria (36).

Infection may also be a source of fever in patients receiving blood products and is more common among platelet transfusions relative to red blood cell transfusions. Transfusion-related bacteremia occurred in 1:100,000 platelet transfusions compared to 1:5,000,000 red blood cell transfusions (37).

Thrombosis

Venous thromboembolism (VTE) is common in patients with cancer, symptomatically occurring in up to 10% of patients (38). However, fever as a presenting symptom of acute pulmonary embolism is rare (<5%) (39). Malignancies most commonly associated with increased risk of thrombosis include pancreatic, brain, lung, ovarian, kidney, as well as lymphoma and myeloma (38). Chemotherapy further increases risk of VTE. VTE may be associated with fever, although rarely. More commonly, VTE present with symptomatic thrombosis (e.g., pulmonary emboli, lower extremity deep vein thrombosis) or incidentally on imaging.

Drugs

Drug-associated fever is an ill-defined syndrome in which fever is the predominant manifestation of an adverse drug reaction. It is normally a diagnosis of exclusion (12). Drugs commonly associated with fever include antibiotics (e.g., nitrofurantoin, minocycline), anticonvulsants (e.g., phenytoin), cytotoxic agents (e.g., bleomycin), kinase inhibitors (e.g., dabrafenib, trametinib), and immunotherapies. Important in the treatment of patients with hematologic malignancy and tumor lysis, allopurinol may be associated with drug fever, often accompanied by hepatotoxicity, renal impairment, rash, and eosinophilia (40). A well-known side effect observed in patients receiving combination targeted therapy for metastatic melanoma with dabrafenib and trametinib, fever may

TABLE 8.4 CYTOTOXIC AGENTS ASSOCIATED WITH FEVER AFTER ADMINISTRATION

Bleomycin	Mustine
Cisplatin	Mithramycin
Cytarabine	Streptozocin
Cyclophosphamide	Thiotepa
Etoposide	Vinblastine
5-Fluorouracil	Vincristine
Methotrexate	

present in up to 60% of patients (41). In some cases of drug fever, the offending drug has been taken by the patient for months to years prior to onset of the febrile reaction, making diagnosis a challenge. Once the offending pharmacologic agent has been stopped, most patients experience defervescence within 72 to 96 hours (Table 8.4).

Immunotherapy

Fever is associated with the use of multiple immunotherapeutic treatments, including immune-modulating antibodies, cytokines, adoptive T-cell therapy, chimeric antigen receptor T cells (CAR-T), and cancer vaccines (42). Fever is thought to result from cytokine release and generalized immune system activation (43).

Cytokine-release syndrome (CRS) is a distinct clinical diagnosis characterized by fever, chills, hypotension, and organ-specific findings (e.g., dyspnea, tachycardia, confusion, headache, erythema, arthralgias, myalgias) and laboratory abnormalities. CRS is commonly associated with CAR-T therapy and infusion of monoclonal or bispecific antibodies (43). Fevers equal or exceed 40°C in up to 80% of patients (44). Commonly, fever is the presenting symptom of CRS (45). Fevers present within hours to days of CAR-T transfusion. Supportive care interventions in the setting of CRS include acetaminophen and cooling blankets (45), as well as appropriate hematologic and infectious disease assessment.

Monoclonal antibodies are rarely associated with fever (46). Similarly, checkpoint inhibitors are rarely associated with fever, either during infusion or in the setting of immune-related adverse event of hepatotoxicity.

Patients treated with IL-2 frequently develop fever within hours of administration of the first or second dose, and can reach as high as 40.5°C. Acetaminophen is included in IL-2 treatment, both prior to and during infusion (47). Use of an NSAID has also been endorsed in this setting, although there have been concerns raised about potential for gastritis and renal impairment (48).

Corticosteroid use should always be discussed with the patient's primary oncologist prior to administration in the setting of immunotherapy. This is particularly important for patients involved in or considering clinical trial, as steroid administration may be included in exclusion criteria.

Interferon alpha (IFNa) is associated with the development of fever in up to 80% of patients (49). Partially purified IFN administered at low doses, intramuscularly, induces a fever (38°C to 40°C) within 6 hours that persists for approximately 4 to 8 hours. More severe side effects are seen with intravenous and intrathecal administration or in patients older than 65. The febrile response is characterized by severe rigors, peripheral cyanosis, vasoconstriction, nausea and vomiting, severe muscle aches, and headaches. In patients receiving IFN daily, associated symptoms usually decrease in intensity and disappear within 7 to 10 days. Fever, however, persists, with intermittent (nondaily) injections resulting in peaks at 6 to 12 hours, and tends to last longer than the normal 4 to 8 hours. The administration of other biologic factors is associated with the onset of fever (e.g., TNF).

Antibiotics

Antibiotics themselves are responsible for approximately one-third of drug-related fevers, with the most common offenders being minocycline, beta-lactams, sulfonamides (especially in the setting of glucose-6-phosphate deficiency), and nitrofurantoin. The antifungal agent amphotericin B has been classically associated with frequent drug-induced dose-dependent fever; however, overall utilization of this medication has notably declined and the use of liposomal amphotericin is associated with a lower incidence of fever than amphotericin alone (50).

Opioids

Intravenous injection of morphine can be associated with sweating and vasodilatation, but not necessarily with fever. Drug withdrawal is associated with a syndrome that may include fever and needs to be suspected in febrile patients with cancer in whom opioids have been suddenly stopped. Withdrawal from benzodiazepines, often coadministered with opioids, may also be associated with fever.

Graft versus Host Disease

Graft versus host disease is a major cause of morbidity in patients following allogeneic hematopoietic stem cell transplant. It is classified temporally into acute (≤100 days after HSCT) or chronic (>100 days after HSCT) and characterized by inflammation and/or fibrosis involving multiple organ systems. Most commonly, the skin, gastrointestinal system, liver, lung, and mucosal surfaces are affected. Fever may be a presenting symptom, although typically only in the setting of acute liver GVHD.

Neuroleptic Malignant Syndrome and Serotonin Syndrome

While rare, neuroleptic malignant syndrome (NMS) is an important differential diagnosis of febrile patients who are taking antipsychotic or neuroleptic agents. NMS is a life-threatening neurological emergency characterized by altered mental status, fever, rigidity, and dysautonomia. While overall incidence is low, palliative patients may be at higher risk given the frequent use of associated drugs including high-potency first-generation antipsychotic agents (e.g., haloperidol), second-generation antipsychotic agents (e.g., olanzapine) and antiemetic drugs (e.g., metoclopramide, prochlorperazine). In patients at risk based on pharmaceutical use, serotonin syndrome must be considered as well (with triad of autonomic dysfunction, neuromuscular excitation, and altered mental status).

Systemic Rheumatic Diseases

Even in patients with active malignancy, fever may be caused by non–malignancy-related medical conditions. This broadened differential should be considered in order to avoid premature closure bias in the diagnosis of new or persistent fever. Due to their chronic inflammatory nature, many of the systemic rheumatic diseases are known to induce a febrile response. Among others, systemic lupus erythematosus, rheumatoid arthritis, and undifferentiated systemic rheumatic diseases are well documented to cause fever. Careful review of the patient's past medical history and current symptom spectrum is essential in order to accurately assess and diagnose the cause of fever in such instances.

DIAGNOSIS

The diagnostic approach to patients with fever in the palliative setting should always take into consideration patient goals, and individual wishes regarding the intensity of medical assessment and intervention. For some patients, complete medical assessment, including laboratory testing, various imaging modalities, invasive testing and procedures, and inpatient consultation, is consistent with the goals of care. Other patients may prefer limited or focused interventions, or a purely supportive approach to febrile symptoms in the palliative setting. In any case, a focused

history and physical examination, as well as careful discussion of therapeutic goals and patient preferences are integral to appropriate management of the patient.

In the case of febrile neutropenia, fever should always be assumed to be infectious until proven otherwise. In addition to history and physical examination, evaluation should include complete blood count including leukocyte differential, serum electrolytes, creatinine, blood urea nitrogen, and serum lactate. Additionally, liver function tests including bilirubin, alkaline phosphatase, and transaminases should be ordered. Prior to antibiotic initiation, two blood cultures should be drawn from separate sites, preferably from a peripheral site as well as central venous catheter, if present. Cultures from other sites may be drawn if clinically indicated. Imaging of the chest should be obtained only if signs or symptoms suggest respiratory tract infection. Finally, respiratory viral panel should be considered where appropriate (3).

Timing of assessment is integral to patient outcomes, particularly in the setting of febrile neutropenia. Guidelines recommend the assessment within 15 minutes of triage for patients presenting with febrile neutropenia within 6 weeks of receiving chemotherapy (3). For patients with febrile neutropenia, one study observed that each hour delay in empiric antibiotic initiation increased 28-day mortality by 18% (51).

The diagnosis of neoplastic fever can theoretically be confirmed with the use of naproxen (52). Proponents of the naproxen test state that it does not result in a decrease in temperature in patients with infection. In this historical study, successful treatment of presumed neoplastic fever was demonstrated in 21 patients with cancer, with 15 responding to a dose of 250 mg of naproxen per day, whereas others responded following an increase in naproxen dose. The true sensitivity and specificity of the naproxen test are uncertain; neoplastic fever should always be considered as a diagnosis of exclusion.

SYMPTOMATIC SUPPORT OF FEBRILE PATIENT

Primary to any treatment of fever in patients with cancer is the treatment of the underlying cause of fever. Antibiotics use is standard of care in the management of patients with febrile neutropenia. However, antibiotics should not be used for the treatment of fever in patients without neutropenia in the absence of evidence of infection. For patients with or without neutropenia, nonsteroidal anti-inflammatory drugs may be useful in the treatment of fever associated with infection.

Aspirin is a commonly used antipyretic, which functions by inhibiting cyclooxygenase, an enzyme involved in prostaglandin synthesis (2). Cyclooxygenase inhibitors allow the anterior hypothalamus to recognize an elevated set-point temperature, which in turn promotes hypothalamic temperature regulation through cooling mechanisms (2).

Physical cooling (e.g., through sponging) alone is likely to be uncomfortable for patients with fever and should be reserved for those in a hot and humid environment that may impede evaporative heat loss or for those with defective heat loss mechanisms (53). Sponging, when it is done, should be with tepid water because the use of cold water will induce shivering, which increases patient discomfort and causes an elevation in temperature (54). Aggressive cooling of critically ill patients through sponging resulted in early closure of a randomized study that studied its effect because of increased mortality in those receiving the aggressive cooling (55).

Agents that lower body temperature (antipyretics) primarily comprise three groups:

1. pure antipyretics that do not work in the absence of pyrogen and do not affect normal temperature at usual therapeutic doses (e.g., acetaminophen)
2. agents that cause hypothermia in afebrile subjects by directly impairing thermoregulatory function
3. those that are antipyretic at lower doses and cause hypothermia at higher doses (e.g., chlorpromazine)

Only salicylates, acetaminophen, and ibuprofen have been approved for antipyretic use in the United States, and none of these agents are likely to cause hypothermia in normothermic patients. Aspirin is not recommended for use in children because of the risk of Reye's syndrome, a disease process that results in liver failure (56). However, aspirin has been the standard of reference in nearly two-thirds of clinical comparisons of antipyretic activity (57).

Aspirin and other NSAIDs are less likely to be utilized for fever control in oncologic settings because of their well-recognized impact on platelet dysfunction, thrombocytopenia, and overall elevated GI bleeding risk. In most areas of clinical practice, acetaminophen is the agent of choice due to its antipyretic efficacy and overall favorable safety profile. For control of fever and sequelae, acetaminophen can be dosed every 6 hours with a 24-hour maximum dose of 3 to 4 g. While patients with chronic liver disease are often advised to avoid acetaminophen entirely, many patients with significant liver impairment can in fact safely administer and process up to 2 g of acetaminophen daily (58).

As such, dose-adjusted acetaminophen remains a worthwhile component of symptomatic relief of fever in patients with liver damage, though attention must be paid to the presence of other factors that increase the risk of acetaminophen-induced hepatotoxicity (e.g., malnutrition, low body weight, advanced age, concurrent use of drugs that interact with acetaminophen metabolism) and lab trending may be warranted (59,60).

Steroids may be particularly effective as antipyretics in patients with both hematologic and oncologic malignancies. In addition to antipyretic properties, steroids are helpful adjuncts in the management of pain (e.g., bone pain, pain related to capsular distention), nausea, bowel obstruction, and cerebral edema. Steroids have numerous, well-known side effects including increased bleeding risk, potential for anxiety and insomnia, and immune suppression, particularly with higher doses and longer-term use. Despite these risks, steroids remain a helpful option for symptomatic support of fever, particularly in patients pursuing a palliative approach to care, and those near end of life.

In pediatric populations, acetaminophen has a dose–response effect, with doses of 5, 10, and 20 mg/kg bringing about a reduction in temperature of 0.3°C, 1.6°C, and 2.5°C, respectively, after 3 hours (53). Aspirin and acetaminophen appear equally effective at approximately 10 mg/kg. Ibuprofen, 0.5 mg/kg, is about as effective as 10 mg/kg of aspirin and 12.5 mg/kg of acetaminophen. Indomethacin (75 mg), naproxen (500 mg), and diclofenac sodium (75 mg) have been found to be equally effective in the management of paraneoplastic fever (61).

More recently, two agents have been explored in the symptomatic management of fever and sweats among oncology patients. A case report shed light on a potential role for the muscarinic antagonist oxybutynin in treating neoplastic fever refractory to first-line intervention. In the case, a patient with advanced cholangiocarcinoma found rapid and lasting relief of bothersome fever and sweats with oxybutynin 2.5 mg b.i.d. Dose can be increased as needed for symptom control up to 5 mg b.i.d. (62). A newly emerging agent for the management of night sweats in patients with cancer is dronabinol. A small study found dronabinol to be effective in persistent, symptomatic paraneoplastic night sweats in a palliative care setting (63). While night sweats are distinct from fever, this offers an interesting approach to symptomatic management of sweating for patients with cancer.

Growth Factors

Granulocyte colony stimulating factors (G-CSFs) are used in the primary or secondary prophylaxis of neutropenic fever. For primary prophylaxis,

G-CSFs are given to decrease the incidence of febrile neutropenia and hospitalization. Guidelines recommend administration if the anticipated risk of febrile neutropenia is 20% or higher (64). Growth factor support is especially important to consider in certain clinical scenarios where risk of neutropenic fever is higher, for example dose-dense or high-intensity chemotherapy regimens, concurrent chemotherapy and radiation, and treatment in patients with history of myelosuppression.

Secondary prophylaxis is the use of G-CSFs in subsequent chemotherapy cycles, after the onset of treatment-related febrile neutropenia. After the initial presentation of febrile neutropenia, the risk of developing febrile neutropenia is increased. Use of G-CSFs reduces the risk of subsequent episodes of febrile neutropenia by nearly 50% (65). Overall, G-CSFs reduce the duration and depth of neutropenia, which can lead to improved clinical outcomes, including reducing the risk of febrile neutropenia.

While G-CSFs are not recommended for routine use in patients presenting with febrile neutropenia (17), use may be considered in patients who are at particularly high risk for infection-associated complications or poor prognosis. Factors to consider include prolonged (>10 days) or profound (<100 cells/μL) neutropenia, age >65, pneumonia or other clinically documented infection, sepsis syndrome, invasive fungal infection, prior episode of febrile neutropenia, or being hospitalized at the time of fever (64).

ETHICAL CONSIDERATIONS FOR TREATMENT OF INFECTIONS

The approach to patients with fever in the palliative setting should always take into consideration patient goals, and individual wishes regarding the intensity of medical assessment and intervention. In some cases, the standard infectious evaluation and antimicrobial management may cause more harm than benefit to patient. Furthermore, inpatient or emergency room care settings may be undesired by the individual patient, particularly those with serious illness or nearing end of life. While some patients may prefer usual medical or medically intensive care, other patients may prefer limited, focused, or purely palliative interventions. A focused history and examination, and careful discussion of therapeutic goals, potential harms and benefits, and patient preferences is key in respecting patient autonomy and appropriate medical decision making. Patients, and, by extension, their surrogate decision makers, must be afforded the opportunity to explore and consider the potential risks and benefits of care decisions.

There is a growing body of research supporting a more palliative approach to antibiotic administration in the end-of-life setting (66,67). Recent research has called into question the survival benefit of antimicrobials at the end of life. One study found no difference in survival among patients nearing the end of life who chose full use of antimicrobials; limited, symptom-directed use; or no use (68). While survival was not associated with antimicrobial choice, symptom palliation of urinary tract infections improved with treatment, while other infectious sites had less effective symptom control with antimicrobials (68). Another study examining antibiotic use at the end of life among oncology patients found that a minority experienced symptom relief with infection-focused treatment (67).

While antimicrobials may palliate symptoms related to some infections, they may also prolong life, or the dying process. Without understanding the individual patient's goals of care, providers may inadvertently cause greater harm than benefit to patients nearing the end of life or make decisions not consistent with patient autonomy. For example, a patient may wish to maintain care at home and avoid emergency department visit or inpatient hospitalization knowing that cancer-related prognosis is poor. Other patients may wish for more aggressive measures, such as central access and intensive care, but to avoid intubation or resuscitation attempts should clinical status decline. Other patients may want full interventions until a particular life event or visitation is able to take place. Importantly, antimicrobial therapy may decrease quality of life or complicate bereavement if not in line with patient goals of care. In summary, management of fever should always respect patient autonomy, and carefully consider the potential harms and benefits associated with care.

REFERENCES

1. Celsus AC. De Medicina. In. *Book VII.* Loeb Classical Library; 30.
2. Costanzo L. *Physiology.* 6th ed. Philadelphia, PA: Wolters Kluwer Health/Lippincott Williams & Wilkins; 2018.
3. Taplitz RA, Kennedy EB, Bow EJ, et al. Outpatient management of fever and neutropenia in adults treated for malignancy: American Society of Clinical Oncology and Infectious Diseases Society of America Clinical Practice Guideline Update. *J Clin Oncol.* 2018;36(14):1443-1453.
4. Petersdorf RG, Beeson PB. Fever of unexplained origin: report on 100 cases. *Medicine (Baltimore).* 1961;40:1-30.
5. Engel A, Kern WV, Murdter G, Kern P. Kinetics and correlation with body temperature of circulating interleukin-6, interleukin-8, tumor necrosis factor alpha and interleukin-1 beta in patients with fever and neutropenia. *Infection.* 1994;22(3):160-164.

6. Porat R, Dinarello CA. Pathophysiology and treatment of fever in adults. In: Weller PF, Sullivan M, eds. *UpToDate*. Waltham, MA: Wolters Kluwer; 2018. https://www.uptodate.com/home/how-use-uptodate-presentation.

7. Ashman RB, Mullbacher A. Host-damaging immune responses in virus infections. *Surv Immunol Res*. 1984;3(1):11-15.

8. Norman DC. Fever in the elderly. *Clin Infect Dis*. 2000;31(1):148-151.

9. Pasikhova Y, Ludlow S, Baluch A. Fever in patients with cancer. *Cancer Control*. 2017;24(2):193-197.

10. Odagiri T, Morita T, Sakurai H, et al. A multicenter cohort study to explore differentiating factors between tumor fever and infection among advanced cancer patients. *J Palliat Med*. 2019;22(11):1331-1336.

11. Zell JA, Chang JC. Neoplastic fever: a neglected paraneoplastic syndrome. *Support Care Cancer*. 2005;13(11): 870-877.

12. Greenberg SB, Taber L. *Fever of Unknown Origin*. New York, NY: Raven Press; 1991.

13. Smith K, Chiu A, Parikh R, Yahalom J, Younes A. Hodgkin lymphoma: clinical manifestations, staging, and therapy. In: Hoffman R, Benz EJ, Silberstein LE, et al., eds. *Hematology: Basic Principles and Practice*. 7th ed. Philadelphia, PA: Elsevier; 2018: Chapter 75.

14. Good GR, DiNubile MJ. Images in clinical medicine. Cyclic fever in Hodgkin's disease (Pel-Ebstein fever). *N Engl J Med*. 1995;332(7):436.

15. Bodey GP, Buckley M, Sathe YS, Freireich EJ. Quantitative relationships between circulating leukocytes and infection in patients with acute leukemia. *Ann Intern Med*. 1966;64(2):328-340.

16. Rice L, Jung M. Neutrophilic leukocytosis, neutropenia, monocytosis, and monocytopenia. In: *Hematology: Basic Principles and Practice*. Philadelphia, PA: Elsevier; 2018: Chapter 48.

17. Freifeld AG, Bow EJ, Sepkowitz KA, et al. Clinical practice guideline for the use of antimicrobial agents in neutropenic patients with cancer: 2010 update by the infectious diseases society of america. *Clin Infect Dis*. 2011;52(4):e56-e93.

18. Palmore TN, Parta M, Cuellar-Rodriguez J, Gea-Banacloche JC. Infections in the cancer patient. In DeVita VT, Lawrence TS, Rosenberg SA, eds. DeVita, Hellman, and Rosenberg's Cancer: Principles and Practice of Oncology. 10th ed. Philadelphia, PA: Lippincott Williams & Wilkins; 2019:2037-2068.

19. Gudiol C, Bodro M, Simonetti A, et al. Changing aetiology, clinical features, antimicrobial resistance, and outcomes of bloodstream infection in neutropenic cancer patients. *Clin Microbiol Infect*. 2013;19(5):474-479.

20. Holland T, Fowler VG Jr, Shelburne SA III. Invasive gram-positive bacterial infection in cancer patients. *Clin Infect Dis*. 2014;59(suppl 5):S331-S334.

21. Carvalho AS, Lagana D, Catford J, Shaw D, Bak N. Bloodstream infections in neutropenic patients with haematological malignancies. *Infect Dis Health*. 2020;25:22-29.

22. Antonio M, Gudiol C, Royo-Cebrecos C, Grillo S, Ardanuy C, Carratala J. Current etiology, clinical features and outcomes of bacteremia in older patients with solid tumors. *J Geriatr Oncol*. 2019;10(2):246-251.

23. Klastersky J, Paesmans M, Rubenstein EB, et al. The multinational association for supportive care in cancer risk index: a multinational scoring system for identifying low-risk febrile neutropenic cancer patients. *J Clin Oncol*. 2000;18(16):3038-3051.

24. Klastersky J, Paesmans M, Georgala A, et al. Outpatient oral antibiotics for febrile neutropenic cancer patients using a score predictive for complications. *J Clin Oncol*. 2006;24(25):4129-4134.

25. Lehrnbecher T, Robinson P, Fisher B, et al. Guideline for the management of fever and neutropenia in children with cancer and hematopoietic stem-cell transplantation recipients: 2017 update. *J Clin Oncol*. 2017;35(18):2082-2094.

26. Lehrnbecher T, Phillips R, Alexander S, et al. Guideline for the management of fever and neutropenia in children with cancer and/or undergoing hematopoietic stem-cell transplantation. *J Clin Oncol*. 2012;30(35): 4427-4438.

27. Orme LM, Babl FE, Barnes C, Barnett P, Donath S, Ashley DM. Outpatient versus inpatient IV antibiotic management for pediatric oncology patients with low risk febrile neutropenia: a randomised trial. *Pediatr Blood Cancer*. 2014;61(8):1427-1433.

28. Brack E, Bodmer N, Simon A, et al. First-day step-down to oral outpatient treatment versus continued standard treatment in children with cancer and low-risk fever in neutropenia. A randomized controlled trial within the multicenter SPOG 2003 FN study. *Pediatr Blood Cancer*. 2012;59(3):423-430.

29. Ahmed N, El-Mahallawy HA, Ahmed IA, Nassif S, El-Beshlawy A, El-Haddad A. Early hospital discharge versus continued hospitalization in febrile pediatric cancer patients with prolonged neutropenia: a randomized, prospective study. *Pediatr Blood Cancer*. 2007;49(6):786-792.

30. Santolaya ME, Alvarez AM, Aviles CL, et al. Early hospital discharge followed by outpatient management versus continued hospitalization of children with cancer, fever, and neutropenia at low risk for invasive bacterial infection. *J Clin Oncol*. 2004;22(18):3784-3789.

31. Anand A, Glatt AE. Clostridium difficile infection associated with antineoplastic chemotherapy: a review. *Clin Infect Dis*. 1993;17(1):109-113.

32. Mead PA, Safdieh JE, Nizza P, Tuma S, Sepkowitz KA. Ommaya reservoir infections: a 16-year retrospective analysis. *J Infect*. 2014;68(3):225-230.

33. Machado M, Salcman M, Kaplan RS, Montgomery E. Expanded role of the cerebrospinal fluid reservoir in neurooncology: indications, causes of revision, and complications. *Neurosurgery*. 1985;17(4):600-603.

34. Siegal T, Pfeffer MR, Steiner I. Antibiotic therapy for infected Ommaya reservoir systems. *Neurosurgery*. 1988;22(1 Pt 1):97-100.

35. Jiang M, Li CL, Pan C, Yu Li. The risk of bloodstream infection associated with totally implantable venous access ports in cancer patient: a systematic review and meta-analysis. *Support Care Cancer*. 2020;28:361-372

36. Carson JL, Guyatt G, Heddle NM, et al. Clinical practice guidelines from the AABB: red blood cell transfusion thresholds and storage. *JAMA*. 2016;316(19):2025-2035.

37. Kuehnert MJ, Roth VR, Haley NR, et al. Transfusion-transmitted bacterial infection in the United States, 1998 through 2000. *Transfusion*. 2001;41(12):1493-1499.

38. Timp JF, Braekkan SK, Versteeg HH, Cannegieter SC. Epidemiology of cancer-associated venous thrombosis. *Blood*. 2013;122(10):1712-1723.

39. Stein PD, Beemath A, Matta F, et al. Clinical characteristics of patients with acute pulmonary embolism: data from PIOPED II. *Am J Med*. 2007;120(10):871-879.

40. Arellano F, Sacristan JA. Allopurinol hypersensitivity syndrome: a review. *Ann Pharmacother*. 1993;27(3): 337-343.

41. Menzies AM, Ashworth MT, Swann S, et al. Characteristics of pyrexia in BRAFV600E/K metastatic melanoma patients treated with combined dabrafenib and trametinib in a phase I/II clinical trial. *Ann Oncol*. 2015;26(2):415-421.

42. Naidoo J, Page DB, Li BT, et al. Toxicities of the anti-PD-1 and anti-PD-L1 immune checkpoint antibodies. *Ann Oncol.* 2015;26(12):2375-2391.

43. Kroschinsky F, Stolzel F, von Bonin S, et al. New drugs, new toxicities: severe side effects of modern targeted and immunotherapy of cancer and their management. *Crit Care.* 2017;21(1):89.

44. Brudno JN, Kochenderfer JN. Toxicities of chimeric antigen receptor T cells: recognition and management. *Blood.* 2016;127(26):3321-3330.

45. Brudno JN, Kochenderfer JN. Recent advances in CAR T-cell toxicity: mechanisms, manifestations and management. *Blood Rev.* 2019;34:45-55.

46. Achkar T, Tarhini AA. The use of immunotherapy in the treatment of melanoma. *J Hematol Oncol.* 2017;10(1):88.

47. Schwartzentruber DJ. Guidelines for the safe administration of high-dose interleukin-2. *J Immunother.* 2001;24(4):287-293.

48. Sundin DJ, Wolin MJ. Toxicity management in patients receiving low-dose aldesleukin therapy. *Ann Pharmacother.* 1998;32(12):1344-1352.

49. Jonasch E, Haluska FG. Interferon in oncological practice: review of interferon biology, clinical applications, and toxicities. *Oncologist.* 2001;6(1):34-55.

50. McDonald M, Sexton DJ. Drug fever. In: Weller PF, Sullivan M, eds. *UpToDate.* Waltham, MA: Wolters Kluwer; 2018. https://www.uptodate.com/home/how-use-uptodate-presentation

51. Rosa RG, Goldani LZ. Factors associated with hospital length of stay among cancer patients with febrile neutropenia. *PLoS One.* 2014;9(10):e108969.

52. Chang JC, Gross HM. Neoplastic fever responds to the treatment of an adequate dose of naproxen. *J Clin Oncol.* 1985;3(4):552-558.

53. Clark WG. Antipyretics. In: Mackowiak P, ed. *Fever: Basic Mechanics and Management.* New York, NY: Raven Press; 1991:297-340.

54. Steele RW, Tanaka PT, Lara RP, Bass JW. Evaluation of sponging and of oral antipyretic therapy to reduce fever. *J Pediatr.* 1970;77(5):824-829.

55. Schulman CI, Namias N, Doherty J, et al. The effect of antipyretic therapy upon outcomes in critically ill patients: a randomized, prospective study. *Surg Infect (Larchmt).* 2005;6(4):369-375.

56. Pinsky PF, Hurwitz ES, Schonberger LB, Gunn WJ. Reye's syndrome and aspirin. Evidence for a dose-response effect. *JAMA.* 1988;260(5):657-661.

57. Seed JC. A clinical comparison of the antipyretic potency of aspirin and sodium salicylate. *Clin Pharmacol Ther.* 1965;6:354-358.

58. Bosilkovska M, Walder B, Besson M, Daali Y, Desmeules J. Analgesics in patients with hepatic impairment: pharmacology and clinical implications. *Drugs.* 2012;72(12):1645-1669.

59. Chandok N, Watt KD. Pain management in the cirrhotic patient: the clinical challenge. *Mayo Clin Proc.* 2010;85(5):451-458.

60. Imani F, Motavaf M, Safari S, Alavian SM. The therapeutic use of analgesics in patients with liver cirrhosis: a literature review and evidence-based recommendations. *Hepat Mon.* 2014;14(10):e23539.

61. Tsavaris N, Zinelis A, Karabelis A, et al. A randomized trial of the effect of three non-steroid anti-inflammatory agents in ameliorating cancer-induced fever. *J Intern Med.* 1990;228(5):451-455.

62. Yarchoan M, Tucker W, Smith TJ. Successful treatment of neoplastic fever with oxybutynin. *J Palliat Med.* 2019;22(12):1491.

63. Carr C, Vertelney H, Fronk J, Trieu S. Dronabinol for the treatment of paraneoplastic night sweats in cancer patients: a report of five cases. *J Palliat Med.* 2019;22(10):1221-1223.

64. Smith TJ, Bohlke K, Lyman GH, et al. Recommendations for the use of WBC growth factors: American Society of Clinical Oncology Clinical practice guideline update. *J Clin Oncol.* 2015;33(28):3199-3212.

65. Crawford J, Ozer H, Stoller R, et al. Reduction by granulocyte colony-stimulating factor of fever and neutropenia induced by chemotherapy in patients with small-cell lung cancer. *N Engl J Med.* 1991;325(3):164-170.

66. Baghban A, Juthani-Mehta M. Antimicrobial use at the end of life. *Infect Dis Clin North Am.* 2017;31(4):639-647.

67. Oh DY, Kim JH, Kim DW, et al. Antibiotic use during the last days of life in cancer patients. *Eur J Cancer Care.* 2005;15(1):74-79.

68. White PH, Kuhlenschmidt HL, Vancura BG, Navari RM. Antimicrobial use in patients with advanced cancer receiving hospice care. *J Pain Symptom Manage.* 2003;25(5):438-443.

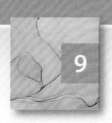

9 Hot Flashes

Cindy S. Tofthagen and Charles L. Loprinzi

Hot flashes are frequently associated with menopause in women; however, hot flashes also affect men undergoing androgen deprivation therapy for prostate cancer. Hot flashes have been reported to occur in up to 70% of men after orchiectomy, 80% of men receiving neoadjuvant hormonal therapy before radical prostatectomy, and 70% to 80% of men receiving long-term androgen deprivation therapy (1–3). Hot flashes can be more substantial in patients with cancer. In many premenopausal women with breast cancer and other gynecologic malignancies, the precipitation of menopause by oophorectomy, chemotherapy, radiotherapy, or hormonal manipulation can lead to the rapid onset of hot flash symptoms that are more frequent and severe than those associated with natural menopause (4). Other reasons for the high frequency of menopausal cancer survivors include age at diagnosis (frequently older than 50 years) and the abrupt withdrawal of hormonal therapy.

Although variable, hot flashes are often characterized as a sudden and disturbing sensation of intense warmth perceived mainly in the upper part of the chest. Red blotches can appear on the skin and the increase in skin temperature can lead to profuse diaphoresis. This feeling of intense warmth can be accompanied by palpitations, irritability, and anxiety. Hot flashes usually last a few minutes but can occur for a few seconds or for 10 minutes or longer. The frequency of hot flashes can also be quite variable, ranging from every 20 minutes to once a month. Nearly one-third of women during perimenopause and three-quarters of women during menopause experience hot flashes (5). However, the prevalence of (or reporting of) hot flashes has been noted to be variable among differing cultures and ethnic groups. African American women, cigarette smoking, low socioeconomic status, and obesity are associated with a higher prevalence of hot flashes (6). Many women experience hot flashes for 6 months to 2 years, although some women have them for 10 years or longer. Hot flash symptoms can have serious detrimental effects on a patient's work, recreation, sleep, and general perception of quality of life (7).

PATHOPHYSIOLOGY OF HOT FLASHES

The pathophysiology of hot flashes is not entirely understood. The thermoregulatory nucleus in the medial preoptic area of the hypothalamus is felt to regulate the mechanism leading to heat loss during hot flashes. The thermoregulatory nucleus activates perspiration and vasodilatation to keep core body temperature within a tightly regulated range, known as the thermoregulatory zone. In menopausal women with hot flashes, the thermoregulatory zone is shifted downward and is narrower than it is in menopausal women who do not have hot flashes (8). Therefore, in women with hot flashes, small changes in body temperature (as low as 0.01°C) may trigger the mechanisms of heat loss and lead to vasomotor symptoms (9).

The relatively rapid dramatic decreases in sexual hormone levels that occur in menopausal women and in men receiving androgen deprivation therapy are thought to be responsible for lowering and narrowing the thermoregulatory zone. However, sexual hormones have profound effects on multiple neuroendocrine pathways; the exact mechanisms by which they affect the thermoregulatory zone continue to be elucidated. Since estrogen withdrawal results in decreased central serotonergic activity and since some of the newer antidepressants have been shown to relieve hot flashes in placebo-controlled, randomized clinical trials (vide infra), serotonin (5-HT) is thought to play an important role in mediating the thermoregulatory effects of estrogen. In particular, the 5-HT_{2A} receptor has been closely associated with thermoregulation in mammals. Multiple animal and human studies have shown that central expression of the 5-HT_{2A} receptor decreases after estrogen withdrawal and that estrogen treatment reverses this change in estrogen-deficient animals and women (10,11). In addition, tamoxifen has been shown to block the positive effects of estrogen on central 5-HT_{2A} receptor expression in ovariectomized rats (12). Since estrogen withdrawal and tamoxifen treatment result in decreased central expression of 5-HT_{2A} receptors, it is possible that the efficacy of the newer antidepressants against hot flashes is due, at least in part, to their ability to cause a "compensatory" increase in central 5-HT$_{2A}$ signaling (13). Similarly, norepinephrine has also been implicated in the pathophysiology of hot flashes. Estrogen withdrawal leads to increased norepinephrine levels in the hypothalamus, which are thought to contribute to the lowering and narrowing of the thermoregulatory zone as well (8).

Another possible mechanism for hot flashes is endogenous opioid peptide withdrawal. In morphine-dependent rats, abrupt opioid withdrawal was associated with rapid temperature changes, which were eliminated with estrogen administration (14). This theory suggests that estrogen increases central opioid peptide activity, and therefore, estrogen deficiency may be associated with decreased endogenous central opioid activity and subsequent thermoregulatory dysfunction. The neuroendocrine pathways that govern thermoregulation in mammals are extraordinarily complex and, as yet, incompletely understood. There is a clear need for further research to clarify the pathophysiology of hot flashes and guide the development of more targeted nonhormonal therapeutic options.

TREATMENT OF HOT FLASHES

It is recommended that hot flashes be routinely assessed during clinical encounters in both cancer and noncancer patients, as a component of systematic symptom surveys. Assessment of frequency, intensity, duration, and potential triggers of hot flashes may be helpful. Self-directed diaries to record these variables can be used to formulate treatment recommendations. The Hot Flash Related Daily Interference Scale (HFR-DIS) is a validated tool utilized in the research setting to monitor hot flash symptomology prior to and following treatment (15). A shortened version of this instrument known as the Hot Flashes Interference Scale (HFI) is derived from the HFRDIS, which contains three items assessing interference with sleep, mood, and cognition (16). Studies are ongoing regarding devices that measure skin conductance as an objective marker for hot flashes; however, these have not been well validated (17). At this time, patient reports of hot flash experiences are the most reasonable measure.

PHARMACOLOGIC INTERVENTIONS

Pharmacologic options for management of hot flashes includes a variety of hormonal and nonhormonal therapies.

Hormonal Therapy

Estrogen

Estrogen therapy is the most established effective treatment option for hot flashes and can reduce symptoms by 80% to 90% (18). However, the use of estrogen is controversial, due to evidence of associated long-term health risks including coronary heart disease, cerebrovascular disease, venous thromboembolism, and breast cancer (19,20). The controversy surrounding its effect on breast cancer has been especially influential on clinical practice. The Woman's Health Initiate trial demonstrated a 26% increased risk of breast cancer in females receiving combination hormonal therapy (estrogen plus progestin) (19). The HABITS (hormonal replacement therapy after breast cancer—is it safe?) trial was stopped prematurely after an interim analysis found an increased risk of new breast cancers in breast cancer survivors (HR = 2.4) with the use of combination hormonal therapy after 2 years (21). However, the Stockholm trial found no such risk at a median follow-up of 4 years (22). The major difference in the Stockholm trial was the use of a lower dose of progestin. Several other prospective and retrospective studies suggest that at least some breast cancer survivors (small tumors, negative lymph node status, long disease-free survival, or estrogen receptor–negative tumors) could be safely treated with estrogen replacement (23). Despite these data, the use of estrogen in women with a history of, or at high risk for, breast cancer remains controversial and is not recommended.

Commonly utilized estrogen formulations include daily oral micronized 17-β-estradiol (1 mg), conjugated equine estrogens (0.625 mg), piperazine estrone sulfate (1.25 mg), and transdermal 17-β-estradiol (50 μg/day). Although the preceding doses are effective, lower doses have also been shown to be efficacious and should be used for the shortest period of time possible. Contraindications to estrogen use include known coronary heart disease, previous venous thromboembolic disease or stroke, active liver disease, history of estrogen-dependent cancer, or those at high risk for these pathologies.

Progesterone Analogs

Progesterone therapy alone is another effective hormonal agent for the treatment of hot flashes. A placebo-controlled, randomized clinical trial of megestrol 40 mg daily in 97 women with a history of breast cancer and 66 men receiving androgen deprivation therapy showed a marked reduction in hot flashes, of 75% to 80%, in the treatment group compared with 20% to 25% in the placebo group (24). Three years after the completion of the trial, one-third of the women who were still taking megestrol reported having less hot flashes than women who had discontinued therapy (25). Similar results were found in another trial utilizing depot intramuscular medroxyprogesterone acetate (DMPA), a progestational agent (26). The use of a single intramuscular dose of MPA was better tolerated and more efficacious than venlafaxine at a target dose of 75 mg daily over a 6-week period (27).

Despite the efficacy of progesterone analogs for the treatment of hot flashes, many physicians are hesitant in using hormonally active agents in patients with a history of breast or prostate cancer. Though there is some evidence that progesterone analogs are active against breast cancer (28), in vitro data suggest that they can increase epithelial cell proliferation, a potentially undesirable effect in patients with a history of breast cancer (29). In addition, megestrol was reported to increase the prostate-specific antigen level in a patient with prostate cancer (30). To address whether MPA had any influence on breast cancer recurrence or survival, 75 patients who received this drug for treating hot flashes, during the years 2005 through 2012, were identified. These were matched with 75 control patients, with regard to age, stage of disease, HER2 status, and the year of diagnosis. The estimated 10-year progression-free survival was 89% in patients who received MPA and 83% in the matched patients. Estimated 10-year survival rates were 92% and 94%, respectively (31).

Despite its efficacy, patients need to be counseled before starting a progesterone analog if they have a history of breast or prostate cancer. Commonly prescribed regimens include oral megestrol acetate 20 to 40 mg daily or intramuscular DMPA 500 mg once. Potential adverse effects of progesterone analogs include vaginal bleeding upon discontinuation of the medication, weight gain, bloating, and thromboembolic phenomena.

Nonhormonal Therapy

The reluctance to use hormonal agents in patients with a history of breast cancer provided an impetus for finding nonhormonal agents that could help alleviate hot flashes. The following is a summary of their clinical development and therapeutic yield (Table 9.1).

TABLE 9.1 EVIDENCE AND ADVERSE EFFECTS OF BENEFICIAL NONESTROGENIC THERAPEUTICS

	Treatment	Evidence[a]	Adverse events
Women	Citalopram	Two large RCTs	Constipation, dry mouth, nausea
	Desvenlafaxine	Two large RCTs	Dizziness, nausea, vomiting
	DMPA	One large RCT Three moderate RCTs One small RCT	Bloating, weight gain, thrombogenic
	Escitalopram	One large RCT	Fatigue, headaches, insomnia, nausea
	Gabapentin	Two large RCT Two moderate RCTs	Dizziness, fatigue, somnolence
	Megestrol acetate	Two moderate RCTs	Bloating, weight gain, thrombogenic
	Oxybutynin	Two moderate RCTs	Dry mouth, urinary difficulties, cognitive troubles
	Paroxetine	Two large RCTs	Insomnia, nausea, sexual dysfunction
	Pregabalin	One moderate RCT	Cognitive difficulty, sleepiness, weight gain
	Venlafaxine	Three large RCTs One moderate RCT	Anorexia, dry mouth, insomnia, nausea
Men on ADT	DMPA	One large RCT One small RCT	Bloating, weight gain, thrombogenic
	Gabapentin	One large RCT	Dizziness, fatigue, somnolence
	Megestrol acetate	One moderate RCT	Bloating, weight gain, thrombogenic
	Paroxetine	One pilot study	Insomnia, nausea, sexual dysfunction
	Venlafaxine	One pilot study One large RCT (not placebo-controlled)	Anorexia, dry mouth, insomnia, nausea

Note: See sections on each therapeutic for further details.
[a]Number of participants in study: large: >100; moderate: 50 to 99; and small: <50.
DMPA, depomedroxyprogesterone acetate; RCT, randomized controlled trial; ADT, androgen deprivation therapy.

Newer Antidepressants

In the 1990s, several authors reported reductions in hot flash frequency and severity in postmenopausal women who were taking four antidepressants for other reasons. Since then, the results of multiple prospective studies of antidepressants for the treatment of hot flashes have been reported. These studies have been reviewed and systematically analyzed in detail elsewhere (32,33). Given the reluctance to use hormonal agents in women with a history of breast cancer, many of these studies were done in this patient population, but some studies have been done in noncancer patients as well as in men with a history of prostate cancer. Self-completed daily hot flash diaries were used to document the frequency and severity of hot flashes in the majority of these studies. Data on toxicity, quality of life, and mood status were commonly obtained. The main efficacy measures used in most studies were the change from baseline in the weekly average number of daily hot flashes and average hot flash score (defined as the number of mild hot flashes plus twice the number of moderate hot flashes plus three times the number of severe hot flashes plus four times the number of very severe hot flashes during a set period of time).

Venlafaxine

Venlafaxine selectively inhibits serotonin, norepinephrine, and dopamine reuptake, in order of decreasing potency and is referred to as a serotonin norepinephrine reuptake inhibitor (SNRI). In 1998, the efficacy of venlafaxine for the treatment of hot flashes was first supported (34). This pilot study included 23 women with a history of breast cancer and 5 men receiving androgen deprivation therapy for prostate cancer. Patients treated with venlafaxine 12.5 mg twice daily had a >50% reduction in median hot flash scores at 4 weeks. Patients also reported significant improvement in fatigue, sweating, and difficulty sleeping, and, at the completion of the study, 64% of the patients chose to continue venlafaxine.

Subsequently, a placebo-controlled, double-blind, randomized clinical trial was conducted to assess the efficacy and toxicity of venlafaxine in women with hot flashes (35). One-hundred and ninety one women were randomized to placebo or one of three target doses of venlafaxine extended release (ER): 37.5 mg daily, 75 mg daily, or 150 mg daily for 4 weeks. After 4 weeks of treatment, the median frequency of hot flashes decreased by 19%, 30%, 46%, and 58% in women in the four study groups, respectively. Dry mouth, nausea, constipation, and decreased appetite were dose-dependent toxicities associated with venlafaxine. Sixty-nine percent of the women were taking tamoxifen, and efficacy was similar whether tamoxifen was being used, or not.

In another placebo-controlled, double-blind, randomized clinical trial, venlafaxine ER at a target dose of 75 mg daily was found to significantly decrease patient-perceived hot flash scores. This trial included 80 postmenopausal women who were treated for a total of 12 weeks. Despite the improvement in subjective hot flash scores, there were no statistically significant differences between the two groups in hot flash frequency or severity. This is likely because the authors of this study did not collect pretreatment baseline measures for hot flash frequencies or severity (36). Dry mouth, insomnia, and decreased appetite were significantly more common in the venlafaxine group. Mental health and vitality were significantly improved in the venlafaxine group and 93% of women in this group chose to continue venlafaxine at the conclusion of the trial.

Venlafaxine has also been compared with gabapentin and DMPA in two separate clinical trials. To compare venlafaxine and gabapentin, a group-sequential, open-label, randomized, crossover clinical trial of 4 weeks on each therapy was constructed (37). When compared with gabapentin at a target dose of 300 mg three times daily, venlafaxine ER 75 mg daily was found to be as effective in reducing hot flash scores (66% reduction in each group). However, women preferred venlafaxine to gabapentin at the end of the trial period (68% vs. 32%). Clinically, since there were approximately one-third of women in this trial who felt that gabapentin worked better for their hot flashes, this can be tried in those where venlafaxine is not helpful.

When compared with a single intramuscular dose of DMPA 400 mg, venlafaxine ER 75 mg daily was found to be less effective and less well tolerated (27). However, there were substantial reductions in hot flash scores in both groups over the 6-week period (79% vs. 55%), respectively.

The efficacy of venlafaxine for the alleviation of hot flashes in men undergoing androgen deprivation therapy was evaluated in two published trials to date. In the first pilot study, 23 men were treated with venlafaxine 12.5 mg twice daily for 4 weeks; however, only 16 completed the study (38). Of these, 10 patients had a >50% reduction in their hot flash scores at the end of the study. Treatment was well tolerated and median weekly hot flash scores decreased by 54%. The average incidence of severe and very severe hot flashes decreased from 2.3 per day at baseline to 0.6 per day at the end of the study. In the second trial, 309 men undergoing androgen deprivation therapy were randomly assigned to either venlafaxine 75 mg daily, oral

MPA 20 mg daily, or cyproterone acetate 100 mg daily over a 1-month period (39). In this double-blind trial, the change in median daily hot flash scores between randomization and 1 month was −47%, −84%, and −95%, respectively. A third trial was also unable to illustrate a benefit of venlafaxine in men with hot flashes (40). This was a three-arm trial that compared a soy protein preparation versus venlafaxine versus both versus a placebo.

Given available data, venlafaxine is a viable treatment option for the treatment of hot flashes in women and might work in men too. When this treatment approach is utilized, therapy should be initiated with venlafaxine ER 37.5 mg daily and increased to 75 mg daily after 1 week, if tolerated. Common adverse effects include loss of appetite, dry mouth, insomnia, and nausea.

Desvenlafaxine

Desvenlafaxine is a related SNRI, being the succinate salt form of the major active metabolite of venlafaxine. Desvenlafaxine has been studied in two large, randomized, placebo-controlled, clinical trials involving women without a history of breast cancer (41,42). In both trials, desvenlafaxine was associated with a 60% to 70% reduction in severity and frequency of hot flashes compared with placebo (~50% reduction). Therapy should be initiated at 50 mg daily and increased to 100 mg daily after 3 days if tolerated. The major adverse effect is dose-dependent nausea, vomiting, and dizziness.

Paroxetine

Paroxetine is a selective serotonin reuptake inhibitor (SSRI), with minimal effects on the reuptake of norepinephrine. The efficacy of paroxetine against hot flashes was initially supported in a pilot study in 2000 (40). In this study, women were treated with paroxetine 10 mg daily for 1 week, followed by 20 mg daily for 4 weeks. After 5 weeks of treatment, the mean hot flash frequency decreased by 67%, while the mean hot flash severity score decreased by 75%. There was also a statistically significant, change from baseline, improvement in depression, sleep, anxiety, and quality of life scores.

Given these positive findings, the authors conducted a placebo-controlled, double-blind, randomized clinical trial evaluating paroxetine controlled release (CR) in women suffering from hot flashes (43). One hundred and sixty-five women were randomized to either placebo, paroxetine CR 12.5 mg daily, or paroxetine CR 25 mg daily for 6 weeks. Among the 139 women who completed the trial, the hot flash score decreased by 62% and 65% in the lower- and higher-dose paroxetine groups, respectively, compared with a 38% reduction in the placebo group. The mean daily hot

flash frequency decreased from 7.1 to 3.8, 6.4 to 3.2, and 6.6 to 4.8 in the three groups, respectively. The improvement in hot flash symptoms was independent of tamoxifen use. Adverse events were reported by 54% of women taking placebo and by 58% of women taking paroxetine. Subsequent to this trial, a placebo-controlled, double-blind, randomized, crossover clinical trial evaluating paroxetine 10 and 20 mg daily was completed (44). In this trial, 151 women were assigned to receive 4 weeks of paroxetine 10 or 20 mg daily followed by placebo or vice versa. Paroxetine 10 mg daily was found to reduce hot flash frequency by 41% compared with 14% with placebo. Paroxetine 20 mg reduced the frequency of hot flashes by 52% compared with 27% with placebo. While doses had relatively similar efficacy, patients taking the 10 mg dose were less likely to discontinue treatment.

Two pilot studies have supported the efficacy of paroxetine for the treatment of hot flashes in men undergoing androgen deprivation therapy. In the first, 26 men were treated with ER paroxetine to a target dose of 37.5 mg daily over 4 weeks (45). Of the 18 patients who completed the study, the median frequency of hot flashes decreased from 6.2 per day at baseline to 2.5 per day and the hot flash scores decreased from 10.6 per day to 3 per day. In the second study, 10 patients treated with paroxetine 10 mg daily had modest improvements in both hot flash frequency (3.5 per day vs. 2 per day) and severity (46).

Paroxetine, the only antidepressant that has obtained a formal FDA approval indication, is, thus, is an effective therapeutic option for the treatment of hot flashes in women and possibly in men. Therapy should be initiated at 10 mg daily with no data to support increased dosing leading to significantly improved outcomes. It is not recommended to use paroxetine in women taking tamoxifen due to concern for reducing tamoxifen's effectiveness (vide infra). Common adverse effects are dose-dependent and include sexual dysfunction, nausea, and insomnia.

Fluoxetine

Fluoxetine is an SSRI with minimal effects on the reuptake of norepinephrine. The efficacy of fluoxetine for the treatment of hot flashes was studied in an 8-week, placebo-controlled, double-blind, crossover clinical trial involving women (47). Patients were randomized to fluoxetine 20 mg daily or placebo, and after 4 weeks, were crossed over. By the end of the first treatment period, a nonsignificant difference was seen in hot flash scores in the fluoxetine arm compared with placebo (50% vs. 36%). However, a cross-over analysis demonstrated a significantly greater improvement in hot flash scores with fluoxetine than with placebo. There was no statistically significant difference in adverse events, and efficacy was similar whether tamoxifen was being used or not.

The long-term efficacy and toxicity of fluoxetine and citalopram were compared in a placebo-controlled, double-blind, randomized clinical trial (48). One hundred and fifty women with a history of breast cancer were randomized to placebo, fluoxetine, or citalopram over a 9-month period. Fluoxetine and citalopram were started at 10 mg and then increased to 20 mg daily at 1 month and further increased to 30 mg daily at 6 months. There were no statistically significant differences among the three groups with respect to hot flashes at any time during the trial. Discontinuation rates were 40% in the placebo group, 34% in the fluoxetine group, and 34% in the citalopram group. Baseline information was obtained on the first day of treatment rather than preceding initiation of therapy. This is a possible confounder, as previous studies have shown efficacy within 1 day of treatment (32).

Common adverse effects include loss of appetite, nausea, and insomnia. Similar to paroxetine, fluoxetine should not be used in patients receiving tamoxifen (vide infra). Given the evidence to date, fluoxetine should not be considered among the current nonhormonal therapies to use in practice.

Citalopram

Citalopram is a potent and specific SSRI. The efficacy of citalopram for hot flashes was first supported in two small pilot studies. In contrast, a large, placebo-controlled, randomized trial evaluating citalopram and fluoxetine at a target dose of 30 mg daily concluded that neither were effective compared with placebo (48). This trial failed to collect baseline data prior to starting the study drug (see Section Fluoxetine). Another double-blind, placebo-controlled, randomized clinical trial evaluated 254 women who were allotted to either placebo or citalopram at target doses of 10, 20, or 30 mg daily over a 6-week period (49). Hot flash frequency decreased by 20%, 46%, 43%, and 50%, respectively. Although reductions in hot flash frequency were relatively similar in all citalopram groups, citalopram 20 mg daily appeared to be more effective than 10 mg daily in regard to beneficial impacts on daily life, including sleep, mood, and enjoyment, as measured by the HFRDIS.

Citalopram is, thus, an effective treatment for women suffering from hot flashes. Therapy should be initiated and continued at 20 mg daily. Common adverse effects include nausea, constipation, and dry mouth. Given the available data, citalopram can be safely utilized in patients receiving tamoxifen (vide infra).

Escitalopram

Escitalopram, being the *S*-enantiomer of racemic citalopram, is also an SSRI. Only one double-blind, placebo-controlled, randomized trial evaluating escitalopram at 10 to 20 mg daily has been published to date (50). Two-hundred and five postmenopausal women without a history of breast cancer were randomized to placebo or escitalopram 10 mg daily for 8 weeks. Escitalopram was found to be modestly more effective than placebo at decreasing the frequency of hot flashes (47% vs. 33%). Adverse events were higher in the placebo group (53% vs. 63%) and only seven patients in the escitalopram arm discontinued therapy due to an adverse event.

Given the available data, escitalopram is a therapeutic option in women suffering from hot flashes. Therapy should be initiated at 10 mg daily and increased to 20 mg daily after 4 weeks if ineffective. Common adverse effects include nausea, headaches, fatigue, and sleeping difficulties.

Sertraline

Sertraline is a potent and specific SSRI. To date, there have been three published trials assessing the efficacy of sertraline in reducing hot flashes with variable results. In the first double-blind, placebo-controlled, randomized, crossover clinical trial, 62 women, with early-stage breast cancer on adjuvant tamoxifen, were randomized to sertraline 50 mg daily or placebo for 6 weeks and then crossed over (51). A nonstatistically significant difference was seen between the sertraline and placebo groups (36% vs. 27%). At the end of 12 weeks, 49% of patients preferred the sertraline period, 11% preferred the placebo period, and 41% had no preference. Another double-blind, placebo-controlled, crossover clinical trial involving 102 women without a history of breast cancer were randomized to sertraline 50 mg daily or placebo for 4 weeks and then crossed over after a 1-week washout period (52). Although the hot flash score was significantly better in the sertraline group, no difference was seen in the severity of symptoms between groups. In a subsequent double-blind, placebo-controlled, randomized clinical trial, sertraline, 50 to 100 mg daily over a 6-week period, was found to be no more effective than placebo in either hot flash frequency or hot flash scores (53).

Given the available evidence, sertraline has not been found to be consistently helpful in alleviating hot flashes and is not recommended.

Interactions between Tamoxifen and the Newer Antidepressants

Tamoxifen is converted to its active metabolite, endoxifen, by the hepatic enzyme cytochrome P450 2D6 (CYP2D6). It has been hypothesized that patients on tamoxifen with reduced CYP2D6 activity, due to genomic variants or by drugs that inhibit CYP2D6 function, might result in poorer outcomes (54,55). SSRIs are an important class of drugs that inhibit CYP2D6 function. Among the SSRIs, paroxetine, a potent CYP2D6 inhibitor, has been associated with an increased risk of death from breast cancer (54). It is important to bear in mind that there is a gradient of potency for inhibition of CYP2D6 among the SSRIs and SNRIs with paroxetine and fluoxetine having greater inhibitory potential compared with citalopram and venlafaxine. Given currently available data, use of venlafaxine or citalopram should be preferentially considered in patients receiving tamoxifen (56,57).

Antiepileptics

Gabapentin. Gabapentin is a γ-aminobutyric acid (GABA) analog that is used in a variety of neurologic and pain syndromes. The exact mechanism of action is unclear, but it is suggested that it reduces noradrenergic hyperactivity. The efficacy of gabapentin for the treatment of hot flashes was first noted serendipitously in a group of six patients at the University of Rochester (58). Since then, four trials, as well as a pooled analysis, have shown the benefit of gabapentin in reducing hot flashes in women (32). The first placebo-controlled, randomized clinical trial involved 59 postmenopausal women without a history of breast cancer who were treated with either gabapentin 900 mg daily or placebo (59). After 12 weeks of therapy, patients receiving gabapentin had a significantly greater reduction in hot flash frequency, compared with placebo (45% vs. 29%). An open-label treatment phase followed during which gabapentin was able to be increased (maximum dose of 2,700 mg daily) and was associated with a greater reduction in hot flash frequency from baseline. Two other placebo-controlled, randomized clinical trials involving a similar population showed similar reductions in hot flash scores compared with placebo (51% vs. 26% and 71% vs. 54%, respectively) (60,61). Gabapentin (900 mg daily) in breast cancer survivors was also effective at reducing hot flashes (62). A placebo-controlled, randomized clinical trial of gabapentin in men receiving androgen deprivation therapy for prostate cancer showed similar but less robust results (63). In this trial, patients receiving gabapentin 900 mg daily had a statistically significant reduction in hot flash frequency from baseline compared with placebo (46% vs. 22%). However, no statistically significant difference was observed in men taking gabapentin at 300 to 600 mg daily.

Gabapentin, thus, is an effective therapeutic option in the treatment of hot flashes in women and men. Therapy should be initiated at 300 mg daily and titrated up to 300 mg three times daily (900 mg daily), if tolerated. The most common adverse effects of gabapentin are dose-dependent and include dizziness, somnolence, and fatigue.

Pregabalin. Pregabalin is a newer generation GABA analog that appears to be a more potent analgesic than gabapentin. A pilot study, consisting of six patients, demonstrated a reduction in hot flashes by 65% with pregabalin 50 to 150 mg daily (64). This was corroborated by a double-blind, placebo-controlled, randomized clinical trial, involving 163 women who received pregabalin at a target dose of 75 mg twice daily, 150 mg twice daily, or placebo (65). After 6 weeks, hot flash scores decreased by 65%, 71%, and 50%, respectively. Therefore, pregabalin is an effective therapeutic option in the treatment of hot flashes in women. Therapy should be initiated at 50 mg at bedtime for the first week, then 50 mg twice daily for the second week, then 75 mg twice daily thereafter, if tolerated. Adverse effects are primarily dose-dependent and include cognitive difficulty, dizziness, weight gain, and sleepiness.

Other Centrally Acting Compounds

Clonidine. Clonidine is a centrally acting α_2-receptor agonist first proposed as a treatment for hot flashes in the 1970s. One purported mechanism of action is that clonidine raises the sweating threshold by reducing norepinephrine release. The efficacy of transdermal clonidine (equivalent to an oral dose of 0.1 mg daily) for the treatment of tamoxifen-induced hot flashes was first shown in a placebo-controlled, randomized clinical trial (66). However, transdermal clonidine was associated with significant adverse effects, including fatigue, dry mouth, and constipation. A similar study in men with postorchiectomy hot flashes failed to demonstrate a significant decrease in hot flash frequency or severity (67). Another placebo-controlled, randomized clinical trial, involving 194 women with tamoxifen-induced hot flashes, demonstrated a decrease in hot flashes in the clonidine group (0.1 mg orally nightly) compared with the placebo group, after 8 weeks of therapy (38% vs. 24%) (62). Patients in the clonidine group had more adverse effects, especially insomnia. Although clonidine decreases hot flashes, its unfavorable toxicity profile, and the availability of other agents, limits its use.

Methyldopa. Methyldopa is a centrally acting α_2-receptor agonist that has been investigated as a treatment for hot flashes. A 2006 systematic review, including three poor-quality crossover trials, found no difference in frequency of hot flashes in patients receiving methyldopa versus placebo

(33). Fatigue, dizziness, and dry mouth occurred more often in the study groups. Due to its limited efficacy and toxicity profile, methyldopa is not recommended as a therapy for hot flashes.

Bellergal. Bellergal Retard is a brand name for a combination product of ergotamine, belladonna alkaloids, and phenobarbital. Although several reports favor its use over placebo, this therapy should not be recommended given marginal reported efficacy, the dose-dependent anticholinergic side effects of belladonna (dizziness, constipation, dry mouth, and blurry vision), and the risk of phenobarbital dependence (68).

Veralipride. Veralipride is a substituted benzamide derivative with antidopaminergic (D_2) properties. There have been two small placebo-controlled reports, suggesting marked improvements in hot flash frequency and severity with the use of veralipride (100 mg daily) (69,70). However, this medication is not approved for use in the United States due to its toxicity profile, which includes mastodynia, galactorrhea, gastrointestinal distress, and tardive dyskinesia.

Complementary and Alternative Therapies

Vitamin E. Based on some case series, vitamin E (α-tocopherol) was first recognized in the 1940s as a potential treatment for hot flashes. In 1998, a placebo-controlled, randomized, crossover clinical trial involving 120 women demonstrated a marginal benefit with an average of one less hot flash per day with vitamin E (800 IU daily) compared with placebo (71). Side effects were similar in both groups. A subsequent prospective, double-blind, placebo-controlled trial also reported positive results; however, the treatment arms were not randomized (all patients received placebos for 4 weeks followed by a washout period and then 4 weeks of vitamin E) (72). Thus, while there is a suggestion that vitamin E may help decrease hot flashes to some extent, there is not yet convincing proof. Although concerns regarding the carcinogenicity of vitamin E have been raised, a 2008 meta-analysis found no effect on cancer incidence or mortality (73). Thus, vitamin E is a reasonable option to try, albeit it has limited efficacy.

Phytoestrogens and Soy. When compared with the United States, the prevalence of hot flashes is significantly less in Asia. One theory for this difference is the predominance of soy-based dietary intake. Phytoestrogens are classified into three main classes: isoflavones, lignins, and coumestans. These compounds are purported to have both estrogenic and antiestrogenic properties. Isoflavone precursors are found in soy, red clover, alfalfa,

and other beans. A 2016 meta-analysis concluded that phytoestrogens showed a modest benefit in treatment of hot flashes (74). There is ongoing debate over whether soy decreases, or increases, the risk of estrogen-dependent tumors. Lignan precursors are found in seeds (flaxseed), whole grains, millet, fruits, and vegetables. A clinical trial involving 188 women failed to show a benefit in hot flash scores with a daily flaxseed bar (providing 410 mg of lignins) compared with placebo over a 6-week period (75).

Black Cohosh. Black cohosh (*Cimicifuga racemosa*) is a herbaceous perennial plant native to North America. Although historical trials suggested improvement in vasomotor symptoms in nonmedication-induced menopause (76), subsequent trials have not shown similar efficacy (74,77–79).

Oxybutynin. Oxybutynin, an anticholinergic typically prescribed for treatment of bladder spasms, has been demonstrated to decrease hot flashes by about 70% to 80% (80,81). A double blind, randomized clinical trial comparing oxybutynin to placebo in menopausal women demonstrated response rates of approximately 70% with improvements in menopausal symptoms and sleep compared to placebo (82). A recent publication, regarding a double-blind, placebo-controlled, trial in women demonstrated that low doses (5 to 10 mg/day) decreased hot flashes by about 80% and improved life quality (83). It may also be helpful in men undergoing androgen deprivation (81) but further study is needed. Dry mouth is the main side effect and results in discontinuation by a small minority of patients (82). Epidemiologic data strongly suggest that anticholinergics can cause moderate declines in neuro-cognitive function and should likely be avoided in senior adults (84–86).

Breast Cancer versus No Breast Cancer

When nonhormonal therapies were initially shown to be helpful in women with a history of breast cancer, many of whom were taking tamoxifen, the question arose as to whether hot flash treatments would work differently in women with a history of breast cancer and/or taking tamoxifen, versus other women. This question was evaluated by looking at data from many randomized double-blinded clinical trials that included women with and without a history of breast cancer and with and without tamoxifen use, concluding that hot flash treatments did not appear to be different in these different groups of women (87).

NONPHARMACOLOGIC INTERVENTIONS

Multiple nonpharmacologic interventions have been purported to alleviate hot flashes. These include the use of air conditioners, cold water, special diets, exercise programs, acupuncture, yoga, relaxation techniques, paced respiration, biofeedback, and more. The evidence to support the use of the majority of these interventions is limited at this time; however, many patients prefer nonpharmacologic treatments that may offer relief with lower risks of side effects and drug interactions.

Acupuncture

Over the last two decades, multiple trials have explored the efficacy of acupuncture in reducing hot flashes. A meta-analysis of 16 randomized clinical trials involving over 1,100 women found that acupuncture was superior to no treatment, not superior to sham acupuncture, and inferior to hormonal therapy (88). More recent trials have demonstrated mixed results (89–91). One explanation for these findings is that the types of sham acupuncture typically used in clinical trials may have therapeutic effects (92). In total, there is suggestive evidence that acupuncture may help hot flashes.

Stellate Ganglion Block

This procedure involves injection of an anesthetic next to a nerve group in the neck (stellate ganglion) and has been used for decades to treat chronic pain. The mechanism of action is not completely understood but may be associated with the neurological connection of the stellate ganglion to the insular cortex, a structure that is known to play a role in the pathophysiology of hot flashes (93). Early studies demonstrated positive results in reducing hot flash severity and frequency (94–96). Comparison of stellate ganglion block versus pregabalin found that stellate ganglion block was more effective than pregabalin 75 mg twice a day (97). Compared to paroxetine, stellate ganglion block has been shown to be equally effective (98). While the data regarding stellate ganglion blocks support that it is effective, large trials have not been completed and it is not commonly used in practice.

Relaxation Techniques and Yoga

Many different modalities of relaxation (e.g., paced breathing and mindfulness-based stress reduction) have been investigated for the treatment of menopausal symptoms. Although small trials have shown positive results, a systematic review from 2017 concluded that further investigation is needed prior to recommending mindfulness, meditation, or relaxation (99). Yoga, which incorporates relaxation techniques and physical posturing, has been studied for hot flashes, although individual study results have been mixed (100). A meta-analysis of eight clinical trials involving over 900 total participants reported that yoga reduces hot flashes and improves mood in peri- or postmenopausal women (101). Yoga and meditation may also be useful for treating menopausal symptoms in breast cancer survivors, although hot flashes were not a specific outcome in a comparison with usual care (102).

Hypnosis

Hypnosis is one of the many mind–body therapies utilized in both cancer and noncancer supportive care. Two randomized controlled trials of hypnosis versus no treatment and hypnosis versus attention control have demonstrated impressive reductions in hot flashes ranging from 68% to 74% (103,104). Results of a four-arm clinical trial showed that hypnosis was equally effective to venlafaxine at reducing hot flashes (105). Despite its apparent efficacy, further data regarding the implementation of this approach is needed, to make it more practical for use in clinical practice. A pilot study demonstrated that self-hypnosis, as opposed to having a hypnotist provide this therapy, was feasible and reduced hot flashes by approximately 75% (106). Randomized controlled studies are ongoing to try to solidify this treatment approach.

Cognitive Behavioral Therapy

Cognitive behavioral therapy may be useful in reducing hot flashes through modifications in cognitive appraisal of symptoms (107). Multiple studies have demonstrated reductions in hot flashes using individual-delivered (108), group-delivered (109), and telephone-delivered (110,111) cognitive behavioral therapy led by nurses (109) and therapists. Cognitive behavioral therapy seems to be effective in both women and men. While this appears to be an effective treatment for hot flashes, the most effective dose, frequency, and delivery methods are yet to be determined.

RECOMMENDATIONS

It is well known that hot flashes can have serious detrimental effects on quality of life. Clinicians should be aware of the prevalence of hot flashes and the multitude of therapeutic options available. Given the available research to date, multiple evidence-based recommendations can be made for treating hot flashes in patients suffering from hot flashes (Table 9.2).

TABLE 9.2 DOSING SCHEDULES AND EXPECTED RESPONSE OF BENEFICIAL NONESTROGENIC THERAPEUTICS

Treatment	Dosing schedule	Expected HF reduction (%)[a]
Citalopram	Initiate and continue at 20 mg daily	50–60
Desvenlafaxine	Initiate at 50 mg daily and increase to goal of 100 mg daily after 3 d	50–60
DMPA	Give 400 mg IM once, can repeat after 3–12 mo, if needed	70–80
Escitalopram	Initiate at 10 mg daily and increase to 20 mg daily after 4 wk if needed	40–50
Gabapentin	Initiate at 300 mg daily and titrate up to 300 mg three times daily if tolerated	50–60
Megestrol acetate	Initiate and continue at 20–40 mg daily	70–80
Oxybutynin	Initiate at 5 mg/d, with potential increase to 10 mg/d	70–80
Paroxetine	Initiate and continue at 10 mg daily	50–60
Pregabalin	Initiate at 50 mg QHS for 1 wk, then 50 mg twice daily for 1 wk, then 75 mg twice daily thereafter	50–60
Vitamin E	Initiate and continue at 800 IU daily	20–30
Venlafaxine	Initiate venlafaxine ER at 37.5 mg daily and increase to 75 mg daily after 1 wk	50–60

See sections on each therapeutic for further details.
[a]Expected percentage reduction is based on HF reduction from patients baseline; placebo effect is ~20%–50%.
HF, hot flash; DMPA, depomedroxy progesterone acetate; QHS, at bedtime; ADT, androgen deprivation therapy.

MANAGEMENT SUMMARY

- If a patient has mild symptoms that do not interfere with his or her daily activities, a trial of vitamin E 800 IU daily is a reasonable option. Despite the marginal benefit seen over placebo, this readily available and inexpensive therapy may allow a patient to get the well-known placebo effect without associated costs and toxicities of other therapeutic options.
- When nonpharmacological options are desired, yoga, cognitive behavioral therapy, or acupuncture should be tried.
- If a patient has more severe symptoms, it is of prime importance to assess the feasibility of hormonal therapy, as hormonal therapy has been shown to have the most significant therapeutic potential. However, if contraindications or patient preferences preclude the use of hormonal therapy, nonhormonal therapy should be considered.
- In women, citalopram, venlafaxine, paroxetine, desvenlafaxine, oxybutynin, gabapentin, and pregabalin should be considered as reasonable therapeutic options. It is of importance to minimize undesired toxicities by utilizing known side effects to their advantages. For example, in women with a history of depressive symptoms,

an antidepressant would be a more reasonable option than gabapentin. Given the randomized trial that compared venlafaxine with gabapentin (37), it seems reasonable to start with an antidepressant first.
- While good cross-study comparisons have not been completed between the antidepressants, citalopram may be the best tolerated among the antidepressants that appear to work well against hot flashes. Oxybutynin, another nonhormonal drug that also markedly decreases hot flashes, is another very reasonable option to employ. For patients who do not want to take the above noted items, progesterone analogs are effective nonestrogenic hormonal options.
- Men undergoing androgen deprivation therapy have been less well studied in clinical trials. Nonetheless, with clonidine appearing to be an exception, it appears that hot flash therapies that work in women usually also work in men (112). Thus, it appears reasonable to try hot flash treatments in men based on what has been learned in women.
- Fortunately, there are many options available for treatment of hot flashes, allowing clinicians to focus on which ones are most appropriate and acceptable to the individual patient.

REFERENCES

1. Buchholz NP, Mattarelli G, Buchholz MM. Post-orchiectomy hot flushes. *Eur Urol.* 1994;26(2):120-122.
2. Lanfrey P, Mottet N, Dagues F, et al. [Hot flashes and hormonal treatment of prostate cancer]. *Prog Urol.* 1996;6(1):17-22.
3. Schow DA, Renfer LG, Rozanski TA, Thompson IM. Prevalence of hot flushes during and after neoadjuvant hormonal therapy for localized prostate cancer. *South Med J.* 1998;91(9):855-857.
4. Carpenter JS, Andrykowski MA, Cordova M, et al. Hot flashes in postmenopausal women treated for breast carcinoma: prevalence, severity, correlates, management, and relation to quality of life. *Cancer.* 1998;82(9):1682-1691.
5. Avis N, Crawford S, McKinlay S. Psychosocial, behavioral, and health factors related to menopause symptomatology. *Womens Health.* 1997;3:103-120.
6. Gold EB, Sternfeld B, Kelsey JL, et al. Relation of demographic and lifestyle factors to symptoms in a multiracial/ethnic population of women 40-55 years of age. *Am J Epidemiol.* 2000;152(5):463-473.
7. Daly E, Gray A, Barlow D, McPherson K, Roche M, Vessey M. Measuring the impact of menopausal symptoms on quality of life. *BMJ.* 1993;307(6908):836-840.
8. Freedman RR, Krell W. Reduced thermoregulatory null zone in postmenopausal women with hot flashes. *Am J Obstet Gynecol.* 1999;181(1):66-70.
9. Freedman RR, Norton D, Woodward S, Cornelissen G. Core body temperature and circadian rhythm of hot flashes in menopausal women. *J Clin Endocrinol Metab.* 1995;80(8):2354-2358.
10. Bethea C, Lu N, Gundlah C. Diverse actions of ovarian steroids in the serotonin neural system. *Front Neuroendocrinol.* 2002;23:4-100.
11. Moses-Kolko EL, Berga SL, et al. Widespread increases of cortical serotonin type 2A receptor availability after hormone therapy in euthymic postmenopausal women. *Fertil Steril.* 2003;80(3):554-559.
12. Sumner BE, Grant KE, Rosie R, Hegele-Hartung C, Fritzemeier KH, Fink G. Effects of tamoxifen on serotonin transporter and 5-hydroxytryptamine(2A) receptor binding sites and mRNA levels in the brain of ovariectomized rats with or without acute estradiol replacement. *Brain Res Mol Brain Res.* 1999;73(1-2):119-128.
13. Sipe K, Leventhal L, Burroughs K, Cosmi S, Johnston GH, Deecher DC. Serotonin 2A receptors modulate tail-skin temperature in two rodent models of estrogen deficiency-related thermoregulatory dysfunction. *Brain Res.* 2004;1028(2):191-202.
14. Merchenthaler I, Funkhouser JM, Carver JM, Lundeen SG, Ghosh K, Winneker RC. The effect of estrogens and antiestrogens in a rat model for hot flush. *Maturitas.* 1998;30(3):307-316.
15. Carpenter JS. The Hot Flash Related Daily Interference Scale: a tool for assessing the impact of hot flashes on quality of life following breast cancer. *J Pain Symptom Manage.* 2001;22(6):979-989.
16. Carpenter JS, Bakoyannis G, Otte JL, et al. Validity, cutpoints, and minimally important differences for two hot flash-related daily interference scales. *Menopause.* 2017;24(8):877-885.
17. Loprinzi CL, Barton DL. Gadgets for measuring hot flashes: have they become the gold standard? *J Support Oncol.* 2009;7(4):136-137.
18. Notelovitz M, Lenihan JP, McDermott M, Kerber IJ, Nanavati N, Arce J. Initial 17beta-estradiol dose for treating vasomotor symptoms. *Obstet Gynecol.* 2000;95(5):726-731.
19. Rossouw JE, Anderson GL, Prentice RL, et al. Risks and benefits of estrogen plus progestin in healthy postmenopausal women: principal results From the Women's Health Initiative randomized controlled trial. *JAMA.* 2002;288(3):321-333.
20. North American Menopause Society. Estrogen and progestogen use in postmenopausal women: 2010 position statement of The North American Menopause Society. *Menopause.* 2010;17(2):242-255.
21. Holmberg L, Iversen OE, Rudenstam CM, et al. Increased risk of recurrence after hormone replacement therapy in breast cancer survivors. *J Natl Cancer Inst.* 2008;100(7):475-482.
22. von Schoultz E, Rutqvist LE. Menopausal hormone therapy after breast cancer: the Stockholm randomized trial. *J Natl Cancer Inst.* 2005;97(7):533-535.
23. Col NF, Hirota LK, Orr RK, Erban JK, Wong JB, Lau J. Hormone replacement therapy after breast cancer: a systematic review and quantitative assessment of risk. *J Clin Oncol.* 2001;19(8):2357-2363.
24. Loprinzi CL, Michalak JC, Quella SK, et al. Megestrol acetate for the prevention of hot flashes. *N Engl J Med.* 1994;331(6):347-352.
25. Quella SK, Loprinzi CL, Sloan JA, et al. Long term use of megestrol acetate by cancer survivors for the treatment of hot flashes. *Cancer.* 1998;82(9):1784-1788.
26. Bertelli G, Venturini M, Del Mastro L, et al. Intramuscular depot medroxyprogesterone versus oral megestrol for the control of postmenopausal hot flashes in breast cancer patients: a randomized study. *Ann Oncol.* 2002;13(6):883-888.
27. Loprinzi CL, Levitt R, Barton D, et al. Phase III comparison of depomedroxyprogesterone acetate to venlafaxine for managing hot flashes: North Central Cancer Treatment Group Trial N99C7. *J Clin Oncol.* 2006;24(9):1409-1414.
28. Dixon AR, Jackson L, Chan S, Haybittle J, Blamey RW. A randomised trial of second-line hormone vs single agent chemotherapy in tamoxifen resistant advanced breast cancer. *Br J Cancer.* 1992;66(2):402-404.
29. Hofseth LJ, Raafat AM, Osuch JR, Pathak DR, Slomski CA, Haslam SZ. Hormone replacement therapy with estrogen or estrogen plus medroxyprogesterone acetate is associated with increased epithelial proliferation in the normal postmenopausal breast. *J Clin Endocrinol Metab.* 1999;84(12):4559-4565.
30. Sartor O, Eastham JA. Progressive prostate cancer associated with use of megestrol acetate administered for control of hot flashes. *South Med J.* 1999;92(4):415-416.
31. Ertz-Archambault NM, Rogoff LB, Kosiorek HE, et al. Depomedroxyprogesterone acetate therapy for hot flashes in survivors of breast cancer: no unfavorable impact on recurrence and survival. *Support Care Cancer.* 2020;28(5):2139-2143.
32. Loprinzi CL, Sloan J, Stearns V, et al. Newer antidepressants and gabapentin for hot flashes: an individual patient pooled analysis. *J Clin Oncol.* 2009;27(17):2831-2837.
33. Nelson HD, Vesco KK, Haney E, et al. Nonhormonal therapies for menopausal hot flashes: systematic review and meta-analysis. *JAMA.* 2006;295(17):2057-2071.
34. Loprinzi CL, Pisansky TM, Fonseca R, et al. Pilot evaluation of venlafaxine hydrochloride for the therapy of hot flashes in cancer survivors. *J Clin Oncol.* 1998;16(7):2377-2381.
35. Loprinzi CL, Kugler JW, Sloan JA, et al. Venlafaxine in management of hot flashes in survivors of breast cancer: a randomised controlled trial. *Lancet.* 2000;356(9247):2059-2063.

36. Evans ML, Pritts E, Vittinghoff E, McClish K, Morgan KS, Jaffe RB. Management of postmenopausal hot flushes with venlafaxine hydrochloride: a randomized, controlled trial. *Obstet Gynecol.* 2005;105(1):161-166.

37. Bordeleau L, Pritchard KI, Loprinzi CL, et al. Multicenter, randomized, cross-over clinical trial of venlafaxine versus gabapentin for the management of hot flashes in breast cancer survivors. *J Clin Oncol.* 2010;28(35): 5147-5152.

38. Quella SK, Loprinzi CL, Sloan J, et al. Pilot evaluation of venlafaxine for the treatment of hot flashes in men undergoing androgen ablation therapy for prostate cancer. *J Urol.* 1999;162(1):98-102.

39. Irani J, Salomon L, Oba R, Bouchard P, Mottet N. Efficacy of venlafaxine, medroxyprogesterone acetate, and cyproterone acetate for the treatment of vasomotor hot flushes in men taking gonadotropin-releasing hormone analogues for prostate cancer: a double-blind, randomised trial. *Lancet Oncol.* 2010;11(2):147-154.

40. Vitolins MZ, Griffin L, Tomlinson WV, et al. Randomized trial to assess the impact of venlafaxine and soy protein on hot flashes and quality of life in men with prostate cancer. *J Clin Oncol.* 2013;31(32):4092-4098.

41. Archer DF, Seidman L, Constantine GD, Pickar JH, Olivier S. A double-blind, randomly assigned, placebo-controlled study of desvenlafaxine efficacy and safety for the treatment of vasomotor symptoms associated with menopause. *Am J Obstet Gynecol.* 2009;200(2): 172.e1-172.e10.

42. Speroff L, Gass M, Constantine G, Olivier S. Efficacy and tolerability of desvenlafaxine succinate treatment for menopausal vasomotor symptoms: a randomized controlled trial. *Obstet Gynecol.* 2008;111(1):77-87.

43. Stearns V, Beebe KL, Iyengar M, Dube E. Paroxetine controlled release in the treatment of menopausal hot flashes: a randomized controlled trial. *JAMA.* 2003;289(21):2827-2834.

44. Stearns V, Slack R, Greep N, et al. Paroxetine is an effective treatment for hot flashes: results from a prospective randomized clinical trial. *J Clin Oncol.* 2005;23(28): 6919-6930.

45. Loprinzi CL, Barton DL, Carpenter LA, et al. Pilot evaluation of paroxetine for treating hot flashes in men. *Mayo Clinic Proc.* 2004;79(10):1247-1251.

46. Naoe M, Ogawa Y, Shichijo T, Fuji K, Fukagai T, Yoshida H. Pilot evaluation of selective serotonin reuptake inhibitor antidepressants in hot flash patients under androgen-deprivation therapy for prostate cancer. *Prostate Cancer Prostatic Dis.* 2006;9(3):275-278.

47. Loprinzi CL, Sloan JA, Perez EA, et al. Phase III evaluation of fluoxetine for treatment of hot flashes. *J Clin Oncol.* 2002;20(6):1578-1583.

48. Suvanto-Luukkonen E, Koivunen R, Sundstrom H, et al. Citalopram and fluoxetine in the treatment of postmenopausal symptoms: a prospective, randomized, 9-month, placebo-controlled, double-blind study. *Menopause.* 2005;12(1):18-26.

49. Barton DL, LaVasseur BI, Sloan JA, et al. Phase III, placebo-controlled trial of three doses of citalopram for the treatment of hot flashes: NCCTG trial N05C9. *J Clin Oncol.* 2010;28(20):3278-3283.

50. Freeman EW, Guthrie KA, Caan B, et al. Efficacy of escitalopram for hot flashes in healthy menopausal women: a randomized controlled trial. *JAMA.* 2011;305(3):267-274.

51. Kimmick GG, Lovato J, McQuellon R, Robinson E, Muss HB. Randomized, double-blind, placebo-controlled, crossover study of sertraline (Zoloft) for the treatment of hot flashes in women with early stage breast cancer taking tamoxifen. *Breast J.* 2006;12(2):114-122.

52. Gordon PR, Kerwin JP, Boesen KG, Senf J. Sertraline to treat hot flashes: a randomized controlled, double-blind, crossover trial in a general population. *Menopause.* 2006;13(4):568-575.

53. Grady D, Cohen B, Tice J, Kristof M, Olyaie A, Sawaya GF. Ineffectiveness of sertraline for treatment of menopausal hot flushes: a randomized controlled trial. *Obstet Gynecol.* 2007;109(4):823-830.

54. Kelly CM, Juurlink DN, Gomes T, et al. Selective serotonin reuptake inhibitors and breast cancer mortality in women receiving tamoxifen: a population based cohort study. *BMJ* 2010;340:c693.

55. Kiyotani K, Mushiroda T, Imamura CK, et al. Significant effect of polymorphisms in CYP2D6 and ABCC2 on clinical outcomes of adjuvant tamoxifen therapy for breast cancer patients. *J Clin Oncol.* 2010;28(8):1287-1293.

56. Desmarais JE, Looper KJ. Interactions between tamoxifen and antidepressants via cytochrome P450 2D6. *J Clin Psychiatry.* 2009;70(12):1688-1697.

57. Lash TL, Cronin-Fenton D, Ahern TP, et al. Breast cancer recurrence risk related to concurrent use of SSRI antidepressants and tamoxifen. *Acta Oncol.* 2010;49(3):305-312.

58. Guttuso TJ Jr. Gabapentin's effects on hot flashes and hypothermia. *Neurology.* 2000;54(11):2161-2163.

59. Guttuso T Jr, Kurlan R, McDermott MP, Kieburtz K. Gabapentin's effects on hot flashes in postmenopausal women: a randomized controlled trial. *Obstet Gynecol.* 2003;101(2):337-345.

60. Butt DA, Lock M, Lewis JE, Ross S, Moineddin R. Gabapentin for the treatment of menopausal hot flashes: a randomized controlled trial. *Menopause.* 2008;15(2):310-318.

61. Reddy SY, Warner H, Guttuso T Jr, et al. Gabapentin, estrogen, and placebo for treating hot flushes: a randomized controlled trial. *Obstet Gynecol.* 2006;108(1):41-48.

62. Pandya KJ, Raubertas RF, Flynn PJ, et al. Oral clonidine in postmenopausal patients with breast cancer experiencing tamoxifen-induced hot flashes: a University of Rochester Cancer Center Community Clinical Oncology Program study. *Ann Intern Med.* 2000;132(10):788-793.

63. Loprinzi CL, Dueck AC, Khoyratty BS, et al. A phase III randomized, double-blind, placebo-controlled trial of gabapentin in the management of hot flashes in men (N00CB). *Ann Oncol.* 2009;20(3):542-549.

64. Present CA, Kelly C. Palliation of vasomotor instability (hot flashes) using pregabalin. *Community Oncol.* 2007;4:83-84.

65. Loprinzi CL, Qin R, Balcueva EP, et al. Phase III, randomized, double-blind, placebo-controlled evaluation of pregabalin for alleviating hot flashes, N07C1. *J Clin Oncol.* 2010;28(4):641-647.

66. Goldberg RM, Loprinzi CL, O'Fallon JR, et al. Transdermal clonidine for ameliorating tamoxifen-induced hot flashes. *J Clin Oncol.* 1994;12(1):155-158.

67. Loprinzi CL, Goldberg RM, O'Fallon JR, et al. Transdermal clonidine for ameliorating post-orchiectomy hot flashes. *J Urol.* 1994;151(3):634-636.

68. Bergmans MG, Merkus JM, Corbey RS, Schellekens LA, Ubachs JM. Effect of Bellergal Retard on climacteric complaints: a double-blind, placebo-controlled study. *Maturitas.* 1987;9(3):227-234.

69. David A, Don R, Tajchner G, Weissglas L. Veralipride: alternative antidopaminergic treatment for menopausal symptoms. *Am J Obstet Gynecol.* 1988;158(5):1107-1115.

70. Melis GB, Gambacciani M, Cagnacci A, Paoletti AM, Mais V, Fioretti P. Effects of the dopamine antagonist veralipride on hot flushes and luteinizing hormone secretion in postmenopausal women. *Obstet Gynecol.* 1988;72(5):688-692.

71. Barton DL, Loprinzi CL, Quella SK, et al. Prospective evaluation of vitamin E for hot flashes in breast cancer survivors. *J Clin Oncol.* 1998;16(2):495-500.

72. Ziaei S, Kazemnejad A, Zareai M. The effect of vitamin E on hot flashes in menopausal women. *Gynecol Obstet Invest.* 2007;64(4):204-207.

73. Bardia A, Tleyjeh IM, Cerhan JR, et al. Efficacy of antioxidant supplementation in reducing primary cancer incidence and mortality: systematic review and meta-analysis. *Mayo Clinic Proc.* 2008;83(1):23-34.

74. Franco OH, Chowdhury R, Troup J, et al. Use of plant-based therapies and menopausal symptoms: a systematic review and meta-analysis. *JAMA.* 2016;315(23):2554-2563.

75. Pruthi S, Qin R, Terstreip SA, et al. A phase III, randomized, placebo-controlled, double-blind trial of flaxseed for the treatment of hot flashes: North Central Cancer Treatment Group N08C7. *Menopause.* 2012;19(1):48-53.

76. Kronenberg F, Fugh-Berman A. Complementary and alternative medicine for menopausal symptoms: a review of randomized, controlled trials. *Ann Intern Med.* 2002;137(10):805-813.

77. Jacobson JS, Troxel AB, Evans J, et al. Randomized trial of black cohosh for the treatment of hot flashes among women with a history of breast cancer. *J Clin Oncol.* 2001;19(10):2739-2745.

78. Geller SE, Shulman LP, van Breemen RB, et al. Safety and efficacy of black cohosh and red clover for the management of vasomotor symptoms: a randomized controlled trial. *Menopause.* 2009;16(6):1156-1166.

79. Pockaj BA, Gallagher JG, Loprinzi CL, et al. Phase III double-blind, randomized, placebo-controlled crossover trial of black cohosh in the management of hot flashes: NCCTG Trial N01CC1. *J Clin Oncol.* 2006;24(18):2836-2841.

80. Sexton T, Younus J, Perera F, Kligman L, Lock M. Oxybutynin for refractory hot flashes in cancer patients. *Menopause.* 2007;14(3 Pt 1):505-509.

81. Smith TJ, Loprinzi CL, Deville C. Oxybutynin for hot flashes due to androgen deprivation in men. *N Engl J Med.* 2018;378(18):1745-1746.

82. Simon JA, Gaines T, LaGuardia KD. Extended-release oxybutynin therapy for vasomotor symptoms in women: a randomized clinical trial. *Menopause.* 2016;23(11):1214-1221.

83. Leon-Ferre RA, Novotny PJ, Wolfe EG, et al. Oxybutynin versus placebo for hot flashes in women with or without cancer: a randomized, double blind clinical trial (ACCRU SC-1603). *JNCI Cancer Spectr.* 2019;4(1):pkz088.

84. Geller EJ, Crane AK, Wells EC, et al. Effect of anticholinergic use for the treatment of overactive bladder on cognitive function in postmenopausal women. *Clin Drug Investig.* 2012;32(10):697-705.

85. Gray SL, Anderson ML, Dublin S, et al. Cumulative use of strong anticholinergics and incident dementia: a prospective cohort study. *JAMA Intern Med.* 2015;175(3):401-407.

86. Grossi CM, Richardson K, Fox C, et al. Anticholinergic and benzodiazepine medication use and risk of incident dementia: a UK cohort study. *BMC Geriatr.* 2019;19(1):276.

87. Bardia A, Novotny P, Sloan J, Barton D, Loprinzi C. Efficacy of nonestrogenic hot flash therapies among women stratified by breast cancer history and tamoxifen use: a pooled analysis. *Menopause.* 2009;16(3):477-483.

88. Dodin S, Blanchet C, Marc I, et al. Acupuncture for menopausal hot flushes. *Cochrane Database Syst Rev.* 2013;(7):CD007410.

89. Liu Z, Ai Y, Wang W, et al. Acupuncture for symptoms in menopause transition: a randomized controlled trial. *Am J Obstet Gynecol.* 2018;219(4):373.e1-373.e310.

90. Lesi G, Razzini G, Musti MA, et al. Acupuncture as an integrative approach for the treatment of hot flashes in women with breast cancer: a prospective multicenter randomized controlled trial (AcCliMaT). *J Clin Oncol.* 2016;34(15):1795-1802.

91. Lee MS, Kim KH, Shin BC, Choi SM, Ernst E. Acupuncture for treating hot flushes in men with prostate cancer: a systematic review. *Support Care Cancer.* 2009;17(7):763-770.

92. Kim TH, Lee MS, Alraek T, Birch S. Acupuncture in sham device controlled trials may not be as effective as acupuncture in the real world: a preliminary network meta-analysis of studies of acupuncture for hot flashes in menopausal women. *Acupunct Med.* 2020;38(1):37-44.

93. Lipov E, Kelzenberg BM. Stellate ganglion block (SGB) to treat perimenopausal hot flashes: clinical evidence and neurobiology. *Maturitas.* 2011;69(2):95-96.

94. Haest K, Kumar A, Leunen K, et al. Does the stellate ganglion block reduce severe hot flushes and sleep disturbances in breast cancer patients? *Cancer Res.* 2009;69(24 suppl):809.

95. Lipov EG, Joshi JR, Sanders S, et al. Effects of stellate-ganglion block on hot flushes and night awakenings in survivors of breast cancer: a pilot study. *Lancet Oncol.* 2008;9(6):523-532.

96. Pachman DR, Barton D, Carns PE, et al. Pilot evaluation of a stellate ganglion block for the treatment of hot flashes. *Support Care Cancer.* 2011;19(7):941-947.

97. Othman AH, Zaky AH. Management of hot flushes in breast cancer survivors: comparison between stellate ganglion block and pregabalin. *Pain Med.* 2014;15(3):410-417.

98. Rahimzadeh P, Imani F, Nafissi N, Ebrahimi B, Faiz SHR. Comparison of the effects of stellate ganglion block and paroxetine on hot flashes and sleep disturbance in breast cancer survivors. *Cancer Manag Res.* 2018;10:4831-4837.

99. Goldstein KM, Shepherd-Banigan M, Coeytaux RR, et al. Use of mindfulness, meditation and relaxation to treat vasomotor symptoms. *Climacteric.* 2017;20(2):178-182.

100. Newton KM, Reed SD, Guthrie KA, et al. Efficacy of yoga for vasomotor symptoms: a randomized controlled trial. *Menopause.* 2014;21(4):339-346.

101. Shepherd-Banigan M, Goldstein KM, Coeytaux RR, et al. Improving vasomotor symptoms; psychological symptoms; and health-related quality of life in peri- or post-menopausal women through yoga: an umbrella systematic review and meta-analysis. *Complementary Ther Med.* 2017;34:156-164.

102. Cramer H, Rabsilber S, Lauche R, Kummel S, Dobos G. Yoga and meditation for menopausal symptoms in breast cancer survivors—a randomized controlled trial. *Cancer.* 2015;121(13):2175-2184.

103. Elkins GR, Fisher WI, Johnson AK, Carpenter JS, Keith TZ. Clinical hypnosis in the treatment of postmenopausal hot flashes: a randomized controlled trial. *Menopause.* 2013;20(3):291-298.

104. Elkins G, Marcus J, Stearns V, et al. Randomized trial of a hypnosis intervention for treatment of hot flashes among breast cancer survivors. *J Clin Oncol.* 2008;26(31):5022-5026.

105. Barton DL, Schroeder KCF, Banerjee T, Wolf S, Keith TZ, Elkins G. Efficacy of a biobehavioral intervention

for hot flashes: a randomized controlled pilot study. *Menopause.* 2017;24(7):774-782.

106. Elkins G, Johnson A, Fisher W, Sliwinski J, Keith T. A pilot investigation of guided self-hypnosis in the treatment of hot flashes among postmenopausal women. *Int J Clin Exp Hypn.* 2013;61(3):342-350.

107. Norton S, Chilcot J, Hunter MS. Cognitive-behavior therapy for menopausal symptoms (hot flushes and night sweats): moderators and mediators of treatment effects. *Menopause.* 2014;21(6):574-578.

108. Hardy C, Griffiths A, Norton S, Hunter MS. Self-help cognitive behavior therapy for working women with problematic hot flushes and night sweats (MENOS@ Work): a multicenter randomized controlled trial. *Menopause.* 2018;25(5):508-519.

109. Fenlon D, Nuttall J, May C, et al. MENOS4 trial: a multicentre randomised controlled trial (RCT) of a breast care nurse delivered cognitive behavioural therapy (CBT) intervention to reduce the impact of hot flushes in women with breast cancer: study protocol. *BMC Womens Health.* 2018;18(1):63.

110. McCurry SM, Guthrie KA, Morin CM, et al. Telephone-based cognitive behavioral therapy for insomnia in perimenopausal and postmenopausal women with vasomotor symptoms: a MsFLASH randomized clinical trial. *JAMA Intern Med.* 2016;176(7):913-920.

111. Stefanopoulou E, Yousaf O, Grunfeld EA, Hunter MS. A randomised controlled trial of a brief cognitive behavioural intervention for men who have hot flushes following prostate cancer treatment (MANCAN). *Psychooncology.* 2015;24(9):1159-1166.

112. Loprinzi CL, Wolf SL. Hot flushes: mostly sex neutral? *Lancet Oncol.* 2010;11(2):107-108.

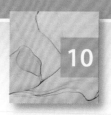

10 Anorexia/Weight Loss

Egidio Del Fabbro and Eduardo Bruera

CACHEXIA

Cancer cachexia is a multifactorial syndrome characterized by involuntary loss of skeletal muscle (with or without fat loss) that leads to progressive, impaired function and cannot be fully reversed by conventional nutritional support (1). Cancer cachexia is common, reported to occur in up to 90% of patients with advanced cancer, and often accompanied by a proinflammatory response and a cluster of symptoms that include fatigue and poor appetite. The clinical implications of cancer cachexia are profound, since weight loss is associated with more chemotherapy-related side effects; fewer completed cycles of chemotherapy; and decreased survival (2,3). Furthermore, severe involuntary weight loss impairs cancer patients' quality of life (QOL) (4) and sense of dignity (5).

EPIDEMIOLOGY

Worldwide, there is wide variation of malnutrition prevalence rates, probably because of the many different tools used for screening and assessment. Up to 70% of patients with cancer are thought to be malnourished, the majority due to reduced food intake (6).

An autopsy series of 816 patients with solid tumors at MD Anderson Cancer Center found that infection was the commonest cause of death, followed by organ failure; however, in 10% of patients no cause could be attributed other than severe emaciation and/or electrolyte imbalance (7). Subsequently, a landmark study by Dewys et al. (8) of more than 3,000 patients reported a shorter median survival in patients with weight loss compared with those without weight loss. Except in patients with pancreatic or gastric cancer, decreased weight correlated with poor performance status, and within each performance status category or tumor stage, weight loss was associated with decreased survival. Up to 70% of patients with breast cancer or acute lymphoblastic leukemia had no evidence of weight loss, but about half of prostate cancer, colon cancer, and lung cancer patients experienced weight loss, and 85% of gastric and pancreatic patients lost weight (one-third >10%). The study also suggested that any weight loss (0% to 5%) was associated with a poorer prognosis, and the prognostic effect of weight loss was greater in patients with a more favorable prognosis (good performance status or early tumor stage).

A prospective study carried out in 1979 at the National Cancer Institute in Milan of 280 patients with a variety of tumors (9) reported that specific cancers and advanced stage were more likely to be associated with weight loss. Patients with upper gastrointestinal tumors (esophagus and stomach) had significantly decreased weight, serum albumin, and triceps skinfold thickness, and treatment with chemotherapy or radiotherapy was associated with an additional decrease in arm muscle circumference. Malnutrition also became progressively more severe as the disease advanced, except in patients with cancer of the breast or cervix.

PROGNOSIS

A number of studies have reported that weight loss is associated with a poor prognosis in patients with advanced cancer. A systematic review of prognostic factors in patients with recently diagnosed incurable cancer showed (10) that weight loss, fatigue, anorexia, nausea, dyspnea, pain, multiple comorbidities, and poor performance status were all associated with decreased survival.

In 1,555 consecutive patients with locally advanced or metastatic gastrointestinal carcinomas (esophagus, stomach, pancreas, and colorectal), weight loss at presentation was more common in men than in women and correlated with decreased tumor response, QOL, and performance status (11). Patients with weight loss received lower chemotherapy doses, but they developed more severe dose-limiting toxicity (plantar–palmar syndrome and stomatitis) and received 1 month less treatment. Another prospective study of 770 lung cancer patients found that weight loss was reported by 59%, 58%, and 76% of patients with small cell lung cancer, non–small cell lung cancer (NSCLC), and mesothelioma, respectively (12), and those patients with weight loss had increased treatment toxicity and decreased survival.

In summary, several aspects of malnutrition in oncology patients are associated with poor prognosis. These include body composition, depletion of skeletal muscle mass, decreased quality of muscle, anorexia, inflammation, baseline body mass index (BMI) and weight loss (13).

MECHANISMS OF CACHEXIA

Starvation versus Cachexia

Unlike starvation, which is characterized by a loss of fat primarily, weight loss due to cachexia is characterized by a loss of both muscle and fat (Table 10.1). Cachexia will occur despite caloric supplementation and can be differentiated from starvation by endocrine abnormalities such as insulin and ghrelin resistance and frequently also by increased resting energy expenditure. Unfortunately, most patients with cancer cachexia will also have a significant component of "starvation" that exacerbates muscle wasting through either a decline in appetite or other symptoms that affect oral intake (e.g., nausea and dysgeusia).

Inflammation

An aberrant proinflammatory response as a result of the tumor–host interaction has detrimental effects on cell metabolism, protein synthesis, hormone action, and the autonomic nervous system (ANS). Specific factors produced by the tumor, for example, tumor-derived leukemia inhibitory factor (14), are responsible in part for a marked increase in serum IL-6 levels. Although increased activity of proinflammatory cytokines is proposed as the principle unifying mechanism causing both anorexia (15) and muscle wasting (16), the pathophysiology of cachexia is complex and multifactorial (Fig. 10.1), so none of the interrelated mechanisms that contribute to this syndrome should be viewed in isolation.

The primary sites of dysregulation are known to be the hypothalamus centrally (producing anorexia) and skeletal muscle and adipose tissue peripherally (increased catabolism and decreased anabolism).

Peripheral

In cancer cachexia, proinflammatory cytokines appear to induce muscle wasting by targeting certain muscle gene products. Skeletal muscle is composed of core myofibrillar proteins, including myosin heavy chain (MyHC), actin, troponin, and tropomyosin. Transcription of the MyHC gene and many other muscle genes is regulated in part by the nuclear transcription factor MyoD. Myogenic cell cultures and animal models of tumor-induced cachexia indicate that MyHC is a selective target for procachectic inflammatory cytokines (TNF-α and IFN-γ) by inhibiting MyoD and increasing the degradation of MyHC via the ligase-dependent ubiquitin–proteasome pathway (by IL-6) (17). The ligase-dependent ubiquitin–proteasome pathway is a major cellular mechanism that degrades proteins and regulates skeletal muscle wasting in cancer and other disease states. An emerging mechanism found to activate both the ubiquitin–proteasome and the autophagy–lysosome pathways is the systemic activation of Toll-like receptor 4 (TLR4) by cancer-released heat shock proteins 70 and 90 (18).

Animal models also indicate that muscle wasting induced by circulating cytokines may be modulated by genetic ablation of adipose triglyceride lipase (ATL) (19). Animals with and without ATL activity were injected with tumor cells, resulting in high circulating levels of inflammatory cytokines such as IL-6, TNF-α, and lipid-mobilizing factor (zinc-α$_2$-glycoprotein). However, only the animals with ATL activity experienced adipose tissue wasting and muscle loss accompanied by an increased expression of the ubiquitin–proteasome pathway. These studies suggest that lipolysis plays an important role in cancer cachexia and that lipases may be important therapeutic targets for the prevention of muscle wasting. Other factors also mediate wasting of adipose tissue. Chronic inflammation (especially that mediated by IL-6) promotes cancer cachexia by regulating white adipose tissue lipolysis in early-stage cachexia and browning in late-stage cachexia (20). Tumor-derived parathyroid-hormone-related protein (PTHrP) also has an important independent role in mediating the browning of fat and driving expression of genes involved in adipose tissue thermogenesis (21).

Central

Systemic proinflammatory cytokines stimulate the production of cytokines within the hypothalamus. Proinflammatory cytokines are implicated in causing anorexia by stimulating neural pathways within the arcuate nucleus of the hypothalamus to secrete

TABLE 10.1 STARVATION VERSUS CACHEXIA

	Starvation	Cachexia
Caloric intake	↓↓	↓
Resting energy expenditure	↓	↓↑ or ↔
Body fat	↓↓	↓
Lean body mass	↓	↔
Inflammatory markers	↔	↑ or ↔
Insulin	↓	↑

↔, unchanged; ↓, reduced; ↓↓, markedly reduced; ↓↑, increased or reduced; ↑, increased.

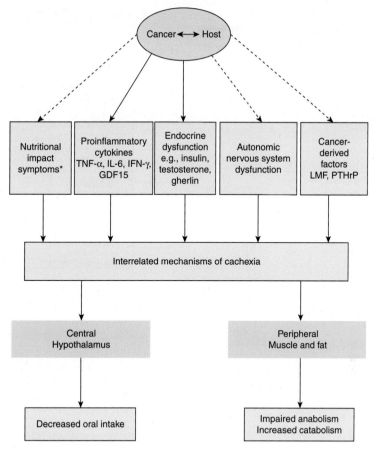

Figure 10.1 Mechanisms of cancer cachexia. PTHrP, parathyroid hormone-related protein; LMF, Lipid-mobilizing factor; TNF-α, tumor necrosis factor alpha; IL-6, interleukin-6; IFN-γ, interferon-gamma; GDF-15, growth differentiating factor 15.

anorexigenic peptides such as α-melanocyte-stimulating hormone (α-MSH), which is derived from proopiomelanocortin. α-MSH inhibits feeding and increases energy expenditure by activating melanocortin receptors, primarily the type 4 melanocortin receptor (MC4-R). In healthy animals, orally administered selective MC4-R antagonists (22) that penetrate the blood–brain barrier increase food intake, and in mice with C26 adenocarcinoma, selective MC4-R antagonists prevent tumor-induced loss of body weight, fat mass, and lean body mass. Inflammatory cytokines also inhibit the release of orexigenic neuropeptides such as agouti-related protein from another set of neurons within the hypothalamus that stimulate feeding.

Cytokines also have other central effects that decrease the oral intake indirectly by producing symptoms such as early satiety (via IL-1) and depression (IL-6) (23).

Although animal models have shown a compelling association between proinflammatory cytokines and cachexia, the evidence in human studies is inconsistent with some studies demonstrating a correlation between serum cytokines and clinical outcomes, for example, weight loss (24,25) or performance status (26,27), and others showing no significant relationship (28–30). It might be that proinflammatory cytokines such as TNF-α act in a paracrine rather than in an endocrine fashion so that serum levels do not accurately reflect tissue concentrations (31). Genetic factors such as single-nucleotide polymorphisms also appear to determine an individual's susceptibility for developing cachexia by influencing factors such as inflammation (32).

Neuroendocrine

Neural pathways within the hypothalamus are also influenced by orexigenic hormones such as ghrelin and testosterone. Ghrelin and insulin levels are elevated in patients with cachexia, suggesting resistance to these hormones, possibly mediated by inflammatory cytokines. In addition, the ANS may

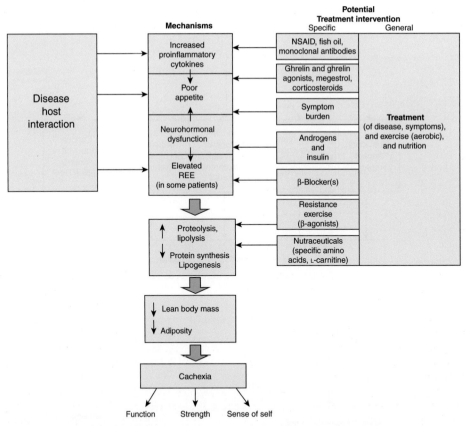

Figure 10.2 A multimodal treatment model. REE, resting energy expenditure; NSAID, nonsteroidal anti-inflammatory drug.

play a role in producing the syndrome of cachexia. Since many patients with advanced cancer have a dysfunctional ANS (33), other chronic sympathetic activation (34,35) or abnormalities of the vagus, which has a role in ghrelin activity (36) and an acute anti-inflammatory effect (37), may amplify the mechanisms causing cachexia (Fig. 10.2).

DIAGNOSIS OF CACHEXIA AND DEFINITIONS OF SARCOPENIA

The clinical diagnosis of cachexia is obvious in patients who present with temporal wasting, anorexia, poor performance status, and a markedly underweight BMI. However, diagnosing patients earlier in the disease trajectory before cachexia becomes "refractory" to intervention is important in order to initiate effective therapy. *Fearon's definition for cancer cachexia* is largely weight based, and emphasizes direct measures of muscularity, requiring >5% weight loss within the last 6 months *or* >2% weight loss in patients with a BMI < 20 kg/m² (1). Alternate criteria for a diagnosis include *sarcopenia* assessed by anthropometry, dual energy x-ray absorptiometry (DEXA), bioelectrical impedance analysis (BIA), or computerized tomography (CT).

In body composition research, the term *sarcopenia* refers to a low skeletal muscle mass, rather than the current clinical definition describing a combination of decreased strength and low muscle mass. In clinical research, *sarcopenia* is considered "muscle failure," rather than purely low muscle mass, and may arise from adverse muscle changes that accumulate across a lifetime, commonly in older adults (38). Sarcopenia is *primary* or age related when no other specific cause is evident and *secondary* when factors other than or in addition to ageing, such as cancer, are evident. Weight loss and anorexia may contribute to the development of sarcopenia but are not used as criteria for the diagnosis.

A history of weight loss is important in oncology patients because of the association with poor clinical outcomes and because an underweight BMI at initial visit is the exception in most outpatients. The increased prevalence of obesity in the general population increases the likelihood of *sarcopenic obesity* (SO), a combination of reduced lean body mass and excess adiposity. SO is associated with decreased survival in several cancer types including pancreatic cancer (39), where up to 25% of patients may have SO. Ninety-five percent of patients referred to a cachexia clinic had a normal or even overweight BMI (40) while a palliative care clinic reported marked weight loss in 71% of patients (30% with significant muscle mass reduction) in spite of a normal or increased BMI (41).

CLASSIFICATION

Ideally, patients should be enrolled in cachexia intervention trials at similar points along their illness trajectory to compare outcomes between the treatment and control arms. Patients enrolled in trials should also be able to complete the full duration of study treatment, given that attrition rates are substantial in PC due to symptom burden, disease progression, or death (42). To address these challenges and improve clinical trial design, a consensus classification of cancer cachexia proposed three stages: cachexia, precachexia, and refractory cachexia (Fig. 10.3). Precachexia is characterized by early clinical and metabolic signs (e.g., anorexia, impaired glucose tolerance, or elevated C-reactive protein [CRP]) that may precede an involuntary weight loss of $\leq$5%. Patients who have >5% loss of body weight over the last 6 months, or a BMI <20 kg/m^2 and ongoing weight loss of >2%, or sarcopenia (skeletal muscle index of males <7.26 kg/m^2 and females <5.45 kg/m^2) and ongoing weight loss of >2% (but have not entered the refractory stage) are classified as having cachexia. The last stage attempts to identify those patients thought to be "refractory" to anticachexia therapy. Patients with cachexia who have a poor performance status (WHO 3 or 4) and a life expectancy of <3 months are placed within this category.

Since the classification of cachexia stages, there is additional progress regarding weight loss and prognostication. There is now substantial evidence that energy reserves are important predictors of prognosis in patients with solid tumors. A retrospective study of >8,000 European and Canadian patients found that greater percentage weight loss in lower-BMI patients was associated with shorter survival. Based on these findings, a grading system combining baseline BMI and weight loss was able to distinguish survival when applied to a variety of specific cancers, stages, ages, and performance statuses (43). Since patients have varying degrees of risk based on their initial BMI, the authors suggest a single weight loss percentage cut-off is no longer appropriate. For example, within all patients with weight loss <10.9%, there are significantly different subsets of patients with median survival times as long as 21.5 months (weight stable with high BMI) and as short as 4.7 months (initial BMI < 20 kg/m^2). The grading system also shows a significant association with QOL, function, and symptom scores (44).

CLINICAL ASSESSMENT

The clinical assessment includes a history focused on nutrition (quantity and composition), symptoms contributing to poor oral intake, weight and body composition, a physical examination, and identification of any reversible metabolic abnormalities.

A clinical approach to cachexia in terms of "primary" and "secondary" cachexia is a useful framework for approaching the clinical management of patients with cancer and involuntary weight loss. Primary cachexia denotes the syndrome (discussed earlier in this chapter) that is characterized by muscle loss (with or without loss of fat). Secondary cachexia includes potentially treatable contributors to the weight loss of primary cachexia such as nutritional impact symptoms (NIS) and comorbid metabolic abnormalities (e.g., hypogonadism, thyroid dysfunction, and vitamin B_{12} and vitamin D deficiency). Other causes of weight loss that have a predominant starvation component such as gastrointestinal obstruction may also be included in this category, especially if they respond to endoscopic or surgical treatment (e.g., stent placement or endoscopic dilatation for esophageal obstruction).

Nutritional Impact Symptoms

Advanced cancer patients with cachexia may have multiple concurrent symptoms that compromise oral intake and contribute to nutritional decline (Table 10.2). NIS are included in the

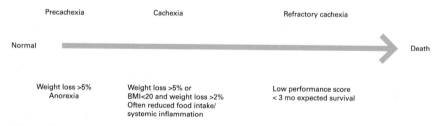

Figure 10.3 Classification of cachexia.

TABLE 10.2 FINDINGS AND INTERVENTIONS FOR SECONDARY NUTRITIONAL IMPACT IN 151 CANCER PATIENTS REFERRED TO A CACHEXIA CLINIC

Nutritional impact symptoms	Number (%)	Corresponding interventions	Number (% treated among affected individuals)
Early satiety	94 (62%)	Metoclopramide	74 (79%)
Constipation	78 (52%)	Laxatives	68 (87%)
Nausea or vomiting	67 (44%)	Antiemetics (mostly metoclopramide)	54 (81%)
Depressed mood	63 (42%)	Antidepressant (mostly mirtazapine)	51 (81%)
Dysgeusia	42 (28%)	Zinc supplement	20 (48%)
Dysphagia	21 (14%)	GI or speech therapy evaluation	5 (24%)
Dry mouth	14 (9%)	Artificial saliva	2 (14%)
Mucositis	11 (7%)	Opioids and topical mouthwash	3 (27%)
Dental pain	8 (5%)	Dental referral	2 (25%)

GI, gastrointestinal.
From Del Fabbro E, Hui D, Dalal S, et al. Clinical outcomes and contributors to weight loss in a cancer cachexia clinic. *J Palliat Med.* 2011;14(9):1004-1008.

Patient-Generated Subjective Global Assessment (PG-SGA) of Nutritional Status, a validated screening tool that includes a patient report of weight and weight change, food intake, symptoms, activities, and function. The PG-SGA short form (SF) can be completed in <5 minutes and is easily implemented in oncology and supportive care practices with sufficient personnel resources, especially those clinics with dieticians. NIS listed in the PG-SGA SF include poor appetite, pain, nausea, vomiting, constipation, altered smell and taste, mouth sores, dry mouth, dysphagia, depression, and diarrhea. The PG-SGA uses a numerical score to provide a global rating: well nourished, moderately nourished, or suspected of being malnourished or severely malnourished. The higher the score, the greater is the risk for malnutrition; for example, a score of ≥9 indicates a critical need for nutrition intervention. Nutrition triage recommendations include patient and family education, symptom management, and nutrition intervention such as additional food, oral nutrition supplements, and enteral nutrition (EN) or parenteral nutrition (PN). In clinical practice, the scored PG-SGA is quick, valid, and a reliable nutrition assessment tool that enables identification of malnourished patients for nutritional support (45).

Two retrospective studies hint at the importance of NIS when managing patients with weight loss. A chart review of patients seen in a cachexia clinic at a comprehensive cancer center found the majority had three or more uncontrolled NIS (40). A combination of nonpharmacological and readily available, inexpensive pharmacological interventions were used to manage symptoms, with a third of patients experiencing weight gain by their second visit. In addition, a second study found that a higher number of NIS in patients with head and

neck cancer are associated with poor clinical outcomes. The aggregate burden of symptoms was a significant independent predictor of reduced intake, weight loss, and survival in 635 patients prior to chemo or radiation (46). Table 10.2 shows the interventions commonly used to treat NIS.

The Edmonton Symptom Assessment Scale (ESAS) is a valid questionnaire used in daily practice to identify the presence and severity of some NIS such as nausea, depression, and fatigue. Unfortunately, the ESAS does not include other NIS such as early satiety, constipation, and dysgeusia. The ESAS does, however, score appetite on a 0 to 10 scale. Using similar numerical rating appetite scales from patient-reported outcomes, a meta-analysis of cooperative group trials found appetite loss to be a significant independent prognostic factor in patients with cancer (47).

Body Composition

Body composition in patients with the same BMI may vary considerably, although typically, both muscle and fat are depleted. Most patients reporting weight loss have normal or elevated BMIs, and a significant proportion of obese cancer patients (20%) are sarcopenic. Muscle wasting may therefore be under recognized and masked by adipose tissue (48). Evidence suggests sarcopenia identified prior to definitive antineoplastic treatment is also associated with poor clinical outcomes. A systematic review of pretherapy sarcopenia found associations with surgery and chemotherapy complications; diminished overall survival during chemotherapy; decreased relapse-free survival after surgery; and decreased progression-free survival after chemotherapy for hepatocellular carcinoma and metastatic breast cancer (49).

The least invasive method to assess body composition is midarm muscle area. Triceps skinfold thickness using calipers (in millimeters) and the midarm circumference (in centimeters) are entered into the following equation: midarm muscle area = (midarm circumference in centimeters) $- \pi \times$ (tricipital skinfold thickness in millimeters)2/ $(4 \times \pi)$ – a correction factor of 10 for men and 6.5 for women. Other measures shown to be useful for prognostication include calf circumference (50). Ultrasound is a promising noninvasive tool shown to be reliable for the assessment of muscle size in older adults. However, more high-quality research is required to confirm these findings in patients with cancer (51).

Bioimpedance analysis (BIA) relies on the different electrical properties of fat and muscle (increased water content). The bioimpedance devices are relatively easy to use and not burdensome to patients but may provide falsely elevated results of muscle mass when patients have edema. Additional information such as the ratio of resistance and reactance (phase angle) provided by BIA is useful for prognostication in patients with advanced cancer (13,52).

Dual-energy x-ray absorptiometry (DEXA) scans are based on the three-component model of body composition. DEXA uses two x-ray energies to measure body fat, muscle, and bone mineral. DEXA is more burdensome to patients (must be in supine position while the image is taken) than BIA and is more expensive. DEXA is the most commonly used modality in clinical trials.

Computed tomography (CT) scan is expensive, used mostly in research settings and not practical for regular clinical use. However, for those patients being routinely evaluated for restaging and follow-up, CT is a useful, opportunistic method to distinguish muscle and adipose tissue (53) and can assess body composition changes longitudinally (54). More recently automated methods of evaluation by CT suggest that body composition research will be accelerated and, eventually, facilitate integration of body composition measures into clinical care (55).

Indirect Calorimetry

Indirect calorimetry (IC) provides information regarding patients' caloric requirements and identifies the presence of hypermetabolism. About half of patients with cachexia will be hypermetabolic (REE > 110% of predicted) (56). Since more than 80% of caloric daily requirements are due to basal energy expenditure (REE), IC provides a more accurate measure of REE for an individual rather than a "predicted estimate," for example, by using a formula such as the Harris Benedict Equation

(HBE). Unfortunately, despite its portability and relative ease of use, the diminished accuracy of bedside IC limits its use for recommending individualized daily caloric goals (57). Metabolic room chambers are noninvasive and accurate (58) but require more time and expense. Because elevated metabolic rates may be modified pharmacologically, IC could be useful in determining the role of therapeutic options. Preliminary studies using β-blockers (59) have demonstrated some success in decreasing the resting energy expenditure of hypermetabolic patients and maintaining lean body mass.

When IC is not practical, energy expenditure can be estimated by using equations such as the HBE or a general estimate of 25 to 30 kcal/kg body weight. These estimates should be used with caution since there are inconsistencies and variations in predicted estimates for energy requirements (60).

Harris Benedict Equation (kcal/day):

$$\text{Males} = 66.5 + (13.7 \times W) + (5.0 \times H) - (6.8 \times A)$$

$$\text{Females} = 65.5 + (9.6 \times W) + (1.7 \times H) - (4.7 \times A)$$

W = usual or adjusted weight in kilograms, H = height in centimeters, and A = age in years.

When using HBE, the total caloric requirements (TCRs) can be estimated by multiplying the REE by the sum of the stress and activity factors, that is, TCR = REE × activity factor × stress factor. The stress factor for cancer is controversial, but depending on the clinical condition of the patient it ranges from 1.1 to 1.3 (61). The activity factors for sedentary patients are usually reported as 1.2.

Laboratory Assessment

Laboratory tests for levels of hormones and vitamins, such as testosterone, thyroid-stimulating hormone, vitamin B_{12}, and vitamin D, may identify secondary causes of weight loss or muscle weakness. A retrospective study of oncology patients referred to a cachexia clinic found that 73% of males were hypogonadal, while 4% of patients were hypothyroid and only 3% were vitamin B_{12} deficient (40). Another study of 100 consecutive patients complaining of moderate fatigue or poor appetite demonstrated a high frequency of low vitamin D levels (70%) (62). Although these vitamin and testosterone deficiencies are associated with muscle weakness and weight loss, their clinical relevance in oncology patients is not yet established. High-quality randomized, placebo-controlled trials will be required to assess their impact on symptoms, function, and QOL.

An elevated serum CRP level is helpful (but not essential) for the diagnosis of cachexia (and precachexia), for directing therapy with an immune modulator (e.g., nonsteroidal anti-inflammatory drugs [NSAIDs]), and as a prognostic and functional marker. A multicenter prospective cohort study of 1,702 patients found high CRP ($\geq$10 mg/dL) was associated with weight loss, anorexia, fatigue, and impaired activities of daily living (ADL). Other laboratory tests that provide indirect evidence of the proinflammatory state and metabolic dysregulation include a decreased hemoglobin, elevated white blood cell count, and hypoalbuminemia. Emerging data suggest that tumor-derived PTHrP promotes fat browning with increased energy expenditure, and is an important predictor of cancer-associated weight loss independent of hypercalcemia, inflammation, tumor burden, and other comorbidities (63).

MANAGEMENT

Cachexia is no longer thought to be an inevitable consequence of cancer's progression, with no effective therapeutic interventions. However, while there have been advances in the management of cancer cachexia, with several trials (see Table 10.3) showing improved clinical outcomes including lean body mass, appetite, and function, it must be emphasized that there is still no standard treatment for cachexia. Because the mechanisms of the cachexia syndrome are multifactorial, a comprehensive multidimensional approach using pharmacologic and nonpharmacologic interventions such as physical therapy and counseling (89) is most likely to be effective in reversing or stabilizing weight loss and muscle wasting (90).

Ideally, treatment should be individualized, taking into account the patients' overall condition, the principal mechanisms of their weight loss, and their goals of care. Although many patients and their families perceive poor appetite as a significant burden, patients with cachexia may have very different priorities, and so the therapeutic options may vary quite considerably. For many, maintaining lean body mass and function may be important, while for others the ability to preserve their appetite in order to enjoy meals with family and friends may be the primary goal. Some patients may be very concerned about their body image and the obvious, visible external manifestation of their illness.

Symptom Management

The foundation of cachexia management begins with the identification and management of NIS contributing to decreased nutritional intake (Table 10.2). Early satiety due to gastroparesis and autonomic dysfunction is the most common gastrointestinal symptom in cachectic patients and can be treated effectively with metoclopramide (10 mg every 4 hours orally) (91). Metoclopramide enables the stomach to accommodate more food and improves motility (92). Patients should be made aware of the risk for extrapyramidal symptoms (particularly within the first 48 hours), which are usually reversible. Tardive dyskinesia, however, is often irreversible, and the duration of treatment and total cumulative dose are associated with an increased risk. The risk versus benefit of metoclopramide treatment beyond 3 months should be discussed in detail with patients. Constipation may also contribute to early satiety and can be effectively managed with laxatives.

Depressed mood leading to decreased oral intake should be managed with counseling and antidepressants if indicated. Mirtazapine and olanzapine (93) are useful agents for both depression and nausea (94). Mirtazapine improves gastric accommodation and like metoclopramide has 5HT$_4$ agonist activity that promotes gastric (95) emptying and intestinal secretions. A retrospective study of low-dose olanzapine (1.5 mg daily) reported increased food intake 3 days after starting the drug in oncology patients without nausea, suggesting olanzapine has an ameliorating effect on cancer-related anorexia that is independent of its antiemetic efficacy (96).

In animal models, orally administered zinc increases appetite and appears to mediate its effects through the vagus to increase expression of orexigenic hypothalamic neuropeptides (97). Zinc supplementation has objectively improved dysgeusia in a study of patients with advanced cancer complaining of taste alteration (98) but was not effective in another placebo-controlled study (99) when administered prior to radiation therapy. In the absence of other effective agents, a trial of zinc sulfate is warranted in patients with dysgeusia since this supplement has few side effects.

Appetite Stimulation

Progestational agents such as megestrol acetate (MA) and medroxyprogesterone improve appetite, body weight (86), and other symptoms such as fatigue and nausea. A systematic review found MA improved weight but not QOL, with more adverse events but no difference in deaths when compared to placebo (85). Because of the increased risk for thromboembolism, inform patients of the potentially serious side effects, and reserve MA for patients placing a high priority on improved appetite, since MA may have an antianabolic effect on muscle. Since some of the adverse effects may be dose related, it seems prudent to start at a low dose (e.g., 160 mg/d) and monitor clinical response.

TABLE 10.3 REVIEW OF SELECTED CACHEXIA TRIALS

Author	Intervention	Methodology	Outcome measures	Intervention duration	Participants	Relevant results
Monoclonal Antibodies						
Golan et al. 2018 (64)	Antimyostatin Antibody 100 mg vs. 300 mg vs. placebo	Phase II RCT	Overall Survival	8 weeks	125 patients on chemo for pancreatic cancer	No benefit for survival Increased anorexia and fatigue in treatment group
Corticosteroids						
Yennu et al. 2013 (65)	Dexamethasone 4 mg b.i.d.	Double blind RCT single center	Appetite Fatigue	2 weeks	Advanced cancer, 84 patients	Improved FACIT fatigue and FAACT
Anamorelin						
Temel et al. 2016 (66)	Anamorelin 100 mg p.o.	Two Phase III RCTs Multicenter	Handgrip LBM	12 weeks	979 patients Inoperable NSCLC (international)	No difference for handgrip Improved LBM, appetite
Katakami et al. 2018 (67)	Anamorelin 110 mg	Multicenter Double-blind Placebo-controlled	LBM	12 weeks	Inoperable NSCLC patients (Japan)	No change in handgrip or 6 MW Improved LBM, appetite
Hamauchi et al. 2019 (68)	Anamorelin 100 mg	Multicenter Open label Single arm	LBM Appetite Weight	12 weeks	Gastrointestinal 50 patients Japan	Improved appetite, LBM, weight
Beta Blocker						
Coats 2016 (69)	Espindolol 2.5 mg b.i.d. 10 mg b.i.d. Placebo	Phase II RCT	Weight loss FFM Handgrip	4 weeks	Colorectal NSCLC	10 mg improved weight loss, FFM, handgrip significantly
Testosterone						
Wright et al. 2018 (70)	Adjunct Testosterone 100 mg weekly	28 males and females Double blind placebo control	Lean body mass, weight, function	7 weeks	Head and neck, cervical cancer On chemo Rx	LBM, weight, function better than placebo
Del Fabbro et al. 2013 (71)	Intramuscular testosterone replacement 150–200 mg every 2nd week	29 males Double blind placebo control	FACT fatigue FAACT	72 days	Advanced cancer	Fatigue score improved day 72, not cachexia

(Continued)

TABLE 10.3 REVIEW OF SELECTED CACHEXIA TRIALS (*Continued*)

Author	Intervention	Methodology	Outcome measures	Intervention duration	Participants	Relevant results
Thalidomide						
Mantovani et al. 2010 (72)	Multimodal dietary supplement, antioxidants, and thalidomide 200 mg, progestin, L-carnitine, fish oil 2.2 g vs. any single agent	Randomized 332 patients	Appetite Lean body mass Strength Physical activity PS REE Inflammatory cytokines	12 weeks	Solid tumors Weight loss >5% Expected survival ≥4 mo	Only combination therapy improved all outcomes Lean body mass REE Physical activity Performance status IL-6 and TNF-α levels
Gordon et al. 2005 (73)	Thalidomide 200 mg	RCT of 50 patients Placebo controlled	Weight Arm muscle	24 weeks	Pancreatic cancer >10%	Improvement in weight and arm muscle mass
Bruera 1999 (74)	Thalidomide 100 mg qhs	Open-label single-arm 37 patients	Appetite Symptoms Caloric intake	10 days	Metastatic cancer, decreased appetite, and weight loss >5%	Improved caloric intake and trend to better appetite
Melatonin						
Del Fabbro et al. 2013 (75)	Melatonin 20 mg	RCT double blind placebo	Appetite score on ESAS FAACT Weight	4 weeks	Advanced solid tumors	No improvement compared to placebo
Lissoni et al. 1996 (76)	Melatonin 20 mg	RCT of 100 patients No placebo Unblinded	Prevention of 10% weight loss	12 weeks	Metastatic solid tumors	Prevented >10% weight loss and decreased TNF-α levels, but no difference in caloric intake
Fish Oil						
Murphy et al. 2011 (77)	Fish oil 2.2 g	RCT of 40 patients, no placebo	Skeletal muscle Total adipose tissue	6 weeks	Advanced cancer	Skeletal muscle improved as measured by CT
Ries et al. 2012 (78)	Fish oil/omega-3-FAs (n-3-FA)/EPA	Systematic review of 38 included studies	Cachexia	2–8 weeks	Advanced cancer	Not enough evidence to support a net benefit of n-3-FA for cachexia in advanced cancer
Dewey et al. 2007 (79)	Fish oil (EPA) 1.5–2.2 g	Systematic review of 5 trials and 587 cancer patients	Effectiveness and safety of EPA in relieving symptoms associated with cachexia	2–8 weeks	Advanced cancer	Insufficient evidence for the use of fish oil (on its own or with other treatments) for weight loss in patients with advanced cancer

Author	Intervention	Methodology	Outcome measures	Intervention duration	Participants	Relevant results
Burns et al. 2004 (80)	High-dose fish oil (4.7 g EPA and 2.8 g DHA as part of 8.5 g omega-3 FAs)	Phase II	Weight	>4 weeks	Advanced cancer >2% weight loss in 1 month	Majority did not gain weight and many had GI side effects, but a small subset of patients had weight stabilization or weight gain
NSAIDs						
Lai et al. 2008 (81)	Celecoxib vs. placebo	RCT of 11 patients	Weight LBM QOL	3 weeks	Head and neck or upper GI cancer with <5% weight loss	Celecoxib arm improved in weight and QOL No change in LBM, REE, and CRP
Mantovani et al. 2006 (82)	Antioxidants Medroxyprogesterone Celecoxib Omega-3 supplement	Single arm of 44 patients	Performance status LBM Appetite REE Proinflammatory cytokines Reactive oxygen Species QOL	16 weeks	Advanced cancer, solid tumors	LBM, QOL, appetite, and proinflammatory cytokines all improved. Grip strength and PS did not
Cerchietti et al. 2004 (83)	Celecoxib plus medroxyprogesterone	Single-arm trial of 15 patients	Symptoms Weight Performance status	4 weeks	Lung cancer, weight loss, anorexia, fatigue, performance status ≥2, and ↑ acute phase	Improved body-weight-change rate, nausea, early satiety, fatigue, appetite, and performance status
Mcmillan et al. 1999 (84)	Ibuprofen plus Megace vs. Megace plus placebo	Randomized double-blind trial of 73 patients	Weight QOL Midarm circumference	12 weeks	Metastatic GI cancers Weight loss >5%	Ibuprofen plus Megace more effective regarding weight preservation QOL Midarm circumference CRP levels No change in appetite
Lundholm et al. 1994 (35)	Indomethacin or prednisone vs. placebo	Double-blind RCT of 135 patients	Survival Weight Arm circumference	Until death	Solid tumors with some weight loss	Indomethacin = better survival Prednisone showed greater weight gain and arm circumference Both groups maintained performance status better than placebo group

(Continued)

TABLE 10.3 REVIEW OF SELECTED CACHEXIA TRIALS (Continued)

Author	Intervention	Methodology	Outcome measures	Intervention duration	Participants	Relevant results
Megestrol						
Ruiz-Garcia et al. 2018 (85)	Megestrol vs. other drugs; megestrol vs. placebo; megestrol vs. no treatment; different doses of megestrol	Systematic review, qualitative studies: 38, quantitative studies: 36	Weight gain QOL Adverse events Death	Varied	Cancer	MA gains weight but not QOL; more adverse events, but no difference in death; no optimal dose identified
Loprinzi et al. 1999 (86)	Megestrol vs. dexamethasone 0.75 mg q.i.d., fluoxymesterone 10 mg orally b.i.d.	Randomized double-blind trial of 475 patients into 3 arms	Appetite Weight Adverse effects	4 weeks	Cancer, lost 5 lb in 2 months and PS 2 or better Advanced cancer	Megestrol and dexamethasone better appetite and weight Nonsignificant trend favoring megestrol More discontinued on dexamethasone but more thrombosis on megestrol
Cannabinoids						
Strasser et al. 2006 (87)	Cannabis extract vs. delta-9-tetrahydrocannabinol vs. placebo	Three arms, double-blind RCT of 243 patients	Weight Appetite QOL	6 weeks	Advanced cancer with 5% weight loss and PS ≥2	No difference in appetite, QOL, or weight
Jatoi et al. 2002 (88)	Megestrol plus dronabinol vs. dronabinol vs. megestrol	Randomized double-blind trial of 469 patients	Appetite Weight	4 weeks	Advanced cancer, weight loss 5 lb in 2 months	Appetite and weight, QOL better with Megace than with dronabinol Impotence worse

PS, pinch strength; REE, resting energy expenditure; RCT, randomized controlled trial; CT, computed tomography; FA, fatty acid; EPA, eicosapentaenoic acid; FFM, fat-free mass; NSCLC, non–small cell lung cancer; DHA, docosahexaenoic acid; GI, gastrointestinal; LBM, lean body mass; QOL, quality of life; CRP, C-reactive protein; NNT, number needed to treat.

Common side effects include hypertension, hyperglycemia, and fluid retention; however, the more serious side effects such as thromboembolism, hypogonadism, and hypoadrenalism often limit the use of these agents. While the risk for thromboembolism appears to be dose dependent, MA < 480 mg/d does not appear to increase the incidence of thrombosis compared with placebo. Avoid MA in patients with a history of deep venous thrombosis, pulmonary embolism, or severe cardiac disease, and never discontinue their medication abruptly, as there is a risk of precipitating adrenal insufficiency. Consider monitoring testosterone levels, since profound hypogonadism is a common but treatable side effect.

Clinical trials using MA in combination with other agents have not demonstrated any additive benefits. Large randomized studies comparing MA to combination therapy with either fish oil (100) or cannabinoids (88) have shown no greater benefit with combination therapy than with MA alone. These trials were of short duration (4 weeks), and outcomes of lean body mass and physical function were not assessed.

Corticosteroids may stimulate appetite, decrease nausea, and improve fatigue in the short term. The effects of corticosteroids on appetite and food intake are usually limited to a couple of weeks, and the side effects such as myopathy, immunosuppression, and hyperglycemia increase over time. Corticosteroids should be reserved for patients with limited life expectancy and a cluster of symptoms that include fatigue and loss of appetite. Based on two double-blind RCTs showing improved fatigue and appetite within 7 to 14 days, it seems reasonable (65,101) to prescribe twice-daily dexamethasone (4 mg) or methylprednisolone (16 mg). The benefit of continuing beyond 2 weeks is unclear, and lower doses or tapering is indicated depending on side effects.

Cannabinoids: Medications containing cannabinoid delta-9-tetrahydrocannabinol (THC) are approved for use in anorexia related to AIDS and chemotherapy-induced nausea and emesis. A large multicenter trial (87) in cancer patients with anorexia showed no benefit of THC or cannabis extract over placebo. The use of THC is also limited by central nervous system side effects at higher doses, such as sedation, confusion, and perceptual disturbances. A small RCT comparing THC 2.5 mg b.i.d. to placebo found THC-treated patients reported improved ($p = 0.026$) and chemosensory perception and food "tasted better" ($p = 0.04$). Patients also consumed a greater proportion of protein in their diet and experienced improved sleep quality (102). Unfortunately, a systematic review found no convincing, unbiased, high-quality evidence suggesting that cannabinoids are of value for anorexia or cachexia in patients with cancer (103).

Ghrelin and ghrelin agonists are the most likely agents to be approved for anorexia and weight loss in the near future. Promising phase III trials of the ghrelin mimetic anamorelin showed improved appetite and gains in lean body mass after 12 weeks of treatment compared to placebo (66). Subsequently, two multicenter studies from Japan reported improved clinical outcomes, supporting the use of anamorelin for cancer cachexia (67). An open-label, single-arm study investigating the efficacy and safety of 100 mg anamorelin daily found rapidly improved anorexia, LBM, and body weight in patients with advanced gastrointestinal cancer (68). A double-blind RCT in 174 patients with stage III/IV NSCLC and cachexia reported a significant improvement in LBM and appetite compared to baseline, in patients on anamorelin.

Immune Modulation

"Sickness behavior" manifested by fatigue and other related symptoms such as poor appetite is likely the result of an aberrant proinflammatory response. Therapy with immune modulators may therefore improve multiple symptoms associated with cachexia and advanced cancer. Nonspecific immune modulators used in clinical trials for cancer cachexia include fish oil, thalidomide, NSAIDs, and melatonin.

Specific monoclonal antibodies targeting receptors such as IL-1, IL-6 (104), PTHrP, inflammatory mediator growth differentiation factor (GDF)15, and Fn14 have demonstrated potential as effective therapies in animal (105) and preliminary clinical studies. PTHrP, GDF15 (106), IL-6, and IL-8 correlate with more severe weight loss in patients with cancer cachexia and are therefore promising future therapies (63). The enormous promise of these therapies should be tempered by previous placebo-controlled trials (64), including TNF-α inhibitors, infliximab (107), and etanercept (108), which showed no weight gain or improved appetite in patients with cancer.

Nonsteroidal Anti-Inflammatory Drugs

NSAIDs, including celecoxib (81), ibuprofen, and indomethacin, have been used in combination with other pharmacologic agents to treat cachexia (see Table 10.3). A systematic literature review identified 11 of 13 trials showing improvement or stabilization in weight or lean body mass (109); however, the evidence was insufficient to recommend use of NSAIDs outside clinical trials. Several trials by the same group of investigators have used indomethacin, often in combination with β-blockers and nutritional support. A double-blind trial of indomethacin (50 mg b.i.d.) or prednisone (10 mg b.i.d.) versus placebo in 135 patients with solid tumors and weight loss showed improved survival in the group administered with indomethacin (35). The prednisone group demonstrated more weight gain and greater arm circumference. Most recently, a multimodal approach (indomethacin, nutritional support, erythropoietin, and β-blockers in selected patients) by this group of investigators was extended to include insulin. The study is discussed in *Hormone Replacement Therapies*.

The only prospective randomized study of an NSAID in combination with a progestin found that ibuprofen (1,200 mg daily in divided doses) and MA increased lean body mass and improved QOL compared with MA alone (84). Notably, individuals on combination therapy did not appear to be at greater risk for major hemorrhage than those on MA alone (800 mg daily). Other preliminary trials combining NSAIDs with progestins (either medroxyprogesterone or megestrol acetate) or with L-carnitine are given in Table 10.3 (82–84).

Thalidomide

Single-agent thalidomide has improved multiple symptoms, including appetite, nausea, and insomnia in patients with advanced cancer (4,74); however, its history of teratogenicity and potential for side effects at high doses may limit its clinical use. Despite some promising preliminary studies, a systematic review concluded that the evidence was insufficient (110) to recommend thalidomide as a cancer-cachexia therapy.

Two early trials with favorable clinical outcomes reported no significant adverse effects. Esophageal cancer (111) patients given 2 weeks of thalidomide (200 mg/d) experienced transitory somnolence and gained lean body mass loss, while a randomized placebo-controlled trial (73) of 50 patients with pancreatic cancer showed that thalidomide (200 mg/d) was well tolerated and effective at attenuating loss of weight and lean body mass after 4 weeks of therapy. There were no significant differences in QOL, survival, strength, or physical function between thalidomide and placebo. A dose escalation study (4) also confirmed the benefits of thalidomide at low doses (see Table 10.3); however, a randomized, controlled study in advanced esophageal cancer using doses of 200 mg daily (112) suggested the drug was poorly tolerated. Only 6 patients on thalidomide and 16 patients on placebo completed the protocol; adverse drug reactions or complications of disease caused withdrawal, and thalidomide showed no benefit over placebo.

Melatonin

Melatonin (76) has shown some benefit as a therapy for cachexia, possibly through its antioxidant, antiapoptosis function, and appears to have few adverse effects, even at doses of 20 mg daily. Systematic reviews (113) and meta-analysis (114) have found melatonin reduces chemotherapy side effects such as weight loss, weakness, anorexia, and fatigue. Unfortunately, the only double-blind, placebo-controlled trial in oncology patients with anorexia showed no improvement in appetite or weight (75). The control group were provided with supportive care by a specialist palliative care team; it is possible that the measured benefit from a specific therapeutic intervention such as melatonin may be not be as marked when accompanied by optimal symptom management in the placebo arm.

Fish Oil

Fish oil has anti-inflammatory and anticarcinogenic effects (115), and a long-term prospective study indicated that fish and long-chain n-3 fatty acids may decrease the risk of colorectal cancer (116). In patients with advanced pancreatic cancer, a protein-dense oral supplement enriched with n-3 fatty acid eicosapentaenoic acid (EPA) was associated with an encouraging increase in physical activity, despite no gain in weight or lean body mass (117). Unfortunately, fish oil appears to be ineffective in patients with advanced cancer. A randomized placebo-controlled trial of 60 patients with advanced cancer showed no improvement in appetite or weight after 2 weeks (118), and systematic reviews by *Cochrane and the European Palliative Care Research Collaborative* (77,78) found insufficient evidence to support the use of oral fish oil (on its own or in the presence of other treatments) for cachexia (79). Despite these negative studies in patients with advanced cancer, fish oil may prove to be useful in some subsets of patients depending on their tumor type, disease trajectory, or ability to tolerate prolonged anticachexia therapy. A randomized controlled trial of 40 patients with NSCLC receiving chemotherapy showed gains in weight and skeletal muscle mass in those patients receiving fish oil (77), and an earlier phase II study suggested that higher doses of fish oil might be more effective in certain patients but limited by an increased frequency of gastrointestinal side effects (80). A meta-analysis (119) evaluated the impact of oral nutritional interventions on a range of outcomes in patients undergoing chemoradiotherapy. A subset analysis of four RCTs found omega-3 fatty acids improved body weight by approximately 2 kg.

Hormone Replacement Therapies

Insulin

Cachexia is associated with insulin resistance, and so exogenous administration may benefit cachectic individuals. Although insulin decreases appetite centrally, it has peripheral anabolic effects particularly with regard to fat metabolism. A Swedish group (120) randomized 138 patients with a variety of gastrointestinal malignancies to receive insulin plus supportive care versus supportive care alone. Once-daily, long-acting insulin at 4 units/d with a stepwise increase of 2 units/wk to a total of 10 to 16 units/d increased retention of body fat, improved metabolic efficiency during a close to maximum work load, and prolonged survival. However, the addition of insulin to the multimodal regimen did not result in weight gain or improved QOL. Supportive care comprised a multimodal regimen of anti-inflammatories (indomethacin), recombinant erythropoietin for prevention of anemia, and specialized nutritional care oral supplements plus home parenteral nutrition (HPN) if intake declined to <80% of expected levels. There were few side effects reported, but the positive clinical outcomes need to be replicated in larger multicenter studies.

Testosterone

Low testosterone is associated with poor appetite (121) in individuals with cancer and decreased survival (62) in those with cancer cachexia. Possible mechanisms for testosterone deficiency include medications (122) (e.g., opioids, megestrol, corticosteroids) chemotherapy, radiation therapy, and chronic inflammation (123). Two small, placebo-controlled trials found some cancer cachexia-related outcomes were improved after intramuscular testosterone injections. A randomized controlled trial (RCT) in 29 men with advanced cancer reported improved Performance Status and Fatigue scores in those given intramuscular testosterone replacement therapy (TRT) compared to a placebo injection. There were no differences in weight, appetite, or adverse effects between the two study arms (71). A double blind, placebo-controlled phase II trial in 28 men *and* women administered weekly injections of adjunct testosterone or placebo for 7 weeks (70). Loss of weight and lean body mass were significantly greater in the placebo group, and physical performance improved in the testosterone group. Larger, adequately powered trials are needed to establish the efficacy of testosterone for improving lean body mass and fatigue in patients with cancer. While testosterone is contraindicated in metastatic prostate or breast cancer (124), there is accumulating evidence (125) that TRT may be safe for patients after *definitive* treatment of prostate cancer, and that addition of androgen therapy improves survival in elderly patients with AML without increasing toxicity (126).

Selective androgen receptor modulators (SARMs) in theory may provide the anabolic effects of testosterone with reduced virilization. Enobosarm showed early promise in otherwise healthy older patients (127), with improved lean body mass and physical function. Although phase II studies showed that patients with cancer cachexia treated with enobosarm experienced significant increases in lean body mass from baseline, there was no significant difference when compared to placebo (128).

Modulating Elevated Metabolic Rate

β-Blockers improve survival and modulate body composition (129) in individuals with congestive heart failure, and they attenuate weight loss in catabolic conditions such as burns (130). A small study of cachectic patients with solid tumors showed that β-blockers decrease resting energy metabolism (59). Randomized controlled trials are required to determine whether β-blockers are effective for cancer patients who are hypermetabolic or have increased sympathetic activity. More recently, a multicenter phase II study found espindolol reversed weight loss compared to placebo and improved fat free mass and hand grip strength in patients with cancer-related cachexia (69).

Exercise

Multiple studies show that exercise attenuates the fatigue experienced by individuals with cancer. Unfortunately, there are no high-quality studies evaluating the effect of exercise on appetite, weight, and body mass in patients with advanced cancer. A recent meta-analysis (131) evaluated RCTs in adults comparing exercise as a sole or adjunct intervention to no treatment or an active control for patients with cancer cachexia. No trials met the inclusion criteria, and the authors remarked that ongoing studies might add to our existing knowledge. Animal models suggest that high-intensity exercise training increases the life span of tumor-bearing rats, promotes a reduction in tumor mass, and prevents indicators of cachexia such as reduced food intake and weight loss (132).

In noncancer conditions such as age-related sarcopenia and HIV-related cachexia, resistance exercise in combination with testosterone (133) increases muscle mass (134). Exercise has the potential to be an important component of cachexia therapy by modulating expression of cytokines and acting in concert with anabolic hormones to improve strength and function (135).

Nutrition

Relying on caloric intake alone will not improve lean body mass or function. Nonetheless, patients may overestimate their daily caloric intake and are unable to appreciate the magnitude of the "starvation" component contributing to their cachexia. A study of 320 patients with advanced cancer and weight loss found the majority of patients consuming diets insufficient to maintain weight even in healthy individuals (136). Nutritionists are able to identify and make recommendations to those patients who have insufficient caloric intake. Although individualized nutritional counseling has not been evaluated in the context of a multimodal strategy, this low-risk intervention is able to improve QOL (137) outcomes and should be used in the comprehensive management of cachectic cancer patients. Nutritional counseling could help patients and their families understand that a shift to conscious control of eating is necessary. A systematic review (138) of nutrition interventions in oncology patients found that counseling with/without ONS was associated with improvements in weight, BMI, energy intake, and PG-SGA score. When IC is unavailable, the TCRs may be estimated by assuming TCR to be some 25 to 30 kcal/kg depending on the patient's performance status. Although the optimal protein requirements for oncology patients has not yet been established, guidelines from the European Society of Clinical Nutrition and Metabolism (ESPEN) recommend a minimum protein supply of 1 g/kg/d and a target of 1.2 to 2 g/kg/d (139).

The addition of specific substrates to the daily diet such as essential and nonessential amino acids as well as branched chain amino acids may be beneficial, although the evidence is derived mostly from animal models of cachexia and preliminary clinical trials. Various studies have suggested the following may be helpful (140), although larger trials are needed to confirm their efficacy in patients with cancer. They include branched-chain amino acids (leucine: 2 to 4 g/day), β-hydroxy β-methyl butyrate (3 g/day), glutamine (0.3 g/kg/day), creatine (5 g/day), and fish oil/eicosapentanoic acid (2.0 to 2.2 g/day EPA and 1.5 g/day DHA). Systemic carnitine depletion characterized by fatigue and muscle weakness is described in several diseases including cancer. L-Carnitine administration to tumor-bearing rats reduces cytokine levels and increases food intake (141), and in cachectic cancer patients, L-carnitine improved lean body mass when used either in combination with celecoxib or as a component of multimodal drug therapy (142).

A systematic review and meta-analysis of 43 studies compared complication rates between cancer patients administered EN or PN (143). Mortality and morbidity were similar, but in adults, the risk of infection was greater in those receiving PN. Since EN is nearly half the cost of PN, these results support the ESPEN guidelines recommending EN over PN in adults, when oral nutrition is inadequate. The authors also concluded that further studies comparing EN and PN for these endpoints appear unnecessary, given the lack of change in meta-conclusion and low publication bias over the past decades. A recent RCT also found more no improvement in HRQoL with PN compared to OF among patients with advanced cancer and malnutrition (144).

Parenteral Nutrition

Families and patients may inquire about the value of PN when the enteral route is impossible or ineffective in stabilizing a patient's weight. Health care professionals need to address the concerns in an empathic manner and relay the risks and benefits of such therapy with a clear understanding. In general, patients at the end of life are unlikely to benefit from PN, and systematic reviews (145) as well as guidelines (146) from the American Society for Parenteral and Enteral Nutrition recommend against the routine use of PN in advanced cancer. A recent systematic review evaluating the effects of PN on health-related QOL, physical function, nutritional status, survival, and adverse events in patients with advanced cancer concluded the evidence was weak and the subject, understudied (147). However, qualitative research (148) suggests that patients and their family might experience social and psychological benefits from HPN treatment. In an earlier study (149), the same group of researchers reported that family members feel powerless and frustrated when facing a loved one's inability to eat. There was also a perception that health care providers neglected nutritional problems. Since patients and family were no longer able to solve the nutritional problems within the family, the offer of HPN was viewed as a "positive" alternative. Counseling patients and their families is especially important to avoid inappropriate use of PN and to prevent any perception of the selective neglect of nutritional issues.

The health care team also needs to be aware that once PN is initiated in the hospital, families may have difficulty accepting the lack of an "alternative" and that withdrawal of PN on discharge could have a considerable psychological impact (150).

In clinical circumstances when the tumor is slow growing and there is mechanical obstruction, PN may be indicated to treat the starvation component of the cachectic patient. However, it should be emphasized that clinical guidelines (151) from the European Association for Palliative Care (EAPC) suggest that PN should be considered only for a small subset of patients with a good performance status who may die of starvation rather than of their cancer. A retrospective review from one center (152) in the United States found that benefits of HPN were confined to a small subset of patients with slow-growing tumors (e.g., carcinoid). Practical guidelines (153) regarding the use of PN are fairly consistent and include the following: PN should be considered if the expected survival of the patient is >3 months and enteral feeding is impossible. Patients must be aware of their diagnosis, desire PN, spend >50% of the time out of bed, and be able to manage intravenous infusions. Patients and family members must be made aware of the potential complications (154) such as sepsis and thrombosis of catheters. As always, the evaluation and treatment of each patient should be individualized, weighing the benefits against potential harm. In addition to the difficult clinical decisions regarding PN, there are reimbursement issues to consider in the United States when a patient is transferred to hospice care. PN might not be covered by health insurance, thereby hindering appropriate transition to hospice care.

Multimodal Interventions

Past efforts to treat cachexia with nutritional or medical interventions may have failed because they focused on a single domain of the syndrome, such as anorexia or muscle wasting, usually with a single therapeutic agent. A more effective approach might be comprehensive multifaceted therapy targeting different pathophysiologic mechanisms simultaneously. One of the earliest trials demonstrating feasibility and efficacy (72) found a combination of multiple therapeutic agents (medroxyprogesterone [500 mg/d] or MA [320 mg/d], EPA, L-carnitine, and thalidomide) was superior to any single arm. Patients had improved appetite, performance status, spontaneous physical activity, and lean body mass. More recently, a phase II multimodal study of exercise, nutrition, and anti-inflammatory treatment for cachexia demonstrated feasibility and safety in patients receiving chemotherapy for incurable lung or pancreatic cancer. The follow-up phase III MENAC intervention is a multimodal, multisite trial (155) comprising ibuprofen (1,200 mg/d), omega-3 fatty acids (2 g EPA and 1 g DHA), ONS contributing 542 kcal and 30 g of protein, and a home-based exercise program consisting of resistance training 3 times/week in addition to aerobic training 2 times/week. Because patients in the early phase of cachexia are more likely to respond, the therapies are given alongside chemotherapy and concomitant symptom management.

A theoretical model of multimodal therapy for cachexia is shown in Figure 10.2. The choice of specific pharmacological agents has varied based on mechanistic considerations or on prior promising single intervention or multimodal trials. Despite the variations in therapy composition, most multimodal regimens share a common purpose in modulating the major mechanisms causing cachexia, identifying patients early in the illness trajectory, and including supportive care measures such as symptom management, exercise, and nutritional counseling/supplementation. Depending on patient goals, the treatment should target the individual's pathophysiology, since the contribution by the different mechanisms of cachexia to an individual's weight loss may vary. In addition, clinical and biologic markers are needed to better identify individuals who may respond to specific interventions so that effective individualized therapeutic regimens can be initiated earlier and with fewer unnecessary side effects (156).

In summary, the evidence for individual pharmacologic interventions (see Table 10.3) remains inconsistent, and ASCO guidelines for cachexia (157) state that no single agent can be recommended as standard of care. Symptom management, nutritional counseling, and exercise when feasible should be the foundation of any multimodal treatment of cancer cachexia. Megestrol and corticosteroids have a beneficial effect on appetite, while thalidomide and NSAIDs have demonstrated improvements in outcomes such as lean body mass and function. Other investigational agents, including anamorelin and monoclonal antibodies targeting cytokines, show most promise in human studies.

CACHEXIA AT THE END OF LIFE

Family members providing care are concerned about nutrition and may perceive the loss of appetite by a loved one as the most burdensome issue at the end of life (158), often more so than pain. For the family, food and eating may be symbolic of nurturing and compassion as well as "not letting go" (159). Although families place high importance on patients' ability to eat and maintain weight, this aspect of care is sometimes neglected by health care providers. A multicenter Japanese study of 702 bereaved family members found high levels of eating-related distress and a need for education and support. About half of family members were distressed, and 1 in 10 felt it was "useless" to consult medical staff about a daily diet (160). Physicians and nurses may not wish to engage in a lengthy discussion about poor appetite and weight loss because of the belief that this is an inevitable outcome of the cancer and no effective therapeutic options are available. Unfortunately, the consequences of avoiding this dialogue could include resentment on the part of families, who might perceive that important aspects of patient care have been neglected. Families in turn may feel frustrated by their failure to increase a patient's oral intake despite the best of efforts. They could also inadvertently worsen symptoms such as early satiety, nausea, abdominal distention, and pain by pressurizing patients to increase their oral intake. Families need to understand that providing more calories or improving oral intake will not reverse cachexia toward the end of life and may in fact cause unnecessary gastrointestinal distress due to bloating, cramping, and nausea. Having to explain this difficult, counterintuitive concept may pose a challenge for many health care providers. Usually, an empathic and straightforward explanation of the widespread, overwhelming nature of the cancer and its effect on muscle and appetite will allay concerns of starvation and reassure families that useful therapy is not being withheld. The body's inability to utilize protein and calories, coupled with the continued breakdown of muscle and fat by tumor products and inflammatory factors, needs to be explained without medical jargon. It helps to remind families that a loved one is not suffering because their calorie intake has declined and that patients almost universally report no hunger at the end of life. To the contrary, aggressive oral feeding as well as tube feeds may exacerbate distressing symptoms such as nausea and increase the risk of aspiration pneumonia.

REFERENCES

1. Fearon K, Strasser F, Anker SD, et al. Definition and classification of cancer cachexia: an international consensus. *Lancet Oncol.* 2011;12(5):489-495.
2. Turner DC, Kondic AG, Anderson KM, et al. Pembrolizumab exposure-response assessments challenged by association of cancer cachexia and catabolic clearance. *Clin Cancer Res.* 2018;24(23):5841-5849.
3. Bachmann J, Heiligensetzer M, Krakowski-Roosen H, Büchler MW, Friess H, Martignoni ME. Cachexia worsens prognosis in patients with resectable pancreatic cancer. *J Gastrointest Surg.* 2008;12(7):1193-1201.
4. Davis M, Lasheen W, Walsh D, Mahmoud F, Bicanovsky L, Lagman R. A phase II dose titration study of thalidomide for cancer-associated anorexia. *J Pain Symptom Manage.* 2012;43(1):78-86.
5. Chochinov HM, Hack T, Hassard T, Kristjanson LJ, McClement S, Harlos M. Dignity in the terminally ill: a cross-sectional, cohort study. *Lancet.* 2002; 360(9350):2026-2030.
6. Schneider SM, Correia MITD. Epidemiology of weight loss, malnutrition and sarcopenia: a transatlantic view. *Nutrition.* 2020;69:110581.
7. Inagaki J, Rodriguez V, Bodey GP. Proceedings: Causes of death in cancer patients. *Cancer.* 1974;33(2): 568-573.
8. Dewys WD, Begg C, Lavin PT, et al. Prognostic effect of weight loss prior to chemotherapy in cancer patients. Eastern Cooperative Oncology Group. *Am J Med.* 1980;69(4): 491-497.
9. Bozzetti F, Migliavacca S, Scotti A, et al. Impact of cancer, type, site, stage and treatment on the nutritional status of patients. *Ann Surg.* 1982;196(2):170-179.
10. Hauser CA, Stockler MR, Tattersall MH. Prognostic factors in patients with recently diagnosed incurable cancer: a systematic review. *Support Care Cancer.* 2006; 14(10):999-1011.
11. Andreyev HJ, Norman AR, Oates J, Cunningham D. Why do patients with weight loss have a worse outcome when undergoing chemotherapy for gastrointestinal malignancies?. *Eur J Cancer.* 1998;34(4):503-509.
12. Ross PJ, Ashley S, Norton A, et al. Do patients with weight loss have a worse outcome when undergoing chemotherapy for lung cancers? *Br J Cancer.* 2004;90(10): 1905-1911.
13. Hui D, Paiva CE, Del Fabbro EG, et al. Prognostication in advanced cancer: update and directions for future research. *Support Care Cancer.* 2019;27(6):1973-1984.
14. Kandarian SC, Nosacka RL, Delitto AE, et al. Tumour-derived leukaemia inhibitory factor is a major driver of cancer cachexia and morbidity in C26 tumour-bearing mice. *J Cachexia Sarcopenia Muscle.* 2018;9(6):1109-1120.
15. Braun TP, Marks DL. Pathophysiology and treatment of inflammatory anorexia in chronic disease. *J Cachexia Sarcopenia Muscle.* 2010;1(2):135-145.
16. Acharyya S, Ladner KJ, Nelsen LL, et al. Cancer cachexia is regulated by selective targeting of skeletal muscle gene products. *J Clin Invest.* 2004;114(3):370-378.
17. Chamberlain JS. Cachexia in cancer--zeroing in on myosin. *N Engl J Med.* 2004;351(20):2124-2125.
18. Sin TK, Zhang G, Zhang Z, Gao S, Li M, Li YP. Cancer takes a toll on skeletal muscle by releasing heat shock proteins—an emerging mechanism of cancer-induced cachexia. *Cancers (Basel).* 2019;11(9):1272.
19. Das SK, Eder S, Schauer S, et al. Adipose triglyceride lipase contributes to cancer-associated cachexia [published correction appears in *Science.* 2011 Sep 16;333(6049):1576]. *Science.* 2011;333(6039):233-238.
20. Han J, Meng Q, Shen L, Wu G. Interleukin-6 induces fat loss in cancer cachexia by promoting white adipose tissue lipolysis and browning. *Lipids Health Dis.* 2018;17(1):14. doi: 10.1186/s12944-018-0657-0.
21. Kir S, White JP, Kleiner S, Kazak L, Cohen P, Baracos VE, Spiegelman BM. Tumour-derived PTH-related protein triggers adipose tissue browning and cancer cachexia. *Nature.* 2014;513(7516):100-104.
22. Weyermann P, Dallmann R, Magyar J, et al. Orally available selective melanocortin-4 receptor antagonists stimulate food intake and reduce cancer-induced cachexia in mice. *PLoS One.* 2009;4(3):e4774.
23. Lutgendorf SK, Weinrib AZ, Penedo F, et al. Interleukin-6, cortisol, and depressive symptoms in ovarian cancer patients. *J Clin Oncol.* 2008;26(29):4820-4827.
24. Pfitzenmaier J, Vessella R, Higano CS, Noteboom JL, Wallace D Jr, Corey E. Elevation of cytokine levels in cachectic patients with prostate carcinoma. *Cancer.* 2003; 97(5):1211-1216.
25. Fortunati N, Manti R, Birocco N, et al. Pro-inflammatory cytokines and oxidative stress/antioxidant parameters characterize the bio-humoral profile of early cachexia in lung cancer patients. *Oncol Rep.* 2007;18(6):1521-1527.
26. Ebrahimi B, Tucker SL, Li D, Abbruzzese JL, Kurzrock R. Cytokines in pancreatic carcinoma: correlation with phenotypic characteristics and prognosis. *Cancer.* 2004;101(12):2727-2736.

27. Martín F, Santolaria F, Batista N, et al. Cytokine levels (IL-6 and IFN-gamma), acute phase response and nutritional status as prognostic factors in lung cancer. *Cytokine.* 1999;11(1):80-86.

28. Maltoni M, Fabbri L, Nanni O, et al. Serum levels of tumour necrosis factor alpha and other cytokines do not correlate with weight loss and anorexia in cancer patients. *Support Care Cancer.* 1997;5(2):130-135.

29. Ramsey ML, Talbert E, Ahn D, et al. Circulating interleukin-6 is associated with disease progression, but not cachexia in pancreatic cancer. *Pancreatology.* 2019;19(1): 80-87.

30. Shibata M, Nezu T, Kanou H, Abe H, Takekawa M, Fukuzawa M. Decreased production of interleukin-12 and type 2 immune responses are marked in cachectic patients with colorectal and gastric cancer. *J Clin Gastroenterol.* 2002;34(4):416-420.

31. Garcia JM, Garcia-Touza M, Hijazi RA, et al. Active ghrelin levels and active to total ghrelin ratio in cancer-induced cachexia. *J Clin Endocrinol Metab.* 2005;90(5):2920-2926.

32. Johns N, Stretch C, Tan BH, et al. New genetic signatures associated with cancer cachexia as defined by low skeletal muscle index and weight loss. *J Cachexia Sarcopenia Muscle.* 2017;8(1):122-130.

33. Fadul N, Strasser F, Palmer JL, et al. The association between autonomic dysfunction and survival in male patients with advanced cancer: a preliminary report. *J Pain Symptom Manage.* 2010;39(2):283-290.

34. Straub RH, Cutolo M, Buttgereit F, Pongratz G. Energy regulation and neuroendocrine-immune control in chronic inflammatory diseases. *J Intern Med.* 2010;267(6):543-560.

35. Lundholm K, Gelin J, Hyltander A, et al. Anti-inflammatory treatment may prolong survival in undernourished patients with metastatic solid tumors. *Cancer Res.* 1994;54(21):5602-5606.

36. Shrestha YB, Wickwire K, Giraudo SQ. Direct effects of nutrients, acetylcholine, CCK, and insulin on ghrelin release from the isolated stomachs of rats. *Peptides.* 2009;30(6):1187-1191.

37. Rosas-Ballina M, Tracey KJ. Cholinergic control of inflammation. *J Intern Med.* 2009;265(6):663-679.

38. Cruz-Jentoft AJ, Bahat G, Bauer J, et al. Sarcopenia: revised European consensus on definition and diagnosis [published correction appears in *Age Ageing.* 2019 Jul 1;48(4):601]. *Age Ageing.* 2019;48(1):16-31.

39. Mintziras I, Miligkos M, Wächter S, Manoharan J, Maurer E, Bartsch DK. Sarcopenia and sarcopenic obesity are significantly associated with poorer overall survival in patients with pancreatic cancer: systematic review and meta-analysis. *Int J Surg.* 2018;59:19-26.

40. Del Fabbro E, Hui D, Dalal S, Dev R, Nooruddin ZI, Bruera E. Clinical outcomes and contributors to weight loss in a cancer cachexia clinic (published correction appears in *J Palliat Med.* 2011 Dec;14(12):1361. Noorhuddin, Zohra [corrected to Nooruddin, Zohra I]). *J Palliat Med.* 2011;14(9):1004-1008.

41. Sarhill N, Mahmoud F, Walsh D, et al. Evaluation of nutritional status in advanced metastatic cancer. *Support Care Cancer.* 2003;11(10):652-659.

42. Palmer JL. Analysis of missing data in palliative care studies. *J Pain Symptom Manage.* 2004;28(6):612-618.

43. Martin L, Senesse P, Gioulbasanis I, et al. Diagnostic criteria for the classification of cancer-associated weight loss [published correction appears in *J Clin Oncol.* 2015 Mar 1;33(7):814]. *J Clin Oncol.* 2015;33(1):90-99.

44. Daly L, Dolan R, Power D, et al. The relationship between the BMI-adjusted weight loss grading system

and quality of life in patients with incurable cancer. *J Cachexia Sarcopenia Muscle.* 2020;11(1):160-168.

45. Bauer J, Capra S, Ferguson M. Use of the scored Patient-Generated Subjective Global Assessment (PG-SGA) as a nutrition assessment tool in patients with cancer. *Eur J Clin Nutr.* 2002;56(8):779-785.

46. Farhangfar A, Makarewicz M, Ghosh S, et al. Nutrition impact symptoms in a population cohort of head and neck cancer patients: multivariate regression analysis of symptoms on oral intake, weight loss and survival. *Oral Oncol.* 2014;50(9):877-883.

47. Ediebah DE, Quinten C, Coens C, et al. Quality of life as a prognostic indicator of survival: a pooled analysis of individual patient data from canadian cancer trials group clinical trials. *Cancer.* 2018;124(16):3409-3416.

48. Prado CM, Lieffers JR, McCargar LJ, et al. Prevalence and clinical implications of sarcopenic obesity in patients with solid tumours of the respiratory and gastrointestinal tracts: a population-based study. *Lancet Oncol.* 2008;9(7):629-635.

49. Pamoukdjian F, Bouillet T, Lévy V, Soussan M, Zelek L, Paillaud E. Prevalence and predictive value of pretherapeutic sarcopenia in cancer patients: a systematic review. *Clin Nutr.* 2018;37(4):1101-1113.

50. da Silva JR Jr, Wiegert EVM, Oliveira L, Calixto-Lima L. Different methods for diagnosis of sarcopenia and its association with nutritional status and survival in patients with advanced cancer in palliative care. *Nutrition.* 2019;60:48-52.

51. Nijholt W, Scafoglieri A, Jager-Wittenaar H, Hobbelen JSM, van der Schans CP. The reliability and validity of ultrasound to quantify muscles in older adults: a systematic review. *J Cachexia Sarcopenia Muscle.* 2017;8(5):702-712.

52. Crawford GB, Robinson JA, Hunt RW, Piller NB, Esterman A. Estimating survival in patients with cancer receiving palliative care: is analysis of body composition using bioimpedance helpful? *J Palliat Med.* 2009;12(11):1009-1014.

53. Prado CM, Birdsell LA, Baracos VE. The emerging role of computerized tomography in assessing cancer cachexia. *Curr Opin Support Palliat Care.* 2009;3(4):269-275.

54. Heymsfield SB, Adamek M, Gonzalez MC, Jia G, Thomas DM. Assessing skeletal muscle mass: historical overview and state of the art. *J Cachexia Sarcopenia Muscle.* 2014;5(1):9-18.

55. Cespedes Feliciano EM, Popuri K, Cobzas D, et al. Evaluation of automated computed tomography segmentation to assess body composition and mortality associations in cancer patients. *J Cachexia Sarcopenia Muscle.* 2020. doi: 10.1002/jcsm.12573.

56. Dev R, Hui D, Chisholm G, et al. Hypermetabolism and symptom burden in advanced cancer patients evaluated in a cachexia clinic. *J Cachexia Sarcopenia Muscle.* 2015;6(1):95-98.

57. Purcell SA, Elliott SA, Ryan AM, Sawyer MB, Prado CM. Accuracy of a portable indirect calorimeter for measuring resting energy expenditure in individuals with cancer. *JPEN J Parenter Enteral Nutr.* 2019;43(1):145-151.

58. Chen S, Wohlers E, Ruud E, Moon J, Ni B, Celi FS. Improving temporal accuracy of human metabolic chambers for dynamic metabolic studies. *PLoS One.* 2018;13(4):e0193467.

59. Hyltander A, Daneryd P, Sandström R, Körner U, Lundholm K. Beta-adrenoceptor activity and resting energy metabolism in weight losing cancer patients. *Eur J Cancer.* 2000;36(3):330-334. doi: 10.1016/s0959-8049(99)00273-7.

60. Reeves MM, Capra S. Predicting energy requirements in the clinical setting: are current methods evidence based?. *Nutr Rev.* 2003;61(4):143-151. doi: 10.1301/nr.2003.apr.143-151.

61. Reeves MM, Battistutta D, Capra S, Bauer J, Davies PS. Resting energy expenditure in patients with solid tumors undergoing anticancer therapy. *Nutrition.* 2006;22(6):609-615.

62. Dev R, Del Fabbro E, Schwartz GG, et al. Preliminary report: vitamin D deficiency in advanced cancer patients with symptoms of fatigue or anorexia. *Oncologist.* 2011;16(11):1637-1641.

63. Hong N, Yoon HJ, Lee YH, et al. Serum PTHrP predicts weight loss in cancer patients independent of hypercalcemia, inflammation, and tumor burden. *J Clin Endocrinol Metab.* 2016;101(3):1207-1214.

64. Golan T, Geva R, Richards D, et al. LY2495655, an antimyostatin antibody, in pancreatic cancer: a randomized, phase 2 trial. *J Cachexia Sarcopenia Muscle.* 2018;9(5):871-879.

65. Yennurajalingam S, Frisbee-Hume S, Palmer JL, et al. Reduction of cancer-related fatigue with dexamethasone: a double-blind, randomized, placebo-controlled trial in patients with advanced cancer. *J Clin Oncol.* 2013;31(25):3076-3082.

66. Temel JS, Abernethy AP, Currow DC, et al. Anamorelin in patients with non-small-cell lung cancer and cachexia (ROMANA 1 and ROMANA 2): results from two randomised, double-blind, phase 3 trials. *Lancet Oncol.* 2016;17(4):519-531.

67. Katakami N, Uchino J, Yokoyama T, et al. Anamorelin (ONO-7643) for the treatment of patients with non-small cell lung cancer and cachexia: results from a randomized, double-blind, placebo-controlled, multicenter study of Japanese patients (ONO-7643-04). *Cancer.* 2018;124(3):606-616.

68. Hamauchi S, Furuse J, Takano T, et al. A multicenter, open-label, single-arm study of anamorelin (ONO-7643) in advanced gastrointestinal cancer patients with cancer cachexia. *Cancer.* 2019;125(23):4294-4302.

69. Stewart Coats AJ, Ho GF, Prabhash K, et al. Espindolol for the treatment and prevention of cachexia in patients with stage III/IV non-small cell lung cancer or colorectal cancer: a randomized, double-blind, placebo-controlled, international multicentre phase II study (the ACT-ONE trial). *J Cachexia Sarcopenia Muscle.* 2016;7(3):355-365.

70. Wright TJ, Dillon EL, Durham WJ, et al. A randomized trial of adjunct testosterone for cancer-related muscle loss in men and women. *J Cachexia Sarcopenia Muscle.* 2018;9(3):482-496.

71. Del Fabbro E, Garcia JM, Dev R, et al. Testosterone replacement for fatigue in hypogonadal ambulatory males with advanced cancer: a preliminary double-blind placebo-controlled trial. *Support Care Cancer.* 2013;21(9):2599-2607.

72. Mantovani G, Macciò A, Madeddu C, et al. Randomized phase III clinical trial of five different arms of treatment in 332 patients with cancer cachexia. *Oncologist.* 2010;15(2):200-211.

73. Gordon JN, Trebble TM, Ellis RD, Duncan HD, Johns T, Goggin PM. Thalidomide in the treatment of cancer cachexia: a randomised placebo controlled trial. *Gut.* 2005;54(4):540-545.

74. Bruera E, Neumann CM, Pituskin E, Calder K, Ball G, Hanson J. Thalidomide in patients with cachexia due to terminal cancer: preliminary report. *Ann Oncol.* 1999;10(7):857-859.

75. Del Fabbro E, Dev R, Hui D, Palmer L, Bruera E. Effects of melatonin on appetite and other symptoms in patients with advanced cancer and cachexia: a double-blind placebo-controlled trial. *J Clin Oncol.* 2013;31(10):1271-1276.

76. Lissoni P, Paolorossi F, Tancini G, et al. Is there a role for melatonin in the treatment of neoplastic cachexia?. *Eur J Cancer.* 1996;32A(8):1340-1343.

77. Murphy RA, Mourtzakis M, Chu QS, Baracos VE, Reiman T, Mazurak VC. Nutritional intervention with fish oil provides a benefit over standard of care for weight and skeletal muscle mass in patients with non-small cell lung cancer receiving chemotherapy. *Cancer.* 2011;117(8):1775-1782.

78. Ries A, Trottenberg P, Elsner F, et al. A systematic review on the role of fish oil for the treatment of cachexia in advanced cancer: an EPCRC cachexia guidelines project. *Palliat Med.* 2012;26(4):294-304.

79. Dewey A, Baughan C, Dean T, Higgins B, Johnson I. Eicosapentaenoic acid (EPA, an omega-3 fatty acid from fish oils) for the treatment of cancer cachexia. *Cochrane Database Syst Rev.* 2007;2007(1):CD004597.

80. Burns CP, Halabi S, Clamon G, et al. Phase II study of high-dose fish oil capsules for patients with cancer-related cachexia. *Cancer.* 2004;101(2):370-378.

81. Lai V, George J, Richey L, et al. Results of a pilot study of the effects of celecoxib on cancer cachexia in patients with cancer of the head, neck, and gastrointestinal tract. *Head Neck.* 2008;30(1):67-74.

82. Mantovani G, Macciò A, Madeddu C, et al. A phase II study with antioxidants, both in the diet and supplemented, pharmaconutritional support, progestagen, and anti-cyclooxygenase-2 showing efficacy and safety in patients with cancer-related anorexia/cachexia and oxidative stress. *Cancer Epidemiol Biomarkers Prev.* 2006;15(5):1030-1034.

83. Cerchietti LC, Navigante AH, Peluffo GD, et al. Effects of celecoxib, medroxyprogesterone, and dietary intervention on systemic syndromes in patients with advanced lung adenocarcinoma: a pilot study. *J Pain Symptom Manage.* 2004;27(1):85-95.

84. McMillan DC, Wigmore SJ, Fearon KC, O'Gorman P, Wright CE, McArdle CS. A prospective randomized study of megestrol acetate and ibuprofen in gastrointestinal cancer patients with weight loss. *Br J Cancer.* 1999;79(3-4):495-500.

85. Ruiz-García V, López-Briz E, Carbonell-Sanchis R, Bort-Martí S, Gonzálvez-Perales JL. Megestrol acetate for cachexia-anorexia syndrome. A systematic review. *J Cachexia Sarcopenia Muscle.* 2018;9(3):444-452.

86. Loprinzi CL, Kugler JW, Sloan JA, et al. Randomized comparison of megestrol acetate versus dexamethasone versus fluoxymesterone for the treatment of cancer anorexia/cachexia. *J Clin Oncol.* 1999;17(10):3299-3306.

87. Cannabis-In-Cachexia-Study-Group; Strasser F, Luftner D, et al. Comparison of orally administered cannabis extract and delta-9-tetrahydrocannabinol in treating patients with cancer-related anorexia-cachexia syndrome: a multicenter, phase III, randomized, double-blind, placebo-controlled clinical trial from the Cannabis-In-Cachexia-Study-Group. *J Clin Oncol.* 2006;24(21):3394-3400.

88. Jatoi A, Windschitl HE, Loprinzi CL, et al. Dronabinol versus megestrol acetate versus combination therapy for cancer-associated anorexia: a North Central Cancer Treatment Group study. *J Clin Oncol.* 2002;20(2):567-573.

89. Del Fabbro E, Orr TA, Stella SM. Practical approaches to managing cancer patients with weight loss. *Curr Opin Support Palliat Care.* 2017;11(4):272-277.

90. Del Fabbro E. More is better: a multimodality approach to cancer cachexia. *Oncologist.* 2010;15(2):119-121.

91. Shivshanker K, Bennett RW Jr, Haynie TP. Tumor-associated gastroparesis: correction with metoclopramide. *Am J Surg.* 1983;145(2):221-225.

92. Walsh D, Davis M, Ripamonti C, Bruera E, Davies A, Molassiotis A. 2016 Updated MASCC/ESMO consensus recommendations: management of nausea and vomiting in advanced cancer. *Support Care Cancer.* 2017;25(1):333-340.

93. Navari RM. Nausea and vomiting in advanced cancer. *Curr Treat Options Oncol.* 2020;21(2):14.

94. Kast RE, Foley KF. Cancer chemotherapy and cachexia: mirtazapine and olanzapine are 5-HT3 antagonists with good antinausea effects. *Eur J Cancer Care (Engl).* 2007;16(4):351-354.

95. Kim SW, Shin IS, Kim JM, et al. Mirtazapine for severe gastroparesis unresponsive to conventional prokinetic treatment. *Psychosomatics.* 2006;47(5):440-442.

96. Okamoto H, Shono K, Nozaki-Taguchi N. Low-dose of olanzapine has ameliorating effects on cancer-related anorexia. *Cancer Manage Res.* 2019;11:2233-2239.

97. Suzuki H, Asakawa A, Li JB, et al. Zinc as an appetite stimulator—the possible role of zinc in the progression of diseases such as cachexia and sarcopenia. *Recent Pat Food Nutr Agric.* 2011;3(3):226-231.

98. Ripamonti C, Zecca E, Brunelli C, et al. A randomized, controlled clinical trial to evaluate the effects of zinc sulfate on cancer patients with taste alterations caused by head and neck irradiation. *Cancer.* 1998;82(10):1938-1945.

99. Halyard MY, Jatoi A, Sloan JA, et al. Does zinc sulfate prevent therapy-induced taste alterations in head and neck cancer patients? Results of phase III double-blind, placebo-controlled trial from the North Central Cancer Treatment Group (N01C4). *Int J Radiat Oncol Biol Phys.* 2007;67(5):1318-1322.

100. Jatoi A, Rowland K, Loprinzi CL, et al. An eicosapentaenoic acid supplement versus megestrol acetate versus both for patients with cancer-associated wasting: a North Central Cancer Treatment Group and National Cancer Institute of Canada collaborative effort. *J Clin Oncol.* 2004;22(12):2469-2476.

101. Paulsen O, Klepstad P, Rosland JH, et al. Efficacy of methylprednisolone on pain, fatigue, and appetite loss in patients with advanced cancer using opioids: a randomized, placebo-controlled, double-blind trial. *J Clin Oncol.* 2014;32(29):3221-3228.

102. Brisbois TD, de Kock IH, Watanabe SM, et al. Delta-9-tetrahydrocannabinol may palliate altered chemosensory perception in cancer patients: results of a randomized, double-blind, placebo-controlled pilot trial. *Ann Oncol.* 2011;22(9):2086-2093.

103. Mücke M, Weier M, Carter C, et al. Systematic review and meta-analysis of cannabinoids in palliative medicine. *J Cachexia Sarcopenia Muscle.* 2018;9(2):220-234.

104. Trikha M, Corringham R, Klein B, Rossi JF. Targeted anti-interleukin-6 monoclonal antibody therapy for cancer: a review of the rationale and clinical evidence. *Clin Cancer Res.* 2003;9(13):4653-4665.

105. Johnston AJ, Murphy KT, Jenkinson L, et al. Targeting of Fn14 prevents cancer-induced cachexia and prolongs survival. *Cell.* 2015;162(6):1365-1378.

106. Lerner L, Hayes TG, Tao N, et al. Plasma growth differentiation factor 15 is associated with weight loss and mortality in cancer patients. *J Cachexia Sarcopenia Muscle.* 2015;6(4):317-324.

107. Wiedenmann B, Malfertheiner P, Friess H, et al. A multicenter, phase II study of infliximab plus gemcitabine in pancreatic cancer cachexia. *J Support Oncol.* 2008;6(1):18-25.

108. Jatoi A, Dakhil SR, Nguyen PL, et al. A placebo-controlled double blind trial of etanercept for the cancer anorexia/weight loss syndrome: results from N00C1 from the North Central Cancer Treatment Group. *Cancer.* 2007;110(6):1396-1403.

109. Solheim TS, Fearon KC, Blum D, Kaasa S. Non-steroidal anti-inflammatory treatment in cancer cachexia: a systematic literature review. *Acta Oncol.* 2013; 52(1):6-17.

110. Reid J, Mills M, Cantwell M, Cardwell CR, Murray LJ, Donnelly M. Thalidomide for managing cancer cachexia. *Cochrane Database Syst Rev.* 2012;2012(4): CD008664.

111. Khan ZH, Simpson EJ, Cole AT, et al. Oesophageal cancer and cachexia: the effect of short-term treatment with thalidomide on weight loss and lean body mass. *Aliment Pharmacol Ther.* 2003;17(5):677-682.

112. Wilkes EA, Selby AL, Cole AT, Freeman JG, Rennie MJ, Khan ZH. Poor tolerability of thalidomide in end-stage oesophageal cancer. *Eur J Cancer Care (Engl).* 2011;20(5):593-600.

113. Najafi M, Hooshangi Shayesteh MR, Mortezaee K, Farhood B, Haghi-Aminjan H. The role of melatonin on doxorubicin-induced cardiotoxicity: a systematic review. *Life Sci.* 2020;241:117173.

114. Wang Y, Wang P, Zheng X, Du X. Therapeutic strategies of melatonin in cancer patients: a systematic review and meta-analysis. *Onco Targets Ther.* 2018;11: 7895-7908.

115. Roynette CE, Calder PC, Dupertuis YM, Pichard C. n-3 polyunsaturated fatty acids and colon cancer prevention. *Clin Nutr.* 2004;23(2):139-151.

116. Hall MN, Chavarro JE, Lee IM, Willett WC, Ma J. A 22-year prospective study of fish, n-3 fatty acid intake, and colorectal cancer risk in men [published correction appears in *Cancer Epidemiol Biomarkers Prev.* 2008 Oct;17(10):2901]. *Cancer Epidemiol Biomarkers Prev.* 2008;17(5):1136-1143.

117. Moses AW, Slater C, Preston T, Barber MD, Fearon KC. Reduced total energy expenditure and physical activity in cachectic patients with pancreatic cancer can be modulated by an energy and protein dense oral supplement enriched with n-3 fatty acids. *Br J Cancer.* 2004;90(5): 996-1002.

118. Bruera E, Strasser F, Palmer JL, et al. Effect of fish oil on appetite and other symptoms in patients with advanced cancer and anorexia/cachexia: a double-blind, placebo-controlled study. *J Clin Oncol.* 2003;21(1):129-134.

119. de van der Schueren MAE, Laviano A, Blanchard H, Jourdan M, Arends J, Baracos VE. Systematic review and meta-analysis of the evidence for oral nutritional intervention on nutritional and clinical outcomes during chemo(radio)therapy: current evidence and guidance for design of future trials. *Ann Oncol.* 2018;29(5):1141-1153.

120. Lundholm K, Körner U, Gunnebo L, et al. Insulin treatment in cancer cachexia: effects on survival, metabolism, and physical functioning. *Clin Cancer Res.* 2007;13(9):2699-2706.

121. Garcia JM, Li H, Mann D, et al. Hypogonadism in male patients with cancer. *Cancer.* 2006;106(12):2583-2591.

122. Dev R, Hui D, Dalal S, et al. Association between serum cortisol and testosterone levels, opioid therapy, and symptom distress in patients with advanced cancer. *J Pain Symptom Manage.* 2011;41(4):788-795.

123. Burney BO, Hayes TG, Smiechowska J, et al. Low testosterone levels and increased inflammatory markers in patients with cancer and relationship with cachexia. *J Clin Endocrinol Metab*. 2012;97(5):E700-E709.

124. Bhasin S, Brito JP, Cunningham GR, et al. Testosterone therapy in men with hypogonadism: an endocrine society clinical practice guideline. *J Clin Endocrinol Metab*. 2018;103(5):1715-1744.

125. Miah S, Tharakan T, Gallagher KA, et al. The effects of testosterone replacement therapy on the prostate: a clinical perspective. *F1000Res*. 2019;8:F1000 Faculty Rev-217.

126. Pigneux A, Béné MC, Guardiola P, et al. Addition of androgens improves survival in elderly patients with acute myeloid leukemia: a GOELAMS study. *J Clin Oncol*. 2017;35(4):387-393.

127. Dalton JT, Barnette KG, Bohl CE, et al. The selective androgen receptor modulator GTx-024 (enobosarm) improves lean body mass and physical function in healthy elderly men and postmenopausal women: results of a double-blind, placebo-controlled phase II trial. *J Cachexia Sarcopenia Muscle*. 2011;2(3):153-161.

128. Dobs AS, Boccia RV, Croot CC, et al. Effects of enobosarm on muscle wasting and physical function in patients with cancer: a double-blind, randomised controlled phase 2 trial. *Lancet Oncol*. 2013;14(4):335-345.

129. Lainscak M, Keber I, Anker SD. Body composition changes in patients with systolic heart failure treated with beta blockers: a pilot study. *Int J Cardiol*. 2006;106(3):319-322.

130. Herndon DN, Hart DW, Wolf SE, Chinkes DL, Wolfe RR. Reversal of catabolism by beta-blockade after severe burns. *N Engl J Med*. 2001;345(17):1223-1229.

131. Grande AJ, Silva V, Riera R, et al. Exercise for cancer cachexia in adults. *Cochrane Database Syst Rev*. 2014;(11):CD010804.

132. Bacurau AV, Belmonte MA, Navarro F, et al. Effect of a high-intensity exercise training on the metabolism and function of macrophages and lymphocytes of walker 256 tumor bearing rats. *Exp Biol Med (Maywood)*. 2007;232(10):1289-1299. doi: 10.3181/0704-RM-93.

133. Lambert CP, Sullivan DH, Freeling SA, Lindquist DM, Evans WJ. Effects of testosterone replacement and/or resistance exercise on the composition of megestrol acetate stimulated weight gain in elderly men: a randomized controlled trial. *J Clin Endocrinol Metab*. 2002;87(5):2100-2106.

134. Grinspoon S, Corcoran C, Parlman K, et al. Effects of testosterone and progressive resistance training in eugonadal men with AIDS wasting. A randomized, controlled trial. *Ann Intern Med*. 2000;133(5):348-355.

135. Lewis MI, Fournier M, Storer TW, et al. Skeletal muscle adaptations to testosterone and resistance training in men with COPD. *J Appl Physiol (1985)*. 2007;103(4):1299-1310.

136. Nasrah R, Kanbalian M, Van Der Borch C, Swinton N, Wing S, Jagoe RT. Defining the role of dietary intake in determining weight change in patients with cancer cachexia. *Clin Nutr*. 2018;37(1):235-241.

137. Ravasco P, Monteiro Grillo I, Camilo M. Cancer wasting and quality of life react to early individualized nutritional counselling!. *Clin Nutr*. 2007;26(1):7-15.

138. Lee JLC, Leong LP, Lim SL. Nutrition intervention approaches to reduce malnutrition in oncology patients: a systematic review. *Support Care Cancer*. 2016;24(1):469-480.

139. Arends J, Bachmann P, Baracos V, et al. ESPEN guidelines on nutrition in cancer patients. *Clin Nutr*. 2017;36(1):11-48.

140. Prado CM, Purcell SA, Laviano A. Nutrition interventions to treat low muscle mass in cancer. *J Cachexia Sarcopenia Muscle*. 2020;11(2):366-380.

141. Laviano A, Molfino A, Seelaender M, et al. Carnitine administration reduces cytokine levels, improves food intake, and ameliorates body composition in tumor-bearing rats. *Cancer Invest*. 2011;29(10):696-700.

142. Ringseis R, Keller J, Eder K. Mechanisms underlying the anti-wasting effect of L-carnitine supplementation under pathologic conditions: evidence from experimental and clinical studies. *Eur J Nutr*. 2013;52(5):1421-1442.

143. Chow R, Bruera E, Arends J, et al. Enteral and parenteral nutrition in cancer patients, a comparison of complication rates: an updated systematic review and (cumulative) meta-analysis [published correction appears in *Support Care Cancer*. 2019 Dec 31]. *Support Care Cancer*. 2020;28(3):979-1010.

144. Bouleuc C, Anota A, Cornet C, et al. Impact on health-related quality of life of parenteral nutrition for patients with advanced cancer cachexia: results from a randomized controlled trial. *Oncologist*. 2020;25(5):e843-e851.

145. Klein S, Simes J, Blackburn GL. Total parenteral nutrition and cancer clinical trials. *Cancer*. 1986;58(6):1378-1386.

146. August DA, Huhmann MB; American Society for Parenteral and Enteral Nutrition (A.S.P.E.N.) Board of Directors. A.S.P.E.N. clinical guidelines: nutrition support therapy during adult anticancer treatment and in hematopoietic cell transplantation. *JPEN J Parenter Enteral Nutr*. 2009;33(5):472-500.

147. Tobberup R, Thoresen L, Falkmer UG, Yilmaz MK, Solheim TS, Balstad TR. Effects of current parenteral nutrition treatment on health-related quality of life, physical function, nutritional status, survival and adverse events exclusively in patients with advanced cancer: a systematic literature review. *Crit Rev Oncol Hematol*. 2019;139:96-107.

148. Orrevall Y, Tishelman C, Permert J. Home parenteral nutrition: a qualitative interview study of the experiences of advanced cancer patients and their families. *Clin Nutr*. 2005;24(6):961-970.

149. Orrevall Y, Tishelman C, Herrington MK, Permert J. The path from oral nutrition to home parenteral nutrition: a qualitative interview study of the experiences of advanced cancer patients and their families. *Clin Nutr*. 2004;23(6):1280-1287.

150. Strasser F. Eating-related disorders in patients with advanced cancer. *Support Care Cancer*. 2003;11(1):11-20.

151. Ripamonti C, Twycross R, Baines M, et al. Clinical-practice recommendations for the management of bowel obstruction in patients with end-stage cancer. *Support Care Cancer*. 2001;9(4):223-233.

152. Hoda D, Jatoi A, Burnes J, Loprinzi C, Kelly D. Should patients with advanced, incurable cancers ever be sent home with total parenteral nutrition? A single institution's 20-year experience. *Cancer*. 2005;103(4):863-868.

153. McKinlay AW. Nutritional support in patients with advanced cancer: permission to fall out? *Proc Nutr Soc*. 2004;63(3):431-435.

154. Mullady DK, O'Keefe SJ. Treatment of intestinal failure: home parenteral nutrition. *Nat Clin Pract Gastroenterol Hepatol*. 2006;3(9):492-504.

155. Solheim TS, Laird BJA, Balstad TR, et al. Cancer cachexia: rationale for the MENAC (Multimodal-Exercise, Nutrition and Anti-inflammatory medication for Cachexia) trial. *BMJ Support Palliat Care*. 2018;8(3):258-265.

156. Del Fabbro E. Combination therapy in cachexia. *Ann Palliat Med*. 2019;8(1):59-66.

157. Roeland EJ, Bohlke K, Baracos VE, et al. Management of cancer cachexia: ASCO Guideline. *J Clin Oncol.* 2020;JCO2000611.

158. Suarez-Almazor ME, Newman C, Hanson J, Bruera E. Attitudes of terminally ill cancer patients about euthanasia and assisted suicide: predominance of psychosocial determinants and beliefs over symptom distress and subsequent survival. *J Clin Oncol.* 2002;20(8):2134-2141.

159. van der Riet P, Good P, Higgins I, Sneesby L. Palliative care professionals' perceptions of nutrition and hydration at the end of life. *Int J Palliat Nurs.* 2008;14(3):145-151.

160. Amano K, Maeda I, Morita T, et al. Eating-related distress and need for nutritional support of families of advanced cancer patients: a nationwide survey of bereaved family members. *J Cachexia Sarcopenia Muscle.* 2016;7(5):527-534.

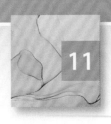

11 Swallowing and Speech Considerations in Palliative Care

Beth I. Solomon and Monique C. King

Many would agree that the ability to eat and communicate are essential to maintaining an individual's overall well-being. Impairments in these functions, can limit one's social, nutritional, cultural, and religious experiences. More often than not, these impairments are encountered with disease diagnosis, with disease progression, or in palliative care. No matter the diagnoses, assessment and management of swallowing and speech issues requires an individualistic approach as a "cook book" method does not address the challenges experienced by patients and families.

Speech–language pathology is a dynamic profession with distinct and valuable contributions to the care of individuals with life-limiting illness. With expertise in the areas of communication, cognition, and swallowing, speech–language pathologists (SLPs) are an indispensable resource for palliative care teams and the global pursuit of relief from suffering. In the pages to follow, this chapter will summarize the role of SLPs in the context of palliative care for adults—with a principal focus on assessment and management of dysphagia (swallowing dysfunction). Additionally, emphasis will be placed on the necessity of SLP collaboration with other fundamental disciplines in order to meet patient and family/caregiver needs while paying homage to the reality that "A good death honors a whole life" (1).

THE SLP PROFESSION

The profession of speech–language pathology is both versatile and complex. SLPs assist individuals at various stages throughout the life span— continually adapting intervention in accordance with changes in one's status. A speech pathologist's academic and clinical training provide the foundation to offer the assessment and treatment of disorders (both progressive and acquired) with an identified impact on one or more of the domains listed in Table 11.1.

REHABILITATION VERSUS PALLIATIVE CARE

As patients transition to palliative care, the focus of speech–language pathology services "is not rehabilitative, but facilitative" (2). Our primary focus shifts away from the goal of *regaining* a patient's prior level of function—a notion that has, at times, caused misunderstanding and disagreement. Frost (2001) maintained that "function is used in therapy to describe an individual's *ability to complete tasks necessary for survival* in the patient's day-to-day environment" with the goal of therapy being to "determine the patient's functional loss, estimate functional potential, and implement a plan to progress from the measured loss to a quantifiable potential" (3). Given that patients qualify for palliative care following the diagnosis of a serious illness without expectation of illness reversal/recovery, SLP services in palliative care aspire to support patients and their families in their changing circumstance. SLPs aim to manage existing symptoms while we "minimize associated complications and optimize quality of life" (4). While the traditional view of rehabilitation is impairment based and driven by a need to fix problems, palliative services are based on a social model contextualized to that which is meaningful to patients/families as they navigate life-limiting illness (5). This distinction in our role within palliative care is critical because it frames the expectations of our patients, their families, other medical disciplines within a treatment team, and our field at large.

As palliative care providers, SLPs seek to understand how each patient/family defines quality of life. Once the patient's priorities are clear, clinicians "can marshal resources to optimize the patient's time…[demonstrating] an openness to their patient's personal and sometime unique views of what they most value" (6). To be successful in the practice of following the patient's lead requires a true understanding that the patient and his/her family/loved ones have the most important voice throughout the palliative care journey. Additionally, SLPs develop comfort with the need to "respond positively and supportively when the patient or family chooses intervention that does not necessarily follow the 'SLP expert' advice prescription" (4). This adjustment in mindset follows SLP recognition of the "physical, social and psychological impact that having a communication or swallowing impairment can have on people with life-limiting conditions and their families" (7).

TABLE 11.1 OVERVIEW OF COMMON DOMAINS ASSESSED (AND TREATED) BY SLPs

Speech	Language	Cognition	Swallowing
Oral Motor/Function	Verbal Expression	Attention	Mentation
Respiratory Coordination	Written Expression	Cognitive Flexibility	Oral Motor/Function
Voice and Resonance	Auditory Comprehension	Memory	Oral Hygiene
Articulation	Reading Comprehension	Planning and Initiation	Dentition
Fluency and Prosody	Pragmatic Language	Problem Solving	Swallowing Phases (Oral Preparatory, Oral, Pharyngeal, Esophageal)

SLP VIEWS OF PALLIATIVE CARE PROVISION

In addressing a previous paucity of published literature outlining SLP-specific services within the hospice care model, Pollens (2004) presented four principal roles of SLPs involved in palliative care—using anecdotal examples from the author's prior experiences within a "home-care based hospice service" (8). Pollens described the roles as follows:

1. To provide consultation to patients, families, and members of the hospice team in the areas of communication, cognition, and swallowing function
2. To develop strategies in the area of communication skills in order to support the patient's role in decision making, to maintain social closeness, and to assist the patient in fulfillment of end-of-life goals
3. To assist in optimizing function related to dysphagia symptoms in order to improve patient comfort and eating satisfaction, and promote positive feeding interactions for family members
4. To communicate with members of the interdisciplinary hospice team, to provide and receive input related to overall patient care (8)

Just over than a decade later, O'Reilly and Walshe (2015) disseminated an open survey to SLPs in the Republic of Ireland, New Zealand, United Kingdom, United States, Canada, and Australia to obtain a preliminary understanding of clinicians' perceptions of their role in the delivery of palliative care. Despite almost two decades of involvement, the integration of SLPs in the palliative care process remains undefined and limited.

SPEECH AND SWALLOWING ETHICAL CONSIDERATIONS

SLPs encounter ethical dilemmas "when the attempts to balance the obligation to benefit the patient (*beneficence*) against the obligation to

minimize unnecessary harm (*no maleficence*) seem to conflict" (9). Sharp and Genesen (1996) explain that systematic resolution of such conflicts is based on four components—one of which is the significance of *patient preferences*—stating "Determining a patient's preferences is critical to good ethical decision-making, based on the principle that patients have the moral right to make decisions that affect their care" (9). Of note: the other three components are *medical indications, quality of life*, and *contextual factors*. In this chapter, particular emphasis is placed on the significance of patient preferences because of the respect for patient autonomy at all stages of health care and especially at end of life. SLPs in palliative care service "advise from their professional perspective of clinical expertise, but will respond positively and supportively when the patient or family chooses intervention that does not necessarily follow the 'SLP expert' advice prescription" (4). As clinicians, we recognize that the patient/family's ultimate decision is based on many factors including "to what level the patient accepts their disease, expectations of therapy and life priorities" (4). As medical professionals, we are obligated to accept a patient's refusal for assessment and treatment while maintaining patient safety.

PALLIATIVE CARE AND TEAMWORK

Palliative care embraces use of a team approach to enhance quality of life. In literature and in practice, highly functional teams are distinguished by their ability to optimize the skills of its members to effectively meet the complex needs of the whole person (10,11). This is especially true of palliative care for dysphagia, which Langmore et al. (2009) aptly described as necessitating "consultation, compassion, and collaborative decision making to help persons face end of life with dignity" (12). As clearly stated by Chin et al. (2019), "No single professional can fulfill all the roles required to care for patients receiving palliative care" (13).

A patient and his/her family/designee(s) are of chief importance to the development of any palliative care team—as the perspectives and wishes of these individuals will direct conversations regarding meaningful quality of life. As Crawford and Price (2003) explain, "In palliative care, the final decision-maker is the patient, and the patient uses many pieces of information, many sources of support, and their own values as a guide" (14). Core and ancillary team members then have a comparable and reciprocal role in structuring patient care and providing education to patients/families/designees(s) to inform their decision-making processes.

Before moving forward in this chapter, it is important to acknowledge ongoing discussions regarding the distinctiveness of the terms "multidisciplinary" and "interdisciplinary." Although often used interchangeably, Jessup (15) contends that multidisciplinary care consists of various disciplines each approaching a patient from a unique point of view in isolation of one another. From this perspective, a multidisciplinary team is analogous to wedges of a pie—with each provider having his/her own defined place on the team (14,16). By contrast, an interdisciplinary team incorporates "separate discipline approaches into a single consultation…often stepping outside of discipline silos to work toward the best outcome for the patient" (15). Interdisciplinary teams work interdependently to address each patient's individual needs (14). An interdisciplinary team is then comparable

to a hand, which is capable of achieving more than the sum of each individual finger (11,14,16).

Terminology preferences aside, comprehensive care occurs neither by chance nor singlehandedly. The combined effort of multiple disciplines recognizes "that the team's goals, which should be aligned with what is best for the patient, are more important than an [individual provider's] goals" (17). The success of a team requires effective, open communication to accomplish targeted goals. Furthermore, team members must migrate from "a parochial view of the world—my function, my values, and my goals are paramount—to a broader view that 'we're all in this together'" (11).

Medicare necessitates that all hospice organizations develop core services as well as ancillary services "as needed for the palliation or comfort care of terminal illness" (8). The ancillary services involved in palliative care for dysphagia can vary by a number of factors (e.g., a patient's diagnosis, prevailing symptoms, patient/family preferences regarding disease management, and regional/geographical access to providers). Further consideration is given to the ideal number of disciplines that will foster a functional, but not overwhelming team size (18).

For the purpose of this chapter, the figure below outlines the principal providers often consulted to assist in the care of patients with dysphagia (see Fig. 11.1). This graphic is by no means exhaustive as each patient/family scenario is individualized

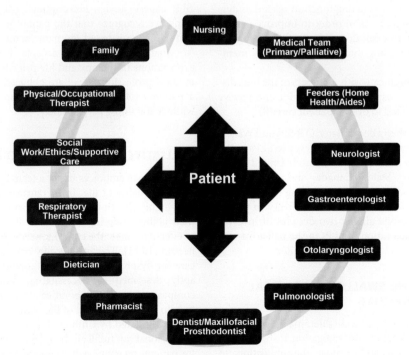

Figure 11.1 Commonly associated disciplines involved in dysphagia management.

and unique. Instead, Figure 11.1 serves as a starting point for understanding and appreciating the breadth of professionals contributing to palliative care of dysphagia.

DYSPHAGIA

Dysphagia (swallowing dysfunction) occurs frequently with a variety of medical conditions and terminal illnesses. Swallowing impairments typically occur in head and neck cancers, progressive neurological diseases, dementia, severe respiratory compromise, and fragility associated with end of life. Consumption of food and liquids is a nutritional necessity in addition to the social pleasures enjoyed by many. The prevalence of dysphagia is unknown; however, some reports indicate up to 22% in individuals over 50 years with over 10 million annual evaluations in the United States (19,20).

The prevalence of patients developing dysphagia during the dying process has been estimated at 28% in long-term care settings and 46% in palliative care settings (21).

When faced with end-of-life issues, the will to eat and/or the ability to eat are frequently impaired. This often is a major frustration and conflict for patient and/or family members. Disinterest with eating or drinking along with the inability to swallow is often pivotal and frequently triggers end of life and or hospice decisions. Additionally dysphagia is often a major factor leading to prolonged hospital stays and comorbidities including pneumonia, asphyxiation, or death. In-hospital mortality is 2.9% higher per year in patients with dysphagia (22).

The need for intervention and management for swallowing problems during palliative care can span over a long period of time with progressive swallowing dysfunction coinciding with physiologic and medical sequelae. The focus herein is on a variety of common causes for stable or progressive swallowing dysfunction. Palliative care for dysphagia is aimed at maximizing swallowing function, maintaining pulmonary patency, and avoiding aspiration and risks of aspiration. Dysphagia, is defined as any difficulty with swallowing food or liquid including medications in tablet, capsule, or liquid formats. Etiologies of dysphagia are numerous and include obstructions such as oropharyngeal tumors, strictures, neurologic impairments affecting motor or sensory function, weakness, fatigue, or respiratory impairment. Common patient complaints of dysphagia include coughing or choking when eating, a sensation of food sticking or stuck in the throat, pain, and weight loss. Any dysfunction in swallowing can influence this enjoyable activity, as well as impair nutrition and hydration thus adding to other medical comorbidities.

SWALLOWING PHYSIOLOGY

The ability to swallow is a well-coordinated activity consisting of >50 paired muscles in the oropharyngeal regions. Cranial function for both sensory input and motor abilities is needed for elicitation of food and liquid transfer to the esophagus (see Table 11.2). Often swallowing is described as a series of both sensory and motor movements occurring with other patterned behaviors such as respiration

TABLE 11.2 CRANIAL NERVES INVOLVED IN SWALLOWING FUNCTION

Cranial nerve		Sensory innervation	Motor innervation
V	Trigeminal (mandibular branch)	Teeth, tongue, buccal cavity lining	Muscles of mastication, mylohyoid and anterior belly of the digastric muscles for hyolaryngeal elevation, tensor veli palatini
VII	Facial	Facial muscles, taste (anterior 2/3rd of tongue)	Muscles of facial expression, labial closure/protrusion/retraction
IX	Glossopharyngeal	Receives input from tonsils, pharynx, and posterior tongue; supplies taste (posterior 1/3rd of tongue)	Stylopharyngeus elevates pharynx and larynx
X	Vagus	Pharynx, larynx, trachea	Muscles of the velopharyngeal mechanism, pharyngeal constrictors including cricopharyngeus, intrinsic muscles of the larynx including vocal folds
XI	Accessory nerve	No sensory component	Sternocleidomastoid, Trapezius Muscles
XII	Hypoglossal nerve	No sensory component	Extrinsic tongue muscles, intrinsic muscles of tongue for articulation and bolus manipulation

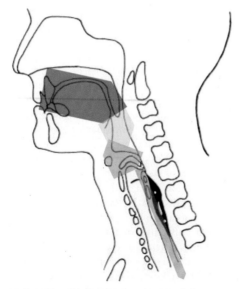

Figure 11.2 Diagram of phases of swallowing (oral, pharyngeal, esophageal).

and cognitive functions. These have neurological control from a central pattern generator within the brainstem with cerebellum involvement (23). For convenience, swallowing is typically divided into phases based on cognitive awareness and the anatomic location of food/liquid bolus. These phases may overlap in their timing and coordination (Fig. 11.2).

PHASES OF SWALLOWING

Cognitive Awareness

Although not always thought of as an actual swallowing phase, an individual's general cognitive *awareness during to the act of eating and or drinking is fundamental.* The ability to see and/or smell food, recognize usage of a utensil, and volitionally initiate mouth opening when food or liquid is presented are components of an individual's overall awareness of the activity of swallowing (24).

Oral Phase

The oral phase begins with the oral preparation of the bolus, which precedes the swallow per se. Volitionally controlled, the oral phase is described frequently as the initial manipulation, mastication, and transit of food or liquid through the oral cavity. The manner in which the bolus is prepared for swallowing varies, depending on the consistency of the material. Liquids are held either between the tongue and palate or in the lingual sulcus, but generally, they pass through the oral cavity in a continuous process. Soft foods are often held immediately between the tongue and anterior hard palate or lateralized for mastication before

resuming a midline position for swallowing. Once the material is small enough and lubricated via salivary flow, the mechanoreceptors for cranial nerve V stimulates and assist with the activation of the central pattern generator for mastication (25).

The bolus is then transported to the posterior oral cavity in a rhythmic coordinated motion for the initiation of the pharyngeal phase of swallowing. The tongue pushes upward and forward in the mouth, contacting the anterior portion of the hard palate. The area of tongue–palate contact expands backward, propelling the bolus through the faucial arches and into the oropharynx.

Pharyngeal Phase

A pharyngeal swallow response is initiated with the movement of bolus. This is a nonvolitional response and occurs with appropriate sensory input to the medullary central pattern generator for swallowing. This is a complex, well-coordinated motor sequence, which assists with the propulsion of the bolus material through the hypopharynx and upper esophageal sphincter (UES) to the esophagus. The pharyngeal sequence of events occurs with approximately a 1-second duration lingual movement posteriorly, soft palate closure, and constrictions in the form of a stripping-like plunger activity at the UES and base of tongue. At the same time, there is anterior superior movement of the larynx to close off the laryngeal inlet with inversion of the epiglottis. A brief cessation of respiration occurs allowing for airway protection and relaxation of the UES. Opening of the UES is a complex process: the cricopharyngeus muscle relaxes, allowing the sphincter to open; the submandibular muscles pull the hyoid bone, the larynx, and the attached anterior wall of the pharynx upward and forward (away from the posterior pharyngeal wall); and the pressure of the descending bolus helps push the sphincter open (26). The pharyngeal constrictors contract sequentially with a peristaltic wave from top to bottom, clearing the pharynx of any residue.

Esophageal Phase

Bolus entry into the esophagus with the relaxation of the UES constitutes the initiation of the esophageal phase. This phase propels the material through the lower esophageal sphincter via a constriction wave occurring between 8 and 15 seconds in the average adult. Motility within the esophagus is also assisted by gravity and requires relaxation of the gastric esophageal sphincter (GES). Reflux of stomach contents is prevented by tonic contraction of the GES and reflex esophageal swallowing that is triggered by esophageal distension (secondary peristalsis) (27).

DYSPHAGIA SIGNS/SYMPTOMS

There are numerous signs and symptoms of swallowing dysfunction that patients, family, or other professionals identify. Most common across the life span are the reports of choking with food/liquid entering the airway. Additionally, patients often complain of globus sensations often described as something may be stuck in their throat or "I feel like a lump or frog is in my throat." Typical signs and symptoms of possible swallowing impairment are included in Table 11.3.

Often, health care providers will highlight aspiration as the pivotal dysphagia sign when in reality other manifestations can be just as worrisome for respiratory sequelae. Laryngeal penetration refers to the liquid or food transit into the laryngeal vestibule that does not pass below the true vocal folds (28). Aspiration refers to a state in which an individual is at risk for entry of gastric secretions, oropharyngeal secretions, solids, or fluids into the tracheobronchial passage (Fig. 11.3). Aspiration of food and/or liquids can have several comorbidities including immediate coughing and choking as well as pulmonary sequelae of bronchitis, pneumonitis, and/or pneumonia following the event. The phenomena of silent aspiration, where food/liquid/saliva enters the upper airway without any overt signs of coughing or choking, is common and thought to have an incidence of 40% in individuals with life-limiting illnesses when multiple causative factors coexist (29). Unfortunately, this cannot be addressed unless instrumental swallowing assess-

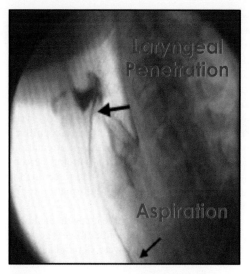

Figure 11.3 X-ray image capture of laryngeal penetration and aspiration during videofluoroscopic assessment of swallowing function.

ments are performed (i.e., videofluoroscopic evaluation of swallowing function [VFSS], fiberoptic endoscopic evaluation of swallowing [FEES]).

ASSESSMENTS

Assessment of swallowing function often occurs when a complaint is reported, observed, or a medical sequela of dysphagia is identified. The overall goals of a swallowing assessment are to identify the pathophysiology of the disorder and determine the relevant interventions while considering the overall health status and the patient and caregivers' wishes regarding nutrition and hydration. Swallowing evaluations should include documentation of swallowing issues, attainment of complete medical history, and physical assessment of cranial nerve functions. Medications for treatment of numerous medical conditions can have effects on swallowing and comorbidities with drug interactions. The following is a non-exhaustive list of pharmacological agents known to have a potential impact on swallowing function: benzodiazepines, neuroleptics, corticosteroids, antihistamines, narcotics, antipsychotics, anticholinergics, antihypertensives, and muscle relaxants. When consulted, SLPs will routinely review prescribed medications at the time of assessment.

Clinical Examination and Bedside Swallow Evaluation

Clinical Examination

A physical examination is essential to look for evidence of cardiopulmonary, gastrointestinal, neurologic, and/or metabolic disease that may impair

TABLE 11.3 FREQUENTLY REPORTED SIGN/SYMPTOMS OF POSSIBLE SWALLOWING IMPAIRMENT

Oral secretions pooling, drooling
Altered tasted or sensation changes
Weight loss
Food liquid backing up into nasal cavity
Difficulty initiating a swallow
Food left in oral cavity or spreading throughout oral cavity
Food or liquid stuck—globus sensation in the neck or chest
Frequent coughing or throat clearing either during or following meals
Wet, gurgly, hoarse voice
Choking
Recurrent upper respiratory infections and or pneumonia
Prolonged eating > 30 minutes
Heartburn and/or pressure in chest
Early satiety during meals

swallowing. This exam includes an assessment of mental status, including the patient's ability to follow directions, and a determination of his/her willingness to participate in therapy. A basic conversation with a patient, if able, can offer a wide array of information including identification of possible disorders of voice (dysphonia), speech (dysarthria, apraxia), and/or spoken or written language (aphasia), in addition to cognitive–communication deficits in the areas of orientation, memory, reasoning, and visual–motor–perceptual function (30). A quick, informal screening for these functions provides useful information to the clinician.

An oral motor cranial nerve assessment should be conducted along with examination of the respiratory system to identify overt signs of obstruction or restriction during breathing. Inspection of the head and neck regions can be performed to assess for abnormal tissue discoloration or tissue changes. Assessment of a dry swallow can be beneficial to note the presence, delays and/or dyscoodination of the hyolaryngeal movement patterns. The presence of primitive reflexes associated with chewing and swallowing (such as the sucking, biting, or snout reflexes) should be noted as these pathologic reflexes are often found in patients with damage to both cerebral hemispheres and can indicate impairments of oral motor control.

Bedside Swallowing Evaluation/Clinical Swallowing Evaluation

The purpose of the bedside swallow evaluation (BSE) or clinical swallow evaluation (CSE) is to screen an individual's swallowing safety. The examinations include observation of a patient eating and drinking to determine if the patient has signs or symptoms of dysphagia, aspiration risks that may further warrant the need of instrumental assessments of swallowing function. Typically, substances that are relatively safe if aspirated are utilized initially with advancement to varied textures (liquid, puree, semisolid, or solid) depending on one's performance. The BSE/CSE is safest when the patient is able to generate a voluntary or reflex cough and is able to follow simple commands. Unstable respiratory status is a relative contraindication. Results of these assessments yield general information of an individual's swallowing ability and safety.

Clinical signs and symptoms of overt aspiration often include: coughing, choking, gurgling, wet or hoarse vocal quality, throat clearing, and stridor following the swallow. More subtle signs of aspiration include teary eyes or sniffling. Other clinical observations include drooling, expectoration of food/liquid, a slow rate of eating, residual food in the mouth after swallowing, impulsive eating or drinking, and abnormal posturing of the head and neck with swallowing. An absence of these overt clinical signs or symptoms *does not* necessarily mean that there is no aspiration. Silent aspiration (i.e., aspiration in the absence of overt signs or symptoms) is common, and a high index of suspicion is imperative (31–33). With silent aspiration estimation up to 40%, it is not confounded that silent aspiration can be missed with the BSE/CSE yielding to the potential of an instrumental assessment (34–36). Silent aspiration can only be definitively confirmed with instrumental assessments (i.e., VFSS and FEES) (37,38).

Instrumental Assessments

The purpose of an instrumental assessment is to determine the mechanism of swallowing dysfunction while maintaining the safest manner for eating and drinking. Additional goals include detection of structural defects, determining which physiologic components are impaired (e.g., bolus preparation, tongue control, initiation of the pharyngeal swallow, tongue base retraction, laryngeal closure, UES opening, esophageal clearance), detecting the presence of and mechanism for aspiration, and testing of therapeutic and compensatory techniques based on the physiologic impairments identified. Relative contraindications include inability to cooperate with the examination and severe respiratory dysfunction. The gold standard to assess oropharyngeal swallow function is the modified barium swallow (MBS) also known as the VFSS. This method is discussed in detail below.

Modified Barium Swallow (Videofluoroscopic Evaluation of Swallowing Function)

The VFSS, otherwise known as the MBS study, is considered the gold standard for evaluation of oral or pharyngeal dysphagia. This evaluation is not to be confused with a routine clinical barium swallow or barium esophagram (evaluation of the esophagus). The goal is to have the patient swallow radiopaque contrast with a variety of liquids and to detect abnormalities of the swallowing mechanism while establishing a safe and efficient method of eating and drinking. An empirical approach is used to identify the factors associated with safe and unsafe swallowing such as the consistency of liquids/food, volume of liquids/food, posture of the patient (especially position of the head and neck), and the means for presenting the food. When abnormalities of swallowing (such as aspiration or retention in the pharynx after swallowing) are recognized compensatory techniques (such as alteration of bolus consistency or posture, or respiratory maneuvers) are attempted (24,39).

In addition to the gold standard of VFSS/MBS, there are other assessments, which can be utilized to provide specific information of structure, physiology, and diagnoses. FEES is a portable procedure that can be completed in both clinical and bedside settings. Utilizing an endoscope transnasally, assessment of swallowing structures prior to and after the swallow can be visualized. Aspiration and retention of material within the hypopharynx can be observed. The barium swallow (esophagram) is an x-ray procedure used to examine the esophagus radiographically with liquid barium to assess for structure and motility issues. For those requiring assessment of esophageal motility with concentration of the force and rhythmic movements of food within the esophagus, esophageal manometry would be recommended. The esophageal pH probe is an outpatient procedure performed to measure the pH or amount of acid that flows into the esophagus from the stomach during a 24-hour period and can assist with diagnoses of reflexive patterning. Table 11.4 offers frequent signs and symptoms of dysphagia with the recommendations of the most minimal assessment and possible associative instrumental evaluations.

Management of Dysphagia

Dysphagia management encompasses decisions regarding one's safety in swallowing and reducing the risk of aspiration, while keeping hydration and nutrition at the forefront. With palliative care, this also includes patient's wishes with the focus on prevention and relief of any suffering. Primary management and care plans should support the patient's condition and wishes with modifications instilled with continuum of palliative support. These may include but are not limited to the following:

- Diet modification with changes in food and or liquid textures
- Changes of bolus delivery, rate of delivery, postural and positioning modifications, and compensations are offered by the speech pathologist
- Enhancing the visual appearance of food as much as possible as many may not want to eat if food is visually unappealing
- Verbal discussions of patients' likes/dislikes with patient, family members, and nutrition/dietary team members
- Often thickening agents, specified rate limiting cups, straws, and spoon delivery are recommended
- Modifications of medication delivery if needed

- Appetite stimulants often are considered in the medical armamentarium for individuals with poor oral intake
- A patient's oral hygiene should be addressed to ensure safe cleaning, maintenance of patient's oral comfort, and avoidance about debris and mucus buildup

Secondary management techniques such as oral motor exercises, vocal exercises, respiratory exercises, and safety compensations such as effortful swallows and supraglottic swallows are often taught to individuals to improve swallowing functions. Speech pathologists and their assistants often help patients with these therapeutic measures.

Education to the patient, family and palliative care team is an essential component of any dysphagia management in palliative care. Discussions of primary goals, nutrition, and hydration with and without modifications are imperative. Teaching tips when one is in distress or having subtle changes during and immediately post eating/drinking is beneficial for the patient family and care providers.

During palliative care, patients and families are often presented with decisions regarding the need for alternative enteral access (e.g., nasogastric feeding tubes, gastrostomy tubes) or total parental nutrition provided intravenously. Patient and family wishes need to be paramount along with comprehensive education provided by the palliative care team.

Numerous diagnoses, treatments, and medical sequelae are often attributed to swallowing dysfunction in patients. Often overlooked is the normal aging process, which frequently causes changes in muscle mass and strength (sarcopenia). Table 11.5 represents many of the more common diagnoses and treatments that have associated swallowing dysfunction.

Communication/Speech Production

Human communication involves the exchange of information and ideas through various processes commonly referred to as speech, language, and cognition. The components of human communication are dynamic and multidimensional, which are continuously influenced by physiological, psychological, and environmental factors. Human communication occurs through a series of autonomic processes mediated by the central neurological system and monitored via a sensory feedback loop (hearing and lip reading). Although complex, the components of communication can be simplified into a four-step process:

- Encoding: the speaker creates the message in his/her mind
- Transmittal: the speaker sends the message
- Reception: the listener receives the message

TABLE 11.4 SIGNS/SYMPTOMS OF POSSIBLE DYSPHAGIA WITH RECOMMENDED ASSESSMENT TOOLS

Signs/symptoms of possible dysphagia	Assessment tools[a]						Other considerations[b]
	BSE/CSE	FEES	VFSS/MBS	Esophagram	Esophageal manometry	Esophageal pH probe	
Pooling of oral secretions/drooling	c						
Altered sensation of taste	c						
Food/liquid backing up into nasal cavity			c				
Bolus pocketing	c		d				
Residue in oral cavity	c		c				
Difficulty initiating a swallow		c	c				
Frequent coughing and/or throat clearing (during or after meals)	d	c	c		d	d	
Choking	d	c	c				
Wet/gurgly/hoarse voice	c	c	c				ENT referral
Prolonged eating (>30 minutes)	c	c	c				Nutritionist referral
Sensation of food/liquid/pills "stuck" in throat or midsternum		c	c	d	d	d	ENT referral (globus) GI referral
Heartburn/pressure in chest during/after meals			d	c	d	d	ENT referral
Early satiety during meals				c			Nutritionist referral
Unexplained weight loss	d	c	c	d			Nutritionist referral

[a]BSE, bedside swallow exam; CSE, clinical swallow evaluation; FEES, fiberoptic endoscopic evaluation of swallowing; VFSS, videofluoroscopic swallow study; MBS, modified barium swallow study.

[b]ENT, ear, nose, and throat specialist; GI, gastroenterologist.

[c]Preferred assessment tool(s) for corresponding signs/symptoms.

[d]Alternative options for assessment pending patient/facility resources and/or findings of preferred assessment tool(s).

TABLE 11.5 DISEASE IMPACT/TREATMENT AND ASSOCIATED SWALLOWING DIFFICULTIES

	Associated swallowing difficulties
Oral cancer— surgical resection	Swallowing dysfunction often is dictated by the amount of resection and the reconstruction of the defect. Lingual movement, muscle strength deficits, and altered sensory input are all factors that will impair both oral and pharyngeal phases of swallow function and can lead to aspiration risks.
Palatal cancers	*Hard Palate Resection:* Patients with hard palate tumor resections that cannot tolerate primary closure of the defect are often are preoperatively referred to prosthodontists for fabrication of a temporary prosthesis. This often is placed intraoperatively or in the postoperative period. Utilization of such device often can alleviate any possible liquid and/or food entering the surgical defect. Individuals typically do not have swallowing difficulties when using these prosthetics.
	Soft Palate Resection: With primary surgical closure, often patients exhibit nasal regurgitation of liquid/food particles secondary to reduced soft palate closure to lateral and pharyngeal walls secondary to edema, and tissue scarring and reduced movement patterns. Extensive resections often require intraoral prosthetics such as a palatal obturator (placed in the surgical defect region).
Oropharyngeal cancer	Resection of tumors of the tonsil and base of tongue affect the bolus transit and initiation of the pharyngeal phase and reduce pharyngeal constriction and hyolaryngeal movements, thus increasing aspiration risks.
Laryngeal cancer	Following total laryngectomy, individuals typically do not have swallowing issues and should be able to eat a normal diet. A small percentage of patients may experience narrowing in the anastomosis region of the base of tongue to the upper esophageal region. With disease recurrence, cervical esophageal strictures can appear and worsen.
Partial laryngectomy	Airway protection is of primary concern with swallowing function with those undergoing partial laryngectomy (e.g., supraglottic resection or hemilaryngectomy). Depending on surgical reconstruction techniques utilized, diminished laryngeal protection with motor and sensory involvement may yield physiologic impairment and aspiration.
Radiation therapy	Radiation treatment to the oral, pharyngeal, and laryngeal cavities often causes early difficulty in swallowing due to edema, mucositis, odynophagia, trismus, loss of taste, and alteration in saliva. Usually an acute effect subsides within a few months. Additionally late effects of treatment with postradiation edema and radiation-induced fibrosis of the oral, pharyngeal, laryngeal, and cervical musculature lead to tissue immobility and diminished musculature movements. These changes result in significant difficulty moving the bolus through the pharynx and closing off of the airway, leaving residue within the pharynx and increasing aspiration.
Chemoradiation protocols for head and neck cancer	Often combination treatments utilizing radiation and various chemotherapeutic agents cause devastating and persistent swallowing impairments with aspiration. High-dose chemoradiation protocols that have the greatest swallowing toxicity. Swallowing disorders may include severely restricted laryngeal elevation and often virtually absent pharyngeal wall contraction. During swallowing, there is little pressure generated on the food to drive it through the pharynx and into the esophagus, leaving most of the food in the pharynx to be aspirated after the swallow.
Chemotherapy	With any malignancy, chemotherapy can have a direct toxicity to the oral, pharyngeal, laryngeal, and esophageal mucosa. Research has shown that the cough reflex is impaired/absent in the irradiated head and neck cancer patient (40). Effects of mucositis can include diminished eating/drinking desire and motoric and sensory change including diminished cough yielding to aspiration risk.
Immunotherapy	Different types of immunotherapy can cause varying morbidities depending on the type of treatment and location of the cancer and an individual's general medical status. Varying symptoms include mucositis, diminished muscle strength/fatigue, mucosal and skin changes, muscular weakness, and pain with swallowing are frequently seen. Often during severe cytokine storms, there can be a plethora of respiratory, muscular and neurologic symptoms can arise acutely and often are treated effectively with speech pathology services.

(Continued)

	Associated swallowing difficulties
Amyotrophic lateral sclerosis	Swallowing disturbances present with upper motor neuron (UMN) degeneration predominate, slowed slurred speech often is the initial symptom, whereas if lower motor neuron (LMN) involvement is dominant, swallowing difficulties may emerge before speech is noticeably worse.
	With disease progression, swallowing impairments worsen and typically, the incidence can be high.
	Standard swallowing assessments for ALS patients rely on a clinical, VFSS/MBS, or FEES to assess the severity of the problem. Standard therapy for dysphagia in ALS emphasizes compensatory interventions such as postural changes and diet modifications. Swallowing exercises are contraindicated due to excess fatigue and the lack of evidence for any benefit. Compensatory techniques are the mainstay until the patient cannot take anything by mouth without choking and aspirating. Both assessment and therapy need to take the cognitive status of the ALS patient into consideration, as approximately 30%–50% of bulbar onset patients have some degree of frontotemporal lobar dementia (FTLD). These patients may not recognize or self-report their swallowing problems, nor will they monitor their ability to swallow safely. It is important to work closely with the caretakers of ALS patients with dementia to guide them in helping the patient compensate for the specific deficits.
Parkinson's disease/ syndromes	The principal symptoms of akinesia, bradykinesia, and rigidity are responsible for swallowing dysfunction in parkinsonian diseases/syndromes. Frequently impairments of inefficient chewing, slow movements, leakage of liquid and/or food in the oral cavity, delayed and impaired movements, delays, and dyscoordination of the pharyngeal swallow response are observed. Pharyngeal food/liquid retention and delays in laryngeal closure bolus clearance are noted. Additionally, assessment of one's cognitive status with these diagnoses is warranted specifically with diagnosis of a parkinsonian syndrome. Diet modification, medication adjustments, adaptive drinking containers and utensil modification, nutritional aids, and strengthening of laryngeal closure can be considered as intervention modifications depending on the impairment. Because the disease progresses slowly, many patients and families opt to continue to eat orally until the end. Some individuals supplement nutrition while maintaining pleasurable feeding with modifications to maintain quality of life.
Dementia	Dysphagia with a dementia diagnosis can have a host of swallowing impairments including difficulty recognizing and holding utensils, mastication issues, retention of food or liquid in the oral cavity, delays in swallowing responses, aspiration, dehydration, and weight loss. With fluctuations in mentation, cognition, and sleep issues, individuals often struggle to swallow safely. Standard management techniques often do not prevent aspiration risk and dehydration and malnutrition. Often, alternative feeding is recommended; however, patients remain at risk for aspiration of saliva and gastroesophageal reflux.
Cerebrovascular disease	Cerebrovascular accidents are devastating occurrences that can have life-altering quality. Swallowing impairments, severity, and prognosis are impacted by the loci of neurological damage. Generally, anterior and subcortical strokes yield a high incidence of dysphagia. Brainstem strokes cause the most severe dysphagia especially when the medulla is affected. Right hemisphere infarctions tend to cause behavioral deficits with reduced ability to utilize strategies. Swallowing manifestations are variable and may include oral food retention, delayed oral transfer, delayed elicitation of a pharyngeal swallow, decreased hyolaryngeal elevation, and aspiration. Generally, swallowing function improves within 6–8 weeks post insult. Brainstem stroke, bilateral hemispheric involvement, or multiple cortical strokes may take longer to recover and may result in a permanent dysphagia. These patients need palliative care when standard treatment fails.
Multiple sclerosis	Multiple sclerosis is a chronic, unpredictable, potentially debilitating inflammatory disease with varying swallowing manifestations, typically the most severe when the brainstem is involved. Impairments with muscle coordination, sensation, and strength contribute to oropharyngeal difficulties. It is thought that up to 40% of patients could have silent aspiration on VFSS. Compensatory therapeutic interventions often are beneficial; however, as with other progressive disorders, the intervention may not be permanent, thus requiring dietary changes and alterations with feeding techniques.
Chronic illness, deconditioning, and frailty	Neuromuscular weakness with critical illness can occur with prolonged acute care hospitalizations and frequent have dysphagia manifestations. Multisystem diseases including chronic obstructive pulmonary disease (COPD), cardiac disorders, and renal failure often have dysphagia as a comorbidity. Coordination of swallowing and respiratory support, muscle weakness, and coordination contribute the swallowing impairment and often can have beneficial outcomes when therapy is initiated.

- Decoding: the listener breaks down the message in his/her mind

Through the well-coordinated, timed, multidimensional group of processes, speech is the system that produces individual sounds, which when placed together develop meaningful messages. It is the verbal means of communication often thought of as the motor vehicle for message delivery. Language may be defined as an arbitrary system of signs or symbols used according to prescribed rules to convey meaning within a linguistic community (41). Cognition refers to the mental processes by which one recognizes, manipulates, and exchanges information to better "understand and make sense of the world" (42). Cognition gives rise to the thoughts and ideas for which one uses speech and language. During the palliative care period, communication processes are met with fluctuations in an individual's overall medical and cognitive status. Although communication can be difficult with care providers and family, one may use additional sensory modalities (visual/auditory) to facilitate the changing communicative needs.

Verbal speech utilizes the systems of respiration, phonation, resonation, articulation, and hearing. Although each system works concurrently with each other, any dysfunction of weakness in one or more systems can compromise the verbal output and meaningful communication exchange. Overall mediation of speech production requires the complex neural networking, regulation, and monitoring of muscle activity of both the central nervous system and peripheral nervous system.

Assessments

Speech pathologists have an extensive collection of assessment tools for evaluation of the various domains involved with communication. To implement successful interventions and treatments, a thorough assessment of the speech domains is needed; however, this may not be possible in the palliative care/end of life settings, often creating the environment for diagnostic therapeutics to foster success with meaningful and functional communicative exchanges. If possible, early consultations with an SLP should be considered to establish baseline functional levels; to gather psychosocial communicative essentials; and to educate patient, family, and caregivers on intervention strategies and potential changes during disease course. Early consultation with our profession can assist with easing communication stress and offer the patients the strategies needed to communicate personal and functional messages along with establishing

TABLE 11.6 COMMUNICATION DEFICITS FREQUENTLY ASSOCIATED WITH MEDICAL DETERIORATION IN PALLIATIVE CARE

Dysarthrias and motor speech disorders
Memory impairment
Reduced judgment/problem solving skills
Comprehension deficits (auditory, written language)
Impairments in word retrieval and naming
Inability to speak
Impairments in breath support and ability to maintain sufficient breath for speech
Vocal and resonance dysfunction

potential communicative alternatives as one's status changes (Table 11.6).

The speech pathologists' assessment toolbox contains both formal standardized and informal measures. Often one's status and overall needs will dictate what measurement tools are utilized. In any case, the primary goals of palliative care should be followed to create communication ease and reduce frustrations. This may require the therapist to quickly determine psychosocial factors influencing a patient's communication needs in addition to the speech, language and cognitive impairments to create successful meaningful exchanges. This requires allowing appropriate time for an individual to communicate the message as well as respecting the individual's cultural, religious, and emotional needs especially during communicative exchange. Educating other interdisciplinary members of these needs will assist with the communication process among all providers. Often coassessment, treatment, and collaboration with palliative care partners (many of whom were previously described) can assist with implementation of therapeutic needs and goals to achieve optimal speech intelligibility. Frequently, speech pathologists work closely with maxillofacial prosthodontics, evaluating needs for prosthetic device fabrication (i.e., palatal lifts, obturators, and/or palatal drops) for both head and neck cancer and neurological diagnoses. Additional collaborations with physical and occupational therapies help to determine appropriateness and ease in use of augmentative alternative communication in cases of complex and progressive disorders (e.g., Amyotrophic lateral sclerosis, severe multiple sclerosis, brain injuries).

Treatment Considerations

The pattern of functional communication decline and speech dysfunction in individuals at the end of life varies depending on the person's diagnosis. In some cases, the decline may be very gradual until the last few months or weeks of life, or may be inconsistent over long periods as in the case of dementias. No matter the situation, effective speech pathology interventions must employ considerations and understanding with one's disease process and anticipated changes in speech, language, and cognition; the individual and his/her communication needs; legal and ethical considerations; and overall patient safety.

Therapeutic intervention and management may involve therapeutic exercise, changes in positioning, facilitation of specific strategies (e.g., increasing volume, over articulation or phrasing), visual cueing and modeling, and utilization of biofeedback to enhance overall intelligibility. Therapists often are the individuals to make the decisions about the appropriateness of treatment for the specific communication disorders, as well as when such treatment is no longer appropriate. Altering therapeutic goals and management at pivotal times during the palliative care and disease process aids clinicians with effective communication modalities between the patient and his/her communication partners (family, health care providers, friends, others). Continuous assessment of functional performance and treatment modifications serves a good model for optimizing one's speech goals for effective communication. The customization of therapy, communication management, and continuous education with all (patients, family, and providers) is paramount for a therapist to be successful with the changing needs of patient in a supportive care status.

Augmentative Alternative Communication

For severely involved speakers whose intelligibility is so poor that they are unable to communicate verbally in some or all situations, the general goal of treatment involves establishing an immediate functional means of communication. This may include use of augmentative approaches. The term *communication augmentation* refers to any device designed to augment, supplement, or replace verbal communication for someone who is not an independent verbal communicator. These augmentative or alternative communication (AAC) systems can be as low tech as writing or communication picture/written word boards, or higher tech such as talk-back switches, phones, tablets, and computer device applications with speech/voice synthesis. The selection of an appropriate augmentation system requires a thorough evaluation of the individual's communication needs. Although one may think they are at the end of their life, these augmentative systems can assist with bridging the need of communication for individuals and families. To determine an individual's needs, the

clinician needs to consider the patient's physical and cognitive capabilities, including cognition, language, memory, physical control, vision, hearing, and overall medical condition. As previously noted, this assessment may require additional coevaluators. Once the individual's capabilities have been ascertained, augmentative system components can be selected, and appropriate system modifications can be implemented and trialed. Although expensive, augmentative devices can greatly enhance one's ability to communicate when they can no longer speak or write. Loaner devices may be available from local agencies, assistive technology centers, specific disease associations, or universities to trial.

For those with moderate impairments in speech intelligibility who are able to use speech as their primary means of communication but whose intelligibility is compromised, the general goal of treatment involves improving intelligibility. Use of compensatory strategies with speech production or augmentative systems is commonly used as a modality if communication situations become problematic or the patient is fatigued or if there is an acute status change. These augmented systems often serve as a second system for individuals to facilitate communication exchanges. Speech pathologists will often provide such communication alternatives that may include pictorial boards, individualized communication books or board, and/or writing tablets.

When early referrals to speech pathology are initiated with patients receiving palliative care support and when one anticipates anticipated speech intelligibility deterioration or an individual's inability to produce speech, speech pathologists can assist with speech and voice recordings of one's natural speech. Again, collaborations with others such as computer engineering will facilitate the mode of retrieval in anticipation of the patient's needs and desires.

Tracheostomy

More often than not, the use of a tracheostomy tube insertion to assist with ventilation and respiratory support occurs within palliative care. The use of tracheostomy tube will alter one's ability to communicate naturally, often requiring specialized management for both speech and swallowing function. Speech pathologists have the working knowledge and toolbox of strategies to facilitate these modalities offering patients, caregivers, and family tricks and tips for effective functionality. Providing education to the patient/and family preoperatively (if feasible) along with facilitation of speech and swallowing postoperatively is within the scope of a speech pathologist's practice.

Teaching finger occlusion to obtain speech and use of speaking valves in isolation and with ventilation are many of the speech pathology goals with tracheostomy patients. Continuous education with tracheostomy use and activities of speech, swallowing, and emergency communication is typically offered by speech pathology to ensure patient safety with all who are involved in an individual's care. Of paramount importance is safety, and secondary alternatives for communication are essential when treating this group of patients such as writing/communication boards and tablet/computer application availability.

As indicated earlier in this chapter, the breadth of intervention and management strategies for varying conditions should be individualistic. Specific diagnoses with treatments and associated deficits in the speech pathology domains with care plan considerations are provided in Table 11.7 below.

Vignettes

History/Background

Patient X is a 45-year-old, left-handed, native English-speaking male who presented to his local emergency room following a week of progressive paresthesia in his right extremities, acute word retrieval difficulties, and subtle slurring of speech. A subsequent brain MRI revealed an enhancing mass in the left precentral gyrus. One week later, he underwent a left parietal craniotomy for tumor resection with pathology results revealing a grade IV glioblastoma. He received inpatient speech services immediately after surgery followed by transfer to an acute inpatient rehabilitation facility. Speech intervention initially targeted mild-to-moderate anomia at the conversational level and mild dysarthria. He was discharged home with outpatient chemoradiation treatments until he was

TABLE 11.7 COMMON MEDICAL DIAGNOSES AND TREATMENT WITH SPEECH, LANGUAGE, AND COGNITIVE ISSUES AND PLAN OF CARE CONSIDERATIONS

Diagnosis	Deficits of speech/language/ cognition	Plan of care considerations
Stroke	Deficits and severity vary by site/size of infarct(s) and potential for aphasia, apraxia, dysarthria, and impaired executive functioning.	Care plans should include methods to maximize auditory comprehension, verbal output, oral motor strengthening, and establishment of the patient's most effective mode of communication.
Brain tumors	Deficits and severity vary by site/size of lesion as well as rate of progression/recurrence and potential for aphasia, apraxia, dysarthria, and impaired executive functioning.	Intervention should be geared toward maximizing functional communication exchanges as well as safety and independence during the completion of familiar activities of daily living.
Dementia	Progressive decline in cognitive–communication function resulting in an inability to communicate basic wants/needs or complete self-care tasks	To the extent tolerated, patients benefit from techniques focused on environmental orientation and compensation of declining memory.
Parkinson's disease/ syndromes	Dysarthria (hypokinetic), dementia	Patients initially benefit from active exercise such as Lee Silverman Voice Treatment (43); with disease progression, voice amplification or augmentative and alternative communication devices may become necessary; implement strategies for functional memory deficits.
Amyotrophic lateral sclerosis (ALS)	Dysarthria (spastic, flaccid), possible dementia	As patient status declines with active exercise, initiate use of augmentative and alternative communication as able/tolerated.
Oral cancer	Dysarthria	Establish exercise program, articulatory strategies, and co-treatments with maxillofacial prosthodontics for fabrication and modification of prosthetic devices.
Partial laryngectomy	Degree of dysphonia is greatest with a hemilaryngectomy and depends on extent of resection/reconstruction.	Emphasize volitional airway protection and use range of motion exercises for residual laryngeal structures (24).
Total laryngectomy	Patients have complete aphonia due to the absence of laryngeal structures.	Use of an artificial larynx, esophageal speech, or tracheoesophageal puncture to facilitate phonation.

diagnosed with further disease progression after several in-home falls and a marked decline in his overall communication skills.

Palliative Care/Food for Thought:

- As Mr. X continues to undergo medical treatment and navigate the malignancy of a glioblastoma, the inclusion of SLP services within his interdisciplinary palliative care team is crucial. Given his existing deficits in the domains of speech and language as well as predicted declines with further disease progression, SLP services would foster successful communication exchanges. The focus of care would include
  - educating the patient, family, and medical team on strategies to enhance current communication and possible communicative changes in the future
  - supporting Mr. X in his ability to convey a range of thoughts, emotions, preferences, and needs
  - increasing his comprehension of the various auditory and visual input provided by family, friends, and staff
  - early identification of augmentative and alternative communication tools to implement with fluctuations in patient status
- Of greatest importance is the guarantee that SLP services will respect Mr. X's autonomy, show deference to the values communicated by the patient and his family, and remain committed to ethical management of his care with every interaction.

History/Background

Patient Y is a 61-year-old, right-handed female with newly diagnosed multiple system atrophy (MSA) consistent with the cerebellar variant. Her clinical presentation includes depression, gait ataxia, complaints of intermittent coughing during meals, and an unintentional 10-lb weight loss within the last 2 months. Screenings of her cognitive function have been unremarkable thus far. In addition, she does not currently exhibit any appreciable changes in speech intelligibility. She is scheduled to have a VFSS/MBS next week. Of note: After receiving initial counseling regarding her diagnosis, Mrs. Y opted to complete an advance directive, which specifies that she does not consent to the insertion/use of feeding tubes if she is deemed unsafe to continue oral intake.

Palliative Care/Food for Thought:

- Findings from the VFSS/MBS and patient's wishes consistent with her advance directive, the focus of care would include
  - patient and family education regarding assessment findings, recommended diet textures, interventions, and evidence-based knowledge regarding expected changes in swallow function with disease progression
  - educating patient/family of diet alternates along with discussion of supplementary feeding tubes to ensure understanding of all options while paying respect to the advance directive
  - thorough patient and family education regarding aspiration—including prevalent symptoms of airway compromise and aspiration precautions; and
  - early collaboration with a dietician to optimize nutritional status
- Throughout the palliative care process, SLPs must continuously engage in honest, transparent dialogue with patients and families regarding safety for oral intake, consequences of repeated aspiration, and all available options for maximizing the enjoyment of eating without compromising overall health.

CONCLUSION

The processes of communication and swallowing appear simplistic and rudimentary to most; however, their dysfunction or loss can be devastating to one's sense of quality. To achieve successful care, the speech language pathology profession is a essential partner within the palliative care team, offering both continuous diagnostic assessments, interventions, strategies for speech and swallowing function, as well as education and support to all interdisciplinary professional team members, the patient, and family. Although often frequently challenging, the scope of practice within the profession offers a continuum of transitions for patient care from independent functioning to palliation and support within the life span for communication and swallowing functions. The speech pathologist's contribution to a patient's empowerment with communication is crucial through life's end easing frustration and providing support to all involved thus defining total palliation.

REFERENCES

1. Saunders C. The evolution of palliative care. *Pharos Alpha Omega Alpha Honor Med Soc.* 2003;66(3):6.
2. American Speech-Language-Hearing Association. *End of Life Resources and References. Secondary End of Life Resources and References*; n.d. https://www.asha.org/SLP/End-of-Life-Resources/
3. Frost M. The role of physical, occupational, and speech therapy in hospice: patient empowerment. *Am J Hosp Palliat Care.* 2001;18(6):397-402. doi: 10.1177/104990910101800609.
4. Roe JW, Leslie P. Beginning of the end? Ending the therapeutic relationship in palliative care. *Int J Speech Lang Pathol.* 2010;12(4):304-308; discussion 29-32. doi: 10.3109/17549507.2010.485330.

5. Pollens RD. Integrating speech-language pathology services in palliative end-of-life care. *Topics Lang Disord.* 2012;32(2):137-148.

6. Wittry SA, Lam NY, McNalley T. The value of rehabilitation medicine for patients receiving palliative care. *Am J Hosp Palliat Care.* 2018;35(6):889-896. doi: 10.1177/1049909117742896.

7. O'Reilly AC, Walshe M. Perspectives on the role of the speech and language therapist in palliative care: an international survey. *Palliat Med.* 2015;29(8):756-761. doi: 10.1177/0269216315575678.

8. Pollens RD. Role of the speech-language pathologist in palliative hospice care. *J Palliat Med.* 2004;7(5):694-702. doi: 10.1089/jpm.2004.7.694.

9. Sharp HM, Genesen LB. Ethical decision-making in dysphagia management. *Am J Speech Lang Pathol.* 1996;5(1):15-22.

10. Mathisen B, Yates P, Crofts P. Palliative care curriculum for speech-language pathology students. *Int J Lang Commun Disord.* 2011;46(3):273-285. doi: 10.3109/13682822.2010.495739.

11. Parker-Oliver D, Bronstein LR, Kurzejeski L. Examining variables related to successful collaboration on the hospice team. *Health Social Work.* 2005;30(4):279-286. doi: 10.1093/hsw/30.4.279.

12. Langmore SE, Grillone G, Elackattu A, Walsh M. Disorders of swallowing: palliative care. *Otolaryngol Clin North Am.* 2009;42(1):87-105, ix. doi: 10.1016/j.otc.2008.09.005.

13. Chin LTL, Lim YJ, Choo WL. Much ado about fried chicken: abetting aspiration or respecting autonomy? *Am J Speech Lang Pathol.* 2019;28(3):1356-1362. doi: 10.1044/2019_ajslp-18-0207.

14. Crawford GB, Price SD. Team working: palliative care as a model of interdisciplinary practice. *Med J Aust.* 2003;179(S6):S32-S34.

15. Jessup RL. Interdisciplinary versus multidisciplinary care teams: do we understand the difference? *Aust Health Rev.* 2007;31(3):330-331. doi: 10.1071/ah070330.

16. Youngwerth J, Twaddle M. Cultures of interdisciplinary teams: how to foster good dynamics. *J Palliat Med.* 2011;14(5):650-654. doi: 10.1089/jpm.2010.0395.

17. Weller J, Boyd M, Cumin D. Teams, tribes and patient safety: overcoming barriers to effective teamwork in healthcare. *Postgrad Med J.* 2014;90(1061):149-154. doi: 10.1136/postgradmedj-2012-131168.

18. Noreika DM, Coyne PJ. Implementing palliative care interdisciplinary teams: consultative versus integrative models. *Crit Care Nurs Clin North Am.* 2015;27(3):297-306. doi: 10.1016/j.cnc.2015.05.006.

19. Domenech E, Kelly J. Swallowing disorders. *Med Clin North Am.* 1999;83(1):97-113, ix. doi: 10.1016/s0025-7125(05)70090-0.

20. Howden CW. Management of acid-related disorders in patients with dysphagia. *Am J Med.* 2004;117(suppl 5A):44s-48s. doi: 10.1016/j.amjmed.2004.07.017.

21. Smith BJ, Chong L, Nam S, Seto R. Dysphagia in a palliative care setting—a coordinated overview of caregivers' responses to dietary changes: the DysCORD qualitative study. *J Palliat Care.* 2015;31(4):221-227. doi: 10.1177/082585971503100403.

22. Patel DA, Krishnaswami S, Steger E, et al. Economic and survival burden of dysphagia among inpatients in the United States. *Dis Esophagus.* 2018;31(1):1-7. doi: 10.1093/dote/dox131.

23. Ludlow CL. Central nervous system control of voice and swallowing. *J Clin Neurophysiol.* 2015;32(4):294-303. doi: 10.1097/wnp.0000000000000186.

24. Logemann JA. *Evaluation and Treatment of Swallowing Disorders.* 2nd ed. Austin, Texa. New York: Pro-Ed; 1998.

25. Corbin-Lewis K, Liss JM. *Clinical Anatomy & Physiology of the Swallow Mechanism.* Cengage Learning; San Diego, CA. 2014.

26. Goyal RK. Disorders of the cricopharyngeus muscle. *Otolaryngol Clin North Am.* 1984;17(1):115-130.

27. Castell DO. Esophageal disorders in the elderly. *Gastroenterol Clin North Am.* 1990;19(2):235-254.

28. Rosenbek JC, Robbins JA, Roecker EB, Coyle JL, Wood JL. A penetration-aspiration scale. *Dysphagia.* 1996;11(2):93-98. doi: 10.1007/bf00417897.

29. Ramsey D, Smithard D, Kalra L. Silent aspiration: what do we know? *Dysphagia.* 2005;20(3):218-225. doi: 10.1007/s00455-005-0018-9.

30. Martin BJ, Corlew MM. The incidence of communication disorders in dysphagic patients. *J Speech Hear Disord.* 1990;55(1):28-32. doi: 10.1044/jshd.5501.28.

31. Nguyen NP, Moltz CC, Frank C, et al. Dysphagia following chemoradiation for locally advanced head and neck cancer. *Ann Oncol.* 2004;15(3):383-388. doi: 10.1093/annonc/mdh101.

32. Ramsey DJ, Smithard DG, Kalra L. Early assessments of dysphagia and aspiration risk in acute stroke patients. *Stroke.* 2003;34(5):1252-1257. doi: 10.1161/01.Str.0000066309.06490.B8.

33. Smith CH, Logemann JA, Colangelo LA, Rademaker AW, Pauloski BR. Incidence and patient characteristics associated with silent aspiration in the acute care setting. *Dysphagia.* 1999;14(1):1-7. doi: 10.1007/pl00009579.

34. Palmer JB, Drennan JC, Baba M. Evaluation and treatment of swallowing impairments. *Am Fam Physician.* 2000;61(8):2453-2462.

35. Palmer JB, DuChane AS. Rehabilitation of swallowing disorders in the elderly. In: Felsenthal G, Garrison SJ, Steinberg FU, eds. *Rehabilitation of the Aging and Older Patient.* Baltimore, MD: Williams & Wilkins; 1994.

36. Wakasugi Y, Tohara H, Hattori F, et al. Screening test for silent aspiration at the bedside. *Dysphagia.* 2008;23(4):364-370. doi: 10.1007/s00455-008-9150-7.

37. Garon BR, Sierzant T, Ormiston C. Silent aspiration: results of 2,000 video fluoroscopic evaluations. *J Neurosci Nurs.* 2009;41(4):178-185; quiz 86-87.

38. Levine MS, Ralls PW, Balfe DM, et al. Imaging recommendations for patients with dysphagia. American College of Radiology. ACR Appropriateness Criteria. *Radiology.* 2000;215(suppl):225-230.

39. Martin-Harris B, Logemann JA, McMahon S, Schleicher M, Sandidge J. Clinical utility of the modified barium swallow. *Dysphagia.* 2000;15(3):136-141. doi: 10.1007/s004550010015.

40. Nguyen NP, Moltz CC, Frank C, et al. Effectiveness of the cough reflex in patients with aspiration following radiation for head and neck cancer. *Lung.* 2007;185(5):243-248. doi: 10.1007/s00408-007-9016-z.

41. Kent R. Normal aspects of articulation. In: Bernthal JE, Bankson NW, eds. *Articulation and Phonological Disorders.* 2nd ed. Englewood Cliffs, NJ: Prentice Hall; 1988.

42. Cherry K. *What is Cognition? Secondary What is Cognition?*; 2020. https://www.verywellmind.com/what-is-cognition-2794982

43. Ramig LO, Fox C, Sapir S. Parkinson's disease: speech and voice disorders and their treatment with the Lee Silverman Voice Treatment. *Semin Speech Lang.* 2004;25(2):169-180. doi: 10.1055/s-2004-825653.

12 Chemotherapy-Related Nausea and Vomiting and Treatment-Related Nausea and Vomiting

Han Le

The ability of chemotherapy to cause nausea and vomiting is legendary and remains a widespread fear among cancer patients. Indeed, nausea and vomiting related to chemotherapy significantly decreases patient quality of life (1). Over the past two decades, however, prevention of chemotherapy-induced nausea and vomiting (CINV) has improved dramatically. This is largely due to new classes of drugs used in prevention. This has meant improvements in quality of life for cancer patients and likely increased compliance in oncologic treatment. Radiation therapy also carries a risk of nausea and vomiting depending on the anatomic location of therapy, though there is less in the way of randomized data to guide therapy.

SYNDROMES OF CINV

CINV can be described as three distinct syndromes: acute, delayed, and anticipatory nausea and vomiting. Though in clinical practice these syndromes can overlap, the terms are helpful to define and categorize CINV. Acute CINV refers to nausea and vomiting that develops within the first 24 hours after chemotherapy administration, often within a couple of hours for most emetogenic chemotherapy agents. Delayed CINV refers to nausea and vomiting that develops more than 24 hours after chemotherapy and is generally considered to last 3 to 5 days following chemotherapy administration, but can vary, depending on many factors, including control of emesis during the acute period. Delayed emesis is considered not as severe as acute emesis (2), though less well understood and may be underappreciated and undertreated by clinicians. Cisplatin has been the most well studied in defining delayed emesis and is the archetype chemotherapy agent in the investigation of antiemetic agents. Without prophylaxis, more than 90% of patients will have some symptoms of nausea or vomiting in the delayed emesis period. Anticipatory CINV occurs when nausea or emesis is triggered by events or settings of prior chemotherapy such as the sights or smells of the infusion room, chemotherapy equipment, or care providers.

RISK OF CINV

The intrinsic emetogenicity of an individual chemotherapy agent appears to be the most important predictive factor for the development of CINV, though CINV is also influenced by patient characteristics. Such characteristics include gender, age, and history of alcohol consumption (3). In addition, experiencing nausea and vomiting with prior chemotherapy is also a risk factor. Consistently, women are more prone to both nausea and vomiting associated with chemotherapy. Older patients are less likely to experience nausea and vomiting compared with younger patients in some series (4). A history of alcohol consumption is protective against the risk of nausea and vomiting associated with chemotherapy. History of motion sickness and hyperemesis gravidarum are not well-established risk factors for CINV.

The emetogenicity of individual chemotherapy agents depends on the type of chemotherapy, dose and route, and rate of administration. Chemotherapeutic agents are classified by their risk of inducing CINV, and the most commonly used classification is modified from the Hesketh classification, originally described as five levels of emetic risk (5). It has now been modified to four levels: high, moderate, low, or minimal risk of inducing emesis (Table 12.1) (6).

RESEARCH IN PREVENTION OF CINV

The prevention of CINV is an area of very solid and consistent clinical research, which has resulted in the development of guidelines that are evidence based. In the research setting, it is useful to distinguish periods of acute and delayed emesis, as well as overall response. Vomiting is more frequently used as an endpoint, because it is a more consistent measure than nausea, which tends to be more subjective. Visual analogue scales do exist for nausea, which can help patients quantify their symptoms. Another endpoint used to judge the effectiveness of antiemetic therapy is the use of rescue medications as a measure of how well or poorly both nausea and emesis are controlled. Complete response or

180

TABLE 12.1 CLASSIFICATION OF EMETIC RISK OF INTRAVENOUS ANTINEOPLASTIC AGENTS

Emetic risk (estimated incidence without prophylaxis)	Antineoplastic agents
High (>90%)	Cisplatin
	Mechlorethamine
	Streptozotocin
	Cyclophosphamide ($\geq$1,500 mg/m^2)
	Carmustine
	Dacarbazine
Moderate (30%–90%)	Oxaliplatin
	Cytarabine (>1 g/m^2)
	Carboplatin
	Ifosfamide
	Cyclophosphamide (<1,500 mg/m^2)
	Doxorubicin
	Daunorubicin
	Epirubicin
	Idarubicin
	Irinotecan
	Azacitidine
	Bendamustine
	Clofarabine
	Alemtuzumab
Low (10%–30%)	Paclitaxel
	Docetaxel
	Mitoxantrone
	Doxorubicin HCl liposome injection
	Ixabepilone
	Topotecan
	Etoposide
	Pemetrexed
	Methotrexate
	Mitomycin
	Gemcitabine
	Cytarabine ($\leq$100 mg/m^2)
	5-Fluorouracil
	Bortezomib
	Cetuximab
	Trastuzumab
	Panitumumab
	Catumaxomab

TABLE 12.1 CLASSIFICATION OF EMETIC RISK OF INTRAVENOUS ANTINEOPLASTIC AGENTS (*Continued*)

Emetic risk (estimated incidence without prophylaxis)	Antineoplastic agents
Minimal (<10%)	Bleomycin
	Busulfan
	2-Chlorodeoxyadenosine
	Fludarabine
	Vinblastine
	Vincristine
	Vinorelbine
	Bevacizumab
	Rituximab

From Roila F, Herrstedt J, Aapro M, et al. Guideline update for MASCC and ESMO in the prevention of chemotherapy- and radiotherapy-induced nausea and vomiting: results of the Perugia consensus conference. *Ann Oncol.* 2010;21:v232-v243, by permission of Oxford University Press.

protection is often defined as no vomiting and no use of rescue medications. Episodes of vomiting and degree of nausea are often captured with the use of a diary or frequent telephone contact.

PATHOPHYSIOLOGY OF CINV

Nausea and vomiting resulting from chemotherapy involves a complicated and multifaceted physiology. Afferent stimulatory input likely comes from several sources, including vagal afferent nerves in the abdomen. These are known to have a number of receptors on their terminal ends, including 5-hydroxytryptamine-3 ($5\text{-}HT_3$), neurokinin (NK)-1, and cholecystokinin-1. Enteroendocrine cells located within the gastrointestinal tract release neurotransmitters in response to chemotherapy, including 5-HT, substance P, and cholecystokinin, which then bind to the vagal afferent nerves in the abdomen. The so-called chemotherapy trigger zone is also thought to provide afferent input in response to chemotherapy. Anatomically, this is the area postrema where the blood–brain barrier is less restrictive and thus may be an area exposed to chemotherapy or chemotherapy by-products. Input then flows into the central nervous system proper to an area termed the "vomiting center," though it is now more widely believed that this represents a number of separate brain stem areas that are connected to coordinate emesis, including the parvocellular reticular formation, the Botzinger complex, and the nucleus tractus solitarius (7).

Key to the process of emesis is the involvement of a number of neurotransmitters. In CINV, the most important neurotransmitters include dopamine, serotonin ($5\text{-}HT_3$), substance P, and the cannabinoids (8). Dopamine antagonists such as phenothiazines have been used for decades for

prevention of CINV, exemplifying the importance of dopamine as an active neurotransmitter. More recently, the importance of 5-HT in CINV has been realized, with the type 3 receptor emerging as the most relevant. This is likely to be mainly at the level of the afferent signals in the gastrointestinal area, though $5\text{-}HT_3$ receptors are found not only in the vagal afferent fibers but also in the area postrema and the nucleus tractus solitarius (8,9).

Substance P is a neuropeptide that also plays an important role in CINV. It belongs to a family of neurotransmitters called tachykinins, which bind to NK receptors. Substance P has an affinity for NK_1 receptors, which are located in the gastrointestinal tract, the area postrema, and the nucleus solitarius—all important areas active in the physiology of emesis (8). It was discovered in the initial animal studies that emesis was prevented by inhibitors of substance P, proving the principle of importance of this neurotransmitter. This occurred with both centrally acting and peripherally acting stimuli (10).

RADIATION THERAPY–INDUCED NAUSEA AND VOMITING

The risk of radiation therapy–induced nausea and vomiting (RINV) is primarily dependent on the area of the body being treated. Depending on the type of radiation, the risk of nausea and vomiting is divided into four categories: high, moderate, low, and minimal (11,12). High risk includes total body irradiation and total nodal irradiation. Moderate risk involves radiation sites in the upper abdomen, half-body irradiation, and upper body irradiation. Low risk includes cranial and craniospinal irradiation as well as head and neck, lower thorax, and pelvis. Minimal risk includes radiation to the extremities and breast.

Animal studies have demonstrated the importance of 5-HT$_3$ in the pathophysiology of RINV, with a better response to inhibition of 5-HT$_3$–mediated pathways than with dopamine pathways (13). It is speculated that the direct toxic effects on areas such as the gastrointestinal tract stimulate afferent fibers and transmit signals to the collective vomiting center. Additional potential stimuli include the tissue breakdown products that occur as a consequence of radiation treatment.

DRUGS USED IN THE PREVENTION OF TREATMENT-RELATED NAUSEA AND VOMITING

The three classes of drugs that have the most relevance in the prevention of treatment-related nausea and vomiting include the 5-HT$_3$ receptor antagonists, the NK$_1$ antagonists, and corticosteroids (Table 12.2). They may be given alone or in combination, depending on the clinical setting. These three classes are now in routine use in the place of dopamine antagonists, which are now mainly used as supplemental medications in cases where standard prophylaxis has not worked.

5-HT$_3$ Antagonists

This class of drugs includes the first-generation agents dolasetron, granisetron, ondansetron, tropisetron, and ramosetron and the second-generation agent palonosetron. They are given as oral, intravenous (IV), and transdermal preparations, with first-generation IV formulations considered equivalent to oral administration (14). Previously, all first-generation agents had been considered to be of equal efficacy and used interchangeably (15),

TABLE 12.2 DOSES OF COMMONLY USED ANTIEMETIC AGENTS

Drug	Prechemotherapy dose	
	Acute emesis prophylaxis	Delayed emesis prophylaxis
Highest therapeutic index		
Aprepitant	125 mg orally	80 mg orally days 2 and 3
	110 mg IV	
Fosaprepitant	150 mg IV	
Dexamethasone		
With aprepitant	12 mg orally or IV	8 mg days 2–4[a]
Without aprepitant	20 mg orally or IV[a]	8 mg b.i.d. days 2–4[a]
	8 mg orally or IV[b]	8 mg days 2 and 3[c]
Ondansetron	24 mg orally[a]; 8 mg orally b.i.d.[b]	
	8 mg or 0.15 mg/kg IV	
Granisetron	2 mg orally	
	1 mg or 0.01 mg/kg IV	
Tropisetron	5 mg orally or IV	
Dolasetron	100 mg orally	
	100 mg or 1.8 mg/kg IV	
Palonosetron	0.25 mg IV	
	0.5 mg orally	
Lower therapeutic index		
Prochlorperazine	10 mg orally or IV	—
Dronabinol	5 mg/m^2 orally	5 mg/m^2 orally q2–4h PRN
Nabilone	1–2 mg orally	1–2 mg b.i.d. or t.i.d. PRN
Olanzapine	5 mg orally daily for 2 d preceding chemotherapy; 10 mg on day 1	10 mg days 2–4

IV, intravenously; b.i.d., twice daily; t.i.d., thrice daily.
[a]When used with highly emetic chemotherapy.
[b]When used with moderately emetic chemotherapy.
[c]When used with moderately emetic chemotherapy with potential for delayed emesis.

though a meta-analysis (16) has suggested that while ondansetron and granisetron are equivalent, granisetron is more effective than tropisetron. Data for ramosetron and dolasetron are more limited. Side effects of 5-HT$_3$ receptor antagonists include constipation, headache, and a transient rise in liver enzymes. The Multinational Association of Supportive Care in Cancer (MASCC)/ European Society for Medical Oncology (ESMO) guidelines laid out several principles in regard to 5-HT$_3$ receptor antagonists: the lowest therapeutic dose should be used; the adverse effects of this class are similar among agents; and the use of a single dose prior to chemotherapy remains the optimal integration of this class of medications.

Prior to the development of 5-HT$_3$ receptor antagonists, high-dose metoclopramide was used for both acute and delayed emesis following cisplatin and other high-risk chemotherapy agents. Early studies showed better control of CINV with 5-HT$_3$ receptor antagonists. One series (17) involved 307 patients being treated with cisplatin of at least 100 mg/m^2 for a variety of cancers, though most patients had either lung or head and neck cancer. Patients were randomized to ondansetron at a dose of 0.15 mg/kg every 4 hours for a total of three doses of metoclopramide 2 mg/kg every 2 hours for three doses, then every 3 hours for three additional doses starting 30 minutes before cisplatin administration. Responses were defined as a complete response if the patient experienced no emesis for the first 24 hours of the study, a major response if one to two episodes of emesis occurred, minor response if three to five episodes occurred, and treatment failure if more than five episodes of emesis occurred or if a patient required rescue emetic therapy with PRN medications. The complete response rate was higher in the ondansetron group, with 54% of patients experiencing no vomiting in the first 24 hours after therapy compared with 41% of patients treated with metoclopramide ($p = 0.70$). In addition, more patients in the metoclopramide arm were considered treatment failures, with 36% in the metoclopramide group compared with 21% in the ondansetron group ($p = 0.007$). The median time to onset of emesis was 20.5 hours in the ondansetron group compared with 4.3 hours in the metoclopramide group. As expected, global satisfaction with nausea and vomiting control was also higher in the ondansetron group (85% vs. 63%, $p = 0.001$). Adverse events in the metoclopramide group included acute dystonic reactions in eight patients versus none in the ondansetron group ($p = 0.005$). Diarrhea was more common in the metoclopramide group, whereas headache and increased liver function abnormalities were more common in the ondansetron group.

Granisetron has been formulated into a transdermal patch called the granisetron transdermal delivery system (GTDS), which delivers granisetron over a period of 7 days. In a phase III trial (18) of 641 patients designed as a noninferiority study, the GTDS patch was compared with oral granisetron given at 2 mg/d for 3 to 5 days. All patients were being treated with chemotherapy regimens that contained multiple days of chemotherapy administration involving either highly or moderately emetogenic chemotherapy. The primary endpoint of noninferiority was met and the patients' global satisfaction with antiemetic therapy was similar in the two groups. The American Society of Clinical Oncology (ASCO) guidelines on the use of antiemetics suggest consideration for use of the GTDS patch during multiple-day regimens of chemotherapy as an alternative to taking a 5-HT$_3$ receptor antagonist on a daily basis (12).

Palonosetron has a longer half-life than first-generation 5-HT$_3$ antagonists and can be given intravenously or orally. Oral palonosetron at a dose of 0.5 mg was found to be equivalent to IV palonosetron at 0.25 mg (19). Several randomized trials have compared first-generation 5-HT$_3$ antagonists to palonosetron. In one trial of patients receiving highly emetogenic chemotherapy (20), palonosetron was compared with ondansetron given at a dose of 32 mg on the day of chemotherapy. In this trial, steroids for delayed emesis were not consistently given or mandated by trial design. In a post hoc subgroup analysis, patients who did receive steroids had improvements in both acute and delayed emesis in the palonosetron group compared with ondansetron. Palonosetron (21) was also compared with granisetron in patients receiving either cisplatin or combination therapy with doxorubicin or epirubicin and cyclophosphamide. Patients were randomized to either a single dose of palonosetron at 0.75 mg or granisetron 40 µg/kg prior to chemotherapy. All patients received steroids for delayed emesis. Palonosetron was found to be similar in efficacy in the acute phase, with a 75.3% response rate in the palonosetron group compared with 73.3% in the granisetron group. However, palonosetron was found to be superior to granisetron for delayed emesis, with 56.8% of patients in the palonosetron group experiencing a complete response compared with 44.5% ($p < 0.0001$) of patients treated with granisetron. Overall, 56.8% of patients experienced no vomiting through the acute and delayed phase compared with 44.5% in the granisetron group ($p < 0.0001$). Complete response was defined as no vomiting or use of rescue medications. In highly emetogenic chemotherapy, palonosetron appears to be more efficacious than first-generation 5-HT$_3$ antagonists, though the antiemetic regimen for highly emetogenic chemotherapy now includes NK$_1$ antagonists, and the comparison of first-generation 5-HT$_3$ antagonists with palonosetron when used with an NK$_1$ antagonist is unknown.

Two large phase III trials (22,23) have compared palonosetron with first-generation 5-HT$_3$ antagonists in moderately emetogenic chemotherapy. These trials were designed as noninferiority studies and in this setting, palonosetron was found to be noninferior to the first-generation 5-HT$_3$ antagonist. In one trial comparing dolasetron 100 mg with palonosetron at 0.25 mg, palonosetron was found in post hoc analysis to have a higher rate of complete response in the delayed emesis setting as well as overall. In the other trial, ondansetron given at a dose of 32 mg was found to have a decreased rate of complete response compared with palonosetron 0.25 mg in both acute and delayed emesis as well as overall. This was also a post hoc analysis.

Corticosteroids

Corticosteroids have been an integral part of the prevention and treatment of nausea and vomiting for decades. A large meta-analysis (24) looked at a select group of 32 studies that used dexamethasone as antiemetic prophylaxis in a comparative setting. More than 5,000 patients were included. The analysis concluded that dexamethasone increased the chances of no vomiting in the acute setting by 25% to 30%. It was also found to be superior to metoclopramide, though comparable to a 5-HT$_3$ receptor antagonist in the acute setting. In the delayed setting, dexamethasone also increased the chances of no vomiting by 25% to 30%. In this setting, a trend toward superior efficacy was noted compared with metoclopramide. One trial compared dexamethasone to a 5-HT$_3$ receptor antagonist and found dexamethasone to be more effective in the delayed emesis setting. Steroids are most often used with additional antiemetics for prevention in highly emetogenic and moderately emetogenic chemotherapy or as a single agent for prevention with the use of mildly emetogenic chemotherapy agents.

NK$_1$ Receptor Antagonists

The newest class of drugs to be used in the prevention of CINV are antagonists of the binding of substance P to the NK$_1$ receptor. In an early study with substance P antagonists (25), 159 patients treated with cisplatin of at least 70 mg/m^2 were randomized to one of three groups. All groups were treated with dexamethasone at a dose of 20 mg and granisetron prior to cisplatin. Delayed emesis was given as rescue medication, but not prophylactically and consisted of oral or IV metoclopramide and/or oral

dexamethasone. Group one was also given the substance P antagonist L-754,030 at 400 mg on days 2 to 5, group two was given L-754,030 on day 1 only and placebo on days 2 to 5, and group three was given placebo on days 1 to 5 in addition to the standard antiemetic prophylaxis. The groups receiving the L-754,030 had the least amount of vomiting, with 93% reporting no vomiting in group one, 94% in group two, and 67% in group three ($p < 0.001$ for the comparison between groups one and two with group three). Patients randomized to the substance P antagonist also fared better during the delayed emesis phase. In patients receiving daily L-754,030, 52% had no emesis and used no rescue medications, compared with 43% of patients in group two and 16% of patients in group three ($p < 0.001$ for the comparison between groups one and three, $p = 0.003$ for the comparison between groups two and three). Nausea was also measured using a visual analogue scale. Nausea scores were lower in group one compared with group three for days 1 to 5 ($p = 0.003$) and in groups one and two compared with placebo on day 2 ($p = 0.002$ for group one vs. group three, $p = 0.005$ for group two vs. group three). L-754,030 has gone on to further study and is now in routine clinical use under the generic name aprepitant. Aprepitant was the first substance P antagonist to enter clinical use. Casopitant is another NK$_1$ antagonist that has similar efficacy to aprepitant but was tested mainly as a single daily dose, either orally or intravenously. The manufacturer of casopitant has decided not to pursue regulatory approval for this medication (26). An IV formulation, fosaprepitant is also in routine clinical use.

The importance of aprepitant was shown in a phase III trial (27) in patients being treated with high-dose cisplatin. In this trial, more than 500 patients were randomized to either aprepitant plus ondansetron and dexamethasone or ondansetron, dexamethasone, and placebo. All patients received delayed emesis protection with dexamethasone on days 1 through 4; patients in the aprepitant group also received aprepitant on days 2 and 3. The groups receiving aprepitant fared better in all categories. For acute emesis, the complete response rate was 89.2% compared with 78.1% ($p < 0.001$), whereas for delayed emesis, the compete response rate was 75.4% compared with 55.8% ($p < 0.001$). Similarly, the overall complete response rate was 72.7% in the aprepitant group compared with 52.3% in the group that received placebo plus ondansetron and dexamethasone. Another phase III trial originating in Latin America and using similar trial design in patients receiving highly emetogenic chemotherapy showed comparable outcomes (28).

Though cyclophosphamide and doxorubicin (AC) are considered moderately emetogenic chemotherapy agents, the combination is considered more emetogenic than other moderately emetogenic combinations. In breast cancer setting where this combination is used most frequently, aprepitant has been studied in addition to an ondansetron- and dexamethasone-containing premedication regimen. In one study (29), aprepitant was used for delayed emesis in the experimental arm, whereas ondansetron was used for delayed emesis in the control arm. During the 5 days studied, the aprepitant-containing regimen was found to offer better protection, with an overall complete response rate of 50.8% compared with 42.5% in the arm treated with ondansetron and dexamethasone alone. The data for the use of aprepitant in other types of moderately emetogenic chemotherapy are not as clear. In a phase III study (30), the addition of aprepitant with different moderately emetogenic chemotherapy regimens including doxorubicin and cyclophosphamide was tested. All patients received ondansetron and dexamethasone. Overall, complete response was better in the aprepitant-containing arm (62.8% vs. 47.1%, $p < 0.01$). However, retrospective analysis considered the doxorubicin/cyclophosphamide-containing regimens separately and found that the aprepitant-containing arms continued to be superior, while complete response rates were similar among other moderately emetogenic regimens regardless of the treatment arm.

Like other chemotherapy side effects, nausea and vomiting can increase with subsequent chemotherapy cycles. There is a suggestion that aprepitant may improve the durability of CINV protection. In one series of approximately 200 patients receiving at least 70 mg/m^2 of cisplatin, patients were given a premedication regimen of ondansetron and dexamethasone on day 1 and dexamethasone on days 2 through 5 and randomized to aprepitant or placebo on days 1 through 3. Antiemetic protection was recorded through six cycles of chemotherapy. In the first cycle, the complete response rate was 64% in the aprepitant group compared with 49% ($p < 0.05$) in the group treated with ondansetron and dexamethasone alone. By cycle 6, the complete response rate was 59% in the aprepitant-containing group but had dropped to 34% in the ondansetron and dexamethasone group ($p < 0.05$) (31).

The effectiveness of aprepitant might raise the question of how much additional contribution is being made by including the 5-HT$_3$ receptor antagonist. One series (32) looked at a regimen of aprepitant, dexamethasone, and granisetron compared with aprepitant, dexamethasone, and placebo in more than 300 patients receiving highly emetogenic chemotherapy. The group with all three active drugs fared the best, with an overall complete response rate of 80% compared with 57% in the placebo-containing group ($p < 0.01$).

The dosing and schedule of aprepitant have evolved with the introduction of the IV preparation fosaprepitant. In a noninferiority study (33), the 3-day oral regimen of aprepitant (125 mg on day 1, 80 mg on days 2 and 3) was compared with a single dose of fosaprepitant of 150 mg. The study included 2,322 patients who were starting treatment with cisplatin at a dose of at least 70 mg/m^2. All patients received dexamethasone for delayed emesis. Similar rates of complete response were seen in both arms, with an overall complete response rate of 71.9% in the fosaprepitant group compared with 72.3% in the aprepitant group. Complete response rates were similar for acute and delayed emesis considered separately, as was the use of rescue medications and nausea.

Side effects of aprepitant are few. Headache and constipation are reported, though in the study that compared aprepitant-containing regimens to those without a 5-HT$_3$ receptor antagonist, no significant difference was noted between the groups (32). Aprepitant is an inhibitor of the cytochrome P450 enzyme CYP3A4, which has implications for interactions with chemotherapy and other medications. Aprepitant decreases the metabolism of dexamethasone and therefore plasma concentrations are higher when given with aprepitant (34). This has led to a reduction in the dose of dexamethasone when it is given with aprepitant from 20 to 12 mg on day 1, and 8 to 4 mg on days 2 and 3. Steroids are not decreased, however, when they are part of an antineoplastic regimen. Aprepitant does not seem to have any clinically meaningful interactions with chemotherapy.

Other Drugs Useful in CINV

Though the mainstay of prevention of CINV includes dexamethasone, 5-HT$_3$ antagonists, and NK$_1$ antagonists, other medications may be useful in cases of intolerance to standard antiemetic therapy or as a supplement when standard preventive regimens fall short. Phenothiazines such as prochlorperazine are often used as single agents to prevent CINV given prior to administration of chemotherapy agents of low emetic risk or as rescue medication for nausea or vomiting that occurs despite prophylaxis. Benzodiazepines are also used for nausea and vomiting that occurs despite prophylaxis, as well as for anticipatory CINV. Cannabinoids may be useful as supplemental agents when standard antiemetic protection fails. They are considered to have weak antiemetic properties but can have significant side effects including sedation, dizziness, and dysphoria.

Olanzapine has antagonist properties against multiple pathways relevant to CINV including dopamine and 5-HT$_3$ receptors (35). It has been studied in combination with a 5-HT$_3$ receptor antagonist and was found to control both acute and delayed emesis (36). It has also been compared with aprepitant directly. In a study (37) of patients undergoing treatment with either high-dose cisplatin or the combination of doxorubicin and cyclophosphamide, the combination of aprepitant (days 1 to 3), palonosetron (day 1), and dexamethasone (days 2 to 4) was compared with olanzapine, palonosetron, and dexamethasone. Palonosetron and dexamethasone were dosed similarly in both arms. Olanzapine was given at a dose of 10 mg orally on days 1 to 4. There was an overall complete response rate of 73% in the aprepitant-containing arm compared with 77% in the olanzapine-containing arm, which was not a statistically significant difference. Nausea, however, was better controlled in the olanzapine arm in both the delayed emesis time period and overall, with 69% of patients on the olanzapine arm reporting no nausea compared with 38% in the aprepitant arm for both parameters ($p < 0.01$). However, new data have since been produced and the ASCO 2020 update now incorporates olanzapine into antiemetic regimens for certain chemotherapy regimens (12).

MANAGEMENT OF CINV

The goal of antiemetic therapy in treatment-related nausea and vomiting is complete prevention; therefore, a guideline-driven approach to choose the optimal antiemetic regimen for the chemotherapy given is important. The level of emetogenicity is defined by the chemotherapeutic agent of greater emetic risk. It may be useful to provide antiemetics for patients to have at home in case nausea or vomiting occurs despite optimal prophylaxis. Nausea and vomiting in the cancer patient may be complex and difficult to discern, as there are multiple potential causes of emesis in addition to chemotherapy that the practitioner needs to consider, such as constipation, small bowel obstruction or ileus, metabolic disturbances, and occult central nervous system metastases.

Highly Emetogenic Chemotherapy

The optimal preventative therapy for highly emetogenic chemotherapy is a four-drug combination of NK$_1$ receptor antagonist, a serotonin (5-HT$_3$) receptor antagonist, dexamethasone, and olanzapine on day 1 (Table 12.3). Dexamethasone and olanzapine should be continued on days 2 to 4 for delayed emesis (12). The addition of olanzapine stems from a phase III study of 705 patients with nonhematologic malignancies from 26 hospitals in Japan who were treated with antiemetics while undergoing cisplatin chemotherapy (38). In this study, all patients were prophylactically treated with a guideline-recommended three-drug antiemetic regimen of aprepitant, palonosetron, and dexamethasone while 354 patients were randomly assigned to also receive 5 mg of olanzapine as part of their antiemetic regimen. Overall, 276 patients (78%; 95% CI 74 to 82) in the olanzapine group achieved a complete response as compared to 223 patients (64%; 95% CI 59 to 69) in the placebo group

TABLE 12.3 RECOMMENDED ANTIEMETIC THERAPY FOR SINGLE-DAY INTRAVENOUS CHEMOTHERAPY

Emetic risk	Prevention of acute emesis	Prevention of delayed emesis
High	5-HT$_3$ receptor antagonists: Granisetron 2 mg oral; 0.01 mg/kg or 1 mg IV Ondansetron 8 mg oral twice daily; 8 mg or 0.15 mg/kg IV Dolasetron 100 mg oral Tropisetron 5 mg oral or IV Ramosetron 0.3 mg IV Palonosetron 0.5 mg oral; 0.25 mg IV Dexamethasone: 12 mg oral or IV Aprepitant: 125 mg oral or Fosaprepitant: 150 mg IV Olanzapine 10 or 5 mg oral	Dexamethasone 8 mg oral or IV days 2–4 plus aprepitant 80 mg days 2 and 3 or dexamethasone 8 mg oral or IV alone if fosaprepitant is used Olanzapine 10 or 5 mg oral on days 2–4
Moderate	Palonosetron 0.5 mg oral; 0.25 mg IV Dexamethasone 12 mg oral or IV	Dexamethasone 8 mg days 2 and 3
Low	Dexamethasone 8 mg or prochlorperazine 10 mg oral or IV	No preventive measures
Minimal	As needed	No preventive measures

($p < 0.0001$). However, complete response was more significant in the delayed phase ($p < 0.0001$) versus the acute phase ($p = 0.0021$).

Anthracyclines combined with cyclophosphamide regimens are considered to be highly emetogenic and thus patients on these regimens should also receive the same four-drug combination. However, only olanzapine should be continued on days 2 to 4.

Moderately Emetogenic Chemotherapy

The optimal preventive regimen for moderately emetogenic chemotherapy is a 5-HT$_3$ receptor antagonist and dexamethasone. Palonosetron has been shown to have superiority over first-generation 5-HT$_3$ receptor antagonists in this setting (Table 12.3). Chemotherapy regimens with moderate-emetic-risk antineoplastic agents known to cause delayed nausea and vomiting (i.e., cyclophosphamide, doxorubicin, oxaliplatin) should be offered dexamethasone on days 2 to 3. The utility of dexamethasone for delayed emesis was looked at in a phase III study (39) of patients receiving a variety of moderately emetogenic chemotherapy regimens including AC. There was no difference in complete response rates in the acute phase between the group receiving 1 day of dexamethasone and the 3-day regimen (88.6% vs. 84.3%; $p = 0.262$) or the delayed phase (68.7% vs. 77.7%; $p = 0.116$). There was a preplanned subset analysis of AC chemotherapy versus non-AC regimens. In the non-AC group, there was no difference in the complete response rates between the two treatment groups in either the acute or delayed phases. Dexamethasone continues to be incorporated into ASCO guidelines for delayed emesis until these data can be validated.

Low and Minimal Emetogenic Chemotherapy

The optimal preventive regimen for low-risk emetogenic chemotherapy is either a single dose of a 5-HT$_3$ receptor antagonist or single 8 mg dose of dexamethasone on day 1 prior to administration (Table 12.3) (12). For minimal risk emetogenic chemotherapy, no prophylaxis is recommended (Table 12.3).

Chemotherapy Given over Multiple Days

The optimal preventive regimen for chemotherapy regimens given over multiple days is more complex, particularly when highly emetogenic chemotherapy is used, and there are little data. One approach is to use a 5-HT$_3$ receptor antagonist daily during chemotherapy followed by dexamethasone for delayed emesis after the chemotherapy is complete (40). The granisetron patch is another option, as its efficacy is designed to last 7 days. The Hoosier Oncology Group incorporated aprepitant daily into a 5-day cisplatin regimen for testicular cancer patients in addition to a 5-HT$_3$ antagonist and dexamethasone. A preliminary report suggests that it is safe and well tolerated (41). ASCO guidelines in 2020 recommend that antiemetics be given according to the emetogenicity of the chemotherapy given on each day and for 2 days after the completion of the chemotherapy (12).

High-Dose Chemotherapy

High-dose chemotherapy in anticipation of transplant also presents a challenge in terms of emesis. ASCO guidelines recommend a three-drug combination of NK$_1$ receptor antagonist, a 5-HT$_3$ receptor antagonist, and dexamethasone for those receiving high-dose chemotherapy in anticipation of hematopoietic stem-cell transplantation. There is new, low quality and weak evidence to suggest the addition of olanzapine to the antiemetic regimen for these adults. A study of 101 patients looked to compare complete response during the overall, acute (chemotherapy days) and delayed phase (5 days after chemotherapy administration) in patients receiving 10 mg of olanzapine in addition to guideline-approved three-drug antiemetic regimen while undergoing high-dose chemotherapy for stem cell transplantation (42). The olanzapine group had significantly more patients with complete response versus the placebo group (55% vs. 26%; $p = 0.003$) for the overall period as well as the delayed period (60.8% vs. 30%; $p = 0.001$). However, no difference was found between the two arms in the acute phase (76% vs. 62%; $p = 0.13$).

Anticipatory Nausea and Vomiting

Anticipatory nausea and vomiting can be difficult to manage. The best preventative measure is insuring that optimal antiemetic prophylaxis is given, starting with the first cycle of chemotherapy. The incidence of anticipatory nausea and vomiting has decreased as antiemetic therapies have improved. If it does develop, potential options or management includes systemic desensitization, hypnosis, or pharmacologic therapy, though often routinely given antiemetics are not effective. Benzodiazepines and a support group showed benefit in one study (43).

Nausea and Vomiting Despite Prophylaxis

At times, despite guideline-driven prophylaxis, patients develop nausea and vomiting during the course of their cancer treatment. The first step in management is an evaluation of the cause of nausea and vomiting to ensure it represents a failure of antiemetic therapy or is the result of another process. Adults with breakthrough nausea despite receiving optimal prophylaxis who did not receive olanzapine prophylactically should be given olanzapine. Those who have breakthrough nausea and have already received olanzapine should be offered an antiemetic of a different class in addition to continuing an antiemetic regimen (12). The addition of a benzodiazepine may be of use. High-dose metoclopramide may also be used in the place of a 5-HT$_3$ receptor antagonist.

ORAL CHEMOTHERAPY

Though nausea and vomiting may be a significant risk with oral chemotherapy, it does not follow the same pattern of acute and delayed emesis that IV chemotherapy does, as oral therapies are often given on a continuous basis. The ESMO/MASCC guidelines (11) include oral chemotherapy, though the risks of emesis are not as well established as with IV therapy (see Table 12.4). The ESMO/MASCC guidelines divide agents into similar high,

TABLE 12.4 ANTIEMETIC CLASSIFICATION OF ORAL CHEMOTHERAPY

Degree of emetogenicity	Agent
High (>90%)	Hexamethylmelamine
	Procarbazine
Moderate (30%–90%)	Cyclophosphamide
	Temozolomide
	Vinorelbine
	Imatinib
Low (10%–30%)	Capecitabine
	Tegafur–uracil
	Fludarabine
	Etoposide
	Sunitinib
	Everolimus
	Lapatinib
	Lenalidomide
	Thalidomide
Minimal (<10%)	Chlorambucil
	Hydroxyurea
	L-Phenylalanine mustard
	6-Thioguanine
	Methotrexate
	Gefitinib
	Erlotinib
	Sorafenib

moderate, low, and minimal risk categories. No recommendation was made regarding antiemetic prophylaxis, though it would seem reasonable to use a well-tolerated phenothiazine or 5-HT$_3$ receptor antagonist prophylactically in patients being treated with highly emetogenic oral chemotherapy or for patients in whom nausea or vomiting develops.

Immune Checkpoint Inhibitors

Immune checkpoint inhibitors (CPIs), which work by disrupting signaling on immune cells to ultimately prime them to attack tumor cells, are now more commonly used and some have even become standard of care in the management of several advanced solid malignancies (44). A concern previously raised was whether guideline-endorsed antiemetic regimens including dexamethasone be modified when CPIs are incorporated. The hypothesis is that concurrent corticosteroid use could adversely affect the therapeutic efficacy of CPIs through their immunosuppressive effects. A systematic review of 27 articles that sought to review the interactions between immune CPIs and corticosteroids did not find definitive evidence to conclude that concomitant use lead to poorer clinical outcomes (45). An expert panel convened by ASCO looked at 10 randomized controlled trials comparing the combination of chemotherapy and a CPI with chemotherapy alone and found several that demonstrated superior overall survival and progression free survival when the combination was used. Of those trials, two specified for corticosteroid-containing antiemetic regimens to be used (46,47). Both were phase III trials comparing the addition of the CPI pembrolizumab to platinum-based, high emetogenic chemotherapy for adult patients with metastatic squamous non–small cell lung cancers. Both trials showed significant overall survival and progression-free survival in the pembrolizumab arm despite the concurrent use of prophylactic antiemetics that included corticosteroids. ASCO guidelines in 2020 concluded that the addition of CPIs to chemotherapy does not change the guideline recommendation for an antiemetic regimen based on the emetogenicity of the agents administered. They also state that CPIs administered alone or in combination with another CPI are minimally emetogenic and do not require the routine use of a prophylactic antiemetic.

RADIATION-INDUCED NAUSEA AND VOMITING

There are less randomized data to base recommendations for RINV compared with CINV. Both ESMO/MASCC (11) and ASCO guidelines (12)

TABLE 12.5 RECOMMENDED ANTIEMETIC THERAPY FOR RADIATION-INDUCED NAUSEA AND VOMITING

Risk level	Irradiated area	Antiemetic guidelines
High (>90%)	Total body irradiation, total nodal irradiation	Prophylaxis with **5-HT₃ receptor antagonists:** Granisetron 2 mg oral; 0.01 mg/kg or 1 mg IV Ondansetron 8 mg oral twice daily; 8 mg or 0.15 mg/kg IV Dolasetron 100 mg oral Tropisetron 5 mg oral or IV Palonosetron 0.5 mg oral; 0.25 mg IV plus **dexamethasone** 4 mg oral or IV days 1–5
Moderate (60%–90%)	Upper abdomen, HBI, UBI	Prophylaxis with **5-HT₃ receptor antagonists:** Granisetron 2 mg oral; 0.01 mg/kg or 1 mg IV Ondansetron 8 mg oral twice daily; 8 mg or 0.15 mg/kg IV Dolasetron 100 mg oral Tropisetron 5 mg oral or IV Palonosetron 0.5 mg oral; 0.25 mg IV plus **dexamethasone** 4 mg oral or IV days 1–5
Low (30%–60%)	Cranium, craniospinal, H&N, lower thorax region, pelvis	Prophylaxis or rescue with **5-HT₃ receptor antagonists:** Granisetron 2 mg oral; 0.01 mg/kg or 1 mg IV Ondansetron 8 mg oral twice daily; 8 mg or 0.15 mg/kg IV Dolasetron 100 mg oral Tropisetron 5 mg oral or IV Palonosetron 0.5 mg oral; 0.25 mg IV
Minimal (<30%)	Extremities, breast	Rescue with **dopamine receptor antagonists** or **5-HT₃ receptor antagonists:** Granisetron 2 mg oral; 0.01 mg/kg or 1 mg IV Ondansetron 8 mg oral twice daily; 8 mg or 0.15 mg/kg IV Dolasetron 100 mg oral Tropisetron 5 mg oral or IV Palonosetron 0.5 mg oral; 0.25 mg IV

HBI, half-body irradiation; UBI, upper body irradiation; H&N, head and neck.
In low or minimal risk situations, if a patient requires rescue antiemetics, therapy should then be used prophylactically for the remainder of treatment.

recommend the use of a 5-HT₃ antagonist with both moderately and highly emetogenic radiation therapy, which includes total body or total nodal irradiation, and moderately emetogenic radiation, which includes the upper abdomen or half-body irradiation (Table 12.5). Dexamethasone is also recommended during fractions 1 to 5 at a dose of 4 mg daily. The addition of dexamethasone is supported by a study of 211 patients undergoing radiation to the upper abdomen (48). In this trial, all patients were treated with a daily prophylactic 5-HT₃ receptor antagonist and randomized to dexamethasone 4 mg daily on fractions 1 to 5 or placebo. During the prophylactic period, while dexamethasone was being given, no difference in complete control of emesis, nausea, or the use of rescue medications was noted. However, parameters were looked at over fractions 1 to 15 and improvements in overall nausea were noted, as well as better complete protection from vomiting (23% vs. 12%, $p = 0.02$) and a trend toward less use of rescue medications (71% vs. 82%, $p = 0.09$). For radiation in the low-risk category, a 5-HT₃ antagonist is recommended as prophylaxis or rescue medication. For minimal risk, rescue therapy only is recommended, though if used, subsequent

prophylaxis is recommended. When treatment involves combined chemotherapy and radiation, antiemetic prophylaxis is given on the basis of the chemotherapeutic agent unless the risk of emesis is higher from the radiation.

COMPLEMENTARY THERAPIES

In addition to standard pharmacologic therapy to prevent treatment-related nausea and vomiting, alternative therapies and techniques have been studied in addition to or in place of antiemetic therapy. Acupuncture has long been reported to decrease nausea and vomiting, and several studies have investigated its use in treatment-related nausea and vomiting. The P6 acupuncture point, which is located three fingerbreadths proximal to the flexor crease of the wrist, is the most commonly used acupuncture point. In a meta-analysis (49) of studies testing acupuncture in CINV, several techniques were investigated including acupuncture (using a needle), electroacupuncture (acupuncture with the addition of an electrical current), non-invasive electrostimulation (using a wrist device without a needle), and acupressure (manual pressure on the acupuncture site). There were mixed results. Overall, acupuncture decreased the rate of vomiting, but many of the studies included did not follow guidelines in terms of antiemetic therapy. In one that did, there was no effect of the acupuncture. While this implies that acupuncture may have an antiemetic effect, how these data should be used in clinical practice is unclear and no major guideline has included acupuncture as a recommended therapy.

Nausea can be a challenging problem both to treat and to study. In one study of 644 patients, those who experienced nausea with prior chemotherapy cycles were randomized to varying doses of ginger or placebo (50). Ginger extract was given for 6 days starting 3 days before chemotherapy. All doses of ginger were found to decrease nausea ($p = 0.003$), with the largest reduction occurring with the lower two doses. This is an intriguing data set that requires validation and further study.

FUTURE DIRECTIONS

Clinical and basic science research in the area of treatment-induced nausea and vomiting continues. Additional research will best define the optimal prophylaxis of moderately emetogenic therapy in both the acute and delayed settings. Current research involves expansion of the various classes of drugs that are in current use for prophylaxis as well as trials of new medications such as olanzapine, whose role continues to evolve. The delivery of antiemetic therapy remains an active area of research, testing newer ways to administer antiemetic therapy such as transdermal methods or as a dissolving tablet. Nausea continues to be a difficult problem for cancer patients and current research is also focusing on this important area. In addition, patient-reported outcomes are more frequently being used in an attempt to more accurately reflect patient's experiences and side effects. As personalized medicine continues to move forward, another active area of research is the influence of genetic makeup on the risk of emesis and degree of protection from particular antiemetic therapies. For example, 5-HT$_3$ receptor antagonists are metabolized by the cytochrome P450 system, of which there are more than 30 types of isoenzymes that participate in metabolism (51).

CONCLUSION

Nausea and vomiting remains a difficult problem and is widely feared by patients receiving cancer treatment. The last several decades have seen tremendous advances with new pharmacologic therapy for the prevention of treatment-related nausea and vomiting. Challenges remain, including

nausea, emesis that occurs despite prophylaxis, and adherence to guidelines. Future directions should address quality measures as they relate to appropriate antiemetic prophylaxis and new therapies to improve upon the gains that have been made.

REFERENCES

1. Martin CG, Rubenstein EB, Elting LS, et al. Measuring chemotherapy-induced nausea and emesis. *Cancer.* 2003;98:645-655.
2. Kris MG, Gralla RJ, Clark RA. Incidence, course and severity of delayed nausea and vomiting following the administration of high-dose cisplatin. *J Clin Oncol.* 1985;3:1379-1384.
3. Osoba D, Zee B, Pater J, et al. Determinants of post-chemotherapy nausea and vomiting in patients with cancer. *J Clin Oncol.* 1997;15:116-123.
4. Pollera CF, Giannarelli D. Prognostic factors influencing cisplatin-induced emesis. *Cancer.* 1989;64: 1117-1122.
5. Hesketh PJ, Kris MJ, Grunberg SM, et al. Proposal for classifying the acute emetogenicity of cancer chemotherapy. *J Clin Oncol.* 1997;15:103-109.
6. Blanchard EM, Hesketh PJ. Management of adverse effects of treatment: nausea and vomiting. In: DeVita VT, et al., eds. *Cancer: Principles and Practice of Oncology.* Philadelphia, PA: Lippincott Williams and Wilkins; 2011:2321-2328.
7. Hesketh PJ. Drug therapy: chemotherapy induced nausea and vomiting. *N Engl J Med.* 2008;358:2482-2494.
8. Hesketh PJ. Understanding the pathobiology of chemotherapy-induced nausea and vomiting. *Oncology.* 2004;18:9-14.
9. Andrews PLR, Sanders GJ. Abdominal afferent neurons: an important target for the treatment of gastrointestinal dysfunction. *Curr Opin Pharmacol.* 2002;2:650-656.
10. Hesketh PJ, van Bells S, Aapro M, et al. Differential involvement of neurotransmitters through the time course of cisplatin-induced emesis as revealed through specific antagonists. *Eur J Cancer.* 2003;39:1074-1080.
11. Roila F, Herrstedt J, Aapro M, et al. Guideline update for MASCC and ESMO in the prevention of chemotherapy- and radiotherapy-induced nausea and vomiting: results of the Perugia consensus conference. *Ann Oncol.* 2010;21:v232-v243.
12. Hesketh PJ, Kris MG, Basch E, et al. Antiemetics: American Society of Clinical Oncology guideline update. *J Clin Oncol.* 2020;38:2782-2797.
13. Miner WD, Sanger GJ, Turner DH. Evidence that 5-hydroxytryptamine 3 receptors mediate cytotoxic drug and radiation-evoked emesis. *Br J Cancer.* 1987;56:159-162.
14. Perez EZ, Hesketh P, Sandbach J, et al. Comparison of single dose oral granisetron versus intravenous ondansetron in the prevention of nausea and vomiting induced by moderately emetogenic chemotherapy: a multicenter, double-blind, randomized parallel study. *J Clin Oncol.* 1998;16:754-760.
15. Kris MG, Hesketh PJ, Somerfield MR, et al. American Society of Clinical Oncology guideline for antiemetics in oncology: update 2006. *J Clin Oncol.* 2006;24:2932-2947.
16. Jordan K, Hinke A, Grothey A, et al. A meta-analysis comparing the efficacy of four 5-HT-3 receptor antagonists for acute chemotherapy-induced emesis. *Support Care Cancer.* 2007;15:1023-1033.
17. Hainsworth J, Harvey W, Pendergrass K, et al. A single-blind comparison of intravenous ondansetron, a

selective serotonin antagonist, with intravenous meto-clopramide in the prevention of nausea and vomiting associated with high-dose cisplatin chemotherapy. *J Clin Oncol.* 1991;9:721-728.

18. Boccia RV, Gordan LN, Clark G, et al. Efficacy and tolerability of transdermal granisetron for the control of chemotherapy-induced nausea and vomiting associated with moderately and highly emetogenic multi-day chemotherapy: a randomized, double blind, phase III study. *Support Care Cancer.* 2011;19:1609-1617.

19. Grunberg S, Voisin E, Zufferli M, Piraccini G. Oral palonosetron is as effective as intravenous palonosetron: a phase 3 dose ranging trial in patients receiving moderately emetogenic chemotherapy. *Eur J Cancer.* 2007;5(suppl 5):155.

20. Aapro MS, Grunberg SM, Manikas GM, et al. A phase II double blind, randomized trial of palonosetron compared with ondansetron in preventing chemotherapy-induced nausea and vomiting following highly emetogenic chemotherapy. *Ann Oncol.* 2006;17:1441-1449.

21. Saito M, Aogi K, Sekine I, et al. Palonosetron plus dexamethasone versus granisetron plus dexamethasone for prevention of nausea and vomiting during chemotherapy: a double-blind, double dummy, randomized, comparative phase III trial. *Lancet Oncol.* 2009;10:115-124.

22. Eisenberg P, Figueroa-Vadillo J, Zamora R, et al. Improved prevention of moderately emetogenic chemotherapy-induced nausea and vomiting with palonosetron, a pharmacologically novel 5-HT3 receptor antagonist: results of a phase III, single-dose trial versus dolasetron. *Cancer.* 2003;93:2473-2482.

23. Gralla R, Lichinitser M, Van Der Vegt S, et al. Palonosetron improves prevention of chemotherapy-induced nausea and vomiting following moderately emetogenic chemotherapy: results of a double-blind randomized phase III trial comparing single doses of palonosetron with ondansetron. *Ann Oncol.* 2003;14:1570-1577.

24. Ioannidis JPA, Hesketh PJ, Lau J. Contribution of dexamethasone to control of chemotherapy-induced nausea and vomiting: a meta-analysis of randomized evidence. *J Clin Oncol.* 2000;18:3409-3422.

25. Navari RM, Reinhardt RR, Gralla RJ, et al. Reduction of cisplatin-induced emesis by a selective neurokinin-1-receptor antagonist. *N Engl J Med.* 1999;340:190-195.

26. Grunberg S, Rolski J, Strausz J, et al. Efficacy and safety of casopitant mesylate, a neurokinin-1 (NK1)-antagonist in the prevention of chemotherapy related nausea and vomiting in patients receiving cisplatin based highly emetogenic chemotherapy: a randomized, double-blind placebo-controlled trial. *Lancet Oncol.* 2009;10:549-558.

27. Hesketh PJ, Grunberg SM, Gralla RJ, et al. The oral neurokinin-1 antagonists aprepitant for the prevention of chemotherapy-induced nausea and vomiting: a multinational, randomized, double-blind, placebo-controlled trial in patients receiving high-dose cisplatin—the aprepitant protocol 052 study group. *J Clin Oncol.* 2003;21:4112-4119.

28. Poli-Bigelli S, Rodrigues-Pereira J, Carides AD, et al. Addition of the neurokinin 1 receptor antagonist aprepitant to standard antiemetic therapy improves control of chemotherapy induced nausea and vomiting. *Cancer.* 2003;97:3090-3098.

29. Warr DG, Hesketh PJ, Gralla RJ, et al. Efficacy and tolerability of aprepitant for the prevention of chemotherapy-induced nausea and vomiting in patients with breast cancer after moderately emetogenic chemotherapy. *J Clin Oncol.* 2005;23:2822-2830.

30. Rapoport BL, Jordan K, Boice JA, et al. Aprepitant for the prevention of chemotherapy-induced nausea and vomiting associated with a broad range of moderately emetogenic chemotherapy and tumor types: a randomized, double blind study. *Support Care Cancer.* 2010;18:423-431.

31. de Wit R, Herrstedt J, Rapoport B, et al. Addition of the oral NK1 antagonist aprepitant to standard antiemetics provides protection against nausea and vomiting during multiple cycles of cisplatin-based chemotherapy. *J Clin Oncol.* 2003;21:4105-4111.

32. Campos D, Pereira JR, Reinhardt RR, et al. Prevention of cisplatin-induced emesis by the oral neurokinin-1 antagonist, MK-869, in combination with granisetron and dexamethasone or with dexamethasone alone. *J Clin Oncol.* 2001;19:1759-1767.

33. Grunberg S, Chua D, Maru A, et al. Single dose fosaprepitant for the prevention of chemotherapy-induced nausea and vomiting associated with cisplatin therapy: randomized, double blind study protocol-EASE. *J Clin Oncol.* 2011;29:1495-1501.

34. McCrea JB, Majumdar AK, Goldberg MR, et al. Effects of the neurokinin 1 antagonist aprepitant on the pharmacokinetics of dexamethasone and methylprednisolone. *Clin Pharmacol Ther.* 2003;74:17-24.

35. Feyer P, Jordan K. Update and new trends in antiemetic therapy: the continuing need for novel therapies. *Ann Oncol.* 2011;22:30-38.

36. Navari RM, Einhorn LH, Passik SD, et al. A phase II trial of olanzapine for the prevention of chemotherapy-induced nausea and vomiting: a Hoosier Oncology Group study. *Support Care Cancer.* 2005;13:529-534.

37. Navari RM, Gray SE, Kerr AC. Olanzapine versus aprepitant for the prevention of chemotherapy induced nausea and vomiting: a randomized phase III trial. *J Support Oncol.* 2011;9:188-195.

38. Hashimoto H, Abe M, Tokuyama O, et al. Olanzapine 5 mg plus standard antiemetic therapy for the prevention of chemotherapy-induced nausea and vomiting (J-FORCE): a multicentre, randomised, double-blind, placebo-controlled, phase 3 trial. *Lancet Oncol.* 2020;21:242-249.

39. Celio L, Frustaci S, Denaro A. Palonosetron in combination with 1-day versus 3-day dexamethasone for prevention of nausea and vomiting following moderately emetogenic chemotherapy: a randomized, multicenter, phase III trial. *Support Care Cancer.* 2011;19:1217-1225.

40. Einhorn LH, Rapoport B, Koeller J, et al. Antiemetic therapy for multiple-day chemotherapy and high dose chemotherapy with stem cell transplant: review and consensus statement. *Support Care Cancer.* 2005;13:112-116.

41. Brames M, Johnston E, Nichols C, et al. Phase III study of granisetron+dexamethasone +/− aprepitant in patients with germ cell tumors undergoing 5 day courses of cisplatin based combination: a Hoosier Oncology Group (H.O.G.) study. *Support Care Cancer.* 2009;17:871-872 (abstract).

42. Clemmons AB, Orr J, Andrick B, et al. Randomized, placebo-controlled, phase III trial of Fosaprepitant, Ondansetron, Dexamethasone (FOND) versus FOND Plus Olanzapine (FOND-O) for the prevention of chemotherapy-induced nausea and vomiting in patients with hematologic malignancies receiving highly emetogenic chemotherapy and hematopoietic cell transplantation regimens: the FOND-O Trial. *Biol Blood Marrow Transplant.* 2018;24:2065-2071.

43. Razavi D, Delvuax N, Farvacques C, et al. Prevention of adjustment disorders and anticipatory nausea

secondary to adjuvant chemotherapy: a double-blind, placebo-controlled study assessing the usefulness of alprazolam. *J Clin Oncol*. 1993;11:1384-1390.

44. Dine J, Gordon R, Shames Y, Kasler MK, Barton-Burke M. Immune checkpoint inhibitors: an innovation in immunotherapy for the treatment and management of patients with cancer. *Asia Pac J Oncol Nurs*. 2017;4(2):127-135.

45. Garant A, Guilbault C, Ekmekjian T, et al. Concomitant use of corticosteroids and immune checkpoint inhibitors in patients with hematologic or solid neoplasms: a systematic review. *Crit Rev Oncol Hematol*. 2017;120:86-92.

46. Gandhi L, Rodríguez-Abreu D, Gadgeel S, et al. Pembrolizumab plus chemotherapy in metastatic non-small-cell lung cancer. *N Engl J Med*. 2018;378:2078-2092.

47. Paz-Ares L, Luft A, Vicente D, et al: Pembrolizumab plus chemotherapy for squamous non-small-cell lung cancer. *N Engl J Med*. 2018;379:2040-2051.

48. Wong RKS, Paul N, Ding K, et al. 5-Hydroxytryptamine-3 receptor antagonist with or without short-course dexamethasone in the prophylaxis of radiation induced emesis: a placebo-controlled randomized trial of the National Cancer Institute of Canada Clinical Trials Group (Sc19). *J Clin Oncol*. 2006;24:3458-3464.

49. Ezzo J, Vickers M, Richardson MA, et al. Acupuncture-point stimulation for chemotherapy-induced nausea and vomiting. *J Clin Oncol*. 2005;23:7188-7198.

50. Ryan JL, Heckler C, Dakhil SR, et al. Ginger for chemotherapy-related nausea in cancer patients: a URCC CCOP randomized, double blind, placebo controlled clinical trial of 644 cancer patients. *J Clin Oncol*. 2009;27:9511 (abstract).

51. Nielson M, Olsen NV. Genetic polymorphisms in the cytochrome P450 system and efficacy of 5-hydroxytryptamine type 3 receptor antagonists for postoperative nausea and vomiting. *Br J Anaesth*. 2008;101:441-445.

13 Assessment and Management of Chronic Nausea and Vomiting

Lakshmi Vaidyanathan

INTRODUCTION

Nausea and vomiting are frequently experienced by patients with cancer, with a prevalence of up to 70% in advanced stages (1,2) and in at least 40% of patients with cancer in the last 6 weeks of life (3). Chronic nausea and vomiting can lead to debility from malnutrition and volume and electrolyte disturbances. In addition to the physical distress, they are a source of psychological and spiritual distress to patients and families.

Nausea is an unpleasant subjective sensation of the need to vomit. It may or may not result in vomiting. Associated autonomic symptoms such as diaphoresis, tachycardia, tachypnea, pallor, and dizziness are common. Vomiting is an objective symptom resulting from the expulsion of gastric contents through the mouth and sometimes the nose. This is a forceful action caused by abdominal muscle contractions and the opening of the gastric cardia. Understanding of the neurophysiology underlying the vomiting reflex has prompted the evolution of the pathophysiology-based approach to treating this symptom.

PATHOPHYSIOLOGY OF NAUSEA AND VOMITING

There are multiple neurophysiological pathways and neurotransmitters involved in the activation of nausea and the vomiting reflex. Once the clinical etiology of nausea and vomiting has been determined, an understanding of the pathophysiological basis can help guide the choice of appropriate antiemetic agents.

The pathophysiology of vomiting is better understood than that of nausea. The vomiting center is not a distinct anatomical structure, but a diffuse neural network in the medulla, that is activated sequentially by a central pattern generator (4–6). Emetogenic stimuli are integrated in this network with parasympathetic and efferent motor activity to produce the vomiting reflex. The main receptors at this VC are muscarinic (AChM) and histamine (H1). Serotonin (5-HT2) receptors are also present. Outlined below are the four pathways that provide input to the vomiting

center, which acts as the final common pathway (5,6). The interrelationship between these afferent inputs and the pathophysiological linkages to the mechanism of action of antiemetics are depicted in Figure 13.1.

1. The chemoreceptor trigger zone (CTZ) is in the floor of the fourth ventricle in an area outside the blood–brain barrier. It has chemoreceptors exposed to the cerebrospinal fluid and fenestrated capillaries exposed to the systemic circulation. Stimulants from the systemic circulation and the CSF can trigger the CTZ. The principal receptors at this site are dopaminergic (D2). Other receptors include serotonin (HT3), opioid, cannabinoid, and neurokinin 1 (NK1).

2. The vestibular system stimulates the vomiting center via cranial nerve VIII (vestibulocochlear nerve). The main receptors in this system are histamine (H1) and muscarinic (AChM). Motion sickness is mediated by this pathway.

3. The gastrointestinal system sends signals to the VC via the vagus nerve, with additional input from the splanchnic nerves, sympathetic ganglia, and the glossopharyngeal nerve. The chemoreceptors and mechanoreceptors in the liver and gut stimulate the vagus in the GI tract, serosa, and viscera. The enterochromaffin cells in the small intestine store serotonin. Irritation or distension of the gut results in stimulation of the 5-HT3 receptors in the GI system, which sends signals to the VC via the vagus.

4. The VC receives afferent signals from the cortex that can stimulate or inhibit the emetic cascade. Meningeal irritation increase in intracranial pressure, psychiatric disorders, emotional stress (anticipatory nausea and vomiting), and unpleasant sensory input (e.g., foul smell) can activate the VC. Recognizing the complex interplay of these physical factors with emotional and existential concerns empathy and attention to all the domains of suffering (physical, emotional and spiritual) are essential to achieve satisfactory symptom control and better quality of life.

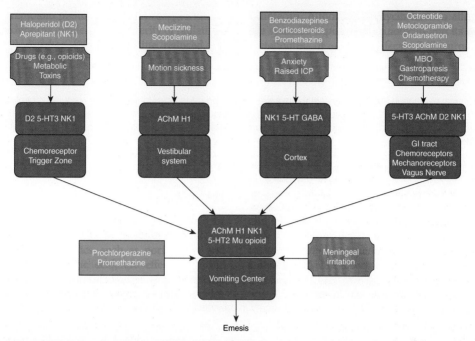

Figure 13.1 Pathophysiology of nausea and vomiting.

Etiology of Chronic Nausea and Vomiting Not Associated with Cancer Treatment

The initial evaluation of any symptom should focus on identifying its cause. In the case of chronic nausea and vomiting, an etiology can be identified 75% of the time, and 25% of cases have more than one identifiable cause (7). Such an approach provides the opportunity to treat potentially reversible causes. In one study, with the use of etiology-based antiemetic drug guidelines, nausea was controlled for 44% of patients at 48 hours and for 56% at 1 week. Vomiting was more effectively controlled with 69% at 48 hours and 89% (7).

CLINICAL EVALUATION OF NAUSEA AND VOMITING

A thorough history and physical examination is the first step to ascertain the etiology of nausea and vomiting. The history should include onset of symptoms, their severity and duration, other associated symptoms (fever, early satiety, abdominal distension, change in bowel habits, abdominal pain), aggravating and alleviating factors, their relationship to other gastrointestinal factors such as bowel irregularities and meal intake, or a lack of relationship. Family or caregiver reports of cognitive impairment or confusion may lead to consideration for metabolic etiology or brain metastases. Recent medication changes, particularly the introduction or change in the dose of opioids is relevant as this is the commonest cause

of medication-induced nausea and vomiting in patients with advanced cancer. Table 13.1 outlines medications that are commonly implicated in nausea and vomiting. The nature and stage of the patient's cancer and symptoms to raise suspicion for brain metastases should be explored. Recent headaches, visual changes, and lack of association to meals and lack of change in bowel pattern should raise suspicion for central nervous system (CNS) cause of nausea and vomiting. The presence of other medical comorbidities such as diabetes, systemic infections, HIV, hypothyroidism, and cardiac disease may cause nausea and vomiting. The history should also include an assessment

TABLE 13.1 MEDICATIONS THAT COMMONLY CAUSE NAUSEA AND VOMITING

Mechanism	Medication
CTZ activation	Opioids
	Digoxin
	Chemotherapy
	Antibiotics
	SSRIs
Decreased gastrointestinal motility	Opioids
	Anticholinergics
Gastrointestinal mucosal irritation	NSAIDs
	Iron
	Antibiotics

The Etiology-based Approach

An etiology-based approach creates a systematic process for managing nausea and vomiting to include not only the choice of antiemetics but the identification of potentially reversible underlying causes. Following is an outline of the general approach (6,8):

- Clinical evaluation (history, physical examination, appropriate testing) to identify the most likely etiologies
- Treat reversible causes if feasible, for example, hypercalcemia, constipation
- Implement relevant nonpharmacological measures and address psychosocial stressors
- Identify the pathway and most likely neurotransmitters by which the cause triggers the emesis reflex
- Choose the antiemetic that is the best fit in terms of the following:
  - The most likely emetic pathway receptors involved
  - Availability of a suitable route of administration
  - Lack of contraindications to use (e.g., drug–drug interactions)
- Administer the antiemetic in a scheduled fashion
- Titrate the dose of the antiemetic to effective symptom relief or toxicity
- Add a second antiemetic with a different mechanism of action if the symptoms remain inadequately controlled after maximization of the first-line medication
- Titrate the second agent to maximum benefit or toxicity before considering another option

The most common causes of nausea and vomiting in patient with advanced cancer are delayed gastric emptying and metabolic/chemical causes (7,9). The following points highlight some of the common causes of nausea and vomiting unrelated to cancer treatment in patients with advanced cancer:

1. **Delayed gastric emptying:** Medications (opioids, anticholinergics, etc.), paraneoplastic syndrome, compressed stomach from ascites, hepatomegaly or splenomegaly, and tumor invasion of the gastrointestinal wall are common causes.
2. **Metabolic/chemical:** Hypercalcemia, hyponatremia and uremia are common metabolic causes of nausea and vomiting. Correction of these metabolic abnormalities can alleviate the symptoms if such correction is feasible and consistent with the patient's overall goals. They may also signify a state of advanced debility, which is why ascertaining the symptom cluster as opposed to evaluating symptoms in isolation is important. Medications such as digoxin and antibiotics can stimulate the CTZ, thereby causing nausea and vomiting.
3. **Visceral:** Malignant bowel obstruction, constipation, gastritis, obstructive uropathy and peritoneal carcinomatosis are notable causes.
4. **Central nervous system causes:** Intracranial metastases and leptomeningeal carcinomatosis can stimulate the vomiting center.

of how these symptoms affect the patient's functionality, psychological state, and perception of quality of life and the caregiver burdens. Patients who are hypovolemic and malnourished may also report dry mouth, weight loss, postural dizziness, and generalized weakness. The weight loss and loss of appetite can be a source of emotional distress for families as well.

Physical examination can help ascertain the etiology and the impact of these symptoms on the patient's overall health. The presence of abdominal distension and absent bowel sounds associated with constipation are highly suggestive of intestinal obstruction. Hepatomegaly, icterus, and/or ascites associated with early satiety indicates gastric stasis or delayed gastric emptying as the cause. The presence of succussion splash on auscultation of the epigastric region with movement suggests gastroparesis. CNS etiologies may be deduced by findings such as cognitive impairment, neck stiffness, cranial nerve abnormalities,

and papilledema. Rectal examination may help identify constipation. Clinical signs of hypovolemia such as tachycardia, hypotension, and orthostasis are relevant towards determining the effects of the symptoms on overall health and influence the overall management of the patient. Muscle wasting, weight loss, and decline in ambulation are markers of disease severity.

Many of the common causes of nausea and vomiting in patients with advanced cancer can be excluded based on history and physical examination alone. Decisions to further the investigation with laboratory and/or radiological tests should be made based on the patient's overall therapeutic goals. Laboratory tests can identify metabolic causes like hypercalcemia, hyponatremia, liver failure, or renal failure. Imaging studies of the abdomen for suspected intra-abdominal etiologies and of the brain for suspected CNS etiologies are appropriate if such information is likely to influence the management plan. For suspected upper gastrointestinal etiologies such as esophagitis or gastric malignancies, an upper endoscopy may be indicated.

Treatment of Nausea and Vomiting Unrelated to Cancer Treatment— Nonpharmacologic

Environmental modification to avoid the smells, sights, and sounds that worsen or exacerbate nausea should be considered. Refining the mealtime experience for patients in accordance with their comfort is an important nonpharmacological consideration especially if the nausea is chronic or long-standing. These strategies also involve the patient's family and support systems. Small, frequent meals may help patients with early satiety due to gastric stasis. Psychological techniques for relaxation may alleviate chemotherapy-induced nausea and vomiting (CINV) and postoperative nausea and vomiting (PONV) (10). These may still be applicable to patients with a significant psychological component to their symptoms. Systematic reviews of acupuncture support its role in CINV and PONV (11). There is evidence to support the possible role of acupressure in CINV and radiation-related nausea and vomiting (12,13). Massage therapy, if feasible, may have a short-term benefit (14). Aromatherapy needs further study (15).

Treatment of Nausea and Vomiting Unrelated to Cancer Treatment— Pharmacological

An approach based on pathophysiology and the most likely neurotransmitters involved (an etiologic approach) to antiemetic use is conventionally taught in the palliative medicine field. Despite the lack of definitive evidence to support the etiologic over the empiric method, the etiologic approach promotes systematic thinking, which can be effective in identifying potentially reversible causes and establishing consistency in practice. Guideline-based antiemetic therapy is appropriate for the management of malignant bowel obstruction (MBO) (16). Limited evidence suggests that both approaches are effective in alleviating the symptoms (17). An open-label study showed that the etiology-based, guideline-directed approach may be superior at 24 hours. This benefit was not sustained at 72 hours (18). Table 13.2 summarizes antiemetic medication classes.

ANTIEMETICS

Dopamine Antagonists

Haloperidol, a butyrophenone, is one of the most potent central D2 receptor antagonists at the CTZ

(6). Antiemetic doses are substantially lower than its doses when used as an antipsychotic. Its long half-life (14 to 36 hours) allows for once or twice daily dosing (19). It is less likely to cause sedation and hypotension than phenothiazines, but more likely to cause extrapyramidal symptoms (17). Patients with Parkinson's disease are more sensitive to its side effects, and it should be avoided in them (17). Other potential adverse effects include QT interval prolongation and neuroleptic malignant syndrome (17). Haloperidol is a substrate of CYP 3A4, so coadministration with carbamazepine, phenytoin, phenobarbital, or rifampicin may alter the clinical pharmacokinetics of haloperidol (20).

Despite its wide use in palliative care, high-quality evidence is not available to substantiate its benefit in the treatment of nausea and vomiting in palliative care patients (21). A prospective uncontrolled clinical trial has shown that haloperidol provides at least partial relief in around 50% of patients with nausea and vomiting not related to chemotherapy or radiotherapy (22).

Phenothiazines are another class of antipsychotic agents that also have antiemetic properties. Unlike haloperidol, their antiemetic effect is not restricted to the D2 receptors in the CTZ. They act on other receptors in the antiemetic pathway, alpha adrenergic, muscarinic, histamine, and 5-HT3 with varying affinities. Their side-effect profile is influenced by the variable receptor site affinity between medications in this class (6). Prochlorperazine is the most widely used phenothiazine antiemetic. It is available in oral and intravenous formulations. It should also be avoided in patients with an absolute neutrophil count of <1,000 cells/μL due to the risk of neutropenia (20). It should be used with caution in those with hepatic impairment (17). Other potential side effects include confusion, respiratory depression, extrapyramidal effects, and anticholinergic effects (20). Chlorpromazine has greater affinity for alpha-adrenergic receptors and therefore has a greater propensity to cause sedation and hypotension compared to prochlorperazine. There is paucity of evidence for the role of phenothiazines in advanced cancer.

Prokinetic Agents

Metoclopramide is categorized as a prokinetic agent. It acts at multiple receptor sites. It stimulates the 5-HT4 receptors, resulting in acetylcholine release from enteric neurons to stimulate the cholinergic system in the gut wall. This mechanism appears to play an important role in reversing gastroparesis and improving upper gastrointestinal peristalsis (17). At high doses, it has anti-D2 activity at the CTZ. It has anti-D2 activity

TABLE 13.2 SUMMARY OF ANTIEMETIC AGENTS

Medication classes	Receptors/Mechanism of action	Uses	Adverse effects	Dose	Route	Comments
Prokinetic						
Metoclopramide	Anti-D2: CTZ (high doses) Anti-5-HT3: GI Pro 5-HT4: GI (prokinetic)	Partial intestinal obstruction, gastroparesis	Extrapyramidal symptoms	5–20 mg before meals and at bedtime or 3–4 times a day	PO/IV/SC	
Dopamine antagonists						
Haloperidol	Anti-D2	Metabolic, medication, and gastrointestinal causes of nausea and vomiting	Extrapyramidal effects, QT prolongation	1.5–2.5 mg oral once or twice a day or 1–2 mg twice or thrice a day SC/IV	PO/SC/IV	
Prochlorperazine	Anti-D2, anti-Ach, anti-H1		Extrapyramidal effects, QT prolongation, sedation	5–10 mg every 6 h PO/IV; 25 mg twice or thrice a day PR	PO/IV/PR	
Chlorpromazine	Anti-D2, alpha 1 adrenergic, anti-H1, anti-Ach		Sedation, hypotension, QT prolongation	10–25 mg every 8 h	PO/IV/PR	IV has to be given slowly to prevent hypotension
Antihistamine						
Diphenhydramine	Anti-H1, anti-Ach	Motion sickness, vestibular disorders, nausea/vomiting from CNS causes	Xerostomia, sedation	1 mg/kg/dose every 4 h up to a max of 100 mg/dose	PO/SQ/IV	
Hydroxyzine			Xerostomia, sedation	0.5–1.0 mg/kg/dose every 4 h to max of 100 mg/dose	PO/IM	
Promethazine			Xerostomia, sedation, dystonia	12.5–25 mg every 4 h	PO/PR	IV administration longer recommended due to the risk of tissue necrosis and gangrene
Serotonin 5-HT3 receptor antagonists						
Ondansetron	Anti-HT3	Chemotherapy or radiation therapy-induced N/V, intractable N/V	Headache, constipation, QT prolongation	4–8 mg every 6 h	PO/IV	

	Mechanism of action	Indication	Side effects	Dose	Route	Comments
Multireceptor site antiemetic						
Olanzapine	Antagonizes multiple dopamine, serotonin and muscarinic receptors. Also, anti-alpha1 adrenergic; anti-H1	Chemotherapy N/V, intractable N/V	Sedation, orthostatic hypotension, appetite stimulation, weight gain, hyperglycemia	2.5–10 mg daily	PO	
Anticholinergic agents						
Scopolamine	Anti-Ach, antiemetic, antisecretory	Motion sickness, malignant bowel obstruction	Dry mouth, sedation, confusion, urinary retention, ileus	1–1.5 mg/h, every 72 h transdermal	Transdermal	
Hyoscyamine		Motion sickness, malignant bowel obstruction	Dry mouth, sedation, confusion, urinary retention, ileus	0.125–0.25 mg PO/SL every 4 h or 0.25–0.50 mg SC/IV every 4 h	PO/SL/SC/IV	
NK1 receptor antagonist						
Aprepitant	Anti-NK1 receptor (substance P)	Chemotherapy-induced N/V		125 mg oral on day 1 followed by 80 mg daily	PO	
Corticosteroids						
Dexamethasone	Unclear, may have multiple mechanisms of action, anti-inflammatory, antiemetic	Malignant bowel obstruction, raised intracranial pressure, chemotherapy-induced N/V	Hyperglycemia, fat redistribution, skin changes, myopathy	For chronic N/V, initial dose 4–8 mg daily followed by a taper. The lowest effective dose should be used	PO/IV	
Cannabinoids						
Dronabinol	Unclear, may be via the endocannabinoid system and mu opioid receptors	Chemotherapy-induced nausea/vomiting	Sedation, dysphoria, hallucinations	2.5 mg twice daily, can be titrated to a maximum of 20 mg oral daily	PO	
Nabilone				0.5–1 mg at night titrated up to 3 mg twice daily	PO	
Somatostatin analogue						
Octreotide	Inhibits secretion of multiple gastrointestinal hormones, antisecretory	Malignant bowel obstruction	Injection site irritation, abdominal cramps, flatulence, diarrhea, hyperglycemia, gallstones	100–200 µg three times daily	SC/IV	Depot preparations available

in the gut and weak peripheral anti-5HT3 receptor activity (19,20). Small studies favor the use of metoclopramide for chronic nausea in advanced cancer (16,23). Metoclopramide is also used to treat nausea and vomiting associated with delayed gastric emptying and partial bowel obstruction without colic (17). Prolonged use beyond 12 weeks is not recommended by the FDA due to the increased risk of developing tardive dyskinesia with longer-term use. Extrapyramidal symptoms (akathisia, acute dystonia, tardive dyskinesia) are a concern especially in frail older patients. Dose reduction is recommended in renal impairment with a 50% reduction for creatinine clearance <40 mL/min and total daily dose not to exceed 10 mg daily for end-stage renal disease with need for dialysis. It should be doses cautiously in the elderly and in the presence of severe liver impairment (20).

Erythromycin is the other prokinetic agent that can be used to treat diabetic gastroparesis. It is a macrolide antibiotic, with agonistic action on the motilin receptors. Motilin is a peptide hormone that activates the smooth muscle in the gut wall (24).

Domperidone and cisapride are D2 antagonists and prokinetic agents that are no longer available in the United States. Domperidone has a lower risk of extrapyramidal side effects than metoclopramide but was taken off the market because of cardiac toxicity. Cisapride, unlike the other prokinetic agents, has activity throughout the gastrointestinal tract. Cardiac arrhythmias with the agent's use led to its withdrawal from the US market (6,24).

Many D2 antagonists prolong QT interval. Caution should be exerted when these medications are used concurrently with other QT prolonging agents.

Antihistamines

Promethazine, dimenhydrinate, meclizine, and diphenhydramine are used, primarily for motion sickness and other vestibular disorders. Their antiemetic effect is via the H1 receptor in the vomiting center and the vestibular system. They also have variable antimuscarinic activity that can be favorable by decreasing gastrointestinal secretions and unfavorable due to dry mouth and CNS side effects like sedation. Promethazine is commonly used as an antiemetic. It is available in oral, rectal, and parenteral formulations. There is a US boxed warning for injectable promethazine due to the risk of severe tissue injury. It may help with emesis due to CNS neoplasms causing raised intracranial pressure (20). The main side effect is sedation.

Anticholinergics

Scopolamine is a muscarinic (M1-5) receptor antagonist (17). It relaxes the gastrointestinal wall smooth muscle and decreases gastrointestinal secretions. It is used as prophylaxis against motion sickness. Drowsiness and xerostomia are the main side effects. Other anticholinergic side effects such as ileus, urinary retention, confusion, and tremors can occur, and caution should be exerted in the elderly. It is used as an antisecretory agent in the palliation of intestinal obstruction. It comes as a 1 mg/3-day transdermal patch (25).

Hyoscyamine is also an anticholinergic agent that blocks the action of acetylcholine at the parasympathetic sites in the smooth muscles, secretory glands, and CNS. It is available for administration orally, sublingually, intravenously, and subcutaneously (26).

The antisecretory effects of these agents in the gastrointestinal tract and their availability in formulations that bypass the gastrointestinal tract make them options for use in managing nausea and vomiting in MBO (16).

Serotonin Antagonists

Serotonin receptor antagonists block the 5-HT3 receptors located peripherally (terminals of vagal afferents in the gut) and centrally (CTZ and the vomiting center) (19). The largest storage site for serotonin is the enterochromaffin cells in the gut. Local insults to the GI tract can lead to release of serotonin and stimulation of the vagal 5-HT3 receptors. There are multiple agents available in the markets. Ondansetron, granisetron, dolasetron, and palonosetron are examples of agents in this class, available in the United States. They have become a mainstay in antiemetic guidelines for CINV (16). They are also used in radiation-induced and PONV. Their role in chronic nausea and vomiting in advanced cancer is less clear. Ondansetron can be used as an adjunct or alternative antiemetic in refractory nausea and vomiting in patients with advanced cancer (26–30). It is available in oral, oral disintegrating, and intravenous formulations.

Headache and constipation are the most common side effects. They have been associated with dose-dependent increases in electrocardiographic QTc intervals and should be used cautiously with other QTc prolonging drugs. Dosage adjustment is recommended in severe hepatic impairment.

Other Agents

Corticosteroids

Corticosteroids are widely prescribed for nausea and vomiting, both as a single agent (for increased intracranial pressure, for example) and for its synergistic effect with serotonin antagonists (for chemotherapy-induced emesis). It is also used for its additive effect (as a component of combination regimens for MBO, for example). The mechanism of antiemetic activity of corticosteroids remains unknown. It has been postulated that corticosteroids reduce the permeability of the blood–brain barrier to emetic toxins, reduce brain stem release of enkephalin, deplete medullary amine γ-aminobutyric acid from medullary antiemetic neurons, and inhibit central prostaglandin synthesis and/or serotonin synthesis and release (6).

Dexamethasone is the recommended steroid of choice because of its limited mineralocorticoid effect and its prolonged half-life, allowing once-daily dosing.

Patients with advanced illness may have multiple symptoms palliated by steroids. However, steroids also have significant toxicity. An initial dose of 4 to 8 mg daily is common, followed by a slow taper once symptoms are adequately controlled. The lowest effective dose should be utilized.

A systematic Cochrane review showed insufficient evidence to either support or refute the role of corticosteroids in the treatment of nausea and vomiting in advanced cancer (8).

Cannabinoids

Synthetic cannabinoids dronabinol and nabilone have been approved for use in CINV. Their mechanism of action may involve the brain stem cannabinoid system and the mu-opioid receptor (31). Side effects include sedation, dizziness, hallucinations, and paranoia. The role of other forms of cannabis in the management of CINV has not been studied in comparison to existing CINV regimens (32). The role of cannabis in chronic nausea and vomiting as compared to traditional antiemetics is not clear. The legalization of "medical marijuana" in multiple states has prompted its use to manage cancer-related nausea and emesis. Long-term cannabis use can cause cannabinoid hyperemesis syndrome, characterized by cyclic episodes of nausea and vomiting.

Olanzapine

Olanzapine is an atypical antipsychotic agent with an affinity for multiple receptor sites in the emetic pathways. It blocks multiple dopamine (D1, D2, D3, D4), serotonin (5-HT2A, 5-HT2C, 5-HT3, 5-HT6), alpha 1 adrenergic, histamine (H1), and cholinergic (M1, M2, M3, M4) receptors. Olanzapine has a higher affinity for the 5HT2 receptor than for D2, resulting in fewer extrapyramidal side effects (33,34). It does not cause QT prolongation

at conventional doses. It is available as an oral tablet and oral disintegrating tablet with similar pharmacokinetics. It can be administered intramuscularly, although this route is generally avoided in palliative care due to discomfort. It has reportedly been given subcutaneously without local skin irritation for the treatment of delirium (34). The most common short-term adverse effects noted in psychiatric populations are postural hypotension, constipation, dizziness, and dry mouth. Somnolence is another commonly reported side effect although one small study noted that careful dose titration over 7 to 10 days in the range of 2.5 to 7.5 mg may prevent excessive sedation. Weight gain and appetite stimulation are other notable side effects, which may be beneficial in cachectic patients (34). Development of glucose intolerance has been associated with olanzapine use. Neuroleptic malignant syndrome can rarely occur, and it can lower seizure threshold. It can be used in the presence of renal and liver dysfunction.

Olanzapine is recommended in the management of breakthrough chemotherapy-induced emesis. It has a role in the management of nausea and vomiting in advanced cancer, refractory to conventional antiemetics such as metoclopramide (16).

Neurokinin 1 (NK1) antagonists: This class of medications is now included in CINV guidelines due to their efficacy in delayed emesis from chemotherapy (16). Delayed CINV is thought to be due to the release of substance P in the brainstem. Substance P, a neuropeptide, may induce nausea by binding to the NK1 receptor in the gut and the CNS. NK1 antagonists inhibit this emetic pathway (17). Aprepitant was the first commercial oral preparation. Fosaprepitant is an injectable formulation. The role of these agents for chronic nausea and vomiting in patients with advanced cancer has yet to be determined. Substance P and other tachykinins are implicated in pain and depression pathways. In the future, the NK1 antagonists may have a role in the management of chronic nausea in patients with advanced cancer (17).

Somatostatin analogue (Octreotide): Octreotide is a synthetic analogue of somatostatin. Octreotide reduces vomiting by inhibiting the release of several gastrointestinal hormones, thereby reducing gastrointestinal secretions, decreasing intestinal motility, decreasing bile flow, decreasing splanchnic blood circulation, and increasing the absorption of water and electrolytes (35). Octreotide may even be effective in relieving partial bowel obstruction by reducing the hypertensive state in the lumen. This hypertensive state promotes the cycle of distension–secretion–distension, which can ultimately lead to total obstruction if not treated (36).

A double-blind placebo-controlled trial did not show a significant reduction in the number of days free of vomiting with the use of octreotide in MBO (37). However other prospective studies have shown a reduction in the volume of GI secretions and the number of episodes of vomiting with the use of octreotide when compared to scopolamine butylbromide (36). Octreotide is generally well tolerated, and there it has been used internationally for many years as an antisecretory antiemetic in MBO. It is recommended in the palliation of MBO when high-output vomiting is noted and can be combined with a conventional antiemetics such as a D2 receptor antagonist (16,36).

Its duration of action is around 8 hours. It is dosed as 100 μg subcutaneously three times daily or 100 to 600 μg/d intravenously or by continuous subcutaneous infusion. The most common side effects are local skin reactions, gastrointestinal effects like abdominal cramping, nausea/vomiting, diarrhea or constipation, and gallstones. Headache, hypothyroidism, and cardiac toxicity including bradycardia and QT prolongation are other potential side effects. The medication is generally well tolerated. It should be used with caution in the presence of diabetes, renal failure, and hepatic impairment due to its effects on insulin and other hormones (20).

Approach to specific clinical syndromes associated with nausea and vomiting: Table 13.3 summarizes the etiological approach to managing nausea and vomiting associated with common clinical syndromes.

TABLE 13.3 SUMMARY OF THE ETIOLOGICAL APPROACH FOR THE TREATMENT OF CHRONIC NAUSEA AND VOMITING ASSOCIATED WITH COMMON CLINICAL SYNDROMES IN CANCER

Clinical syndromes	Associated signs and symptoms	Pathophysiology	Treatment
Toxin-induced nausea/ vomiting Medications (e.g., opioids, digoxin) Metabolic (e.g., hypercalcemia)	Other features of drug toxicity or the metabolic abnormality	CTZ (D2)	Haloperidol/ prochlorperazine
			Discontinue offending medication if feasible
			Treat metabolic derangement
Impaired gastric motility Medications (e.g., opioids, anticholinergics), diabetes, malignant ascites	Postprandial nausea/ vomiting, early satiety, hiccups, abdominal fullness, reflux	Vagal afferents to VC (H1, Ach)	Metoclopramide (prokinetic)
			Manage underlying cause
			Anti-H1 blocker or proton pump inhibitor for reflux symptoms
Malignant bowel obstruction	Nausea/vomiting, altered bowel pattern, abdominal distension, abdominal pain, colic, decreased oral intake	GI mechanoreceptors via vagal afferents to the vomiting center (H1, Ach)	Octreotide and haloperidol and/or anticholinergic & steroid
			Metoclopramide for partial obstruction and no colic
		Toxins from ischemic bowel and tumor products activate the CTZ (D2)(5-HT3)	Venting NG tube or gastrostomy tube
			Cancer-directed surgery/ treatment if feasible
CNS metastases	Headache, neck stiffness, other focal neurologic signs, no change in bowel pattern	Stimulation of the VC (H1, Ach) and meningeal mechanoreceptors (H1)	Corticosteroids to decrease cerebral edema and/or inflammation
			Cyclizine/promethazine for nausea if needed
			Treat underlying cause (e.g., radiation therapy)

OPIOID-INDUCED NAUSEA AND VOMITING

Opioid-induced nausea and vomiting is experienced by up to 40% of patients with cancer with no prior emesis (38). These symptoms typically resolve after 3 to 5 days of opioid continuation, a fact that is important to share with patients to set expectations and prevent premature discontinuation of effective pain management. Prompt treatment of this side effect is an important step. A small fraction of patients on opioids will continue to experience persistent nausea and vomiting, it is reasonable to attempt scheduled antiemetics for these patients if pain control with the offending opioid is effective. Alternatively, dose reduction can be tried if pain control is effective. Lastly, opioid rotation can be attempted if the side effect is intolerable or persists despite opioid reduction (26). The basis of opioid rotation is that a new opioid with variable opioid receptor affinity may be less likely to cause nausea.

There are multiple mechanisms causing opioid-induced nausea and vomiting. They include stimulation of the CTZ, decrease in gastric motility, and increase in vestibular sensitivity. Associated symptoms may clarify the predominant mechanism of action. There is no evidence to support a specific approach, mechanistic or empiric, to treat this. Cost and existence of other comorbidities may influence the antiemetic choice. Haloperidol and prochlorperazine are first line antiemetics for this purpose by palliative care experts due to their predominant effect on the D2 receptors of the CTZ. Metoclopramide is another consideration due to its effect on the CTZ dopaminergic sites and its additional prokinetic effects, which are relevant if gastrointestinal dysmotility is a feature (6,26). If the patient describes movement-sensitive nausea and vomiting, an antihistamine or anticholinergic that would act on the vestibular pathway may be tried. Prophylactic antiemetic medication is not recommended at the initiation of opioid therapy (16).

Delayed Gastric Emptying

Gastroparesis is a chronic motility disorder of the stomach characterized by delayed gastric emptying in the absence of gastric outlet obstruction. It causes nausea, vomiting, early satiety, bloating, abdominal pain, and reduced oral intake. Diabetes mellitus is the most common cause of gastroparesis in the general population (24). Malignant gastroparesis can be due to direct and indirect effects of the cancer or the effects of treatments. It occurs most commonly with gastrointestinal cancers such as pancreatic or gastric cancer. It occurs in as many as 60% of patients with pancreatic cancer (39,40).

Massive ascites, hepatomegaly, and intra-abdominal tumor progression can delay gastric emptying. Paraneoplastic syndrome is another etiology. Medications such as opioids cause dysmotility. Abdominal radiation may be a possible contributory factor (6).

Pharmacological agents that promote gastric and intestinal motility are the treatment of choice. Metoclopramide sensitizes tissues to the effects of acetylcholine in the gut. Small trials have demonstrated improvement in gastroparesis-related symptoms (23,41). Erythromycin is a macrolide antibiotic that has prokinetic properties. A meta-analysis suggested that erythromycin improved gastric motility by 43% (42). Other interventions such as small frequent meals, low in fat, should be adopted to maintain nutritional intake and decrease the symptom burden (24). In patients with diabetes, regulation of blood glucose levels reduces gastroparesis symptoms if such regulation is feasible and consistent with the overall goals.

Cisapride and domperidone are prokinetic agents that are unavailable in the United States due to their cardiac toxicity.

Malignant Bowel Obstruction

MBO is a common complication in advanced cancers, particularly with ovarian and colon primary. The clinical features of MBO vary with the site and severity of the obstruction. Abdominal pain is common, particularly when the obstruction is gastric or proximal small intestinal. Intermittent colic can result from superimposed intestinal segmental activity to overcome the obstruction in the small or large intestine. Nausea and vomiting are more prominent in gastric and small intestinal obstruction. Change in bowel habits and reduction in oral intake are other reported symptoms (35,36).

The management of this syndrome is based not only on the site and severity of obstruction but also the patient's performance status, prognosis, and goals. Surgery may be appropriate for some patients with good performance status if the benefits outweigh the burdens and if such an approach aligns with the patient's goals. For many patients, this complication occurs in the more advanced stages of the disease trajectory when surgery is typically not recommended. The role of other cancer-specific treatment options should also be evaluated based on the benefits and burdens in the context of the patient's prognosis and goals.

The insertion of expandable metallic stents via endoscopy or colonoscopy in the gastric outlet, small intestine, or colon can result in rapid palliation of symptoms. This approach can be helpful in patients who are not surgical candidates or when further workup is warranted to determine surgical candidacy (35,36).

Pharmacological management to alleviate nausea, vomiting, and pain is indicated both for immediate symptom relief and as a long-term strategy for patients who are not candidates for surgery or other disease-directed treatments. The triple strategy of an antisecretory agent, antiemetic, and analgesic helps alleviate vomiting, nausea, and abdominal pain. Sometimes an antiemetic without an antisecretory agent may suffice. Antisecretory agents such as octreotide, a somatostatin analogue, or anticholinergic agents have been shown in small studies to decrease gastrointestinal secretions, distension of the gut lumen, and vomiting.

Octreotide can be administered subcutaneously; the typical dose is 100 μg every 8 hours subcutaneously. Cost of octreotide can be a limiting factor. Anticholinergic agents available for this purpose in the United States include transdermal scopolamine 1 to 1.5 mg/h, to be changed every 3 days, and hyoscyamine, which can be administered orally, sublingually, subcutaneously, or intravenously. Opioids are the mainstay of treatment for pain. If an antiemetic is needed, a central dopamine antagonist such as haloperidol or prochlorperazine is reasonable. Despite the paucity of evidence, dexamethasone is frequently used as an antiemetic and its effect may be predominantly due to its anti-inflammatory effect that might alleviate bowel wall inflammation. Pharmacological therapy alone without the use of a nasogastric tube or gastrostomy tube for decompression can be effective. The 2016 Multinational Association of Supportive Care in Cancer (MASCC) and European Society of Medical Oncology (ESMO) guidelines recommend octreotide with a conventional antiemetic such as haloperidol to alleviate nausea and vomiting due to malignant intestinal obstruction. If the first line is suboptimal, the addition of or change to an anticholinergic antisecretory agent and/or corticosteroid is recommended (16).

Metoclopramide can be used as an antiemetic for functional obstruction due to tumor infiltration of the intestinal wall, nerves, and/or mesentery. Gut dysmotility can also be a result of paraneoplastic syndrome. Metoclopramide should be avoided in complete intestinal obstruction as its prokinetic effects can worsen or cause colicky pain (35,36).

Temporary gastric decompression with a nasogastric tube may be reasonable in symptomatic gastric outlet or small intestinal obstruction with discomfort and large-volume emesis from gastric distension. Nasogastric tube insertion is intrusive and should only be used as a short-term intervention until medications take effect. For patients who are deemed candidates for longer-term decompression, the insertion of a percutaneous gastrostomy tube (PEG) can be considered. Patients who tolerate intermittent venting via a PEG tube can return home, continue limited oral intake, and maintain an active lifestyle. The presence of ascites, active gastric ulceration, coagulopathy, and previous gastrectomy are relative contraindications to PEG tube insertion (35,36).

Patients with persistent malignant intestinal obstruction who are not surgical candidates are unable to maintain natural nutrition and hydration. Parenteral nutrition is only appropriate for a small subset of patients with good performance status, slow-growing tumors of the gastrointestinal tract, and sparing of vital organs.

Psychosocial and existential support is important for patients and families who are struggling with issues related to nutrition and hydration and the prognosis associated with decline in nutritional intake.

Metabolic or Chemical Causes

These are mediated by the chemical action of toxins on the CTZ or gastrointestinal irritation causing serotonin release or both. Medications such as opioids, digoxin, antimicrobials, NSAIDs, and chemotherapeutic agents among others have been implicated. Metabolic derangements such as hypercalcemia, uremia, hyponatremia, and liver failure can cause these symptoms as well (43). Other coexisting symptoms and signs may point to the causative etiology (17). For example, hypercalcemia can also cause confusion and constipation. Treatment of the underlying cause if feasible and use of a D2 receptor antagonist such as haloperidol can alleviate nausea and vomiting in these scenarios (9,17). CINV is managed with combination, guideline-based antiemetics, which include 5-HT3 receptor antagonists, corticosteroids, and NK1 receptor antagonists (9,17,44).

CNS Metastases

Meningeal irritation and raised intracranial pressure from primary or metastatic neoplasms of the brain can cause nausea and vomiting. There may be no change in eating pattern or bowel movements. The treatment of choice is systemic corticosteroids, typically dexamethasone, which can be dosed once or twice daily. If nausea and vomiting persist despite corticosteroids, the use of an antiemetic that targets the vomiting center (e.g., promethazine) is a consideration.

Intractable Nausea and Vomiting

Nausea and vomiting are labeled "intractable" when they persist or are not adequately alleviated despite the use of multiple antiemetics in series or in combination. A history and physical examination are the first step in assessing symptom severity and the potential contributing factors. A thorough medication history is relevant as opioids, antibiotics and antidepressants are frequent contributors to nausea and vomiting in patients with advanced disease. Medical testing to identify metabolic causes, malignant intestinal obstruction, and CNS disease should be based on the patient's overall goals. Reversible causes or contributors such as constipation and hypercalcemia should be corrected. The choice of antiemetic agents should consider comorbid illnesses, potential drug–drug interactions, and potential efficacy. The route of administration is a consideration as well. In the absence of the ability to tolerate the oral route, subcutaneous, intravenous, or rectal administration should be considered. If the patient has refractory symptoms despite the use of appropriate scheduled doses of one or more antiemetics, an empiric trial of multiple antiemetics acting on different emetic pathways via tolerable routes should be attempted. Simultaneously, reversible factors such as constipation and opioid dose or type should be addressed.

Atypical antiemetics may have to be considered and combined with more commonly used antiemetics to alleviate the symptoms. For example, corticosteroids are used in this scenario despite the lack of data. Olanzapine is an antipsychotic that acts on multiple receptor sites (33,34). Mirtazapine may have some antiemetic properties due to its anti-HT3 effect. Cannabinoids may be a consideration, but their psychomimetic side effects can be limiting particularly in the elderly. Megestrol acetate is a synthetic pregestational agent used as an appetite stimulant that may also alleviate nausea, although it is rarely prescribed for this indication. 5-HT3 receptor antagonists can be used orally or intravenously in combination with other antiemetics with different mechanisms of action (26,29,30).

CONCLUSION

Nausea and vomiting are common causes of physical discomfort and psychological distress among patients with cancer. These symptoms increase in frequency with cancer progression. An understanding of the pathophysiology of nausea and vomiting and the mechanism of action of antiemetics allows for effective medication management while limiting toxicity, irrespective of whether the empiric or mechanism-based approach is adopted. A comprehensive and relevant clinical evaluation will facilitate diagnosis and an understanding of the relationship between physical symptoms and psychosocial challenges.

In addition to the use of antiemetic medications, the overall approach should include elimination of reversible causes when possible, lifestyle measures (including dietary modification, relaxation techniques, massage) that can alleviate symptoms and ongoing emotional support.

REFERENCES

1. Solano JP, Gomes B, Higginson I. A comparison of symptom prevalence in far advanced cancer, AIDS, heart disease, chronic obstructive pulmonary disease and renal disease. *J Pain Symptom Manage.* 2006;31:58-69.
2. Tranmer JE, Heyland D, Dudgeon D, et al. Measuring the symptom experience of seriously ill cancer and noncancer hospitalized patients near the end of life with the memorial symptom assessment scale. *J Pain Symptom Manage.* 2003;25:420-429.
3. Reuben DB, Mor V. Nausea and vomiting in terminal cancer patients. *Arch Intern Med.* 1986;146(10):2021-2023.
4. Smith HS, Smith EJ, Smith AR. Pathophysiology of nausea and vomiting in palliative medicine. *Ann Palliat Med.* 2012;1(2):87-93.
5. Cherny NI, Fallon MT, Kaasa S, Portenoy RK, Currow DC, eds. *Oxford Textbook of Palliative Medicine.* 5th ed. 661-674.
6. Von Roenn JH. *Principles and Practice of Palliative Care and Supportive Oncology.* 4th ed.
7. Stephenson J, Davies A. An assessment of etiology-based guidelines for the management of nausea and vomiting in patients with advanced cancer. *Support Care Cancer.* 2006;14:348. doi: 10.1007/s00520-005-0897-1.
8. Vayne-Bossert P, Haywood A, Good P, Khan S, Rickett K, Hardy JR. Corticosteroids for adult patients with advanced cancer who have nausea and vomiting (not related to chemotherapy, radiotherapy, or surgery). *Cochrane Database Syst Rev.* 2017;(7). Art No: CD012002.
9. Kim S, Shoemaker LK, Davis MP. Nausea and vomiting in advanced cancer. *Am J Hosp Palliat Care.* 2010;27(3):219-225. doi: 10.1177/1049909110361228.
10. Burish TG, Tope DM. Psychological techniques for controlling the adverse side effects of cancer chemotherapy: findings from a decade of research. *J Pain Symptom Manage.* 1992;7(5):287-301.
11. Ernst E. Acupuncture: what does the most reliable evidence tell us? *J Pain Symptom Manage.* 2009;37(4):709-714.
12. Roscoe JA, Bushnow P, Jean-Pierre P, et al. Acupressure bands are effective in reducing radiation therapy-related nausea. *J Pain Symptom Manage.* 2009;38(3):81-389.
13. Lee, J, Dodd M, Dibble S, Abrams D. Review of acupressure studies for chemotherapy-induced nausea and vomiting control. *J Pain Symptom Manage.* 2008;36(5):529-544.
14. Cassileth BR, Vickers AJ. Massage therapy for symptom control: outcome study at a major cancer center. *J Pain Symptom Manage.* 2004;28(3):244-249.
15. Shin ES, Seo Kh, Lee SH, Jung YM, Kim MJ, Yeon JY. Massage with or without aromatherapy for symptom relief in people with cancer. *Cochrane Database Syst Rev.* 2016;(6). Art No.: CD009873. doi:10.1002/14651858. CD009873.pub3.
16. Roila F, et al. 2016 MASCC and ESMO guideline update for the prevention of chemotherapy and radiotherapy-induced nausea and vomiting and of nausea and vomiting in advanced cancer patients. *Ann Oncol.* 2016;27(suppl 5):v119-v133.

17. Glare PA, et al. Treatment of nausea and vomiting in terminally ill cancer patients. *Drugs*. 2008;68(18):2575-2590.

18. Hardy J, et al. A randomized open-label study of guideline-driven antiemetic therapy versus single agent antiemetic therapy in patients with advanced cancer and nausea not related to anticancer treatment. *BMC Cancer*. 2018;18(1):510.

19. Davis MP, Walsh D. Treatment of nausea and vomiting in advanced cancer. *Support Care Cancer*. 2000;8:444-452.

20. Glare P, Miller J, Nikolova, T, Tickoo R. Treating nausea and vomiting in palliative care: a review. *Clin Interv Aging*. 2011;6:243-259.

21. Murray-Brown F, Dorman S. Haloperidol for the treatment of nausea and vomiting in palliative care patients (Review). *Cochrane Database Syst Rev*. 2015;(11). Art No.: CD006271.

22. Hardy JR, et al. The efficacy of haloperidol in the management of nausea and vomiting in patients with cancer. *J Pain Symptom Manage*. 2010;40(1):111-116.

23. Bruera E, et al. A double-blind, crossover study of controlled-release metoclopramide and placebo for the chronic nausea and dyspepsia of advanced cancer. *J Pain Symptom Manage*. 2000;19(6):427-435.

24. Liu N, Abell T. Gastroparesis updates on Pathogenesis and Management. *Gut Liver*. 2017;11(5):579-589.

25. LeGrand SB, Walsh D. Scopolamine for cancer-related nausea and vomiting. *J Pain Symptom Manage*. 2010;40(1):136-141.

26. Wood GJ, Shega JW, Von Roenn J. Management of intractable nausea and vomiting in patients at the end of life. "I was feeling Nauseous All of the Time…. Nothing was working. *JAMA*. 2007;298(10):1196-1207.

27. Mystakidou K, Befon S, Liossi C, Vlachos L. Comparison of tropisetron and chlorpromazine combinations in the control of nausea and vomiting in patients with advanced cancer. *J Pain Symptom Manage*. 1998;15(3):176-184.

28. Mystakidou K, Befon S, Liossi C, Vlachos L. Comparison of the efficacy and safety of tropisetron, metoclopramide and chlorpromazine in the treatment of emesis associated with far advanced cancer. *Cancer*. 1998;83(6):1214-1221.

29. Cole RM, Robinson F, Harvey L, Trethowan K, Murdoch V. Successful control of intractable nausea and vomiting requiring combined ondansetron and haloperidol in a patient with advanced cancer. *J Pain Symptom Manage*. 1994;9(1):48-50.

30. Currow DC, et al. Use of ondansetron in palliative medicine. *J Pain Symptom Manage*. 1997;13(5):302-307.

31. Harris DG. Nausea and vomiting in advanced cancer. *Br Med Bull*. 2010;96:175-185.

32. Wilkie G, Sakr B, Rizack T. Medical marijuana use in oncology: a review. *JAMA Oncol*. 2016;2(5):670-675.

33. Srivastava M, Brito-Dellan N, Mellar D, Leach M, Lagman, R. Olanzapine as an antiemetic in refractory nausea and vomiting in advanced cancer. *J Pain Symptom Manage*. 2003;25(6):578-582.

34. Prommer E. Olanzapine: palliative medicine update. *Am J Hosp Palliat Care*. 2012;30(1):75-82.

35. Ripamonti C, et al. Clinical-practice recommendations for the management of bowel obstruction in patients with end-stage cancer. *Support Care Cancer*. 2001;9:223-233.

36. Ripamonti CI, Easson AM, Gerdes H. Management of malignant bowel obstruction. *Eur J Cancer*. 2008;44(8):1105-1115.

37. Currow DC, et al. Double-blind, placebo-controlled, randomized trial of octreotide in malignant bowel obstruction. *J Pain Symptom Manage*. 2015;49(5):814-821.

38. Laugsand EA, Kaasa S, Klepstad P. Management of opioid-induced nausea and vomiting in cancer patients: systematic review and evidence-based recommendations. *Palliat Med*. 2011;25(5):442-453.

39. Barkin JS, Goldberg RI, Sfakianakis GN, Levi J. Pancreatic carcinoma is associated with delayed gastric emptying. *Dig Dis Sci*. 1986;31:265.

40. Dearbhla K, et al. Malignancy-associated gastroparesis: an important and overlooked cause of chronic nausea and vomiting. *BMJ Case Rep*. 2014;2014:bcr2013201815.

41. Bruera E, et al. Chronic nausea in advanced cancer patients: a retrospective assessment of a metoclopramide-based antiemetic regimen. *J Pain Symptom Manage*. 1996;11(3):147-153.

42. Maganti K, Onyemere K, Jones MP. Oral erythromycin and symptomatic relief of gastroparesis: a systematic review. *Am J Gastroenterol*. 2003;98:259.

43. Gordon P, LeGrand SB, Walsh D. Nausea and vomiting in advanced cancer. *Eur J Pharmacol*. 2014;722:187-191.

44. Collis E, Mather H. Nausea and vomiting in palliative care. *BMJ*. 2015;351:h6249. doi: 10.1136/bmj.h6249 (published December 3, 2015). Pages 1–11.

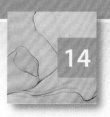

14 Diarrhea, Malabsorption, and Constipation

Erica Schockett and Pallavi Doddakashi

The pathophysiology of the gastrointestinal (GI) tract leading to changes in normal activity is complex. The GI function is mediated through endocrine, paracrine, and neural forms of cellular communication. The GI tract has its own intrinsic nervous system in the form of myenteric and submucosal plexuses, receiving an extrinsic input from the central nervous system via the autonomic nervous system. Furthermore, the GI tract has its own pacemaker cells, which generate rhythmic electrical activity. Complex communication and coordination are required to produce segmental and peristaltic contractions that mix and move the endoluminal content forward. Many neurotransmitters mediate this communication. Any damage occurring at the different levels of this complex system may result in changes of GI mobility and activity.

DIARRHEA

Diarrhea is generally defined as the frequent passage of loose stools with urgency, commonly more than three unformed stools in 24 hours (1). Diarrhea is a common and significant problem among patients with cancer, occurring in 5% to 10% of patients with advanced disease, and is seen as a major treatment complication in patients receiving chemotherapy, particularly with some agents (2). Diarrhea is also included among the top 10 consequences of adverse drug reactions in hospitalized patients with cancer (3). The consequences of diarrhea can be troublesome and include loss of water, electrolytes, and albumin, failure to reach nutritional goals, declining immune function, and the risk of bedsores or systemic infection. Diarrhea also brings additional work for the staff or family who have to prevent maceration and bedsores. Moreover, losses of comfort and dignity have to be considered. Severe diarrhea, other than being debilitating, can be a costly complication in cancer patients (4).

Although a practical definition is lacking, diarrhea is commonly diagnosed when there is an abnormal increase in daily stool weight, water content, or frequency as a consequence of incomplete absorption of electrolytes and water from luminal content. There may also be symptoms of urgency, perianal discomfort, or incontinence.

Pathophysiology

Osmotic Diarrhea

Absorption of water in the intestines is dependent on adequate absorption of solutes. Retention of nonabsorbable compounds within the lumen triggers an osmotic shift of water into the lumen (5).

The proximal small bowel is highly permeable to water; sodium and water influx across the duodenum rapidly adjusting the osmolarity of luminal fluid toward that of plasma. This can lead to water secretion despite similar osmolarity values between luminal contents and plasma.

On the contrary, the mucosa of the ileum and colon have low permeability to sodium and solutes. There is an effective action ion transport mechanism that allows the reabsorption of electrolytes and water even against electrochemical gradients.

Osmotic diarrhea typically results from one of two situations; ingestion of a poorly absorbed substrate or malabsorption. When large amounts of lactulose are ingested, an unabsorbable sugar in the small intestines, the protective role of colonic bacteria may be exhausted, producing diarrhea proportional to the osmotic force of the malabsorbed saccharide (6). There is an unaccounted gap between the stool water electrolytes and measured osmolality (7). The gap is due to poorly absorbed molecules that draw fluid into the lumen. Similarly, carbohydrate malabsorption may induce osmotic diarrhea characterized by a low stool pH, and high stool osmolarity. The ingestion of other substances, such as magnesium and sulfate, may also produce osmotic diarrhea. However, there will be a normal pH, unlike in carbohydrate-induced diarrhea. In general, osmotic diarrhea commonly subsides as the patient discontinues the poorly absorbable agent.

Moreover, reversible chemotherapy-related hypolactasia and lactose intolerance are not infrequent in patients treated with 5-fluorouracil (5-FU)–based adjuvant chemotherapy for colorectal cancer. There are limited data that avoidance of lactose during chemotherapy may improve treatment tolerability in these patients (8).

Secretory Diarrhea

Secretory diarrhea is rarely present as the sole mechanism and is often associated with other mechanisms (6). It is associated with abnormal ion transport in intestinal epithelial cells, resulting in excessive secretion and/or impaired absorption of fluid and electrolytes (9). Unlike in osmotic diarrhea, the osmotic gap is small and diarrhea usually persists despite fasting.

Many factors affect ion transport in epithelial cells of the gut. These include bacterial toxins, intraluminal secretagogues (such as bile acids or laxatives), or circulating secretagogues (such as hormones, drugs, and poisons). In addition, medical problems that compromise regulation of intestinal function or reduce absorptive surface area (by disease or resection) can induce secretory diarrhea (10).

Endocrine tumors may cause diarrhea through the release of secretagogue transmitters (11). Diarrhea is a common manifestation of carcinoid syndrome, occurring in approximately 80% of patients, and is largely a consequence of excess secretion of serotonin (12). Excess serotonin increases peristalsis, which results in reduced absorption of water and electrolytes, leading to diarrhea. Reduction in serotonin production is associated with improvement in carcinoid syndrome diarrhea. In the Zollinger-Ellison syndrome, secretory diarrhea is the consequence of gastric hypersecretion caused by a high concentration of circulating gastrin, overwhelming the intestinal absorptive capacity. In medullary carcinoma of the thyroid, circulating calcitonin is the major mediator of intestinal secretion (13). Malabsorption due to different mechanisms may equally produce diarrhea (see Section Malabsorption).

Chemotherapy-Induced Diarrhea

Chemotherapy-related diarrhea is common and most often described with fluoropyrimidines (particularly fluorouracil and capecitabine), irinotecan, and several molecular targeted agents (such as tyrosine kinase inhibitors, vascular endothelial growth factor [VEGF] inhibitors). In addition, small molecule monoclonal antibodies (such as ipilimumab and cetuximab) can cause severe diarrhea and immune-mediated colitis. Grade 3 to 4 diarrhea secondary to chemotherapy has been reported with a frequency of 5% to 47% (14). Patients who experienced chemotherapy-induced diarrhea often require changes in their regimen, including dose reductions, delays in therapy, reduction in dose intensity, and discontinuation of therapy (2). These agents cause acute and chronic damage to the intestinal mucosa, necrosis, and extensive inflammation of the bowel wall. Mucosal and submucosal factors, produced directly or indirectly by the inflamed intestine, stimulate the secretion of intestinal fluid and electrolytes. Similar anatomic changes have been observed in patients with graft-versus-host disease (GVHD)–induced diarrhea, as well as with radiation enteritis (15). Acute radiation enteritis is thought to be a consequence of direct exposure of rapidly dividing intestinal epithelium, to the cytotoxic effects of radiation (16). In patients treated with concurrent pelvic radiation therapy and fluorouracil, 53% developed diarrhea (17). The incidence of grade 3 diarrhea is correlated with the volume of small bowel receiving at least 15 Gy of radiation (18). Chronic radiation enteritis is less common and is usually associated with radiation doses >45 Gy. The underlying pathology is progressive obliterative endarteritis causing tissue ischemia leading to submucosal fibrosis (16).

Infectious Diarrhea

Intestinal mucositis also increases the risk of superinfection by opportunistic pathogens such as *Clostridium difficile*, *Clostridium perfringens*, *Bacillus cereus*, *Giardia lamblia*, *Cryptosporidium*, *Salmonella*, *Shigella*, *Campylobacter*, and *Rotavirus*, particularly in patients who may be neutropenic or immunosuppressed. Bacterial enterotoxins or other infective agents induce secretion by a local nervous reflex mediated by enteroendocrine cells or inflammation (1). The incidence of *C. difficile*–induced diarrhea is very high—almost half a million infections in 2011 (19).

Medication-Induced Diarrhea

Finally, many drugs may cause diarrhea. Diuretics, caffeine, theophylline, antacids, poorly absorbable laxative agents, and osmotically active solutes, often chronically administered in a palliative care setting, likely produce reflex nervous secretion or directly activate secretory cellular mechanism (1).

The use of long-term antibiotics is also associated with diarrhea, with an incidence ranging between 15% and 25% of all cases (20). Agents more frequently causing diarrhea include fluoroquinolones, clindamycin, broad-spectrum penicillins, or cephalosporins, because of the disruption of the normal flora and facilitation of the overgrowth of pathogens. *C. difficile*, an anaerobic organism, produces two toxins that mediate colitis and diarrhea. The potent enterotoxin of *C. difficile* can induce pseudomembranous enterocolitis, which presents as a severe microbial diarrhea. Other infectious agents include *C. perfringens*, *Staphylococcus aureus*, *Klebsiella oxytoca*, *Candida* species, and *Salmonella* species (21).

Diarrhea can also be induced by enteral feeding is via nasogastric tube or gastroenterostomies. It is a common problem that is observable in 10% to

60% of patients. Formula osmolarity, rate of delivery, and contamination with other medications are determinants (22).

Deranged Motility

Deranged motility may reduce the contact time between luminal contents and epithelial cells. This commonly occurs in patients with cancer with postsurgical disorders, such as postgastrectomy dumping syndrome, postvagotomy, ileocecal valve resection, or neoplastic and chronic diseases such as malignant carcinoid syndrome, medullary carcinoma of the thyroid, and diabetes. The mechanism by which diabetic neuropathy causes dysmotility is attributed to sympathetic denervation of the bowel with a prevalence of cholinergic innervation (21). Similarly, procedures such as celiac plexus block can produce sympathetic denervation of the bowel leading to unopposed cholinergic activity. This results in increased intestinal motility and diarrhea until adaptation mechanisms develop (22).

Spinal cord damage may reduce intestinal mobility favoring bacterial overgrowth, inducing deconjugation of bile acids in the small bowel and thereby causing diarrhea and steatorrhea. Diarrhea secondary to dysmotility disorders commonly subsides after a 1- to 2-day fast, resulting in small stool volume and osmolality in the range of 250 to 300 mOsm.

Assessment

The assessment includes a detailed medical history, dietary history, previous surgery, medication review, physical examination, and description of stools. Frequency, amount, and consistency of the stools should be carefully obtained. When the stools are consistently large, light in color, watery or greasy, free of blood, or contain undigested food particles, the underlying disorder is likely to be in the small bowel or the proximal colon. Indeed, diarrhea, in which frequent but small quantities of feces are dark in color and often contain mucus or blood in spite of a sense of urgency, is associated with a disorder of the left colon or rectum (22). Widespread inflammation may simultaneously produce both patterns of diarrhea, confirmed by the passage of nonbloody diarrheal fluid, pus, or exudates. Other useful information includes fecal incontinence, change in stool caliber, rectal bleeding, and small, frequent, but otherwise normal stools.

Timing and spontaneous recovery are also important. Although osmotic diarrhea typically stops or reduces after fasting or stopping the drug previously used, secretory diarrhea persists in spite of fasting. Chemotherapy-induced diarrhea typically occurs 2 to 14 days after therapy. Radiation colitis is probable in patients who have recently received pelvic radiation for malignancies of the urogenital tract and of the prostate.

A physical examination should precede any further investigation. Signs of anemia, fever, postural hypotension, lymphadenopathy, neuropathy, hepatosplenomegaly, ascites, gaseous abdominal distention or lymphadenopathy, reduced anal sphincter tone, rectal mass or impaction, and deterioration of nutritional status are of paramount importance in defining the type of diarrhea. Some etiologies may have a typical clinical pattern. For example, carbohydrate malabsorption is typically associated with excessive flatus and mushy stools, whereas intermittent diarrhea and constipation are frequent in diabetic neuropathy, as well as in irritable bowel syndrome or subobstructive disorders. Autonomic neuropathy or anal sphincter dysfunction may be characterized by nocturnal diarrhea and fecal soiling. Alternating diarrhea and constipation suggests fixed colonic obstruction. Fecal impaction may cause apparent diarrhea because only liquids pass a partial obstruction. Secretory diarrhea combined with upper GI symptoms caused by refractory peptic ulcer disease is suggestive of a gastrin-secreting tumor. High circulating serotonin levels in carcinoid syndrome cause other effects besides diarrhea, including hypotension, sweating, flushing, palpitations, and wheezing (21). The association of heat intolerance, palpitations, and weight loss suggests possible hyperthyroidism. Intestinal dysmotility or bacterial overgrowth due to diabetes, neoplastic conditions, or postoperative conditions should be suspected, excluding other causes.

Chronic bowel ischemia should be considered in elderly patients with the clinical features of diffuse atherosclerotic disease. Rectal examination and abdominal palpation should be performed to look for fecal masses and to exclude fecal impaction and intestinal obstruction, as well as for perianal fistula or abscess. Rectal involvement is probable in the presence of *tenesmus*, commonly defined as the passing of a little or no stool in spite of a sense of rectal urgency.

Of course, the site of neoplasm and metastases is important. The location of the tumor can be verified by abdominal x-ray, computed tomography scan, magnetic resonance imaging, angiography, or laparoscopy.

Laboratory findings should complete the investigation. If feasible, the collected stool specimen should be submitted for qualitative study. A positive finding in either the stool guaiac or the leukocyte test leads to a suspicion of an exudative mechanism, as in radiation colitis, colonic neoplasm, or infective diarrhea. Stool cultures for bacterial, fungal, and viral pathogens, as well as a formal evaluation of the GI tract, should complete the initial assessment (15). Gram stain of the stool can diagnose the presence of *Staphylococcus, Campylobacter,* or *Candida* infection. Multiple stool cultures should be obtained from patients with secretory diarrhea to rule out microorganisms producing enterotoxins that stimulate intestinal secretion. The presence of a microorganism in the stool is diagnostic.

An osmotic gap of >100 mmol/L due to a reduction of stool content in sodium and potassium suggests osmotic diarrhea, whereas lower values (<50 mmol/L) indicate secretory diarrhea due to active secretion of salts and water.

Treatment

As a general rule, current medication should be reviewed, evaluating for any use of laxatives, antacids, theophylline preparations, central nervous system drugs, antiarrhythmics, or antibiotics. Evidence-based dietary advice is limited and often difficult to follow by most patients with cancer, but it may be helpful in some circumstances. Binders of osmotically active substances (kaolin–pectin) give a thicker consistency to loose stools, producing a viscous, colloidal, and absorbent solution, but their antidiarrheal effectiveness is disputable. Apples without the peel are particularly rich in pectin. Other dietary advice includes avoiding cold meals, milk, vegetables rich in fibers, fatty meat, and fish, coffee, and alcohol.

As diarrhea is associated with the occurrence of dehydration, the patient should be rehydrated, possibly by oral solutions containing glucose, electrolytes, and water. However, clinical signs of dehydration, such as orthostatic hypotension, decreased skin turgor, and a dry mouth, suggest the need for intensive hydration through intravenous route, especially in patients suffering from nausea and vomiting in whom oral therapy is ineffective. Patients may experience electrolyte imbalance, particularly hypokalemia (1).

Considering the different mechanisms involved in determining diarrhea in patients with cancer, there are no broadly accepted treatment protocols. Particular strategies have been anecdotally suggested for specific etiologies (Table 14.1). The most common treatment medications and doses used for diarrhea are given in Table 14.2. Agents with oral opiates (such as loperamide) and bile acid sequestrants (such as cholestyramine) have been favorably used in radiation-induced diarrhea (23). The rationale for the use of bile acid sequestrants is the prevalence of bile salt malabsorption in patients with a history of pelvic radiotherapy. However, their use is limited by associated GI side effects including

TABLE 14.1 ETIOLOGY-BASED TREATMENT

Etiology	Treatment
All conditions	Dietary advice and adequate hydration
Radiation-induced diarrhea	Hypofractionated–accelerated radiotherapy and amifostine Cholestyramine, aspirin, sucralfate, silicate smectite, and steroids
Bacterial overgrowth–related diarrhea	Antibiotics
Antibiotic-associated diarrhea	Discontinuation of antibiotics and start with metronidazole Probiotic bacteria
Chemotherapy-induced diarrhea	Alkalization, activated charcoal, loperamide, and octreotide
Hormonal gastrointestinal tumors	Octreotide
Diabetic diarrhea	Clonidine

bloating, flatulence, and abdominal discomfort. It is important to note that symptoms can often stop after completion of radiation treatment. In gynecologic malignancies, prior operation with low pelvic fields and prior operation with small volume were significantly protective factors for overall diarrhea. Conversely, large volume was a significant factor of overall and moderate to severe diarrhea in patients with large-field operations (24). Amifostine is a cytoprotective adjuvant used in cancer che-

TABLE 14.2 TREATMENT MEDICATIONS FOR DIARRHEA

Bile acid sequestrant	
Cholestyramine	4–12 g
Antibiotics	
Vancomycin	125–250 mg 8 hourly
Metronidazole	250–500 mg 8 hourly
Mucosal prostaglandin inhibitors	
Aspirin	300 mg 4 hourly
Opioid agents	
Codeine	10–60 mg 4 hourly
Loperamide	4 mg stat, then 2 mg 6 hourly and after each loose
Somatostatin analogs	
Octreotide	0.3–0.6 mg/d (continuous infusion) 0.1 mg 8 hourly

motherapy, and preliminary studies suggest that it may reduce the incidence and severity of radiation-induced diarrhea (25). Amifostine reduced the incidence and severity of diarrhea associated with 5-fluorouracil, although its use may be associated with hypotension (26).

Steroids may exert a positive effect on several conditions associated with diarrhea, including secretory diarrhea, intestinal pseudo-obstruction, radiation-induced enteritis, and endocrine tumors due to anti-inflammatory effects. They are capable of reducing the release and effect of inflammation mediators; thereby promoting salt and water absorption. In addition, systemic glucocorticoids plus oral nonabsorbable steroids can be used for GVHD-induced diarrhea without infection (27).

Systemic antibiotics, such as norfloxacin and amoxicillin–clavulanic acid, are effective in the treatment of bacterial overgrowth–related diarrhea (28). Rifaximin, a nonsystemic antibiotic has also demonstrated efficacy in eradicating small intestinal bacterial overgrowth (SIBO). However, diagnostic tests, interpretation, dosing, and duration of Rifaximin varied across study populations warranting further investigation (29). On the contrary, antibiotic-associated diarrhea (pseudomembranous enterocolitis) requires the discontinuation of antibiotics and the start of either oral fidaxomicin or oral vancomycin, both of which are more effective than oral metronidazole (30). Bismuth subsalicylate in doses of 30 to 60 mL every 30 minutes for eight doses may bring mild symptomatic relief in patients with acute infectious diarrhea with an unknown effect. Probiotic bacteria (i.e., live bacteria that survive passage through the GI tract) alongside rehydration may have beneficial effects on the host with infectious diarrhea (31). Live *Lactobacillus acidophilus* plus *Bifidobacterium bifidum* reduced the incidence of radiation-induced diarrhea and the need for antidiarrheal medication and had a significant benefits on stool consistency (32).

Alkalization of the intestinal tract by oral administration of sodium bicarbonate has been reported to be a promising method for preventing delayed diarrhea, a dose-limiting toxicity in patients receiving chemotherapy with irinotecan, without decreasing the blood levels of irinotecan and its active metabolites, thereby improving the tolerability of long-term chemotherapy without reducing the efficacy (33). Activated charcoal, given the evening before the irinotecan dose and then t.i.d. for 48 hours after the dose, reduced irinotecan-induced diarrhea and optimized its dose intensity, possibly by adsorbing free luminal SN-38, the irinotecan-active moiety that has a direct effect on mucosal topoisomerase-I (34). Broad-spectrum antibiotics may influence the intestinal toxicity of irinotecan. Although neomycin had no effect on the systemic exposure of irinotecan and its major metabolites, it changed fecal β-glucuronidase activity and decreased fecal concentrations of the pharmacologically active metabolite SN-38. It was associated with an improvement in diarrhea and not with hematologic toxicity, suggesting that bacterial β-glucuronidase plays a crucial role in irinotecan-induced diarrhea without affecting heterocyclic and systemic SN-38 levels (35).

Opioids have been traditionally used for their antidiarrheal properties owing to the widespread presence of opioid receptors at different peripheral sites, including smooth muscle, myenteric plexus, and spinal cord. It is well known that their activation increases ileocecal tone and decreases small intestine and colon peristalsis (increasing electrolyte and water absorption). It also impairs the defecation reflex by inhibiting anorectal sphincter relaxation and diminishing anorectal sensitivity to distention. As a consequence, the contact time between the intestinal mucosa and luminal contents is enhanced by the reduction of colonic propulsive activity, resulting in greater fluid absorption (36). Antidiarrheal effects can be obtained by both oral and parenteral opioids. Loperamide (Imodium) and diphenoxylate–atropine (Lomotil) are the most commonly used, and both are FDA approved for chemotherapy-related diarrhea. Among opioids, loperamide is more specific because of the prevalent peripheral effect due to the inability to cross the blood–brain barrier. Loperamide shows the highest antidiarrheal/analgesic ratio among the opioid-like agents and is proved to be the drug of choice because of its few adverse effects. However, life threatening toxicity (such as cardiac arrest, ventricular fibrillation, prolonged QTC) can result at high doses from loperamide-induced cardiac toxicity (37). The standard dose of loperamide is 4 mg followed by 2 mg after every unformed stool. The dosage is titrated against the effect and higher doses of 2 mg every 2 hours have been recommended (up to 16 mg/day in conjunction with chemotherapeutic agents associated with a high incidence of diarrhea (38). Loperamide-simethicone combination was significantly more effective than the drugs taken alone in the treatment of acute diarrhea with gas-related abdominal discomfort (39). However, the risk of developing paralytic ileus in the presence of continuous secretion should be considered as a life-threatening complication. Of note, opioids may paradoxically cause diarrhea secondary to fecal impaction.

Despite the absence of literature supporting efficacy in cancer treatment–induced diarrhea, deodorized tincture of opium (DTO) is widely used in the treatment of diarrhea. DTO contains the equivalent of 10 mg/mL morphine. Recommended dose is 10 to 15 drops every 3 to 4 hours (23). It is available in liquid form only, requiring measurement with a dropper.

Data from several clinical trials suggest that octreotide may be useful in the symptomatic treatment of diarrhea refractory to other medications (36,38). The mechanism by which octreotide produces these beneficial effects are multifactorial, as it reduces the secretion of many pancreatic and GI hormones, prolongs intestinal transit time and thereby promotes absorption of electrolytes (40). Octreotide has been found to control diarrhea in several conditions, such as carcinoid tumors, vipoma, gastrinoma, small cell lung cancer, and acquired immunodeficiency syndrome–related diarrhea (41). However, hormonal responses to the somatostatin analog do not always parallel clinical responses, probably because of the effects of cosecreted peptides. A dose–response effect of octreotide has been demonstrated. Octreotide seems to be an effective agent in the management of chemotherapy-related diarrhea and refractory GVHD-associated diarrhea (42,43). Doses of 0.3 to 1.2 mg/d subcutaneously are commonly effective. Octreotide was also effective in the treatment of radiation-induced diarrhea (23).

The long-acting, biodegradable, and microsphere formulation of octreotide for monthly subcutaneous administration (30 mg) has been evaluated for the prophylaxis of diarrhea, speeding the resolution of diarrhea and preventing further episodes during subsequent cycles of chemotherapy (44). A preventive strategy with octreotide long acting release (LAR) as prophylaxis has also been proposed for patients with a prior cycle of chemotherapy complicated by persistent diarrhea (39,45). Studies regarding efficacy of octreotide LAR in the prevention of CID remain inconsistent. One reason that might explain the absence of benefit seen in studies that used octreotide LAR for diarrhea induced by cancer treatment is the pharmacokinetic profile (46).

MALABSORPTION

Ineffective absorption of breakdown products in the small intestine may occur because a disorder interferes with the digestion of food or directly with the absorption of nutrients. The digestive and absorptive processes are inextricably linked. The series of events include the reduction of particle size, solubilization of hydrophobic lipids, and enzymatic digestion of nutrients to small fragments, absorption of the products of digestion across the intestinal cells, and transport through lymphatics.

Pathophysiology of Digestion

The pancreatic secretion of lipase, amylase, and proteases break down fat to monoglycerides and fatty acids, carbohydrates to monosaccharides and disaccharides, and proteins to peptides and amino acids. Several processes have been recognized to facilitate the absorption of fat from the aqueous luminal environment. Triglycerides are emulsified together with phospholipids, bile salts, and monoglycerides and diglycerides and dispersed into a variety of phases and particles. Lipid digestion begins in the mouth and in the stomach, active at a low pH, promoting emulsion stability, and facilitating the action of pancreatic lipases. Gastric and pyloric motility further promote emulsification of lipids. This effect is amplified by bile salts and biliary phospholipids, which influence the absorption of cholesterol and sterol vitamins. Lipolysis to fatty acids and monoglycerides is mediated by pancreatic lipases (36). Protein digestion begins in the stomach. Acid denaturation leads to proteolysis, which is promoted by endopeptidases activated by an acidic environment, cleaving the internal bonds of large proteins to form nonabsorbable peptides. Pancreatic peptidases convert proteins and polypeptides into amino acids and oligopeptides. Hormonal and neural stimulation stimulate the release of proenzymes by the pancreas. Enteropeptidases and trypsin activate a cascade of events that promote the activation of chymotrypsin, elastase, and carboxypeptidases A and B in the duodenum. The hydrolysis of fat, protein, and carbohydrate by pancreatic enzymes, and the solubilization of fat by bile salts, may be altered by several conditions (13,36). In pancreatic carcinoma or following pancreatic resection, decreased pancreatic enzymes and bicarbonate release may limit the digestion of fat and protein leading to pancreatic insufficiency. These disorders may also be associated with malabsorption of fat-soluble vitamins. The Zollinger-Ellison syndrome is characterized by an extreme acid hypersecretion, causing a low luminal pH, which inactivates pancreatic enzymes with consequent fat malabsorption. A decrease in intraluminal bile salts due to disruption of the enterohepatic circulation is also seen in patients with Zollinger-Ellison syndrome. Biliary tract obstruction, terminal ileal resection, or cholestatic liver disease results in decreased formation of bile salts or delivery to the duodenum (47). Many postsurgical disorders have been associated with a marked proliferation of intraluminal microorganisms, including an afferent loop of a Billroth II partial gastrectomy, a surgical blind loop with end-to-side anastomosis, or a recirculating loop with side-to-side anastomosis. The final consequence depends on the extension of resection. With limited small bowel resections, malabsorbed bile acids pass into the colon and increase colon motility, while decreasing water and electrolyte absorption, resulting in diarrhea. In contrast, after massive small bowel resection, the bile acid pool will decrease because of the loss of intestinal bile salts. This phenomenon is associated with a loss of the absorptive intestinal surface and bacterial overgrowth. These processes will result in steatorrhea. Bacterial overgrowth causes catabolism of carbohydrates by gram-negative aerobes, deconjugation of bile salts by anaerobes, and the binding of cobalamin by anaerobes. Other than massive resection involving the ileocecal calve, causes of bacterial overgrowth include obstruction or strictures and autonomic neuropathy (13).

Pathophysiology of Absorption

Products of digestion are normally absorbed from the lumen through the enterocyte to appear in the lymphatics or the portal vein. This passage is specific for each digested substance, according to the circumstances. Active transport requires energy to move nutrients against a gradient, whereas passive diffusion allows nutrients to pass according to gradient differentials. Facilitated diffusion is an intermediate mechanism, similar to passive diffusion, but carrier-mediated and subject to competitive inhibition. Endocytosis is a process in which parts of a cell membrane engulf nutrients.

Absorption of monosaccharides occurs predominantly in the proximal small intestine, although not all the dietary carbohydrate is absorbed. The simple diffusion of monosaccharides across membranes is slow, but it is important in the presence of high luminal concentrations of glucose. When luminal concentrations of glucose are low, specific active transport systems, especially through sodium-coupled transporters, mediate efficient transport of these substances. Monosaccharides may also enter enterocytes by facilitated diffusion. However, the uptake may be limited by enzyme activity, for example, lactase. Xylose is not digested and has a low affinity for carriers. Some of the carbohydrates reach the colon and are fermented by bacteria into short-chain fatty acids with the production of gases such as hydrogen and methane. Short-chain fatty acids are subsequently absorbed by colonic epithelial cells.

Fat products rapidly and passively diffuse into enterocytes, with the rate of transfer depending on the chain length. Fatty acids and monoglycerides are metabolized into triglycerides and assembled with phospholipids and cholesteryl esters into chylomicrons. Short-chain and medium-chain fatty acids have a less complex absorptive mechanism. They may be absorbed intact by passive diffusion or completely hydrolyzed, but they are not reesterified

inside the enterocytes. Lipid absorption is highly efficient; only small amounts of lipids enter the colon. These may be absorbed by the colonic mucosa or undergo bacterial metabolism.

Bile salts are synthesized from cholesterol in the liver, conjugated with amino acids, secreted into the bile, and recycled back to the liver through the portal system. Minimal daily losses are balanced by hepatic synthesis. Passive diffusion and active transport are involved in bile salt transport in the small intestine to limit fecal loss. A certain amount of bile salt in the colonic lumen is essential for normal colonic function. In the colon, bile salts are not absorbed, but they stimulate colonic motility and secretion of sodium chloride and water. In contrast, bile salt deficiency may cause constipation (36).

Amino acids are absorbed by enterocytes and oligopeptides are digested by the enterocyte and oligopeptidases and dipeptidases of the brush border. A specific transport mechanism exists for the intracellular transport of amino acids and dipeptides. Protein absorption is efficient and occurs mainly in the jejunum and ileum (48).

Mucosal damage, as observed with radiation enteritis, may impair epithelial cell transport. Other than extensive mucosal damage, lymphatic obstruction and bacterial overgrowth are the principal mechanisms of radiation-induced malabsorption (49).

A large surgical resection of the small intestine reduces the epithelial surface area available for absorption. After a gastrectomy, low levels of vitamin E and total cholesterol were found as a consequence of loss of passage through the duodenum (50). The extent and specific level of resection are predictive of severe malabsorption and short bowel syndrome. Most patients with short bowel syndrome have either a high jejunostomy with a residual jejunal length <100 cm or a jejunocolic anastomosis. The recovery from massive small bowel resection depends on the adaptive response of the remaining mucosa (48). Resection of >50% of the small intestine still results in significant malabsorption. The inclusion of the distal two-thirds of the ileum and ileocecal sphincter in the resected section increases the risk of malabsorption. Preservation of the ileocecal sphincter is important, because it may prevent small bowel contamination from colonic flora and may increase the transit time of the intraluminal content.

After intestinal resections, increased amount of bile salts reach the colon promoting water and electrolyte secretion, unless liver production compensates the losses as in limited resections. The consequent lack of solubilization of intraluminal fat will worsen the effects of bile salts on the colon mucosa. Enterostomy or intestinal fistulae may also result in a reduced absorption due to the loss of intestinal surface area.

Diabetic neuropathy may also result in intestinal dysmotility and bacterial overgrowth and, as a consequence, in malabsorption. Lymphatic transport of chylomicrons and proteins is limited by lymphatic obstruction leading to dilatation and potential rupture of intestinal lymphatic vessels that cause intestinal leakage of proteins, chylomicrons, and small lymphocytes. Localized ileal tumors, diffuse intestinal lymphomas, metastatic carcinoma, and metastatic carcinoid disease may all lead to lymphatic obstruction, fat malabsorption, and protein-losing enteropathy (36).

Assessment

Patients with malabsorption usually lose weight. If fats are not absorbed properly, the stools are light colored, soft, bulky, and foul smelling. Documentation of steatorrhea is the cornerstone of the diagnostic evaluation. Malabsorption can cause deficiencies of all nutrients or proteins, fats, vitamins, or minerals selectively. Certain physical signs are frequently associated with specific deficiency states secondary to malabsorption, such as glossitis in folate or vitamin B_{12} deficiency and hyperkeratosis, ecchymoses, and hematuria due to fat-soluble vitamin deficiency (vitamins A and K). Anemia (chronic blood loss or malabsorption of iron, folate, or vitamin B_{12}), leukocytosis with eosinophilia, low serum levels of albumin, iron, cholesterol, and an extension of the prothrombin time are the most common laboratory findings in malabsorption (36). Impaired absorption of calcium and magnesium may induce weakness, paresthesias, and tetany. Osteopenia and bone pain, spontaneous fractures, and vertebral collapse may develop from vitamin D and calcium deficiency. Peripheral neuropathy may occur after gastric resection because of vitamin B_{12} deficiency. Weakness, severe weight loss, and fatigue result from caloric deprivation. In pancreatic carcinoma, floating, bulky, and malodorous stools and increased gas production are often associated with anorexia. Steatorrhea, peripheral lymphocytopenia, hypoalbuminemia, chylous ascites, and peripheral edema are the hallmarks of abnormalities of lymphatic transport. Symptoms of dumping syndrome after gastrectomy include early nausea, abdominal distention, weakness, and diarrhea after a meal, followed by hypoglycemia, sweating, dizziness, and tachycardia. Obstruction may also result in malabsorption, an obstructed bile duct could result in jaundice.

Overall, malabsorption should be suspected when an individual loses weight and has diarrhea and nutritional deficiencies despite eating well.

Reviewing current drugs is important in the diagnostic evaluation. Colchicine, and neomycin, are the most common drugs causing malabsorption, although the pathophysiologic mechanisms are unknown. Dietary phosphate absorption may be limited by the use of aluminum-containing antacids, resulting in hypophosphatemia and hypercalciuria.

Laboratory tests can help confirm the diagnosis. Tests that directly measure fat in stool samples are the most reliable ones for diagnosing malabsorption of fat. Other laboratory tests can detect malabsorption of other specific substances, such as lactose or vitamin B_{12}. Undigested food fragments may mean that food passes through the intestine too rapidly. Such fragments can indicate an anatomically abnormal intestinal pathway, such as a direct connection between the stomach and the large intestine that bypasses the small intestine. Small intestinal barium x-rays may define anatomic abnormalities after massive resection. Biochemical examination of the fecal material may give information about the origin of a fistula (pancreatic or enteric). Liver function tests and imaging of the liver or biliary tract may demonstrate parenchymal liver disease as a cause of decreased production of bile salts or a biliary tract obstruction (Table 14.3).

Treatment

After assessing the causes of malabsorption, therapy should be directed to correct the deficiencies, including enzyme replacement, bicarbonate supplements, vitamins, calcium, magnesium, and iron. For example, vitamin B_{12} replacement is necessary

---

TABLE 14.3 MALABSORPTION: SIGNS AND SYMPTOMS

- Steatorrhea
- Weight loss, weakness, and fatigue (caloric deprivation)
- Glossitis (folate or vitamin B_{12} deficiency)
- Hyperkeratosis, ecchymoses, and hematuria (vitamins A and K deficiency)
- Weakness, paresthesias, and tetany (calcium and magnesium deficiencies)
- Early nausea, abdominal distention, weakness, and diarrhea after a meal, followed by hypoglycemia, sweating, dizziness, and tachycardia (after gastric resection)
- Osteopenia and bone pain, spontaneous fractures (vitamin D and calcium deficiencies)
- Chylous ascites—peripheral edema (abnormalities of lymphatic transport)
- Peripheral neuropathy (vitamin B_{12} deficiency)
- Laboratory findings: anemia (iron, folate, or vitamin B_{12} deficiencies), leukocytosis with eosinophilia, peripheral lymphocytopenia, and hypoalbuminemia

after terminal ileal resection. Pancreatic enzyme replacement along with a low-fat, high-protein diet is indicated in the case of malabsorption due to pancreatic insufficiency. The effectiveness of enzyme replacements is variable and, in part, depends on a high enough gastric pH to prevent their degradation in the stomach (51). Large doses of pancreatic extract are required with each meal. Sodium and bicarbonate or anti-H_2 inhibitors and hydrogen pump inhibitors are mainly added to raise the duodenal pH.

Fat intake should be strictly limited, especially in short bowel syndrome. Medium-chain triglycerides may be substituted for long-chain triglycerides to improve fat absorption after a small intestinal resection, as they are useful in the presence of lymphatic obstruction because they do not require intestinal lymphatic transport. Oxalate should also be restricted in short bowel syndrome sparing the colon.

For patients with prominent dumping, dietary modification comprising frequent small, dry meals that are high in protein and low in carbohydrates, along with ingestion of substances that prolong the absorption of carbohydrates, such as fiber (such as pectin), may be useful (36).

An aggressive approach should be reserved in the presence of severe malnutrition and dehydration, especially after surgery. Parenteral nutrition is strongly indicated in the immediate postoperative period after massive intestinal resection. The duration of parenteral nutrition is inversely proportional to the length of the remaining intestine. The weaning to oral nutrition depends on several variables, including the preoperative nutritional state, the absorptive deficit, and the tolerance to oral intake. Oral feeding should be started as soon as possible, as adaptation of the remaining bowel to resection is facilitated by the early introduction of oral or enteral nutrients. Moreover, intraluminal nutrients stimulate trophic GI hormones regulating mucosal repair. H_2-blocking agents may also favorably influence the rate of adaptation of the remaining intestine after massive resection, possibly by a mucosal trophic effect improving nutrient absorption. Nutrients requiring minimal digestion for absorption should be chosen, such as commercial preparations containing simple sugars, amino acids, or oligopeptides, as well as medium-chain triglycerides. An excessive osmolar load should be avoided to prevent the occurrence of diarrhea. More complex food should be added gradually.

Drugs that Limit Acid Secretion

H_2 blockers and proton pump inhibitors are used to treat the transient acid hypersecretion after extensive bowel resection or the acid hypersecretion state in patients with gastrinoma (Zollinger-Ellison syndrome). The use of cholestyramine should be carefully considered. It may be indicated in limited intestinal resections, because it binds bile salts and prevents their irritant effects on the colon. However, in short bowel syndrome after massive intestinal resection, it may reduce the bile salt pool, thereby increasing fat malabsorption. Aluminum hydroxide exerts similar effects.

Drugs that Limit Secretions or Transit Time

In patients affected by malabsorption due to short bowel syndrome, it is useful to reduce the intestinal output or the transit time. Loperamide can delay the transit time or reduce secretions (36). Octreotide has been used because of its ability to reduce gastric, pancreatic, and biliary secretions, as well as intestinal transit time (48). Octreotide is often indicated for those who continue to have high fluid losses, and patients requiring intravenous fluid >3 L/day (52). It may reduce or shorten the use of parenteral administration in several postoperative conditions, such as enterocutaneous or pancreatic fistulae. Its use in terminally ill patients has been favorably reported (36). Clonidine and exenatide can also be used in patients with high fluid losses that are refractory to other measures (53,54).

Antibiotic Use

Antibiotic-associated malnutrition requires discontinuation of any implicated antimicrobial agents. However, if there is stasis with bacterial overgrowth caused by impaired motility or stricture, such as in radiation enteritis or blind loop syndrome, broad-spectrum antibiotics should be administered. A 7 to 10 days course of rifaximin or metronidazole plus a cephalosporin seems to be effective in suppressing the flora and correcting malabsorption. However, cyclic therapy may be needed (42).

Reversal of a short segment of the bowel or construction of a recirculating loop has been advocated in patients with life-threatening malabsorption and uncontrolled weight loss. However, such operations may have negative consequences, as they can lead to stasis and bacterial overgrowth, further compromising intestinal absorption. More often the benefit is of limited value (36).

CONSTIPATION

In the general population, the prevalence of constipation is significant and increases with age. In advanced cancer patients, the combination of underlying disease and medication often leads to a dramatic increase in occurrence. The range of prevalence in hospitalized patients receiving cancer treatment varies from 10% to 70% and is reported by approximately 50% of hospice patients at admission (55) and 72% of patients receiving oral morphine for cancer pain (56). Moreover, constipation is considered the first cause of adverse drug reactions in hospitalized patients with cancer (3).

In addition to causing discomfort, constipation affects daily living and nutritional intake compromising quality of life. Moreover, synergism of constipation with other abdominal processes such as ascites or tumor may increase pain and can limit diaphragmatic excursion worsening dyspnea. Untreated constipation may progress to obstipation, which may potentially lead to life-threatening complications associated with bowel obstruction.

Pathophysiology

There are many, often concomitant, causes of constipation in patients with cancer (Table 14.4). Constipation may be secondary to systemic diseases or those solely afflicting the GI tract. It may be directly due to cancer or secondary effects of cancer. Furthermore, a great number of medication and treatments are known to cause constipation. For example, opioid-induced constipation is caused by the linkage of the opioid-to-opioid receptors in the bowel and the central nervous system (55).

Neurogenic

Constipation is frequently noted in patients with various neurologic disorders. A visceral neuropathy seems to be present in most patients with severe slow-transit constipation. Disturbance in the extrinsic nerve supply to the colon has been found in these patients, along with a lack of inhibitory innervation of colonic circular muscle and a diminished release of acetylcholine. Patients with advanced cancer frequently complain of GI symptoms, including anorexia, chronic nausea, and early satiety—a symptom complex often associated with physical signs of an autonomic neuropathy. Autonomic neuropathy may also be manifested as severe constipation, including postural hypotension and resting tachycardia. It is a multifactorial syndrome with many possible causative factors including malnutrition, decreased activity, diabetes, and drugs such as vinca alkaloids, opioids, and tricyclic antidepressants) (36).

Diabetic dysmotility has traditionally been thought to reflect a generalized autonomic neuropathy. However, secretions of GI hormones may also be important.

Peripheral neuropathy is a common complication of cancer chemotherapy. Patients receiving a high cumulative dose of vincristine or cisplatin seem to be at a significantly elevated risk for the development of long-term side effects (1). These drugs have been shown to cause symptoms of autonomic polyneuropathy with constipation, bladder atony, and hypotension. Whereas many reports describe acute neurologic side effects during therapy, there is no consensus about persistent and late damage to the peripheral nervous system. Chemotherapy-induced peripheral neuropathy (CIPN) can persist from months to years. The long-term neurologic side effects in patients with curable malignancies, such as Hodgkin's disease and testicular cancer, may be particularly troublesome.

Ogilvie's syndrome describes a variety of states with a similar clinical picture due to intrinsic defects in the intestinal smooth muscle, with a massive colonic dilatation in the absence of an obstruction or inflammatory process. Also termed as *pseudo-obstruction*, this syndrome can be categorized into those with myopathic and those with neuropathic features. Several conditions involving the intestinal smooth muscle are associated

TABLE 14.4 CAUSES OF CONSTIPATION IN PATIENTS WITH CANCER

Neurogenic disorders
Periphery
  Ganglionopathy
  Autonomic neuropathy
Central nervous system
  Spinal cord lesions
    Parkinson's disease
Metabolic and endocrine diseases
Diabetes
Uremia
Hypokalemia
Hypothyroidism
Hypercalcemia
Pheochromocytoma
Enteric glucagon excess
Malignancy
Direct effects
  Cerebral or spinal cord tumors
  Intestinal obstruction
  Hypercalcemia
Secondary effects
  Inadequate food intake and low-fiber diet
  Poor fluid intake
  Reduced activity
  Previous bowel surgery
  Autonomic neuropathy
  Radiotherapy
  Sedation, low level of consciousness
Drugs
Opioids
Nonsteroidal anti-inflammatory drugs
Anticholinergics
Anticonvulsants
Antidepressants
Diuretics
Antacids
Anti-Parkinson drugs
Antihypertensive agents
Vinca alkaloids

with colonic pseudo-obstruction, including endocrine and metabolic disorders, neurologic diseases, nonoperative trauma, surgery, nonintestinal inflammatory processes, infections, malignancy, radiation therapy, drugs, and cardiovascular and respiratory diseases.

Long-term denervation abolishes the normal pelvic floor muscle activity. This neurologic impairment may be produced by nerve damage not only following chemotherapy but also as a consequence of radiotherapy, pelvic surgery, compression, or invasion by neoplastic growth or during prolonged chronic opioid therapy. Loss of the normal rectal muscle tone is also a consequence of prolonged immobility that is often seen in debilitated patients with cancer. Rectal sensation may be reduced, and the rectal capacity of distention may be increased after vincristine treatment or as a consequence of neoplastic involvement of the pelvic sacral nerves. The rectosigmoid junction is a key area in the mechanism of constipation. Rectal outlet obstruction and failure of the puborectalis and anal sphincter muscles to relax are frequent findings in patients with neurologic diseases with intractable constipation. Several mechanisms are possible for constipation by outlet obstruction, including a hyperactive rectosigmoid junction, increased storage capacity of the rectum, spasticity, and hypertonicity of the anal canal with incoordination of the reflex between the rectum and anus. Anismus is a spastic pelvic floor syndrome, recently termed *rectosphincteric dyssynergia* for its similarity with vesicourethral dyssynergia. Similar extrinsic innervation of the bladder and the rectum has been observed, explaining why patients with severe slow-transit constipation often complain of urologic symptoms (55).

The integrity of the spinal cord neurons is essential to maintain normal defecation. In patients with spinal cord lesions above the lumbosacral area, incontinence is controlled but defecation is impaired. This is due to the interruption of the cortical pathways, demonstrating the importance of supraspinal control of distal colonic function and defecation. Moreover, colonic response to a meal is reduced. However, appropriate stimuli may be sufficient to result in an evacuation. In patients with damage to the cauda equina, transit time is prolonged and the recto–anal inhibitory reflex is weaker, offering little protection against fecal incontinence.

In patients with cancer having Parkinson's disease, constipation is probably caused by the degeneration of the autonomic nervous system, particularly the myenteric plexus. Psychiatric and neurologic diseases are frequently associated with colonic dysmotility (57).

Metabolic

A large variety of metabolic disorders predispose to constipation. Of particular relevance to patients with cancer are dehydration, hypercalcemia, hypokalemia, and uremia. Chronic dehydration can also result in dry stools that are difficult to expel.

Medication-Induced Constipation

Many drugs can induce constipation. Some examples include anticholinergics, antiemetics, and diuretics. Patients treated with carbamazepine may develop severe constipation that is not dose related but is refractory to the concomitant use of oral laxatives, requiring drug discontinuation. Selective 5-HT$_3$ receptor antagonists can also cause constipation. They antagonize the ability of 5-hydroxytryptamine (5-HT) to evoke cholinergic mediated contractions of the intestinal longitudinal muscle (58).

One of the most striking pharmacologic features of opioids is their ability to cause constipation. Opioid-induced constipation (OIC) occurs in 51% to 87% of patients receiving opioids for cancer and between 41% and 57% patients receiving opioids for chronic noncancer pain (59). Opioids affect the intestines by different mechanisms. They affect GI motility, secreto-absorptive function, and sphincter performance. Opioids bind to specific opioid receptors in the enteric and central nervous systems. Receptors have been identified on gut smooth muscle, suggesting that there is a local effect of opioid drugs, although central opioid effects cannot be excluded. In the gut, opioids inhibit the release of neurotransmitters, which results in an increased muscular tone and decrease in propulsive activity leading to an increased transit time. Opioids bind to receptors on secretomotor neurons in the submucosa and suppress acetylcholine and vasoactive intestinal peptide release, resulting in decreased chloride and water secretion into the lumen. Moreover, the prolonged bowel transit on its own may facilitate the increased intestinal absorption of fluid and electrolytes. Opioid use may lead to fecal impaction, spurious diarrhea, and bowel pseudo-obstruction, causing abdominal pain, nausea, and vomiting, and interference with drug administration and absorption (60).

Oral morphine invariably causes constipation when used in repeated doses to treat cancer pain. Although other common unwanted effects, such as sedation, nausea, and vomiting, tend to improve with continued use and often resolve completely, opioid-induced constipation does not get better with repeated administration. It is likely that other factors can contribute to slow intestinal transit, such as immobility, concomitant medications, or disease-related factors. The importance of other factors in the development of constipation is demonstrated by the fact that approximately 50% of hospice patients not on opioids required regular oral laxatives.

In a population receiving oral morphine for cancer pain, constipation affected 72% of patients, although an interindividual variation was observed (56). Postoperative pain relief by both parenteral and intraspinal opioids is often associated with adynamic ileus. Gastric emptying and small bowel transit are inhibited. This is an important consideration for patients with cancer undergoing surgical procedures in which the ileus is likely to be a severe problem. Epidural anesthesia with local anesthetics appears to disrupt GI motility less than systemic opioids (55).

Assessment

There are challenges associated with defining constipation in cancer patients. The subjective assessment is often different from the objective view assessed by a health care professional.

It is important to first establish what the patient means by constipation—if the stools are too small, too hard, too difficult to expel, or too infrequent or if the patients have a feeling of incomplete evacuation after defecation. A variety of definitions have been used by patients and health care providers—straining, hard stools, the desire but inability to defecate, infrequent stools, and abdominal discomfort. Stool weight, consistency, and possible parameters to measure may be unreliable because of the wide range in healthy subjects.

Constipation is commonly defined as a decrease in the frequency of the passage of formed stools and characterized by stools that are hard and difficult to pass (61). A frequency of at least three bowel movements per week is viewed as an objective indicator of normality.

Different tools have been proposed to assess constipation. The Rome IV Criteria highlights the physical characteristics of the stool, frequency of bowel movements, and subjective perceptions of distress as important to the definition, as well as component of chronicity, including six elements: straining, hard stool, the sensation of incomplete evacuation, the sensation of anorectal obstruction, fewer than three bowel movements per week. Constipation can be diagnosed if the criteria has been present for the last 3 months with symptom onset at least 6 months prior to diagnosis. The development of the bowel function index was based on established criteria of known assessment tool for opioid-induced constipation. This index is a subjective scale assessment, including three simple questions to be rated from 0 to 100 during the last 7 days: ease of defecation, feeling of incomplete bowel evacuation, and personal judgment regarding constipation (62). The Victoria Hospice Bowel Performance scale uses images to describe stool consistency and has been found to be meaningful for patients (63). The Patient Assessment Constipation Symptoms is composed of three domains: abdominal symptoms (4 items), rectal symptoms (3 items), and stool symptoms (5 items) and is validated for opioid-induced constipation (64).

A careful history and physical examination will be helpful. History should be taken regarding the onset of constipation, bowel habits, current bowel performance, and use of laxatives. Patients who develop progressive constipation in the absence of any clear precipitating cause should be considered for an evaluation looking at electrolytes, renal, and hepatic function tests.

Impaction with overflow should be excluded by performing a rectal examination. Therefore, the first step is to completely evacuate the bowel. Multiple enemas may be needed. Digital fragmentation is unpleasant, but it may permit most of the fecal impaction in the rectum to be diagnosed. A pseudo-diarrhea in the presence of impaired anal sphincter function may be discovered. Gentle digital examination of the rectum may reveal a hard mass, tumor, ulcer, anal stenosis, anismus, or a lax anal sphincter. Patients with spinal cord lesions may have reduced sensation, but the anal tone is preserved, whereas patients with sacral nerve root infiltration will have a reduced anal tone. The examination of the abdomen may reveal fecal masses in the left iliac fossa. Fecal masses are usually not tender, relatively mobile, and can be indented with pressure (55).

Imaging with an abdominal radiograph may distinguish between constipation and obstruction. Examination after a barium meal may help distinguish between paralytic ileus and mechanical obstruction. Barium studies may help reveal a small intestine motility dysfunction in chronic intestinal pseudo-obstruction. In visceral myopathy, intestinal contractions are infrequent, whereas with a visceral neuropathy, patients tend to have less distension and faster intestinal transit time due to uncoordinated contractions (55).

When constipation is due to ineffective colonic musculature, measurement of colonic transit time may be a useful tool to detect specific areas of the bowel that are not functioning properly. A study of transit time may demonstrate delayed transit in the colon, storage of feces in the rectum, or retrograde movement due to a distal spasm. A radiologic constipation score has been proposed, assessing the amount of stool in each of the four abdominal quadrants (65). However, no concordant correlation has been found (66).

Treatment

Recommendations from expert groups (63,67) have confirmed the lack of existing scientific evidence and the ongoing need for controlled studies in the field. General recommendations suggest that it would be useful to synergize pharmacologic interventions and principal mechanism considered to be responsible for constipation. Thus, an extensive effort should be made to find the cause of constipation and treatment should be directed at that specific cause.

The management of constipation should be divided into general interventions and therapeutic measures. Etiologic factors, such as physiologic consequences of cancer-associated debility, biochemical abnormalities, including hypercalcemia and hyperkalemia, and drug use, should be identified and reversed wherever possible. Adequate fluid intake is helpful in increasing the stool water content.

Fluids, fruit, juice, and bran are all recommended. However, fiber deficiency is unlikely to account for a lower stool weight, and there is no justification for the claim that treatment with bran can return stool output and transit time to normal. In patients with far-advanced cancer, the use of high amounts of fiber is beyond the capacity of most patients. Fiber consumption may decrease fluid intake relatively, thereby paradoxically worsening the situation. Since an unfavorable toilet environment, such as lack of privacy or inappropriate posture, may lead to constipation, patients should be provided privacy and appropriate facilities in the hospital setting.

When there are irreversible causes of constipation, symptomatic relief should be provided. Moreover, in spite of prophylaxis, most of these patients will require chronic laxatives, especially in the advanced stage of their disease or when treated with chronic opioid therapy. It is appropriate to begin prophylactic laxative treatment in patients with risk factors for constipation, including the elderly, those who are bedridden, or those requiring drugs that are known to cause constipation.

Low-rectal impaction should be removed manually. Appropriate sedation and analgesics are usually required to make this procedure comfortable. A more proximal mass can be broken by a sigmoidoscope or by delivering a pulsating stream of water against the stool. The use of enemas and rectal interventions is limited to the acute short-term management of more severe episodes.

Laxatives

Therapeutic interventions for the management of constipation are based on the administration of laxatives, either orally or rectally. Laxatives will promote active electrolyte secretion, decrease water and electrolyte absorption, increase intraluminal osmolarity, and increase hydrostatic pressure in the gut. Although laxatives can be divided into several groups, no agent acts purely to soften the stool or stimulate peristalsis. Clinical criteria, responsiveness, acceptability, and the patient's preference should guide the selection of the drug. Table 14.5 outlines different medications that are useful in constipation.

According to their modes of action, they are divided into bulk-forming laxatives, osmotic laxatives, stimulant laxatives, lubricating agents, and others.

Bulk-forming agents are high-fiber foods containing polysaccharides or cellulose derivatives that are resistant to bacterial breakdown. Bulk-forming laxatives are not recommended for use in palliative care patients, since such patients are normally not able to take in the required amount of fluids. These agents increase stool bulk and correct its consistency by increasing the mass and the water content of the stool. Evidence of their effect may be observed after 24 hours or more.

Emollient laxatives are surfactant substances that are not absorbed in the gut, acting as a detergent and facilitating the mixture of water and fat. They also promote water and electrolyte secretion.

Stimulant laxatives are the most commonly used drugs to treat constipation. They are represented by the anthraquinone derivatives, such as senna, cascara, and danthron, and the diphenylmethane derivatives, such as bisacodyl and phenolphthalein. This class of drugs acts at the level of the colon and distal ileum by directly stimulating the myenteric plexus. Senna is converted to an active form by colonic bacteria. As a consequence, its site of action is primarily the colon. An increase in myoelectric colonic activity has been observed after the administration of oral senna. Danthron and the polyphenolic agents bisacodyl and sodium picosulfate undergo glucuronidation and are secreted in the bile (68). The enterohepatic circulation may prolong their effect. Bisacodyl stimulates the mucosal nerve plexus, producing contractions of the entire colon and decreasing water absorption in the small and large intestine. Castor oil is metabolized into ricinoleic acid that has stimulant secretory properties and an effect on glucose absorption. All of these drugs may cause severe cramping. The cathartic action occurs within 1 to 3 days. Proposed doses start at 15 mg of senna daily, 50 mg of danthron daily, or 5 mg of bisacodyl daily. Bisacodyl suppositories promote colonic peristalsis with a short onset due to rapid conversion to its active metabolite by the rectal flora. Docusate, alone or in combination with danthron,

TABLE 14.5 LAXATIVES USED FOR CONSTIPATION

Class–drugs–doses	Onset	Medication Considerations
Lubricant laxatives		
Liquid paraffin (10 mL/d)	1–3 d	Paraffin inhalation
Surfactant laxatives		
Docusate (300 mg)	1–3 d	Avoid with mineral oil
Bulk-forming agents	2–4 d	
Bran (8 g)		If taken with inadequate amount of water can precipitate fecal impaction in intestinal obstruction
Methylcellulose and ispaghula (4 g)		
Osmotic laxatives	1–2 d	
Lactulose (15 mL b.i.d.)		Side effects include dose related cramps and gaseous distention. Can be useful in hepatic encephalopathy
Mannitol		
Sorbitol		
Amidotrizoate (50 mL)		
Polyethylene glycol (two sachets daily in water)		High volumes of water needed to be ingested
Anthracenes (6–12 h) 6–12		Colicky pain
Senna (15 mg)		Urine pink discoloration
Dantron (50 mg)		
Polyphenolics (6–12 h)		Colicky pain
Bisacodyl (10 mg)		
Sodium picosulfate (5 mg)		
Opioid antagonists		
Naloxone (dose titration)	1-2 hours	Possible withdrawal
Methylnaltrexone SC (8 or 12 mg every other day)		
Naldemedine (0.2 mg)		
Lubiprostone (24 µg b.i.d.)		

is most commonly used at doses of 100 to 300 mg every 8 hours. The effectiveness of docusate has been questioned (55).

Lubricant laxatives are represented by mineral oil. They may be useful in the management of transient acute constipation or fecal impaction, but they have little role in the management of chronic constipation. They lubricate the stool surface, allowing the coated feces to pass more easily. There may also be a decrease in colonic absorption of water and fat vitamins. Absorption of small amounts may cause foreign body reactions in the bowel lymphoid tissue. Liquid paraffin, 15 to 45 mL in 24 hours, may be given orally or rectally, with an effect noted in 8 to 24 hours.

Saline laxatives exert an osmotic effect by increasing the intraluminal volume. They also appear to directly stimulate peristalsis and increase water secretion. The dose can be given as 195 to 300 mL given once or in divided doses. Magnesium, sulfate, phosphate, and citrate ions are the ingredients in saline laxatives. Saline laxatives usually produce results in a few hours. Their use may lead to electrolyte imbalances with accumulation of magnesium in patients with renal dysfunction or an excessive load of sodium in patients with hypertension. Administered rectally, they stimulate rectal peristalsis within 15 minutes. Repeated use of a phosphate enema may cause hypocalcemia and hyperphosphatemia or rectal gangrene in patients with hemorrhoids. Glycerin can be used rectally as an osmotic and as a lubricant. Magnesium salts tend to cause urgent liquid stools, making them less convenient for many patients, other than leading to toxicity with continuing use, especially in patients with renal insufficiency.

Hyperosmotic laxatives are not broken down or absorbed in the small bowel, drawing fluid into the bowel lumen. They pull water along with luminal contents to keep the stool softer and more voluminous. Lactulose increases fecal weight and frequency, but it may result in bloating, colic, and flatulence due to bacterial metabolization when it reaches the colon. Moreover, it is expensive in comparison with other preparations. The latency of action is 1 to 2 days. Starting doses are 15 to 30 mL daily. Orally administered macrogol is not metabolized, and pH value and bowel flora remain unchanged resulting in less gas bloating. Polyethylene glycol (PEG) hydrates hardened stools, increases stool volume, decreases the duration of colon passage, and dilates the bowel wall, which then triggers the defecation reflex. Even when given for some time, the effectiveness of PEG will not decrease (69). Limited studies and reviews demonstrate treatment of constipation resistant to laxatives in advanced cancer with amidotrizoate and diatrizoate meglumine (Gastrografin); however, further research is required to understand safety and effectiveness (70,71).

Patients with advanced cancer are likely to have chronic constipation and will need continuous laxative treatment. No data exist to guide the clinician or patient in the optimal choice of laxatives, as there have been no adequate comparative studies of long-term management of opioid-induced constipation. One of the main limitations of such trials is the lack of reliable clinical assessment tools. A 2015 Cochrane review found that laxatives were of similar effectiveness, but overall evidence remains limited due to insufficient data from a few small RCT's (72). In a comparative study conducted with the objective of determining treatment and cost efficiency for senna and lactulose in patients with terminal cancer treated with opioids, no difference was found in defecation-free intervals or in days with defecation between the laxatives (73). In a recent systematic review, the use of docusate for constipation in palliative care was found to be based on inadequate experimental evidence (74). In a study of healthy volunteers, in which constipation was induced by loperamide, a combination of stimulant and softening laxatives was most likely to maintain normal bowel function at the lowest dose and least adverse effects (75).

Opioid Antagonists and Opioid Therapy Modification

Opioid-induced constipation can be severe and refractory to therapy with conventional laxatives. Opioid receptor agonists cause constipation by disrupting neurotransmission in the enteric nervous system. Opioid concentration in the enteric nervous system correlates better with opioid-induced, prolonged, intestinal transit time than concentrations in the central nervous system (76). Peripherally acting mu-opioid receptor antagonists (PAMORAs) are an evidence-based treatment for refractory OIC.

Subcutaneous methylnaltrexone is the first FDA-approved peripheral opioid receptor antagonist for OIC in patients with noncancer pain and for patients with any advanced illness receiving palliative care who have had an inadequate response to traditional laxatives. The oral formulation has only been FDA approved for OIC in patients with noncancer pain and is currently under clinical investigation. Methylnaltrexone is an opioid antagonist that cannot penetrate the blood–brain barrier and therefore does not induce symptoms of opioid withdrawal or interfere with analgesia. Current evidence, although limited, demonstrates slightly better efficacy with subcutaneous methylnaltrexone than oral methylnaltrexone (77). Methylnaltrexone, administered every second day for 2 weeks at a dosage of 0.15 mg/kg subcutaneously, produced a faster time to bowel movement laxation in comparison with placebo, with most patients having a bowel movement within the first 2 hours after administration (78). Failure rate, observed in about half the patients, may be due to other concomitant causes of constipation and/or to the possible central constipating effect exerted by opioids at level of spinal dorsal horn (79).

Naloxone is a competitive antagonist of opioid receptors inside and outside the central nervous system and, after systemic administration, it reverses both centrally and peripherally mediated opioid effects. The naloxone dose of 20% of the daily morphine dose demonstrated a clinical laxative effect (80). Naloxone has a low oral bioavailability of <2%. It undergoes extensive hepatic metabolism to form the partly active metabolite 6β-naloxol and glucuronide of naloxone and 6β-naloxol. Oral administration theoretically allows selective blocking of intestinal opioid receptors without blocking the desired opioid effects, as long as hepatic first-pass capacity is not exceeded. The low systemic bioavailability due to marked hepatic first-pass metabolism allows for the low plasma levels and high enteric wall concentration. According to this observation, oral administration of naloxone should reverse opioid-induced constipation, without causing systemic opioid withdrawal in most patients. Reversal of analgesia does not seem to be an early symptom of systemic opioid antagonism, but some studies have demonstrated increased opioid requirements for analgesia while on naloxone that were only decreased after stopping naloxone (81).

Current research is investigating the use of sustained release naloxone as a way to reverse peripheral effects on the gut without altering central analgesic effects of opioids (82). This formulation is not available or approved in any country as of yet.

In recent years, coadministration of slow-release oxycodone and naloxone in a ratio of 2:1 has been found to be associated with a significant improvement in bowel function compared with slow-release oxycodone alone, with no reduction in the analgesic efficacy of naloxone, in a dose range of 20 to 80 mg (83). It is likely that the slow absorption of naloxone avoids possible peaks overlapping the extracting capacity of liver. A long-acting formulation, Targiniq ER (oxycodone plus naloxone), is approved in the United States for the treatment of moderate to severe pain for which alternative treatment options are inadequate. Canada has approved this drug combination for relief or prevention of OIC in patients who require an opioid.

Naldemedine is an oral medication that is well tolerated. Studies have shown a significantly higher response rate than placebo (84). There were no signs of opioid withdrawal, and the analgesic effect of the opioid was not significantly affected. Naldemedine was FDA approved for OIC in adult patients with noncancer pain. However, efficacy was also seen in treatment for OIC in patients with cancer (85), and the drug can be used off-label in the cancer population.

Other Drugs

Lubiprostone is a type 2 chloride channel activator that induces secretion of fluid in the intestine. Several large trials have been done, with efficacy confirmed in two randomized controlled trials (86,87). Patients receiving lubiprostone had improved bowel movements and abdominal discomfort compared to placebo. Overall effectiveness was higher than placebo during 11 of the 12 weeks, and side effects were tolerable. However, in a third identical trial, efficacy for lubiprostone could not be shown for patients with chronic noncancer pain (88). In the United States, it is approved for the treatment of OIC in patients receiving opioid therapy for chronic noncancer pain.

Metoclopramide given by the subcutaneous route, but not by the oral route, seems to be effective in narcotic bowel syndrome. Given its prokinetic profile, it can be considered in those with delayed gastric emptying and constipation. Effects of metoclopramide are mediated by a central and peripheral antidopaminergic effect and a stimulation of cholinergic receptors (3).

Neostigmine given by subcutaneous route has been proposed for refractory constipation, ileus, or acute colonic pseudo-obstruction (Ogilvie's syndrome) for its cholinergic activity (89). Use should be avoided in patients with new-onset heart block, history of second-degree heart block, or following bowel resection with primary anastomosis.

Linaclotide, a guanylyl cyclase C agonist, is used for the treatment of irritable bowel syndrome and chronic idiopathic constipation. Prucalopride, a selective 5-HT$_4$ receptor agonist, acts as a prokinetic in the gut and is also approved for chronic idiopathic constipation. A trial of either medication could be considered for those with OIC.

Opioid Rotation

Constipation may require modification of opioid therapy (90). Opioid rotation is a strategy for maintaining or improving analgesic quality directed toward decreasing the effects of previous opiates on the GI tract. Among opioids, there may be differences in the analgesia/constipation ratio. Present research indicates that there is a relationship between the type of opioid and the degree of constipation. For example, treatment with transdermal fentanyl or methadone tends to cause less constipation compared with morphine or hydromorphone. Among opioids, there may be differences in the analgesia/constipation ratio. Although an algorithm-guided opioid rotation may be effective, prospective randomized trials regarding the efficacy and cost of this strategy are lacking and caution is necessary because equianalgesic doses can vary from person to person. Clinical studies have revealed that at doses of oral morphine and transdermal fentanyl that yield equivalent pain relief, constipation differs significantly between the two drugs. Recent trials are remarkably consistent in that transdermal fentanyl causes less constipation than oral, sustained morphine at the same level of analgesia (55). Differences in pharmacologic profiles, such as affinity to opioid receptors and higher exposure of opioid-binding receptors in the GI tract, may offer an explanation for the clinically observed variations in the constipation-inducing potentials of equipotent doses of morphine and fentanyl. The lipophilicity profile of fentanyl allows for the ease with which fentanyl penetrates the brain. As less opioid is required to produce a central analgesic effect, less opioid is available in the peripheral circulation to induce constipation.

Methadone has a high oral bioavailability and a rapid and extensive distribution phase, followed by a slow elimination. The end of the distribution phase is at or below the minimum effective concentration necessary for an effect. This may result in limiting the continuous bathing of intestinal receptors. The high lipophilicity of methadone also allows for the maintenance of a low plasma concentration with a relevant clinical effect. In a retrospective analysis, the laxative/opioid dose ratio was lower in patients receiving methadone than in patients on morphine.

Constipation seems to be the symptom that improves the most after opioid switching. This could be simply due to difference in tolerance of different opioids at the level of receptors located in the bowel.

Therapeutic Strategy

The treatment consists of basic measures and the application of laxatives. Although there is no correlation between the dose of opioid and the dose of laxative, an upward titration of laxatives was seen with increasing doses of morphine (55). Approximate equivalents of laxatives and typical requirements of opioid therapy have been proposed, but there is a large individual patient variation. Proportionally less laxative is required at higher opioid doses.

In a constipated patient, after excluding bowel obstruction, it is mandatory to promote a bowel movement. Local measures to soften fecal mass are necessary in cases of rectal impaction. The short latency of action of rectal laxatives may be useful to remove hard feces impacted in the rectum. Glycerin suppositories or sorbitol enemas soften the stool by osmosis, also lubricating the rectal wall. Water penetration may be facilitated by a stool softener. Saline enemas cannot be regularly administered and should be used as a last resort if suppositories fail. Any patient requiring an enema should be reevaluated for a possible laxative dose titration. PAMORAs, such as methylnaltrexone, are recommended for patients on opioids who have failed to respond to optimal laxative therapy (63). These agents should be avoided if a bowel obstruction is suspected. Practical and economic considerations may influence the choice of drug for chronic constipation, according to the setting (home, hospital, hospice, or palliative care unit). Laxatives are the mainstay of pharmacologic intervention. Although stimulant agents may cause painful colic, peristaltic stimulants are indicated in patients who are unable to pass soft stool. Senna is the most useful drug in the presence of soft feces in the rectum. Stool softeners may be useful in the presence of hard stool. All patients who are started on opioid analgesia should have a prophylactic laxative unless a contraindication exists. Periodic laxative-free intervals have been advocated for patients with a relatively long prognosis to avoid tolerance (55).

The laxative dose should be titrated according to the response and not according to the dose of opioids. The opioid dose increments do not determine laxative efficacy, indicating that the constipating effect of opioids is not a function of the dose. Combination therapy with different mechanisms may be useful when high doses of one laxative are required. In patients suspected of having intestinal obstruction, laxatives with a softening action should be tried. However, treatment should be immediately interrupted if transit stops.

Patients with colostomies require the same approach to treatment. Before using stimulating agents, an obstruction should be excluded in the absence of feces in a colostomy. Patients with paraplegia often require regular manual evacuation. Glycerin and bisacodyl suppositories should be given to patients with cauda equina syndrome.

Opioid switching may be indicated in cases in which there are serious therapeutic difficulties in maintaining bowel transit. Some slow-release formulations of opioid antagonist, such as oxycodone–naloxone, may improve the bowel transit.

REFERENCES

1. Solomon R, Cherny NI. Constipation and diarrhea in patients with cancer. *Cancer J.* 2006;12(5):355-364.
2. Arnold RJ, et al. Clinical implications of chemotherapy-induced diarrhea in patients with cancer. *J Support Oncol.* 2005;3(3):227-232.
3. Lau PM, Stewart K, Dooley M. The ten most common adverse drug reactions (ADRs) in oncology patients: do they matter to you? *Support Care Cancer.* 2004;12(9):626-633.
4. Dranitsaris G, Maroun J, Shah A. Severe chemotherapy-induced diarrhea in patients with colorectal cancer: a cost of illness analysis. *Support Care Cancer.* 2005;13(5): 318-324.
5. McQuade RM, et al. Chemotherapy-induced constipation and diarrhea: pathophysiology, current and emerging treatments. *Front Pharmacol.* 2016;7:414.
6. Clausen MR, Jorgensen J, Mortensen PB. Comparison of diarrhea induced by ingestion of fructooligosaccharide Idolax and disaccharide lactulose: role of osmolarity versus fermentation of malabsorbed carbohydrate. *Dig Dis Sci.* 1998;43(12):2696-2707.
7. Camilleri M, Sellin JH, Barrett KE. Pathophysiology, evaluation, and management of chronic watery diarrhea. *Gastroenterology.* 2017;152(3):515-532.e2.
8. Osterlund P, et al. Lactose intolerance associated with adjuvant 5-fluorouracil-based chemotherapy for colorectal cancer. *Clin Gastroenterol Hepatol.* 2004;2(8): 696-703.
9. Thiagarajah JR, Donowitz M, Verkman AS. Secretory diarrhoea: mechanisms and emerging therapies. *Nat Rev Gastroenterol Hepatol.* 2015;12(8):446-457.
10. Schiller LR. Secretory diarrhea. *Curr Gastroenterol Rep.* 1999;1(5):389-397.
11. Jensen RT. Overview of chronic diarrhea caused by functional neuroendocrine neoplasms. *Semin Gastrointest Dis.* 1999;10(4):156-172.
12. Naraev BG, et al. Management of diarrhea in patients with carcinoid syndrome. *Pancreas.* 2019;48(8):961-972.

13. Sleisenger MH, Fordtran JS. *Gastrointestinal Disease: Pathophysiology, Diagnosis, Management.* 5th ed. Philadelphia, PA: Saunders; 1993.

14. Andreyev J, et al. Guidance on the management of diarrhoea during cancer chemotherapy. *Lancet Oncol.* 2014;15(10):e447-e460.

15. Kornblau S, et al. Management of cancer treatment-related diarrhea. Issues and therapeutic strategies. *J Pain Symptom Manage.* 2000;19(2):118-129.

16. Harb AH, Abou Fadel C, Sharara AI. Radiation enteritis. *Curr Gastroenterol Rep.* 2014;16(5):383.

17. Martenson JA, et al. Phase III, double-blind study of depot octreotide versus placebo in the prevention of acute diarrhea in patients receiving pelvic radiation therapy: results of North Central Cancer Treatment Group N00CA. *J Clin Oncol.* 2008;26(32):5248-5253.

18. Robertson JM, Sohn M, Yan D. Predicting grade 3 acute diarrhea during radiation therapy for rectal cancer using a cutoff-dose logistic regression normal tissue complication probability model. *Int J Radiat Oncol Biol Phys.* 2010;77(1):66-72.

19. Lessa FC, et al. Burden of Clostridium difficile infection in the United States. *N Engl J Med.* 2015;372(9):825-834.

20. Depestel DD, Aronoff DM. Epidemiology of Clostridium difficile infection. *J Pharm Pract.* 2013;26(5):464-475.

21. Schiller LR. Diarrhea. *Med Clin North Am.* 2000;84(5):1259-1274, x.

22. Cherny NI. Evaluation and management of treatment-related diarrhea in patients with advanced cancer: a review. *J Pain Symptom Manage.* 2008;36(4):413-423.

23. Benson AB III, et al. Recommended guidelines for the treatment of cancer treatment-induced diarrhea. *J Clin Oncol.* 2004;22(14):2918-2926.

24. Huang EY, et al. Acute diarrhea during pelvic irradiation: is small-bowel volume effect different in gynecologic patients with prior abdomen operation or not? *Gynecol Oncol.* 2005;97(1):118-125.

25. Stacey R, Green JT. Radiation-induced small bowel disease: latest developments and clinical guidance. *Ther Adv Chronic Dis.* 2014;5(1):15-29.

26. Tsavaris N, et al. Amifostine, in a reduced dose, protects against severe diarrhea associated with weekly fluorouracil and folinic acid chemotherapy in advanced colorectal cancer: a pilot study. *J Pain Symptom Manage.* 2003;26(3):849-854.

27. Ruutu T, et al. Prophylaxis and treatment of GVHD: EBMT-ELN working group recommendations for a standardized practice. *Bone Marrow Transplant.* 2014;49(2):168-173.

28. Attar A, et al. Antibiotic efficacy in small intestinal bacterial overgrowth-related chronic diarrhea: a crossover, randomized trial. *Gastroenterology.* 1999;117(4):794-797.

29. Rao SSC, Bhagatwala J. Small intestinal bacterial overgrowth: clinical features and therapeutic management. *Clin Transl Gastroenterol.* 2019;10(10):e00078.

30. Nelson RL, Suda KJ, Evans CT. Antibiotic treatment for Clostridium difficile-associated diarrhoea in adults. *Cochrane Database Syst Rev.* 2017;3:CD004610.

31. Saavedra J. Probiotics and infectious diarrhea. *Am J Gastroenterol.* 2000;95(1 suppl):S16-S18.

32. Chitapanarux I, et al. Randomized controlled trial of live lactobacillus acidophilus plus bifidobacterium bifidum in prophylaxis of diarrhea during radiotherapy in cervical cancer patients. *Radiat Oncol.* 2010;5:31.

33. Valenti Moreno V, et al. Prevention of irinotecan associated diarrhea by intestinal alkalization. A pilot study in gastrointestinal cancer patients. *Clin Transl Oncol.* 2006;8(3):208-212.

34. Michael M, et al. Phase II study of activated charcoal to prevent irinotecan-induced diarrhea. *J Clin Oncol.* 2004;22(21):4410-4417.

35. Kehrer DF, et al. Modulation of irinotecan-induced diarrhea by cotreatment with neomycin in cancer patients. *Clin Cancer Res.* 2001;7(5):1136-1141.

36. Mercadante S. Diarrhea in terminally ill patients: pathophysiology and treatment. *J Pain Symptom Manage.* 1995;10(4):298-309.

37. Wu PE, Juurlink DN. Clinical review: loperamide toxicity. *Ann Emerg Med.* 2017;70(2):245-252.

38. Cascinu S, et al. High-dose loperamide in the treatment of 5-fluorouracil-induced diarrhea in colorectal cancer patients. *Support Care Cancer.* 2000;8(1):65-67.

39. Kaplan MA, et al. Loperamide-simethicone vs loperamide alone, simethicone alone, and placebo in the treatment of acute diarrhea with gas-related abdominal discomfort. A randomized controlled trial. *Arch Fam Med.* 1999;8(3):243-248.

40. Mercadante S. The role of octreotide in palliative care. *J Pain Symptom Manage.* 1994;9(6):406-411.

41. Cello JP, et al. Effect of octreotide on refractory AIDS-associated diarrhea. A prospective, multicenter clinical trial. *Ann Intern Med.* 1991;115(9):705-710.

42. Ippoliti C, et al. Use of octreotide in the symptomatic management of diarrhea induced by graft-versus-host disease in patients with hematologic malignancies. *J Clin Oncol.* 1997;15(11):3350-3354.

43. Wasserman E, et al. Octreotide (SMS 201–995) for hematopoietic support-dependent high-dose chemotherapy (HSD-HDC)-related diarrhoea: dose finding study and evaluation of efficacy. *Bone Marrow Transplant.* 1997;20(9):711-714.

44. Rosenoff SH. Octreotide LAR resolves severe chemotherapy-induced diarrhoea (CID) and allows continuation of full-dose therapy. *Eur J Cancer Care (Engl).* 2004;13(4):380-383.

45. Anthony L. New strategies for the prevention and reduction of cancer treatment-induced diarrhea. *Semin Oncol Nurs.* 2003;19(4 suppl 3):17-21.

46. Hoff PM, et al. Randomized phase III trial exploring the use of long-acting release octreotide in the prevention of chemotherapy-induced diarrhea in patients with colorectal cancer: the LARCID trial. *J Clin Oncol.* 2014;32(10):1006-1011.

47. Ung KA, et al. Impact of bile acid malabsorption on steatorrhoea and symptoms in patients with chronic diarrhoea. *Eur J Gastroenterol Hepatol.* 2000;12(5):541-547.

48. Cecil RL, Bennett JC, Plum F. *Cecil Textbook of Medicine.* 20th ed. Philadelphia, PA: Saunders; 1996.

49. Vistad I, et al. Intestinal malabsorption in long-term survivors of cervical cancer treated with radiotherapy. *Int J Radiat Oncol Biol Phys.* 2009;73(4):1141-1147.

50. Rino Y, et al. Vitamin E malabsorption and neurological consequences after gastrectomy for gastric cancer. *Hepatogastroenterology.* 2007;54(78):1858-1861.

51. Harewood GC, Murray JA. Approaching the patient with chronic malabsorption syndrome. *Semin Gastrointest Dis.* 1999;10(4):138-144.

52. Buchman AL, Scolapio J, Fryer J. AGA technical review on short bowel syndrome and intestinal transplantation. *Gastroenterology.* 2003;124(4):1111-1134.

53. Buchman AL, et al. Clonidine reduces diarrhea and sodium loss in patients with proximal jejunostomy: a controlled study. *JPEN J Parenter Enteral Nutr.* 2006;30(6):487-491.

54. Kunkel D, et al. Efficacy of the glucagon-like peptide-1 agonist exenatide in the treatment of short bowel syndrome. *Neurogastroenterol Motil.* 2011;23(8):739-e328.

55. Berger A, Shuster JL, Von Roenn JH. *Principles and Practice of Palliative Care and Supportive Oncology.* 4th ed. Philadelphia, PA: Wolters Kluwer Health/Lippincott Williams & Wilkins; 2013:942, xvii.

56. Droney J, et al. Constipation in cancer patients on morphine. *Support Care Cancer.* 2008;16(5):453-459.

57. Voltz R. *Palliative Care in Neurology. Contemporary Neurology Series.* Oxford, New York: Oxford University Press; 2004:448, xxviii.

58. Gershon MD. Review article: serotonin receptors and transporters—roles in normal and abnormal gastrointestinal motility. *Aliment Pharmacol Ther.* 2004;20(suppl 7):3-14.

59. Farmer AD, et al. Pathophysiology and management of opioid-induced constipation: European expert consensus statement. *United European Gastroenterol J.* 2019;7(1):7-20.

60. Kurz A, Sessler DI. Opioid-induced bowel dysfunction: pathophysiology and potential new therapies. *Drugs.* 2003;63(7):649-671.

61. McMillan SC. Assessing and managing opiate-induced constipation in adults with cancer. *Cancer Control.* 2004;11(3 Suppl):3-9.

62. Rentz AM, et al. Validation of the Bowel Function Index to detect clinically meaningful changes in opioid-induced constipation. *J Med Econ.* 2009;12(4):371-383.

63. Librach SL, et al. Consensus recommendations for the management of constipation in patients with advanced, progressive illness. *J Pain Symptom Manage.* 2010;40(5):761-773.

64. Slappendel R, et al. Validation of the PAC-SYM questionnaire for opioid-induced constipation in patients with chronic low back pain. *Eur J Pain.* 2006;10(3):209-217.

65. Bruera E, et al. The assessment of constipation in terminal cancer patients admitted to a palliative care unit: a retrospective review. *J Pain Symptom Manage.* 1994;9(8):515-519.

66. Nagaviroj K, et al. Comparison of the Constipation Assessment Scale and plain abdominal radiography in the assessment of constipation in advanced cancer patients. *J Pain Symptom Manage.* 2011;42(2):222-228.

67. Larkin PJ, et al. The management of constipation in palliative care: clinical practice recommendations. *Palliat Med.* 2008;22(7):796-807.

68. Twycross RG, et al. Sodium picosulfate in opioid-induced constipation: results of an open-label, prospective, dose-ranging study. *Palliat Med.* 2006;20(4):419-423.

69. Klaschik E, Nauck F, Ostgathe C. Constipation—modern laxative therapy. *Support Care Cancer.* 2003;11(11):679-685.

70. Mercadante S, Ferrera P, Casuccio A. Effectiveness and tolerability of amidotrizoate for the treatment of constipation resistant to laxatives in advanced cancer patients. *J Pain Symptom Manage.* 2011;41(2):421-425.

71. Heng S, Hardy J, Good P. A retrospective audit on usage of Diatrizoate Meglumine (Gastrografin) for intestinal obstruction or constipation in patients with advanced neoplasms. *Palliat Med.* 2018;32(1):294-298.

72. Candy B, et al. Laxatives for the management of constipation in people receiving palliative care. *Cochrane Database Syst Rev.* 2015;(5):CD003448.

73. Agra Y, et al. Efficacy of senna versus lactulose in terminal cancer patients treated with opioids. *J Pain Symptom Manage.* 1998;15(1):1-7.

74. Hurdon V, Viola R, Schroder C. How useful is docusate in patients at risk for constipation? A systematic review of the evidence in the chronically ill. *J Pain Symptom Manage.* 2000;19(2):130-136.

75. Sykes NP. A volunteer model for the comparison of laxatives in opioid-related constipation. *J Pain Symptom Manage.* 1996;11(6):363-369.

76. Culpepper-Morgan JA, et al. Treatment of opioid-induced constipation with oral naloxone: a pilot study. *Clin Pharmacol Ther.* 1992;52(1):90-95.

77. Sridharan K, Sivaramakrishnan G. Drugs for treating opioid-induced constipation: a mixed treatment comparison network meta-analysis of randomized controlled clinical trials. *J Pain Symptom Manage.* 2018;55(2):468-479.e1.

78. Chappell D, Rehm M, Conzen P. Methylnaltrexone for opioid-induced constipation in advanced illness. *N Engl J Med.* 2008;359(10):1071; author reply 1071.

79. Berde C, Nurko S. Opioid side effects—mechanism-based therapy. *N Engl J Med.* 2008;358(22):2400-2402.

80. Sykes NP. An investigation of the ability of oral naloxone to correct opioid-related constipation in patients with advanced cancer. *Palliat Med.* 1996;10(2):135-144.

81. Liu M, Wittbrodt E. Low-dose oral naloxone reverses opioid-induced constipation and analgesia. *J Pain Symptom Manage.* 2002;23(1):48-53.

82. Sanders M, et al. New formulation of sustained release naloxone can reverse opioid induced constipation without compromising the desired opioid effects. *Pain Med.* 2015;16(8):1540-1550.

83. Meissner W, et al. A randomised controlled trial with prolonged-release oral oxycodone and naloxone to prevent and reverse opioid-induced constipation. *Eur J Pain.* 2009;13(1):56-64.

84. Hale M, et al. Naldemedine versus placebo for opioid-induced constipation (COMPOSE-1 and COMPOSE-2): two multicentre, phase 3, double-blind, randomised, parallel-group trials. *Lancet Gastroenterol Hepatol.* 2017;2(8):555-564.

85. Katakami N, et al. Randomized phase III and extension studies of naldemedine in patients with opioid-induced constipation and cancer. *J Clin Oncol.* 2017;35(34):3859-3866.

86. Cryer B, et al. A randomized study of lubiprostone for opioid-induced constipation in patients with chronic noncancer pain. *Pain Med.* 2014;15(11):1825-1834.

87. Jamal MM, et al. A randomized, placebo-controlled trial of lubiprostone for opioid-induced constipation in chronic noncancer pain. *Am J Gastroenterol.* 2015;110(5):725-732.

88. Spierings ELH, et al. Efficacy and safety of lubiprostone in patients with opioid-induced constipation: phase 3 study results and pooled analysis of the effect of concomitant methadone use on clinical outcomes. *Pain Med.* 2018;19(6):1184-1194.

89. Rubiales AS, et al. Neostigmine for refractory constipation in advanced cancer patients. *J Pain Symptom Manage.* 2006;32(3):204-205.

90. Ketwaroo GA, Cheng V, Lembo A. Opioid-induced bowel dysfunction. *Curr Gastroenterol Rep.* 2013;15(9):344.

15 Bowel Obstruction

Maria Pia Morelli

DEFINITION AND EPIDEMIOLOGY

Malignant bowel obstruction (MBO) was defined using the following criteria: clinical evidence of bowel obstruction (history/physical/radiologic examination); bowel obstruction beyond the ligament of Treitz, in the setting of a diagnosis of intra-abdominal cancer with incurable disease; or a diagnosis of non–intra-abdominal primary cancer with clear intraperitoneal disease (1,2). However, in cancer patients, the small bowel obstruction could be also a consequence of a benign process as adhesions due to multiple abdominal surgeries, intussusception of the bowel, or prior radiation therapy. Some reports suggest that benign causes are responsible for obstruction in about 48% of the patients with colorectal cancer (2–6). Regardless of the etiology, management of bowel obstruction in patients with advanced cancers is a common and difficult scenario, which in about 40% of the cases requires surgical consultations, which requires a careful weighing of risks and benefits.

MBO is a common complication in patients with abdominal or pelvic cancers, such as those arising from colon, ovary, and stomach. Bowel obstruction occurs in patients with a diagnosis of advanced primary or metastatic intra-abdominal malignancy such as ovarian cancer (5.5% to 42%) and colorectal cancer (4.4% to 24%) (3,7). Colon cancer arising at the splenic flexure can cause bowel obstruction in 49% of cases, tumors of right and left colon in 25% of cases, and tumors of the rectum and rectosigmoid junction in 6% of cases (4). Other intra-abdominal cancers as pancreatic, bladder, and prostate cancers can cause bowel obstruction through local infiltration of the adjacent intestine (4).

MBO has also been reported in patients with non–intra-abdominal cancers, such as melanoma, breast cancer, and lung cancer (8). The interval from diagnosis of cancer to onset of MBO is significantly longer between intra-abdominal (mean 22.4 months) and extra-abdominal primary tumors (mean 57.5 months) (8–13).

Bowel obstruction may be partial or complete, and at single or multiple sites. In a large cohort study of 490 cancer patients from MD Anderson,

the anatomic sites of obstruction were classified as gastric outlet, small bowel, and large bowel in 16%, 64%, and 20%, respectively.

Cancer patients may develop bowel obstruction at any time in their clinical history: at the time of the initial diagnosis, as often happens in the case of colorectal cancers, or as part of a recurrence or more advanced disease, and the management of each case should be addressed individually with a multidisciplinary approach and decided in consideration of the disease stage and therapeutic option available.

PATHOPHYSIOLOGY

Several physiopathologic mechanisms and causes may be involved in the onset of bowel obstruction, and there is variability in both presentation and etiology.

Mechanical obstruction is caused by the following: (a) *extrinsic occlusion of the lumen* due to an enlargement of the primary tumor or recurrence, mesenteric and omental masses, or postsurgical complications. Malignant etiologies are more likely to result in a large bowel obstruction while postsurgical adhesions more often result in small bowel obstructions; (b) *post-radiation enteritis* can result in fibrotic changes and intestinal damage, and in serositis that can cause bowel narrowing and dysmotility. Radiation treatment complications can occur acutely, around the time of treatment, and/or even years after treatment is completed as a tardive and more chronic side effects; (c) *intraluminal occlusion of the lumen* due to neoplastic mass, polypoidal lesions, or annular tumoral dissemination; and (d) *intramural occlusion of the lumen* due to intestinal linitis plastica, as is often seen in tumor of the stomach.

Functional obstruction (or adynamic ileus) is caused by intestinal motility disorders consequent to: (a) *tumor infiltration of the mesentery or bowel muscle and nerves (peritoneal carcinomatosis),* malignant involvement of the celiac plexus; (b) *paraneoplastic neuropathy* and paraneoplastic pseudo-obstruction; (c) *chronic intestinal pseudo-obstruction* mainly due to diabetes mellitus, previous gastric surgery, and other neurologic disorders; and (d) opioid-induced bowel dysmotilities.

At least four factors occur in bowel obstruction: (a) accumulation of gastric, pancreatic, and biliary secretions that are a potent stimulus for further intestinal secretions; (b) decreased absorption of water and sodium from the intestinal lumen; (c) increased secretion of water and sodium into the lumen as distension increases; and (d) bowel wall edema proximal to the level of the obstruction secondary to inflammation (Fig. 15.1). These factors produce a vicious circle of secretion–distension–secretion–motor hyperactivity. Depletion of water and salt in the lumen is considered the most important "toxic factor" in bowel obstruction (4,6).

Clinical and Radiologic Diagnosis

In cancer patients, the symptoms from bowel obstruction occur in different combinations and intensity depending on the site of obstruction. Although the clinical presentation is typically characterized by abdominal pain, loss of appetite, nausea, vomiting, inability to have a bowel movement or pass flatus, and abdominal distension, the proximal obstruction at the level of the gastric outlet or proximal small bowel can have an abrupt onset characterized by the cycle of pain,

nausea, and vomiting, which often relieve the pain. Distal small bowel, colon, and rectum obstructions usually have a more insidious clinical presentation with progressively worsening constipation and abdominal distension. In this case compression of the bowel lumen develops slowly and often remains partial, and symptoms become more frequent and last longer until near to complete obstruction results. Intestinal obstruction may progress rapidly and cause life-threatening conditions as intestinal ischemia, perforation, and peritonitis. Initial management includes a clinical assessment to rule out acute presentation of obstruction and to ensure that the patient does not have a surgical emergency. Gastrointestinal (GI) symptoms such as pain at the tumor site, abdominal cramps, nausea and vomiting, and abdominal distension are caused by the sequence of distension–secretion–motor activity of the obstructed bowel. Moreover, vomiting and dehydration induce electrolytes, acid–base, and kidney function abnormalities that should be closely monitored (Fig. 15.1; Table 15.1) (4,6,12–14). In order to be able to diagnose the condition in a proper manner, a complete clinical history, physical examination, and blood work are mandatory before any investigation is ordered. Once the

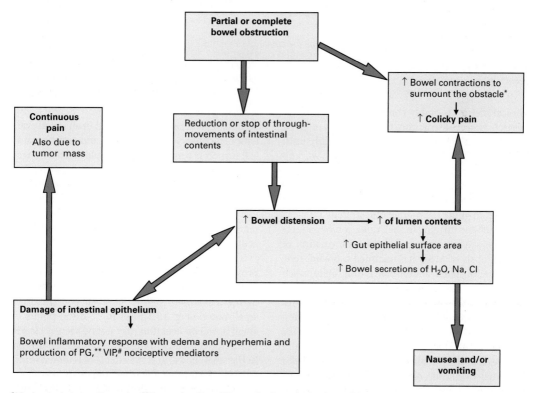

*Mechanical obstruction only, **Prostaglandins, #Vasoactive intestinal polypeptide

Figure 15.1 Pathophysiology of bowel obstruction.

TABLE 15.1 COMMON SYMPTOMS IN CANCER PATIENTS WITH MALIGNANT BOWEL OBSTRUCTION

Vomiting	Intermittent or continuous	It develops early and in great amounts in gastric, duodenum, and small bowel obstructions and develops later in large bowel obstruction.	Biliary vomiting is almost odorless and indicates an obstruction in the upper part of the abdomen. The presence of bad-smelling and fecaloid vomiting can be the first sign of an ileal or colic obstruction.
Nausea	Intermittent or continuous		
Colicky pain	Variable intensity and localization due to distension proximal to the obstruction; secondary to gas and fluid accumulation most of which are produced by the gut	If it is intense, periumbilical, and occurring at brief intervals, may be an indication of an obstruction at the jejunum–ileal level. In large bowel obstruction, the pain is less intense, deeper, and occurring at longer intervals, and spreads toward the colon wall.	An overall acute pain that begins intensely and becomes stronger or a pain that is specifically localized, may be a symptom of a perforation or an ileal or colic strangulation. A pain that increases with palpation may be due to peritoneal irritation or the beginning of a perforation.
Continuous pain	Variable intensity and localization	It is due to abdominal distension, tumor mass, and/or hepatomegaly.	
Dry mouth		It is due to severe dehydration, metabolic alterations, and above all the use of drugs with anticholinergic properties and poor mouth care.	
Constipation	Intermittent or complete	In case of complete obstruction, there is no evacuation of feces and no flatus.	In case of partial obstruction, the symptom is intermittent.
Overflow diarrhea		It is the result of bacterial liquefaction of the fecal material.	

clinical picture is highly consistent with the diagnoses of bowel obstruction, the symptoms referred to by the patient should be monitored daily until resolution. Furthermore, a diagnostic workup should be performed to establish the diagnoses, identify the level of the obstruction, and assess tumor burden, and all together, this information will help to guide the therapeutic strategy.

Radiologic imaging in the evaluation of patients with the acute abdomen and the confirmation of the diagnosis of MBO has assumed a pivotal role. For decades, plain abdominal radiography taken in the supine and standing positions has been the standard in the initial evaluation of patients with acute abdominal pain or suspected obstruction (Fig. 15.2). Plain radiography can document the air-filled dilated loops of bowel and differential air–fluid levels, which makes it a very useful exam for an initial diagnosis. Additionally, plain radiography can identify signs of bowel obstruction complication as "free air"; pneumoperitoneum, in case of perforated viscus; and loss of haustration as in the case of toxic megacolon and the accuracy for

localizing the point and cause of obstruction is low. Although plain radiology is useful in an initial evaluation, it comes with limitations, and once the clinical suspect is confirmed more sophisticated images should be used to tackle details of the diagnosis. The sensitivity of plain films in making a diagnosis of small bowel obstruction has been reported to be as low as 66% (15). Despite this, it remains an important first step in the evaluation of most patients with acute and chronic abdominal symptoms.

Contrast GI series using barium suspensions provide excellent radiologic definition of the mucosal pattern and luminal patency, particularly in the assessment of the stomach and proximal small bowel (Fig. 15.3), but more distal points of small bowel obstruction may not be seen as clearly due to the difficulty in the barium reaching this far in the small bowel and the effects of retained luminal fluid. As it is not absorbed, the retention of barium in the lumen, and the inability to subsequently eliminate it in the setting of obstruction, can then interfere with subsequent radiographic studies. For these reasons, barium small bowel series

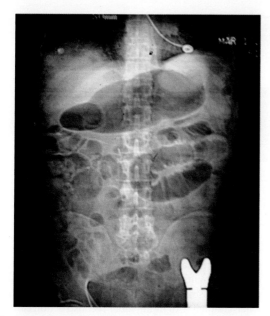

Figure 15.2 Plain abdominal x-ray image of a patient with obstructing metastasis from renal cancer. Dilated small bowel loop seen, but cause or severity not clearly determined. (Image kindly provided by Dr. Mark Gollub, MSKCC.)

should be used selectively, and preferably, for evaluating more chronic symptoms or for searching the cause of persistent intestinal symptoms when acute obstruction has already been ruled out.

In the evaluation of large bowel obstruction, barium enema provides a quick, accurate, and inexpensive assessment of the location and cause of obstruction. This, however, should be performed with caution to avoid excessive insertion of barium proximal to the point of obstruction, as this can lead to retention of the barium proximal to the obstruction leading to dehydration of the barium and potential impaction. This is especially a problem in patients with incomplete and inoperable large bowel obstruction. Similarly, if large bowel obstruction is suspected on initial plain abdominal x-rays, a small bowel series should not be performed to avoid the barium from becoming trapped in the proximal obstructed regions of the colon.

Gastrografin (diatrizoate meglumine) may also be useful in evaluating small and large bowel obstructions (Fig. 15.4), but it usually only provides good visualization of proximal small bowel obstruction as the water-soluble nature of the Gastrografin will result in it being diluted by the excess fluid retained in the distal small bowel.

Enteroclysis (the small bowel enema) requires the insertion of a long nasoenteric tube, which is manipulated under fluoroscopy guidance beyond the stomach by the radiologist. The contrast is then inserted under pressure resulting in full distension of the loops of small bowel, permitting better assessment of the mucosal pattern and patency, and improving the accuracy of diagnosis in small bowel obstruction. The discomfort associated with the procedure results in the need for it to be done with

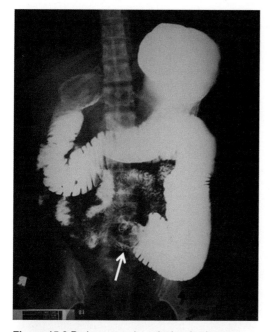

Figure 15.3 Barium gastrointestinal series image demonstrating high-grade, malignant-appearing, small bowel obstruction from a primary jejunal cancer (*arrow*). (Image kindly provided by Dr. Mark Gollub, MSKCC.)

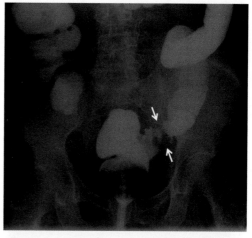

Figure 15.4 Gastrografin enema image of a patient with ovarian cancer causing partial sigmoid colon obstruction, shown between the *arrows*.

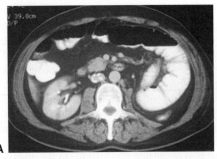 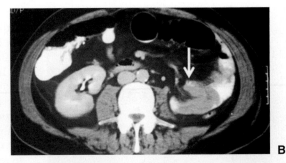

A   **B**

Figure 15.5 A: Computed tomography scan image of a patient with malignant bowel obstruction caused by metastasis from renal cancer (same patient as in Fig. 15.2) showing the dilated jejunal loop. **B:** Subsequent image showing obstructing mass causing intussusceptions (*arrow*). (Images kindly provided by Dr. Marc Gollub, MSKCC.)

the use of sedatives. Unfortunately, as it requires radiologists with expertise in the technique, it is not widely available. Transcutaneous ultrasonography has been used successfully in making the diagnosis of MBO, but it has limited usefulness when bowel loops are filled with air, and it is also more operator dependent and is therefore less utilized.

Although these techniques are available, once the clinical diagnoses of bowel obstruction is suspected and reinforced by a plain radiography, abdominopelvic cross-sectional imaging by computed tomography (CT) scanning should be performed for the evaluation of patients presenting with acute abdominal symptoms without unnecessary delays (16). In case of contraindication for CT scan (Fig. 15.5), magnetic resonance imaging (MRI) has now been shown to be a valid optimal option in the assessment of abdominal symptoms and in the diagnosis of bowel obstruction.

Comparative studies have demonstrated superior results with cross-sectional imaging in accurately predicting the cause of symptoms. The diagnostic accuracy for determining the cause of obstruction was reported to be 87% for CT, 23%

for ultrasound, and 7% for plain film radiography (17). Newer technology in CT scanning such as spiral and multidetector scanners provides a better global assessment of the abdomen and pelvis and when coupled with multiplanar reconstruction can help focus on the transition point in bowel obstruction, thereby helping determine the site, cause, and the administration of intravenous and oral contrast will provide more detailed information about the severity of obstruction that can lead to changes in management (Fig. 15.6) (18). CT scanning also provides a greater appreciation for the integrity of the bowel wall proximal to the obstruction, helping to predict the existence of ischemia, pneumatosis, or early perforation with greater accuracy than other modalities, and is considered the best modality for determining which patients would benefit from immediate surgical intervention versus conservative management [16].

A recent report by Angelilli et al. (19) demonstrated a sensitivity, specificity, and accuracy for CT scan of 74%, 100%, and 92%, respectively, in confirming a neoplastic cause of MBO. Multidetector CT scanning has also been shown to be

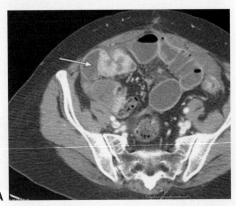 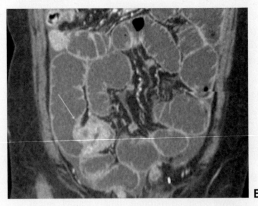

A   **B**

Figure 15.6 A and B: Axial and coronal reconstruction images of a computed tomography scan in a patient with malignant small bowel obstruction from an ovarian cancer implant (*arrow*). (Images kindly provided by Dr. Mark Gollub, MSKCC.)

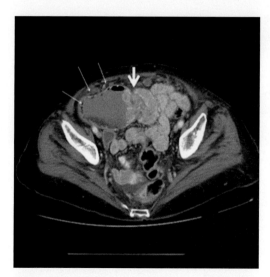

Figure 15.7 Computed tomography scan image of an obstructing small bowel metastasis (*large arrow*) with edema and pneumatosis (*small arrows*) of the jejunal wall. (Image kindly provided by Dr. Mark Gollub, MSKCC.)

highly accurate in identifying the malignant cause of colonic obstruction and in identifying specific features such as the presence of air–fluid levels in the colonic lumen, mural pneumatosis, and a right colon diameter of >10 cm as poor prognostic features (Fig. 15.7) (20). These features help expedite making a decision on management, which can sometimes be critical in the overall prognosis for patients with strangulating bowel obstruction.

MRI may also provide similar diagnostic information, but it is not as widely available as CT scanning and local expertise in its use in the assessment of bowel obstruction is limited. The strength of MRI is the absence of radiation exposure, so in the pediatric population, especially in those with chronic or recurrent GI symptoms, such as patients with inflammatory bowel disease, it is becoming the preferred modality of repeated imaging. The expected results with MRI should be similar to those with CT scanning, but the data on the sensitivity, specificity, and accuracy are still awaited.

THERAPIES

The management of patients with MBO is one of the greatest challenges for physicians who care for cancer patients. Especially in those patients who have a good performance status, MBO is often the first significant and most significant sign of clinical deterioration, but dramatically impacts quality of life (QOL) and outcome. Its management can be quite challenging. For this reason, the approaches to management of the patient with MBO should

be "tailored" for each specific situation. Although MBO is usually associated with advanced-stage disease when it occurs at the time of initial diagnosis, regardless of the primary site of malignancy, management generally proceeds with curative intent and each patient should be managed according to appropriate principles/guidelines for the underlying malignancy. On the other hand, MBO as part of recurrent disease is often managed with palliative intent; in this context, different factors should be considered to determine the most appropriate treatment.

For patients with recurrent disease, MBO generally occurs in a chronic and slow fashion that results in narrowing of the diameter of the small or large bowel (or both simultaneously).

In the face of a clearly incurable situation, significant patient discomfort and suffering must be balanced with the need to simplify the care of those patients with a short time to live. The goal in any decision we make needs to impact the QOL of the affected person in a positive way, and each assessment and management needs to be tailored to the specific needs of the patients. Figure 15.8 shows the algorithm for assessing and managing a patient with MBO. The physicians need to consider a series of questions when faced with terminal cancer patients (patients are no longer responsive to specific oncologic therapies) with bowel obstruction: Is the patient fit for surgery? Is there a place for stenting? Is it necessary to use a venting nasogastric tube (NGT) in inoperable patients? When should a venting gastrostomy be considered? What drugs are indicated for symptom control? What is the proper route for drug administration? What is the role of parenteral hydration and total parenteral nutrition (PN)? Figure 15.8 shows the algorithm for assessing and managing a patient with MBO.

Endoscopic Management of Gastroduodenal and Proximal Jejunal Obstruction

Gastric outlet obstruction (GOO) and small bowel obstruction are very debilitating presentations of malignancy that are commonly seen in patients with pancreatic cancer, distal gastric cancer, gallbladder cancer, and cholangiocarcinoma. This can also result from metastases of a variety of extra-abdominal malignancies, such as breast cancer and lung cancer. Although GOO is technically not considered MBO, it will be discussed here as it is a common source of morbidity in cancer patients and is managed in a manner similar to other forms of MBO. Advances in endoscopic techniques have now permitted the treatment of this problem to be readily accomplished with the endoscopic insertion of a self-expanding metal stent (SEMS)

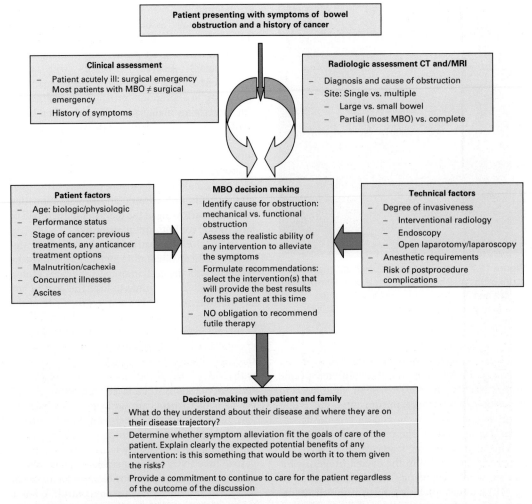

Figure 15.8 Algorithm for assessing and managing a patient with malignant bowel obstruction. MBO, malignant bowel obstruction; CT, computed tomography; MRI, magnetic resonance imaging.

(Fig. 15.9) or gastric venting via a percutaneously placed gastrostomy (drainage percutaneous endoscopic gastrostomy [PEG]). These approaches are particularly useful for patients with limited expected survival.

The procedure is easily performed using techniques similar to those used for inserting bile duct stents in patients with obstructive jaundice. The technical success rates for placement of enteral stents have been reported to be >90%, and clinical success for resolution of nausea and vomiting with improved ability to consume food orally is reported to be over 75% (21–25) (Table 15.2).

In the limited comparative studies published, endoscopic stent placement has been associated with shorter hospital stay and lower periprocedural mortality in patients with GOO secondary to pancreatic cancer (26,27) and with more rapid food intake compared with surgical bypass (26,28).

Stent placement has even been shown to be effective in palliating symptoms from obstruction in the setting of limited degrees of peritoneal carcinomatosis (29).

Delayed stent failure can occur, however, from food impaction or reobstruction caused by tumor ingrowth. Stent migration also can occur, sometimes in association with cancer treatment, if there is reduction in the size of the tumor. In most cases, reobstruction due to tumor ingrowth can be managed with the placement of a second stent or tumor ablation by Nd:YAG laser or argon plasma coagulator (30). In comparative studies, those managed with stent did just as well initially as patients managed with surgical bypass, but they had a greater need for reintervention because of delayed stent occlusion (28,31).

The effect of palliative treatments on the patient's QOL in malignant GOO has been limited

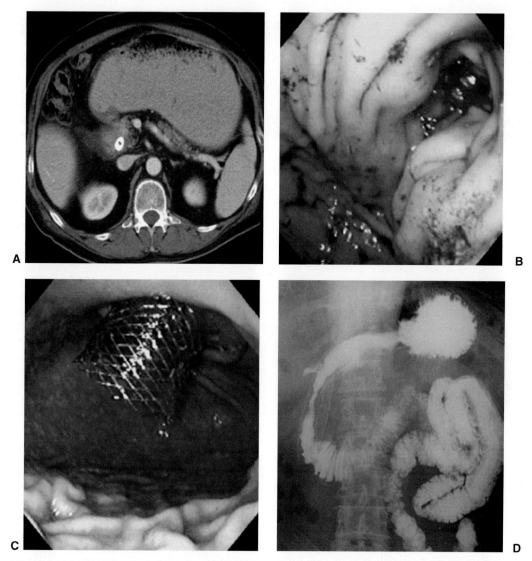

Figure 15.9 Radiographic and endoscopic images of a patient with malignant duodenal obstruction treated with endoscopic stenting. **A:** Computed tomography scan demonstrating dilated stomach and transition point in duodenum. **B:** Endoscopy showing obstructed pylorus. **C:** Endoscopy image after insertion of stent. **D:** Barium gastrointestinal series after stent insertion demonstrating relief of obstruction.

TABLE 15.2 SUMMARY RESULTS FROM TWO MULTICENTER STUDIES OF ENDOSCOPIC STENT PLACEMENT FOR TREATMENT OF MALIGNANT GASTRODUODENAL OBSTRUCTION

	Dorman et al. (23)	Telford et al. (22)
Number of cases	606	176
Study design	Pooled analysis	Multicenter study
Technical success	97%	98%
Clinical success	87%	84%
Perforation/bleeding	1.2%	2%
Migration	5%	6%
Reobstruction	18%	20%

or absent from most studies (32,33). In a prospective, nonrandomized study, Schmidt et al. showed that stent placement was associated with a shorter hospital stay than surgical bypass, but both the procedures were associated with improvements in nausea, vomiting, ability to eat, and several measures of QOL (33). In another prospective study examining QOL in patients with malignant GOO, Mehta et al. randomized 27 patients to receive laparoscopic gastrojejunostomy or endoscopic stent placement for malignant GOO. Stent placement was associated with less pain and shorter hospital stay, with a greater improvement in physical health following stent placement relative to those managed surgically (32).

We presently consider surgical bypass to be the preferred option for patients with a good performance status, a slowly progressive disease, and a relatively longer life expectancy (>60 days). Furthermore, if the site of obstruction is more distal in the jejunum or if there are multiple sites of obstruction, endoscopic stenting is likely to have a lower rate of technical success, so surgical intervention or drainage gastrostomy should be considered. We estimated that the patients who are best suited for endoscopic stenting are those with a short length of tumor and a single site of obstruction that is located at the pylorus or in the proximal two-thirds of the duodenum, with an intermediate to high performance status and an intermediate life expectancy of >30 days. Patients with a poor performance status, a rapidly progressive disease, an evidence of advanced carcinomatosis with moderate to severe ascites or multiple levels of obstruction on cross-sectional imaging, and a very short life expectancy of <30 days are best served by medical palliation of symptoms or the insertion of a drainage PEG.

Endoscopic Management of Malignant Small Bowel Obstruction

Much of the experience with endoscopic management of small bowel obstruction comes from that which has just been reviewed in the setting of gastroduodenal obstruction above. Most gastroscopes are unable to reach beyond the ligament of Treitz and colonoscopes are unable to reach very far retrograde up into the terminal ileum, so most cases of small bowel obstruction have not been amenable to endoscopic stenting.

The recent development of long enteroscopes that can be advanced far into the small intestine through an overtube, which permits the pleating of the small bowel, has permitted some investigators to report success in stenting areas of the small intestine not previously accessible to standard

endoscopes. Most of these reports are anecdotal, but with time, increasing interventional endoscopist experience, and further development of the enteroscopes, stents, and manipulating tools, the ability to treat mid-jejunal and ileal points of malignant obstruction may become more available and such patients will have another option for treatment (34,35). The selection of patients appropriate for such interventions will, however, remain challenging.

Endoscopic Management of Malignant Colorectal Obstruction

The endoscopic management of malignant large bowel obstruction has paralleled the experience reported with the treatment of malignant esophageal and gastroduodenal obstruction. Although initially approached with thermal ablative techniques such as Nd:YAG laser, greater success has been noted with the ability to insert SEMS in the colon (Fig. 15.10). The technical success rates for insertion of metallic stents have ranged from 80% to 100%, with clinical improvement in symptoms reported to be in >75% of patients (36–38). Many patients treated with stents have a durable relief of symptoms until death from progression of disease, but as has been seen with the use of stents in other parts of the body, restenosis, usually caused by tumor ingrowth through the interstices of the stent or stent migration, can cause delayed failure. This can usually be managed with insertion of another stent, endoscopic dilation, or laser ablation (36,37,39,40).

Two analyses of pooled data from the multiple reported case series have been published (41,42) (Table 15.3). Both analyses report clinical success rates of 88% and 91%, defined as a resolution of obstructive symptoms following the insertion of stents. The limitations to success are a very proximal location of obstruction with a higher rate of failure in the proximal colon in some reported series and the ability to traverse a tightly obstructing tumor with the endoscope or a guidewire. A greater success with stenting primary colorectal cancer has been noted, with lesser success for obstruction caused by extrinsic compression from metastatic or locally invasive pelvic tumors such as ovarian cancer, but some good results have also been reported for such patients (40,43,44). Limited data on cost effectiveness of colorectal stenting are available in published reports, with some calculations suggesting a potential reduction of approximately 50% in the estimated cost of palliation for such patients compared with surgical patients. This is predominantly attributed to a reduced hospital stay with stenting (41).

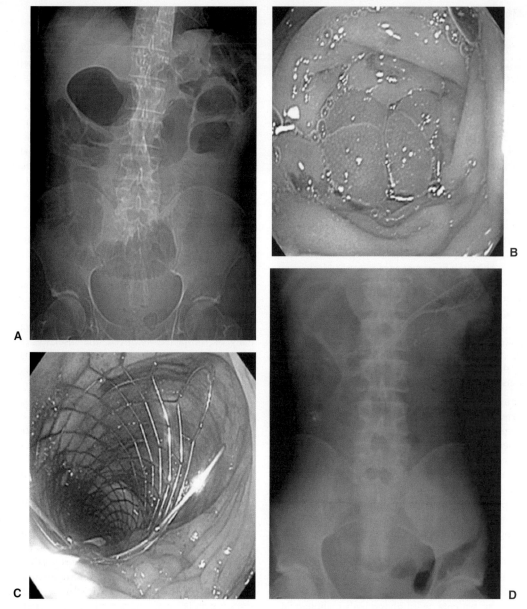

Figure 15.10 Endoscopic and radiographic images of a patient with malignant obstruction of the transverse colon, treated with stent placement. **A:** Abdominal x-ray showing dilated right colon. **B:** Endoscopy image showing obstructed colon. **C:** Endoscopy image after stent insertion. **D:** Abdominal x-ray showing the decompressed right colon, and partially expanded transverse colon stent.

TABLE 15.3 RESULTS OF SYSTEMATIC REVIEWS OF EFFICACY AND SAFETY OF COLORECTAL STENTING IN THE MANAGEMENT OF ACUTE MALIGNANT COLORECTAL OBSTRUCTION

	Khot et al. (41)	Sebastian et al. (42)
Technical success	551 (92%)	1,198 (94%)
Clinical success	525 (88%)	1,198 (91%)
Palliative success	301/336 (90%)	791 (93%)
Deaths	3 (1%)	7 (0.6%)
Perforation	22 (4%)	45 (3.8%)
Stent migration	54 (10%)	132 (11.8%)
Reobstruction	53 (10%)	82 (7.3%)

A recent multicenter study was completed demonstrating similar results with a newer generation of nitinol SEMS, the Wallflex (45). This study, like most others, demonstrates the ease of use, high technical and short-term clinical efficacy, and low overall and serious complication rate.

The proper evaluation of the efficacy of palliative treatments requires a careful assessment of the effect of the treatment on symptoms and the QOL and less attention on survival. In one prospective, nonrandomized series evaluating the effect of endoscopic stenting and surgical diversion in palliating malignant colorectal obstruction, symptoms improved significantly after either treatment, but were more durable after stenting than after surgery. Although there was a trend toward improved QOL, neither treatment had a significant effect on overall QOL (45). This and other studies demonstrate how difficult it is to actually quantify the benefits of therapeutic interventions in the dying patient.

Drainage Percutaneous Endoscopic Gastrostomy in Bowel Obstruction

Often all efforts to completely reconstitute the patency of the GI tract will fail or be considered inappropriate due to the extent of intraperitoneal disease or the realization of the medical futility of such attempts. In this setting in a patient with intractable nausea and vomiting, the insertion of an NGT will often immediately stop the vomiting, but it may be associated with severe nasopharyngeal discomfort or pain associated with swallowing or coughing, or be cosmetically unacceptable, confining the patient at home.

Gastric venting with PEG tube placement has become widely acceptable, in this setting, for palliation of nausea and vomiting due to GI obstruction in patients with abdominal malignancies (46,47). Drainage PEG tube placement provides a rapid and safe method of achieving symptomatic relief without the risks of a surgical procedure or the discomfort of an NGT.

Clinical guidelines following the early experience with PEG tubes for nutritional support suggested that patients with advanced abdominal malignancies or prior surgery were contraindicated for PEG placement due to the presence of ascites, adhesions, or tumor infiltration of the stomach, but published data have shown that endoscopic PEG placement can be safely performed and can provide meaningful palliation of the severe nausea and vomiting occurring with such irreversible forms of bowel obstruction (47).

In an early series, Campagnutta et al. (46) reported on 34 patients with bowel obstruction from gynecologic malignancies that were palliated with drainage PEG. Using 15- and 20-Fr tubes, 94% had PEGs successfully placed and 84.4% had resolution of symptoms, with return of the ability to consume liquids or soft food for a median of 74 days.

In a retrospective study, 28-Fr PEG tube placement was feasible in 98% of patients with advanced recurrent ovarian cancer, even in patients with tumor encasing the stomach, diffuse carcinomatosis, and ascites (47). This approach has also been used to temporarily palliate symptoms in patients still undergoing systemic anticancer therapy with curative intent. However, for most patients with MBO from advanced peritoneal carcinomatosis, drainage PEG tubes only help reduce some of the symptoms associated with MBO such as nausea and vomiting, but often will require additional treatments to control pain from the distension associated with ascites, direct tumor effect in the abdomen, and elsewhere.

In some cases where the stomach has been partially or completely removed, the insertion of a venting PEG becomes impossible, so a drainage PEJ (jejunostomy) tube can be inserted and serve the same purpose (48).

Surgical Procedures

Surgical interventions, either open or laparoscopically, may benefit select patients with MBO. The best surgical procedure that is most likely to relieve symptoms for the greatest length of time with reasonable operative morbidity is chosen (49).

Complete surgical resection of a tumor is most desirable. However, it is only worthwhile if the entire tumor in that area can be resected with negative margins. The exception can be ovarian or some GI cancers, where intraperitoneal chemotherapy can treat the residual disease after a "debulking" operation of all obvious disease. Otherwise, debulking of a tumor is generally not beneficial, as the tumor will only grow back in the absence of anticancer therapy.

If the tumor cannot be resected, but there is a healthy nonobstructed bowel before and after the site of obstruction, a side-to-side bypass can be performed. This will restore bowel continuity and allow the patients to eat and maintain their nutritional status. In the case of distal obstruction, a stoma can be created out of the most distal unaffected bowel segment. In order to maintain one's nutrition orally, it is necessary to have a minimum of 100 cm of proximal bowel before a stoma, so the length of proximal bowel should be measured prior to creating a proximal stoma. Proximal stomas also have high outputs and may cause significant fluid balance problems.

Finally, in the absence of any other option, a gastrostomy tube may be placed to avoid the need for an NGT. A venting gastrostomy tube may provide significant symptomatic relief for the patients with intractable nausea and vomiting not controlled by antiemetics and may allow discharge from hospital and death at home (50). These tubes can be inserted by endoscopic procedures, by interventional radiology, or by open surgery. They can only be placed if the stomach can be brought up freely to the adjacent abdominal wall that is free of tumor. Ascites is a relative contraindication; however, they may still be successful if the ascites is drained prior and after placement to allow the stomach and abdominal wall to be brought together. Symptomatic relief from an NGT suggests that the tube will be effective to relieve symptoms. However, placement of a percutaneous tube is an invasive procedure and is associated with discomfort, complications, and a failure rate and should be offered only to patients with poorly controlled symptoms on aggressive medications and those who are not imminently dying.

The likelihood of success depends on the location of the bowel obstruction, with large bowel obstruction successfully relieved in 80% of cases versus 25% if both large and small bowels are involved (51). The number of obstructed sites also affects the likelihood of success; a single site of obstruction has a high likelihood of success as compared with multiple sites of obstruction. It is worth emphasizing that MBO from generalized carcinomatosis is a distinct entity that responds poorly, or not at all, to surgical intervention and these patients are not surgical candidates (6,52,53).

Surgical Decision-Making

In addition to the technical factors already described, surgical decision-making must take into account individual patient and disease factors. Performance status remains one of the best predictors of low complication rates and survival (54); patient factors associated with poor surgical outcomes include advanced age (both physiologic and chronologic), poor nutritional status (see below), ascites, concurrent illness and comorbidities, previous and future anticancer treatment, psychological health, and social support (55–57).

Disease factors such as etiology, time from primary presentation, tumor grade, and tumor extent and available anticancer treatment options also affect decision-making. Slow-growing, well-differentiated tumors are more likely to be associated with better outcomes and longer survival. The best predictor of the future is the pace of the disease in the past and its response to treatment prior to the presentation of obstruction, due to the biology and inherent growth characteristics of the tumor. Patients with bulky liver or lung metastatic disease will die much sooner than will those with localized pelvic or intraperitoneal disease and are therefore less likely to benefit from surgery.

The selection of patients who will benefit from these procedures is an ongoing challenge and can be done only by individualizing management. Because the management of MBO is rarely an emergency, time can and should be taken into account to come up with an appropriate individualized treatment plan. In the face of an incurable, progressive illness, the balance between honesty and maintaining hope and optimism can be difficult to achieve, but it is necessary to avoid the use of futile treatments and harm to the patient (58). A futile treatment is carried out when it is unlikely to produce the desired benefit (59). It may be easier to offer a treatment just to do something; the more difficult decision may be not to do something when it is not going to help. However, there is little guidance on what should be considered a futile treatment as the definition will vary from patient to patient and/or clinician to clinician based on previous personal experiences and expectations. Most clinicians agree, however, that palliative surgery in oncology patients should not be offered to meet emotional, existential, and/or psychological needs (60).

An approach to this decision-making can be outlined as follows. The clinician first needs to decide which, if any, treatments are appropriate or feasible. This can only be done through a thorough preoperative evaluation to avoid intraoperative surprises or emergencies. The patients are asked what they understand about where they are on their disease trajectory and what their expectations are. Their current medical condition and expected prognosis are discussed. All treatment options including surgery, interventional radiology, and medications should be discussed; along with the complication rates and the expected success of each intervention. Reasonable treatment goals are set, whether this is continued curative therapy, withdrawal of inappropriate therapies, or vigorous palliative care. The goals addressed include relief of suffering and improvement of QOL and may vary between similar patients as they are based on the patients' perceptions and life experiences. Questions are answered, and a plan is developed with the patient. This may take several visits as the patient comes to terms with his or her disease.

With careful preoperative planning, it is possible to determine before the operation in most cases which option is most likely; however, the final decision must always be made in the operating room. The possibility that no surgical procedure may be possible must also be discussed, and the patient and family must be prepared for that option. Finally, there must be a commitment to ongoing care with a clear care plan whatever the outcome of the surgery. Several recent papers from large cancer centers have followed patients prospectively with MBO. Significant symptom relief can be obtained by selecting appropriate patients for either surgery or stenting with minimal procedural mortality (54,57,61,62).

Nutritional Considerations

Any malignancy will influence patients' nutritional status, whether due to the disease itself or due to cancer-related treatments. Nutritional status may be further impaired due to decreased oral intake of patients with MBO, which affects the course of disease and therefore the prognosis of a patient (63).

Cachexia is a catabolic metabolic state that is commonly seen in advanced end-stage cancer, where the patient is metabolically breaking down intrinsic muscle, protein, and fat (64). Cachexia is associated with inflammation, hypercatabolism, hormonal changes, and production of tumor factors. There is no consensus in the literature on how to best diagnose cachexia. It is important to try to distinguish cachexia from malnutrition caused by inadequate oral intake due to MBO. Cachexia is not reversible by increasing nutritional intake, it represents end-stage disease, and therefore interventions to improve oral intake will not be helpful. Unfortunately, in advanced cancer patients, cachexia, MBO, and poor nutritional status are often seen together.

The European Society for Clinical Nutrition and Metabolism (ESPEN) defined severe malnutrition as existing when patients have at least one of the following risk factors: weight loss $\geq 10\%$ to 15% within 6 months, body mass index ≤ 18 kg/m², and serum albumin ≤ 30 g/L (without evidence of renal and/or liver dysfunction) (65).

The use of PN in advanced cancer remains controversial. Recent guidelines by ESPEN were published for the use of PN in patients who will undergo a surgical procedure (65) and for those who will not undergo a surgical intervention (66). For those patients who meet the ESPEN definition for severe malnutrition or undernourishment (body mass index <18.5 to 22 kg/m² depending on age), in whom a surgery is planned, and who cannot be enterally fed, ESPEN recommends starting PN 7 to 10 days preoperatively to decrease the rate of postoperative infections, length of stay in hospital, and postoperative mortality. Postoperative

PN is indicated for malnourished patients who required emergency surgery and therefore could not receive PN preoperatively (65).

For those patients with advanced cancer and poor nutritional status who do not require surgery, PN is considered ineffective if the reason for the poor nutritional status is not located in the GI tract. Also, PN does not have a role as a supplement while patients are on chemotherapy, radiation treatment, or both therapies simultaneously and also are able to receive oral or enteral nutrition adequately (66).

One recently published study evaluated the effectiveness of a home PN program in 38 patients with advanced malignant disease. The most common indication for home PN in this group was MBO. Patients who started on PN with a Karnofsky Performance Status ≥ 50 did have a longer survival compared with those patients who had a score ≤ 50 at the time of the beginning of PN (67). There may therefore be a role for PN for select patients with MBO for whom some improvement in QOL and extension of life may be expected.

Pharmacologic Treatment of Symptoms

Symptomatic pharmacologic approach *should* be used in inoperable patients with the following aims: (a) to relieve continuous abdominal pain and intestinal colic; (b) to reduce vomiting to an acceptable level for the patient (e.g., 1 to 2 times in 24 hours) with medical therapy and without the use of the NGT, which use could cause more discomfort than benefit; (c) to relieve nausea; (d) to achieve hospital discharge; and (e) to allow for care at home/hospice if otherwise possible (14). Clinical practice recommendations for the management of MBO in patients with end-stage cancer have been published by the Working Group of the European Association for Palliative Care (6).

The drugs of choice may vary between different countries and different centers, based on the clinical experience, drug availability, cost, and fashion. Medication should be tailored to each patient with regard to both the drugs to be administered and the route of administration (Fig. 15.11) (6). Dosage and choice of drug should be highly personalized. Most MBO patients are not able to use the oral route and therefore alternative routes should be considered. If a central venous catheter has been previously inserted, this can be used to administer drugs for symptom control. Continuous subcutaneous infusion of drugs using a portable syringe driver allows the parenteral administration of different drug combinations, produces minimal discomfort for the patient, and is easy to use in a home setting. Rectal and sublingual administration can

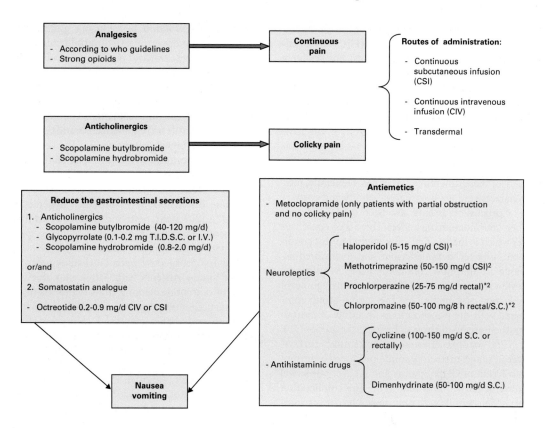

Figure 15.11 Symptomatic pharmacologic approach.

[1] Butyrophenones
[2] Phenothiazines
*Skin irritation when administered subcutaneously (S.C.)

occasionally be used. Finally, some drugs, such as fentanyl and scopolamine, may also be administered by the transdermal route.

Pain

Opioid analgesics, administered according to the World Health Organization (WHO) and European Society of Medical Oncology (ESMO) guidelines (68,69), are the most effective drugs in the management of abdominal, continuous, and colicky, pain associated with bowel obstruction. The dose of opioids should be titrated against the effect and most usually be administered parenterally. In patients with subsequent episodes of subacute obstruction to which opioids may negatively contribute, it may be useful to choose the drug on the basis of presumed selectivity of distribution at the intestinal sites. Morphine tends to accumulate in intestinal tissues, interacting with local opioid receptors. It has been reported that more lipophilic drugs, like methadone and fentanyl, may limit their presence at the opioid intestinal receptors (70,71). Somatostatin analogues have shown more benefit and fewer side effects than anticholinergics in decreasing secretions and controlling vomiting (Fig. 15.11).

Nausea and Vomiting

Nausea and vomiting can be managed using two different pharmacologic approaches (Fig. 15.11):

1. Administration of drugs that reduce GI secretions such as anticholinergics (hyoscine, scopolamine, hydrobromide, hyoscine butylbromide, and glycopyrrolate) and/or somatostatin analogues (octreotide) (6,70,72–78). Some clinicians prefer glycopyrrolate as it is a quaternary amine, less easily crosses the blood–brain barrier than tertiary amines like hyoscine or scopolamine, and therefore is less likely to cause cognitive side effects.

2. Administration of antiemetics acting on the central nervous system, alone or in association with drugs to reduce GI secretions. Metoclopramide is the drug of choice in functional intestinal obstruction; it is not recommended in the presence of complete bowel obstruction as it may increase nausea, vomiting, and colicky pain. It is a prokinetic acting at the level of acetylcholine and dopamine receptors, thus stimulating the musculature of the GI tract. Other antiemetics are the butyrophenones, antihistaminic–

antiemetics, and phenothiazines (prochlorperazine and chlorpromazine (6)) (Fig. 15.11). Haloperidol, a dopamine antagonist and a potent suppressor of the chemoreceptor trigger zone, is considered to be the antiemetic drug of first choice when the obstruction is complete. Haloperidol can be combined with scopolamine butylbromide and opioid analgesic in the same syringe.

There are no comparative studies on the efficacy of these different approaches. Generally, physicians are guided by drug availability and costs.

Corticosteroids have also been used because of their anti-inflammatory effect. There is no consensus on which is the most effective steroid in this condition; however, dexamethasone and methylprednisolone are the most commonly used. A systematic review showed a tendency but no definite significant reduction of symptoms in the steroid group compared with the placebo group. In terms of mortality, there are no differences between the groups (79).

The coadministration of octreotide, corticosteroids, and metoclopramide produced a prompt resolution of GI symptoms and recovery of bowel movements within 5 days (72). The combination of corticosteroids with granisetron has been evaluated in a study of 24 patients refractory to other antiemetic treatment showing nausea and vomiting control in more than 80% of the patients (84).

A meta-analysis compared the effectiveness of histamine-2 receptor antagonists and proton pump inhibitors (PPI) in reducing gastric secretions in patients with MBO. It was done based on seven randomized controlled trials. In total, 445 patients were included, of which 223 received ranitidine and 222 different PPIs (omeprazole, lansoprazole, pantoprazole, and rabeprazole). Both drugs were able to reduce the gastric secretions and between them, the histamine-2 receptor antagonist was the most potent (80). Considering the recent withdrawal from the market of ranitidine, which was used in this study, we recommend the use of a different histamine-2 receptor antagonist such as famotidine or cimetidine. Based on this report, we cannot make final conclusions, but these findings represent another tool available in the management of this condition and something that needs further investigation.

Octreotide, a synthetic analogue of somatostatin that has a more potent biologic activity and a longer half-life, has also been used to manage the symptoms of bowel obstruction. It may be administered subcutaneously or intravenously either as a bolus or as a continuous infusion. Somatostatin and its analogues have been shown to inhibit the release and activity of GI hormones,

modulate GI function by reducing gastric acid secretion, slow down intestinal motility, decrease bile flow, increase mucous production, and reduce splanchnic blood flow. It reduces GI contents and increases absorption of water and electrolytes at the intracellular level, via cyclic adenosine monophosphate and calcium regulation. The inhibitory effect of octreotide on both peristalsis and GI secretions reduces bowel distension and the secretion of water and sodium by the intestinal epithelium, thereby reducing vomiting and pain. The drug may therefore break the vicious circle represented by secretion, distension, and contractile hyperactivity (81). Additionally, octreotide indirectly inhibits submucosal excitatory nerves, thus reducing spastic activity responsible for colicky pain.

The first prospective open-label study was performed on 14 patients with MBO who received doses of octreotide ranging from 0.3 to 0.6 mg/d after unsuccessful symptom control of nausea and vomiting with haloperidol and chlorpromazine. All the patients had a reduction in nausea and quantity of vomiting at different levels, and in two patients the NGT was removed (82).

Many studies, although uncontrolled, strongly support the use of octreotide for reducing GI secretions, nausea, and vomiting in patients with MBO (3,4,6,13,14,83,84). In many cases, the NGT can be removed. Reported effective doses range from 100 to 600 μg/d, either as a continuous infusion or as intermittent subcutaneous boluses. Octreotide has been coadministered with numerous other agents, including morphine, haloperidol, and scopolamine butylbromide.

The combination of the two drugs (octreotide and scopolamine butylbromide) may reduce GI secretions and vomiting whenever the use of one drug alone is ineffective (77,78).

Three randomized trials have compared octreotide with hyoscine butylbromide (77,78,85). In all of these trials, octreotide was superior in the control of symptoms compared with hyoscine butylbromide.

Two randomized, prospective studies were carried out by Ripamonti et al. to compare the antisecretory effects of octreotide (0.3 mg/d) and scopolamine butylbromide (SB) (60 mg/d) that were administered by continuous subcutaneous infusion for 3 days in 17 patients with inoperable bowel obstruction having an NGT (77) and in 15 patients without NGT (78). In both the studies, half of the patients were cared for at home and the other half were admitted to surgical wards. In both the studies, the hospitalized patients received significantly more parenteral hydration per day (2,000 vs. 500 mL) than did the patients cared for at home.

In the study of Ripamonti et al. (77), the NGT could be removed in all 10 home care patients and in 3 hospitalized patients without changing the dosage of the drugs. Octreotide significantly reduced the amount of GI secretions already at T2 ($p = 0.016$) and T3 ($p = 0.020$). Pain relief was obtained in all 17 patients, and only 2 patients required an increase in the morphine dose at T1. In the second study (78), octreotide treatment induced a significantly more rapid reduction in the number of daily episodes of vomiting and intensity of nausea when compared with scopolamine butylbromide treatment at the different time intervals examined.

In the third randomized controlled trial, Mystakidou et al. (85) evaluated the efficacy of octreotide in the management of nausea, vomiting, and abdominal pain secondary to MBO in inoperable cancer patients. Sixty-eight terminally ill patients were enrolled, and the patients were randomly assigned into two equal groups. One group received scopolamine butylbromide 60 to 80 mg/d and chlorpromazine 15 to 25 mg/d, and the comparative group received octreotide 0.6 to 0.8 mg/d and chlorpromazine 15 to 25 mg/d. The drugs were administered via continuous subcutaneous infusion. Patients on octreotide presented significant less intensity of nausea and quantity of vomiting episodes. The survival time ranged from 7 to 61 days (85).

Mercadante et al. (86) studied 15 consecutive advanced cancer patients with inoperable MBO receiving octreotide in combination with metoclopramide, corticosteroids, and an initial bolus of amidotrizoatoate (a mixture of sodium diatrizoate, meglumine diatrizoate, and a wetting agent [polysorbate 80]). Recovery of bowel transit appeared in 1 to 5 days in 14 of 15 patients till death.

Few studies have addressed the use of long-acting octreotide in patients with advanced malignancies who developed MBO at some point during the course of the disease (87,88). The efficacy and safety of octreotide long-acting release (LAR) at a dose of 30 mg on day 1 and octreotide for 2 weeks were evaluated in a pilot study of 15 patients with advanced ovarian cancer. Of 13 evaluable patients, 3 had a major efficacy to LAR treatment with reduction in GI symptoms, 2 had minor response, 4 had no response, and 4 had progressive symptoms. No significant toxicities were due to LAR (87).

A meta-analysis from Mercadante et al. (89) did an extensive review of randomized control trials or reports or review articles evaluating the activity of octreotide for the treatment of MBO in patients who are not candidates for any additional treatment published between June 1993 and June 2011 on electronic database, including MEDLINE, PUBMED, CANCERLIY, and EMBASE. Among the studies analyzed, 3 were randomized controlled trials comparing octreotide with scopolamine butylbromide, 3 were retrospective analysis, and 10 were observational studies including two performed with sustained-release octreotide (LAR). Based on their analysis, the control of vomiting was obtained in more than 60% treated with octreotide, and octreotide seems to be significantly more effective and faster than hyoscine butylbromide in reducing the amount of GI secretions in patients having an NGT and in reducing the intensity of nausea and the number of vomiting episodes in patients without NGT.

Recently, an Australian study from Currow et al. (90) reported the results from a double-blind, placebo-controlled, randomized study evaluating the activity of octreotide compared to placebo in patients receiving best supportive care treatment for MBO including ranitidine infusion 200 mg/24 hours, dexamethasone (8 mg/24 hours), and parenteral hydration (10 to 20 mg/24 hours). The study involved 12 palliative care service across Australia and enrolled a total of 87 patients (45, octreotide arm). Although the study didn't show any reduction in number of days free of vomiting, it did suggest a reduced number of episodes of vomiting in patients receiving octreotide. Surprisingly, the study showed that patients receiving octreotide were two times more likely to receive hyoscine (scopolamine) butylbromide as well.

We do think this is an interesting finding, but based on only a small number of patients, we are unable to make further conclusions at the present time. It will be interesting to see more research in this area, because this drug might be used potentially in the ambulatory setting. Considering the fact that the goal of the treatment is improvement in the QOL of the patient and based on the strong evidence available in the literature that supports a real benefit with the use of this medication, the authors of this chapter consider that octreotide should be part of the treatment once the patient is diagnosed.

CONCLUSION

MBO is a common feature of patients with abdominal and pelvic cancers, especially in those with ovarian, peritoneal, colorectal, and gastric cancers. This clinical condition, which usually presents as the inability to have bowel movement, passing gas, abdominal pain, and vomiting, can be either the initial presentation or a late event related to an advanced stage of disease, and for this reason its management strategy should take into considerations the overall goal of care for each individual patient. Contrast-enhanced helical multidetector row CT scan should be used to evaluate the extension and degree of the MBO to better plan a therapeutic strategy including surgery and medical management. Patients who are surgical candidates should receive surgery with optimal surgical debulking intent, especially those with a newly diagnosed disease, good performance status, and effective therapeutic option available. For those patients who are deemed not to be good candidates, the goal should be symptoms relief, comfort, and good QOL. Stent placement and endoscopically placed gastrostomy tube should be considered in addition to medical management. NGT placement should be limited as it can cause more discomfort than benefit. Although data are limited by the lack of large randomized trials, data suggest that haloperidol should be considered the first antiemetic choice, and that octreotide has a better antisecretory effect compared with anticholinergics and should be started promptly to improve nausea and vomiting control. Corticosteroids and other antiemetic drugs, such as antihistamine H_2 and H_3, can be used to provide additional benefit for nausea and vomiting control. Overall, MBO is a severe condition and should be treated with a multidisciplinary approach with the ultimate goal of controlling symptoms and improving patient's QoL regardless whether the obstruction is resolved or not (91).

REFERENCES

1. Anthony T, Baron T, Mercadante S, et al. Report of the clinical protocol committee: development of randomized trials for malignant bowel obstruction. *J Pain Symptom Manage.* 2007;34:S49-S59.
2. Krouse RS. The international conference on malignant bowel obstruction: a meeting of the minds to advance palliative care research. *J Pain Symptom Manage.* 2007;34: S1-S6.
3. Correa R, Ripamonti CI, Dodge JE, Easson AM. Malignant bowel obstruction. In: Davis M, et al., eds. *Supportive Oncology.* Elsevier; Vol. 30; 2011:326-341.
4. Ripamonti C, Mercadante S. How to use octreotide for malignant bowel obstruction. *J Support Oncol.* 2004;2(4): 357-364.
5. Krebs HB, Goplerud DR. Mechanical intestinal obstruction in patients with gynecologic disease: a review of 368 patients. *Am J Obstet Gynecol.* 1987;157:577-583.
6. Ripamonti C, Twycross R, Baines M, et al. Clinical-practice recommendations for the management of bowel obstruction in patients with end-stage cancer. *Support Care Cancer.* 2001;9:223-233.
7. Tunca JC, Buchler DA, Mack EA, Ruzicka FF, Crowley JJ, Carr WF. The management of ovarian-cancer-caused bowel obstruction. *Gynecol Oncol.* 1981;12:186-192.
8. Idelevich E, Kashtan H, Mavor E, Brenner B. Small bowel obstruction caused by secondary tumors. *Surg Oncol.* 2006;15:29-32.
9. Turnbull ADM, Guerra J, Starners HF. Results for surgery for obstructing carcinomatosis of gastrointestinal, pancreatic, or biliary origin. *J Clin Oncol.* 1989;7:381-386.
10. Aabo K, Pedersen H, Bach F, Knudsen J. Surgical management of intestinal obstruction in the late course of malignant disease. *Acta Chir Scand.* 1984;150:173-176.
11. Phillips RKS, Hittinger R, Fry JS, Fielding LP. Malignant large bowel obstruction. *Br J Surg.* 1985;72:296-302.
12. Ripamonti C, De Conno F, Ventafridda V, Rossi B, Baines MJ. Management of bowel obstruction in advanced and terminal cancer patients. *Ann Oncol.* 1993;4:15-21.
13. Ripamonti C, Bruera E. Palliative management of malignant bowel obstruction. *Int J Gynecol Cancer.* 2002; 12:135-143.
14. Ripamonti C, Easson A, Gerdes H. Management of malignant bowel obstruction. *Eur J Cancer.* 2008;44: 1105-1115.
15. Shrake PD, Rex DK, Lappas JC, et al. Radiographic evaluation of suspected small-bowel obstruction. *Am J Gastroenterol.* 1991;86:175-178.
16. Maglinte DDT, Balthazar EJ, Kelvin FM, et al. The role of radiology in the diagnosis of small-bowel obstruction. *Am J Radiol.* 1997;168:1171-1180.
17. Suri S, Gupta S, Sudhakar PJ, et al. Comparative evaluation of plain films, ultrasound and CT in the diagnosis of intestinal obstruction. *Acta Radiol.* 1999;40(4): 422-428.
18. Caoili EM, Paulson EK. CT of small-bowel obstruction: another perspective using multiplanar reformations. *AJR Am J Roentgenol.* 2000;174:993-998.
19. Angelilli G, Moschetta M, Sabato L, et al. Value of "protruding lips" sign in malignant bowel obstructions. *Eur J Radiol.* 2011;80(3):681-685.
20. Angelilli G, Moschetta M, Binetti F, et al. Prognostic value of MDCT in malignant large-bowel obstructions. *Radiol Med.* 2010;115:747-757.
21. Lowe AS, Beckett CG, Jowett S, et al. Self-expandable metal stent placement for the palliation of malignant gastroduodenal obstruction: experience in a large, single, UK centre. *Clin Radiol.* 2007;62:738-744.
22. Telford JJ, Carr-Locke DL, Baron TH, et al. Palliation of patients with malignant gastric outlet obstruction with the enteral Wallstent: outcomes from a multicenter study. *Gastrointest Endosc.* 2004;60:916-920.
23. Dormann A, Meisner S, Verin N, et al. Self-expanding metal stents for gastroduodenal malignancies: systematic review of their clinical effectiveness. *Endoscopy.* 2004;36:543-550.
24. Nassif T, Prat F, Meduri B, et al. Endoscopic palliation of malignant gastric outlet obstruction using self-expandable metallic stents: results of a multicenter study. *Endoscopy.* 2003;35:483-489.
25. Costamagna G, Tringali A, Spicak J, et al. Treatment of malignant gastroduodenal obstruction with a nitinol self-expanding metal stent: an international prospective multicentre registry. *Dig Liver Dis.* 2012;44(1): 37-43.
26. Espinel J, Sanz O, Vivas S, et al. Malignant gastrointestinal obstruction: endoscopic stenting versus surgical palliation. *Surg Endosc.* 2006;20:1083-1087.
27. Lillemoe KD, Cameron JL, Hardacre JM, et al. Is prophylactic gastrojejunostomy indicated for unresectable periampullary cancer? A prospective randomized trial. *Ann Surg.* 1999;230:322-328; discussion 328-330.
28. Jeurnink SM, Steyerberg EW, Hof GV, et al. Gastrojejunostomy versus stent placement in patients with malignant gastric outlet obstruction: a comparison in 95 patients. *J Surg Oncol.* 2007;96(5):389-396.
29. Mendelsohn RB, Gerdes H, Markowitz AJ, Dimaio CJ, Schattner MA. Carcinomatosis is not a contraindication to enteral stenting in selected patients with malignant gastric outlet obstruction. *Gastrointest Endosc.* 2011;73(6):1135-1140.

30. Holt AP, Patel M, Ahmed MM. Palliation of patients with malignant gastroduodenal obstruction with self-expanding metallic stents: the treatment of choice? *Gastrointest Endosc.* 2004;60:1010-1017.

31. Wong YT, Brams DM, Munson L, et al. Gastric outlet obstruction secondary to pancreatic cancer: surgical vs endoscopic palliation. *Surg Endosc.* 2002;16:310-312.

32. Mehta S, Hindmarsh A, Cheong E, et al. Prospective randomized trial of laparoscopic gastrojejunostomy versus duodenal stenting for malignant gastric outflow obstruction. *Surg Endosc.* 2006;20:239-242.

33. Schmidt C, Gerdes H, Hawkins W, et al. A prospective observational study examining quality of life in patients with malignant gastric outlet obstruction. *Am J Surg.* 2009;198:92-99.

34. Lennon AM, Chandrasekhara V, Shin EJ, et al. Spiral-enteroscopy-assisted enteral stent placement for palliation of malignant small-bowel obstruction. *Gastrointest Endosc.* 2010;71(2):422-425.

35. Ross AS, Semrad C, Waxman I, et al. Enteral stent placement by double balloon enteroscopy for palliation of malignant small bowel obstruction. *Gastrointest Endosc.* 2006;65(5):835-837.

36. Camunez F, Echenagusia A, Simo G, et al. Malignant colorectal obstruction treated by means of self-expanding metallic stents: effectiveness before surgery and in palliation. *Radiology.* 2000;216:492-497.

37. Law WL, Chu KW, Ho JW, et al. Self-expanding metallic stent in the treatment of colonic obstruction caused by advanced malignancies. *Dis Colon Rectum.* 2000;43:1522-1527.

38. Mainar A, De Gregorio MA, Tejero E, et al. Acute colorectal obstruction: treatment with self-expandable metallic stents before scheduled surgery—results of a multicenter study. *Radiology.* 1999;210:65-69.

39. Nash CL, Markowitz AJ, Schattner M, et al. Colorectal stents for the management of malignant large bowel obstruction. *Gastrointest Endosc.* 2002;55:AB216.

40. Pothuri B, Guiguis A, Gerdes H, et al. The use of colorectal stents for palliation of large bowel obstruction due to recurrent gynecologic cancer. *Gynecol Oncol.* 2004;95:513-517.

41. Khot UP, Wenk Lang A, Murali K, et al. Systematic review of the efficacy and safety of colorectal stents. *Br J Surg.* 2002;89:1096-1102.

42. Sebastian S, Johnston S, Geoghegan T, et al. Pooled analysis of the efficacy and safety of self-expanding metal stenting in malignant colorectal obstruction. *Am J Gastroenterol.* 2004;99:2051-2057.

43. Caceres A, Zhou Q, Iasonos A, Gerdes H, Chi DS, Barakat RR. Colorectal stents for palliation of large-bowel obstructions in recurrent gynecologic cancer: an updated series. *Gynecol Oncol.* 2008;108(3):482-485.

44. Nagula S, Ishil N, Nash C, et al. Quality of life and symptom control after stent placement or surgical palliation of malignant colorectal obstruction. *J Am Coll Surg.* 2010;210:45-53.

45. Meisner S, Gonzalez-Huix F, Vandervoort JG, et al. Self-expandable metal stents for relieving malignant colorectal obstruction: short-term safety and efficacy within 30 days of stent procedure in 447 patients. *Gastrointest Endosc.* 2011;74(4):876-884.

46. Campagnutta E, Cannizzaro R, Gallo A, et al. Palliative treatment of upper intestinal obstruction by gynecological malignancy: the usefulness of percutaneous endoscopic gastrostomy. *Gynecol Oncol.* 1996;62:103-105.

47. Pothuri B, Montemarano M, Gerardi M, et al. Percutaneous endoscopic gastrostomy tube placement in patients with malignant bowel obstruction due to ovarian carcinoma. *Gynecol Oncol.* 2005;96:330-334.

48. Piccinni G, Angrisano A, Testini M, et al. Venting direct percutaneous jejunostomy (DPEJ) for drainage of malignant bowel obstruction in patients operated on for gastric cancer. *Support Care Cancer.* 2005;13:535-539.

49. Krouse RS, McCahill LE, Easson AM, Dunn GP. When the sun can set on an unoperated bowel obstruction: management of malignant bowel obstruction. *J Am Coll Surg.* 2002;195:117-128.

50. Brooksbank M, Game P, Ashby M. Palliative venting gastrostomy in malignant intestinal obstruction. *Palliat Med.* 2002;16:520.

51. Bryan D, Radbod R, Berek J. An analysis of surgical versus chemotherapeutic intervention for the management of intestinal obstruction in advanced ovarian cancer. *Int J Gynecol Cancer.* 2006;16:125-134.

52. Helyer LK, Law CH, Butler M, et al. Surgery as a bridge to palliative chemotherapy in patients with malignant bowel obstruction from colorectal cancer. *Ann Surg Oncol.* 2007;14:1264-1271.

53. Abbas SM, Merrie AE. Resection of peritoneal metastases causing malignant small bowel obstruction. *World J Surg Oncol.* 2007;5:122.

54. Wright FC, Chakraborty A, Helyer L, Moravan V, Selby DJ. Predictors of survival in patients with non-curative stage IV cancer and malignant bowel obstruction. *Surg Oncol.* 2010;101(5):425-429.

55. Weiss SM, Skibber JM, Rosato FE. Bowel obstruction in cancer patients: performance status as a predictor of survival. *J Surg Oncol.* 1984;25:15-17.

56. Medina-Franco H, García-Alvarez MN, Ortiz-López LJ, Cuairán JZ. Predictors of adverse surgical outcome in the management of malignant bowel obstruction. *Rev Invest Clin.* 2008;60(3):212-216.

57. Imai K, Yasuda H, Koda K, et al. An analysis of palliative surgery for the patients with malignant bowel obstruction. *Gan To Kagaku Ryoho.* 2010;37(suppl 2):264-267.

58. Tattersall MH, Butow PN, Clayton JM. Insights from cancer patient communication research. *Hematol Oncol Clin North Am.* 2002;16:731-743.

59. Schneiderman LJ, Jecker N. Futility in practice. *Arch Intern Med.* 1993;153(4):437-441.

60. Hofmann B, Håheim LL, Søreide JA. Ethics of palliative surgery in patients with cancer. *Br J Surg.* 2005;92:802-809.

61. Dalal KM, Gollub MJ, Miner TJ, et al. Management of patients with malignant bowel obstruction and stage IV colorectal cancer. *J Palliat Med.* 2011;14(7):822-828.

62. Chakraborty A, Selby D, Gardiner K, et al. Malignant bowel obstruction: natural history of a heterogeneous patient population followed prospectively over two years. *J Pain Symptom Manage.* 2011;41(2):412-420.

63. Andreyev HJ, Norman AR, Oates J, Cunningham D. Why do patients with weight loss have a worse outcome when undergoing chemotherapy for gastrointestinal malignancies? *Eur J Cancer.* 1998;34(4):503-509.

64. MacDonald N, Easson AM, Mazurak VC, Dunn GP, Baracos VE. Understanding and managing cancer cachexia. *J Am Coll Surg.* 2003;197(1):143-161.

65. Braga M, Ljungqvist O, Soeters P, Fearon K, Weimann A, Bozzetti F. ESPEN guidelines on parenteral nutrition: surgery. *Clin Nutr.* 2009;28(4):378-386.

66. Bozzetti F, Arends J, Lundholm K, Micklewright A, Zurcher G, Muscaritoli M. ESPEN guidelines on parenteral nutrition: non-surgical oncology. *Clin Nutr.* 2009;28(4):445-454.

67. Soo I, Gramlich L. Use of parenteral nutrition in patients with advanced cancer. *Appl Physiol Nutr Metab.* 2008;33(1):102-106.

68. World Health Organization. *Cancer Pain Relief.* 2nd ed. Geneva, Switzerland: WHO; 1996.

69. Ripamonti CI, Bandieri E, Roila F; on behalf of the ESMO Guidelines Working Group. Management of cancer pain: ESMO Clinical Practice Guidelines. *Ann Oncol*. 2011;22(suppl 6):vi69-vi77.

70. Mercadante S. Pain in inoperable bowel obstruction. *Pain Digest*. 1995;5:9-13.

71. Haazen L, Noorduin H, Megens A, Meert T. The constipation-inducing potential of morphine and transdermal fentanyl. *Eur J Pain*. 1999;3(suppl A):9-15.

72. Porzio G, Aielli F, Verna L, et al. Can malignant bowel obstruction in advanced cancer patients be treated at home? *Support Care Cancer*. 2011;19:431-433.

73. Ventafridda V, Ripamonti C, Caraceni A, et al. The management of inoperable gastrointestinal obstruction in terminal cancer patients. *Tumori*. 1990;76:389-393.

74. De Conno F, Caraceni A, Zecca E, Spoldi E, Ventafridda V. Continuous subcutaneous infusion of hyoscine butylbromide reduces secretions in patients with gastrointestinal obstruction. *J Pain Symptom Manage*. 1991;6:484-486.

75. Fainsinger RL, Spachynski K, Hanson J, et al. Symptom control in terminally ill patients with malignant bowel obstruction. *J Pain Symptom Manage*. 1994;9:12-18.

76. Mercadante S, Sapio M, Serretta R. Treatment of pain in chronic bowel subobstruction with self-administration of methadone. *Support Care Cancer*. 1997;5:327-329.

77. Ripamonti C, Mercadante S, Groff L, Zecca E, De Conno F, Casuccio A. Role of octreotide, scopolamine butylbromide and hydration in symptom control of patients with inoperable bowel obstruction having a nasogastric tube. A prospective, randomized clinical trial. *J Pain Symptom Manage*. 2000;19:23-34.

78. Mercadante S, Ripamonti C, Casuccio A, Zecca E, Groff L. Comparison of octreotide and hyoscine butylbromide in controlling gastrointestinal symptoms due to malignant inoperable bowel obstruction. *Support Care Cancer*. 2000;8:188-191.

79. Feuer DJ, Broadley KE. Systematic review and meta-analysis of corticosteroids for the resolution of malignant bowel obstruction in advanced gynaecological and gastrointestinal cancers. Systematic Review Steering Committee. *Ann Oncol*. 1999;10:1035-1041.

80. Clark K, Lam L, Currow D. Reducing gastric secretions—a role for histamine 2 antagonists or proton pump inhibitors in malignant bowel obstruction? *Support Care Cancer*. 2009;17(12):1463-1468.

81. Riley J, Fallon MT. Octreotide in terminal malignant obstruction of the gastrointestinal tract. *Eur J Palliat Care*. 1994;1:23-28.

82. Mercadante S, Spoldi E, Caraceni A, Maddaloni S, Simonetti MT. Octreotide in relieving gastrointestinal symptoms due to bowel obstruction. *Palliat Med*. 1993;7:295-299.

83. Shima Y, Ohtsu A, Shirao K, Sasaki Y. Clinical efficacy and safety of octreotide (SMS201-995) in terminally ill Japanese cancer patients with malignant bowel obstruction. *Jpn J Clin Oncol*. 2008;38:354-359.

84. Hisanaga T, Shinjo T, Morita T, et al. Multicenter prospective study on efficacy and safety of octreotide for inoperable malignant bowel obstruction. *Jpn J Clin Oncol*. 2010;40:739-745.

85. Mystakidou K, Tsilika E, Kalaidopoulou O, Chondros K, Georgaki S, Papadimitriou L. Comparison of octreotide administration vs conservative treatment in the management of inoperable bowel obstruction in patients with far advanced cancer: a randomized, double-blind, controlled clinical trial. *Anticancer Res*. 2002;22(2B):1187-1192.

86. Mercadante S, Ferrera P, Villari P, Maeeazzo A. Aggressive pharmacological treatment for reversing bowel obstruction. *J Pain Symptom Manage*. 2004;28:412-416.

87. Matulonis UA, Seiden MV, Roche M, et al. Long-acting octreotide for the treatment and symptomatic relief of bowel obstruction in advanced ovarian cancer. *J Pain Symptom Manage*. 2005;30:563-569.

88. Massacesi C, Galeazzi G. Sustained release octreotide may have a role in the treatment of malignant bowel obstruction. *Palliat Med*. 2006;20:715-716.

89. Mercadante S, Porzio G. Octreotide for malignant bowel obstruction: twenty years after. *Crit Rev Oncol Hematol*. 2012;83(3):388-392.

90. Currow DC, Quinn S, Agar M, et al. Double blind, placebo-controlled, randomized trial of octreotide in malignant bowel obstruction. *J Pain Symptom Manage*. 2015;49(5):814-821.

91. Laval G, Mercelin-Benazech B, Guirimand F, et al. Recommendations for bowel obstruction with peritoneal carcinomatosis. *J Pain Symptom Manage*. 2014;48(1):75-91.

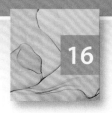

16 Diagnosis and Management of Effusions

Gary T. Buckholz and Charles F. von Gunten

DIAGNOSIS AND MANAGEMENT OF ASCITES

Ascites, the accumulation of fluid in the abdomen, is common. Its formation may be a direct result of a malignant process or secondary to liver cirrhosis or other comorbidities. Because the pathophysiology of fluid collection varies, treatment strategies differ. Clinical distinction between the causes of ascites is therefore important.

Of all patients with ascites, approximately 80% have cirrhosis (1). Other causes of nonmalignant ascites include the following: heart failure, 3%; tuberculosis, 2%; nephrogenic ascites related to hemodialysis, 1%; pancreatic disease, 1%; and miscellaneous entities such as hepatic vein thrombosis (Budd-Chiari syndrome), pericardial disease, and the nephrotic syndrome account for approximately 2% (1). Only 10% of patients who have ascites have malignancy as the primary cause (1). In these patients, epithelial malignancies, particularly ovarian, endometrial, breast, colon, gastric, and pancreatic carcinomas, cause over 80% of malignant ascites. The remaining 20% are due to malignancies of unknown origin (2). In one study, Runyon has shown that 53.3% of malignant ascites is associated with peritoneal carcinomatosis, 13.3% is associated with massive liver metastases, 13.3% is associated with peritoneal carcinomatosis and massive liver metastases, 13.3% is associated with hepatocellular carcinoma with portal hypertension, and 6.7% is associated with chylous ascites (3).

In general, the presence of ascites portends a poor prognosis, regardless of the cause. Patients with nonmalignant ascites related to cirrhosis have a survival rate of approximately 50% at 2 years (1). The mean survival in patients with malignant ascites is generally <4 months (4). However, with ascites due to a malignancy that is relatively sensitive to chemotherapy, such as newly diagnosed ovarian cancer or lymphoma, the mean survival may improve significantly (4).

Pathophysiology

Nonmalignant Ascites

The mechanisms that lead to the development of ascites are many, and controversy still exists regarding which factors are most important. The most common cause of nonmalignant ascites is cirrhosis of the liver. In cirrhotic ascites, abnormal sodium retention is mediated by various hormonal and neural mechanisms, similar to those responsible for excess fluid retention in congestive heart failure (CHF). A hemodynamic state exists where total blood volume is increased, cardiac output is increased, and systemic vascular resistance is low. Studies have implicated nitric oxide as one of the potential mediators of this arterial vasodilation (5). In response, the vasoconstrictors of the renin–angiotensin–aldosterone system and the sympathetic nervous system are activated. Although atrial natriuretic peptide levels are increased, there is reduced renal responsiveness (6). In addition, arginine vasopressin, a potent vasoconstrictor, is activated in a manner independent of the osmotic state (7). The net result is an increase in total body sodium and water. In conjunction with cirrhosis, which has caused increased hepatic venous and lymphatic resistance, severe portal hypertension ensues. The increase in hepatic venous sinusoidal and portal pressures causes the excess fluid volume to localize to the peritoneal cavity secondary to fluid transudation from the splanchnic capillary bed. Ascites accumulation is also exacerbated by diminished intravascular oncotic pressure, resulting from hypoalbuminemia due to decreased synthetic capacity of the cirrhotic liver.

Malignant Ascites

Malignant ascites arises through pathophysiologic mechanisms different from those of nonmalignant ascites. First, in peritoneal carcinomatosis, neovascularization and subsequent "leak" from vessels is thought to play a prime role in ascites development. Researchers have identified a vascular growth and permeability factor that increases fluid leak from peritoneal vasculature; vascular endothelial growth factor (VEGF) is a prime candidate for this activity (8). Compared with cirrhotic ascites, high levels of VEGF are present in malignant ascites from gastric, colon, and ovarian cancers (9). In animal models, inhibiting the tyrosine kinase activity of VEGF receptors reduced ascites formation (10). Matrix metalloproteinases (MMPs) also appear to be involved in this process. Breaking down the extracellular matrix is an important step in neovascularization and metastatic spread. In animal models, MMP inhibitors significantly reduced malignant ascites (11). Second, portal pressures may be raised by direct tumor invasion of the liver with resultant hepatic venous obstruction. The resultant portal hypertension leads to transudation of fluid across the splanchnic bed into the abdominal cavity similar to cirrhotic ascites. A final mechanism of ascites formation is due to lymphatic obstruction, commonly caused by lymphoma, resulting in chylous ascites.

Diagnosis

History

Patients with ascites commonly notice an increase in abdominal girth, a sensation of fullness or bloating, and early satiety. Other useful historical features include recent weight gain and ankle swelling. Patients may describe vague, generalized abdominal discomfort, or a feeling of heaviness with ambulation. They may also note indigestion, nausea, and vomiting due to delayed gastric emptying, esophageal reflux symptoms due to increased intra-abdominal pressure, or protrusion of the umbilicus.

Physical Examination

Physical examination for ascites includes inspection for bulging flanks, percussion for flank dullness, a test for shifting dullness, and a test for a fluid wave. Jugular venous distention should also be assessed, as it may indicate a potentially reversible cardiac cause of ascites.

When significant ascites is present, the abdominal flanks bulge due to the weight of abdominal free fluid. The examiner should look for bulging flanks when the patient is supine. The distinction between excess adipose tissue and ascites may be made by percussing the flanks to assess for dullness (Fig. 16.1). To detect flank dullness in the supine patient, approximately 1,500 mL of fluid must be present (12).

If dullness to percussion is found, examination for shifting dullness is a useful maneuver. The flank is tapped and a mark is made on the skin at the location where the tone changes. The patient is then turned partially toward the side that has been percussed. If the location of the dullness shifts upward toward the umbilicus, it is further evidence of intra-abdominal ascites (Fig. 16.2).

The elicitation of a fluid wave may also help to confirm the diagnosis. The test is performed by having an assistant place the medial edges of both hands firmly down the midline of the abdomen to block transmission of a wave through

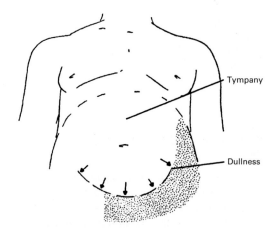

Figure 16.1 Shifting dullness.

subcutaneous fat. The examiner places his/her hands on the flanks and then taps one flank sharply while simultaneously using the fingertips of the opposite hand to feel for an impulse transmitted through the ascites to the other flank. This test is 90% specific, but it is only 62% sensitive (13).

Several additional aspects of the physical examination may also be helpful. The liver may be ballotable, if it is enlarged and ascites is present. If ascites is severe, the examiner may discern umbilical, abdominal, or inguinal hernias; scrotal or lower extremity edema; or abdominal wall venous engorgement. The umbilicus may be flattened or slightly protuberant. The puddle sign and auscultatory percussion, the two additional maneuvers that have been described for the physical diagnosis of ascites, are not recommended (13).

Several diagnostic tests may be useful, particularly if the physical examination is equivocal. A plain radiograph of the abdomen may demonstrate a hazy or ground glass pattern. Ultrasonography or computed tomography (CT) of the abdomen readily identifies as little as 100 mL of free fluid. These latter tests are most helpful in making the diagnosis when there is a relatively small amount of fluid or when loculation is present.

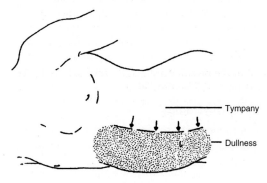

Figure 16.2 Tympany and dullness.

Laboratory Abnormalities

A diagnostic paracentesis of 10 to 20 mL of fluid is useful to confirm the presence of ascites. More importantly, it is essential to help determine its cause. Identifying the cause has profound implications for what treatment is attempted.

To perform paracentesis, one of the two locations is chosen. The first is a midline location 2 cm inferior to the umbilicus. This location is over the linea alba, which is typically avascular. The second is a location 2 cm superior and medial to the anterior iliac spine and lateral to the edge of the rectus sheath, avoiding entry into the inferior epigastric artery. Ultrasonography may be performed if the fluid is difficult to obtain, loculation is suspected, or surgical scarring is present. Previous surgery in the area of the procedure increases the possibility that the bowel may be adherent to the abdominal wall.

After careful cleansing and local anesthetizing, a 2-in 20-G angiocatheter is attached to a 20-mL syringe. To minimize the risk of fluid leaking after the procedure, the Z technique is performed. The skin is displaced 2 cm relative to the deep fascia. The needle is slowly advanced while a small amount of negative pressure is intermittently applied through the syringe until ascitic fluid is obtained. The intermittent pressure helps to avoid trapping omentum or bowel against the needle tip. After the necessary amount of fluid has been obtained, the needle is withdrawn. The fascial planes overlap to prevent fluid leakage, a common complication with a more direct approach.

The color of the fluid should be noted. A white milky fluid is characteristic of chylous ascites. Bloody fluid is almost always malignant in origin, although it may be due to abdominal tuberculosis. Initial bloody fluid that clears is more likely related to the trauma of the procedure.

The fluid should undergo cytologic analysis, determination of cell counts with a differential, and determination of albumin and total protein concentrations. A Gram's stain with culture can be performed if infection is suspected, but it has a low sensitivity. Inoculation of ascites directly into blood culture bottles increases the sensitivity of detecting infection up to 85% (14). The cell count, particularly the absolute neutrophil count, is useful in the presumptive diagnosis of bacterial peritonitis. If the neutrophil count is >250 cells/mL, bacterial peritonitis is presumed and empiric antibiotics should be started.

Cytology is the most specific test to demonstrate that the ascites is due to malignancy. Cytology is approximately 97% sensitive with peritoneal carcinomatosis (3), but it is not helpful in the detection of other types of malignant ascites such as massive hepatic metastasis or lymphomatous obstruction of lymph vessels. Therefore, the absence of malignant cells does not exclude malignancy as a cause.

In the past, the total protein concentration has been used to classify ascites into the broad categories of exudate (total protein >25 g/L) and transudate (total protein <25 g/L). However, this classification system has limitations and sometimes fails to lead to optimal treatment. It has been superseded by the serum-ascites albumin gradient (SAAG). It is defined as the serum albumin concentration minus the ascitic fluid albumin concentration. The SAAG directly correlates with the portal pressure (15). Patients with an SAAG of 1.1 g/dL or more have ascites that is due in part to increased portal pressures, with an accuracy of 97%. Patients with an SAAG <1.1 g/dL do not have portal hypertension, with an accuracy of 97% (16).

The superiority of the SAAG to the exudate/transudate characterization is shown using two examples. Cardiac ascites is associated with portal hypertension and would be expected to be transudative; however, the total protein levels in cardiac ascites are often exudative (16,17). In this example, although total protein is not useful for primary categorization, it may be useful to identify some forms of ascites. Furthermore, ascites associated with spontaneous bacterial peritonitis (SBP) would be expected to be exudative consistent with an infection. However, SBP almost exclusively develops in low protein content ascites associated with portal hypertension, and total protein levels are typically in the transudative range (16).

Management

Overall goals for patient care should be considered before specific choices for managing ascites are made. The prognosis, expected response to management of the underlying conditions, and preferences for treatment should be established with the patient and family before any treatment plan is instituted. Each ascites treatment modality has associated burdens and benefits that deserve to be considered and discussed.

Whether ascites has a low or a high SAAG is critical in determining the overall management plan. Ascites due to portal hypertension *is* in equilibrium with total body fluid. The most common cause of nonmalignant ascites, cirrhosis, falls within this category. Efforts to restrict salt and to affect fluid balance with diuretics are often successful. Malignant ascites may or may not be responsive to these efforts, depending on its cause. In peritoneal carcinomatosis, the SAAG is low, there is no portal hypertension, and the ascites *is not* in equilibrium with total body fluid (18). Consequently, salt and fluid restriction and diuretics may be of little use.

Their injudicious use may result in intravascular volume depletion, diminished renal perfusion, azotemia, hypotension, and fatigue (2). However, there are high SAAG forms of malignant ascites that are responsive to salt restriction and diuretics. For example, in cases of massive hepatic metastasis, portal hypertension is present and salt restriction and diuretics are indicated (18). One exception to this rule is nephrotic syndrome in which the SAAG is low but the ascites is diuretic responsive (19). The total protein is also low (<25 g/L) in nephrotic syndrome and thus is helpful in identifying this form of ascites (see Table 16.1 for a summary).

Interventions for ascites management in the supportive or palliative care setting should generally be reserved for patients who are symptomatic. The following ascites-related symptoms may spur intervention:

- Dyspnea
- Fatigue
- Anorexia or early satiety
- Nausea/vomiting
- Pain
- Diminished exercise tolerance

Dietary Management

The dietary management of ascites with a high SAAG begins with sodium restriction. Patients with cirrhosis may excrete as little as 5 to 10 mEq of sodium/d in their urine. Limiting sodium intake to 88 mmol or 2 g/d (equivalent to 5 g of sodium chloride/d) is an attainable goal for a motivated patient, but it does make food less palatable. Considering a patient's goals of care, it may be better to liberalize the sodium intake and control ascites through other methods.

Patients are also prone to develop dilutional hyponatremia. The management of this condition has typically been by fluid restriction to 1 L/d. In the patient with advanced disease, when treatment goals are purely palliative, fluid restriction is usually intolerably burdensome. Judicious medical management may be less burdensome. For patients with cirrhotic ascites, serum sodium levels as low as 120 mmol/L are well tolerated and rarely dictate intervention (1).

Pharmacologic Management

For the majority of patients, the pharmacologic management of ascites is palliative. That is, the goal of therapy is to minimize symptoms and optimize quality of life without the expectation that the underlying cause can be reversed.

Systemic chemotherapy may be an effective management strategy for patients with malignant ascites due to a responsive cancer (e.g., lymphoma,

TABLE 16.1 CAUSES OF ASCITES AND DIURETIC RESPONSIVENESS

Cause of ascites	Serum-ascites albumin gradient	Typical diuretic response
Cirrhosis	High (≥1.1 g/dL)	Yes
Alcoholic hepatitis	High (≥1.1 g/dL)	Yes
Cardiac ascites	High (≥1.1 g/dL)	Yes
Fulminant hepatic failure	High (≥1.1 g/dL)	Yes
Budd-Chiari syndrome	High (≥1.1 g/dL)	Yes
Portal vein thrombosis	High (≥1.1 g/dL)	Yes
Venoocclusive disease	High (≥1.1 g/dL)	Yes
Acute fatty liver of pregnancy	High (≥1.1 g/dL)	Yes
Myxedema	High (≥1.1 g/dL)	Yes
Tuberculosis (without cirrhosis)	Low (≤1.1 g/dL)	No
Pancreatic ascites (without cirrhosis)	Low (≤1.1 g/dL)	No
Biliary ascites (without cirrhosis)	Low (≤1.1 g/dL)	No
Nephrotic syndrome	Low (≤1.1 g/dL)	Yes
Serositis from connective tissue disease	Low (≤1.1 g/dL)	No
Bowel obstruction/ infarction	Low (≤1.1 g/dL)	No
Mixed ascites (i.e., cirrhosis plus infection or cancer)	High (≥1.1 g/dL)	Yes
Peritoneal carcinomatosis	Low (≤1.1 g/dL)	No
Massive hepatic metastasis	High (≥1.1 g/dL)	Yes

breast, or ovarian cancer). In addition to systemic chemotherapy, intraperitoneal chemotherapy is an option. In theory, intraperitoneal chemotherapy can deliver high doses to peritoneal sites with minimal systemic side effects. In practice, intraperitoneal chemotherapy is often limited by uneven distribution and poor tissue penetration. Hyperthermic intracavitary chemotherapy after surgical debulking may overcome some of these limitations and enhance the cytotoxicity of chemotherapy (20,21). Biologically active agents have also been used intraperitoneally to treat malignant ascites. Early clinical trials have used interferon (IFN)-α, IFN-β, and IFN-γ, tumor necrosis factor, interleukin-2, anti-VEGF antibodies, anti-VEGF receptor antibodies, VEGF receptor tyrosine kinase inhibitors, and metalloproteinase inhibitors. To date, no phase III clinical trials have been performed. Overall, the efficacy and role of intraperitoneal chemotherapeutic and biologic agents in both curative and palliative care remain to be determined.

Diuretic therapy could be useful in patients whose ascites has a high SAAG, as opposed to low SAAG ascites that is typically diuretic unresponsive. As with any drug therapy in the supportive care setting, the patient's symptoms should first be ascertained and the benefit versus the burden of therapy considered. The goal of diuretic therapy is to reduce extravascular fluid accumulation. Diuretic therapy should be directed to achieve a slow and gradual diuresis that does not exceed the capacity for mobilization of ascitic fluid. In the patient with ascites and edema, edema acts as a fluid reservoir to buffer the effects of a rapid contraction of plasma volume. Approximately 1 L/d (net) can safely be diuresed. In patients with ascites but without edema, diuresis may be achieved at the expense of the intravascular volume, leading to symptomatic orthostatic hypotension. In these patients, a more modest goal is to achieve net diuresis of 500 mL/d. Diuretics should not be administered with the goal to render the patient free of edema and ascites. Rather, only enough fluid should be mobilized to promote the patient's comfort. Overly aggressive diuretic therapy for ascites in a patient with high SAAG ascites has been associated with the hepatorenal syndrome and death (22).

For patients with high SAAG ascites in whom diuretics may be helpful, the renin–angiotensin–aldosterone system is activated. Therefore, the initial diuretic of choice for management is one that acts at the distal nephron to block the effect of increased aldosterone activity (23,24). Spirono-lactone, an aldosterone receptor antagonist, is a first-line therapy. Dosing begins at 100 mg/d and can be titrated up to effect or a maximum of 400 mg/d (Table 16.2). Given spironolactone's long half-life, daily dosing is sufficient. Spironolactone may cause painful gynecomastia (25). Amiloride hydrochloride, 10 mg/d, is an alternative. It acts faster and does not cause gynecomastia. It can be titrated up to a dose of 40 mg/d. Because these diuretics are relatively potassium sparing, patients should be advised not to use salt substitutes, as these are usually preparations of potassium chloride. If patients have a suboptimal response despite maximal use of the distal diuretics, a loop diuretic may be added, beginning at low doses (e.g., furosemide, 40 mg orally daily). There is evidence to support the combined use of a distal tubule diuretic and a loop diuretic at the beginning of therapy (24). This combination may effect a more rapid diuresis while maintaining potassium homeostasis. A ratio of 100 mg of spironolactone to 40 mg of furosemide is recommended as a starting point (1). The ratio can be adjusted to maintain normokalemia. The dosages can be increased in parallel until the goals of therapy have been attained, up to a maximum of spironolactone, 400 mg/d, and furosemide, 160 mg/d, or until therapy is limited by side effects (1). If there is no response to this level of therapy, the ascites is considered refractory to diuretic therapy if the following are true: (a) salt intake is appropriately limited and (b) nonsteroidal anti-inflammatory medications, which can affect glomerular filtration, are not being used.

Aquaretics comprise a new class of agents that can enhance water excretion. There are two types that are in the early stages of clinical evaluation in cirrhotic ascites—κ-opioid agonists and vasopressin receptor antagonists. In advanced cirrhosis, hyponatremia and hypoosmolality are in part due to elevated vasopressin levels that are independent of osmolality. Although the mechanism of action is not clear, κ-opioid agonists can increase free water excretion and raise the plasma sodium concentration (26). Renal V2 vasopressin receptors mediate the insertion of water channels into renal tubules,

TABLE 16.2 DIURETICS

Diuretics	Major site of action	Dosage range (mg/d)	Comments
Spironolactone	Distal tubule	100–400	Long half-life and gynecomastia
Amiloride hydrochloride	Distal tubule	10–40	—
Triamterene	Distal tubule	100–300	—
Furosemide	Loop of Henle	40–160	—
Ethacrynic acid	Loop of Henle	50–200	Can be used for sulfa allergy

thereby rendering them permeable to water. A specific V2 receptor antagonist has been effective in promoting water excretion and correcting hyponatremia (27). The clinical utility of these agents remains to be established.

In the patient who has limited mobility, urinary tract outflow symptoms such as hesitancy and frequency, poor appetite, and poor oral intake or who has difficulties related to polypharmacy, diuretic therapy may be excessively burdensome. Injudicious diuretic therapy can result in incontinence (with attendant self-esteem and skin care issues), sleep deprivation from frequent urination, fatigue from hyponatremia or hypokalemia, and falls from postural hypotension.

SBP Prophylaxis

Patients with cirrhotic ascites with low protein content are at increased risk for SBP (28). This increased risk may be due to decreased opsonin levels in the ascites (29). Patients with SBP may be asymptomatic or may observe fever, abdominal pain, nausea/vomiting, or mental status changes. Studies have indicated that antibiotic prophylaxis is effective in preventing SBP. Norfloxacin (400 mg/d), ciprofloxacin (750 mg/wk), or one trimethoprim and sulfamethoxazole (Septra DS) per day Monday through Friday as primary prophylaxis significantly decreases the risk of developing SBP (30–32). Liver transplant protocols call for the routine use of SBP prophylaxis (33). Prophylaxis raises the concern of drug-resistant organisms. The long-term clinical significance remains unknown, but after 6 months on once a week ciprofloxacin there was no evidence of resistance (31). The use of prophylaxis in an individual case is dependent on the overall treatment goals and the disease context.

Invasive Interventions

Therapeutic Paracentesis

Large-volume therapeutic paracentesis (≥5 L) of high SAAG ascites with concurrent colloid infusion is a simple procedure and is associated with minimal morbidity or mortality (34,35). The symptom response is much faster than when diuretics are used alone. In the patient with refractory ascites, it may be the only therapeutic modality that is effective. In fact, total paracentesis (mean, 10.7 L) associated with colloid infusion has been shown to be safe (36). If the ascites is in equilibrium with the systemic circulation, as is the case with portal hypertension, there is a risk of hemodynamic compromise. Colloid plasma volume expansion (e.g., 6 to 8 g of albumin/L of ascites removed) has been used to avoid this complication; recent

meta-analysis suggests it is superior to other approaches to volume expansion (35). However, the choice for albumin infusions should be judicious. Most patients with paracentesis-induced circulatory dysfunction are asymptomatic, though increased renin levels are predictive of worse outcome (37). Albumin is expensive, but it is not known to cause harm. There are no reports of hepatorenal syndrome associated with paracentesis for low SAAG malignant ascites.

Surgical Procedures

Liver transplantation offers cure for a subset of patients with cirrhosis (33) and a subset of patients with small hepatocellular carcinoma (38).

Other surgical techniques offer palliation. Peritoneovenous shunts have been reported for management of malignant and nonmalignant ascites. They are placed surgically during a 30- to 60-minute procedure while the patient is under local anesthesia. Their purpose is to drain ascites from the peritoneal space via a one-way valve into the thoracic venous system. Unfortunately, the rate of complications is high, including shunt occlusion, heart failure due to fluid overload, infection, and disseminated intravascular coagulation. Stanley et al. (39) and Gines et al. (40) compared serial paracentesis with peritoneovenous shunts in patients with cirrhosis. There was no survival improvement, but there was a high rate of complications with the peritoneovenous shunts. Similarly, Gough and Balderson (41) compared peritoneovenous shunts with nonoperative management in patients with malignant ascites. They found no difference in survival or quality of life. Thus, although there may be specific cases in which peritoneovenous shunting is advantageous in either nonmalignant or malignant ascites, serial paracentesis remains the first-line therapy.

Externally draining, implanted abdominal catheters may be beneficial for selected patients who require repeated large-volume paracentesis for comfort and whose prognosis warrants a surgical procedure. The catheter is surgically placed in the peritoneal cavity with an external drain, which can be accessed intermittently by physicians, nurses, or even trained family members (42). There are no comparative studies between these implanted catheters and serial paracentesis in patients with cirrhotic or malignant ascites. A study of 17 patients with an implanted catheter and abdominal carcinoma was complicated by 2 cases of cellulitis, 1 case of peritonitis, and 8 cases of asymptomatic culture-positive ascites (43). With no guidance from the literature, use of implanted catheters must be individualized.

The transjugular intrahepatic portosystemic shunt (TIPS) is a procedure performed by interventional radiologists that creates a side-to-side shunt that effectively relieves portal hypertension. The role of TIPS in patients with cirrhosis and refractory ascites remains controversial, potentially due to studies on differing populations. Rössle et al. showed that in comparison with serial large-volume paracentesis, TIPS led to a higher rate of ascites resolution and improved survival without transplantation (44). However, Sanyal et al. found that although TIPS improved ascites control versus paracentesis, there was no improvement in quality of life or survival (45). Given the rate of shunt complications and trend of increased frequency of worse encephalopathy, these authors recommend against TIPS as a first-line therapy. TIPS has also been employed in a few cases of malignant ascites associated with portal hypertension. In two cases of malignant portal and hepatic vein occlusion, TIPS improved ascites and quality of life (46). Whether to pursue any of the above invasive surgical procedures is dependent on the patient's goals and the disease context, and the decision must be individualized.

DIAGNOSIS AND MANAGEMENT OF PLEURAL EFFUSIONS

The pleural space is bordered by the parietal and visceral pleuras. The visceral pleura covers all lung surfaces including the intralobar fissures. The parietal pleura covers the inner surfaces of the thoracic cavity including the mediastinum, diaphragm, and chest wall. Fluid accumulates in this space from systemic capillaries through a pressure gradient and is drained by a network of lymphatics along the diaphragm and parietal pleura to the mediastinal lymph nodes. The pleural space is important as it couples movement of the chest wall with the lungs by creating a vacuum to keep the pleural spaces close and the small amount of fluid collected in this space acts as a lubricant. A pleural effusion is created when a wide range of diseases create excessive fluid collection through a variety of mechanisms.

Pleural effusions are common with approximately 1.5 million cases occurring annually in the United States (47). Internationally, in industrialized countries, the prevalence is thought to be approximately 320 cases per 100,000 people (48). The incidence of pleural effusions between sexes is equal; however, two-thirds of malignant pleural effusions occur in women and are often associated with breast and gynecologic malignancies. Malignant effusions in men are most common in lung cancer. Effusions associated with mesothelioma are more common in men, likely due to occupational exposure. Additionally, effusions associated with chronic pancreatitis and rheumatoid arthritis are more common in men.

It is critical to determine the underlying mechanism and disease process as there are significant prognostic implications. Morbidity and mortality correlate with the underlying disease process. Patients with nonmalignant pleural effusions experience less morbidity and mortality when effusions and causes are recognized and treated promptly. Most parapneumonic effusions or empyemas occur in patients with a predisposition to aspiration and systemic or local immunocompromised status, such as malignancy, chronic lung disease, or diabetes mellitus (49). Empyema has a mortality of up to 20% and is associated with high hospital cost (50,51). Radiologic characteristics (as defined by The American College of Chest Physicians) associated with poor prognosis are effusions that occupy more than 50% of the hemithorax, are loculated, or are associated with a thickened parietal pleura (51).

Approximately, 25% of all pleural effusions identified in the hospital setting are due to malignancy and the finding of a malignant effusion means that the primary tumor is likely not resectable as it implies disseminated disease (52). Median survival depends on the site and stage of the primary tumor (3 to 12 months, with the shortest in lung and the longest in breast primaries) (53). When the effusion is due to malignancy, laboratory work-up of the fluid and the serum also yield helpful prognostic information.

Pathophysiology

The normal amount of fluid in the pleural space is between 7 and 14 mL (54). Excessive fluid can be created in this space through a variety of mechanisms. Mechanisms that cause an increased hydrostatic pressure gradient generally cause a transudate with low protein content. Transudative mechanisms include the following:

- Increased pulmonary capillary pressure (e.g., CHF)
- Decreased intrapleural pressure (e.g., atelectasis)
- Decreased plasma oncotic pressure causing excess leakage from pulmonary vessels as well as leakage across the diaphragm and pleural membranes (e.g., low albumin)

Mechanisms that increase permeability of the pleural vessels or obstruct lymphatic drainage generally cause an exudate with high protein content. Examples that cause this include malignancy and infection. Distinguishing between a transudate and an exudate is important to establish a working differential diagnosis.

Diagnosis

History

When a pleural effusion is present, history and physical examination can begin to establish the likelihood of transudate versus exudate and what further work-up may be needed (55). It will also be important to establish whether the patient is critically ill, the severity of their symptoms, and their goals of care especially given the invasiveness of further work-up and potential management.

Important components of history include constitutional symptoms such as weight loss, night sweats, and asthenia, which are associated with exudative causes. Cough productive of purulent sputum may suggest an infectious etiology. Patients may have dyspnea with or without orthopnea. Pleural effusions will decrease chest wall compliance, depress the diaphragm, and decrease lung volume resulting in shortness of breath. Dyspnea itself is nonspecific; however, presence of orthopnea may suggest a transudate caused by CHF. If the pleura, ribs, or chest walls are involved (e.g., exudate caused by infection, malignancy, or pulmonary embolism), then pleuritic pain can be a presenting symptom. Patients with pulmonary embolism often have pleuritic pain and the high severity of their dyspnea is often out of proportion to the size of the effusion elicited by examination or imaging. They may also have a history of recent leg swelling. Skin, eye, or joint issues may suggest collagen vascular disease.

Past medical history for chronic or recent illnesses listed in Table 16.3 will be helpful. For example, a recent or recurrent diagnosis of pneumonia may suggest parapneumonic effusion or empyema. A recent history of deep vein thrombosis may suggest pulmonary embolism.

A medication history may reveal medications associated with toxicities that may cause exudative pleural effusions. While this is not a common adverse effect, some of the more common medications where this can be encountered are listed in Table 16.3. An occupational history may elicit asbestos exposure and risk of mesothelioma from occupations such as shipbuilding, electrical work, construction, carpentry, and insulation work.

Physical Examination

Upon examination, it is important to note the presence of labored breathing (use of accessory muscles and/or intercostal retractions in a child or thin adult), tachypnea, and anxiety (potentially caused by dyspnea). With severe effusions, there may be decreased chest wall movement on

TABLE 16.3 UNILATERAL PLEURAL EFFUSIONS: DIFFERENTIAL DIAGNOSIS OF TRANSUDATES AND EXUDATES

Transudative effusions	
Congestive heart failure[a]	Atelectasis[a]
Cirrhosis[a]	Myxedema
Nephrotic syndrome[a]	Pulmonary embolism
Peritoneal dialysis[a]	Urinothorax

Exudative effusions	
Malignancy[a]	*Other inflammatory*
Lung	Pulmonary embolism with infarction[a]
Lymphoma	Dressler's syndrome
Mesothelioma	Asbestosis
Metastatic	Uremia
	Trapped lung
Infectious	Radiation therapy
Parapneumonic[a]	Meigs syndrome
Tuberculous[a]	
Fungal	*Lymphatic disease*
Viral	Chylothorax
Parasitic	Lymphangiomyomatosis
Abdominal abscess	Yellow nail syndrome
Hepatitis	
	Drug induced
Noninfectious gastrointestinal	Drug-induced lupus
Pancreatitis	Nitrofurantoin
Esophageal rupture	Dantrolene
Abdominal surgery	Amiodarone
Variceal sclerotherapy	Methysergide
	Procarbazine
Collagen vascular disease	Practolol
Lupus erythematosus	Bromocriptine
Rheumatoid arthritis	Minoxidil
Wegener's granulomatosis	Bleomycin
Churg-Strauss syndrome	Methotrexate
Familial Mediterranean fever	Mitomycin
Sjögren's syndrome	
Immunoblastic lymphadenopathy	

[a]Common causes of unilateral pleural effusions.
From Bartter T, Santarelli R, Akers SM, Pratter MR. The evaluation of pleural effusion. *Chest.* 1994;106(4):1209-1214; Rahman NM, Chapman SJ, Davies RJ. Pleural effusion: a structured approach to care. *Br Med Bull.* 2004;72:31-47; Maskell NA, Butland RJ. BTS guidelines for the investigation of a unilateral pleural effusion in adults. *Thorax.* 2003;58(suppl 2):ii8-ii17. Ref. (56).

the affected side. Generally upon auscultation, there are decreased or absent breath sounds over the effusion area and a pleural friction rub may be present. Dullness to percussion over the area of effusion is the most accurate examination finding for diagnosing pleural effusion while the absence of reduced tactile vocal fremitus made pleural effusion less likely (57). Additionally, pleural effusion and ascites together are common in patients with malignant disease (58), and this is associated with spread of malignant disease to the pleura and peritoneum.

Laboratory Abnormalities

If pleural effusion is suspected by history and physical examination, confirmation of the diagnosis can be made by imaging. If at least 200 to 300 mL of fluid is present, an erect posteroanterior chest radiograph may detect effusions with blunting of the costophrenic angles. Pleural thickening can be distinguished from fluid by using the decubitus view, as gravity will pull fluid to the dependent part of the lung. Therefore, decubitus views are more sensitive and can detect as little as 50 mL of fluid (59); however, to attain 100% sensitivity with chest radiographs, the amount of fluid must exceed 500 mL (60). Chest radiographs may also show consolidation, tumor, or pleural calcification.

Ultrasound is very sensitive, as it can also detect fluid levels as little as 50 mL; however, for 100% sensitivity, the amount of fluid must exceed only 100 mL (60). Therefore, ultrasound is more sensitive than radiographs. If available, ultrasound can be helpful to diagnose relatively small or loculated effusions and can be extremely helpful in performing diagnostic or therapeutic thoracentesis with lower complication rates.

While chest radiographs and/or ultrasound are usually the first step(s) and are often sufficient to guide further work-up, CT of the chest is the best imaging study to see the entire pleural space as well as the pulmonary parenchyma and mediastinum (61). This could be especially helpful if exudative causes are suspected and fluid analysis does not lead to immediate diagnosis.

Between physical examination and imaging, distinguishing between unilateral and bilateral effusions is important. The differential for unilateral effusion is extensive and is encompassed in Table 16.3. Massive unilateral effusions with near "white-out" are often due to malignancy (62). Bilateral effusions are usually limited to the transudative causes listed in Table 16.3.

A diagnostic thoracentesis can be performed to help narrow the differential diagnosis and determine the specific cause. Relative contraindications include a small volume of fluid, the inability of the

patient to cooperate, a bleeding diathesis, a systemic anticoagulation, a mechanical ventilation, and a cutaneous disease such as herpes zoster at the needle entry site (63).

Since major complication rates of thoracentesis are significant, it is critical to consider the overall context of the individual patient's situation (medical, psychosocial, and spiritual) and their goals of care prior to thoracentesis and other invasive work-up. Major complication rates of thoracentesis done by house officers have ranged from 11.6% to 30.3%, with pneumothorax being the most common complication with 3.9% to 6.1% of patients requiring a chest tube. In addition, up to 14% of diagnostic thoracenteses yielded inadequate fluid for analysis (52). Ultrasound guidance and experienced clinicians decrease the rate of complications. Aside from the goals of care, which may not include invasive tests, if the clinical course is typical and includes pleural effusion, sampling may not be necessary. For example, bilateral pleural effusion consistent with CHF can be observed with ongoing traditional and/or supportive therapies.

If fluid is obtained, the appearance and odor of the fluid may indicate certain illnesses (see Table 16.4 (64)). Most often it is straw yellow in color, which is nonspecific and is caused by many disease states. The pleural fluid should be sent for laboratory analysis and initially include pH, protein, lactate dehydrogenase (LDH), glucose,

TABLE 16.4 RELATIONSHIP BETWEEN PLEURAL FLUID APPEARANCE AND CAUSES

Cause	Fluid appearance/ odor
Pseudochylothorax and chylothorax	Milky white
Urinothorax	Urine
Anaerobic empyema	Putrid
Chylothorax	Bile stained
Aspergillus infection	Black
Empyema	Turbid
Amebic liver abscess	"Anchovy" brown
Esophageal rupture	Food particles
Trauma, pulmonary embolism, benign asbestos-related effusion, pneumonia, malignant neoplasm, after myocardial infarction syndrome	Blood stained

From Maskell NA, Butland RJ. BTS guidelines for the investigation of a unilateral pleural effusion in adults. *Thorax.* 2003;58(suppl 2):ii8-ii17; McGrath EE, Anderson PB. Diagnosis of pleural effusion: a systematic approach. *Am J Crit Care.* 2011;20(2):119-127; quiz 128.

cytology, Gram stain, and acid-fast bacillus stains with culture and sensitivities. While several techniques have been put forth to help distinguish between transudates and exudates, the Light's criteria have been the gold standard for approximately 40 years (65). The fluid is considered an exudate if one or more of the following criteria are met:

- Ratio of pleural fluid LDH to serum level of LDH is >0.6.
- Pleural fluid level of LDH is >200.
- Ratio of pleural fluid level of protein to serum level of protein is >0.5.

Light's criteria have high sensitivity and specificity for differentiating between transudates and exudates. When used alone, these have an accuracy of 96% (66). However, they may lose accuracy for transudates due to CHF after a patient has been diuresed (52). In this scenario, a pleural fluid cholesterol level >55 mg/dL (67,68) and/or serum albumin minus pleural fluid albumin of >1.2 mg/dL (69) may help diagnose an exudate.

A pH < 7.2 in infected effusions indicates an empyema that in turn necessitates prompt chest tube drainage. A low pH can also occur in esophageal rupture, rheumatoid arthritis, and malignancy associated with poor outcome. A low pH and a low glucose level are both associated with more extensive pleural involvement with tumor, a higher yield on fluid cytology, decreased success rates of pleural sclerosis, and shorter survival times (52). In one study, mean survival was 2.1 months for low-pH malignant effusions and 9.8 months for normal-pH malignant effusions (70). If malignancy is suspected, cytology is important and positive in 60% of patients with neoplasm. If the first sample is negative, a second sample increases the chance of diagnosing malignancy to about 72% (64,71).

In the rare case that fluid analysis and a CT imaging do not yield a diagnosis, an expanded pleural fluid analysis including polymerase chain reaction for *Streptococcus pneumoniae* and tuberculosis, specific tumor markers, and complement levels (low levels in rheumatoid arthritis and systemic lupus) may help establish a diagnosis (64). Bronchoscopy may be helpful if the patient has parenchymal abnormalities or hemoptysis, but negative fluid cytology (52). Finally, a pleural biopsy (radiologically or with thoracoscopy) can be considered (64).

Management

Management of pleural effusions depends on the underlying illness. Generally, this means that the use of conventional therapies to treat the underlying illness, if possible, will also treat the pleural effusion. For example, once the diagnosis of tuberculous pleural effusion is made, the best way to treat the effusion is to treat the patient appropriately for pulmonary tuberculosis. If a patient has a malignancy that is responsive to chemotherapy, such as breast or small cell lung cancer, then the malignant pleural effusion may resolve with traditional anticancer therapies. Radiation may suffice for the malignant pleural effusion associated with lymphoma.

Patients with empyema or complicated parapneumonic effusion should be managed with antibiotics and prompt drainage of the infected pleural effusion. Some guidelines also add the intrapleural administration of fibrinolytic medications (50,51). However, there is a wide variation in the management and it is questionable that the addition of fibrinolytics change outcomes significantly (72). Video-assisted thoracoscopic surgery (VATS) may be utilized, but it is usually reserved for empyema that is refractory to thoracostomy or fibrinolytic therapy. Further studies are needed to clarify the role of VATS.

Symptomatic management of malignant pleural effusion does not improve survival, and it primarily focuses on the relief of dyspnea. Removal of the fluid by therapeutic thoracentesis can achieve dramatic and prompt relief of dyspnea. However, in nearly 100% of cases, the fluid reaccumulates within 30 days (73) and one study showed symptoms recurring within an average of 4.2 days (74). Also, up to 50% of patients may not achieve significant improvement in dyspnea or exercise tolerance secondary to comorbid conditions, general debility from the malignancy, or trapped lung (75). With repeated therapeutic thoracentesis, there is an increased risk of adhesions, loculations, and infection (76). In spite of this, patients who achieve significant symptomatic relief and have a limited prognosis of days to weeks may benefit from repeated thoracentesis. The best volume of pleural fluid to drain while avoiding reexpansion pulmonary edema and maintaining best symptomatic relief is not known; however, 1 to 1.5 L/thoracentesis is recommended (77).

If symptomatic relief is achieved with therapeutic thoracentesis and the patient's prognosis is months to years, they may benefit from chest tube thoracostomy and chemical pleurodesis. It is important to evaluate the patient's goals of care and describe the procedure, which usually requires a hospital stay. A chest catheter is inserted into the pleural space with the patient under local anesthesia or conscious sedation. After drainage of fluid, chemical agents are instilled that cause inflammation with fibrin deposition and adhesion between the layers of pleura. This may produce significant pain and fever. Numerous clinical trials have been performed to help determine the best chemical agent and talc appears to be favored (78,79). Talc may also be instilled via thoracoscopy with insufflation. This is performed by a trained pulmonologist or thoracic surgeon with a flexible pleuroscope. This has a success rate of up to 90% and a recent meta-analysis showed that the relative risk of nonrecurrence of effusion is 1.19 in favor of thoracoscopic pleurodesis compared with tube thoracostomy pleurodesis (79). VATS with talc poudrage has also yielded high success rates; however, it is more invasive and requires surgical expertise and more ancillary and logistical support (75).

If chemical pleurodesis is not recommended, is not within the patient's goals of care, or is not successful, a long-term, indwelling, tunneled pleural catheter may be a good option, particularly if the patient's prognosis is at least many weeks to months. Generally, the procedure is performed under conscious sedation as an outpatient. This allows the fluid to be drained at home with nursing assistance or sometimes the patient or family can be trained to do it as well. Cost effectiveness depends on prognosis, with one study showing an indwelling pleural catheter becoming more cost effective when prognosis was 6 weeks or less (80). Safety, efficacy, and survival appear to be similar between the two therapies (81).

Finally, a pleuroperitoneal shunt where the fluid is manually pumped from the pleural space to the peritoneal cavity can be an option especially in the case where trapped lung makes lung expansion inadequate for pleurodesis. While this intervention is often successful, shunt clotting, risk of infection, and manual operation are factors that have made this intervention fall out of favor for the majority of patients (75).

REFERENCES

1. Runyon B. Current concepts: care of patients with ascites. *N Engl J Med.* 1994;330(5):337-342.
2. Sharma S, Walsh D. Management of symptomatic malignant ascites with diuretics: two case reports and a review of the literature. *J Pain Symptom Manage.* 1995;10(3):237-242.
3. Runyon B, Hoefs J, Morgan T. Ascitic fluid analysis in malignancy related ascites. *Hepatology.* 1988;8:1104-1109.
4. Garrison R, Kaelin L, Galloway R, et al. Malignant ascites: clinical and experimental observations. *Ann Surg.* 1986;203:644-649.
5. Martin P, Gines P, Schrier RW. Nitric oxide as a mediator of hemodynamic abnormalities and sodium and water retention in cirrhosis. *N Engl J Med.* 1998;339(8):533-541.
6. Gines P, Jimenez W, Arroyo V, et al. Atrial natriuretic factor in cirrhosis with ascites; plasma levels, cardiac release and splanchnic extraction. *Hepatology.* 1988;8(3):636-642.
7. Bichet D, Szatalowicz V, Chaimovitz C, Schrier RW. Role of vasopressin in abnormal water excretion in cirrhotic patients. *Ann Intern Med.* 1982;96:413-417.
8. Senger DR, Galli SJ, Dvorak AM, et al. Tumor cells secrete a vascular permeability factor that promotes accumulation of ascites fluid. *Science.* 1983;219:983-985.
9. Zebrowski BK, Liu W, Ramirez K, et al. Markedly elevated levels of vascular endothelial growth factor in malignant ascites. *Ann Surg Oncol.* 1999;6(4):373-378.
10. Xu L, Yoneda J, Herrera C, et al. Inhibition of malignant ascites and growth of human ovarian carcinoma by oral administration of a potent inhibitor of the vascular endothelial growth factor receptor tyrosine kinases. *Int J Oncol.* 2000;16(3):445-454.
11. Watson SA, Morris TM, Robinson G, et al. Inhibition of organ invasion by the matrix metalloproteinase inhibitor batimastat (BB-94) in two human colon carcinoma metastasis models. *Cancer Res.* 1995;55(16):3629-3633.
12. Cattau EL Jr, Benjamin SB, Knuff TE, et al. The accuracy of the physical exam in the diagnosis of suspected ascites. *JAMA.* 1982;247(8):1164-1166.
13. Williams JW Jr, Simel DI. Does this patient have ascites? How to divine fluid in the abdomen. *JAMA.* 1992;267(19): 2645-2648.
14. Runyon BA, Antillon MR, Akriviadis EA, et al. Bedside inoculation of blood culture bottles with ascitic fluid is superior to delayed inoculation in the detection of spontaneous bacterial peritonitis. *J Clin Microbiol.* 1990;28:2811-2812.
15. Hoefs JC. Serum protein concentration and portal pressure determine the ascitic fluid protein concentration in patients with chronic liver disease. *J Lab Clin Med.* 1983;102:260-273.
16. Runyon BA, Montano AA, Akriviadis EA, et al. The serum-ascites albumin gradient is superior to the exudate–transudate concept in the differential diagnosis of ascites. *Ann Intern Med.* 1992;117:215-220.
17. Runyon BA. Cardiac ascites: a characterization. *J Clin Gastroenterol.* 1988;10(4):410-412.
18. Pockros PJ, Esrason KT, Nguyen C, et al. Mobilization of malignant ascites with diuretics is dependent on ascitic fluid characteristics. *Gastroenterology.* 1992;103(4): 1302-1306.
19. Ackerman Z. Ascites in nephrotic syndrome: incidence, patients' characteristics, and complications. *J Clin Gastroenterol.* 1996;22:31-34.
20. Loggie BW, Perini M, Fleming RA, et al. Treatment and prevention of malignant ascites associated with disseminated intraperitoneal malignancies by aggressive combined-modality therapy. *Am Surg.* 1997;63(2):137-143.
21. Shen P, Hawksworth J, Lovato J, et al. Cytoreductive surgery and intraperitoneal hyperthermic chemotherapy with mitomycin C for peritoneal carcinomatosis from nonappendiceal colorectal carcinoma. *Ann Surg Oncol.* 2004;11(2):178-186.
22. Roberts LR, Kamath PS. Ascites and hepatorenal syndrome: pathophysiology and management. *Mayo Clin Proc.* 1996;71(9):874-881.
23. Pérez-Ayuso RM, Arroyo V, Planas R, et al. Randomized comparative study of efficacy of furosemide versus spironolactone in nonazotemic cirrhosis with ascites: relationship between the diuretic response and the activity of the renin–aldosterone system. *Gastroenterology.* 1983;84:961-968.
24. Fogel MR, Sawhney VK, Neal EA, et al. Diuresis in the ascitic patient: a randomized controlled trial of three regimens. *J Clin Gastroenterol.* 1981;3(suppl 1):73-80.
25. Mantero F, Lucarelli G. Aldosterone antagonists in hypertension and heart failure. *Ann Endocrinol.* 2000;61(1): 52-60.
26. Gadano A, Moreau R, Pessione F, et al. Aquaretic effects of niravoline, a kappa-opioid agonist, in patients with cirrhosis. *J Hepatol.* 2000;32(1):38-42.

27. Wong F, Blei AT, Blendis LM, et al. A vasopressin receptor antagonist (VPA-985) improves serum sodium concentration in patients with hyponatremia: a multicenter, randomized, placebo-controlled trial. *Hepatology.* 2003;37(1):182-191.

28. Runyon BA. Low-protein concentration ascitic fluid is predisposed to spontaneous bacterial peritonitis. *Gastroenterology.* 1986;91(6):1343-1346.

29. Runyon BA. Patients with deficient ascitic fluid opsonic activity are predisposed to spontaneous bacterial peritonitis. *Hepatology.* 1988;8(3):632-635.

30. Grangé JD, Roulot D, Pelletier G, et al. Norfloxacin primary prophylaxis of bacterial infections in cirrhotic patients with ascites: a double-blind randomized trial. *J Hepatol.* 1998;29(3):430-436.

31. Rolachon A, Cordier L, Bacq Y, et al. Ciprofloxacin and long-term prevention of spontaneous bacterial peritonitis: results of a prospective controlled trial. *Hepatology.* 1995;22:1171-1174.

32. Singh N, Gayowski T, Yu VL, et al. Trimethoprim-sulfamethoxazole for the prevention of spontaneous bacterial peritonitis in cirrhosis: a randomized trial. *Ann Intern Med.* 1995;122(8):595-598.

33. Saab S, Han SH, Martin P. Liver transplantation: selection, listing criteria, and preoperative management. *Clin Liver Dis.* 2000;4(3):513-532.

34. Ginés P, Arroyo V, Quintero E, et al. Comparison of paracentesis and diuretics in the treatment of cirrhotics with tense ascites: results of a randomized study. *Gastroenterology.* 1987;93(2):234-241.

35. Bernardi M, Caraceni P, Navickis RJ, Wilkes MM. Albumin infusion in patients undergoing large-volume paracentesis: a meta-analysis of randomized trials. *Hepatology.* 2012;55(4):1172-1181.

36. Tító L, Ginès P, Arroyo V, et al. Total paracentesis associated with intravenous albumin management of patients with cirrhosis and ascites. *Gastroenterology.* 1990;98(1):146-151.

37. Gines A, Fernandez-Esparrach G, Monescillo A, et al. Randomized trial comparing albumin, dextran 70, and polygeline in cirrhotic patients with ascites treated by paracentesis. *Gastroenterology.* 1996;111(4):1002-1010.

38. Llovet JM, Bruix J, Fuster J, et al. Liver transplantation for small hepatocellular carcinoma: the tumor-node-metastasis classification does not have prognostic power. *Hepatology.* 1998;27(6):1572-1577.

39. Stanley MM, Ochi S, Lee KK, et al. Peritoneovenous shunting as compared with medical treatment in patients with alcoholic cirrhosis and massive ascites: Veterans Administration Cooperative Study on Treatment of Alcoholic Cirrhosis with Ascites. *N Engl J Med.* 1989;321(24):1632-1638.

40. Gines P, Arroyo V, Vargas B, et al. Paracentesis with intravenous infusion of albumin as compared with peritoneovenous shunting in cirrhosis with refractory ascites. *N Engl J Med.* 1991;325:829-835.

41. Gough IR, Balderson GA. Malignant ascites: a comparison of peritoneovenous shunting and nonoperative management. *Cancer.* 1993;71(7):2377-2382.

42. Murphy M, Rossi M. Managing ascites via the Tenckhoff catheter. *Med Surg Nurs.* 1995;4:468-471.

43. Belfort MA, Stevens PJ, DeHaek K, et al. A new approach to the management of malignant ascites: a permanently implanted abdominal drain. *Eur J Surg Oncol.* 1990;16(1):47-53.

44. Rössle M, Ochs A, Gülberg V, et al. A comparison of paracentesis and transjugular intrahepatic portosystemic shunting in patients with ascites. *N Engl J Med.* 2000;342(23):1701-1707.

45. Sanyal AJ, Genning C, Reddy KR, et al. The North American study for the treatment of refractory ascites. *Gastroenterology.* 2003;124(3):634-641.

46. Burger JA, Ochs A, Wirth K, et al. The transjugular stent implantation for the treatment of malignant portal and hepatic vein obstruction in cancer patients. *Ann Oncol.* 1997;8(2):200-202.

47. Sahn SA. The value of pleural fluid analysis. *Am J Med Sci.* 2008;335(1):7-15.

48. Sahn SA. Pleural effusions of extravascular origin. *Clin Chest Med.* 2006;27(2):285-308.

49. Bartlett JG. Anaerobic bacterial infections of the lung and pleural space. *Clin Infect Dis.* 1993;16(suppl 4): S248-S255.

50. Colice GL, Curtis A, Deslauriers J, et al. Medical and surgical treatment of parapneumonic effusions: an evidence-based guideline. *Chest.* 2000;118(4):1158-1171.

51. Davies CW, Gleeson FV, Davies RJ. BTS guidelines for the management of pleural infection. *Thorax.* 2003;58(suppl 2):ii18-ii28.

52. Bartter T, Santarelli R, Akers SM, Pratter MR. The evaluation of pleural effusion. *Chest.* 1994;106(4):1209-1214.

53. Rahman NM, Chapman SJ, Davies RJ. Pleural effusion: a structured approach to care. *Br Med Bull.* 2004;72:31-47.

54. Sahn SA. State of the art. The pleura. *Am Rev Respir Dis.* 1988;138(1):184-234.

55. Scheurich JW, Keuer SP, Graham DY. Pleural effusion: comparison of clinical judgment and Light's criteria in determining the cause. *South Med J.* 1989;82(12): 1487-1491.

56. Maskell NA, Butland RJ. BTS guidelines for the investigation of a unilateral pleural effusion in adults. *Thorax.* 2003;58(suppl 2):ii8-ii17.

57. Wong CL, Holroyd-Leduc J, Straus SE. Does this patient have a pleural effusion? *JAMA.* 2009;301(3):309-317.

58. Covey AM. Management of malignant pleural effusions and ascites. *J Support Oncol.* 2005;3(2):169-173, 176.

59. Blackmore CC, Black WC, Dallas RV, Crow HC. Pleural fluid volume estimation: a chest radiograph prediction rule. *Acad Radiol.* 1996;3(2):103-109.

60. Gryminski J, Krakowka P, Lypacewicz G. The diagnosis of pleural effusion by ultrasonic and radiologic techniques. *Chest.* 1976;70(1):33-37.

61. McLoud TC, Flower CD. Imaging the pleura: sonography, CT, and MR imaging. *AJR Am J Roentgenol.* 1991;156(6):1145-1153.

62. Maher GG, Berger HW. Massive pleural effusion: malignant and nonmalignant causes in 46 patients. *Am Rev Respir Dis.* 1972;105(3):458-460.

63. Sokolowski JW Jr, Burgher LW, Jones FL Jr, Patterson JR, Selecky PA. Guidelines for thoracentesis and needle biopsy of the pleura. This position paper of the American Thoracic Society was adopted by the ATS Board of Directors, June 1988. *Am Rev Respir Dis.* 1989;140(1):257-258.

64. McGrath EE, Anderson PB. Diagnosis of pleural effusion: a systematic approach. *Am J Crit Care.* 2011;20(2):119-127; quiz 128.

65. Light RW, Macgregor MI, Luchsinger PC, Ball WC Jr. Pleural effusions: the diagnostic separation of transudates and exudates. *Ann Intern Med.* 1972;77(4):507-513.

66. Romero S, Martinez A, Hernandez L, et al. Light's criteria revisited: consistency and comparison with new proposed alternative criteria for separating pleural transudates from exudates. *Respiration.* 2000;67(1):18-23.

67. Hamm H, Brohan U, Bohmer R, Missmahl HP. Cholesterol in pleural effusions. A diagnostic aid. *Chest.* 1987;92(2):296-302.

68. Valdes L, Pose A, Suarez J, et al. Cholesterol: a useful parameter for distinguishing between pleural exudates and transudates. *Chest*. 1991;99(5):1097-1102.

69. Roth BJ, O'Meara TF, Cragun WH. The serum-effusion albumin gradient in the evaluation of pleural effusions. *Chest*. 1990;98(3):546-549.

70. Sahn SA, Good JT Jr. Pleural fluid pH in malignant effusions. Diagnostic, prognostic, and therapeutic implications. *Ann Intern Med*. 1988;108(3):345-349.

71. Ryan CJ, Rodgers RF, Unni KK, Hepper NG. The outcome of patients with pleural effusion of indeterminate cause at thoracotomy. *Mayo Clin Proc*. 1981;56(3): 145-149.

72. Schiza S, Siafakas NM. Clinical presentation and management of empyema, lung abscess and pleural effusion. *Curr Opin Pulm Med*. 2006;12(3):205-211.

73. Antunes G, Neville E, Duffy J, Ali N. BTS guidelines for the management of malignant pleural effusions. *Thorax*. 2003;58(suppl 2):ii29-ii38.

74. Rodriguez-Panadero F, Janssen JP, Astoul P. Thoracoscopy: general overview and place in the diagnosis and management of pleural effusion. *Eur Respir J*. 2006;28(2):409-422.

75. Musani AI. Treatment options for malignant pleural effusion. *Curr Opin Pulm Med*. 2009;15(4):380-387.

76. Lombardi G, Zustovich F, Nicoletto MO, Donach M, Artioli G, Pastorelli D. Diagnosis and treatment of malignant pleural effusion: a systematic literature review and new approaches. *Am J Clin Oncol*. 2010;33(4):420-423.

77. Antony VB, Loddenkemper R, Astoul P, et al. Management of malignant pleural effusions. *Eur Respir J*. 2001;18(2):402-419.

78. Tan C, Sedrakyan A, Browne J, Swift S, Treasure T. The evidence on the effectiveness of management for malignant pleural effusion: a systematic review. *Eur J Cardiothorac Surg*. 2006;29(5):829-838.

79. Shaw P, Agarwal R. Pleurodesis for malignant pleural effusions. *Cochrane Database Syst Rev*. 2004;(1): CD002916.

80. Olden AM, Holloway R. Treatment of malignant pleural effusion: PleuRx catheter or talc pleurodesis? A cost-effectiveness analysis. *J Palliat Med*. 2010;13(1):59-65.

81. Putnam JB Jr, Light RW, Rodriguez RM, et al. A randomized comparison of indwelling pleural catheter and doxycycline pleurodesis in the management of malignant pleural effusions. *Cancer*. 1999;86(10):1992-1999.

17 Hiccups and Other Gastrointestinal Symptoms

Nabeel Sarhill, Fade Mahmoud, and Donato G. Dumlao

Gastrointestinal (GI) symptoms are commonly seen in patients with cancer, regardless of the disease site. These symptoms are experienced during the course of the illness or as a result of therapy. Any physician experienced in caring for patients with advanced cancer knows that many of the symptoms discussed in this chapter such as hiccups, dyspepsia, heartburn, and early satiety are commonly associated with other symptoms such as nausea, anorexia, cachexia, and abdominal pain and that such clusters of symptoms are often similar regardless of the primary cancer diagnosis.

Patients with advanced pancreatic, biliary, neuroendocrine, gynecologic, genitourinary, or breast cancers that have peritoneal or pelvic involvement, typically present with a set of symptoms including hiccups, dyspepsia, heartburn, early satiety, belatedness, excessive gas, food intolerance, and/or malabsorption. These symptoms are, moreover, almost always associated with nausea, vomiting and abdominal pain—additional symptoms that themselves often have multiple etiologies. Many GI problems seen in patients with cancer are not caused by the cancer and are not life threatening. They can, however, cause significant distress if the patient or family believes they are cancer related and may be markers of disease progression.

HICCUPS

Definition/Incidence

Hiccup is a spasmodic, involuntary contraction of the inspiratory (external) intercostal muscles and the diaphragm associated with a strong, sudden inspiration and abrupt glottic closure (1). The medical term for hiccups, singultus, is of Latin origin and means to gasp or sigh. Hiccups were first attributed to phrenic nerve irritation by Shortt in 1833 (2). Hiccups can be classified by their duration as acute (up to 48 hours), persistent or protracted (longer than 48 hours), and intractable (>1 month) (1,2).

Pathophysiology/Etiology

Hiccup is a primitive reflex that contains three parts. The afferent portion consists of branches of the vagus nerve, the phrenic nerve, and the sympathetic chain from T6 to T12. The hiccup center is located in the spinal cord between C3 and C5. The efferent limb is primarily the phrenic nerve with involvement of the efferents to the glottis and accessory muscles of respiration (1).

In addition to the neural pathways, numerous anatomic structures are involved in the mechanism of hiccup (epiglottis, larynx, hyoid muscles, superior constrictor of the pharynx, esophagus, stomach, diaphragm, and exterior intercostal, sternocleidomastoid, anterior serratus, and scalene muscles). Given this extensive list, it is not surprising that hiccup has been associated with many conditions affecting the central nervous system (CNS), thorax, mediastinum, and abdominal viscera, although a cause-and-effect relationship has not always been clear. One report listed over 100 causes, the most common being an overdistended stomach (3). Some cancer-related causes of persistent and intractable hiccups are listed in Table 17.1.

Treatment/Management

Management is usually aimed at inhibiting or interrupting the irritated reflex arc. Nonpharmacologic therapies (4) include the Valsalva maneuver (expiring forcefully against a closed glottis), ocular compression, carotid sinus massage, ice water gargles, breath holding, rebreathing into a paper bag, gagging, ingesting granulated sugar, biting a lemon wedge, sipping vinegar, or inducing emesis. Physical changes that may help stop hiccups include pulling the knees to the chest, leaning forward to compress the chest, or tapping over the fifth cervical vertebra. Although these measures have not been subjected to controlled clinical trials, most are worth a try.

Acupuncture may be a clinically useful, safe, and low-cost therapy for persistent hiccups in patients with cancer. In a case series, 16 adult male patients aged 27 to 71 with persistent cancer-related hiccups received one to three acupuncture sessions over a 1- to 7-day period. Thirteen patients experienced complete remission of persistent hiccups ($p < 0.0001$), and three patients experienced decreased hiccups severity. Significant improvement was observed in discomfort ($p < 0.0001$), distress ($p < 0.0001$), and fatigue ($p = 0.0078$) (5).

TABLE 17.1 CAUSES OF HICCUPS IN THE PATIENT WITH CANCER

Uremia

Alcohol

Hyponatremia, hypokalemia, and hypocalcemia

Fever

Diaphragmatic irritation (diaphragmatic tumors and pericarditis)

Pleuritis

Esophageal obstruction

Pericarditis

Hepatomegaly

Subphrenic abscess

Esophageal cancer

Mediastinal tumors

Herpes zoster

Lung cancer

Gastric distension

Gastric cancer

Pancreatic cancer

Intra-abdominal abscess

Bowel obstruction

Gastrointestinal hemorrhage

Short-acting barbiturates

Dexamethasone

Diazepam and chlordiazepoxide

Infections (meningitis)

Grief reaction

Psychosis

A comprehensive list of the causes of hiccups can be found in Launois S, Bizec JL, Whitelaw WA, et al. Hiccup in adults: an overview. *Eur Respir J.* 1993;6:563-575.

The only medication approved by the US Food and Drug Administration for hiccups is the antipsychotic phenothiazine chlorpromazine (25 to 50 mg through i.v., orally, or rectally three to four times a day) (6). Chlorpromazine is less attractive in patients with cancer due to side effects of hypotension and sedation. Gabapentin, an anticonvulsant, may modulate diaphragmatic excitability by blocking neural calcium channels and increasing the release of γ-aminobutyric acid (GABA). Case series have shown gabapentin (300 mg p.o. three times daily with dose titration) to be effective in intractable hiccups (7). In a retrospective study of patients with advanced cancer; 37 (3.9%) of 944 in-hospital patients and 6 (4.5%) of 134 patients observed at home presented with severe chronic hiccups. Gabapentin (300 mg three times a day

with dose titration) was effective in these cases. Responses were observed in 32 patients (74.4%) with gabapentin at a dosage of 900 mg/d and in 9 patients (20.93%) at a dosage of 1,200 mg/d (8). Gabapentin is not hepatically metabolized and has a relatively safe side-effect profile making it a potentially useful agent in the advanced cancer setting, especially among patients requiring adjuvant analgesia due to neuropathic cancer pain (8). Midazolam has been successfully utilized in patients with terminal hiccups (9). Midazolam infusion may be especially useful if intractable hiccups occur in the setting of refractory terminal delirium or agitation. Other medical therapies to treat hiccups are listed in Table 17.2 (10–18).

Various invasive methods have been tried. As gastric distension is the most common cause of hiccups in patients with cancer, initial treatment should be aimed at relieving the distension and increasing gastric emptying. The insertion of a nasogastric tube may also serve the purpose by stimulating the pharynx or causing gagging. High-pressure oxygen inhalation has been tried. Percutaneous stimulation of the phrenic nerve has also been reported. Phrenic nerve injection may be a reasonable option for drug refractory hiccups if an experienced practitioner is available. In a case series, 1% lidocaine solution was administered via ultrasonographic guidance to the area of the phrenic nerve to five cancer patients with intractable hiccups. Hiccups ceased in all five patients within 5 minutes. Hiccups did not recur in three patients, and there were no adverse effects (19). A surgical approach consists of an attack on the phrenic nerve (by a crush technique), usually first attempted on the left. Regardless of the treatment, in most cases, hiccups stop because of, or in spite of, therapeutic measures (20,21).

It is important to remember that hiccups in cancer may be extremely distressing and affect the quality of life by interfering with food intake, causing insomnia, or exacerbating pain and other symptoms. For this reason, it may be advisable to pursue diagnosis and treatment more aggressively than in the general population (22).

DYSPEPSIA

Definition/Incidence

Dyspepsia consists of episodic or persistent symptoms that include abdominal pain or discomfort, postprandial fullness, abdominal bloating, belching, early satiety, anorexia, nausea, vomiting, heartburn, and regurgitation. There is considerable overlap between this constellation of symptoms and those of gastroesophageal reflux disease (GERD), biliary tract disease, irritable bowel syndrome, and

TABLE 17.2 COMMONLY USED DRUGS IN THE TREATMENT OF HICCUPS

Drug	Dose	Side Effects
Chlorpromazine	25–50 mg i.v. three to four times daily, infused slowly 25–50 mg p.o. three times daily	Sedation, hypotension, and extrapyramidal symptoms
Metoclopramide	10 mg p.o. or i.v. three to four times daily	Extrapyramidal symptoms[a]
Gabapentin	300 mg p.o. three times daily	Drowsiness, headache, fatigue, blurred vision, tremor, anxiety, skin rash, itching, fever, flu-like symptoms, and seizures
Haloperidol	1–5 mg p.o. three times daily or s.c. q12h	Sedation and extrapyramidal symptoms
Baclofen	10–20 mg p.o. three times daily	Sedation, confusion, and less commonly, nausea and fatigue
Nifedipine	10 mg p.o. three times daily	Hypotension; use with caution in patients with coronary artery disease
Amitriptyline	10 mg p.o. three times daily	Cardiac arrhythmias, blurred vision, urinary retention, dry mouth, constipation, and dizziness
Carbamazepine	200 mg three times daily	Dizziness, drowsiness, nausea or vomiting, and low red and white blood cell counts
Diphenylhydantoin	200 mg i.v. once and then 100 mg p.o. four times daily	Enlarged gums, unsteadiness, confusion, lymphadenopathy, fever, muscle pain, skin rash or itching, slurred speech, sore throat, and nervousness or irritability
Valproic acid	15 mg/kg p.o. daily in one to three divided doses	Dizziness, drowsiness, nervousness, upset stomach, vomiting, diarrhea, tremor, sore throat, and drug-induced hepatitis
Ketamine (Ketalar)	0.4 mg/kg (one-fifth of the usual anesthetic dose) i.v.; supplemental dose of one-third to half initial dose may be given for maintenance	Resuscitative equipment should be immediately available during administration of medication
Lidocaine	1 mg/kg i.v. loading dose followed by an infusion of 2 mg/min i.v.	May increase risk of adverse central nervous system and cardiac effects in elderly; high plasma concentrations can cause seizures, heart block, and atrioventricular conduction abnormalities
Ephedrine	25 mg i.m. q6h	Headache, restlessness, anxiety, tremor, weakness, dizziness, confusion, delirium, hallucinations, palpitations, sweating, nausea or vomiting, and urinary retention
		Serious side effects include severe hypertension that may lead to cerebral hemorrhage or cardiac ischemia
Methylphenidate (Ritalin)	5 mg p.o. daily or divided b.i.d.; not to exceed 60 mg/d	Insomnia, anorexia, irritability, nervousness, upset stomach, headaches, dry mouth, blurry vision, nausea, hypersensitivity, palpitations, and cardiac arrhythmias
Other therapies	Behavioral conditioning (including other members of the family unit) Hypnosis Acupuncture Phrenic nerve or diaphragmatic pacing	

[a]More common in younger women.
Adapted from Liu FC, Chen CA, Yang SS, et al. Acupuncture therapy rapidly terminates intractable hiccups complicating acute myocardial infarction. *South Med J.* 2005;98(3):385-387; Schiff E, River Y, Oliven A, et al. Acupuncture therapy for persistent hiccups. *Am J Med Sci.* 2002;323(3):166-168.

chronic pancreatitis. This condition is reported in approximately 25% of the population each year, but most do not seek medical care (23,24).

Pathophysiology/Etiology

Results of upper GI endoscopy in 3,667 general medical patients with dyspepsia were as follows: normal (34%), gastroesophageal reflux (24%), inflammation (20%), ulcer (20%), and cancer (2%) (23). Dyspepsia is divided into two categories: organic dyspepsia and functional dyspepsia. Patients in the first group have anatomical abnormalities (e.g., peptic ulcer disease, GERD, or gastric or esophageal cancer). Patients in the second category have symptoms for which no focal lesion can be found (Table 17.3). Delayed gastric emptying reported in approximately 30% of patients with functional dyspepsia is associated with postprandial fullness, early satiety, nausea, and vomiting. Hypersensitivity to gastric distension is observed in 37% of patients with functional dyspepsia and is associated with postprandial pain, belching, and weight loss. Psychosocial factors have also been identified as pathophysiologic mechanisms (25,26).

Patients with advance malignancies who present with a cluster of GI symptoms also present with some form of malignancy-related dysmotility syndrome, which is commonly known as malignant gastroparesis with or without pseudo-obstruction (functional obstruction). By definition, gastroparesis is a disorder of the stomach caused by delayed gastric emptying in the absence of mechanical obstruction. Patients can present with esophageal dysmotility, gastroparesis, intestinal pseudo-obstruction, and constipation. Patients may present with a dominant symptom like nausea, early satiety, or dyspepsia. Some patients may present with pan-gut involvement.

Dysmotility-like dyspepsia, or gastroparesis, is particularly common in those with upper GI tumors and seen in 60% of patients with advanced pancreatic cancer (27). The pathogenesis of malignant gastroparesis is unclear, but it is believed to be due to either the cancer itself by infiltrating the celiac plexus or vagus nerve, or a complication of its treatment such as the toxic effects of chemotherapy and radiation therapy (28). Gastroparesis has also been linked to disruption of the interstitial cells of Cajal (ICC). Hu autoantibodies have been identified to affect the ICC also called the intrinsic pacemaker of the GI tract or myenteric plexus. By generating electrical slow waves, the ICC are intercalated between the intramural neurons and the effector smooth muscular cells to form a gastroenteric pacemaker system. Loss of ICC causes dysmotility-like symptoms in vivo. A loss of these cells has been detected in patients with paraneoplastic gastroparesis (29).

Other causes of cancer-induced dyspepsia include gastric cancer or lymphoma, gastritis secondary to radiotherapy/chemotherapy, gastric compression secondary to intra-abdominal tumor, hepatomegaly, splenomegaly, ascites, or gastric outlet obstruction due to tumor. Medications that have been associated with dyspepsia include acarbose, alcohol, alendronate, codeine, iron, metformin, nonsteroidal anti-inflammatory drugs, erythromycin, potassium, corticosteroids, and theophylline. Dosage reduction or discontinuation of the offending agent may relieve dyspepsia.

Gastroparesis with or without intestinal pseudo-obstruction is one of the most underdiagnosed problems in cancer patients and is often overlooked as a cause of dyspepsia. The exact prevalence of gastroparesis is unknown. A patient may present with symptoms consistent with small bowel obstruction that spontaneously resolves with bowel rest, nasogastric drainage of gastric and intestinal contents, hydration, and steroids. In these cases a CT scan of abdomen may or may not show gastric distention and small bowel dilatation without a clear cutoff point. Patients with gastroparesis can have a normal scan of the abdomen and pelvis if they just vomited. An EGD that demonstrates substantial fluid and food after an overnight fast suggests gastroparesis. Clinical conditions such as

TABLE 17.3 CLASSIFICATION OF NONULCER DYSPEPSIA BY SYMPTOM TYPE AND THEIR TREATMENTS

Classification	Symptoms	Treatment
Reflux-like	Heartburn and regurgitation without esophagitis	Antacid, H_2-blocker, and proton pump inhibitor
Ulcer-like	Epigastric pain relieved by food and antacids, relapse, and remission, without ulcer	As above
Dysmotility-like	Abdominal bloating, distension, early satiety, nausea, and vomiting	Prokinetic agent and antiflatulence agent
Nonspecific	Symptoms do not fall into one of the three categories in the preceding text	Start simple: antacid and antiflatulence agent (simethicone)

diabetes mellitus, hypothyroidism, neuromuscular and autoimmune disorders, and medications like anticholinergics and opioids can aggravate functional gastroparesis.

Gastroparesis, if left untreated, can cause significant morbidity and mortality. Patients can experience bloating, abdominal distention, flatulence, and nausea and can have premature satiety with resultant epigastric heaviness or fullness even after the consumption of small meals (30). Gastroparesis can contribute to electrolyte or acid–base disturbances, volume depletion, and frequent hospitalizations.

The diagnosis of paraneoplastic dyspepsia requires a high index of clinical suspicion. A panel of serologic tests for paraneoplastic autoantibodies, scintigraphic gastric emptying, and esophageal manometry are useful as first-line screening tests. Nuclear scintigraphy is considered the gold standard for diagnosing and quantifying delayed gastric emptying. Seropositivity for type 1 antineuronal nuclear antibody, Purkinje cell cytoplasmic antibody, or N-type calcium channel–binding antibodies has been detected in patients with paraneoplastic gastroparesis, but its diagnostic value is under investigation (31).

Management/Treatment

The management of organic dyspepsia should be directed at the cause. Treatment may be based on previous history (e.g., obstructing lesion responding to primary tumor treatment) or recent endoscopy findings. In functional dyspepsia, treatment should be based on symptoms (Table 17.3). Nutrition support in gastroparesis begins with encouraging smaller volume, low-fat, low-fiber meals and, if necessary, liquid caloric supplements. Metoclopramide is now the prokinetic drug of choice (32). Controlled-release metoclopramide (20 to 80 mg q12h) is effective in ameliorating symptoms of the cancer-induced dyspepsia such as nausea, vomiting, loss of appetite, and bloating (33).

Subcutaneous administration of metoclopramide is useful as it allows for continued guaranteed absorption. Low-dosage erythromycin also has a prokinetic role, either alone or in combination with metoclopramide.

Antiemetics should be used for nausea, and there should be a low threshold for placing a jejunal feeding tube (either by laparoscopy or by mini-laparotomy). Parenteral nutrition can be employed but should be used only briefly during hospitalization and not encouraged or sustained in an outpatient.

Gastric electrical stimulation (GES) has been proven to be beneficial for drug-refractory gastroparesis (34), and can be useful for patients who do not respond to standard medical therapy. The

dramatic decrease in nausea and vomiting, as well as a sustained evidence of improved quality of life, gastric emptying, nutritional status, and decreased hospitalizations by this device, is documented by a long-term follow-up of more than a year (34).

Botulinum injection in the pylorus has not been shown to be effective in 2 randomized trials. Finally, 2% to 5% of patients will have refractory gastroparesis or intestinal pseudo-obstruction. In these cases, venting gastrostomy/jejunostomy is indicated.

HEARTBURN

Definition/Incidence

Heartburn (pyrosis) is the most common GI complaint in the western population; 33% to 44% of the population complain of heartburn at least monthly, and 7% to 13% may have it daily (35). Heartburn is a retrosternal burning sensation that usually radiates proximally from the xiphoid process to the neck. It is caused by the reflux of the gastric content into the esophagus. GERD occurs when the amount of gastric content that refluxes into the esophagus exceeds the normal limit, causing symptoms with or without esophagitis. Although there is no clear evidence that GERD is more common in those with cancer, certain conditions in this population may increase their risk, such as intra-abdominal lesions, which increase pressure on the stomach. In addition to the typical symptoms (heartburn, regurgitation, and dysphagia), abnormal reflux can cause atypical symptoms such as coughing, chest pain, and wheezing and also damage to the lungs (pneumonia, asthma, and idiopathic pulmonary fibrosis), vocal cords (laryngitis and cancer), ear (otitis media), and teeth (enamel decay). Approximately 50% of the patients with reflux develop esophagitis, which is classified on the basis of severity.

Pathophysiology/Etiology

The most important pathophysiologic factor in GERD is frequent transient relaxation of the lower esophageal sphincter (LES). Other factors include anatomic disruption of the LES as in hiatal hernia, transient increase in intra-abdominal pressure, abnormal esophageal peristalsis with impaired clearance of acid, and gastroparesis.

A number of foods, drugs, and neurohumoral factors reduce basal LES pressure, making patients prone to gastroesophageal reflux and heartburn (Table 17.4). Avoiding these foods and medications often constitutes the initial treatment of GERD. Some common agents that increase LES pressure include a protein meal, bethanechol, metoclopramide, and α-adrenergic agonists.

TABLE 17.4 AGGRAVATING FACTORS FOR HEARTBURN

Low LES Pressure	Direct Mucosal Irritant	Increased Intra-abdominal Pressure	Others
Certain foods	Certain foods	Bending over	Supine position
Fats	Citrus products	Lifting	Lying on right side
Sugars	Tomato-based products	Straining at stool	Red wine
Chocolate	Spicy foods	Exercise	Emotions
Onions	Coffee		
Coffee	Medications		
Alcohol	Aspirin		
Cigarettes	Nonsteroidal anti-inflammatory drug		
Medications	Tetracycline		
Progesterone	Quinidine sulfate		
Theophylline	Potassium chloride tablets		
Anticholinergic agents	Iron salts		
Adrenergic agonists			
Adrenergic antagonists			
Diazepam			
Estrogens			
Mint, anise, and dill			
Benzodiazepines			
Meperidine hydrochloride			
Nitrates			
Calcium channel blockers			

LES, lower esophageal sphincter.

Heartburn is most frequently noted within 1 hour of eating, particularly after the largest meal of the day. Patients may note a variety of presentations: Wine drinkers, for example, may have heartburn after hearty consumption of red, but not white, wine. Lying down, especially after a late meal, causes heartburn within 1 to 2 hours (in contrast to peptic ulcer disease heartburn tends not to awaken patients in the early morning). Heartburn may be accompanied by regurgitation, a bitter acidic fluid in the mouth that is common at night or when the patient bends over. The regurgitated material comes from the stomach and is yellow or green in color, suggesting the presence of bile.

Many disorders cause epigastric or substernal pain similar to heartburn, making it important to determine the cause in each patient. Causes include collagen vascular disorders, scleroderma, mixed connective tissue disorders, raised intra-abdominal pressure, gastroparesis, nasogastric tube, prolonged recumbent position, persistent vomiting, pregnancy, hypothyroidism, Zollinger-Ellison syndrome, medications, and some surgical procedures (e.g., myotomy and esophagogastrectomy).

Finally, the absence of nausea, retching, and abdominal contractions suggests regurgitation rather than vomiting. This is a clinically important distinction: The regurgitation of bland material is atypical for acid reflux disease and suggests the presence of an esophageal motility disorder (i.e., achalasia) or delayed gastric emptying.

Treatment/Management

The goal of treatment is to control symptoms, to heal esophagitis, and to prevent recurrent esophagitis or complications. Treatment should be undertaken in a stepwise manner and be based on lifestyle modification and control of gastric acid secretion. Lifestyle modification includes losing weight and avoiding precipitating factors such as chocolate, spicy food, alcohol, citrus juice, and tomato-based products. The patient is asked to eat several small meals during the day and avoid large ones and elevate the head of the bed. Antacids are effective in mild symptoms if given after each meal and at bedtime. More aggressive therapy includes H_2-receptor blockers, sucralfate, or omeprazole. Metoclopramide works very well in GERD among patients with cancer who commonly have gastroparesis. It increases the LES pressure and enhances gastric emptying. Long-term therapy is usually necessary. Approximately 80% of patients have a recurrent but nonprogressive GERD that is controlled with medications. In 20% of patients, the disease is progressive and severe complications may occur, such as strictures or Barrett's esophagus. Laparoscopic fundoplication or other palliative procedures should be considered and discussed with patients having cancer. Over the last decade, a new noninvasive endoscopic technique, called *Enteryx*, has been developed to treat GERD (36). This procedure involves the injection of a compound called *ethylene polyvinyl alcohol* into the LES, just within the stomach. The injection is administered with guidance from real-time x-ray. The compound is in liquid form outside the body, but when it comes in contact with the tissues inside the body, it turns into an expanding, spongy material. The procedure may cause a sore throat or chest pain. Although this treatment resulted in a highly significant improvement at 6 and 12 months, longer follow-up is needed to better assess the duration of efficacy of these positive effects.

EARLY SATIETY

Definition/Incidence

Early satiety is the desire to eat combined with an inability to consume more than an unusually small amount of food. This is in contrast to anorexia, in which there is a reduced desire to eat. Early satiety should be distinguished not only from anorexia but also from nausea, bloating, postprandial filling, pyrosis, food aversion, and dyspepsia. However, all of these symptoms may be due to the same physiologic abnormality—delayed gastric emptying. Patients generally do not report this symptom unless questioned. The incidence of cancer-related early satiety varies from 13% to 62% depending on the study and population being evaluated (37–39).

Pathophysiology/Etiology

Satiety and its consequent effect on food intake are caused by overlapping stimuli from the CNS and the GI tract. Ingested nutrients and peptide hormones (insulin, glucagon, and norepinephrine-stimulating α_2-adrenergic receptors in the medial hypothalamus), along with serotonin and dopaminergic-α-adrenergic receptors in the lateral hypothalamus, affect satiety. Cholecystokinin may also have primary effects on satiety as it is known that exogenous administration of peptides like cholecystokinin and bombesin affect satiety both centrally and peripherally and inhibit feeding activity in animals.

Early satiety can be caused by tumor encroachment on the GI tract, inappropriate satiety signals from oropharyngeal receptors, hyperglycemia, or gastric muscle atrophy. Reduced upper GI motility due to autonomic nervous system dysfunction, possibly a paraneoplastic syndrome, has also been implicated (40). Tumor type and previous chemotherapy treatment have not been shown to affect the incidence of early satiety in cancer. However, patients with taste aversions appear to have a higher incidence of early satiety than do those without (41).

Treatment/Management

It is important to distinguish early satiety from other GI symptoms, and if bloating, pyrosis, anorexia, or nausea not due to gastric status is present, it should be treated appropriately. If there is pressure on the stomach ("squashed stomach"), it should be reduced if possible, although in many cases it is not. Problems such as ascites may be amenable to paracentesis, which can provide temporary relief. Those with gastroduodenal ulcers should be treated with appropriate therapy (H_2-blocker, proton pump inhibitor, and antibiotics). In patients with cicatrization at the pyloric outlet, balloon dilatation may afford relief for variable periods.

Patients with early satiety should be instructed to eat frequent, small meals, with the bulk of their daily intake consumed early, as gastric stasis increases as the day progresses. They should also be instructed to eat sitting up and avoid liquids at mealtimes, as liquids promote gastric distension and a sense of fullness. Prokinetic agents (e.g., metoclopramide and domperidone) may be helpful. The rationale for prokinetic agent use in early satiety is based on the assumption that the symptom(s) is due to delayed gastric emptying. Metoclopramide is the drug of choice in the United States (32). It is a dopamine antagonist that increases LES pressure and enhances gastric antral contractility. It is generally well-tolerated orally, but extrapyramidal reactions, which appear to be more common in young women, do occur; insomnia (often noted to be "jumpy legs" on further questioning) and sedation have also been reported. Metoclopramide, 10 mg three times daily orally, is an effective treatment for many and enhances food intake. The central effects of metoclopramide may have a direct effect on anorexia to improve appetite in addition to the peripheral effects on gastric contractility. The other prokinetic agents, cisapride

TABLE 17.5 TREATMENT OF DYSPEPSIA, HEARTBURN, AND EARLY SATIETY

Dyspepsia	1. Antacids (aluminum hydroxide, magnesium hydroxide, and simethicone): 10–20 mL or 2–4 tablets p.o. four to six times daily between meals and at bedtime 2. Treat *Helicobacter pylori* 3. Treat peptic ulcer disease with proton pump inhibitors 4. Prokinetic drug: Metoclopramide: 10 mg p.o. or i.v. three to four times daily Controlled-release metoclopramide: 20–80 mg p.o. q12h Domperidone: 10–20 mg p.o. three to four times daily, 15–30 min before meals (not available in the United States) Cisapride: 5–20 mg p.o. four times daily at least 15 min before meals and at bedtime (not available in the United States) Erythromycin: 30–50 mg/kg p.o. daily in two to four divided doses; maximum 2 g daily
Early satiety	1. Eat frequent, small meals, with the bulk of their daily intake consumed early 2. Eat sitting up and avoid liquids at mealtimes 3. Prokinetic drug (e.g., metoclopramide, domperidone, and erythromycin) (see preceding text for doses)
Heartburn	1. Lifestyle modification: Weight loss Avoid chocolate, spicy food, alcohol, citrus juice, and tomato-based products Eat several small meals during the day Elevate the head of the bed 2. Antacids (aluminum hydroxide, magnesium hydroxide, and simethicone): 10–20 mL or 2–4 tablets p.o. four to six times daily between meals and at bedtime 3. H_2-receptor antagonist: Cimetidine 300 mg p.o. four times daily or 800 mg p.o. at bedtime or 400 mg p.o. twice daily for up to 8 wk i.m., i.v.: 300 mg every 6 h Ranitidine 150 mg twice daily or 300 mg once daily at bedtime 4. Proton pump inhibitors: omeprazole 20 mg p.o. daily

and domperidone, are not available in the United States. Cisapride has been removed from the market due to drug interactions causing cardiac abnormalities. Domperidone, also a dopamine antagonist, does not cross the blood–brain barrier, and hence its side-effect profile is superior to that of metoclopramide; unfortunately, it has not yet been approved in the United States. Erythromycin is another prokinetic agent, but it is less useful in cancer-related gastroparesis as it causes gastric dumping, (which is useful in acute gastric stasis e.g., diabetic gastroparesis). Treatments for early satiety, dyspepsia, and heartburn are listed in Table 17.5.

GI HEMORRHAGE

Definition/Incidence

GI bleeding may originate at any site from the mouth to the anus. It can be occult or overt, with varying degrees of severity. A careful history and physical examination often suggest the site as well as the cause of the bleeding. Although controversial, most agree that 20% loss of circulating volume produces hemodynamic changes and >30% produces shock with organ damage. In the debilitated patient with cancer, the ability to tolerate a GI hemorrhage is compromised and these may occur with far less blood loss.

The overall incidence of acute upper GI hemorrhage is 100 hospitalizations per 100,000 adults per year (42). In a study of over 15 million people, there was an overall mortality rate of 14% (43). However, in patients younger than 60 without malignancy or organ failure, the mortality was only 0.6%. In 800 admissions to a palliative home care program, the incidence of GI bleeding was 2.3%; those with liver cancer or hepatic metastases were at higher risk (44).

Pathophysiology/Etiology

GI bleeding can be multifactorial, and one should not assume that a tumor is the source of bleeding. In a general population of 2,225 patients, duodenal ulcer (24%), gastric erosions (23%), and gastric ulcer (21%) accounted for most of the upper GI bleeding (45). In cancer, gastritis (36%), peptic or stress ulceration (26%), and tumor necrosis (23%) are the most common causes. *Candida* esophagitis, particularly during chemotherapy administration, Mallory-Weiss mucosal tears with significant bleeding in the setting of thrombocytopenia (46), and inflammatory conditions (e.g., radiation therapy) are less common (47). In the general population, 43% of lower GI bleeding is due to diverticulosis (48). Massive lower GI bleeding can be a late complication of the high-dose radiation therapy used for treatment of GI, gynecologic, or genitourinary cancer.

Other causes of bleeding in patients with cancer include thrombocytopenia and coagulopathies secondary to the disease or the treatment. Aggressive chemotherapy may cause stress-related ulceration of the mucosa or suppress bone marrow production. The incidence of GI perforation after chemotherapy is 10%, most of whom are patients with lymphoma. GI lymphomas are more common sources of tumor bleeding than other intra-abdominal malignancies. Bleeding is the presenting symptom in 15% to 28% of patients, but only 3% to 4% have perforation (49). Hemorrhage has been reported in 27% of those receiving chemotherapy for unresected lymphoma. Resection before treatment may reduce the bleeding and perforation by 50%. Cytosine arabinoside can cause bowel necrosis, and hepatic arterial infusion of fluorodeoxyuridine may cause upper GI toxicity, resulting in gastritis and peptic ulcers. The initiation of chemotherapy has been reported to trigger or accelerate disseminated intravascular coagulation in lymphoma, presumably due to release of thromboplastin-like or other clot-promoting agents (50).

Medications may be responsible for GI bleeding. Drugs usually implicated are corticosteroids, nonsteroidal anti-inflammatory drugs, and aspirin (51). Cephalosporins, streptomycin, isoniazid, penicillin, β-lactam, and amphotericin B may cause bleeding due to their ability to inhibit clotting factor or impair platelet function.

Upper GI Bleeding—Diagnostic Evaluation

Hematemesis is the vomiting of blood, either bright red or dark, with a "coffee grounds" appearance. Melena is foul-smelling stool with a coal black, sticky, tar-like appearance. Hematemesis and melena indicate that the bleeding may be from the nasopharynx, esophagus, stomach, duodenum, or, rarely, the proximal jejunum. Endoscopy is used to evaluate upper GI bleeding. Hemodynamically unstable patients should undergo emergent endoscopy, as they may benefit from both diagnosis and therapy (e.g., ligation for variceal bleeding).

Lower GI Bleeding—Diagnostic Evaluation

Hematochezia is the passage of red blood from the anus. Blood from the distal colon, rectum, or anus is fresh and usually bright red, whereas blood from the proximal colon is likely to be darker. Bleeding from the cecum or ascending colon may appear black, but it is not as shiny or tar-like as in melena. Early colonoscopy for the detection of lower lesions may be the first diagnostic step (52). However, when the bleeding is significant it is often difficult to identify the source. A technetium 99–labeled red cell scan may identify the general location of bleeding; however, results are variable. If the source remains unknown, the next step is typically angiography. It can detect the bleeding site as well as allow treatment with intra-arterial infusion of vasopressin or embolization (53).

Treatment/Management

General

It is important to understand the status of the primary disease, the expected survival, the potential for cure, and goals of care in cancer patients with GI hemorrhage. If the long-term survival rate is poor or of goals of care are inconsistent with possible therapies, patients should not be subjected to unnecessary tests and procedures.

If workup and treatment are appropriate, the first objective is to determine the source of the hemorrhage, stop the bleeding, and prevent recurrence. A quick assessment of the hemodynamic status including vital signs and postural blood pressure should be made. A sudden increase in pulse or postural hypotension may be the first indication of bleeding. The hematocrit should follow; however, it may take hours to equilibrate. Packed red blood cells should be transfused until the hematocrit is >25%. A coagulopathy should initially be corrected with four units of fresh frozen plasma; thrombocytopenia <50,000/mm^3 requires platelet transfusions.

Upper GI Bleeding Treatment

To prevent stress ulceration and recurrent bleeding several medications are now available, although there is no evidence of their benefit in the immediate posttreatment period (Table 17.6) (54). Endotracheal intubation to prevent aspiration may be necessary in massive upper GI bleeding. Supportive measures with antacids, H$_2$-receptor blockers, and blood products control the bleeding in 60% of patients with gastritis or ulceration. Endoscopic control using bipolar system of electrocoagulation (BICAP), yttrium–aluminum–garnet laser, and other modalities may provide temporary control of bleeding ulceration or tumors. If medical management fails, surgery should be considered. The decision to operate should also be based on the patient's goals of care, potential quality of life, and disease prognosis, as surgery is associated with high morbidity and mortality (55).

Variceal bleeding may be treated with endoscopic sclerotherapy or variceal ligation. Medical management is less effective, but octreotide acetate, a long-acting synthetic analog of somatostatin (50 to 100 µg i.v. bolus followed by an infusion at 25 to 50 µg/h) may reduce portal hypertension in acute variceal hemorrhage. Balloon tamponade

TABLE 17.6 DRUGS USED TO PREVENT RECURRENT UPPER GASTROINTESTINAL BLEEDING

Drug	Dose
Antacid	Two tablespoons of high-potency liquid, after meals (heartburn)
H₂-blocker	Ranitidine hydrochloride, 150 mg p.o. twice daily
	Famotidine, 40 mg, at bedtime
	Nizatidine, 150 mg, at bedtime (duodenal)/150 mg p.o. b.i.d. (gastric ulcer)
Proton pump inhibitor	Omeprazole, 20 mg p.o. daily
Sucralfate	1 g twice daily
Prokinetic	Metoclopramide, 5–15 mg p.o. four times daily

may temporize bleeding until more definitive therapy is begun. However, it is associated with a high rate of complications and mortality. Splenorenal and portosystemic shunts control variceal bleeding in a very select group of patients (56).

Lower GI Bleeding—Treatment

For lower GI bleeding, colonoscopy, radionuclide imaging, or mesenteric angiography may be required to identify the source. It may be difficult, however, to determine the source of significant bleeding when performing colonoscopy. If the bleeding rate is >1 mL/min, selective mesenteric arteriography is the best procedure to localize the source. When it is not possible to localize the source, subtotal colectomy should be performed. In poor-risk patients, therapy with selective infusion of vasopressin or embolization of the bleeding vessel can be performed, but there is a risk of bowel infarction (57).

The Dying Patient

GI hemorrhage may be a terminal event in advanced cancer, and the family and professional team should be prepared as this can be a very distressing time. Bleeding may occur very rapidly, and the patient could die immediately of asphyxiation (upper GI bleed) or a precipitous drop in blood pressure resulting in cardiac arrest due to massive lower GI bleed. GI hemorrhage prevented a peaceful death in 2% of patients in a study of 200 hospice patients (58). The key to successful symptom management in the final days, particularly in the home, is preparation. It is important to have a plan to control these symptoms. If a nursing staff is available then midazolam should be given at 10 mg i.v. if an existing access is already available or i.m. preferably deltoid muscle. If a nursing staff is not available such as a catastrophic bleeding occurred at home, then the caregiver may administer diazepam 10 mg per rectum, midazolam 10 mg/1 mL buccal, or lorazepam 4 mg/1 mL sublingual (59,60). It is helpful to have dark sheets and towels available to camouflage the bleeding. Although

symptoms can be managed well in most, poor preparation precludes a comfortable death.

BILIARY OBSTRUCTION

Definition/Incidence

Biliary obstruction is the blockage of the flow of bile resulting in increased pressure in the biliary system. Malignant obstruction can occur anywhere in the biliary tree, but it most often affects the extrahepatic biliary tree or liver hilum. Its incidence in malignant disease varies depending on the etiology and the stage of disease. Extrahepatic biliary obstruction is common in carcinoma of the head of the pancreas. Less common tumors are in the ampulla, bile duct, gallbladder, or liver. Cholangiocarcinoma, metastatic tumor, or enlarged lymphatic nodes are other causes of biliary obstruction (61).

Pathophysiology/Etiology

Normally, the hepatocyte secretes bile. Blocking the flow raises pressure in the biliary system rendering the hepatocyte unable to secrete more. The pressure needed to stop secretion is 300 mm Hg of H_2O, but there is evidence of cholestasis with lesser pressure. A neural or hormonal mechanism may be responsible for cholestasis before the necessary biliary pressure is reached.

Treatment/Management

Patients usually present in the advanced stage of the disease, and surgical resection is rarely possible. Patients with symptomatic biliary obstruction should be evaluated for some type of biliary bypass procedure (62). Although survival is often limited, the symptoms, particularly pruritus, are quite distressing and less amenable to other treatments. Open surgical procedures have not been shown to prolong survival and are associated with greater morbidity and mortality than endoscopically placed stents (63). Unless the patient is moribund, a stenting procedure should be considered, as it may offer dramatic relief.

Stent placement with biliary drainage results in decreased serum bilirubin, and symptoms of pruritus usually resolve within 24 to 48 hours. The duration of palliation afforded by stenting depends on the underlying disease and the type of stent used to relieve the obstruction (64).

There are two types of endoscopically placed stents: self-expanding metallic stents (SEMSs) and plastic stents. The major drawback of plastic stents is occlusion with a bacterial biofilm. This results in occlusion and recurrence of jaundice and requires one or more stent changes in 30% to 60% of patients. In randomized trials comparing plastic stents with SEMS in malignant bile duct occlusion, SEMS provided longer patency rates but had no survival advantage. In a three-arm study comparing plastic stent left in place until dysfunction occurred versus plastic stent routinely changed every 3 months versus SEMS, an initial success rate of 97% was obtained. The plastic stent not routinely changed had the poorest complication-free survival rate. The SEMSs were the most cost-effective when life expectancy was >6 months (65,66). Endoscopic ultrasound-guided biliary drainage (EUSBD) has been shown to be effective for palliation of biliary obstruction and a viable alternative to percutaneous transhepatic cholangiography in patients in whom endoscopic retrograde cholangiopancreatography (ERCP) has been unsuccessful. A case series of eight patients presented with biliary obstruction from inoperable pancreatic cancer or cholangiocarcinoma underwent transduodenal EUSBD after a failed ERCP. EUS was used to access the common bile duct from the duodenum after which a guidewire was advanced upward toward the liver hilum. The metal stent was then advanced into the biliary tree. Technical success (correct stent placement) and clinical success (a 50% decrease in serum bilirubin level within 2 weeks after the stent placement) were achieved in all eight patients. No stent malfunction or occlusion was observed. Complications included one case of duodenal perforation, which required surgery, and one case of self-limiting abdominal pain (67).

The method to control symptoms that are associated with biliary obstruction depends on the performance status of the patient, tumor type, and local professional expertise. It is important to remember that patients may appear gravely ill due to infection and obstruction, yet may improve dramatically with antibiotics and a procedure to relieve the obstruction.

HEPATIC FAILURE

Definition/Incidence

Hepatic failure is the severe inability of the liver to function normally, as evidenced by jaundice and abnormal plasma levels of ammonia, bilirubin, alkaline phosphatase, glutamic oxaloacetic transaminase, lactic dehydrogenase, and reversal of the albumin/globulin ratio. It quickly leads to failure of other organs. The hallmark of acute hepatic failure is hepatic encephalopathy and coagulopathy (68).

Pathophysiology/Etiology

Most hepatic failure, regardless of cause, results from massive coagulative necrosis of hepatocytes. Viral hepatitis accounts for approximately 70%, and drug ingestion (primarily acetaminophen) accounts for most of the remaining 30%. Malignant causes are associated with metastatic gastric carcinoma, carcinoid, breast cancer, small cell lung cancer, melanoma, leukemia, and lymphoma. Hepatic failure may be the presenting sign of malignancy in some cases (69). Sinusoidal obstruction with subsequent ischemia has been reported in metastatic liver disease. Occlusion of hepatic venous outflow may occur in the setting of intensive chemotherapy or bone marrow transplantation or recrudescence of hepatitis B virus after treatment.

Clinical Manifestations

Regardless of the cause, hepatic failure begins with nausea and malaise. It proceeds to accumulation of ammonia as a result of diminished urea formation, hepatic encephalopathy, cerebral edema, prolonged prothrombin time, rapidly rising bilirubin, metabolic changes, GI bleeding, sepsis, respiratory failure, renal failure, and cardiovascular collapse (70).

Hepatic Encephalopathy

Hepatic encephalopathy is a complex neuropsychiatric syndrome characterized by cognitive changes, fluctuating neurologic signs, and electroencephalographic changes. In severe cases, irreversible coma and death occur (71). It results from severe hepatocellular dysfunction or intrahepatic and extrahepatic shunting of portal venous blood into the systemic circulation bypassing the liver. Toxic substances are not detoxified by the liver; this leads to metabolic abnormalities in the CNS. Most patients have elevated blood ammonia levels (72). Cognitive changes are due to excessive concentrations of GABA. The role of endogenous benzodiazepine agonists is unclear, but these may contribute to hepatic encephalopathy. A partial response has been observed in some after the administration of a benzodiazepine antagonist (flumazenil) (73). The most common predisposing factor is GI bleeding, which leads to an increase in ammonia production. Hypokalemic alkalosis, hypoxia, CNS-depressing drugs (e.g., barbiturates and benzodiazepines), and acute infection may also trigger hepatic encephalopathy (74).

Reversal of the sleep/wake cycle is among the earliest signs of encephalopathy. Mood disturbances, confusion, alterations in personality, deterioration in self-care and handwriting, and daytime somnolence are also seen. The diagnosis of hepatic encephalopathy is usually one of exclusion (75). There are no diagnostic liver function test abnormalities, although an elevated serum ammonia level is highly suggestive of the diagnosis (75). It is sometimes difficult to distinguish hepatic encephalopathy from other forms of delirium.

Portal Hypertension

Tumor burden may compress the hepatic blood vessels; this can result in portal hypertension, which causes collateral vessels in the esophagus and the stomach to become enlarged and tortuous (varices). Bleeding of the varices is likely, because the liver is unable to synthesize vitamin K and clotting factors. Procedures to reduce the pressure include a portal–systemic shunt, and β-adrenergic blockade (e.g., propranolol hydrochloride), if not contraindicated (76).

Spontaneous Bacterial Peritonitis

Spontaneous bacterial peritonitis occurs with ascites without an obvious primary source of infection. The ascitic fluid has low concentrations of opsonic proteins, which normally provide protection against bacteria. Paracentesis reveals cloudy fluid with a white cell count of >500 cells/μL (>250 polymorphonuclear leukocytes). Common isolates are *Escherichia coli*, pneumococci, and, to a lesser extent, anaerobes. Empirical therapy with intravenous cefotaxime sodium (2 g every 8 hours for at least 5 days) and an aminoglycoside should be initiated if clinically appropriate (75).

Hepatorenal Syndrome

Hepatorenal syndrome is a disorder characterized by worsening azotemia, oliguria, hyponatremia, low urinary sodium, and hypotension, with structurally intact kidneys. It is diagnosed only in the absence of identifiable causes of renal dysfunction. Treatment is usually ineffective. Some patients with hypotension and decreased plasma volume may respond to volume expansion, but care must be taken to rehydrate slowly to avoid variceal bleeding (77).

Treatment/Management

Whenever possible, the inciting agent should be treated or eliminated. There is little role for liver transplant in the patient with cancer. For most, treatment of the underlying disease provides the best method to reverse the process of hepatic failure. It may be useful to review adverse prognostic

TABLE 17.7 ADVERSE PROGNOSTIC INDICATORS IN HEPATIC FAILURE

Indicator	Value
Age	<10 y, >40 y
Cause	Idiosyncratic drug reaction, halothane, non-A, non-B hepatitis
Jaundice	>7 d before onset of encephalopathy
Bilirubin	>300 μmol/L (18 mg/dL)
Prothrombin time	>100 s
Factor V level	<20%
Clinical status	Respiratory failure
	Rapid reduction in liver size
	Coma

indicators in hepatic encephalopathy (Table 17.7) before embarking on intensive, supportive therapy in those who survive.

Stenting biliary obstructions may provide relief from jaundice and pruritus. Paracentesis helps control symptomatic ascites. Neuropsychiatric symptoms are distressing and should be controlled with appropriate medications. Flumazenil, a short-acting benzodiazepine antagonist, may have a role in the management of hepatic encephalopathy (71). Reducing oral protein intake in advanced cancer is rarely necessary. Administering lactulose, a nonabsorbable laxative sugar, may help. The initial dose is 30 to 50 mL every hour until diarrhea occurs; thereafter the dose is adjusted (15 to 30 mL three times daily) so that the patient has two to four soft stools daily (75).

In the terminal state, it may be appropriate to allow a deteriorating level of consciousness to progress and to forgo treatment. The neuropsychiatric symptoms are controlled with neuroleptics (if hallucinating, chlorpromazine 50 to 200 mg every 2 to 3 hours) or with diazepam (if agitated). The goal is to relieve distress without concern for the adverse effect of major tranquilizers on the mental status.

TENESMUS

Definition/Incidence

Tenesmus is a painful spasm of the anal sphincter with a sensation of the urgent need to defecate, with involuntary straining, but with little bowel movement if any. Patients complain of an abnormally frequent desire to defecate and a sensation that evacuation is incomplete. Rectal pain is not commonly caused by organic lesions, which more frequently result in tenesmus. It is a distressing, difficult to control problem. In the patient with cancer, it occurs most commonly in cancer of the rectum or after pelvic radiation.

Pathophysiology/Etiology

Tenesmus is thought to be a motility disorder of the rectum, with decreased compliance and high-amplitude pressure waves in the rectal wall. This results in an increased sensitivity to distension of the rectum. Rectal causes of tenesmus include impacted feces, carcinoma, rectal prolapse, rectal polyps, adenoma, hemorrhoids, fissure, proctitis, foreign body, and abscess. Infectious causes include *Shigella*, *Campylobacter*, and *Clostridium difficile*.

In the patient with rectal cancer, tenesmus is usually an ominous sign indicating circumferential growth or ulceration involving the sphincter muscle. Tenesmus typically occurs in the morning on waking and subsides as the day progresses. Accompanying perineal or buttock pain suggests involvement of the sacral nerve plexus. Patients presenting with this symptom complex are unlikely to be candidates for sphincter-saving procedures. Tenesmus can also be caused by damage from radiation therapy (acute and late effects) for rectal cancer or other pelvic structures (e.g., cervix, prostate, bladder, and testes).

Treatment/Management

Treatment is based on the cause and is variably effective. Infectious causes should be treated with appropriate antibiotics. Radiation-induced tenesmus is a difficult problem. Symptoms usually resolve spontaneously within 2 to 6 months (78). Tenesmus and rectal bleeding have been treated with oral sulfasalazine combined with steroid enemas or sucralfate enemas (2 g in 20 mL of tap water) (79).

Curative intent pelvic exenteration effectively controlled pain and tenesmus in 89% and palliative intent in 67% of patients with rectal cancer (80). However, this is a procedure associated with significant morbidity and should not be performed for the sole purpose of controlling pain. Radiotherapy may also provide symptomatic relief, but the primary purpose is to control the disease; and it may be most useful in those who have not received chemotherapy (81). Metal expandable stents have been used successfully and are associated with little morbidity, but these may migrate (82). Lumbar sympathectomy produced complete relief of tenesmus in 10 of 12 patients with cancers in the pelvic region. Duration of relief was 3 days to 7 months (mean, 53 days). In this small series, the only complication was transient hypotension responding to intravenous fluids (83); however, mild, reversible bruising and stiffness at the needle insertion site often occur. Up to 20% of patients have limb pain, which develops after a 10- to 14-day latent period and spontaneously resolves after a few weeks. Major neurologic deficits are uncommon when lumbar sympathectomy is performed by experienced pain practitioners, making it one of the most important treatment modes currently available.

A general treatment plan should include a laxative and stool softener unless diarrhea is the prominent symptom, in which case an obstructing lesion should be ruled out. Care should be taken when prescribing roughage in those with previous radiation, as the bowel/rectal wall can be traumatized. Dexamethasone (4 to 16 mg daily) may provide some relief through its anti-inflammatory actions. The calcium channel antagonist nifedipine (10 to 20 mg two to three times daily) may help to relieve spasms. Epidural opioids and local anesthetics may also be helpful. Systemic opioids should be tried, but these are less effective, as in other forms of neuropathic pain. Traditional neuropathic pain treatment such as tricyclic antidepressants (e.g., amitriptyline hydrochloride) should be used with caution, as one of the main side effects is constipation.

CONCLUSIONS

GI symptoms are so common in the general, healthy population that it may be more difficult to evaluate them in those with cancer. Common symptoms may be disease-related or a comorbidity unrelated to the cancer. Both may represent potentially life-threatening problems, and yet the decision to treat may not be clear if based on management guidelines for the general population. Decisions regarding treatment must be evaluated with an understanding of the goals of therapy, potential quality of life, and life expectancy. Consultation with GI specialists and ongoing communication with the patient and family help to provide the framework in which to make these often difficult decisions.

REFERENCES

1. Askenasy JJM. About the mechanism of hiccup. *Eur Neurol.* 1992;32:159-163.
2. Marinella MA. Diagnosis and management of hiccups in the patient with advanced cancer. *J Support Oncol.* 2009;7(4):122-127, 130.
3. Lewis JH. Hiccups: causes and cures. *J Clin Gastroenterol.* 1985;7:539-552.
4. Launois S, Bizec JL, Whitelaw WA, et al. Hiccup in adults: an overview. *Eur Respir J.* 1993;6:563-575.
5. Ge AX, Ryan ME, Giaccone G, Hughes MS, Pavletic SZ. Acupuncture treatment for persistent hiccups in patients with cancer. *J Altern Complement Med.* 2010;16(7):811-816.

6. Friedgood CE, Ripstein CB. Chlorpromazine (thorazine) in the treatment of intractable hiccups. *JAMA.* 1955;157:309-310.

7. Alonso-Navarro H, Rubio L, Jiménez-Jiménez FJ. Refractory hiccup: successful treatment with gabapentin. *Clin Neuropharmacol.* 2007;30(3):186-187.

8. Porzio G, Aielli F, Verna L, Aloisi P, Galletti B, Ficorella C. Gabapentin in the treatment of hiccups in patients with advanced cancer: a 5-year experience. *Clin Neuropharmacol.* 2010;33(4):179-180.

9. Moro C, Sironi P, Berardi E, Beretta G, Labianca R. Midazolam for long-term treatment of intractable hiccup. *J Pain Symptom Manage.* 2005;29(3):221-223.

10. Ives TJ, Flemming MF, Weart CW, et al. Treatment of intractable hiccup with intramuscular haloperidol. *Am J Psychiatry.* 1985;142:1368-1369.

11. Lipps DC, Jabbari B, Mitchel MH, et al. Nifedipine for intractable hiccups. *Neurology.* 1990;40:531-532.

12. Madanagopolan N. Metoclopramide in hiccup. *Curr Med Res Opin.* 1975;3:371-374.

13. Walker P, Watanabe S, Bruera E. Baclofen, a treatment for chronic hiccup. *J Pain Symptom Manage.* 1998;16:125-132.

14. Parvin R, Milo R, Klein C, et al. Amitriptyline for intractable hiccup. *Am J Gastroenterol.* 1988;63:1007-1008.

15. McFarling DA, Susac JO. Carbamazepine for hiccoughs. *JAMA.* 1974;230:962.

16. Petroski D, Patel AN. Diphenylhydantoin for intractable hiccups. *Lancet.* 1974;1:739.

17. Jacobson PL, Messenheimer JA, Farmer TW. Treatment of intractable hiccups with valproic acid. *Neurology.* 1981;31:1458-1460.

18. Marechal R, Berghmans T, Sculier P. Successful treatment of intractable hiccup with methylphenidate in a lung cancer patient. *Support Care Cancer.* 2003;11(2):126.

19. Calvo E, Fernandez-Torre F, Brugarolas A. Cervical phrenic nerve block for intractable hiccups in cancer patients. *J Natl Cancer Inst.* 2002;94(15):1175-1176.

20. Aravot DJ, Wright G, Rees A, et al. Non-invasive phrenic nerve stimulation for intractable hiccups. *Lancet.* 1989;2:1047.

21. Salem MR. Treatment of hiccups by pharyngeal stimulation in anesthetized and conscious subjects. *JAMA.* 1967;202:126-130.

22. Smith HS, Busracamwongs A. Management of hiccups in the palliative care population. *Am J Hosp Palliat Care.* 2003;20(2):149-154.

23. Heading RC. Definitions of dyspepsia. *Scand J Gastroenterol.* 1991;26(suppl 182):1-6.

24. Ofman JJ, Etchason J, Fullerton S, et al. Management strategies for *Helicobacter pylori* seropositive patients with dyspepsia: clinical and economic consequences. *Ann Intern Med.* 1997;126:280-291.

25. Tack J, Lee KJ. Pathophysiology and treatment of functional dyspepsia. *J Clin Gastroenterol.* 2005;39(5 suppl):S211-S216.

26. Fisher RS, Parkman HP. Management of nonulcer dyspepsia. *N Engl J Med.* 1998;339:1376-1381.

27. Barkin JS, Goldberg RI, Sfakianakis GN, Levi J. Pancreatic carcinoma is associated with delayed gastric emptying. *Dig Dis Sci.* 1986;31(3):265-267.

28. Donthireddy KR, Ailawadhi S, Nasser E, et al. Malignant gastroparesis: pathogenesis and management of an underrecognized disorder. *J Support Oncol.* 2007;5(8):355-363.

29. Pardi DS, Miller SM, Miller DL, et al. Paraneoplastic dysmotility: loss of interstitial cells of Cajal. *Am J Gastroenterol.* 2002;97(7):1828-1833.

30. Talley NJ. Nonulcer dyspepsia: current approaches to diagnosis and management. *Am Fam Physician.* 1993;47:1407-1416.

31. Lee HR, Lennon VA, Camilleri M, et al. Paraneoplastic gastrointestinal motor dysfunction: clinical and laboratory characteristics. *Am J Gastroenterol.* 2001;96(2):373-379.

32. Nelson KA, Walsh TD. The use of metoclopramide in anorexia due to the cancer-associated dyspepsia syndrome (CADS). *J Palliat Care.* 1993;9:14-18.

33. Wilson J, Plourde JY, Marshall D, et al. Long-term safety and clinical effectiveness of controlled-release metoclopramide in cancer-associated dyspepsia syndrome: a multicenter evaluation. *J Palliat Care.* 2002;18(2):84-91.

34. Forster J, Sarosiek I, Delcore R, et al. Gastric pacing is a new surgical treatment for gastroparesis. *Am J Surg.* 2001;182(6):676-681.

35. Abell T, Lou J, Tabbaa M, et al. Gastric electrical stimulation for gastroparesis improves nutritional parameters at short, intermediate, and long-term follow-up. *JPEN J Parenter Enteral Nutr.* 2003;27(4):277-281.

36. Nebel OT, Fornes MF, Castell DO. Symptomatic gastroesophageal reflux: incidence and precipitating factors. *Dig Dis Sci.* 1976;21:953-964.

37. Johnson DA, Ganz R, Aisenberg J, et al. Endoscopic implantation of Enteryx for treatment of GERD: 12-month results of a prospective, multicenter trial. *Am J Gastroenterol.* 2003;98(9):1921-1930.

38. Donnelly S, Walsh D. The symptom of advanced cancer. *Semin Oncol.* 1995;22(2 suppl 3):67-72.

39. Dunlop GM. A study of the relative frequency and importance of gastrointestinal symptoms, and weakness in patients with far advanced cancer. *Palliat Med.* 1989;4:37-43.

40. Armes PJ, Plant HJ, Allbright A, et al. A study to investigate the incidence of early satiety in patients with advanced cancer. *Br J Cancer.* 1992;65:481-484.

41. Nelson KA, Walsh DT, Sheehan FG, et al. Assessment of upper gastrointestinal motility in the cancer-associated dyspepsia syndrome. *J Palliat Care.* 1993;9(1):27-31.

42. Neilson SS, Theologides A, Vickers ZM. Influence of food odors on food aversions and preferences in patients with cancer. *Am J Clin Nutr.* 1980;33:2253-2261.

43. Longstreth GF. Epidemiology for hospitalization for acute upper gastrointestinal hemorrhage: a population based study. *Am J Gastroenterol.* 1995;90:206-210.

44. Rockall TA, Logan RFA, Devlin HB, et al. Incidence of and mortality from acute upper gastrointestinal haemorrhage in the United Kingdom. *BMJ.* 1995;311:222.

45. Mercadante S, Baressi L, Casuccio A, et al. Gastrointestinal bleeding in advanced cancer patients. *J Pain Symptom Manage.* 2000;19:160-162.

46. Silverstein FE, Gilbert DA, Tedesco FJ. The national ASGE survey on upper gastrointestinal bleeding. *Gastrointest Endosc.* 1981;27:73.

47. Spencer GD, Hackman RC, McDonald GB, et al. A prospective study of unexplained nausea and vomiting after marrow transplantation. *Transplantation.* 1986;42:602-607.

48. Kemeny MM, Brennan MF. The surgical complications of chemotherapy in the cancer patient. *Curr Probl Surg.* 1987;24:613-675.

49. Boley SJ, DiBiase A, Brandt LJ, et al. Lower intestinal bleeding in the elderly. *Am J Surg.* 1979;137:57.

50. Weingrad DN, Decosse JJ, Sherlock P, et al. Primary gastrointestinal lymphoma. *Cancer.* 1982;49:1258-1265.

51. Gabriel SE, Jaakkimaenen L, Bombardier C. Risk for serious gastrointestinal complications related to the use of nonsteroidal anti-inflammatory drugs: a meta-analysis. *Ann Intern Med.* 1991;115:787-797.

52. Jensen DM, Machicado GA. Diagnosis and treatment of severe hematochezia. The role of urgent colonoscopy after purge. *Gastroenterology.* 1988;95:1569-1574.

53. Nusbaum M, Baum S. Radiographic demonstration of unknown sites of gastrointestinal bleeding. *Surg Forum.* 1963;14:374-375.

54. Lind T, Aadland E, Eriksson S, et al. Beneficial effects of I.V. omeprazole in patients with peptic ulcer bleeding. *Gastroenterology.* 1995;108:A150.

55. Cotlon RB, Rosenberg MT, Waldram RPL, et al. Early endoscopy of esophagus, stomach, and duodenal bulb in patients with hematemesis and melena. *BMJ.* 1973;2: 505-509.

56. Graham D, Smith JL. The course of patients after variceal hemorrhage. *Gastroenterology.* 1981;80:800-809.

57. Jensen DM. Current management of severe lower gastrointestinal tract bleeding. *Gastrointest Endosc.* 1995;41:171-173.

58. Lichter I, Hunt E. The last 48 hours of life. *J Palliat Care.* 1990;6:7-15.

59. Pereira J, Phan T. Management of bleeding in patients with advanced cancer. *Oncologist.* 2004;9:561-570.

60. Regnard C, Makin W. Management of bleeding in advanced cancer—a flow diagram. *Palliat Med.* 1992;6: 74-78.

61. Stellato TA, Zollinger RM, Shuck JM. Metastatic malignant biliary obstruction. *Am Surg.* 1989;157:381-385.

62. Bear HD, Turner MA, Parker GA, et al. Treatment of biliary obstruction caused by metastatic cancer. *Am J Surg.* 1989;157:381-385.

63. Smith AC, Dowsett JF, Russell RCG, et al. Randomized trial of endoscopic stenting versus surgical bypass in malignant low bile duct obstruction. *Lancet.* 1994;334:1655-1660.

64. Earnshaw JJ, Hayter JP, Teasdale C, et al. Should endoscopic stenting be the initial treatment of malignant biliary obstruction? *Ann R Coll Surg Engl.* 1992;74: 338-341.

65. Wagner HJ, Knyrim K, Vakil N, et al. Polyethylene endoprostheses versus metal stents in the palliative treatment of malignant hilar obstruction. A prospective and randomized trial. *Endoscopy.* 1993;25:213-218.

66. Schmassmann A, von Gunten E, Knuchel J, et al. Wall stents versus plastic stents in malignant biliary obstruction: effects of stent patency of the first and second stent on patient compliance and survival. *Am J Gastroenterol.* 1996;91:654-659.

67. Siddiqui AA, Sreenarasimhaiah J, Lara LF, Harford W, Lee C, Eloubeidi MA. Endoscopic ultrasound-guided transduodenal placement of a fully covered metal stent for palliative biliary drainage in patients with malignant biliary obstruction. *Surg Endosc.* 2011;25(2):549-555.

68. O'Grady JG, Schalm SW, Williams R. Acute liver failure: redefining the syndromes. *Lancet.* 1993;342:273-275.

69. McGuire BM, Cherwitz DL, Rabe KM, et al. Small cell carcinoma of the lung manifesting as acute hepatic failure. *Mayo Clin Proc.* 1997;72:133-139.

70. Fingerote RJ. Fulminant hepatic failure. *Am J Gastroenterol.* 1993;88:1000-1010.

71. Butterworth RF. Pathogenesis and treatment of portal-systemic encephalopathy: an update. *Dig Dis Sci.* 1992;37:321-340.

72. Lockwood AH. Hepatic encephalopathy. *Neurol Clin.* 2002;20:241-246.

73. Howard CD, Seifert CF. Flumazenil in the treatment of hepatic encephalopathy. *Ann Pharmacother.* 1993;27:46-48.

74. Hoyumpa AM, Desmond PV, Avant GR, et al. Clinical conference: hepatic encephalopathy. *Gastroenterology.* 1979;78:184.

75. Hoofnagle JH, Carithers RL, Shapiro C, et al. Fulminant hepatic failure: summary of a workshop. *Hepatology.* 1995;21:240.

76. D'Amico G, Pagliaco L, Bosch J. The treatment of portal hypertension: a meta-analysis review. *Hepatology.* 1995;22:332-354.

77. Wilkinson SP, Portmann B, Hurst D, et al. Pathogenesis of renal failure in cirrhosis and fulminant hepatic failure. *Postgrad Med J.* 1975;51:503.

78. Sedwick DM, Howard GC, Ferguson A. Pathogenesis of acute radiation injury to the rectum. A prospective study in patients. *Int J Colorectal Dis.* 1994;9:23-30.

79. Regnard CFB. Control of bleeding in advanced cancer. *Lancet.* 1991;337:974.

80. Yeung RS, Moffat FL, Falk RE. Pelvic exenteration for recurrent and extensive primary colorectal adenocarcinoma. *Cancer.* 1993;72:1853-1858.

81. Midgley R, Kerr D. Colorectal cancer. *Lancet.* 1999;353:391-399.

82. Rey JF, Romanczyk T, Graff M. Metal stents for palliation of rectal carcinoma: a preliminary report on 12 patients. *Endoscopy.* 1995;27:501-504.

83. Bristow A, Foster JMG. Lumbar sympathectomy in the management of rectal tenesmoid pain. *Ann R Coll Surg Engl.* 1988;70:38-39.

18 Oral Manifestations and Complications of Cancer Therapy

Jane M. Fall-Dickson, Madeline R. Kozak, and Ann M. Berger

INTRODUCTION

Efficacy of cancer treatment protocols designed to increase cure rates and to extend disease-free survival and survival time, including chemotherapy (CT), radiation therapy (RT), and hematopoietic stem cell transplantation (HSCT), is tempered by treatment-related side effects and associated symptoms. Oral complications comprise one such treatment-related side effect category and include oral mucositis and oral chronic graft versus host disease (cGVHD) with related oropharyngeal pain, oral sensitivity, and xerostomia, often leading to impaired health-related quality of life (HRQOL). Complex pathogenesis of and evidence-based management strategies for these oral complications and related oral symptoms, as well as, future clinical research directions, are presented in this chapter.

ORAL MUCOSITIS

Oral mucositis is an inflammation of the mucous membranes of the oral cavity and oropharynx characterized by tissue erythema, edema, and atrophy, often progressing to ulceration (1). The clinical significance of CT- and RT-related oral mucositis as a dose- and treatment-limiting side effect is associated significantly with oropharyngeal pain, impaired HRQOL, and decreased functional status (2–4). Oral mucositis presents clinically with asymptomatic erythema and progresses from solitary, white, elevated desquamative patches that are mildly painful to large, contiguous, pseudomembranous, painful ulcers. Oral sequelae of stomatogenic CT agents' mechanism of action typically include epithelial hyperplasia, collagen and glandular degeneration, epithelial dysplasia, atrophy, and localized or diffuse mucosal ulceration. Nonkeratinized mucosal areas are most affected. The loss of basement membrane epithelial cells exposes underlying connective, innervated tissue stroma, which leads to severe oropharyngeal pain intensity. Healing of oral lesions in nonmyelosuppressed patients occurs 2 to 3 weeks after cancer treatment, with decreasing oropharyngeal pain reported in parallel with mucosal healing.

Frequency and severity of oral mucositis are influenced by patient- and treatment-related risk factors (Table 18.1) (5,6). Risk factors for CT-related oral mucositis are complex. Although women have reported more frequent severe oral mucositis than men, and children are three times more likely than adults to develop mucositis, Driezen (7) reported no age or gender-related risk for this oral condition. Dodd et al. reported in a study of 332 patients receiving CT no increased risk for oral mucositis related to smoking history or previous oral lesions, presence of dental appliances, or type of oral care regimens used (6). Conflicting study results may reflect inconsistent inclusion criteria regarding risk factors in clinical trials (5). Treatment-related risk factors include CT continuous infusion for breast and colon cancer (5-fluorouracil [5-FU] and leucovorin); selected anthracyclines, alkylating agents, taxanes, vinca alkaloids, antimetabolites, and antitumor antibiotics; myeloablative HSCT conditioning regimens including high-dose melphalan or carmustine, cytarabine, and melphalan (BEAM) (8–10); and RT targeted to the head and neck. Individual patient's unique drug metabolism also affects oral mucositis incidence and severity.

CHEMOTHERAPY-INDUCED MUCOSITIS

Clinically significant oral mucositis has been reported to range from 15% in patients who are receiving low-risk treatments to 60% to 100% in the high-dose CT, RT, and HSCT settings (11). Ulcerative oral mucositis is reported in 78% of patients in the HSCT setting (12) with approximately half of these patients requiring parenteral analgesia and/or total parenteral nutrition (TPN) (13). Oral mucositis is a risk factor for life-threatening infections in neutropenic patients. Oral infections, such as herpes simplex virus (HSV), may increase oral mucositis severity. Importantly, a four times greater relative risk of septicemia is reported in patients with oral mucositis and oral infections due to mucosal barrier injury.

The association between severe oral mucositis and clinical outcomes in patients who receive conditioning CT is well known (14,15). McCann et al. (14) conducted a descriptive study with 197

TABLE 18.1 PATIENT- AND TREATMENT-RELATED RISK FACTORS FOR ORAL MUCOSITIS

Patient Related

Demographic
  Age: >65 y; <20 y
  Gender
Oral Cavity Specific
  Periodontal diseases
  Microbial flora
  Chronic low-grade oral infections
  Herpes simplex virus infection
  Ill-fitting dental prostheses
Systemic
  Salivary gland secretory dysfunction
  Inborn inability to metabolize chemotherapeutic
  agents effectively
  Inadequate nutritional status
Behavioral
  Exposure to oral stressors including alcohol and
  smoking
  Inadequate oral health and hygiene practices

Treatment Related

Cancer Treatment
  Radiation therapy: dose, schedule
  Chemotherapy: agent, dose, schedule
Cancer Treatment Related
  Myelosuppression, neutropenia,
  immunosuppression
Medication Usage
  Antidepressants, opiates, antihypertensives,
  antihistamines, diuretics, and sedatives
Oral Cavity
  Inadequate oral care during treatment
  Oral infections of bacterial, viral, or fungal origin
  Xerostomia
Systemic
  Impairment of renal or hepatic function
  Protein or calorie malnutrition
  Dehydration

Adapted from Barasch A, Peterson DE. Risk factors for ulcerative mucositis in cancer patients: unanswered questions. *Oral Oncol.* 2003;39:91-100; Dodd MJ, Miaskowski C, Shiba GH, et al. Risk factors for CT-induced oral mucositis: dental appliances, oral hygiene, previous oral lesion, and a history of smoking. *Cancer Invest.* 1999;17:278-284.

patients diagnosed with multiple myeloma (MM) or non-Hodgkin's lymphoma treated with either high-dose melphalan or BEAM, respectively. Severe oral mucositis, defined as World Health Organization (WHO) grades 3 and 4, increased TPN duration by 2.7 days, opioid use by 4.6 days, and antibiotic use by 2.4 days.

RADIATION-INDUCED MUCOSITIS

Oral mucositis is almost always observed when RT targets the oropharyngeal area, with severity dependent upon type of ionizing radiation, volume of tissue irradiated, daily and cumulative dose, and treatment duration. Oral mucositis is a dose- and rate-limiting toxicity for RT delivered to the head and neck, with hyperfractionated RT, and

in combined RT and CT treatment protocols. Atrophic changes in the oral epithelium are observed usually at total doses of 1,600 to 2,000 cGy, administered at a rate of 200 cGy/d (16). Doses >6,000 cGy or combination RT + CT are risk factors for permanent salivary gland damage (16,17). Addition of total-body irradiation (TBI) to the HSCT conditioning regimen increases oral mucositis severity via direct mucosal damage and indirectly through xerostomia. Negative oral/dental effects of RT result from salivary glands and teeth included in the treatment field. Teeth may become desensitized with related risk for asymptomatic early caries, thus, requiring daily fluoride application.

Health care costs and resource use are increased significantly for patients with head and neck cancer who develop oral mucositis (18,19). A prospective, longitudinal study of 75 patients with head and neck cancer receiving RT with/without CT reported that 76% of participants had severe oral pain requiring increased health care visits, 51% required feeding tube placement, and 37% required hospitalization for an average of 4.9 days (19).

RADIATION THERAPY–RELATED COMPLICATIONS

Chronic effects of RT delivered to the head and neck include soft tissue fibrosis, trismus, none or slow healing of mucosal ulcerations, and slow healing dental extraction sites. RT-induced fibrotic changes may occur in masticatory muscles or the temporal mandibular joint up to 1 year post-RT. Early phases of RT-associated fibrogenesis are characterized as wound healing with up-regulation of tumor necrosis factor-alpha (TNF-α) and other proinflammatory cytokines (20). As RT-related fibrogenesis continues, it functions biologically as a nonhealing wound (20).

Osteoradionecrosis is a relatively uncommon condition related to hypocellularity, hypovascularity, and tissue ischemia. Higher incidences are reported with RT to the bone with total doses of >65 Gy (21). Osteoradionecrosis is usually trauma related, for example, tooth extractions not timed to allow extraction site healing for 10 to 14 days before the start of RT. Osteonecrosis of the jaw bone is strongly associated with bisphosphonate use (22,23).

PATHOGENESIS OF CHEMOTHERAPY- AND RADIATION THERAPY–INDUCED ORAL MUCOSITIS

Cancer therapy is designed to target rapidly dividing cells, and thus, affects not only cancer cells but also rapidly dividing normal cells including oral basal epithelium that has a 7- to 14-day cell turnover rate. Understanding of the complex pathogenesis of oral mucositis is being advanced rapidly by the current intense research interest focused on elucidating mechanisms of mucosal injury. Basic and translational research multidisciplinary efforts are applying advanced molecular–genetic techniques, cell biology, and our understanding of host–microbiome cross-talk to this oral condition (24,25). In 2004, Sonis (26) described a comprehensive five-phase oral mucositis pathogenesis model including initiation, message generation, signaling and amplification, ulceration, and healing. Initiation occurs following CT administration through DNA damage and generation of reactive oxygen species. The acute inflammatory or vascular phase occurs shortly following CT or RT administration (12). Message generation involves up-regulation of transcription factors, including nuclear factor-kappa B (NF-κB), and activation of cytokines and stress response genes. Signaling and amplification of proinflammatory cytokines within epithelial tissue includes TNF-α, which is related to tissue damage, and interleukin (IL)-1, which induces an inflammatory response and increases subepithelial vascularity with potential increase in local CT levels. Epithelial renewal and atrophy typically begin 4 to 5 days after CT administration. This phase is driven efficiently by cell cycle S phase–specific agents, including methotrexate, 5-FU, and cytarabine. Oropharyngeal ulceration may begin about 1 week post-CT at the time of maximum neutropenia (12) and is probably not related to a specific CT agent classification. This most complex, symptomatic ulceration phase, during which patients often report acute oropharyngeal pain, requires expert pain management to avoid dysphagia, decreased oral intake, and difficulty speaking. Bacterial colonization of mucosal ulceration may occur with gram-negative organisms that release endotoxins inducing release of IL-1 and TNF and production of nitric oxide increasing local mucosal injury. RT and CT likely amplify and prolong this cytokine release with related exacerbated tissue response. Transcription factors may modify genetic expression of cytokines and enzymes critical in tissue damage (12).

Clinical research that is currently focusing on the role of host–microbiome cross-talk is examining its role in the pathogenesis of oral mucositis, oral inflammatory changes across the oral mucositis trajectory, and healing (25). Importance of this research focus was supported by the recent systematic review conducted between January 2011 and June 2016 by the Mucositis Study Group of the Multinational Association of Supportive Care in Cancer/International Society of Oral Oncology (MASCC/ISOO) (27). This review stressed

importance of recognizing the impact of the microbiota throughout all phases of oral mucositis: pretreatment; initiation; signaling; amplification; ulceration; and healing. Future research directions included defining the role of the microbiome in oral mucositis, discovering new targets for mucosal protective agents, and discovering similarities between animal and human models of oral mucositis (24).

Analysis of immunologic activity throughout the oral mucositis biological process using saliva analysis has proved both efficient and effective. Avivi et al. (28) evaluated salivary antioxidant and immunologic activity in 25 patients with MM treated with conditioning melphalan and HSCT who developed oral mucositis. Oral mucositis was associated with a reduction in secretory immunoglobulin A and antioxidant activity. The increase in salivary albumin and carbonyl indicated mucosal and oxidative damage, respectively.

Clinical research regarding the relationship between oral mucositis–related tissue injury and reported symptoms is ongoing. For example, Fall-Dickson et al. (29) described oral mucositis-related oropharyngeal pain intensity in patients undergoing HSCT with conditioning CT and measured TNF-α concentration in blood, saliva, and oral epithelial cells obtained by buccal brushing. Oral mucositis severity significantly correlated with overall intensity of oral pain. TNF-α RNA content in oral buccal epithelial cell samples correlated with greatest intensity of oral pain with swallowing.

CHRONIC GRAFT-VERSUS-HOST DISEASE ORAL MANIFESTATIONS

Patients who have undergone allogeneic HSCT (alloHSCT) frequently develop GVHD, an alloimmune condition derived from an immune attack mediated by donor T cells recognizing antigens expressed on normal tissues (30). GVHD occurs after alloHSCT due to disparities in minor histocompatibility antigens between donor and recipient, inherited independently of human leucocyte antigen (HLA) genes (30). Systemic corticosteroids are the primary treatment for cGVHD. In 2017, the US Food and Drug Administration (FDA) approved Imbruvica (ibrutinib) for cGVHD treatment in adult patients after failure of one or more systemic treatments (31). Current research interest is focused on testing emerging therapeutics, which include the JAK family of nonreceptor tyrosine kinases (30).

Chronic GVHD was historically defined as occurring >100 days post-HSCT (32) and is now classified based on characteristic clinical presentation. Chronic GVHD is reported to occur in 30% to 60% of patients 100 days post-alloHSCT (33). Approximately 80% of patients with extensive cGVHD have oral involvement (34) that is a major contributing factor to patient morbidity after alloHSCT. Although oral lesions are most commonly seen with extensive cGVHD organ involvement, patients may also present with only oral cGHVD, thus making comprehensive oral examination important. Oral cGVHD presents with tissue atrophy and erythema, lichenoid changes, angular stomatitis, and pseudomembranous ulcerations that occur typically on buccal and labial mucosa and the lateral tongue, and xerostomia (34). Treister et al. (35) correlated the distribution, type, and extent of oral cGVHD lesions with oral pain and discomfort. The buccal and labial mucosa and tongue were the frequently reported oral sites of ulcerations (93%), erythematous lesions (72%), and reticular lesions (76%). Ulcerations in the soft palate, although uncommon, were associated with increased pain intensity. Functional impact was significant with restriction of oral intake due to discomfort. Decreased oral intake leads to weight loss and malnutrition, which remain serious clinical problems with cGVHD.

Although oral cGVHD is appreciated to be a serious long-term complication of alloHSCT, little is known about its pathogenesis. Imanguli et al. (36) proposed a model of cGVHD pathogenesis in which the production of type 1 interferon by plasmacytoid dendritic cells plays a central role in cGVHD initiation and continuation. Fall-Dickson et al. (37) examined associations among clinical characteristics of oral cGVHD and related oral pain and perceived oral dryness, salivary proinflammatory cytokine IL-6 and IL-1α concentrations, and HR-QOL. Salivary IL-6 correlated with oral cGVHD severity, oral ulceration, and erythema, suggesting its utility as a biomarker for active oral cGVHD. Fall-Dickson et al. have presented a complex pathobiology model describing iterative steps of the progression from activation of antigen presenting cells (APCs) to oral ulceration (30).

The clinical importance of oral cGVHD has been recognized through the National Institutes of Health (NIH) Consensus Development Project on Criteria for Clinical Trials in cGVHD (38) and through reported outcomes of the 2009 conference sponsored by the German-Austrian-Swiss working party for bone marrow and blood stem cell transplantation held in Regensburg, Germany (39). These outcomes included a summary of the evidence for diagnosis, first- and second-line therapies, topical treatments, and practical treatment guidelines. The authors concurred that a comprehensive, interdisciplinary treatment approach for oral cGVHD must include assessment of mucosa, salivary glands, musculoskeletal tissues, teeth, periodontium, and oral function (39).

The importance of using valid and reliable assessment tools for oral cGVHD has been recognized for decades. The Schubert Oral Mucositis Rating Scale was validated through the NIH Consensus Development Project (38). Treister et al. (40) analyzed inter- and intraobserver variability in component and composite scores of the NIH oral cGVHD Activity Assessment Instrument. Twenty-four clinicians from six major HSCT centers scored high-quality intraoral photographs of 12 patients followed 1 week later by a second evaluation. Although mean interrater reliability (IRR) scores ranged from poor to moderate, and thus, were unacceptable for the clinical trial setting, greater concordance was observed among the participating oral medicine experts. These results and participant feedback suggest formal training may decrease variability. Bassim et al. (41) examined construct validity and internal consistency of the NIH Oral Mucosal Score (OMS) and its discrete components of erythema, lichenoid, ulcers, and mucoceles, as well as, measures of oral pain and function, and related QOL, nutrition, and laboratory parameters in 198 patients diagnosed with cGVHD. The NIH OMS is based solely on clinician assessment of oral mucosa in the patient who has undergone peripheral blood stem cell transplantation/bone marrow transplant (BMT). Results supported construct validity of the discrete components of the NIH OMS through strong associations between erythema and lichenoid and impaired oral QOL, function, and nutrition, and lower serum albumin levels. Oral cGVHD ulceration correlated primarily with oral pain. Valid and reliable assessment tools for oral cGVHD such as the NIH OMS are needed to measure efficacy of agents in the clinical trial setting to advance the science of oral cGVHD and to increase treatment options.

SEQUELAE OF ORAL COMPLICATIONS

Oropharyngeal Pain

Oral mucositis is the principal etiology of most pain experienced during the 3-week post-BMT time period. Patients have described this oral pain as the most unforgettable ordeal of BMT. McGuire et al. (42) reported in patients undergoing autologous and alloBMT that oral pain was reported before observed oral mucositis, that pain intensity did not correlate directly with extent of mucosal injury, and that some patients reported limited or no pain after BMT. A descriptive, cross-sectional study of women with breast cancer undergoing autologous HSCT conducted by Fall-Dickson et al. (43) showed a significant positive correlation between oral pain intensity and oral mucositis severity.

The sensory dimension of oral mucositis–related pain reported with general mucosal inflammation and breakdown ranges from mild discomfort to severe and debilitating pain requiring opioids (44). Oral pain is associated significantly with cGVHD and has been described as severe, burning, and irritating with associated oral dryness and loss of taste. Mucositis-related oral pain reported with CT is usually of <3 months' duration, contrasting with the usually chronic oral pain accompanying oral cGVHD.

Gender differences have been reported for oral mucositis–related pain. Women reported higher pain intensity scores in a study examining capsaicin efficacy for oral mucositis–related pain. Pain management is critical to avoid suffering and psychological distress (45). Adequate assessment of oral pain requires a comprehensive pain assessment tool such as the Painometer (Dola Health Systems, Baltimore, MD) (46) that assesses overall intensity, sensory, and affective dimensions of pain.

Xerostomia

Xerostomia is a major clinical challenge experienced by patients who receive head and neck RT, with severity dependent on RT dosage and volume of exposed salivary glands in the treatment field. Patients may also develop xerostomia as a late oral complication of HSCT. Xerostomia can affect taste, oral comfort, prosthetic fit, speech, swallowing, and promotes caries-producing organisms.

Brand et al. (47) reported in a cross-sectional study of patients with a history of autologous or alloHSCT significantly higher levels of xerostomia than seen in the comparison group. Xerostomia severity was not significantly associated with either RT given before HSCT or the type of HSCT. A cross-sectional study by Imanguli et al. (48) evaluated sicca signs and symptoms in 101 patients with cGVHD with assessment tools used for Sjögren's syndrome. Of the 77% of patients reporting xerostomia, those with salivary dysfunction showed histopathologic changes consisting of mononuclear infiltration and fibrosis or atrophy, suggesting that salivary gland involvement is common in cGVHD. Salivary antioxidant capacity and function were assessed in 30 patients after HSCT by Nagler et al. (49). Salivary gland function was assessed through measuring total protein, secretory immunoglobulin A, antioxidant peroxidase, uric acid, and total antioxidant status in a saliva sample. In patients who developed GVHD after HSCT, there was a significant decrease in salivary flow rate pre- and post-HSCT with no recovery and a reduction in salivary protein content and salivary antioxidant capacity. In patients without GVHD after HSCT, salivary flow rates returned to normal in 3 to 5 months. Decreased salivary flow rate with related decrease in its protective functions for oral mucosa contribute to oral cGVHD severity. Bassim et al. (50) tested the feasibility of using liquid chromatography tandem mass spectrometry to identify protein biomarkers related to oral cGVHD. Pooled saliva from five patients with moderate or severe oral cGVHD was compared to saliva from a gender- and age-matched pool of five patients with GVHD without oral mucosal findings. Reported reduction in salivary lactoperoxidase, lactotransferrin, and several cysteine proteinase inhibitor family proteins suggests impaired oral antimicrobial host immunity in oral cGVHD (50).

STRATEGIES FOR PREVENTION AND TREATMENT OF ORAL COMPLICATIONS

The need for standardized treatment for prevention and treatment of oral mucositis was supported by the recent systematic review published between January 2011 and June 2016 by the Mucositis Study Group of the Multinational Association of Supportive Care in Cancer/International Society of Oral Oncology (27). This systematic review identified research progress since the previous review and highlighted useful research directions and potential new targets for further investigation (27). The guideline update systematically reviewed new literature since the 2011 cutoff date of the previous guidelines and also merged previously published and newly published clinical trials. Results from these systematic reviews will be presented throughout the following sections.

Pretherapy Dental Evaluation and Intervention

Oral and dental stabilization prior to CT or RT are critically important to avoid serious sequelae and require an experienced dental team and informed patients working together for appropriate oral hygiene and elimination of oral infection.

Patients scheduled for CT or head and neck RT should undergo a dental screening to promote optimal mucosal health before, during, and following cancer treatment. Ideally this should occur at least 2 weeks before therapy starts to allow for recovery from soft tissue manipulations, restoration of teeth, and proper healing of potential extraction sites. The initial dental appointment includes examination of dentition for caries and defective restorations, the periodontium, pulp vitality, and denture fit to avoid ill-fitting dentures causing irritation of irradiated tissue and ulceration extending to underlying bone (51–53).

A panoramic radiograph combined with intraoral radiographs as needed is necessary to screen for periodontal disease, periapical infections, cysts, third-molar pathology, unerupted or partially erupted teeth, and residual root tips. Dental caries, repair of defective restorations, removal of orthodontic appliances, remediation of ill-fitting prostheses, and periapical or third molar pathologies need to be addressed before cancer treatment begins. Bacterial load should be reduced prior to cancer treatment via root planing, scaling, and prophylaxis, excluding visible tumor located at the site of anticipated dental manipulation. The decision to extract asymptomatic teeth prior to the start of RT is based on radiation exposure, type, portal field, fractionization, and total dosage in addition to tumor prognosis and expediency of control of the cancer (51,52). Teeth with class II or III mobility without use as abutment teeth for prosthetic retention should also be considered for extraction before RT. Extractions of residual root tips and impacted teeth should be performed atraumatically. Alveolectomy and primary wound closure eliminate sharp ridges and bone spicules that could project to the overlying soft tissues. This is important for prosthetic consideration because negligible bone remodeling is anticipated after RT. Patients need written instructions for use of oral care agents and instruments for effective daily plaque removal, use of prescribed fluoride treatments, and reportable oral observations and symptoms.

Assessment of the Oral Mucosa

Consistent and frequently scheduled oral cavity assessment is needed to assess clinical signs before, during, and after treatment. No standard grading system for severity of oral complications of cancer treatment exists, and available oral complications grading tools are based often on two or more clinical parameters combined with functional status, such as eating ability. One commonly used tool is the National Cancer Institute Common Terminology Criteria for Adverse Events v.4.0, which includes descriptive terminology and a severity grading scale for each reportable adverse event (54). Frequently used oral mucosal assessment tools include those that capture both objective and subjective data—the Oral Assessment Guide (55) and the World Health Organization Index (56)— and instruments that assess only observed oral changes—the Oral Mucositis Rating Scale (57), the

Oral Mucositis Index (58), and the Oral Mucositis Assessment Scale (OMAS) (59,60).

The OMAS was developed as a scoring system for anatomic extent and severity of oral mucositis in clinical research studies (59,60). Nine regions of the oral cavity are clinically assessed for erythema or ulceration, namely lip (upper and lower), cheek (right and left), right and left ventral and lateral tongue, floor of mouth, soft palate/fauces, and hard palate. Erythema is rated on a scale from 0 to 2 (0 = none, 1 = not severe, and 2 = severe), and ulceration or pseudomembrane is a combined category rated on scores based on estimated surface area involved (0 = no lesion, 1 = <1 cm², 2 = 1 to 3 cm², and 3 = >3 cm²). The total mucositis score is the sum of contributions from the nine regions with a possible range from 0 to 45; the mean mucositis score is the sum of the mean erythema and ulceration scores; the mucositis score is the summation of the maximum ulceration and erythema scores across all sites. Validity and reliability have been demonstrated for the OMAS through clinical research studies (60,61).

Treatment Strategies

The optimal treatment strategies for oral complications and related sequelae are unknown. Treatment strategies for oral mucositis and related oropharyngeal pain are mainly empirical, and testing is needed in the randomized controlled clinical trial setting (Table 18.2). Fall-Dickson Cordes, and Berger (62) presented a comprehensive review of clinical research regarding treatment strategies for oral complications of cancer strategies demonstrating conflicting study results. The most recent 2019 MASCC/ISOO systematic review of basic oral care for the management of oral mucositis in cancer patients (63) has now replaced earlier reviews (64,65). Based on the 17 new papers across 6 interventions that were merged with prior MASCC/ISOO guidelines, the review panel suggested that oral care is useful to prevent oral mucositis during CT, head and neck RT, and HSCT (63). Chlorhexidine was not recommended to prevent oral mucositis in the head and neck cancer RT setting. Guidelines were not possible from this systematic review for professional oral care, patient education, saline, and sodium bicarbonate (63).

RADIOPROTECTORS

Vitamins and Other Antioxidants

Vitamin E has been tested in CT-induced oral mucositis because it stabilizes cellular membranes and may improve herpetic gingivitis, possibly through antioxidant activity. Wadleigh et al.

TABLE 18.2 FORMULARY OF STANDARD TREATMENTS FOR ORAL COMPLICATIONS OF CANCER TREATMENTS[a]

Therapeutic or prevention treatments	Instructions
Prevention of oral mucositis	
Amifostine	200 mg/m² daily, as 3-min IV infusion 15–30 min before radiation therapy. Hydrate adequately, monitor blood pressure, and use antiemetics.
Cryotherapy Distilled water, 1 gallon	Place ice chips in mouth for 30 min beginning 5 min prior to bolus administration of chemotherapy.
NAHCO₃ powder, 3 tablespoons or 11.6 g	Rinse mouth twice a day for 30 s. Do not swallow.
NaCl powder, 3 tablespoons or 11.6 g	Combine all ingredients. Rinse mouth 2–4 times daily. Do not swallow.
Povidone iodine 0.5% oral rinse	Rinse mouth 2–4 times daily. Do not swallow.
Treatment of oral mucositis–related pain	
Carafate suspension, 1 g	Rinse mouth 4 times daily. Do not swallow.
Diphenhydramine (Benadryl, McNEIL-PPC, Inc., Fort Washington, PA), 12.5 mg/5 mL; kaolin and pectin (Kaopectate, Chattem, Inc., Chattanooga, TN)	Use equal amounts of each. Rinse mouth with 10–15 mL 4–6 times daily. Do not swallow.
Diphenhydramine (Benadryl), 12.5 mg/5 mL: 30 mL; Maalox (Norvartis, Basel, Switzerland), 30 mL; nystatin, 100,000 units/mL: 30 mL	Combine all ingredients. Rinse mouth with 15 mL 4–6 times per day. Do not swallow.
Diphenhydramine (Benadryl), 12.5 mg/5 mL: 30 mL; viscous lidocaine (xylocaine) 2%, 30 mL; Maalox, 30 mL	Combine all ingredients. Rinse mouth with 15 mL 4–6 times per day. Do not swallow.
Diphenhydramine (Benadryl), 12.5 mg/5 mL: 30 mL; tetracycline, 125 mg/5 mL suspension 60 mL; nystatin oral suspension, 100,000 units/mL 45 mL; viscous lidocaine (xylocaine) 2%, 30 mL; hydrocortisone suspension, 10 mg/5 mL: 30 mL; sterile water for irrigation, 45 mL	Combine all ingredients. Rinse mouth with 15 mL 4–6 times per day. Do not swallow.
Dyclonine hydrochloride 0.5% or 1.0% solution	Rinse mouth with 10–15 mL every 2–3 h. Do not swallow.
Gelclair (Sinclair Pharmaceuticals, Surrey, England)	Mix one Gelclair packet per manufacturer's directions with 40 mL or 3 tablespoons of water. Stir and rinse immediately for at least 1 min, gargle, and spit out at least 3 times a day.
Opiates	Oral, transdermal, or parenteral opiates may be used, such as patient controlled analgesia (PCA). Use tablet form of oral analgesics. Do not use elixir because alcohol exacerbates oral mucositis.
Viscous lidocaine (xylocaine) 2% solution	Rinse mouth with 10–15 mL every 2–3 h. Do not swallow.
Xerostomia	
Biotene chewing gum (GlaxoSmithKline, Brentford, England)	Use as needed.
Pilocarpine	5 mg oral 3 times a day
Salivart synthetic saliva spray (Gebauer Company, Cleveland, OH)	Spray mouth 4–6 times per day.
Xerolube salivary substitute (Colgate-Palmolive Company, New York, NY)	Rinse mouth 4–6 times per day.

IV, intravenous; NaCl, sodium chloride; NAHCO₃, sodium bicarbonate.
[a]Many of the medications listed have been used alone or in combination to treat oral mucositis.
Adapted from Fall-Dickson JM, Cordes S, Berger AM. Management of adverse effects of treatment: oral complications. In: DeVita VT, Lawrence TS, Rosenberg SA, eds. *Cancer: Principles & Practice of Oncology.* 11th ed. Philadelphia, PA: Lippincott Williams & Wilkins; 2019.

(66) reported efficacy of vitamin E in a sample of 18 patients undergoing CT, who were randomized to receive topical vitamin E or placebo. A recent meta-analysis by Chaitanya et al. (67) analyzed 8 studies (6 in adults; 2 in children) and showed that topical use of vitamin E significantly reduced mucositis ($p < 0.001$).

Other antioxidants that have been tested for efficacy with oral mucositis include vitamin C and glutathione. Osaki et al. (68) reported results from a study of 63 patients with head and neck cancer who were treated with chemoradiation. Twenty-six patients received regimen 1 (vitamins C and E and glutathione) and 37 patients received regimen 2 (regimen 1 + azelastine). In the azelastine arm, 21 patients remained at grade 1 or 2 oral mucositis, 6 patients had grade 3 oral mucositis, and 10 patients had grade 4 oral mucositis. In the control group, grade 3 or 4 oral mucositis was observed in more than half the patients. Watanabe et al. (69) investigated the effect of polaprezinc on CT- and RT-induced oral mucositis, oral pain, xerostomia, and taste disturbance in patients with head and neck cancer. Thirty-one patients were randomly assigned to polaprezinc or azulene solution as a control for 3 minutes four times daily until therapy completion. A marked decrease was seen in incidence of oral mucositis, pain, xerostomia, taste disturbance, and analgesic requirement, as well as, a significant increase in food intake in the polaprezinc group.

Zinc sulfate has not shown efficacy in the prevention of RT- and CT-induced oral mucositis when compared to placebo (70,71) In a randomized, double-blind, placebo-controlled trial, Sangthawan et al. (71) tested efficacy of zinc sulfate supplementation in reducing RT-induced oral mucositis and pharyngitis in patients with head and neck cancer. A total of 144 patients with head and neck cancer receiving RT alone or postoperative RT were enrolled. Zinc sulfate (50 mg) and placebo were administered three times a day at mealtime, on the first day of RT and continued until RT completion. This intervention showed no benefit in relieving radiation-induced oral mucositis and pharyngitis, when compared to placebo.

Amifostine

Amifostine is a thiol compound, selective cytoprotective agent that has been approved by the US FDA for salivary gland protection in patients receiving RT. A retrospective study conducted by Kouloulias et al. (72) reported reduced severity of oral and esophageal toxicity in a sample of 177 patients with diverse tumor types who received amifostine before RT. Based on a meta-analysis that included patients who received amifostine

before RT, there was significant reduction in oral mucositis severity at doses >300 mg/m^2 (73). A multicenter, open-label, randomized controlled trial analyzed the use of amifostine in patients with MM who received conditioning CT with melphalan prior to autologous HSCT (74). Ninety patients were randomized to receive or not receive amifostine (910 mg/m^2). The use of amifostine was associated with a reduction in median grade and frequency of severe oral mucositis. However, there was no reduction in parenteral nutrition and analgesics use and no significant difference between the median progression-free or overall survival times. A recent systematic review of 31 papers literature from 1966 to 2010 by Nicolatou-Galitis et al. (75) found insufficient evidence to support the use of amifostine with any cancer treatment.

Glutamine

Glutamine is an amino acid, immunomodulator, and mucosal protective agent that has been studied in multiple clinical trials with conflicting results. An extensive literature review performed by Savarese et al. (76) reported that glutamine supplementation may have an impact on incidence and severity of anthracycline-associated oral mucositis. A randomized, double-blind, placebo-controlled trial of glutamine supplementation in patients who underwent autologous HSCT reported an increase in severe oral mucositis and opioid use, as well as, prolonged length of hospital stay (77). Another randomized controlled study comparing oral glutamine supplementation (30 g/d) versus placebo in 58 patients undergoing HSCT reported no difference in length of hospital stay, nutrition, oral mucositis and diarrhea severity, engraftment time, survival, and relapse between both groups (78). Other clinical trials have reported more promising data on the use of glutamine (79,80). A retrospective cohort study including 117 patients treated with RT for head and neck cancer or chest tested if oral glutamine prevents oral mucositis or acute radiation-induced esophagitis and improves nutritional status (81). Overall, glutamine was associated with significant reduction of mucositis, weight loss, and enteral nutrition use. The risk difference for developing oral mucositis in patients receiving glutamine when compared with controls was −9.0% (95% confidence interval = −18.0% to −1.0%). The majority of patients not receiving glutamine developed severe malnutrition. No differences were seen in interruption of RT, hospitalization, opioid use, or death during RT.

In a double-blind, randomized, placebo-controlled trial of oral glutamine for the prevention of oral mucositis in children undergoing HSCT, 120 patients were randomized to receive glutamine or glycine twice a day until 28 days post-HSCT. The glutamine group showed a significant reduction in days of intravenous opioid use and TPN, but no difference in toxicity was observed between the two groups (82).

Yarom et al. (83) reported from their review group for the 2019 MASCC/ISOO systematic review a new suggestion for the use of oral glutamine for the prevention of oral mucositis in the RT setting for head and neck cancer. They also reported that no guideline was possible for zinc as a preventive agent in the head and neck cancer setting when patients were treated with RT or CT.

Anti-inflammatory Agents

Prostaglandins are a family of naturally occurring eicosanoids, some of which have shown cytoprotective activity. Misoprostol, a synthetic analog of prostaglandin E1, has been studied as a prevention and treatment option for oral mucositis related to its anti-inflammatory and mucosa-protecting properties. A randomized, double-blind, placebo-controlled, parallel-group study conducted by Lalla et al. (84) tested efficacy of misoprostol oral rinse in reducing the severity of oral mucosal injury caused by high-dose CT. Forty-eight patients receiving myeloablative high-dose CT were randomized to misoprostol ($n = 22$) or placebo rinse ($n = 26$). Results showed no significant effect of misoprostol rinse in oral mucositis.

Topical dinoprostone was administered four times daily in a nonblinded study to 10 patients with oral carcinomas who were receiving 5-FU and mitomycin with concomitant RT (85). The control group comprised 14 patients who were receiving identical cancer treatment. Eight of the ten subjects who received dinoprostone were evaluable; no patient developed severe oral mucositis as compared with six episodes in the control arm. A second pilot study was conducted with 15 patients who received RT to the head and neck, showing that an inflammatory reaction was detected in 5 patients in the vicinity of their tumor when treated with topically applied PGE_2, and that no patients developed any bullous or desquamating inflammatory lesions (86). A double-blind, placebo-controlled study of PGE_2 in 60 patients undergoing BMT showed no significant differences in incidence, severity, or duration of oral mucositis. However, incidence of HSV was higher in the PGE_2 arm, and increased oral mucositis severity was seen in patients who developed HSV (87).

Benzydamine is a nonsteroidal anti-inflammatory drug with reported analgesic, anesthetic, and antimicrobial properties without activity on arachidonic acid metabolism. This agent has been shown to reduce the severity of oral mucositis and related oral pain in patients who undergo RT. Epstein and Stevenson-Moore (88) reported in a double-blind, placebo-controlled trial that benzydamine produced statistically significant decrease in pain from RT-induced oral mucositis and a reduction in both total surface area and the size of oral ulceration. Positive responses to benzydamine have been reported in three other studies (89,90). In a small prospective, double-blind, randomized study comparing the efficacy of chlorhexidine gluconate and benzydamine hydrochloride oral rinse in patients with head and neck cancer to prevent and to treat RT-induced oropharyngeal mucositis, a trend showed decrease in mucositis, oropharyngeal pain, and dysphagia in those receiving benzydamine (91).

Ariyawardana et al. reported from their review group for the 2019 MASCC/ISOO systematic review on 11 new papers and 5 interventions. They confirmed the existing guideline on the use of benzydamine mouthwash for prevention of oral mucositis in the RT setting for head and neck cancer (92). The review panel also recommended the use of benzydamine mouthwash for treatment in the RT setting for head and neck cancer.

BIOLOGIC RESPONSE MODIFIERS

Epidermal Growth Factors

Studies of epidermal growth factor (EGF) as a treatment option for CT- and RT-induced oral mucositis have reported conflicting data. EGF may function as a marker of mucosal damage and could facilitate the healing process (93). In a phase 1 trial conducted by Girdler et al. (94), EGF mouthwash used by patients treated with CT showed onset delay and severity reduction of recurrent ulcerations. No statistical difference was seen in resolution of established ulcers. A double-blind, placebo-controlled, prospective phase 2 study reported potential benefit from EGF oral spray for oral mucositis in patients treated with RT for head and neck cancer. One hundred and thirteen patients were randomized into one of four arms: EGF treatment groups (10, 50, and 100 µg/mL doses twice daily) and placebo. The 50 µg/mL dose showed the best efficacy (95). Kim et al. (96) evaluated efficacy and safety of recombinant human EGF (rhEGF) oral spray for CT-induced oral mucositis with HSCT. Fifty-eight patients were randomly assigned to either the rhEGF group or placebo group. The incidence of National Cancer Institute (NCI) assessment tool grade ≥2 oral mucositis was higher in rhEGF than placebo group (78.6% vs. 50%; $p = 0.0496$), respectively. Mucositis duration with the NCI assessment tool grade ≥2 was shorter in the rhEGF group (8.5 vs. 14.5 days).

rhEGF significantly reduced limitations in swallowing and drinking, and reduced hospitalization duration, administration of TPN, and opioid usage, in patients with grade ≥3. Results were better for patients with advanced oral mucositis in the rhEGF group for several secondary end points. The final analysis of this study was recently released (97). In this randomized, controlled phase 2 study, a total of 138 patients were enrolled; in the intention-to-treat analysis, rhEGF reduced neither the incidence of grade ≥2 oral mucositis ($p = 0.717$) nor its duration ($p = 0.725$); however, in the per-protocol analysis, the duration of use and cumulative dose of opioids was shorter in the rhEGF group ($p = 0.046$).

Hematopoietic Growth Factors

Hematologic growth factors are standard treatment for patients who are treated with high-dose CT because of their well-established efficacy to decrease the duration of CT-induced neutropenia. Gabrilove et al. (98) reported on 27 patients with bladder cancer who received escalating doses of granulocyte colony-stimulating factor (G-CSF) during treatment with methotrexate, vinblastine, doxorubicin, and cisplatin. The patients received the G-CSF during the first of two cycles of CT. Although significantly less oral mucositis was seen during cycle one of G-CSF, positive results may be biased related to possible cumulative CT toxicity with resultant increase in oral mucositis severity. Conversely, Bronchud et al. (99) reported from a study of 17 patients with breast or ovarian carcinoma treated with escalating doses of doxorubicin with G-CSF that G-CSF did not prevent severe oral mucositis. A third study compared clinical outcomes in 55 adult patients who received CT for non-Hodgkin's lymphoma and G-CSF with clinical outcomes in 39 patients who received CT alone. Patients who did not receive G-CSF had neutropenia as the primary cause of treatment delay compared with those patients who received G-CSF and experienced oral mucositis as the main cause of treatment delay (100). Granulocyte-macrophage colony-stimulating factor (GM-CSF) has demonstrated conflicting results in patients who received diverse cancer treatments (101–104). An open, randomized controlled phase 3 trial conducted by Masucci et al. (101) analyzed the efficacy of GM-CSF in patients with head and neck cancer who experienced RT-induced oral mucositis. A significant reduction in oral mucositis severity was observed in the GM-CSF treatment group. Conversely, results from a Radiation Therapy Oncology Group double-blind, placebo-controlled, randomized study ($N = 121$) designed to analyze efficacy and safety of GM-CSF in reducing severity and duration of oral mucositis and related pain in patients with head and neck cancer receiving RT (103), GM-CSF had no significant effect on severity or duration of oral mucositis. Raber-Durlacher et al. (105) systematically reviewed two randomized, controlled trials with GM-CSF mouthwashes and suggested against the use of GM-CSF mouthwash in the setting of high-dose CT followed by HSCT. This systematic review also examined the use of systemic GM-CSF and on the basis of five studies concluded that there was not enough evidence to recommend the use of systemic GM-CSF in patients receiving CT or RT.

Keratinocyte Growth Factors

Palifermin, a recombinant human keratinocyte growth factor and member of the fibroblast growth factor family, has shown efficacy in reducing oral mucosal injury related to CT (106). Spielberger et al. (106) reported from a double-blind study comparing the effect of palifermin with a placebo on development of oral mucositis in 212 patients with hematologic cancers. Palifermin or placebo was administered intravenously for 3 consecutive days immediately before initiating conditioning therapy with fractionated total-body radiation plus high-dose CT. The palifermin group had significant reductions in grade 4 oral mucositis, soreness of the mouth and throat, opioid use, and incidence of TPN use. Luthi et al. (107) reported lower grade 3 or 4 oral mucositis in 34 patients who received melphalan or BEAM with HSCT and were treated with palifermin (0.06 mg/kg) injections 3 days before conditioning CT and 3 days after HSCT compared with controls. Nasilowska-Adamska et al. (108) reported palifermin 60 µg/kg/d for 3 consecutive days before and after conditioning therapy for HSCT significantly reduced incidence, severity, and duration of oral mucositis in 106 patients. In a subsequent study (109), 53 patients with hematologic diseases used the same regimen and also showed a significant reduction in incidence and median duration of oral mucositis, decreased incidence of opioid and TPN use, and less prevalence of acute GVHD.

A randomized, placebo-controlled, double-blind study conducted by Le et al. (110) evaluated efficacy and safety of palifermin to reduce CT-induced oral mucositis in patients with locally advanced head and neck cancer. A total of 188 patients received palifermin (180 µg/kg) or placebo before chemoradiotherapy and then weekly for 7 weeks. The palifermin group showed a lower incidence of severe oral mucositis when compared with the placebo group (54% and 69%, $p = 0.041$). However, opioid use, average mouth and throat soreness, and chemoradiotherapy compliance were not significantly different between the treatment arms. After median follow-up of 26 months, overall survival and progression-free survival and other secondary outcomes such as opioid use were similar between the treatment arms.

A multicenter, double-blind, randomized study investigated the effectiveness of palifermin in reducing severe oral mucositis in patients with postoperative chemoradiotherapy for head and neck cancer (111). A total of 186 patients with carcinoma of the oral cavity, oropharynx, hypopharynx, or larynx (stages II to IVB) were randomly assigned to receive weekly palifermin (120 μg/kg) or placebo from 3 days before and throughout radiochemotherapy. Forty-seven of ninety two patients (51%) in the palifermin group developed severe oral mucositis versus 63 (67%) of 94 in the placebo group ($p = 0.027$). In addition, palifermin decreased the duration and prolonged the time to develop severe oral mucositis. Although palifermin reduced the occurrence of severe oral mucositis, its role in the management of patients with head and neck cancer undergoing postoperative chemoradiotherapy remains to be confirmed.

Palifermin has also been studied in patients with solid tumors. In a randomized controlled trial conducted by Rosen et al. (112), 64 patients with metastatic colorectal cancer who received 5-FU and leucovorin were randomized to receive palifermin (40 μg/kg) for 3 consecutive days before each of two cycles of CT. The incidence of oral mucositis WHO grade 2 or higher was significantly lower, and patients reported less severe symptoms in the treatment arm. Brizel et al. (113) compared palifermin (60 μg/kg) versus placebo in patients with locally advanced head and neck cancer treated with chemoradiation. Patients received two types of RT—standard (total dose of 70 Gy delivered in 2-Gy daily fractions) and hyperfractionated (total dose 72 Gy delivered in 1.25-Gy fractions twice a day for 7 weeks)—and CT including cisplatin (20 mg/m^2 for 4 days) and continuous infusion of 5-FU (1,000 mg/m^2/d for 4 days in weeks 1 and 5 of RT). Palifermin was well tolerated with decreased incidence of oral mucositis, dysphagia, and xerostomia in patients treated with hyperfractionated RT but not standard RT. However, palifermin did not reduce the morbidity of concurrent chemoradiotherapy.

A randomized, double-blind, placebo-controlled trial conducted by Vadhan-Raj et al. (114) evaluated efficacy of palifermin as a single dose before each cycle in patients receiving multicycle CT. Forty-four patients with sarcoma were randomized in a 2:1 ratio to receive palifermin (180 μg/kg), single dose 3 days before each CT cycle (maximum of six cycles), or placebo.

Palifermin decreased the incidence of moderate to severe mucositis (44% vs. 88%, $p < 0.001$) and severe mucositis (13% vs. 51%, $p = 0.002$). Reported adverse effects included thickening of oral mucosa and altered taste. Eighty-eight percent (seven of eight) patients with severe mucositis in the placebo group received palifermin in an open-label fashion. Palifermin as a single dose before each CT cycle reduced incidence and severity of oral mucositis in patients with sarcoma. In their systematic review of five randomized, controlled trials' results, Raber-Durlacher et al. (105) recommended the use of palifermin at a dose of ≥60 g/kg/d for 3 days prior to conditioning therapy and for 3 days after HSCT to prevent oral mucositis.

Antimicrobials

Antimicrobial approaches have included systemic administration of antibiotics, antivirals (acyclovir, valacyclovir, ganciclovir), antifungal (fluconazole), as well as, topical therapy. Donnelly et al. (115) evaluated the evidence base for the role of infection in the pathophysiology of oral mucositis through a comprehensive review of 31 prospective randomized trials. No clear pattern of patient type, cancer treatment, or type of antimicrobial agent used was reported, and there oral mucositis assessment was not consistent.

Oral candidiasis is a common acute and chronic oral sequela of head and neck RT. Lesions present as chronic removable white or nonmovable hyperplasia and also chronic diffused patchy erythema with angular cheilitis. Treatment approaches for oral candidiasis include mycostatin (troche; Bristol-Myers Squibb Company, New York, NY), nystatin (liquid or ointment), or clotrimazole. Pseudomembranous candidiasis is successfully treated topically. Chronic candidiasis usually requires much longer treatment, and it may be necessary to use oral ketoconazole, fluconazole, or intravenous amphotericin B.

Acyclovir prophylaxis is accepted treatment for HSV for patients who are cytomegalovirus seropositive and undergoing HSCT. A randomized controlled clinical trial in patients undergoing HSCT compared fluconazole with placebo and showed that fluconazole prevented systemic fungal infections (7% fluconazole vs. 18% placebo) and significantly reduced the incidence of mucosal infection and oropharyngeal colonization by *Candida albicans* (116).

Conflicting reports exist regarding chlorhexidine mouthwash for alleviating oral mucositis and reducing oral colonization by gram-positive, gram-negative, and *Candida* species in patients receiving CT, RT, or HSCT. Most studies have not demonstrated efficacy of chlorhexidine mouthwash for oral mucositis reduction in patients receiving intensive CT (117). Dodd et al. (118) tested the efficacy of the PRO-SELF Mouth Aware (PSMA) program combined with randomization to one of two mouthwashes (0.12% chlorhexidine or sterile water) for prevention of CT-related oral mucositis in 222 patients. Although chlorhexidine was no more effective than water for oral mucositis incidence, days to onset, and severity, the PSMA program appeared to reduce oral mucositis incidence. A double-blind, placebo-controlled, randomized study of chlorhexidine prophylaxis for 5-FU–based CT-induced oral mucositis in patients with gastrointestinal malignancies conducted by Sorensen et al. (119) suggested a role for chlorhexidine in prevention of oral mucositis. A total of 225 patients were randomized to chlorhexidine mouth rinse three times a day for 3 weeks versus placebo or cryotherapy with ice 45 minutes during CT. The frequency and duration of oral mucositis were significantly improved in the chlorhexidine and cryotherapy arms.

Sutherland and Browman (120) reviewed 59 studies assessing prophylaxis of RT-induced oral mucositis in patients with head and neck cancer. Interventions chosen based on the biologic etiology of oral mucositis were effective. Spijkervet et al. (121) evaluated efficacy of lozenges containing polymyxin E_2 2 mg, tobramycin 1.8 mg, and amphotericin B 10 mg taken four times daily for oropharyngeal flora related to oral mucositis. These researchers compared 15 patients receiving RT using polymyxin E_2 2 mg, tobramycin 1.8 mg, and amphotericin B 10 mg, and two other groups of 15 patients each, one using 0.1% chlorhexidine and the other using placebo. The selectively decontaminated group had significantly reduced oral mucositis severity and extent when compared with the chlorhexidine and placebo groups.

A randomized, double-blind study conducted by Sharma et al. (122) evaluated the effects of administering *Lactobacillus brevis* CD2 lozenges on incidence and severity of oral mucositis and tolerance to chemoradiotherapy in patients with head and neck squamous cell carcinoma. Two hundred patients received daily treatment with lozenge containing either *L. brevis* CD2 or placebo during and for 1 week after completion of chemoradiotherapy. Severe oral mucositis (grades 3 and 4) developed in 52% and 77% of patients in the treatment and placebo arms, respectively ($p < 0.001$). A significant difference in cancer treatment completion rates was seen among groups ($p = 0.001$). *L. brevis* CD2 lozenges were associated with a lower incidence of CT-/RT-induced severe oral mucositis and a higher rate of treatment completion.

Triclosan, an antibacterial agent used commonly in periodontal therapy, has also been evaluated in the management of RT-induced oral mucositis. Satheeshkumar et al. (123) conducted a randomized study to determine triclosan effectiveness in the management of RT-induced oral mucositis. Twenty-four patients with oral cancer with RT-induced grade 1 oral mucositis were randomized to either triclosan mouthwash (0.03%) or sodium bicarbonate (2 mg) mouthwash. Triclosan reduced progression to grade 4 oral mucositis in most patients. Triclosan mouthwash effectively reduced the severity of RT-induced oral mucositis.

Cryotherapy

Cryotherapy, which is administered as ice chips and flavored ice products, has been used to prevent oral mucositis and to improve patient's overall QOL by decreasing its severity and improving nutritional status. A 2015 Cochrane Review concluded that "...oral cryotherapy leads to large reduction in oral mucositis of all severities in adults receiving 5FU for solid cancers" (124). This review also stated that oral cryotherapy leads to an appreciable reduction in oral mucositis in adults receiving high-dose melphalan before HSCT (124).

Efficacy of cryotherapy for the reduction of 5-FU–induced oral mucositis severity was shown through a North Central Cancer Treatment Group and Mayo Clinic–sponsored controlled randomized trial (125). In contrast, a study with 178 patients who were randomized to 30 versus 60 minutes of oral cryotherapy reported similar severity of oral mucositis in both groups (126). This study recommended use of 30 minutes of oral cryotherapy prior to bolus administration of 5-FU–based CT. Additional studies have confirmed these results (127–129). Cryotherapy used to induce vasoconstriction should be considered for patients receiving 5-FU or melphalan (130) administered for short infusion times.

Effectiveness of aggressive oral care in combination with cryotherapy has also been evaluated. In a pilot randomized controlled study, 46 patients admitted for autologous HSCT were randomly assigned to the experimental arm ($n = 23$) receiving 1-hour oral cryotherapy or usual care ($n = 23$) (131). Overall mean of oral mucositis severity for the treatment arm was significantly lower than for the control arm: 0.43 versus 1.14, on a 0 to 4 scale ($p < 0.001$). The mean pain score in the treatment arm was significantly lower: 0.30 versus 1.64 ($p < 0.001$). Results suggest that oral cryotherapy + aggressive oral care protocols reduce oral mucositis and related oral pain intensity compared with oral care alone.

Use of intravenous opioids has become a common clinical practice for patients with CT- and RT-induced oral mucositis. Cryotherapy is an important adjuvant technique to opiate analgesia. A randomized controlled trial conducted by Svanberg et al. (132) showed that this technique may alleviate development of oral mucositis and related oral pain, resulting in decreased days and total dose of intravenous opiates in patients treated with autologous BMT.

Laser

Several studies have confirmed the effectiveness of low-energy laser for prevention and treatment of CT- or RT-induced oral mucositis (133–138). A phase 3 double-blind, placebo-controlled randomized study compared two different low level GaA1As diode lasers (650 and 780 nm) to prevent oral mucositis in patients undergoing HSCT treated with either CT or chemoradiotherapy (136). Seventy patients were randomized to treatment with 650 nm laser, 780 nm laser, or placebo. Low-level laser therapy was safe and more effective for decreasing oral mucositis and related oral pain. The efficacy of low-energy He/Ne laser was studied in a sample of 30 and 24 patients in two randomized controlled clinical trials (134,139). Low-energy He/Ne laser demonstrated a reduction in the severity and duration of oral mucositis.

In a triple-blinded randomized controlled trial conducted by Gautam et al. (140), prophylactic low-level laser therapy was tested to prevent CT-induced oral mucositis. A total of 221 patients with head and neck cancer scheduled to undergo chemoradiation were randomized into laser ($n = 111$) or placebo ($n = 110$) groups. The laser group received (HeNe) $\lambda = 632.8$ nm, power density = 24 mW, dosage = 3.0 J/point, total dosage/session = 36 to 40 J, spot size = 1 cm², five sessions per week; the placebo group received sham treatment daily prior to RT. In the laser group, there was significant reduction in incidence of severe oral mucositis ($p < 0.0001$), associated pain ($p < 0.0001$), dysphagia ($p < 0.0001$), and opioid use ($p < 0.0001$) when compared to the placebo group. These investigators also reported effect of low-level laser therapy to improve subjective experience of oral mucositis and QOL in patients with head and neck cancer (141).

Zadik et al. (142) reported from their review group for the 2019 MASCC/ISOO systematic review that the use of photobiomodulation for prevention of oral mucositis and related oral pain was recommended for patients treated with HSCT, and RT for head and neck cancer with and without CT.

Miscellaneous Agents

Tao et al. (143) reported on the use of a different heparin sulfate, RTG-OTD70DERM, in a multicenter, randomized, double-blind, placebo-controlled trial of 76 patients with head and neck cancers treated with RT. No significant difference was observed in the incidence and duration of grade ≥2 radiodermitis. Clinical trials testing whether heparin mimetics reduce oral mucositis are still needed.

A prospective, randomized, multicenter study conducted by Wu et al. (144) investigated the role of Actovegin (Nycomed Austria GmbH, Linz, Austria), a deproteinized extract of calf blood, in the prevention and treatment of CT-induced oral mucositis in patients with nasopharyngeal carcinoma. A total of 156 patients were randomized to receive Actovegin for prevention ($n = 53$) or treatment ($n = 51$) or to a control group ($n = 52$). Actovegin 30 mL/daily (5 days/week) was given for the duration of the radiotherapy for group 1 and from the onset of grade 2 mucositis for group 2. The incidence of grade 3 mucositis was lower in group 1 versus group 2 ($p = 0.002$), and group 2 had a lower progression rate of mucositis (grade 2 to 3) when compared to the placebo group ($p = 0.035$). Thus, Actovegin showed efficacy in the prevention and treatment of CT-/RT-induced oral mucositis.

Rhodiola algida, a traditional Chinese medicine widely used to stimulate the immune system, also has been tested as a treatment option for cancer patients with oral ulcers. Loo et al. (145) investigated the effect of *R. algida* on healthy lymphocytes in vitro, the homeostasis of patients with cancer, and the healing time of oral ulcers. A total of 462 subjects were treated with 100 μg/mL *R. algida* for 48 hours. Lymphocytes were isolated, and the level of several cytokines and mRNA content were determined. A total of 138 patients with breast cancer were randomized to receive *Rhodiola* (for 14 days after each cycle) and placebo after modified total mastectomy with adjuvant CT. *R. algida* favored the proliferation of lymphocytes, as well as, an increase of IL-2, IL-4, GM-CSF, and the mRNA content of these cytokines. The white blood cell count increased faster in the treatment group. The patients also presented with smaller and fewer oral ulcers. This study suggests that *R. algida* increases immunity of patients receiving adjuvant CT and decreases the quantity of oral ulcers.

Other therapies such as phenylbutyrate mouthwash and visible-light therapy have also mitigated oral mucositis during CT/RT in patients with head-and-neck cancer or in patients undergoing HSCT, respectively (146,147). Larger randomized trials are needed to confirm these results.

Treatment for Oral Chronic Graft Versus Host Disease

Almost all patients with extensive cGVHD require systemic immunosuppressive therapy. Thus, there is a critical need for adjuvant therapies that are both efficacious and avoid the long-term consequences of these corticosteroid therapies. In general, advances in the treatment of cGVHD have been modest, and no standard therapy exists for cGVHD that fails to respond to initial therapy or recurs. Granitto et al. (33), Imanguli et al. (148), and Mays et al. (149) have presented comprehensive reviews of available therapies for oral cGVHD. The most commonly recommended therapies for the management of mucosal involvement of oral cGVHD are topical high and ultrahigh potency corticosteroids, calcineurin inhibitors, and analgesics for related oral pain (149). The most common systemic therapy is corticosteroids with or without cyclosporine. Other agents such as tacrolimus, sirolimus, pentostatin, mycophenolate mofetil, and hydroxychloroquine have been used as salvage treatment (148). Emerging systemic therapies include monoclonal antibodies such as infliximab, etanercept, daclizumab, and rituximab (148,150). Extracorporeal photophoresis, a process that separates a patient's mononuclear cells through apheresis and exposes them to ultraviolet light A, has shown promise.

Patients with symptomatic disease limited to the oral cavity have benefited from topical steroids such as dexamethasone elixir (0.5 mg/mL) as a mouth rinse (10 mL) for 2 to 3 minutes at least four times daily (151). Clobetasol 0.05%, which is a topical high-potency steroid, has been administered four times daily for 2 to 3 weeks depending on the severity of the ulcerative oral cGVHD to decrease inflammation and oral pain. If local steroids alone are not adequate to control oral disease, then topical cyclosporine (152) or topical tacrolimus may be tried (153,154). Intraoral psoralen plus ultraviolet A irradiation may be appropriate based on the patient's condition (45). Although topical and local therapy for oral cGVHD offers several advantages to systemic therapy, including fewer side effects, there currently exists no evidence that one topical therapy is superior to another. Most trials have been open label with very small numbers of subjects. Oral topical treatments need further evaluation in multicenter randomized clinical trials such as reported by Elad et al. (155) who reported that a new mouthwash formulation using effervescent tablets of budesonide (3 mg/10 mL) improved oral cGVHD severity and reduced oral pain in all four treatment arms ($n = 18$).

St. John et al. (156) examined the efficacy of topical thalidomide gel 20 mg in patients with oral ulcerative cGVHD through a phase 2, randomized, placebo-controlled, double-blind clinical trial. Results suggested that topical thalidomide gel 20 mg has single-agent activity for oral ulcerative cGVHD. This therapy also decreased cGVHD-related oropharyngeal pain and decreased TNF-α and IL-6 expression levels in oral saliva and oral ulcer exudate.

A small randomized, double-blind, placebo-controlled pilot study was recently conducted to test the safety and efficacy of a clobetasol oral rinse in oral cGVHD at the NIH Clinical Center, Bethesda, Maryland (clinicaltrials.gov) (157). Subjects were randomized to clobetasol 0.05% rinse or placebo.

SYMPTOM MANAGEMENT

Oropharyngeal Pain

Oral mucositis is the principal etiology of most pain experienced during the 3-week post-HSCT time period. This pain is often described as the most unforgettable ordeal of HSCT. Oral mucositis–related oropharyngeal pain is multidimensional. The sensory dimension of this oral pain has been described with general mucosal inflammation and breakdown as ranging from mild discomfort to severe and debilitating pain, requiring opioids for pain management (56). Immunocompromised patients with cancer who are also HIV positive develop larger, more painful lesions than those experienced by patients without cancer. Oral pain associated with cGVHD has been described as severe, with symptoms of burning, irritation, dryness, and loss of taste being reported. In contrast to the often long-lasting oral pain with oral cGVHD, oral mucositis–related oral pain with CT is usually of <3 months' duration.

Sucralfate

Sucralfate is an aluminum salt of a sulfated disaccharide that has shown efficacy in the treatment of gastrointestinal ulcerations and has been tested as a mouthwash for the prevention and treatment of oral mucositis. Sucralfate creates a protective barrier at the ulcer site via the formation of an ionic bond to proteins. Study results with sucralfate are conflicting. A phase 3 study conducted by the North Central Cancer Treatment Group compared sucralfate suspension versus placebo for 5-FU–related oral mucositis. Results demonstrated that in the 50 patients who experienced oral mucositis, the sucralfate suspension provided no beneficial reduction in 5-FU–induced oral mucositis severity or duration and also had considerable additional gastrointestinal toxicity (158). Additionally, no efficacy was demonstrated for a sucralfate mouthwash for prevention and treatment of 5-FU–induced oral mucositis in a randomized controlled clinical trial with 81 patients with colorectal cancer who received either sucralfate suspension or placebo four times daily during their first cycle of 5-FU and leucovorin (159).

A prospective, double-blind study compared the effectiveness of sucralfate suspension to a formulation of diphenhydramine hydrochloride syrup plus kaolin-pectin for RT-induced oral mucositis in patients with head and neck cancer. Results showed no statistically significant differences between the two groups. In a study comparing outcomes between 21 patients who received standard oral care and 24 patients who received sucralfate suspension four times daily, the sucralfate group had a significant difference in mucosal edema, oral pain, dysphagia, and weight loss (160). Conversely, a double-blind, placebo-controlled study with sucralfate in 33 patients who received RT to the head and neck showed no statistically significant differences in oral mucositis (159). However, the sucralfate group did experience less oral pain and required a later start of topical and systemic analgesics throughout RT (161). Dodd et al. (162) used a pilot randomized controlled clinical trial to evaluate the efficacy of a micronized sucralfate mouthwash compared with a salt and soda mouthwash in 30 patients who received RT. All patients also used PSMA, which is a systematic oral hygiene program. Results demonstrated no significant difference in efficacy between the two groups.

The MASCC/ISOO Clinical Practice Guidelines now recommend that based on the evidence (a) sucralfate mouthwash not be used to treat oral mucositis in patients receiving CT or in patients receiving RT for head and neck cancer and (b) sucralfate not be used to prevent oral mucositis in patients receiving CT or RT for head neck cancer (163).

Gelclair

Gelclair (Sinclair Pharmaceuticals, Surrey, England) is a concentrated, bioadherent gel that has received US Food and Drug Administration approval as a 510(k) medical device indicated for the management of oral mucositis–related pain. Gelclair adheres to the oral surface, creating a protective barrier for irritated tissue and sensitized nociceptors. The safety and efficacy have been evaluated in small clinical trials with mixed results. Innocenti et al. (164) reported a 92% decrease in oral pain from baseline 5 to 7 hours after Gelclair administration in patients with oral mucositis, severe diffuse oral aphthous lesions, and postoral

surgery pain. More than half of these patients reported that the maximum effect of Gelclair lasted longer than 3 hours, and 87% of patients reported overall improvements from baseline for pain with swallowing food, liquids, and saliva following 1 week of treatment. DeCordi et al. (165) reported from a clinical study in which Gelclair was administered to patients with oral mucositis three times daily before meals as a 2- to 3-minute swish and spit for 3 to 10 days. Significant improvements were reported for pain, oral mucositis severity, and function. No adverse effects were reported during either trial. Patients reported that the taste, smell, texture, and use of Gelclair were acceptable. Barber et al. (166) conducted a prospective, randomized controlled trial comparing Gelclair versus standard therapy with sucralfate and oxethazaine (Mucaine, Wyeth, Dallas, TX) in patients with RT-induced oral mucositis. This study showed no significant difference between both therapies in terms of general pain. Gelclair can be an important adjuvant to opiate therapy in the management of oral mucositis–related oral pain, with the caveat that more research in the clinical setting is needed.

Anesthetic Cocktails

Anesthetic cocktails, composed of agents such as viscous lidocaine or dyclonine hydrochloride, have been used with some success for oral mucositis–related oral pain for temporary pain relief. These agents may alter taste perception, which may decrease oral intake. Other analgesics and mucosal-coating agents used for pain control include kaolin–pectin, diphenhydramine, Orabase (Colgate-Palmolive Company, New York, NY), and Oratect Gel (MGI Pharma, Woodcliffe Lake, NJ). Hospital-based pharmacies commonly formulate and dispense topical mixtures containing an analgesic, an anti-inflammatory agent, and a coating agent for use as an oral comfort measure for patients during cancer treatment. One large clinical research center uses a topical formulation containing viscous lidocaine 2% (40 mL), diphenhydramine 12.5 mg/5 mL (40 mL), and Maalox (Norvartis, Basel, Switzerland) 10 mg (40 mL) and prescribes its use every 3 to 4 hours as needed.

Doxepin

Doxepin is a tricyclic antidepressant used for many years in the management of patients with chronic benign or malignant pain. Its topical application is prescribed for pruritus and neuropathic pain. Pilot studies on topical doxepin rinse in patients with oral mucositis pain have shown adequate analgesia for up to 4 hours after application (167,168). Epstein et al. (169) assessed the effectiveness of oral doxepin rinse for oral mucositis–related pain in patients with head and neck cancer in the RT or HSCT setting. Nine patients rinsed with doxepin (5 mL) three to six times per day for 1 week and returned for a follow-up visit. Oral mucositis was scored using the OMAS and oral pain was assessed using a visual analog scale (VAS). There was a statistically significant reduction in VAS scores for 2 hours following doxepin rinse at the initial visit and also over a 1-week period, showing that repeated dosing continues to bring significant pain relief. Further randomized controlled trials are needed to confirm these results.

Opioids

Severe oral mucositis–related oropharyngeal pain may interfere with hydration and nutritional intake and affect QOL. Management of this pain may require use of opioids, often administered at high doses by patient-controlled analgesia pumps. Other routes of administration are oral, transmucosal, transdermal, and parenteral. The efficacy of oral transmucosal fentanyl citrate was compared with morphine sulfate immediate release in a randomized, controlled clinical trial for the treatment of breakthrough cancer pain in 134 adult ambulatory patients with cancer (170). Study results showed that oral transmucosal fentanyl was more effective than morphine sulfate immediate release in treating breakthrough pain. Darwish et al. (171) conducted a phase 1 open-label study to investigate the absorption profile of fentanyl buccal tablets in patients with or without oral mucositis. Sixteen patients (50% with oral mucositis) received a single 200 µg dose of fentanyl buccal tablet, which was well tolerated and showed a similar absorption profile within both groups. Transdermal fentanyl has also shown to be an effective, convenient, and well-tolerated treatment in patients with oral mucositis pain in the RT and in the HSCT setting (172,173).

Topical morphine for mucositis-related pain was evaluated in 26 patients following chemoradiation for head and neck cancer (169). Patients were randomized to morphine mouthwash (1 mL 2% morphine solution) or magic mouthwash (equal parts of lidocaine, diphenhydramine, and magnesium aluminum hydroxide). Patients in the morphine mouth group demonstrated both significantly shorter duration and lower intensity of oral pain than the magic mouthwash group. Swisher et al. (174) described an oral mucositis pain management algorithm to promote symptom management for patients undergoing HSCT who are transitioning from inpatient to ambulatory care. A key component of this successful program was use of a multidisciplinary team who could respond to the report of oral pain. No standard treatment

has been defined for the prevention or treatment of oral mucositis–related pain; thus, it is essential to continue clinical trials testing promising agents such as sublingual methadone, transdermal buprenorphine, and ketamine mouthwash (175–177).

Xerostomia

Xerostomia is a major negative sequela for patients who receive RT to the head and neck. Xerostomia severity depends on radiation dosage, location, and volume of exposed salivary glands. Significant xerostomia has not been shown with CT alone. The severity of xerostomia can affect oral comfort, fit of prostheses, speech, and swallowing. Many of the enzymes (mucin) found in patients with xerostomia contribute to the growth of caries-producing organisms. Oral hygiene regimens that include the use of water/saline and daily fluoride application with brushing teeth at least three times daily may reduce colonization of oral pathogens.

Treatment guidelines for the management of xerostomia are designed to increase patient comfort (178). Mercadante et al. reported from a 2017 systematic review and meta analysis of 1,732 patients from 20 studies that pilocarpine and cevimeline should be the first line of therapy in head and neck cancer survivors with RT-induced xerostomia and hyposalivation (179). Sialagogues have been investigated as stimulants for the residual salivary parenchyma (pilocarpine, 5- and 10-mg doses), with reported subjective improvement in some patients (180). Extreme caution with the use of pilocarpine is warranted because of reported side effects of glaucoma and cardiac problems. A randomized, controlled trial tested the efficacy of amifostine in a sample of 315 patients with head and neck cancer (181). The patients received standard fractionated radiation with or without amifostine, administered at 200 mg/m^2 as a 3-minute intravenous infusion 15 to 30 minutes before each treatment fraction. Patient eligibility criteria required that the radiation field encompassed at least 75% of both parotid glands. The Radiation Therapy Oncology Group Acute and Late Morbidity Score and Criteria was used to rate the severity of xerostomia. The incidence of grade ≥2 acute xerostomia (90 days from start of radiotherapy) and late xerostomia (9 to 12 months after radiotherapy) was significantly reduced in patients receiving amifostine. Whole saliva collection 1 year following RT showed in the amifostine group that more patients produced 0.1 g of saliva (72% vs. 49%) and that median saliva production was greater (0.26 g vs. 0.1 g). Stimulated saliva collections showed no difference between the treatment arms. Supporting these improvements in saliva production were subjects' reports of oral dryness. Artificial saliva has not demonstrated increased oral cavity comfort. Patients have reported subjective improvement in comfort levels through the frequent use of sugarless gum, mints, or candies.

REFERENCES

1. Raber-Durlacher JE, Elad S, Barasch A. Oral mucositis. *Oral Oncol.* 2010;46:452-456.
2. National Institutes of Health Consensus Development Panel. Consensus statement: oral complications of cancer therapies. *NCI Monogr.* 1989;9:3-8.
3. Cheng KK, Leung SF, Liang RH, et al. Severe oral mucositis associated with cancer therapy: impact on oral functional status and quality of life. *Support Care Cancer.* 2009;18:1477-1485.
4. Elting LS, Keefe DM, Sonis ST, et al. Patient-reported measurements of oral mucositis in head and neck cancer patients treated with radiotherapy with or without chemotherapy: demonstration of increased frequency, severity, resistance to palliation, and impact on quality of life. *Cancer.* 2008;113:2704-2713.
5. Barasch A, Peterson DE. Risk factors for ulcerative mucositis in cancer patients: unanswered questions. *Oral Oncol.* 2003;39:91-100.
6. Dodd MJ, Miaskowski C, Shiba GH, et al. Risk factors for CT-induced oral mucositis: dental appliances, oral hygiene, previous oral lesion, and a history of smoking. *Cancer Invest.* 1999;17:278-284.
7. Driezen S. Description and incidence of oral complications. *NCI Monogr.* 1990;9:11-15.
8. Grazziutti ML, Dong L, Miceli MH, et al. Oral mucositis in myeloma patients undergoing melphalan-based autologous stem cell transplantation: incidence, risk factors and a severity predictive model. *Bone Marrow Transplant.* 2006;38:501-506.
9. Vokurka S, Steinerova K, Karas M, et al. Characteristics and risk factors of oral mucositis after allogenic stem cell transplantation with FLU/MEL conditioning regimen in context with BU/CY2. *Bone Marrow Transplant.* 2009;44:601-605.
10. Blijlevens N, Schwenkglenks M, Bacon P, et al. Prospective oral mucositis audit: oral mucositis in patients receiving high-dose melphalan or BEAM conditioning chemotherapy—European Blood and Marrow Transplantation Mucositis Advisory Group. *J Clin Oncol.* 2008;26:1519-1525.
11. Cinausero M, Aprile G, Ermacora P, et al. New frontiers in the pathobiology and treatment of cancer regimen-related mucosal injury. *Front Pharmacol.* 2017;8:1-16.
12. Woo SB, Sonis ST, Monopoli MM, et al. A longitudinal study of oral ulcerative mucositis in bone marrow transplant recipients. *Cancer.* 1993;72:1612-1617.
13. Sonis ST. Mucositis as a biological process: a new hypothesis for the development of CT-induced stomatotoxicity. *Oral Oncol.* 1998;34:39-43.
14. McCann S, Schwenkglenks M, Bacon P, et al. The prospective oral mucositis audit: relationship of severe oral mucositis with clinical and medical resource use outcomes in patients receiving high-dose melphalan or BEAM-conditioning chemotherapy and autologous SCT. *Bone Marrow Transplant.* 2009;43:141-147.
15. Vera-Llonch M, Oster G, Ford CM, et al. Oral mucositis and outcomes of allogeneic hematopoietic stem-cell transplantation in patients with hematologic malignancies. *Support Care Cancer.* 2007;15:491-496.
16. Shih A, Miaskowshi C, Dodd MJ, et al. Mechanisms for radiation-induced oral mucositis and the consequences. *Cancer Nurs.* 2003;26:222-229.
17. Vera-Llonch M, Oster G, Hagiwara M, et al. Oral mucositis in patients undergoing radiation treatment for head and neck carcinoma: risk factors and clinical consequences. *Cancer.* 2006;106:329-336.
18. Elting LS, Cooksley CD, Chambers MS, et al. Risk outcomes, and costs of radiation-induced oral mucositis among patients with head-and-neck malignancies. *Int J Radiat Oncol Biol Phys.* 2007;68:1110-1120.
19. Murphy BA, Beaumont JL, Isitt J, et al. Mucositis-related morbidity and resource utilization in head and neck cancer patients receiving radiation therapy with or without chemotherapy. *J Pain Symptom Manage.* 2009;38:522-532.
20. Bentzen SM. Preventing or reducing late side effects of RT: radiobiology meets molecular pathology. *Nat Rev Cancer.* 2006;6:702-713.
21. Vissink A, Jansma J, Spijkervet FK, et al. Oral sequelae of head and neck radiotherapy. *Crit Rev Oral Biol Med.* 2003;14:199-212.
22. Merigo E, Manfredi M, Meleti M, et al. Jaw bone necrosis without previous dental extractions associated with the use of biphosphonates (pamidronate and zoledronate): a four-case report. *J Oral Pathol Med.* 2005;34:613-617.
23. Ruggiero SL, Mehrotra B, Rosenberg TJ, et al. Osteonecrosis of the jaws associated with the use of biphosphonates: a review of 63 cases. *J Oral Maxillofac Surg.* 2004;62:527-534.
24. Bowen J, Al-Dasooqi, Bossi P, et al. On behalf of the Mucositis Study Group of the Multinational Association of Supportive Care in Cancer/International Society of Oral Oncology (MASCC/ISOO). The pathogenesis of mucositis: updated perspectives and emerging targets. *Support Care Cancer.* 2019;27:4023-4033.
25. Vasconcelos RM, Sanfillippo N, Paster BJ, et al. Host-microbiome cross-talk in oral mucositis. *J Dent Res.* 2016;95:725-733.
26. Sonis ST. The pathobiology of mucositis. *Nat Rev Cancer.* 2004;4:277-284.
27. Ranna V, Cheng KKF, Castillo DA, et al. On behalf of the Mucositis Study group of the Multinational Association of Supportive Care in Cancer/International Society for Oral Oncology (MASCC/ISOO). Development of the MASCC/ISOO clinical practice guidelines for mucositis: an overview of the methods. *Support Care Cancer.* 2019;27:3933-3948.
28. Avivi I, Avraham S, Koren-Michowitz M, et al. Oral integrity and salivary profile in myeloma patients undergoing high-dose therapy followed by autologous SCT. *Bone Marrow Transplant.* 2009;43:801-806.
29. Fall-Dickson JM, Ramsay ES, Castro K, et al. Oral mucositis–related oropharyngeal pain and correlative tumor necrosis factor-a expression in adult oncology patients undergoing hematopoietic stem cell transplantation. *Clin Ther.* 2007;29:2547-2561.
30. Fall-Dickson JM, Pavletic SZ, Mays JW, Schubert MM. Oral complications of chronic graft-versus-host disease. *J Natl Cancer Inst Monogr.* 2019;53:lgz007. doi: 10.1093/jncimonographs/Igz00.
31. IMBRUVICA, US Prescribing Information. August 2017. https://www.accessdata.fda.gov/drugsatfda_docs/label/2017/205552s017lbl.pdf
32. Mays JW, Sarmadi M, Moutsopoulos NM. Oral manifestations of systemic autoimmune and inflammatory diseases: diagnosis and clinical management. *J Evid Based Dent Pract.* 2012;12:265-282.
33. Granitto MH, Fall-Dickson JM, Norton CK, et al. Review of therapies for the treatment of oral chronic graft-versus-host disease. *Clin J Oncol Nurs.* 2013;18:76-81.
34. Lloid ME. Oral medicine concerns of the BMT patient. In: Buchsel PC, Whedon MB, eds. *Bone Marrow Transplantation Administrative and Clinical Strategies.* Boston, MA: Jones and Bartlett; 1995:257.

35. Treister NS, Cook EF, Antin J, et al. Clinical evaluation of oral chronic graft-versus-host disease. *Biol Blood Marrow Transplant.* 2008;14:110-115.

36. Imanguli MM, Swaim WD, League SC, et al. Increased T-bet+ cytotoxic effectors and type 1 interferon-mediated processes in chronic graft-versus-host disease of the oral mucosa. *Blood.* 2009;113:3620-3630.

37. Fall-Dickson JM, Mitchell SA, Marden S, et al. Oral symptom intensity, health-related quality of life, and correlative salivary cytokines in adult survivors of hematopoietic stem cell transplantation with oral chronic graft-versus-host disease. *Biol Blood Marrow Transplant.* 2010;16:948-956.

38. Pavletic SZ, Martin P, Lee SJ, et al. Measuring therapeutic response in chronic graft-versus-host-disease: National Institutes of Health Consensus Development Project on Criteria for Clinical Trials in Chronic Graft-versus-Host Disease: IV. Response criteria working group report. *Biol Blood Marrow Transplant.* 2006;12:252-266.

39. Meier JK, Wolff D, Pavletic S, et al. Oral chronic graft-versus-host disease: report from the International Consensus Conference on clinical practice in cGVHD. *Clin Oral Investig.* 2011;15:127-139.

40. Treister NS, Stevenson K, Kim H, et al. Oral chronic graft-versus-host disease scoring using the NIH Consensus Criteria. *Biol Blood Marrow Transplant.* 2010;16:108-114.

41. Bassim CW, Fassil ZH, Mays JW, et al. Validation of the National Institutes of Health chronic GVHD oral mucosal score using component-specific measures. *Bone Marrow Transplant.* 2014;49:116-121.

42. McGuire DB, Altomonte V, Peterson DE, et al. Patterns of mucositis and pain in patients receiving preparative chemotherapy and bone marrow transplantation. *Oncol Nurs Forum.* 1993;20:1493-1502.

43. Fall-Dickson JM, Mock V, Berk RA, et al. Stomatitis-related pain in women with breast cancer undergoing autologous hematopoietic stem cell transplant. *Cancer Nurs.* 2008;31:452-461.

44. Schubert MM, Williams BE, Lloid ME, et al. Clinical assessment scale for the rating of oral mucosal changes associated with bone marrow transplantation. Development of an oral mucositis index. *Cancer.* 1992;69:2469-2477.

45. Vogelsang GB. How I treat chronic graft-versus-host disease. *Blood.* 2001;97:1196-1201.

46. Gaston-Johnasson F. Measurement of pain: the psychometric properties of the Pain-O-Meter, a simple, inexpensive pain assessment tool that could change health care practices. *J Pain Symptom Manage.* 1996;12:172-181.

47. Brand HS, Bots CP, Raber-Durlacher JE. Xerostomia and chronic oral complications among patients treated with haematopoietic stem cell transplantation. *Br Dent J.* 2009;207:E17.

48. Imanguli MM, Atkinson JC, Mitchell SA, et al. Salivary gland involvement by chronic graft-versus-host disease: prevalence, clinical significance and recommendations for evaluation. *Biol Blood Marrow Transplant.* 2010;16:1362-1369.

49. Nagler R, Barness-Hadar L, Lieba M, et al. Salivary antioxidant capacity in graft versus host disease. *Cancer Invest.* 2006;24:269-277.

50. Bassim CW, Ambatipudi KS, Mays JW, et al. Quantitative salivary proteomic differences in oral chronic graft-versus-host disease. *J Clin Immunol.* 2012;32:1390-1399.

51. Beumer J, Curtis, T, Morris LR. Radiation complications in edentulous patients. *J Prosthet Dent.* 1976;36:193-203.

52. Beumer J, Sung EC, Kagan R, et al. *Oral Management of Patients Treated with Radiation Therapy and/or Chemoradiation. Maxillofacial Rehabilitation: Prosthodontic and Surgical Management of Cancer-Related, Acquired and Congenital Defects of the Head and Neck.* 3rd ed. Quintessence Publishing Co, Inc: USA; 2011:1-59.

53. Margalit DN, Losi SM, Tishler RB, et al. Ensuring head and neck oncology patients receive recommended pretreatment dental evaluations. *J Oncol Pract.* 2015;11(2):151-154. doi: 10.1200/Jop.2014.000414.

54. National Cancer Institute; Division of Cancer Treatment & Diagnosis. *Cancer Therapy Evaluation Program: Common Terminology Criteria for Adverse Events (CTCAE) v5.0*; 2017. https://ctep.cancer.gov/protocolDevelopment/electronic_applications/ctc.htm

55. Eilers J, Berger AM, Petersen MC. Development, testing, and application of the oral assessment guide. *Oncol Nurs Forum.* 1988;15:325-330.

56. World Health Organization. *WHO Handbook for Reporting Results of Cancer Treatment. Offset Publication No. 48.* Geneva, Switzerland: World Health Organization; 1979:15.

57. Schubert MM, Sullivan KM, Morton TH, et al. Oral manifestations of chronic graft-versus-host disease. *Arch Intern Med.* 1984;144:1591-1595.

58. McGuire DB, Peterson DE, Muller S, et al. The 20 item oral mucositis index: reliability and validity in bone marrow and stem cell transplant patients. *Cancer Invest.* 2002;20:893-903.

59. Sonis ST, Eilers JP, Epstein JB, et al. Validation of a new scoring system for the assessment of clinical trial research of oral mucositis induced by radiation or CT. *Cancer.* 1999;85:2103-2113.

60. Sonis ST, Oster G, Fuchs H, et al. Oral mucositis and the clinical and economic outcomes of hematopoietic stem-cell transplantation. *J Clin Oncol.* 2001;19:2201-2205.

61. Elad S, Ackerstein A, Bitan M, et al. A prospective, double-blind phase two study evaluating the safety and efficacy of a topical histamine gel for the prophylaxis of oral mucositis in patients post hematopoietic stem cell transplantation. *Bone Marrow Transplant.* 2006;37:757-762.

62. Fall-Dickson JM, Cordes S, Berger AM. Management of adverse effects of treatment: oral complications. In: DeVita VT, Lawrence TS, Rosenberg SA, eds. *Cancer: Principles & Practice of Oncology.* 11th ed. Philadelphia, PA: Lippincott Williams & Wilkins; 2019.

63. Hong CHL, Gueiros LA, Fulton JS, et al. On behalf for the Mucositis Study Group of the Multinational Association of Supportive Care in Cancer/International Society for Oral Oncology. Systematic review of basic oral care for the management of oral mucositis in cancer patents and clinical practice guidelines. *Support Care Cancer.* 2019;27:3949-3967.

64. Rubenstein EB, Peterson DE, Schubert M, et al. Clinical practice guidelines for the prevention and treatment of cancer therapy-induced oral and gastrointestinal mucositis. *Cancer.* 2004;100:2026-2046.

65. Lalla RV, Bowen J, Barasch A, et al. MASCC/ISOO clinical practice guidelines for the management of mucositis secondary to cancer therapy. *Cancer.* 2014;120:1453-1461. doi: 10.1002/cncr.29174.

66. Wadleigh RG, Redman RS, Graham MI, et al. Vitamin E in the treatment of chemotherapy-induced mucositis. *Am J Med.* 1992;92:481-484.

67. Chaitanya NC, Muthukrishnan A, Babu DBG, et al. Role of vitamin E and vitamin A in oral mucositis induced by cancer chemo/radiotherapy—a meta-analysis. *J Clin Diagn Res.* 2017;11(5):ZE06-ZE09. doi: 10.7860/Jcdr/2017/26845.9905.

68. Osaki T, Ueta E, Yoneda K, et al. Prophylaxis of oral mucositis associated with chemoradiotherapy for oral carcinoma by Azelastine hydrochloride (azelastine) with other antioxidants. *Head Neck.* 1994;16:331-339.

69. Watanabe T, Ishihara M, Matsuura K. Polaprezinc prevents oral mucositis associated with radiochemotherapy in patients with head and neck cancer. *Int J Cancer.* 2010;127:1984-1990.

70. Mansouri A, Hadjibabaie M, Iravani M, et al. The effect of zinc sulfate in the prevention of high-dose chemotherapy-induced mucositis: a double-blind, randomized, placebo-controlled study. *Hematol Oncol.* 2012;30:22-26.

71. Sangthawan D, Phungrassami T, Sinkitjarurnchai W. A randomized double-blind, placebo-controlled trial of zinc sulfate supplementation for alleviation of radiation-induced oral mucositis and pharyngitis in head and neck cancer patients. *J Med Assoc Thai.* 2013;96:69-76.

72. Kouloulias V, Kouvaris JR, Kokakis JD, et al. Impact on cytoprotective efficacy of intermediate interval between amifostine administration and radiotherapy: a retrospective analysis. *Int J Radiat Oncol Biol Phys.* 2004;59:1148-1156.

73. Sasse AD, Clark LG, Sasse EC, et al. Amifostine reduces side effects and improves complete response rate during radiotherapy: results of a meta-analysis. *Int J Radiat Oncol Biol Phys.* 2006;64:784-791.

74. Spencer A, Horvath N, Gibson J, et al. Prospective randomised trial of amifostine cytoprotection in myeloma patients undergoing high-dose melphalan conditioned autologous stem cell transplantation. *Bone Marrow Transplant.* 2005;35:971-977.

75. Nicolatou-Galitis O, Sarri T, Bowen J, et al. Systematic review of amifostine for the management of oral mucositis in cancer patients. *Support Care Cancer.* 2013;21(1):357-364. doi: 10.1007/s00520-012-1613-6.

76. Savarese DM, Savy G, Vahdat L, et al. Prevention of chemotherapy and radiation toxicity with glutamine. *Cancer Treat Rev.* 2003;29:501-513.

77. Pytlik R, Benes P, Patorkova M, et al. Standardized parenteral alanyl-glutamine dipeptide supplementation is not beneficial in autologus transplant patients: a randomized, double-blind, placebo-controlled study. *Bone Marrow Transplant.* 2002;30:953-961.

78. Coughlin-Dickson TM, Wong RM, Negrin RS, et al. Effect of oral glutamine supplementation during bone marrow transplantation. *JPEN J Parenter Enteral Nutr.* 2000;24:61-66.

79. Anderson PM, Ramsey NK, Shy Xo, et al. Effect of low-dose oral glutamine on painful stomatitis during bone marrow transplantation. *Bone Marrow Transplant.* 1998;22:339-344.

80. Peterson DE, Jones JB, Pettit RG. Randomized, placebo-controlled trial of safaris for prevention and treatment of oral mucositis in breast cancer patients receiving anthracycline-based chemotherapy. *Cancer.* 2007;109:322-331.

81. Vidal-Casariego A, Calleja-Fernández A, Ballesteros-Pomar MD, et al. Efficacy of glutamine in the prevention of oral mucositis and acute radiation-induced esophagitis: a retrospective study. *Nutr Cancer.* 2013;65:424-429.

82. Aquino VM, Harvey AR, Garvin JH, et al. A double-blind randomized placebo-controlled study of oral glutamine in the prevention of mucositis in children undergoing hematopoietic stem cell transplantation: a pediatric blood and marrow transplant consortium study. *Bone Marrow Transplant.* 2005;36:611-616.

83. Yarom N, Hovan A, Bossi P, et al. On behalf of the Multinational Association of Supportive Care in Cancer/International Society for Oral Oncology. Systemic review of natural and miscellaneous agents for the management of oral mucositis in cancer patients and clinical practice guideline—part 1: vitamins, mineral and nutritional supplements. *Support Care Cancer.* 2019;27:3997-4010.

84. Lalla RV, Gordon GB, Schubert M, et al. A randomized, double-blind, placebo-controlled trial of misoprostol for oral mucositis secondary to high-dose chemotherapy. *Support Care Cancer.* 2012;20:1797-1804.

85. Porteder H, Rausch E, Kment G, et al. Local prostaglandin E2 in patients with oral malignancies undergoing chemo and radiotherapy. *J Craniomaxillofac Surg.* 1988;16:371-374.

86. Matejka M, Nell A, Kment G, et al. Local benefit of prostaglandin E2 in radioCT-induced oral mucositis. *Br J Oral Maxillofac Surg.* 1990;28:89-91.

87. Labor B, Mrsic M, Pavleric A, et al. Prostaglandin E2 for prophylaxis of oral mucositis following BMT. *Bone Marrow Transplant.* 1993;11:379-382.

88. Epstein JB, Stevenson-Moore P. Benzydamine hydrochloride in prevention and management of pain in mucositis associated with RT. *Oral Surg Oral Med Oral Pathol.* 1986;62:145-148.

89. Epstein JB, Silverman S, Paggiarino DA, et al. Benzydamine HCl for prophylaxis of radiation-induced oral mucositis: results from a multicenter, randomized, double-blind, placebo-controlled clinical trial. *Cancer.* 2001;92:875-885.

90. Epstein JB, Stevenson-Moore P, Jackson S, et al. Prevention of oral mucositis in RT: a controlled study with benzydamine hydrochloride rinse. *Int J Radiat Oncol Biol Phys.* 1989;16:1571-1575.

91. Kin-Fong Cheng K, Ka Tsui Yuen J. A pilot study of chlorhexidine and benzydamine oral rinses for the prevention and treatment of irradiation mucositis in patients with head and neck cancer. *Cancer Nurs.* 2006;29(5):423-430.

92. Ariyawardana A, Cheng KKF, Kandwal A, et al. On behalf of the Mucositis Study Group of the Multinational Association of Supportive Care in Cancer/International Society for Oral Oncology (MASCC/ISOO). Systematic review of anti-inflammatory agents for the management of oral mucositis in cancer patients and clinical practice guidelines. *Support Care Cancer.* 2019;27:3985-3995.

93. Hong JP, Lee SW, Song SY, et al. Recombinant human epidermal growth factor treatment of radiation-induced severe oral mucositis in patients with head and neck malignancies. *Eur J Cancer Care.* 2009;18:636-641.

94. Girdler NM, Mcgurk M, Aqual S, et al. The effect of epidermal growth factor mouthwash on cytotoxic-induced oral ulceration: a phase I clinical trial. *Am J Clin Oncol.* 1995;18:403-406.

95. Wu HG, Song SY, Kim YS, et al. Therapeutic effect of recombinant human epidermal growth factor (RhEGF) on mucositis in patients undergoing radiotherapy, with or without chemotherapy, for head and neck cancer: a double-blind, placebo-controlled prospective phase 2 multi-institutional clinical trial. *Cancer.* 2009;115:3699-3708.

96. Kim KI, Kim JW, Lee HJ, et al. Recombinant human epidermal growth factor on oral mucositis induced by intensive chemotherapy with stem cell transplantation. *Am J Hematol.* 2013;88:107-112.

97. Kim JW, Kim MG, Lee HJ, et al. Topical recombinant human epidermal growth factor for oral mucositis induced by intensive chemotherapy with hematopoietic stem cell transplantation: final analysis of a randomized, double-blind, placebo-controlled, phase 2 trial. *PLoS One.* 2017;12(1):e0168854. doi: ARTN e0168854.

98. Gabrilove JL, Jakubowski A, Scher H, et al. Effect of granulocyte colony-stimulating factor on neutropenia and associated morbidity due to CT for transitional-cell carcinoma of the urothelium. *N Engl J Med*. 1988;318:1414-1422.

99. Bronchud MH, Howell A, Crowther D, et al. The use of granulocyte colony-stimulating factor to increase the intensity of treatment with doxorubicin in patients with advanced breast and ovarian cancer. *Br J Cancer*. 1989;60:121-125.

100. Pettengell R, Gurney H, Radford JA, et al. Granulocyte colony-stimulating factor to prevent dose-limiting neutropenia in non-Hodgkin's lymphoma: a randomized controlled trial. *Blood*. 1992;80:1430-1436.

101. Masucci B, Broman P, Kelly C, et al. Therapeutic efficacy by recombinant human granulocyte/monocyte-colony stimulating factor on mucositis occurring in patients with oral and oropharynx tumors treated with curative radiotherapy: a multicenter open randomized phase III study. *Med Oncol*. 2005;22:247-256.

102. Mcaleese JJ, Bishop KM, A'Hern R, et al. Randomized phase II study of GM-CSF to reduce mucositis caused by accelerated radiotherapy of laryngeal cancer. *Br J Radiol*. 2006;79:608-613.

103. Ryu JK, Swann S, LeVeque F, et al. The impact of concurrent granulocyte macrophage-colony stimulating factor on radiation-induced mucositis in head and neck cancer patients: a double-blind placebo-controlled prospective phase III study by Radiation Therapy Oncology Group 9901. *Int J Radiat Oncol Biol Phys*. 2007;67:643-650.

104. Saarilahti K, Kajanti M, Joensuu T. Comparison of granulocyte-macrophage colony-stimulating factor and sucralfate mouthwashes in the prevention of radiation-induced mucositis: a double-blind prospective randomized phase III study. *Int J Radiat Oncol Biol Phys*. 2002;2:479-485.

105. Raber-Durlacher JE, von Bultzingslowen I, Logan RM, et al. Systematic review of cytokines and growth factors for the management of oral mucositis in cancer patients. *Support Care Cancer*. 2013;21(1):343-355. doi: 10.1007/s00520-012-1594-5.

106. Spielberger R, Stiff P, Bensinger W, et al. Palifermin for oral mucositis after intensive therapy for hematologic cancers. *N Engl J Med*. 2004;351:2590-2598.

107. Luthi F, Berwert L, Frosasard V. Prevention of oral mucositis with palifermin in patients treated with high-dose CT and autologous stem cell transplantation: a single center experience. *Blood*. 2006;108:843.

108. Nasilowska-Adamska B, Rzepecki P, Manko J, et al. The significance of palifermin (Kepivance) in reduction of oral mucositis (OM) incidence and acute graft versus host disease (aGVHD) in a patient with hematological disease undergoing HSCT. *Blood*. 2006;108:840.

109. Nasilowska-Adamska B, Rzepecki P, Manko J, et al. The influence of palifermin (Kepivance) on oral mucositis and acute graft versus host disease in patients with hematological diseases undergoing hematopoietic stem cell transplantation. *Bone Marrow Transplant*. 2007;40:983-988.

110. Le QT, Kim HE, Schneider CJ, et al. Palifermin reduces severe mucositis in definitive chemoradiotherapy of locally advanced head and neck cancer: a randomized, placebo-controlled study. *J Clin Oncol*. 2011;29:2808-2814.

111. Henke M, Alfonsi M, Foa P, et al. Palifermin decreases severe oral mucositis of patients undergoing postoperative radiochemotherapy for head and neck cancer: a randomized, placebo-controlled trial. *J Clin Oncol*. 2011;29:2815-2820.

112. Rosen LS, Abdi E, David ID, et al. Palifermin reduces the incidence of oral mucositis in patients with metastatic colorectal cancer treated with fluorouracil-based chemotherapy. *J Clin Oncol*. 2006;24:5194-5200.

113. Brizel DM, Murphy BA, Rosenthal DI, et al. Phase II study of palifermin and concurrent chemoradiation in head and neck squamous cell carcinoma. *J Clin Oncol*. 2008;26:2489-2496.

114. Vadhan-Raj S, Trent J, Patel S, et al. Single-dose palifermin prevents severe oral mucositis during multicycle chemotherapy in patients with cancer: a randomized trial. *Ann Intern Med*. 2010;153:358-367.

115. Donnelly JP, Bellm LA, Epstein JB, et al. Antimicrobial therapy to prevent or treat oral mucositis. *Lancet Infect Dis*. 2003;3:405-412.

116. Slavin MA, Osborne B, Adams R, et al. Efficacy and safety of fluconazole prophylaxis for fungal infections after marrow transplantation—a prospective, randomized, double-blind study. *J Infect Dis*. 1995;171:1545-1552.

117. Wahlin BY. Effects of chlorhexidine mouth rinse on oral health in patients with acute leukemia. *Oral Surg Oral Med Oral Pathol*. 1989;68:279-287.

118. Dodd MJ, Larson PL, Dibble SL, et al. Randomized clinical trial of chlorhexidine versus placebo for prevention of oral mucositis in patients receiving chemotherapy. *Oncol Nurs Forum*. 1996;23:921-927.

119. Sorensen JB, Skovsgaard T, Bork E, et al. Double-blind, placebo-controlled, randomized study of chlorhexidine prophylaxis for 5-fluorouracil-based chemotherapy-induced oral mucositis with non-blinded randomized comparison to oral cooling (cryotherapy) in gastrointestinal malignancies. *Cancer*. 2008;112:1600-1606.

120. Sutherland SE, Browman GP. Prophylaxis of oral mucositis in irradiated head-and-neck cancer patients: a proposed classification scheme of interventions and meta-analysis of randomized controlled trials. *Int J Radiat Oncol Biol Phys*. 2001;4:917-930.

121. Spijkervet FK, Saene HK, van Saene JJ, et al. Effect of selective elimination of the oral flora on mucositis in irradiated head and neck cancer patients. *J Surg Oncol*. 1991;46:167-173.

122. Sharma A, Rath GK, Chaudhary SP, et al. Lactobacillus brevis CD2 lozenges reduce radiation- and chemotherapy-induced mucositis in patients with head and neck cancer: a randomized double-blind placebo-controlled study. *Eur J Cancer*. 2012;48:875-881.

123. Satheeshkumar PS, Chamba MS, Balan A, et al. Effectiveness of triclosan in the management of radiation-induced oral mucositis: a randomized clinical trial. *J Cancer Res Ther*. 2010;6:466-472.

124. Riley P, Glenny AM, Worthington HV, Littlewood A, Clarkson JE, McCabe MG. Interventions for preventing oral mucositis in patients with cancer receiving oral cryotherapy (Review). *Cochrane Database Syst Rev*. 2015;(12):CD011552.

125. Mahoud DJ, Dose AM, Loprinzi CL, et al. Inhibition of fluorouracil-induced stomatitis by oral cryotherapy. *J Clin Oncol*. 1991;9:449-452.

126. Rocke LK, Loprinzi CL, Lee JK, et al. A randomized clinical trial of two different durations of oral cryotherapy for prevention of 5-FU–related stomatitis. *Cancer*. 1993;72:2234-2238.

127. Cascinu S, Fedeli A, Fedeli SL, et al. Oral cooling (cryotherapy), an effective treatment for the prevention of

5-FU–induced stomatitis. *Eur J Cancer B Oral Oncol.* 1994;30:234-236.

128. Papadeas E, Naxakis S, Riga M, et al. Prevention of 5-fluorouracil–related stomatitis by oral cryotherapy: a randomized controlled study. *Eur J Oncol Nurs.* 2007;11:60-65.

129. Katrancı N, Ovayolu N, Ovayolu O, et al. Evaluation of the effect of cryotherapy in preventing oral mucositis associated with chemotherapy—a randomized controlled trial. *Eur J Oncol Nurs.* 2012;16:339-344.

130. Lilleby K, Garcia P, Gooley T, et al. A prospective, randomized study of cryotherapy during administration of high-dose melphalan to decrease the severity and duration of oral mucositis in patients with multiple myeloma undergoing autologous peripheral blood stem cell transplantation. *Bone Marrow Transplant.* 2006;37:1031-1035.

131. Salvador P, Azusano C, Wang L, et al. A pilot randomized controlled trial of an oral care intervention to reduce mucositis severity in stem cell transplant patients. *J Pain Symptom Manage.* 2012;44: 64-73.

132. Svanberg A, Birgegård G, Öhrn K. Oral cryotherapy reduces mucositis and opioid use after myeloablative therapy: a randomized controlled trial. *Support Care Cancer.* 2007;15:1155-1161.

133. Bensadoun RJ, Ciais G. Radiation- and chemotherapy-induced mucositis in oncology: results of multicenter phase III studies. *J Oral Laser Appl.* 2002;2:115-120.

134. Bensadoun RJ, Ciais G, Schubert MM, et al. Low-energy He/Ne laser in the prevention of radiation-induced mucositis. A multicenter phase III randomized study in patients with head and neck cancer. *Support Care Cancer.* 1999;7:244-252.

135. Cowen D, Tardieu C, Schubert M, et al. Low energy helium-neon laser in the prevention of oral mucositis in patients undergoing bone-marrow transplant: results of a double-blind randomized trial. *Int J Radiat Oncol Biol Phys.* 1997;38:697-703.

136. Borst GR, Sonke JJ, den Hollander S, et al. Clinical results of image-guided deep inspiration breath hold breast irradiation. *Int J Radiat Oncol Biol Phys.* 2010;78:1345-1351.

137. Genot-Klastersky MT, Klastersky J, Awada F, et al. The use of lower-energy laser (LEL) for the prevention of chemotherapy- and/or radiotherapy-induced oral mucositis in cancer patients: results from two prospective studies. *Support Care Cancer.* 2008;16:1381-1387.

138. Zanin T, Zanin F, Carvalhosa AA, et al. Use of 660-nm diode laser in the prevention and treatment of human oral mucositis induced by radiotherapy and chemotherapy. *Photomed Laser Surg.* 2010;26:233-237.

139. Arora H, Pai KM, Maiya A, et al. Efficacy of He-Ne Laser in the prevention and treatment of radiotherapy-induced oral mucositis in oral cancer patients. *Oral Surg Oral Med Oral Pathol Oral Radiol Endod.* 2008;105:180-186.

140. Gautam AP, Fernandes DJ, Vidyasagar MS, et al. Effect of low-level laser therapy on patient reported measures of oral mucositis and quality of life in head and neck cancer patients receiving chemoradiotherapy— a randomized controlled trial. *Support Care Cancer.* 2013;21:1421-1428.

141. Gautam AP, Fernandes DJ, Vidyasagar MS, et al. Low level laser therapy for concurrent chemoradiotherapy induced oral mucositis in head and neck cancer patients a triple blinded randomized controlled trial. *Radiother Oncol.* 2012;104:349-354.

142. Zadik Y, Arany PR, Fregnani ER, et al. Systematic review of photobiomodulation for the management of oral mucositis in cancer patients and clinical practice guidelines. *Support Care Cancer.* 2019;27:3969-3983.

143. Tao YG, Auperin A, Sire C, et al. Multicenter randomized double-blind, placebo-controlled trial GORTEC (Groupe Oncologie Radiotherapie Tete et Cou) 2009-01 evaluating the effect of the regenerating agent on radiodermatitis of head and neck cancer patients. *Int J Radiat Oncol Biol Phys.* 2017;99(3):590-595. doi: 10.1016/j.ijrobp.2017.07.019.

144. Wu SX, Cui TT, Zhao C, et al. A prospective, randomized, multi-center trial to investigate Actovegin in prevention and treatment of acute oral mucositis caused by chemoradiotherapy for nasopharyngeal carcinoma. *Radiother Oncol.* 2010;97:113-118.

145. Loo WT, Jin LJ, Chow LW, et al. Rhodiola algida improves chemotherapy-induced oral mucositis in breast cancer patients. *Expert Opin Investig Drugs.* 2010;19:S91-S100.

146. Elad S, Luboshitz-Shon N, Cohen T, et al. A randomized controlled trial of visible-light therapy for the prevention of oral mucositis. *Oral Oncol.* 2011;47:125-130.

147. Yen SH, Wang LW, Lin YH, et al. Phenylbutyrate mouthwash mitigates oral mucositis during radiotherapy or chemoradiotherapy in patients with head-and-neck cancer. *Int J Radiat Oncol Biol Phys.* 2012;82:1463-1470.

148. Imanguli M, Pavletic SZ, Guadagnini JP, et al. Chronic graft versus host disease of oral mucosa: review of available therapies. *Oral Surg Oral Med Oral Pathol Oral Radiol Endod.* 2006;101:175-183.

149. Mays JW, Fassil H, Edwards DA, et al. Oral chronic graft-versus-host disease: current pathogenesis, therapy, and research. *Oral Dis.* 2013;9:327-346.

150. Zaja F, Bacigalupo A, Patriarca F, et al. Treatment of refractory chronic GVHD with rituximab: a GITMO study. *Bone Marrow Transplant.* 2007;40:273-277.

151. Wolff D, Anders V, Corio R, et al. Oral PUVA and topical steroids for treatment of oral manifestations of chronic graft-vs-host disease. *Photodermatol Photoimmunol Photomed.* 2004;20:184-190.

152. Epstein JB, Reece DE. Topical cyclosporine A for treatment of oral chronic graft-versus-host disease. *Bone Marrow Transplant.* 1994;13:81-86.

153. Albert MH, Becker B, Schuster FR, et al. Oral graft vs host disease in children: treatment with topical tacrolimus ointment. *Pediatr Transplant.* 2007;11:306-311.

154. Eckardt A, Starke O, Stadler M, et al. Severe oral chronic graft-versus-host disease following allogenic bone marrow transplantation: highly effective treatment with topical tacrolimus. *Oral Oncol.* 2004;40:811-814.

155. Elad S, Zeevi I, Finke ZJ, et al. Improvement in oral chronic graft-versus-host disease with the administration of effervescent tablets of topical budesonide—an open, randomized, multicenter study. *Biol Blood Marrow Transplant.* 2012;18:134-140.

156. St.John L, Gordon SM, Childs R, et al. Topical thalidomide gel in oral chronic GVHD, and role of *in situ* cytokine expression in monitoring biological activity. *Bone Marrow Transplant.* 2013;48:610-611.

157. National Institutes of Health Clinical Center, National Cancer Institute. Clobetasol for oral graft-versus-host disease. http://clinicaltrials.gov/ct2/show/NCT01557517

158. Loprinzi CL, Ghosh C, Camoriani J, et al. Phase III controlled evaluation of sucralfate to alleviate stomatitis in patients receiving fluorouracil-based CT. *J Clin Oncol.* 1997;15:1235-1238.

159. Nottage M, McLachlan SA, Brittain MA, et al. Sucralfate mouthwash for prevention and treatment of 5-FU–induced mucositis: a randomized, placebo-controlled trial. *Support Care Cancer*. 2003;11:41-47.

160. Scherlacher A, Beaufort-Spontin E. Radiotherapy of head-neck neoplasms: prevention of inflammation of the mucosa by sucralfate treatment. *HNO*. 1990;38:24-28.

161. Epstein JB, Wong FLW. The efficacy of sucralfate suspension in the prevention of oral mucositis due to RT. *Int J Radiat Oncol Biol Phys*. 1994;28:693-698.

162. Dodd M, Miaskowski C, Greenspan D. Radiation-induced mucositis: a randomized clinical trial of micronized sucralfate versus salt and soda mouthwashes. *Cancer Invest*. 2003;21:21-33.

163. Kubota K, Kobayashi W, Sakaki H, et al. Professional oral health care reduces oral mucositis pain in patients treated by superselective intra-arterial chemotherapy concurrent with radiotherapy for oral cancer. *Support Care Cancer*. 2015;23:3323-3329.

164. Innocenti M, Moscatelli G, Lopez S. Efficacy of Gelclair in reducing pain in palliative care patients with oral lesions. Preliminary findings from an open pilot study. *J Pain Symptom Manage*. 2001;24:456-457.

165. DeCordi SD, Giorgutti E, Martina S, et al. Gelclair: potentially an efficacious treatment for CT-induced mucositis. *Proceedings from the Italian Anti-tumor League III Congress of Professional Oncology Nurses*. October 10-12, 2001, Congliano, Italy (abst).

166. Barber C, Powell R, Ellis A, et al. Comparing pain control and ability to eat and drink with standard therapy vs Gelclair: a preliminary, double centre, randomised controlled trial on patients with radiotherapy-induced oral mucositis. *Support Care Cancer*. 2007;15:427-440.

167. Epstein JB, Truelove EL, Oien H, et al. Oral topical doxepin rinse: analgesic effect in patients with oral mucosal pain due to cancer or cancer therapy. *Oral Oncol*. 2001;37:632-637.

168. Epstein JD, Epstein JB, Epstein MS, et al. Oral topical doxepin rinse: analgesic effect and duration of pain reduction in patients with oral mucositis due to cancer therapy. *Anesth Analg*. 2006;103:465-470.

169. Epstein JB, Epstein JD, Epstein MS, et al. Doxepin rinse for management of mucositis pain in patients with cancer: one week follow-up of tropical therapy. *Spec Care Dentist*. 2009;28:73-77.

170. Coluzzi PH, Schwartzberg L, Conroy JD, et al. Breakthrough cancer pain: a randomized trial comparing oral transmucosal fentanyl (OTFC) and morphine sulfate immediate release (MSIR). *Pain*. 2001;91:123-130.

171. Darwish M, Kirby M, Robertson P, et al. Absorption of fentanyl from fentanyl buccal tablet in cancer patients with or without oral mucositis. *Clin Drug Investig*. 2007;27:605-611.

172. Kim JG, Sohn SK, Kim DH, et al. Effectiveness of transdermal fentanyl patch for treatment of acute pain due to oral mucositis in patients receiving stem cell transplantation. *Transplant Proc*. 2005;37:4488-4491.

173. Cerchietti LC, Navigante AH, Bonomi MR, et al. Effect of topical morphine for mucositis-associated pain following concomitant chemoradiotherapy for head and neck cancer. *Cancer*. 2002;95:2230-2236.

174. Swisher ME, Scheidler VR, Kennedy MJ. A mucositis pain management algorithm: a creative strategy to enhance the transition to ambulatory care. *Oncol Nurs Forum*. 1998.

175. Gupta A, Duckles B, Giordano J. Use of sublingual methadone for treating pain of chemotherapy-induced oral mucositis. *J Opioid Manag*. 2010;6:67–69..

176. Joseph-Ryan A, Lin F, Samady R. Ketamine mouthwash for mucositis pain. *J Palliat Med*. 2009;12:989–991..

177. Huscher A, De Stefani A, Smussi I. Transdermal buprenorphine for oropharyngeal mucositis–associated pain in patients treated with radiotherapy for head and neck cancer. *J Palliat Med*. 2010;13:357–358.

178. Atkinson JC, Grisius M, Massey W. Salivary hypofunction and xerostomia: diagnosis and treatment. *Dent Clin North Am*. 2005;49:309–326.

179. Mercadante, V., Hamad, A.A., Lodi, G., Porter, S., Fedele, S. (2017). Interventions for the management of radiotherapy-induced xerostomia and hyposalivation: a systematic review and meta-analysis. *Oral Oncology*. 2017;66:64–74.

180. Agha-Hosseini F, Mirzaii-Dizgah I, Ghavamzadeh L, et al. Effect of pilocarpine hydrochloride on unstimulated whole saliva flow rate and composition in patients with chronic graft-versus-host disease (cGVHD). *Bone Marrow Transplant*. 2007;39:431–434.

181. Brizel DM, Wasserman TH, Strnad V, et al. Final report of a phase III randomized trial of amifostine as a radioprotectant in head and neck cancer. Proceedings of the American Society for Therapeutic Radiology and Oncology 41st Annual Meeting. *Int J Red One Biol Phys*. 1999, San Antonio, Texas, Oct. 31–Nov. 4, Texas. (abst).

19 Pruritus

Ivy Akid and Ambereen K. Mehta

PRURITUS

The Latin term "prurire" means "burning." In patients with cancer, pruritus may be attributable to a primary skin disease, a coexisting medical condition, medication adverse effect, or the cancer itself. It can significantly diminish patient quality of life as much as the sensation of pain can in palliative care patients. Physician awareness of its importance and skilled management may relieve patients of additional physical and emotional burden and distress. This chapter reviews the etiologies, diagnostic workup, and management of clinical pruritus. To quote Krajnik and Zylicz, "There is no one cure for all pruritic symptoms. Better understanding of mechanisms of pruritus may help develop better treatments" (1).

PRURITUS SENSATIONS

In simple terms, pruritus is the sensation that provokes scratching. It can be categorized as acute or chronic and graded between mild and intractable. Chronic itch is a state of persistent itch in which the cause cannot be removed or treated. It can be mild or persistent. Objective analysis often cannot easily confirm the presence or severity of pruritus. Nevertheless, patients are generally thought to be reliable in their assessment of pruritus severity. Scratch marks (excoriations), skin thickening (lichenification), and other visible cutaneous sequelae of the subjective sensation often support patients' subjective complaints on physical exam.

In addition to, or in lieu of, classic itch descriptions of the sensation include burning, stinging, tingling, tickling, or a crawling sensation. These descriptions have similar pathogenic mechanisms and therefore are treated identically. Bernhard summarized this notion by stating "one man's itch is another man's tickle… one man's sting is another man's pain." (2) Itch is readily distinguished from pain and many patients with severe pruritus would prefer pain instead. Perhaps more importantly, evidence suggests that itch degrades quality of life and may also negatively impact survival as well. For example, pruritus in patients on hemodialysis may be associated with poor sleep quality and a 17% higher mortality rate (3). Severe pruritus may also portend poor prognosis such as in Hodgkin's disease (4).

Pruritus is a distinct, complex sensation considered to be a primary sensory modality (5). Itch was reclassified into several overlapping categories in a recently published paper from the International Forum for the Study of Itch. They grouped it into several overlapping categories in an attempt to optimize diagnosis and treatment of itch. They envisioned three groups of conditions: (a) pruritus on inflamed skin; (b) pruritus on noninflamed skin; and (c) pruritus presenting with severe secondary skin changes. Any underlying disease is thus defined as a dermatologic disease, neurologic disease, a systemic disease, or a psychiatric disease. These underlying diseases are likely to drive the sensation of itch.

MECHANISMS

The cause of human itch can be divided into four groups: (a) `pruritoceptive (dermatological); (b) neurogenic (systemic); (c) neuropathic; and (d) psychogenic mechanisms. Pruritoceptive itch occurs from the cellular layers of the skin and produces a somatic sensation of itch. This is the most common cause of pruritus in dermatology and histamine is its most explored pruritogen. Neurogenic itch originates from organs other than the skin without peripheral nerve damage. Neurogenic itch is linked to hematological disease, hepatobiliary disease, and chronic kidney disease. Neuropathic itch refers to itch of neuronal origin and is due to damaged central afferent nerves or peripheral afferent nerves. This type of itch is often accompanied by localized neuropathic symptoms. Psychogenic itch is a diagnosis of exclusion in the presence of mental health symptoms (6).

While new data on the origin and propagators of itch are constantly being elucidated, it is known that at least a portion of the cutaneous itch response is carried by unique sensory histamine-sensitive mechano-insensitive C fibers (7). These unmyelinated fibers carry pruritic sensations along the spinothalamic tract to the thalamus and subthalamus. Experimental injections of histamine into the skin induced itch or pain and systemic antihistamine administration suppressed itch or pain (8). Electrophysiologically, pain receptors and itch fibers can be clearly distinguished from one another, in spite of their nearly identical histologic characteristics. Even still, the way in which they exert their phenotypic responses shows considerable commonality. For example, patients with chronic itch have shown an increase in skin innervation and central sensitization of itch-signaling spinal neurons in the same way that patients with chronic pain have been found to have central sensitization of nerve endings (9,10).

Histamine alone is unable to explain the myriad of situations in which itch occurs. Many patients with pruritus do not demonstrate signs of histamine release such as cutaneous wheal and flare. Additionally, the histamine pathway cannot explain itch caused by mechanical properties. Many pruritic conditions do not improve with antihistamines, which further suggest that histamine may only be a minor pruritus mediator. Therefore, other elements such as cytokines and neuropeptides may cause a substantial portion of pruritus (11,12). Recent evidence suggests opiates, serotonin, prostaglandins, kinins, proteases, other neuropeptides, and physical stimuli all contribute to pruritus. Tumor necrosis factor-α (TNF-α), though it may not have a direct pruritogenic effect, is elevated in many diseases that are characteristically associated with itch (13). Similarly, patients with prurigo nodularis have been found to have increased expression of TRPV1, a vanilloid receptor (14). Protease-activated receptor 2 (PAR-2) is a specific receptor on primary afferent nerves that has been found to be elevated in patients with atopic dermatitis (15). Each of these agents can trigger pruritus independently or through a secondary mediator.

Another pathway causing itch was described in the 1950s. The seed pods of the tropical plant *Mucuna pruriens* was used to produce an itch powder called cowhage, which contains the protease mucunain (16). It causes itch without any associated flare with what has since been identified to be an erythematous reaction transmitted by mechano-insensitive C fibers (17). Recently, it was discovered that mucunain induces itch by activating a group of "polymodal" C fibers that respond to mechanical stimuli rather than histamine. This supports a distinctly different population of C fibers from those triggered by histamine, which when stimulated result in the same end result of itch (18,19). It is not yet fully understood what the role of this alternate pathway is though there is speculation that "polymodal" C fibers are the most frequent type of afferent C fibers in human skin

nerves (20). Any advances in our understanding of the propagators of itch bring about hope for novel potential treatments for pruritus.

Pruritic sensations may also arise within the central nervous system (CNS). This pathway is thought to occur following the use of opioids, which have been known to induce pruritus, as well as opioid antagonists, which have been used to decrease pruritus in liver diseases (21,22). Administration of exogenous opioids at spinal levels in spinal anesthesia may relieve pain but stimulate itching (23). Plasma removed from patients with cholestatic itching and injected into murine models leads to scratching behavior that can be abolished with administration of the opioid receptor antagonist naloxone hydrochloride (24). Clinical conditions such as phantom limb itch after mastectomy are thought to be the result of centrally mediated insults (25–27).

DERMATOLOGIC DISEASES AND PRURITUS

Pruritus is a common manifestation of several skin diseases. The most common skin disease to cause pruritus is xerosis, or dry skin. Patients with cancer who have undergone chemotherapy, radiation therapy, or experienced weight loss with dramatic loss of subcutaneous fat may experience this. Xerosis can also cause the skin to become more sensitive, making it susceptible to irritation from environmental assault propagating the cycle (28).

A wide array of dermatologic diseases presents with pruritus symptomatology including scabies, atopic dermatitis, dermatitis, bullous pemphigoid, miliaria, pediculosis, urticaria, and dermatitis herpetiformis (29). A thorough history and physical examination are key to diagnosing and treating pruritus. Signs of systemic diseases may be subtle or nonspecific, particularly in the immunocompromised host. A notable example published as a case report showed eczema and intense pruritus as the first sign of acute myeloid leukemia (AML). The patient was admitted to the ICU with anaphylactic shock and subsequently died (30). Pruritus as an unusual symptom of disease may provide the astute practitioner with early clues for swift clinical management.

PRURITUS AND MALIGNANCY

Pruritus has been found to be an associated symptom with multiple types of malignancies. Certain neoplasms are more frequently associated with pruritus, such as polycythemia, Hodgkin's disease, and other hematologic malignancies. Another class of malignancies with a well-established connection to pruritus is cutaneous lymphomas such as cutaneous T-cell lymphoma and peripheral T-cell lymphoma (Table 19.1) (4,31–46). While it is still being investigated, a connection has been noted between endogenous opioids and lymphoma-induced pruritus. This connection is further established by

TABLE 19.1 SYSTEMIC CONDITIONS REPORTED TO BE ASSOCIATED WITH GENERALIZED PRURITUS

Organ systems and etiologies	Example
Autoimmune	Sjögren's syndrome Progressive systemic sclerosis Lupus erythematosus Sicca syndrome
Endocrine	Hyperthyroidism Hypothyroidism Parathyroid disease
Central nervous system	Cerebrovascular accident Delusions of parasitosis Depression Multiple sclerosis Neurodermatitis Psychosis Syrinx Brain tumor
Hematopoietic	Paraproteinemia Iron deficiency anemia Mastocytosis
Liver malignancy	Primary biliary cirrhosis Extrahepatic biliary obstruction Hepatitis Breast carcinoma Carcinoid syndrome Cutaneous T-cell lymphoma Gastrointestinal tract cancers: tongue, stomach, and colon Hodgkin's disease Insulinoma Leukemia Lung cancer Multiple myeloma Non-Hodgkin's lymphoma Polycythemia vera Prostatic carcinoma Thyroid carcinoma Uterine carcinoma
Iatrogenic	Drug ingestion Drug-induced cholestasis Injection site reaction
Infectious	Human immunodeficiency virus Parasitic diseases Scabies Syphilis
Renal	Chronic renal insufficiency and renal failure Dialysis dermatosis

the efficacy of butorphanol, which is a K agonist and μ antagonist, in treating non-Hodgkin's lymphoma–related pruritus (47). The cytokines interleukin-6 (IL-6) and interleukin-8 (IL-8) have been found to be closely related to the pathophysiology of lymphoma-induced itch (48–50). Neurokinin-1 (NK-1) is another neuropeptide believed to contribute to malignancy-related itch. Since its dominant ligand is substance P and an increase in the number of NK-1 receptors has been noted on keratinocytes of patients with chronic pruritus (51–53).

Pruritus is a common presenting symptom for cancers, whether they are solid cancers or hematologic cancers (54,55). If a malignancy is physically obstructing the biliary system, regardless of whether from a primary or malignant tumor, pruritus can be a presenting symptom (44). Solid tumors causing pruritus are believed to be connected to local immune phenomenon and, thus, the pruritus sensation may be generalized or localized. For example, prostate cancer can lead to scrotal itch (56). Increased blood levels of alkaline phosphatase (ALP) have been associated with pruritus such as in patients with primary biliary cholangitis.

One prospective study found that superficial lesions such as basal cell carcinoma are more likely to cause itching when compared to deeper lesions such as squamous cell carcinoma, which are more closely associated with pain. The amount of inflammation and the presence of neutrophils and eosinophils are contributing factors to the level of itch or pain. Cutaneous T-cell lymphomas are known to have severe pruritus, most commonly Sezary syndrome and mycosis fungoides. In Sezary syndrome, the chronic pruritus is generalized, thought to be linked with IL-3 and abnormal T cells in the peripheral blood and lymph nodes (57). A cross-sectional study of 16,925 patients found that those with pruritus were more likely to have concomitant malignancy than those who did not have pruritus. Cancers of the liver, hematopoietic system, gallbladder, biliary tract, and skin were most strongly associated with pruritus (58).

PRURITUS AS AN ADVERSE EFFECT

Pruritus is a potential adverse reaction of radiation therapy, chemotherapy, or pharmacological therapy (Table 19.2) (51,59–65). Radiation therapy resulting in acute radiodermatitis may cause erythema and pruritus. Chemotherapeutic agents can also cause anemia or other metabolic disturbances, which can also lead to pruritus. Newer chemotherapeutic medications and high-dose combinations have an increased risk of cutaneous toxicity and pruritic reactions.

TABLE 19.2 ANTITUMOR AGENTS ASSOCIATED WITH PRURITUS

Interferon-α

Bacille Calmette-Guérin

Bleomycin sulfate

Carboplatin

Carmustine

Chlorambucil

Cisplatin

Cyclophosphamide

Cytosine arabinoside and daunomycin

Daunomycin

Docetaxel

Doxorubicin

Gemcitabine hydrochloride

Hydroxyurea

Imatinib

Interleukin-2 with levamisole hydrochloride or interferon-α

L-Asparaginase

Mechlorethamine hydrochloride

Megestrol acetate

Methotrexate

Mitomycin

Oxaliplatin

Paclitaxel

Procarbazine hydrochloride

EGFR inhibitors (e.g., erlotinib)

EGFR, epidermal growth factor receptor.

Targeted anticancer medications either act on biological pathways or specifically target abnormal tissue to preserve normal tissue. While these treatments have decreased systemic toxicity, they have increased cutaneous side effects such as pruritus. Epidermal growth factor receptor (EGFR) inhibitors developed for lung cancer treatment have been found to cause debilitating pruritus through mast cell accumulation within skin lesions being treated with these medication (66). Patients using EGFR inhibitors have a high prevalence of itching among cancer patients receiving anticancer medications (67). These patients were found to develop intense, long-lasting itching that led to sleep disturbances as well as severe itching at specific body sites. A survey of 110 oncologists revealed that 76% temporarily held EGFR inhibitor therapy due to development of rash and pruritus (68). Gefitinib is used to treat non–small cell lung cancer (NSCLC) with increased levels of mutations of EGFR but has a very high incidence of rash and pruritus. Conversely, aprepitant, an NK-1 antagonist, has antipruritic activity and has been shown to improve refractory pruritus caused by medications such a gefitinib (68).

Oncologic immunotherapy agents such as those that target the programmed death 1 protein (PD-1) and programmed death-ligand 1 (PD-L1) are used to treat multiple cancer types such as NSCLC, melanoma, and Hodgkin's lymphoma. A meta-analysis of phase II/III randomized controlled trials of PD-1 and PD-L1 inhibitors found pruritus to be a common adverse effect after treatment. Pruritus was noted to range from mild severity to severe with significant decreases in quality of life. Pruritus was also found to be a predictor of development of bullous pemphigoid (69). Managing and preventing, as possible, common dermatological side effects of these targeted medications may improve survival and quality of life.

Rash may or may not be seen with many pharmacologic agents used to treat oncologic adverse effects. The most common presentation of rash is a typical morbilliform drug rash. Pain relief medications such as opioids, especially when administered intravenously, have also been found to cause pruritus (70). Discontinuing these therapies, if possible, often improves or resolves pruritus. The mechanism of pruritus due to opiates involves the central nervous system. Estrogens and ketoconazole precipitate pruritus by causing cholestasis. Over 100 medications have been recorded as causing pruritus without a rash (60). When treating a patient with pruritus, careful medication reconciliation and simplification of the patients' drug regimen are critical to alleviating the pruritic reaction.

NEUROPSYCHIATRY

Pruritus and the psych are closely related. Patients with underlying psychiatric disease have reported pruritus, known as psychocutaneous disease, and patients with chronic pruritus have reported psychiatric disease such as anxiety and depression (71,72). Itch may be heightened or triggered by pyschosocial stressors that result from severe disease burden with generalized pruritus (73). Edwards and colleagues reported that a high level of psychological stress enhances a person's ability to perceive intense itch stimuli (74). In an experimental, placebo study, positive verbal suggestions influenced subjects' expectations for itch reduction under both closed label and open label placebo (75). Recent theories identify that cognitive factors play a more dynamic and complex role in chronic itch, including factors of "attention, affect, and expectancies" that shape the "experience of itch by altered perceptions and interpretations." (76) Drug therapies can be targeted to improve mood and psychiatric conditions using psychoactive pharmacotherapies including H1 antihistamines, antidepressants, antiepileptics, opioid agonists, antipsychotics, and NK-1 receptor antagonists (77). Recognition of neuropsychiatric disease is a crucial piece to curtail management and provide optimal relief of pruritus.

EVALUATION

The diagnostic workup to evaluate a patient with pruritus includes obtaining a detailed history, review of symptoms, and a focused clinical examination. A medication reconciliation can identify pharmaceutical agents that could induce or exacerbate pruritus. A temporal history of the pruritus and any therapeutic changes especially is important to identify possible causes. Other historic points of value include others in the family or household with similar symptoms or signs, an abnormal or excessive bathing history, new or changed household products, new or changed personal care products, and new or changed symptoms of neuropsychiatric disease. A complete dermatologic clinical examination can quickly identify or exclude common dermatological diseases such as urticaria and scabies. Scabies preparations, fungal examinations, and skin biopsies may be needed to diagnose specific dermatologic diseases. A more complex evaluation is necessary for patients with long-standing generalized pruritus including necessary laboratory tests. Extensive, undirected evaluation of these patients rarely leads to a specific attributable cause (78). There is neither a single list nor specific guidelines for tests to perform in any individual patient placing more importance on a thorough and thoughtful evaluation

TREATMENT

Treating pruritus in the patient with cancer can take many forms. In general, the primary approaches to management should involve removal of the cause of itch, if possible, in conjunction with control of symptoms. Although there are some specific issues to consider in this population of patients, most of the management is similar to other forms of itch. It is important to devote adequate time to a given therapy to obtain optimum results although, there are few guidelines regarding the appropriate duration of therapy for chronic pruritus resulting in variations in clinical practice that rely on individual experience.

Topical Treatment

Some topical treatments are able to treat the underlying disease causing pruritus, such as topical permethrin for scabies infestation. More commonly, this is not the case especially when the cause is less specific or itch is chronic. In this case, providers

TABLE 19.3 ADVANTAGES AND DISADVANTAGES OF TOPICAL AGENTS

Topical agent	Examples	Advantages	Disadvantages
Emollients and moisturizers	Petrolatum Moisturizing lotions	Inexpensive and reduces irritant dermatitis	May be too greasy and insufficient in inflammatory diseases
Corticosteroids	Hydrocortisone Desonide Triamcinolone Fluocinonide Clobetasol	Effective for inflammatory dermatoses and mainstay of topical therapy	May cause atrophy, sensitivity, and adrenal suppression
Topical calcineurin inhibitors	Tacrolimus Pimecrolimus	Effective for inflammatory dermatoses and no atrophy	May cause itch or burn on application
Anesthetics	Camphor Pramoxine Benzocaine Prilocaine (EMLA) Menthol	Excellent pruritus relief and no atrophy or adrenal suppression	Potentially sensitizing and short-transient activity
Antihistamines	Diphenhydramine hydrochloride Doxepin hydrochloride	Modest relief and no atrophy or adrenal suppression	Potentially sedating and sensitizing
Cooling agents	Calamine Alcohol	May be soothing and cooling	Calamine leaves visible film Alcohol dries the skin
Miscellaneous	Coal tar	Coal tar is anti-inflammatory in nature	Tar is not elegant and stains
	Capsaicin	Capsaicin works differently than other agents	Capsaicin often burns

EMLA, eutectic mixture of topical anesthetics.

must weigh the risks and benefits of each topical agent before selecting one (Table 19.3).

A key aspect to consider with regard to skin therapy is hydration and lubrication of the surface of the skin (28,79). Applying emollients such as lotions, creams, and ointments twice daily are effective for maintaining or treating severely dry skin. Some emollients such as camphor, phenol, menthol, pramoxine, and benzocaine have local anesthetic effects that provide relief through cooling and numbing of the affected skin. Other efficacious topical treatment options are cool compresses and shake lotions (calamine), which have been used for years as home remedies for pruritus.

Topical anti-inflammatory medications prove useful for cancer patients with pruritus. Topical corticosteroids are used as adjunctive agents for pruritus control. Table 19.4 provides information regarding prescribing quantity information. The amount of topical corticosteroid prescribed should be enough to cover the affected skin. While any topical corticosteroid may be beneficial, for widespread pruritus hydrocortisone 1% or 2.5% or triamcinolone 0.1% are prescribed. Long-term use of halogenated corticosteroids should be used with caution in patients with thin skin, as seen in some cancer patients, over certain areas of the body, or in the elderly. Overuse of corticosteroids can lead to dermatologic iatrogenic disease. Some patients who are high risk of overutilization may not be candidates for this treatment or may require supervision when using topical steroids (80). Emollients should be remembered to be included in the treatment plan if appropriate, even if topical corticosteroids are required (81,82).

Nonsteroidal anti-inflammatory topical treatments are available for patients who are unable to use or have not found relief with topical steroids. Topical tacrolimus 0.1% ointment (Protopic) can cause short-lived burning and stinging with topical application; however, it can be used for long periods of time on any skin site without the risk of atrophy. Pimecrolimus cream (Elidel) is less effective than tacrolimus but is also known to be safe and effective for long-term use. Both tacrolimus and pimecrolimus are known for not causing long-term atrophy and neither is known to suppress systemic immune function (83,84). Pruritus associated with atopic dermatitis can be treated with topical crisaborole 2% ointment, which is a nonsteroidal phosphodiesterase-4 inhibitor. It has been shown to quickly alleviate pruritus in a timeframe similar to topical corticosteroids (TCSs) and topical calcineurin inhibitors (TCIs). Crisaborole also has a favorable safety profile making it a safe alternative to TCS or TCI treatment. Studies have shown that ceramides, pseudoceramides, or ceramide precursors increase skin hydration and improve the severity of flare ups in a manner similar to corticosteroids but with the ability to be used indefinitely. This is due to the ability of ceramides to decrease skin dryness by restoring the skin's barrier function. This is specifically beneficial in the treatment of atopic dermatitis. Another potent antipruritic agent is topical pine tar. This has been used since the age of Hippocrates and has provided relief from itch and inflammation even though the exact mechanism of action is not known. Pine tar has been found to improve atopic dermatitis scoring and, again, sparing the need for steroids (85).

Capsaicin cream is of limited help in select patients with a wide range of inflammatory and noninflammatory dermatoses but should not be used for generalized pruritus. Topical capsaicin cream (Zostrix) needs to be applied three times a day and may be used indefinitely. Topical application of capsaicin can produce significant burning and stinging sensations and thus requires careful patient instructions. Often the burning sensation diminishes after 1 or more weeks of use and then relief from pruritus may occur (86–88).

Other topical agents only have modest efficacy for relieving pruritus. A mixture of local anesthetics (lidocaine and prilocaine) has been shown to be useful in treating experimentally induced pruritus and may be beneficial in recalcitrant pruritic conditions (89). However, this combination has not been shown to offer any additional advantages over other anesthetic methods mentioned. Topical doxepin hydrochloride (Zonalon), which is an antihistamine and antidepressant, has been shown to have modest efficacy (90). Topical use of doxepin hydrochloride has been shown to cause sedation

TABLE 19.4 AMOUNTS OF TOPICAL AGENT PRESCRIBING INFORMATION

Location	One application (g)	Twice daily for 1 wk[a]	Twice daily for 1 mo[a]
Hands, scalp, genitalia, or face	2	30 g (1 oz)	120 g (4 oz)
Upper extremity or one side of trunk	3	45 g (1.5 oz)	180 g (6 oz)
One lower extremity	4	60 g (2 oz)	240 g (8 oz)
Entire body	30–60	540 g (1 lb)	2,700 g (5 lb)

[a]Although the twice-daily dosing of topical agents is appropriate for many patients, clinicians employ these agents from daily to four times daily.

and allergic contact dermatitis making it a therapy less frequently utilized. Generally, all topical agents have sensitizing potential and may induce allergic contact dermatitis. When topical therapies are not appropriate, systemic therapies are necessary.

Systemic Treatment

The process of decreased bile flow and poor formation of bile, both consequences of primary liver disease, is described as cholestasis. The process of scarring, or fibrosis, of the liver is described as cirrhosis. Oral systemic agents for the relief of pruritus are generally indicated for moderate to severe pruritus, such as when it begins to have a significant impact on quality of life such as interfering with sleep or with a significant neuropsychiatric component (Table 19.5). Primary biliary cirrhosis (PBC) and primary sclerosing cholangitis (PSC), both chronic, cholestatic liver diseases, cause pruritus in more than two-thirds of patients with these disorders (103,104). Other causes of cholestasis include obstructive cholestasis such as cholangiocarcinoma

or chronic hepatitis C infections. Some chronic liver diseases rarely result in pruritus such as nonalcoholic fatty liver disease, nonalcoholic steatohepatitis, biliary hamartomas, or parenteral nutrition-induced cholestasis (105). Treatment of cholestatic-induced pruritus includes rifampicin, opioid antagonists, selective serotonin reuptake inhibitors (SSRIs), or removal from the systemic circulation such as with plasmapheresis. Evidence for rifampicin includes randomized controlled trials and cohort studies. Sertraline, an SSRI, is recommended as a first-line treatment for pruritus due to cholestasis.

A review of the pharmacologic control of pruritus nearly three decades ago found the most effective antihistamines are centrally acting first-generation H1 blockers such as hydroxyzine (Atarax) and diphenhydramine hydrochloride (Benadryl) (106). Moreover, the side effect of sedation may be an added benefit for patients suffering from pruritus-induced insomnia (107). Caution with antihistamines should be practiced in the elderly due to undesirable anticholinergic side effects leading

TABLE 19.5 SYSTEMIC OR PHYSICAL PRURITUS TREATMENT MODALITY FOR SPECIFIC CONDITIONS

Drug or modality	Dosage range	Reference
Ultraviolet B phototherapy	N/A	(74,91,92)
Activated charcoal	50 g every 4 h	(93)
Rifampin	300 mg b.i.d.	(94,95)
Ondansetron	8 mg t.i.d.	(95,96)
Cholestyramine	4–6 g t.i.d. with meals	(94)
Nalmefene	2–10 mg b.i.d.	(33,34)
Naltrexone	25–50 mg daily	
Prednisone	5–60 mg daily	(7–10,12,13)
Phototherapy	N/A	(91,92,97)
Thalidomide	100–300 mg daily	(98)
Antihistamines		(13,99)
Cetirizine	10–20 mg daily	
Chlorpheniramine	4–12 mg q8-12h	
Desloratadine	50–10 mg daily	
Diphenhydramine	25–50 mg q6-8h	
Fexofenadine	60–180 mg daily	
Hydroxyzine	10–100 mg q6h	
Loratadine	10–20 mg daily	
Doxepin	10–150 mg qhs	(100)
Paroxetine	10–50 mg daily	(101)
Gabapentin	300–1,500 mg daily	
Aspirin	81–325 mg daily	(60)
Mirtazapine	15 mg qhs	(102–104)

N/A, not applicable.

to memory impairment or impaired psychomotor function (108,109). Cetirizine hydrochloride (Zyrtec) is an antihistamine that is less sedating than hydroxyzine, but more sedating than the typically nonsedating antihistamines (e.g., desloratadine and fexofenadine hydrochloride). There are conflicting data on the antipruritic efficacy of terfenadine and acrivastine in atopic dermatitis (12,110). Doxepin hydrochloride, a tricyclic antidepressant with antihistamine activity, may be an effective agent for the treatment of refractory pruritus (111).

With regard to urticaria, nonsedating antihistamines may be quite useful. Unfortunately, nonsedating antihistamines are of limited value in nonurticarial conditions. For patients with cancer, the role of histamine in itch mediation is uncertain. Burtin and colleagues found that histamine injections lead to a decreased skin response in cancer patients without additional effects. They theorized that, in some way, tumors recreate the effect of histamine H1-antagonists in the skin response to histamine thus limiting the usefulness of antihistamines in relieving cancer-related itch (112).

One highly effective treatment of pruritus is systemic corticosteroids. Systemic corticosteroids are best used in short duration for morbilliform drug eruptions or contact dermatitis, either allergic or irritant. Prolonged use of systemic corticosteroids often induces significant adverse sequelae such as hypertension, diabetes, fluid retention, and osteoporosis. Additionally, patients with cancer receiving immunotherapy may not be candidates for systemic steroids.

These limitations of the use of steroids for pruritus result in the need for other systemic therapeutic agents (Table 19.5). Activated charcoal, naloxone hydrochloride, naltrexone hydrochloride, sertraline, and cholestyramine, for instance, have been demonstrated to be effective in the treatment of pruritus of biliary cirrhosis (21,22,113–115). Sertraline has been found to be effective with fewer side effects than rifampin. The use of opioid antagonists may be inappropriate in certain populations, especially when optimizing end-of-life care. Sertraline, a serotonin reuptake inhibitor, has been found to be an effective treatment for chronic liver disease with pruritus (116), with fewer side effects (117) than rifampin.

Rifampin may be effective in the treatment of pruritus of primary biliary cirrhosis (115,118). Aspirin occasionally exacerbates pruritus (43), but it has been reported to be helpful in the treatment of pruritus associated with polycythemia rubra vera. Interferon-α has been used with some success in intractable pruritic conditions, especially polycythemia vera, but its cost and side effects demand careful consideration (45,46). Another confounding factor is that 30% of patients with melanoma receiving interferon-α experienced treatment-related pruritus (119). Thalidomide, a teratogenic anti-inflammatory agent, has had success in treating intractable pruritus when skin inflammation is present (120,121). More recently, the antiemetic, aprepitant, has been shown to be an effective treatment of EGFR inhibitor–induced pruritus (122). Gabapentin has achieved modest success in the treatment of pruritus in conditions such as brachioradial pruritus (91,121). The serotonin agents, paroxetine hydrochloride and ondansetron, have shown some effect with intractable pruritus, but their effects may be short lived (92–94,121). A recent advance in the treatment of refractory pruritus was found with the antidepressant drug, mirtazapine, due to its favorable safety profile compared with other antidepressants (95,96,121).

It is important to remind patients and practitioners that although pruritus may not be relieved with a systemic medication, and additional therapies may be necessary such as physical treatment modalities.

Physical Treatment Modalities

A wide range of pruritic disorders from atopic dermatitis to systemic disease have been treated with physical modalities. Examples of these treatments are phototherapy using ultraviolet radiation (ultraviolet A [UVA], ultraviolet B [UVB]) and psoralen photochemotherapy (97–99). UV therapy begins with three weekly doses and is titrated until effect or signs of erythema (100). Several rounds of treatment may be necessary to achieve relief with subsequent ongoing weekly maintenance therapy. UVB is often considered for uremic pruritus given its high degree of efficacy. Dialysis therapy may mitigate cutaneous pruritus indirectly by resolving the underlying cause of uremia. In a study performed in China, peritoneal dialysis and high-flux hemofiltration provided better relief of cutaneous pruritus in elderly uremic patients than the general low-flux hemodialysis utilized in developing countries. This was demonstrated by subjective data reported by patients, in addition to objective lab values of lower iPTH and beta-microglobulin serum levels (101). Other nonpharmacological physical modalities such as transcutaneous electrical nerve stimulation may bring relief for generalized itch associated with hematologic malignancies (102).

CONCLUSIONS

In conclusion, pruritus in patients with cancer is common and provides a diagnostic and therapeutic challenge for the physician. Evaluation includes obtaining an excellent history and physical examination. A thorough search to rule out systemic disease may occasionally be indicated. The physician should address the therapeutic intervention to correct the underlying cutaneous disease. Systemic antipruritics are often beneficial and well tolerated, but they have well-known side effects. Above all, diagnosis and management should be curtailed for the individual. Future studies to study pharmacological and non-pharmacological interventions are necessary for this specific patient population.

With regard to pruritus, there has been a dearth of new original studies since the last publication. Additionally, many of the published articles have been review papers. Furthermore, the strength and quality of the evidence provided by the existing studies is unknown due to the scarcity of data on pruritus. There is a potential for future studies to bridge the current gaps of knowledge surrounding pruritus, such as an increase in the number and quality of randomized controlled trials will further strengthen our understanding of this unique symptom.

REFERENCES

1. Krajnik M, Zylicz Z (Ben). Pain assessment, recognising clinical patterns, and cancer pain syndromes. In: Hanna M, Zylicz Z (Ben), eds. *Cancer Pain.* London, UK: Springer London; 2013:95-108. doi: 10.1007/978-0-85729-230-8_7.

2. Bernhard J. Itches, pains, and other strange sensations. *Curr Chall Dermatol.* 1991:1-10.

3. Pisoni RL, Wikström B, Elder SJ, et al. Pruritus in haemodialysis patients: international results from the Dialysis Outcomes and Practice Patterns Study (DOPPS). *Nephrol Dial Transplant.* 2006;21(12):3495-3505. doi: 10.1093/ndt/gfl461.

4. Gobbi PG, Attardo-Parrinello G, Lattanzio G, Rizzo SC, Ascari E. Severe pruritus should be a B-symptom in Hodgkin's disease. *Cancer.* 1983;51(10):1934-1936. doi: 10.1002/1097-0142(19830515)51:10<1934::aid-cncr2820511030>3.0.co;2-r.

5. Denman ST. A review of pruritus. *J Am Acad Dermatol.* 1986;14(3):375-392. doi: 10.1016/s0190-9622(86)70047-9.

6. Rinaldi G. The itch-scratch cycle: a review of the mechanisms. *Dermatol Pract Concept.* 2019;9(2):90-97. doi: 10.5826/dpc.0902a03.

7. Schmelz M, Schmidt R, Bickel A, Handwerker HO, Torebjörk HE. Specific C-receptors for itch in human skin. *J Neurosci.* 1997;17(20):8003-8008. http://www.ncbi.nlm.nih.gov/pubmed/9315918

8. Arnold AJ, Simpson JG, Jones HE, Ahmed AR. Suppression of histamine-induced pruritus by hydroxyzine and various neuroleptics. *J Am Acad Dermatol.* 1979;1(6):509-512. doi: 10.1016/s0190-9622(79)80094-8.

9. Yosipovitch G, Carstens E, McGlone F. Chronic itch and chronic pain: analogous mechanisms. *Pain.* 2007;131(1-2):4-7. doi: 10.1016/j.pain.2007.04.017.

10. Toyoda M, Nakamura M, Makino T, Hino T, Kagoura M, Morohashi M. Nerve growth factor and substance P are useful plasma markers of disease activity in atopic dermatitis. *Br J Dermatol.* 2002;147(1):71-79. doi: 10.1046/j.1365-2133.2002.04803.x.

11. Krause L, Shuster S. Mechanism of action of antipruritic drugs. *Br Med J (Clin Res Ed).* 1983;287(6400):1199-1200. doi: 10.1136/bmj.287.6400.1199.

12. Berth-Jones J, Graham-Brown RA. Failure of terfenadine in relieving the pruritus of atopic dermatitis. *Br J Dermatol.* 1989;121(5):635-637. doi: 10.1111/j.1365-2133.1989.tb08196.x.

13. Lober CW. Pruritus and malignancy. *Clin Dermatol.* 1993;11(1):125-128. doi: 10.1016/0738-081x(93)90108-o.

14. Ständer S, Moormann C, Schumacher M, et al. Expression of vanilloid receptor subtype 1 in cutaneous sensory nerve fibers, mast cells, and epithelial cells of appendage structures. *Exp Dermatol.* 2004;13(3):129-139. doi: 10.1111/j.0906-6705.2004.0178.x.

15. Steinhoff M, Neisius U, Ikoma A, et al. Proteinase-activated receptor-2 mediates itch: a novel pathway for pruritus in human skin. *J Neurosci.* 2003;23(15):6176-6180.

16. Shelley W, Arthur R. Mucanain, the active pruritogenic proteinase of cowhage. *Science.* 1955;80:469-470.

17. Schmelz M, Michael K, Weidner C, Schmidt R, Torebjörk H, Handwerker H. Which nerve fibers mediate the axon reflex flare in human skin? *Neuroreport.* 2000;11(3):645-648.

18. Davidson S, Zhang X, Yoon CH, Khasabov SG, Simone DA, Giesler GJ. The itch-producing agents histamine and cowhage activate separate populations of primate spinothalamic tract neurons. *J Neurosci.* 2007;27(37):10007-10014. doi: 10.1523/JNEUROSCI.2862-07.2007.

19. Namer B, Carr R, Johanek LM, Schmelz M, Handwerker HO, Ringkamp M. Separate peripheral pathways for pruritus in man. *J Neurophysiol.* 2008;100(4):2062-2069. doi: 10.1152/jn.90482.2008.

20. Schmidt R, Schmelz M, Forster C, Ringkamp M, Torebjörk E, Handwerker H. Novel classes of responsive and unresponsive C nociceptors in human skin. *J Neurosci.* 1995;15(1 Pt 1):333-341. http://www.ncbi.nlm.nih.gov/pubmed/7823139

21. Bernstein JE, Swift RM, Soltani K, Lorincz AL. Antipruritic effect of an opiate antagonist, naloxone hydrochloride. *J Invest Dermatol.* 1982;78(1):82-83. doi: 10.1111/1523-1747.ep12497974.

22. Bernstein JE, Swift R. Relief of intractable pruritus with naloxone. *Arch Dermatol.* 1979;115(11):1366-1367. http://www.ncbi.nlm.nih.gov/pubmed/389168

23. Fischer HB, Scott PV. Spinal opiate analgesia and facial pruritus. *Anaesthesia.* 1982;37(7):777-778. doi: 10.1111/j.1365-2044.1982.tb01326.x.

24. Bergasa NV, Thomas DA, Vergalla J, Turner ML, Jones EA. Plasma from patients with the pruritus of cholestasis induces opioid receptor-mediated scratching in monkeys. *Life Sci.* 1993;53(16):1253-1257. doi: 10.1016/0024-3205(93)90569-o.

25. King CA, Huff FJ, Jorizzo JL. Unilateral neurogenic pruritus: paroxysmal itching associated with central nervous system lesions. *Ann Intern Med.* 1982;97(2):222-223. doi: 10.7326/0003-4819-97-2-222.

26. Bernhard JD. Phantom itch, pseudophantom itch, and senile pruritus. *Int J Dermatol.* 1992;31(12):856-857. doi: 10.1111/j.1365-4362.1992.tb03541.x.

27. Lierman LM. Phantom breast experiences after mastectomy. *Oncol Nurs Forum.* 1988;15(1):41-44. http://www.ncbi.nlm.nih.gov/pubmed/3344245

28. Hannuksela A, Kinnunen T. Moisturizers prevent irritant dermatitis. *Acta Derm Venereol.* 1992;72(1):42-44. http://www.ncbi.nlm.nih.gov/pubmed/1350143

29. Gilchrest BA. Pruritus: pathogenesis, therapy, and significance in systemic disease states. *Arch Intern Med.* 1982;142(1):101-105. doi: 10.1001/archinte.142.1.101.

30. Jin X, Li F, Li X, et al. Cutaneous presentation preceding acute monocytic leukemia. *Medicine (Baltimore).* 2017;96(10):e6269. doi: 10.1097/MD.0000000000006269.

31. Rosenberg FW. Cutaneous manifestations of internal malignancy. *Cutis.* 1977;20(2):227-234. http://www.ncbi.nlm.nih.gov/pubmed/408101

32. Cormia FE. Pruritus, an uncommon but important symptom of systemic carcinoma. *Arch Dermatol.* 1965;92(1):36-39. http://www.ncbi.nlm.nih.gov/pubmed/11850949

33. Erskine JG, Rowan RM, Alexander JO, Sekoni GA. Pruritus as a presentation of myelomatosis. *Br Med J.* 1977;1(6062):687-688. doi: 10.1136/bmj.1.6062.687.

34. Mengel CE. Cutaneous manifestations of the malignant carcinoid syndrome. *Ann Intern Med.* 1963;58(6):989. doi: 10.7326/0003-4819-58-6-989.

35. Beeaff DE. Pruritus as a sign of systemic disease. Report of metastatic small cell carcinoma. *Ariz Med.* 1980;37(12):831-833. http://www.ncbi.nlm.nih.gov/pubmed/6257210

36. Thomas S, Harrington CI. Intractable pruritus as the presenting symptom of carcinoma of the bronchus: a case report and review of the literature. *Clin Exp Dermatol.* 1983;8(5):459-461. doi: 10.1111/j.1365-2230.1983.tb01813.x.

37. Shoenfeld Y, Weiberger A, Ben-Bassat M, Pinkhas J. Generalized pruritus in metastatic adenocarcinoma of the stomach. *Dermatologica.* 1977;155(2):122-124. doi: 10.1159/000250965.

38. Degos R, Civatte J, Blanchet P, Duterque M. [Pruritus, only symptom of Hodgkin's disease for 5 years]. *Ann Med Interne (Paris).* 1973;124(3):235-238. http://www.ncbi.nlm.nih.gov/pubmed/4716717

39. Alexander LL. Pruritus and Hodgkin's disease. *JAMA.* 1979;241(24):2598-2599. http://www.ncbi.nlm.nih.gov/pubmed/439350

40. Bluefarb S. *Cutaneous Manifestations of the Malignant Lymphomas.* Springfield, IL: Charles C. Thomas; 1959.

41. Stock H. Cutaneous paraneoplastic syndromes. *Med Klin.* 1976;71:356-372.

42. Curth HO. A spectrum of organ systems that respond to the presence of cancer. How and why the skin reacts. *Ann N Y Acad Sci.* 1974;230:435-442. doi: 10.1111/j.1749-6632.1974.tb14477.x.

43. Fjellner B, Hägermark O. Pruritus in polycythemia vera: treatment with aspirin and possibility of platelet involvement. *Acta Derm Venereol.* 1979;59(6):505-512. http://www.ncbi.nlm.nih.gov/pubmed/94209

44. Ballinger AB, McHugh M, Catnach SM, Alstead EM, Clark ML. Symptom relief and quality of life after stenting for malignant bile duct obstruction. *Gut.* 1994;35(4):467-470. doi: 10.1136/gut.35.4.467.

45. de Wolf JT, Hendriks DW, Egger RC, Esselink MT, Halie MR, Vellenga E. Alpha-interferon for intractable pruritus in polycythaemia vera. *Lancet (London, Engl).* 1991;337(8735):241. doi: 10.1016/0140-6736(91)92206-h.

46. Flecknoe-Brown S. Relief of itch associated with myeloproliferative disease by alpha-interferon. *Aust N Z J Med.* 1991;21(1):81. doi: 10.1111/j.1445-5994.1991.tb03012.x.

47. Dawn AG, Yosipovitch G. Butorphanol for treatment of intractable pruritus. *J Am Acad Dermatol.* 2006;54(3):527-531. doi: 10.1016/j.jaad.2005.12.010.

48. Wang H, Yosipovitch G. New insights into the pathophysiology and treatment of chronic itch in patients with end-stage renal disease, chronic liver disease, and lymphoma. *Int J Dermatol.* 2010;49(1):1-11. doi: 10.1111/j.1365-4632.2009.04249.x.

49. Biggar RJ, Johansen JS, Smedby KE, et al. Serum YKL-40 and interleukin 6 levels in Hodgkin lymphoma. *Clin Cancer Res.* 2008;14(21):6974-6978. doi: 10.1158/1078-0432.CCR-08-1026.

50. Lee HL, Eom H-S, Yun T, et al. Serum and urine levels of interleukin-8 in patients with non-Hodgkin's lymphoma. *Cytokine.* 2008;43(1):71-75. doi: 10.1016/j.cyto.2008.04.004.

51. Vincenzi B, Tonini G, Santini D. Aprepitant for erlotinib-induced pruritus. *N Engl J Med.* 2010;363(4):397-398. doi: 10.1056/NEJMc1003937.

52. Sankhala KK, Pandya DM, Sarantopoulos J, Soefje SA, Giles FJ, Chawla SP. Prevention of chemotherapy induced nausea and vomiting: a focus on aprepitant. *Expert Opin Drug Metab Toxicol.* 2009;5(12):1607-1614. doi: 10.1517/17425250903451675.

53. Curran MP, Robinson DM. Aprepitant: a review of its use in the prevention of nausea and vomiting. *Drugs.* 2009;69(13):1853-1878. doi: 10.2165/11203680-000000000-00000.

54. Johnson RE, Kanigsberg ND, Jimenez CL. Localized pruritus: a presenting symptom of a spinal cord tumor in a child with features of neurofibromatosis. *J Am Acad Dermatol.* 2000;43(5 Pt 2):958-961. doi: 10.1067/mjd.2000.104000.

55. King NKK, Siriwardana HPP, Coyne JD, Siriwardena AK. Intractable pruritus associated with insulinoma in the absence of multiple endocrine neoplasia: a novel paraneoplastic phenomenon. *Scand J Gastroenterol.* 2003;38(6):678-680. doi: 10.1080/00365520310001950.

56. Seccareccia D, Gebara N. Pruritus in palliative care: getting up to scratch. *Can Fam Physician.* 2011;57(9):1010-1013, e316-e319. http://www.ncbi.nlm.nih.gov/pubmed/21918143

57. Larson VA, Tang O, Ständer S, Kang S, Kwatra SG. Association between itch and cancer in 16,925 patients with pruritus: experience at a tertiary care center. *J Am Acad Dermatol.* 2019;80(4):931-937. doi: 10.1016/j.jaad.2018.08.044.

58. Shevchenko A, Valdes-Rodriguez R, Yosipovitch G. Causes, pathophysiology, and treatment of pruritus in the mature patient. *Clin Dermatol.* 2018;36(2):140-151. doi: 10.1016/j.clindermatol.2017.10.005.

59. Breathnach SM, Hinter H. *Adverse Reactions and the Skin.* Oxford, UK: Blackwell Science; 1992.

60. Bork C. *Cutaneous Side Effects of Drugs.* Philadelphia, PA: WB Saunders; 1988.

61. Call TG, Creagan ET, Frytak S, et al. Phase I trial of combined recombinant interleukin-2 with levamisole in patients with advanced malignant disease. *Am J Clin Oncol.* 1994;17(4):344-347. doi: 10.1097/00000421-199408000-00013.

62. Hortobagyi GN, Richman SP, Dandridge K, Gutterman JU, Blumenschein GR, Hersh EM. Immunotherapy with BCG administered by scarification: standardization of reactions and management of side effects. *Cancer.* 1978;42(5):2293-2303. doi: 10.1002/1097-0142(197811)42:5<2293::aid-cncr2820420529>3.0.co;2-o.

63. Ogilvie GK, Richardson RC, Curtis CR, et al. Acute and short-term toxicoses associated with the administration of doxorubicin to dogs with malignant tumors. *J Am Vet Med Assoc.* 1989;195(11):1584-1587. http://www.ncbi.nlm.nih.gov/pubmed/2599942

64. Valeyrie L, Bastuji-Garin S, Revuz J, et al. Adverse cutaneous reactions to imatinib (STI571) in Philadelphia chromosome-positive leukemias: a prospective study of 54 patients. *J Am Acad Dermatol.* 2003;48(2):201-206. doi: 10.1067/mjd.2003.44.

65. Bhargava P, Gammon D, McCormick MJ. Hypersensitivity and idiosyncratic reactions to oxaliplatin. *Cancer.* 2004;100(1):211-212. doi: 10.1002/cncr.11901.

66. Gerber PA, Buhren BA, Cevikbas F, Bölke E, Steinhoff M, Homey B. Preliminary evidence for a role of mast

cells in epidermal growth factor receptor inhibitor-induced pruritus. *J Am Acad Dermatol.* 2010;63(1):163-165. doi: 10.1016/j.jaad.2009.09.023.

67. Cho S, Lee J, Lim J, et al. Pruritus in patients under targeted anticancer therapy: a multidimensional analysis using the 5-D itch scale. *Acta Derm Venereol.* 2019;99(4):435-441. doi: 10.2340/00015555-3129.

68. Qin H, Wang F, Wang K, et al. Aprepitant for gefitinib-induced refractory pruritus in Chinese malignancy population. *Ann Transl Med.* 2019;7(3):54. doi: 10.21037/atm.2019.01.02.

69. Yang W, Li S, Yang Q. Risk of dermatologic and mucosal adverse events associated with PD-1/PD-L1 inhibitors in cancer patients. *Medicine (Baltimore).* 2019;98(20):e15731. doi: 10.1097/MD.0000000000015731.

70. Georgieva J, Steinhoff M, Orfanos CE, Treudler R. Ethylene-oxide-induced pruritus associated with extracorporeal photochemotherapy. *Transfusion.* 2004;44(10):1532-1533. doi: 10.1111/j.1537-2995.2004.00433.x.

71. Lee HG, Stull C, Yosipovitch G. Psychiatric disorders and pruritus. *Clin Dermatol.* 2017;35(3):273-280. doi: 10.1016/j.clindermatol.2017.01.008.

72. Kuhn H, Mennella C, Magid M, Stamu-O'Brien C, Kroumpouzos G. Psychocutaneous disease: clinical perspectives. *J Am Acad Dermatol.* 2017;76(5):779-791. doi: 10.1016/j.jaad.2016.11.013.

73. Calnan C, O'Neill D. Itching in tension states. *Br J Dermatol.* 1952;64(7-8):274-280. doi: 10.1111/j.1365-2133.1952.tb15806.x.

74. Edwards AE, Shellow WV, Wright ET, Dignam TF. Pruritic skin diseases, psychological stress, and the itch sensation. A reliable method for the induction of experimental pruritus. *Arch Dermatol.* 1976;112(3):339-343. http://www.ncbi.nlm.nih.gov/pubmed/1259446

75. Meeuwis SH, van Middendorp H, van Laarhoven AIM, Veldhuijzen DS, Lavrijsen APM, Evers AWM. Effects of open- and closed-label nocebo and placebo suggestions on itch and itch expectations. *Front Psychiatry.* 2019;10. doi: 10.3389/fpsyt.2019.00436.

76. Evers AWM, Peerdeman KJ, van Laarhoven AIM. What is new in the psychology of chronic itch? *Exp Dermatol.* 2019;28(12):1442-1447. doi: 10.1111/exd.13992.

77. Reszke R, Szepietowski JC. Can we use psychoactive drugs to treat pruritus? *Exp Dermatol.* 2019;28(12):1422-1431. doi: 10.1111/exd.13959.

78. Fleischer AB. Pruritus in the elderly: management by senior dermatologists. *J Am Acad Dermatol.* 1993;28(4):603-609. doi: 10.1016/0190-9622(93)70081-4.

79. Ghadially R, Halkier-Sorensen L, Elias PM. Effects of petrolatum on stratum corneum structure and function. *J Am Acad Dermatol.* 1992;26(3 Pt 2):387-396. doi: 10.1016/0190-9622(92)70060-s.

80. Fransway AF, Winkelmann RK. Treatment of pruritus. *Semin Dermatol.* 1988;7(4):310-325. http://www.ncbi.nlm.nih.gov/pubmed/2908675

81. Watsky KL, Freije L, Leneveu MC, Wenck HA, Leffell DJ. Water-in-oil emollients as steroid-sparing adjunctive therapy in the treatment of psoriasis. *Cutis.* 1992;50(5):383-386. http://www.ncbi.nlm.nih.gov/pubmed/1468261

82. Ronayne C, Bray G, Robertson G. The use of aqueous cream to relieve pruritus in patients with liver disease. *Br J Nurs.* 1993;2(10):527-528. http://www.ncbi.nlm.nih.gov/pubmed/8324350

83. Fleischer AB. Treatment of atopic dermatitis: role of tacrolimus ointment as a topical noncorticosteroidal

therapy. *J Allergy Clin Immunol.* 1999;104(3 Pt 2):S126-S130. doi: 10.1016/s0091-6749(99)70055-2.

84. Kang S, Lucky AW, Pariser D, Lawrence I, Hanifin JM. Long-term safety and efficacy of tacrolimus ointment for the treatment of atopic dermatitis in children. *J Am Acad Dermatol.* 2001;44(1 suppl):S58-S64. doi: 10.1067/mjd.2001.109812.

85. Harrison IP, Spada F. Breaking the itch-scratch cycle: topical options for the management of chronic cutaneous itch in atopic dermatitis. *Medicines (Basel).* 2019;6(3):76. doi: 10.3390/medicines6030076.

86. Breneman DL, Cardone JS, Blumsack RF, Lather RM, Searle EA, Pollack VE. Topical capsaicin for treatment of hemodialysis-related pruritus. *J Am Acad Dermatol.* 1992;26(1):91-94. doi: 10.1016/0190-9622(92)70013-6.

87. Leibsohn E. Treatment of notalgia paresthetica with capsaicin. *Cutis.* 1992;49(5):335-336. http://www.ncbi.nlm.nih.gov/pubmed/1521492

88. Fusco BM, Giacovazzo M. Peppers and pain. The promise of capsaicin. *Drugs.* 1997;53(6):909-914. doi: 10.2165/00003495-199753060-00001.

89. Shuttleworth D, Hill S, Marks R, Connelly DM. Relief of experimentally induced pruritus with a novel eutectic mixture of local anaesthetic agents. *Br J Dermatol.* 1988;119(4):535-540. doi: 10.1111/j.1365-2133.1988.tb03259.x.

90. Drake L, Breneman D, Greene S, et al. Effects of topical doxepin 5% cream on pruritic eczema. *J Invest Dermatol.* 1992;98:605.

91. Winhoven SM, Coulson IH, Bottomley WW. Brachioradial pruritus: response to treatment with gabapentin. *Br J Dermatol.* 2004;150(4):786-787. doi: 10.1111/j.0007-0963.2004.05889.x.

92. Müller C, Pongratz S, Pidlich J, et al. Treatment of pruritus in chronic liver disease with the 5-hydroxytryptamine receptor type 3 antagonist ondansetron: a randomized, placebo-controlled, double-blind crossover trial. *Eur J Gastroenterol Hepatol.* 1998;10(10):865-870. doi: 10.1097/00042737-199810000-00010.

93. Zylicz Z, Smits C, Krajnik M. Paroxetine for pruritus in advanced cancer. *J Pain Symptom Manage.* 1998;16(2):121-124. doi: 10.1016/s0885-3924(98)00048-7.

94. Krajnik M, Zylicz Z. Understanding pruritus in systemic disease. *J Pain Symptom Manage.* 2001;21(2):151-168. doi: 10.1016/s0885-3924(00)00256-6.

95. Davis MP, Frandsen JL, Walsh D, Andresen S, Taylor S. Mirtazapine for pruritus. *J Pain Symptom Manage.* 2003;25(3):288-291. doi: 10.1016/s0885-3924(02)00645-0.

96. Hundley JL, Yosipovitch G. Mirtazapine for reducing nocturnal itch in patients with chronic pruritus: a pilot study. *J Am Acad Dermatol.* 2004;50(6):889-891. doi: 10.1016/j.jaad.2004.01.045.

97. Gilchrest BA, Rowe JW, Brown RS, Steinman TI, Arndt KA. Ultraviolet phototherapy of uremic pruritus. Long-term results and possible mechanism of action. *Ann Intern Med.* 1979;91(1):17-21. doi: 10.7326/0003-4819-91-1-17.

98. Morison WL, Parrish J, Fitzpatrick TB. Oral psoralen photochemotherapy of atopic eczema. *Br J Dermatol.* 1978;98(1):25-30. doi: 10.1111/j.1365-2133.1978.tb07329.x.

99. Jekler J, Larkö O. UVA solarium versus UVB phototherapy of atopic dermatitis: a paired-comparison study. *Br J Dermatol.* 1991;125(6):569-572. doi: 10.1111/j.1365-2133.1991.tb14796.x.

100. Zanolli MD, Feldman SR, Clark AR, et al. *Phototherapy and Psoriasis Treatment Protocols.* New York, NY: Parthenon Publishers; 2000.

101. Jin D, Shen H, Feng S, et al. Treatment effects of different incident dialysis modalities on pruritus in elderly uremic patients. *Int J Gerontol.* 2014;8(4):223-227. doi: 10.1016/j.ijge.2014.06.002.

102. Tinegate H, McLelland J. Transcutaneous electrical nerve stimulation may improve pruritus associated with haematological disorders. *Clin Lab Haematol.* 2002;24(6):389-390. doi: 10.1046/j.1365-2257.2002.00472.x.

103. Kremer AE, Namer B, Bolier R, Fischer MJ, Oude Elferink RP, Beuers U. Pathogenesis and management of pruritus in PBC and PSC. *Dig Dis.* 2015;33(suppl 2):164-175. doi: 10.1159/000440829.

104. Beuers U, Kremer AE, Bolier R, Elferink RP. Pruritus in cholestasis: facts and fiction. *Hepatology.* 2014;60(1):399-407. doi: 10.1002/hep.26909.

105. Kremer AE, Bolier R, van Dijk R, Elferink RPJO, Beuers U. Advances in pathogenesis and management of pruritus in cholestasis. *Dig Dis.* 2014;32(5):637-645. doi: 10.1159/000360518.

106. Winkelmann RK. Pharmacologic control of pruritus. *Med Clin North Am.* 1982;66(5):1119-1133. doi: 10.1016/s0025-7125(16)31386-4.

107. Aoki T, Kushimoto H, Hishikawa Y, Savin JA. Nocturnal scratching and its relationship to the disturbed sleep of itchy subjects. *Clin Exp Dermatol.* 1991;16(4):268-272. doi: 10.1111/j.1365-2230.1991.tb00372.x.

108. Higgins EM, du Vivier AW. Cutaneous manifestations of malignant disease. *Br J Hosp Med.* 1992;48(9):552-554, 558-561. http://www.ncbi.nlm.nih.gov/pubmed/1477711

109. De Conno F, Ventafridda V, Saita L. Skin problems in advanced and terminal cancer patients. *J Pain Symptom Manage.* 1991;6(4):247-256. doi: 10.1016/0885-3924(91)90015-v.

110. Doherty V, Sylvester DG, Kennedy CT, Harvey SG, Calthrop JG, Gibson JR. Treatment of itching in atopic eczema with antihistamines with a low sedative profile. *BMJ.* 1989;298(6666):96. doi: 10.1136/bmj.298.6666.96.

111. Richelson E. Tricyclic antidepressants block histamine H1 receptors of mouse neuroblastoma cells. *Nature.* 1978;274(5667):176-177. doi: 10.1038/274176a0.

112. Burtin C, Noirot C, Giroux C, Scheinmann P. Decreased skin response to intradermal histamine in cancer patients. *J Allergy Clin Immunol.* 1986;78(1 Pt 1):83-89. doi: 10.1016/0091-6749(86)90118-1.

113. Pederson JA, Matter BJ, Czerwinski AW, Llach F. Relief of idiopathic generalized pruritus in dialysis patients treated with activated oral charcoal. *Ann Intern Med.* 1980;93(3):446-448. doi: 10.7326/0003-4819-93-3-446.

114. Terra SG, Tsunoda SM. Opioid antagonists in the treatment of pruritus from cholestatic liver disease. *Ann Pharmacother.* 1998;32(11):1228-1230. doi: 10.1345/aph.18115.

115. Ghent CN, Carruthers SG. Treatment of pruritus in primary biliary cirrhosis with rifampin. Results of a double-blind, crossover, randomized trial. *Gastroenterology.* 1988;94(2):488-493. doi: 10.1016/0016-5085(88)90442-8.

116. Mayo MJ, Handem I, Saldana S, Jacobe H, Getachew Y, Rush AJ. Sertraline as a first-line treatment for cholestatic pruritus. *Hepatology.* 2007;45(3):666-674. doi: 10.1002/hep.21553.

117. Ataei S, Kord L, Larki A, et al. Comparison of sertraline with rifampin in the treatment of cholestatic pruritus: a randomized clinical trial. *Rev Recent Clin Trials.* 2019;14(3):217-223. doi: 10.2174/1574887114666190328130720.

118. Bergasa NV. The pruritus of cholestasis. *Semin Dermatol.* 1995;14(4):302-312. http://www.ncbi.nlm.nih.gov/pubmed/8679436

119. Guillot B, Blazquez L, Bessis D, Dereure O, Guilhou JJ. A prospective study of cutaneous adverse events induced by low-dose alpha-interferon treatment for malignant melanoma. *Dermatology.* 2004;208(1):49-54. doi: 10.1159/000075046.

120. Calabrese L, Fleischer AB. Thalidomide: current and potential clinical applications. *Am J Med.* 2000;108(6):487-495. doi: 10.1016/s0002-9343(99)00408-8.

121. Summey BT, Yosipovitch G. Pharmacologic advances in the systemic treatment of itch. *Dermatol Ther.* 2005;18(4):328-332. doi: 10.1111/j.1529-8019.2005.00035.x.

122. Levêque D. Aprepitant for erlotinib-induced pruritus. *N Engl J Med.* 2010;363(17):1680-1681; author reply 1681. doi: 10.1056/NEJMc1009698.

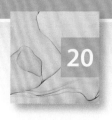

20 Management of Tumor-Related Skin Disorders

Shali Zhang

The skin offers clues to internal health. Many different cutaneous signs can manifest in the setting of underlying malignancies. In some cases, the skin manifestations of a tumor-related skin disorder (TRSD) may even allow for early detection of an occult problem. Proper management of these dermatologic conditions can also improve quality of life for patients. In this chapter, we review select TRSDs with respect to their presentation, commonly associated malignancies (Table 20.1), and potential management strategies.

TRSDs can be divided into two groups:

1. Generalized eruptions associated with internal malignancy
2. Cancer-related genodermatoses.

The former are paraneoplastic dermatoses, where a nonmalignant skin disorder occurs in association with an underlying cancer. The latter are heritable skin conditions with cancer associations. More common examples of these uncommon conditions will be discussed.

GENERALIZED ERUPTIONS ASSOCIATED WITH INTERNAL MALIGNANCY

Pruritus

Pruritus, or itch, is a common, nonspecific skin complaint that is often the result of abnormally dry skin. However, chronic, intractable pruritus accompanied by severe excoriations may be an indicator of underlying malignancy (1). This type of pruritus is most frequently seen in patients with cancers of the hematopoietic system (2), but may be observed with any internal malignancy. Classically, paraneoplastic itch has been described with Hodgkin's lymphoma, and itch severity may be correlated with a poor prognosis (3), especially if associated with fever or weight loss.

Unlike primary skin conditions that are pruritic, there are usually no true primary lesions on physical examination. Upon inspection, secondary changes including excoriations, lichenification, and pigmentary changes can be significant (Fig. 20.1A).

Intractable pruritus is best evaluated by a dermatologist, who can distinguish primary pruritus from pruritus secondary to another condition.

Other systemic causes of pruritus should be ruled out including cholestatic liver disease, renal disease, human immunodeficiency virus disease, thyroid disorders, or diabetes. Infestation with scabies should also be considered in the differential diagnosis. In contrast to the localized nature of nonmalignant pruritus, malignancy-associated pruritus tends to be generalized.

In cases where the index of suspicion is high for a malignancy, a workup should include a thorough history and physical examination with evaluation of complete blood count (CBC), liver function tests (LFTs), and a chest x-ray. In addition, age-appropriate and symptom-directed cancer screening should be performed.

While traditional itch relievers such as oral antihistamines (especially, sedating antihistamines), topical corticosteroids, and ultraviolet light therapy can be effective for pruritus due to systemic diseases, these treatments are unable to provide satisfactory relief for itch associated with lymphomas (Table 20.2). Malignancy-associated pruritus usually requires treatment of the underlying cancer. However, support for the use of low-dose mirtazapine (7.5 to 15 mg) with gabapentin (300 mg at night up to 900 to 2,400 mg/d), paroxetine (4), butorphanol (3 to 4 mg/d) (5), and thalidomide (6) has been documented. Oral prednisone (40 mg/d tapering down gradually in 3 weeks) has also been found to be helpful for the itch of lymphoma (7). Recently, off-label use of aprepitant has been shown to be promising for intractable, paraneoplastic pruritus (8).

Sign of Leser-Trélat

The sign of Leser-Trélat is the sudden and rapid increase in the number or size of seborrheic keratoses (SKs) in association with internal malignancy. While there is some controversy over the validity of this sign as a paraneoplastic syndrome (9), it has been described in association with a variety of cancers. The most frequently associated cancers are carcinomas of the gastrointestinal tract, particularly gastric carcinomas followed by colorectal cancer (10,11). It has also been documented in a variety of other malignancies, including breast (12), lung (13), lymphoma (14), melanoma (15)

TABLE 20.1 TUMOR-ASSOCIATED SKIN DISORDERS

Tumor-associated disorder	Major features	Most commonly associated cancer(s)
Pruritus	Secondary excoriations, lichenification, and hyperpigmentation	Hodgkin's lymphoma
Leser-Trélat	Eruptive seborrheic keratosis	Gastric adenocarcinoma
Erythema gyratum repens	Scaly, expanding erythematous "wood grain" pattern on trunk and extremities	Lung cancer
Hypertrichosis lanuginosa acquisita	Downy facial hair growth	Lung cancer, colorectal carcinoma
Necrolytic migratory erythema	Blistering, erythematous rash with stomatitis	Glucagonoma
Paraneoplastic pemphigus	Stomatitis, mucocutaneous ulcerations, and polymorphous skin lesions	Non-Hodgkin's lymphoma, chronic lymphocytic leukemia
Bazex syndrome	Psoriasiform lesions of ears and acral sites with nail dystrophy	Aerodigestive tract carcinoma
Acanthosis nigricans	Velvety hyperpigmentation of intertriginous regions	Gastric adenocarcinoma
Dermatomyositis	Proximal myopathy, heliotrope rash, Gottron's papules	Ovarian carcinoma
Sweet's syndrome	Painful, erythematous plaques with blisters, pyrexia, and neutrophilia	Leukemia
Muir-Torre syndrome	Sebaceous adenomas and keratoacanthomas	Colorectal adenocarcinoma
Cowden's syndrome	Multiple hamartomas	Breast carcinoma, follicular thyroid carcinoma
Multiple endocrine neoplasia IIB	Lip, tongue, oral neuromas	Medullary thyroid carcinoma, Pheochromocytoma
Peutz-Jeghers syndrome	Mucocutaneous pigmentation	Colonic adenocarcinoma

and cancers of the urinary tract (16). While the pathogenesis of Leser-Trélat remains unclear, evidence suggests that increases in tumor-derived growth factors may play a role (11).

On physical examination, SKs are waxy, hyperpigmented, verruciform papules or plaques (Fig. 20.2) that appear to be "stuck on." At times they can look as though they might be easily peeled away from the surface of the skin. Even though the lesions in Leser-Trélat frequently affect the back, chest, and extremities, the face and groin may also be involved (17). The concomitant presence of acanthosis nigricans (discussed later in this chapter) may raise suspicion of an underlying malignancy (11).

The differential diagnosis of the individual lesions includes benign, premalignant, and malignant lesions, including lentigines, nevi, actinic keratoses, atypical nevi, pigmented Bowen's disease, and melanoma. Diagnosis is usually clinical, and can be aided by the use of dermoscopy. Confirmation can be obtained by a skin biopsy.

Although SKs are very common especially in older individuals, the sudden, explosive eruption of numerous lesions or their onset before the third decade is unusual and should prompt further investigation. A workup consists of a complete history and physical examination, routine blood studies (CBC and LFTs), chest x-ray, and age- and gender-specific cancer screening (i.e., mammogram and Pap smear for women, and prostate-specific antigen [PSA] for men). Endoscopic evaluation of the gastrointestinal tract should also be considered, along with any symptom-directed diagnostic studies.

While pruritus may be a prominent feature in some cases, the presence of SKs itself is not dangerous to the patient, and providing reassurance of this is important.

SKs that are particularly irritating or cosmetically bothersome may be treated by a number of different destructive methods. Cryosurgery with liquid nitrogen is the most common treatment modality. SKs may also be removed using curettage and cautery under local anesthesia, chemical cauterization with topical application of 70% trichloroacetic acid, or with laser treatments. Larger lesions can be treated by shave removal.

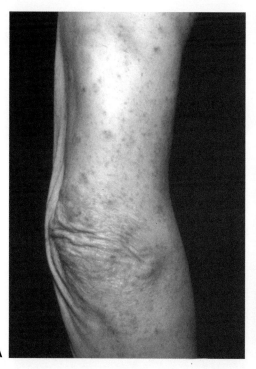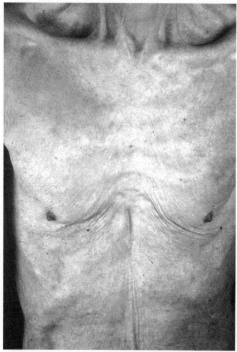

Figure 20.1 A: Pruritus in Hodgkin's disease. **B:** Pruritus associated with xerosis. (NYU Langone Medical Center, Ronald O. Perelman Department of Dermatology slide collection.)

TABLE 20.2 SELECT SYMPTOMATIC TREATMENT OF PRURITUS

Medication	Notes
Antihistamines • Hydroxyzine • H₁ Antagonists	• Reduces itching by reducing skin inflammation. • Sedating antihistamine is antipruritic partly due to its soporific effects.
Topical corticosteroids • Triamcinolone • Clobetasol	• Reduces itching by controlling the inflammatory response. • Risk of skin atrophy. Avoid using for prolonged periods.
Ultraviolet light therapy (UVA and UVB)	• Nonpharmacologic treatment option. Can be used in patients with contraindications to systemic agents. • Adverse side effects include erythema, burning, photoaging, and potential increased risk of skin cancers.
Antidepressants (SSRIs and SNRIs) • Paroxetine • Mirtazapine	• SNRIs and SSRIs are indicated in paraneoplastic pruritus. • Mirtazapine may cause increased appetite and weight gain.
Neuroleptics • Gabapentin	• Structural analogues of GABA neurotransmitter. • Precise antipruritic mechanism is unknown
Tricyclic antidepressants • Doxepin • Amitriptyline	• Doxepin treats depression and anxiety at high doses and has antipruritic effects at lower concentrations.
Opioid receptor antagonists and agonists • Naltrexone • Butorphanol	• Considered in patients refractory to regular antipruritic therapy. • Common side effects may include dizziness, nausea, vomiting, headache, drowsiness, and dry mouth.

UVA, ultraviolet light A; UVB, ultraviolet light B; SSRIs, serotonin reuptake inhibitors; SNRIs, selective norepinephrine reuptake inhibitors; GABA, gamma-aminobutyric acid.

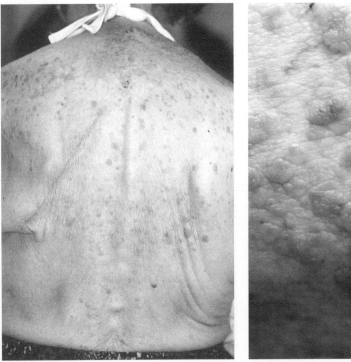

A   B

Figure 20.2 A: Leser-Trélat associated with lung cancer—note pneumonectomy scar. **B:** Close-up view of seborrheic keratoses in Leser-Trélat. (Yale Department of Dermatology Residents' slide collection.)

Erythema Gyratum Repens

Erythema gyratum repens is a rare, inflammatory dermatoses that is associated with an underlying malignancy approximately 70% to 84% of the time (18,19). Gammel first described erythema gyratum repens in 1952 in association with breast carcinoma (20). Since that time, this reactive eruption has been described in a variety of other cancers, including notably that of the lung (21) and esophagus (22).

The rash of erythema gyratum repens is distinct and visually striking. On clinical examination, multiple, concentric and serpiginous bands take on a "wood grain" appearance (Fig. 20.3). They tend to affect the trunk and proximal extremities (19) while sparing the hands, feet, and face (23). There is mild scaling associated with the lesions, and patients may complain of pruritus. Lesions are rapidly advancing, migrating over the course of hours. Unlike the characteristic clinical picture, histopathologic findings are nonspecific and may include hyperkeratosis, acanthosis, spongiosis, and a superficial perivascular lymphohistiocytic infiltrate (24). Because deposits of immunoglobulin (Ig)G and C3 have been found at the basement membrane of lesional skin, erythema gyratum repens is thought to be mediated by an immune response to the presence of tumor antigens (25).

On suspicion of erythema gyratum repens, dermatologic consultation is advised for confirmation. Because of the high likelihood of association with underlying cancer, an extensive search for malignancy is indicated. Standard screening laboratory and imaging studies should be performed

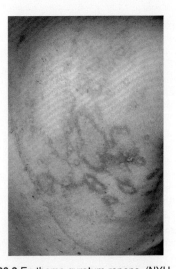

Figure 20.3 Erythema gyratum repens. (NYU Langone Medical Center, Ronald O. Perelman Department of Dermatology slide collection.)

with special attention toward ruling out cancer of the lung (19,25). While it has been found in the absence of malignancy (26), the cutaneous eruption can precede the onset of malignancy, so it is important to repeat screening tests periodically.

The most effective treatment of cutaneous lesions is therapy targeting the underlying tumor (19). Skin manifestations may resolve after removal of localized tumors but can persist until death in widespread disease. Associated pruritus and inflammation can be treated with oral antihistamines and topical and systemic corticosteroids (Table 20.2).

Hypertrichosis Lanuginosa Acquisita

Hypertrichosis lanuginosa acquisita (HLA), also known as malignant down, is characterized by the growth of fine, nonpigmented hair that occurs primarily on the face (22). It is most commonly associated with cancers of the lung (27) and colorectal cancers (28) but has also been reported with carcinomas of the breast (29), kidney (30), and pancreas (31).

HLA frequently appears after the tumor has already metastasized, and its presence usually implies poor prognosis with a survival time of <2 years (22). However, lanugo hair growth can appear before the tumor is diagnosed (29). Thus, for patients presenting with HLA, blood examination, chest x-ray, and colonoscopy are advised (32).

The most effective treatment for HLA is successful removal of the underlying tumor. Cosmetic management may be attempted through electrolysis, depilatories, or shaving. Because the hairs are not pigmented, treatment with hair removal laser have limited efficacy as lasers target melanin in the hair follicle. Treatment with 13.9% eflornithine HCl cream applied to the affected area twice daily can be helpful to slow down hair growth. This agent inhibits ornithine decarboxylase, a key hair cycle enzyme (33). When combined with microneedling (a procedure where small needles puncture the topmost layer, allowing enhanced permeation of agent to the skin), the hair growth inhibitory activity of eflornithine is potentially increased (34).

Necrolytic Migratory Erythema

Necrolytic migratory erythema (NME) is present in almost 70% of patients with glucagonoma, a condition caused by a rare neuroendocrine tumor of pancreatic islet α-cells (35,36). The eruption of NME begins as an erythematous patch involving the groin and spreads to the buttocks (particularly the intergluteal cleft), perineum, thighs, and lower extremities (Fig. 20.4).

The erythematous areas may have scalloped borders and will eventually undergo scaling and blister formation. Upon rupture of the blisters, superficial crusting and erosions occur with eventual healing and pigmentary change over the course of several weeks. This may follow a relapsing and remitting course and occur in association with stomatitis (Fig. 20.4B) (37). Laboratory abnormalities will show elevated plasma glucagon levels, which is a diagnostic finding. Anemia and elevated glucose levels often accompany this condition (36).

NME can clinically resemble dermatoses of other nutritional deficiencies (36). The differential diagnosis also includes intertrigo, superficial candidiasis, bullous drug eruption, and pemphigus. Consultation with dermatology and a skin biopsy can help clarify the diagnosis. The most specific histologic findings of NME are vacuolated dyskeratotic epidermal cells leading to a superficial epidermal necrosis (Fig. 20.4D) (36).

As with other paraneoplastic syndromes, treatment of the underlying tumor results in the significant amelioration, and even resolution of cutaneous symptoms (38). Unfortunately, patients with NME may already have metastatic disease at the time of diagnosis (39).

In these cases, palliative treatment with the somatostatin analog octreotide has been promising (40,41). Improvement may be noted as early as 1 week after beginning therapy, but resistance can develop. While waiting for response, denuded areas should be gently cleansed twice daily, covered with a bland emollient such as petroleum jelly, and dressed with a nonadherent bandage. Monitoring for secondary infection is important, especially in the hospitalized patient.

NME has occasionally been reported in patients without glucagonoma or evidence of pancreatic disease (42,43).

Paraneoplastic Pemphigus

Paraneoplastic pemphigus (PNP) is a potentially life-threatening, immunologically mediated blistering skin disorder that can occur in association with lymphoproliferative malignancies (44). PNP is characterized by severe, hemorrhagic stomatitis, painful oral pharyngeal ulcers, and skin lesions with variable morphology (Fig. 20.5) (45–47). Though most commonly seen with non-Hodgkin's lymphoma and chronic lymphocytic leukemia (48), PNP has also been associated with Castleman's disease, thymoma, Waldenstrom's macroglobulinemia, and various carcinomas and sarcomas (49).

The pathogenesis of PNP centers on production of autoantibodies that attack components of the hemidesmosome and desmosome that adhere epidermal cells to their basement membrane and to one another (46). These pathogenic autoantibodies recognize desmoglein-1, desmoglein-3,

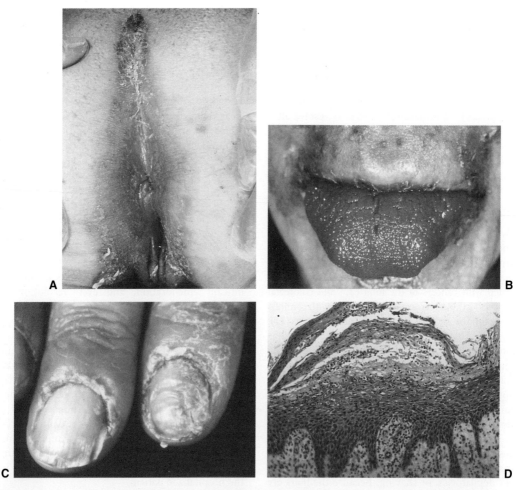

Figure 20.4 Necrolytic migratory erythema in the glucagonoma syndrome. **A:** Perianal blistering. **B:** Stomatitis. **C:** Characteristic periungual involvement. **D:** Histologic findings include superficial epidermal necrosis and dyskeratotic cells. (NYU Langone Medical Center, Ronald O. Perelman Department of Dermatology slide collection.)

hemidesmosomal antigen BP230 (BPAg1), and the plakin proteins (44). Targeting such components weakens the scaffolding system of the skin and renders the epidermal cells more susceptible to shearing forces, causing formation of blisters. These blisters rupture and result in erosive stomatitis, ulceration of the oral mucosa, and cutaneous erosions (46,47).

Microscopically, findings can be varied (46,47). A perilesional biopsy will show suprabasilar acantholysis of oral epithelium or skin epidermis. Necrotic keratinocytes along with a scant lymphocytic infiltrate may also be seen. Direct immunofluorescence studies may demonstrate deposition of IgG and C3 on epidermal surfaces and variably along the basement membrane. Indirect immunofluorescence studies have shown the presence of antibodies that recognize antigens on monkey esophagus as well as transitional epithelium from

rat bladder (50). Immunoprecipitation studies will demonstrate the presence of autoantibodies to desmogleins 1 and 3, envoplakins, periplakins, desmoplakins, or BPAg1 (48). Because of the complex nature of the disease and its diagnosis, the consideration of PNP necessitates consultation with a dermatologist.

PNP can be recalcitrant to therapy. The concomitant treatment of the underlying condition associated with PNP offers the best chance at success (49). To reduce symptoms, oral steroids have traditionally been used as first-line treatment (49,51). High-potency topical steroid gels twice daily can also provide some relief to affected oral mucosa. To decrease steroid dosage, potent immunosuppressive drugs such as azathioprine, cyclosporine, cyclophosphamide, and mycophenolate can also added in combination (49,51). More recently, rituximab (a chimeric anti-CD20 monoclonal antibody)

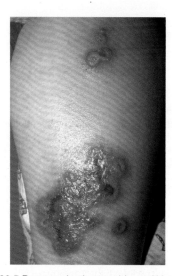

Figure 20.5 Paraneoplastic pemphigus. Although paraneoplastic pemphigus commonly affects the oral mucosa, other areas may present with superficial blisters as seen in this patient. (NYU Langone Medical Center, Ronald O. Perelman Department of Dermatology slide collection.)

has emerged as a preferred therapy given its superior effectiveness and reduced tumorigenicity risk (49). For those that do not respond, intravenous immunoglobulin (IVIG) can be added (49). Antimicrobial therapy is also recommended, because of the risk of sepsis following loss of skin integrity and iatrogenic immunosuppression (52). Analgesics should be considered to reduce the pain caused by extensive erosions (52).

Unfortunately, the mortality of PNP is very high (57% to 90%), and most deaths occur within the first year of diagnosis (48,49,52).

Bazex Syndrome

Bazex syndrome, also known as acrokeratosis paraneoplastica, refers to a cutaneous eruption of psoriasiform lesions on the ears, nose, fingers, and toes (Fig. 20.6), with keratoderma and nail

changes that occur in setting of an internal malignancy (53). It disproportionally affects males, and the most common associated malignancy is squamous cell carcinoma of the upper aerodigestive tract (53).

The skin lesions typically precede the diagnosis of malignancy (54) and may evolve through three stages (55). In the initial stage, there is vesicle formation with thickening of the periungual skin, subungual hyperkeratosis, and nail dystrophy. Erythematous, scaly plaques develop on the helices of the ears, the dorsal aspects of the digits, and the toes. This stage is usually asymptomatic (53). The second stage ensues if the tumor remains undiagnosed and untreated. This is characterized by violaceous color changes on the palms and soles, which are resistant to local therapy. If the tumor remains unrecognized, the skin lesions spread to the trunk, extremities, and scalp in the final stage.

The biopsy findings of Bazex syndrome are a combination of nonspecific features including hyperkeratosis, acanthosis, parakeratosis, and specific features of other disorders with dyskeratotic keratinocytes, vacuolar degeneration, and pigment incontinence (53). A mononuclear perivascular cell infiltrate may also be present in the superficial dermis (53). In one report of Bazex syndrome associated with SCC of the tonsil, direct immunofluorescence studies showed deposition of IgA, IgM, IgG, and C3 on the basement membrane (56), supporting an immunologically mediated pathogenic mechanism.

Since the most commonly associated malignancies are SCCs of the aerodigestive track, a full social history detailing risk factors of tobacco use and alcohol consumption should be elicited. The physical examination should include a thorough inspection of the head and neck (57). An exhaustive workup for underlying malignancy with serologic and radiologic studies is indicated.

The skin lesions of Bazex syndrome are generally resistant to topical therapy including corticosteroids, salicylic acid, and vitamin D analogues (54).

Figure 20.6 Bazex syndrome. **A:** Psoriasiform dermatitis. **B:** Foot involvement. (NYU Langone Medical Center, Ronald O. Perelman Department of Dermatology slide collection.)

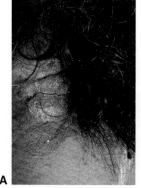

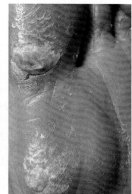

A   B

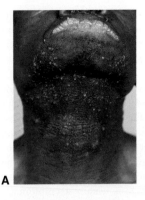
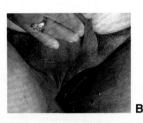

A   **B**

Figure 20.7 Acanthosis nigricans, characterized by velvety, hyperpigmented plaques involving intertriginous areas. **A:** Acanthosis nigricans of the neck. **B:** Acanthosis nigricans of the groin. (NYU Langone Medical Center, Ronald O. Perelman Department of Dermatology slide collection.)

However, treatment of the underlying tumor can result in resolution of cutaneous symptoms (54,58).

Malignant Acanthosis Nigricans

Acanthosis nigricans is a reactive skin condition that is commonly linked to obesity, insulin resistance, and endocrinopathies (59). More rarely, acanthosis nigricans can be a cutaneous sign of an internal malignancy.

In malignancy-associated acanthosis nigricans (MAN), the typical velvet-like, hyperpigmented skin thickenings usually seen on the neck and intertriginous areas (Fig. 20.7) take on a more striking appearance and present in less typical locations such as the oral mucosa (60), areolae of the nipple (61), or palms and soles (61). The development of such lesions can be sudden in onset, rapidly progressive, and extensive (61). Soft papillomas and warty nodules may even stud the affected surface (59). Those affected with MAN are generally older and nonobese (59).

MAN is most frequently associated with adenocarcinoma of the stomach (62) but may be seen with almost any internal cancers including cancers of the liver (63), lung (64), kidney (65), ovary (66), and breast (61). Interestingly, the coexistence of acanthosis nigricans and Leser-Trélat was reported in a patient with advanced gastric adenocarcinoma (11). In this case, appearance of both conditions preceded other manifestations of the malignancy by 6 months. Acanthosis nigricans presenting with rugose thickenings of the palms ("tripe palms") has also been reported as a marker for internal malignancy (67).

In patients presenting with acanthosis nigricans, a full history and examination should be conducted. Laboratory studies such as fasting glucose and insulin levels should help rule out obesity-associated acanthosis nigricans. In patients where an underlying malignancy is suspected, screening tests for common gastrointestinal cancers should be considered and workup and imaging studies should be directed by clinical symptoms.

First-line treatment for MAN is treating the underlying cancer (68). Anderson et al. report a case of MAN with complete resolution after combination chemotherapy (69). There is a case report of MAN resolving with cyproheptadine (70). Extensive MAN with severe itching may benefit from psoralen and ultraviolet light A treatment (PUVA) (71).

Dermatomyositis

Dermatomyositis (DM) is an idiopathic, autoimmune, inflammatory disease that is characterized by proximal muscle weakness, and characteristic cutaneous findings. The estimated prevalence of internal malignancy in adult patients with DM is approximately 20%, with the risk of developing an internal malignancy highest in the first year following diagnosis and 5 years thereafter (72).

Clinically, DM may manifest with proximal muscle weakness resulting in difficulty performing daily activities such as combing hair, putting on a shirt, or rising from a seated position. Cutaneous findings can vary, but the features considered pathognomonic include a heliotrope rash and Gottron's papules (Fig. 20.8). The heliotrope rash is a pink to violet dermatitis involving the eyelids and periorbital skin. Gottron's papules are raised lesions present on the joints of the hands. The "shawl sign" is also a common feature, and it refers to poikiloderma (blotchy erythema with telangiectasias, atrophy, and hypopigmentation), involving the upper chest, shoulders, and upper back (73,74).

Laboratory values of creatine phosphokinase (CPK) and aldolase are commonly elevated in DM. Anti-Jo-1 and antinuclear antibodies may also be present (73). A skin biopsy showing epidermal atrophy, vacuolar interface changes in the basal keratinocytes, superficial and deep perivascular infiltrate, mucin deposition, and thickening of the basement membrane can help support the diagnosis (73,74).

DM may be associated with any malignancy, but particularly with gynecological cancers such as breast and ovary followed by cancers of the colon (75,76). DM has also been reported with hematologic and prostate cancers (76).

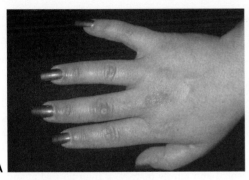
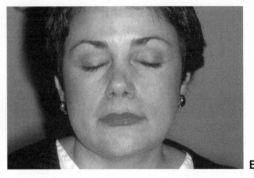

A   **B**

Figure 20.8 Dermatomyositis. **A:** Gottron's papule. **B:** Characteristic heliotrope rash. (Yale Department of Dermatology Resident slide collection.)

Recent developments in understanding of myositis-specific antibodies can help direct workup. Anti-TIF1 (previously anti-p155/140) is strongly associated with malignancy. Except in children, the finding of anti-NXP2 antibodies is also correlated with an increased risk of malignancy (74). Any adult patient with newly diagnosed DM and Anti-TIF1 or anti-NXP2 must be evaluated for the presence of a visceral malignancy. History and physical, including a pelvic examination, age-appropriate screening, symptom-targeted screening, and whole body imaging (CT, MRI) should be performed and repeated annually for 5 years (77).

Treatment of the cutaneous manifestations of DM consists of topical steroids, topical calcineurin inhibitors (tacrolimus), and systemic glucocorticoids in combination with steroid-sparing agents such as methotrexate and mycophenolate mofetil (77). Prevention with sunscreen (SPF30+), protective clothing, and avoidance of sunlight are crucial since cutaneous eruptions in DM are photosensitive. In patients with refractory disease, rituximab and IVIG have been effective (77,78). Most recently, tofacitinib, an oral Janus kinase (JAK)-1/3 inhibitor, seemed promising in refractory cutaneous disease (79). If pruritus is significant, antihistamines such as hydroxyzine and systemic antidepressants such as doxepin and amitriptyline can be added for symptomatic relief (80).

Sweet's Syndrome

Sweet's syndrome, also known as acute febrile neutrophilic dermatosis, is named after Dr. Robert Sweet, who first described this inflammatory skin disorder in 1964 (81,82). It is characterized by the abrupt onset of painful erythematous to violaceous plaques or nodules with fever and leukocytosis (83). The cutaneous lesions, which may ulcerate, involve the face, neck, and extremities (Fig. 20.9) (84). In addition to the cutaneous lesions, involvement of the eyes, lung, heart, kidneys, liver, gastrointestinal tract, and central nervous system has been described (83).

Sweet's syndrome may be malignancy-associated, drug-induced, or secondary to infectious or inflammatory conditions (83,84). In rare cases, it has even been associated with pregnancy (85). Clinical features that raise the index of suspicious for an underlying malignancy include advanced age, vesiculobullous morphology, anemia, elevated erythrocyte sedimentation rate, and absence of arthralgias (83).

In malignancy-associated Sweet's syndrome, the most frequently reported malignancies are hematologic, notably acute myelogenous leukemia (84). Less commonly, Sweet's syndrome has been reported with solid malignant tumors (86). In a study of cases of Sweet's syndrome associated with solid tumors, the most commonly associated malignancies were genitourinary carcinomas (37%), breast carcinomas (23%), and cancers of the gastrointestinal tract (17%) (86).

There is no consensus on the particular workup for underlying associated conditions in patients diagnosed with Sweet's syndrome. However, given the malignancy associations, a full history and physical plus age-appropriate malignancy screening is important. Because of the frequency of hematologic disorders, a peripheral blood smear, testing for paraproteinemia, and a

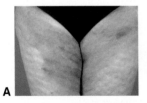
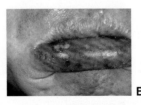

A   **B**

Figure 20.9 Sweet's syndrome. **A:** An indurated plaque in a patient with Sweet's syndrome. Involvement of oral mucosa. (NYU Langone Medical Center, Ronald O. Perelman Department of Dermatology slide collection.) **B:** Involvement of oral mucosa.

bone marrow biopsy should be considered, (83). Additional testing for associated diseases (e.g., inflammatory bowel disease, other autoimmune disorders) should be conducted based on index of suspicion (83).

The mainstay treatment of Sweet's syndrome is systemic corticosteroids, with an effective response being a minor diagnostic criterion. Symptoms usually resolve with oral prednisone at 0.5 to 1 mg/kg/d, or pulse intravenous methylprednisolone in refractory cases (83). Intralesional corticosteroid injections and high-potency topical corticosteroids (clobetasol propionate 0.05%) can also be effective (86). Alternative first-line treatments include potassium iodide and colchicine (87). The successful use of indomethacin, dapsone, clofazimine, and cyclosporine has also been reported (87).

CANCER-RELATED GENODERMATOSES

Muir-Torre Syndrome

The Muir-Torre syndrome (MTS) was first described by Muir et al. in 1967 (88), and by Torre in 1968 (89), who noted an association of sebaceous adenomas of the skin with internal cancers.

These malignancies are most commonly colorectal adenocarcinomas, followed by tumors of the urogenital system (endometrium, ovary, bladder, kidney, and ureter) (90). Less commonly, CNS malignancies and various sarcomas have also been reported (91).

While the majority of cases of MTS are transmitted in an autosomal dominant manner, as a result of defects in mismatch repair genes leading to microsatellite instability, some cases may be sporadic (91). A less common autosomal recessive subtype of MTS does not demonstrate microsatellite instability and results from defective base excision repair (92).

The skin lesions most often associated with MTS are sebaceous adenomas, sebaceous epitheliomas, sebaceous carcinomas, and keratoacanthomas (KAs) (91). On physical examination, sebaceous adenomas appear as pink- to yellow-colored papules, usually measuring <5 mm. They are commonly located on the face but can occur anywhere. Sebaceous epitheliomas can take on a cystic appearance, whereas sebaceous carcinomas typically appear as a papule on the eyelid and can be overlooked in the early stages. Sebaceous carcinomas are common on the eyelid but may appear as cystic lesions on the extremities (Fig. 20.10). KAs usually occur as a rapidly growing dome-shaped nodule with a keratinaceous central core.

The presence of sebaceous neoplasms or multiple KAs should prompt a thorough review of personal and family history of internal malignancies (91). Cystic sebaceous neoplasms have also been reported as specific markers of MTS (93). After informed consent, these skin lesions should be sent for immunohistochemical analysis.

The treatment of choice for sebaceous carcinoma and KA-like SCC on the face is Mohs micrographic surgery (MMS) (94). MMS offers the highest rate of cure and the advantage of tissue conservation due to superior margin control. Sebaceous epitheliomas can be excised with clear margins, whereas sebaceous adenomas can be removed by tangential (shave) excision. Incomplete removal is likely to result in local recurrence.

Management of MTS must proceed beyond treatment of the primary skin lesions and should include a collaboration of dermatologists, gastroenterologists, geneticists, oncologists, and surgeons. Appropriate cancer screening should be performed on patients and their family members.

Cowden's Syndrome

Cowden's syndrome (CS) is an autosomal dominant disorder characterized by multi-organ hamartomatous neoplasms and an increased risk of malignancy, particularly of the breast, thyroid, and endometrium (95). While generally associated with benign colonic polyps, CS may carry more of a risk for GI malignancy than previously thought (96).

Although it was widely reported that 80% of patients with CS have a mutation in the PTEN tumor suppressor gene, larger cohort studies with

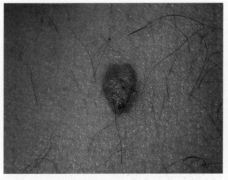 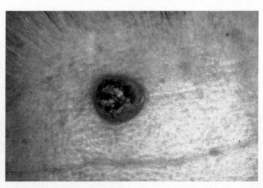

A   **B**

Figure 20.10 Muir-Torre syndrome. **A:** Sebaceous carcinomas as shown here are seen in Muir-Torre syndrome. (Photo by John Carucci.) **B:** Keratoacanthomas may be associated with Muir-Torre syndrome.

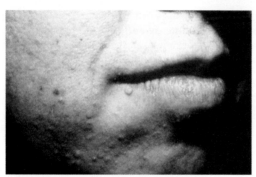

Figure 20.11 Cowden's syndrome. Perioral trichilemmomas are characteristic in Cowden's syndrome. (Yale Department of Dermatology Residents' slide collection.)

revised diagnostic criteria now suggests about 30% to 35% of people actually have the inherited mutation (96).

Skin manifestations are almost always present in this condition and they include facial trichilemmomas (which sometimes can be mistaken for warts) (Fig. 20.11) and oral papillomas, which give a "cobblestone appearance" to the tongue and oral mucosa (97). Mucocutaneous neuromas, acral keratotic papules, palmoplantar pits, and penile pigmentation (in males) may also be present (96,97).

When CS is suspected, dermatologic consultation is important for confirmation. Skin biopsy of a facial papule showing trichilemmoma is one of the major diagnostic criteria (96). Management of this condition requires a multidisciplinary effort with many specialists. Appropriate cancer screening should be performed for breast and thyroid carcinomas, with regular, close follow-ups for ongoing surveillance. Genetic counseling should also be offered.

Trichilemmomas are benign lesions; however, trichilemmomal carcinoma has been reported in CS (98). Treatment of skin lesions is through destructive modalities such as laser ablation, dermabrasion, or shave excision, but recurrences are common. Oral retinoids such as acitretin have also been proposed but were found to be only temporarily helpful, as mucocutaneous lesions reoccur upon drug withdrawal (99). Because inactivating mutations in the *PTEN* allow for unrestrained Akt and downstream mTOR signaling, sirolimus, an inhibitor of mTOR, has garnered

interest. Recently, a pilot study in humans evaluating sirolimus in the treatment of Cowden's disease showed some evidence of improvement in skin and GI lesions (100).

Multiple Endocrine Neoplasia

Multiple endocrine neoplasia (MEN) IIb is also known as multiple mucosal neuroma syndrome (101). It is due to an activating mutation in the *RET* protooncogene (102). Although inherited in an autosomal dominant manner, it can also occur sporadically (103).

Mucocutaneous signs are almost always present and include neuromas on the tongue, lips, and oral mucosa (104). These appear as papules or nodules and may involve the palatal, nasal, and laryngeal mucosa (101).

Patients usually present early in childhood; the appearance of mucosal lesions may be as early as the first year of life and precede development of internal cancers by decades (104). Skeletal abnormalities are also seen in an overwhelming majority of patients with MEN IIb, typically exhibiting a marfanoid habitus (104).

Nearly everyone with MEN IIb has medullary carcinoma of the thyroid, followed by pheochromocytoma in up to 50% of individuals (104,105). Gastrointestinal involvement is present in majority of the patients, and GI neuroma may lead to diarrhea, constipation, and megacolon (104,106).

If MEN is suspected, consultation with a dermatologist and geneticist is indicated. Workup should include urine catecholamine level, thyroid scan, thyroid function tests, and CT scan of the abdomen. Because of the hereditary nature and high penetrance of MEN IIb, *RET* molecular genetic testing is considered in individuals with clinical diagnosis. Screening for malignancies and periodic examination of patients and their relatives at high risk may lead to early diagnosis and curative treatment of associated internal cancers (104).

Unfortunately, treatment of neuromas by excision often results in recurrence.

Peutz-Jeghers Syndrome

Peutz-Jeghers syndrome (PJS) is an autosomal dominant condition characterized by mucocutaneous pigmentation and hamartomatous intestinal

Figure 20.12 A: Peutz-Jeghers syndrome periorificial lentiginosis in a patient with Peutz-Jeghers syndrome. **B:** Involvement of digits. (NYU Langone Medical Center, Ronald O. Perelman Department of Dermatology slide collection.)

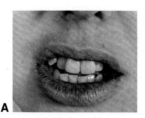

A

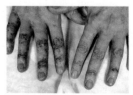

B

polyps that have malignant potential (107). The genetic defect is due to loss of function mutations in the tumor suppressor gene serine/threonine kinase 11 (STK11) (108). Inheritance represents over 70% of the cases, with approximately 25% to 30% of cases occurring sporadically (107,109).

Mucocutaneous freckling is a characteristic feature of PJS in 90% to 95% of cases (107,109). The pigmented macules appear in infancy around the mouth, particularly at the vermilion border of the lip (107,109). These 2 to 5 mm uniformly brown to black macules can also occur on the face, buccal mucosa, palms, soles, digits (Fig. 20.12), perianal area, intestinal mucosa, and nail plate (107).

GI polyps are predominantly in the small intestines and colon and occur in 88% to 100% of PJS patients. Larger polyps can cause recurrent intussusception, leading to bleeding and abdominal pain (107,110). These hamartomas of the colon also have the potential to develop into adenocarcinoma.

While colorectal cancers are most frequently reported associated malignancy (39%), there is also increased risk of breast, ovarian, uterine, lung, small bowel, gastric, and pancreatic carcinoma (107,111). The lifetime cumulative cancer risk for a person with PJS can approach 80% by 70 years of age (107). Adequate periodic screening is thus essential for patients with PJS.

Consensus surveillance guidelines recommend upper gastrointestinal endoscopy, video capsule endoscopy, and colonoscopy, starting at 8 years of age (or sooner if symptomatic) and repeated every 3 years if polyps are found. In the absence of polyps, subsequent endoscopy should be done at age 18 (109,112). Screening for breast and gynecologic cancers should begin at age 25 and for pancreatic cancers at age 30. Lung cancer screening in PJS smokers is also recommended (107).

When PJS is diagnosed, consultation with a geneticist and close follow-up with gastroenterology is indicated.

No treatment is necessary for skin and mucosal melanotic macules. Over time, the lentigines on the lips may resolve without intervention; however, those on the buccal mucosa can persist. If a source of cosmetic concern, the lentigines can be successfully treated with Q-switched alexandrite lasers (113).

CONCLUSION

The skin can play an important role in the detection of internal malignancies. Tumor-associated skin disorders may appear in many forms with varying degrees of severity. Managing the skin conditions can greatly increase patients' comfort. In select cases, prompt diagnosis and effective management can lead to early detection of cancer

and alter prognosis. Since skin abnormalities may be the presenting sign of an occult malignancy, it is essential that any suspected case be evaluated by a dermatologist. Individuals presenting with these cutaneous paraneoplastic dermatoses should have a thorough workup for the associated malignancy. Symptomatic relief should be provided. Often, only treatment of the underlying disease permits complete resolution of its cutaneous manifestations.

REFERENCES

1. Yosipovitch G. Chronic pruritus: a paraneoplastic sign. *Dermatol Ther*. 2010;23(6):590-596.
2. Larson VA, Tang O, Stander S, Kang S, Kwatra SG. Association between itch and cancer in 16,925 patients with pruritus: experience at a tertiary care center. *J Am Acad Dermatol*. 2019;80(4):931-937.
3. Gobbi PG, Attardo-Parrinello G, Lattanzio G, Rizzo SC, Ascari E. Severe pruritus should be a B-symptom in Hodgkin's disease. *Cancer*. 1983;51(10):1934-1936.
4. Stander S, Bockenholt B, Schurmeyer-Horst F, et al. Treatment of chronic pruritus with the selective serotonin re-uptake inhibitors paroxetine and fluvoxamine: results of an open-labelled, two-arm proof-of-concept study. *Acta Derm Venereol*. 2009;89(1):45-51.
5. Dawn AG, Yosipovitch G. Butorphanol for treatment of intractable pruritus. *J Am Acad Dermatol*. 2006;54(3):527-531.
6. Goncalves F. Thalidomide for the control of severe paraneoplastic pruritus associated with Hodgkin's disease. *Am J Hosp Palliat Care*. 2010;27(7):486-487.
7. Wang H, Yosipovitch G. New insights into the pathophysiology and treatment of chronic itch in patients with end-stage renal disease, chronic liver disease, and lymphoma. *Int J Dermatol*. 2010;49(1):1-11.
8. He A, Alhariri JM, Sweren RJ, Kwatra MM, Kwatra SG. Aprepitant for the treatment of chronic refractory pruritus. *Biomed Res Int*. 2017;2017:4790810.
9. Turan E, Yesilova Y, Yurt N, Kocarslan S. Leser-Trelat sign: does it really exist? *Acta Dermatovenerol Croat*. 2013;21(2):123-127.
10. Chakradeo K, Narsinghpura K, Ekladious A. Sign of Leser-Trelat. *BMJ Case Rep*. 2016;2016:bcr2016215316.
11. Yeh JS, Munn SE, Plunkett TA, Harper PG, Hopster DJ, du Vivier AW. Coexistence of acanthosis nigricans and the sign of Leser-Trelat in a patient with gastric adenocarcinoma: a case report and literature review. *J Am Acad Dermatol*. 2000;42(2 Pt 2):357-362.
12. Bernett CN, Schmieder GJ. Leser Trelat sign. In: *StatPearls*. Treasure Island, FL: StatPearls Publishing; 2020.
13. Heaphy MR Jr, Millns JL, Schroeter AL. The sign of Leser-Trelat in a case of adenocarcinoma of the lung. *J Am Acad Dermatol*. 2000;43(2 Pt 2):386-390.
14. Wagner RF, Wagner KD. Malignant neoplasms and the Leser-Trelat sign. *Arch Dermatol*. 1981;117(9):598-599.
15. Gori N, Esposito I, Del Regno L, D'Amore A, Peris K, Di Stefani A. Leser-Trelat sign as a rare manifestation of cutaneous melanoma. *Dermatol Reports*. 2020;12(1):8665.
16. Stollmeier A, Rosario BA, Mayer BL, Frandoloso GA, Magalhaes FL, Marques GL. Seborrheic keratoses as the first sign of bladder carcinoma: case report of Leser-Trelat sign in a rare association with urinary tract cancer. *Case Rep Med*. 2016;2016:4259190.
17. Schwartz RA. Sign of Leser-Trelat. *J Am Acad Dermatol*. 1996;35(1):88-95.

18. Rongioletti F, Fausti V, Parodi A. Erythema gyratum repens is not an obligate paraneoplastic disease: a systematic review of the literature and personal experience. *J Eur Acad Dermatol Venereol.* 2014;28(1):112-115.

19. Boyd AS, Neldner KH, Menter A. Erythema gyratum repens: a paraneoplastic eruption. *J Am Acad Dermatol.* 1992;26(5 Pt 1):757-762.

20. Gammel JA. Erythema gyratum repens; skin manifestations in patient with carcinoma of breast. *AMA Arch Derm Syphilol.* 1952;66(4):494-505.

21. Eubanks LE, McBurney E, Reed R. Erythema gyratum repens. *Am J Med Sci.* 2001;321(5):302-305.

22. Kurzrock R, Cohen PR. Cutaneous paraneoplastic syndromes in solid tumors. *Am J Med.* 1995;99(6):662-671.

23. Votquenne N, Richert B. Erythema gyratum repens. *JAMA Dermatol.* 2020;156:912.

24. Calonje E, McKee PH. *McKee's Pathology of the Skin: With Clinical Correlations.* New York, NY: Elsevier; 2020.

25. Holt PJ, Davies MG. Erythema gyratum repens—an immunologically mediated dermatosis? *Br J Dermatol.* 1977;96(4):343-347.

26. Kawakami T, Saito R. Erythema gyratum repens unassociated with underlying malignancy. *J Dermatol.* 1995;22(8):587-589.

27. Russell P, Floridis J. Hypertrichosis lanuginosa acquisita: a rare dermatological disorder. *Lancet.* 2016;387(10032):2035.

28. Brinkmann J, Breier B, Goos M. [Hypertrichosis lanuginosa acquisita in ulcerative colitis with colon cancer]. *Hautarzt.* 1992;43(11):714-716.

29. Levine D, Miller S, Al-Dawsari N, Barak O, Gottlieb AB. Paraneoplastic dermatoses associated with gynecologic and breast malignancies. *Obstet Gynecol Surv.* 2010;65(7):455-461.

30. Duncan LE, Hemming JD. Renal cell carcinoma of the kidney and hypertrichosis lanuginosa acquisita. *Br J Urol.* 1994;74(5):678-679.

31. McLean DI, Macaulay JC. Hypertrichosis lanuginosa acquisita associated with pancreatic carcinoma. *Br J Dermatol.* 1977;96(3):313-316.

32. Cohen PR, Kurzrock R. Mucocutaneous paraneoplastic syndromes. *Semin Oncol.* 1997;24(3):334-359.

33. Hickman JG, Huber F, Palmisano M. Human dermal safety studies with eflornithine HCl 13.9% cream (Vaniqa), a novel treatment for excessive facial hair. *Curr Med Res Opin.* 2001;16(4):235-244.

34. Kumar A, Naguib YW, Shi YC, Cui Z. A method to improve the efficacy of topical eflornithine hydrochloride cream. *Drug Deliv.* 2016;23(5):1495-1501.

35. Wei J, Lin S, Wang C, et al. Glucagonoma syndrome: a case report. *Oncol Lett.* 2015;10(2):1113-1116.

36. van Beek AP, de Haas ER, van Vloten WA, Lips CJ, Roijers JF, Canninga-van Dijk MR. The glucagonoma syndrome and necrolytic migratory erythema: a clinical review. *Eur J Endocrinol.* 2004;151(5):531-537.

37. Toberer F, Hartschuh W, Wiedemeyer K. Glucagonoma-associated necrolytic migratory erythema: the broad spectrum of the clinical and histopathological findings and clues to the diagnosis. *Am J Dermatopathol.* 2019;41(3):e29-e32.

38. V'Lckova-Laskoska M, Balabanova-Stefanova M, Arsovska-Bezhoska I, Caca-Biljanovska N, Laskoski D. Necrolytic migratory erythema: complete healing after surgical removal of pancreatic carcinoma. *Acta Dermatovenerol Croat.* 2018;26(4):329-332.

39. Pujol RM, Wang CY, el-Azhary RA, Su WP, Gibson LE, Schroeter AL. Necrolytic migratory erythema: clinicopathologic study of 13 cases. *Int J Dermatol.* 2004;43(1):12-18.

40. Poggi G, Villani L, Bernardo G. Multimodality treatment of unresectable hepatic metastases from pancreatic glucagonoma. *Rare Tumors.* 2009;1(1):e6.

41. Saavedra C, Lamarca A, Hubner RA. Resolution of necrolytic migratory erythema with somatostatin analogue in a patient diagnosed with pancreatic glucagonoma. *BMJ Case Rep.* 2019;12(8):e229115.

42. Technau K, Renkl A, Norgauer J, Ziemer M. Necrolytic migratory erythema with myelodysplastic syndrome without glucagonoma. *Eur J Dermatol.* 2005;15(2):110-112.

43. Nakashima H, Komine M, Sasaki K, et al. Necrolytic migratory erythema without glucagonoma in a patient with short bowel syndrome. *J Dermatol.* 2006;33(8):557-562.

44. Zhu X, Zhang B. Paraneoplastic pemphigus. *J Dermatol.* 2007;34(8):503-511.

45. Allen CM, Camisa C. Paraneoplastic pemphigus: a review of the literature. *Oral Dis.* 2000;6(4):208-214.

46. Anhalt GJ. Paraneoplastic pemphigus. *Adv Dermatol.* 1997;12:77-96; discussion 97.

47. Sklavounou A, Laskaris G. Paraneoplastic pemphigus: a review. *Oral Oncol.* 1998;34(6):437-440.

48. Ouedraogo E, Gottlieb J, de Masson A, et al. Risk factors for death and survival in paraneoplastic pemphigus associated with hematologic malignancies in adults. *J Am Acad Dermatol.* 2019;80(6):1544-1549.

49. Wieczorek M, Czernik A. Paraneoplastic pemphigus: a short review. *Clin Cosmet Investig Dermatol.* 2016;9:291-295.

50. Morrison LH. When to request immunofluorescence: practical hints. *Semin Cutan Med Surg.* 1999;18(1):36-42.

51. Cizenski JD, Michel P, Watson IT, et al. Spectrum of orocutaneous disease associations: immune-mediated conditions. *J Am Acad Dermatol.* 2017;77(5):795-806.

52. Paolino G, Didona D, Magliulo G, et al. Paraneoplastic pemphigus: insight into the autoimmune pathogenesis, clinical features and therapy. *Int J Mol Sci.* 2017;18(12):2532.

53. Bolognia JL, Brewer YP, Cooper DL. Bazex syndrome (acrokeratosis paraneoplastica). An analytic review. *Medicine (Baltimore).* 1991;70(4):269-280.

54. Rassler F, Goetze S, Elsner P. Acrokeratosis paraneoplastica (Bazex syndrome)—a systematic review on risk factors, diagnosis, prognosis and management. *J Eur Acad Dermatol Venereol.* 2017;31(7):1119-1136.

55. Bolognia JL. Bazex syndrome: acrokeratosis paraneoplastica. *Semin Dermatol.* 1995;14(2):84-89.

56. Pecora AL, Landsman L, Imgrund SP, Lambert WC. Acrokeratosis paraneoplastica (Bazex' syndrome). Report of a case and review of the literature. *Arch Dermatol.* 1983;119(10):820-826.

57. Abreu Velez AM, Howard MS. Diagnosis and treatment of cutaneous paraneoplastic disorders. *Dermatol Ther.* 2010;23(6):662-675.

58. Hara M, Hunayama M, Aiba S, et al. Acrokeratosis paraneoplastica (Bazex syndrome) associated with primary cutaneous squamous cell carcinoma of the lower leg, vitiligo and alopecia areata. *Br J Dermatol.* 1995;133(1):121-124.

59. Schwartz RA. Acanthosis nigricans. *J Am Acad Dermatol.* 1994;31(1):1-19; quiz 20-12.

60. Ramirez-Amador V, Esquivel-Pedraza L, Caballero-Mendoza E, Berumen-Campos J, Orozco-Topete R, Angeles-Angeles A. Oral manifestations as a hallmark of malignant acanthosis nigricans. *J Oral Pathol Med.* 1999;28(6):278-281.

61. Arellano J, Iglesias P, Suarez C, Corredoira Y, Schnettler K. Malignant acanthosis nigricans as a paraneoplastic

manifestation of metastatic breast cancer. *Int J Womens Dermatol*. 2019;5(3):183-186.

62. Yu Q, Li XL, Ji G, et al. Malignant acanthosis nigricans: an early diagnostic clue for gastric adenocarcinoma. *World J Surg Oncol*. 2017;15(1):208.

63. Kaminska-Winciorek G, Brzezinska-Wcislo L, Lis-Swiety A, Krauze E. Paraneoplastic type of acanthosis nigricans in patient with hepatocellular carcinoma. *Adv Med Sci*. 2007;52:254-256.

64. Serap D, Ozlem S, Melike Y, et al. Acanthosis nigricans in a patient with lung cancer: a case report. *Case Rep Med*. 2010;2010:412159.

65. Ferraz de Campos FP, Narvaez MR, Reis PV, et al. Acanthosis Nigricans associated with clear-cell renal cell carcinoma. *Autops Case Rep*. 2016;6(1):33-40.

66. Oh CW, Yoon J, Kim CY. Malignant acanthosis nigricans associated with ovarian cancer. *Case Rep Dermatol*. 2010;2(2):103-109.

67. Barman B, Devi LP, Thakur BK, Raphael V. Tripe palms and acanthosis nigricans: a clue for diagnosis of advanced pancreatic adenocarcinoma. *Indian Dermatol Online J*. 2019;10(4):453-455.

68. Phiske MM. An approach to acanthosis nigricans. *Indian Dermatol Online J*. 2014;5(3):239-249.

69. Anderson SH, Hudson-Peacock M, Muller AF. Malignant acanthosis nigricans: potential role of chemotherapy. *Br J Dermatol*. 1999;141(4):714-716.

70. Greenwood R, Tring FC. Treatment of malignant acanthosis nigricans with cyproheptadine. *Br J Dermatol*. 1982;106(6):697-698.

71. Bonnekoh B, Thiele B, Merk H, Mahrle G. [Systemic photochemotherapy (PUVA) in acanthosis nigricans maligna: regression of keratosis, hyperpigmentation and pruritus]. *Z Hautkr*. 1989;64(12):1059-1062.

72. Qiang JK, Kim WB, Baibergenova A, Alhusayen R. Risk of malignancy in dermatomyositis and polymyositis. *J Cutan Med Surg*. 2017;21(2):131-136.

73. Callen JP. Dermatomyositis. *Lancet*. 2000;355(9197): 53-57.

74. DeWane ME, Waldman R, Lu J. Dermatomyositis: clinical features and pathogenesis. *J Am Acad Dermatol*. 2020;82(2):267-281.

75. Cherin P, Piette JC, Herson S, et al. Dermatomyositis and ovarian cancer: a report of 7 cases and literature review. *J Rheumatol*. 1993;20(11):1897-1899.

76. Leatham H, Schadt C, Chisolm S, et al. Evidence supports blind screening for internal malignancy in dermatomyositis: data from 2 large US dermatology cohorts. *Medicine (Baltimore)*. 2018;97(2):e9639.

77. Waldman R, DeWane ME, Lu J. Dermatomyositis: diagnosis and treatment. *J Am Acad Dermatol*. 2020;82(2):283-296.

78. Femia AN, Eastham AB, Lam C, Merola JF, Qureshi AA, Vleugels RA. Intravenous immunoglobulin for refractory cutaneous dermatomyositis: a retrospective analysis from an academic medical center. *J Am Acad Dermatol*. 2013;69(4):654-657.

79. Kurtzman DJ, Wright NA, Lin J, et al. Tofacitinib citrate for refractory cutaneous dermatomyositis: an alternative treatment. *JAMA Dermatol*. 2016;152(8): 944-945.

80. Vleugels RA, Callen JP. Dermatomyositis: current and future treatments. *Exp Rev Dermatol*. 2009;4(6): 581-594.

81. Sweet RD. Further observations on acute febrile neutrophilic dermatosis. *Br J Dermatol*. 1968;80(12): 800-805.

82. Sweet RD. Acute febrile neutrophilic dermatosis—1978. *Br J Dermatol*. 1979;100(1):93-99.

83. Nelson CA, Stephen S, Ashchyan HJ, James WD, Micheletti RG, Rosenbach M. Neutrophilic dermatoses: pathogenesis, sweet syndrome, neutrophilic eccrine hidradenitis, and Behcet disease. *J Am Acad Dermatol*. 2018;79(6):987-1006.

84. Cohen PR. Sweet's syndrome—a comprehensive review of an acute febrile neutrophilic dermatosis. *Orphanet J Rare Dis*. 2007;2:34.

85. Satra K, Zalka A, Cohen PR, Grossman ME. Sweet's syndrome and pregnancy. *J Am Acad Dermatol*. 1994; 30(2 Pt 2):297-300.

86. Cohen PR, Holder WR, Tucker SB, Kono S, Kurzrock R. Sweet syndrome in patients with solid tumors. *Cancer*. 1993;72(9):2723-2731.

87. Cohen PR. Neutrophilic dermatoses: a review of current treatment options. *Am J Clin Dermatol*. 2009;10(5): 301-312.

88. Muir EG, Bell AJ, Barlow KA. Multiple primary carcinomata of the colon, duodenum, and larynx associated with kerato-acanthomata of the face. *Br J Surg*. 1967;54(3):191-195.

89. Torre D. Multiple sebaceous tumors. *Arch Dermatol*. 1968;98(5):549-551.

90. Ponti G, Ponz de Leon M. Muir-Torre syndrome. *Lancet Oncol*. 2005;6(12):980-987.

91. John AM, Schwartz RA. Muir-Torre syndrome (MTS): an update and approach to diagnosis and management. *J Am Acad Dermatol*. 2016;74(3):558-566.

92. Kim RH, Nagler AR, Meehan SA. Universal immunohistochemical screening of sebaceous neoplasms for Muir-Torre syndrome: putting the cart before the horse? *J Am Acad Dermatol*. 2016;75(5):1078-1079.

93. Lachiewicz AM, Wilkinson TM, Groben P, Ollila DW, Thomas NE. Muir-Torre syndrome. *Am J Clin Dermatol*. 2007;8(5):315-319.

94. Leslie DF, Greenway HT. Mohs Micrographic Surgery for skin cancer. *Australas J Dermatol*. 1991;32(3): 159-164.

95. Pilarski R. PTEN Hamartoma Tumor syndrome: a clinical overview. *Cancers (Basel)*. 2019;11(6):844.

96. Pilarski R, Burt R, Kohlman W, Pho L, Shannon KM, Swisher E. Cowden syndrome and the PTEN hamartoma tumor syndrome: systematic review and revised diagnostic criteria. *J Natl Cancer Inst*. 2013;105(21):1607-1616.

97. Lopes S, Vide J, Moreira E, Azevedo F. Cowden syndrome: clinical case and a brief review. *Dermatol Online J*. 2017;23(8):13030.

98. O'Hare AM, Cooper PH, Parlette HL III. Trichilemmomal carcinoma in a patient with Cowden's disease (multiple hamartoma syndrome). *J Am Acad Dermatol*. 1997;36(6 Pt 1):1021-1023.

99. Masmoudi A, Chermi ZM, Marrekchi S, et al. Cowden syndrome. *J Dermatol Case Rep*. 2011;5(1):8-13.

100. Komiya T, Blumenthal GM, DeChowdhury R, et al. A pilot study of sirolimus in subjects with Cowden syndrome or other syndromes characterized by germline mutations in PTEN. *Oncologist*. 2019;24(12): 1510-e1265.

101. Holloway KB, Flowers FP. Multiple endocrine neoplasia 2B (MEN 2B)/MEN 3. *Dermatol Clin*. 1995;13(1): 99-103.

102. Goodfellow PJ, Wells SA Jr. RET gene and its implications for cancer. *J Natl Cancer Inst*. 1995;87(20):1515-1523.

103. Znaczko A, Donnelly DE, Morrison PJ. Epidemiology, clinical features, and genetics of multiple endocrine neoplasia type 2B in a complete population. *Oncologist*. 2014;19(12):1284-1286.

104. Vasen HF, van der Feltz M, Raue F, et al. The natural course of multiple endocrine neoplasia type IIb. A study of 18 cases. *Arch Intern Med*. 1992;152(6):1250-1252.

105. Moline J, Eng C. Multiple endocrine neoplasia type 2: an overview. *Genet Med*. 2011;13(9):755-764.

106. Carney JA, Go VL, Sizemore GW, Hayles AB. Alimentary-tract ganglioneuromatosis. A major component of the syndrome of multiple endocrine neoplasia, type 2b. *N Engl J Med*. 1976;295(23):1287-1291.

107. Wilder EG, Frieder J, Sulhan S, et al. Spectrum of orocutaneous disease associations: genodermatoses and inflammatory conditions. *J Am Acad Dermatol*. 2017; 77(5):809-830.

108. Hemminki A, Markie D, Tomlinson I, et al. A serine/threonine kinase gene defective in Peutz-Jeghers syndrome. *Nature*. 1998;391(6663):184-187.

109. Achatz MI, Porter CC, Brugieres L, et al. Cancer screening recommendations and clinical management of inherited gastrointestinal cancer syndromes in childhood. *Clin Cancer Res*. 2017;23(13):e107-e114.

110. Ponti G, Tomasi A, Manfredini M, Pellacani G. Oral mucosal stigmata in hereditary-cancer syndromes: from germline mutations to distinctive clinical phenotypes and tailored therapies. *Gene*. 2016;582(1):23-32.

111. van Lier MG, Wagner A, Mathus-Vliegen EM, Kuipers EJ, Steyerberg EW, van Leerdam ME. High cancer risk in Peutz-Jeghers syndrome: a systematic review and surveillance recommendations. *Am J Gastroenterol*. 2010;105(6):1258-1264; author reply 1265.

112. Beggs AD, Latchford AR, Vasen HF, et al. Peutz-Jeghers syndrome: a systematic review and recommendations for management. *Gut*. 2010;59(7):975-986.

113. Li Y, Tong X, Yang J, Yang L, Tao J, Tu Y. Q-switched alexandrite laser treatment of facial and labial lentigines associated with Peutz-Jeghers syndrome. *Photodermatol Photoimmunol Photomed*. 2012;28(4):196-199.

21 Dermatologic Adverse Events during Treatment

Brianna Olamiju, Sara Yumeen, Yevgeniy Balagula, Alyx Rosen Aigen, and Jonathan Scott Leventhal

INTRODUCTION

Chemotherapy and radiation have been standard anticancer treatment regimens for decades, and the advent of newer targeted agents has revolutionized the management of patients with various malignancies. However, these anticancer therapies are associated with a wide range of adverse events (AEs), with dermatologic toxicities that affect the skin, hair, and nails being the most common. When severe, these therapies can prompt alteration of oncologic therapy, leading to dose reduction or cessation. Timely diagnosis and management of such toxicities is essential to the overall care of patients with cancer. This chapter will introduce practitioners to the grading scale, basic pathophysiology, clinical appearance, and management of the most common skin, hair, and nail AEs in oncology.

TRADITIONAL CHEMOTHERAPY

Alopecia

Chemotherapy-induced alopecia (CIA) is a prevalent, emotionally distressing toxicity associated with multiple chemotherapeutic agents (1). It usually occurs within a few weeks after the first round of chemotherapy and manifests as a patchy anagen effluvium, often first noticeable in the crown and temporo-occipital scalp with subsequent diffuse alopecia of the entire scalp (2). In addition to the scalp, CIA may occur on other body areas including the eyebrows, eyelashes, and axillae. The incidence of CIA has been reported as >80% for taxanes (paclitaxel), 60% to 100% for topoisomerase inhibitors (doxorubicin), >60% for alkylators (cyclophosphamide), and in 10% to 50% of cases treated with antimetabolites (3). CIA usually reverts within 2 to 6 months after chemotherapy is halted. Importantly, studies have demonstrated that CIA is associated with negative impact on quality of life, including poor body image and affecting psychosocial health (4).

CIA typically begins within days to weeks and peaks at 1 to 2 months following chemotherapy initiation (Fig. 21.1). Eyebrows, eyelashes, beard, axillary, and pubic hair have a lower percentage of anagen hairs but may also be affected by chemotherapy, especially at higher doses. New hair growth typically occurs once the biologic effect of the treatment process is removed and may present with a different texture or color. Chemotherapy-induced anagen effluvium is the most common form of CIA. However, telogen effluvium can also occur and is characterized by thinning or a decrease in hair density rather than total baldness. It is frequently associated with methotrexate, 5-fluorouracil, and retinoid (5).

Though not life threatening, CIA has been a documented traumatic aspect of chemotherapy for over 50 years since the introduction of anticancer therapy, yet no completely effective means of prevention or treatment have been established. Scalp cooling is the only FDA-approved tool that may result in lower rates of CIA (6). It works by triggering diminished blood flow to the scalp prompting decreased drug delivery to the area (3). Of note, this intervention is contraindicated in patients with hematologic malignancies or an existing history of scalp metastasis (7). Other contraindications include pediatric patients, cancers of the head and neck, central nervous system malignancies, cold sensitivity or cold agglutin disease, imminent bone marrow ablation chemotherapy or skull irradiation, severe liver or renal disease, skin cancer, and small cell or squamous cell carcinoma of the lung (7).

During chemotherapy, if alopecia develops, use of wigs, head scarves, or hats/turbans is a common camouflage approach. Oncologists can provide prescriptions for wigs, which are then often paid for by insurance companies, and some cancer hospitals may even have hair salons that are staffed with wig specialists. The most notable treatment for acceleration of hair regrowth following chemotherapy is 2% topical minoxidil. In a double-blind, randomized trial, patients who applied 1 mL of 2% topical minoxidil solution to their scalps twice daily throughout chemotherapy and up to 4 months postchemotherapy experienced hair regrowth on average of 50.2 days sooner than did patients in the placebo group (8).

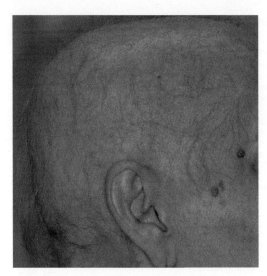

Figure 21.1 Chemotherapy-induced alopecia.

There is a small cohort of patients who may experience persistent postchemotherapy alopecia (pCIA), defined as incomplete hair regrowth 6 months after termination of chemotherapy. It has been reported in breast cancer survivors treated with taxanes and cyclophosphamide-based therapeutics (9). Incidence rates are documented to be as high as 30% for patients previously on taxanes (10).

Hand–Foot Syndrome

Hand–foot syndrome (HFS), also known as palmar–plantar erythrodysesthesia, presents clinically as bilateral erythema, edema, and tenderness of the palms and soles. In severe cases, blistering may even occur (11). The predilection for the palms and soles is thought to be due to drug transport to the skin's surface via the vasculature and high proliferation of keratinocytes (12). HFS from conventional chemotherapies occurs frequently in patients treated with capecitabine, 5-fluorouracil (particularly with continuous infusion), doxorubicin or PEGylated doxorubicin (PLD), cytarabine, methotrexate, and docetaxel. Taxane-induced HFS may manifest uniquely as scaly, erythematous lesions on the dorsal hands and thenar eminences (13), and is referred to as periarticular thenar erythema with onycholysis (PATEO) syndrome. It typically has an onset between 2 and 21 days, but can occur as late as 10 months in patients on chemotherapy drugs that last longer in the body (14). The term "toxic erythema of chemotherapy" (TEC) is used to describe a similar clinical phenomenon that consists of inflammatory eruptions involving intertriginous zones, elbows, knees, and ears usually occurring 2 days to 3 weeks after initiation of chemotherapy (15). TEC is postulated to be caused by a toxic insult to the straight portion of the eccrine ducts as chemotherapy drugs are excreted by the eccrine glands and is documented most frequently with cytarabine, anthracyclines, 5-flourouracil, capecitabine, taxanes, and methotrexate (15). See Figure 21.2 for detailed treatment algorithm for HFS based on severity.

Oral Mucositis

Numerous chemotherapy agents such as paclitaxel, doclitaxel, 5 fluorouracil, epirubicin, cisplatin, and cyclophosphamide are documented to cause dose-dependent oral mucositis. This adverse effect classically presents as erythema that progresses to localized ulcerations within the buccal mucosa (16). Understandably, patients often describe these lesions as very painful and may report more severe discomfort when eating spicy foods. Treatment for oral mucositis secondary to chemotherapy is typically supportive and may include topical steroids, as needed. There is also evidence to support the efficacy of palifermin, cryotherapy, and low-power laser to decrease the incidence and severity of this condition (17). In addition to being associated with chemotherapy, oral mucositis can occur as an adverse effect of radiation therapy, especially for cancers of the head and neck.

Nail Changes

Significant nail changes can occur in the setting of traditional chemotherapy including onycholysis, paronychia, brittle nails, subungual hemorrhage, nail pigmentation, splinter hemorrhage, Mees' lines, and Beau's lines. Taxanes, including docetaxel and paclitaxel, are the most common class of cancer chemotherapeutics that lead to nail toxicities. Nail changes associated with chemotherapy drugs may lead to pain, infection, and negative impact on quality of life (13). Onycholysis with underlying hemorrhage occurs due to toxicity to the nail bed epithelium and results in separation of the nail plate from the nail bed (Fig. 21.3). Aside from taxanes, bleomycin, capecitabine, doxorubicin, etoposide, 5-fluorouracil, and methotrexate have also been reported to cause onycholysis (18). Prevention and management of onycholysis is similar to paronychia and includes keeping nails short, applying topical antimicrobial solutions, and avoiding contact irritants. Vinegar soaks appropriately diluted with water may also be helpful.

Other—Inflammation of Actinic and Seborrheic Keratoses, Maculopapular Rash, Hyperpigmentation

Several chemotherapeutic drugs have been implicated in causing inflamed actinic keratoses, including fluorouracil or its prodrug, capecitabine,

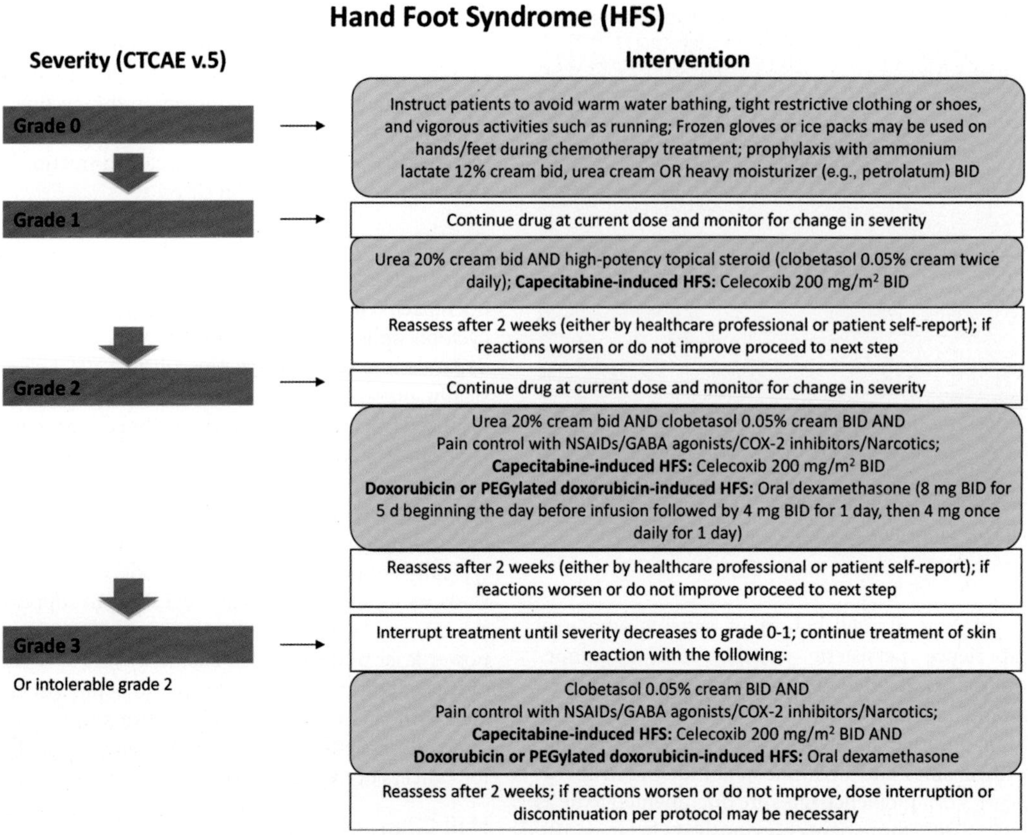

Hand Foot Syndrome (HFS)

Severity (CTCAE v.5)		Intervention

Grade 0 → Instruct patients to avoid warm water bathing, tight restrictive clothing or shoes, and vigorous activities such as running; Frozen gloves or ice packs may be used on hands/feet during chemotherapy treatment; prophylaxis with ammonium lactate 12% cream bid, urea cream OR heavy moisturizer (e.g., petrolatum) BID

Grade 1 → Continue drug at current dose and monitor for change in severity

Urea 20% cream bid AND high-potency topical steroid (clobetasol 0.05% cream twice daily); **Capecitabine-induced HFS:** Celecoxib 200 mg/m^2 BID

Reassess after 2 weeks (either by healthcare professional or patient self-report); if reactions worsen or do not improve proceed to next step

Grade 2 → Continue drug at current dose and monitor for change in severity

Urea 20% cream bid AND clobetasol 0.05% cream BID AND Pain control with NSAIDs/GABA agonists/COX-2 inhibitors/Narcotics; **Capecitabine-induced HFS:** Celecoxib 200 mg/m^2 BID **Doxorubicin or PEGylated doxorubicin-induced HFS:** Oral dexamethasone (8 mg BID for 5 d beginning the day before infusion followed by 4 mg BID for 1 day, then 4 mg once daily for 1 day)

Reassess after 2 weeks (either by healthcare professional or patient self-report); if reactions worsen or do not improve proceed to next step

Grade 3

Or intolerable grade 2

→ Interrupt treatment until severity decreases to grade 0-1; continue treatment of skin reaction with the following:

Clobetasol 0.05% cream BID AND Pain control with NSAIDs/GABA agonists/COX-2 inhibitors/Narcotics; **Capecitabine-induced HFS:** Celecoxib 200 mg/m^2 BID AND **Doxorubicin or PEGylated doxorubicin-induced HFS:** Oral dexamethasone

Reassess after 2 weeks; if reactions worsen or do not improve, dose interruption or discontinuation per protocol may be necessary

Figure 21.2 Algorithm for the management of hand–foot syndrome. (Adapted from Freites-Martinez A, Lacouture ME. Dermatologic adverse events. In: Olver IN, ed. *The MASCC Textbook of Cancer Supportive Care and Survivorship*. 2nd ed. New York, NY: Springer; 2018:597-620.)

and less commonly docetaxel (19). There are also reports of chemotherapy-induced inflamed seborrheic keratoses, particularly on sun-exposed areas such as the neck and chest (20). Recognition of this benign condition is important to avoid unnecessary cessation of chemotherapy. Maculopapular rash has been associated with some

chemotherapeutic agents and typically manifests as an exanthematous reaction similar to a morbilliform drug eruption to antibiotics (21). Finally, diffuse or localized pigmentary changes of the skin, nails, and mucous membranes may also occur with chemotherapy treatment (22). For example, bleomycin has been associated with flagellate hyperpigmentation, fluorouracil has been associated with serpentine hyperpigmentation that usually resolves weeks to months after treatment has ended (23), and busulfan is known to cause hyperpigmentation in a cutaneous presentation that may resemble Addison's disease (24).

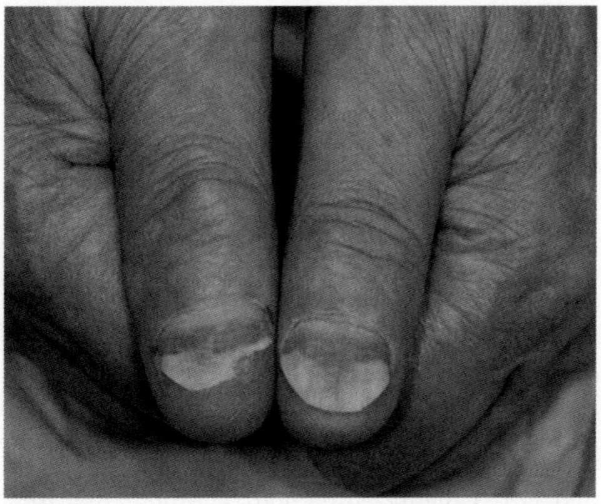

TARGETED THERAPY

Papulopustular Rash

The papulopustular rash (PPR) is the most common dermatologic AE occurring in patients treated with epidermal growth factor receptor (EGFR) inhibitors. Its occurrence is most common with monoclonal antibodies such as cetuximab and panitumumab, and less common with small molecule oral inhibitors including erlotinib. It typically

Figure 21.3 Taxane-induced onycholysis.

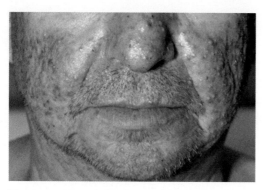

Figure 21.4 EGFR inhibitor–induced papulopustular (acneiform) rash on the face.

occurs in a dose-dependent manner in >75% of patients after 1 to 2 weeks of therapy (25). The etiology of the PPR is likely a result of inhibition of EGFR, as has been described for erlotinib, cetuximab, and panitumumab (25). The rash is characterized by erythematous papules and/or pustules affecting the seborrheic-rich areas, including the face, specifically the cheeks, nose, forehead, chin, perioral regions, and the scalp and upper trunk (Fig. 21.4) (26). Physical symptoms often associated with the PPR include pain, pruritus, burning, and irritation in up to 62% of patients, all of which negatively impact a patient's QoL (27). MEK inhibitors and anti-HER2 therapies for breast cancer may also manifest with PPR.

Grade severity of the rash is based on the body surface area (BSA) involved and degree of limitation to performing activities of daily living (ADLs), shown in Table 21.1. Prophylaxis and management strategies are shown in Figure 21.5.

Nail Changes

Anticancer agents can cause a wide range of nail toxicities. They can damage the nail bed and cause onycholysis or subungual hemorrhage, or cause inflammation of the proximal nail folds, also known as paronychia. Additional nail changes include nail ridging, brittleness, and alterations in pigmentation.

Paronychia

All patients who receive treatment with EGFR inhibitors are at risk for developing nail changes, with incidence up to 72.5% (28). Paronychia is characterized by painful erythema, edema, and tenderness of the nail folds (Fig. 21.6). With increased severity, painful pyogenic granuloma–like lesions may develop, which bleed with minimal trauma and mimic ingrown nails in patients with no preceding history of ingrown nails. Multiple fingers may be affected with a predilection for

the great toes and thumbs. Panitumumab-treated patients experience the greatest incidence of all-grade (26.5%) paronychia in comparison to the other EGFR inhibitors. Infection is not the primary event in paronychia development, but identification of microorganisms in lesions is common. Management strategies (shown in Fig. 21.7) are aimed at minimizing periungual trauma, preventing superinfection, and eliminating excessive granulation tissue. Promising new treatments include topical timolol and topical povidone–iodine. Topical timolol, 0.5% gel twice daily under occlusion for 1 month has resulted in partial to complete response in patients with paronychia and pseudopyogenic granuloma (29). Topical povidone solution, composed of 2% povidone–iodine in a dimethylsulfoxide vehicle also results in partial to complete resolution of paronychia (30).

Hair Changes

With the advent of novel targeted therapies, including EGFR inhibitors, hair changes as a side effect of therapy have been observed. These include trichomegaly and curling of the eyebrows and eyelashes, hypertrichosis and hirsutism of the face and female lip, and curlier, finer, and more brittle hair on the scalp and extremities after prolonged treatment. In men, fewer shavings of the beard may be seen. Alopecia may occur and is generally mild and usually manifests as an androgenetic hair loss pattern, however erlotinib-induced cicatricial alopecia and inflammatory nonscarring alopecia have been described (31). Although these hair changes are seen less frequently than other common EGFR inhibitor cutaneous AEs, occurring in only 5% to 6% of patients (32), they may be associated with significant psychosocial discomfort. Multikinase inhibitors have been associated with hair changes characterized by alterations of hair texture, density, and color. Alopecia has been reported most commonly with sorafenib (44%), sunitinib (5% to 21%), and pazopanib (8% to 10%) [33]. Reversible hair depigmentation has also been reported to occur with sunitinib (7% to 14%) and pazopanib (27% to 44%) (33). Tyrosine kinase inhibitor imatinib has also been reported to induce depigmentation of skin as well as eyebrow and scalp hairs, resulting in leukotrichia (34). Management of scalp hair changes includes frequent hair brushing, which can loosen hair kinking and reduce its brittleness (35). Regular eyelash trimming or even electrolysis may be necessary and can prevent keratitis. Wax depilation, threading, laser, or bleaching of undesired facial hair offers good cosmetic results, but gentle skin care is recommended in conjunction to avoid irritating adverse effects of these treatments.

TABLE 21.1 GRADING OF DERMATOLOGIC ADVERSE EVENTS

AE term	Grade 1	Grade 2	Grade 3	Grade 4	Grade 5
Alopecia	Hair loss of <50% of normal for that individual that is not obvious from a distance but only on close inspection; a different hairstyle may be required to cover the hair loss but it does not require a wig to camouflage	Hair loss of ≥50% normal for that individual that is readily apparent to others; a wig is necessary to completely camouflage the hair loss; associated with psychosocial impact	—	—	—
Radiation dermatitis	Faint erythema or dry desquamation	Moderate to brisk erythema; patchy moist desquamation, mostly confined to skin folds and creases; moderate edema	Moist desquamation in areas other than skin folds and creases; bleeding induced by minor trauma or abrasion	Life-threatening consequences; skin necrosis or ulceration of full-thickness dermis; spontaneous bleeding from involved site; skin graft indicated	
Dry skin	Covering <10% BSA and no associated erythema or pruritus	Covering 10%–30% BSA and associated with erythema or pruritus; limiting instrumental ADL	Covering >30% BSA and associated with pruritus; limiting self-care ADL		
Hypertrichosis	Increase in length, thickness or density of hair that the patient either is able to camouflage by periodic shaving or removal of hairs or is not concerned enough about the overgrowth to use any form of hair removal	Increase in length, thickness or density of hair at least on the usual exposed areas of the body that requires shaving or use of hair removal to camouflage; associated with psychosocial impact			
Oral mucositis	Asymptomatic or mild symptoms; intervention not indicated	Moderate pain or ulcer that does not interfere with oral intake; modified diet indicated	Severe pain; interfering with oral intake	Life-threatening consequences; urgent intervention indicated	Death
Palmar–plantar erythrodysesthesia syndrome	Minimal skin changes or dermatitis (e.g., erythema, edema, or hyperkeratosis) without pain	Skin changes (e.g., peeling, blisters, bleeding, fissures, edema, or hyperkeratosis) with pain; limiting instrumental ADL	Severe skin changes (e.g., peeling, blisters, bleeding, fissures, edema, or hyperkeratosis) with pain; limiting self-care ADL	—	—

				Life-threatening consequences	Death
Papulopustular rash	Papules and/or pustules covering <10% BSA, which may or may not be associated with symptoms of pruritus or tenderness	Papules and/or pustules covering 10%–30% BSA, which may or may not be associated with symptoms of pruritus or tenderness; associated with psychosocial impact; limiting instrumental ADL; papules and/or pustules covering >30% BSA with or without mild symptoms	Papules and/or pustules covering >30% BSA with moderate or severe symptoms; limiting self-care ADL; IV antibiotics indicated	Papules and/or pustules covering >30% BSA with moderate or severe symptoms; limiting self-care ADL; IV antibiotics indicated	—
Paronychia	Nail fold edema or erythema; disruption of the cuticle	Localized or oral (e.g., antibiotic, antifungal, antiviral) intervention indicated; edema or erythema with pain; associated discharge or nail plate separation; limiting instrumental ADL	Surgical intervention or IV antibiotics indicated; limiting self-care ADL	—	—
Pruritus	Mild or localized; topical intervention indicated	Widespread and intermittent; skin changes from scratching (e.g., edema, papulation, excoriations, lichenification, oozing/crusts); oral intervention indicated; limiting instrumental ADL	Widespread and constant; limiting self-care ADL or sleep; systemic corticosteroid or immunosuppressive therapy indicated	—	—
Rash maculopapular	Macules/papules covering <10% BSA with or without symptoms (e.g., pruritus, burning, tightness)	Macules/papules covering 10%–30% BSA with or without symptoms (e.g., pruritus, burning, tightness); limiting instrumental ADL; rash covering >30% BSA with or without mild symptoms	Macules/papules covering >30% BSA with or without symptoms; limiting self-care ADL	—	—
Acute graft versus host disease	<25% BSA	25%–50% BSA	Generalized erythroderma	Erythroderma, bullous lesions, +/– desquamation	—
Chronic graft versus host disease	1%–18% BSA	19%–50% BDS	>50% BSA with presence of sclerotic features	>50% BSA with presence of deep sclerotic features, hidebound quality, impaired mobility secondary to sclerosis, ulceration	—

Adapted from Common Terminology Criteria for Adverse Events version 5.0—Selected Skin and Subcutaneous Tissue Disorders.

Papulopustular (Acneiform) Rash

Severity (CTCAE v.5)	Intervention

Grade 0 →

Prophylactic therapy with Sunscreen SPF 30; moisturizing creams; gentle skin care. Prophylactic therapy with doxycycline or minocycline 100 mg daily and low potency topical steroid for the first 6 weeks of therapy.

Grade 1 →

Continue drug at current dose and monitor for change in severity

Topical low/moderate strength steroid daily AND
Topical antibiotic BID (clindamycin 1–2%, erythromycin 1–2%, metronidazole 1%)

Reassess after 2 weeks (either by healthcare professional or patient self-report); if reactions worsen or do not improve proceed to next step

Grade 2 →

Continue drug at current dose and monitor for change in severity

Oral antibiotics* for 6 weeks (doxycycline or minocycline 100 mg BID) AND Topical antibiotic*, topical low/moderate strength steroids AND Consider prednisone 0.5 mg/kg taper for intolerable rash or if inadequate response to therapy.

Reassess after 2 weeks (either by healthcare professional or patient self-report); if reactions worsen or do not improve proceed to next step

Grade ≥3
Or intolerable grade 2 →

Dose modify as per protocol; obtain bacterial/viral cultures if infection is suspected; continue treatment of skin reaction with the following:

Oral antibiotics* with doxycycline or minocycline 100 mg BID AND
Topical moderate/high strength steroids AND
Prednisone 0.5 mg/kg taper AND
Consider low dose isotretinoin (20–30 mg daily) for recalcitrant cases.

Reassess after 2 weeks; if reactions worsen or do not improve, dose interruption or discontinuation per protocol may be necessary

*Tailor antibiotics to superficial wound culture

Figure 21.5 Algorithm for the management of papulopustular (acneiform) rash. (Adapted from Freites-Martinez A, Lacouture ME. Dermatologic adverse events. In: Olver IN, ed. *The MASCC Textbook of Cancer Supportive Care and Survivorship*. 2nd ed. New York, NY: Springer; 2018:597-620.)

Xerosis, Pruritus, and Fissures

Xerosis (skin dryness) is a late reaction seen with cetuximab and other EGFR inhibitors as well as the MKIs sorafenib and sunitinib. Gefitinib can also cause xerosis of the face and distal fingers or toes. It commonly occurs following the appearance of the PPR and is frequently reported with pruritus (36). Between 33% and 100% of patients treated with EGFR inhibitors for more than 6 months develop xerosis (37). Xerosis appears as scaling or even fine desquamation. Pruritus associated with xerosis can lead to widespread excoriations and an increased risk of secondary skin infections, in particular *Staphylococcus aureus.* Extreme dryness of the hands and feet can lead to fissures or tiny cracks on the fingertips, toes, and dorsal aspects of interphalangeal joints, which can be extremely painful and bleed. Preventative measures include minimizing exposure to hot water during bathing or dish washing and using alcohol-free emollients to moisturize the skin (Table 21.2). See Figures 21.8 and 21.9 for detailed algorithms for the management of xerosis and pruritus.

Hand–Foot Skin Reaction

Hand–foot skin reaction (HFSR) is the most common dose-limiting side effect of targeted MKIs, including pazopanib, sorafenib, and sunitinib. HSFR also occurs with anti-VEGFR therapies and with BRAF inhibitors. Overall incidence of HSFR with MKIs has been reported as 2% with pazopanib, 4% to 12% with sunitinib, and 2% to 26% with

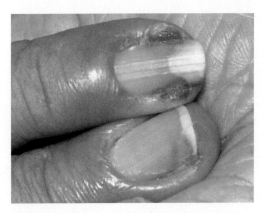

Figure 21.6 EGFR inhibitor–induced paronychia.

Paronychia

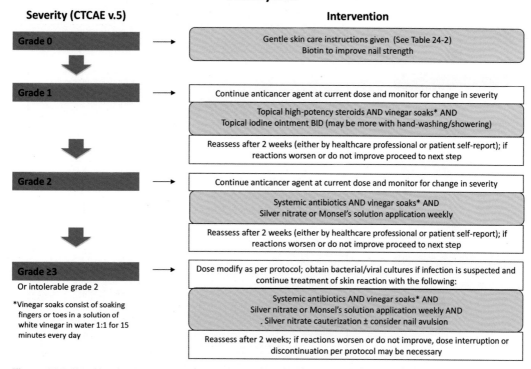

Severity (CTCAE v.5)		Intervention

Grade 0 → Gentle skin care instructions given (See Table 24-2)
Biotin to improve nail strength

Grade 1 → Continue anticancer agent at current dose and monitor for change in severity

Topical high-potency steroids AND vinegar soaks* AND
Topical iodine ointment BID (may be more with hand-washing/showering)

Reassess after 2 weeks (either by healthcare professional or patient self-report); if
reactions worsen or do not improve proceed to next step

Grade 2 → Continue anticancer agent at current dose and monitor for change in severity

Systemic antibiotics AND vinegar soaks* AND
Silver nitrate or Monsel's solution application weekly

Reassess after 2 weeks (either by healthcare professional or patient self-report); if
reactions worsen or do not improve proceed to next step

Grade ≥3
Or intolerable grade 2 → Dose modify as per protocol; obtain bacterial/viral cultures if infection is suspected and
continue treatment of skin reaction with the following:

*Vinegar soaks consist of soaking
fingers or toes in a solution of
white vinegar in water 1:1 for 15
minutes every day

Systemic antibiotics AND vinegar soaks* AND
Silver nitrate or Monsel's solution application weekly AND
Silver nitrate cauterization ± consider nail avulsion

Reassess after 2 weeks; if reactions worsen or do not improve, dose interruption or
discontinuation per protocol may be necessary

Figure 21.7 Algorithm for the management of paronychia. (Adapted from Freites-Martinez A, Lacouture ME. Dermatologic adverse events. In: Olver IN, ed. *The MASCC Textbook of Cancer Supportive Care and Survivorship*. 2nd ed. New York, NY: Springer; 2018:597-620.)

sorafenib (38). Clinically, patients with HFSR present within the first 2 to 4 weeks of treatment with tender, scaly lesions with surrounding erythema localized to areas of pressure or friction including the tips of fingers and toes, heels, and metatarsophalangeal joints (39). Lesions progress to thickened, hyperkeratotic, painful skin that impairs function and movement (39) (Fig. 21.10). Uncommonly, large painful bullae in areas of friction can also be seen. The condition appears to be dose dependent and typically subsides within several weeks after treatment discontinuation. HFSR differs both clinically and mechanistically from classical HFS. HFSR may be the result of the combined

TABLE 21.2 PREVENTATIVE STRATEGIES FOR DERMATOLOGIC TOXICITIES OF TARGETED ANTICANCER THERAPIES

Papulopustular rash	Hand–foot syndrome/ hand–foot skin reaction	Xerosis/Pruritus	Paronychia
Broad-spectrum (UVA/ UVB) sunscreen with SPF ≥ 15 Physical blockers (zinc oxide, titanium dioxide)	Wear thick cotton gloves/ socks and shoes with padded insoles	Minimize the frequency and duration of hot showers or baths	Avoid wearing tight-fitting shoes
Limit excessive sun exposure	Avoid trauma/friction to hands/feet	Use lukewarm water to shower and wash dishes	Keep nails short
Alcohol-free emollients to moisturize dry skin twice a day	Avoid hot water when bathing or dish washing	Alcohol-free emollients to moisturize dry skin twice a day	Avoid hot water when bathing or dish washing
	Moisturize with creams containing keratolytics (ammonium lactate or urea)		Moisturize periungual areas

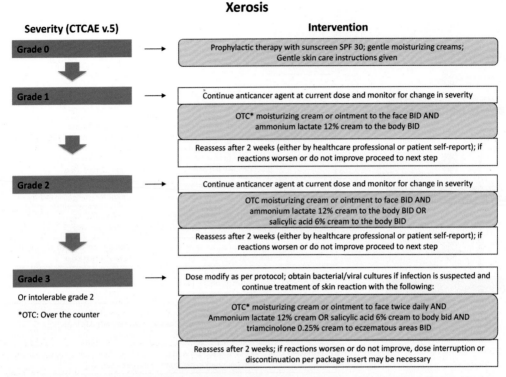

Figure 21.8 Algorithm for the management of xerosis. OTC, over the counter. (Adapted from Freites-Martinez A, Lacouture ME. Dermatologic adverse events. In: Olver IN, ed. *The MASCC Textbook of Cancer Supportive Care and Survivorship*. 2nd ed. New York, NY: Springer; 2018:597-620.)

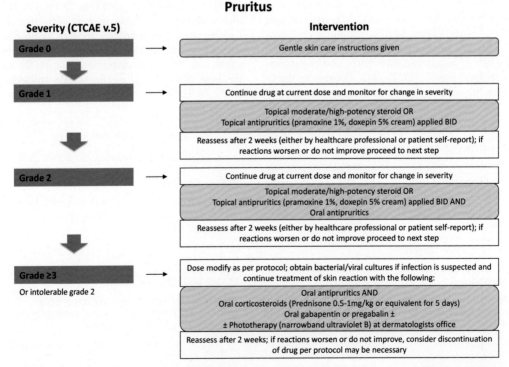

Figure 21.9 Algorithm for the management of pruritus. (Adapted from Balagula E, Lacouture ME. Dermatologic toxicities. In: Olver IN, ed. *The MASCC Textbook of Cancer Supportive Care and Survivorship*. New York, NY: Springer; 2011:361-380.)

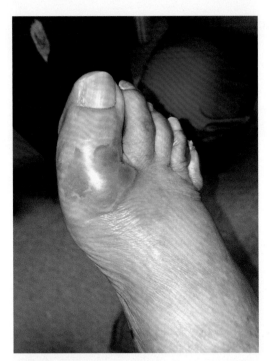

Figure 21.10 Multikinase inhibitor–induced hand–foot skin reaction.

inhibition of vascular endothelial growth factor receptor and platelet-derived growth factor receptor that potentially prevents proper functioning of vascular repair mechanisms leading to drug leakage from capillaries damaged by subclinical trauma (39). Preventative measures are similar to those implemented for HFS and are most important during the first 2 to 4 weeks of treatment (Table 21.2). Treatment recommendations are based on the CTCAE v5.0 grades (Fig. 21.2).

CHECKPOINT INHIBITOR THERAPY

Maculopapular Rash

Maculopapular rash is the most common dermatologic adverse effect associated with checkpoint inhibitor therapy, with an incidence rate of 14% to 40% of patients depending on the specific agent (40). It is most frequently observed in anti-CTLA-4 monotherapy and anti-PD-1/CTLA-4 combination therapy (41). Clinically, these lesions present as pruritic erythematous macules and papules, most commonly found on the trunk and upper limbs, and may worsen with each subsequent treatment (42). In the majority of cases, these lesions are low grade and should not prompt cessation of treatment. When appropriate, the rash can be treated with topical steroids, and severe presentations may require systemic corticosteroids. The CTCAE is used to stratify severity

of the maculopapular rash (see Table 21.1). Mild maculopapular rash should not cause cessation of the immune checkpoint inhibitor (ICPi) and can be treated with mild topical corticosteroids and/or oral antihistamines. If severe, anticancer therapy should be held and systemic steroids should be administered until the rash resolves to Grade 1.

Vitiligo-Like Depigmentation

Vitiligo-like depigmentation may occur from ICPis (Fig. 21.11), in addition to other forms of melanocyte alteration, including regression of melanocytic nevi. This AE is strongly associated with melanoma patients on ICPis, but may occur in other tumors less commonly (43). Such treatment-induced vitiligo usually presents months after initiation of treatment and is not presumed to be dose related (44). Interestingly, some studies have demonstrated that the manifestation of vitiligo in patients on ICPis may be associated with greater survival outcomes (45).

Severe Cutaneous Adverse Reactions

Severe cutaneous adverse reactions (SCARs) have been reported in rare cases with ICPis. Stevens-Johnson syndrome/toxic epidermal necrolysis (SJS/TEN) is a grade 4 exfoliative dermatitis reaction that constitutes <1% of cutaneous AEs from ICPis (46). The skin classically presents with dusky macules or papules with possible associated mucosal involvement. SJS/TEN can be a very severe reaction that necessitates the cessation of the causative drug, urgent hospitalization, and treatment typically with intravenous systemic corticosteroids or IVIG (47). Drug reaction with eosinophilia and systemic symptoms (DRESS) has also been reported with ICPis, usually between 2 and 8 weeks after initiation of the culprit drug, with a documented mortality close to 10% (48).

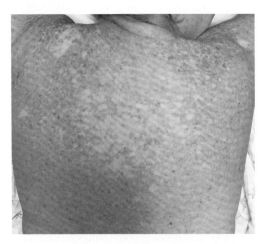

Figure 21.11 Vitiligo-like depigmentation.

Finally, acute generalized exanthematous pustulosis (AGEP) has infrequently been associated with ICPis, and is classically characterized by fever, diffuse erythema with predilection to intertriginous sites with nonfollicular pustules, and neutropenia 48 to 72 hours after the initiation of a new medication. Similar to other SCARs, its management consists of cessation of the culprit agent and systemic corticosteroids.

Other—Lichenoid, Psoriasiform, Immunobullous, Sarcoidosis

A pruritic lichenoid reaction may be observed in patients on anti-PD-1/PD-L1 agents. This rash typically occurs at a later onset in comparison to the maculopapular rash and clinically manifests similarly to lichen planus with pruritic, pink-violaceous papules and/or plaques and may also involve the mucosal surfaces (Fig. 21.12). The mainstay of treatment for this condition involves topical and/or oral corticosteroids for severe presentations. The addition of phototherapy in these patients may also be helpful for mitigating the rash (49). Psoriasiform reactions can also occur, especially in patients with a preexisting history of psoriasis (50). Most commonly, patients present with plaque psoriasis, though other forms of psoriasis such as palmoplantar, pustular, and erythrodermic presentations have been reported (51).

Immunobullous reactions, in particular bullous pemphigoid, have been increasingly documented as adverse reactions to PD-1 and PD-L1 ICPis (52). These reactions can be very severe, and they occur in approximately 1% of patients on these agents. Clinically, this reaction presents as either scattered vesicles or widespread bullae and

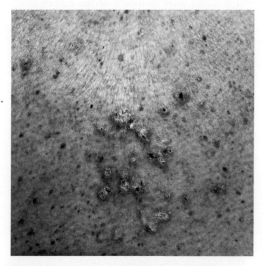

Figure 21.12 Lichenoid reaction from anti PD-1 therapy.

erosions with denuded skin and mucosal ulceration (52). Immunobullous disorders more commonly prompt a pause or cessation of the ICPi and in suspected cases, direct immunofluorescence (DIF) studies and BP 180/230 blood antigens should be collected. Treating this condition may require systemic drugs such as prednisone, omalizumab, or rituximab for recalcitrant cases (53).

Finally, though rare, cutaneous and systemic sarcoidosis has been reported in patients on ICPi therapy. Skin lesions present most typically as periorificial papules, annular plaques, or subcutaneous lesions (54). It is advised that clinicians consider sarcoidosis in patients on an ICPi with new-onset hilar lymphadenopathy. This condition typically responds well to treatment with topical or systemic corticosteroids depending on the severity.

ENDOCRINE THERAPY

Alopecia

The reported incidence of all-grade alopecia from endocrine therapy ranges from 0% to 25.4% (55). Lowest incidences of alopecia have been reported with antiandrogen therapy such as flutamide, with no alopecia associated with its use (56). Highest incidences have been associated with SERM therapy, in particular tamoxifen (25.4%), and also aromatase inhibitors, especially anastrozole (14.7%) (57). The risk of alopecia incidence is increased with combined endocrine therapies in contrast with monotherapy. Alopecia clinically manifests as female pattern/androgenetic alopecia. There is more often prominent recession of the frontotemporal area than of the mid-anterior hairline. Additionally, mild–moderate alopecia is typically seen on the crown of the scalp (58). Even with low-grade alopecia, patients have reported a high negative emotion score on quality of life questionnaires (40). Management and prevention include application of topical 2% to 5% minoxidil to promote hair regrowth, which has shown moderate to significant improvement in alopecia. As with alopecia resulting from traditional chemotherapies, camouflaging with wigs, scarves, hat, turbans, or camouflage sprays may be employed.

Flushing

Vasomotor symptoms and cutaneous flushing have been implicated as side effects of various endocrine therapies. Hot flashes are among the most common and bothersome side effects associated with SERM therapy, aromatase inhibitor, and androgen deprivation therapy. Hot flashes occur as sensations of warmth and appearance of visible redness in the face and upper body and can be associated with nausea and sweating. Mainstays of therapy for endocrine therapy associated flushing in women include selective serotonin reuptake inhibitors (SSRIs) and selective noradrenalin reuptake inhibitors (SNRIs), and gabapentin. In men, therapeutic options include SSRIs/SNRIs, medroxyprogesterone, cyproterone acetate, and gabapentin.

RADIATION THERAPY

Radiation Dermatitis

Dermatitis occurs in the vast majority of patients receiving radiotherapy. It can be seen within the first few weeks of radiation treatment and mild symptoms include erythema, pruritus, edema, and dry desquamation. Lesions may progress to blisters with moist desquamation (Fig. 21.13). Grade 4 radiation dermatitis, characterized by skin necrosis or ulceration of full thickness dermis, is rare, while impetiginization of open wounds is common. The addition of EGFR inhibitors to chemoradiation therapy protocols is associated with an increased risk of high-grade radiation dermatitis, p (59). The most important step in preventing radiation dermatitis is cleaning and drying the skin in the irradiation field prior to radiation therapy sessions, even when ulcerated. Patients should

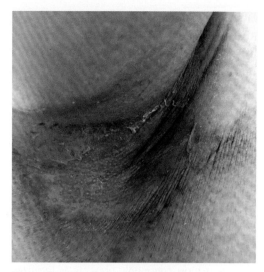

Figure 21.13 Radiation dermatitis desquamation.

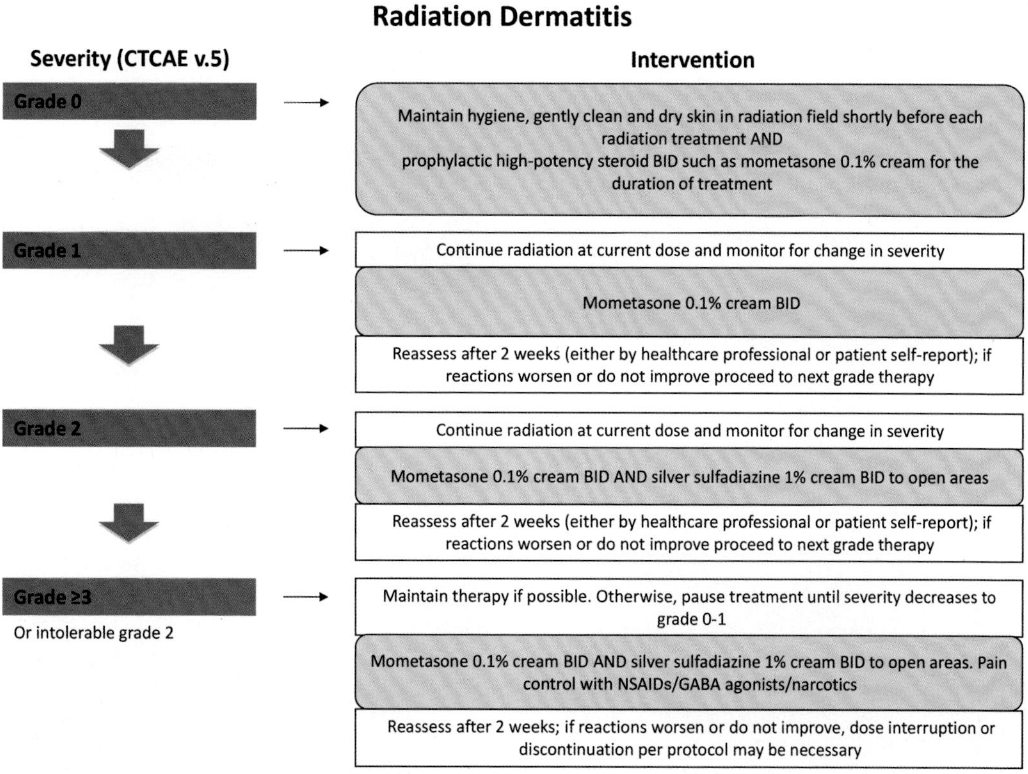

avoid using any topical products (i.e., ointments, emollients, creams, etc.) during the 4 hours prior to treatment. A detailed algorithm for the management of radiation dermatitis can be found in Figure 21.14.

Radiation Dermatitis

Severity (CTCAE v.5)	Intervention
Grade 0	Maintain hygiene, gently clean and dry skin in radiation field shortly before each radiation treatment AND prophylactic high-potency steroid BID such as mometasone 0.1% cream for the duration of treatment
Grade 1	Continue radiation at current dose and monitor for change in severity
	Mometasone 0.1% cream BID
	Reassess after 2 weeks (either by healthcare professional or patient self-report); if reactions worsen or do not improve proceed to next grade therapy
Grade 2	Continue radiation at current dose and monitor for change in severity
	Mometasone 0.1% cream BID AND silver sulfadiazine 1% cream BID to open areas
	Reassess after 2 weeks (either by healthcare professional or patient self-report); if reactions worsen or do not improve proceed to next grade therapy
Grade ≥3 Or intolerable grade 2	Maintain therapy if possible. Otherwise, pause treatment until severity decreases to grade 0-1
	Mometasone 0.1% cream BID AND silver sulfadiazine 1% cream BID to open areas. Pain control with NSAIDs/GABA agonists/narcotics
	Reassess after 2 weeks; if reactions worsen or do not improve, dose interruption or discontinuation per protocol may be necessary

Figure 21.14 Algorithm for the management of radiation dermatitis. (Adapted from Freites-Martinez A, Lacouture ME. Dermatologic adverse events. In: Olver IN, ed. *The MASCC Textbook of Cancer Supportive Care and Survivorship*. 2nd ed. New York, NY: Springer; 2018:597-620.)

Fibrosis

Radiation fibrosis of the skin is most commonly seen in patients treated for breast cancer. Symptoms include skin retraction and induration, pain, necrosis and ulceration, restricted arm and neck movement, lymphedema, and brachial or cervical plexopathy. It is typically a late side effect of radiation therapy, similar to hyperpigmentation, telangiectasias, or hair loss, and typically occurs between 6 months and 10 years later (60). The risk of developing radiation fibrosis appears to be dose dependent (60).

Morphea

Radiation-induced morphea (RIM), also known as localized scleroderma, is an uncommon and often misdiagnosed cutaneous complication of radiotherapy. It most commonly presents as localized scleroderma in patients with a history of breast cancer with a general latency of onset ranging from 1 month to several years after radiotherapy (61) (Fig. 21.15). Biopsy is commonly indicated to rule out carcinoma and other diagnoses such as radiation-induced fibrosis, infection, or fat necrosis. Multiple agents have been used for treatment including topical steroids, phototherapy, and systemic drugs such as methotrexate, mycophenolate, and extracorporeal photopheresis (ECP) (62).

Increased Skin Cancer Risk

Patients who have been previously treated with radiation therapy experience an increased risk of skin cancer, among other neoplasms, later in life. Adult survivors of childhood cancer under 35 years previously treated with radiation therapy have an approximately 40-fold elevated risk of nonmelanoma skin cancer and 2.5-fold elevated risk of melanoma compared to individuals who were not treated with radiation in childhood (63). Radiation has also been shown to increase the risk of angiosarcomas, an aggressive neoplasm with a predilection for skin and soft tissue (64). These cases typically present as painless multifocal erythematous patches and plaques. It is important to distinguish radiation-induced angiosarcoma from atypical vascular lesions, a benign condition that can be also be prompted by radiation.

STEM CELL TRANSPLANTATION

Graft versus Host Disease

The curative potential of allogenic stem cell transplantation is limited by occurrence of graft versus host disease (GVHD). Acute GVHD (aGVHD) presents as an exanthem characterized by a rash with a morbilliform appearance, occurring on the nape of neck, ears, shoulders, palms, and soles (65). It is often pruritic and painful. It is staged by body surface area (BSA) involved and degree of erythroderma, shown in Table 21.1 (65). The differential diagnosis of aGVHD includes fixed drug eruption, poikiloderma, skin toxicity from radiation, viral exanthem, and lymphocyte recovery eruptions. Chronic GVHD (cGVHD) can have many presentations, including lichenoid, morpheaform, fasciitis, and sclerotic (Fig. 21.16). The grading, as for

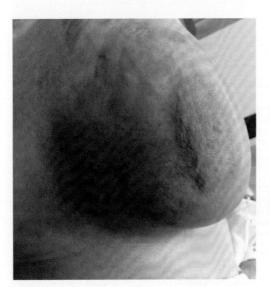

Figure 21.15 Radiation-induced morphea.

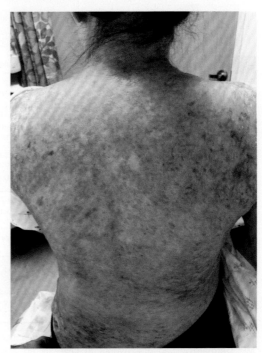

Figure 21.16 Sclerodermoid chronic GVHD.

acute, is based on BSA involved, but also considers presence of sclerotic features (65) (Table 21.1).

Corticosteroids are the first-line treatment for GVHD, and other systemic immunosuppressants such as cyclosporine, tacrolimus, or sirolimus may be used for cGVHD. Steroid-refractory GVHD accounts for up to one-third of deaths in patients receiving allogenic stem cell transplants (65). Ibrutinib, a small molecule inhibitor of Bruton's tyrosine kinase (BTK), has been approved by the FDA for second-line treatment of steroid-refractory cGVHD. Since May 2019, ruxolitinib has been approved for use of steroid-refractory aGVHD in adult and pediatric patients 12 years and older. Ruxolitinib is administered as an oral medication at a dose of 5 mg twice daily, and the dose can be increased to 10 mg twice daily after 3 days in the absence of toxicity (66).

An additional, often late-implemented, therapeutic tool for GVHD is ECP. While its use has reliable response rates, its late implementation may hamper its effects. There is evidence to suggest towards progression of earlier adoption of ECP—toward first-line therapy in clinical trials and even prophylaxis before onset.

REFERENCES

1. McGowan D. Chemo-induced hair loss: prevention of a distressing side-effect. *Br J Nurs.* 2013;22(10):S12.
2. Yun SJ, Kim SJ. Hair loss pattern due to chemotherapy-induced anagen effluvium: a cross-sectional observation. *Dermatology.* 2007;215(1):36-40.
3. Trueb RM. Chemotherapy-induced alopecia. *Semin Cutan Med Surg.* 2009;28(1):11-14.
4. Choi EK, Kim I-R, Chang O, et al. Impact of chemotherapy-induced alopecia distress on body image, psychosocial well-being, and depression in breast cancer patients. *Psychooncology.* 2014;23(10):1103-1110.
5. Olsen EA. Chemotherapy-induced alopecia: overview and methodology for characterizing hair changes and regrowth. In: Oliver IN, ed. *The MASCC Textbook of Cancer Supportive Care and Survivorship.* New York, NY: Springer; 2011:381-386.
6. Shin H, Jo SJ, Kim DH, Kwon O, Myung SK. Efficacy of interventions for prevention of chemotherapy-induced alopecia: a systematic review and meta-analysis. *Int J Cancer.* 2015;136(5):E442-E454.
7. Forsberg SA. Scalp cooling therapy and cytotoxic treatment. *Lancet.* 2001;357(9262):1134.
8. Duvic M, Lemak NA, Valero V, et al. A randomized trial of minoxidil in chemotherapy-induced alopecia. *J Am Acad Dermatol.* 1996;35(1):74-78.
9. Kluger N, Jacot W, Frouin E, et al. Permanent scalp alopecia related to breast cancer chemotherapy by sequential fluorouracil/epirubicin/cyclophosphamide (FEC) and docetaxel: a prospective study of 20 patients. *Ann Oncol.* 2012;23(11):2879-2884.
10. Kang D, Kim IR, Choi EK, et al. Permanent chemotherapy-induced alopecia in patients with breast cancer: a 3-year prospective cohort study. *Oncologist.* 2019;24(3):414-420.
11. Miller KK, Gorcey L, McLellan BN. Chemotherapy-induced hand-foot syndrome and nail changes: a review

12. Martschick A, Sehouli J, Patzelt A, et al. The pathogenetic mechanism of anthracycline-induced palmar-plantar erythrodysesthesia. *Anticancer Res.* 2009;29(6):2307-2313.
13. Poi MJ, Berger M, Lustberg M, et al. Docetaxel-induced skin toxicities in breast cancer patients subsequent to paclitaxel shortage: a case series and literature review. *Support Care Cancer.* 2013;21(10):2679-2686.
14. Degen A, Alter M, Schenck F, et al. The hand-foot-syndrome associated with medical tumor therapy—classification and management. *J Dtsch Dermatol Ges.* 2010;8(9):652-661.
15. Bolognia JL, Cooper DL, Glusac EJ. Toxic erythema of chemotherapy: a useful clinical term. *J Am Acad Dermatol.* 2008;59(3):524-529.
16. Scully C, Sonis S, Diz PD. Oral mucositis. *Oral Dis.* 2006;12(3):229-241.
17. Chaveli-Lopez B, Bagan-Sebastian JV. Treatment of oral mucositis due to chemotherapy. *J Clin Exp Dent.* 2016;8(2):e201-e209.
18. Reyes-Habito CM, Roh EK. Cutaneous reactions to chemotherapeutic drugs and targeted therapies for cancer: Part I. Conventional chemotherapeutic drugs. *J Am Acad Dermatol.* 2014;71(2):203.e1-203.e12.
19. Wyatt AJ, Leonard GD, Sachs DL. Cutaneous reactions to chemotherapy and their management. *Am J Clin Dermatol.* 2006;7(1):45-63.
20. Matsudate Y, Murao K, Kubo Y. Chemotherapy-induced inflammation of seborrheic keratoses due to pemetrexed treatment. *J Dermatol.* 2017;44(5):602-603.
21. Heidary N, Naik H, Burgin S. Chemotherapeutic agents and the skin: An update. *J Am Acad Dermatol.* 2008;58(4):545-570.
22. Singal R, Tunnessen WW Jr, Wiley JM, Hood AF. Discrete pigmentation after chemotherapy. *Pediatr Dermatol.* 1991;8(3):231-235.
23. Jain V, Bhandary S, Prasad GN, Shenoi SD. Serpentine supravenous streaks induced by 5-fluorouracil. *J Am Acad Dermatol.* 2005;53(3):529-530.
24. Adam BA, Ismail R, Sivanesan S. Busulfan hyperpigmentation: light and electron microscopic studies. *J Dermatol.* 1980;7(6):405-411.
25. Lacouture ME. Mechanisms of cutaneous toxicities to EGFR inhibitors. *Nat Rev Cancer.* 2006;6(10):803-812.
26. Agero AL, Dusza SW, Benvenuto-Andrade C, Busam KJ, Myskowski P, Halpern AC. Dermatologic side effects associated with the epidermal growth factor receptor inhibitors. *J Am Acad Dermatol.* 2006;55(4):657-670.
27. Li T, Perez-Soler R. Skin toxicities associated with epidermal growth factor receptor inhibitors. *Target Oncol.* 2009;4(2):107-119.
28. Amador ML, Hidalgo M. Epidermal growth factor receptor as a therapeutic target for the treatment of colorectal cancer. *Clin Colorectal Cancer.* 2004;4(1):51-62.
29. Cubiro X, Planas-Ciudad S, Garcia-Muret MP, Puig L. Topical timolol for paronychia and pseudopyogenic granuloma in patients treated with epidermal growth factor receptor inhibitors and capecitabine. *JAMA Dermatol.* 2018;154(1):99-100.
30. Capriotti K, Capriotti J, Pelletier J, Stewart K. Chemotherapy-associated paronychia treated with 2% povidone-iodine: a series of cases. *Cancer Manag Res.* 2017;9:225-228.
31. Segaert S, Chiritescu G, Lemmens L, Dumon K, Van Cutsem E, Tejpar S. Skin toxicities of targeted therapies. *Eur J Cancer.* 2009;45(suppl 1):295-308.

32. Lynch TJ Jr, Kim ES, Eaby B, Garey J, West DP, Lacouture ME. Epidermal growth factor receptor inhibitor-associated cutaneous toxicities: an evolving paradigm in clinical management. *Oncologist*. 2007;12(5): 610-621.

33. Lee WJ, Lee JL, Chang SE, et al. Cutaneous adverse effects in patients treated with the multitargeted kinase inhibitors sorafenib and sunitinib. *Br J Dermatol*. 2009;161(5):1045-1051.

34. Campbell T, Felsten L, Moore J. Disappearance of lentigines in a patient receiving imatinib treatment for familial gastrointestinal stromal tumor syndrome. *Arch Dermatol*. 2009;145(11):1313-1316.

35. Macdonald JB, Macdonald B, Golitz LE, LoRusso P, Sekulic A. Cutaneous adverse effects of targeted therapies: Part I: Inhibitors of the cellular membrane. *J Am Acad Dermatol*. 2015;72(2):203-218; quiz 19-20.

36. Balagula Y, Lacouture ME, Cotliar JA. Dermatologic toxicities of targeted anticancer therapies. *J Support Oncol*. 2010;8(4):149-161.

37. Osio A, Mateus C, Soria JC, et al. Cutaneous side-effects in patients on long-term treatment with epidermal growth factor receptor inhibitors. *Br J Dermatol*. 2009;161(3):515-521.

38. Hurwitz HI, Dowlati A, Saini S, et al. Phase I trial of pazopanib in patients with advanced cancer. *Clin Cancer Res*. 2009;15(12):4220-4227.

39. Lacouture ME, Wu S, Robert C, et al. Evolving strategies for the management of hand-foot skin reaction associated with the multitargeted kinase inhibitors sorafenib and sunitinib. *Oncologist*. 2008;13(9):1001-1011.

40. Freites-Martinez A, Chan D, Sibaud V, et al. Assessment of quality of life and treatment outcomes of patients with persistent postchemotherapy alopecia. *JAMA Dermatol*. 2019;155(6):724-728.

41. Belum VR, Benhuri B, Postow MA, et al. Characterisation and management of dermatologic adverse events to agents targeting the PD-1 receptor. *Eur J Cancer*. 2016;60:12-25.

42. Sibaud V. Dermatologic reactions to immune checkpoint inhibitors: skin toxicities and immunotherapy. *Am J Clin Dermatol*. 2018;19(3):345-361.

43. Curry JL, Tetzlaff MT, Nagarajan P, et al. Diverse types of dermatologic toxicities from immune checkpoint blockade therapy. *J Cutan Pathol*. 2017;44(2):158-176.

44. Sibaud V, Meyer N, Lamant L, Vigarios E, Mazieres J, Delord JP. Dermatologic complications of anti-PD-1/PD-L1 immune checkpoint antibodies. *Curr Opin Oncol*. 2016;28(4):254-263.

45. Hua C, Boussemart L, Mateus C, et al. Association of vitiligo with tumor response in patients with metastatic melanoma treated with pembrolizumab. *JAMA Dermatol*. 2016;152(1):45-51.

46. Wang PF, Chen Y, Song SY, et al. Immune-related adverse events associated with anti-PD-1/PD-L1 treatment for malignancies: a meta-analysis. *Front Pharmacol*. 2017;8:730.

47. Brahmer JR, Lacchetti C, Thompson JA. Management of immune-related adverse events in patients treated with immune checkpoint inhibitor therapy: American Society of Clinical Oncology clinical practice guideline summary. *J Oncol Pract*. 2018;14(4):247-249.

48. Kardaun SH, Sekula P, Valeyrie-Allanore L, et al. Drug reaction with eosinophilia and systemic symptoms (DRESS): an original multisystem adverse drug reaction. Results from the prospective RegiSCAR study. *Br J Dermatol*. 2013;169(5):1071-1080.

49. Coleman EL, Olamiju B, Leventhal JS. The life-threatening eruptions of immune checkpoint inhibitor therapy. *Clin Dermatol*. 2020;38(1):94-104.

50. Chia PL, John T. Severe psoriasis flare after anti-programmed death ligand 1 (PD-L1) therapy for metastatic non-small cell lung cancer (NSCLC). *J Immunother*. 2016;39(5):202-204.

51. Bonigen J, Raynaud-Donzel C, Hureaux J, et al. Anti-PD1-induced psoriasis: a study of 21 patients. *J Eur Acad Dermatol Venereol*. 2017;31(5):e254-e257.

52. Siegel J, Totonchy M, Damsky W, et al. Bullous disorders associated with anti-PD-1 and anti-PD-L1 therapy: a retrospective analysis evaluating the clinical and histopathologic features, frequency, and impact on cancer therapy. *J Am Acad Dermatol*. 2018;79(6):1081-1088.

53. Sowerby L, Dewan AK, Granter S, Gandhi L, LeBoeuf NR. Rituximab treatment of nivolumab-induced bullous pemphigoid. *JAMA Dermatol*. 2017;153(6): 603-605.

54. Suozzi KC, Stahl M, Ko CJ, et al. Immune-related sarcoidosis observed in combination ipilimumab and nivolumab therapy. *JAAD Case Rep*. 2016;2(3):264-268.

55. Saggar V, Wu S, Dickler MN, Lacouture ME. Alopecia with endocrine therapies in patients with cancer. *Oncologist*. 2013;18(10):1126-1134.

56. Chao Y, Chan WK, Huang YS, et al. Phase II study of flutamide in the treatment of hepatocellular carcinoma. *Cancer*. 1996;77(4):635-639.

57. Schomburg A, Kirchner II, Fenner M, Menzel T, Poliwoda H, Atzpodien J. Lack of therapeutic efficacy of tamoxifen in advanced renal cell carcinoma. *Eur J Cancer*. 1993;29A(5):737-740.

58. Freites-Martinez A, Shapiro J, Chan D, et al. Endocrine therapy-induced alopecia in patients with breast cancer. *JAMA Dermatol*. 2018;154(6):670-675.

59. Tejwani A, Wu S, Jia Y, Agulnik M, Millender L, Lacouture ME. Increased risk of high-grade dermatologic toxicities with radiation plus epidermal growth factor receptor inhibitor therapy. *Cancer*. 2009;115(6):1286-1299.

60. Miller RC, Schwartz DJ, Sloan JA, et al. Mometasone furoate effect on acute skin toxicity in breast cancer patients receiving radiotherapy: a phase III double-blind, randomized trial from the North Central Cancer Treatment Group N06C4. *Int J Radiat Oncol Biol Phys*. 2011;79(5):1460-1466.

61. Dyer BA, Hodges MG, Mayadev JS. Radiation-induced morphea: an under-recognized complication of breast irradiation. *Clin Breast Cancer*. 2016;16(4):e141-e143.

62. Spalek M, Jonska-Gmyrek J, Galecki J. Radiation-induced morphea—a literature review. *J Eur Acad Dermatol Venereol*. 2015;29(2):197-202.

63. Pappo AS, Armstrong GT, Liu W, et al. Melanoma as a subsequent neoplasm in adult survivors of childhood cancer: a report from the childhood cancer survivor study. *Pediatr Blood Cancer*. 2013;60(3):461-466.

64. Fineberg S, Rosen PP. Cutaneous angiosarcoma and atypical vascular lesions of the skin and breast after radiation therapy for breast carcinoma. *Am J Clin Pathol*. 1994;102(6):757-763.

65. Filipovich AH, Weisdorf D, Pavletic S, et al. National Institutes of Health consensus development project on criteria for clinical trials in chronic graft-versus-host disease: I. Diagnosis and staging working group report. *Biol Blood Marrow Transplant*. 2005;11(12):945-956.

66. Jagasia M, Zeiser R, Arbushites M, Delaite P, Gadbaw B, Bubnoff NV. Ruxolitinib for the treatment of patients with steroid-refractory GVHD: an introduction to the REACH trials. *Immunotherapy*. 2018;10(5):391-402.

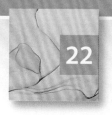

Management of Pressure Injury, Fungating Malignant Wounds, Fistulas, and Stomas

Sonika Pandey and Linda J. Stricker

The skin is a vital human organ with highly developed physiology and several essential functions in the regulation of homeostasis and immunity. Normal wound healing involves a sequence of overlapping physiological phases that include inflammation, cellular migration, proliferation, matrix deposition, and remodeling. Slow healing may occur due to impaired cellular and tissue responses and lead to chronic wounds. Multiple systemic and local risk factors are associated with impaired wound healing (Table 22.1). Examples of chronic wounds include diabetic foot ulcers, infected wounds, ischemic ulcers, pressure injuries, and malignant ulcers.

For patients with advanced cancer, particularly the elderly, pressure and fungating tumor masses are the most common causes of chronic wounds. The wound healing is often impaired in this population due to multiple risk factors and comorbidities. Patients with chronic wounds may also struggle with poor body image, loneliness, depression, and decreased intimacy.

ASSESSMENT OF A PATIENT WITH WOUND

In any patient with cancer who has developed a wound or is at risk of developing one, a comprehensive assessment should be done, including the illness context, wound characteristics, condition of surrounding skin, risk of pressure injury, and associated signs and symptoms such as pain, odor, and psychosocial impact of the wound.

1. Illness context: The context of the patient's illness includes factors such as cancer type, stage, and prognosis; functional status (e.g., as measured by Karnofsky or Palliative Performance Scale); nutritional, fluid, and cognitive status; decision-making capacity; and goals of care (Table 22.2).
2. Wound assessment:
   a. Wound description should include etiology (e.g., pressure, vascular), location (Fig. 22.1), and duration. Each wound description should include length, width, depth, character of wound base, presence of undermining or tunneling, drainage, odor, and bleeding. Labeled photographs or diagrams are helpful for documentation and ongoing assessments (Fig. 22.2 and Table 22.3).
   b. The surrounding skin of the wound should be assessed for any contamination, maceration, signs of infection, and edema and for the blood supply, particularly in lower extremity wounds.
3. Wound-related goals of care: Effective communication with the patient or surrogate decision maker about the context of the patient's illness, the patient's personal goals of care, and possible therapeutic options including their benefits and risks of harm and burden is important. Goals of wound care might range from attempts towards complete wound healing to a more palliative approach where the objective is to improve quality of life and relieve suffering by addressing odor, exudate bleeding, pain, and other distressing symptoms. Decisions about palliative wound care should not be solely based on patient diagnosis as many patients with limited life expectancy may have wounds that are expected to heal. Palliative wound care is a reasonable option for patients when the wound is not responding to treatment, wound healing is not expected, or goals of care are focused exclusively on comfort.

PRESSURE INJURY

Pressure injuries (previously known as pressure ulcers) are an important problem worldwide. An estimated 2.5 million pressure injuries are treated each year in acute care facilities in the United States (1). The overall prevalence of pressure injuries in hospitalized patients ranges from 5% to 15% but is significantly higher in intensive care units. Pressure injuries are also common in long-term care settings (2). Pressure-induced skin injury is

TABLE 22.1 RISK FACTORS FOR IMPAIRED WOUND HEALING

Immobilization
Malnutrition
Arterial insufficiency
Smoking
Diabetes
Autoimmune disorders
Wounds from malignancy
Infection
Smoking
Medications—steroids, immunosuppressive
   therapies, anticoagulants, chemotherapy
Venous insufficiency ulcers
Foreign bodies

frequently encountered in patients with cancer, particularly those who are debilitated by their illness or by treatment (3,4).

Definition of Pressure Injury

In 2016, National Pressure Ulcer Advisory Panel (NPUAP) changed the terminology to "pressure injury" instead of "pressure ulcer" to recognize the fact that not all skin damage due to pressure results into skin ulceration. For example, stage I pressure injury and deep tissue injury can occur without skin ulceration.

Pressure injury is defined as localized damage to the skin and underlying soft tissue usually over a bony prominence. The injury can present as intact skin or an open ulcer and may be painful. The injury occurs when skin integrity is overwhelmed by intense and/or prolonged pressure or pressure often in combination with shear forces (5). Pressure injury may also occur in the setting of circulatory collapse as in sepsis.

Pressure injury develops when pressure exceeds arterial capillary perfusion pressure resulting in ischemia and eventual tissue necrosis. Tissues differ in their susceptibility to pressure-related injury. Muscle tissue is highly susceptible while skin is less vulnerable. Evidence of pressure injury on the skin surface is a telltale sign of much larger and deeper damage underneath. Normal skin can withstand 30 to 60 minutes of poor perfusion. When the pressure and hypoxia are sustained, ischemia and necrosis can develop rapidly (6,7). Pressure injuries most often develop at bony prominences where the pressure is highest. Approximately 70% of pressure injuries occur over the sacrum, ischial tuberosity, or greater trochanter, while 15% to 25% occur on the lower extremities, typically the heel or lateral malleolus. Though these locations are the most classic, pressure injuries can occur at any site of prolonged pressure, including the elbow, ear, nose, chest, and back.

Immobility is a major risk factor for pressure injury because it causes sustained pressure, which

TABLE 22.2 CONTEXT ASSESSMENT

Issue	Examples
Cancer type, stage, prognosis	Stage IV breast cancer with metastases to liver, lungs, bone; prognosis 1–2 mo
Comorbidities	Rheumatoid arthritis
	Autoimmune disorders, for example, systemic lupus, vasculitis
Functional status, for example, KPS or PPS	KPS or PPS = 50%
Nutritional/fluid status	Appetite, for example, anorectic
	Degree of cachexia, for example, 20-lb weight loss, albumin 2.1 g/dL
	Mild dehydration with orthostatic hypotension and 1+ pitting ankle edema
Cognitive status	Alert, oriented ×3, normal Mini-Mental Status
Decision-making capacity	Has capacity
Medications that could delay healing	Steroids
	Nonsteroidal anti-inflammatory drugs
	Immunosuppressive medications
Goals of care	Maintain function
	Minimize symptoms
	Interact clearly with family and friends

KPS, Karnofsky Performance Scale; PPS, Palliative Performance Scale.

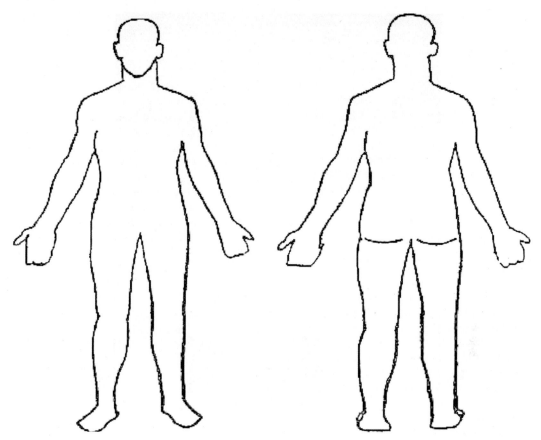

Figure 22.1 Wound location. Mark the location of each wound on the body diagrams. Label sites as A, B, C, and D.

in turn leads to tissue ischemia. Other factors include shear and friction forces that occur when lying at an incline; these may stress local capillary beds and contribute to tissue hypoxia (8). Excess moisture from perspiration or incontinence can render skin more susceptible to breakdown with friction. Other factors such as poor nutritional status, sensory loss, reduced skin perfusion, and medical comorbidities reduce the ability of soft tissues to withstand pressure and shear forces.

Pressure Injury Risk Assessment

The risk of developing a pressure injury increases as cancer advances, particularly when patients are debilitated (9). Risk should be periodically assessed using either a Braden (10) (http://www.bradenscale.com/) or a Norton (11) risk assessment tool. Both tools examine the most significant risk factors for developing a pressure injury including sensory perception, moisture, activity, mobility, nutrition, and friction/shear. Evidence of clinical efficacy of these risk assessment tools in lowering the incidence of pressure injury is lacking (12,13).

Staging of Pressure Injuries

Staging criteria have been developed by the National Pressure Ulcer Advisory Panel (NPUAP) and are used to guide management (14):

- Stage 1 pressure injury: Intact skin with localized area of nonblanchable erythema, which may appear differently in darkly pigmented skin. Presence of blanchable erythema or changes in sensation, temperature, or firmness may precede visual changes.
- Stage 2 pressure injury: Partial-thickness skin loss with exposed dermis. The wound bed is viable, pink or red, and moist and may also present as intact or open/ruptured serum-filled blister.
- Stage 3 pressure injury: Full-thickness loss of skin, in which adipose (fat) is visible in the ulcer and granulation tissue and epibole (rolled wound edges) are often present. Slough and/or eschar may be visible. The depth of tissue damage varies by anatomical location; areas of significant adiposity can develop deep wounds. Undermining and tunneling may occur. Fascia, muscle, tendon, ligament, cartilage, and/or bone are not exposed.

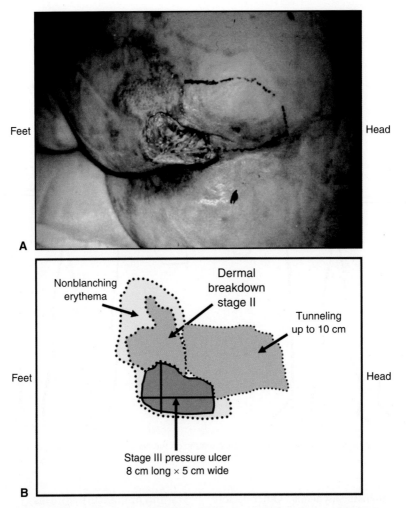

Figure 22.2 Description of a sacral pressure injury. **(A)** Photograph or **(B)** trace the circumference of the wound and damage to surrounding skin onto a transparency or plastic page protector, including areas of tracking or tunneling (indicating measurements, usually in centimeters). Use plastic wrap next to the skin to avoid bacterial or body fluid contamination.

- Stage 4 pressure injury: Full-thickness skin and tissue loss with exposed or directly palpable fascia, muscle, tendon, ligament, cartilage, or bone in the ulcer. Slough and/or eschar may be visible. Epibole (rolled wound edges), undermining, and/or tunneling often occur. Depth varies by anatomical location. If slough or eschar obscures the extent of tissue loss this is an unstageable pressure injury.
- Unstageable pressure injury: Obscured full-thickness skin and tissue loss. Full-thickness skin and tissue loss in which the extent of tissue damage within the ulcer cannot be confirmed because it is obscured by slough or eschar. If slough or eschar is removed, a stage 3 or stage 4 pressure injury will be revealed.

- Deep tissue pressure injury: Persistent nonblanchable deep red, maroon, or purple discoloration. Intact or nonintact skin with localized area of persistent nonblanchable deep red, maroon, purple discoloration or epidermal separation revealing a dark wound bed or blood-filled blister. Pain and temperature change often precede skin color changes. Discoloration may appear differently in darkly pigmented skin. If necrotic tissue, subcutaneous tissue, granulation tissue, fascia, muscle, or other underlying structures are visible, this indicates a full-thickness pressure injury (unstageable, stage 3, or stage 4). Do not use DTPI to describe vascular, traumatic, neuropathic, or dermatologic conditions.

TABLE 22.3 WOUND ASSESSMENT

	Examples
Type of wound (etiology)	Pressure, malignant cavitating or fungating, chemotherapy extravasation, radiation reaction, diabetic, neurotrophic, arterial, venous, acute surgical, acute trauma
Location	Precise location, ideally placing the wound on a body diagram (Fig. 22.1)
Duration	How long the patient has had it
Description of pressure injury	Nonblanching erythema of dermis, no breakdown or disruption of epidermis Dermal breakdown Cavity with breakdown extending to subcutaneous fat, muscle, bone
Description of malignant fungating wound	Nodular, cauliflower, cavitating Percent necrosis
Base/surface	Color, for example, black if eschar, red if granulation tissue, or yellow if fibrous tissue or slough Friability, for example, tissue breaking down on contact Exposed structures, for example, tendon, nerve, major blood vessel
Dimensions (Fig. 22.2)	Greatest vertical (head to toe) and horizontal dimensions at right angles Greatest depth of open wound using a probe, or height of a raised fungating wound Depth of any tracks (e.g., overhanging skin) or tunnels that extend underneath the skin through soft tissue and either dead end (e.g., sinus tracts) or open onto the skin in another location (e.g., fistula)
Exudate	Color, for example, serous, sanguineous, serosanguineous Purulence Volume, for example, none, mild, moderate, copious
Bleeding	Oozing or frank bleeding
Strikethrough, that is, drainage on the outside of an old dressing	Color, for example, serous, sanguineous, serosanguineous Purulence Volume, for example, spotting, soaked

The pressure injury should be staged according to its maximum depth. NPUAP has advised against "reverse staging" of the wound. For example, a healing stage 4 wound should not be reclassified to lower stages but should be labeled as *healing stage 4 pressure injury*.

The Pressure Ulcer Scale for Healing (PUSH) tool is a validated scale that gives a score based on wound size, amount of exudate, and tissue type (15) and is used for monitoring wound progress over time.

Management of Pressure Injury

Early recognition and initiation of treatment of pressure injury are key. When pressure injury is recognized early, progression can be arrested and significant morbidity preempted. Some patients are such high risk (due to unmodifiable risk factors such as hemodynamic instability, advanced illness with skin failure) that pressure injuries cannot be avoided despite implementation of best preventive strategies (16). Pressure redistribution is the cornerstone of pressure injury prevention. Other important factors include frequent repositioning, proper nutrition, and moisture management.

Wound care should always involve an interdisciplinary team that includes a nurse and physician at a minimum and may include an enterostomal therapist who is an expert in wound care, a pharmacist, a social worker, a chaplain, a physiotherapist, and a dietitian, especially when the patient's issues are more complex.

Pressure Injury—When the Goal Is to Heal

Person-centered pressure injury evaluation should include assessment of patient's overall health, psychosocial needs, and potentially reversible conditions. Particular attention should be paid to identify the source of pressure, underlying risk factors, and elements affecting wound healing. Additionally, assessment of patient's cognition, functional status, resources, caregiver time, and values and goals are important to overall care planning. Laboratory tests and radiological imaging should be done on a case-by-case basis in alignment with the patient's goals of care and prognosis.

Important elements of pressure injury management include reducing underlying causes of tissue damage by providing pressure redistribution with proper positioning and support surfaces, optimizing nutrition, controlling pain and infection, and providing appropriate wound care.

Wound care should focus on preparing a clean and moist wound bed by cleansing and débriding when there is necrotic tissue or slough with pre-emptive anesthesia/analgesia, and controlling infection and bleeding (17–20). Also, selection of appropriate wound dressing is the key to promote moist interactive healing. If there is a risk of significant shearing, tearing, or regular contamination with exudate, urine, or stool that could cause maceration, protect surrounding skin. Pack all dead spaces to keep them open and draining.

Pressure Redistribution. Continuous pressure, particularly over bony prominences, increases the risk of ischemia, skin breakdown, and pain (9,21). Pressure injuries can develop within hours if the circulation remains compromised. Pressure redistribution is an important component of pressure injury prevention and treatment. Pressure redistribution is achieved by proper repositioning and use of specialized support surfaces to avoid long periods of sustained pressure over bony prominences.

Proper Positioning. Proper positioning and repositioning of a bedridden patient is widely recommended and used in practice. In order to minimize sacral pressure in patients who are bedridden, it is recommended that the head of the bed should be as low as possible, ideally at <30°. The head of the bed may be raised for short periods of time for social interaction.

When a patient is unable to move by herself/himself, turning should be done from back to side, to one side, and then to the other. In addition to reducing pressure, this helps to relieve joint position fatigue in immobilized patients. As patients approach death, the need for turning lessens as the concern for skin breakdown becomes less important.

Although traditionally a 2-hour interval has been suggested for repositioning, evidence behind this practice from high-quality studies is lacking (22). It is unclear whether 2-hour repositioning frequency is better than longer intervals especially if the patient is on high-quality support surface (23). High-quality, adequately powered trials are needed to assess the effects of position and optimal frequency of repositioning on pressure injury incidence.

Support Surfaces. Patients with reduced mobility who are at risk of pressure injury or who already have a wound benefit from off-loading of pressure points or redistributing pressure through use of special support surfaces. Therapeutic static or dynamic support surfaces that reduce pressure include specially mattresses, beds, mattress overlays, and cushions. Static refers to nonpowered and dynamic to powered devices.

There is evidence to suggest that static support surfaces (foam, gel, or air mattresses) are superior to standard hospital beds in preventing pressure injuries in high-risk patients. Evidence regarding effectiveness of one class of support surface over another is lacking (1,24,25). Decisions regarding selection of devices are usually based on ease of use, device availability, nursing preferences, cost, and overall goals.

Three groups of mattresses/beds have demonstrated efficacy:

Group 1. Nonpowered devices made of gel, foam, or water are designed to replace a standard mattress or serve as an overlay on the top of the mattress. If employed early enough in patients at risk (e.g., bed-bound, limited mobility, cachexia), they will help prevent pressure injuries.

Group 2. Alternating air-loss or low-air-loss beds are used for patients at high risk of developing a pressure injury or who have already developed pressure injury. The goal is to prevent worsening and promote healing.

Group 3. Complete bed systems such as air-fluidized beds are expensive and are usually reserved for patients who need extensive pressure relief. Patients frequently describe them as overly confining.

Several pressure-reducing cushions are available for chairs and wheelchairs. A professional assessment for customized pressure-reducing cushions may be useful for chairfast patients who will use a chair or a wheelchair for a prolonged time. Round cushions commonly called *donut* are not recommended as they may restrict blood supply to vulnerable areas.

Nutrition and Fluid Replacement. Patients may be able to tolerate frequent small meals or between-meal supplements, particularly if the diet is liberalized and accommodates personal food preferences.

- Calories: Provide 30 to 35 kcal/kg/d.
- Hydration: Ensure adequate electrolyte-containing fluid intake noting that hypervolemia can delay healing. Strive for euvolemia.
- Protein: Daily allowance of up to 1.5 g/kg/d may delay onset of pressure injuries and promote healing.
- Vitamins: Deficiency of vitamin C and zinc can delay healing, but there is little evidence to support routine supplementation. If diet is poor in fruits and vegetables and deficiency is suspected or confirmed, offer a mineral and vitamin supplement.

Vigorous attempts to replete nutritional stores may not be appropriate for terminally ill patients in whom skin failure is due to their advanced illness. Under such circumstances, the emphasis may be better placed on optimizing quality of life and comfort, with meals and hydration offered as desired by patients and without rigid caloric or other nutrient goals.

Control Pain and Infection. Pain should also be assessed and treated appropriately. Opioid and/or nonopioid pain medications should be used based on severity of the pain. Pain should be assessed using standardized pain scales. Special attention should be given to control pain prior to dressing changes and débridement. Patients may need scheduled pain medicines for persistent wound pain. Local factors causing infection or underlying ischemia should be considered if the patient reports worsening pain.

All wounds are colonized by bacteria, fungi, and other infective agents, but this does not mean they are infected. Signs suggestive of infections include poorly healing wound, increased foul-smelling exudate, cellulitis, and necrotic muscle. Only clinically significant infections should be evaluated with appropriate laboratory imaging if needed and treated with antibiotics. If the infection is superficial, cleanse the wound with saline or water and apply a topical antibiotic with each change of dressing (26). Honey is known for its antimicrobial activity, but there are no clear guidelines for use of honey for specific wound types. Medical-grade honey-impregnated dressings are now available for wound care. Clear evidence is lacking, but in studies, honey appears to heal partial-thickness burns more quickly than does conventional treatment (27). If there is infection in the surrounding tissues or if wound healing is delayed, consider adding a systemic antibiotic until the infection is cleared.

Wound Care. Preparation of wound bed to promote healthy granulation tissue is an important element of wound care. This is achieved by management of moisture and exudate, bacterial balance, and débridement. Important elements of wound care include cleansing, débridement of necrotic tissue or slough, and use of appropriate dressings to–promote granulation tissue (17–20).

Cleanse. Prepare the wound bed by cleansing and rinsing away exudate, slough, and debris. Normal saline or sterile water or commercially available cleanser can be used for cleansing the wound bed. Use of hydrogen peroxide, povidone–iodine, or sodium hypochlorite is not recommended as topical wound cleanser as these agents are cytotoxic to granulation tissues and delay healing (28)

Débride. Necrotic tissue (eschar or slough) and contaminated and foreign material can delay wound healing and harbor infections. Optimal wound healing will not occur until these are removed. There are several débridement techniques, for example, surgical/sharp, autolytic, enzymatic/chemical, mechanical, or larval.

Débridement technique should be selected based on a thorough assessment of wound and the goals of care for the patient (Table 22.4).

Dress the Wound and Surrounding Tissue. This section aims to present the principles and suggest a strategy for dressing chronic wounds, not recommend specific dressings. Any reference to commercial products is only to illustrate a point, not to recommend products. Contact manufacturers for detailed information about their products and how to use them.

There are different classes of dressing: foams, alginates, hydrogels, hydrocolloids, films, gauze, petroleum, silver, and nonstick dressings (Table 22.5). They are distinguished by their absorbency, wear time, and occlusiveness. Within each class, specific products also vary by size, user friendliness, cost/accessibility, adhesive used, and impact on the wound margin and surrounding skin. As studies of different types of moist wound dressings showed no difference in pressure injury healing outcomes, use clinical judgment to select a type of dressing most appropriate for a given wound (29,34).

Dressing Strategy. If healing is the goal, use a dressing strategy that enables the following:

1. Keep the wound bed continuously moist.
2. Control exudate. This should be done without desiccating the wound bed. Wound exudates can be substantial, especially from stage 4 pressure injuries and malignant wounds. When there are copious exudates, consider uncontrolled edema or increased bacterial burden or infection as possible causes.
3. Keep surrounding skin dry. In addition to cleansing surrounding skin, zinc oxide or barrier creams or sprays may help protect the skin from prolonged contact or contamination with fluids. Some sprays may also increase adherence of adjacent dressing. When the risk is expected to be ongoing, thin film or hydrocolloid dressings placed around the wound with a cutout for the wound dressings can provide further protection.
4. Eliminate dead space. Loosely fill all cavities with nonadherent dressing materials (e.g., alginates or hydrogel-soaked gauze).
5. Consider caregiver time, skill, and burden. Do not create a plan that is not physically or financially possible for the patient and caregivers to adhere to.
6. Dress in layers. The primary or first layer goes next to the surface of the wound. It can include a hydrogel, an antibiotic, and/or thromboplastin. Subsequent layers rest one on top of the other. Finally, the top or outer layer typically holds the dressing in place and serves as the "aesthetic" covering.

TABLE 22.4 DÉBRIDEMENT TECHNIQUES

Technique	Mechanism	Precautions	Comments
Surgical/sharp	Use of curved scissors, curette, or scalpel	Make sure there is adequate blood supply for healing to occur: ABI > 0.5 Toe pressure >40 mm Hg Transcutaneous oxygen saturation >30%	Fastest, most effective technique for large areas of necrosis, a high degree of contamination, or frank infection Requires a skilled clinician Manage procedural pain with preemptive anesthesia (e.g., topical lidocaine cream or spray, EMLA)
Autolytic	Use of moist interactive dressings (e.g., hydrogels, hydrocolloids, alginates, films) to liquefy necrotic tissue	Remove as much loose debris as possible when changing dressings (usually q24–48h initially)	Gentlest technique. Results should be seen within 72 h Occlusive dressings facilitate autolysis by maintaining a moist environment Monitor for overhydration and infection
Enzymic/chemical	Use of collagenase or papain to digest damaged collagen, but not newly formed granulation tissue	Bacterial infection and bacteremia can occur. Detergents, bleach, hexachlorophene, and heavy metals (e.g., silver, mercury) may inactivate enzymes	Faster than autolytic débridement (29). To facilitate the process, score eschar without causing bleeding Do not use on normal or granulation tissue. Enzymes do not facilitate the granulation and re-epithelialization phases of wound care. They may damage normal tissues
Mechanical	Use of gentle irrigation to remove necrotic tissue. Use an 18–20G Angiocath on a 30- to 60-mL syringe to keep pressure under 15 PSI	Excessive force may flush away migrating epithelial cells or damage normal tissue	Saline wet-to-dry gauze dressings, irrigation, and whirlpool therapy are alternate mechanical débriding techniques. The latter is not recommended as it may cause pain or bleeding and damage normal or granulation tissue that sticks to the dry gauze when the dressing is removed
Larval	Use of larvae to consume necrotic tissue (30–33)	Use larvae cultured for this purpose Enclose them within the wound. Monitor their activity closely. Remove them between 48 and 72 h	Relatively rapid technique to débride large volumes of necrotic tissue May be offensive to patients, families, or staff Generally painless

ABI, ankle–brachial index; EMLA, eutectic mixture of long-acting anesthetics; PSI, pounds per square inch.

Adjuvant Therapies. In addition to standard wound preparation and dressing strategies, for more challenging wounds, there are a number of adjunctive therapies that could help stimulate the granulation process, for example, negative pressure wound therapy (NPWT), hyperbaric oxygen, therapeutic ultrasound, and electrical stimulation. However, specific indications for their use remain uncertain.

Pressure Injuries—When the Goal Is to Stabilize

When the pressure injury appears unlikely to heal and overall prognosis is poor, the goal is to stabilize the wound. The plan of care is based on the assessment of the wound and the surrounding tissues. Assess and stage the pressure injury as discussed earlier.

Reduce Interface Pressure. Always reduce the interface pressure using the techniques described earlier. This will minimize the risk of further progression of the existing pressure injuries and reduce the risk that new injuries will develop.

Cleanse, Débride, Dress. *Dry Wounds.* If the wound is covered with a dry eschar and there is no sign of pain, odor, or infection in the wound, the eschar, or the surrounding tissues, leave the wound alone. The dry eschar may be the most effective barrier against infections. To reduce bacterial burden, intermittently paint the eschar and the surrounding tissues with an aseptic iodine solution and let it air-dry. While it is contraindicated for healing wounds, the cytotoxicity of iodine can minimize the risk of infection and the need for a more complex wound management strategy (18). If the wound needs to be covered to protect it, or for aesthetic reasons, cover it with a nonstick, nonocclusive dressing.

Wet Wound. If the wound is open, wet, or infected in the wound bed or surrounding tissues, pursue a conservative wound management

TABLE 22.5 DRESSINGS

Class	Absorbency	Wear time	Types	Comments
1. Foams	4+/4	24 h–7 d	Mesh sponges	Ideal for copious exudate May macerate surrounding skin Either protect the surrounding skin with petrolatum or zinc oxide ointment or cut the foam to the inside dimensions of the wound and wick the exudate to secondary dressings
2. Alginates	3+/4	12–48 or more hours	Sheets, ribbons, or ropes	Seaweed derivative Hemostatic Rope wicks vertically—ideal for packing tracks and tunnels Convert to gel on contact with fluid; can wash off in the shower
3. Hydrogels	Variable, depending on the tonicity of the gel	24–72 h	Several different bases used in different products, for example, hydrocolloid, propylene glycol, sodium chloride	Facilitate autolytic débridement Use to hydrate
4. Hydrocolloids	Minimal 1–2+/4	24–48 h for débridement 3–7 d for protection	Millimeter-thick pads consisting of a membrane or other backing with a hydrophilic layer (e.g., gelatin, pectin) and a hydrophobic layer (e.g., carboxymethylcellulose) Gelatin layer liquefies on contact with fluids, minimizing trauma on removal Usually self-adhesive	Facilitate autolytic débridement Protect bony prominences and areas of potential skin breakdown Occlusive barrier for fluids (e.g., urine, feces) and for showering and swimming Occasional allergies to adhesives Must avoid leakage channels, which can introduce bacteria, and rippling, which can result in new pressure points
5. Transparent films/membranes	None	Up to 7 d	Both adhesive and nonadhesive films	Protect fragile skin from shearing and tearing Permit visualization Oxygen permeable Facilitate re-epithelialization Avoid leakage channels, which can introduce bacteria Barrier for showering and swimming
6. Gauze	Variable 1–2+/4	Variable, depending on strikethrough Up to 7 d	Pads, tapes, nets	Ideal outer dressings Hold dressing in place Cosmetic
7. Nonstick	None	Up to 7 d	Petroleum-coated pads, inert pads, inert mesh	Facilitate nonadherence
8. Silicone mesh	None	Indefinite	—	Apply as a second skin. Can use topical treatments over mesh
9. Petroleum impregnated	Minimal	48–72 h	Gauze	Nonadherent, retains moisture. Use with larger wounds with minimal necrosis and slough
10. Silver	Variable. Impregnated foams, hydrofiber, alginates. Also available in paste	Variable	Gauze, sponge, strips	Ideal for heavily colonized wounds or clinical signs of infection. Discontinue after 2 wk if no improvement

strategy to stabilize the wound; control infection, exudate, odors and bleeding; and maintain the best possible body image.

MALIGNANT FUNGATING WOUNDS

Malignant wounds occur in up to 10% of patients with advanced or metastatic cancer, usually in the last 6 months of life (12). They can evolve from a primary tumor of skin or an invasive underlying mass, a recurrence along a surgical suture line, or a metastasis. They can be both erosive injuries and/or expanding nodules. If many nodules confluence, the result can be a cauliflower-like wound. They are commonly associated with cancers that start in the breast, particularly when they reoccur locally (50% or more). Other common sites include the head and neck (up to 30%) and axilla or groin (approximately 5%) (13–15).

Although a tumor initially stimulates neovascularization, a rapidly growing tumor can outstrip its available blood supply and necrose centrally. When the process involves the skin, it frequently becomes friable and produces significant exudate, becomes malodorous as the tissue putrefies and/or becomes infected with anaerobes, and frequently bleeds.

Patients with malignant wounds suffer devastating physical symptoms that often lead to psychosocial and spiritual distress (30). Patients report debilitating pain, pruritus, malodor, exudate and bleeding, and these symptoms often lead to shame, humiliation, fear, guilt, depression, anxiety, and social isolation (31).The management of malignant wounds is basically the same as for advanced pressure injuries (12–15,32,33).

For some patients, antineoplastic treatments may offer significant palliation of the symptoms associated with a malignant wound. Radiation therapy may decrease bleeding, pain, and exudate. Chemotherapy or hormonal therapy may even promote wound healing in patients with responsive disease. Surgery may be an option for some malignant wounds if consistent with patient's goals of care. However, decisions about these treatments should be individualized with careful consideration of burden and benefits of such interventions.

Assessment, Staging

Use the assessment tool described earlier (Table 22.1). There is no specific staging system for malignant wounds.

Management of Malignant Fungating Wounds

Establish Goals of Care

Ensure that everyone is clear about the goals of care. If there exists chemotherapy or radiation therapy that could treat the underlying cancer and cause it to shrink or disappear, it may be possible to heal the malignant wound. Otherwise, if there is no effective therapy for the underlying disease, then malignant wounds are unlikely to heal. Focus goals on stabilizing the wound; controlling infection, exudate, odors, and bleeding; and maintaining the best possible body image.

Reduce Interface Pressure

To minimize the risk of developing or extending any pressure injury, reduce the interface pressure as much as possible by repositioning, turning, and supporting on pressure-reducing surfaces.

Cleanse

To remove necrotic debris and exudate, flush gently with normal saline or water at low pressures, as underlying necrotic tissue may be friable and bleed easily. Avoid cytotoxic wound cleansers.

Débride

Débride using autolysis or a very gentle surgical/sharp technique. Cautiously remove as much of the putrefying necrotic tissue that may be infected as possible, particularly if there is an associated foul odor. Use caution when approaching the tumor surface that may be friable, painful, and bleed easily, particularly if there is a lot of neovascularization close to the surface.

Control Infection

Most frequently, anaerobes infect the necrotic tissues associated with a malignant wound and produce a foul/putrid odor and a purulent exudate. If the infection is superficial, cleanse the wound with normal saline or water, débride cautiously, and apply a topical antibiotic with each dressing change (26). Metronidazole and silver sulfadiazine are the preferred antimicrobials to control anaerobic infections in tumors. They will usually control superficial infections within 5 to 7 days. If the infection is deep into the tumor or invades surrounding tissues, add systemic metronidazole.

Control Bleeding

Bleeding is a common problem in malignant wounds. As tumors outgrow their blood supply, their surfaces become friable, coagulation is frequently impaired, and they become predisposed to oozing from microvascular fragmentation or frank bleeding if a small or large blood vessel is involved.

When wound surfaces are particularly friable, apply an inert, nonstick, nonabsorbent dressing such as silicone mesh or Vaseline gauze as the first dressing layer. If oozing is significant, during each dressing change apply 5 to 10 mL of low-dose topical thromboplastin as a spray across the wound surface to stimulate coagulation (100 or 1,000 units/mL solution is as effective as higher concentration solutions and is less expensive). A 0.5% to 1% silver nitrate solution may be equally effective.

Other hemostatic agents such as Mohs' paste (zinc chloride paste) can be dabbed over large areas, and there have been a few case series reporting its use to control bleeding in malignant wounds as well (35). Alginate dressings are hemostatic and can be left in place as the primary dressing layer for several days. Alginates are only effective if wound has minimal bleeding. Hemostatic surgical sponges may be equally effective. A short course of high dose per fraction palliative radiation therapy (typically 250 to 800 cGy/fraction/d) will sclerose most vessels and stop bleeding from a malignant wound in just a few days (36). For frank bleeding, try silver nitrate sticks and electrocautery and/or apply gentle pressure for 10 to 15 minutes. Interventional radiology may be able to stop bleeding from a larger blood vessel by sclerosing it.

In all situations where bleeding is a significant risk, discuss the situation with the patient, family, and caregivers and decide on how and in what setting everyone will cope with a major catastrophic bleed. If bleeding occurs uncontrollably, dark towels lessen the sight of blood and reduce anxiety of the family, caregiver, and staff. If the patient is aware and distressed by the protracted bleeding, sedation with a rapid-acting benzodiazepine (e.g., midazolam or lorazepam) may be warranted.

Associated Issues

Odor. Odor from malignant fungating wound can be very distressing to patient, family, and their caregivers and severely affect quality of life. It can lead to embarrassment, depression and social isolation (37). Odor emanating from wounds is caused by putrefying tissue and/or infection. Odor can be pervasive and may permeate the clothes, furniture, and the room.

Odor management is achieved by careful débridement of necrotic tissue, which helps decrease the bacterial burden. If "healing" is not the goal of wound care, cytotoxic soaks of acetic acid and Dakin solution can help minimize the odor in addition to a topical antimicrobial therapy (e.g., metronidazole).

Also, there are multiple environmental changes that will help patients and families cope with foul odors, including the following:
a. *Ventilate adequately.* Open windows to allow fresh air into the environment. Run a fan on a low speed so that it circulates air around the room without chilling the patient.

b. *Absorb odors.* Place inexpensive kitty litter or activated charcoal in a flat container with a large surface area under the patient's bed. As long as the air in the room is circulating freely, odors will diminish rapidly. Alternately, burn a flame, for example, a candle, to combust the chemicals causing the odor.
For particularly odorous wounds, place an occlusive dressing that contains charcoal or a disposable diaper over the wound to contain the odor.

c. *Alternate odors.* Introduce an alternate odor that is tolerable to the patient and family, for example, aromatherapy, coffee, vanilla, or vinegar. Avoid commercial fragrances and perfumes as many are not tolerated by patients with advanced cancer.

Pain. Pressure injuries and malignant wounds are often painful unless the patient is paraplegic or has an altered sensorium (38–41). Malignant fungating wounds can cause pain due to multiple reasons, for example, tumor compression of an organ, dermal erosion and exposure of nerve endings, damage of nerve due to tumor invasion, edema secondary to impaired lymphatic drainage or wound infection (42).

The pain can be constant with or without breakthrough pain, or acute. Constant pain can be the result of a local tissue reaction, underlying cancer, infection, the products of inflammation, or increased pressure at a bony prominence. Intermittent acute pain occurs with specific procedures, for example, débridement. Cyclic acute pain occurs with recurring dressing changes (43–45).

To appropriately treat wound-related pain, it is important to know if the pain is nociceptive in origin, that is, the result of normal nociception and nerve function; neuropathic in origin, that is, the result of abnormal nerve function; or mixed.

Pain management follows standard pain management principles:

1. *Treat the underlying cause.* Where possible treat the cancer, control infections, heal the wound, and/or move the patient to a pressure-reducing or relieving surface.
2. *For constant pain.* Provide oral analgesics around the clock. If pain is nociceptive in origin, particularly if it is associated with inflammation, it will likely respond to a nonsteroidal anti-inflammatory drug (NSAID) and/or an opioid analgesic dosed once every half-life. If the pain is neuropathic in origin, analgesic antidepressants or an anticonvulsant may be needed as an effective coanalgesic. For breakthrough pain, provide 10% of the total 24-hour

oral dose of opioid every 1 hour as needed. There is some evidence that topical morphine mixed into a hydrogel placed against the wound surface in the primary dressing layer may reduce constant wound pain (46,47).

3. *For both intermittent and cyclic acute pain.* Provide preemptive anesthesia and/or analgesia. Ensure that the pharmacokinetics of the medication closely follow the temporal profile of the pain.

Careful selection of dressings to minimize tissue adherence, for example, hydrogels, alginates, and nonstick dressings, will minimize pain during dressing changes. If pain persists, consider reducing the frequency of dressing changes.

FISTULA MANAGEMENT

Fistula formation in people with cancer is not an uncommon complication. Predisposing factors relate fistula formation to the type and extent of the malignancy, comorbid conditions, immunosuppression, and radiation-related damage to tissues and vessels (48–50).

Patients presenting with a fistula face immeasurable physical, psychological, social, and financial challenges (48,49). Even in patients without a terminal disease, mortality rates associated with an enterocutaneous fistula (ECF) range from 5% to 15% (50,51).

A fistula is an abnormal communication from one epithelial surface to another epithelial surface (48,49,52). This includes internal connections from one organ to another organ or from an organ to the surface of the skin (48,49,52). Signs of an impending fistula include localized erythema and pain with increasing discomfort, leukocytosis (which may not be evident with immunosuppressed patients), fever, fluid and electrolyte imbalances,

altered mental state, and general malaise. The specific name of the fistula is according to origin to exit points (48,49,53).

Medical Management

Medical management for a patient with a fistula centers on controlling sepsis, stabilizing fluids and electrolytes, and optimizing nutritional status (48–50,54–56). Radiography will identify the origin of fistulae, and computerized tomography (CT) scan will aid in making the diagnosis (54). Depending on the type and extent of the fistula, intravenous fluids, antibiotic therapy, and enteral or parenteral nutritional support are considered in the management plan. Conservative therapy may elicit spontaneous closure of a fistula but only under optimum conditions (48,49,57). Once epithelialization (also known as somatization) of a fistula tract has occurred, it will not close without surgical intervention (48,54,58).

Medical management of fistulae has the primary goal of spontaneous closure. Using conservative methods such as nutritional management, fluid and electrolyte balance, and containment provides options for care. In cases where fistulae output is high, using medications (Table 22.6) such as H2 antagonists, somatostatin-14, or octreotide to decrease secretions combined with placing the patient NPO with nutritional support can create an environment for spontaneous closure (49,59).

Topical Management

Topical management of fistulae is an applied science. The goals of topical therapy in fistula care include containing effluent to quantify and control odor, facilitate comfort, assist in pain management, and restore and maintain integrity of the perifistular skin (48–50,53). Wound, ostomy, continence (WOC) nurses can be a tremendous asset

TABLE 22.6 MEDICATIONS FOR DECREASING SECRETIONS IN FISTULAS WHEN OUTPUT IS HIGH

Histamine receptor antagonists (H2)	Cimetidine
	Acts to reduce gastric secretions by decreasing histamine's affect on H2 receptors in gastric cells No effect on spontaneous fistula closure, but does reduce gastric output to improve management (2)
Somatostatin-14	Hormone naturally produced by pancreas octreotide/synthetic form of somatostatin
	Decreases intestinal output Has a short half-life (1–3 min) Slows gastric and gastrointestinal motility Improves fluid and electrolyte absorption Synthetic form is best when used with total parenteral administration (TPN) Octreotide has longer half-life (2 h) Octreotide administration is every 8 h by subcutaneous injection Monitor fistula output for decreased output; discontinue if no response (9)

in developing a plan of care for the patient with a fistula (51,59–61).

Negative Pressure Wound Therapy

Selective use of NPWT in patients with an ECF promotes closure in a nonepithelialized ECF and helps to manage effluent (48,49,57,58,62,63). It is essential for the clinician to follow the manufacturer's guidelines because NPWT systems on the market are not all approved for this use. Application of a contact layer to the base of the wound, protection of perifistular skin, and use of low suction is the standard approach in carefully selected patients (48,49,57,58).

Additional Topical Therapies

A myriad of wound, ostomy, and draining wound/fistula products may be useful in assisting the clinician in achieving the goals of topical therapy. Use of pouches, solid wafer skin barriers, topical wound dressings, catheter holders, and odor controlling agents may be appropriate (48,49,51,52,64). Creative combinations of these products significantly improve the quality of life for a patient with a fistula (53). Determining which combinations of product to use in a given situation requires a careful analysis of the skin planes adjacent to the fistulae (48,49,61).

A holistic approach to the care of these individuals is important. Many patients require one or more people to assist with care, and because of changes in the fistula size and configuration, frequent modifications of the plan are common (48,52,53). Financial considerations are significant. Establishment of a set protocol and expected wear time are useful in determining anticipated costs. Involvement of a care manager, social services, and financial specialist will support the patient and family to maximize reimbursement for supplies (52,65).

An effective and economical approach to fistula care is a plan that includes pouching. The main goals of topical fistula management are realized when an effective and predictable pouch seal is achieved (48,49,53,61,64). If the fistula is not too large, a standard ostomy pouch can provide a secure, straightforward, and cost-effective option (48,51,53). Unlike pouching a stoma, managing a fistula with a pouch usually requires several additional steps beyond sizing and application of the pouch. The aperture of an ostomy pouch is sized to one-eighth inch larger than the base of the stoma, but the opening for a fistula may need to extend beyond the margins of the opening to a more even skin surface (51,53,64). This leaves the potential for skin exposed to chemical erosion from fistula effluent. Protect exposed skin with skin barrier pastes and powders, and fill uneven skin creases with skin barrier (wafers, paste, strips, washers, or rings) to even out the skin contours before the pouch is applied (48,49,51,53,64). For copious drainage, connection to constant drainage or use of suction to collect the effluent is helpful (50,57,59).

OSTOMY MANAGEMENT

The palliative care patient with an ostomy requires special considerations to maintain a secure pouch seal, maintain or restore peristomal skin integrity, and conserve energy with the application and removal process (48,51,53,64,66).

The patient with an established ostomy usually has a preferred stoma management method. However, changes in body contour, stoma size, abdominal firmness, skin changes, anemia, and tendency toward mucosal bleeding may necessitate recommendation of a new pouching system (51,53).

Fecal diversions are usually best managed with a drainable pouching system (67). Selection of a pouching system depends on the location of the stoma, as well as the patient's preference and ability to manage the colostomy. In some cases, use of a closed end pouch with a descending or sigmoid colostomy with thick stool and once or twice daily function may be an option. Colostomy irrigation can be used in selected cases. Colostomy irrigation reduces frequency of stool evacuation from left-sided colostomies resulting in more predictable bowel elimination patterns. There is some evidence that it reduces flatus and odor compared to spontaneous evacuation and may improve quality of life (68). Appropriate patient selection is the key if colostomy irrigation is used as there are risks associated with this procedure and one has to make sure that there are no contraindications. Also, there is strong need for staff and patient education on this procedure (69). Consultation with WOC nurse is extremely helpful in selecting the appropriate pouching system.

Efforts made to simplify the pouching procedure will minimize fatigue and ease the process for the patient and caregiver (52,53,66). Establishing a predictable wear time is essential and adds continuity to the plan of care. A pouch should not be left on until it leaks because undermining of the seal can leave the skin exposed to damage from effluent (64,65).

Urinary or fecal diversions not only result in an alteration in elimination but also can cause profound impact on body image (65,67). Counseling focused on encouraging the patient to verbalize feelings and concerns will provide important clues that individualize the plan to address those issues (53,66).

Advances in the manufacturing of ostomy pouches offer secure, odor-proof, and discreet care for the person with an ostomy (64,65). Even with modern technology, nothing promotes effective ostomy management like a well-sited, well-constructed stoma (61,64,65,67). Consultation with a WOC nurse preoperatively, postoperatively, and after discharge provides the patient and family specialized ostomy care teaching, counseling, and follow-up.

CONCLUSION

Chronic wounds are relatively common in patients with advanced cancer. After doing a comprehensive, whole-person assessment, consider what the goals of care and treatment plan for the wound will be in light of the context of the patient's underlying cancer (and other comorbidities).

Care of patients presenting with fistulae or ostomies can be challenging for the patient, family, and health care team. A systematic, multidisciplinary approach with collaboration of a wound nurse can support the plan of care and improve the patient's quality of life (66).

Also, patients living with chronic wounds are inevitably "wounded" far beyond their physical wound. Anxiety and depression are common, particularly in the face of multiple unexpected losses. Changes in intimacy, relationships, and finances can be dramatic and even lead to social isolation.

ACKNOWLEDGMENT

The authors would like to acknowledge the contribution of Dr. Frank D. Ferris, Dr. Susan K. Bodtke, Dr. Paula Erwin-Toth and Dr. Linda J. Stricker on the previous edition.

REFERENCES

1. Reddy M, Gill SS, Rochon PA. Preventing pressure ulcers: a systematic review. *JAMA.* 2006;296(8):974.
2. Mervis JS, Phillips TJ. Pressure ulcers: pathophysiology, epidemiology, risk factors, and presentation. *J Am Acad Dermatol.* 2019;81(4):881-890.
3. Walker P. *Update on Pressure Ulcers. Principles & Practice of Supportive Oncology Updates. Vol. 3. No. 6.* 2nd ed. New York, NY: Lippincott Williams & Wilkins; 2000:1-11.
4. Brem H, Lyder C. Protocol for the successful treatment of pressure ulcers. *Am J Surg.* 2004;188(suppl 1A):9-17. Review.
5. NPUAP. https://cdn.ymaws.com/npuap.site.com/resource/resmgr/npuap_pressure_injury_stages.pdf
6. Leigh I, Bennett G. Pressure ulcers: prevalence, etiology, and treatment modalities, a review. *Am J Surg.* 1994;167:25S-30S.
7. Eachempati SR, Hydo LJ, Barie PS. Factors influencing the development of decubitus ulcers in critically ill surgical patients. *Crit Care Med.* 2001;29(9):1678-1682.
8. Pressure ulcers: pathophysiology, epidemiology, risk factors, and presentation. *J Am Acad Dermatol.* 2019;81(4):881-890.
9. Agency for Health Care Policy and Research. *Pressure Ulcers in Adults Prediction and Prevention, Clinical Guideline No. 3.* Rockville, MD: AHCPR; 1992. http://www.ncbi.nlm.nih.gov/books/NBK63854/. Accessed October 10, 2011.
10. Bergstrom N, Braden BJ, Laguzza A, et al. The Braden scale for predicting pressure ulcer sore risk. *Nurs Res.* 1987;36:205-210.
11. Norton D, McLaren R, Exton-Smith AN. *An Investigation of Geriatric Nursing Problems in Hospitals.* London, UK: National Corporation for the Care of Old People; 1962.
12. Moore ZE, Patton D. Risk assessment tools for the prevention of pressure ulcers. *Cochrane Database Syst Rev.* 2019;(1):CD006471.
13. Chou R, Dana T, Bougatsos C, et al. Pressure ulcer risk assessment and prevention: a systematic comparative effectiveness review. *Ann Intern Med.* 2013;159(1):28-38.
14. *Updated Pressure Ulcer Staging System Revised 2016.* https://cdn.ymaws.com/npuap.site-ym.com/resource/resmgr/npuap_pressure_injury_stages.pdf
15. *Pressure Ulcer Scale for Healing (PUSH) v 3.0. National Pressure Ulcer Advisory Panel 2007.* http://www.npuap.org/PDF/push3.pdf. Accessed October 10, 2011.
16. Black JM, Edsberg LE, Baharestani MM, et al. Pressure ulcers: avoidable or unavoidable? Results of the National Pressure Ulcer Advisory Panel Consensus Conference. National Pressure Ulcer Advisory Panel. *Ostomy Wound Manage.* 2011;57(2):24-37.
17. Walker P. Management of pressure ulcers. *Oncology (Williston Park).* 2001;15(11):1499-1508, 1511.
18. Sibbald RG, Williamson D, Orsted HL, et al. Preparing the wound bed—debridement, bacterial balance, and moisture balance. *Ostomy Wound Manage.* 2000;46(11):14-22, 24-28, 30-35.
19. Krasner DL. How to prepare the wound bed. *Ostomy Wound Manage.* 2001;47(4):59-61.
20. Vowden K, Vowden P. Wound bed preparation. *World Wide Wounds*; March 2002. http://www.worldwidewounds.com/2002/april/Vowden/Wound-Bed-Preparation.html. Accessed October 10, 2011.
21. Walker P. The pathophysiology and management of pressure ulcers. In: Portenoy RK, Bruera E, eds. *Topics in Palliative Care.* Vol. 3. New York, NY: Oxford University Press; 1998:253-270.
22. Knox DM, Anderson TM, Anderson PS. Effects of different turn intervals on skin of healthy older adults. *Adv Wound Care.* 1994;7(1):48.
23. Gillespie BM, Chaboyer WP, McInnes E, Kent B, Whitty JA, Thalib L. Repositioning for pressure ulcer prevention in adults. *Cochrane Database Syst Rev.* 2014;(4):CD009958.
24. Shi C, Dumville JC, Cullum N. Support surfaces for pressure ulcer prevention: a network meta-analysis. *PLoS One.* 2018;13(2):e0192707.
25. McInnes E, Jammali-Blasi A, Bell-Syer SE, Dumville JC, Middleton V, Cullum N. Support surfaces for pressure ulcer prevention. *Cochrane Database Syst Rev.* 2015;(9):CD001735.
26. Spann CT, Tutrone WD, Weinberg JM, et al. Topical antibacterial agents for wound care: a primer. *Dermatol Surg.* 2003;29(6):620-626.
27. Jull AB, Cullum N, Dumville JC, Westby MJ, Deshpande S, Walker N. Honey as a topical treatment for wounds. *Cochrane Database Syst Rev.* 2015;(3):CD005083.
28. Rodeheaver GT. Wound cleansing, wound irrigation, wound disinfection. In: Krasner DL, Rodeheaver GT, Sibbald RG, eds. *Chronic Wound Care: A Clinical Source Book for Healthcare Professionals.* 3rd ed. Wayne, PA: HMP Communications; 2001:369-383.

29. Ovington L, Peirce B. Wound dressings: form, function, feasibility, and facts. In: Krasner DL, Rodeheaver GT, Sibbald RG, eds. *Chronic Wound Care: A Clinical Sourcebook for Healthcare Professionals.* 3rd ed. Wayne, PA: HMP Communications; 2001:311-319.

30. Lo S-F, Hu W-Y, Hayter M, Chan S-C, Hsu M-Y, Wu L-Y. Experiences of living with a malignant fungating wound: a qualitative study. *J Clin Nurs.* 2008;17(20): 2699-2708.

31. Probst S, Arber A, Faithfull S. Coping with an exulcerated breast carcinoma: an interpretative phenomenological study. *J Wound Care.* 2013;22(7):352-360.

32. Barton P, Parslow N. Malignant wounds: holistic assessment and management. In: Krasner DL, Rodeheaver GT, Sibbald RG, eds. *Chronic Wound Care: A Clinical Sourcebook for Healthcare Professionals.* 3rd ed. Wayne, PA: HMP Communications; 2001:699-710.

33. Grocott P. The palliative management of fungating malignant wounds. *J Wound Care.* 2000;9(1):4-9.

34. Ovington LG. Dressings and adjunctive therapies: AHCPR guidelines revisited. *Ostomy Wound Manage.* 1999;45(suppl 1A):94S-106S.

35. Beers EH. Palliative wound care: less is more. *Surg Clin North Am.* 2019;99(5):899-919.

36. Ferris FD, Bezjak A, Rosenthal SG. The palliative uses of radiation therapy in surgical oncology patients. *Surg Oncol Clin N Am.* 2001;10(1):185-201.

37. Piggin C. Malodorous fungating wounds: uncertain concepts underlying the management of social isolation. *Int J Palliat Nurs.* 2003;9(5):216-221.

38. Krasner D. Using a gentler hand: reflections on patients with pressure ulcers who experience pain. *Ostomy Wound Manage.* 1996;42(3):20-22.

39. Reddy M, Keast D, Fowler E, et al. Pain in pressure ulcers. *Ostomy Wound Manage.* 2003;49(suppl 4):30-35.

40. Popescu A, Salcido RS. Wound pain: a challenge for the patient and the wound care specialist. *Adv Skin Wound Care.* 2004;17(1):14-20.

41. Naylor W. Assessment and management of pain in fungating wounds. *Br J Nurs.* 2001;10(suppl 22):S33-S36.

42. Tilley, Charles. Palliative wound care for malignant fungating wounds: holistic considerations at end-of-life. *Nurs Clin North Am.* 2016;51(3):513-531.

43. Moffatt C, Briggs M, Hollinworth H, et al. *Pain at Wound Dressing Changes. EWMA Position Document.* London, UK: Medical Education Partnership; 2002.

44. Reddy M, Kohr R, Queen D, et al. Practical treatment of wound pain and trauma: a patient-centered approach. An overview. *Ostomy Wound Manage.* 2003;49(suppl 4):2-15.

45. Krasner D. The chronic wound pain experience: a conceptual model. *Ostomy Wound Manage.* 1995;41(3):20-25.

46. Twillman RK, Long TD, Cathers TA, et al. Treatment of painful skin ulcers with topical opioids. *J Pain Symptom Manage.* 1999;17(4):288-292.

47. Zeppetella G, Paul J, Ribeiro MD. Analgesic efficacy of morphine applied topically to painful ulcers. *J Pain Symptom Manage.* 2003;25(6):555-558.

48. Erwin-Toth P, Stricker L. Drain, tube, & fistula management. In: Baranoski S, Ayello E, eds. *Wound Care Essentials: Practice Principles.* 3rd ed. Philadelphia, PA: Wolters Kluwer Health/Lippincott Williams & Wilkins; 2012:19;477-490.

49. Bryant R, Rolstad B. Management of draining wounds & fistulas. In: Bryant R, Nix D, eds. *Acute & Chronic Wounds: Current Management Concepts.* 4th ed. St. Louis, MO: Mosby/Elsevier; 2012:490-516.

50. Martinez A, Ferron G, Le Gal M, Torrent J, Capdet J, Querleu D. Management of ileocutaneous fistulae using TNP after surgery for abdominal malignancy. *J Wound Care.* 2009;18(7):282-288.

51. Brindle C, Blankenship J. Management complex abdominal wounds with small bowel fistulae: isolation techniques and exudate control to improve outcomes. *J Wound Ostomy Continence Nurs.* 2009;36(4):396-403.

52. Slater R. Supporting patients with enterocutaneous fistula: from hospital to home. *Br J Community Nurs.* 2011;16(2):66-73.

53. Phillips J, Walton M. Caring for patients with enterocutaneous fistula. *Br J Nurs.* 1993;2(9):496-500.

54. Schecter WP, Hirshberg A, Chang DS, et al. Enteric fistulas: principles of management. *J Am Coll Surg.* 2009;209(4):484-491.

55. Mawdsley J, Hollington P, Bassett P, et al. An analysis of predictive factors for healing and mortality in patients with enterocutaneous fistula. *Aliment Pharmacol Ther.* 2008;28:1111-1121.

56. Austin T. Nutrition management of enterocutaneous fistula. *Support Line.* 2006;28(6):10-16.

57. Bovill E, Banwell P, Teot L, et al. Topical negative pressure wound therapy: a review of its role and guidelines for its use in the management of acute wounds. *Int Wound J.* 2008;5(4):511-529.

58. Schein M. What's new in postoperative enterocutaneous fistula. *World J Surg.* 2008;32:336-338.

59. Kordasiewicz L. Abdominal wound with a fistula and large amount of drainage status after incarcerated hernia. *J Wound Ostomy Continence Nurs.* 2004;31(3):150-153.

60. Davis M, Dere K, Hadley G. Options for managing an open wound with draining enterocutaneous fistula. *J Wound Ostomy Continence Nurs.* 2000;27(2):118-123.

61. Geiger-Jones E, Harbit M. Management of an ileostomy and mucous fistula located in a dehisced wound in a patient with morbid obesity. *J Wound Ostomy Continence Nurs.* 2003;30(6):351-356.

62. Wainstein D, Fernandez E, Gonzales D, et al. Treatment of high-output enterocutaneous fistula with a vacuum-compaction device. *World J Surg.* 2008;32:430-435.

63. Gunn LA, Follmar KE, Wong MS, Lettieri SC, Levin LS, Erdmann D. Management of enterocutaneous fistulas using negative-pressure dressings. *Ann Plast Surg.* 2006;57(6):621-625.

64. Erwin-Toth P, Stricker L, van Rijswijk L. Peristomal skin complications. *Am J Nurs.* 2010;110(2):43-48.

65. Skovgaard R, Keiding H. A cost-effectiveness analysis of fistula treatment in the abdominal region using a new integrated fistula and wound management system. *J Wound Ostomy Continence Nurs.* 2008;35(6): 592-595.

66. Floruta C, Berschorner J, Hull T. Gastrointestinal cancers: medical management. In: Colwell J, Goldberg M, Carmel J, eds. *Fecal & Urinary Diversions: Management Principles.* St. Louis, MO: Mosby/Elsevier; 2004:102-125.

67. Colwell J. Principles of stoma management. In: Colwell J, Goldberg M, Carmel J, eds. *Fecal & Urinary Diversions: Management Principles.* St. Louis, MO: Mosby/Elsevier; 2004:240-262.

68. Carole A-L, Mary K, Dea J. Colostomy irrigation to maintain continence: an old method revived Bauer. *Nursing.* 2016;46(8):59-62.

69. Cobb MD, Grant M, Tallman NJ, et al. Colostomy irrigation: current knowledge and practice of WOC nurses. *J Wound Ostomy Continence Nurs.* 2015;42(1):65-70.

23 Lymphedema

Vaughan L. Keeley

Lymphedema can occur as an aftermath of cancer treatment, and it can also be a feature of advanced disease. The approaches to management of these two groups may be different. In the former, "supportive" treatment would aim to minimize the edema and enable the patient, with successfully treated cancer, to live as normally as possible with the problem. Methods for the early detection and possible prevention of lymphedema in this group are being investigated. In the latter, a "palliative" approach would aim to alleviate symptoms as much as possible while ensuring that any burden of treatment would be outweighed by the benefits. Edema in patients with advanced cancer may be only one of a number of problems that are experienced and would therefore need to be considered in this context.

PATHOPHYSIOLOGY

Lymphedema is traditionally defined as the accumulation of a relatively protein-rich fluid in the interstitial space of tissues due to a low-output failure of the lymphatic system, that is, lymph transport is reduced (1).

It is usually classified into "primary," which is an umbrella term describing lymphedema arising from lymphatic dysplasia usually of genetic origin, and "secondary," in which extrinsic factors damage previously apparently normal lymphatics. Lymphedema associated with cancer and its treatment is therefore "secondary lymphedema."

However, the cause of edema in patients with advanced cancer is usually more complex and multifactorial in nature. It is helpful, therefore, to consider the mechanisms involved in edema formation.

The Formation of Edema

Edema is the accumulation of excessive fluid in the interstitial space and results from an imbalance between the formation and drainage of interstitial fluid.

Fluid enters the interstitial space by capillary filtration. The amount of filtrate is determined by Starling's forces acting across the capillary wall. These are the hydrostatic pressure gradient, which tends to push fluid from the capillary into the interstitial space, and the colloid osmotic pressure gradient due to plasma proteins that are retained in the capillary, which tends to draw water from the interstitial space into the capillary. The volume of filtrate will also be determined by the permeability of the capillary wall.

In the past, it was felt that the process of filtration occurred largely in the arterial end of the capillary and 90% of the filtered fluid was reabsorbed by the venous end of the capillary. The remaining 10% was thought to be drained by the lymph vessels. However, more recent evidence indicates that once fluid reaches the interstitial space, the route of exit for all of it is through the freely permeable initial lymphatic capillary, that is, by lymphatic drainage (2). Therefore, edema occurs whenever capillary filtration exceeds lymphatic drainage and failure of lymphatic drainage is a feature of all types of chronic edema.

Table 23.1 shows the changes in capillary filtration and lymphatic drainage in different patterns of chronic edema

In venous edema, for example, in chronic venous insufficiency of the leg, capillary filtration is raised because of increased hydrostatic pressure in the capillaries, but this results in increased lymphatic drainage due to the spare capacity of the lymphatic system to transport fluid. When this capacity is exceeded, then edema occurs (high-output failure of the lymphatics). If high-output failure of the lymphatic system persists, then there is a gradual deterioration in lymphatic transport capacity and worsening edema develops. In this situation, the edema has both venous and lymphatic components (sometimes known as phlebolymphedema).

In patients with reduced mobility, particularly those who spend a lot of time sitting in a chair, so-called dependency edema can occur. Again, there are venous and lymphatic components: poor mobility results in failure of the calf muscle pump that aids both venous and lymphatic drainage, and therefore, capillary filtration is increased and lymphatic drainage is reduced.

In patients with hypoalbuminemia, the colloid osmotic pressure in the plasma is reduced, and

TABLE 23.1 CHRONIC EDEMAS

Type	Pathology	Capillary filtration	Lymphatic drainage
Primary lymphedema	Lymphatic dysplasia	Normal	↓
Secondary lymphedema	Lymphatic damage	Probably normal	↓
Venous edema	High-output failure	↑↑	Initial ↑ then ↓
Lymphovenous edema	Reduced venous and lymphatic drainage	↑↑	↓
Advanced cancer	Lymphatic obstruction, venous obstruction, hypoalbuminemia, immobility	↑↑	↓

therefore, capillary filtration is increased, and edema occurs when lymphatic drainage is unable to remove the extra fluid.

Post–Cancer Treatment Edema

It has long been assumed that axillary lymphadenectomy and radiotherapy carried out to treat breast cancer leads to lymphedema of the arm in some women because of simple damage to the lymphatics. However, it has now become clear that this is perhaps too simplistic a view. Studies have shown that, contrary to predictions, lymph flow is *increased* in both the "at-risk" and contralateral arm in women who go on to develop lymphedema compared with those who do not (3). Once the edema has developed, however, lymph flow is reduced. This suggests that there may be a constitutional (possibly genetic) tendency to lymphedema in some women possibly mediated by raised capillary filtration and lymphatic drainage (high-output failure) (4). In addition, the role of inflammation in the pathophysiology of lymphedema is being increasingly recognized (4).

Edema in Advanced Cancer

In patients with advanced cancer, the edema usually arises because of a number of factors (Table 23.2). A patient may have lymphatic obstruction due to metastatic disease in the lymph nodes or due to previous treatment. There may be extrinsic venous compression causing venous hypertension or even venous thrombosis. In advanced disease, hypoalbuminemia is common, and finally, in association with the cachexia of advanced disease, weakness and immobility may result. These factors will lead to increased capillary filtration and reduced lymphatic drainage. This situation is often seen in patients with advanced pelvic malignancies.

INCIDENCE

The precise incidence of lymphedema following treatment for cancer is difficult to determine. There is a lack of international agreement about the definition of the degree of swelling that constitutes lymphedema, and there are different ways of measuring it. Furthermore, it is recognized that lymphedema may take years to develop after cancer treatment, so a long duration of follow-up is essential to capture all cases.

Cancer treatment–related lymphedema is most commonly seen in patients who have been treated for breast cancer, gynecologic cancers, genitourinary cancers, melanoma, and head and neck cancers.

Breast Cancer–Related Lymphedema

Breast cancer–related lymphedema (BCRL) is the type that has been studied most, but even in this group there remain a number of uncertainties about the true incidence and cause (4). A study using different definitions of BCRL with a 5-year follow-up illustrates these challenges. The incidence at 5 years ranged from 43% based on

TABLE 23.2 CAUSES OF EDEMA IN ADVANCED CANCER

General
- Cardiac failure (which may be secondary to or exacerbated by anemia)
- Hypoalbuminemia
- Late-stage chronic renal failure
- Drugs:
  Nonsteroidal anti-inflammatory drugs and corticosteroids (salt and water retention)
  Calcium channel blockers (vasodilation and impaired lymphatic pump)
- Malignant ascites

Local
- Lymphatic obstruction/damage
  Due to surgery/radiotherapy, metastatic tumor in lymph nodes or skin lymphatics, and recurrent infections
- Venous obstruction
  For example, deep vein thrombosis, superior vena caval obstruction, inferior vena caval obstruction, extrinsic venous compression by tumor, and thrombophlebitis migrans
- Lymphovenous edema
  Due to immobility and dependency or localized weakness due to neurologic deficit

self-reported symptoms to 94% based on a 2-cm change in circumference from baseline at any point in the arm (5).

The most robust data on the incidence of BCRL have been derived from a complex systematic review of 30 prospective cohort studies (6). The overall incidence was 21.4% with the vast majority (18.9%) having developed BCRL within 2 years, and 5.6% of those who had had sentinel node biopsies developed BCRL compared with 19.9% of those who had had axillary node clearance (ANC).

This review also examined the risk factors for developing BCRL and found a strong level of evidence for the following:

- Extensive surgery (ANC, greater number of lymph nodes removed and mastectomy)
- Being overweight or obese

Other studies have shown that other factors including the number of positive nodes removed and taxane chemotherapy contribute to the risk.

Attempts have therefore been made to reduce the incidence of BCRL by modifications of surgical and radiotherapy techniques. The following factors should help with this:

- Wide local excision rather than mastectomy
- Sentinel node biopsy (SNB) rather than axillary node sampling
- Avoidance of axillary radiotherapy following ANC
- Modification of radiotherapy techniques
- Avoidance of arm infections and inflammation

Breast lymphedema is a relatively neglected aftermath of breast cancer treatment. It may occur following wide local excision of the tumor and postoperative radiotherapy. A systematic review of 28 papers that represented 4,011 patients found a great variation in the reported incidence of breast edema (0% to 90.4%) (7).

Gynecologic Cancer

The prevalence of lower limb lymphedema after treatment for gynecologic cancers depends upon the type of cancer and surgery carried out. Nevertheless, one study has shown an overall prevalence of 18% in women treated for all gynecologic cancers (8). In 16% of these women, the edema developed between 1 and 5 years following treatment. The prevalence was 47% in women treated for vulval cancer with lymphadenectomy and radiotherapy.

In a recent prospective single-center study using bioimpedance spectroscopy (BIS) to define lymphedema, 27% of women had lymphedema prior to the surgery but a further 37% developed new lymphedema by 2 years following treatment (9). Some of the lymphedema was transient, but in

60% it was persistent. BIS measures extracellular fluid and has been investigated as a tool for the early detection of lymphedema. The reason for the high incidence of preoperative lymphedema in this study is not clear, but a raised body mass index (BMI) was again found to be a risk factor for the development of lymphedema. People with a high BMI can develop lymphedema in the absence of cancer or its treatment.

Genitourinary Cancers

In a systematic review, which included 8 studies involving patients with genitourinary cancer, the incidence of lymphedema following genitourinary cancer was 10% (10).

Melanoma

In a single-center cross-sectional study of lymphedema after surgery for melanoma, 5% developed lymphedema after axillary SNB compared with 31% after ANC (11). Thirty-five percent developed lymphedema after inguinal SNB compared with 83% after completion inguinal node dissection. The high incidence after inguinal node surgery raises important issues of information provision and surveillance in this group.

Head and Neck Cancer

The incidence of moderate to severe internal or external lymphedema after the treatment of head and neck cancer has been reported as 75% in a single-center prospective study with careful examination with nasal endoscopy to detect internal lymphedema and clinical examination to detect external lymphedema after radiotherapy (12). This novel approach has drawn attention to a significant problem.

Incidence of Edema in Advanced Cancer

Edema has been estimated to occur in 19% of people with advanced cancer (13). It is associated with a poor prognosis and is a factor in a number of palliative care prognostic indicators (14).

CLINICAL FEATURES

Lymphedema due to Cancer Treatments

Symptoms and Signs

Lymphedema is often described as a firm nonpitting edema. However, in the early stages of its development, the swelling may be soft and "pit" easily on pressure. As the condition progresses, the swelling becomes firmer because of the deposition of adipose tissue and fibrosis in the subcutaneous space and a reduction in the proportion of fluid present.

The development of the typical skin changes of lymphedema takes a variable amount of time and seems to be more prominent in leg edema than in arm edema.

These changes include the following:

- An increase in skin thickness
- Hyperkeratosis: a buildup of horny scale on the skin surface
- A deepening of skin creases, especially round the ankle and base of toes (Fig. 23.1)
- A warty appearance to the skin as hyperkeratosis worsens
- Lymphangiectasia: small blisters due to dilated lymph vessels. These may burst and cause significant leakage (lymphorrhea). These are said to occur particularly following radiotherapy, which causes fibrosis and obstruction of the deep collecting lymphatics.
- Papillomatosis: with papules consisting of dilated skin lymphatics surrounded by rigid fibrous tissue, which may give a "cobblestone" appearance to areas of skin, particularly on the legs

The physical sign, Stemmer's sign, is the inability to pick up a fold of skin over the proximal phalanx of the second toe, and its presence is said to be diagnostic of lymphedema (15). However, it may be negative in some types of chronic edema for example lymphedema, which mainly affects the proximal part of the leg such as that which follows inguinal node dissection for melanoma.

Pain may be a feature of lymphedema. In one study of various types of lymphedema, 57% of patients reported pain, while 32% described "tightness." Patients with active cancer were more likely to report both tightness and pain (16). Four types of pain were described: tissue pressure, muscle stretch, neurologic, and inflammation. Neurologic pain tended to occur in patients with advanced cancer. When lymphedema first appears, particularly if the swelling develops quickly, pain may occur, which subsequently subsides.

In the early stages of the development of lymphedema, limb function and mobility may be normal, but as swelling develops, particularly around the joints, mobility is reduced and this may in turn exacerbate the swelling due to the reduced action of the muscle pump. As a result, the limb can become increasingly heavy and cause further pain and discomfort at the shoulder or hip in the case of arm and leg edema, respectively.

Lymphedema after Breast Cancer Treatment

Patients may often develop symptoms before any objective evidence of lymphedema (17). These symptoms may include a feeling of fullness, tightness, or heaviness of the arm. Some patients may develop symptoms shortly after the initial treatment, and it may be that these are transient changes that will resolve. In women who have had treatment for breast cancer and who develop edema of the arm or worsening of existing lymphedema despite appropriate treatment, it is important to consider whether there may be recurrence of the breast cancer or evidence of an acute deep vein thrombosis (DVT).

Psychosocial Aspects

Lymphedema, especially following cancer treatment, can be associated with significant psychological morbidity and a reduction in quality of life (17). These may relate to issues of altered body image, disability, and the fear of cancer recurrence. The development of arm swelling can be particularly distressing for women who have had to cope with surgery, radiotherapy, and chemotherapy for breast cancer, and their consequences. To have undergone all these treatments and then be left with persistent arm edema as a constant reminder of previous breast cancer can be traumatic. There is also a negative impact on work and career (18).

Complications

The most common complications of lymphedema are cellulitis and lymphorrhea. DVT may occur

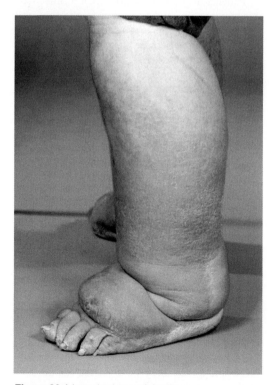

Figure 23.1 Lymphedema of the leg.

in immobile limbs and in recurrent cancer. New malignancies, especially lymphangiosarcoma, are very rare.

Cellulitis

In lymphedematous limbs, there is an altered local immune response (19). This leads to a predisposition to developing infections and, rarely, new malignancies in the affected area. The most important infection is cellulitis, which can not only be very unpleasant for the sufferer but may also lead to further damage to the lymphatic system and worsening edema, particularly in those patients who experience recurrent episodes, which is quite common in lymphedema.

Cellulitis in lymphedema is generally believed to be due to infection by β-hemolytic streptococci, although sometimes other bacteria such as staphylococci may be involved.

The usual clinical picture is the development of a flu-like illness with fever, muscular aches, and sometimes headache and vomiting. This is followed by the appearance of red inflamed painful tender areas in the skin of the lymphedematous limb. The skin changes can be very variable ranging from the whole limb being extremely inflamed to a relatively mild patchy rash.

Proving bacterial infection in all cases is difficult. Sometimes it is clear that bacterial infection has entered the tissues through cuts, broken skin, and ruptured lymphangiectasia or papillomata. In the feet, the skin between the toes may be cracked because of tinea pedis (fungal) infections, to which people with lymphedema are predisposed.

Lymphorrhea

This is the leakage of lymph through the skin at sites of laceration or ruptured cutaneous lymph blisters (lymphangiectasia). This can be particularly distressing if it affects the legs, as large volumes of fluid can leak out. There is an associated increased risk of infection.

Deep Vein Thrombosis

Patients with lymphedema are at risk for DVT in the affected limb, particularly if the limb is very edematous and immobile or if there is an associated abnormality of venous flow because of treatment for malignancy. A DVT can occur even when a patient is wearing a compression garment as treatment for lymphedema. However, if this is the case, recurrence of cancer should be considered.

Malignancy

Although very rare, malignancies can arise in the skin of affected limbs. The most important of these is lymphangiosarcoma. The term *Stewart-Treves* *syndrome* is used to describe its occurrence in postmastectomy lymphedema. In this situation, the incidence is <0.45% and the mean time from the surgery to onset is approximately 10 years.

Lymphangiosarcoma presents as single or multiple bluish-red nodules in the skin, which spread rapidly locally often forming satellite lesions that may become confluent and ulcerate.

Edema of Advanced Cancer

Symptoms and Signs

The general symptoms and signs of edema in advanced cancer may be similar to those described in the previous section. However, as the cause is often more complex, the clinical picture may also vary (Table 23.2). Pure lymphedema is unusual in advanced disease, and if it does occur, because of the short prognosis there is usually no time for the more chronic skin changes to develop. Therefore, edema in advanced cancer is often very soft and pitting. The skin can look stretched and shiny rather than thickened as in chronic lymphedema.

Pain is more likely to be a problem in patients with advanced cancer, particularly neuropathic pain resulting from nerve compression or destruction by tumor. This is often severe with tingling, burning, or stabbing features and altered sensation in the area of the pain. Light touch might be more painful than deep pressure (touch-evoked allodynia).

Patients may also be more prone to infections due to poor skin condition (often fragile, thin, and dry), skin tumors, ulceration, and reduced resistance to infection because of treatment or as a feature of advanced disease.

Ulceration of the skin is generally uncommon in pure lymphedema in comparison with venous disease but can occur in patients with edema in advanced malignancy. There can be significant associated lymphorrhea that can cause distress to patients. Superimposed infection by anaerobic bacteria can lead to unpleasant malodorous discharge and increased pain.

Immobility may be worse in patients with advanced malignancy because of generalized weakness or local nerve injury caused by tumor, such as brachial plexus infiltration in breast cancer.

The psychosocial aspects of edema in these situations are often greater, with patients having to cope with progressive disease and impending death, as well as the problems of lymphedema.

Specific Situations

Locally Advanced Breast Cancer

In locally advanced breast cancer, a particularly severe and intractable type of edema can develop. In this situation, the deep lymphatic drainage of the arm may have already been damaged by surgery and radiotherapy, but this can be worsened by the recurrence of disease in axillary lymph nodes and the development of metastatic disease in the skin of the upper arm and chest wall with infiltration of the skin lymphatics. The arm can become extremely swollen. The problem may be exacerbated by brachial plexopathy, resulting in immobility of the arm and DVT because of extrinsic venous compression by tumor. In the latter, distended collateral veins may be seen around the shoulder.

The arm can become very heavy, swollen, painful, and dysfunctional. Blisters are common, and breakdown of the skin may lead to ulceration and persistent lymphorrhea. The hand and fingers may swell to such an extent as to give the appearance of "a boxing glove" (Fig. 23.2).

Advanced Pelvic Malignant Disease

Patients with advanced cancers of the uterus, ovary, prostate, bladder, or rectum may have gross edema of the legs and trunk, often of mixed cause as follows:

- Lymphatic obstruction from metastatic disease in lymph nodes
- Extrinsic venous compression
- Inferior vena caval obstruction (IVCO)
- DVT
- Hypoalbuminemia
- Fluid-retaining drugs
- Ascites

Ascites

Malignant ascites is common in advanced ovarian, colorectal, gastric, pancreatic, and uterine cancers and is associated with a poor prognosis (median survival, 2 to 3 months). Leg edema often occurs in the presence of ascites.

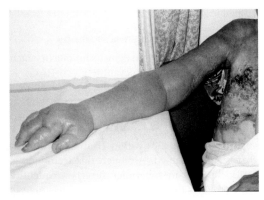

Figure 23.2 Lymphedema of the arm in locally advanced breast cancer.

Hypoalbuminemia

Hypoalbuminemia is common in advanced cancer because of the cachexia–anorexia syndrome, which causes a reduction in hepatic protein synthesis. Hypoalbuminemia may cause edema on its own but is usually seen in the context of other factors as described in the preceding text.

Superior Vena Caval Obstruction

Superior vena caval obstruction (SVCO) is usually seen in patients with extrinsic compression of the vena cava by metastases in the upper mediastinal lymph nodes. It should be approached as an emergent situation when diagnosed (cross reference). It is particularly common in lung cancer. The features may develop very quickly perhaps because of secondary venous thrombosis. The most common presenting symptoms are as follows:

- Dyspnea
- Neck and facial swelling
- Trunk and arm swelling
- A sensation of choking
- A feeling of fullness in the head
- Headache

On examination, the following may be present:

- Thoracic vein distension
- Neck vein distension
- Facial edema
- Tachypnea
- Facial plethora
- Cyanosis
- Arm edema

The condition can be very distressing for patients and, if untreated, may lead to death.

Inferior Vena Caval Obstruction

IVCO usually occurs because of extrinsic compression by retroperitoneal lymphadenopathy or hepatomegaly due to metastatic disease. Patients develop edema of the legs, abdomen, and genitalia, and if the obstruction is above the level of the hepatic veins, ascites may occur as well. Dilated collateral veins are often seen on the abdominal wall.

Complications

Although the complications of edema in advanced cancer may be similar to those of lymphedema described in the preceding text, patients with advanced disease are particularly prone to venous thrombosis due to the increased coagulability of their blood. They are also more prone to lymphorrhea and infections, but the short prognosis means that the development of lymphangiosarcomas is not an issue.

DIFFERENTIAL DIAGNOSIS AND INVESTIGATIONS

In patients with cancer treatment–related lymphedema, the diagnosis is usually based on the clinical history and examination. However, the possibility of DVT or recurrence of malignant disease does need to be borne in mind.

In patients with advanced malignancy, elucidating potentially reversible contributory factors is an important part of the management of edema (Table 23.2).

Investigations

Specific investigations may include the following:

- Computed tomography scan/magnetic resonance imaging/ultrasound scan to look for recurrent disease
- Full blood count to look for anemia
- Plasma B–type natriuretic peptide (BNP) and echocardiogram to look for evidence of heart failure
- Serum albumin to detect hypoalbuminemia
- Plasma urea and creatinine to look for evidence of renal failure

Deep Vein Thrombosis

In the United Kingdom, current diagnostic practice for DVT of the lower limb relies on the use of an algorithm based on signs and symptoms (Wells' score (20)—see Table 23.3) together with D-dimer levels in the blood and an ultrasound examination of the leg to assess deep vein blood flow. Unfortunately, in patients with advanced malignancy the level of D-dimers may be elevated in the absence of DVT, so this element of the assessment may not be particularly helpful.

A "Wells' score" of 2 or higher indicates that the probability of DVT is "likely"; a score of <2 indicates the probability of DVT is "unlikely." In patients with symptoms in both legs, the more symptomatic leg is used.

DVT can be ruled out in a patient who is scored in the "unlikely" category and who has a negative D-dimer test (20). In those with positive D-dimers, a Wells' score in the "likely" category, further investigation with ultrasound imaging of the leg is recommended.

DVT of the arm can occur in recurrent breast cancer and can be investigated by ultrasound.

Lymphoscintigraphy

Lymphoscintigraphy is a specific examination for lymphedema (21). A subcutaneous or intradermal injection of a radioactively labeled macromolecule, for example, ^{99m}Tc-labelled protein or colloid, is used. This is taken up by the lymphatics, which can

TABLE 23.3 WELL'S SCORE

Clinical model for predicting the pretest probability of deep vein thrombosis

Clinical characteristics	Score
Active cancer (patient receiving treatment for cancer within the previous 6 months or currently receiving palliative treatment)	1
Paralysis, paresis, or recent plaster immobilization of the lower extremities	1
Recently bedridden for 3 days or more or major surgery within the previous 12 weeks requiring general or regional anesthesia	1
Localized tenderness along the distribution of the deep venous system	1
Entire leg swollen	1
Calf swelling at least 3 cm larger than that on the asymptomatic side (measured 10 cm below tibial tuberosity)	1
Pitting edema confined to the symptomatic leg	1
Collateral superficial veins (nonvaricose)	1
Previously documented deep vein thrombosis	1
Alternative diagnosis at least as likely as deep vein thrombosis	−2

then be detected using an external gamma camera. Although this is a useful technique in the assessment of patients with primary lymphedema, its place in patients who have cancer-related lymphedema is limited. However, practice does vary around the world. In the United Kingdom, lymphoscintigraphy is rarely done in this situation, as it is felt it is unlikely to affect management, and the diagnosis is usually clear on clinical grounds. However, in other countries, isotope lymphoscintigraphy is more commonly performed in cancer-related lymphedema.

Indocyanine Green Lymphography

This is a relatively new imaging technique in which the fluorescent dye, indocyanine green (ICG), is injected intradermally into the peripheral part of the limb. The dye binds to protein, which is absorbed by the lymphatics and can be imaged using an infrared camera. Real-time images of the superficial lymphatics within 10 mm of the skin surface are obtained. Although this technique is routinely used in supermicrosurgery to identify lymph vessels for lymphaticovenular anastomosis (LVA), it has also been used in the research setting to look for the early detection of BCRL (22).

MANAGEMENT

Early Detection and Prevention of BCRL

In recent years, there has been a growing interest in the prevention of BCRL (4). Prevention can be considered in a number of ways:

- preventing BCRL from developing altogether, for example by changing surgical and radiotherapy techniques
- preventing the progression of early subclinical lymphedema into established BCRL by early detection and intervention
- preventing the progression and complications of established BCRL

The latter two depend upon having clear diagnostic criteria for clinical lymphedema, ways of measuring subclinical lymphedema, and successful interventions. As stated above, there are no internationally agreed diagnostic criteria for clinical lymphedema, but measures that are commonly reported in the literature include a relative arm volume change (RAVC) from baseline of >10% or a change in bioimpedance (BIS) of L-Dex of 10 or more. Both of these approaches require preoperative measurements to give a baseline.

There is conflicting opinion on which of these techniques is superior. In some clinical guidelines BIS is favored (23), but other research shows RAVC is superior (24). Normatively determined circumference and BIS thresholds have been proposed as alternatives (25).

There is even greater difficulty in defining diagnostic criteria for subclinical lymphedema, where intervention may possibly prevent progression to established lymphedema (26). What does seem to be clear from clinical experience, however, is that early intervention with compression treatment in mild lymphedema reduces the likelihood of progression.

Studies have shown that manual lymphatic drainage (MLD) (see below) does not prevent lymphedema (27) but exercise programs may help (28,29). A microsurgical technique (LYMPHA) of LVA at the time of breast surgery with a 4-year follow-up reported BCRL in 3/74 patients (30).

Finally, it seems reasonable for patients to take sensible precautions to minimize the risk of infection or overload of the lymphatics that may cause further damage to lymph vessels and precipitate overt edema. Examples of these are given in Tables 23.4 and 23.5.

Management of Treatment-Related Edema

The mainstay of cancer treatment–related edema is a combination of physical treatments that together

TABLE 23.4 RECOMMENDATIONS TO REDUCE THE RISK OF LYMPHEDEMA AFTER BREAST CANCER TREATMENT

- Avoid injuries including cuts and abrasions, for example, wear gloves when gardening
- Use a thimble when sewing
- Use an oven glove when cooking
- Take care when ironing
- Avoid tight clothing, including tight bra straps
- Avoid irritating cosmetics/soaps
- Avoid sunburn
- Avoid insect bites/cat scratches
- Use an electric razor for shaving
- Avoid obesity
- Avoid injections or venipuncture in the "at-risk" arm (but see text)
- Avoid blood pressure measurement in the "at-risk" arm (but see text)
- Seek medical advice if "at-risk" arm becomes inflamed or swollen

are known as complex decongestive therapy, CDT, complex physical therapy, CPT, or *decongestive lymphedema therapy* (DLT) (31).

The treatment comprises four elements:

- Compression
- Skin care
- Exercise
- Massage: MLD or simple lymphatic drainage (SLD).

Compression is carried out in the form of a specific multilayer lymphedema bandage (MLLB), Velcro compression wraps, or elastic compression garments.

Skin care typically involves the use of a moisturizing cream such as aqueous cream, but also looks at ways of protecting the skin such as avoiding cuts and abrasions, avoiding sun burn, avoiding venipuncture, intravenous infusions, and treating conditions such as eczema. It is often also recommended to avoid having blood pressure measured

TABLE 23.5 RECOMMENDATIONS TO PATIENTS AT RISK FOR DEVELOPING LEG LYMPHEDEMA

- Avoid standing for several hours
- Maintain skin hygiene especially feet
- Avoid tight shoes, socks, other clothing
- Avoid walking barefoot outdoors
- Avoid irritating cosmetics or soaps
- Avoid injections in the "at-risk" limb
- Avoid insect bites/cat scratches/cuts/injuries
- Treat fungal infections, for example, tinea pedis, early
- Avoid sunburn
- Avoid surgery, for example, for varicose veins, if possible
- Avoid obesity
- Use an electric razor for shaving
- Seek medical advice if "at-risk" leg becomes inflamed or swollen

in the lymphedematous arm. The aim of these recommendations is to improve the skin condition and reduce the likelihood of infections. However, recent literature raises the issue of whether these recommendations are too cautious as there is little evidence that ipsilateral blood draws, injections, blood pressure measurements, and air travel are significant risk factors for the development of BCRL (32).

Exercise encourages lymphatic drainage, but some patients may require specific physiotherapy/exercises to improve function if joints have become stiff.

MLD is a type of gentle skin massage applied by trained therapists, which is designed to improve lymph drainage. SLD is based on the principles of MLD, but is carried out by the patients themselves or by a carer.

MLD is said to stimulate contraction of the lymph collectors and enhance protein resorption. The massage technique is designed to improve drainage from congested areas. It includes breathing exercises to improve thoracic duct drainage and gentle superficial massage working distal to proximal, for example, commencing on the trunk, then the proximal part of the limb, and then the distal area, to encourage proximal flow. There are a number of different "schools" of MLD, for example, Vodder, Leduc, Földi, Casley-Smith, and the recently developed "Fill and Flush" technique (33). Although different techniques are employed, the basic principles are shared by all schools.

For patients with moderate to severe edema, an intensive phase of treatment over a period of approximately 2 weeks involving compression bandaging (with or without MLD) to reduce the swelling and improve the shape of the limb is carried out. Patients who have associated truncal edema usually require MLD together with compression bandaging. This intensive phase of treatment is followed by the application of compression garments, that is, an elastic stocking or arm sleeve, which is then worn daily indefinitely.

Some patients require repeated courses of bandaging treatment over a period of time. Other patients with more mild edema may be managed with skin care and compression garments alone.

Patients with "midline" edema, that is, truncal, breast, genital, or head and neck edema, are best treated with MLD and SLD as these are not areas to which compression garments can be easily applied. Specialist garments for these areas, however, are available and may be helpful in some situations. Adhesive skin tapes (e.g., Kinesio tape) may also be useful in "midline" edema.

Evidence for Effectiveness of Treatments

The combination of physical treatments has been shown to produce a sustained improvement in limb volume and a reduction in the incidence of episodes of cellulitis (34). However, there is little robust evidence in the literature to validate the individual components of these treatment regimes. A Cochrane review found that MLD is safe and may offer additional benefit to compression bandaging for swelling reduction in those with mild to moderate BCRL but recommended that this finding needed to be confirmed by randomized data (35).

Other Treatments

Intermittent Pneumatic Compression (IPC) Pumps

A variety of these devices is available, ranging from single-chambered sleeves providing intermittent compression to a limb to multichambered devices (e.g., 5 to 10 chambers) that produce an intermittent sequential (peristaltic) compression massaging fluid from the distal to the proximal part of the limb. There has been renewed interest in the use of IPC in treating lymphedema with the development of more sophisticated devices that produce a massage-like effect rather than simply compressing. IPC is increasingly being used as part of a multimodal management regimen.

Surgery for Cancer-Related Lymphedema

There are two main types of surgery that are currently being used: reductive for example liposuction and reconstructive for example lymphaticovenous anastomosis (LVA) and vascularized lymph node transfer (VLNT). However, in most countries including the United Kingdom, surgery is not currently routine practice in the treatment of cancer-related lymphedema.

Liposuction has been used for patients with advanced, severe BCRL where adipose tissue and fibrosis predominate in the swelling (36). Although the reduction in limb volume is good and sustained with this technique, patients have to wear compression hosiery 24 hours per day indefinitely following surgery to maintain the benefit.

LVA, a supermicrosurgical technique where lymphatics are anastomosed to venules to bypass obstruction, has been increasingly used to treat early cancer-related lymphedema. A systematic review showed that the effects of LVA for BCRL were variable although overall it seemed effective in early-stage BCRL. The number of patients who experienced symptom relief ranges from 50% to 100% (37).

In VLNT, lymph nodes are transferred from another area of the body to replace those removed as part of cancer treatment, with the concept that new lymph vessels will regenerate and replace the damaged ones. In a small randomized controlled study (n = 36), in women with BCRL, half the women were randomized to receiving 6 months' treatment with compression and physiotherapy and the other half to having this same treatment following free lymph-node transfer (38). After 18 months, there was a 57% reduction in limb volume in those who had lymph-node transfer compared with 18% in the control group.

Drug Treatments

Drug treatments for lymphedema are generally disappointing. Diuretics seem to have no role in the treatment of pure lymphedema, although they can be helpful if fluid retention is present as well. There is new interest and early promising results in the use of anti-inflammatories such as ketoprofen (39).

Treatment of Infection

Local fungal infections such as tinea pedis are treated with topical antifungals such as terbinafine cream. Fungal nail infections are more difficult to eradicate and may require treatment with oral terbinafine.

Treatment of cellulitis is aimed at β-hemolytic streptococci and depending upon the severity of the problem may be managed at home with oral antibiotics, but may require admission to hospital for intravenous therapy (Table 23.6) (40).

Bed rest and elevation of the lymphedematous limb is part of the management. Compression garments are not worn until they can be tolerated comfortably.

If intravenous antibiotics are required, then flucloxacillin 2 g 6 hourly may be used. If there is no response after 48 hours to this management, then clindamycin 600 mg 6 hourly i.v. could be substituted. Once the patient's condition begins to improve, a switch can be made to oral antibiotics.

In patients who develop recurrent cellulitis, that is, who have two or more attacks of cellulitis per year, prophylactic antibiotics may be considered.

TABLE 23.6 ORAL ANTIBIOTICS FOR THE TREATMENT OF CELLULITIS

1. Amoxicillin 500 mg t.i.d. for at least 14 days
2. Flucloxacillin 500 mg q.i.d. if evidence of staphylococcal infections, for example, folliculitis
3. Clindamycin 300 mg q.i.d. to be substituted for the amoxicillin if there is a poor response to oral antibiotics after 48 hours. This is recommended for patients who are allergic to penicillin as the first-line treatment

However, reduction in limb volume by treatment and improvement of skin condition should reduce the incidence of infection. A suggested antibiotic regimen is phenoxymethylpenicillin 250 mg twice daily. The duration of prophylaxis is dependent on individual circumstances, but patients in whom attempts to withdraw it after successful treatment of the lymphedema have resulted in recurrence of cellulitis may need this therapy lifelong.

Management of Patients with Advanced Cancer

The general principles of management are as for patients with lymphedema caused by cancer treatment, but they may have to be modified in the light of circumstances (41). In view of the complex cause, it is helpful to identify potentially reversible factors as described in the preceding text and treat these accordingly, for example, blood transfusion for anemia.

When uncontrolled tumor is the main cause of the edema, this is unlikely to respond very well to treatment and an emphasis should be placed on enhancing the patient's quality of life, respecting the patient's choices and priorities, and providing psychological support to the patient and the family. It is important that any burden of treatment should not exceed the benefit gained.

Skin Care

Skin care remains important in advanced disease, and the avoidance of trauma is particularly relevant. The shearing forces when putting on and taking off a compression garment may cause damage to the skin, and a light support bandage may be more appropriate in these circumstances. Where there is skin breakdown, nonadherent dressings may have to be applied. Occasionally, hemostatic dressings may be needed to control bleeding (e.g., calcium alginate) or topical epinephrine solution 1 in 1,000 (1 mg in 1 mL) used when dressings are changed.

Fungating Lesions

Fungating lesions, for example, on the chest wall or upper arm, in locally advanced breast cancer may become malodorous because of superadded anaerobic bacterial infection. Topical metronidazole 0.8% gel daily or oral metronidazole 400 mg b.i.d. for 2 weeks is often helpful. Topical metronidazole is relatively free from adverse effects, but sometimes it is difficult to apply the gel to deeper crevices, and in some situations in which there is profuse discharge the gel is flushed away or diluted, thereby making it less effective. In these circumstances, oral metronidazole may be helpful.

Support and Positioning

In very ill patients, support and positioning of swollen limbs using pillows and so on may relieve discomfort. It is important to try to avoid the use of an arm sling for people with arm edema, as this may cause pooling of fluid of the elbow and stiffness of the elbow joint. However, in some patients with severe arm edema and weakness from brachial plexopathy, a sling that can take the weight away from the shoulders and distribute it across the back may help with comfort and improve steadiness on movement (e.g., Lancaster sling).

Exercise

Exercises need to be adjusted to the patients' abilities and condition. Passive movements may be helpful to reduce stiffness and discomfort, but more active exercise regimes are usually inappropriate.

Massage

The presence of active cancer is often considered to be a contraindication to massage techniques such as MLD and SLD. It is argued that stimulation of lymph flow around the site of a tumor may lead to metastasis. There is no evidence either way to support or refute this in the literature, but in the presence of advanced metastatic disease the potential benefits of massage, particularly for truncal edema, outweigh any risk of inducing further metastatic spread. It is important that the patient makes an informed choice in this situation.

Compression

The aim of management in advanced cancer is often to relieve discomfort rather than to aggressively try to reduce limb volume. The skin may be too fragile to tolerate significant compression, and therefore modifications of bandaging techniques to provide support from light bandages or from light compression garments or Velcro compression wraps are often needed. Velcro compression wraps have the advantage of bandages in avoiding shearing forces on fragile skin while being more easily applied and removed by patients or their carers. Shaped Tubigrip is a useful alternative to compression garments. In all circumstances, the skin condition needs to be checked regularly, particularly if there is impaired skin sensation, to confirm that the bandage or garment is not causing additional problems (42).

Lymphorrhea is helped by bandaging. A sterile pad or gauze is used to absorb the lymph and the gentle pressure applied by bandage often stops lymphorrhea in 24 to 48 hours. Sometimes, however, the bandage may need changing several times a day initially because of the rapid leakage of lymph.

In certain circumstances, compression bandaging may increase the amount of fluid leakage. For example, in patients with fungating breast tumors in the axilla or chest wall, the application of a bandage to the ipsilateral swollen arm may result in an increased discharge from the lesion. This is believed to be due to the increased flow of lymph through "open" lymphatics near the skin surface.

High levels of compression (>30 mm Hg) of the legs should be avoided in patients with acute heart failure, which may be contributing to their edema in advanced disease. Because of the multifactorial nature of the edema, those with bilateral leg swelling, genital edema, and truncal edema often do not tolerate compression bandaging of the legs. This may be ineffective or, particularly where there is hypoalbuminemia, simply push fluid onto the abdominal wall and genital areas making the edema there worse.

Appliances to Aid Mobility and Function

Various aids that may help with walking, dressing, use of swollen hands and arms, and so on may be provided by an occupational therapist.

Drug Treatments

Corticosteroids

Systemic corticosteroids are often used for a variety of symptoms in advanced cancer. They work by reducing inflammation and peritumor edema and thereby can relieve pressure on neighboring structures such as lymphatics, veins, and nerves. They can therefore have a role in reducing pain and swelling.

Dexamethasone is commonly used as a starting dose of 8 to 16 mg daily. This is usually given as a trial for 1 week to determine whether it is effective. If the drug is ineffective, it is discontinued at this stage. If it is effective, then the dose is gradually reduced until the lowest level that relieves the symptoms is reached. This usually takes a period of weeks, over which time adverse effects such as fluid retention, gastrointestinal disturbance, weight gain, proximal myopathy, diabetes, and psychosis may develop. Should these occur, the balance of benefit versus the side effects of the drugs should be reviewed with the patient and a decision made whether to continue or gradually withdraw the treatment.

Diuretics

Diuretics may be helpful in the management of edema of advanced cancer if fluid retention, for example, due to drugs, or heart failure is present. Furosemide is commonly used and the dose adjusted according to effect.

Analgesics

Pain associated with edema in advanced cancer may respond to opioid analgesics, but if neuropathic pain is present other approaches such as the use of amitriptyline or one of the anticonvulsant drugs such as gabapentin may be helpful (see Chapter 2).

Treatment of Specific Potentially Reversible Factors

Potentially reversible factors should be treated in the light of a patient's general condition. Aggressive invasive treatment may not be appropriate in patients with a very short prognosis. A detailed description of all the treatment regimes is beyond the scope of this chapter, but a brief summary is given in Table 23.7.

The management of DVT with anticoagulants in patients with advanced cancer is not easy. The presence of existing bleeding from tumors such as fungating breast lesions would represent a contraindication. Although patients with advanced cancer are more prone to thrombosis, they are also more prone to hemorrhage if anticoagulated with warfarin. Drug interactions between warfarin and other medications that the person may be taking are common. Furthermore, patients who are anticoagulated to a "routine" level with warfarin, that is, international normalized ratio = 2 to 2.5, may still develop further thromboembolic events. Anticoagulation to a higher level is sometimes used but has an associated increased risk of bleeding. Low-molecular-weight heparins, for example, enoxaparin, may be a more appropriate alternative but are more expensive and require daily subcutaneous injections. The use of newer direct oral anticoagulants (DOACs) for example apixaban can also circumvent some of the problems with warfarin. The likely risks and benefits of anticoagulation should be considered and an informed decision made with the patient.

Needle Drainage of Edema in Advanced Disease

There has been renewed interest in subcutaneous needle drainage of severe edema in advanced cancer. In a recent multicenter, nonrandomized, observational study of 32 procedures in 31 patients, quality of life as measured by a validated lymphedema specific tool, improved significantly at 2 weeks. The average volume drained was 5.5 L and the cellulitis rate was 6% (43). This suggests that this approach is worth considering in patients with severe edema where other treatments have been unsuccessful.

Other Approaches

A recently reported case series used intravenous infusion of furosemide in hypertonic saline combined with multilayer compression bandaging over 3 days in resistant limb edema in advanced disease in 19 patients (44). They reported a clinically meaningful reduction in limb volume of 1.52 L combined with a reduction in symptoms but stable blood and performance parameters.

Effectiveness of Treatments for Lymphedema in Advanced Cancer

A systematic review highlighted the lack of good-quality evidence for the techniques used in this setting (45). However, it is not an easy area in which to carry out research. However, in a small study of 12 patients with lymphedema in advanced cancer with a median survival of 40 days, who received three or more CDT interventions, limb volume was reduced and quality of life increased following the treatment (46). The International Lymphoedema Framework produced a "position document" on lymphedema in advanced cancer and edema at the end of life (47).

MANAGEMENT SUMMARY

The management of cancer treatment–related lymphedema is not curative but can help control the significant symptoms experienced by patients and reduce the risk of cellulitis.

- Compression is currently the mainstay of treatment.

TABLE 23.7 TREATMENT OF POTENTIALLY REVERSIBLE FACTORS IN ADVANCED CANCER

Condition	Treatment
Anemia	Blood transfusion
Heart failure	Diuretics, digoxin, angiotensin-converting enzyme inhibitors
Fluid-retaining drugs	Withdraw if possible or use diuretics
Hypoalbuminemia	Treatment generally unrewarding
Malignant ascites	Paracentesis Diuretic therapy, for example, with spironolactone with or without furosemide Anticancer therapy, for example, in ovarian cancer
Superior vena caval obstruction	Metal stent High-dose corticosteroids plus radiotherapy Chemotherapy
Inferior vena caval obstruction	Corticosteroids Metal stent
Deep vein thrombosis	Anticoagulation, for example with low-molecular-weight heparin, direct oral anticoagulant (DOAC), or warfarin

- The situation in patients with edema in advanced cancer is different and the treatment is more "palliative" in nature. In all situations, the balance of benefit versus burden should be weighed up.

REFERENCES

1. The diagnosis and treatment of peripheral lymphedema: 2016 consensus document of the International Society of Lymphology. *Lymphology*. 2016;49:170-184.
2. Levick JR, Michel CC. Microvascular fluid exchange and the revised Starling principle. *Cardiovasc Res*. 2010;87:198-210.
3. Stanton AWB, Modi S, Bennett Britton TM, et al. Lymphatic drainage in the muscle and sucutis of the arm after breast cancer treatment. *Breast Cancer Res Treat*. 2009;117(3):549-557.
4. Rockson S, Keeley V, Kilbreath S, et al. Cancer- associated secondary lymphedema. *Nat Rev Dis Primers*. 2019;5:22. doi:10.1038/s41572-019-0072-5.
5. Armer JM, Stewart BR. Post-breast cancer lymphedema: incidence increases from 12 to 30 to 60 months. *Lymphology*. 2010;43:118-127.
6. Disipio T, Rye S, Newman B, Hayes S. Incidence of unilateral arm lymphoedema after breast cancer: a systematic review and meta- analysis. *Lancet Oncol*. 2013;14:500-515.
7. Verbelen H, Gebruers N, Beyers T, et al. Breast edema in breast cancer patients following breast-conserving surgery and radiotherapy: a systematic review. *Breast Cancer Res Treat*. 2014;147(3):463-471. doi:10.1007/s10549-014-3110-8.
8. Ryan M, Stainton MC, Slaytor EK, et al. Aetiology and prevalence of lower limb lymphoedema following treatment for gynaecological cancer. *Aust N Z J Obstet Gynaecol*. 2003;43:148-151.
9. Hayes SC, Janda M, Ward LC, et al. Lymphedema following gynecological cancer: results from a prospective, longitudinal cohort study on prevalence, incidence and risk factors. *Gynecol Oncol*. 2017;146:623-629. doi:10.1016/j.ygyno.2017.06.004.
10. Cormier JN, Askew RL, Mungovan KS, Xing Y, Ross MI, Armer J. Lymphedema beyond breast cancer. a systematic review and meta-analysis of cancer-related secondary lymphedema. *Cancer*. 2010;116:5138-5149.
11. Gjorup C. Melanoma related limb lymphoedema and associated risk factors. PhD thesis 2017 University of Copenhagen, Denmark.
12. Ridner SH, Dietrich MS, Niermann K, et al. A prospective study of the lymphedema and fibrosis continuum in patients with head and neck cancer. *Lymphat Res Biol*. 2016;14:198-205
13. Teunissen SCCM, Wesker W, Kruitwagen C, et al. Symptom prevalence in patients with incurable cancer: a systematic review. *J Pain Symptom Manage*. 2007;34(1):94-104.
14. Gwilliam B, Keeley V, Todd C, et al. Development of Prognosis in Palliative care Study (PiPS) predictor models to improve prognostication in advanced cancer: prospective cohort study. *BMJ*. 2011;343:d4920.
15. Stemmer R. Ein klinisches Zeichen zur Früh-und differential-diagnose des Lymphödems. *Vasa*. 1976;5: 261-262.
16. Badger CM, Mortimer PS, Regnard CFB, et al. Pain in the chronically swollen limb. *Prog Lymphol*. 1998;11:243-246.
17. Wanchai A, Armer JN, Stewart BR, Lasinski BB. Breast cancer-related lymphedema: a literature review for clinical practice. *Int J Nurs Sci*. 2016;3:202-207.
18. Boyages J, Kalfa S, Xu Y, et al. Worse and worse off: the impact of lymphedema on work and career after breast cancer. *Springerplus*. 2016;5:657. doi:10.1186/s40064-016-2300-8.
19. Mallon E, Powell S, Mortimer P, et al. Evidence of altered cell mediated immunity in post-mastectomy lymphoedema. *Br J Dermatol*. 1997;137:928-933.
20. Wells PS, Anderson DR, Rodger M, et al. Evaluation of D-dimer in the diagnosis of suspected deep-vein thrombosis. *N Engl J Med*. 2003;349:1227-1235.
21. Keeley V. The role of lymphoscintigraphy in the management of chronic oedema. *J Lymphoedema*. 2006;1(1): 42-57.
22. Mihara M, Hara H, Araki J, et al. Indocyanine green (ICG) lymphography is superior to lymphoscintigraphy for diagnostic imaging of early lymphedema of the upper limbs. *PLoS One*. 2012;7(6):e38182. doi:10.1371/journal.pone.0038182.
23. Levenhagen K, Davies C, Perdomo M, Ryans K, Gilchrist L. Diagnosis of upper quadrant lymphedema secondary to cancer: clinical practice guideline from the Oncology Section of the American Physical Therapy Association. *Phys Ther*. 2017;97:729-745. doi:10.1093/ptj/pzx050.
24. Bundred NJ, Stockton C, Keeley V, et al. Comparison of multi-frequency bioimpedance with perometry for the early detection of lymphoedema after axillary node clearance for breast cancer. *Breast Cancer Res Treat*. 2015;151:121-129. doi:10.1007/s10549-015-3357-8.
25. Dylke ES, Schembri GP, Bailey DL, et al. Diagnosis of upper limb lymphedema: development of an evidence-based approach. *Acta Oncol*. 2016;55(12):1477-1483.
26. Ridner S, Dietrich M, Cowher M, et al. A randomized trial evaluating bioimpedance spectroscopy versus tape measurement for the prevention of lymphedema following treatment for breast cancer: interim analysis. *Ann Surg Oncol*. 2019;26(10):3250-3259. doi:10.1245/s10434-019-07344-5.
27. Devoogdt N, Christiaens MR, Geraerts I, et al. Effect of manual lymph drainage in addition to guidelines and exercise therapy on arm lymphoedema related to breast cancer: randomized controlled trial. *BMJ*. 2011;343:d5326.
28. Box RC, Reul-Hirche HM, Bullock-Saxton JE, Furnival CM. Physiotherapy after breast cancer surgery: results of a randomized controlled study to minimize lymphoedema. *Breast Cancer Res Treat*. 2002;75(1):51-64.
29. Torres Lacomba M, Yuste Sanchez MJ, Zapico Coni A, et al. Effectiveness of early physiotherapy to prevent lymphoedema after surgery for breast cancer: randomized, single blinded, clinical trial. *BMJ*. 2010;340:b5396.
30. Boccardo F, Casabona F, Decian F, et al. Lymphatic microsurgical preventing healing approach (LYMPHA) for primary surgical prevention of breast cancer- related lymphedema: over 4 years follow- up. *Microsurgery*. 2014;34:421-424.
31. Lymphoedema Framework. *Best Practice for the Management of Lymphoedema. International Consensus*. London: MEP Ltd; 2006.
32. Ferguson C, Swaroop M, Horick N, et al. Impact of ipsilateral blood draws, injections, blood pressure measurements, and air travel on the risk of lymphedema for patients treated for breast cancer. *J Clin Oncol*. 2016;34:691-698. doi:10.1200/jco.2015.61.5948.
33. Belgrado J-P, Vandermeeren L, Vankerckhove S, et al. Near-infrared fluorescence lymphatic imaging to reconsider occlusion pressure of superficial lymphatic collectors in upper extremities of healthy volunteers. *Lymphat Res Biol*. 2016;14(2):70-77. doi:10.1089/lrb.2015.0040.

34. Ko DSC, Lerner R, Klose G, et al. Effective treatment of lymphoedema of the extremities. *Arch Surg.* 1998;133:452-458.

35. Ezzo J, Manheimer E, McNeely ML, et al. Manual lymphatic drainage for lymphedema following breast cancer treatment. *Cochrane Database Syst Rev.* 2015;(5):CD003475. doi:10.1002/14651858.CD003475.pub2.

36. Schaverien M, Munnoch, A, Brorson H. Liposuction treatment of lymphedema. *Semin Plast Surg.* 2018;32(1):42-47. doi:10.1055/s-0038-1635116.

37. Cornelissen A, Beugels I, Ewalds L, et al. Effect of lymphaticovenous anastomosis in breast cancer-related lymphedema: a review of the literature. *Lymphat Res Biol.* 2018;16(5):426-434. doi:10.1089/lrb.2017.0067.

38. Dionyssiou D, Demiri E, Tsimponis A, et al. A randomized control study of treating secondary stage II breast cancer-related lymphoedema with free lymph node transfer. *Breast Cancer Res Treat.* 2016;156:73-79. doi:10.1007/s10549-016-3716-0.

39. Rockson S, Tian W, Jiang X, et al. Pilot studies demonstrate the potential benefits of antiinflammatory therapy in human lymphedema. *JCI Insight.* 2018;3(20):e123775.

40. BLS/LSN Consensus Guidelines on the Management of Cellulitis in Lymphoedema. 2019. www.thebls.com

41. Towers A, Hodgson P, Shay C, Keeley V. Care of palliative patients with cancer-related lymphoedema. *J Lymphoedema.* 2010;5(1):72-80.

42. Crooks S, Locke J, Walker J, Keeley V. Palliative bandaging in breast cancer related arm oedema. *J Lymphoedema.* 2007;2(1):50-54.

43. Landers A, Holyoake J. Lymphoedema in advanced cancer: does subcutaneous needle drainage improve quality of life? *BMJ Support Palliat Care.* 2019. Epub ahead of print. doi:10.1136/bmjspcare-2019-001924.

44. Gradalski T. Diuretics combined with compression in resistant limb edema of advanced disease—A case series report. *J Pain Symptom Manage.* 2018;55:1179-1183.

45. Beck M, Wanchai A, Stewart BR, Cormier JN, Armer JM. Palliative care for cancer-related lymphoedema: a systematic review. *J Palliat Med.* 2012;15(7):821-827.

46. Cobbe S, Nugent K, Real S. Pilot study: the effectiveness of complex decongestive therapy for lymphedema in palliative care patients with advanced cancer. *J Palliat Med.* 2018;21(4):473-478. doi:10.1089/jpm.2017.0235.

47. International Lymphoedema Framework. Position Document. The management of lymphoedema in advanced cancer and oedema at the end of life. 2010. www.lympho.org

24 Dyspnea in the Cancer Patient

Ann M. Berger

INTRODUCTION

Dyspnea, an unpleasant awareness of breathing, is a very common symptom that is often unrecognized in people with cancer. It is a complex and distressing symptom that can impact people's daily functioning (1) and result in impaired quality of life (2,3), social isolation (4), and prompt terminal sedation (5). Patients with breathlessness are more likely to visit the emergency department (6) and die in the hospital than at home (7).

Despite the fact that breathlessness is very common in people with cancer (8–13), it is often not well controlled. Studies show that unlike pain that is usually improved with current interventions, the intensity of dyspnea is not impacted (14,15). Higginson and McCarthy (14) found that in a group of terminally ill cancer patients cared for at home, pain scores decreased, but there was no change in dyspnea scores over time. In a convenience sample of patients admitted to an acute care palliative care unit, Dudgeon et al. (15) also found that for patients who had scores >50 mm on a 100-mm visual analog scale after 7 days of intervention, the median score for breathlessness remained at 50 mm while pain decreased to 30 mm. A recent study found that 27% and 39% of cancer outpatients with moderate to severe pain and dyspnea, respectively, had no evidence of a comprehensive assessment (16).

To optimally manage this distressing symptom, it is necessary to have an understanding of its prevalence and impact; the multidimensional nature of the symptom; the underlying pathophysiology and associated factors; components of a thorough assessment; the clinical syndromes common in cancer patients; and the indications and limitations of current therapeutic approaches.

PREVALENCE

In a large, geographically based cohort with a full scope of cancer diagnoses, over one-half of the patients reported shortness of breath, with half of them having scores on the Edmonton Symptom Assessment System (ESAS) in the moderate to severe range (13). In another study of an outpatient general population, 46% reported breathlessness with only 15% describing the intensity as moderate to severe (8). The differences in intensity may be related to cancer type and/or proximity to death. The first study found that patients with lung cancer had higher intensity scores than other diagnoses and patients with lung cancer composed 19% of the patients as opposed to 4% in the second study. Seow et al. found that patients with lung cancer had 50% greater chance of reporting moderate to severe breathlessness and that the intensity of dyspnea increased over the last 6 months of life (17). Muers and Round found breathlessness to be present at diagnosis in 60% of 298 patients with non–small cell lung cancer and in nearly 90% just prior to death (10). In a radiation oncology community setting, Lutz et al. found that 73% of patients with locally advanced lung cancer presented with breathlessness and the severity was worse in the group that survived <3 months (18). Two studies examined the trajectory of breathlessness in patients with advanced cancer (11,12). In a study of 5,386 cancer patients, Currow et al. showed that the intensity of breathlessness and the prevalence of severe breathlessness increased as death approached, with a significant increase in the rate of change between 3 and 10 days before death (11). Bausewein et al. prospectively followed the intensity of breathlessness in 49 advanced cancer patients and found that breathlessness increased over time and there were four different trajectories for individual patients, with fluctuating breathlessness being the most common (12).

IMPACT OF DYSPNEA

Breathlessness is one of the most distressing symptoms for patients (3) and can severely impair their quality of life. In a study of 70 patients with advanced cancer, Reddy et al. identified that patients experienced two types of dyspnea: continuous and breakthrough. The majority of patients had breakthrough dyspnea alone (61%), with 39% experiencing constant dyspnea and 20% also having episodes of breakthrough breathlessness (2). Breakthrough dyspnea occurred on an average five to six times a day with a median intensity of 5/10 on ESAS. The median intensity of breathlessness in patients with constant dyspnea was 7/10. Those who experienced continuous dyspnea had a worse quality of life than those with breakthrough dyspnea only, with significant differences in their general activity, mood, walking ability, normal work, and enjoyment of life (2). In a study of late-stage cancer patients, Roberts et al. (1) found that various activities intensified dyspnea for patients: climbing stairs—95.6%, walking slowly—47.8%, getting dressed—52.2%, talking or eating—56.5%, and at rest—26.1% (1). This study showed that the patients decreased their activity to whatever degree would relieve their breathlessness. Sixty-two percent of the patients with dyspnea had been short of breath for >3 months and most had received no assistance from nurses or physicians, leaving them to cope in isolation. Other studies of patients with lung cancer showed that 97% had decreased their activities, 80% had socially isolated themselves from friends and family (4), 36% were housebound, and 10% largely chair bound because of their breathlessness (19). In a study of terminally ill cancer patients, the willingness to live was directly related to the intensity of breathlessness (20). Uncontrolled dyspnea prompted terminal sedation in 25% to 53% of patients requiring sedation for uncontrolled symptoms (5).

MULTIDIMENSIONAL NATURE OF DYSPNEA

Dyspnea is a complex subjective experience that depends on the integration of respiratory afferent activity, respiratory motor drive, affective state, attention, experience, and learning (21).

Ventilation results from activation of the respiratory motor drive that is generated in the brainstem respiratory neural network. Receptors in the upper airway, lower airway, lung parenchyma and respiratory muscles, and peripheral and central chemoreceptors provide sensory input to the brainstem respiratory network as well as to higher brain centers (somatosensory and association cortices) (see Fig. 24.1). Normally breathing is not uncomfortable, but if the magnitude of the stimulus from one or more of these sensory afferents is great enough, then changes in breathing effort are perceived. Attention, experience/learning, and the person's affective state further modulate respiratory sensation and perception (21). Recent brain imaging studies suggest that the unpleasantness of dyspnea is processed cortically in the anterior insula and amygdala areas of the brain (22). These neural networks for processing dyspnea are shared with other unpleasant sensations such as pain (23).

Abernethy and Wheeler proposed a new conceptual model of breathlessness that they named "Total Dyspnea" (24). This model of Total Dyspnea encompasses four domains: physical, psychological, interpersonal, and existential that contribute to a patient's distress and suffering. They suggest that "Total Dyspnea" provides a more comprehensive, integrated, conceptual framework to help

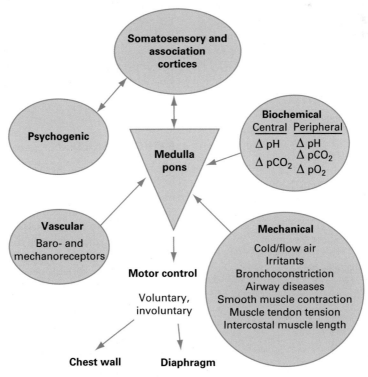

Figure 24.1 Brainstem respiratory network.

clinicians understand breathlessness and the suffering of patients and families.

FACTORS ASSOCIATED WITH DYSPNEA IN THE CANCER PATIENT

A number of authors have examined the factors that are associated with dyspnea in patients with cancer (Table 24.1) (2,8,9,25–31). In two different studies, investigators found that dyspnea in cancer patients had diverse etiologies, commonly with more than one factor contributing to the breathlessness (26,31). In another study, the presence and intensity of dyspnea were strongly related to the number of risk factors a patient had (8). Primary or metastatic involvement of the lung or pleura with cancer was associated with the presence of dyspnea in most studies (2,8,9,25,26,31). In a study of 923 cancer outpatients, Dudgeon et al. found that the risk factors significantly related to the presence of dyspnea were a history of smoking, asthma, or chronic obstructive pulmonary disease (COPD), and lung irradiation; or a history of exposure to asbestos, coal dust, cotton dust, or grain dust (8). They also found that the intensity of shortness of breath was significantly associated with the presence of hilar, mediastinal, and rib metastases, and surprisingly, the presence of mediastinal or hilar metastases was associated with a higher intensity of dyspnea than was the presence of lung metastases (8).

The general debility of terminal cancer (9), respiratory muscle weakness (26–28), and the presence of the hyperventilation syndrome (25) have been associated with the presence of dyspnea in cancer patients. Interestingly, the presence or severity of dyspnea could not be predicted by the level of oxygen saturation, air flow obstruction, or the type or severity of abnormal spirometry (26–28).

The intensity of fatigue, sleep, anxiety, depression, and sense of well-being were significantly associated with ESAS shortness of breath scores in univariate analyses in a prospective observational study of 70 cancer patients with dyspnea (2). In multivariate analyses, ESAS dyspnea was associated with fatigue, forced expiratory volume in 1 minute (FEV_1), pain, and depression.

In another study of 171 consecutive outpatients with lung cancer, psychological distress, the presence of organic causes, cough, and pain were significantly correlated with total dyspnea as measured by the Cancer Dyspnea Scale (CDS) (30). In this study, heart rate significantly correlated with the "sense of effort" subscale, and psychological distress and pain significantly correlated with the "sense of anxiety" factor.

Anxiety is significantly correlated with the intensity of dyspnea in a number of studies in cancer patients (2,25–28,30). These correlations are significant ($p = 0.03$ to 0.001) but low ($r = 0.26$ to 0.32), with anxiety explaining only 9% of the variance in the intensity of dyspnea. Tanaka et al. also found significant correlations with the intensity of dyspnea and depression scores as measured by the Hospital Anxiety and Depression Scale (HADS) (30). When they combined the HADS anxiety and depression scores, the correlation coefficient was $r = 0.63$ ($p < 0.01$), explaining 36% of variance in the intensity of dyspnea. Reddy et al. found HADS depression, but not anxiety, to be significantly correlated in univariate and multivariate analyses with the Oxygen Cost Diagram, an instrument that evaluates the effect of shortness of breath on the person's activities of daily living (2).

PATHOPHYSIOLOGY

The pathophysiologic mechanisms of dyspnea can be categorized as increased ventilatory demand, impaired mechanical responses, or a combination of these two mechanisms. Spirometry and other pulmonary function tests (PFTs) are useful in determining the underlying etiology of dyspnea. Table 24.2 outlines the pathophysiologic mechanisms of dyspnea with the potential clinical causes in a person with cancer.

Increased Ventilatory Demand

The brainstem respiratory neural network will activate the respiratory motor drive and ventilation if there is an increase in physiologic dead space in the lung, hypoxia from any cause, severe

---

TABLE 24.1 FACTORS ASSOCIATED WITH DYSPNEA IN CANCER PATIENTS

A. Dyspnea Due Directly to Cancer
- Lung involvement (primary or metastatic)
- Pleural involvement (primary or metastatic)
- Hilar or mediastinal metastases
- Rib metastases

B. Dyspnea Due Indirectly to Cancer
- General debility
- Fatigue
- Respiratory muscle weakness

C. Dyspnea Due to Cancer Treatment
- Lung included in the radiation field

D. Dyspnea Unrelated to Cancer
- History of smoking
- Chronic obstructive pulmonary disease
- Asthma
- History of exposure to: asbestos, coal dust, cotton dust, and grain dust
- Anxiety
- Depression
- Poor sleep

TABLE 24.2 PATHOPHYSIOLOGIC AND CLINICAL MECHANISMS OF DYSPNEA IN THE CANCER PATIENT

A. Impaired Mechanical Response

(a) Restrictive ventilatory deficit
  (i) Pleural or parenchymal disease
    • Primary or metastatic
    • Pleural effusion
  (ii) Reduced movement of diaphragm
    • Ascites
    • Hepatomegaly
  (iii) Reduced chest wall compliance
    • Pain
    • Hilar/mediastinal involvement
    • Chest wall invasion with tumor
    • Deconditioning
    • Neuromuscular
    • Neurohumoral
  (iv) Respiratory muscle weakness
    • Phrenic nerve paralysis
    • Cachexia
    • Electrolyte abnormalities
    • Steroid use
    • Deconditioning
(b) Obstructive ventilatory deficit
  (i) Tumor obstruction
  (ii) Asthma
  (iii) COPD
(c) Mixed Obstructive/Restrictive Disease (any combination of factors)

B. Increased Ventilatory Demand

(a) Increased physiologic dead space
  (i) Thromboemboli
  (ii) Tumor emboli
  (iii) Vascular obstruction
  (iv) Radiation pneumonitis
  (v) Chemotherapy-induced pneumonitis
(b) Severe deconditioning
(c) Hypoxemia—anemia
(d) Change in V_{CO_2} or arterial P_{CO_2} set point
(e) Increased neural reflex activity
(f) Psychological causes
  (i) Anxiety
  (ii) Depression

COPD, chronic obstructive pulmonary disease.
Modified from Booth S, Dudgeon D. *Dyspnea in Advanced Disease: A Guide to Clinical Management.* New York, NY: Oxford University Press; 2006.

deconditioning with early and accelerated rise in blood lactate levels, changes in V_{CO_2} or arterial P_{CO_2} set points, and psychological causes such as anxiety and depression. Increased physiologic dead space can occur as a result of thromboemboli, tumor emboli, vascular obstruction, or chemo- or radiation acute or chronic pneumonitis.

When dyspnea is secondary to an increased ventilatory demand spirometry is usually normal.

Impaired Mechanical Responses

Impaired mechanical responses result in restrictive or obstructive ventilatory deficits or a combination of both.

Restrictive Ventilatory Deficit

A restrictive ventilatory deficit results from decreased distensibility of the lung parenchyma, pleura, or chest wall; from reduced movement of the diaphragm; or from a reduction in the maximum force exerted by the respiratory muscles. The principal diagnostic features of a restrictive ventilatory deficit are a concurrent reduction in both FEV_1 and vital capacity (FVC), decreased total lung capacity (TLC) and residual volume (RV), and often decreased diffusing capacity as well.

Obstructive Ventilatory Deficit

An obstructive ventilatory deficit refers to impedance to the flow of air within the lung. Progressive narrowing of the airways can result from structural changes from external compression or obstruction within the lumen of the airway by tumor, mucus, inflammation, or edema. Bronchoconstriction, a functional change which causes narrowing of the airways, results from increased bronchomotor tone from the release of histamine, leukotrienes, and other mediators. The hallmarks of an obstructive ventilatory deficit are a reduced FEV_1/FVC and an increased TLC, RV, and functional residual capacity.

MULTIDIMENSIONAL ASSESSMENT OF DYSPNEA

As dyspnea is a complex subjective experience a comprehensive assessment requires a qualitative appraisal, clinical assessment, and measurement of the different factors that impact on the perception of breathlessness and the effects of shortness of breath on the individual.

Qualitative Aspects of Dyspnea

The majority of scientists studying dyspnea accept that dyspnea is not a single sensation (32). They have found that there are a variety of sensations of breathing discomfort that differ in the quality of the experience, the stimuli that evoke them, and the afferent pathways (32). In COPD patients, there are at least four different "qualities" of uncomfortable breathing sensations: air hunger, work, unsatisfied inspiration, and tightness (21). In a study of 131 patients with primary or secondary lung cancer, Wilcock et al. found that there were clusters of words that were associated with the underlying cause of breathlessness (collapse, metastases, and pleural thickening) but that the overlap in the clusters between groups was too great to be useful in differential diagnosis (33).

Others suggest that to adequately characterize dyspnea, measurement of both the sensory intensity and affective intensity or unpleasantness of dyspnea is necessary. There is growing evidence to support that there are different/separate dimensions of sensory intensity and affective intensity or unpleasantness and that the ratio of sensory intensity to affective rating varies among subjects (32). In addition, there is cognitive evaluation and an emotional response to the sensation that will be affected by the person's life experiences and personal situation and perhaps personality (32). There is great variation in the "dyspnea" experienced by different patients with similar disease states. Lansing et al. (32) suggest that knowing whether a therapy works by decreasing intensity or reducing the affective response can help determine which patients are most likely to benefit. Better measurement/assessment could provide a more sophisticated assessment of how potential therapies work and lead to appropriate choice of treatments for individuals in whom affect is a major component of respiratory discomfort.

Clinical Assessment

Clinical assessments are usually directed to determine the underlying pathophysiology and appropriate treatments and to evaluate response to therapy.

History

As in all areas of medicine, a thorough history is central to determining the underlying etiology of a person's breathlessness. This should include its temporal onset (acute or chronic), whether it is affected by positions, qualities, associated symptoms, precipitating and relieving events or activities, and response to medications. A past history of smoking, underlying lung or cardiac disease, concurrent medical conditions, allergy history, and details of previous medications or treatments should be elicited (34,35).

The initial approach to assessment and possible treatment is greatly affected by whether the breathlessness is an acute, subacute, or chronic problem (36). The differential diagnosis of acute shortness of breath is relatively narrow: pneumonia, pulmonary embolism, congestive heart failure, or myocardial infarction. This knowledge should guide further questioning, the physical examination, and possible investigations. In the setting of advanced disease, it is important to determine if the breathlessness is related to the underlying disease and potentially irreversible or whether it is completely unrelated and potentially curable.

To determine if dyspnea is present, it is important to ask more than the question, "Are you short of breath?" Patients universally respond to breathlessness by decreasing their activity. It is therefore helpful to ask about shortness of breath in relation to activities such as "walking at the same speed as someone of your age," "stopping to catch your breath when walking upstairs," or "eating." It is also important to quantify the amount of exercise, or lack of, that is needed for the person to become breathless, as this will provide a baseline for comparison to assess progression or improvement (37).

It can be helpful in establishing a diagnosis to inquire in which position dyspnea occurs (37). Positional dyspnea common in cancer patients includes orthopnea (difficulty in breathing while lying flat) with superior vena cava syndrome, pericardial effusion; platypnea (difficulty in breathing while sitting up and relieved by lying flat) is rare, but it occurs status post-pneumonectomy; and trepopnea (when patients are more comfortable breathing while lying on one side) occurs in people with a large pleural effusion (37).

Physical Examination

A careful physical examination focused on possible underlying causes of dyspnea should be performed. Particular attention should be directed to identify signs that are associated with the clinical syndromes identified in the history or common in people with cancer (see Table 24.3).

It is important to recognize that dyspnea, like pain, is a subjective experience that may not be evident to an observer. Tachypnea, a rapid respiratory rate, is not dyspnea. Medical personnel must learn to ask and accept the patient's assessments, often without measurable physical correlates. When patients say that they are having discomfort with breathing, we must believe they are dyspneic. In a study of patients with COPD with high, medium, and low levels of breathlessness, Gift et al. (38) found that there were no significant differences in respiratory rate, depth of respiration, or peak expiratory flow rates at the three levels of dyspnea. There was, however, a significant difference in the use of accessory muscles between patients with high and low levels of dyspnea suggesting that the extent of use of accessory muscles is a physical finding that is helpful when assessing the intensity of breathlessness.

Laboratory Evaluation

There are a number of tests that can help determine the etiology of a person's dyspnea, but the choice of the appropriate diagnostic tests should be guided by the stage of the disease, the prognosis, the risk/benefit ratios of any proposed tests or interventions, and the desires of the patient and family.

Possible blood tests include a hemoglobin, white blood cell count and differential, and serum calcium, potassium, magnesium, and phosphate.

If appropriate, radiologic examinations may include a chest radiograph, ventilation/perfusion scan, computed tomography (CT) scan, CT

TABLE 24.3 CAUSES OF DYSPNEA IN CANCER PATIENTS

A. Dyspnea Due Directly to Cancer
- Lung involvement (primary or metastatic)
- Lymphangitic carcinomatosis
- Intrinsic or extrinsic airway obstruction by tumor
- Pleural effusion
- Pericardial effusion
- Ascites
- Hepatomegaly
- Phrenic nerve paralysis
- Tumor microemboli
- Pulmonary leukostasis
- Superior vena cava syndrome

B. Dyspnea Due Indirectly to Cancer
- Cachexia
- Na, K, Mg, PO_4 abnormalities
- Anemia
- Pneumonia
- Pulmonary aspiration
- Pulmonary emboli
- Neurologic paraneoplastic syndromes

C. Dyspnea Due to Cancer Treatment
- Surgery
- Radiation pneumonitis/fibrosis
- Chemotherapy-induced pulmonary disease
- Chemotherapy-induced cardiomyopathy
- Radiation-induced pericardial disease

D. Dyspnea Unrelated to Cancer
- Chronic obstructive pulmonary disease
- Asthma
- Congestive heart failure
- Interstitial lung disease
- Pneumothorax
- Anxiety
- Chest wall deformity
- Obesity
- Neuromuscular disorders
- Pulmonary vascular disease

Modified from Dudgeon D, Rosenthal S. Management of dyspnea and cough in patients with cancer. In: Cherny NI, Foley KM, eds. *Hematology/Oncology Clinics of North America: Pain and Palliative Care*, Vol. 10(1). Philadelphia, PA: W.B. Saunders Co.; 1996:157-171.

angiogram, magnetic resonance imaging, or an echocardiogram.

A pulse oximeter measures oxygen saturation noninvasively. At high saturations, pulse oximeters are reasonably accurate (+/− 3%), but less accurate below saturations of about 80% (39). Measures of oxygen saturation while walking are helpful in unmasking hypoxia with exercise. It should be remembered that oxygen saturation does not indicate whether the person has adequate ventilation. A person who is retaining carbon dioxide can have normal or near-normal oxygen saturations, so arterial blood gas analysis should be considered in situations where information about not only oxygenation (Po_2) but also ventilation (Pco_2) and/or acid–base balance (pH) would be helpful (39).

Lung function tests vary from simple spirometry with handheld electronic devices to more complicated tests that require sophisticated equipment in a lung function laboratory. Standardized PFTs are helpful to determine the underlying diagnosis, its severity, and response to treatment. Two basic patterns of disorder are demonstrated with spirometry: obstructive and restrictive (see Table 2.1). Results of PFTs do not necessarily reflect the intensity of a person's dyspnea (40). Maximum inspiratory and expiratory measurements are helpful in assessing respiratory muscle strength, but they are dependent on patient effort. Unlike others (26,27), Bruera et al. (28) found that in cancer patients with moderate to severe dyspnea, multivariate analysis showed that maximum inspiratory pressure (PI_{max}) ($p = 0.02$) was an independent correlate of the intensity of dyspnea.

Exercise testing with increasing workloads on either a cycle ergometer or treadmill is performed to identify a cardiac or respiratory cause for exercise limitation, quantify functional disability, and assess the response to treatment (39). Simpler measures of exercise capacity include the 6- or 12-minute walking test and the shuttle walking test. The walking tests correlate with measures of both dyspnea and exercise capacity (38). The shuttle walking test was validated in comparison with the treadmill exercise test (41) and is a reproducible test of functional capacity in ambulatory advanced cancer patients (42).

MEASUREMENT

Measurement instruments bring objectivity and precision to the evaluation of clinical assessments or interventions and to research questions. Which instrument is appropriate depends on the question, the setting, the acuity of the symptom, the functional status of the patient, and what dimensions you wish to examine. Most of the measurement instruments for breathlessness were developed for use in patients with COPD, only a few have been validated in patients with cancer (see Table 24.4).

Unidimensional Instruments

Three types of unidimensional scales are commonly used to measure breathlessness: Visual Analog Scale (VAS), Numerical Rating Scale (NRS), and the Modified Borg Scale (43). Unidimensional scales are self-administered and quick to complete. They can measure breathlessness in general or in relation to exercise. The VAS and NRS are anchored by words such as "no breathlessness" or "worst possible breathlessness." These scales can be used as an initial assessment to monitor progress and to evaluate effectiveness of treatment in an individual patient (44). Magnitude estimation scales use a ratio scaling technique that measures the relationship between the intensity of a physical stimulus and its perceived magnitude (45,46). This type of scale allows comparisons within individuals and across population groups (47). The Borg scale (48) and Oxygen Cost Diagram (49) are examples.

Multidimensional Assessment Instruments

The Dyspnea Assessment Questionnaire (DAQ) (25) and the CDS (50) are examples of scales developed to assess the multidimensional nature of dyspnea in cancer patients. The DAQ measures both qualitative and quantitative components of breathlessness (25). The CDS measures three factors: sense of effort, sense of anxiety, and sense of discomfort (50).

Quality of Life Instruments

Measurement of quality of life attempts to provide standardized estimates of the *overall* impact on the individual. The Lung Cancer Symptom Scale (LCSS) (51,52) has six items that measure major symptoms of people with lung cancer and three related to symptomatic distress, activity status, and overall quality of life. The European Organization for Research and Treatment Quality of Life Questionnaire and Lung Cancer Module assesses the physical, emotional, social, and cognitive dimension of the person's life (53,54). The Functional Assessment of Cancer Therapy—Lung Cancer Quality of Life Instrument measures five dimension of quality of life: physical, social and family, emotional well-being, and functional well-being, and relationship with physician (55).

CAUSES AND MANAGEMENT OF DYSPNEA

The causes of dyspnea in the cancer patient fall into four clinical categories: direct tumor effects, indirect tumor effects, treatment-related causes, and problems unrelated to the cancer (Table 24.2).

Direct Tumor Effects

The causes of dyspnea due directly to cancer include parenchymal involvement by tumor (primary or metastatic), lymphangitic carcinomatosis, extrinsic or intrinsic obstruction of airways by tumor, pleural tumor, pleural effusion, pericardial effusion, ascites, hepatomegaly, phrenic nerve paralysis, superior vena cava obstruction, multiple tumor microemboli, and pulmonary leukostasis.

If the tumor is the cause of the shortness of breath, then chemotherapy, external beam radiation, brachytherapy, or surgery should be considered if appropriate to the stage of disease and the overall condition and wishes of the patient. Chapter 30 address management of airway obstruction, pleural and pericardial effusions, and superior vena cava obstruction.

Dyspnea Due to Cancer Treatment

Dyspnea can result from surgery, radiation therapy, and/or systemic therapy. The management of toxicity related to radiation and systemic therapy is discussed in Chapter 32.

Surgery

Pneumonectomy or lobectomy can result in shortness of breath in patients with preexisting impairment of pulmonary function. In a study examining the long-term effects, 5 or more years, after pneumonectomy for lung cancer, Deslauriers et al. found that 37% had moderate to severe dyspnea (56).

Dyspnea Indirectly Due to Cancer

Dyspnea can result from indirect consequences of the cancer such as malnutrition, mineral and electrolyte deficiencies, infection, anemia, pulmonary emboli, aspiration, neurologic paraneoplastic syndromes, and severe deconditioning. These underlying causes of dyspnea should be treated if appropriate to the person's stage of disease, prognosis, and wishes.

Muscle Weakness

Studies demonstrate that there is an association between dyspnea and respiratory (26–28,57) and generalized (9,58) muscle weakness in the advanced cancer patient. Both generalized and ventilatory muscle weaknesses can result from severe deconditioning, but other factors that can affect muscle function are hypocalcemia, hypokalemia, hypomagnesemia, severe hypophosphatemia, malnutrition, and possibly the cancer or its treatment (59,60). There is evidence that pulmonary rehabilitation programs improve dyspnea and functional capacity in patients who participate preoperatively, during aggressive chemotherapy and/or radiation treatments (61), or in the palliative phase of their illness (62). Although there are no studies in cancer patients, there is evidence in COPD patients that refeeding and anabolic steroids improve exercise tolerance (63–65).

Infection

Patients with cancer are at an increased risk for pneumonia due to immunosuppression from the disease or its treatment and also from the tumor causing mucosal erosion or an abscess, fistula, or obstruction.

Pulmonary Emboli

Cancer patients have a fourfold to sevenfold higher risk of developing a venous thromboembolism than patients without cancer. The risk depends on the extent and type of tumor with pancreatic, brain, myeloproliferative, and gastric cancers at the highest risk. Surgery, chemotherapy, radiation therapy, growth factors, immobility, and the presence of central venous catheters increase the risk of a pulmonary embolism for patients (66). Typically, patients with acute pulmonary embolic disease describe a single or multiple episodes of acute shortness of breath. Less commonly, multiple small emboli produce pulmonary hypertension with no history of acute episodes (67). It is possible that an episode of acute shortness of breath just prior to death is a result of a large pulmonary embolus. Chapter 32 addresses this issue.

Dyspnea Unrelated to the Cancer

Risk factors for dyspnea unrelated to cancer include preexisting COPD, cardiovascular disease, asthma, interstitial lung disease, pneumothorax, anxiety, chest wall deformity, obesity, neuromuscular disorders, and pulmonary vascular disease.

PHARMACOLOGIC MANAGEMENT

Opioids

There are three systematic reviews that examined the effectiveness of oral or parenteral opioids for the management of dyspnea, two for palliation in cancer patients (68,69) and one in all patient groups (70).

In the *Cochrane Review* (70), the authors identified 18 randomized double-blind, controlled trials comparing the use of any opioid drug against placebo for the treatment of breathlessness in patients with any illness (only two studies conducted with cancer patients met the inclusion criteria for review [one parenteral and one nebulized]). There was statistically strong evidence for a small effect of oral and parenteral opioids for the treatment of breathlessness in the studies (71–78) involving the nonnebulized route of administration (70).

Opioid receptors are located throughout the respiratory tract, and it is hypothesized that if the receptors are interrupted directly, lower doses, with fewer systemic side effects, would be required to control breathlessness (79). The *Cochrane Review* (70) identified nine randomized double-blind, controlled trials comparing the use of nebulized opioids or placebo for the control of breathlessness (80–88). One of these trials (82) included only cancer patients. The authors concluded that there was no evidence that nebulized opioids were more effective than nebulized saline in relieving breathlessness (70).

There are eight randomized trials that include only cancer patients (69,77,82,89–93). Two placebo-controlled crossover trials (77,89) showed that a single bolus dose of morphine significantly improved dyspnea.

Allard et al. (90) studied the effectiveness of supplemental doses of opioids, equivalent to 25% or 50% of their regular 4-hourly dose of opioids, to improve breathlessness in terminally ill cancer patients. They found significant decrements relative to baseline for mean dyspnea ($p < 0.0001$) and respiratory frequency ($p = 0.004$) in all patients. They concluded that a 25% dose of the 4-hourly opioid was sufficient to improve dyspnea.

One randomized, 2-day, crossover study of only 11 patients of the planned 100 compared subcutaneous versus nebulized morphine (93). Both treatments improved dyspnea 1 hour posttreatment with no differences between the effect of the two treatments, but the sample size was not large enough to make meaningful conclusions.

A double-blind, randomized, crossover, controlled trial of 20 cancer patients comparing the effects of nebulized hydromorphone, systemic hydromorphone, and nebulized saline for the relief of acute episodic breathlessness showed that all treatments resulted in statistically significant improvements in breathlessness (92). Only the nebulized hydromorphone resulted in what was considered a clinically significant change (1 cm VAS). The authors, however, suggested that nebulized saline provided significant relief of incident breathlessness that was not significantly different from the effect of opioids.

Sedatives and Tranquilizers

Chlorpromazine decreases breathlessness without affecting ventilation or producing sedation in healthy subjects (94). There are conflicting results from trials studying the effectiveness of promethazine, a phenothiazine antiemetic, in reducing dyspnea (94–96). In an open-labeled trial, McIver et al. found chlorpromazine effective for relief of dyspnea in advanced cancer (97).

In a double-blind, placebo-controlled, randomized trial, Light et al. studied the effectiveness of morphine alone, morphine and promethazine, and morphine and prochlorperazine for the treatment of breathlessness in COPD patients (74). The combination of morphine and promethazine significantly improved exercise tolerance without worsening dyspnea compared with placebo, morphine alone, or the combination of morphine and prochlorperazine (74). Ventafridda et al. have also found the combination of morphine and chlorpromazine to be effective (98). In their systematic review, Viola et al. suggested that phenothiazines could be used as an alternative when systemic opioids could not be used or in addition to systemic opioids (68).

In a *Cochrane Review*, Simon et al. examined the efficacy of benzodiazepines for the relief of breathlessness in patients with advanced disease (99). They identified 7 studies including 200 participants with advanced cancer and COPD. Analysis of the seven studies, and meta-analysis of six, did not show a significant beneficial effect of benzodiazepines for relief of breathlessness in patients with advanced COPD and cancer. No significant effect on prevention of breakthrough dyspnea in cancer patients was found. They observed that there was a slight but nonsignificant trend toward a beneficial effect. They suggested that benzodiazepines could be considered as second-line or third-line options in an individual therapeutic trial if opioids and nonpharmacologic agents had failed.

Navigante et al. (91) in a single-blinded 2-day study compared subcutaneous morphine with subcutaneous midazolam or a combination of both morphine and midazolam to alleviate severe dyspnea in terminally ill cancer patients. Significant improvements in dyspnea intensity occurred in all three arms. Significantly, more patients in the combined group reported relief of dyspnea at 24 and 48 hours and had less episodes of breakthrough dyspnea than the other groups.

Navigante et al. (100) randomized 63 ambulatory advanced cancer patients to receive oral morphine or oral midazolam using a fast drug titration followed by an ambulatory 5-day period. During the titration period, all patients had their dyspnea improve by at least 50%. On the second day, dyspnea intensity decreased in both the morphine and midazolam groups and on subsequent days maintained this level or continued to drop. During the ambulatory phase, midazolam was superior to morphine in controlling baseline and breakthrough dyspnea.

Oxygen

Oxygen in the hypoxic patient with COPD is associated with improved survival, quality of life, and neuropsychologic functioning (101). The benefits in cancer patients are unfortunately less clear. In a systematic review and meta-analysis of all randomized controlled studies on the use of oxygen for the relief of dyspnea in chronic terminal illness,

Cranston et al. identified 4 papers involving a total of 97 patients with cancer (102). Two studies of a total of 52 participants at rest who received 4 to 5 L/min of oxygen for up to 15 minutes resulted in a reduction of shortness of breath over the baseline (77,103). The meta-analysis, however, failed to show a significant improvement in their dyspnea when oxygen inhalation was compared with air inhalation. The change in dyspnea with oxygen inhalation was inconsistent and appeared to be independent of resting hypoxia (102). The meta-analysis showed that participants appeared to perceive an improvement in their dyspnea at rest and during exercise. In the two studies that examined the effect of oxygen inhalation during exercise, oxygen did neither appear to reduce exercise-induced dyspnea nor increase the distance walked (102).

In another systematic review and meta-analysis, Uronis et al. identified five randomized controlled trials comparing oxygen and air in people with cancer who were mildly hypoxemic or nonhypoxemic (104). One hundred and thirty-four people were included in the analysis. Oxygen did not improve dyspnea and only two or four studies detected a statistically significant individual preference for oxygen. In a large cohort study of 1,239 patients, most of whom had cancer and were prescribed oxygen, approximately one-third had an improvement in their breathlessness. It was not possible to predict the responders from demographic factors, baseline breathlessness, or underlying diagnosis (105). Despite the lack of clear evidence of benefit, some terminally ill patients reported a marked improvement in both their breathlessness and quality of life with supplemental oxygen and, therefore, most palliative care physicians would suggest a therapeutic trial.

NONPHARMACOLOGIC MANAGEMENT

A *Cochrane Review* by Bausewein et al. identified 47 studies that tested a variety of interventions mostly in COPD patients. The interventions with the highest strength of evidence were all conducted in COPD patients and included neuromuscular electrical stimulation, chest wall vibration, walking aids, and breathing training (106).

Numerous small studies in healthy males (107) and patients with COPD have demonstrated that a fan directed against the cheek improved breathlessness (107,108) and improved exercise time (109,110). Galbraith et al. examined the effectiveness of a handheld fan to reduce the sensation of breathlessness in 50 patients, 11 with primary or secondary lung cancer (111). They found that a fan directed at the face for 5 minutes significantly reduced the score on the VAS breathless scale more than if it was directed at the leg (111).

GUIDES TO MORE PRACTICE

Cancer Care Ontario's Web site (112) has a number of useful tools to help clinicians manage dyspnea effectively. In their Web site under CCO Toolbox, there is a section called Symptom Management Tools. These include a Dyspnea Algorithm (Fig. 24.2), Pocket Guide, Guide to Practice, Video Series on Managing Shortness of Breath, and iPhone and Windows Phone7 apps.

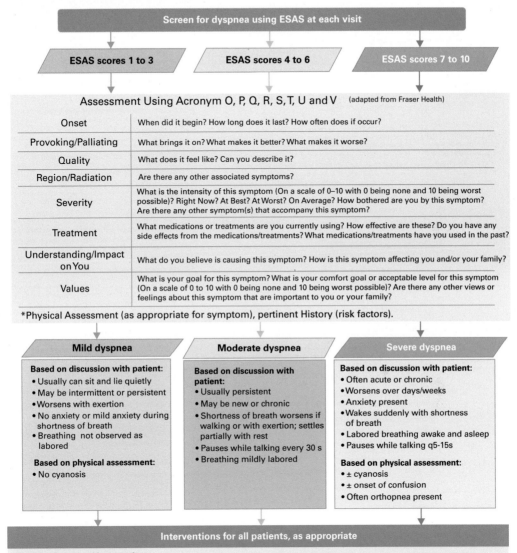

Figure 24.2 Dyspnea algorithm. ESAS, Edmonton Symptom Assessment System; PPS, Palliative Performance Scale; CCO, Cancer Care Ontario.

Dyspnea in Adults with Cancer: Care Map

Mild Dyspnea Care pathway 1	Moderate Dyspnea Care pathway 2	Severe Dyspnea Care pathway 3

PHARMACOLOGIC
- Supplemental oxygen is recommended for hypoxic patients experiencing dyspnea.

- Supplemental oxygen is _not_ recommended for nonhypoxic, dyspneic patients.

- Systemic opioids, by the oral or parenteral routes, can be used to manage dyspnea in advanced cancer patients.

PHARMACOLOGIC
For Patients with PPS 100%–10%:

Nonopioids
- May use benzodiazepines for anxiety.
- There is no evidence for the use of systemic corticosteroids.

Systemic Opioids
For opioid-native patients:
- Morphine (or equivalent dose of alternate immediate-release opioid) 5 mg po q4th regularly and 2.5 mg po q2h prn for breakthrough dyspnea.
- If the oral route is not available or reliable, morphine 3 mg subcut q4h regularly and 1.5 mg subcut q1h prn for breakthrough dyspnea.

For patients already taking systemic opioids:
- Increase the patient's regular dose by 25%, guided by the total breakthrough doses used in the previous 24 h.
- The breakthrough dose is 10% of the total 24-h regular opioid dose, using the same opioid by the same route.
  - Oral breakthrough doses q2h as needed.
  - Subcutaneous breakthrough doses q1h as needed, due to more rapid peak effect.
- Do not use nebulized opioids, nebulized furosemide, nebulized lidocaine, or benzodiazepines.

NON-PHARMACOLOGIC
- Attend to the meaning of the symptom (or attend to fear/anxiety).
- If dyspnea is acute or there is an unexpected change, further assessment may be required to identify potentially treatable causes.

PHARMACOLOGIC
For Patients with PPS 100%–10%:
Systemic Opioids
For opioid-naïve patients:
- Give a subcut bolus of morphine 2.5 mg (or an equivalent dose of an alternate opioid).
  - If tolerated, repeat dose every 30 min if needed.
  - Consider doubling dose if two doses fail to produce an adequater reduction in dyspnea and are tolerated.
  - Monitor the patient's respiratory rate closely, since the time to peak effect of a subcut dose of morphine may be longer than 30 min.
- If intravenous access is available, consider giving an IV bolus of morphine 2.5 mg (or an equivalent dose of an alternate opioid) to achieve a more rapid effect.
  - If tolerated, repeat dose every 30 min if needed.
  - Consider doubling dose if two doses fail to produce an adequate reduction in dyspnea and are tolerated.
  - Monitor the patient's respiratory rate closely, since IV boluses of morphine result in faster and higher peak effects.
- Start a regular dose of an immediate-release opioid, guided by the bolus doses used.
  - For the breakthrough opioid dose, consider using the subcut route initially for severe dyspnea until the symptom comes under control.

For patients already taking systemic opioids:
- Follow the same suggestions as above for opioid naïve patients, with the following changes.
  - Give a subcut bolus of the patient's current opioid using a dose equal to 10% of the regular, 24-h, parenteral-dose-equivalent of the patient's current opioid (a parenteral dose is equivalent to half the oral dose).
  - Consider giving an IV bolus of the patient's current opioid, using a dose equal to 10% of the regular, 24-h, parenteral-dose-equivalent of the patient's current opioid.
  - Increase the regular opioid dose by 25%, guided by the bolus doses used.

Psychoactive medications
- Consider a trial of chlorpromazine or methotrimeprazine, if severe dyspnea persists despite other therapies.
- Methotrimeprazine 2.5–10 mg po or subcut q6-8h regularly or as needed.
- Chlorpromazine 7.5–25 mg po or IV q6-8h regularly or as needed.
- Consider benzodiazepine for coexisting anxiety.

For Patients with PPS 100%–20%:
- If patient has or may have COPD, consider a 5-d trial of a corticosteroid
  - Dexamethasone 8 mg/d po or subcut or IV
  - Prednisone 50 mg/d po
  - Discontinue corticosteroid if there is no obvious benefit after 5 d.
- If the patient does not have COPD, but has known or suspected lung involvement by the cancer, weight the risks before commencing a 5-d trial.
  - Other potential benefits, such as for appetite stimulation or pain management, may justify a 5-d trial of a corticosteroid.
- Do not start prophylactic gastric mucosal protection therapy during a 5-d trial of a corticosteroid, but consider such therapy if the corticosteroid is continued past the trial.
- Prochlorperazine is not recommended as a therapy for managing dyspnea.
- No comparative trials are available to support or refute the use of other phenothiazines, such as chlorpromazine and methotrimeprazine, however oral promethazine may be used as a second-line agent if systemic opioids cannot be used or in addition to systemic opioids.

For Patients with PPS 30%–10%:
- Consider a trial of chlorpromazine or methotrimeprazine, if dyspnea persists despite other therapies.
  - Methotrimeprazine 2.5–10 mg po or subcut q6-8h regularly or as needed.
  - Chlorpromazine 7.5–25 mg po q6-8h regularly or as needed
- Anxiety, nausea, or agitation, may justify a trial of chlorpromazine or methotrimeprazine.

Follow-Up and Ongoing Monitoring
If dyspnea remains unrelieved despite the approaches outlined above, request the assistance of a palliative care consultation team.

For full references and more information please refer to *CCO's Symptom Management Guide-to-Practice: Dyspnea* document.

Disclaimer: Care has been taken by Cancer Care Ontario's Algorithm Development group in the preparation of the information contained in this Guide-to-Practice document. Nonetheless, any person seeking to apply or consult the Guide-to-Practice document is expected to use independent clinical judgment and skills in the context of individual clinical circumstances or seek out the supervision of a qualified specialist clinician. CCO makes no representation or warranties of any kind whatsoever regarding their content or use or application and disclaims any responsibility for their application or use in any way.

Figure 24.2 *(Continued)*

SUMMARY

Dyspnea is a very common symptom in patients with cancer. Despite breathlessness' profound effect on people's quality of life, it is often unrecognized, and therefore, people often receive little assistance in managing this distressing symptom. Effective management requires an understanding of its prevalence and impact; the multidimensional nature of the symptom; the underlying pathophysiology and associated factors; components of a thorough assessment; the clinical syndromes common in cancer patients; and the indications and limitations of current therapeutic approaches. More research is necessary to further optimize the available treatment options.

ACKNOWLEDGMENT

This chapter, originally authored by Dr. Deborah Dudgeon, was rerun for the 5th edition of Principles and Practice of Palliative Care and Supportive Oncology after a careful review by Dr. Ann Berger

REFERENCES

1. Roberts DK, Thorne SE, Pearson C. The experience of dyspnea in late-stage cancer. Patients' and nurses' perspectives. *Cancer Nurs.* 1993;16(4):310-320.
2. Reddy SK, Parsons HA, Elsayem A, Palmer JL, Bruera E. Characteristics and correlates of dyspnea in patients with advanced cancer. *J Palliat Med.* 2009;12(1):29-35.
3. Tishelman C, Petersson L-M, Degner LF, Sprangers MAG. Symptom prevalence, intensity, and distress in patients with inoperable lung cancer in relation to time of death. *J Clin Oncol.* 2007;25(34):5381-5389.
4. Brown ML, Carrieri V, Janson-Bjerklie S, Dodd MJ. Lung cancer and dyspnea: the patient's perception. *Oncol Nurs Forum.* 1986;13(5):19-24.
5. Fainsinger R, Waller A, Bercovici M, et al. A multicentre international study of sedation for uncontrolled symptoms in terminally ill patients. *Palliat Med.* 2000;14(4):257-265.
6. Barbera L, Taylor C, Dudgeon D. Why do patients with cancer visit the emergency department near the end of life? *CMAJ.* 2010;182(6):563-568.
7. Edmonds P, Higginson I, Altmann D, Sen-Gupta G, McDonnell M. Is the presence of dyspnea a risk factor for morbidity in cancer patients? *J Pain Symptom Manage.* 2000;19(1):15-22.
8. Dudgeon DJ, Kristjanson L, Sloan JA, Lertzman M, Clement K. Dyspnea in cancer patients: prevalence and associated factors. *J Pain Symptom Manage.* 2001;21(2):95-102.
9. Reuben DB, Mor V. Dyspnea in terminally ill cancer patients. *Chest.* 1986;89:234-236.
10. Muers MF, Round CE. Palliation of symptoms in non-small cell lung cancer: a study by the Yorkshire Regional Cancer Organisation Thoracic Group. *Thorax.* 1993;48:339-343.
11. Currow D, Davidson PM, Agar MR, et al. Do the trajectories of dyspnea differ in prevalence and intensity by diagnosis at the end of life? A consecutive cohort study. *J Pain Symptom Manage.* 2010;39(4):680-690.
12. Bausewein C, Booth S, Gysels M, Kulkarni AG, Haberland B, Higginson IJ. Individual breathlessness trajectories do not match summary trajectories in advanced cancer and chronic obstructive pulmonary disease: results from a longitudinal study. *Palliat Med.* 2010;24(8):777-786.
13. Barbera L, Hsien S, Howell D, et al. Symptom burden and performance status in a population-based cohort of ambulatory cancer patients. *Cancer.* 2010;116(24):5767-5776.
14. Higginson I, McCarthy M. Measuring symptoms in terminal cancer: are pain and dyspnoea controlled? *J Royal Soc Med.* 1989;82:264-267.
15. Dudgeon D, Harlos M, Clinch JJ. The Edmonton Symptom Assessment Scale (ESAS) as an audit tool. *J Palliat Care.* 1999;15(3):14-19.
16. Dudgeon D, King S, Hughes E, et al. Improving the quality of care and decreasing the morbidity of patients with lung cancer through routine symptom screening. *Am Soc Clin Oncol.* 2008;26(suppl):abstr 9621.
17. Seow H, Barbera L, Sutradhar R, et al. Trajectory of performance status and symptom scores for patients with cancer during the last six months of life. *J Clin Oncol.* 2011;29(9):1151-1158.
18. Lutz S, Norrell R, Bertucio C, et al. Symptom frequency and severity in patients with metastatic or locally recurrent lung cancer: a prospective study using the Lung Cancer Symptom Scale in a community hospital. *J Palliat Med.* 2001;4(2):157-165.
19. Gore JM, Brophy CJ, Greenstone MA. How well do we care for patients with end stage chronic obstructive pulmonary disease (COPD)? A comparison of palliative care and quality of life in COPD and lung cancer. *Thorax.* 2000;55:1000-1006.
20. Chochinov MH, Tataryn D, Clinch JJ, Dudgeon D. Will to live in the terminally ill. *Lancet.* 1999;354(9181):816-819.
21. O'Donnell DE, Banzett RB, Carrieri-Kohlman V, et al. Pathophysiology of dyspnea in chronic obstructive pulmonary disease. A roundtable. *Proc Am Thoracic Soc.* 2007;4:145-168.
22. von Leupoldt A Sommer T, Kegat S, et al. The unpleasantness of perceived dyspnea is processed in the anterior insula and amygdala. *Am J Respir Crit Care Med.* 2008;177(9):1026-1032.
23. Peiffer C. Dyspnea and emotion: what can we learn from functional brain imaging? *Am J Respir Crit Care Med.* 2008;177:937-939.
24. Abernethy AP, Wheeler JL. Total dyspnoea. *Curr Opin Support Palliat Care.* 2008;2:110-113.
25. Heyse-Moore LH. *On Dyspnoea in Advanced Cancer.* Southampton: Southampton University; 1993.
26. Dudgeon D, Lertzman M. Dyspnea in the advanced cancer patient. *J Pain Symptom Manage.* 1998;16(4):212-219.
27. Dudgeon DJ, Lertzman M, Askew GR. Physiological changes and clinical correlations of dyspnea in cancer outpatients. *J Pain Symptom Manage.* 2001;21(5):373-379.
28. Bruera E, Schmitz B, Pither J, Neumann CM, Hanson J. The frequency and correlates of dyspnea in patients with advanced cancer. *J Pain Symptom Manage.* 2000;19(5):357-362.
29. Dudgeon DJ, Webb KA, O'Donnell DE. Unexplained dyspnea and exercise intolerance in patients with cancer: physiological correlates. *Am Soc Clin Oncol.* 2001;20:303b.
30. Tanaka K, Akechi T, Okuyama T, Nishiwaki Y, Uchitomi Y. Factors correlated with dyspnea in advanced lung cancer patients: organic causes and what else? *J Pain Symptom Manage.* 2002;23(6):490-500.
31. Escalante CP, Martin CG, Elting LS, et al. Dyspnea in cancer patients. Etiology, resource utilization, and survival—implications in a managed care world. *Cancer.* 1996;78(6):1314-1319.
32. Lansing RW, Gracely RH, Banzett RB. The multiple dimensions of dyspnea: review and hypotheses. *Respir Physiol Neurobiol.* 2009;167(1):53-60.
33. Wilcock A, Crosby V, Hughes AC, Fielding K, Corcoran R, Tattersfield AE. Descriptors of breathlessness in patients with cancer and other cardiorespiratory diseases. *J Pain Symptom Manage.* 2002;23(3):182-189.
34. Silvestri GA, Mahler DA. Evaluation of dyspnea in the elderly patient. *Clin Chest Med.* 1993;14(3):393-404.

35. Ferrin MS, Tino G. Acute dyspnea. *Am Assoc Crit Care Nurs Clin Issues.* 1997;8(3):398-410.

36. Man GCW, Hsu K, Sproule BJ. Effect of alprazolam on exercise and dyspnea in patients with chronic obstructive pulmonary disease. *Chest.* 1986;90(6):832-836.

37. Swartz MH. *Textbook of Physical Diagnosis: History and Examination.* 4th ed. Philadelphia, PA: W.B. Saunders Company; 2002.

38. Gift AG, Plaut SM, Jacox A. Psychologic and physiologic factors related to dyspnea in subjects with chronic obstructive pulmonary disease. *Heart Lung.* 1986;15:595-601.

39. Hancox B, Whyte K. *McGraw-Hill's Pocket Guide to Lung Function Tests.* Roseville, NSW: McGraw-Hill; 2001.

40. Heyse-Moore LH, Beynon T, Ross V. Does spirometry predict dyspnoea in advanced cancer? *Palliat Med.* 2000;14(3):189-195.

41. Singh SJ, Morgan MD, Hardman AE, Rowe C, Bardsley PA. Comparison of oxygen uptake during a conventional treadmill test and the shuttle walking test in chronic airflow limitation. *Eur Respir J.* 1994;7(11):2016-2020.

42. Booth S, Adams L. The shuttle walking test: a reproducible method for evaluating the impact of shortness of breath on functional capacity in patients with advanced cancer. *Thorax.* 2001;56(2):146-150.

43. Bausewein C, Farquhar M, Booth S, Gysels M, Higginson IJ. Measurement of breathlessness in advanced disease: a systematic review. *Respir Med.* 2006;101: 399-410.

44. Gift AG. Clinical measurement of dyspnea. *Dimens Crit Care Nurs.* 1989;8(4):210-216.

45. Wilcock A, Corcoran R, Tattersfield AE. Safety and efficacy of nebulized lignocaine in patients with cancer and breathlessness. *Palliat Med.* 1994;8:35-38.

46. van der Molen, B. Dyspnoea: a study of measurement instruments for the assessment of dyspnoea and their application for patients with advanced cancer. *J Adv Nurs.* 1995;22:948-956.

47. Killian KJ. Assessment of dyspnoea. *Eur Respir J.* 1988;1(3):195-197.

48. Borg GAV. Psychophysical basis of perceived exertion. *Med Sci Sports Exerc.* 1982;14(5):377-381.

49. McGavin CR, Artvinli M, Naoe H, McHardy G. Dyspnoea, disability and distance walked: comparison of estimates of exercise performance in respiratory disease. *Br Med J.* 1978; 2:241-243.

50. Tanaka K, Akechi T, Okuyama T, Nishiwaki Y, Uchitomi Y. Development and validation of the cancer dyspnoea scale: a multidimensional, brief, self-rating scale. *Br J Cancer.* 2000;82(4):800-805.

51. Hollen PJ, Gralla RJ, Kris MG, Potanovich LM. Quality of life assessment in individuals with lung cancer: testing the Lung Cancer Symptom Scale (LCSS). *Eur J Cancer.* 1993;29A:S51-S58.

52. Hollen PJ, Gralla RJ. Comparison of instruments for measuring quality of life in patients with lung cancer. *Semin Oncol.* 1996;23(2 suppl 5):31-40.

53. Aaronson NK, Ahmedzai S, Bergman B. The European Organization for Research and Treatment of Cancer QLQ-C30: a quality-of-life instrument for use in international clinical trials in oncology. *J Natl Cancer Inst.* 1993;85:365-376.

54. Bergman B, Aaronson NK, Ahmedzai S. The EORTC QLQ-LC13: a modular supplement to the EORTC core Quality of Life Questionnaire (QLQ-C30) for use in lung cancer clinical trials. *Eur J Cancer.* 1994;30A: 635-642.

55. Cella DF, Bonomi AE, Lloyd SR, Tulsky DS, Kaplan E, Bonomi P. Reliability and validity of the Functional Assessment of Cancer Therapy-Lung (FACT-L) quality of life instrument. *Lung Cancer.* 1995;12:199-220.

56. Deslauriers J, Ugalde P, Miro S, et al. Adjustments in cardiorespiratory function after pneumonectomy: results of the pneumonectomy project. *J Thoracic Cardiovasc Surg.* 2010;141(1):7-15.

57. Travers J, Dudgeon D, Amjadi K, et al. Mechanisms of exertional dyspnea in patients with cancer. *J Appl Physiol.* 2007;104(1):57-66.

58. Dudgeon, DJ, O'Donnell DE, Day A, Webb KA, McBride I, Dillon K. Mechanisms of exertional dyspnea in patients with cancer: a case-matched control study. *J Palliat Care.* 2002;18(3):207.

59. Lewis MI, Belman MJ. Nutrition and the respiratory muscles. *Clin Chest Med.* 1988;9(2):337-347.

60. Rochester DF, Arora NS. Respiratory muscle failure. *Med Clin North Am.* 1983;67(3):573-597.

61. Shannon VR. Role of pulmonary rehabilitation in the management of patients with lung cancer. *Curr Opin Pulm Med.* 2010;16(4):334-339.

62. Oldervoll LM, Loge JH, Paltiel H, et al. The effect of a physical exercise program in palliative care: a phase II study. *J Pain Symptom Manage.* 2006;31(5):421-430.

63. Whittaker JS, Ryan CF, Buckley PA, Road JD. The effects of refeeding on peripheral and respiratory muscle function in malnourished chronic obstructive pulmonary disease patients. *Am Rev Respir Dis.* 1990;142:283-288.

64. O'Donnell DE, McGuire M, Samis L, Webb KA. The impact of exercise reconditioning on breathlessness in severe chronic airflow limitation. *Am J Respir Crit Care Med.* 1995;152:2005-2013.

65. Schols AM, Soeters PB, Mostert R, Pluymers RJ, Wouters EF. Physiologic effects of nutritional support and anabolic steroids in patients with chronic obstructive pulmonary disease. A placebo-controlled randomized trial. *Am J Respir Crit Care Med.* 1995;152(4 Pt 1):1268-1274.

66. Streiff MB. Anticoagulation in the management of venous thromboembolism in the cancer patient. *J Thromb Thrombolysis.* 2011;31(3):282-294.

67. Scully RE, Mark EJ, McNeely WF, McNeely BU. Case record of the Massachusetts General Hospital (Case 30-1987). *N Engl J Med.* 1987;317(4):225-235.

68. Viola R, Kiteley C, Lloyd NS, Mackay JA, Wilson J, Wong RKS. The management of dyspnea in cancer patients: a systematic review. *Support Care Cancer.* 2008;16:329-337.

69. Ben-Aharon I, Gafter-Gvili A, Leibovici L, Stemmer SM. Interventions for alleviating cancer-related dyspnea: a systematic review. *J Clin Oncol.* 2008;26(14):2396-2404.

70. Jennings AL, Davies A, Higgins JPT, Broadley K. *Opioids for the Palliation of Breathlessness in Terminal Illness (Cochrane Review). The Cochrane Library [4].* Oxford: Update Software; 2001.

71. Woodcock AA, Johnson MA, Geddes DM. Breathlessness, alcohol and opiates. *N Engl J Med.* 1982;306:1363-1364.

72. Woodcock AA, Gross ER, Gellert A, Shah S, Johnson M, Geddes DM. Effects of dihydrocodeine, alcohol, and caffeine on breathlessness and exercise tolerance in patients with chronic obstructive lung disease and normal blood gases. *N Engl J Med.* 1981;305(27): 1611-1616.

73. Poole PJ, Veale AG, Black PN. The effect of sustained-release morphine on breathlessness and quality of life in severe chronic obstructive pulmonary disease. *Am J Respir Crit Care Med.* 1998;157(6 Pt 1):1877-1880.

74. Light RW, Stansbury DW, Webster JS. Effect of 30 mg of morphine alone or with promethazine or prochlorperazine on the exercise capacity of patients with COPD. *Chest.* 1996;109(4):975-981.

75. Johnson MA, Woodcock AA, Geddes DM. Dihydrocodeine for breathlessness in "pink puffers." *Br Med J.* 1983;286:675-677.

76. Eiser N, Denman WT, West C, Luce P. Oral diamorphine: lack of effect on dyspnoea and exercise tolerance in the "pink puffer" syndrome. *Eur Respir J.* 1991;4(8):926-931.

77. Bruera E, MacEachern T, Ripamonti C, Hanson J. Subcutaneous morphine for dyspnea in cancer patients. *Ann Intern Med.* 1993;119(9):906-907.

78. Chua TP, Harrington D, Ponikowski P, Webb-Peploe K, Poole-Wilson PA, Coats AJ. Effects of dihydrocodeine on chemosensitivity and exercise tolerance in patients with chronic heart failure. *J Am Coll Cardiol.* 1997;29(1):147-152.

79. Zebraski SE, Kochenash SM, Raffa RB. Lung opioid receptors: pharmacology and possible target for nebulized morphine in dyspnea. *Life Sci.* 2000;66(23):2221-2231.

80. Beauford W, Saylor TT, Stansbury DW, Avalos K, Light RW. Effects of nebulized morphine sulfate on the exercise tolerance of the ventilatory limited COPD patient. *Chest.* 1993;104(1):175-178.

81. Davis CL, Hodder C, Love S, Shah R, Slevin M, Wedzicha J. Effect of nebulised morphine and morphine 6-glucuronide on exercise endurance in patients with chronic obstructive pulmonary disease. *Thorax.* 1994;49:393P.

82. Davis CL, Penn K, A'Hern R, Daniels J, Slevin M. Single dose randomised controlled trial of nebulised morphine in patients with cancer related breathlessness. *Palliat Med.* 1996;10(1):64-65.

83. Harris-Eze AO, Sridhar G, Clemens RE, Zintel TA, Gallagher CG, Marciniuk DD. Low-dose nebulized morphine does not improve exercise in interstitial lung disease. *Am J Respir Crit Care Med.* 1995;152:1940-1945.

84. Jankelson D, Hosseini K, Mather LE, Seale JP, Young IH. Lack of effect of high doses of inhaled morphine on exercise endurance in chronic obstructive pulmonary disease. *Eur Respir J.* 1997;10(10):2270-2274.

85. Leung R, Hill P, Burdon JGW. Effect of inhaled morphine on the development of breathlessness during exercise in patients with chronic lung disease. *Thorax.* 1996;51(6):596-600.

86. Masood AR, Reed JW, Thomas SHL. Lack of effect of inhaled morphine on exercise-induced breathlessness in chronic obstructive pulmonary disease. *Thorax.* 1995;50(6):629-634.

87. Noseda A, Carpiaux JP, Markstein C, Meyvaert A, de Maertelaer V. Disabling dyspnoea in patients with advanced disease: lack of effect of nebulized morphine. *Eur Respir J.* 1997;10(5):1079-1083.

88. Young IH, Daviskas E, Keena VA. Effect of low dose nebulised morphine on exercise endurance in patients with chronic lung disease. *Thorax.* 1989;44:387-390.

89. Mazzocato C, Buclin T, Rapin CH. The effects of morphine on dyspnea and ventilatory function in elderly patients with advanced cancer: a randomized double-blind controlled trial. *Ann Oncol.* 1999;10(12):1511-1514.

90. Allard P, Lamontagne C, Bernard P, Tremblay C. How effective are supplementary doses of opioids for dyspnea in terminally ill cancer patients? A randomized continuous sequential clinical trial. *J Pain Symptom Manage.* 1999;17(4):256-265.

91. Navigante AH, Cerchietti LCA, Castro MA, Lutteral MA, Cabalar ME. Midazolam as adjunct therapy to morphine in the alleviation of severe dyspnea perception in patients with advanced cancer. *J Pain Symptom Manage.* 2006;31(1):38-47.

92. Charles MA, Reymond L, Israel F. Relief of incident dyspnea in palliative cancer patients: a pilot, randomized, controlled trial comparing nebulized hydromorphone, systemic hydromorphone, and nebulized saline. *J Pain Symptom Manage.* 2008;36(1):29-38.

93. Bruera E, Sala R, Spruyt O, Palmer JL, Zhang T, Willey J. Nebulized versus subcutaneous morphine for patients with cancer dyspnea: a preliminary study. *J Pain Symptom Manage.* 2005;29(6):613-618.

94. O'Neill PA, Morton PB, Stark RD. Chlorpromazine—a specific effect on breathlessness? *Br J Clin Pharmacol.* 1985;19:793-797.

95. Woodcock AA, Gross ER, Geddes DM. Drug treatment of breathlessness: contrasting effects of diazepam and promethazine in pink puffers. *Br Med J.* 1981;283:343-346.

96. Rice KL, Kronenberg RS, Hedemark LL, Niewoehner DE. Effects of chronic administration of codeine and promethazine on breathlessness and exercise tolerance in patients with chronic airflow obstruction. *Br J Dis Chest.* 1987;81:287-292.

97. McIver B, Walsh D, Nelson K. The use of chlorpromazine for symptom control in dying cancer patients. *J Pain Symptom Manage.* 1994;9(5):341-345.

98. Ventafridda V, Spoldi E, De Conno F. Control of dyspnea in advanced cancer patients. *Chest.* 1990;98:1544-1545.

99. Simon ST, Higginson IJ, Booth S, Harding R, Bausewein C. *Benzodiazepines for the Relief of Breathlessness in Advanced Malignant and Non-malignant Diseases in Adults (Review).* Cochrane Pain, Palliative and Supportive Care Group: Canada: John Wiley & Sons Ltd; 2011.

100. Navigante AH, Castro MA, Cerchietti LC. Morphine versus midazolam as upfront therapy to control dyspnea perception in cancer patients while its underlying cause is sought or treated. *J Pain Symptom Manage.* 2010;39(5):820-830.

101. Philip J, Gold M, Milner A, Di Iulio J, Miller B, Spruyt O. A randomized, double-blind, crossover trial of the effect of oxygen on dyspnea in patients with advanced cancer. *J Pain Symptom Manage.* 2006;32(6):541-550.

102. Cranston JM, Crockett A, Currow D. Oxygen therapy for dyspnoea in adults (review). *Cochrane Libr.* 2008;3(4):1-54.

103. Booth S, Kelly M, Cox NP, Adams L, Guz A. Does oxygen help dyspnea in patients with cancer? *Am J Respir Crit Care Med.* 1996;153:1515-1518.

104. Uronis H, Abernethy AP. Oxygen for relief of dyspnea: what is the evidence? *Curr Opin Support Palliat Care.* 2008;2(2):89-94.

105. Currow DC, Agar M, Smith J, Abernethy AP. Does palliative home oxygen improve dyspnoea? A consecutive cohort study. *Palliat Med.* 2009;23(4):309-316.

106. Bausewein C, Booth S, Higginson GM. *Non-pharmacological Interventions for Breathlessness in Advanced Stages of Malignant and Non-malignant Diseases (Review).* Cochrane Pain, Palliative and Supportive Care Group: Canada: John Wiley & Sons Ltd; 2008.

107. Schwartzstein RM, Lahive K, Pope A, Weinberger SE, Weiss JW. Cold facial stimulation reduces breathlessness induced in normal subjects. *Am Rev Respir Dis.* 1987;136:58-61.

108. Baltzan, M, Alter A, Rotaple M, Kamel H, Wolkove N. Fan to palliate exercise-induced dyspnea with severe COPD. *Am J Respir Crit Care Med.* 2000;161(suppl 3):A59.

109. Marchetti N, Travaline JM, Criner JL. Air current applied to the face of COPD patients enhances leg ergometry performance. *Am J Respir Crit Care Med.* 2004;169:A773.

110. Spence DP, Graham DR, Ahmed J, Rees K, Pearson MG, Calverley PM. Does cold air affect exercise capacity and dyspnoea in stable COPD? *Chest.* 1993;103:693-696.

111. Galbraith S, Fagan P, Perkins P, Lynch A, Booth S. Does the use of a handheld fan improve chronic dyspnea? A randomized, controlled, crossover trial. *J Pain Symptom Manage.* 2009;39(5):831-838.

112. Cancer Care Ontario. *Symptom Management Tools* [Internet]. Toronto: Cancer Care Ontario; 2010. https://www.cancercare.on.ca/toolbox/symptools/

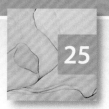
Hemoptysis, Airway Obstruction, Bronchospasm, Cough, and Pulmonary Complications/Symptoms of Cancer and Its Treatment

Sebastian Cousins, Hunter Groninger, and Jaya Vijayan

INTRODUCTION

Complications from malignancies in and around the chest cavity, including the pulmonary tree, are common and associated with significant symptoms and morbidity. Nearly any malignancy (excepting primary brain malignancies) has the capacity to wreak havoc in these vital organs, circulatory structures, and potential spaces. Complications in the chest cavity or pulmonary tree typically suggest incurable malignancy. From the perspective of palliative care and supportive oncology, the clinical approach to the patient with such complications should reflect both evaluation of disease-modifying treatment options and management of symptom burden, always considering the patient's goals. Finally, many of these complications correlate with worsened functional status and shortened prognosis and can lead directly to death. In addition to a comprehensive approach to managing these clinical situations, the supportive oncology or palliative care expert should be prepared to counsel patients and families and provide the best end-of-life care.

This chapter provides an overview of some of the more common malignancy-related complications that arise in the chest cavity and corresponding management strategies. It also broaches common symptoms arising in the pulmonary system (except for dyspnea, which is discussed elsewhere). Finally, we summarize discussion points regarding noninvasive positive pressure ventilation (NIPPV), a treatment option that may be overlooked in the palliative care setting. Although by no means exhaustive, this chapter should provide a sense of the breadth and depth to which malignancy can affect these critical organ systems.

PLEURAL EFFUSIONS

Incidence

Malignant pleural effusions (MPEs) are relatively common and associated with significant management challenges. In any given general hospital patient population, up to 60% of all pleural effusions are malignant, the highest incidence seen in patients over 50 years old (1–4). In up to 50% of patients, MPE is the initial manifestation of cancer (4,5) but eventually about half of all patients with disseminated cancer develop a one (4). Table 25.1 lists the frequency of the various tumor types that are associated with MPEs.

Diagnosis

The approach to the diagnosis and management of a patient with a suspected MPE is shown in Figure 25.1. Initial diagnosis typically begins with the posterior-anterior chest radiograph with decubitus views. Blunting of the costophrenic angle may suggest 175 to 500 mL of free fluid; a decubitus view may show as little as 100 mL (6). Computed tomography (CT) scans may be necessary if the hemithorax is opaque on chest radiograph, when a mesothelioma is suspected, or when the underlying primary tumor is unknown. Occasionally, chest ultrasonography can be employed to differentiate pleural fluid and pleural thickening (7), but this modality is more commonly used to localize smaller effusions en route to diagnostic or therapeutic thoracentesis (8). Using color Doppler to distinguish pleural thickening from minimal pleural effusions is an effective technique, with a sensitivity of 91% and accuracy of 95% (9).

If the patient is symptomatic, enough fluid should be drained by thoracentesis to relieve symptoms. Rapid removal of a large amount of fluid (especially over 1,500 mL) may result in life-threatening reexpansion pulmonary edema (10). MPEs are frequently hemorrhagic (erythrocyte count >100,000/mm), but this is nonspecific and occurs in only one-third of cases (5). Elevated levels of lactate dehydrogenase (LDH) or protein in the pleural fluid, and ratios of fluid to concurrent serum levels of LDH and protein, distinguish transudate from an exudate (11). If findings suggest transudate, malignancy may be reasonably excluded. However, an exudate with a negative cytology result necessitates a second diagnostic

TABLE 25.1 TUMOR CAUSES OF MALIGNANT PLEURAL EFFUSIONS FROM COLLECTED SERIES

Tumor type	Incidence (%)
Lung	35
Breast	23
Lymphoma/leukemia	10
Adenocarcinoma (unknown primary)	12
Reproductive tract	6
Gastrointestinal tract	5
Genitourinary tract	3
Primary unknown	3
Other cancers	5

From Hausheer FH, Yarbro JW. Diagnosis and treatment of malignant pleural effusion. *Semin Oncol*. 1985;12:54-75, with permission.

thoracentesis with cytology to improve sensitivity by another 10% (3). Cytology remains the cornerstone to diagnosing a malignant effusion, although important variables contribute to its efficacy: tumor type, cytopathologist experience, and the volume of fluid sent for analysis (12). With some cell types, such as Hodgkin's disease, the rate of positive cytology results may prove as low as 23%, while with others, such a breast or lung cancer, remain as high as 73% (3).

When two exudative pleural fluid cytology results are negative for malignancy in the face of high clinical suspicion for malignancy, moving to video-assisted thoracoscopy surgery (VATS) is reasonable, a technique that permits visually directed pleural biopsy and directed therapeutic intervention including lysis of adhesions, mechanical or chemical pleurodesis, or pleurectomy (13).

Prognosis

Most patients with MPE have incurable cancer. Treatment should be targeted to the most effective palliation for maximal comfortable time outside the hospital if this is consistent with the patient's goals. For all patients, the overall mean survival time is 3 to 6 months. In general, mortality is high: from 54% at 1 month to 84% at 6 months (14–16).

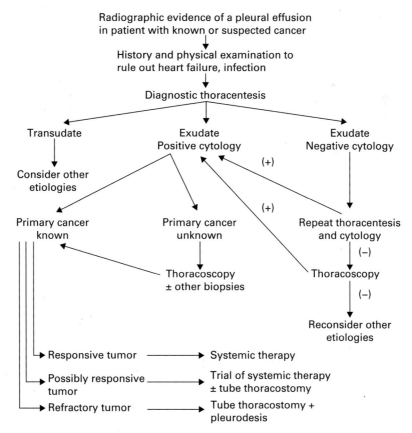

Figure 25.1 Approach to the diagnosis and treatment of malignant pleural effusions. +, study result is positive; –, study result is negative. (From Ruckdeschel JC. Management of malignant pleural effusion: an overview. *Semin Oncol*. 1988;15:24-28, with permission.)

Management

Management of Underlying Malignancy

Whenever indicated, a therapeutic thoracentesis should be followed by appropriate disease-modifying therapies such as systemic chemotherapy or hormonal therapy (17,18). If the malignancy is resistant to systemic therapies, then tube thoracostomy followed by intrapleural therapy may be appropriate, if the patient has a reasonable life expectancy. If the patient's performance status is significantly reduced, simple prolonged drainage by an indwelling catheter may be more appropriate.

Management of Fluid Accumulation

While thoracentesis typically relieves symptoms briefly, fluid usually reaccumulates quickly—in up to 97% of patients by 1 month (19). Tube thoracostomy has a role in draining the pleural cavity and maintaining opposition of the pleural surfaces when a therapeutic agent is infused into the chest cavity for sclerotherapy.

Soft indwelling catheters made of silicone and plastic (Silastic) may be placed under local anesthesia, allow patient or caregiver to periodically drain the pleural space for symptomatic relief. When employed more than 6 weeks, these catheters facilitate spontaneous pleurodesis between 40% and 46% of the time (20–22).

Fibrinolytic Agents Intrapleural instillation of a fibrinolytic agent, such as urokinase, may help to break up more gelatinous or fibrous fluid accumulations (23,24).

Pleurodesis Drainage of the pleural space with reexpansion of the lung, followed by instillation of a chemical agent into the pleural cavity, remains the most common management strategy for MPEs. This mechanism, called *pleural sclerotherapy* or *pleurodesis*, is thought to be the creation of an inflammatory pleuritis between visceral and parietal pleura that facilitates more permanent closing of the potential space.

Pleuroperitoneal Shunt Internal drainage of the malignant effusion into the abdomen using an implanted, valved, manually operated pump is occasionally an option in motivated patients with good performance status who have a trapped lung and an intractable effusion (5,18,25).

Recurrent Effusions A refractory pleural effusion in which the first attempt of pleural sclerotherapy has failed is a clinical challenge. At times, a second tube thoracostomy, followed by intrapleural sclerotherapy, is attempted, usually using a different sclerosing agent. If this second attempt fails and the patient has a good performance status and a reasonable estimated life span, then VATS talc poudrage may be considered. In many instances, the placement of a Silastic catheter with prolonged external drainage has become the treatment of choice.

Summary

Patients with MPEs generally have terminal disease with a limited life span—often a few months. Choice to pursue disease-modifying therapy should reflect the clinician's understanding of the patient's overall prognosis along with motivation to provide the maximum quality of life and function. A suggested treatment algorithm for MPEs is shown in Figure 25.2.

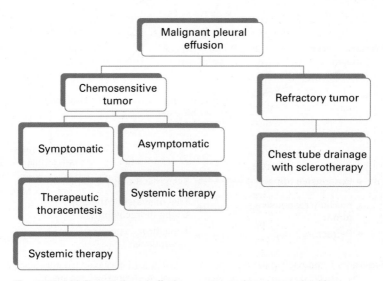

Figure 25.2 Malignant pleural effusion—suggested treatment algorithm.

PERICARDIAL EFFUSIONS

Incidence

In a collection of autopsy studies of patients with disseminated cancer, involvement of the heart and pericardium with metastatic malignancy is seen in up to 21% of cases (25–30), with the highest incidence occurring in patients with leukemia (69%), melanoma (64%), and lymphoma (24%) (30).

Etiology

Nearly any primary malignancy can metastasize to the pericardium and cause an effusion (30) except for primary brain tumors. As with MPEs, the most common perpetrators are malignancies of the lung and breast and lymphoma or leukemia: together, these account for almost 75% of all pericardial malignant events (31). Elucidating the cause of such an effusion is critically important, since approximately 40% of patients with an underlying cancer have a nonmalignant etiology (32).

Pathophysiology

The increase in pericardial fluid, threatening to cause tamponade, typically results from obstruction of the mediastinal lymphatic system, especially by cancers that commonly involve the mediastinal lymph nodes (27). With slow accumulation of fluid, the pericardium can distend to contain up to 2 L. Rapid accumulation does not allow such tissue distension and hemodynamic compromise may occur with as little as 200 mL of fluid in the pericardial space (33). The critical outcome is impaired diastolic filling of the right side of the heart, which eventually overwhelms compensatory mechanisms, leading to hemodynamic instability (*cardiac tamponade*) (34).

Clinical Presentation

The most common presenting symptom is dyspnea on exertion, which may progress to dyspnea at rest as cardiac function becomes more compromised (27,32,34). Other common symptoms include chest pain or heaviness (63%), cough (30% to 43%), and weakness or fatigue (26%). Less common symptoms include peripheral edema, low grade fevers, dizziness, nausea, diaphoresis, and peripheral venous constriction.

On examination, the classic signs associated with cardiac tamponade are often referred to as *Beck's triad*: faint heart sounds, hypotension, and venous distention (34). These criteria are not always helpful in the diagnosis of pericardial effusions. In one series of 153 patients, 37.5% of patients with pericardial effusions had none of these symptoms and none of the patients had all three elements (35). Hypotension may be found in over 60% of patients, elevated venous pressure is seen in 50% to 60%,

and resting tachycardia occurs in up to 90% (27). A central venous pressure >15 mm Hg along with hypotension is highly suggestive of tamponade. The pathophysiologic effects of cardiac tamponade tend to exaggerate the normal fall in systolic blood pressure with inspiration, a phenomenon termed *pulsus paradoxus*. Other less frequent signs that may be present include a narrower pulse pressure, a visible increase in venous pressure on inspiration (Kussmaul's sign), hepatomegaly, hepatojugular reflux, peripheral edema, cyanosis, pericardial friction rub, arrhythmias, cold clammy extremities, low-grade fever, and ascites.

Diagnosis

Radiographic

In any patient with cancer, a change in the size and contour of the heart in the setting of clear lung fields on a chest x-ray should prompt consideration of a pericardial effusion. The cardiac silhouette might resemble the so-called "water-bottle heart" with bulging of the normal contours. However, a normal-size heart shadow does not exclude the presence of a pericardial effusion or even a life-threatening tamponade. A chest CT scan is more sensitive and may suggest a malignant pericardial process if the effusion has a high density, there is pericardial thickening, masses are contiguous with the pericardium, or there is an obliteration of the tissue planes between the mass and the heart (27).

A more invasive (but more accurate) diagnostic procedure is right heart catheterization. Findings from this procedure in true tamponade are a depressed cardiac output and the equalization of diastolic pressure in all heart chambers (34).

Electrocardiography

Electrocardiography (ECG) changes—including sinus tachycardia, atrial and ventricular arrhythmias, low voltage QRS, and diffuse nonspecific ST and T-wave abnormalities—may reflect presence of an effusion. Electrical alternans (alternating large and small P wave and QRS complexes) is occasionally seen and generally resolves immediately with drainage of the effusion (28,34).

Echocardiography

Echocardiography may detect as little as 15 mL of pericardial fluid as well as identifying myocardial masses and even loculations of fluid.

Pericardial Fluid Examination

Percutaneous, ultrasound-guided pericardiocentesis can safely be performed in patients with larger effusions (>1 cm anterior clear space on echocardiogram), yielding fluid sample for examination in approximately 90% of patients and temporary tamponade relief (27,36). In a malignant effusion, the result of cytology will be positive for malignant cells in 65% to 90% of cases (37). False-negative cytologic results can frequently be seen with lymphoma and mesothelioma. Negative cytology alone does not exclude neoplastic pericarditis, and it may be necessary to obtain pericardial tissue for histology if clinical suspicion remains high.

Differential Diagnosis of Pericardial Effusion

Up to 40% of patients with symptomatic pericardial effusions and cancer will have a benign etiology of the effusion (32). Generally, the pericardial fluid analysis together with the patient's history will exclude many of the potential diagnoses and may identify the actual cause of the effusion.

Prognosis

Quality of life and functional status associated with malignant pericardial effusions depend largely on the malignancy cell type and stage. In general terms, prognosis is limited at best; for example, after surgical drainage of an effusion, patients with breast cancer have a mean survival of 8 to 18 months (38,39), patients with lymphoma have a mean survival of 10 months (38), and patients with lung cancer have a mean survival of 3 to 5 months (38,40).

Management

Pericardiocentesis

This is the initial procedure of choice in the emergency management of life-threatening pericardial effusion (tamponade). When combined with echocardiography, the success rate in obtaining fluid for diagnosis and relieving symptoms rises to almost 97% with a decrease in the complication rate from 2.4% (27,39). Most (39% to 56%) malignant effusions will recur even after single or repeated drainage (27,39). During initial drainage, insertion of a small pigtail catheter into the pericardial space can facilitate intermittent drainage over several days (27).

Intrapericardial Sclerosis

A logical extension of pericardiocentesis with catheter drainage is injection of a sclerosing agent into the pericardium through the indwelling catheter to prevent a recurrence of the effusion, much like that practiced with MPE. Agents used in small studies include tetracycline, doxycycline, minocycline, bleomycin, and talc.

Radiotherapy

External beam radiotherapy has been advocated for a variety of tumors with cardiac and pericardial involvement (41). Generally, this strategy is reserved for radiotherapy-naive patients with radiosensitive tumors (27).

Surgical Approaches

The most popular approach to surgical treatment of a malignant pericardial effusion is the *subxiphoid pericardiectomy* (i.e., "pericardial window"), which offers the distinct advantages of very low mortality (1% or less), 1% major morbidity, and 100% immediate efficacy in relieving tamponade. The long-term effusion recurrence rate is low (3% to 7%) (27,42–45). Diagnostic accuracy approaches 100% because fluid and pericardial tissue are both removed and sent for pathologic evaluation. If necessary, a *left anterior thoracotomy* for pericardiectomy has a low morbidity and mortality and allows examination and biopsy of the contents of the left pleural cavity if desired. More extensively, the *median sternotomy with pericardiectomy* gives very wide exposure to most of the pericardium. The advent of VATS has allowed a minimally invasive option for pericardiectomy; one series of 28 patients demonstrate 100% long-term success, no significant morbidity, and 0% mortality (46). Finally, more novel attempts to maximize fluid drainage, while minimizing surgical risks include the pericardioperitoneal shunt (47) and percutaneous balloon pericardiotomy (48).

Summary

Malignant pericardial effusion is not uncommon in advanced cancers, especially with cancers of the lung and breast and with leukemia or lymphoma. In general, these patients have incurable cancer. Nonetheless, most patients with symptomatic effusions deserve treatment evaluation, as they may respond rapidly to pericardial decompression. Therapy must be individualized, taking into consideration the tumor cell type and sensitivity to disease-modifying therapies, patient performance status and prognosis, and presence/absence of pericardial tamponade, leading to some meaningful period of palliation. A suggested treatment algorithm for patients with chemosensitive tumor is shown in Figure 25.3.

SUPERIOR VENA CAVA SYNDROME

Primary or metastatic tumors can cause superior vena cava (SVC) obstruction, also known as *SVC syndrome* (49). Cancers classically associated with SVC syndrome include lung cancer (particularly right-sided), breast cancer, primary mediastinal lymphoma, lymphoblastic lymphoma, thymoma, and germ cell tumors (either primary or metastatic to mediastinum).

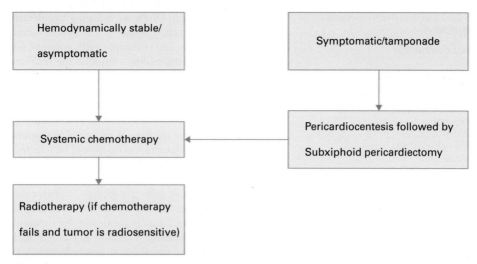

Figure 25.3 Malignant pericardial effusion treatment algorithm for patients with chemosensitive tumor.

Presentation

The patient's clinical presentation varies based on the extent of obstruction and acuity of its development. Blockage is better tolerated when there has been time for collateral veins to develop in adjacent venous systems like the azygous and internal mammary, a process that usually takes weeks. The veins on the patient's chest wall may be visibly distended. Edema in the arms, facial plethora, chemosis, and periorbital edema may also occur. Stridor is an alarming sign that edema is narrowing the luminal diameter of the pharynx and larynx. Hoarseness and dysphagia can result from edema around the airway and digestive tract. Presyncope or syncope is more common earlier in the disease course when cardiac output declines without compensation. Headaches stem from distension of cerebral vessels against the dura, and confusion may indicate cerebral edema. These symptoms may be more noticeable when the patient is supine.

Diagnosis

Imaging is crucial to diagnosis and treatment planning. While the gold standard for localizing obstruction remains selective venography, multidetector CT and magnetic resonance imaging (MRI) are usually preferable for their noninvasiveness, easier availability, and decreased contrast load. In one small study (47 patients), CT evidence of collateral vessels was correlated with the patients who had symptoms of SVC syndrome (sensitivity of 96% and specificity of 92%) (50).

Treatment

SVC syndrome requires prompt recognition and treatment, but the clinical course typically permits completion of appropriate diagnostic studies before definitive therapy (51). Patients who have

neurologic symptoms or airway compromise need immediate treatment. *Endovascular stenting* is the treatment of choice and generally relieves symptoms more quickly than chemoradiation (52). *Chemotherapy* may be the only necessary treatment in patient presenting nonemergently with small cell lung cancer, lymphoma, or germ cell tumors. Changes in the SVC lumen following mediastinal *radiation* may be disproportionately small relative to the magnitude of symptom improvement. Cases of catheter-related thrombosis have been successfully treated with instillation of *thrombolytics* into the device (53), but fibrinolytic therapy should be administered carefully in cases in which brain metastases are known or have not been excluded.

TRACHEOBRONCHIAL OBSTRUCTION

Tracheobronchial obstruction may be intrinsic or extrinsic. *Intrinsic* obstruction is usually caused by primary lung malignancies or from metastases arising from the airway epithelium (most commonly renal cell, colon, rectum, cervical, breast carcinomas, and malignant melanomas) (54,55). *Extrinsic* obstruction occurs when the airways are surrounded by solid tumor or are encased by enlarged lymph nodes. This scenario usually results from locally advanced disease arising from the lung, esophagus, thyroid, or lymphoma. Table 25.2 lists common etiologies of airway obstruction.

Clinical Presentation

Patients with proximal airway obstruction usually present with dyspnea, hemoptysis, wheezing, or stridor and sometimes with pneumonia or atelectasis. Distal airway obstruction, on the other hand, tends to present with obstructive pneumonitis (56).

TABLE 25.2 ETIOLOGIES OF AIRWAY OBSTRUCTION

Intrinsic obstruction
Malignant
- Primary tumors
  - Tracheal
    - Squamous carcinoma
    - Adenoid cystic carcinoma
  - Bronchogenic
  - Squamous
  - Adenocarcinoma
  - Small cell
  - Mixed morphology
- Metastatic
  - Breast cancer
  - Melanoma
  - Larynx
  - Esophagus
  - Renal cell
  - Colon

Extrinsic obstruction
- Rectal
- Cervical
- Kaposi sarcoma (rarely obstructing)

Benign
- Papillomas
- Chondromas
- Hamartoma
- Lipoma
- Leiomyoma
- Granular cell myoblastoma
- Granuloma 2 retained foreign body
- Hemangiomas
- Postintubation strictures

Low-grade malignancy
- Carcinoid

Malignant
- Lung
- Lymphoma
- Esophageal
- Thyroid

Benign
- Fungal infection
- Reactive lymphadenopathy
- Bronchomalacia
- Mediastinal fibrosis
- Vascular compression
- Goiter

Evaluation

A grossly abnormal radiograph with a large central parenchymal mass or mediastinal mass/adenopathy causing tracheal narrowing or deviation raises concern for airway patency. Often, abnormalities become more evident on the lateral x-ray view.

CT scan of the neck and chest better defines airway anatomy (54,56). In medically stable patients, pulmonary function testing (including spirometry and flow-volume loops) may be an inexpensive and noninvasive method to identify upper airway obstruction. Often, such testing can determine if the obstructing lesion is intrinsic or extrinsic. A more complete evaluation, with potential for tissue biopsy, includes direct visualization with laryngoscopy or bronchoscopy.

Management

Patients who have airway obstruction because of primary tracheal or laryngeal malignancies or benign strictures/lesions should be referred to the appropriate specialist (otolaryngologist, oncologist, and/or radiation oncologist) for evaluation and possible definitive therapy. Palliative therapeutic options (Table 25.3) for airway management in patients who are not candidates for definitive therapeutic procedures include airway stents, thermal treatments, cryotherapy, brachytherapy, photodynamic therapy (PDT), and tracheostomy. Patients with either obstructions that are laryngeal or high in the tracheobronchial tree may require tracheostomy to maintain airway patency.

Management of Intrinsic Obstruction

Any palliative therapy necessitates an adequate diameter for passage of a bronchoscope while maintaining adequate oxygenation and ventilation. For large exophytic intraluminal masses, *rigid bronchoscopy* with a *microdebrider* can be used selectively to "core out" the obstructing tumor (54,57–59). In one series (58), 51 of 56 patients had significant improvement in airway obstruction after bronchoscopic "core out," and only 2 patients required a repeat procedure.

Another option for palliative resection of intrinsic obstructing lesions of the large airways are thermal (heat) treatments such as *laser endobronchial resection* (56), *contact electrocautery*, or *argon plasma coagulation (APC)* (59). Most patients demonstrate relief of symptoms and/or reexpansion of

TABLE 25.3 SELECT TREATMENT OPTIONS FOR CENTRAL OBSTRUCTING MALIGNANT AIRWAY LESIONS

Intrinsic	Extrinsic
	External beam radiation
Mechanical debulking (microdebrider)	Stent
Thermal therapy (laser, electrocautery, APC) Stent Cryotherapy	
Brachytherapy External beam radiation	
Photodynamic therapy	

Combination of treatment plans is often necessary.

the obstructed lung. In one study, it was found to be a fair alternative to tracheostomy (60).

Bronchoscopic brachytherapy involves the placement of a radiation source near an endobronchial tumor. This therapy can improve symptoms of dyspnea and hemoptysis in up to 90% of patients with stable airway disease (61).

PDT is another option for the obstructed airway secondary to a malignant lesion. Studies have found PDT to be effective in treating endobronchial tumors (62,63). Complications from PDT can include airway edema and mucous plugging with atelectasis.

Freezing endoluminal tumor through *cryotherapy* is another option to palliate airway obstruction. A major drawback to brachytherapy or PDT is the lack of immediate tumor response (58,64).

Airway stents may also be used to treat intrinsic obstruction. There are various types of stents, including self-expanding metallic stents (SEMS) and Silastic (silicone) stents (59).

Management of Extrinsic Obstruction

Over the last two decades, insertion of *airway stents* has gained popularity has an effective palliative treatment for extrinsic compression. The most impressive benefit is in the immediate palliation of airway obstruction on placement of the stent. Figure 25.4 gives an algorithm for the management of central airway obstruction.

STRIDOR

Stridor is loud, harsh breathing, noticed particularly on inspiration, generated from obstructed airflow in the upper airway and large intrathoracic central airways. Treatment depends on the location of the obstruction and etiology. When evaluating patients presenting with stridor, it is useful to consider the airway as three zones (64–66): the *supraglottic zone* (nose, oral cavity, pharynx, and supraglottic larynx), the *extrathoracic tracheal zone* (glottis and subglottis), and the *intrathoracic tracheal zone*. Stridor originating from the supraglottic zone tends to occur on inspiration. Lesions of the extrathoracic tracheal zone tend to produce biphasic stridor (on both inspiration and expiration). Stridor from the intrathoracic tracheal zone may be more expiratory, often mistook for wheezing and distal airways. Some causes of stridor are listed in Table 25.4.

Evaluation

If a patient presents in severe respiratory distress with inadequate oxygenation or ventilation, establishment of an airway comes first. In the stable patient, history may help determine the cause. Gradual onset of symptoms over weeks or months, especially if accompanied by constitutional symptoms, may suggest neoplasm. Stridor manifesting for hours to days, especially in a febrile patient, is suspicious for infectious etiology (e.g., epiglottitis, croup, or abscess).

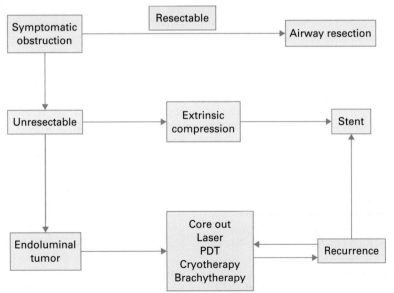

Algorithm for management of malignant central airway obstruction

Figure 25.4 Algorithm for the management of central airway obstruction. PDT, photodynamic therapy. (Adapted from Wood D. Management of malignant tracheobronchial obstruction. *Surg Clin North Am.* 2002;82(3):640:Figure 6.)

TABLE 25.4 CAUSES OF STRIDOR

Infection
Tracheitis: bacterial or viral
Epiglottitis
Abscess: peritonsillar or retropharyngeal
Viral laryngotracheobronchitis

Neoplasm
See Table 25.3

Congenital
Laryngomalacia
Tracheomalacia/tracheal stenosis
Vocal cord cysts/paralysis
Webs

Trauma
Facial
Ingestion
Inhalation injury

Postintubation
Airway fracture
Postsurgical

Neurologic
Central nervous system malformation
Hypoxic encephalopathy

Other
Foreign bodies (airway and esophageal)
Psychogenic
Exercise

A history of previous prolonged or traumatic intubation may suggest subglottic stenosis (67).

Physical examination demonstrates loud, noisy breathing. Respiratory rate, depth of respiration, use of accessory muscles of respiration, level of alertness, and evidence of cyanosis should be evaluated. Intense pain or inability to handle oral secretions may suggest peritonsillar abscess, retropharyngeal hematoma or abscess, epiglottitis, or foreign body. Crepitation on airway palpation suggests subcutaneous emphysema. A displaced trachea or firm mass could indicate tumor or goiter. Lymphadenopathy may suggest neoplasm.

Radiologic studies of the neck and chest can be obtained, but CT scans will provide more definitive anatomic information. Spirometry with flow volume loops may be beneficial in the evaluation of stridor as there are certain characteristics on these loops that are consistent with fixed upper airway obstructions.

Management

Stridor secondary to infectious etiologies requires treatment with appropriate antimicrobial therapy depending on the suspected cause of the stridor (epiglottitis, pharyngitis, tracheitis, croup). Several pharmacologic therapies are available to stabilize the stridorous patient who is clinically decompensated. *Heliox*, a mixture of helium and oxygen available in different proportions, has been useful in improving oxygenation, ventilation, and decreasing work of breathing in patients with stridor from various etiologies (68–72), including status asthmaticus, postextubation edema, and extrinsic compression from tumor. Although somewhat nonspecific, intravenous *corticosteroids* can be beneficial. *Racemic epinephrine* may be used, especially for postextubation stridor (64).

Although no specific trials comment on this, in more extreme cases, NIPPV may decrease the work of breathing and overcome large airway obstruction, although currently no studies have evaluated the efficacy of this treatment. Finally, endotracheal intubation or tracheostomy must be considered in appropriate clinical situations.

BRONCHOSPASM

Bronchospasm, defined as abnormal narrowing of the airways, is usually episodic and can occur in a variety of pulmonary disorders. Patients complain of dyspnea, wheezing, chest tightness, or pressure, although occasionally cough is the only symptom. Exacerbation of symptoms may frequently occur in the early hours of the morning, when the bronchial tone is normally increased. Auscultation of the chest reveals wheezing, usually with prolonged expiration.

Evaluation

A patient may have multiple etiologies of bronchospasm. The differential diagnosis includes asthma, chronic obstructive pulmonary disease (COPD), upper/large airway obstruction (see previous Section on Tracheobronchial Obstruction), congestive heart failure, gastroesophageal reflux disease (GERD), bronchiectasis, bronchiolitis (infectious or inflammatory, medication induced), lymphangitic tumor spread, or, rarely, pulmonary embolism.

Chest radiographs may demonstrate bronchial wall thickening, flattened diaphragms, and increased retrosternal air space, consistent with hyper-expansion and air trapping and would support the diagnosis of asthma or COPD. An unchanged chest radiograph or one with atelectasis or small pleural effusion should alert the clinician to possible pulmonary embolism.

Therapy

Relief of bronchospasm is aimed at dilation of distal airways and reducing inflammation. Many pharmacologic agents are available to treat bronchospasm (Table 25.5). *β-Agonists* promote airway smooth muscle relaxation, increase mucociliary clearance, and increase the secretion of electrolytes by the airways. Side effects include tremor, tachycardia, palpitations, hypokalemia, and hyperglycemia. In general, to prevent tachyphylaxis, patients

TABLE 25.5 SELECT THERAPY FOR BRONCHOSPASM

Medications

β-Agonists

Albuterol (Proventil and Ventolin)	MDI	Two to three puffs up to q.i.d.
	Neb	0.5–0.75 mL in 2.5-mL saline q.i.d.
Levalbuterol (Xopenex)	MDI	One to two puffs q.i.d.
Pirbuterol	MDI	Two to three puffs q.i.d.

Anticholinergics

Ipratropium bromide (Atrovent)	MDI	Two puffs up to q.i.d.
	Neb	500 µg in 2.5-mL saline t.i.d. to q.i.d.
Tiotropium (Spiriva)	DPI	18 µg or one capsule once daily

Nonsteroidal anti-inflammatory

Cromolyn sodium (Intal)	MDI	Two to four puffs b.i.d. to q.i.d.
	Neb	1–2 mL (10–20 mg) b.i.d. to q.i.d.
Nedocromil sodium (Tilade)	MDI	Two puffs b.i.d. to q.i.d.

Long-acting β-agonist

Formoterol (Foradil)	DPI	12 µg b.i.d.
Salmeterol (Serevent)	DPI	50 µg b.i.d.

Inhaled corticosteroids

Beclomethasone (QVAR)	MDI	40, 80 µg one to two inhalations b.i.d.
Budesonide (Pulmicort)	Neb	0.25–0.50 mg b.i.d.
	DPI	Two to four inhalations b.i.d.
Flunisolide (Aerobid)	MDI	Two to four inhalations b.i.d.
Fluticasone (Flovent)	DPI	44, 110, 220 µg strengths, one to two inhalations b.i.d.
Mometasone (Asmanex)	Spray DPI	One to two inhalations b.i.d.
Triamcinolone (Azmacort)	MDI	Two to four puffs t.i.d. to q.i.d.

Combination medications

Advair (Fluticasone/Salmeterol)	DPI	100/50, 250/50, 500/50 One inhalation b.i.d.
Combivent (Albuterol/Ipratropium)	MDI	One to two inhalations q.i.d. 3 mL q.i.d.

Leukotriene receptor antagonists

Montelukast (Singulair)	Oral	10 mg daily
Zafirlukast (Accolate)	Oral	20 mg b.i.d.
Zileuton (Zyflo)	Oral	600 mg up to q.i.d. monitor LFTs

MDI, metered-dose inhaler; Neb, through nebulizer; DPI, dry powder inhaler; LFTs, liver function tests.

are advised not to use β-agonists more than four to five times a day. The Global Initiative for Asthma (GINA) does not recommend asthma treatment with short-acting β_2-agonists (SABA) alone, as this treatment does not protect patients from severe exacerbations. Instead, GINA recommends that all adults and adolescents with asthma should receive either symptom-driven (in mild asthma) or daily low-dose ICS-containing controller treatment to reduce the risk of serious exacerbations (73).

Anticholinergic agents act by decreasing the parasympathetic bronchoconstriction of the airways. Ipratropium bromide and dry powder tiotropium are the anticholinergic agents available for inhalational use in the United States. Because of studies showing that ipratropium bromide may be more effective than β-agonists in promoting bronchodilation in patients with COPD, it is now the first agent used in maintenance therapy in COPD with persistent airway obstruction (74–76).

Corticosteroids are widely used in the treatment of bronchospasm (77). Even patients with mild to moderate symptoms may benefit from inhaled corticosteroids. Patients should be cautioned that these medications must be used regularly and may take weeks for therapeutic effect and should always be combined with a short-acting agent for breakthrough relief. Patients with more serious symptoms or those in respiratory distress may require systemic corticosteroids. Besides corticosteroids, other pharmacologic *anti-inflammatory agents* may be employed to stem the inflammatory pathways leading to bronchospasm. Cromolyn sulfate and nedocromil sodium appear to work as mast cell stabilizers. *Leukotriene receptor antagonists* work to block additional components of inflammation and allow mild bronchodilation (77,78).

HEMOPTYSIS

Hemoptysis, the expectoration of blood originating in the lung, can range in presentation from blood-tinged sputum to massive hemoptysis (defined as blood loss of 400 to 600 mL/d). While massive hemoptysis occurs in fewer than 5% of cases, it carries a mortality rate of up to 85% if surgical intervention is not possible (79,80). Given such stakes, management of hemoptysis necessitates careful consideration of etiology and severity in the context of the patient's functional status and goals. Table 25.6 lists causes of hemoptysis.

Diagnosis

A diagnosis of hemoptysis is established by localization of bleeding to the lower respiratory tract. Nasopharyngeal, laryngeal, or gastrointestinal tract bleeding may be difficult to clinically distinguish from frank hemoptysis. Bleeding from these sources may result in bloody cough, which can be misinterpreted as hemoptysis. A thorough examination of the nasopharynx, larynx, and upper gastrointestinal tract should be included in evaluation.

The next step is bleeding site localization within the pulmonary tree. A chest x-ray is often helpful in revealing a tumor or abscess. Bronchoscopy may allow direct visualization of the source or lung segment and allows tissue sampling for cytologic, histologic, and microbiologic testing (81,82). CT remains superior to bronchoscopy in identifying bronchiectasis, lung abscess, aspergilloma, and distal parenchymal abnormalities.

Management

The severity of hemoptysis determines the pace of workup and management. A review of a decade of experience at an academic medical center, the general mortality rate was 9% if blood loss was <1,000 mL/24 hours, but it was 58% if the blood loss was >1,000 mL/24 hours (79). Here, a malignant cause for hemoptysis >1,000 mL/24 hours increased the mortality rate to 80%.

TABLE 25.6 CAUSES OF HEMOPTYSIS

Pulmonary	Traumatic
Bronchitis	Blunt/penetrating chest injury
Bronchiectasis	Ruptured bronchus
Pulmonary embolism	**Systemic disease**
Cystic fibrosis	Goodpasture's syndrome
Infectious	Vasculitis
Lung abscess	Systemic lupus erythematosus
Mycetoma	**Drugs/toxins**
Necrotizing pneumonia	Aspirin
Viral	Anticoagulation
Fungal	Penicillamine
Parasitic	Solvents
Septic embolism	Crack cocaine
Cardiac	**Drugs/toxins**
Mitral stenosis	Aspirin
Congestive heart failure	Anticoagulation
Neoplastic	Penicillamine
Bronchogenic carcinoma	Solvents
Bronchial adenoma	Crack cocaine
Endobronchial hamartoma	**Miscellaneous**
Metastatic disease	Foreign body
Tracheal tumors	Endometriosis
Hematologic	Broncholithiasis
Coagulopathy	Cryptogenic hemoptysis
Platelet dysfunction	**Iatrogenic**
Thrombocytopenia	Lung biopsy
Disseminated intravascular coagulation	Pulmonary artery catheterization
Vascular	Lymphangiography
Pulmonary hypertension	Transtracheal aspirate
Arteriovenous malformation	
Aortic aneurysm	

Modified from Cahill BC, Ingbar DH. Massive hemoptysis: assessment and management. *Clin Chest Med.* 1994;15:147, with permission.

Bronchoscopy

If bronchoscopy identifies the site of bleeding, concomitant local therapies may be employed. A pulmonary tamponade balloon can be inflated in the segmental bronchus leading to the site of bleeding, allowing time for stabilization of the patient and potentially more definitive therapy (83). Bleeding from visible lesions in the trachea and proximal bronchi can be coagulated with a laser.

Radiotherapy

External beam radiation for 6 to 7 weeks is usually employed to attempt a cure for inoperable nonsmall cell carcinoma. In the palliative setting, therapy is delivered in the shortest time possible, with lower doses to achieve symptom relief while minimizing side effects. *Endobronchial brachytherapy* with ^{192}Ir is another alternative, alone or in combination with bronchoscopic laser therapy. In recent years, high dose rates have been favored to decrease the time of treatment and permit outpatient rather than inpatient therapy. Potential complications of brachytherapy include mucositis, fistula formation, and fatal hemoptysis (84).

Angiographic and Surgical Intervention

After angiographic identification of the vessels in question, a variety of agents (e.g., Gelfoam, polyvinyl alcohol particles, and metallic coils) can be injection selectively to stem bleeding. Reported success rates vary between 75% and 90%, with a rebleeding rate of 15% to 30% (85). The definitive therapy for massive hemoptysis is resection of the diseased portion of the lung, but this intervention depends on specific anatomy and residual lung function, as well as overall comorbidities and functional status.

Other Modalities

Other modalities can be used to manage hemoptysis of varying degrees, including neodymium yttrium aluminum garnet (Nd:YAG) laser photocoagulation, electrocautery, cryotherapy, APC, and PDT.

Exsanguination and End-of-Life Care

If oxygenation is compromised or the patient continues to bleed vigorously, endotracheal intubation may become necessary. Goals of care should ideally be clarified before such extreme situations. Deciding to intubate a patient with a terminal illness can be challenging. If bleeding can be localized and controlled quickly, a short period of ventilator support may be quite reasonable if it allows for improved quality of life. This may be unlikely for a patient in the later stages of a terminal illness, especially in the setting of massive hemoptysis. In the setting of fatal hemoptysis, exsanguination usually occurs within seconds to minutes with a rapid loss of consciousness. In such situations, intravenous opioids and benzodiazepines can be administered to control dyspnea and anxiety. Attention and emotional support need to be paid to the family members as well. While use of continuous oral suction and judicious placement of dark towels or blankets may help obscure the blood loss, many family members may be disturbed by frank blood loss associated with exsanguination.

BRONCHORRHEA/SECRETIONS

Bronchial secretion is observed in 44% of terminally ill cancer patients and can cause significant distress for both patients and family members.

Etiology

Primary lung cancer, pneumonia, and dysphagia are significantly associated with the development of bronchial secretions (86). The hypothesized pathophysiology is the inability to expectorate the products in the respiratory system. Classical "death rattle" (type 1) corresponds to a combined syndrome of aspiration due to dysphagia and inability to expectorate. Theoretically, this is caused by aspiration of saliva related to terminal consciousness disturbance and/or neurologic complications and antimuscarinic medications are assumed to be effective when the products are saliva. "Pseudo" death rattle (type II) is a syndrome of inability to expectorate increased pulmonary secretion from tumor, infection, edema, and bleeding. This type does not always occur near death and antimuscarinic medications are assumed to be less effective.

Clinical Presentation

Bronchial secretion is defined as sounds audible at the bedside produced by movement of secretions in the hypopharynx or the bronchial tree in association with respiration. Morita et al., as part of a prospective observational study to investigate the incidence and underlying etiologies of bronchial secretion, proposed criteria for classifying the severity: inaudible (*Grade 0*), audible only very close to the patient (*Grade 1*), clearly audible at the end of the bed in a quiet room (*Grade 2*), and clearly audible at about 6 m or at the door of the room (*Grade 3*) (86). Bronchial secretion is regarded as present when patients have a score of Grade 1 or higher.

Treatment

Treatment of bronchorrhea in palliative care is limited by a lack of clinical trials. Antimuscarinic medications are used for as many as 73% of patients with bronchial secretions with 79% effectiveness, but 10% of all dying patients have refractory secretion or received palliative sedation therapy (86). A 2010 *Cochrane Review* of four studies comparing atropine, glycopyrrolate, hyoscine butylbromide, and scopolamine (hyoscine hydrobromide) found no conclusive evidence of one drug being superior to another (87).

COUGH

Etiology

A protective, complex reflex that helps clear the airways of foreign material or excessive secretions, cough is common in patients with advanced malignancy. Etiologies may stem from the malignancy itself—such as endobronchial tumor burden, pericardial disease, vocal cord paralysis, or aspiration—or from its treatments—such as radiation pneumonitis or chemotherapy-induced interstitial lung disease (88). Additionally, patients with underlying cancer may have the same causes of cough found in the general population. The most common etiologies of chronic cough remain upper airway cough syndrome (previously postnasal drip syndrome), asthma, and GERD (89,90).

A detailed history and physical examination are important to determine the cause of chronic cough (91). Chest radiographs should be obtained early in the evaluation (92). In patients who chronically produce sputum or in whom there is a suspicion of interstitial lung disease, a high-resolution chest CT scan may be helpful. Notably, among patients with interstitial lung disease, up to 10% to 15% have normal chest radiograph.

If the evaluation points toward sinus etiology, radiographs and CT scans may be indicated. Some experts recommend a trial of antihistamine decongestants before pursuing sinus radiographic studies (93). Spirometry, before and after inhaled bronchodilators and methacholine challenge, evaluates for asthma or chronic obstructive lung disease. Barium esophagography or 24-hour esophageal pH monitoring can be used to evaluate for GERD. Finally, bronchoscopy may be considered to evaluate for occult foreign body aspiration or small endobronchial lesions, although studies have found this to be of low yield (89).

Management

Treatment of cough is most successful when tailored to a specific etiology (asthma, GERD, upper airway cough syndrome, etc.). In patients for whom no cause is found for their cough or it is due to airway involvement with tumor, empiric pharmacologic therapy with a β-agonists or corticosteroid is reasonable.

Opioids continue to be used as effective antitussives (94,95). To date, there is no evidence of superiority of one opioid over another for this indication. Codeine, 15 to 30 mg every 4 to 6 hours, is a reasonable starting dose, with titration upward to control symptoms if the side effects are tolerable. Nonopioid cough preparations, including guaifenesin, dextromethorphan, and benzonatate, may be tried, although studies show them to be only weakly beneficial. Studies of over-the-counter antitussive preparations demonstrate wide variability in efficacy (95–97).

Lidocaine appears to have an antitussive effect when inhaled through a nebulizer, likely acting on afferent C fibers in the larynx and trachea (88,94). When administered, patients should be cautioned regarding anesthesia of the oropharynx and larynx and potential buccal injuries or aspiration. There are currently no specific guidelines for this treatment.

Noninvasive Positive Pressure Ventilation

NIPPV can be used to palliate dyspnea in terminally ill patients. The cost and experience needed to initiate NIPPV generally limits its use to the hospital setting, although it can be used at home or a hospice facility provided adequate nursing, respiratory therapy, and physician support are available to use it safely. Continuing NIPPV for palliation in patients/families who are already comfortable managing home NIPPV (e.g., for COPD or amyotrophic lateral sclerosis) can be practical in the home or hospice facility setting, if it is consistent with the care goals (98). A shared approach between the patient, family, and medical team, in which clinical information is exchanged and patient preferences are elucidated is vital for decision-making. Table 25.7 lists some helpful phrases that can be used when communicating with the patient and family about the goals of care using NIPPV.

Monitoring of pulse oximetry and arterial blood gases are not needed for patients using NIPPV at the end of life for symptom control. Rather, the effect of NIPPV should be assessed based on improvement of dyspnea and decrease in respiratory rate. For a more detailed discussion on the practical aspects and settings of NIPPV, please see the Chapter on *Palliative Care in the ICU*.

NIPPV should be discontinued if it does not provide relief from dyspnea within an hour of the maximally tolerated setting, once a patient is no longer alert, or at any point when it is no longer meeting a patient's goals. If the patient does not tolerate the mask, or feels claustrophobic, a small dose of an opioid or benzodiazepine can be administered to alleviate anxiety. If the patient is still uncomfortable, then NIPPV should be stopped;

TABLE 25.7 HELPFUL PHRASES TO USE IN COMMUNICATING WITH FAMILY ABOUT THE GOALS OF CARE USING NONINVASIVE POSITIVE PRESSURE VENTILATION

	Primary goals of care	Potentially helpful phrases to clarify goals with family and/or patient
Category 1	Restore health; will use intubation if necessary and indicated	We can use the mask (NIPPV) to try to get him over this without having to put the breathing tube in his throat. If this does not improve things or is too uncomfortable for him, we will use the breathing tube.
Category 2	Restore health without using endotracheal intubation and without causing unacceptable discomfort	We can use the mask (NIPPV) to try to get him over this. He has been very clear that he does not want the breathing tube, so if the mask does not improve things or is too uncomfortable for him, we will plan to stop using it and focus on keeping him comfortable. In this situation, it would mean that he would likely die, although we would make it as comfortable as possible for him.
Category 3	Maximize comfort while minimizing adverse effects of opiates	It may be reasonable to try the mask (NIPPV) to see if it makes him more comfortable. We know that it would not fix the underlying problem, but it might improve his breathing temporarily. If it does not make him more comfortable, we will stop it and try something else so his death will be as comfortable as possible.

NIPPV, noninvasive positive pressure ventilation.
Adapted from Curtis JR, Cook DJ, Sinuff T, et al. Noninvasive positive pressure ventilation in critical and palliative care settings: understanding the goals of therapy. *Crit Care Med*. 2007;35(3):932-939.

after revisiting goals of care, other symptom management avenues may be pursued (98).

REFERENCES

1. Light RW, MacGregor MI, Luchsinger PC, et al. Pleural effusions: the diagnostic separation of transudates and exudates. *Ann Intern Med*. 1972;77:507-513.
2. Tinney WS, Olsen AM. The significance of fluid in the pleural space: a study of 274 cases. *J Thorac Surg*. 1943;14:248-252.
3. Hausheer FH, Yarbro JW. Diagnosis and treatment of malignant pleural effusion. *Semin Oncol*. 1985;12:54-75.
4. Matthay RA, Coppage L, Shaw C, et al. Malignancies metastatic to the pleura. *Invest Radiol*. 1990;23:601-619.
5. Fenton KN, Richardson JD. Diagnosis and management of malignant pleural effusions. *Am J Surg*. 1995;170:69-74.
6. Woodring JH. Recognition of a pleural effusion on supine radiographs: how much fluid is required? *Am J Roentgenol*. 1984;142:59-64.
7. Doust BD, Baum JK, Maklad NF, et al. Ultrasonic evaluation of pleural opacities. *Radiology*. 1975;114:135-140.
8. Ravin CE. Thoracentesis of located pleural effusions using grey scale ultrasonic guidance. *Chest*. 1977;71:666-668.
9. Hasan A, Makhlouf H, Mahmoud A. Discrimination between pleural thickening and minimal pleural effusion using color doppler chest ultrasonography. *Eur Respir J*. 2013;42:P2256.
10. Ratliff JL, Chavez CM, Jamchuk A, et al. Re-expansion pulmonary edema. *Chest*. 1973;64:634-636.
11. Health and Public Policy Committee, American College of Physicians. Diagnostic thoracentesis and pleural biopsy in pleural effusions. *Ann Intern Med*. 1985;103:799-802.
12. Leff A, Hopewell PC, Costello J. Pleural effusion from malignancy. *Ann Intern Med*. 1978;88:532-537.
13. LoCicero J III. Thoracoscopic management of malignant pleural effusion. *Ann Thorac Surg*. 1993;36:641-643.
14. Chernow B, Sahn SA. Carcinomatous involvement of the pleura. *Am J Med*. 1977;63:693-702.
15. Roy RH, Can DT, Payne WS. The problem of chylothorax. *Mayo Clin Proc*. 1967;42:437-467.
16. Van de Molengraft FJ, Vooijs GP. Survival of patients with malignancy-associated effusion. *Acta Cytol*. 1989;33:911-916.
17. Ruckdeschel JC. Management of malignant pleural effusion: an overview. *Semin Oncol*. 1988;15:24-28.
18. Olopade OI, Ultmann JE. Malignant effusions. *CA Cancer J Clin*. 1991;41:166-179.
19. Anderson CB, Philpott GW, Ferguson TB. The treatment of malignant pleural effusions. *Cancer*. 1974;33:916-922.
20. Patz EF Jr, McAdams HP, Erasmus JJ, et al. Sclerotherapy for malignant pleural effusions: a prospective randomized trial of bleomycin vs doxycycline with small bore catheter drainage. *Chest*. 1998;113(5):1305-1311.
21. Pllak JS, Burdge CM, Rosenblatt M, et al. Treatment of malignant pleural effusions with tunneled long-term drainage catheters. *J Vasc Interv Radiol*. 2001;12(2):201-208.
22. Putnam JB Jr, Light RW, Rodriguez RM, et al. A randomized comparison of indwelling pleural catheter and doxycycline pleurodesis in the management of malignant pleural effusions. *Cancer*. 1999;86(10):1992-1996.
23. Robinson LA, Fleming WH, Galbraith TA. Intrapleural doxycycline control of malignant pleural effusions. *Ann Thorac Surg*. 1993;55:1115-1122.
24. Robinson LA, Moulton AL, Fleming WH, et al. Intrapleural fibrinolytic treatment of multiloculated thoracic empyemas. *Ann Thorac Surg*. 1994;57:803-814.
25. Pass HI. Treatment of malignant pleural and pericardial effusion. In: DeVita VT Jr, Hellman S, Rosenberg SA, eds. *Cancer: Principles and Practice of Oncology*. 4th ed. Philadelphia, PA: JB Lippincott Co; 1993:2246-2253.
26. Hawkins JW, Vacek JL. What constitutes definitive therapy of malignant pericardial effusion? "Medical" versus surgical treatment. *Am Heart J*. 1989;118:428-432.
27. Theologides A. Neoplastic cardiac tamponade. *Semin Oncol*. 1978;3:181-192.

28. Thurber DL, Edwards JE, Achor RWP. Secondary malignant tumors of the pericardium. *Circulation.* 1962;26:228-241.

29. Lokich JJ. The management of malignant pericardial effusions. *JAMA.* 1973;224:1401-1404.

30. Buzaid AC, Garewal HS, Greenberg BR. Managing malignant pericardial effusion. *West J Med.* 1989;150: 174-179.

31. Spodick DH. Macrophysiology, microphysiology, and anatomy of the pericardium: a synopsis. *Am Heart J.* 1992;124:1046-1051.

32. Posner MR, Cohen GI, Skarin AT. Pericardial disease in patients with cancer—the differentiation of malignant from idiopathic and radiation-induced pericarditis. *Am J Med.* 1981;71:407-413.

33. Spodick DH. The normal and diseased pericardium: current concepts of pericardial physiology, diagnosis and treatment. *J Am Coll Cardiol.* 1983;1:240-251.

34. Beck CS. Acute and chronic compression of the heart. *Am Heart J.* 1937;14:515-525.

35. Stolz L, Valenzuela J, Situ-LaCasse E, et al. Clinical and historical features of emergency department patients with pericardial effusions. *World J Emerg Med.* 2017;8(1):29-33.

36. Eisenberg MJ, Oken NK, Guerrero S, et al. Prognostic value of echocardiography in hospitalized patients with pericardial effusion. *Am J Cardiol.* 1992;70:934-939.

37. Reyes VC, Strinden C, Banerji M. The role of cytology in neoplastic cardiac tamponade. *Acta Cytol.* 1982;26:299-302.

38. Miller JI Jr. Surgical management of pericardial disease. In: Schlant RC, Alexander RW, O'Roiurke RA, et al., eds. *The Heart, Arteries and Veins.* 8th ed. New York, NY: McGraw-Hill; 1994:1675-1680.

39. Press OW, Livingston R. Management of malignant pericardial effusion and tamponade. *JAMA.* 1987;257:1088-1092.

40. Palatianos GM, Thurer RJ, Pompeo MQ, et al. Clinical experience with subxiphoid drainage of pericardial effusions. *Ann Thorac Surg.* 1989;48:381-385.

41. Cham WC, Freiman AH, Carstens HB, et al. Radiation therapy of cardiac and pericardial metastases. *Radiology.* 1975;114:701-704.

42. Sanchez-Armegol A, Rodriguez-Panadero F. Survival and talc pleurodesis in metastatic pleural carcinoma, revisited. *Chest.* 1993;104:1482-1485.

43. Ruckdeschel JC, Chang P, Martin RG, et al. Radiation-related pericardial effusions in patients with Hodgkin's disease. *Medicine (Baltimore).* 1975;54:245-270.

44. Zwischenberger JB, Bradford DW. Management of malignant pericardial effusion. In: Pass HI, Mitchell JB, Johnson DH, et al., eds. *Lung Cancer: Principles and Practice.* Philadelphia, PA: Lippincott–Raven; 1996:655-662.

45. Moores DWO, Allen KB, Faber LP, et al. Subxiphoid pericardial drainage for pericardial tamponade. *J Thorac Cardiovasc Surg.* 1995;109:546-552.

46. Liu H-P, Chang C-H, Lin PJ, et al. Thoracoscopic management of effusive pericardial disease: indications and technique. *Ann Thorac Surg.* 1994;58:1695-1697.

47. Wang N, Feikes JR, Mogensen T, et al. Pericardioperitoneal shunt: an alternative treatment for malignant pericardial effusion. *Ann Thorac Surg.* 1994;57:289-292.

48. Ziskind AA, Pearce AC, Lemmon CC, et al. Percutaneous balloon pericardiotomy for the treatment of cardiac tamponade and large pericardial effusions: description of techniques and report of first 50 cases. *J Am Coll Cardiol.* 1993;21:1-5.

49. Lewis MA, Hendrickson AW, Moynihan TJ. Oncologic emergencies: pathophysiology, presentation, diagnosis, and treatment. *Cancer J Clin.* 2011;61:287-314.

50. Kim HJ, Kim HS, Chung SH. CT Diagnosis of superior vena cava syndrome: importance of collateral vessels. *Am J Roentgenol.* 1993;161(3):539-542.

51. Schraufnagel DE, Hill R, Leech JA, Pare JA. Superior vena caval obstruction. Is it a medical emergency? *Am J Med.* 1981;70:1169-1174.

52. Ganeshan A, Hon LQ, Warakaulle DR, Morgan R, Uberoi R. Superior vena caval stenting for SVC obstruction: current status. *Eur J Radiol.* 2009;71:343-349.

53. Guijarro EJF, Anton RF, Colmenarejo RA, et al. Superior vena cava syndrome with central venous catheter for chemotherapy treated successfully with fibrinolysis. *Clin Transl Oncol.* 2007;9:198-200.

54. Wood D. Management of malignant tracheobronchial obstruction. *Surg Clin North Am.* 2002;82:621-642.

55. Braman SS, Whitcomb ME. Endobronchial metastasis. *Arch Intern Med.* 1995;135:543.

56. Chen K, Vawn J, Wenker O. Malignant airway obstruction: recognition and management. *J Emerg Med.* 1998;16(1):83-92.

57. Mathisen DJ. Surgical management of tracheobronchial disease. *Clin Chest Med.* 1992;13:151.

58. Mathisen DJ, Grillo HC. Endoscopic relief of malignant airway obstruction. *Ann Thorac Surg.* 1989;48:469.

59. Mudambi L, Miller R, Eapen GA. Malignant central airway obstruction. *J Thorac Dis.* 2017;9(suppl 10): S1087-S1110.

60. Paleri V, Stafford FW, Sammut MS. Laser debulking in malignant upper airway obstruction. *Head Neck.* 2005;27:296-301.

61. Marsh BR. Bronchoscopic brachytherapy. *Laryngoscope.* 1989;99:1.

62. Diaz-Jimenez J, Martinez-Ballaren J, Llunell A, et al. Efficacy and safety of photodynamic therapy versus Nd-YAG laser resection in NSCLC with airway obstruction. *Eur Respir J.* 1999;14:800-855.

63. McCaughan J, Williams T. Photodynamic therapy for endobronchial malignant disease: a prospective fourteen year study. *J Thorac Cardiovasc Surg.* 1997;114:940-946.

64. Lee P, Temm M, Chhajed P. Advances in bronchoscopy—therapeutic bronchoscopy. *J Assoc Physicians India.* 2004;52:905-914.

65. Santamaria JP, Schafermeyer R. Stridor: a review. *Pediatr Emerg Care.* 1992;8:229.

66. Stool SE. Stridor. *Int Anesthesiol Clin.* 1988;26:19.

67. O'Hollaren MT, Everts EC. Evaluating the patient with stridor. *Ann Allergy.* 1991;67:301.

68. Curtis JL, Mahlmeister M, Fink JB, et al. Helium–oxygen gas therapy use and availability for the emergency treatment of inoperable airway obstruction. *Chest.* 1986;90:455.

69. Orr JB. Helium–oxygen gas mixtures in the management of patients with airway obstruction. *Ear Nose Throat J.* 1988;67:866.

70. Skrinskas GJ, Hyland RH, Hutcheon MA. Using helium–oxygen mixtures in the management of acute airway obstruction. *Can Med Assoc J.* 1983;R8:555.

71. Gluck E, Onorato DJ, Castriotta R. Helium–oxygen mixtures in intubated patients with status asthmaticus and respiratory acidosis. *Chest.* 1990;98:693.

72. Gupta V, Cheifetz I. Heliox administration in the pediatric intensive care unit: an evidence-based review. *Pediatr Crit Care Med.* 2005;6:204.

73. Global Initiative for Asthma. *Pocket Guide for Asthma Management and Prevention (for Adults and Children Older than 5 Years).* https://ginasthma.org/wp-content/uploads/2019/04/GINA-2019-main-Pocket-Guide-wms.pdf. Accessed November 10, 2019.

74. Tashkin DP, Ashutosh K, Bleecker ER, et al. Comparison of the anticholinergic bronchodilator ipratropium

bromide with metaproterenol in chronic obstructive pulmonary disease. *Am J Med.* 1986;81:81.

75. Marlin GE, Bush DE, Berent N. Comparison of ipratropium bromide and fenoterol in asthma and chronic bronchitis. *Br J Clin Pharmacol.* 1978;6:547.

76. Braun SR, Levy SF. Comparison of ipratropium bromide and albuterol in chronic obstructive lung disease: a three-center study. *Am J Med.* 1991;91(4):S28-S32.

77. National Asthma Education and Prevention Program. *Expert Panel Report 2.* Bethesda, MD: National Institute of Health, Publication No. 97–405; April 1997.

78. Kamada AK, Szefler SJ, Martin RJ, et al. Issues in the use of inhaled glucocorticoids. *Am J Respir Crit Care Med.* 1996;153:1739-1748.

79. Corey R, Hla KM. Major and massive hemoptysis: reassessment of conservative management. *Am J Med Sci.* 1987;294:301-309.

80. Thompson AB, Teschler H, Rennard SI. Pathogenesis, evaluation, and therapy for massive hemoptysis. *Clin Chest Med.* 1992;13:69-82.

81. Set PA, Flower CDR, Smith IE, et al. Hemoptysis: comparative study of the role of CT and fiberoptic bronchoscopy. *Radiology.* 1993;189:677-680.

82. McGuinness G, Beacher JR, Harkin TJ, et al. Hemoptysis: prospective high-resolution CT/bronchoscopic correlation. *Chest.* 1994;105:1155-1162.

83. Saw EC, Gottlieb LS, Yokayama T, et al. Flexible fiberoptic bronchoscopy and endobronchial tamponade in the management of massive hemoptysis. *Chest.* 1976;70: 589-591.

84. Khanavkar B, Stern P, Alberti W, et al. Complications associated with brachytherapy alone or with laser in lung cancer. *Chest.* 1991;99:1062-1065.

85. Menchini L, Remy-Jardin M, Faivre JB, et al. Cryptogenic haemoptysis in smokers: angiography and results of embolisation in 35 patients. *Eur Respir J.* 2009;34(5):1031

86. Morita T, Hyodo I, Yoshimi T, et al. Incidence and underlying etiologies of bronchial secretion in terminally ill cancer patients: a multicenter, prospective, observational study. *J Pain Symptom Manage.* 2004;27(6):533-539.

87. Wee B, Hillier R. Interventions for noisy breathing in patients near to death. *Cochrane Database Syst Rev.* 2008;(1):CD005177.

88. Cowcher K, Hank GW. Long-term management of respiratory symptoms in advanced cancer. *J Pain Symptom Manage.* 1990;5:320.

89. Poe RH, Israel RH, Utell MJ, et al. Chronic cough: bronchoscopy or pulmonary function testing? *Am Rev Respir Dis.* 1982;126:160.

90. Irwin RS, Curley FJ, French CL. Chronic cough. *Am Rev Respir Dis.* 1990;141:640.

91. Shuttair MF, Braun SR. Contemporary management of chronic persistent cough. *Mo Med.* 1992;89:795.

92. Irwin RS, Curley FJ. The treatment of cough. A comprehensive review. *Chest.* 1991;99:1477.

93. Pratter MR, Bartter T, Akers S, et al. An algorithmic approach to chronic cough. *Ann Intern Med.* 1993;119:977.

94. Fuller RW, Jackson DM. Physiology and treatment of cough. *Thorax.* 1990;45:425.

95. Irwin RS, Curley FJ, Bennett FM. Appropriate use of antitussives and protussives. A practical review. *Drugs.* 1993;46:80.

96. Irwin RS, Baumann MN, Bolser DC, et al. Diagnosis and management of cough: ACCP evidence-based clinical practice guidelines. *Chest.* 2006;129:1S-23S.

97. Smith MB, Feldman W. Over-the-counter cold medications. A critical review of clinical trials between 1950 and 1991. *JAMA.* 1993;269:2258.

98. Yeow ME, Szmuilowicz E. Practical aspects of using noninvasive positive pressure ventilation at the end of life #231. *J Palliat Med.* 2010;13(9):1150-1151.

26 Prevention, Assessment, and Management of Treatment-Induced Cardiac Disease in Cancer Patients

Krishna Upadhyaya, Sarah C. Hull, Ben A. Lin, Elizabeth Prsic, Mariana Henry, and Lauren A. Baldassarre

INTRODUCTION

During the last half century, the development of effective detection and treatment strategies for many malignancies has led to a significant population of cancer survivors (1). According to the Surveillance, Epidemiology and End Results Program (SEER) from the National Institutes of Health (NIH), it is estimated that approximately 67% of adults newly diagnosed with cancer will survive for 5 or more years beyond the time of diagnosis. Furthermore, in 2016, the NIH estimated that there were more than 15 million cancer survivors in the United States and that number is expected to grow to 20 million by 2026 (2). The impact of cancer and cancer treatment on the overall health of a survivor is substantial. Effects include organ damage and functional disabilities that occur as a consequence of the disease and/or the treatments. The recognition of these effects is increasing, and there is accumulating evidence available to guide the physician caring for these patients. Additionally, as a consequence of improved survival in cancer patients, they are reaching an age at which cardiovascular disease typically manifests, including myocardial ischemia and/or infarction, hypertension, congestive heart failure, and stroke. Long-term cancer survivors are at risk for a variety of cardiac sequelae.

The care of a patient with cardiovascular disease is often challenging and complex. Caring for a patient with a malignancy multiplies these complexities and requires strong collaboration and evidence-based decision-making. As the complexity of cancer therapeutics continues to rise, increasingly collaborative management of multiple comorbidities will be required. These treatments may have significant adverse effects on the cardiovascular system. As such, it becomes imperative for specialists to understand the prevention, identification, and treatment of cardiac disease in cancer patients in order to avoid or prevent adverse cardiovascular effects and provide optimal care and outcomes.

Cancer therapy–related cardiovascular toxicity traditionally has included cardiomyopathy

with or without overt congestive heart failure, endothelial dysfunction, and arrhythmias. While doxorubicin cardiomyopathy is the most studied form of chemotherapy-induced cardiotoxicity, newer classes of cancer treatments such as tyrosine kinase inhibitors (TKIs) and immune checkpoint inhibitors (ICIs) have been approved by the FDA within the last few decades and have been found to have cardiotoxic effects as well. Radiotherapy can also cause significant cardiac complications. Cancer patients represent a rapidly expanding patient population at risk for cardiovascular disease, potentially leading to an increase in cardiovascular-related mortality that may offset the advancements in cancer survival. This chapter will attempt to elucidate these challenges and provide a framework to approach these issues.

CANCER THERAPEUTICS–RELATED CARDIAC DYSFUNCTION

Definitions

Chemotherapy-related cardiotoxicity was originally described in the 1960s as toxicity observed with the use of anthracyclines in cancer therapy. In the 1970s, Von Hoff and colleagues described a dose-dependent toxicity, by defining a curve plotting the probability of developing congestive heart failure as a function of the cumulative dose of doxorubicin in approximately 4,000 patients who had received the drug on a 3-week administration schedule (3,4). They found that patients who received a cumulative dose of 400, 550, and 700 mg/m^2 had a 3%, 7%, and 18% incidence of cardiotoxicity, respectively. Cancer therapeutics–related cardiac dysfunction (CTRCD) has since been recognized as a major side effect of anthracyclines and other chemotherapeutic agents (5,6). Due to high rates of mortality in chemotherapy-exposed patients who develop heart failure, there has been a focus on early detection of cardiotoxicity. In one study by Felker and colleagues that looked at long-term survival in patients with doxorubicin-related cardiotoxicity, mortality rates were as high as 60% (7). Different professional societies have used slightly different definitions of CTRCD. Per expert consensus from the American Society of Echocardiography and European Association of Cardiovascular Imaging (ASE/EACVI), the definition of CTRCD is a decrease in LVEF by >10% to below 53%, which should be confirmed with repeat cardiac imaging in 2 to 3 weeks. The European Society for Medical Oncology (ESMO) incorporates symptoms and defines CTRCD as a decrease of left ventricular ejection fraction (LVEF) by 5% or more to <55% in the presence of symptoms of heart failure or an asymptomatic decrease in LVEF by 10% or more to <55% (8). CTRCD is classified as type I and type II, based on the mechanism of toxicity (5,9). Type I is generally thought to cause irreversible, dose-dependent damage at the cellular level, whereas type II is thought to be reversible, not due to direct cellular damage and not dose dependent. Type I is typically associated with anthracyclines and type II with trastuzumab. While this classification has utility in organizing chemotherapeutic agents by toxicity mechanism, it does not have strong evidence behind it as there can be overlap depending on acuity of exposure; furthermore, new agents including TKIs and ICIs do not necessarily fall into those generalized categories.

Presentation and Diagnosis

Patients with CTRCD may not experience symptoms until the cardiac damage is established. Manifestations may include tachycardia or a slow return of the heart rate to baseline after minimal activity, which suggests limited cardiac reserve. Other common symptoms include dyspnea while performing activities that did not previously elicit this symptom or fatigue out of proportion to the activity level, both of which may also indicate limited cardiac reserve. As cardiac dysfunction progresses, the patient may experience exertional dyspnea, orthopnea, weight gain, fluid retention, and a diastolic gallop (S3). Modalities such as transthoracic echocardiography (TTE) and multigated acquisition (MUGA) radionuclide angiography have traditionally been used to evaluate cardiac function and LVEF. MUGA scans, however, are now rarely performed since these require radiation exposure, while other reliable alternatives do not. Advanced TTE techniques (including myocardial strain and 3D LV imaging) are preferred, and cardiac magnetic resonance (CMR) imaging can be performed when further evaluation is needed. TTE advantages include low cost, portability, and the ability to assess valvular as well as ventricular function. Patients should get a baseline TTE that includes global longitudinal strain (GLS) and 3D LVEF measurements prior to the initiation of chemotherapy. The follow-up schedule of TTEs generally follow a pattern of repeat TTE within 1 to 3 months of chemotherapy initiation or at the end of therapy, and then again 6 months after therapy is completed. Recommended follow-up schedules vary slightly based on chemotherapeutic agent (see "Selected Cancer Therapies" for specific categories).

Clinical symptoms and even asymptomatic LVEF reductions, however, may not occur until late in the course of cardiotoxicity, so there has been growing interest in early subclinical markers of dysfunction. One approach that has shown promise is myocardial strain imaging, specifically GLS measurement by TTE. Strain can be defined as the change in length along a cardiac coordinate axis (longitudinal, radial, or circumferential) of a myocardial segment during systole as a percentage of its original length at end-diastole. Yingchoncharoen et al. performed a meta-analysis that showed normal GLS to be an overall mean of −19.7% but with variability across 24 studies that included healthy subjects (10). A consensus statement from the American and European echocardiography societies points out that there is no currently recognized lower limit (of magnitude) for normal GLS since measurements are affected by vendor, analysis software version, age, gender, and load dependency (5). It is recommended to perform serial TTE studies with a consistent hardware and software platform. A relative reduction in GLS magnitude of <8% from baseline is likely not significant, whereas >15% from baseline is likely abnormal and suggests LV dysfunction. Global radial strain (GRS) and global circumferential strain (GCS), however, have not been predictive of LV dysfunction. GLS also has higher reproducibility when compared with GRS/GCS, with putative mechanism related to the longitudinal axis being aligned with the axial ultrasound beam direction in the apical views and, therefore, having better spatial resolution for myocardial segment displacements in that direction (11). While GLS does forecast future changes in LVEF, the prognostic value of abnormal GLS in cancer survivors with normal LVEF and how this finding should impact treatment are currently unknown (12).

CMR has developed tremendously over recent years and is becoming integral to the evaluation of patients with CTRCD. It has become the gold standard for evaluation of LVEF, right ventricular EF, LV mass, and LV and RV volumes (13,14). CMR is also able to provide information regarding tissue characterization for the detection of inflammation, edema, and fibrosis without patient exposure to radiation. The limitations to widespread use are cost and availability. Therefore, TTE remains the preferred initial imaging modality for assessing CTRCD, whereas CMR can be used in patients in whom body habitus limitations preclude adequate TTE windows or 3D LVEF assessment is not feasible (15). CMR should also be utilized to confirm an abnormal LVEF and performed as part of the cardiomyopathy workup. CMR protocols utilize gadolinium-based contrast agents that enhance in fibrotic or inflamed tissue but not in normal myocardium, which helps aid in the detection of pathologies such as myocarditis (16). Stress perfusion imaging can potentially be added to the CMR protocol, allowing concurrent evaluation for myocardial ischemia as well as LVEF and myocardial tissue characterization (17).

Risk Factors and Screening

There has also been interest in using biomarkers as predictive tools to determine which patients will develop cardiac dysfunction. Studies have explored using cardiac biomarkers such as troponin and brain natriuretic peptide (BNP) in the early detection of cardiotoxicity. Cardinale and colleagues checked troponin on 703 patients with cancer following each dose of chemotherapy and 1 month afterward (18). Patients with initially or persistently positive troponin were at higher risk of developing CTRCD. The optimal timing of troponin measurement is still unclear, but it is recommended to check a baseline troponin and then at the completion of therapy, unless there are symptoms in the intervening period (5). The data behind BNP, however, are conflicting and less robust. An elevated level may be indicative of high filling pressures and raises the concern for CTRCD, but further studies need to be completed in this area (19). Still, it may be reasonable to check BNP levels at baseline and completion of therapy in high-risk patients. Endomyocardial biopsy has been shown to detect early cardiotoxicity even after low anthracycline doses, but this examination is expensive and invasive with risks such as cardiac perforation and tamponade (20).

Factors associated with increased risk of cardiotoxicity include exposure to multiple anthracyclines and nonanthracycline agents, cumulative anthracycline dosage, radiation exposure, extremes of age, and preexisting heart disease (21,22). Significant data related to susceptibility to cardiovascular injury have evolved from the study of children with cancer who received anthracycline-based therapy for hematologic malignancies such as leukemia, lymphoma, and sarcomas. In a study of 14,358 pediatric cancer survivors followed up to 30 years, compared with their siblings, they were three times more likely to experience a chronic cardiovascular disease (1). There is no ideal algorithm to avoid CTRCD, and the oncologic benefit must be weighed against the cardiotoxic risks.

However, the goal is to maximize survival and minimize mortality and morbidity from both cancer and the cardiotoxicity of cancer therapy by controlling cardiac risk factors. Clinical judgment is critical in the decision-making process, and it is important to remain vigilant in screening for cardiovascular disease even after cancer therapy has been completed.

Management

The first goal of cardioprotection is to allow cancer therapy to be administered with maximum effectiveness and minimum cardiotoxicity. A second goal is to preserve the structural and functional integrity of the heart, so that there is sufficient reserve when exposed to additional stressors later in life. These stressors include additional chemotherapy exposure, radiation, hypertension, valvular heart disease, and ischemic heart disease. There are multiple methods that have evolved for preventive cardioprotection. These include dose limitation, schedule modification, innovative delivery systems, analogues, and chemical cardioprotection. The principles of intervention for patients who have experienced cardiotoxicity include symptom amelioration, reduction of workload, improvement of cardiac output through optimization of hemodynamics, revascularization if necessary, and possible organ transplantation in severe cases. It is critical to consider avoidance of additional exposure to the toxic agent after cardiotoxicity has been detected, though this may not always be necessary. It is also important to be sure that the patient's symptoms are due to cardiac dysfunction and not due to other causes. Symptoms such as dyspnea, fatigue, and lightheadedness are often nonspecific and may be related to other conditions such as pulmonary pathology (including infiltrates or pleural effusions), metastatic disease progression, endocrine abnormalities, infections, deconditioning, neurologic conditions, and anemia. Furthermore, if the patient is of advanced age and has coronary artery disease (CAD) risk factors, concurrent ischemic cardiomyopathy is high on the differential diagnosis of cardiac dysfunction and must be assessed accordingly. This is important because potentially lifesaving chemotherapeutics should not be held if the cardiotoxicity is from another source. After withdrawal of the offending agent, if cardiomyopathy persists, the physician should follow standard guidelines for the treatment of heart failure that have been well publicized by the American Heart Association (AHA) and the American College of Cardiology (ACC) (23,24). There are four stages of heart failure: stage A being at-risk individuals with structurally normal hearts, stage B being patients with structurally abnormal hearts with some degree of cardiomyopathy but asymptomatic, stage C being patients with structural cardiac disease and clinical (symptomatic) heart failure, and stage D being refractory heart failure with significant symptom burden despite optimal medical management. Individuals at stage A should have risk factor modification such as hypertension, diabetes, or lipid management, as detailed in later sections. Patients at stage B and C who have reduced LVEF should initiate guideline-directed medical therapy (GDMT) whether they are symptomatic or not.

Commonly used agents include beta-blockers such as carvedilol and metoprolol succinate. Angiotensin converting enzyme inhibitors (ACEi), such as lisinopril, and angiotensin receptor blockers (ARBs), such as losartan, should be initiated to help prevent adverse remodeling and decrease afterload. Spironolactone should also be part of GDMT in patients with reduced LVEF and NYHA class II symptoms or more. More recently, these patients should also be considered for initiation of a neprilysin inhibitor–ARB combination, such as sacubitril–valsartan. In the landmark PARADIGM HF trial, patients on this therapy had a reduction in the primary outcome of cardiovascular mortality or heart failure hospitalization compared to enalapril (21.8% vs. 26.5%) (25). The drugs should be administered at low doses and titrated according to the patient's clinical response, including blood pressure, since these agents may lead to hypotension. This is particularly important in the cancer patient who is receiving therapy and may be intermittently volume depleted. Patients with advanced stage D heart failure should be managed by an experienced team of cardiologists including an advanced heart failure specialist. These patients may require intravenous inotropic agents, biventricular pacing, implantable cardioverter–defibrillators, left ventricular assist devices, or even consideration for heart transplant.

SELECTED CANCER THERAPIES

Anthracyclines

The original anthracycline was isolated from the bacteria *Streptomyces peucetius* and was subsequently named daunorubicin. Adriamycin was developed as a derivative and later designated as doxorubicin. This agent serves as one of the gold standards of oncologic treatment, particularly because of its broad spectrum of activity.

The mechanism of oncologic action for anthracyclines has not been fully defined. There appear to be multiple mechanisms that play a role in tumor destruction. These include inhibition of DNA and RNA synthesis (22,26,27). There may also be an interaction with topoisomerase II and direct reaction with the cellular membrane, which leads to alteration of function (28). Anthracyclines have been shown to induce breaks in double-stranded DNA and free radical formation, which can lead to intracellular accumulation of mutated or oxidatively modified proteins. These proteins can in turn induce activation of caspases that subsequently lead to apoptosis (cell death). Induction of autophagy, an evolutionary mechanism of protein/organelle recycling, has also been implicated in how anthracyclines can promote cell death and lead to heart failure (29).

Doxorubicin and other anthracyclines classically fall into type I CTRCD but can cause acute or chronic cardiotoxicity. The acute form typically occurs within days of administration and may manifest as myo-pericarditis, arrhythmia, or chest pain. Rarely, it may cause a drop in LVEF, but this is generally reversible with prompt supportive treatment. The chronic form of toxicity, which may occur within a month of administration or many years later, leads to cardiomyopathy with reduced LVEF that is often irreversible due to cellular damage. The reported incidence of chronic cardiotoxicity has varied among different studies but has been reported as <2%, which is related to cumulative lifetime total dose, whereas incidence of acute toxicity has been reported as approximately 11% (22). The FDA has a black box warning for doxorubicin, which cautions a 1% to 2% risk of cardiotoxicity at a cumulative dose of 300 mg/m^2, 3% to 5% risk at a dose of 400 mg/m^2, 5% to 8% risk at 450 mg/m^2, and 6% to 20% risk at 500 mg/m^2. There is a rapidly increasing risk of cardiomyopathy above 400 mg/m^2, and it is recommended not to exceed 550 mg/m^2 cumulative dose (30). In addition to a baseline TTE, it is recommended to obtain a follow-up TTE at the completion of treatment and 6 months later, even in the absence of symptoms (5).

A number of pharmacologic agents for cardioprotection have been explored, with dexrazoxane showing efficacy in reducing doxorubicin cardiotoxicity. This compound belongs to a class of agents which, when hydrolyzed, yield a compound that is similar to a metal ion chelating agent. It is postulated that dexrazoxane may enter the cell by diffusion and chelate free iron or iron bound to iron–anthracycline complexes, thereby reducing oxygen radical production (31,32). Two large multicenter trials conducted by Swain et al. (33,34) evaluated the ability of dexrazoxane to confer cardioprotection in patients with metastatic breast cancer who were anthracycline naive. From these trials, it was found that dexrazoxane is cardioprotective for patients who receive it from the initiation of chemotherapy onward. However, one of the trials brought up a concern that dexrazoxane may interfere with tumor response, due to the finding of a lower response rate of the breast cancer to chemotherapy. A more recent Cochrane review looked at several trials that evaluated the use of dexrazoxane and found that there was significant cardio-protective benefit without interference with chemotherapy (35). However, there is significant variability between the studies as well as some concern for adverse effects from dexrazoxane use. Therefore, its use remains controversial, but in patients with high risk of cardiac damage, it may be considered. Additional studies are needed to define the role of this drug in cancer patients receiving anthracyclines.

Trastuzumab

Trastuzumab is a monoclonal antibody against epidermal growth factor 2 (HER2) and is used mainly for breast cancer but other oncologic conditions as well. It has specific activity against breast cancers that express HER2, binds to it on cancer cells, and triggers tumor suppressive action through antibody-dependent cell-mediated cytotoxicity. While the benefits of trastuzumab have been demonstrated, it carries with it significant cardiotoxicity risk, especially when used with other chemotherapies (36). The phase III trial by Slamon et al. showed that trastuzumab with concurrent anthracycline and cyclophosphamide or trastuzumab with concurrent paclitaxel (in patients that had a history of anthracyclines use) caused heart failure in up to 27% and 13% of patients, respectively, as compared to only 8% in the anthracycline group alone (37). The HERA Trial showed a rate of cardiotoxicity of 4% with 1 year of use and up to 7% with 2 years of use, of trastuzumab alone as adjuvant chemotherapy (38). Trastuzumab has classically been categorized as a type II CTRCD, because of the lack of myocyte injury and largely reversible nature of cardiac dysfunction, though there has been some conflicting evidence in long-term use. It is clear, however, that use of trastuzumab with other chemotherapeutics potentiates the risk of cardiotoxicity. In addition to a baseline TTE, surveillance TTEs are recommended every 3 months during active treatment (5).

Tyrosine Kinase Inhibitors

Tyrosine kinase is an enzyme that plays a key role in signal transduction cascades. Its activation leads to transferring of a phosphate from adenosine triphosphate to the tyrosine residue of certain proteins, which in turn activates cell signaling. In cancer cells, these proteins can become mutated, which may result in overexpression leading to inhibition of apoptosis and increased cell proliferation.

TKIs block this enzyme from activating and thus inhibit the phosphorylation event, which triggers cell signaling (39). It can be misleading to consider TKIs as a single class of drugs, since individual molecules act on different targets and, hence, can have very different effects. Some can target one molecule, while others can target multiple ones. In general, there are two classes of TKIs: monoclonal TKIs, such as bevacizumab, and small molecule TKIs, such as sunitinib. Furthermore, they can also be subdivided into receptor tyrosine kinases and nonreceptor tyrosine kinases, of which some agents can have activity on both (40). TKI cardiotoxicity may manifest as heart failure, conduction abnormalities, QT prolongation, thromboembolism, acute coronary syndromes (ACSs), and hypertension (41,42).

Certain subgroups of TKIs deserve special mention. One subgroup includes vascular endothelial growth factor (VEGF) inhibitors such as bevacizumab. These agents work by blocking endothelial cell proliferation and angiogenesis, which is a key mechanism by which cancer cells maintain adequate blood supply for nourishment and growth. Importantly, these agents present a significant risk of hypertension (42). In one small, phase I/II study of 75 patients treated with sunitinib by Chu et al., 47% of patients developed hypertension (defined as >150/100 mm Hg) (43). Therefore, providers must remain vigilant about monitoring and controlling hypertension in these patients.

Sorafenib and sunitinib in particular are multitargeted TKIs, that is, they target multiple different receptor tyrosine and nonreceptor tyrosine kinases, including VEGF, PDGFR, cKIT, etc. Therefore, their cardiotoxic side effects are more varied than specific agents such as bevacizumab. These include myocardial infarction and heart failure in up to 11% of patients as seen in the above-mentioned study by Chu et al. with sunitinib, as well as significant hypertension. Clinicians must pay close attention to patients with preexisting CAD or hypertension, as these comorbidities may be exacerbated by these agents.

Lastly, drugs that are specific to certain non-receptor TKIs are worth mentioning, including imatinib, dasatinib, and nilotinib. These agents target Abl, which is associated with the Philadelphia chromosome in chronic lymphocytic leukemia, as well as other nonreceptor tyrosine kinases. Nilotinib can prolong the QT interval and provoke arterial thrombosis. Dasatinib, which in addition to Abl, also binds the Src family of kinases and can cause pleural and pericardial effusions, though the mechanism is unknown, in addition to pulmonary arterial hypertension (42). Less commonly, dasatinib can cause heart failure, which was reported in

1.6% of 258 patients as published in the Warnings and Precautions of its FDA package insert (44).

There are no data showing ideal monitoring intervals, but an approach similar to that used for trastuzumab may be reasonable. Patients would then have a baseline TTE and surveillance TTEs every 3 months while on therapy (5).

Immune Checkpoint Inhibitors

ICIs are a new class of cancer therapeutics that have emerged in the last decade and have revolutionized the field of oncology. The first agent introduced in 2010 was ipilimumab, a monoclonal antibody against cytotoxic T lymphocyte–associated antigen 4 (CTLA-4). Since then several other agents have been approved that target programmed cell death protein 1 (PD-1), such as pembrolizumab and nivolumab, and programmed cell death ligand 1 (PDL-1), such as atezolizumab and durvalumab. Normally, these pathways function to prevent T cells from attacking self and to protect against autoimmune disease. When these drugs are used to inhibit checkpoint pathways, T cells are disinhibited and thus able to function as antitumor cells (45). Patients with solid tumors and hematologic malignancies have seen very promising results in terms of prognosis since the introduction of these new agents. However, these agents have shown immune-related adverse events (IRAEs) across a range of organs, including the heart (46). The incidence of cardiotoxicity in safety databases is less compared with other organs, but toxicities are broad and can include conduction abnormalities, pericardial disease, and heart failure. The most significant and potentially fatal cardiotoxicity, however, is myocarditis. This can range from asymptomatic structural or electrical changes to fulminant myocarditis with cardiogenic shock, multiorgan failure, arrhythmia, and death. Post mortem studies have shown infiltration of immune cells in the myocardium, but the exact mechanism is not fully understood (46). While cardiac side effects are generally uncommon, myocarditis is the most common and the most dangerous among these. Troponin should be checked should there be any suspicion of myocarditis, with a low threshold for CMR to evaluate for myocardial inflammation. In studies looking at safety databases of over 20,000 patients, there were 18 patients who developed myocarditis, or 0.09%. There is increased risk of myocarditis with simultaneous use of more than one agent, up to 0.27% risk (47). More recent studies by Mahmood and colleagues have shown even higher rates of myocarditis, up to over 1%, with a median time of within 34 days of initiation of an ICI (48). Management of these patients includes first stopping the ICI, and then considering use of steroids, immunosuppressive medications, or intravenous immunoglobulin. Care in this setting should be coordinated in conjunction with a hematology oncology specialist. There are no data on screening guidelines for patients on ICIs, but a baseline TTE is recommended. It is unknown how often to screen these patients during therapy or long-term follow-up.

Antimetabolites

The group of antimetabolite chemotherapeutics have a unique cardiotoxicity profile. These agents include 5-fluorouracil (5-FU), capecitabine, cytarabine, and more. They typically function to inhibit DNA synthesis, which in turn limits tumor growth. Cardiotoxic effects of this class include chest pain, ACS, and less commonly arrhythmia, pericarditis, or myocarditis (49). Patients who present with ACS should be treated with typical GDMT, and consideration of coronary angiography if clinically indicated. The mechanism of action is thought to be due to coronary vasospasm, so vasodilators such as nitroglycerin and calcium channel blockers should be administered, in addition to stopping the drug infusion. Patients with high pretest probability of CAD may warrant risk stratification with stress testing prior to drug administration (5). In patients with known underlying CAD, discussion of risks and benefits should include consideration of alternative agents. If a patient develops ACS with 5-FU and is subsequently revascularized (indicated for plaque rupture or critical stenosis rather than transient vasospasm), rechallenging with 5-FU may be considered, but there is a high rate of recurrent vasospasm (49).

Radiation

Radiation-induced vasculopathy has been associated with the treatment of a number of malignancies including lymphoma, breast cancer, head and neck cancer, and thoracic tumors. Interestingly, the incidence of ischemic heart disease and stroke associated with radiation therapy has not been shown to increase until years after treatment (50–52). Surgical wounds within previously irradiated tissues are also prone to vascular alterations, associated with increased incidence of microvascular occlusion and delayed wound healing (52). The adverse effects of radiation on tissues can be acute, such as pericardial effusion, usually occurring within 4 to 6 weeks after exposure, and late, such as CAD, that may manifest years after irradiation. These effects indicate an ongoing, progressive process. The evidence for late adverse effects is primarily derived from epidemiological studies. Most experimental studies have focused on the acute effects in cell culture experiments. Radiation sensitivity of the vasculature has been linked to endothelial dysfunction, which may lead to atherosclerosis and a prothrombotic state over time (53–57).

The clinical consequences of radiation injury to the blood vessels are significant. A retrospective cohort study of the Childhood Cancer Survivor Study showed that survivors of childhood malignancies into adulthood that had radiation exposure had a 15-fold higher rate of heart failure and a 10-fold higher rate of cardiovascular disease as compared to their siblings (58). This risk is further amplified in the presence of traditional cardiovascular risk factors. Most cardiac events occur more than 10 years after completing radiotherapy; therefore, the proof of causality is complicated (59). It is estimated that 3 million cancer survivors worldwide have received radiation therapy as a component of their therapy (60). Therefore, clinicians must be aware of the potential cardiovascular risk and manage the risk factors appropriately. In the ASE guidelines, screening TTE is recommended 5 years after exposure for patients that are high risk, and 10 years after exposure for all other patients, with continued reassessment every 5 years as long as patients remain asymptomatic (61).

The potential cardiotoxicity of selected chemotherapy drugs is summarized in Table 26.1.

TABLE 26.1 CARDIOTOXICITY OF SELECTED NONANTHRACYCLINE CANCER CHEMOTHERAPY AGENTS

Drug/therapy	Comments and potential associated cardiovascular toxicities
Androgen deprivation therapy	Accelerated atherosclerosis, metabolic syndrome (62)
Antimetabolites	
Fluorouracil	Coronary vasospasm, angina, myocardial infarction, arrhythmias, pericarditis, myocarditis, and pulmonary embolism (49)
Capecitabine	Similar to fluorouracil (47)
Fludarabine	Hypotension, chest pain, and severe cardiotoxicity in combination with melphalan (63)
Cytarabine	Pericarditis, pericardial effusion, tamponade (64)
Microtubule-targeting agents	
Vinca alkaloids	Hypertension, myocardial ischemia, vaso-occlusive events (65)
Paclitaxel	Bradycardia, heart block (66)
Alkylating agents	
Cyclophosphamide	Arrhythmia, heart failure, myopericarditis (67)
Ifosfamide	Arrhythmias, ST-T wave segment changes, generally reversible heart failure (68)
Cisplatin	Sustained ventricular tachycardia, bradycardia, ST-T wave segment changes, bundle branch block, myocardial infarction, ischemic cardiomyopathy (69)
Thalidomide	Bradycardia (70)
Monoclonal antibodies	
Trastuzumab	Reversible cardiac dysfunction, heart failure (36)
Rituximab	Arrhythmias, angina (71)
Alemtuzumab	Arrhythmias, heart failure (72)
VEGF inhibitors	
Bevacizumab	Angina, myocardial infarction, heart failure, significant hypertension, thromboembolic events (42)
Topoisomerase inhibitors	
Etoposide	Myocardial infarction, vasospastic angina (73,74)
Biologic response modifiers	
Interferon alpha	Myocardial infarction, arrhythmias, cardiomyopathy with prolonged administration (75)
Interleukin 2	Arrhythmias, hypotension, capillary leak syndrome (76)
Differentiation agents	
All-trans retinoic acid	Pericardial effusion, myocardial infarction (77)
Tyrosine kinase inhibitors	
Sorafenib and sunitinib	Heart failure, reversible cardiac injury, hypertension (42)
Imatinib	Small risk of cardiomyopathy (40)

TABLE 26.1 CARDIOTOXICITY OF SELECTED NONANTHRACYCLINE CANCER CHEMOTHERAPY AGENTS *(Continued)*

Drug/therapy	Comments and potential associated cardiovascular toxicities
Nilotinib	QT interval prolongation, occlusive arterial disease including coronary thrombosis (42)
Ponatinib	Similar to nilotinib (78)
Dasatinib	Angina, pericardial and pleural effusion, QT prolongation, pulmonary arterial hypertension, heart failure (42)
Ibrutinib	Atrial fibrillation (60)
Immune checkpoint inhibitors	
Pembrolizumab, nivolumab, ipilimumab	Myocarditis, heart failure, arrhythmias, pericardial disease (46)
Proteasome inhibitors	
Carfilzomib	Cardiomyopathy, arrhythmia, hypertension, pulmonary arterial hypertension (79–81)
Bortezomib	Similar to carfilzomib but with lower event rate (81)

CLINICAL PRESENTATIONS AND MANAGEMENT OF CARDIOVASCULAR TOXICITIES

Arrhythmias

A number of arrhythmias are associated with chemotherapeutic agents. In most instances, treatment may continue with careful monitoring. In a minority of cases, such as when patients develop bradycardia, the patient may require a temporary and/or permanent pacer to allow cancer therapy to continue. A few agents in particular, are associated with increased risk of atrial fibrillation, including ibrutinib, cisplatin, interleukin-2, and anthracyclines (82,83).

QT Interval Prolongation

The QT interval is an ECG measure of ventricular repolarization. Abnormalities of repolarization may lead to an increased risk of ventricular arrhythmias. The incidence of QTc prolongation in a systematic review was as high as 22%, including patients both on targeted and nontargeted therapies (84). In addition, cancer patients have many comorbidities such as structural heart disease, coronary heart disease, hepatic and renal dysfunction, as well as concomitant medications that are known to prolong the QT interval. These include antiemetics, antifungals, antiarrhythmics, methadone, quinolone, and macrolides. This risk can be exacerbated by electrolyte abnormalities and dehydration in cancer patients who commonly experience nausea, vomiting, and diarrhea (85).

Hypertension

There is a significant interest in hypertension in patients with malignancy. This focus has surged due to the increased prevalence of hypertension related to the use of angiogenesis inhibitors in targeted cancer therapy, although it has been described with more traditional therapies as well. Hypertension is also common and may be a pre-existing condition exacerbated by these therapies. In fact, it is the most common reported comorbid condition in cancer registries, in one study by Kuriakose and colleagues up to 30%, and may adversely affect prognosis (86–88). The link between hypertension and doxorubicin-related cardiotoxicity was first suggested by Van Hoff and colleagues in 1979, where a higher probability of developing heart failure was seen in patients with cardiac disease, hypertension, or both as compared to all other patients in the study (3). In a more recent study by Jain and colleagues, it was found that patients had a 58% greater risk of developing heart failure if they had hypertension, compared to patients who did not (87). Theoretically, in patients who develop damage to the myocardium from cardiotoxicity, hypertension can add a second stressor, or hit, which can further exacerbate the damage. It is therefore important that hypertension be diagnosed and managed effectively to reduce cardiotoxicity from cancer therapy.

Imperative in the treatment of hypertension in any population is to reduce morbidity and mortality by reducing the incidence of target organ damage, such as myocardial ischemia, infarction, stroke, and renal failure. The treatment modalities are those recommended by the guidelines developed by the Joint National Committee (JNC8) of the NIH as well as the ACC/AHA Clinical Performance and Quality Measures for Adults With High Blood Pressure (89). The choice of an antihypertensive agent should take into consideration the mechanism and pathophysiology of the blood pressure elevation, the potential drug–drug interactions, and indications or contraindications for particular agents. According to ACC/AHA guidelines, blood pressure goal is <130/80 mm Hg for patients that require pharmacologic therapy for hypertension. Blood pressure goals in cancer patients are not clearly identified due to the lack of data, but extrapolating from the ACC/AHA guidelines, target blood pressure is <130/80 mm Hg. Initial treatment strategy in the general population as per the JNC8 guidelines is calcium channel blocker, thiazide diuretic, ACEi, or ARB. In patients with cardiotoxicity, however, the preferred first-line agents are usually ACEi/ARB or beta-blockers, which is extrapolated from strong data in noncancer patients with ischemic/nonischemic cardiomyopathy, wherein ACEi/ARBs and beta-blockers are shown to promote adverse remodeling and improve mortality (90–93).

Patients with hypertension associated with antiangiogenic agents such as bevacizumab, sorafenib, and sunitinib may require multiple antihypertensive medications. The patient will need to be monitored carefully during therapy and appropriate adjustments made as the blood pressure may vary. Physicians must be cognizant of possible drug–drug interactions such as with sorafenib, which is metabolized by the cytochrome P-450 system (CYP3A4) in the liver. Drugs such as verapamil and diltiazem are inhibitors of the CYP3A4 isoenzyme and may lead to increased sorafenib levels. Therefore, oncology patients may not necessarily follow all of the same guidelines for hypertension as for the general population.

Ischemic Heart Disease and Cancer

Ischemic heart disease is primarily due to obstruction of the coronary arteries, which is usually a consequence of atherosclerosis. The pathogenesis of atherosclerosis is multifactorial and is related to the accumulation of lipid-laden plaque within the coronary arteries and further mediated by inflammation. CAD leads to more deaths, disability, and economic loss in developed nations than any other disease. The economic costs are in the multibillion dollar range, which entail both health expenditures and loss of productivity. The patient with cancer and the patient with ischemic heart disease represent two groups with diseases that together compound the above effects by several-fold.

There is a tremendous focus on the primary prevention of CAD, with emphasis on behavioral and environmental changes that reduce the risk of adverse events in patients at risk for CAD. Preventive measures should be directed at the establishment of healthy lifestyles as early in life as possible,

including smoking cessation, healthy eating, and being active. The initial approach should include identification of the high-risk patient and implementation of a successful preventive program.

Patients should be screened for risk factors such as hypertension and hyperlipidemia. Timely recognition and treatment of hypertension becomes extremely important in the cancer patient who is receiving targeted therapy with VEGF inhibitors. These agents lead to an increase in the incidence of hypertension. While there are no specific cholesterol guidelines in patients with chemotherapy-related cardiotoxicity, the general cholesterol recommendations should be diligently followed for these patients in order to reduce the risk for cardiovascular events. The AHA/ACC have published updated guidelines in 2018 for the treatment of patients with hyperlipidemia. Patients with a known history of atherosclerotic cardiovascular disease (ASCVD) less than the age of 75 should be on a high dose statin to reduce cholesterol by 50%, with a goal LDL of <70 mg/dL if they have high risk (which includes age >65 years, hypertension, diabetes, family history, chronic kidney disease, heart failure, or smoking). For primary prevention, patients should have their 10-year ASCVD risk calculated, and if more than intermediate risk (>7.5%), then they should be on a moderate dose statin with goal reduction in LDL by 30%, or if they are high risk (>20%), then they should be on a high-intensity statin with goal LDL reduction of 50%. Additional interventions include the appropriate diagnosis and treatment of diabetes, smoking cessation, a reduction in saturated fat with adoption of a Mediterranean-type diet, weight control, and an increase in physical activity (94).

The diagnosis of coronary disease includes an initial history and physical examination and an electrocardiogram. Adjunctive imaging plays a significant role in the evaluation since this increases the sensitivity and specificity of detection of disease. This includes TTE, myocardial perfusion imaging with radioisotopes, and CMR when indicated. Coronary CT angiography is also an established noninvasive screening method to risk stratify patients for CAD. This modality has the ability to delineate the coronary anatomy and define both nonobstructive and obstructive plaques.

The optimal treatment of CAD requires behavioral and environmental interventions, pharmacologic therapy, and sometimes coronary revascularization. Among the agents commonly used are antiplatelet agents, beta-blocking agents, nitrates (short- and long-acting), lipid-lowering agents, neuro-hormonal blocking agents (ACEi/

ARBs), and late sodium (Na) channel antagonists. Revascularization procedures include percutaneous transluminal coronary angioplasty, coronary artery stents, coronary artery bypass surgery, and hybrid procedures. Many patients with CAD and/or cancer also have arrhythmias that require pharmacologic intervention and possible ablative procedures. The decisions for implementation of these interventions should be collaborative between the cardiologist, oncologist, and surgeon.

The patient with CAD may be asymptomatic or present with clinical symptoms of ischemia. This can manifest as stable angina or ACS. ACS is subcategorized as unstable angina, non–ST-segment elevation myocardial infarction, and ST-segment elevation myocardial infarction. The clinical presentation of patients with cancer and ACS is generally the same as patients in the noncancer population. It is well established that patients who have survived cancer are at risk for CAD (95). The pathophysiology of ACS involves unstable atherosclerotic plaques, inflammation, platelet aggregation, and thrombosis. Individuals with cancer are also prothrombotic and may be vulnerable to similar mechanisms including platelet activation, aggregation, and an increase in procoagulant factors. The AHA/ACA guidelines recommend use of dual antiplatelet therapy (DAPT) for patients with ACS with or without stenting (96). However, there is further consideration in cancer patients, as they may have other comorbidities that noncancer patients may not have such as hematologic abnormalities including thrombocytopenia and anemia. Thrombocytopenia is not protective for ACS or percutaneous coronary interventions, but in fact increases risk of thrombosis and bleeding. Major guidelines and large trials unfortunately exclude patients with cancer or low platelets, and so data are either in small studies or must be extrapolated to oncology patients. Sarkiss et al. demonstrated that in cancer patients with ACS and thrombocytopenia (platelets <100,000), those who did not receive ASA had a 7-day survival rate of 6% compared with 90% in those who received ASA. Patients with a platelet count >100,000 who received ASA had a 7-day survival of 88% compared with 45% in those who did not receive ASA (97). There was increased bleeding risk in the low platelet group, but no significant increased risk between aspirin versus no-aspirin group. The Society for Cardiovascular Angiography and Interventions (SCAI) released an expert consensus in 2016 to provide guidance in this setting (98). If cancer patients with ACS status post stenting have a platelet count of >10,000, they may take aspirin monotherapy.

If their counts are 30,000 to 50,000, then they can be maintained on DAPT with aspirin and clopidogrel, with close monitoring and potentially scaling back to monotherapy after 6 months. If the count is >50,000, patients can be maintained on DAPT with any agent (including ticagrelor or prasugrel), and if >100,000 then can be treated similar to a noncancer patient. In patients with stable coronary disease and thrombocytopenia, patients should be preferentially medically managed unless there is no other option, at which point a multidisciplinary risk/benefit discussion is required.

Preoperative Assessment of the Cancer Patient with Heart Disease for Noncardiac Surgery

Preoperative assessment of the cancer patient with heart disease is vital to a successful outcome after noncardiac surgery. Most clinicians feel that detailed assessment and management and appropriate interventions will lead to a successful outcome. This is particularly important since there are significant changes in physiologic status for these patients in the operating room and postoperatively.

The initial step in this process involves assessment by the anesthesiologist in a preoperative clinic before the procedure with a thorough review of the patient's medical record and leading to cardiovascular risk assessment or additional investigation by other specialists when indicated. There is general consensus that previous treatment for malignancy (chemotherapy, radiotherapy, and surgery) may affect the patient's subsequent response to anesthesia and surgery. In addition, many tumors are associated with physiologic disturbances. They may have secretory properties, paraneoplastic syndromes, and endocrine effects. The clinical manifestations may include bronchospasm, fever secondary to cytokine release, hypotension, hypertension, hypercalcemia, and hypermetabolic syndromes.

The cardiologist will typically be involved in risk stratification of these patients when they have existing coronary or structural heart disease, or possibly if they have been treated for their cancer with potentially cardiotoxic chemotherapy and radiotherapy. There are a number of tools available for the risk stratification process. In addition to the history, physical examination, ECG, and risk factor assessment, there are a number of adjunctive techniques that are available. These must take into account patient symptoms and activity level. Risk factor assessment may be done with the Revised Cardiac Risk Index, wherein patients receive points for a history of ischemic heart disease, history of congestive heart failure, history of cerebrovascular event, diabetes on insulin, chronic kidney disease with creatinine >2, and high-risk surgery (76). A score of 0 or 1 is considered low risk, and ≥2 suggests increased risk. If a patient is asymptomatic, has good functional capacity, and low risk score, then they can proceed without any further workup. If a patient is symptomatic, has unknown functional capacity, or is moderate to high risk and further workup would change management, then one should consider risk stratification with stress testing (or anatomic coronary evaluation) and proceed based on the results. However, there are emerging data that suggests that the RCRI score may underestimate risk, so the clinician must take into account the whole patient when determining risk and not rely on just one tool (99).

Further investigation with stress testing or coronary angiography (which may be invasive with fluoroscopy or occasionally noninvasive by CT) may be required prior to surgery in order to reduce the perioperative risk of major cardiac events, especially if the patient is symptomatic or has low activity level and cannot reliably describe symptoms. The highest risk patients are those with congestive heart failure, unstable angina, significant arrhythmias, and recent myocardial infarction. One must also consider the type and length of surgery, mode of anesthesia, expected blood loss, and fluid balance concerns. At times, a multidisciplinary discussion is warranted to determine whether or not the surgical procedure can be delayed to allow coronary revascularization by either percutaneous coronary intervention (with uninterrupted DAPT afterward) or coronary artery bypass graft surgery.

In summary, the preoperative evaluation of cancer patients, particularly if they have heart disease, must take into account the type of cancer, the type of heart disease and the current level of activity, previous chemotherapy, radiation exposure, and comorbid conditions. Given that the proposed procedure may be a part of a continuum of cancer therapy, there must be careful collaboration to achieve the best outcomes in both short- and long-term settings (73).

ETHICAL CONSIDERATIONS

There are several ethical considerations that are particularly salient in the cardiac care of cancer patients. Not surprisingly, given that cardiovascular disease and malignancy are the leading causes of mortality in the United States, cardio-oncology specialists must be skilled and sensitive in discussing end-of-life issues. Simply eliciting "Do Not Resuscitate" status, for example, is woefully insufficient in older patients struggling with a high burden of both cardiac and oncologic morbidity. Rather than asking what specific treatments patients might want, physicians should seek to understand patient goals as well as fears, and propose treatment strategies accordingly in order to best serve patient values and priorities. For example, a patient with ischemic cardiomyopathy and stage IV malignancy with a life expectancy of 18 months might understandably desire to proceed with angioplasty in order to relieve refractory angina, though might find it less desirable to undergo defibrillator implantation (even if strictly within guideline-supported indications) because this procedure does not provide symptomatic benefit but rather only detects and treats lethal arrhythmia, which would otherwise result in an immediate and painless death, with a painful shock. Simply asking a patient if he or she is willing or not to undergo invasive procedures is often insufficient to tease out important nuances. It is critical to understand whether patient goals of care prioritize maximum longevity, preserved functional status, avoidance of suffering, or even a context-specific combination of these.

Shared decision-making is an important strategy in navigating many decisions facing patients with cardiac disease and cancer. For example, a patient with moderate leukemia-related thrombocytopenia and significant CAD might struggle with the decision to take aspirin or other antiplatelet medications, and it is important to help him or her understand the risks and benefits of both options. Some patients may worry more about avoiding bleeding risk, while others may fear another ischemic cardiovascular event above all else. Of course, some treatments are more amenable to shared decision-making than others. For example, a cardio-oncology specialist should urge a young woman with breast cancer and uncontrolled hypertension to initiate aggressive therapy with beta-blockade and renin–angiotensin–aldosterone system blockade in order to significantly reduce the risk of cardiotoxicity before initiating treatment with doxorubicin. This recommendation is less appropriately framed as a shared decision; of course, the patient may decline any treatment she does not desire, but the physician should make clear that this is the best option given our current understanding of how profoundly hypertension potentiates the risk of cardiotoxicity in this case.

Finally, in order to provide comprehensive and compassionate care within this framework, it is critical to ensure adequate time during office visits in order to allow thoughtful and unhurried conversations with ample time for questions.

CONCLUSION

Today's oncology and palliative care providers must be fully aware of cardiovascular risks in order to prevent or mitigate adverse cardiac outcomes, and cardiologists must be ready to assist oncologists by performing evaluations relevant to their choice of therapy. The coordination of patient care with the goal of optimizing outcomes is built around robust communication. This includes close working relationships among various clinicians, multidisciplinary conferences, multidisciplinary care clinics, development of oncology multispecialty groups, development of guideline-based care, and a central society for the development of research and clinical guideline development.

Cardio-oncology (and onco-cardiology) are terms used to describe this relatively new field of interdisciplinary medicine between specialists in cardiovascular disease and oncology. This evolving subspecialty involves evaluation and treatment of the cardiotoxic effects of chemotherapy, radiation therapy, targeted therapies, and immunotherapy. These include, but are not limited to thrombosis, hypertension, congestive heart failure, ischemic heart disease, and arrhythmia. The care of a patient with heart disease and cancer can be immensely challenging, often requiring a delicate balance in order to achieve the best possible outcome for each individual patient.

ACKNOWLEDGMENTS

The authors would like to thank David Slosky for contributions to the prior version of this chapter.

REFERENCES

1. Krischer JP, et al. Clinical cardiotoxicity following anthracycline treatment for childhood cancer: the Pediatric Oncology Group experience. *J Clin Oncol.* 1997;15(4):1544-1552.
2. Cancer Stat Facts. 2019. https://seer.cancer.gov/statfacts/
3. Von Hoff DD, et al. Risk factors for doxorubicin-induced congestive heart failure. *Ann Intern Med.* 1979;91(5):710-717.
4. Von Hoff DD, et al. Daunomycin-induced cardiotoxicity in children and adults. A review of 110 cases. *Am J Med.* 1977;62(2):200-208.
5. Plana JC, et al. Expert consensus for multimodality imaging evaluation of adult patients during and after cancer therapy: a report from the American Society of Echocardiography and the European Association of Cardiovascular Imaging. *J Am Soc Echocardiogr.* 2014;27(9):911-939.
6. Zamorano JL, et al. 2016 ESC Position Paper on cancer treatments and cardiovascular toxicity developed under the auspices of the ESC Committee for Practice Guidelines: the Task Force for cancer treatments and cardiovascular toxicity of the European Society of Cardiology (ESC). *Eur J Heart Fail.* 2017;19(1):9-42.
7. Felker GM, et al. Underlying causes and long-term survival in patients with initially unexplained cardiomyopathy. *N Engl J Med.* 2000;342(15):1077-1084.
8. Curigliano G, et al. Cardiovascular toxicity induced by chemotherapy, targeted agents and radiotherapy: ESMO Clinical Practice Guidelines. *Ann Oncol.* 2012;23(suppl 7):vii155-vii166.
9. Suter TM, Ewer MS. Cancer drugs and the heart: importance and management. *Eur Heart J.* 2013;34(15):1102-1111.
10. Yingchoncharoen T, et al. Normal ranges of left ventricular strain: a meta-analysis. *J Am Soc Echocardiogr.* 2013;26(2):185-191.
11. Mor-Avi V, et al. Current and evolving echocardiographic techniques for the quantitative evaluation of cardiac mechanics: ASE/EAE consensus statement on methodology and indications endorsed by the Japanese Society of Echocardiography. *Eur J Echocardiogr.* 2011;12(3):167-205.
12. Thavendiranathan P, et al. Use of myocardial strain imaging by echocardiography for the early detection of cardiotoxicity in patients during and after cancer chemotherapy: a systematic review. *J Am Coll Cardiol.* 2014;63(25 Pt A):2751-2768.
13. Bellenger NG, et al. Comparison of left ventricular ejection fraction and volumes in heart failure by echocardiography, radionuclide ventriculography and cardiovascular magnetic resonance; are they interchangeable? *Eur Heart J.* 2000;21(16):1387-1396.
14. Walker J, et al. Role of three-dimensional echocardiography in breast cancer: comparison with two-dimensional echocardiography, multiple-gated acquisition scans, and cardiac magnetic resonance imaging. *J Clin Oncol.* 2010;28(21):3429-3436.
15. Thiele H, et al. Improved accuracy of quantitative assessment of left ventricular volume and ejection fraction by geometric models with steady-state free precession. *J Cardiovasc Magn Reson.* 2002;4(3):327-339.
16. Soufer A, Baldassarre LA. The role of cardiac magnetic resonance imaging to detect cardiac toxicity from cancer therapeutics. *Curr Treat Options Cardiovasc Med.* 2019;21(6):28.
17. Lipinski MJ, et al. Prognostic value of stress cardiac magnetic resonance imaging in patients with known or suspected coronary artery disease: a systematic review and meta-analysis. *J Am Coll Cardiol.* 2013;62(9):826-838.
18. Cardinale D, et al. Prognostic value of troponin I in cardiac risk stratification of cancer patients undergoing high-dose chemotherapy. *Circulation.* 2004;109(22):2749-2754.
19. Michel L, Rassaf T, Totzeck M. Biomarkers for the detection of apparent and subclinical cancer therapy-related cardiotoxicity. *J Thorac Dis.* 2018;10(suppl 35):S4282-S4295.
20. Friedman MA, et al. Doxorubicin cardiotoxicity. Serial endomyocardial biopsies and systolic time intervals. *JAMA.* 1978;240(15):1603-1606.
21. Minow RA, et al. Adriamycin cardiomyopathy—risk factors. *Cancer.* 1977;39(4):1397-1402.
22. Cai F, et al. Anthracycline-induced cardiotoxicity in the chemotherapy treatment of breast cancer: preventive strategies and treatment. *Mol Clin Oncol.* 2019;11(1):15-23.
23. Yancy CW, et al. 2013 ACCF/AHA guideline for the management of heart failure: executive summary: a report of the American College of Cardiology Foundation/American Heart Association Task Force on practice guidelines. *Circulation.* 2013;128(16):1810-1852.
24. Yancy CW, et al. 2017 ACC/AHA/HFSA focused update of the 2013 ACCF/AHA guideline for the management of heart failure: a report of the American College of

Cardiology/American Heart Association Task Force on Clinical Practice Guidelines and the Heart Failure Society of America. *J Card Fail*. 2017;23(8):628-651.

25. McMurray JJ, et al. Angiotensin-neprilysin inhibition versus enalapril in heart failure. *N Engl J Med*. 2014;371(11):993-1004.

26. Chaires JB. Biophysical chemistry of the daunomycin-DNA interaction. *Biophys Chem*. 1990;35(2-3):191-202.

27. Chatterjee K, et al. Doxorubicin cardiomyopathy. *Cardiology*. 2010;115(2):155-162.

28. Tritton TR, Yee G, Wingard LB Jr. Immobilized adriamycin: a tool for separating cell surface from intracellular mechanisms. *Fed Proc*. 1983;42(2):284-287.

29. Zhu H, et al. Cardiac autophagy is a maladaptive response to hemodynamic stress. *J Clin Invest*. 2007;117(7):1782-1793.

30. Adriamycin Package Insert. 2012. https://www.accessdata.fda.gov/drugsatfda_docs/label/2012/062921s022lbl.pdf

31. Hellmann K. Overview and historical development of dexrazoxane. *Semin Oncol*. 1998;25(4 suppl 10):48-54.

32. Hasinoff BB. Chemistry of dexrazoxane and analogues. *Semin Oncol*. 1998;25(4 suppl 10):3-9.

33. Swain SM, et al. Cardioprotection with dexrazoxane for doxorubicin-containing therapy in advanced breast cancer. *J Clin Oncol*. 1997;15(4):1318-1332.

34. Swain SM, et al. Delayed administration of dexrazoxane provides cardioprotection for patients with advanced breast cancer treated with doxorubicin-containing therapy. *J Clin Oncol*. 1997;15(4):1333-1340.

35. van Dalen EC, et al. Cardioprotective interventions for cancer patients receiving anthracyclines. *Cochrane Database Syst Rev*. 2011;(6):CD003917.

36. Mohan N, et al. Trastuzumab-mediated cardiotoxicity: current understanding, challenges, and frontiers. *Antib Ther*. 2018;1(1):13-17.

37. Slamon DJ, et al. Use of chemotherapy plus a monoclonal antibody against HER2 for metastatic breast cancer that overexpresses HER2. *N Engl J Med*. 2001;344(11):783-792.

38. Cameron D, et al. 11 years' follow-up of trastuzumab after adjuvant chemotherapy in HER2-positive early breast cancer: final analysis of the HERceptin Adjuvant (HERA) trial. *Lancet*. 2017;389(10075):1195-1205.

39. Lee W-S, Kim J. Cardiotoxicity associated with tyrosine kinase-targeted anticancer therapy. *Mol Cell Toxicol*. 2018;14(3):247-254.

40. Orphanos GS, Ioannidis GN, Ardavanis AG. Cardiotoxicity induced by tyrosine kinase inhibitors. *Acta Oncol*. 2009;48(7):964-970.

41. Chaar M, Kamta J, Ait-Oudhia S. Mechanisms, monitoring, and management of tyrosine kinase inhibitors-associated cardiovascular toxicities. *Onco Targets Ther*. 2018;11:6227-6237.

42. Chen MH, Kerkela R, Force T. Mechanisms of cardiac dysfunction associated with tyrosine kinase inhibitor cancer therapeutics. *Circulation*. 2008;118(1):84-95.

43. Chu TF, et al. Cardiotoxicity associated with tyrosine kinase inhibitor sunitinib. *Lancet*. 2007;370(9604):2011-2019.

44. Sprycel (dasatinib) Package Insert. 2010. https://www.accessdata.fda.gov/drugsatfda_docs/label/2010/021986s7s8lbl.pdf

45. Varricchi G, et al. Cardiotoxicity of immune checkpoint inhibitors. *ESMO Open*. 2017;2(4):e000247.

46. Upadhrasta S, et al. Managing cardiotoxicity associated with immune checkpoint inhibitors. *Chronic Dis Transl Med*. 2019;5(1):6-14.

47. Lyon AR, et al. Immune checkpoint inhibitors and cardiovascular toxicity. *Lancet Oncol*. 2018;19(9):e447-e458.

48. Mahmood SS, et al. Myocarditis in patients treated with immune checkpoint inhibitors. *J Am Coll Cardiol*. 2018;71(16):1755-1764.

49. Sara JD, et al. 5-fluorouracil and cardiotoxicity: a review. *Ther Adv Med Oncol*. 2018;10:1758835918780140.

50. Favourable and unfavourable effects on long-term survival of radiotherapy for early breast cancer: an overview of the randomised trials. Early Breast Cancer Trialists' Collaborative Group. *Lancet*. 2000;355(9217):1757-1770.

51. Clarke M, et al. Effects of radiotherapy and of differences in the extent of surgery for early breast cancer on local recurrence and 15-year survival: an overview of the randomised trials. *Lancet*. 2005;366(9503):2087-2106.

52. Rutqvist LE, Rose C, Cavallin-Stahl E. A systematic overview of radiation therapy effects in breast cancer. *Acta Oncol*. 2003;42(5-6):532-545.

53. Fisher B, et al. Lumpectomy compared with lumpectomy and radiation therapy for the treatment of intraductal breast cancer. *N Engl J Med*. 1993;328(22):1581-1586.

54. Fisher B, et al. Lumpectomy and radiation therapy for the treatment of intraductal breast cancer: findings from National Surgical Adjuvant Breast and Bowel Project B-17. *J Clin Oncol*. 1998;16(2):441-452.

55. Taylor CW, et al. Cardiac exposures in breast cancer radiotherapy: 1950s-1990s. *Int J Radiat Oncol Biol Phys*. 2007;69(5):1484-1495.

56. Taylor CW, et al. Cardiac dose from tangential breast cancer radiotherapy in the year 2006. *Int J Radiat Oncol Biol Phys*. 2008;72(2):501-507.

57. Gyenes G, et al. Myocardial damage in breast cancer patients treated with adjuvant radiotherapy: a prospective study. *Int J Radiat Oncol Biol Phys*. 1996;36(4):899-905.

58. Oeffinger KC, et al. Chronic health conditions in adult survivors of childhood cancer. *N Engl J Med*. 2006;355(15):1572-1582.

59. Darby S, et al. Radon in homes and risk of lung cancer: collaborative analysis of individual data from 13 European case–control studies. *BMJ*. 2005;330(7485):223.

60. Bryant AK, et al. Trends in radiation therapy among cancer survivors in the United States, 2000–2030. *Cancer Epidemiol Biomarkers Prev*. 2017;26(6):963-970.

61. Lancellotti P, et al. Expert consensus for multi-modality imaging evaluation of cardiovascular complications of radiotherapy in adults: a report from the European Association of Cardiovascular Imaging and the American Society of Echocardiography. *Eur Heart J Cardiovasc Imaging*. 2013;14(8):721-740.

62. Bhatia N, et al. Cardiovascular effects of androgen deprivation therapy for the treatment of prostate cancer: ABCDE steps to reduce cardiovascular disease in patients with prostate cancer. *Circulation*. 2016;133(5):537-541.

63. Van Besien K, et al. Regimen-related toxicity after fludarabine-melphalan conditioning: a prospective study of 31 patients with hematologic malignancies. *Bone Marrow Transplant*. 2003;32(5):471-476.

64. Reykdal S, Sham R, Kouides P. Cytarabine-induced pericarditis: a case report and review of the literature of the cardio-pulmonary complications of cytarabine therapy. *Leuk Res*. 1995;19(2):141-144.

65. Mandel EM, Lewinski U, Djaldetti M. Vincristine-induced myocardial infarction. *Cancer*. 1975;36(6):1979-1982.

66. Rowinsky EK, et al. Cardiac disturbances during the administration of taxol. *J Clin Oncol*. 1991;9(9):1704-1712.

67. Dhesi S, et al. Cyclophosphamide-induced cardiomyopathy: a case report, review, and recommendations for management. *J Investig Med High Impact Case Rep*. 2013;1(1):2324709613480346.

68. Kandylis K, et al. Ifosfamide cardiotoxicity in humans. *Cancer Chemother Pharmacol*. 1989;24(6):395-396.

69. Hu Y, et al. Cisplatin-induced cardiotoxicity with mid-range ejection fraction: a case report and review of the literature. *Medicine (Baltimore).* 2018;97(52):e13807.

70. Moudgil R, Yeh ET. Mechanisms of cardiotoxicity of cancer chemotherapeutic agents: cardiomyopathy and beyond. *Can J Cardiol.* 2016;32(7):863-870.e5.

71. Cersosimo RJ. Monoclonal antibodies in the treatment of cancer, Part 1. *Am J Health Syst Pharm.* 2003;60(15):1531-1548.

72. Lenihan DJ, et al. Cardiac toxicity of alemtuzumab in patients with mycosis fungoides/Sezary syndrome. *Blood.* 2004;104(3):655-658.

73. Schwarzer S, et al. Non-Q-wave myocardial infarction associated with bleomycin and etoposide chemotherapy. *Eur Heart J.* 1991;12(6):748-750.

74. Yano S, Shimada K. Vasospastic angina after chemotherapy by with carboplatin and etoposide in a patient with lung cancer. *Jpn Circ J.* 1996;60(3):185-188.

75. Sonnenblick M, Rosin A. Cardiotoxicity of interferon. A review of 44 cases. *Chest.* 1991;99(3):557-561.

76. Lee RE, et al. Cardiorespiratory effects of immunotherapy with interleukin-2. *J Clin Oncol.* 1989;7(1):7-20.

77. Montesinos P, et al. Differentiation syndrome in patients with acute promyelocytic leukemia treated with all-trans retinoic acid and anthracycline chemotherapy: characteristics, outcome, and prognostic factors. *Blood.* 2009;113(4):775-783.

78. Moslehi JJ, Deininger M. Tyrosine kinase inhibitor-associated cardiovascular toxicity in chronic myeloid leukemia. *J Clin Oncol.* 2015;33(35):4210-4218.

79. Hrustanovic-Kadic M, Jalil B, El-Kersh K. Carfilzomib-Induced Pulmonary Hypertension. *Am J Ther.* 2019.

80. Chari A, Hajje D. Case series discussion of cardiac and vascular events following carfilzomib treatment: possible mechanism, screening, and monitoring. *BMC Cancer.* 2014;14:915.

81. Chen JH, et al. Cardiac events during treatment with proteasome inhibitor therapy for multiple myeloma. *Cardiooncology.* 2017;3(1):4.

82. Yang X, et al. Anticancer therapy-induced atrial fibrillation: electrophysiology and related mechanisms. *Front Pharmacol.* 2018;9:1058.

83. Kaakeh Y, et al. Drug-induced atrial fibrillation. *Drugs.* 2012;72(12):1617-1630.

84. Porta-Sanchez A, et al. Incidence, diagnosis, and management of QT prolongation induced by cancer therapies: a systematic review. *J Am Heart Assoc.* 2017;6(12):e007724.

85. Strevel EL, Ing DJ, Siu LL. Molecularly targeted oncology therapeutics and prolongation of the QT interval. *J Clin Oncol.* 2007;25(22):3362-3371.

86. Kuriakose RK, Kukreja RC, Xi L. Potential therapeutic strategies for hypertension-exacerbated cardiotoxicity of anticancer drugs. *Oxid Med Cell Longev.* 2016;2016:8139861.

87. Jain M, Townsend RR. Chemotherapy agents and hypertension: a focus on angiogenesis blockade. *Curr Hypertens Rep.* 2007;9(4):320-328.

88. Ray A, Ray S, Koner B. Hypertension, cancer and angiogenesis: Relevant epidemiological and pharmacological aspects. *Indian J Pharmacol.* 2004;36(6):341.

89. Whelton PK, et al. 2017 ACC/AHA/AAPA/ABC/ACPM/AGS/APhA/ASH/ASPC/NMA/PCNA guideline for the prevention, detection, evaluation, and management of high blood pressure in adults: executive summary: a report of the American College of Cardiology/American Heart Association Task Force on Clinical Practice Guidelines. *Circulation.* 2018;138(17):e426-e483.

90. SOLVD Investigators, et al. Effect of enalapril on survival in patients with reduced left ventricular ejection fractions and congestive heart failure. *N Engl J Med.* 1991;325(5):293-302.

91. CONSENSUS Trial Study Group. Effects of enalapril on mortality in severe congestive heart failure. Results of the Cooperative North Scandinavian Enalapril Survival Study (CONSENSUS). *N Engl J Med.* 1987;316(23):1429-1435.

92. Poole-Wilson PA, et al. Comparison of carvedilol and metoprolol on clinical outcomes in patients with chronic heart failure in the Carvedilol Or Metoprolol European Trial (COMET): randomised controlled trial. *Lancet.* 2003;362(9377):7-13.

93. Young JB, et al. Mortality and morbidity reduction with Candesartan in patients with chronic heart failure and left ventricular systolic dysfunction: results of the CHARM low-left ventricular ejection fraction trials. *Circulation.* 2004;110(17):2618-2626.

94. Grundy SM, et al. 2018 AHA/ACC/AACVPR/AAPA/ABC/ACPM/ADA/AGS/APhA/ASPC/NLA/PCNA guideline on the management of blood cholesterol: executive summary: a report of the American College of Cardiology/American Heart Association Task Force on Clinical Practice Guidelines. *Circulation.* 2019;139(25):e1046-e1081.

95. Hull MC, et al. Valvular dysfunction and carotid, subclavian, and coronary artery disease in survivors of Hodgkin lymphoma treated with radiation therapy. *JAMA.* 2003;290(21):2831-2837.

96. Amsterdam EA, et al. 2014 AHA/ACC guideline for the management of patients with Non-ST-Elevation acute coronary syndromes: a report of the American College of Cardiology/American Heart Association Task Force on Practice Guidelines. *J Am Coll Cardiol.* 2014;64(24):e139-e228.

97. Sarkiss MG, et al. Impact of aspirin therapy in cancer patients with thrombocytopenia and acute coronary syndromes. *Cancer.* 2007;109(3):621-627.

98. Iliescu C, et al. SCAI expert consensus statement: evaluation, management, and special considerations of cardio-oncology patients in the cardiac catheterization laboratory (Endorsed by the Cardiological Society of India, and Sociedad Latino Americana de Cardiologia Intervencionista). *Catheter Cardiovasc Interv.* 2016;87(5):895-899.

99. Duceppe E, et al. Canadian cardiovascular society guidelines on perioperative cardiac risk assessment and management for patients who undergo noncardiac surgery. *Can J Cardiol.* 2017;33(1):17-32.

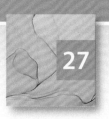

John R. Bach and Liping Wang

"(ALS) has not prevented me from having a very attractive family, and being successful in my work… I have been lucky that my condition has progressed more slowly than is often the case, but it shows that one need not lose hope."—Professor Steven Hawking, communicated via a speech-generating device, initially operated by finger control but ultimately by using a single cheek muscle.

INTRODUCTION AND OBJECTIVES

Palliative care can be defined as the treatment of symptoms including dyspnea, pain, and stress associated with a serious chronic illness irrespective of "prognosis." It does not replace treatments directed to the primary pathology. Its goal is to ease disability and suffering to preserve quality of life for the patient and family. While this is readily understandable, as are medical and psychological interventions for patients with metastatic cancer and other "terminal diseases," palliative care plays a far wider role for patients with generalized muscle weakness and deconditioning who lose the ability to ventilate their lungs and lose physical function to perform activities of daily living (ADL). Besides the fact that general rehabilitation principles apply, which can preserve or restore ADL, respiratory palliative care interventions, by relieving dyspnea and other respiratory symptoms, can greatly prolong life and maintain its quality. These interventions apply to all patients with ventilatory pump failure (VPF). These include ventilator unweanable patients with critical care deconditioning, patients with deconditioning from medical interventions such as repeated chemotherapy, and patients with neuromuscular disease (NMD).

There are 45 muscles involved in respiration. All of these muscles can be weakened to the point of total paralysis for patients with the pediatric- and adult-onset diagnoses considered in Table 27.1. The most common neuromuscular diseases that result in patients requiring the use of noninvasive respiratory muscle aids are spinal muscular atrophy (SMA), muscular dystrophy, and amyotrophic lateral sclerosis/motor neuron disease (ALS/MND), which typically result in acute respiratory failure (ARF) or chronic respiratory failure and translaryngeal intubation in intensive care units without

palliative care they progress to tracheotomy or death. While tracheotomy for up to continuous tracheostomy mechanical ventilation (CTMV) eases symptoms such as dyspnea and can prolong life, as it did for 33 years for Dr. Stephen Hawking who lived with ALS/MND for 55 of his 76 years, up to 80% of TMV users die from complications of the tubes rather than from their diseases per se (1,2). This is the reason why patients with Duchenne muscular dystrophy (DMD) live almost 10 years longer using noninvasive respiratory management and avoid tracheotomy (3).

The use of assistive equipment such as canes and wheelchairs to optimize mobility is widely appreciated. Less well known is the variety of assistive equipment that can provide patients retaining only trace residual muscle activity of any muscle with the ability to operate motorized wheelchairs, computer systems for voice-generated communication, environmental control systems, and robot arms to feed, shave, and assist with transfers. For those who are otherwise locked in, systems are now being developed that allow brain waves to permit simple communication and even operate motorized wheelchairs. The reader is directed to other sources for more information (4,5).

"The first step to wisdom is to call something by what is really is."— Ancient Chinese proverb

WITHOUT RESPIRATORY PALLIATIVE CARE

None of the new medications for neuromuscular disorders (NMDs) are even nearly curative, just as patients debilitated by cancer are rarely cured by medical treatments. Since respiratory muscle weakness initially presents with symptoms due to sleep hypoventilation, patients are typically referred for polysomnograms and treated by continuous positive airway pressure (CPAP) or bilevel PAP at minimal settings, which provide no significant rest for respiratory muscles and are inadequate for respiratory support. In fact, apnea–hypopnea indices are typically normalized by polysomnographic titration without achieving normalization of CO_2 levels, so patients often remain symptomatic for hypercapnia. Indeed, polysomnographs are

TABLE 27.1 CONDITIONS WITH VENTILATORY PUMP FAILURE

Critical care neuromyopathies/deconditioning and chronic debility

Congenital, inflammatory, and metabolic myopathies

Muscular dystrophies

Spinal muscular atrophies

Motor neuron diseases including amyotrophic lateral sclerosis

Postpoliomyelitis

Neuropathies including Guillain-Barré syndrome

Multiple sclerosis

Myasthenia gravis

Traumatic tetraplegia and other myelopathies

Morbid obesity

Chest wall disease

Chronic obstructive pulmonary disease and other lung disorders

programmed to interpret all apneas and hypopneas as either obstructive or central in nature and do not identify or consider respiratory muscle weakness as a cause. This incorrectly attributes the problem to the brain or throat rather than the respiratory muscles. The problem must be correctly identified before it can be treated. Routine polysomnography is not useful for identifying respiratory muscle weakness as the cause of hypoventilation unless CO_2 is monitored, which is rarely the case.

As a weak cough turns otherwise benign upper respiratory tract infections into pneumonia (URI-pneumonia) and ARF, patients are sent for pulmonary function testing (PFT), which do not measure cough flows and is just as inadequate as polysomnography. Prognosis is conventionally thought to parallel decreasing vital capacity (VC), defined as the greatest breath one can inhale then exhale into a spirometer. This indicates approaching death for clinicians unaware of the respiratory muscle aids described in this chapter.

Patients with decreasing respiratory muscle function who require increasing physical assistance with ADL are also frequently encouraged to turn to hospice services, which invariably petition physicians to approve orders for supplemental oxygen (O_2) and narcotics, just as they do for cancer patients, without informing the patients that these medications can severely exacerbate lung hypoventilation, lead to ARF, and hasten death (6).

The Physical Medicine Respiratory Muscle Aids of Noninvasive Respiratory Management

The respiratory muscles include inspiratory muscles, expiratory muscles for coughing to clear airway debris, and bulbar-innervated muscles (BIM) to protect the airways. The inspiratory and expiratory muscles can be entirely substituted for by noninvasive aids, but only patient positioning can prevent aspiration of secretions and render BIM function unnecessary.

Inspiratory and expiratory muscle aids are devices and techniques that involve the manual or mechanical application of forces to the body or intermittent pressure changes to the airways to assist or support inspiratory and expiratory muscle function. Devices primarily acting on the body include negative pressure body ventilators (NPBVs), which no longer have a significant role in therapy, and ventilation corsets that apply force directly to the abdomen to mechanically displace the diaphragm. Negative pressure applied to the airways (forced exsufflation) assists or replaces the coughing function of the expiratory muscles just as positive pressure applied to the airways for inhalation (noninvasive ventilatory support or "NVS") assists or replaces inspiratory muscle function.

The Intervention Objectives

To meet the palliative care goals of easing symptoms, providing ventilatory assistance or support, and maintaining quality of life without resort to tracheotomy, the following are necessary: (a) maintenance of lung and chest wall elasticity by lung volume recruitment (LVR), (b) maintenance of normal lung ventilation around-the-clock, and (c) maximization of cough flows. These can be attained by a specifically focused evaluation of patients with VPF and then equipping them with and training them in the use of respiratory muscle aids, usually in the outpatient setting and at home.

Clinical Assessment

Patients are assessed for symptoms of hypercapnia due to VPF. These include morning headaches, fatigue, sleep disturbances, hypersomnolence, and others (7). Diaphragm weakness can be identified by orthopnea measured as reduced VC supine when compared to that when seated. Respiratory muscle weakness presents with tachypnea, paradoxical breathing, hypophonia, nasal flaring, use of accessory respiratory muscles, and hypercapnia and can result in cyanosis, flushing or pallor, CO_2 narcosis, airway congestion, and ARF. With respiratory orthopnea, the seated position VC can be 25% to 60% greater than supine VC. For infants, paradoxical breathing can be accompanied by flushing, perspiration, and frequent arousals for sleep.

PFTs are designed to assess lung and airways diseases and do not include VC supine, cough flows, end-tidal CO_2, BIM, or LVR assessments, all of which, along with oximetry, must be monitored on a routine basis (8). Arterial blood gases are typically unnecessary because oximetry and capnography can provide the needed information. All symptomatic patients with diminished pulmonary function deserve a trial of nocturnal NVS. However, if pretreatment symptoms are not obvious, CO_2 and O_2 saturation levels are monitored during sleep to further suggest possible benefit from using nocturnal NVS to alleviate daytime symptoms. The LVR and BIM assessments are done by training the patient in air stacking (active LVR), during which the patient retains multiple sequentially delivered volumes of air to the maximum that the glottis can hold. The air is delivered by manual resuscitator or portable ventilator with preset volumes. The maximum volume that can be held is termed the "maximum insufflation capacity (MIC)" (9,10). The MIC minus the VC is a measure of the integrity of the glottis and, since the glottis is the most important BIM to protect the airways, it is an objective, quantifiable, reproducible measure of BIM function.

Nocturnal Support

Patients begin with nocturnal NVS for relief of symptoms. Lip cover, nasal, and oronasal interfaces can be used to deliver the typical inspiratory volumes of 800 to 1,500 mL or pressures of 18 to 25 cm H_2O for NVS during sleep as during waking hours when needed (Figs. 27.1 to 27.3), with

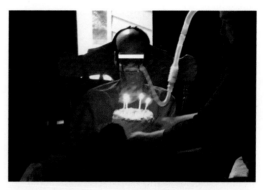

Figure 27.2 Patient with amyotrophic lateral sclerosis dependent on CNVS via nasal interface day and night ongoing now for 14 years.

a physiologic back-up rate of 12 to 14 breaths per minute. The large volumes compensate for air leakage and permit users to physiologically vary tidal volumes; they facilitate active LVR and rest inspiratory muscles (3,8). While a large range is prescribed for the patient to choose from, the choice is usually 1,200 to 1,300 mL.

Excessive air leakage can make NVS ineffective but is generally precluded by avoiding supplemental O_2 and heavily sedating medications. An unsedated ventilatory drive reflexively prevents excessive leakage during sleep via repeated transient low-level arousals, which do not consciously disrupt the patient's sleep (11). This is done without apparent harm since numerous patients have now been dependent on continuous NVS (CNVS) for over 65 years (Fig. 27.4) without barotrauma or other difficulties. A passive mechanism that prevents excessive leakage is the NVS passing via the nose and propelling the soft palate against the posterior surface of the tongue to seal

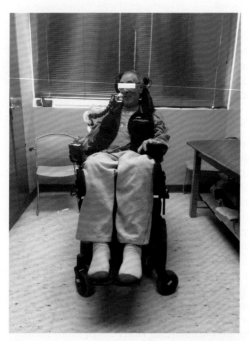

Figure 27.1 Patient with amyotrophic lateral sclerosis dependent on continuous noninvasive ventilatory support (CNVS) via angled mouthpiece set up on flexible metal support arm during the day and nasal CNVS for sleep.

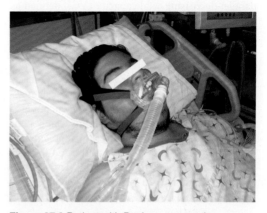

Figure 27.3 Patient with Duchenne muscular dystrophy transferred to be extubated to CNVS after failing multiple extubation attempts to bilevel positive airway pressure and supplemental O_2, using oronasal NVS for sleep.

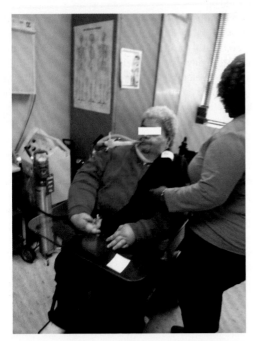

Figure 27.4 Patient dependent on CNVS via angled mouthpiece during the day and lip cover phalange for sleep for 65 years, since 1954, who is employed full time as a rehabilitation counselor despite tetraplegia.

off the oropharynx (12). Occasionally, however, air leakage can be excessive and disrupt sleep, causing prolonged severe O_2 desaturation and conscious arousals with dyspnea. This is treated by switching from nasal to oronasal interfaces (Fig. 27.3) (11).

The nasal and oronasal interfaces for NVS can be vented or non-vented. Vented interfaces have open portals or areas that allow interface leakage to avoid CO_2 rebreathing. These vented interfaces are used with "passive" ventilator circuits that deliver CPAP and bilevel PAP. Non-vented interfaces do not have open portals or leak areas and are used with "active" circuits, circuits with exhalation valves. Active circuits should be used with non-vented interfaces or vented interfaces with all open areas covered or blocked by tape (12).

Humidity is another factor to consider when using nocturnal NVS. Dry nasal mucous membranes can cause vasodilation and nasal congestion. In the case of nasal NVS, the unidirectional airflow with expiration through the mouth can cause loss of humidity and increase airflow resistance, which can be alleviated with the use of a hot water bath humidifier (13). Other options include the use of decongestants.

Normal gastroesophageal sphincter pressure is 25 cm H_2O but is often lower in patients with NMD; thus, there is a predisposition to bloating and abdominal distension even without NVS. The

addition of NVS can exacerbate the abdominal distension and, at times, necessitate placement of an indwelling gastrostomy tube to "burp out" the air. This is always preferable to tracheotomy.

NVS is contraindicated in conditions that prevent reliable access to the NVS interface, such as with depressed cognitive function, some facial orthopedic conditions, pulmonary diseases that necessitate a high fraction of O_2 (fiO_2), uncontrolled seizures, and substance abuse. Diaphragm and phrenic nerve pacing are never indicated for patients with VPF other than for certain patients with high level spinal cord injury (SCI) and no ventilator-free breathing ability (14). Pacing requires presence of a tracheostomy tube or CPAP administration because of the obstructive apneas it causes, whereas NVS ventilates the lungs and prevents obstructive apneas as well.

Daytime Noninvasive Ventilatory Support

The most important interfaces for daytime NVS are 15- and 22-mm mouthpieces and straws (Figs. 27.1, 27.4 to 27.6) (1). Mouthpiece NVS is often initially used for daytime support to aid with eating (15). Patients with decreasing inspiratory muscle strength can become tachypneic, reaching breathing rates over 40 breaths per minute. This permits about 1 second for swallowing food. The use of NVS provides breaths of 1 L or more, main-

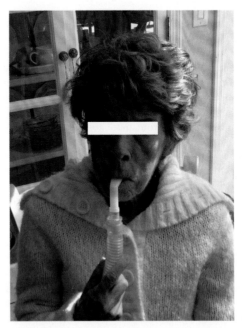

Figure 27.5 Patient with bilateral diaphragm paralysis associated with metastatic thymoma dependent on continuous mouthpiece (diurnal) and nasal (sleep) noninvasive ventilatory support.

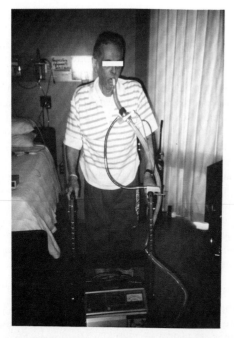

Figure 27.6 Patient with severe lung disease from an explosion. He had been CO_2 narcotic and comatose with agonal breathing and was DNR and refusing re-intubation. While comatose we manually ventilated him via a lip cover phalange which normalized his $PaCO_2$ from 140 mm. He awoke and remained dependent on CNVS at home for 11 months before dying there.

taining minute ventilation and increasing time for swallowing to 10 seconds or more (15).

Patients using sleep NVS who become dyspneic when disconnected from it in the morning or who continue to exhibit symptoms of hypoventilation/hypercapnia tend to continue nasal or oronasal NVS into daytime hours. At this point, patients are transitioned from nasal to mouthpiece NVS. NVS mouthpieces can also be mounted onto a wheelchair with the mouthpiece fixed adjacent to the mouth for easy access (Figs. 27.1 and 27.4). Some neck and lip function is required to grab the mouthpiece for NVS. In addition, the soft palate must be capable of sealing off the nasopharynx to prevent excessive air leakage from the nose, and the reflex opening of the glottis at onset of inspiration must be intact. This sometimes has to be relearned for patients whose glottis had remained closed while receiving TMV (16). As for sleep NVS, 800 to 1,500 mL delivered volumes are also used for daytime NVS and for the same reasons: to compensate for air leakage, to allow for varied tidal volumes, to permit active LVF, and to provide deep breaths to increase cough peak flows (CPF) and louder and longer speech.

For those whose lips or neck muscles are too weak or jaw opening insufficient to grab a mouthpiece, nasal prongs or other nasal interfaces are used for daytime NVS (Fig. 24.2). Nasal NVS is always preferable to tracheotomy. When using nasal NVS around-the-clock, it is important to alternate two or more nasal interfaces for daytime and sleep use. Often nasal prongs are preferred for daytime use.

The intermittent abdominal pressure ventilator (IAPV) is effective for daytime ventilatory support and is often preferred over using facial interfaces (Fig. 27.7). It consists of a girdle or corset worn under the clothing with an elastic air bladder in it that, when inflated by a portable ventilator set up on the back of a wheelchair, raises the diaphragm so that gravity can bring it back down to cause air to enter the airways. The IAPV can augment tidal volumes by 300 to 1,200 mL and is a cosmetic and comfortable alternative for daytime support (17).

ANCILLARY INTERVENTIONS

Glossopharyngeal breathing (GPB) involves the movement of the tongue and pharynx to piston boluses of air into the lungs. Most tidal breaths are accomplished by about seven such boluses. The pistoning can supplement autonomous breathing or completely substitute for it for patients with

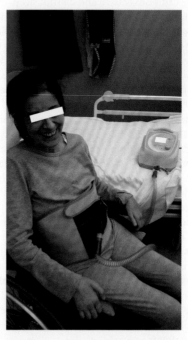

Figure 27.7 Patient with amyotrophic lateral sclerosis using an intermittent abdominal pressure ventilator (IAPV) for daytime ventilatory support and wearing the corset of the IAPV over the clothing for demonstration purposes only.

little or no VC. Progress in mastering it can be spirometrically measured. The GPB or "frog breathing" can assist or support both inspiratory and expiratory functions (18,19). It can often permit patients with little or no VC to breathe free of ventilatory support for as long as all day. Patients who master it do not need to worry about ventilator failure during the day or during sleep because they awaken using it if their ventilators fail suddenly overnight (20–22). Patients with good BIM function are the best candidates to master GPB (16,23), but about 30% of patients with DMD master it as well (19).

LVR can be active or passive and serves to preserve or increase pulmonary compliance. The latter decreases with inability to breathe deeply and expand the lungs to predicted normal lung volumes. Lung expansion can be measured by the lung insufflation capacity (LIC), a measure of passive LVR (24), or the MIC, a measure of active LVR. These correlates inversely with the extent of chest wall contractures and lung and chest wall restriction (25). Thus, LVR can maintain lung and chest wall compliance, promote lung and chest wall growth, and maximize lung inflation volumes (23,26).

Active LVR is performed by GPB or by the air stacking of consecutively delivered volumes of air delivered by volume preset ventilation or manual resuscitator as noted previously. For patients with weak lips, air stacking can be done via nasal, lip cover, or oronasal interfaces, but glottis function is always required to hold the air for active LVR. LVR can increase VC and CPF while reducing atelectasis (9,10,23). It can also permit patients to speak louder and longer phrases. For any patient using NVS or capable of performing active LVR or "air stacking," and who is subsequently intubated for any reason, transitioning from extubation to CNVS will be easier. The LVR can be provided via mouthpiece, lip cover, or nasal/oronasal interfaces.

For patients who cannot air stack because they cannot close the glottis, passive LVR is performed by using a manual resuscitator with blocked exhalation valve to prevent exhalation until maximum lung volumes are attained, the LIC. Adequate delivery can be noted by feeling the resistance of lung recoil while squeezing the manual resuscitator to inflate the lungs. Passive LVR can also be provided by the mechanical insufflation of MIE to pressures of 55 to 70 cm H_2O or more (8,26).

Assisted Coughing and Mechanical Insufflation–Exsufflation

Manually Assisted Coughing

Manually assisted coughing is performed by taking a deep inspiration to at least 1,500 mL, or by air stacking, then having an abdominal thrust timed to glottis opening for the cough. A study showed that with manually assisted coughing, subjects' CPF increased from 150 ± 120 to 255 ± 100 L/min (27). Increased flows can more effectively prevent URI–pneumonias and ARF (28). If patients are unable to air stack, likely due to inability to close the glottis, they can still have manually assisted coughing with abdominal thrusts following deep insufflations. This typically increases CPF well over 180 L/min.

Mechanical Insufflation–Exsufflation

Mechanical insufflation–exsufflation (MIE) is usually used via oronasal interfaces or simple mouthpieces. Pressures of 40 and −40 mm Hg (54.1 cm H_2O), to fully inflate then rapidly deflate the lungs, are optimal. MIE is also used via translaryngeal and tracheostomy tubes at pressures of 60 to 70 cm H_2O due to the severe pressure drop-off and decreased air flows across the tubes (29).

MIE is used to prevent URI–pneumonias as well as to prepare even ventilator unweanable patients for extubation or decannulation if they get pneumonia and develop ARF or require general anesthesia (30,31). About 20% of the time, MIE-exsufflation flows (MIE-EF) can be increased by applying a manual thrust during the exsufflation phase. MIE treatments typically last until secretions are no longer expelled and secretion-related O_2 desaturations resolve. During chest infections or 36 hours postextubation or decannulation, MIE can be used as often as every 20 to 30 minutes around-the-clock to maintain O_2 sat ≥95% in ambient air to avert extubation/decannulation failure.

In comparing MIE to invasive airway suctioning, the left main stem bronchus is missed with routine airway suctioning about 90% of the time (32), while MIE-EF can clear both left and right airways without the discomfort or airway trauma of suctioning. Patients prefer MIE to airway suctioning (33). Effective clearance of airway secretions with MIE improves VC, pulmonary flow rates, and O_2 saturation. In 67 patients with "obstructive dyspnea," increases in VC of 15% to 40% were reported. In patients with NMDs, an increase of 55% in VC was noted without adverse effects (34). More recently, for patients with NMD during chest infections, an improvement of 15% to 400% in VC and normalization of O_2 saturation can occur with the use of MIE (35).

For patients with central nervous system (CNS) or upper MND, such as many hypertonic ALS patients, upper airways eventually collapse too much for effective MIE-EF (36,37). When the MIE-EF are <100 L/min, tracheotomy is typically necessary (36). An MIE-EF of >200 L/min usually very effectively clears secretions and is achievable by all with NMD except for some cases of advanced ALS, which is why tracheostomy tubes are generally only required by CNS and ALS patients. Patients with the ability to air stack but inability to achieve MIE-EF >180 to 200 L/min should be evaluated for upper airway obstruction with laryngoscopy to assess for reversible lesions.

Long-term Domiciliary Prevention of Respiratory Complications by the Oximetry Feedback Protocol

Oximetry feedback using CNVS and MIE is used all day during URIs or multiple times daily for patients with a tendency to aspirate upper airway secretions to prevent URI–pneumonias and ARF. It is also important for successful extubation and decannulation. An O_2 saturation alarm can be set to 94% so that decreases in O_2 sat alert the patient and care providers to use NVS and/or MIE to clear airway secretions to renormalize O_2 sat levels. Oxygen desaturation below 95% during URIs is typically due to bronchial mucous plugs, which can lead to atelectasis, pneumonia, and lung collapse, all preventable by oximetry feedback for effective use of NVS and MIE. The importance of O_2 sat for queuing the use of NVS and MIE is a strong argument against the habitual use of supplemental O_2 in these patients, as it can mask the signs of mucous plugging and hypoventilation.

CRITICAL CARE MANAGEMENT

Conventional management with O_2 and low span bilevel PAP instead of NVS and MIE typically results in CO_2 narcosis and respiratory arrest, as neither intervention may reverse hypercapnia for patients needing ventilatory support (6). Patients with severe and progressive VPF are assumed to be "terminal" and need recourse to palliative care in the form of supplemental O_2 and morphine to ease the dyspnea caused by their VPF. Over a 5-year period, the *New England Journal of Medicine* published 12 papers on euthanasia for ALS without a single mention of the ability of CNVS to relieve their symptoms or prolong their lives (38). All too often, O_2 and narcotics greatly hasten the deaths without the patients being told that this is likely to be the case. This is, in essence, uninformed euthanasia (38). Unfortunately, their physicians simply do not know any less deadly palliative alternatives.

Figure 27.6 is of a man with severe lung disease due to an explosion and inhaled flames that greatly damaged his lung tissues. He underwent intubation for ARF 18 times over a 19-year period and signed an advance directive to never again suffer placement of an invasive airway tube. During his next episode of ARF, unresponsive with agonal breathing although receiving fiO_2 100%, it was pointed out to his pulmonologist that NVS might lower his CO_2 and resuscitate him. Having no objection to this, nasal NVS was first tried but all the air leaked out of his mouth. When the air was delivered via a lip cover interface (Fig. 27.8), his CO_2 decreased and eventually normalized, he awoke, and several days later was discharged home. He walked with the ventilator on a rolling walker and survived 11 months before dying peacefully at home. Besides assuaging his symptoms, the nasal NVS for sleep and mouthpiece NVS for waking hours gave him 11 additional months of life for which he was grateful.

Once patients are intubated, ventilator weaning parameters and spontaneous breathing trials must conventionally be passed before any attempt is made at extubation, which is typically to supplemental O_2 and low span bilevel PAP rather than palliative care measures of noninvasive respiratory management. However, ventilator unweanable patients need to be extubated to CNVS and MIE rather than be weaned to be extubated to O_2 and bilevel PAP.

Table 27.2 demonstrates the criteria for extubating ventilator unweanable patients (30,31). The O_2 sat must be normal, that is >94%, in ambient air. Even a fiO_2 as low as 25% can prevent an oximeter from alerting the physician to airway secretion congestion and marked hypercapnia. Chances of extubation success are decreased if CO_2 and ambient air O_2 sat are not normalized prior to extubation and if airway secretions are not effectively expulsed and lung pathology not corrected by using MIE hourly via the translaryngeal tube. An ambient air O_2 sat <95% points to these abnormalities. Oxygen administration can result in an artificially normalized O_2 sat in the presence of one or all three, and so extubation fails. Extubation of these patients whose O_2 sat in ambient air is <95% should rarely be attempted. Instead of clinicians thinking that patients with advanced ALS, muscular dystrophy,

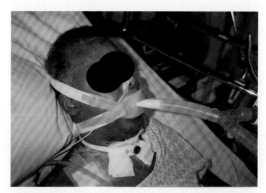

Figure 27.8 Patients with 180 mL of vital capacity and no ventilator-free breathing ability being transitioned from tracheostomy to CNVS, using a lip cover interface for sleep NVS.

TABLE 27.2 CRITERIA FOR EXTUBATION OF VENTILATOR UNWEANABLE PATIENTS

- Must be fully alert and cooperative
- No O_2 and sedating medications minimized
- Failure of respiratory function alone with other organs functional
- Afebrile
- Normal white blood cell count
- Chest x-rays indicating resolving abnormalities
- CO_2 tension <44 mm Hg or end-tidal CO_2 normal
- Oxyhemoglobin sat $\geq$95% for at least 12 hours
- With translaryngeal tube cuff deflation air leakage through the vocal cords (positive leak test)
- Any O_2 desats below 95% reversed by using MIE via translaryngeal tube

MIE, mechanical insufflation–exsufflation; O_2 sat, oxyhemoglobin saturation.

SMA types 1 to 4, or other such conditions would require tracheostomy tubes if they are intubated and, so, morphine and O_2 are warranted, extubation to CNVS and MIE is almost always successful provided that Table 27.2 criteria are met (30,31).

Once criteria are met, any orogastric/nasogastric tubes are removed to facilitate postextubation nasal NVS. The patient is then extubated directly to CNVS on assist/control mode with preset pressures of about 20 cm H_2O or volumes of 800 to 1,500 mL at a rate of 10 to 14 per minute in ambient air. If the patient was using NVS prior to intubation, he or she is extubated to the same settings and interfaces. Once ventilation via nasal interface is achieved, mouthpiece NVS is instituted and then air stacking (30,31).

Patients keep 15-mm angled mouthpieces within easy access to their mouths and wean themselves by taking fewer and fewer intermittent positive pressure ventilations. Diurnal nasal NVS is used for those who cannot grab and use a mouthpiece properly. If O_2 sat decreases to <95%, ventilator positive inspiratory pressures (PIPs), interface or tubing air leakage, CO_2 retention, modification of ventilator settings, and MIE are considered to reverse the desaturation. Low ventilator PIPs indicate air leakage or inadequate settings. MIE is applied via oronasal interfaces at 50 to 60 cm H_2O to correct any decreases in O_2 sat due to airway mucus. This is done by the patients' family or care providers up to every 20 minutes postextubation and for all O_2 desaturations below 95%. Critical care is an ideal setting for family members to learn MIE and NVS management. Hospital staff will not be able to administer MIE at this frequency for the first 36 postextubation hours to optimize chances for its success.

If postextubation oral intake is unsafe or inadequate, a gastrostomy tube is needed. This is typically radiographically inserted (39), an open gastrostomy by general surgery (40) or by percutaneous endoscopic gastrostomy with trochanter passed via an orifice in an oronasal interface used for NVS during the procedure. These methods permit gastrostomy tube placement without intubation or general anesthesia (41).

DECANNULATION

In 1996, decannulation for ventilator-dependent SCI patients and 50 unweanable NMD patients was reported (42). Decannulation is recommended for any patient whose BIM is sufficient such that saliva aspiration does not cause a continuous decrease in baseline O_2 sat below 95% and MIE-EF are over about 180 L/min with the ostomy covered (42). Patients are decannulated to CNVS in ambient air as their care providers use MIE up to every 20 to 30 minutes to maintain O_2 sat >94% for the first 36 hours following decannulation. Patients with tracheostomy tubes who have no ventilator-free breathing ability but who have VCs of 250 mL or greater invariably wean to less than CNVS, typically to sleep-only NVS, after decannulation. These patients' VCs increase, and many wean to nocturnal-only NVS within 3 weeks of decannulation. Only patients with severe glottis dysfunction that results in O_2 desat are poor candidates for decannulation (42). Even patients with little to no VC can be safely decannulated and safe even in the event of disconnection from NVS by using GPB.

Reasons why TMV increases ventilator dependence include tube-triggered airway secretions, which block respiratory exchange membranes, bypassing of upper airway afferents, and respiratory muscle deconditioning (43). Removal of the tube facilitates speech and swallowing and VCs increase.

OUTCOMES

An April 2010 consensus of clinicians with 760 CNVS-dependent patients with ALS and other NMDs noted that patients with DMD live 10 years longer when using CNVS rather than CTMV (3,8). In another study, patients preferred CNVS over TMV for safety, convenience, swallowing, speech, appearance, and comfort (44). For patients with DMD, 101 became CNVS dependent for 7.4 ± 6.1 years to a mean of 30.1 ± 6.1 years of age with 56 still alive. Twenty-six of the original 101 patients became CNVS dependent without hospitalization or any episode of ARF (45,46). At least 81 intubated DMD patients who could not pass spontaneous breathing trials before or after extubation have now been successfully extubated to CNVS and MIE (30,31,46). CNVS is also an alternative to TMV in the perioperative management of flaccid neuromuscular scoliosis (47). Thus, CNVS provides more favorable results in terms of morbidity, mortality, and quality of life compared to TMV, and tracheostomies should be avoided or reversed as described (48,49).

MEDICAL/ONCOLOGY PATIENTS

ARF can develop from progressive hypoventilation or from inadequate CPF during chest infections for increasingly debilitated patients with severe medical or neurological conditions. Thirty percent of otherwise healthy elderly nursing home residents die from pneumonia in part because they become too weak to cough effectively (50). NVS can be implemented to re-normalize CO_2, O_2 sat, and bicarbonate levels and reverse alveolar hypoventilation, as well as permit the extubation of ventilator unweanable medical patients without resorting to tracheotomy (30,31). Only VPF patients with upper motor neuron/CNS disorders such as ALS may eventually require tracheostomy tubes when the O_2 saturation baseline remains below 95% due to inability to expel saliva and airway debris (2,46). Cognitively intact elderly debilitated patients with critical care deconditioning do not require tracheostomy tubes when intubated to CNVS despite being ventilator unweanable (30,31). While it may be

argued that the conclusions of this review are "not evidence based" due to the lack of case–control parameters, it should be noted that it is not ethically plausible to perform a placebo controlled trial when the invention replaces either the function of a vital organ or the vital organ itself (51). A patient with the airway secretions of bronchitis who cannot cough and does not have cough flows provided for them would survive no more than a few hours, just as a patient with a VC of 0 mL would not survive more than a few minutes without full ventilatory support, whether invasive or noninvasive (51). While it has not been demonstrated other than by historical controls that noninvasive management prolongs life more than invasive management (3), the contrary has also not been demonstrated. However, noninvasive management should always be favored to preserve quality of life until it is demonstrated to be inferior to invasive management. At any rate, invasive management is not considered to be palliative. Therefore, it is time for a paradigm shift.

Case Studies

A 66-year-old woman first diagnosed with thymoma in 2001 had five periods of chemotherapy, which reduced her initial cancer burden by one-third. In 2005, 7 lb of tumor were removed from her thorax, after which she failed ventilator weaning parameters and remained intubated for 3 weeks. Radiation therapy was initiated as was fentanyl patch application, which exacerbated her preexisting hypercapnia. In 2014, she was hospitalized four times for CO_2 narcosis, with $PaCO_2$ increasing to 130 mm Hg while treated with supplemental O_2. In May 2014, she failed two extubation attempts, refused tracheotomy, and was transferred to a www.breatheNVS.com center for extubation to CNVS and MIE. Following extubation to CNVS, VC increased from 250 to 550 mL (predicted normal would have been 2,350 mL). She was extubated to mouthpiece CNVS via portable ventilator set to assist control mode volume preset to 750 mL via active ventilator circuit. Her medications included fentanyl and chemotherapeutic agents. The patient had good BIM function and normal articulation and deglutition. She weaned from CNVS in 3 weeks and discontinued NVS as her VC increased to 660 mL seated and 560 mL supine. Cognition and motor power remained intact. Although daytime O_2 sat and CO_2 were normal, sleep end-tidal CO_2 rose to 69 mm Hg with O_2 sats ranging from 79% to 91% and, so, she had discontinued sleep NVS. She also had a productive cough secondary to bronchial tumor invasion. Since CPF of 180 L/min were inadequate, MIE was implemented at 60 cm H_2O to expel airway debris. MIE-EF was over 240 L/min. She returned to using sleep NVS on assist/control mode at 1,000 mL, rate 12 and used mouthpiece NVS on the same settings for dyspnea when walking and to relieve dyspnea during meals. She used NVS for 15 months until dying suddenly at home.

In another example, a 34-year-old woman, quadriplegic from metastatic breast cancer to the cervical spine levels 1 to 2 and 5 to 6 and pons, post-multiple rounds of chemotherapy and whole body radiation twice, had dysarthria and

right-sided hemiparesis secondary to an enlarging thalamic lesion with mass effect from surrounding edema for which she was receiving dexamethasone. She also had a posterior right lung nodule, pseudocirrhosis with ascites due to metastases to the liver, splenomegaly, enlarged left paraaortic lymph nodes, and a lobulated vascular lesion in the left gluteus medius. She was intubated for pneumonia and ARF and failed one extubation attempt, then extubated to low span bilevel PAP and supplemental O_2 on which she developed CO_2 narcosis, and was readmitted and reintubated. Refusing tracheotomy, she was then transferred for extubation to CNVS and MIE with a VC of 170 mL before, which improved to 500 mL following extubation the day after transfer. She weaned to primarily sleep NVS but used mouthpiece NVS for periods during the day. She had a stroke and died 3 months later.

These cases illustrate the parallels in management of acute and chronic pulmonary deterioration between medical/cancer and primary VPF patients for whom acute or chronic debilitation can result in need for respiratory support. This should always be NVS rather than TMV for the amenable cooperative patient. Oxygen therapy is not a substitute for NVS and MIE and can cause ARF. The NVS relieves symptoms of hypoventilation, normalizes CO_2, permits patients to avoid hospitalizations for hypercapnic obtundation, and can prolong life. Implementation of NVS and MIE can be critical in palliative management to avoid hospitalizations, intubations, and tracheostomy tubes for patients with critical care deconditioning as well as advanced cancer and neuromuscular and chest wall pathology. As most end-stage cancer patients choose to live out their days at home, NVS and MIE can spare their throats from invasive tubes, permit continued ambulation when possible (52), and preserve quality of life while simultaneously prolonging life. Twenty of the 254 reported ventilator unweanable patients extubated successfully to CNVS and MIE had cancer/critical care myopathies (30,31).

REFERENCES

1. Bach JR, Alba AS, Saporito LR. Intermittent positive pressure ventilation via the mouth as an alternative to tracheostomy for 257 ventilator users. *Chest.* 1993;103(1):174-182.
2. Bach JR. Amyotrophic lateral sclerosis: communication status and survival with ventilatory support. *Am J Phys Med Rehabil.* 1993;72(6):343-349.
3. Ishikawa Y, Miura T, Ishikawa Y, et al. Duchenne muscular dystrophy: survival by cardio-respiratory interventions. *Neuromusc Disord.* 2011;21:47–51
4. Bach JR, ed. *Pulmonary Rehabilitation: The Obstructive and Paralytic Conditions.* Philadelphia, PA: Hanley & Belfus; 1996:430.
5. Bach JR, Chiou M, eds. *Interventions for Skeletal and Cardiorespiratory Muscle Dysfunction.* Ventilamed. com. Union City, New Jersey. 2020.
6. Chiou M, Bach JR, Saporito LR, Albert O. Quantitation of oxygen induced hypercapnia in respiratory pump failure. *Rev Port Pneumol [Port J Pulmonol].* 2016;22(5):262-265.
7. Bach JR, Alba AS. Management of chronic alveolar hypoventilation by nasal ventilation. *Chest.* 1990;97(1):52-57.
8. Bach JR, Gonçalves MR, Hon AJ, et al. Changing trends in the management of end-stage respiratory muscle failure in neuromuscular disease: current recommendations of an international consensus. *Am J Phys Med Rehabil.* 2013;92(3):267-277.
9. Kang SW, Bach JR. Maximum insufflation capacity: vital capacity and cough flows in neuromuscular disease. *Am J Phys Med Rehabil.* 2000;79(3):222-227.
10. Kang SW, Bach JR. Maximum insufflation capacity. *Chest.* 2000;118(1):61-65.
11. Bach JR, Robert D, Leger P, Langevin B. Sleep fragmentation in kyphoscoliotic individuals with alveolar hypoventilation treated by NIPPV. *Chest.* 1995;107:1552-1558.
12. Bach JR, Alba A, Mosher R, Delaubier A. Intermittent positive pressure ventilation via nasal access in the management of respiratory insufficiency. *Chest.* 1987;92:168-170.
13. Richards GN, Cistulli PA, Ungar RG, Berthon-Jones M, Sullivan CE. Mouth leak with nasal continuous positive airway pressure increases nasal airway resistance. *Am J Respir Crit Care Med.* 1996;154:182-186.
14. Bach JR, O'Connor K. Electrophrenic ventilation: a different perspective. *J Am Paraplegia Soc.* 1991;14(1):9-17.
15. Deo P, Bach JR. Noninvasive ventilatory support to reverse weight loss in Duchenne muscular dystrophy: a case series. *Pulmonology.* 2018;25(2):R34.
16. Bach JR, Alba AS. Noninvasive options for ventilatory support of the traumatic high level quadriplegic patient. *Chest.* 1990;98:613-619.
17. Bach JR, Alba AS. Intermittent abdominal pressure ventilator in a regimen of noninvasive ventilatory support. *Chest.* 1991;99(3):630-636.
18. Bach JR, Alba AS, Bodofsky E, Curran FJ, Schultheiss M. Glossopharyngeal breathing and noninvasive aids in the management of post-polio respiratory insufficiency. *Birth Defects Orig Artic Ser.* 1987;23:99-113.
19. Bach JR, Bianchi C, Vidigal-Lopes M, Turi S, Felisari G. Lung inflation by glossopharyngeal breathing and "air stacking" in Duchenne muscular dystrophy. *Am J Phys Med Rehabil.* 2007;86(4):295-300.
20. Dail C, Rodgers M, Guess V, Adkins HV. *Glossopharyngeal Breathing.* Downey, CA: Rancho Los Amigos Hospital, Department of Physical Therapy; 1979.
21. Dail CW, Affeldt JE. *Glossopharyngeal Breathing [Video].* Los Angeles, CA: College of Medical Evangelists, Department of Visual Education; 1954.
22. Webber B, Higgens J. *Glossopharyngeal Breathing What, When and How? [Video].* West Sussex, UK: Aslan Studios Ltd.; 1999.
23. Bach JR, Kang SW. Disorders of ventilation: weakness, stiffness, and mobilization. *Chest.* 2000;117:301-303.
24. Bach JR, Mahajan K, Lipa B, Saporito L, Komaroff E. Lung insufflation capacity in neuromuscular disease. *Am J Phys Med Rehabil.* 2008;87(9):720-725.
25. Bach JR, Bianchi C. Prevention of pectus excavatum for children with spinal muscular atrophy type 1. *Am J Phys Med Rehabil.* 2003;82:815-819.
26. Bach JR. Update and perspectives on noninvasive respiratory muscle aids: part 2—the expiratory muscle aids. *Chest.* 1994;105(5):1538-1544.
27. Chiou M, Bach JR, Jethani L, Gallagher MF. Active lung volume recruitment to preserve vital capacity in Duchenne muscular dystrophy. *J Rehabil Med.* 2017;49:49-53.
28. Gomez-Merino E, Bach JR. Duchenne muscular dystrophy: prolongation of life by noninvasive ventilation and mechanically assisted coughing. *Am J Phys Med Rehabil.* 2002;81:411-415.
29. Guerin C, Bourdin G, Leray V, et al. Performance of the coughassist insufflation-exsufflation device in the presence of an endotracheal tube or tracheostomy tube: a bench study. *Respir Care.* 2011;56:1108-1114.
30. Bach JR, Goncalves MR, Hamdani I, Winck JC. Extubation of patients with neuromuscular weakness: a new management paradigm. *Chest.* 2010;137:1033-1039.
31. Bach JR, Sinquee DM, Saporito LR, Botticello AL. Efficacy of mechanical insufflation-exsufflation in extubating unweanable subjects with restrictive pulmonary disorders. *Respir Care.* 2015;60:477-483.
32. Fishburn MJ, Marino RJ, Ditunno JF Jr. Atelectasis and pneumonia in acute spinal cord injury. *Arch Phys Med Rehabil.* 1990;71:197-200.
33. Garstang SV, Kirshblum SC, Wood KE. Patient preference for in-exsufflation for secretion management with spinal cord injury. *J Spinal Cord Med.* 2000;23:80-85.
34. Barach AL, Beck GJ. Exsufflation with negative pressure; physiologic and clinical studies in poliomyelitis, bronchial asthma, pulmonary emphysema, and bronchiectasis. *AMA Arch Intern Med.* 1954;93:825-841.
35. Bach JR. Mechanical insufflation-exsufflation: comparison of peak expiratory flows with manually assisted and unassisted coughing techniques. *Chest.* 1993;104:1553-1562.
36. Bach JR, Upadhyaya N. Association of need for tracheotomy with decreasing mechanical in-exsufflation flows in amyotrophic lateral sclerosis: a case report. *Am J Phys Med Rehabil.* 2018;97(4):e20-e22.
37. Andersen T, Sandnes A, Brekka AK, et al. Laryngeal response patterns influence the efficacy of mechanical assisted cough in amyotrophic lateral sclerosis. *Thorax.* 2017;72:221-229.
38. Bach JR. Palliative care becomes "uninformed euthanasia" when patients are not offered noninvasive life preserving options. *J Palliat Care.* 2007;23:181-184.
39. Chesoni SA, Bach JR, Okamura EM. Massive reflux and aspiration after radiographically inserted gastrostomy tube placement. *Am J Phys Med Rehabil.* 2015;94:e6-e9.
40. Bach JR, Gonzalez M, Sharma A, Swan K, Patel A. Open gastrostomy for noninvasive ventilation users with neuromuscular disease. *Am J Phys Med Rehabil.* 2010;89:1-6.
41. Bach JR, Saporito LR, Shah HR, Sinquee D. Decanulation of patients with severe respiratory muscle

insufficiency: efficacy of mechanical insufflation-exsufflation. *J Rehabil Med.* 2014;46:1037-1041.

42. Bach JR, Saporito LR. Criteria for extubation and tracheostomy tube removal for patients with ventilatory failure: a different approach to weaning. *Chest.* 1996;110:156-171.

43. Bach JR. Conventional approaches to managing neuromuscular ventilation failure. In: Bach JR, ed. *Pulmonary Rehabilitation: The Obstructive and Paralytic Conditions.* Philadelphia, PA: Hanley & Belfus; 1996:285-301.

44. Bach JR. A comparison of long-term ventilatory support alternatives from the perspective of the patient and care giver. *Chest.* 1993;104(6):1702-1706.

45. Bach JR, Tran J, Durante S. Cost and physician effort analysis of invasive vs. noninvasive respiratory management of Duchenne muscular dystrophy. *Am J Phys Med Rehabil.* 2015;94(6):474-482.

46. Goncalves MR, Bach JR, Ishikawa Y, Saporito L, Winck JC. Continuous noninvasive ventilatory support outcomes for neuromuscular disease: a multicenter collaboration and literature review. *Pulmonology.* 2019. doi: 10.1016/j.pulmoe.2019.05.006 [Epub ahead of print].

47. Bach JR, Sabharwal S. High pulmonary risk scoliosis surgery: role of noninvasive ventilation and related techniques. *J Spinal Disord Tech.* 2005;18(6):527-530.

48. Bach JR, Rajaraman R, Ballanger F, et al. Neuromuscular ventilatory insufficiency: effect of home mechanical ventilator use v oxygen therapy on pneumonia and hospitalization rates. *Am J Phys Med Rehabil.* 1998;77:8-19.

49. Toussaint M, Steens M, Wasteels G, Soudon P. Diurnal ventilation via mouthpiece: survival in end-stage Duchenne patients. *Eur Respir J.* 2006;28:549-555.

50. Wang TG, Bach JR. Pulmonary dysfunction in residents of chronic care facilities. *Taiwan J Rehabil.* 1993;21:67-73.

51. Bach JR, Chiou M. Limitations of evidence-based medicine. *Rev Port Pneumol [Port J Pulmonol].* 2016;22(1):4-5.

52. Pinto TC, Winck JC, Gonçalves MR. Ventilatory support via mouthpiece to facilitate ambulation. *Am J Phys Med Rehabil.* 2019;98(9):789-793. doi: 10.1097/PHM.0000000000001193.

28 Urologic Issues in Palliative Care

Hiren V. Patel, Brian Shinder, Adam R. Metwalli, Peter A. Pinto, and Eric A. Singer

INTRODUCTION

Urologic malignancies account for nearly 20% of all new cancer diagnoses and 11% of all cancer deaths in the United States in 2020 (1). In addition to these primary sites of disease, metastases from other malignancies and the side effects of the surgery, radiation and chemotherapy, can all deleteriously impact the genitourinary system. This chapter will review many of the most common urologic issues cancer patients experience and provide a schema for their evaluation and management.

It is our belief that palliative care and supportive oncology should be incorporated into the treatment plan early, if not from the time of diagnosis, for many patients. The work of the American Urological Association's web-based ethics curriculum, American College of Surgeons' ethics curriculum and guide to surgical palliative care, and Northwestern University's Education in Palliative and End-of-Life Care (EPEC) program have increased surgeon awareness regarding the importance of interventions that are designed to improve patient quality of life (QOL) even though they may not prolong survival (2–4). Two recent publications have shown that early supportive oncology involvement improves QOL, which is not surprising, but that structured palliative care in addition to routine cancer treatment can actually improve survival when compared to standard oncologic therapy alone, which will certainly stimulate further research on the possible synergy between curative and supportive care (5,6).

SURGICAL PALLIATIVE CARE

Just as palliative care has evolved in scope and practice within the field of internal medicine, the concept of surgical palliative care has matured along with it (7). The definition of surgical palliative care can now be understood as any procedure whose primary intent is to improve QOL or mitigate symptoms caused by advanced disease (2). The efficacy of surgical palliation should be evaluated by the magnitude and duration of improvement in patient-reported symptoms (2).

The American College of Surgeons has outlined three key components that must be addressed prior to undertaking a palliative intervention. These include (a) understanding the patient's symptoms and goals of care, (b) estimating the likely impact the proposed intervention will have on the patient's symptoms, (c) and the patient's prognosis and trajectory of disease (2). While not an exhaustive list, using these points to frame discussions with patients and their families about potential procedures/surgery can help develop realistic expectations, respect patient autonomy, and avoid the harms of unnecessary surgery (7,8). Another specific issue that should be discussed prior to palliative surgery is whether an advance directive such as a do-not-resuscitate order (DNR) has been completed, and how it should be handled during the perioperative period (9).

The American Society of Anesthesiologists, American College of Surgeons, and the Association of Operating Room Nurses have stated that it is inappropriate to automatically discontinue a patient's DNR order upon entry into the operating room (9,10). Instead, they advocate for "required reconsideration" when a patient with a DNR needs a surgical intervention. For this, the patient and/or caregivers, surgeon, and anesthesiologist review the goals of care and proposed treatment plan in order to determine the best course of action. The DNR order may then be maintained, suspended, or revised during the perioperative period based on these discussions. Advance directives are reviewed in detail in Chapter 50 of this textbook.

URINARY OBSTRUCTION

Obstruction of the urinary tract can occur due to a wide range of pathophysiology. It can be chronic and cause a slow deterioration of renal function, or as the result of an acute process resulting in significant discomfort and life-threatening illness. Common causes of upper urinary obstruction include kidney and ureteral stones, strictures of the ureter, and extrinsic compression of the ureter from abdominal or retroperitoneal masses. Lower urinary tract obstruction may be due to benign prostatic obstruction, bladder stones, urethral strictures, and extrinsic compression from pelvic masses. The etiology of obstruction may be secondary to prior disease treatment, the consequence

421

of progressive disease, or even age-related patho-physiology unrelated to the primary diagnosis.

Treatment plans for each patient should be individualized and take into consideration life expectancy, anesthesia risk, and social support systems. As with any medical workup, the first step is still a detailed history and physical to assess the possible location(s) and acuity of the obstruction. The treatment of urinary tract obstruction is variable, and the treatment of choice may change as the patient's goals of care evolve.

Upper Urinary Tract Obstruction

Acute obstruction of the upper urinary tract typically presents with classic symptoms such as flank pain, dysuria, and hematuria. These symptoms can be caused by intrinsic and extrinsic obstructive processes. Intrinsic obstruction can be caused by urinary stones, blood clots, and strictures, whereas extrinsic obstruction can occur when any abdominal or pelvic structure compresses the ureter or renal pelvis. Common causes of extrinsic obstruction include tumors, fibrosis, and enlarged lymph nodes.

Imaging is a mainstay in evaluation of upper tract obstruction. Dilation of the renal pelvis/ureters and intrarenal stones can be visualized very well on ultrasound; however, identifying the cause of obstruction below the renal pelvis may be difficult to assess because the entire length of the ureter may not be well visualized with ultrasound alone. The quality of the images is also dependent on patient body habitus as well as the skill of the technician. Abdominal x-ray without the use of intravenous contrast has virtually no value in evaluating upper urinary tract obstruction. An intravenous pyelogram (IVP), which consists of serial abdominal x-rays shot in a timed fashion after the injection of intravenous contrast, helps delineate the renal shadow and the drainage patterns of the ureters. The IVP was the standard radiologic evaluation for the upper urinary tract until recently but has been supplanted by CT-urogram or CT-IVP due to increased sensitivity as well as additional anatomic information provided by the CT images.

A CT-urogram consists of a noncontrast CT scan followed by a CT scan with intravenous contrast in three phases (arterial, venous, and delayed) is now considered the standard of care by most urologists. Urolithiasis and renal masses are readily identified and characterized, a basic assessment of renal function can be done, and filling defects within the renal pelvis and ureters can be seen. The primary limitation of CT urography in this patient population is the prevalence of renal insufficiency/failure, which often precludes the use of intravenous contrast.

Magnetic resonance imaging (MRI) delineates soft tissue better than CT but tends to be used more as a secondary test to clarify questions posed by the original scan (11). MRI is the study of choice when evaluating for tumor involvement in the renal vein or vena cava (12). Magnetic resonance urography (MRU) also allows for visualization of all anatomic components of the urinary tract using heavily T2-weighted sequences or gadolinium-enhanced T1 images. Since there is no ionizing radiation, it is especially useful for pediatric and/or pregnant patients. However, there are a few disadvantages to MRU that keep it from being a first-line test. MRU is still limited in its ability to visualize stone; compared to CT the availability of the test itself is limited; the time needed to perform a MRU is significantly longer than a CT urogram (30 to 60 minutes vs. 10 to 15, respectively) (11).

After obtaining a detailed history, general lab work (serum chemistries and urine analysis) and appropriate imaging, urologic consultation may be needed for a more in-depth evaluation and treatment plan. More invasive evaluation with cystoscopy/ureteroscopy may be warranted if a questionable filling defect were to be seen on delayed CT images for example.

Nonsurgical Treatment

The treatment of extrinsic compression of the upper urinary tract will vary depending on the etiology, symptoms, and the effect on renal function. If caused by extrinsic compression from malignancy, the primary goal is to treat the underlying disease when possible. Obstruction due to a primary genitourinary malignancy may be treated with either local surgical treatment or systemic therapy, depending on the stage of disease. Obstruction caused by iatrogenic injury or treatment side effect can be temporized with a percutaneous nephrostomy tube or ureteral stent until the inciting factor resolves or definitive surgical treatment/repair is safe to attempt.

Surgical Treatment

Internal ureteral stenting has long been a mainstay for the treatment of upper tract obstruction. Urinary stents are not permanent; and, if left in too long, stents may become encrusted and eventually fail. Traditionally, urologists have recommended replacing stents every 3 to 6 months. It is preferred to place ureteral stents endoscopically in a retrograde fashion in the operating room under general anesthesia. Chung et al. described their 15-year experience with internal ureteral stents for management of extrinsic obstruction and showed a 40.6% failure rate within the first 11 months. Predictors of stent failure include a diagnosis of cancer (regardless of type), baseline creatinine more than 1.3 mg/dL, and poststenting radiation or chemotherapy (13). Limited data exist to suggest ureteral decompression impacts the overall survival of patients with malignant obstruction (14,15). Thus, the benefit is often in the relief of symptoms and improvement of renal function to facilitate further therapy (16).

The Resonance metallic ureteral stent (Cook Medical, Bloomington, Indiana, USA) is a stent designed for the long-term management of extrinsic ureteral obstruction and may remain in place up to 12 months. The metal stent has greater tensile strength than the usual plastic stents and does not compress as readily. Liatsikos et al. performed a prospective study of 50 patients, consisting of both malignant extrinsic obstruction as well as intrinsic stricture disease, and in the patients with malignant extrinsic obstruction showed patency rates of 100% with a mean follow-up time of 8.5 months, while patients with intrinsic stricture disease had a patency rate of 44%. Failure was noted within the first 2 weeks in the latter group (17).

Thermo-expandable stents such as the Memokath (PNN Medical, Denmark) have also been developed as an alternative solution for long-term management of ureteric obstruction. Agrawal et al. performed a prospective study on 55 patients, a mix of malignant extrinsic compression and intrinsic stricture disease, who had a Memokath placed with a mean follow-up of 16 months (range 4 to 98). Fourteen patients required reinsertion over a mean of 7.1 months for migration, encrustation, stricture progression, or incorrect length. The remaining patients maintained their stents between 8 and 12 months and then they were routinely replaced (18). Like the Resonance and Memokath stents, many new innovations in ureteral stents are in development, but the long-term efficacy of all stents is not well defined, and more data are needed.

Tandem ureteral stents have also been used to relieve malignant ureteral obstruction. This technique utilizes two separate double pigtail polymeric stents that are placed in the same ureter, allowing for improved extraluminal flow around the stents. These may serve as a favorable alternative to the placement of nephrostomy tubes without the use of any unfamiliar methods or materials for a urologist. Elsamra et al. reviewed their experience of 178 tandem ureteral stent placements in 40 patients with a median follow-up of 24 months and median stent duration of 129 days (19). Two patients underwent stent exchanges after 1 year, 5 patients after longer than 300 days, and 10 patients after longer than 200 days. Tandem ureteral stent failure evidenced by worsening renal function,

hydronephrosis, flank pain, or evidence of obstruction was seen in only six patients and managed at that point with percutaneous nephrostomy tube placement. Although, the use of tandem ureteral stents for malignant obstruction has mostly been reported in smaller case series, they appear to provide an excellent method for managing malignant extrinsic ureteral compression.

Percutaneous nephrostomy tubes drain urine directly from the kidney through the patient's back and into an external collection device. These tubes are often placed under local anesthesia with sedation by an interventional radiologist under ultrasound guidance, with fluoroscopy, or CT guidance for the most difficult cases. However, patients will be required to be prone for the procedure which may be difficult in elderly and obese patients and those with respiratory compromise. Like ureteral stents, nephrostomy tubes should be exchanged every 3 to 6 months. The advent of external/internal drainage systems (nephroureteral stents) have allowed for temporary nephrostomy tube placement with the ability to later convert to anterogradely placed internal ureteral stents.

In acute obstruction with clinical signs of sepsis (e.g., fever, tachycardia, hypotension), percutaneous nephrostomy tube placement is the recommended intervention. Retrograde instrumentation with cystoscopy and ureteral stent placement in the setting of an active infection puts patients at significant risk of urosepsis, which can be life-threatening (20). Other times, nephrostomy tubes are used as a last resort after failed attempts to place a ureteral stent endoscopically. Ku et al. described a recent retrospective analysis of complications in 148 patients with malignant extrinsic ureteral obstruction who underwent either nephrostomy tube or ureteral stent placement. The study noted no significant differences in fevers, acute pyelonephritis, or catheter-related complications between the two groups (20). When considering primary palliative treatment for obstruction, the risks of anesthesia and the procedure itself as well as the impact of the nephrostomy tube/stent on QOL must be discussed with the patient or his or her health care proxy.

Given the fact that nephrostomy tubes involve direct puncture of the kidney, there is a small risk of bleeding, which is not seen in ureteral stenting. A review of a single center experience with 500 percutaneous nephrostomy tube placements revealed a major complication rate of 0.45% and a minor complication rate of 14.2% (21). Major complication was defined as gross hematuria and hemodynamic instability requiring surgical intervention and/or blood transfusion. Minor complications were tube complications (e.g., dislodgement, kinking) or gross hematuria for >48 hours without clinical symptoms. Given the risk of bleeding, an anticoagulated or thrombocytopenic patient is rarely a candidate for immediate diversion with a percutaneous nephrostomy tube.

QOL has not been well studied comparing nephrostomy tubes directly to ureteral stents. It is well known that the tolerability of living with stents varies from patient to patient. The percentage of patients describing their stents as "terrible" or having a "serious impact on daily life" reach as high as 66% in some QOL studies (22). QOL studies using standardized methods for nephrostomy tubes are few. Of the studies that do exist, the most common complaints involve tube dislodgement, urine leakage around tube, and skin excoriation at the tube exit site (22). Although hard to objectively measure, the concept of extra medical devices (e.g., nephrostomy with external drainage bag) is anecdotally always a concern to patients and their caregivers. When discussing options for patients with malignant ureteral obstruction, providers should keep in mind that overall differences in QOL has not been shown for indwelling stents versus percutaneous tubes (16). Ultimately, the decision for ureteral stent versus percutaneous nephrostomy will be unique to each patient.

In general, surgical treatments for obstructive uropathy in a palliative care setting are temporizing measures and aggressive surgical approaches are generally not indicated. However, advanced prostate and/or bladder cancer can cause obstruction due to local tumor extension occluding the distal ureters. In cases where it is difficult to pass internal stents, percutaneous nephrostomy tube failure, or QOL choice by the patient, pelvic exenteration can be considered. Palliative exenteration is a poorly studied area, but several small series have reported 5 year life expectancy ranging from 25% to 40% in well-selected metastasis-free patients (23). Select palliative exenteration patients show life expectancy ranging from 18 to 24 months with improved QOL (23). Given the morbidity of any exenterative surgery, it is important to ensure that the patient has a good estimated life expectancy. In addition, patients should be counseled extensively on the long recovery process, high likelihood of perioperative complications, and no guarantee of extending life or improving QOL.

Lower Urinary Tract Obstruction

Stones in the lower urinary tract are far more common in men due to prostatic outlet obstruction leading to elevated residual urine in the bladder, although women can also develop them. Advanced prostate cancer can cause bladder outlet obstruction as well, regardless of the actual overall size of the prostate. Transitional cell tumors of the bladder can obstruct outflow as well. Urethral stricture disease is more common in patients who have had long-term urinary catheters, recurrent cystoscopy, sexually transmitted infections, or pelvic trauma.

The male lower urinary tract is generally defined as the bladder, bladder neck, prostatic urethra, and the penile urethra. A detailed medical history, including past surgeries, plus a validated questionnaire (e.g., International Prostate System Score) will be the basis for evaluating obstruction of the lower urinary tract. Benign prostatic hyperplasia (BPH) will affect many men as they age. While always recommended, a digital rectal examination (DRE) assessment of "prostate size" does not always correlate with symptoms of obstruction. "Small" prostates on DRE can still cause significant obstruction due to anatomic variations such as an enlarged prostatic median lobe, which can act as a ball valve causing outlet obstruction.

The female lower urinary tract has a much shorter urethra due to the lack of a prostate; consequently, lower urinary tract obstruction in females is far less common. Extrinsic compression of the bladder from pelvic malignancies and pelvic organ prolapse can cause dysfunctional voiding such as incomplete emptying, urinary frequency and urgency, and incontinence. Iatrogenic causes such as pelvic/vaginal/urologic surgery in the past can also cause lower urinary tract obstruction, which reinforces need for a detailed history. Therefore, a pelvic speculum examination is a key component to the physical assessment. Abdominal ultrasound is a safe and effective way of evaluating lower urinary tract obstruction. Using ultrasonography, a postvoid residual can be calculated, and larger bladder stones can be imaged. Urinalysis can also help rule out the presence of infection, which can exacerbate symptoms of lower urinary tract obstruction. A serum creatinine will also help assess overall renal function, which can dictate the type and timing of treatment. These basic evaluations should be completed prior to urologic consultation for urinary obstruction.

Nonsurgical Treatment

Fortunately, lower urinary tract obstruction can often be managed without surgical interventions (Table 28.1). Maximal medical therapy, as defined in the Medical Therapy of Prostatic Symptoms (MTOPS) trial, found significant improvement in American Urological Association symptom scores in men with BPH when patients were given a combination of alpha blockade (doxazosin) and 5-alpha-reductase inhibitor (finasteride) together compared to either drug alone. The study was double blinded with a mean follow-up of 4.5 years

TABLE 28.1 MANAGEMENT OPTIONS FOR URINARY TRACT OBSTRUCTION

Upper tract	Lower tract
Steroid therapy (retroperitoneal fibrosis)	Alpha blockers (e.g., doxazosin, tamsulosin)
Internal ureteral stent (various types)	5-Alpha-reductase inhibitors (e.g., finasteride)
Percutaneous nephrostomy tube	Clean intermittent catheterization
Surgical urinary diversion	Indwelling urethral catheter
	Suprapubic catheter
	Transurethral surgery (e.g., TURP, PVP, UroLift, Rezum)

and involved 3,047 patients (24). If a patient is assessed by DRE or ultrasound to have a prostate larger than 30 g, combination therapy of an alpha-blocker with a 5-alpha-reductase inhibitor (e.g., finasteride, dutasteride) can be instituted (25). It should be noted that the effects of alpha blockers are often appreciated within several days, while 5-alpha-reductase inhibitors take months to improve urinary symptoms. Additionally, 5-alpha-reductase inhibitors decrease serum PSA values, and the use of this medication must be taken into account for men undergoing prostate cancer screening, although screening may no longer be appropriate for many men in the palliative care/supportive oncology population (26).

Although medical therapy significantly improves the voiding function of many patients, its effects are limited. Many patients with voiding difficulties are older and may have baseline mobility issues. This may be especially true of patients with advanced malignancy who have decreased performance status and spend considerable time in bed. Normal voiding function is difficult to achieve in a recumbent position.

When manual dexterity is preserved, clean intermittent catheterization (CIC) is a reasonable option. First described by Lapides in 1971, CIC education and training allows patients to empty their bladder on a schedule. This is still the simplest form of intervention for outlet obstruction. The key caveat being that patients are required to have the mental and manual dexterity to be able to do this for themselves or have a reliable caregiver assume this responsibility.

When a patient is not a candidate for CIC, an indwelling urinary catheter is a very common intervention for lower urinary tract obstruction. A semipermanent catheter creates a pathway for bacteria to enter the urinary tract; therefore, bacteriuria is a common problem in chronically catheterized patients. If asymptomatic, treatment for bacteriuria is usually discouraged to avoid the creation of drug resistant organisms (27). Indwelling catheters should routinely be changed every 10 to 12 weeks (27). Often, the immobilized patient may benefit most from an endoscopically placed suprapubic catheter. By removing the catheter from the urethra, the risk of urethral erosion or stricture is decreased, and general comfort is improved.

Surgical Treatment

In the palliative care setting, a major goal of surgery for bladder outlet obstruction should be to improve QOL while minimizing the risk of morbidity from the surgery. Over the years, surgical approaches have varied, and techniques continue to evolve. The gold standard is still the traditional electrosurgical transurethral resection of the prostate (TURP). Although the approach is endoscopic, a TURP is not without morbidity. Irrigation solutions such as glycine or mannitol were used in the past putting patients at risk of dilutional hyponatremia if too much fluid was absorbed through open venous sinuses during resection. Today, most cases are done using normal saline, but a patient can still become fluid overloaded from the absorption of irrigant (28). As with any surgical procedure, anesthesia risk and blood loss are also a concern. Caution still needs to be used when considering TURP for patients with significant cardiopulmonary history.

Specific to the palliative care setting, the concept of the "channel TURP" has become more popular. Rather than subjecting patients to complete resection, which increases the risk of morbidity, the goal of the "channel TURP" is to remove enough tissue to allow successful bladder emptying while minimizing the amount of time spent under anesthesia and the amount of fluid absorbed by the patient during the procedure. Patients' with significant comorbidities or even with prostate cancer that may be invading the bladder can be considered candidates for a channel TURP. Marszalek et al. described a rate of 25% repeat TURP, 11% requiring permanent catheters, and 10% with some incontinence in a series of 89 prostate cancer patients who underwent a "channel TURP" (26).

Laser photovaporization of the prostate (PVP) is one of the newer tools at the disposal of urologists for managing benign prostatic hypertrophy (BPH). The "greenlight laser" (AMS Medical systems) energy is selectively absorbed within tissue by hemoglobin. This selective absorption improves the hemostatic effect of the laser while vaporizing prostatic tissue. Multiple studies have been done showing that the PVP compares favorably with the TURP with significantly less blood loss and shorter catheterization time (29).

The improvement in blood loss has led many urologists to expand the indications of PVP use. With many older patients on oral anticoagulant or antiplatelet therapy, PVP is being used to relieve bladder outlet obstruction in patients who are not candidates for TURP due to increased risk of bleeding. Woo et al. recently described his or her experience with the PVP in 43 men who were on Coumadin during their procedure. No patient needed a blood transfusion and only 6 (14%) patients required a catheter for more than 24 hours (30). Thus, in the palliative care and supportive oncology population, the PVP is a reasonable option to consider in patients who may have more significant medical comorbidities or require long-term thromboprophylaxis due to blood clots associated with malignancy.

More recently, prostatic urethral lift or Uro-Lift (NeoTract) has emerged as a minimally invasive therapy for bladder outlet obstruction that can be done in the office or outpatient setting. The delivery system applies a nonabsorbable monofilament suture through the prostatic urethra into the obstructing prostatic lobe, thereby creating a continuous anterior channel. Patients with obstructive median lobes, history of urinary retention, previous BPH surgery, prostatitis within 1-year, active urinary tract infections, and PSA > 10 ng/mL are excluded from receiving the UroLift treatment. Roehrborn et al. has shown improved QOL, flow rate, and urinary symptoms up to 5 years after treatment (31). However, a retreatment rate of 2% to 3% per year for UroLift compared to 1% to 2% per year after TURP is notable, as multiple procedures can be burdensome on patients.

Another procedure that has been used with success in the outpatient setting, the Rezum system (Boston Scientific) utilizes water vapor to ablate obstructive prostatic tissue. Cystoscopically, water vapor is injected into prostatic tissue and the thermal energy is used to create instant cell necrosis. Patients with enlarged median lobes are not excluded from this therapy. A 3-year prospective multicenter randomized controlled trial found a significant improvement (160%, $p < 0.0001$) in symptoms, $\geq 50\%$ improvement in QOL, and flow rate for at least 3 years in 197 men over the age of 50 (32). Additionally, this therapy did not cause any significant decline in sexual function. Overall, Rezum provides long-term efficacy and similar to the UroLift procedure, can be done in an outpatient setting, which is beneficial to the palliative care and supportive oncology population.

HEMATURIA

While there are many benign causes of hematuria, including glomerulonephritis, cystitis, renal trauma, BPH, kidney, ureteral and bladder stones, radiation cystitis, bacterial and viral infections, hematuria, whether gross or microscopic, may also be an indicator of a malignant process within the urinary collecting system. Therefore, depending upon goals of care, a thorough investigation of the entire upper and lower urinary tract should always be considered. The two most common tests used for detection of blood in the urine are the urine dipstick and microscopy. Urine dipsticks can have false-positive reactions in the presence of hemoglobin or myoglobin; consequently, when a dipstick is positive, microscopy is usually necessary to verify the presence of red blood cells (RBCs) and assess RBC morphology.

Once hematuria is confirmed, then a urine culture should be done to eliminate infection as the etiology of bleeding. In the absence of infection or after resolution of infection, a second positive urinalysis/microscopy would indicate the need for a complete urinary tract evaluation (33). If an MRI urogram or CT urogram is performed adequately, then the evaluation is complete after cystoscopy. However, if an ultrasound or cross-sectional imaging with incomplete or absent delayed phase images of the upper urinary tract is used for evaluation, then cystoscopy with bilateral retrograde pyelograms is indicated.

Gross hematuria refers to the presence of blood in the urine that can be seen with the unaided eye. It is important to confirm the presence of RBCs once dark urine is seen. There are multiple other potential causes of discoloration within a urine specimen. Some of the more common causes of discolored urine include concentrated urine and systemic administration of flutamide, phenazopyridine, sulfasalazine, phenolphthalein (seen with the use of some over-the-counter laxatives), nitrofurantoin, metronidazole, methylene blue, bilirubinuria, and vitamin B complex. When a patient presents with a history of gross hematuria and no evidence of infection, the hematuria workup may be done without confirmatory testing of the urine. Anticoagulated patients with hematuria should not be excluded from the workup since the anticoagulation may unmask a previously unidentified lesion in as many as 25% of patients (26).

Causes of asymptomatic microscopic hematuria (Table 28.2) range from minor, clinically insignificant findings that require no intervention to lesions that could be life threatening. When presented with a patient with asymptomatic hematuria, it is important to distinguish whether the

TABLE 28.2 CAUSES OF HEMATURIA

Glomerular causes
Primary glomerulonephritis
  Focal glomerular sclerosis
  IgA nephropathy
  Membranoproliferative glomerulonephritis
  Postinfectious glomerulonephritis
  Rapidly progressive glomerulonephritis
Secondary glomerulonephritis renal tumors
  Cryoglobulinemia
  Hemolytic-uremic syndrome
  Medication-induced nephritis
  Systemic lupus erythematosus
  Thrombotic thrombocytopenic purpura
  Vasculitis
Hereditary
  Alport's syndrome
  Fabry's disease
  Thin glomerular basement membrane disease

Renal causes
Arteriovenous malformations/fistulas
Infarct
Medullary sponge kidney
Papillary necrosis
Polycystic kidney disease
Renal trauma
Renal tumors
Renal vein thrombosis

Extrarenal causes
Benign prostatic enlargement
Calculus disease
Cyclophosphamide cystitis
Foreign body
Indwelling ureteral stent
Indwelling urethral catheter
Lower urinary tract infection
Radiation cystitis
Trauma to ureter, bladder, urethra
Tumor of ureter, bladder, prostate, urethra

bleeding originates from the lower urinary tract (urethra/prostate/bladder) or the upper urinary tract (ureters/kidneys). Often the history and physical examination may identify the location of the hematuria.

The appropriate evaluation (Fig. 28.1) includes a history and physical examination, laboratory analysis of the urine, upper tract evaluation of the ureters and kidney with a CT, lower tract evaluation by cystoscopy, and urine cytology. A flexible cystoscopy can be done in most urologists' office. With a thorough cystoscopy, the urethra, prostate, bladder, and ureteral orifices can be carefully examined, and the source of bleeding often identified. Observation of the ureteral orifices may demonstrate bloody efflux from one side, further aiding in the identification of the laterality of an upper urinary tract source. In patients with microscopic hematuria as many as 16% will have a malignancy identified through this evaluation and 3% of patients with a negative hematuria will have malignancy found on subsequent workup

(35). Lateralizing hematuria requires a retrograde pyelogram or delayed imaging with CT to properly visualize the ureters. The finding of a filling defect may necessitate ureteroscopy and fulguration, biopsy, or resection, as well as the treatment of nonmalignant causes of upper tract hematuria.

When symptomatic, lower urinary tract bleeding may present with dysuria, frequency, urgency, lower abdominal pain, and urinary retention. As the symptoms can sometimes be severe, it is important to treat them while awaiting results from the urine tests. When lateralizing hematuria is found on cystoscopy, one should begin with a radiographic study. Retrograde pyelography or delayed imaging of an abdominal CT scan with oral and IV contrast may be sufficient to identify filling defects and masses in the ureters and kidneys.

Symptomatic upper tract hematuria usually presents with lateralizing flank or abdominal pain caused by obstruction, or if brisk bleeding from the upper tract is present, the patient may also have lower urinary tract symptoms and urinary retention secondary to clots.

Management of Lower Urinary Tract Hematuria

The initial management of all hematuria is dependent on the patient's hemodynamic stability. When hemodynamically unstable, the patient should be aggressively hydrated, transfused, and coagulopathies reversed as needed. Once stabilized, the source of bleeding can be found and treated. If the patient is stable and bleeding is not profuse, the patient may be allowed to hydrate themselves to dilute the blood in their urine and should limit physical exertion as that may exacerbate bleeding. A careful medication review for NSAIDs, aspirin, antiplatelet agents, low-molecular weight heparins, warfarin, and other drugs that can potentiate bleeding is also critical. These should not be stopped until the reason for their use and the risk of halting them has been carefully determined. A summary of management of gross hematuria is show in Table 28.3.

When lower urinary tract obstruction secondary to clots occurs, a large bore three-way catheter should be placed and the bladder aggressively hand-irrigated to remove all clot. Once the clots are removed, continuous bladder irrigation (CBI) may be initiated in order to prevent further clot formation. Alternatively, the patient may be observed without CBI if the resulting urine is clear, indicating that the bleeding was self-limited. Should persistent catheter obstruction occur due to recurrent or persistent clots, a Couvelaire catheter can be used as these catheters have a larger channel through which to hand-irrigate out large

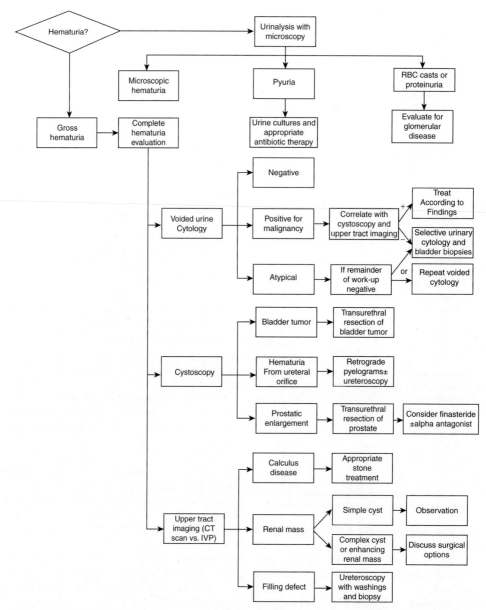

Figure 28.1 Evaluation and management of hematuria. (Reproduced from Kunkle DA, Hirshberg SJ, Greenberg RE. Urologic issues in palliative care. In: Berger AM, Shuster JL Jr, Von Roenn JH, eds. *Principles and Practice of Palliative Care and Supportive Oncology*. Baltimore, MD: Lippincott Williams & Wilkins; 2007:357-370, with permission). Ref. (34).

volumes of clots and are therefore less likely to obstruct. If these measures fail, then the patient may be taken to the operating room for clot evacuation and resection or fulguration of the bleeding source.

Once the conservative treatment of hematuria fails, there are several adjunctive treatments that may be used for protracted bleeding in the bladder. If the bleeding is from the prostate, placing a Foley catheter with a 30-cc balloon on gentle traction may be sufficient to tamponade the bleeding.

Alternatively, 5-alpha reductase inhibitors have been used and have shown to be effective in reducing bleeding (36). For severe cases of prostatic bleeding, transurethral fulguration or resection of the prostate can be effective in halting the bleeding. ε-Aminocaproic acid, an inhibitor of fibrinolytic enzymes like plasmin can be given intravenously at a loading dose of 5 g followed by hourly doses of 1.00 to 1.25 g. Once the patient responds, usually within 6 to 8 hours, the dosing can be changed to oral. Alternatively, ε-aminocaproic acid can

TABLE 28.3 MANAGEMENT OF GROSS HEMATURIA

History and physical examination

Hydrate and transfuse as necessary to stabilize hemodynamics

Stop anticoagulants as necessary

If no clot retention, patient may potentially avoid having catheter placed

3-Way Foley catheter with hand irrigation +/– continuous bladder irrigation (CBI)

Cystoscopy and clot evacuation +/– fulguration

Prostate-related bleeding
  Traction on Foley catheter
  Continuous bladder irrigation
  Prostate fulguration or resection
  5-Alpha-reductase inhibitor may be used

Bladder-related bleeding
  3-Way foley catheter and hand irrigation
  Continuous bladder irrigation
  Cystoscopy and clot evacuation +/– fulguration (resection as necessary)
  Intravesical agents
  Aminocaproic acid (0.1% intravesical)—inhibits plasmin. Contraindicated in patients with DIC. May be given i.v., p.o., or intravesically
    Patient will need clot evacuation before treatment
  Alum (1%)
    Promotes clotting in bladder
    Bladder should be free of clot before using
    Patient should be monitored for aluminum toxicity
    Contraindicated in patients with renal compromise
  Silver nitrate (0.5%–1%) precipitates protein and induces clotting
    Kept in bladder for 15 min
  Formalin (1% intravesical)
    Needs cystogram to determine reflux
    Painful; anesthesia needed
    Resolution within 48 h
    Bladder function impaired after treatment
  Hyperbaric oxygen (best for hemorrhagic cystitis and radiation cystitis). May require up to 60 treatments
    70%–80% improvement or resolution of bleeding
  Transurethral resection and/or fulguration
    Best for discreet bleeding/bladder mass
  Embolization—may manage or stop bleeding
  Percutaneous nephrostomy—may divert urine and allow bleeding to tamponade
  Cystectomy—for intractable bleeding

Upper tract–related bleeding
  Kidney bleeding may be embolized if discreet or vascular source of bleeding found
  Ureteral stent may allow urine to pass source of obstruction
  Ureteroscopy for identification and possible treatment of upper tract bleeding
  Percutaneous nephrostomy may allow bypass of urine into the bladder
  Nephrectomy may be required for intractable bleeding from kidney

be given intravesically as 200 mg/L of normal saline solution through CBI and is continued until 24 hours after bleeding has stopped with a observed 91% of resolution of hematuria (37). This approach should be employed with great caution since an increase in thromboembolic events has been observed and the formation of large intravesical clots is a risk when ε-aminocaproic acid is used (38).

Other intravesical agents commonly used are alum, silver nitrate, and formalin. Alum precipitates proteins and may quickly stop bleeding by forming clots at the source of bleeding. It is important to minimize clot formation in the bladder when using alum as it also forms large amorphous clots that are difficult to remove even endoscopically (39). Serum aluminum levels should be monitored in patients with renal insufficiency, as high levels may cause encephalopathy secondary to acute neurotoxicity. Treatment of acute systemic aluminum toxicity involves chelation with deferoxamine (40). An intravesical solution of 0.5% to 1.0% silver nitrate causes chemical coagulation at the bleeding sites but may also cause renal failure in patients with reflux, necessitating a pretreatment cystogram to assess for the presence of vesicoureteral reflux (41). Formalin can also be used in cases of severe, intractable hematuria. It permanently precipitates the bladder proteins as well as proteins in the small vessels of the bladder. This may causes fibrosis and in some cases, a small capacity bladder, and may cause severe renal injury in patients with vesicoureteral reflux, so pretreatment cystogram is again mandatory (42). Intravesical formalin is painful and requires general anesthesia to administer. Selective embolization of vesicle arteries by interventional radiology has been used with success in patients with severe intractable bleeding that was refractory to most other treatments (39). Hyperbaric oxygen has been used for hemorrhagic cystitis with an observed 82% response rate. However, as many as sixty treatments may be needed before the desired effect is seen, and this therapy is not widely available at most institutions (43). In severe cases of hematuria originating from the bladder, a cystectomy may be necessary to stop bleeding.

Radiation cystitis is seen in as many as 8% of patients who have received radiation therapy for prostate cancer. The management of radiation cystitis may involve many of the treatments discussed above, as it is often recurrent and refractory. Similarly, treatment with chemotherapeutic agents such as cyclophosphamide and ifosfamide may result in hemorrhagic cystitis, a problem that may be avoided if pretreated with Mesna during chemotherapy. Careful surveillance for the presence of malignancy should be done in these patients as the bleeding may represent a secondary malignancy. Treatment of radiation cystitis and hemorrhagic cystitis secondary to chemotherapeutic agents should follow previous guidelines for treatment of hematuria, being as conservative as possible yet aggressive enough to prevent clot retention and further discomfort. Hyperbaric treatment of recurrent radiation cystitis works by increasing oxygenation of the bladder mucosa and may also cause vasoconstriction, resulting in decreased hematuria and healing (43).

Management of Upper Urinary Tract Hematuria

The management of upper tract bleeding is similar to that of the lower tract bleeding. Conservative measures should be used whenever possible. However, when signs of obstruction are present, a percutaneous nephrostomy may be needed to divert the urine, or a ureteral stent may be placed from below to allow drainage past the obstruction. In addition, ε-aminocaproic acid may be used for intractable bleeding, but, again, it should be used with caution as noted previously (44). Biopsy and fulguration of the area of bleeding through endoscopic means may be diagnostic as well as therapeutic. Pseudoaneurysms, arteriovenous malformations, and renal masses may be treated by embolization with good effect after identification by an arteriogram. Total nephrectomy may be needed in extreme cases.

ANDROGEN DEPRIVATION THERAPY

Adenocarcinoma of the prostate is the most common cancer in males and has an age-dependent incidence. Some autopsy series indicate 60% to 80% of men in their 80s will have detectable prostate cancer (45–47). Given the multiple comorbidities found in older patients, this malignancy is often managed with active surveillance or androgen deprivation therapy (ADT) alone as the likelihood of death resulting from prostate cancer is often quite low in this patient population (48).

Long-term treatment with ADT is associated with a variety of metabolic complications. Well-known complications of ADT include weight gain, loss of muscle mass, fatigue, decreased libido, erectile dysfunction, and hot flushes. However, longer-term therapy can result in more serious complications that are less well known (Table 28.4). In addition, the short- and long-term cardiovascular impact of ADT has been characterized more clearly recently and has been shown to contribute to the small but significant rate of cardiovascular mortality associated with

TABLE 28.4 COMMON SIDE EFFECTS ASSOCIATED WITH ANDROGEN DEPRIVATION THERAPY

Early onset	Later onset
Hot flushes	Osteopenia/osteoporosis
Fatigue	Weight gain from increased adiposity
Erectile dysfunction/diminished libido	Loss of muscle mass
Mildly decreased cognition/memory	Elevation of serum cholesterol
QT prolongation/cardiac arrhythmia	Increased insulin resistance

ADT. In the setting of palliative care and supportive oncology, the impact of ADT can be quite significant and deserves careful evaluation in every patient in order to appropriately manage side effects, prevent avoidable long-term complications and, perhaps most important, confirm the need for continued use.

More recent clinical trials have added a new paradigm for treating both nonmetastatic, castration-resistant and metastatic castration-sensitive prostate cancer using selective androgen-receptor inhibitors, such as apalutamide and enzalutamide. Chi et al. demonstrated that in patients with metastatic, castration-sensitive prostate cancer, the addition of apalutamide to ADT significantly increased radiographic progression-free survival (68.2% apalutamide vs. 47.5% ADT only) and overall survival (82.4% apalutamide vs. 73.5% ADT only, $p = 0.005$) compared to ADT only (49). Apalutamide was well tolerated by most patients, with rash as the most common adverse event. Furthermore, a phase III trial in men with nonmetastatic castration-resistant prostate cancer demonstrated that metastasis-free survival (40.5 vs. 16.2 months, $p < 0.0001$) and time to symptomatic progression (HR 0.45, $p < 0.001$) were significantly increased in the apalutamide group (50). Similarly, trials with enzalutamide demonstrated decreased risk of metastatic progression and death in patients with metastatic castration-sensitive prostate cancer (51) and increase in metastasis-free survival in men with nonmetastatic castration-resistant prostate cancer (52). The use of apalutamide and enzalutamide has greatly expanded the therapeutic arsenal for treating prostate cancer, and considerations for treating these patients will need to be reassessed as overall longevity, and life span is increased in these select patient populations.

Palliative Benefits of ADT

The use of ADT in advanced prostate cancer has been practiced since the seminal article by

Huggins et al. demonstrated the link between prostate cancer and androgen signaling in 1941 (53). The clinical benefits were widely known but had not been well quantified until the publication of the Medical Research Council randomized trial of early versus delayed ADT in locally advanced or asymptomatic metastatic disease (54). This landmark study demonstrated statistically significant improvements in pathological fractures, spinal cord compression, and ureteral obstruction favoring early initiation of ADT. It also demonstrated a survival advantage for early treatment which is contrary to prior reports (55).

The duration of therapy for most patients with metastatic disease ranges from 14 to 20 months and patients often receive continued ADT with standard luteinizing hormone-releasing hormone (LHRH) agonists or gonadotrophin-releasing hormone (GnRH) antagonists during chemotherapy even after the disease has progressed to endocrine refractory state. Thus, the long-term impact of ADT in advanced prostate cancer patients becomes increasingly relevant in the management of these patients as the disease continues to progress.

Castrate levels of testosterone can be achieved by different methods (Table 28.5). The original standard treatment was bilateral simple orchiectomy. Over time, chemical castration has become the standard treatment with LHRH agonists, GnRH antagonists, and oral steroidal and non-steroidal antiandrogens. Studies have shown that patients prefer chemical castration over surgical castration because it is less disfiguring, and it can be reversed if desired (56). The available data suggest that chemical castration is equivalent to surgical castration with respect to disease control (57,58). More recently, some data have emerged suggesting that lowering testosterone levels below which LHRH agonists alone typically achieve may have added benefit (59). This may explain the benefits of secondary hormonal ablative therapies such as ketoconazole, which ablates not only gonadal androgens but also adrenal androgen synthesis (60,61). To that end, new agents that more selectively target the adrenal androgen synthesis pathways have been developed and recently approved (62). As such, the clinical application of these new therapies will undoubtedly prolong the duration of ADT for advanced prostate cancer patients. Consequently, the long-term impact of this therapy may potentially become even more of a clinical management dilemma as these patients live longer with the disease.

Early Onset Adverse Effects of ADT

The most common side effect of ADT is hot flushes, which occur in as many as 80% of treated men and often significantly affects their QOL (63). This side effect is exceedingly common and bothersome but does not, by itself, have any long-term or compounded deleterious impact. A randomized controlled trial of megestrol in breast cancer and prostate cancer patients being treated with ADT showed a significant reduction in hot flushes, but this is not commonly used among urologists due to concerns about impact on therapeutic efficacy since PSA levels sometimes actually increase when megestrol is added to ADT (64,65). A few small trials have evaluated antidepressant medications (selective serotonin reuptake inhibitors) for the treatment of hot flushes resulting from ADT, but these data are not strong, and this practice has not been widely adopted to treat this side effect.

Diminished libido is a common early-onset adverse effect of ADT. Testosterone is critical in the maintenance of a healthy libido so the ablation of androgen production logically results in a marked decrease in sexual interest and sexual function in men treated with ADT (66). The Prostate Cancer Outcomes Study (PCOS) showed an increase in men reporting a total lack of sexual interest to 60% after surgical or medical castration. The incidence of severe erectile dysfunction (ED) was reported in over 70% of men in these groups and the cessation of sexual activity was reported in over 80% of men (67). Of course, phosphodiesterase inhibitors (PDEi) can be used to treat erectile dysfunction in men who maintain sexual interest, but if the erectile dysfunction is secondary to diminished libido then PDEi therapy is unlikely to be successful. There are no data systematically evaluating these medications or other ED treatments in this clinical situation.

The impact of ADT on cognition and mood has recently become an area of intense study as conflicting evidence has emerged. A randomized study of men with prostate cancer who treated with ADT compared to men who were observed demonstrated decreased attention span and memory in the patients on ADT (68). However, other studies have shown little or no deleterious impact of ADT with decreases occurring only in selected cognitive and memory domains and, in fact, subjects demonstrated some improvement in object recall (69,70). These data indicate that the effects of ADT are as much physical as cognitive with slowing of reaction times and visuomotor responses as well as decreased performance on vigilance and attention testing.

The impact of ADT on memory has been purported to result from decreased estradiol rather than decreased testosterone (71). In a study by Salminen and colleagues, cognitive decreases were significantly associated with lower estradiol

TABLE 28.5 METHODS TO ACHIEVE ANDROGEN SUPPRESSION

Method	Products	Mechanism of action	Route of administration	Effect on hypothalamic–pituitary–gonadal axis	Advantages	Disadvantages
Simple orchiectomy	N/A	Removal of majority of testosterone-producing tissue	Trans-scrotal surgery	↓Testosterone ↓Estrogens ↑LH ↑LHRH	Single treatment, low morbidity, inexpensive	Irreversible, psychological impact of castration
Estrogens	Diethylstilbestrol (DES)	Feedback inhibition of LH production	Oral	↓Testosterone ↑Estrogens ↓LH ↓LHRH	Inexpensive, avoids loss of bone mineral density	Increased risk of thromboembolic events, gynecomastia
LHRH agonists	Leuprolide Goserelin Triptorelin	Feedback inhibition of LHRH production	Injections or implants (subcutaneous or intramuscular)	↓Testosterone ↓Estrogens ↓LH ↑LHRH	Effective reversible testosterone suppression, longer-acting depot formulation (3, 4, 6, and 12 mo)	Multiple repeat injections, expensive, induces initial testosterone surge
LHRH antagonists	Degarelix	Feedback inhibition of LHRH production	Injection (subcutaneous)	↓Testosterone ↓Estrogens ↓LH ↓LHRH	Immediate reversible testosterone suppression, no surge or flare phenomena	Multiple repeat injections required; expensive; only 1-mo depot available currently
Nonsteroidal antiandrogens (NSAA)	Bicalutamide Flutamide Nilutamide Enzalutamide Apalutamide	Competitive blockade of testosterone receptor binding	Oral	↑Testosterone ↑Estrogens ↔LH ↔LHRH	Preserves libido and erectile function, preserves bone density, may prevent flare phenomenon when used in combination with LHRH agonist	Not proven equally effective as monotherapy, gynecomastia, expensive, rash
Steroidal antiandrogens (SAA)	Cyproterone acetate	Competitive blockade of testosterone receptor binding	Oral	↓Testosterone ↑Estrogens ↔LH ↔LHRH	Preserves libido and erectile function, preserves bone density, may prevent flare phenomenon when used in combination with LHRH agonist	Increased cardiovascular risk, may not be as effective as NSAAs, gynecomastia, expensive, not available in United States
General adrenal Androgen ablation	Ketoconazole	Nonspecific blockade of androgen biosynthesis in the testis and adrenal via P-450 enzymes	Oral	↓Testosterone ↓Estrogens ↑LH ↑LHRH	May be effective in patients who fail initial ADT, inexpensive, can reverse DIC associated with disseminated prostate cancer	Requires oral corticosteroids to prevent adrenal crisis
Selective adrenal androgen ablation	Abiraterone	Inhibition of CYP17A1 enzyme that converts pregnenolone and progesterone to androgen precursors	Oral	↓Testosterone ↓Estrogens ↑LH ↑LHRH	Reduces tissue and serum testosterone levels to nearly undetectable levels, shows activity in patients who have failed ADT and chemotherapy	Newly approved by the FDA, approved for use after chemotherapy, also used with corticosteroids although this may not be physiologically necessary

levels rather than testosterone, and the negatively affected domains included reduced speed of number recognition and decreased visual memory of figures (71). However, verbal fluency improved over the year-long evaluation. The magnitude of the decrease of estradiol dictated the extent of the changes in cognition. Conversely, Almeida and colleagues followed patients treated with ADT for 9 months and evaluated them eight times over a 1-year period and found a paradoxical increase in verbal memory and visual memory using the Cambridge Examination for Mental Disorders of the Elderly-Cognitive Battery (CAMCO-G) (72). However, given the frequency of the evaluations, this study has been criticized because patients are likely to improve over time if administered the same examination repetitively (73).

Clearly, this area of research into the cognitive impact of ADT is still evolving and the data as a whole are limited largely by small sample sizes and some conflicting results. An overall review of the available literature demonstrated that between 47% and 69% of men treated with ADT demonstrated decreased function in at least one cognitive parameter evaluated and that the affected domains are typically visuospatial capability as well as higher-order cognitive skills such as problem solving, abstract concept initiation, cognitive flexibility, and self-regulation required for functional independence and social integration (73,74). Thus, the impact of ADT on cognition is subtle, and the effects are not global in elderly patients. Furthermore, the impact of confounding factors such as depression has not been adequately addressed yet. Unlike the treatment for standard age-related hypogonadism, testosterone replacement is at best highly controversial and generally regarded as absolutely contraindicated in the setting of advanced prostate cancer.

Later Onset Adverse Effects of ADT

The long-term use of ADT results in significant decreases in bone mineral density (BMD) compared to men not receiving ADT. The data from a number of prospective trials have demonstrated that this loss of BMD is substantially greater than that seen in menopausal women (75). The cumulative loss of BMD over the first year of therapy is so significant that men receiving ADT are at higher risk for skeletal fractures. This risk appears to increase in proportion with the number of doses of ADT received (76). The loss of BMD can be treated with bisphosphonate therapy, which prevents additional bone loss but has not been demonstrated to prevent fractures. The Food and Drug Administration (FDA) recently approved the use of denosumab, a monoclonal antibody against RANK ligand, which has been shown in prospective randomized trials to not only prevent loss of BMD but also prevent skeletal related events compared to intravenous bisphosphonate therapy (77,78). The National Osteoporosis Foundation recommends pretreatment assessment of osteoporotic fracture risk using the World Health Organization Fracture Risk Assessment (FRAX) calculator. The FRAX score includes risk factors such as family history of osteoporosis, smoking, glucocorticoid use, low vitamin D levels, low body weight, and history of prior fractures. This calculator has been shown to identify more men at high risk for skeletal-related events than traditional assessments that rely primarily on DEXA scan results.

Cardiovascular Impact of ADT

The use of ADT in advanced prostate cancer has been standard of care for many years, and the primacy of cardiovascular mortality among causes of death in the United States has long been known. However, ADT has recently been associated with an increased risk of coronary artery disease, myocardial infarction, and sudden cardiac death (79). A SEER database analysis also revealed that men who were treated with ADT had a 20% increased risk of cardiovascular morbidity (80). In fact, cardiovascular mortality is the most common noncancer cause of death for men with prostate cancer (81,82).

The adverse impact of hypogonadal levels of testosterone on coronary artery disease may be due to increased arterial rigidity (83). Testosterone replacement therapy has been shown to improve the symptoms of acute angina pectoris as well as have beneficial effects on myocardial infarction (84). Other studies have shown that testosterone supplementation has beneficial effect on exercise-induced cardiac ischemia (85,86). Given the anabolic characteristics of testosterone and the predominantly muscular composition of the heart, it logically stands to reason that ADT may result in some measure of cardiac dysfunction.

Most recently, a population-based analysis of patients with newly diagnosed prostate cancer registered in the United Kingdom's General Practice Research Database revealed an increased risk of CVA and transient ischemic attacks (TIA) for patients treated with ADT (87). This database study included 15,375 men who received ADT during the follow-up period of 3 years and preexisting cardiovascular risk factors at baseline did not alter the correlation between ADT and CVA/TIA risk. Interestingly, patients under 65 or older than 75 years of age appeared to be at a higher risk for CVA/TIA than the intermediate cohort of 65 to 75 years old. These data are similar to the findings of two previously published studies evaluating the risk of ADT and CVA (88,89). However, two other reports suggest that the association between ADT and CVA is weak or nonexistent. In the published study from the Longitudinal Health Insurance Database (LHID) in Taiwan did not demonstrate any increased risk of CVA in patients with a prostate cancer treated with ADT (90). This study may be limited by smaller numbers ($n = 365$) compared to the larger database analyses, but the 1.7% difference found between the groups in this analysis is not likely to be clinically significant regardless of the power of the study. The other report suggesting no correlation between ADT and CVA did not suffer from a small sample size ($n = 19,079$), but this evaluation of the Ontario Cancer Registry may have had a selection bias that could have influenced the findings.

The available data suggest that ADT may have an impact on cardiovascular and cerebrovascular function, but it is evident that the degree of impact is yet to be clearly defined. Furthermore, the physiological mechanisms for this increased risk are also unclear, so the appropriate tests to identify patients at high risk for these life-threatening outcomes have not been identified nor have the appropriate preventive measures been definitively elucidated.

Metabolic Impact of ADT

Recent research has revealed that hypogonadal levels of testosterone leads to a metabolic syndrome characterized by increasing insulin resistance (91,92). This phenomenon appears to occur peripherally rather than as a direct effect on the islet cells of the pancreas. Other associated metabolic abnormalities include hypertriglyceridemia, hypercholesterolemia, hypertension, and obesity. The definition for classic metabolic syndrome includes any three of the following diagnostic findings: blood pressure ≥130/85, waist circumference >102 cm, ≥ triglycerides ≥ 150 mg/100 mL, high-density lipoproteins <40 mg/100 mL, and fasting glucose ≥110 mg/100 mL (93). Given the association of many of these criteria with advancing age in Western society, many men with prostate cancer may meet the definition of classic metabolic syndrome prior to starting ADT. However, these can be markedly worsened by the initiation of ADT. In addition, the metabolic syndrome associated with ADT has some distinct differences relative to the definition of classic metabolic syndrome. Table 28.6 outlines the criteria for diagnosing ADT-induced metabolic syndrome in men in comparison to the findings of classic metabolic syndrome. Interestingly, in men who are already taking cholesterol-lowering medications such as statins still demonstrate negative changes in their lipid profiles after starting ADT (94). Other studies have demon-

TABLE 28.6 CHARACTERISTICS OF ADT-INDUCED METABOLIC SYNDROME COMPARED TO CLASSIC METABOLIC SYNDROME

	ADT-induced metabolic syndrome	Classic metabolic syndrome
Blood pressure	↔	↑
Waist circumference	↑	↑
Ratio of waist–hip measurements	↔	↑
Triglycerides	↑	↑
High-density lipoprotein	↓	↑
Fasting glucose	↑	↑
Fat accumulation	Truncal, subcutaneous	Internal, visceral

strated that ADT worsens insulin resistance, which has been correlated with cardiovascular mortality.

Therefore, in this patient population with many preexisting comorbidities that may be exacerbated by the initiation of ADT, it is imperative to establish a baseline for these parameters prior to starting ADT and continuous regular monitoring of these factors over time is important to detect and treat the onset of ADT-induced metabolic syndrome. Furthermore, a recently completed randomized controlled trial demonstrated significant improvements in abdominal girth measurements, weight, body mass index, and systolic blood pressure for men treated with ADT who were concomitantly started on an exercise program compared to men who received ADT alone (95). Thus, lifestyle changes that includes regular physical activity can improve several parameters that define metabolic syndrome and should be recommended for patients starting ADT.

Quality of Life Impact of ADT

Especially in the palliative care setting, the impact on a patient's quality-of-life (QOL) is often paramount when deciding on treatment options. The general perception among urologists regarding ADT is that it minimally impacts QOL for most patients. However, when this issue has been studied, the data suggest that patients on ADT have statistically significantly decreased physical function and general health (96). In this evaluation of 96 men, there were no significant differences between men on ADT for <6 months and those on ADT for longer than 6 months. There were no differences between men on ADT and healthy controls with respect to the mental health component, but men on ADT scored significantly lower in physical functioning and general health. Total testosterone was significantly associated the physical health component with lower testosterone levels corresponding with lower physical health component scores, whereas preexisting comorbidities understandably correlated inversely with physical health component summary score. These data are somewhat in contrast with other data, which suggests that ADT has negative effect not only on physical functioning but also on emotional and overall QOL measures as well. In men with locally advanced prostate cancer, ADT was shown to lower overall QOL scores and increase emotional distress compared to delayed treatment (97).

An earlier evaluation of the QOL effect of ADT enrolled over 700 patients with advanced prostate cancer in a QOL survey protocol that was administered at 1, 3, and 6 months after ADT was started (98). The comparison groups were ADT with simple orchiectomy plus flutamide, a nonsteroidal antiandrogen (NSAA), or placebo. Response rates were in excess of 80% for the entire study, and interestingly, the expected difference in body image between the two groups was not noted despite higher incidence of gynecomastia in the flutamide group. In general, the addition of flutamide produced a negative QOL difference between the groups with respect to treatment-specific symptoms such as diarrhea as well as physical and emotional functioning. These data indicate that the QOL impact of combined androgen blockade, whether it is with LHRH agonist and NSAA or with orchiectomy and NSAA, has a greater impact on QOL than monotherapy. Therefore, it is important not only to discuss the potential impact of ADT on QOL with patients but also to note that the different types of ADT may have different impacts on QOL.

ERECTILE DYSFUNCTION

The issue of sexual function in elderly men was not a major focus of urologists and gerontologists until the last four or five decades when men began living substantially longer. Even after the average life expectancy exceeded 70 years old, a common misperception was that erectile dysfunction (ED) was part of the normal aging process. As a result, very little effort was expended on characterizing and treating sexual dysfunction in geriatric populations. However, with the advent of geriatric medicine as a specific discipline and with improvements in overall medical care, the performance status and physiological condition of many elder men has improved, and a greater proportion of elderly men desire continued sexual activity throughout their life span. Furthermore, the proportion of men older than 65 years of age is expected to more than double by 2025. As a result, more interest and resources are being focused on the prevention and treatment

of ED in the elderly. The classic definition of erectile dysfunction is persistent and recurrent difficulty to achieve and/or maintain an erection adequate for the completion of intercourse (99).

Erectile dysfunction is not a single complaint but is a spectrum of dysfunction that can be somewhat difficult to quantify. The Massachusetts Male Aging Study provided data on the effect of advancing age on sexual function as well as other health-related QOL measures. In this report, ED was characterized as minimal, moderate, or complete, and the prevalence of ED varied dramatically depending on the definition. For all three degrees of ED, the prevalence was over 50% for the entire cohort of men (ages 40 to 70), but the prevalence of complete ED was only 5% in the youngest group and 15% in the oldest set indicating that the incidence and prevalence of severe ED is far less common than lesser degrees.

Diagnosing ED

Given the multifactorial nature of ED (Table 28.7), a broad evaluation of a patient presenting with ED is mandatory. A complete medical, sexual, and psychosocial history should be obtained in order to identify the specific erectile problem (i.e., difficulty maintaining an erection vs. difficulty achieving an erection vs. lack of interest in sex) as well as recognize reversible contributing comorbidities such as metabolic syndrome, hypogonadism, diabetes, or obesity. In addition, it is very important that the patient clearly expresses his or her expectations

TABLE 28.7 COMMON RISK FACTORS FOR ERECTILE DYSFUNCTION AND ATHEROSCLEROSIS

Erectile dysfunction	Atherosclerosis
Hypogonadism	Hypertension
Diabetes mellitus	Diabetes mellitus
Atherosclerosis/hyperlipidemia	Hyperlipidemia (*elevated triglycerides and low-density lipoproteins*)
Obesity	Obesity
Advanced age	Advanced age (*>45 y of age*)
Cigarette smoking/alcohol use	Cigarette smoking
Physical deconditioning	Physical deconditioning
Depression	Family history (*father or brother diagnosed younger than 55 years old*)
Medications/drugs	Low high-density lipoproteins (HDLs)
Spinal cord injury	Gender (*male > female*)
Prostate surgery	Erectile dysfunction

and values so that a satisfactory, patient-centered treatment plan can be implemented.

A complete medication list is critical to the assessment of ED because many commonly used drugs can cause or worsen ED. Furthermore, drug interactions between commonly used cardiac medications and ED medications can be life threatening. Specifically, nitrate-based medications such as nitroglycerine or isosorbide dinitrate are specifically contraindicated with use of phosphodiesterase 5 inhibitors (PDE5i) due to a resulting severe refractory hypotension that is extremely difficult to treat (100). While this class interaction is well known, many others are less well known which emphasizes the importance of a complete and thorough documentation of all medications (prescription and over-the-counter), supplements, and herbal preparations being used. In addition, the presence of antidepressants may contribute to complaints of anorgasmia, whereas new prescriptions or increases in antihypertensive medications may unmask or exacerbate subclinical ED.

A detailed sexual history should include information about the onset of ED, alleviating and aggravating factors as well as emotional and physical status of the patient, the patient's sexual partner(s) and the exact complaint. The patient should clearly describe the physical factors associated with ED including presence or absence of nocturnal erections, rigidity of erections, differences in erections with sexual arousal, masturbation, and nocturnal erections. The interpersonal impact of ED is significant, and this information should be obtained not only from the patient but also from the patient's sexual partner as sexual satisfaction of both parties is often an important factor in seeking medical advice. Furthermore, the perception of the contributing factors may differ substantially between the patient and his or her partner. Consequently, open dialogue between the patient and his or her partner is an important part of the diagnosis and treatment of ED, and it is the role of the treating physician to facilitate that aspect as well.

In order to quantify baseline erectile function as well as to assess the efficacy of any treatments, standardized measurement tools such as the Sexual Health Inventory for Men (SHIM) are extremely helpful for the physician and the patient. The questionnaire is a useful adjunct to a thorough history, but it does not provide enough detail to be the sole evaluation initially or in follow-up.

The typical portions of a complete history have significance in the evaluation of ED, in particular, the past surgical history can be extremely informative given the prevalence of prostate interventions among elderly men. ED can be a side effect after prostatectomy performed for prostate cancer but ED can also develop after multiple prostate biopsies intended to diagnose prostate cancer. Furthermore, surgeries for benign prostate disease such as TURP may also be associated with ED as well.

The performance of a complete physical examination is important in the evaluation of ED, but it rarely reveals the cause of ED. Rather the physical examination often provides a myriad of clues suggesting the contributing medical disorders that manifest as ED. The general evaluation must include cardiovascular, neurologic, and metabolic assessments with focus on the genitourinary examination. Careful inspection for secondary sex characteristics and testicular size may suggest the presence of hypogonadism. Physical examination may reveal genital abnormalities both physical (i.e., Peyronie's disease) and neurological (i.e., decreased penile sensation or absent bulbocavernosal reflex) that may be the primary cause of the ED.

Laboratory evaluation must include fasting glucose, lipid profile, hormonal levels in order to identify the presence of androgen deficiency, metabolic syndrome, or diabetes. There is virtually no role for imaging modalities in the initial evaluation of ED. A penile duplex ultrasound to evaluate cavernosal blood flow is a useful study but is typically utilized by specialists after initial treatments are unsuccessful. More invasive studies such as infusion cavernosometry, arteriography, and neurophysiologic testing are rarely indicated in the geriatric population.

Medical Treatment of ED

Detailed counseling of patients is necessary not only to educate the patient and his or her partner as to the cause of the ED but also to establish realistic expectations with respect to the effectiveness of any treatment program. For example, in most elderly patients, ED is due to a constellation of contributing comorbidities, and therefore, the patient needs to be clearly informed that oral medical therapy may improve the symptom of ED somewhat but that oral medications are unlikely to produce the rigid erections of his or her youth. In addition, the physician should address other forms of sexual activity that do not rely upon penetrative sexual intercourse in the context of both partners' sexual satisfaction and the limitations of the patient's overall physical condition. This portion of the counseling may be uncomfortable for the physician and the patient but, given the link between sexual satisfaction and mental health, if the patient can accept the fact that sexual satisfaction can be achieved with alternative forms of intimacy, then improvements in overall mental health may occur as well (101). A detailed discussion of the various treatments for ED should be undertaken and the choice of treatment should be made by the patient in conjunction with his or her partner. Table 28.8

TABLE 28.8 ERECTILE DYSFUNCTION TREATMENT OPTIONS

Category	Products	Mechanism of action	Route of administration	Advantages	Disadvantages
Phosphodiesterase 5 inhibitors (PDE5i)	Sildenafil Vardenafil Tadalafil Avanafil	Inhibits degradation of cGMP promoting smooth muscle relaxation and penile blood flow	Oral	Oral administration, effective, available on demand	Expensive, headaches, facial flushing, nasal congestion, myalgia, back pain, visual changes, requires intact neurovascular pathways
Injectable medication	Caverject Tri-Mix	Vasodilatation of cavernous arteries	Injection	Immediate onset, not dependent on intact nerve function	Injection into penis difficult for patients psychologically, local pain or bruising/hematoma at injection site, expensive, not spontaneous
Transurethral medication	MUSE	Vasodilatation of cavernous arteries through absorption of medication	Intraurethral suppository	Immediate onset, not dependent on intact nerve function, no injection/ needles	Urethral burning or discomfort, expensive, variable absorption, not spontaneous
External mechanical	Vacuum erection device (VED) Actis Band	Negative pressure draws venous blood into corpora cavernosa, restriction band prevents outflow	External application of device	No medication interactions, not dependent on intact nerve function, no refractory period	Cumbersome equipment, not spontaneous, low rate of continued usage over time
Internal mechanical	Penile prosthesis	Surgically implanted device that can achieve rigidity through inflation or malleable rods	Surgical implantation of device	Erection on demand, very high satisfaction rate, not dependent on intact nerves	Surgical intervention, expensive, irreversible, risk of infection of prosthetic materials requiring explantation

outlines the pharmacological and mechanical treatment choices for patients with erectile dysfunction. In addition, continued observation should be offered as an option and the patient should be informed that spontaneous remission of ED does occur in a small percentage of patients who are followed expectantly without intervention.

Lifestyle modification can have beneficial effects on ED, and patients should be strongly encouraged to implement durable changes not only to improve their erections but also to lower their risk of cardiovascular disease in the future. The addition of statin medication has been shown to improve ED and should be considered for men with elevated cholesterol and ED. Many antihypertensive medications may induce or exacerbate ED and consideration of changing types of medications may improve ED. Specifically, thiazide diuretics as well as alpha- and beta-blockers have been implicated in the worsening of ED. While depression can cause ED, tricyclic antidepressants can also induce diminished libido and orgasmic dysfunction in addition to classic ED (102,103). Thus, a discussion with the prescribing physician about a change in class of drug may be helpful in improving ED in a patient on these medications. For example, calcium-channel blockers, angiotensin receptor blockers, and ACE inhibitors may improve ED while maintaining hypertensive control. Alternatively, changing from a nonspecific alpha-blocker to a subtype-specific alpha-blocker such as doxazosin or tamsulosin may minimize the ED-inducing potential of alpha blockade for the treatment of hypertension or BPH. Finally, polypharmacy is a major problem among the geriatric population and a review of medications with the intent of discontinuing nonessential medications may have broadly beneficial effects over and above any improvement in ED that may result.

Pharmacotherapy for ED has improved recently with the development of selective phosphodiesterase 5 inhibitors (PDE5i). These drugs are analogs of cGMP that competitively bind to the PDE5 enzyme. This slows the degradation of cGMP thereby prolonging smooth muscle relaxation in the cavernous arteries (104). While these medications have been wildly successful physiologically and commercially, their mechanism of action is dependent upon endogenous production of NO, which is impaired not only by advancing age but also by the numerous comorbidities discussed previously. As such, these medications demonstrate decreasing efficacy with increasing age (104). However, due to their relative ease of use and demonstrable clinical safety, these medications are unquestionably the first-line treatment option for men in whom no contraindication exists (105). Of

note, the PDE5i tadalafil taken once a day is FDA approved for the treatment of both ED and BPH, making it an attractive choice for elderly patients afflicted by both conditions (106).

Patient education is critical to the successful use of PDE5i medications because sexual stimulation is absolutely required, and the efficacy may be affected by factors such as alcohol consumption. The success rates with these medications are in excess of 60% for first-time users applying on-demand therapeutic regimens and up to 50% of nonresponders can be converted to responders with adequate counseling of the patient and his or her partner (107,108). In men for whom episodic dosing is ineffective, a low-dose daily regimen may be beneficial (109,110). And for men with clinical hypogonadism and no contraindication to testosterone supplementation, the effectiveness of PDE5i therapy may be improved with concomitant testosterone replacement because this enhances endogenous NO production (111). The side effects for this class of medication includes facial flushing, headaches, nasal congestion, muscle aches, and back pain. Visual changes may occur frequently as well due to the presence of phosphodiesterase 6 (PDE6) in the retina.

Apomorphine SL is a sublingual preparation of a nonselective dopamine agonist and acts centrally to promote erectogenic signals. This is absorbed quickly, and many patients can achieve erections in 20 minutes. Common side effects are headache, nausea, and dizziness and are so frequent that clinical utility of this compound is limited. The advantage of this therapy is that no interaction with nitrates exists so apomorphine is considered front line oral therapy in patients who take nitrates for chest pain or hypertension (112).

Prior to the advent of PDE5i therapy, vasoactive compounds were the primary medical therapy for ED; these medications are now the primary nonsurgical treatment options for patients in whom PDE5i therapy fails or is contraindicated. The efficacy and safety profiles of these agents are excellent, and the onset of action is rapid. Prostaglandin E1 (PGE1) and papaverine induce vasodilatation as a result of cGMP and cyclic adenosine monophosphate (cAMP) mediate arterial smooth muscle relaxation. The other medication commonly used is phentolamine, which blocks sympathetic vasoconstriction signals. Endogenous NO production does not affect the efficacy of these medications which is why these drugs are effective in men for whom PDE5i medications are unsuccessful. Each of these medications can be administered via intracavernosal injection and PGE1 can also be given as an intraurethral suppository. The duration of erection is dose-dependent, but the onset of erection is typically within a few minutes. Priapism, defined as an erection lasting longer than 4 hours, is a significant side effect and requires immediate medical attention to prevent penile fibrosis. Injection site reactions such as pain or bruising are common and penile fibrosis may develop over time with prolonged use. Intraurethral suppositories of PGE1 may also cause hypotension, dizziness, syncope, urethrodynia, and genital irritation in the partner. Satisfaction rates for this therapy are very high but a bleeding disorder and a history of priapism are relative contraindications for use.

The vacuum erection device is a mechanical apparatus designed to create negative pressure within a cylinder placed around the penis. This negative pressure draws venous blood into the corpora cavernosa resulting in the passive generation of an erection. A constriction band is placed around the penile shaft at the penopubic junction to prevent outflow and allow maintenance of the erection. This mechanism is extremely effective with usable erections in nearly 9 out of 10 men, but it is cumbersome and produces an erection that many patients find unnatural. Since the erection is from venous blood and the constriction band limits penile blood flow, the penis appears cyanotic and is cool to the touch and there is a fulcrum at the constriction band with a rigid penis distal to the band and flaccid penis proximal which alters functionality somewhat as well. Side effects are minimal and limited primarily to local bruising and anejaculation due to mechanical obstruction, but patients must be instructed to remove the constriction band as soon as possible or within 30 minutes to prevent permanent damage including penile necrosis. Patients with bleeding diatheses or on anticoagulation therapy should use the VED with caution (112).

For patients with an excessive venous outflow but normal or slightly low arterial inflow, a condition known as a "venous leak", the use of a constriction band alone may allow for usable erections. These patients typically present with the primary complaint of early loss of erection, often during intercourse. The constriction band is available alone without having to purchase the entire VED and is far less cumbersome than the VED. The clinical diagnosis of venous leak is made after a penile Doppler ultrasound study has been performed and interpreted by a specialist, but since the constriction band is noninvasive and inexpensive, it is reasonable to try this based upon a clinical history that is consistent with venous leak.

Surgical Treatment of ED

Surgical treatments of ED should be reserved for patients who are healthy enough for sexual activity and have failed medical therapy. Penile prostheses may be inflatable or malleable. Malleable or semirigid prostheses are implanted into the cavernosa and have enough rigidity to facilitate penetrative intercourse. These devices can be bent downward when not in use and simply straightened when needed. This model is ideal for patients with limited manual dexterity and the implant can be placed under local anesthetic. Inflatable prostheses are, in general, the primary choice for surgeons and consist of a pump placed into the scrotum and an inflatable cylinder inserted into each cavernosal space. An erection is produced by squeezing the scrotal pump mechanism and a release valve on the pump deflates the cylinders once penile rigidity is no longer desired. Patient satisfaction rates are extremely high, in excess of 90% for patients and their partners (113). Detailed counseling prior to implantation of a penile prosthesis is critical in order to manage patient and partner expectations and minimizes subsequent dissatisfaction.

Complications rates are low but can be quite significant when they do occur. Infection rates are typically less than 2%, and newer prosthesis materials have been imbedded with antibiotics and other novel coatings to further decrease this rate. Another potential complication of the inflatable prosthesis is auto-inflation due to increased pressure or fibrosis around the reservoir or pump valve failure, both of which may require surgical revision to correct. Patients may also complain of loss of penile length with full erection, which may be due to longstanding preexisting intracorporal fibrosis, Peyronie's disease, or the fact that only the penile shaft is rigid with an inflatable penile prosthesis so glans engorgement typically does not occur resulting in the perception of lost length. These complaints can generally be addressed and mitigated preoperatively with adequate counseling from the surgeon. Overall, nearly 60% of men will still have a functional prosthesis in place 15 years after initial implantation (113).

CONCLUSION

Early palliative care and supportive oncology can provide significant benefits to patients and their families. The genitourinary system can be affected by multiple malignant and benign disease processes and their therapies. Thorough history taking and physical examination coupled with an appropriate laboratory evaluation, judicious imaging, and early urology consultation can help maximize patient QOL and survival.

ACKNOWLEDGMENT

This research was funded by the Intramural Research Program of the NIH, National Cancer Institute, Center for Cancer Research and is supported by a grant from the National Cancer Institute (P30CA072720).

REFERENCES

1. Siegel RL, Miller KD, Jemal A. Cancer statistics, 2020. *CA Cancer J Clin.* 2020;70(1):7-30.
2. Dunn GP, Martensen R, Weissman D, eds. *Surgical Palliative Care: A Resident's Guide.* Chicago, IL: American College of Surgeons; 2009:278.
3. American Urological Association. *Clinical Ethics for Urologists.* 2008 [cited 2011 September 26]. http://www.auanet.org/eforms/cme/modules.cfm?ID=407
4. EPEC. *Education in Palliative and End-of-Life Care for Oncology.* 2011 [cited 2011 October 17]. http://epec.net/epec_oncology.php.
5. Temel JS, et al. Early palliative care for patients with metastatic non-small-cell lung cancer. *N Engl J Med.* 2010;363(8):733-742.
6. Bakitas M, et al. Effects of a palliative care intervention on clinical outcomes in patients with advanced cancer: the Project ENABLE II randomized controlled trial. *JAMA.* 2009;302(7):741-749.
7. Hofmann B, Haheim LL, Soreide JA. Ethics of palliative surgery in patients with cancer. *Br J Surg.* 2005;92(7):802-809.
8. Kwok AC, et al. The intensity and variation of surgical care at the end of life: a retrospective cohort study. *Lancet.* 2011;378(9800):1408-1413.
9. Demme RA, et al. Ethical issues in palliative care. *Anesthesiol Clin.* 2006;24(1):129-144.
10. Shapiro ME, Singer EA. Perioperative advance directives: do not resuscitate in the operating room. *Surg Clin North Am.* 2019;99(5):859-865.
11. O'Donoghue PM, McSweeney SE, Jhaveri K. Genitourinary imaging: current and emerging applications. *J Postgrad Med.* 2010;56(2):131-139.
12. Choyke PL, Walther MM, Wagner JR, Rayford W, Lyne JC, Linehan WM. Renal cancer: preoperative evaluation with dual-phase three-dimensional MR angiography. *Radiology.* 1997;205:767-771.
13. Chung SY, et al. 15-year experience with the management of extrinsic ureteral obstruction with indwelling ureteral stents. *J Urol.* 2004;172(2):592-595.
14. Lapitan MC, Buckley BS. Impact of palliative urinary diversion by percutaneous nephrostomy drainage and ureteral stenting among patients with advanced cervical cancer and obstructive uropathy: a prospective cohort. *J Obstet Gynaecol Res.* 2011;37(8):1061-1070.
15. Cordeiro MD, et al. A prognostic model for survival after palliative urinary diversion for malignant ureteric obstruction: a prospective study of 208 patients. *BJU Int.* 2016;117(2):266-271.
16. Farber N, Salib A, Shinder B, Modi PK, Elsamra SE, Singer EA. *American College of Surgeons Evidence-Based Decisions in Surgery: Management of Malignant Upper Urinary Tract Obstruction.* 2017. http://ebds.facs.org/topics
17. Liatsikos E, et al. Ureteral obstruction: is the full metallic double-pigtail stent the way to go? *Eur Urol.* 2010;57(3):480-486.
18. Agrawal S, et al. The thermo-expandable metallic ureteric stent: an 11-year follow-up. *BJU Int.* 2009;103(3):372-376.
19. Elsamra SE, et al. Stenting for malignant ureteral obstruction: Tandem, metal or metal-mesh stents. *Int J Urol.* 2015;22(7):629-636.
20. Ku JH, et al. Percutaneous nephrostomy versus indwelling ureteral stents in the management of extrinsic ureteral obstruction in advanced malignancies: are there differences? *Urology.* 2004;64(5):895-899.
21. Montvilas P, Solvig J, Johansen TE. Single-centre review of radiologically guided percutaneous nephrostomy using "mixed" technique: success and complication rates. *Eur J Radiol.* 2011;80(2):553-558.
22. Kouba E, Wallen EM, Pruthi RS. Management of ureteral obstruction due to advanced malignancy: optimizing therapeutic and palliative outcomes. *J Urol.* 2008;180(2):444-450.
23. Boustead GB Feneley MR. Pelvic exenterative surgery for palliation of malignant disease in the robotic era. *Clin Oncol (R Coll Radiol).* 2010;22(9):740-746.
24. McConnell J, Roehrborn CG, Bautista OM, et al. The long-term effect of doxazosin, finasteride, and combination therapy on the clinical progression of benign prostatic hyperplasia. *N Engl J Med.* 2003;349(25):2387-2398.
25. Djavan B, Margreiter M, Dianat SS. An algorithm for medical management in male lower urinary tract symptoms. *Curr Opin Urol.* 2011;21(1):5-12.
26. Sima C, Panageas, KS., Schrag, D., Cancer screening among patients with advanced cancer. *Journal of American Medical Association.* 2010;304(14):1584-1591.
27. Trautner BW, Darouiche RO. Role of biofilm in catheter-associated urinary tract infection. *Am J Infect Control.* 2004;32(3):177-183.
28. Fitzpatrick J. Minimally invasive and endoscopic management of benign prostatic hyperplasia. In: AJ Wein, et al., eds. *Campbell-Walsh Urology.* 10th ed. 2010:2655-2694, Chapter 93.
29. Gravas S, et al. Critical review of lasers in benign prostatic hyperplasia (BPH). *BJU Int.* 2011;107(7):1030-1043.
30. Woo HH, Hossack TA. Photoselective vaporization of the prostate with the 120-w lithium triborate laser in men taking coumadin. *Urology.* 2011;78(1):142-145.
31. Roehrborn CG, et al. Five year results of the prospective randomized controlled prostatic urethral L.I.F.T. study. *Can J Urol.* 2017;24(3):8802-8813.
32. McVary KT, Roehrborn CG. Three-Year Outcomes of the Prospective, Randomized Controlled Rezum System Study: convective radiofrequency thermal therapy for treatment of lower urinary tract symptoms due to benign prostatic hyperplasia. *Urology.* 2018;111:1-9.
33. Grossfeld GD, et al. Asymptomatic microscopic hematuria in adults: summary of the AUA best practice policy recommendations. *Am Fam Physician.* 2001;63(6):1145-1154.
34. Kunkle DA, Hirshberg SJ, Greenberg RE. Urologic issues in palliative care. In: Berger AM, Shuster JL Jr, Von Roenn JH, eds. *Principles and Practice of Palliative Care and Supportive Oncology.* Baltimore, MD: Lippincott Williams & Wilkins; 2007:357-370.
35. Grossfeld GD, et al. Evaluation of asymptomatic microscopic hematuria in adults: the American Urological Association best practice policy—part II: patient evaluation, cytology, voided markers, imaging, cystoscopy, nephrology evaluation, and follow-up. *Urology.* 2001;57(4):604-610.
36. Foley SJ, et al. A prospective study of the natural history of hematuria associated with benign prostatic hyperplasia and the effect of finasteride. *J Urol.* 2000;163(2):496-498.
37. Singh I, Laungani GB. Intravesical epsilon aminocaproic acid in management of intractable bladder hemorrhage. *Urology.* 1992;40(3):227-229.
38. Gralnick HR, Greipp P. Thrombosis with epsilon aminocaproic acid therapy. *Am J Clin Pathol.* 1971;56(2):151-154.
39. Choong SK, Walkden M, Kirby R. The management of intractable haematuria. *BJU Int.* 2000;86(9):951-959.
40. Perazella M, Brown E. Acute aluminum toxicity and alum bladder irrigation in patients with renal failure. *Am J Kidney Dis.* 1993;21(1):44-46.
41. Raghavaiah NV, Soloway MS. Anuria following silver nitrate irrigation for intractable bladder hemorrhage. *J Urol.* 1977;118(4):681-682.
42. Rastinehad AR, et al. Persistent prostatic hematuria. *Nat Clin Pract Urol.* 2008;5(3):159-165.

43. Corman JM, et al. Treatment of radiation induced hemorrhagic cystitis with hyperbaric oxygen. *J Urol.* 2003; 169(6):2200-2202.

44. Kaye JD, et al. Preliminary experience with epsilon aminocaproic acid for treatment of intractable upper tract hematuria in children with hematological disorders. *J Urol.* 2010;184(3):1152-1157.

45. Soos G, et al. The prevalence of prostate carcinoma and its precursor in Hungary: an autopsy study. *Eur Urol.* 2005;48(5):739-744.

46. Stemmermann GN, et al. A prospective comparison of prostate cancer at autopsy and as a clinical event: the Hawaii Japanese experience. *Cancer Epidemiol Biomarkers Prev.* 1992;1(3):189-193.

47. Rullis I, Shaeffer JA, Lilien OM. Incidence of prostatic carcinoma in the elderly. *Urology.* 1975;6(3):295-297.

48. Borre M, et al. Survival of prostate cancer patients in central and northern Denmark, 1998-2009. *Clin Epidemiol.* 2011;3(suppl 1):41-46.

49. Chi KN, et al. Apalutamide for metastatic, castration-sensitive prostate cancer. *N Engl J Med.* 2019;381(1):13-24.

50. Smith MR, et al. Apalutamide treatment and metastasis-free survival in prostate cancer. *N Engl J Med.* 2018;378(15):1408-1418.

51. Armstrong AJ, et al. ARCHES: a randomized, phase III study of androgen deprivation therapy with enzalutamide or placebo in men with metastatic hormone-sensitive prostate cancer. *J Clin Oncol.* 2019;37(32):2974-2986.

52. Hussain M, et al. Enzalutamide in men with nonmetastatic, castration-resistant prostate cancer. *N Engl J Med.* 2018;378(26):2465-2474.

53. Huggins C, Hodges C. Studies on prostate cancer. I. *Cancer Res.* 1941;1:293-297.

54. Immediate versus deferred treatment for advanced prostatic cancer: initial results of the Medical Research Council Trial. The Medical Research Council Prostate Cancer Working Party Investigators Group. *Br J Urol.* 1997;79(2):235-246.

55. Byar DP. Proceedings: The Veterans Administration Cooperative Urological Research Group's studies of cancer of the prostate. *Cancer.* 1973;32(5):1126-1130.

56. Nyman CR, et al. The patient's choice of androgen-deprivation therapy in locally advanced prostate cancer: bicalutamide, a gonadotrophin-releasing hormone analogue or orchidectomy. *BJU Int.* 2005;96(7):1014-1018.

57. Seidenfeld J, et al. Single-therapy androgen suppression in men with advanced prostate cancer: a systematic review and meta-analysis. *Ann Intern Med.* 2000;132(7): 566-577.

58. Novara G, et al. Impact of surgical and medical castration on serum testosterone level in prostate cancer patients. *Urol Int.* 2009;82(3):249-255.

59. Morote J, et al. Redefining clinically significant castration levels in patients with prostate cancer receiving continuous androgen deprivation therapy. *J Urol.* 2007;178(4 Pt 1):1290-1295.

60. Small EJ, et al. Ketoconazole retains activity in advanced prostate cancer patients with progression despite flutamide withdrawal. *J Urol.* 1997;157(4):1204-1207.

61. Millikan R, et al. Randomized phase 2 trial of ketoconazole and ketoconazole/doxorubicin in androgen independent prostate cancer. *Urol Oncol.* 2001;6(3):111-115.

62. Thompson CA. FDA approves prostate cancer treatment that inhibits testosterone synthesis. *Am J Health Syst Pharm.* 2011;68(11):960.

63. Holzbeierlein JM, McLaughlin MD, Thrasher JB. Complications of androgen deprivation therapy for prostate cancer. *Curr Opin Urol.* 2004;14(3):177-183.

64. Loprinzi CL, et al. Megestrol acetate for the prevention of hot flashes. *N Engl J Med.* 1994;331(6):347-352.

65. Dawson NA, McLeod DG. Dramatic prostate specific antigen decrease in response to discontinuation of megestrol acetate in advanced prostate cancer: expansion of the antiandrogen withdrawal syndrome. *J Urol.* 1995;153(6):1946-1947.

66. Fowler FJ, Jr, et al. The impact of androgen deprivation on quality of life after radical prostatectomy for prostate carcinoma. *Cancer.* 2002;95(2):287-295.

67. Potosky AL, et al. Quality-of-life outcomes after primary androgen deprivation therapy: results from the Prostate Cancer Outcomes Study. *J Clin Oncol.* 2001;19(17):3750-3757.

68. Green HJ, et al. Altered cognitive function in men treated for prostate cancer with luteinizing hormone-releasing hormone analogues and cyproterone acetate: a randomized controlled trial. *BJU Int.* 2002;90(4):427-432.

69. Salminen EK, et al. Associations between serum testosterone fall and cognitive function in prostate cancer patients. *Clin Cancer Res.* 2004;10(22):7575-7582.

70. Salminen E, et al. Androgen deprivation and cognition in prostate cancer. *Br J Cancer.* 2003;89(6):971-976.

71. Salminen EK, et al. Estradiol and cognition during androgen deprivation in men with prostate carcinoma. *Cancer.* 2005;103(7):1381-1387.

72. Almeida OP, et al. One year follow-up study of the association between chemical castration, sex hormones, beta-amyloid, memory and depression in men. *Psychoneuroendocrinology.* 2004;29(8):1071-1081.

73. Nelson CJ, et al. Cognitive effects of hormone therapy in men with prostate cancer: a review. *Cancer.* 2008;113(5):1097-1106.

74. Hanks RA, et al. Measures of executive functioning as predictors of functional ability and social integration in a rehabilitation sample. *Arch Phys Med Rehabil.* 1999;80(9):1030-1037.

75. Higano CS. Bone loss and the evolving role of bisphosphonate therapy in prostate cancer. *Urol Oncol.* 2003;21(5):392-398.

76. Shahinian VB, et al. Risk of fracture after androgen deprivation for prostate cancer. *N Engl J Med.* 2005; 352(2):154-164.

77. Fizazi K, et al. Denosumab versus zoledronic acid for treatment of bone metastases in men with castration-resistant prostate cancer: a randomised, double-blind study. *Lancet.* 2011;377(9768):813-822.

78. Smith MR, et al. Effects of denosumab on bone mineral density in men receiving androgen deprivation therapy for prostate cancer. *J Urol.* 2009;182(6):2670-2675.

79. Keating NL, O'Malley AJ, Smith MR. Diabetes and cardiovascular disease during androgen deprivation therapy for prostate cancer. *J Clin Oncol.* 2006; 24(27):4448-4456.

80. Saigal CS, et al. Androgen deprivation therapy increases cardiovascular morbidity in men with prostate cancer. *Cancer.* 2007;110(7):1493-1500.

81. Lu-Yao G, Stukel TA, Yao SL. Changing patterns in competing causes of death in men with prostate cancer: a population based study. *J Urol.* 2004;171(6 Pt 1): 2285-2290.

82. Newschaffer CJ, et al. Causes of death in elderly prostate cancer patients and in a comparison nonprostate cancer cohort. *J Natl Cancer Inst.* 2000;92(8):613-621.

83. Dockery F, et al. Testosterone suppression in men with prostate cancer leads to an increase in arterial stiffness and hyperinsulinaemia. *Clin Sci (Lond).* 2003;104(2):195-201.

84. English KM, et al. Low-dose transdermal testosterone therapy improves angina threshold in men with chronic stable angina: a randomized, double-blind, placebo-controlled study. *Circulation.* 2000;102(16):1906-1911.

85. Webb CM, et al. Effect of acute testosterone on myocardial ischemia in men with coronary artery disease. *Am J Cardiol.* 1999;83(3):437-439, A9.

86. Rosano GM, et al. Acute anti-ischemic effect of testosterone in men with coronary artery disease. *Circulation.* 1999;99(13):1666-1670.

87. Azoulay L, et al. Androgen-deprivation therapy and the risk of stroke in patients with prostate cancer. *Eur Urol.* 2011;60(6):1244-1250.

88. Keating NL, et al. Diabetes and cardiovascular disease during androgen deprivation therapy: observational study of veterans with prostate cancer. *J Natl Cancer Inst.* 2010;102(1):39-46.

89. Van Hemelrijck M, et al. Absolute and relative risk of cardiovascular disease in men with prostate cancer: results from the Population-Based PCBaSe Sweden. *J Clin Oncol.* 2010;28(21):3448-3456.

90. Chung SD, et al. Hormone therapy for prostate cancer and the risk of stroke: a 5-year follow-up study. *BJU Int.* 2012;109(7):1001-1005.

91. Pitteloud N, et al. Relationship between testosterone levels, insulin sensitivity, and mitochondrial function in men. *Diabetes Care.* 2005;28(7):1636-1642.

92. Braga-Basaria M, et al. Metabolic syndrome in men with prostate cancer undergoing long-term androgen-deprivation therapy. *J Clin Oncol.* 2006;24(24):3979-3983.

93. Executive Summary of The Third Report of The National Cholesterol Education Program (NCEP) Expert Panel on Detection, Evaluation, And Treatment of High Blood Cholesterol In Adults (Adult Treatment Panel III). *JAMA.* 2001;285(19):2486-2497.

94. Yannucci J, et al. The effect of androgen deprivation therapy on fasting serum lipid and glucose parameters. *J Urol.* 2006;176(2):520-525.

95. Nobes JP, et al. A prospective, randomized pilot study evaluating the effects of metformin and lifestyle intervention on patients with prostate cancer receiving androgen deprivation therapy. *BJU Int.* 2012;109(10):1495-1502.

96. Dacal K, Sereika SM, Greenspan SL. Quality of life in prostate cancer patients taking androgen deprivation therapy. *J Am Geriatr Soc.* 2006;54(1):85-90.

97. Herr HW, O'Sullivan M. Quality of life of asymptomatic men with nonmetastatic prostate cancer on androgen deprivation therapy. *J Urol.* 2000;163(6):1743-1746.

98. Moinpour CM, et al. Quality of life in advanced prostate cancer: results of a randomized therapeutic trial. *J Natl Cancer Inst.* 1998;90(20):1537-1544.

99. NIH Consensus Conference. Impotence. NIH Consensus Development Panel on Impotence. *JAMA.* 1993;270(1):83-90.

100. Kloner RA. Pharmacology and drug interaction effects of the phosphodiesterase 5 inhibitors: focus on alpha-blocker interactions. *Am J Cardiol.* 2005;96(12B):42M-46M.

101. Korfage IJ, et al. Erectile dysfunction and mental health in a general population of older men. *J Sex Med.* 2009;6(2):505-512.

102. Montejo-Gonzalez AL, et al. SSRI-induced sexual dysfunction: fluoxetine, paroxetine, sertraline, and fluvoxamine in a prospective, multicenter, and descriptive clinical study of 344 patients. *J Sex Marital Ther.* 1997;23(3):176-194.

103. Rosen RC, Lane RM, Menza M. Effects of SSRIs on sexual function: a critical review. *J Clin Psychopharmacol.* 1999;19(1):67-85.

104. Albersen M, et al. The future is today: emerging drugs for the treatment of erectile dysfunction. *Expert Opin Emerg Drugs.* 2010;15(3):467-480.

105. Fujisawa M, Sawada K. Clinical efficacy and safety of sildenafil in elderly patients with erectile dysfunction. *Arch Androl.* 2004;50(4):255-260. https://wayback. archive-it.org/7993/20170114063354/http://www.fda. gov/NewsEvents/Newsroom/PressAnnouncements/ ucm274642.htm

106. U.F.D. Administration. FDA approves Cialis to treat benign prostatic hyperplasia. 2011.

107. Hatzimouratidis K, Hatzichristou DG. A comparative review of the options for treatment of erectile dysfunction: which treatment for which patient? *Drugs.* 2005;65(12):1621-1650.

108. Albersen M, Orabi H, Lue TF. Evaluation and treatment of erectile dysfunction in the aging male: a mini-review. *Gerontology.* 2012;58(1):3-14.

109. Bella AJ, et al. Daily administration of phosphodiesterase type 5 inhibitors for urological and nonurological indications. *Eur Urol.* 2007;52(4):990-1005.

110. Shindel AW. 2009 update on phosphodiesterase type 5 inhibitor therapy part 1: recent studies on routine dosing for penile rehabilitation, lower urinary tract symptoms, and other indications (CME). *J Sex Med.* 2009;6(7):1794-1808; quiz 1793, 1809-1810.

111. Shabsigh R, et al. Randomized study of testosterone gel as adjunctive therapy to sildenafil in hypogonadal men with erectile dysfunction who do not respond to sildenafil alone. *J Urol.* 2004;172(2):658-663.

112. Hatzimouratidis K, et al. Guidelines on male sexual dysfunction: erectile dysfunction and premature ejaculation. *Eur Urol.* 2010;57(5):804-814.

113. Hellstrom WJ, et al. Implants, mechanical devices, and vascular surgery for erectile dysfunction. *J Sex Med.* 2010;7(1 Pt 2):501-523.

29 Impact of Hepatic and Renal Dysfunction on Pharmacology of Palliative Care Drugs

Katelyn Stepanyan and Thomas Strouse

OVERVIEW

Diminished liver and kidney function are common in palliative care patients. These alterations may be transient, as in the patient with cancer who suffers reversible renal injury from nephrotoxic chemotherapy, or permanent and worsening, such as in the patient with a progressing malignancy metastatic to the liver. Although this chapter is limited to reviewing how hepatic and renal dysfunction affect the pharmacology of common palliative care drugs, it is important to note that a host of other variables are also relevant to the pharmacokinetic (how drugs are absorbed, biotransformed, and excreted) and pharmacodynamic (how drugs work at their target site and the relationship between [drug] and clinical effects) balance in the patient. The reader can consult comprehensive pharmacology textbooks for a more complete picture (1,2).

OPIOIDS

Although the opioid epidemic has left many prescribers rightfully cautious, opioids remain the cornerstone for pain management in palliative care. In the hands of a competent prescriber and responsible patient, they are also quite safe: by contrast to many of the nonopioid analgesics described below, opioids lack organotoxicity, they are broadly effective for a variety of pain states, and there are sufficient data to guide prescribing them in an informed way in end-organ failure.

For the interested reader, many comprehensive reviews of opioid metabolism and pharmacokinetics well beyond the scope of this chapter are available (3–10). For the purposes of this overview, it is useful to divide opioids into two broad metabolic categories: those that undergo little or no hepatic oxidative metabolism, requiring instead the uridine diphosphate glucuronosyltransferases (UGTs), and those that undergo primary or exclusive metabolism via CYP450/hepatic oxidative biotransformation (see also Table 29.1).

The primary UGT group is composed of morphine, hydromorphone, and oxymorphone, while the CYP450 group includes methadone, fentanyl, oxycodone, hydrocodone, codeine, tramadol, tapentadol, and buprenorphine. Normal metabolism of the UGT group, particularly morphine and dilaudid, are more susceptible to embarrassment as a result of changes in renal function due to the buildup of active metabolites that depend on the kidneys for clearance. All opioids are subject to pharmacokinetic variability as a result of anomalies in hepatic function, though the CYP450 group may be more vulnerable. Serum levels of drugs in this latter group are also more vulnerable to the inhibitory or inductive effects on liver isoenzyme activity conferred by starting, stopping, or dose changes of other agents.

In the most general sense, the addition of potent CYP inhibitor drugs to a regimen that already includes regular dosing of an opioid that is primarily a CYP substrate (codeine, hydrocodone, oxycodone, methadone, fentanyl, tramadol, tapentadol, and buprenorphine) is likely to result in higher peak plasma concentrations of the opioid parent molecule and a longer duration of action of that molecule, compared with circumstances before the addition of the inhibitor. Decrements in hepatic oxidative function will likely have similar consequences. Conversely, the addition of drugs that are potent CYP inducers may lower peak plasma concentrations of relevant opioids and shorten their duration of action, just as recovery in hepatic function from an impaired baseline will do the same.

NONOPIOID ANALGESICS

Anticonvulsants

Nearly every commercially available anticonvulsant has been demonstrated to have at least modest analgesic efficacy (11,12). Clinician choice from among them tends to be determined by perceived ease of use: side-effect profile, dosing convenience, monitoring requirements, and increasingly whether or not the manufacturer has obtained an FDA indication for pain. Two of the most commonly prescribed anticonvulsant analgesics, gabapentin and its congener pregabalin, are mediators of the alpha-2-delta subunit of the calcium channel and show broad efficacy in neuropathic pain states. Gabapentin is FDA approved for the treatment of postherpetic neuralgia and pregabalin for diabetic neuropathic pain, fibromyalgia, and postherpetic neuralgia. Both drugs are biologically inert:

443

TABLE 29.1 METABOLIC PATHWAYS OF COMMONLY PRESCRIBED OPIOIDS

Drug category/name	Uses	Primary route of metabolism	Renal notes	Hepatic notes	Comments
Opioids					
Morphine	Analgesic	UGT2B7	M3G metabolite neuroexcitatory, antianalgesic		Avoid, and consider switching in new-onset renal insufficiency
Hydromorphone		UGT2B7	H3G in rodents neuroexcitatory, antianalgesic; human data inconclusive		In renal insufficiency, monitor patient for toxicities; otherwise no change
Oxymorphone		UGT2B7	O3G measurable but has no known pharmacologic activity		No changes unless symptoms emerge
Codeine		CYP2D6	UGT2B7 secondary		Prodrug; 2D6-mediated biotransformation to morphine required
Hydrocodone		CYP2D6, 3A4			Lower doses in new-onset hepatic failure
Oxycodone		CYP2D6, 3A4	UGT2B7 secondary		Lower doses in new-onset hepatic failure
Methadone		CYP2C8/9/19, 2D6, 1A2			P-gp inhibitors may ↑ potency
Fentanyl		CYP3A4, 2B6	UGT secondary		Lower doses in new-onset hepatic and renal failure
Tramadol		CYP2D6	CrCl < 30: max 200 mg/d immediate-release formulation only	Cirrhosis: max 100 mg/d immediate release only	
Tapentadol		CYP2C9/19,	PI: avoid use in "severe renal insufficiency" UGT secondary	PI: 50 mg q8h in "moderate" impairment; "avoid use" in severe impairment	
Buprenorphine		CYP3A4, 2C8 UGT 1A1, 2B7 secondary	Considered safe in renal insufficiency and dialysis UGT secondary	Caution in liver disease	

CYP, cytochrome P450 isoenzyme systems, with trailing roman numeral/letter/numeral denoting family, subfamily, etc; UGT, uridine diphosphate glucuronosyltransferase family/subfamily/etc; p-gp, p-glycoprotein cellular membrane ion pumps; CrCl, creatinine clearance; PI, package insert.
Adapted from Strouse TB. Pharmacokinetic drug interactions in palliative care: focus on opioids. *J Palliat Med.* 2009;12:1043–1050. Reprinted/amended with publisher's permission.

they do not undergo oxidative metabolism and are excreted in urine unchanged, making them particularly well suited for use in patients with complex medical illness, polypharmacy issues, and organ failure. Table 29.2 provides summary data on routes of metabolism and dosing considerations in renal and hepatic dysfunction for commonly prescribed anticonvulsants.

Antidepressants

Not all drugs marketed as "antidepressants" have analgesic efficacy. Despite early optimism, investigations into the possible pain-relieving properties of the selective serotonin reuptake inhibitors were mostly disappointing (13). Clinical research supports the view that among the "modern" antidepressants, the serotonin–norepinephrine reuptake inhibitors (SNRIs) duloxetine, venlafaxine, and milnacipran reliably demonstrate analgesic efficacy. The older tricyclic antidepressants (TCAs), which display some SNRI-like mechanisms of action, are also effective for pain.

Significant differences in safety and side effects separate the older tricyclics from the modern SNRIs, however, and these differences may be magnified in the setting of polypharmacy, concomitant medical illness, end-organ dysfunction, and frank organ failure. What makes the "posttricyclic" antidepressants so much safer than their predecessors is the absence of fast sodium channel membrane-

TABLE 29.2 METABOLIC PATHWAYS OF COMMONLY PRESCRIBED ANTICONVULSANTS

Drug category/ name	Uses	Primary route of metabolism	Renal notes	Hepatic notes	Comments
Anticonvulsants	Seizure prophylaxis Analgesia Anxiolysis				
Gabapentin		Exclusively renal; inert	CrCl 30–60: 200–700 mg b.i.d. CrCl 16–29: 200–700 mg q.d. CrCl 15: 100–300 mg q.d. CrCl < 15: dose proportionately to CrCl	None	Like lithium, may be given once orally after dialysis in patients getting renal replacement therapy at regular intervals: 125–350 mg/dose
Pregabalin		Exclusively renal; inert	CrCl 30–60: 75–300 mg/d b.i.d. or t.i.d. CrCl 15–30: 25–150 mg/d in one or two doses CrCl < 15: 25–75 mg/d	None	Like lithium, may be given once orally after dialysis in patients getting renal replacement therapy at regular intervals: 2× calculated mg/d for CrCl < 15
Lamotrigine		Glucuronidation	Limited data; use with caution	No dose adjustment in mild hepatic impairment; 25% reduction in moderate/ severe; 50% in severe with ascites	Maintenance dose after dialysis in patients getting it at regular intervals
Levetiracetam		Nonenzymatic hydrolysis and renal excretion	Linear relationship to CrCl; dose decrement suggested	No impact	Dose after dialysis

All data referenced in this table are abstracted from the package insert for the indicated drug and is thus consistent with FDA's most current analysis of these agents. Many of the older drugs (e.g., phenytoin and primidone) were approved long before the CYP450 system had been identified. For these, there is often a paucity of what by today's standards would be considered "basic" metabolic information required for approval.

HD, hemodialysis; recs, recommendations; PI, package insert; DPH, diphenylhydantoin (dilantin); FB, felbamate.

stabilizing effects—the mechanism by which clinical doses of the tricyclics may sometimes cause benign cardiac conduction abnormalities and by which intentional or accidental overingestion can cause cardiac arrest and death. It has been repeatedly demonstrated that in renal failure, the hydroxylated metabolites of TCA parent molecules accumulate at concentrations of hundreds to thousands of times what is found in normals; these unmeasured hydroxy-metabolites may be arrhythmogenic and are present in higher than expected concentrations even after dialysis (14). Tricyclics are likely best avoided entirely in patients with renal insufficiency or dialysis dependence (15).

In one of the few prospective trials available, sertraline was compared to placebo in a 12-week antidepressant efficacy trial for patients with depression and chronic kidney disease (16). There were no differences among groups in terms of adverse events or tolerability. Unfortunately, there was also no statistically significant evidence of antidepressant efficacy comparing active drug to placebo.

As a function of the FDA's more stringent requirements in recent years for testing in "special populations," the package inserts for the modern agents duloxetine, venlafaxine, desmethylvenlafaxine, vortioxetine, vilazodone, milnacipran, and levomilnacipran contain recommendations for dose decrements in hepatic and renal insufficiency. It is worth pointing out that these recommendations are empirically based and do not necessarily reflect evidence of toxicity or increased side-effect burden, but rather are simply a response to measurements of elevated serum concentrations of the drugs.

NSAIDs/ASA/Acetaminophen

The potential toxicities of nonsteroidal antiinflammatory drugs (NSAIDs)—both COX-2 specific and nonselective—are well known. There is general consensus that NSAIDs should be avoided in patients with impaired renal function since their effect on renal arteriolar tone can worsen renal insufficiency or precipitate frank renal failure. NSAIDs can be used safely and effectively in patients with static renal failure who are receiving renal replacement therapies.

End-organ toxicities of acetaminophen, particularly hepatotoxicity, are often neglected in palliative care settings. Acetaminophen is the most common coanalgesic included in short-acting compounded opioid products, and it is common for patients to inadvertently exceed the recommended maximum of 4 g of acetaminophen/24 hours due to escalating opioid requirements. It is unknown whether acetaminophen exposure confers added risk to patients with established hepatic

dysfunction, but common sense suggests it should be avoided. Most of the opioid molecules commonly compounded with coanalgesics are also available as single products and can be prescribed that way. Hydrocodone is the exception in North America: it is only available in compounded forms.

Salicylates are effective analgesics but, like NSAIDs, carry the risks of gastric irritation and antiplatelet properties that can cause or exacerbate bleeding. These risks may be compounded in patients with progressive hepatic dysfunction, who often have attendant coagulopathy due to synthetic impairment. Coupled with thrombocytopenia or prescribed anticoagulants, NSAID or acetylsalicylic acid–associated mild gastritis can become a life-threatening bleeding problem.

Misoprostol, H2 blockers (ranitidine and others), and proton pump inhibitors (omeprazole and others) confer some protection.

Ketamine and Lidocaine

Ketamine and lidocaine are both used in the field of palliative care for complex cancer and noncancer pain syndromes, particularly neuropathic pain. Ketamine has additional uses for depression. Both ketamine and lidocaine undergo the majority of their metabolism by the CYP450 enzymes in the liver (17,18). Thus, increased levels may be expected if combined with CYP inhibitors or in the setting of reduced hepatic oxidative function. This is likely more clinically relevant for lidocaine given its narrow therapeutic index, though the data on the influence of renal and hepatic function on both ketamine and lidocaine pharmacokinetics are limited. There are some studies of ketamine suggesting that serum levels are minimally affected by renal dysfunction and dialysis (17).

STIMULANTS

Psychostimulants can be helpful in palliative care patients for the management of fatigue, somnolence, low mood, and other symptoms. The conventional stimulants (methylphenidate and various forms of amphetamine) are best studied and have been used for decades. They appear to work within hours of first doses. There is no evidence for toxic accumulation in renal or liver failure, and they can be prescribed in immediate-release formulations at very low doses and used as needed. Modafinil and armodafinil are also used, and recently published studies support their effectiveness for fatigue and sleepiness in patients with advanced disease. In contrast to the inotropic and chronotropic effects of conventional stimulants, the newer agents have little or no impact on cardiac myocardial oxygen requirements. There is emerging evidence that

TABLE 29.3 METABOLIC PATHWAYS OF COMMONLY PRESCRIBED STIMULANTS/ WAKEFULNESS-PROMOTING AGENTS

Drug category/name	Uses	Primary route of metabolism	Renal notes	Hepatic notes	Comments
Stimulants	Fatigue/ wakefulness promoting/ antidepressant augmentation				
Methylphenidate		Hepatic	Case reports: lack of accumulation in dialysis	None	
Dextroamphetamine		Hepatic	No		
Modafinil		Hepatic	Modafinil acid (inert metabolite) accumulates in CRI	↑ [SS] in cirrhotics	PI recommends dose decrement
Armodafinil		Hepatic	Same as modafinil	Same as modafinil	Same as modafinil

CRI, chronic renal insufficiency; PI, package insert; SS, steady state.
From Stiebel VG. Methylphenidate plasma levels in depressed patients with renal failure. *Psychosomatics*. 1994;35(5):498-500.

modafinil and armodafinil may take weeks to exert their optimal effects, however (19,20). Since the decision to use stimulants for fatigue, lethargy, or somnolence is often taken in the last days or weeks of life, such a delayed effect may prove to limit utility. This is compounded by high per-pill costs and by the absence of an FDA indication for their use as palliative agents. Insurers therefore tend to be recalcitrant about approving payment for modafinil and armodafinil, hospice programs generally cannot afford them, and patients are understandably reluctant to pay out of pocket for agents that may take weeks to work. Modest dose decrements are recommended in organ failure (Table 29.3).

ANTIEMETICS

5-HT₃ Antagonists

Ondansetron revolutionized the management of chemotherapy-related nausea and vomiting. Related compounds available in North America are dolasetron, granisetron, and palonosetron. Ondansetron is almost exclusively biotransformed by the liver and has biologically inactive metabolites. Not surprisingly, steady-state levels are significantly increased in liver failure, without apparent clinical consequence, though it is recommended to limit the maximum daily dose in severe liver failure (Child-Pugh Class C). Interestingly, these drugs have shown promise in managing "renal itch," an intractable symptom common to patients on chronic hemodialysis. Their off-label use in patients receiving renal replacement therapies suggests safety and effectiveness.

Dopamine (D2) Antagonists

Anti-emetics targeting the dopamine receptor include the butyrophenones (haloperidol), benzamides (metoclopramide), and the phenothiazines (prochlorperazine, chlorpromazine), which have antihistaminergic and anticholinergic actions as well (21). Olanzapine is another dopamine antagonist with affinity for other receptors, and is associated with less extrapyramidal side effects than the other dopamine antagonists. With the exception of metoclopramide, there are no FDA recommendations about usage in renal or hepatic failure. Because metoclopramide is excreted principally through the kidneys, dose adjustment in renal disease is warranted.

Antihistamines and Anticholinergics

Drugs in the antihistaminergic and anticholinergic classes include promethazine, diphenhydramine, and hyoscine (scopolamine). Similar to the other antiemetic agents, there are no formal recommendations for dose adjustment in organ dysfunction, though caution is advised in the elderly given the sedative and anticholinergic side effects, as noted in the American Geriatrics Society Beers Criteria (21).

NK1 Receptor Antagonists

Aprepitant is a selective neurokinin/substance P receptor antagonist indicated for preventing chemotherapy-related nausea and vomiting. It is extensively metabolized by hepatic CYP450 enzymes and inhibits P450 3A3/4 in a dose-dependent manner. The package insert (22) asserts that there are no data regarding the impact of advanced liver disease on aprepitant pharmacokinetics or pharmacodynamics. Similarly, fosaprepitant is an NK receptor antagonist available as an injectable formulation.

Synthetic Cannabinoids

Dronabinol was the first cannabinoid approved by the FDA to treat chemotherapy-related nausea. It is predominantly metabolized in the liver and has only recently been the subject of careful pharmacokinetic study (23). There are no recommendations regarding dose modification in organ failure, but empiric dose reduction is prudent. Nabilone is structurally similar to delta-9-tetrahydrocannabinol and also has utility in treatment-resistant nausea. Like dronabinol, it appears to be exclusively hepatically metabolized, but at the time of its approval there were no data submitted to the FDA on the impact of hepatic or renal impairment on its pharmacokinetics. The cannabis plant derived "pure" cannabidiol (CBD) agent Epidiolex was approved by the FDA in 2018 for treatment of childhood epilepsies and can only be used for that purpose, despite potential interest in off-label prescribing for symptom management in palliative care.

APPETITE STIMULANTS

Megestrol acetate is the most widely used and effective agent available for appetite stimulation and the attenuation of the cachexia/anorexia syndrome in patients with cancer or HIV/AIDS. After oxidation by gut mucosa and the liver, megestrol's metabolites are excreted predominantly in urine. There is no guidance in the package insert for dosing adjustments in hepatic or renal failure.

The anti–tumor necrosis factor agents thalidomide and pentoxifylline have been studied as alternate agents to attenuate wasting. Thalidomide has shown promise in controlled trials (24,25) and possesses an FDA indication for use in advanced HIV. Its metabolism is complex, relying both on nonenzymatic hydrolysis and on oxidative biotransformation via CYP2C19 (26). There are no published guidelines for dose adjustment in renal or hepatic dysfunction.

The tetracyclic antidepressant mirtazapine has been noted to cause weight gain in medically well patients treated for depressive illness. A recent phase II trial supports the off-label clinical practice of using mirtazapine to stimulate appetite and promote weight gain in patients with advanced malignancies (27). Mirtazapine's label promotes use "with caution" in renal and hepatic disease, suggesting dose decrements may be indicated. There are no specific known pharmacokinetic drug interactions warranting concern, however. Olanzapine has also

been studied due to both its potent antinauseal and possible anticachexic properties, but results have been mixed (28). There are no special considerations for its use in organ failure.

CORTICOSTEROIDS

Corticosteroids are used widely in the management of malignancies and other life-limiting illnesses. They are a frequent component of the palliative care pharmacopoeia for the management of pain, fatigue, nausea/appetite stimulation, itching, inflammatory processes, and other symptoms. There is essentially no evidence of toxic accumulation of corticosteroid metabolites in renal or liver failure, while at the same time the risks of adrenal insufficiency in critically ill patients continue to be elucidated (29). For the patient receiving outpatient or home-based palliative care services who has been chronically exposed to corticosteroids, it seems prudent to continue physiologic doses in order to avoid an iatrogenic crisis of acute insufficiency and to taper carefully if the eventual goal is discontinuation.

BISPHOSPHONATES AND DENOSUMAB

Bisphosphonates (pamidronate, alendronate, clodronate, zoledronic acid) have revolutionized the prevention and management of skeletal complications of metastatic malignancies and the management of bone pain associated with these complications. Bisphosphonates undergo no hepatic biotransformation and are excreted unchanged in urine; occasionally, they have been implicated in acute renal injury. There are specific published drug-by-drug guidelines for dosage based on creatinine clearance (30). There are no recommendations related to hepatic dysfunction.

Denosumab, a human monoclonal antibody that inhibits RANKL and therefore inhibits osteoclasts, is a useful alternative to bisphosphonates for patients with renal dysfunction, and it is now FDA approved for the prevention of skeletal related events in patients with cancer (31).

STOOL SOFTENERS/LAXATIVES

Most of the stool softeners/laxatives used in palliative care are nonabsorbed and act within the lumen of the gut to alter the water content of stool and/or to affect motility. As such, recommendations regarding use in renal or hepatic failure are moot. It is worthwhile to keep in mind that these agents are less effective in patients who are dehydrated and hypercalcemic or have other metabolic embarrassments associated with decreased bowel motility.

The osmotic laxative lactulose has long been recognized for its therapeutic effect on porto-systemic encephalopathy, making it an excellent choice for the constipated patient with hepatic failure. Polyethylene glycol powder, when mixed with water, is tasteless and textureless, making it more palatable than many of the other osmotic agents.

The newer class of peripheral opioid receptor antagonists includes methylnatrexone, an injectable that does not reverse opioid analgesia centrally and provides rapid, reliable laxation for opioid-induced constipation. It is recommended that the dose be reduced by 50% for patients with creatinine clearance of <30. There are no published recommendations for patients on renal replacement therapies or who have advanced liver failure. Alvimopan should be avoided in patients with Child-Pugh class C or worse hepatic disease. Naldemidine and naloxegol do not carry warnings regarding use in organ dysfunction.

OCTREOTIDE

Octreotide is a somatostatin analogue used to treat neuroendocrine tumor (carcinoid). In palliative care, it is often used for symptomatic management of bowel obstruction. Its putative mechanism(s) of action involve reducing bowel contractility against a fixed obstruction, thus reducing pain and related distress; it also reduces intestinal secretions via its somatostatin-like properties. The only published guidelines pertaining to renal or hepatic insufficiency are intended to govern repeated dosing over time in patients with carcinoid or VIPoma. Octreotide's use in a palliative care setting is much more likely to be short term, for example, in the management of acute bowel obstruction near the end of life. Under such circumstances, conservative mg/kg dosing should be chosen from the nomogram in the package insert.

SEDATIVE–HYPNOTICS

Many palliative care patients will require agents that can broadly be considered sedative–hypnotics. These can be further separated into distinct groups based on structure or mechanism of action: sedating antihistaminic anticholinergics, benzodiazepines, nonbenzodiazepine sleep medicines, sedating antidepressants, sedating atypical antipsychotics, and others.

Sedating antihistaminic anticholinergics are frequently chosen because they are cheap, are available without prescription, and are perceived as safe and effective. They include diphenhydramine, chlorpheniramine, and cyproheptadine. All require some degree of hepatic oxidative metabolism and

their metabolites can accumulate in patients with renal insufficiency. Because these agents have been available without prescription for decades, there has been little scientific attention paid to their pharmacokinetics. Evidence-based recommendations are scarce. General clinical caution—"start low and go slow"—is a reasonable strategy.

For the purposes of this chapter, benzodiazepines can be subdivided into two major metabolic categories: those that undergo extensive hepatic oxidative metabolism and have multiple active metabolites and/or long serum half-lives (diazepam, chlordiazepoxide, and alprazolam) and those without active metabolites (lorazepam, clonazepam, oxazepam, and temazepam) (32). It makes sense to rely on the latter group in patients with known or suspected end-organ failure. Many palliative care patients have been exposed chronically to benzodiazepines, which are prescribed routinely as part of the antiemetic regimen for most cancer chemotherapies, and may therefore have developed significant pharmacologic tolerance. Additionally, benzodiazepines confer anticonvulsant benefits, are effective anxiolytics, and are useful for insomnia with short-term use. The clinician should remain alert, however, to the potential for benzodiazepines to have new, undesirable side effects in organ failure patients: they can mimic or worsen hepatic encephalopathy in patients with liver failure (33) and can contribute to sedation, lethargy, and, in combination with opioids, to life-threatening respiratory depression. Though there is little by way of written recommendations, it is prudent in patients with organ failure to use lowest possible doses of the "no active metabolites" benzodiazepines listed above or to stop them entirely if one can rule out the possibility of withdrawal seizures or rebound anxiety.

The nonbenzodiazepine sedative–hypnotics (eszopiclone, zolpidem, zaleplon in the United States) are distinct from conventional benzodiazepines by virtue of their selectivity for the GABA-A (gamma-aminobutyric acid A) subtype of the BZD receptor in the human central nervous system. It is asserted that this specificity makes them "purer" sedative–hypnotics, lacking in the anxiolytic and anticonvulsant properties of the conventional benzodiazepines and allegedly minimizing the potential for the development by users of tolerance, physiological dependence, and abuse/misuse. Clinical experience challenges some of these assertions. By virtue of their arrival to the marketplace within the last few decades, there are a few more data about metabolism in organ failure: broadly, caution is warranted in patients who develop new-onset renal failure or hepatic failure and lowest possible doses should be sought.

REFERENCES

1. Atkinson AJ, Abnerthy DR, Daniels CE, Dedrick RL, Markey SP, eds. *Principles of Clinical Pharmacology.* New York, NY: Elsevier Academic Press; 2010.
2. Bunton L, Chabner B, Knollman B, eds. *Goodman and Gillman's the Pharmacological Basis of Therapeutics.* New York, NY: McGraw Hill; 2010.
3. Kharasch ED. Opioid analgesics. In: Levy R, Thummel KE, Trager WF, Hansten PD, Eichelbaum M, eds. *Metabolic Drug Interactions.* Philadelphia, PA: Lippincott Williams & Wilkins; 2000:297-320.
4. Holmquist G. Opioid metabolism and the effects of cytochrome P450. *Pain Med.* 2009;10:S20-S29.
5. Osborne R, Joel S, Grebenik K, Trew D, Slevin M. The pharmacokinetics of morphine and morphine glucuronides in kidney failure. *Clin Pharmacol Ther.* 1993;54:158-167.
6. Aureta K, Goucke CR, Ilett KF, Page-Sharp M, Boyd F, Ooh TE. Pharmacokinetics and pharmacodynamics of methadone enantiomers in hospice patients with cancer pain. *Ther Drug Monit.* 2006;28:359-366.
7. Shaiova L, Berger A, Blinderman CD, et al. Consensus guidelines on parenteral methadone use in pain and palliative care. *Palliat Support Care.* 2008;6:165-176.
8. Weschules DJ, Bain KT, Richeimer S. Actual and potential drug interactions associated with methadone. *Pain Med.* 2008;3:315-344.
9. Strouse TB. Pharmacokinetic drug interactions in palliative care: focus on opioids. *J Palliat Med.* 2009;12:1043-1050.
10. Prommer E. Buprenorphine for cancer pain: is it ready for prime time? *Am J Hosp Palliat Care.* 2015;32(8):881-889.
11. Martin WJ, Forouzanfar T. Efficacy of anticonvulsants in orofacial pain states: a systematic review. *Oral Surg Oral Med Oral Pathol Oral Radiol Endod.* 2011;111:627-633.
12. Brill V, England J, Franklin GM, et al. Evidence-based guidelines: treatment of painful diabetic neuropathy. Report of the American Academy of Neurology, the American Association of Neuromuscular and Electrodiagnostic Medicine, and the American Academy of Physical Medicine and Rehabilitation. *Neurology.* 2011;76(20):1758-1765.
13. Max MB, Lynch SA, Muir J, Shoaf SE, Smoller B, Dubner R. Effects of desipramine, amitryptyline, and fluoxetine on pain in diabetic neuropathy. *N Engl J Med.* 1992;326:1250-1256.
14. Cohen LM, Tessier EG, Germain MJ, Levy NB. Update on psychotropic medication use in renal disease. *Psychosomatics.* 2004;45:34-48.
15. McIntyre RS, Baghdady NT, Suman B, Swartz SA. The use of psychotropic drugs in patients with impaired renal function. *Prim Psychiatry.* 2008;15:73-88.
16. Hedayati SS, Gregg LP, Carmody T, Jain N, et al. Effect of sertraline on depressive symptoms in patients with chronic kidney disease without dialysis dependence. *JAMA.* 2017;318:1876-1890.
17. Mion G, Villevielle T. Ketamine pharmacology: an update (pharmacodynamics and molecular aspects, recent findings). *CNS Neurosci Ther.* 2013;19(6):370-380.
18. Daykin H. The efficacy and safety of intravenous lidocaine for analgesia in the older adult: a literature review. *Br J Pain.* 2017;11(1):23-31.
19. Cooper MR, Bird HM, Steinberg M. Efficacy and safety of modafinil in treatment of cancer-related fatigue. *Ann Pharmacother.* 2009;43:721-725.
20. Breitbart W, Alici Y. Psychostimulants for cancer-related fatigue. *J Natl Compr Can Netw.* 2010;8:933-942.
21. Cherny NI, Fallon MT, Kaasa S, Portenoy RK, Currow DC. *Oxford Textbook of Palliative Medicine.* 5th ed. Oxford, United Kingdom: Oxford University Press; 2015.
22. EMEND (Aprepitant) Package insert, FDA website. 2015. Last accessed September 20, 2020. https://www.accessdata.fda.gov/drugsatfda_docs/label/2015/207865lbl.pdf
23. Huestis MA. Pharmacokinetics and metabolism of the plant cannabinoids, Delta9-THC, cannabidiol and cannabinol. *Handb Exp Pharmacol.* 2005;168:657-690.
24. Kaplan G, Thomas S, Fierer DS, et al. Thalidomide for the Treatment of AIDS-associated Wasting. *AIDS Res Hum Retroviruses.* 2000;16(14):1345-1355.
25. Gordon JN, Trebble TM, Ellis RD, Duncan HD, Johns T, Goggin PM. Thalidomide in the treatment of cancer cachexia: a randomized placebo controlled trial. *Gut.* 2005;54:540-545.
26. Lepper ER, Smith NF, Cox MC, Scipture CD, Figg WD. Thalidomide metabolism and hydrolysis: mechanisms and implications. *Curr Drug Metab.* 2006;7:677-685.
27. Riechelmann RP, Burman D, Tannock IF, Rodin G, Zimmermann C. Phase II trial of mirtazapine for cancer-related cachexia and anorexia. *Am J Hosp Palliat Med.* 2010;27:106-110.
28. Naing A, Dalal S, Abdelrahim M, et al. Olanzapine for cachexia in patients with advanced cancer: an exploratory study of effects on weight and metabolic cytokines. *Support Care Cancer.* 2015;23:2649-2654.
29. Mark PE, Pastores SM, Annane D, et al. Recommendations for the diagnosis and management of corticosteroid insufficiency in critically ill adult patients: consensus statements from an international task force by the American College of Critical Care Medicine. *Crit Care Med.* 2008;36:1937-1949.
30. Hillner BE, Ingle JN, Berenson JR, et al. American Society of Clinical Oncology guidelines on the role of bisphosphonates in breast cancer. *J Clin Oncol.* 2000;18:1378-1391.
31. Prommer E. Palliative oncology: denosumab. *Am J Hosp Palliat Care.* 2015;32(5):568-572.
32. Ballenger JC. Benzodiazepines. In: Schatzberg AF and Nemeroff CB, eds. Essentials of Clinical Psychopharmacology. *American Psychiatric Publishing*; 2001:75-92.
33. Butterworth RF. Complications of cirrhosis III: hepatic encephalopathy. *J Hepatol.* 2000;32:171-180.

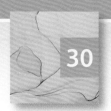

30 Metabolic Disorders in the Cancer Patient

Victoria Anderson and Jaydira Del Rivero

Endocrine disorders occur in individuals with advanced malignancy under various circumstances through the excess production of hormones, cytokines, and growth factors not derived from the anticipated organ or tissue of origin in what is termed a paraneoplastic syndrome (1–3) (Table 30.1).

Conversely, cancer or its metastases may interfere with the normal function of endocrine organs, resulting in hormone-deficiency states. Cancer patients may have metabolic disorders, such as diabetes, thyroid dysfunction, hypercalcemia, etc. that predate the diagnosis of their malignancy. This chapter discusses the most common paraneoplastic syndromes and hormone-deficiency states associated with malignancy, as well as the management of diabetes and thyroid disease in the patient with cancer.

PARANEOPLASTIC SYNDROMES

Hypercalcemia

Hypercalcemia of malignancy (HCM), initially recognized in the late 1940s, is the leading, life-threatening malignancy-related metabolic complication. HCM occurs in 20% to 40% in patients with cancer (1) and results from widely metastatic disease. Moreover, the 30-day mortality rate after onset is >50% (2,3).

Mechanisms of Disease

Malignancies produce hypercalcemia by (a) humoral cause of increased secretion of parathyroid hormone-related protein (PTHrP) or (b) osteoclastic activity causes by extensive localized bone destruction or (c) releasing osteoclast-activating cytokines; another mechanism is the excess production of 1-25-dihydroxy $(OH)_2$ vitamin D3 (1,5) in lymphomas and malignant lymphoproliferative disease (6). HCM is primarily caused by increased osteoclast-mediated bone resorption, that is, osteoclasts activation by cell-to-cell contact with osteoblasts and bone marrow stromal cells (5). Moreover, tumor cells produce circulating soluble factors such as PTHrP, tumor necrosis factor-α, and prostaglandin E (7); along with the macrophage colony-stimulating factor. These factors induce osteoblasts and stromal cells to express the receptor activator of nuclear factor kappa B (RANK) ligand (RANKL) (8). Membrane-bound RANKL then binds to, stimulates RANK expressed by osteoclast progenitors, and promotes osteoclast differentiation and activation (7). Subsequently, osteoclast activity degrades bone and increases the release of calcium and several soluble growth factors, including interleukin-6 (IL-6) and transforming growth factor-β. These factors stimulate tumor cell growth perpetuating a cycle of bone destruction. Interference with renal tubular calcium reabsorption by PTHrP further contributes to elevated serum calcium levels (7). Furthermore, IL-6 stimulates osteoclast formation and causes mild hypercalcemia by downstream effects on PTH that promotes PTHrP-mediated hypercalcemia and bone resorption at later stages in the osteoclast lineage (9,10).

Cancers that commonly produce PTHrP are squamous cell cancers (head, neck, lung, and esophagus), renal cell carcinoma, genitourinary (ovary, testes) multiple myeloma, chronic lymphocytic leukemia, small cell lung cancer, colorectal, GI-neuroendocrine, and breast cancer (3).

Extensive localized bone destruction from metastases and hematologic neoplasms (e.g., multiple myeloma and lymphoma) cause hypercalcemia by releasing osteoclast-activating cytokines, and occasionally (in lymphomas), 1-25-dihydroxyvitamin $(OH)_2$ vitamin D3, calcitriol. Secretion of calcitriol in a variety of B-cell malignancies causes most cases of hypercalcemia in Hodgkin's disease and approximately one-third of cases in non-Hodgkin's lymphoma and lymphoid leukemia's (10). Calcitriol may also be associated with hypercalcemia in the setting of chronic granulomatous diseases. This aspect is of therapeutic interest because glucocorticoids and noncalcemic vitamin D analogues may be possible treatment options for countering this pathophysiologic mechanism.

Patients with malignancy may also have hypercalcemia from a cause unrelated to their cancer. Contrarily, hypercalcemia, from primary hyperparathyroidism, is a common disorder in the general population.

TABLE 30.1 COMMON PARANEOPLASTIC SYNDROMES AND OTHER ENDOCRINE SYNDROME IN CANCER (3,4)

Syndrome	Tumor type
Syndrome of inappropriate antidiuresis (hormone vasopressin)-SIADH	• Lung: squamous, small cell, large cell, bronchial carcinoids • Prostate • Breast • Adrenal • GI
Cushing's syndrome (adrenocorticotropic hormone, corticotropic hormone)	• Lung (small cell, bronchial carcinoids, large cell) • Thymus • Medullary thyroid carcinoma • Pancreatic neuroendocrine tumors • Pheochromocytomas • Paragangliomas • Neuroblastomas
Hypercalcemia	• Bone metastases • Squamous cell head and neck, skin • Breast • Genitourinary (ovary, testis) • Lymphomas • Renal • Multiple myeloma • Chronic lymphocytic leukemia • Lung (small cell), squamous cell • Colorectal, GI-NETs
Hyperthyroidism (human chorionic gonadotropin)	• Ectopic pituitary adenomas, struma ovarii
Gynecomastia (estrogens, follicle-stimulating hormone, luteinizing hormone)	• Lung (SCLC, bronchial carcinoids) • Giant cell tumors (seminomas, teratomas, choriocarcinomas, yolk sac) • Pancreatic neuroendocrine tumors

Diagnosis

Typically, HCM occurs in patients diagnosed with advanced cancer. HCM is rarely a primary symptom of an occult malignancy, but in patients with unexplained hypercalcemia and a low serum PTH concentration <20 mg/dL, the differential diagnosis includes malignancy (Fig. 30.1). Hypercalcemia is the corrected serum calcium (CSC) [serum calcium + 0.8 × (4 − serum albumin)] often >14 mg/dL (10). This is typically higher than in primary hyperparathyroidism and is more likely to cause nausea, vomiting, dehydration, and changes in mentation (hypercalcemic crisis).

Testing for (PTHrP, a normal gene product expressed in a wide variety of neuroendocrine, epithelial, and mesoderm-derived tissues), diagnoses humoral HCM as compared to patients with primary hyperparathyroidism and normal subjects whose serum PTHrP concentrations are low or undetectable respectively. A high serum concentration of PTHrP (>12 pmol/L) diagnoses HCM (11). A simple calculation to differentiate HCM from primary hyperthyroidism using serum chloride, phosphate, and albumin: (chloride-84) × (albumin-15)/phosphate can differentiate malignancy from a parathyroid origin. Calculated values under 400 predict a malignancy whereas values over 500 predict a parathyroid origin. This formula

enables one to classify 97% of patients with cancer and 96% of patients with primary hyperparathyroidism, after excluding 5% of patients of borderline hypercalcemia that fall between the values of 400 and 500. The use of the formula is an inexpensive and easy tool to screen for a preliminary cause of HCM (12).

Clinical Presentation

Clinically, HCM presents heterogeneously with either subtle or dramatic symptoms, the symptom development and severity do not always strictly correlate with serum calcium levels, but may depend more on the briskness with which HCM develops in the patient (11).

The clinical presentation is nausea, vomiting, dehydration, and mental status changes. Cardiovascular changes may include a shortened ST segments and QT intervals, depressed ST segments, widened T waves, prolonged PR and QRS intervals, arrhythmias, ventricular tachycardias, and cardiac arrest (11). Dehydration occurs from the excess of serum calcium resulting in polyuria and gastrointestinal disturbances. Polyuria impairs reabsorption of sodium, potassium, and magnesium by the proximal tubules, causing hypovolemia and dehydration, which further compromise the glomerular filtration rate.

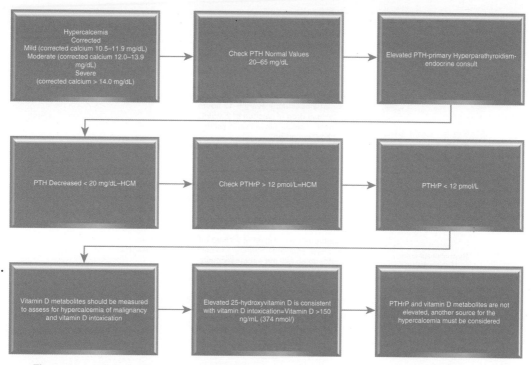

Figure 30.1 Differential diagnostic evaluation of hypercalcemia.

The decreased glomerular filtration rate then leads to increased sodium resorption (and associated increased calcium resorption) in the proximal tubule, creating a positive feedback cycle of compromised kidney function and increasing serum calcium (11).

Above the normal corrected calcium range (8.0 to 10.8 mg/dL), patients can demonstrate subtle symptoms of anorexia, nausea, constipation, and altered mental status. Moderate elevations of CSC levels at approximately 12 mg/dL can lead to renal insufficiency and deposit of excess calcium in tissues. Severe HCM (CSC levels of ≥15 mg/dL) may present with severe nausea and vomiting, dehydration, renal insufficiency, and clouding or loss of consciousness. This condition requires immediate intervention to prevent coma and cardiac arrest that may occur at these levels.

Median survival in the setting of HCM with high serum PTHrP concentrations generally ranges from 1 to 3 months. Patients have a shorter median survival times (4) when serum PTHrP concentration is above 12 mg/dL. In this scenario, it is often associated with a decreased response rate to bisphosphonate therapy and a rapid recurrence of hypercalcemia (10,13). Those who respond to intravenous (IV) bisphosphonate therapy may have a significantly better outcome, although survival duration remains short (53 vs. 19 days) (13).

Treatment

When possible, treatment is directed toward the primary tumor. When surgical resection is not a reasonable medical management is not a reasonable medical management to treat a hypercalcemic crisis the focus shifts to intense IV hydration, to increase urine excretion of calcium and administration of calcitonin, and bisphosphonates (10,14) (Fig. 30.2). Algorithm for Hypercalcemia Treatment (Table 30.2). Other therapies used in selected cases of hypercalcemia include, for example, glucocorticoids that are useful as calcium-lowering agents in hematologic malignancies and in hypercalcemia mediated by vitamin D intoxication (2,11,14).

Intravenous Hydration

Adequate hydration with normal saline is the key to the initial management of HCM. High serum calcium levels lead to inadequate urine concentrating ability by the nephron tubules; this results in polyuria, hypovolemia, and dehydration. Restoring normal blood volume through aggressive IV rehydration 200/300 mL/h is critical. This improves the glomerular filtration rate and, along with sodium, and increases renal excretion of excess serum calcium (6). Use of loop diuretics to counteract fluid overload can be judiciously used especially in those patients who are also at the risk of developing congestive heart failure (6). Careful monitoring of serum and urine electrolytes is also necessary in

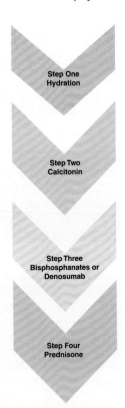

Step One
Hydration

- Titrate carefully based on fluid status 200–300 mL/h of 0.9% normal saline
- A loop diuretic (Furosemide, Toresemide) can be added for patients who develop signs and symptoms of fluid overload during hydration.

Step Two
Calcitonin

- 4–8 international unit per kg to IU/kg subcutaneously or intramuscularly every 6–12 hours
- Maximal drop in calcium of 2 mg/dL
- Onset of calcitonin action is within 4 hours of administration.
- Tachyphylaxis develops after 48 hours

Step Three
Bisphosphanates or
Denosumab

- Zoledronic acid 4 mg administered I.V. over 15 minutes
or
- Pamidronate 60–90 mg administered I.V. over 2–24 hours
or
- ibandronate 2–6 mg administered I.V. over 1–2 hours
or if Hypercalcemia refractory to above bisphosphanates:
- Denosumab 120 mg subcutaneously

Step Four
Prednisone

- In hematologic malignancies and vitamin D toxicity
- 60 mg daily by mouth
- Suitable for outpatient

Figure 30.2 Treatment of hypercalcemia.

these patients, as they often require replacement during IV hydration and diuretic therapies. However, given that HCM tends to worsen with the progression of the underlying cancer, increased calcium diuresis provides only transient relief. Effective treatment of HCM also requires pharmacologic agents to treat the underlying cause of increased calcium release from bone (1,2,6,9).

Early Inhibitors of Osteoclast-Mediated Bone Resorption

The primary pharmacologic approach for the treatment of HCM has been to decrease the rate of bone resorption. Bisphosphonates and calcitonin are agents used in the emergency treatment of HCM. Calcitonin counteracts hypercalcemia by interfering with osteoclast maturation at several points in the differentiation pathway and by simultaneously increasing renal calcium excretion (4). Calcitonin dosing is 4 to 8 IU/kg injected subcutaneously or intramuscularly (5). The onset of the action of calcitonin is approximately 4 hours from administration and the response tends to abate within 48 hours due to down-regulation of the calcitonin receptors by osteoclasts. The most common side effects include nausea, rhinitis, and hypersensitivity reactions (5).

In addition, corticosteroids are highly effective in treating calcitriol-mediated hypercalcemia, particularly among patients with Hodgkin's disease and non-Hodgkin's lymphomas with HCM. Time to response is generally within 1 to 4 days. However, corticosteroids are not as effective to treat HCM in solid tumor cancers (13).

Bisphosphonates

Bisphosphonates are the current standard of care in the treatment of HCM (Table 30.2). They bind strongly to bone mineral and inhibit the effects of mature osteoclasts (14).

Bisphosphonates are nonhydrolyzable analogues of inorganic pyrophosphate that bind avidly to hydroxyapatite crystals and subsequently release during the process of bone resorption. Osteoclasts take up the released cytotoxic bisphosphonate which then inhibit the cell's activity and survival through interference of intracellular signaling pathways required for osteoclast activity and survival. The first-generation bisphosphonates—sodium clodronate, disodium etidronate are non–nitrogen-containing bisphosphonates from cytotoxic adenosine triphosphate (ATP) analogue that were introduced clinically more than three decades ago (4). Newer compounds, alendronate, ibandronic acid, pamidronate disodium, and

TABLE 30.2 BISPHOSPHONATES

Drug	Dose (mg)	Mode of administration	Precautions	Adverse effects
Alendronate Alendronate. Micromedex Solutions. Truven Health Analytics, Inc. Ann Arbor, MI. Available at: http://www.micromedexsolutions.com. Accessed November 5, 2019	5, 10, or 15 mg	IV over 2 h	Renal: use is not recommended in patients with CrCl <35 mL/min	Hepatotoxicity Hypersensitivity reaction Arthralgia Bone pain Fever Osteonecrosis of the jaw *Multiple GI side effects with oral preparations
Clodronate Clodronate. Micromedex Solutions. Truven Health Analytics, Inc. Ann Arbor, MI. Available at: http://www.micromedexsolutions.com. Accessed November 5, 2019	1,500	IV over 2 h with ample hydration followed by 300 mg daily × 5 d	Renal insufficiency may require dosage adjustments	Hypersensitivity, hypocalcemia, hyperkalemia, hyperparathyroidism, hypocalcemia, abdominal pain, arthralgia Osteonecrosis of the jaw
Etidronate Etidronate. Micromedex Solutions. Truven Health Analytics, Inc. Ann Arbor, MI. Available at: http://www.micromedexsolutions.com. Accessed November 5, 2019	20 mg/kg/d	ORALLY for 30–90 d; therapy longer than 90 d is not recommended	Clinically overt osteomalacia Esophageal abnormalities (e.g., stricture or achalasia) that delay esophageal emptying Hypersensitivity to etidronate disodium	Gastritis Leg cramp Headache Heart failure Esophageal erosions Esophageal perforation Esophageal stricture Esophagitis Ulcer of esophagus Arthralgia Bone pain Musculoskeletal pain Myalgia Osteomalacia Osteonecrosis of jaw
Pamidronate Pamidronate. Micromedex Solutions. Truven Health Analytics, Inc. Ann Arbor, MI. Available at: http://www.micromedexsolutions.com. Accessed November 5, 2019	90	2 h i.v.	Do not use if glomerular filtration rate is <30; no need for hepatic adjustment	Fever hypophosphatemia, hypocalcemia, hypomagnesemia, loss of appetite, nausea, vomiting Osteonecrosis of the Jaw
Ibandronate Ibandronate. Micromedex Solutions. Truven Health Analytics, Inc. Ann Arbor, MI. Available at: http://www.micromedexsolutions.com. Accessed November 5, 2019	6/50	1 h i.v. Oral	Do not use if glomerular filtration rate is <30; no need for hepatic adjustment	Rash, abdominal pain, constipation, diarrhea, dyspepsia, nausea, arthralgia, back pain, dizziness, headache Osteonecrosis of the jaw
Zoledronic acid Zoledronic acid. Micromedex Solutions. Truven Health Analytics, Inc. Ann Arbor, MI. Available at: http://www.micromedexsolutions.com. Accessed November 5, 2019	4	15 min i.v.	Do not use in patients with creatinine >4.5 mg/dL (consider increasing the infusion duration in patients with kidney disease); no need for hepatic adjustment	Minor; fever, rarely hypocalcemia, hypophosphatemia, loss of appetite, nausea, vomiting Osteonecrosis of the jaw

zoledronic acid are nitrogen-containing bisphosphonates that inhibit the mevalonate pathway, which is vital for de novo synthesis of cholesterol and other molecules essential for many cellular functions (e.g., vesicular trafficking, cell signaling, cytoskeleton function) (15,16).

The American Association of Clinical Endocrinologists and American College of Endocrinology (AACE/ACE) recommends first-line therapy for moderate fracture risk, alendronate, risedronate, zoledronic acid, or denosumab; while ibandronate and raloxifene are considered alternatives. In those with prior fragility fractures or indicators of high fracture risk, denosumab, teriparatide, and zoledronic acid are recommended for first-line use, with alendronate and risedronate as alternatives (17).

Zoledronic acid (Zometa) gained FDA approval in 2001 for treatment of osteoporosis and in 2008 was approved for HCM, multiple myeloma, and solid tumor bone metastases (prostate resistant to hormone therapy). This approval was based on a large randomized control trial (RCT) (18) demonstrating that zoledronic acid (4 or 8 mg) is superior to pamidronate disodium (90 mg) in treating patients with moderate to severe HCM. Dosing at 4 mg I.V. normalizes calcium levels in 90% of patients in 4 to 7 days and lasts for at least 4 weeks. In comparison, pamidronate disodium and ibandronate acid response rate is 70% to 75% in 4 to 7 days and duration of effect is 2.5 weeks or 5 weeks for higher dose (8 mg) ibandronate (15).

The most commonly reported adverse events of zoledronic acid included fever, anemia, nausea, constipation, and diarrhea. These occurred with similar frequency between the zoledronic acid and pamidronate disodium groups. Renal impairment occurs rarely with the bisphosphonates; however, the risks increase with coadministration of other nephrotoxic drugs, dehydration, preexisting renal insufficiency, and aging. Acute tubular necrosis and renal failure has been reported more frequently in the zoledronic group than in the pamidronate disodium group.

Denosumab

Denosumab is a monoclonal antibody that inhibits the receptor activator of nuclear factor kappa b ligand (RANKL). First approved by the FDA in 2010 for the prevention of osteoporosis in high-risk men and women due to menopause or glucocorticoid use. It is also indicated for men receiving androgen deprivation therapy for nonmetastatic prostate cancer and to increase bone mass in women at high risk for fracture receiving adjuvant aromatase inhibitor therapy for breast cancer. The FDA approved a second labeling for treating bisphosphonate refractory HCM in 2016

at a dose of 120 mg and administered subcutaneously every 4 weeks with additional 120 mg doses on days 8 and 15 of the first month of therapy. It is administered subcutaneously in the upper arm, upper thigh, or abdomen. Denosumab is not eliminated by the kidney and thus does not require dosage adjustments in renal insufficiency, nor has there been reports of renal failure. However, denosumab's potential side effect profile includes hypersensitivity reactions, hypocalcemia, and osteonecrosis of the jaw. Atypical femoral fractures and severe rebound hypercalcemia while rare have been reported. The AACE/ACE recommends denosumab for first-line osteoporosis treatment in severe fracture risk men and women who cannot tolerate oral agents (17).

Medication-Related Osteonecrosis of the Jaw

Diagnosis of medication-related osteonecrosis of the jaw (MRONJ) requires the following criteria as defined by the American Association of Oral and Maxillofacial Surgeons (AAOMS):

1. "Current or previous treatment with antiresorptive or antiangiogenic agents
2. Exposed bone or bone that can be probed through an intraoral or extraoral fistula(e) in the maxillofacial region that has persisted for more than 8 weeks
3. No history of radiation therapy to the jaws or obvious metastatic disease to the jaws" (19).

Medicine-induced osteonecrosis of the jaw is a complication reported by the use of bisphosphonates and denosumab (19). MRONJ occurrence in patients with cancer receiving bisphosphonate therapy is 0.7% to 6.7%, as compared to 0% to 0.7% in cancer patients not receiving bisphosphonates, thus representing a 50% to 100% greater risk (19). Risk factors for MRONJ include denture use, dental alveolar surgery, and concomitant periodontal or periapical disease (19). Osteonecrosis of the jaw can present in the mandible (73%) and maxillae (22.5) or in both (4.5%) (19). Once osteonecrosis occurs discontinuation of the bisphosphonate or replacement with other bisphosphonates does not changes the course disease (19). Therefore, the current recommendation for patients requiring bisphosphonates treatments is a baseline dental evaluation and regular reevaluations during their treatment; aggressive management of dental problems and education and reinforcement of dental hygiene.

Bisphosphonate in the Hospice Setting

There is a paucity of studies on the benefits of bisphosphonate use for palliation of bone pain. The literature discourages use of bisphosphonates in hospice patients for prevention of osteoporosis (20,21). However, O'Carrigan et al. in a Cochrane review supports the use of bisphosphonates in late-stage breast cancer to palliate bone pain and decrease fracture rate (22). Similar findings in the Cochrane review found the use of bisphosphonate in the multiple myeloma population reduces vertebra fractures and pain. However, in this population there was a with a 1/1,000 risk of osteonecrosis of the jaw (23). Use of bisphosphonates has been reported to palliate bone pain in children with Langerhans histiocytosis, and in Ewing's sarcoma (21,24).

HCM is a serious, often life-threatening skeletal complication. The goals of treatment for HCM are to control the underlying disorder, restore adequate hydration, increase urinary excretion of calcium, and inhibit osteoclast activity in bone (Fig. 30.1).

SYNDROME OF INAPPROPRIATE ANTIDIURETIC HORMONE

In the syndrome of inappropriate antidiuretic hormone (SIADH), hyponatremia results from (a) the overproduction of AVP by the posterior pituitary gland in response to a stimulus by tumor cells or (b) by the actual production of AVP or AVP-like peptides by tumor cells or (c) as a side effect of medications that are able to stimulate AVP production. Most cases of SIADH are asymptomatic, the diagnosis is usually first suspected by noticing a low serum sodium on routine chemistries. Diagnosis of SIADH occurs after excluding other causes of hyponatremia, such as hypovolemia, hypervolemia (occurring in renal or hepatic disease or cardiac failure), hypothyroidism, and adrenal insufficiency (25–27). The urine chemistries in SIADH show urinary osmolality that is greater than serum osmolality and a high urinary sodium concentration (Table 30.2) (27). Syndrome of inappropriate antidiuretic hormone (SIADH) occurs frequently in small cell lung cancer and carcinoid tumors and in cancers of the esophagus, pancreas, duodenum, colon, adrenal cortex, prostate, thymomas, and lymphomas. In one series, the incidence of clinically significant SIADH was 9% among 523 patients with small cell lung cancer. A large fraction of patients have milder abnormalities in arginine vasopressin (AVP) metabolism without hyponatremia. Therefore, approximately one-half of patients with abnormal renal handling of water loads have subclinical presentations subclinical (1,2). Another study found that 41% of patients with all types of lung cancers and 43% of patients with colon cancer had significantly elevated levels of AVP without evidence of clinically

significant SIADH (3). Hyponatremia is also a common electrolyte disorder in patients hospitalized with acquired immunodeficiency syndrome (AIDS) and AIDS-related complex. Often it is associated with gastrointestinal losses or SIADH with an increase in morbidity and mortality (5). Medications commonly used by patients with cancer associated with SIADH include diuretics, morphine sulfate, vincristine sulfate, cyclophosphamide, phenothiazine's, and tricyclic antidepressants (Fig. 30.3). Most drugs cause SIADH by stimulating posterior pituitary secretion of AVP.

Diagnosis

Determining the cause of hyponatremia in the cancer patient does not differ from the non-cancer patient. hyponatremia in the patient with cancer does not differ from. Workup includes hepatic and cardiac failure, renal disease, over diuresis, factitious hyponatremia associated with hyperglycemia, and other conditions (Fig. 30.4).

Clinical Presentation

The clinical features of hyponatremia depend on the degree of hyponatremia and the rate of its development. Most patients with chronic hyponatremia are asymptomatic. Generally, symptoms do not occur until the serum sodium falls below 115 to 120 mEq/L (26). Similarly, the signs and symptoms of SIADH caused by water intoxication (i.e., hypoosmolality and hyponatremia) include confusion, lethargy, seizures, and coma. Occasionally, patients present with focal neurologic deficits (26,27).

Treatment

The treatment of SIADH relies on the rate of development of hyponatremia and the presence of neurologic sequelae (Table 30.3). If the patient is symptomatic and has a serum sodium level below 130 mEq/L, fluid restriction to 800 to 1,000 mL per 24 hours is effective in slowly raising serum osmolality over a period of 3 to 10 days (26,27). Acute hyponatremia with neurologic symptoms has a mortality rate of 5% to 8% and warrants aggressive treatment. In patients with severe hyponatremia, (Na <115 and neurologic symptoms) treating with IV administration of hypertonic saline (3% saline at a rate of 0.1 mg/kg/min) may be necessary (26,28). Administered as a 2 mL/kg bolus (maximum 150 mL) of 3% NaCl over 10 minutes followed by a repeat bolus one to two times as needed until symptoms improve (27). Therapeutic goal is a 5 to 6 mEq/L increase in serum sodium (SNa) in 2 hours with monitoring of the serum Na after each bolus of 3% saline or at least every 2 hours (26,28). The 3% NaCl boluses are discontinued

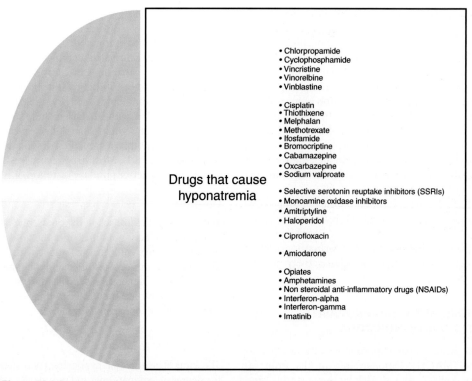

Figure 30.3 Drugs associated with causing hyponatremia.

when the patient is awake and back to his baseline alertness and responsiveness and denies headache and nausea or when the serum sodium increases by 10mEq/L in the first 5 hours (27,28).

During treatment, patient monitoring includes short interval vital signs and neurologic sign checks. Sodium correction should occur slowly and not to exceed 15 to 20 mEq/L. Rapid correction

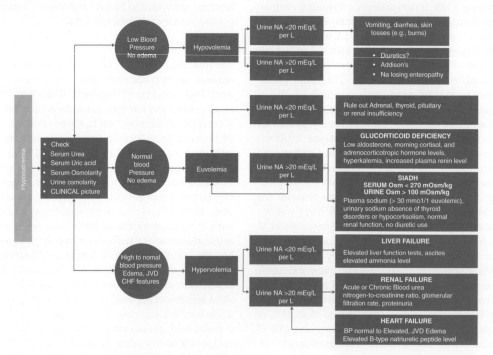

Figure 30.4 Differential diagnosis for hyponatremia.

TABLE 30.3 USUAL TREATMENT OF HYPONATREMIA

Treatment	Dosage	Uses
Fluid restriction	800–1,000 mL limit/24 h	Serum sodium < 130 mEq/L and symptomatic Acute and chronic hyponatremia
Vasopressin 2-receptors: Nonpeptide inhibitors V2R without intrinsic activity Tolvaptan, Conivaptan Vasopressin. Micromedex Solutions. Truven Health Analytics, Inc. Ann Arbor, MI. Available at: http://www.micromedexsolutions.com. Accessed January 18,2020	Tolvaptan: (SAMSCA) The recommended starting dose is 15 mg once daily. Dosage may be increased at intervals ≥24 h to 30 mg once daily and to a maximum of 60 mg once daily as needed to raise serum sodium (2.1) Conivaptan (VAPRISOL) 20-mg i.v. loading dose administered over 30 min, followed by a continuous infusion of 20 mg administered over 24 h	Bradyarrhythmia, tachyarrhythmia hyponatremia
Hypertonic saline (3% saline)	0.1 mg/kg/min 2 mL/kg bolus (maximum 150 mL) of 3% NaCl over 10 min followed by a repeat bolus one to two times	Rarely used Acute severe hyponatremia (mental status changes, coma)
Demeclocycline	Initial dose: 900–1,200 mg/d in divided doses Maintenance: 600–900 mg/d	Chronic hyponatremia
Lithium carbonate (rarely used)	600–900 mg p.o. daily	Chronic hyponatremia Significant toxicity
Urea (rarely used)	30 g in 100 mL orange juice or water daily	Chronic hyponatremia

of severe hyponatremia has been associated with central pontine myelinolysis, with quadriparesis and bulbar palsy 1 to 2 days after hyponatremia is corrected (27). A safe rate of correction in severe hyponatremia is 0.5 to 1.0 mEq/L/h until the sodium concentration reaches 125 mEq/L (27,28). Hyponatremic encephalopathy can occur if after an acute increase in serum sodium of 5 to 6 mEq/ there is no clinical improvement. In patients with more severe hyponatremia.

Expecting compliance with fluid restriction in patients who require chronic treatment of SIADH is unreasonable and the clinician can consider alternatives to include demeclocycline hydrochloride, lithium carbonate, and urea. Demeclocycline is a tetracycline derivative and causes partial nephrogenic diabetes insipidus by inhibiting the formation of AVP-induced cyclic adenosine monophosphate in distal tubules (25,26). Administered orally in divided doses of 900 to 1,200 mg/d and then reduced to maintenance doses of 600 to 900 mg/d. Side effects are mainly gastrointestinal, although hypersensitivity and nephrotoxicity can occur (25). Like demeclocycline, lithium carbonate can cause a reversible, partial form of nephrogenic diabetes insipidus but is less effective. Urea acts as an osmotic diuretic and allows the patient to maintain a normal fluid intake. Urea administered as a once-daily dose of 15 to 30 g of urea in an adult appears to be effective and well tolerated. Ure-Na is a commercially available lemon-flavored urea powder drink in 15 g powder packs that are mixed in orange juice or water and given once daily (29). The usual dosing is 30 g of urea dissolved in 100 mL of orange juice or water once daily (29).

The FDA approval of two vasopressin V2 receptor antagonists or Vaptans, Tolvaptan and Conivaptan to correct hyponatremia secondary to SIADH, is an option. Tolvaptan, an oral formulation, and Conivaptan, an IV preparation are vasopressin V2 receptor antagonists that bind and block the V2 receptor thereby increasing free water clearance via the vasopressin-mediated activation of this receptor (25). Vaptans address the underlying mechanism of water retention without inducing significant electrolyte losses and obviate the need for fluid restriction. Overcorrection is unlikely if serum [Na$^+$] is frequently measured and, to date, there have been no reported cases of osmotic demyelination associated with its use (25).

The serum sodium response to Vaptans is variable for each patient with an approximate increase of 5 to 7 mEq/L within the first 24 hours of administration (25). The most common side effects of Vaptans are increased thirst, polyuria, and dry mouth (25). Vaptans use in euvolemic patients and in conjunction with other hyponatremia treatments is discouraged as it often leads to overcorrection (25). Coadministration of cytochrome-CYP3A4 or cytochrome P-450 inhibitors such as ketoconazole, diltiazem, macrolides, rifampicin, and barbiturates can interfere with the response to Vaptans, whereas grapefruit juice increases bioavailability of Tolvaptan (30). Sedated or patients with a poor Glasgow coma score who cannot maintain oral hydration might be at higher risk for overcorrection. Overcorrection is of concern in neurologically impaired or critically ill children with restricted access to water, and hypertonic saline is preferred over Vaptans (30).

Vaptans are associated with alanine aminotransferase elevation and severe hepatotoxicity with long-term use (30). Vaptans are not a first-line agent in the management of SIADH, because they are expensive, not always necessary, and has substantial risk to Na overcorrection (30). Evidence supports Vaptans as a second-line agent for short-term use in patients with SIADH after conservative measures have failed (30).

CUSHING'S SYNDROME

Cushing syndrome caused by elevated levels of cortisol either produced endogenously by an ectopic source or iatrogenically from drugs. The most common cause of Cushing's syndrome occurs from high doses of glucocorticoids to treat autoimmune and/or inflammatory disorders or neoplasm. Endogenous Cushing's rarely occurs; it is estimated at an incidence of 0.7 to 2.4 per million population per year (31). Cushing's syndrome can be presented either as adrenocorticotropic hormone (ACTH) dependent or ACTH independent. Pituitary adenomas account for 80% to 85% of ACTH-dependent tumors and 15% to 20% are from ectopic sources. ACTH-independent tumors result almost exclusively from adrenal adenomas and rarely from adrenocortical carcinoma or from rare genetic disease such as McCune-Albright, or Carney complex (31). Thymomas, medullary thyroid cancer, GI, pancreatic, adrenal, and ovarian tumors can also secrete ectopic ACTH (32).

Diagnosis

Cushing's syndrome is diagnosed by an elevated 24-hour urinary-free cortisol when it is greater than three times the normal upper limit or at least >100 ng/dL (31). Other screening tests include late night salivary cortisol (>145 ng/dL) and/or an overnight low-dose dexamethasone suppression test; the latter is positive when 1 mg of dexamethasone given at midnight is unable to suppress the following 8:00 AM cortisol to <5 μg/dL.

Determining the cause of Cushing's that is ACTH independent versus dependent begins with measurement of plasma ACTH. Elevated ACTH suggests a dependent cause, conversely a normal to low ACTH suggest an independent cause. Primary adrenal tumors secrete ACTH levels usually below 20 pg/mL, whereas in ectopic source of ACTH, levels are generally >100 to 200 pg/mL (more frequently are elevated above 1,000 pg/mL) (31).

Clinical Presentation

Manifestations of the ectopic ACTH syndrome include hypokalemia, hyperglycemia, edema, muscle weakness (especially proximal) and atrophy, hypertension, and weight loss. Features typically seen in long-standing pituitary or adrenal Cushing's syndrome (e.g., central obesity, plethoric facies, cutaneous striae, "buffalo hump," and hyperpigmentation) are less common in highly malignant tumors such as small cell lung carcinoma but occur more frequently in indolent tumors such as carcinoids, thymomas, and pheochromocytomas (31).

Treatment of Ectopic ACTH Syndromes

Where possible, the treatment of ectopic ACTH syndrome should be directed primarily at the surgical resection of the secreting tumor. Medical management for nonsurgical candidates as palliative treatment in the setting of sepsis or psychosis the is to aim inhibit steroid synthesis. Aminoglutethimide, metyrapone, mitotane, ketoconazole, and octreotide acetate all successfully block steroid synthesis and treat the symptoms of ectopic Cushing's (33,34). While rare, if these drugs fail, bilateral adrenalectomy is considered.

Treatment to achieve eucortisolism may include a combined approach with focused on antisteroidogenesis tumor-directed drugs, glucocorticoid receptor antagonists, or combination drugs might be necessary (31).

HYPOCALCEMIA OF MALIGNANCY

Hypocalcemia of malignancy is rare, and often associated with renal failure and in patients receiving bisphosphonate therapy for bone metastasis (2). It occurs most commonly in association with osteoblastic metastases of the breast, prostate, and lung; its incidence is approximately 16% (18). The etiology of the hypocalcemia is not well understood; however, it is important to consider vitamin D deficiency, as well as malnutrition, hypomagnesemia, and calcium deficiency.

TABLE 30.4 MANAGEMENT OF HYPOCALCEMIA

Acute Symptomatic Hypocalcemia (Tetany)
1. 10% calcium gluconate (90 mg of elemental calcium/10 mL ampule)
   - Dilute 2 × 10 mL ampules of calcium gluconate in 50–100 mL of D5 solution. Infuse 2 mg/kg body weight over 5–10 min or 10% calcium chloride (272 mg of elemental calcium/10 mL ampule)
   - Dilute 1 × 10 mL ampule in 50–100 mL of D5 solution. Infuse 2 mg/kg over 5–10 min.
2. Following rapid loading infusion, reduce to a slower infusion of 15 mg/kg of calcium gluconate mixed with D5 infused over 6–12 h.

Chronic Hypocalcemia
1. Oral elemental calcium 1–2 g in 2–3 divided doses
2. Vitamin D replacement (approximate doses only)
   - 1,25-Dihydroxyvitamin D: 0.25–2.0 µg/d
   - Vitamin D: 25,000–100,000 IU/d

Neck dissection and radiation can cause hypoparathyroidism leading to hypocalcemia, and certain chemotherapeutic agents are also associated with electrolyte imbalance causing PTH resistance, hence hypocalcemia. Moreover, ectopic calcitonin secretion from the underlying tumor has been rarely implicated. Tetany is a rare complication of tumor-associated hypocalcemia. The two well-known clinical findings are Trousseau's and Chvostek's signs. Vitamin D deficiency can present with muscle weakness and hypotonia. Due to the variety of signs and symptoms, it is necessary to check 25-hydroxy vitamin D, calcium, magnesium, phosphorus, and PTH in a patient with suspected hypocalcemia. Vitamin D and calcium supplements are the therapeutic mainstays of all forms of chronic hypocalcemia. Acute hypocalcemia is treated by i.v. calcium gluconate or calcium chloride (Table 30.4).

MANAGEMENT OF ENDOCRINE ISSUES AT THE END OF LIFE

Malignancies and the treatment thereof often occurs in patients with preexisting medical conditions such as diabetes mellitus and thyroid disease. Treatment of these conditions must continue during and after treatment of the malignancy and extended to palliative care. Goals of treatment rely on underlying of the malignancy and its prognosis (35).

HYPERGLYCEMIA/HYPOGLYCEMIA

The absence of strong evidence-based practice guidelines for diabetic management at the end of life necessitates the practitioner to rely on standard guidelines for the treatment of both type 1 and type 2 diabetes mellitus. Patient comfort is the essential goal in preventing hyperglycemic or hypoglycemic events, maintaining glucose levels between 180 and 360 is acceptable (34–37).

The Concomitant use of glucocorticoids with chemotherapy the standard care in most cancer treatments can increase insulin needs in diabetics by 20 to 100%, and in the non-diabetic patient up to 64% will develop steroid induced diabetes (36). The treatment of diabetes in this setting usually requires dietary management often made impossible by emetic effects of chemotherapy on oral intake. Medication treatment of steroid-induced diabetes can includes oral agents, but most often require insulin administration with the expert input of an endocrinologist.

In the cancer population with suboptimal nutrition, recent weight loss, or impaired kidney or liver function, tight management of blood glucose often results in hypoglycemia. Symptoms of hypoglycemia result from neuroglycopenia (confusion, seizures, and coma) or from activation of the adrenergic nervous system (sweating, palpitations, hunger, and tremors). The primary treatment is nutritional support, either oral or IV. Severe hypoglycemia is defined when blood glucose is <50 mg/dL. End-of-life treatment with an IV bolus of 50% dextrose and then continued as a drip of 10% glucose is recommended.

Patients with poor appetite and decreased oral intake require liberalized diets from the traditional "diabetic diet." Patients experiencing early satiety or mechanical problems with chewing and swallowing can benefit from nutritional supplementation and consultation with a registered dietitian to devise an appropriate diet.

In summary, when choosing an appropriate treatment for patients who have preexisting diabetes mellitus or steroid-induced diabetes and cancer, setting reasonable goals to avoid symptomatic hyperglycemia, decrease the risk of hypoglycemia, provide the patient with as many dietary choices as possible and ultimately maintain quality of life.

Euthyroid Sick Syndrome

Euthyroid sick syndrome (ESS) is also known as nonthyroidal illness syndrome or low triiodothyronine (T3) syndrome. ESS is characterized by alterations in the levels of thyroid hormones due to nonthyroidal diseases in the absence of any disorder related to the hypothalamic–hypophysial axis or thyroid gland. Severe illness, whether acute or chronic, can cause changes in thyroid physiology. Changes can occur in levels of total thyroxine (T_4) and, to a lesser extent, free thyroxine and TSH levels. T_4 is decreased because of its decreased binding to its serum transport proteins. The decrease in triiodothyronine (T_3) results from inhibition of 5′-deiodinase, the enzyme that converts T_4 to T_3. Low T_4 levels are associated with a higher mortality rate; TSH levels are generally helpful in distinguishing ESS from pituitary hypothyroidism. In addition, free thyroxine levels are usually normal. ESS has been studied in critically ill patients and in adult cancer patients. Cengiz et al. found that in 35% of patients with non–small-cell lung cancer had ESS (3). Loss of appetite, increased catabolism, feeding disorders, and nutritional insufficiencies are thought to be responsible for the development of ESS in cancer patients, and rarely the need of replacement is needed (5).

ENDOCRINE-RELATED ADVERSE EVENTS RELAYED TO IMMUNOTHERAPY

Immune checkpoint inhibitors are monoclonal antibodies that block the inhibitory molecules programmed death receptor-1 (PD-1) and cytotoxic T lymphocyte-associated protein 4 (CTLA-4). These deactivate and induce apoptosis of activated T cells and are revolutionizing cancer treatment. CTLA-4 is a molecule expressed on T cells in central lymphoid organs and regulates T-cell activation at its early stages and effects receptor-ligand binding between T cells and tumor cells, in draining lymph nodes, and in the tumor microenvironment. As a checkpoint inhibitor, it binds with CD80 and inhibits activated T cells. CTLA-4 inhibitor ipilimumab gained FDA approval in 2011 for the treatment of metastatic melanoma and CTLA-4 drug tremelimumab although available in the United States to treat mesothelioma does not yet FDA indication to treat cancer outside of clinical trials (38–40).

PD-1 and its ligand receptor PDL-1 has a role in tumorigenesis and tumor suppression, which involves the paired effect in the presence of tumor-infiltrating lymphocytes. PD-1 up-regulates interferon gamma expression and stimulates the emergence of PDL-1 on tumor cell surfaces. PDL-1 binds PD-1 and exerts pressure on antigen presenting cells to also express PDL-1. This sends a suppressive signal to T cells and an antiapoptotic signal to tumor cells and finally leads to T-cell dysfunction and tumor survival (38–40).

Drugs aimed at inhibiting PD-1 and PDL-1 to modulate the tumor site immunity; target-tumor induced immune defects and repair ongoing tumor immunity. The FDA has approved six drugs to treat a variety of solid tumors and Hodgkin's lymphoma: Nivolumab PD-1 in 2014, Pembrolizumab PD-1 in 2014, Atezolizumab PDL-1 in 2016, Avelumab PDL-1 in 2017, Durvalumab PDL-1 in 2017, and most recently PD-1 inhibitor Cemiplimab in 2018 (39,40).

The effect of the checkpoint inhibitors on the endocrine system can lead to significant morbidity and in rare cases death. The most endocrine immune-related adverse effects (irAEs) include thyroiditis, hypophysitis, and adrenal insufficiency, and rarely diabetes insipidus, diabetes mellitus, hypocalcemia, and hypoparathyroidism has been reported. The pathogenesis events, while not specifically known, are presumed from autoimmune reactions from unchecked T-cell proliferation.

Surveillance of thyroid, cortisol, and ACTH hormones at baseline and periodically for early diagnosis and management is necessary to prevents crisis. The treatment for these endocrine irAEs includes supportive care, hormone replacement, oral or parenteral glucocorticoids, and brain imaging to rule out other causes. Interrupting immunotherapy is rarely necessary. Discussed earlier in this chapter are the management of thyroid disorders and diabetes, leaving a need for further discourse on adrenocortical insufficiency.

Because of the vascular nature of the adrenal cortex, the adrenal glands are common sites of metastatic disease. Typically, adrenal metastases are found incidentally during abdominal computed tomography and magnetic resonance imaging scans and are usually of no functional significance. In a minority of cases, bilateral adrenal cortical destruction in advanced stages can impair normal functioning and result in deficient production of cortisol (40).

Symptoms of adrenocortical deficiency regardless of the source, either from metastasis or from irAEs, overlap with typical symptoms of advanced malignancy and include weight loss, fatigue, nausea, anorexia, and hypotension. Either hyponatremia or hyperkalemia heightens suspicion for the presence of adrenal insufficiency (40).

The ACTH stimulation test is the most direct diagnostic study used to exclude adrenocortical insufficiency. A normal test contains the following three elements: a morning basal cortisol of at least 7 to 9 µg/dL, an increase >7 µg/dL 30 minutes after administration of 0.25 mg IV ACTH, and a maximum response to IV ACTH of 18 to 20 µg/dL or higher (40).

Severely symptomatic adrenal insufficiency (*adrenal crisis*) is treated with IV saline and stress doses of hydrocortisone with 100 mg intravenously every 8 hours, tapered to a chronic oral maintenance dose of 20 mg every morning and 10 mg every evening. In the cases where concomitant aldosterone deficiency resulting in hyperkalemia may also require the addition of the oral aldosterone analog fludrocortisone acetate (0.05 to 0.20 mg daily) (Fig. 30.5) (40).

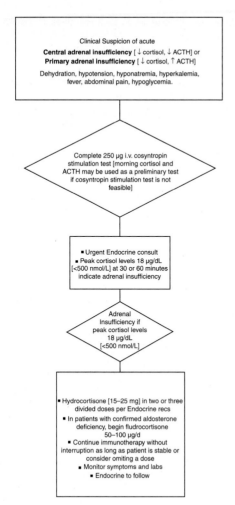

Figure 30.5 Treatment algorithm for adrenal insufficiency.

REFERENCES

1. Goldner W. Cancer related hypercalcemia. *J Oncol Pract.* 2016;12(5):426-432.
2. Reagan PP. Approach to diagnosis and treatment of hypercalcemia in a patient with malignancy. *Am J Kidney Dis.* 2014;63(1):141-147.
3. Dimitriadis GA. Paraneoplastic endocrine syndromes. *Endocr Relat Cancer.* 2017;24:R173-R190.
4. Ralston SH, Gallacher SJ, Patel U, et al. Cancer-associated hypercalcemia: morbidity and mortality. *Ann Intern Med.* 1990;112(7):499-504.
5. Tebben PJ, Singh RJ, Kumar R. Vitamin D-mediated hypercalcemia: mechanisms, diagnosis, and treatment. *Endocr Rev.* 2016;37(5):521-547. doi: 10.1210/er.2016-1070.
6. Mirrakhimov A. Hypercalcemia of malignancy: an update on pathogenesis management. *N Am J Med Sci.* 2015;7(11):483-493.
7. Fisken RA, Heath DA, Bold AM. Hypercalcemia: a hospital survey. *Q J Med.* 1980;49:405-418.
8. Firkin F, Seymour JF, Watson AM, et al. Parathyroid hormone-related protein in hypercalcemia associated with hematological malignancy. *Br J Haematol.* 1996;94(3):486-492.
9. Poe CM, Radford AI. The challenge of hypercalcemia in cancer. *Oncol Nurs Forum.* 1985;12:29-34.
10. Feldner KL, Sarno J. Hypercalcemia of malignancy. *J Adv Pract Oncol.* 2018;9(5):496-504.
11. Horwitz MJ. *Hypercalcemia of Malignancy: Mechanisms.* Up to Date; May 22, 2018. https://www.uptodate.com/contents/hypercalcemia-of-malignancy-mechanisms?search=PTHrP&source=search_result&selectedTitle=1~43&usage_type=default&display_rank=1. Accessed November 4, 2019.
12. Lind L, Ljunghall S. Serum chloride in the differential diagnosis of hypercalcemia. *Exp Clin Endocrinol.* 1991;98(3):179-184.
13. Migliorati CA. Bisphosphonates and oral cavity avascular bone necrosis. *J Clin Oncol.* 2003;21:42-53.
14. Baron RF. Denosumab and bisphosphonates: different mechanisms of action and effects. *Bone.* 2011;48:677-692.
15. Wilcock A. Bisphosphonates. *J Pain Symptom Manage.* 2019;57(7):1018-1030.
16. Yeganeh BW. Targeting the Mevalonate cascade as a new therapeutic approach in heart disease, cancer and pulmonary disease. *Pharmacol Ther.* 2014;143(1):87-110.
17. Tu KL. Osteoporosis: a review of treatment options. *P T.* 2018;43(2):92-104.
18. Dhillon S. Zoledronic acid (Reclast, Aclasta): a review in osteoporosis. *Drugs.* 2016;76:1683-1697.
19. American Association of Oral and Maxillofacial Surgeons. *Medication-Related Osteonecrosis of the Jaw—2014 Update.* American Association of Oral and Maxillofacial Surgeons. Retrieved September 22, 2019 https://www.aaoms.org/docs/govt_affairs/advocacy_white_papers/mronj_position_paper.pdf
20. Maddison AR. Preventive medication use among persons with limited life expectancy. *Prog Palliat Care.* 2011;19(1):15-21.
21. Seiden H. The boy who refused an IV: a case report of subcutaneous clodronate for bone pain in a child with Ewing Sarcoma. *J Med Case Reports.* 2007;1(7):1-4.
22. O'Carrigan BW. Bisphosphonates and other bone agents for breast cancer. *Cochrane Database Syst Rev.* 2017;10(10):CD003474.
23. Mhaskar RK. Bisphosphonates in multiple myeloma: an updated network meta-analysis. *Cochrane Database Syst Rev.* 2017;12(12):CD003188.
24. Chellapandian DM. Bisphosphonates in Langerhans Cell Histiocytosis: an International retrospective case series. *Mediterr J Hematol Infect Dis.* 2016;8(1):e2016033.
25. Cuesta M, Garahay A, Thompson CJ. SIAD: practical recommendations for diagnosis and management. *J Endocrinol Invest.* 2016;39:991-1001.
26. Cuesta M, Thompson CJ. Syndrome of inappropriate antidiuresis (SAID). *Best Pract Res Clin Endocrinol Metab.* 2016;30:175-187.
27. Grohe C, Berardi R, Burst V. Hyponatraemia—SIADH in lung cancer diagnostic and treatment algorithms. *Crit Rev Oncol Hematol.* 2015;96:1-8.
28. Gross P. Clinical management of SIADH. *Ther Adv Endocrinol Metab.* 2012;3(2):61-73.
29. Moritz ML. Syndrome of inappropriate antidiuresis. *Pediatr Clin North Am.* 2019;66:209-226.
30. Peri A. The use of Vaptans in clinical Endocrinology. *J Clin Endocrinol Metab.* 2013;98(4):1321-1332.
31. Sharma ST, Neiman LK, Feelders RA. Cushing's syndrome: epidemiology and developments in disease management. *Clin Epidemiol.* 2015;7:281-293.
32. Pelosof LC, Gerber DE. Paraneoplastic syndromes: an approach to diagnosis and treatment. *Mayo Clin Proc.* 2010;85(9):838-854.

33. Lacroix A, Feelders RA, Stratakis CA, Nieman LK. Cushing's syndrome. *Lancet*. 2015;386:913-927.

34. Sharma A, Skola L, Harvey-Bush S. Management of diabetes mellitus in adults at the end of life: a review of recent literature and guidelines. *J Palliat Med*. 2019;22(9):1113-1138.

35. Angelo M, Ruchalski C, Sproge BJ. An approach to diabetes mellitus in hospice and Palliative Medicine. *J Palliat Med*. 2011;14(1):83-87.

36. Hershey DS. Importance of glycemic control in cancer patients with diabetes: treatment through end of life. *Asia Pac J Oncol Nurs*. 2017;4(4):314-318.

37. Healy SJ, Dungan KM. Hyperglycemia in patients with hematologic malignancies. *Curr Diab Rep*. 2015;15(8):1-9.

38. Gonzales-Rodrieguez E, Rodrigez-Abreu D. Immune checkpoint inhibitors: review and management of endocrine adverse events. *Oncologist*. 2016;21:804-817.

39. Corsello SM, Barnabei A, Marchetti P, Vecchis LD, Salvatori R, Torino F. Endocrine side effects induced by immune checkpoint inhibitors. *J Clin Endocrinol Metab*. 2013;98(4):1361-1375.

40. Del-Rivero J, Cordes LM, Klubo-Gwiedzinska J, Madan RA, Neiman LK, Gulley J. Endocrine related adverse events related to immune check point inhibitors: proposed algorithms for management. *Oncologist*. 2019;24:1-11.

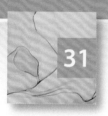

31 Infectious Complications/Management

Juan C. Gea-Banacloche and Jennifer M. Cuellar-Rodríguez

Cancer patients have a significantly increased risk of infections (1,2). Risk factors for this increased susceptibility to infection are directly related to the underlying malignancy or to its treatment (Table 31.1) (3–5).

RISK FACTORS FOR INFECTIONS IN PATIENTS WITH CANCER

Intrinsic Host Factors

Underlying Malignancy

Some hematologic malignancies are associated with specific immune abnormalities that result in increased frequency of infections even in the absence of treatment (see Table 31.1). For instance, the rate of mycobacterial disease seems to be increased in hairy cell leukemia and Hodgkin's lymphoma. Encapsulated bacterial infections are common in patients with multiple myeloma and chronic lymphocytic leukemia, due to impaired B-cell immunity. Few studies have looked at the incidence and type of infections in non-neutropenic patients with solid tumors. Some well-recognized risk factors are related to the anatomic location of the tumor, for example, head and neck tumors predispose to serious infections by oral flora and they also increase the risk of aspiration pneumonia. Endobronchial tumors may cause postobstructive pneumonia. Neoplasias of the biliary tract significantly increase the risk of cholangitis, colon cancer increases the risk of sepsis secondary to enteric organisms and of anorectal infections, etc. (6,7). There is also a specific association of colon cancer with bacteremia caused by streptococci, in particular *Streptococcus gallolyticus* (formerly *Streptococcus bovis*) and anaerobes like *Clostridium septicum*. Tumors of the genitourinary tract may predispose to pyelonephritis. Breast tumors increase the risk of mastitis and abscess formation, usually by *Staphylococcus aureus*. Corticosteroid-producing tumors and corticotrophin hormone–secreting tumors are associated with an increased risk of bacterial and opportunistic infections. *Pneumocystis jirovecii* and *Nocardia* infections have been reported in patients with Cushing's disease.

Other Intrinsic Host Factors

Functional asplenia is present after splenectomy and splenic irradiation and with chronic graft versus host disease (GVHD) (8). Functionally, asplenic patients are at risk for overwhelming sepsis by *Streptococcus pneumoniae*, *Haemophilus influenzae*, and *Neisseria meningitidis*. In asplenic patients with a history of exposure to dogs, *Capnocytophaga canimorsus* should be considered. Other pathogens of concern include *Babesia* that causes babesiosis, *Plasmodium* that causes malaria, and *Salmonella* species.

In addition to the above-mentioned risk factors, other risk factors of particular importance in advanced cancer patients include immobility and poor nutritional status.

Treatment-Related Factors

Neutropenia

Many infections in cancer arise from treatment-induced neutropenia. Lack of granulocytes facilitates bacterial and fungal infections and blunts the inflammatory response allowing infections to progress much faster. The risk of infection is proportional to the degree and duration of neutropenia. There are detailed guidelines for the use of antimicrobial agents in the setting of chemotherapy-induced neutropenic fever (see below) (9).

Mucositis

Chemotherapy and radiation therapy disrupt mucosal integrity. Mucosal linings constitute the first line of host defense against a variety of pathogens, both by providing a physical barrier and by secreting a variety of antimicrobial peptides, including lactoferrin, lysozyme, proteases, phospholipases, and defensins. Chronic GVHD may also compromise mucosal immunity, including defective salivary immunoglobulin secretion. Disruption of the epithelial lining may result in local disease and bloodstream infections by local flora (i.e., aerobic and anaerobic bacteria and yeast). Palifermin, a recombinant human keratinocyte growth factor, may result in decreased infections by reduction in severity of mucositis (10–13).

TABLE 31.1 SELECTED RISK FACTORS FOR INFECTION IN PATIENTS WITH ADVANCED CANCER

Risk factor	Type of infection
Related to underlying malignancy	
AML	Bacterial, fungal, and viral
CLL/MM	Encapsulated bacteria
ALL	PJP
Hairy cell leukemia and Hodgkin's lymphoma	Mycobacterial and viral
ATCL	PJP, *Cryptococcus neoformans*, viral, and *Strongyloides stercoralis*
Obstructive pathology from local growth of the tumor	Bacterial
Colon cancer	Enteric bacterial sepsis, in particular *Streptococcus gallolyticus* and *Clostridium septicum*
Corticosteroid-producing tumors	PJP and *Nocardia* sp.
Related to Treatment	
Neutropenia	Bacterial (mainly gastrointestinal tract) and fungal
Mucositis	Oral flora, including gram-positive and anaerobic bacteria
Corticosteroid	PJP, bacterial, fungal, and herpes viruses
Nucleoside analogs	PJP, bacterial, fungal, and herpes viruses
Monoclonal Ab	Wide range of infections: bacterial, fungal, viral, parasitic—agent specific
GVHD prophylaxis/treatment	PJP, VZV
Miscellaneous	
Immobility	Bacterial—usually related to decubitus ulcers and atelectasis
Nutritional status	Bacterial and yeast infections
Biliary stents, ureteral ostomy tubes, and tracheostomy	Bacterial and yeast
Peripherally inserted central or central venous catheters	Bacterial and yeast

AML, acute myelogenous leukemia; CLL, chronic lymphocytic leukemia; MM, multiple myeloma; ALL, acute lymphocytic leukemia; PJP, pneumocystic jirovecii pneumonia; ATCL, adult T-cell leukemia/lymphoma; Ab, antibodies; GVHD, graft versus host disease; VZV, varicella zoster virus.

Hematopoietic Stem Cell Transplantation

Preparative regimens, GVHD, and GVHD prophylaxis and treatment in hematopoietic stem cell transplantation (HSCT) recipients are significant drivers of infection. There are detailed guidelines for the prevention and treatment of infections in this patient population (14).

Autologous stem cell transplant may be considered a form of intensive chemotherapy. As such, it is typically associated with a few days or weeks of neutropenia and mucositis, followed by a few weeks or months of defective T-cell–mediated immunity. Allogeneic transplant is a more complex procedure, and there are many variants (i.e., conditioning regimen, degree of human leukocyte antigen matching, source of stem cells, and GVHD prophylaxis) that result in very different infectious

disease risk profiles. Early after HSCT, neutropenia and mucositis are the main host defense defects. Following engraftment, the most important risk factor for infection is the occurrence of severe GVHD and its treatment. Active GVHD is associated with immune dysregulation, may be accompanied by cytomegalovirus (CMV) reactivation or disease, and it is also an independent risk factor for mold infection (15). CMV disease delays immune reconstitution and is associated with an increased risk of bacterial and fungal infections (16).

Defects in cell-mediated immunity persist for several months even in uncomplicated allogeneic HSCT, predisposing to opportunistic infections, including candidiasis, *P. jirovecii*, CMV, and herpes zoster (HZ). Repopulation of specific T-cell subsets occurs at different rates. In addition to low

T-cell number, T-cell receptor diversity is reduced (17). In the absence of chronic GVHD, T-cell and B-cell functions are usually reconstituted by 1 to 2 years after engraftment. Chronic GVHD is associated with persistently depressed cell-mediated and humoral immunity, as well as functional asplenia.

Defective reconstitution of humoral immunity is a major factor contributing to increased infection susceptibility in the late transplant period. Invasive pneumococcal disease is relatively common, particularly in patients with chronic GVHD (18).

Immunomodulatory Agents and Infectious Risk

Corticosteroids

Corticosteroids are used as part of some anticancer treatment, as well as powerful anti-inflammatory agents required to palliate the effects of treatments and sometimes symptoms of tumor progression. High-dose corticosteroids have profound effects on the distribution and function of neutrophils, monocytes, and lymphocytes. They blunt fever and local signs of infection. Patients treated with corticosteroids have impaired phagocytic function and cell-mediated immunity. Infections are a frequent complication of corticosteroid use, and differences in the type and frequency of infections are dependent on the dose and duration of treatment (19). Bacterial infections are most common (20); but opportunistic fungal, viral, and mycobacterial infections are also seen, particularly with high doses and long durations of systemic corticosteroids.

Fludarabine

Fludarabine is a fluorinated analog of adenine that is lymphotoxic, primarily affecting $CD4^+$ lymphocytes. Particularly when combined with corticosteroids or cyclophosphamide, fludarabine results in a profound depression of $CD4^+$ cells that may persist for several months after completion of therapy, resulting in opportunistic infections like *P. jirovecii* pneumonia (PJP) or listeriosis, sometimes more than a year after treatment. Mycobacterial and herpes virus infections have also been described.

Interleukin-2

High-dose interleukin-2 (IL-2), sometimes used for metastatic melanoma, is a significant risk factor for bacterial infections, possibly due to a profound but reversible defect in neutrophil chemotaxis. *S. aureus* and coagulase-negative staphylococci are common pathogens, and prophylactic oxacillin can lead to a reduction in central venous catheter (CVC)-associated staphylococcal bacteremia (21).

Alemtuzumab

Alemtuzumab (Campath-1H) is a humanized monoclonal antibody that targets CD52, a glycoprotein abundantly expressed on most B and T lymphocytes, macrophages, and natural killer cells. Alemtuzumab treatment results in prolonged and severe lymphopenia, and it can also cause neutropenia in up to one-third of patients. Infections, both opportunistic and nonopportunistic, have been reported in a significant fraction of patients receiving alemtuzumab (22). Bacterial, viral, fungal, mycobacterial, and *P. jirovecii* infections are observed. CMV reactivation is seen in up to two-thirds of alemtuzumab recipients, although CMV disease seems to be uncommon.

Rituximab, Veltuzumab, and Ofatumumab

Rituximab is a chimeric human/murine monoclonal antibody directed against the B-cell marker CD20. The increased risk of infection with rituximab seems to be low and related to repeated administration (23) and host cofactors (e.g., advanced HIV disease, HSCT, and specific chemotherapeutic regimen) (24). Hepatitis B virus (HBV) reactivation occurs with rituximab treatment. There have been reports of fulminant hepatitis and even death in patients that experienced hepatitis B flare. Also a "reverse seroconversion" phenomenon has been described, with loss of protective HBV surface antibodies and reactivation (25,26). Rarely, rituximab treatment for malignant and nonmalignant conditions can be complicated by progressive multifocal leukoencephalopathy, a chronic encephalitis caused by the John Cunningham (JC) virus (27). There have been several reports of pneumocystic jirovecii pneumonia (PCP) following rituximab, but most patients received other immunosuppressants. Other rare infections that have been described in the setting of rituximab use are enteroviral meningoencephalitis, CMV disease, disseminated varicella zoster virus, refractory babesiosis, parvovirus B19, and nocardiosis (24). Veltuzumab and ofatumumab are next-generation anti-CD20 monoclonal antibodies (humanized and fully human, respectively) expected to be associated with similar infectious risk.

Immunosuppressive Agents for the Prevention and Treatment of GVHD

Immunosuppressive agents to prevent and treat GVHD all involve suppression of T-cell activation to inhibit donor alloreactive T-cell responses. The calcineurin inhibitors (cyclosporine A and tacrolimus), mycophenolate mofetil, sirolimus, and methotrexate are commonly used and are associated with an increased risk of common bacterial and opportunistic infections. Corticosteroids are the mainstay of therapy for GVHD. More intensive immunosuppressive therapy is used in steroid-refractory GVHD, resulting in very high risk for common and opportunistic bacterial, viral, and fungal diseases. Ruxolitinib has been associated with tuberculosis, PJP, hepatitis B reactivation, and fungal infections (28).

There is a growing list of anticytokine antibodies including the IL-2 receptor antagonist, basiliximab, the anti-IL6 antibody tocilizumab and tumor necrosis factor (TNF)-α inhibiting agents, infliximab, etanercept, and adalimumab. Daclizumab in steroid-refractory GVHD is associated with a significant risk of bacterial sepsis. TNF-α is a principal mediator of neutrophil and monocyte activation and inflammation. In patients with autoimmune diseases, agents that deplete TNF-α or inhibit TNF-α signaling are principally associated with an increased risk of tuberculosis and histoplasmosis. In HSCT recipients with refractory GVHD, infliximab was associated with an increased risk of invasive molds (29). Tocilizumab is frequently used to treat the cytokine storm sometimes associated with CAR-T cell therapy and may increase the risk of subsequent bacterial infections (30,31).

Additional Risk Factors for Infection in Advanced Cancer Patients

Although there are only scarce data on the risk factors for infection in advanced cancer patients that require palliative care (32–34), some recognized risk factors include long-term use of invasive devices such as peripherally inserted or CVCs, indwelling urinary catheters, ostomy tubes, biliary stents, and ureteral stents. Other risk factors include immobility, poor nutritional status, and palliative chemotherapy.

PREVENTION OF INFECTION

Preventing infections is preferable to treating them. In the case of cancer patients receiving palliative care, an acute infection may result in extreme loss of quality of life and in very difficult decisions regarding management, including the need to return to the hospital and the appropriateness of invasive diagnostic procedures. In this regard, it may be reasonable to continue prophylactic measures that are adequate to the clinical condition (e.g., antibiotics during neutropenia and opportunistic infection prophylaxis in recipients of stem cell transplantation) and administer the immunizations recommended by the American College of Physicians (ACP) to both patients and caregivers

(https://www.acponline.org/clinical-information/clinical-resources-products/adult-immunization).

Regarding immunizations, it is important to be aware that the recombinant, adjuvanted zoster vaccine much more effective than the attenuated virus vaccine, and it is safe and immunogenic in immunocompromised patients. Both the ACP and the Centers for Disease Control (CDC) (http://www.cdc.gov/vaccines/) offer up to date recommendations and answer to both common and unusual questions.

SPECIAL CONSIDERATIONS FOR ADVANCED CANCER PATIENTS

There are limited data on the incidence of infections, their management, and their effects in advanced cancer patients (32–34). Most studies have focused on current practice relating to antibiotic use in terminal cancer (34–41). There are scarce data on the impact on the quality of life of patients who receive treatment of known or suspected infections.

In general, antibiotics are not perceived as aggressive treatment such as cardiopulmonary resuscitation and artificial nutrition. Their use and possible side effects are often trivialized, and therefore there appears to be no great ethical debate on their use or nonuse in terminal care patients (41–43). However, treatment of infection may indeed be considered a life-sustaining therapy that can serve to prolong life without reversing the underlying medical condition, which at times conflicts with the goals and objectives of palliative care. At the same time, treatment of active infections can help control symptoms and in fact be an extremely important palliative intervention. However, it is possible that at some point an acute infection may be considered by the patient and the care providers as a merciful terminal event that should not be treated. In these cases, initiating or interrupting potentially life-prolonging treatment may present a true ethical dilemma (Fig. 31.1). Ideally, before deciding to treat an episode of infection, it is necessary to reassess the goals of treatment (i.e., palliation vs. curative intent), to determine the potential benefits and burdens of treatment, and to determine the availability of alternative and adjunctive treatments that can effectively palliate infection-related symptoms, such as morphine for shortness of breath and antipyretics for fever. Once specific antimicrobial treatment is instituted, it is recommended to frequently reassess the effectiveness of the intervention on the control of symptoms. Additionally, new symptoms may develop that may be directly related to the use of antimicrobials and therefore affect the overall quality of life (44).

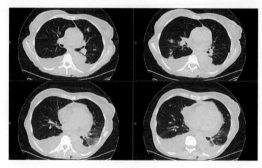

Figure 31.1 A patient with terminal multiple myeloma developed sudden respiratory insufficiency while in the hospital. A computed tomography of the chest showed worsening pleural effusions and multiple pulmonary infiltrates. A bronchoscopy with bronchoalveolar lavage was performed and was initially nondiagnostic. The patient received oxygen, morphine, and corticosteroids and her respiratory distress improved. Seventeen days later, the bronchoalveolar lavage culture was positive for *Mycobacterium tuberculosis*. Treatment for tuberculosis was recommended, but the patient and her family decided against it and she remained quarantined until she passed away 1 week later.

Currently, there are no guidelines or clinical consensus on the treatment of infections in advanced cancer patients. There are no data on antimicrobial selection, efficacy, and safety profile in this susceptible population of patients, and most recommendations are based on extrapolations from other groups.

INCIDENCE AND TYPE OF INFECTIONS IN ADVANCED CANCER PATIENTS

The true incidence of infections in advanced cancer patients is difficult to discern, as many patients treated for suspected infections may not be infected. As an example, the rate of infection was as low as 29% in a study that required a positive culture for the definition of infection, but 83% in a retrospective review of infection based on a clinical diagnosis (32,34). The most common sites of infections are the urinary tract, respiratory tract, bloodstream, and skin and soft tissue. A descriptive review of published reports describing infections in 957 patients with advanced cancer in diverse settings such as palliative care unit, hospice, teaching hospital, hematology/oncology unit, and home found that 42% of terminally ill cancer patients developed infections in the final phase of their care (35). The overall frequencies of infection by organ system were as follows: urinary tract 30.5%, respiratory tract 17.9%, skin 15.7%, and blood 14.4%. The most frequent microbiologic isolates were *S. aureus*, *Escherichia coli*, and other Enterobacteriaceae and *Pseudomonas aeruginosa*.

Candida species were the most commonly isolated fungal pathogen in the urinary tract (35).

CLINICAL EVALUATION

Typical signs and symptoms of infection may or may not be present. Fever, the cardinal sign of infection, may be nonspecific in this patient population or suppressed by advanced age, malnutrition, comorbidities, or the use of corticosteroids. Conversely, fever may be caused by noninfectious processes, including the underlying malignancy, deep venous thrombosis, and drugs. Nonspecific signs of infection may predominate; these include decline in the functional status, confusion, and reduced oral intake. A thorough clinical examination will frequently obviate the need for extensive diagnostic workup.

DIAGNOSTIC TESTS

The use of diagnostic tests for patients with terminal cancer is controversial. A decision to pursue diagnostic workup is usually influenced by the setting in which the patients are been evaluated. Some centers will have limited diagnostic capabilities, as is the case of many palliative care units; however, advanced cancer patients are frequently hospitalized in acute care hospitals (45). A full summary of the diagnostic workup of each possible infection is beyond the scope of this chapter. However, given that the urinary tract, the respiratory tract, and blood are frequent sites of infection, the following initial workup seems reasonable, provided that the resources are available:

1. *A complete blood cell count (CBC) and differential cell counts.* The presence of an elevated white blood cell count or neutrophilia increases the probability of an ongoing bacterial infection. The presence of neutropenia significantly increases the risk of bacterial or fungal infection.
2. *Urinalysis, and if abnormal a urine culture.* Urine culture should be ordered in patients with unexplained fever, altered mental status, and/or typical signs and symptoms of urinary tract infection such as pyuria, hematuria, dysuria, worsening urinary incontinence, and/or suprapubic pain (45). Asymptomatic bacteriuria does not require treatment. A dipstick urine test with a positive leukocyte esterase, nitrites, and/or pyuria should also prompt a urine culture, but the decision to treat is based on the presence of symptoms attributable to the UTI, not just on the urinalysis or urine culture. Appropriately collected urine culture specimens include a midstream or clean catch

urine, or in patients with urethral catheters, cultures should be drawn after the removal of the catheter and insertion of a new one (46).

3. *Blood cultures.* When available, blood cultures should be drawn in all advanced cancer patients in whom an infection is suspected (2). Although, in general peripherally drawn blood cultures are more reliable, if a catheter is in place, blood for culture should be drawn from the catheter. Blood from peripheral sticks should be obtained in individualized cases in which the suspicion of a catheter-related infection is very high, and positive results would impact the management of the patient.

4. *Pulse oximetry and chest X-ray.* To evaluate for pneumonia, heart failure, and pulmonary embolism.

SPECIFIC INFECTIOUS SYNDROMES

Neutropenic Fever

Fever during chemotherapy-induced neutropenia occurs in 10% to 50% of patients with solid tumors and in >80% of those with hematologic malignancies (9). Common sites of infection include the gastrointestinal tract, lung, and skin; bacteremia occurs in up to 25% of patients. Common blood isolates include coagulase-negative staphylococci, Enterobacteriaceae, and nonfermenting gram-negative rods (e.g., *P. aeruginosa*) (9). Invasive yeast (usually *Candida* spp.) infections are more commonly seen in patients with severe mucositis and neutropenia. Invasive mold infections (e.g., *Aspergillus* sp.) typically occur after prolonged neutropenia (>2 weeks). There are International guidelines for the use of antimicrobial agents in the setting of chemotherapy-induced neutropenic fever (9), and these should be consulted for specific questions. The following section discusses the most important principles.

The first step in the evaluation of cancer patients with fever and neutropenia is to assess the risk of severe infection. Risk assessment may help determine the most appropriate initial management of patients with neutropenic fever (see Table 31.2). Low-risk patients are clinically defined as those with anticipated duration of neutropenia of <7 days, are clinically stable, and have no other comorbid conditions than the underlying malignancy (9). In general terms, most consider high-risk patients as those with anticipated prolonged (>7 days) and profound neutropenia (absolute neutrophil count [ANC] ≤ 100 cells/mm^3 following cytotoxic chemotherapy) and/or significant medical comorbidities, including but not limited to hemodynamic instability, inability to take oral medication due to oral or gastrointestinal mucositis, nausea, vomiting, diarrhea, new pulmonary infiltrates, hypoxia or underlying chronic lung disease, new onset abdominal pain, neurologic or mental status changes, and suspected intravascular infection, especially catheter tunnel infection, or significant laboratory abnormalities such as aminotransferase levels >5× normal or creatinine clearance of <30 mL/min. Formal risk classification may also be performed using the Multinational Association for Supportive Care in Cancer (MASCC) risk index scoring system, which uses the summation of weighted risk factors, including age, history, inpatient or outpatient status, acute clinical signs, the presence of medical conditions, and severity of the febrile neutropenic episode (47,48). An MASCC score of <21 is considered to be high risk. High-risk patients should initially receive empiric antibiotic intravenous (i.v.) therapy in the hospital (Table 31.2) (9).

During neutropenia, fever is the best and often the only sign of underlying infection. However, other signs or symptoms (pain and erythema) may also indicate that an infection is present. The physical examination should target commonly infected areas such as the skin (in particular around sites of existing or previous procedures or catheters), oropharynx, perineum, respiratory tract, and abdomen. Additional useful diagnostic tools include blood work, cultures, and radiologic studies.

In all patients being evaluated for neutropenic fever, two sets of blood cultures should be obtained. In patients with a CVC, one set of blood cultures should be obtained from all the lumens, and if feasible an additional set should be obtained from a peripheral vein. If fever persists after the initial antimicrobial therapy, blood cultures should be obtained daily for the next 2 days, beyond this, blood cultures should be obtained only when there is a change in the clinical picture. Cultures from other sites should not routinely be obtained, unless there are clinical signs and symptoms to suggest their need.

Imaging studies should not be performed routinely unless clinically indicated. A chest radiograph should be obtained for patients with respiratory symptoms, bearing in mind that a negative chest radiograph does not rule out pneumonia. Computed tomography (CT) is the preferred method to evaluate all other areas (e.g., sinuses, abdomen, and pelvis), and a chest CT should also be obtained when the suspicion of pneumonia is high and the chest X-ray unrevealing.

Other laboratory analysis useful in planning supportive care and monitoring toxicity include CBC, levels of creatinine and urea nitrogen every 3 days, and weekly monitoring of serum transaminases.

TABLE 31.2 INITIAL EVALUATION AND MANAGEMENT IN NEUTROPENIC FEVER

Assessment of risk
High versus low risk*a*

Diagnostic workup

- Laboratory
  - CBC + differential
  - Serum creatinine and BUN
  - Hepatic transaminases and bilirubin
  - Electrolytes
- Blood cultures (at least two sets), and culture specimens from other sites if suspicious
- Chest radiograph if respiratory signs or symptoms

Initial Treatment High Risk

- Monotherapy with:
  - Ceftazidime or cefepime
  - Imipenem or meropenem
  - Piperacillin-tazobactam
- Consider an additional antimicrobial if resistance is suspected or hemodynamic instability:
  - Aminoglycoside
  - Fluoroquinolone
  - Vancomycin

Initial Treatment Low Risk

- Ciprofloxacin + amoxicillin/clavulanic acid (preferred)
- Ciprofloxacin or levofloxacin
- Ciprofloxacin + clindamycin

*a*High risk: anticipated prolonged (>7 d) and profound (≤100 cells/mm³) neutropenia following cytotoxic chemotherapy and/or significant comorbidities.
CBC, complete blood count; BUN, blood urea nitrogen.

Initial empirical therapy for fever and neutropenia in high-risk patients include monotherapy with an antipseudomonal β-lactam (Table 31.2). Other antibacterial agents may be added for the management of complications such as hypotension, pneumonia, or skin and soft tissue infection (e.g., aminoglycosides, fluoroquinolones for suspected gram-negative infection, and/or vancomycin, daptomycin, or linezolid to cover gram-positive bacteria) or other agents as needed if antimicrobial resistance is suspected based on prior known colonization with resistant bacteria or local patterns of resistance (9).

Patients who meet stringent criteria to be considered at low risk of complications may be treated initially with oral broad-spectrum antibiotics. The regimen of choice is ciprofloxacin and amoxicillin–clavulanate (49). However, in areas where gram-negative resistance to quinolones is >20%, this strategy may not be ideal (50). An outpatient course may be considered after a brief inpatient stay, during which the first dose of antibiotics is initiated, rapidly progressing infection is excluded, and prompt access to medical care can be ensured (preferably patients should be able to reach their medical facility within 1 hour). Readmission to the hospital requires that patients be treated as high-risk patients (9).

Modifications to the initial regimen should be guided by clinical and microbiologic data. Patients who remain or become hemodynamically unstable after initiation of treatment should have their therapy broadened to include coverage for resistant gram-negative, gram-positive, anaerobic bacteria and fungi. Patients with persistent fever, but otherwise asymptomatic, only require a change in antimicrobials to treat identified infections. In clinically stable patients with adequate gastrointestinal absorption, antibiotics may be switched to oral. Empiric gram-positive coverage (i.e., vancomycin) may be stopped in patients with no gram-positive bacteria identified after 2 days of therapy. Empiric antifungal therapy with an antimold active agent (i.e., echinocandin, voriconazole, posaconazole, isavuconazole, or amphotericin B preparation) should be considered in high-risk patients who have persistent fever after 4 to 7 days of broad-spectrum antibacterial coverage and in whom myeloid recovery is not imminent; in these patients, a CT of the chest or sinuses may reveal an occult fungal infection (9).

In high-risk patients who become afebrile after the initiation of empiric antimicrobial therapy, antimicrobial coverage should be continued for at least the duration of neutropenia; in patients with documented infections, duration of therapy should be appropriate for effective eradication of the particular infection, whichever comes last (9). In low-risk patients who have defervesced after 3 days of therapy, broad-spectrum antibiotics may be stopped before reaching an ANC > 500 cells/mm³, when there is no documented infection and there is evidence imminent marrow recovery. The ideal duration of antimicrobial therapy in patients who remain afebrile, but in whom neutropenia recovery is not expected (e.g., refractory aplastic anemia), is unknown. A reasonable approach in patients with no identified source of infection is to give antimicrobial therapy for at least 10 to 14 days.

There are no specific recommendations for the management of neutropenic fever in palliative care patients. Risk assessment and determination goals of therapy should proceed simultaneously. Many patients with terminal cancer may not be considered "low risk" and often the automatic approach would be to admit them to an acute care facility for i.v. therapy. This may not always be in the best interest of quality of life. An approach that may be considered if the patient does not have i.v. access would be to start therapy with an oral combination regimen, similar to the one recommended for low-risk neutropenic patients (i.e., ciprofloxacin plus clindamycin or levofloxacin plus amoxicillin–clavulanic acid) (Table 31.2). If i.v. access is available, then similar recommendations as in other cancer patients seem reasonable; however, the diagnostic workup should be less aggressive and limited to blood work, urinary samples, and limited imaging.

Catheter-Related Bloodstream Infections

The frequency of catheter-related bloodstream infections varies among different cancer populations (51). Definitive diagnosis usually requires that blood cultures be drawn simultaneously from the catheter and the periphery. Differential time to positivity of >2 hours from the cultures drawn from the catheter and those drawn from the periphery is a convincing evidence that the source of bacteremia is the catheter (52,53). However, peripheral blood cultures may not always be available, and deciding when the infection is secondary to an infected catheter may be problematic. Some authors have suggested that the differential time to positivity be applied to cultures drawn simultaneously from different lumens of a multilumen catheter. Infected nonpermanent catheters should be removed whenever feasible. Surgically implanted catheters can be salvaged when there is a rapid clearance of bacteremia after initiation of treatment and when dealing with low virulence organisms such as coagulase-negative staphylococci. In other scenarios, catheter removal should be strongly considered, although this may not always be feasible. Whenever catheter salvage is attempted in addition to i.v. antibiotics, antibiotic lock therapy has been recommended (53).

The duration of systemic antimicrobial therapy depends on several factors, including whether the catheter was removed or not, response to antimicrobial therapy within 48 to 72 hours (resolution of bacteremia and fever), and whether a complicated infection (e.g., endovascular infection or deep tissue infection) is present. In general, other than staphylococcal infections, a 14-day course of systemic antimicrobials is adequate if the catheter is removed and the patient responds to antimicrobial therapy within 72 hours. A 7-day course is adequate in patients with coagulase-negative staphylococcal infections. Cancer patients with *S. aureus* catheter–related bloodstream infections may require longer than 2 weeks of therapy. Complicated catheter-related bloodstream infection caused by any pathogen requires 4 to 6 weeks of antimicrobial therapy (53).

Respiratory Tract Infections

Upper Respiratory Tract Infection

Most upper respiratory tract infections in cancer patients are viral in origin (54,55). If available, a nasopharyngeal swab or wash should be obtained for diagnosis; during influenza season, empiric anti-influenza treatment should be strongly considered. The choice of antiviral treatment (neuraminidase inhibitors like oseltamivir, endonuclease inhibitors like baloxavir or the adamantanes, amantadine, and rimantadine) should be guided by the yearly recommendations provided by the CDC, as different strains of the influenza virus exhibit different susceptibilities.

Bacterial sinusitis is common in both neutropenic and non-neutropenic cancer patients. Mold invasive infections are of particular concern in prolonged and profound neutropenia or in patients receiving high-dose steroids (56,57). Diagnosis usually requires a CT of the sinuses and an otorhinolaryngologist consultation. Suspicious lesions should be biopsied and tissue should be sent for both culture and histopathology (58).

Treatment recommendations for sinusitis in non-neutropenic patients include amoxicillin/clavulanate, azithromycin, cefdinir, cefprozil, or cefpodoxime. The initial treatment in neutropenic patients in whom bacterial sinusitis is suspected should include agents effective against *P. aeruginosa* and Enterobacteriaceae. *S. aureus* infection can occur and the use of an agent active against it should be considered (9). If community-acquired methicillin-resistant *S. aureus* (community-acquired MRSA) is a consideration, the antibiotic options include clindamycin, trimethoprim–sulfamethoxazole (TMP–SMX), and doxycycline. A standard approach is to start with the same agents used in fever and neutropenia (see Table 31.2), keeping in mind that MRSA is not covered by this combination and vancomycin should be added if there is a high suspicion for MRSA. When fungal sinusitis is suspected, maximal efforts should be made to establish the etiologic diagnosis because of significant differences in toxicity and convenience between amphotericin B formulations (treatment of choice for mucormycosis, but available only intravenously and quite toxic) and voriconazole (treatment of choice for aspergillosis and most other invasive fungal infections, available by mouth or i.v. and better tolerated). Pending definitive diagnosis, most experts would recommend empiric amphotericin B, in one of its lipid formulations to minimize toxicity. Once an etiologic diagnosis is established, therapy should be tailored for the specific isolate. Surgical debridement is always required for invasive fungal sinusitis in neutropenic patients.

Lower Respiratory Tract Infection

There are detailed guidelines for the treatment of community-acquired and hospital-acquired pneumonia (59). Non-neutropenic patients with cancer should follow similar recommendations. Many times cancer patients will be in a category where sputum Gram stain and culture, as well as blood cultures, should be obtained. Acceptable oral regimens that are also adequate for palliative care in advanced cancer patients with community-acquired pneumonia are monotherapy with a fluoroquinolone (i.e., levofloxacin) or combination therapy with a β-lactam and a macrolide (azithromycin or clarithromycin) (59). First-line i.v. therapy for patients that require admission hospitalization, but do not require admission to the intensive care unit, include a third-generation cephalosporin (i.e., ceftriaxone) and a macrolide or monotherapy with a fluoroquinolone. Of note, extra antianaerobic coverage is recommended only for lung abscess and empyema. In patients admitted to the intensive care unit or in neutropenic patients, a fluoroquinolone and an antipseudomonal β-lactam agent should be used; anti-MRSA treatment should be considered, in particular in those that are known to be colonized with MRSA (59). If available, an MRSA nasal swab polymerase chain reaction (PCR) has very good negative predictive value for MRSA pneumonia and may allow discontinuation of the vancomycin (60). During influenza season, cancer patients with lower respiratory tract infection should be considered at risk for infection; rapid institution of empiric treatment should be strongly considered, and if available a nasal swab/wash for influenza PCR should be obtained (61,62).

The current guidelines for the management of hospital-acquired and ventilator-associated pneumonia in adults (63) have discarded the category of health care–associated pneumonia and emphasize the necessity for each hospital to develop their own antibiogram and use this to determine the need for using dual gram-negative (for *Pseudomonas aeruginosa*) and empiric MRSA antibiotic treatment. Cancer patients with septic shock or severe sepsis should probably receive dual or triple coverage. Whether hemodynamically stable, nosocomial pneumonia patients require such wide coverage is questionable but, if instituted, de-escalation should be the goal (64). In palliative care hospitalized advanced cancer patients, it seems reasonable to initiate broad-spectrum antimicrobial coverage and to frequently reassess the goal of therapy (i.e., symptom control).

A wider range of microorganisms can cause pulmonary infiltrates in neutropenic and/or highly immunocompromised cancer patients (65–68). Bacterial pathogens are most common, but other opportunistic pathogens are also a concern and the need for etiologic diagnosis becomes more pressing. When suspicion of pneumonia arises, a chest CT can reveal infiltrates that were missed on the chest radiograph or can help to better define known lesions. Unless the etiologic diagnosis is obvious, strong consideration should be given to early bronchoalveolar lavage (BAL) and/or lung biopsy (percutaneous, transbronchial, video-assisted thoracic surgery, or even open lung biopsy) (69). When the resources are available, samples should be sent for bacterial, mycobacterial, *Nocardia*, and fungal stains and culture, as well as either viral culture or PCR. Adjunctive test for those at risk for fungal pneumonia are galactomannan on the BAL and serum (70,71); for those at risk for PCP (i.e., defective T-cell immunity, such as high-dose steroids or HSCT recipients), special stains for PJP on BAL fluid or tissue and/or PCR. Serum β-D-glucan is a very sensitive test for PJP; a negative result may be used to rule out *Pneumocystis* (72). Initial antimicrobial therapy should include broad antibacterial coverage, as outlined above, and depending on the pattern of infiltrates, risk factors, and severity of infections, strong consideration should be given to additional agents like trimethoprim–sulfamethoxazole for PJP. In neutropenic patients that are not responding to broad antibacterial coverage or in those with nodular lung lesions, in particular in the absence of prophylaxis, the addition of voriconazole or a lipid formulation of amphotericin B is recommended (73,74). Besides mold infections, nodular and cavitated lesions in patients receiving corticosteroids should bring to mind *Nocardia*.

Intra-abdominal Infections

Intra-abdominal tumors, depending on their location, may lead to an obstructive cholangitis (e.g., pancreatic and hepatobiliary tumors) or erosion through a viscus. In some instances, tumor may replace most of the bowel wall, with perforation or bacteremia following initiation of chemotherapy.

Neutropenic enterocolitis (typhlitis—inflammation of the cecum) results from a combination of neutropenia and defects in the bowel mucosa related to cytotoxic chemotherapy and in patients with solid tumors receiving taxanes (75,76). Pathologically, typhlitis is characterized by ulceration and necrosis of the bowel wall, hemorrhage, and masses of organisms inside the bowel wall. Suggestive signs include fever, abdominal pain and tenderness, and radiologic evidence of right colonic inflammation. Nausea, vomiting, and diarrhea are the most common symptoms. Abdominal distension, tenderness, and a right lower quadrant fullness or mass reflect thickened bowel. Bacteremia with enteric flora, *P. aeruginosa,* or polymicrobial may occur. Clostridial species are the most common anaerobic pathogens. A CT scan should be performed in patients with suspected typhlitis or undiagnosed abdominal pain in the setting of neutropenia. The differential diagnosis includes *Clostridium difficile* colitis, GVHD of the bowel, CMV colitis (rarely observed during neutropenia), and bowel ischemia (77).

Treatment of typhlitis requires broad-spectrum antibiotics with activity against aerobic gram-negative bacilli and anaerobes (e.g., ceftazidime or cefepime + metronidazole, imipenem, meropenem, or piperacillin/tazobactam) and supportive care, including i.v. fluids and bowel rest. The majority of patients will respond to antibiotic therapy and supportive care. Surgical indications include (a) persistent gastrointestinal bleeding after resolution of neutropenia, thrombocytopenia, and clotting abnormalities; (b) free intraperitoneal air, suggestive of perforation; (c) uncontrolled sepsis despite fluid and vasopressor support; and (d) an intra-abdominal process (such as appendicitis) that would require surgery in the absence of neutropenia (78).

Clostridium difficile Colitis

Patients with cancer are at high risk for *C. difficile* colitis due to prolonged hospitalization where environmental transmission is likely to occur and frequent use of broad-spectrum antibiotics. Both antibiotic and chemotherapy administration can result in a clinical episode of *C. difficile* colitis. The clinical spectrum ranges from asymptomatic carriage to fulminant colitis with toxic megacolon. In severe *C. difficile* disease, paralytic ileus, toxic dilatation of the colon, and bowel perforation may occur. It is important to think of it not only when patients have diarrhea but also in cases of abdominal pain or tenderness, cramping, and fever of unclear etiology. The mainstay of diagnosis is the detection of *C. difficile* toxin A, toxin B, or both in the stool with a cytotoxin test or enzyme immunoassay or PCR for the toxin gene (79,80).

Traditional options for the treatment of *C. difficile* disease include oral or i.v. metronidazole and oral vancomycin. A comparative trial suggests that oral vancomycin may be more efficacious in severe cases (81). Novel antibiotics that have been shown to be effective in *C. difficile* colitis are tigecycline, fidaxomicin, and ramoplanin (50,82,83). Fidaxomicin may be associated with less relapses.

Nitazoxanide, which had efficacy similar to metronidazole in a randomized trial (84), may be considered for milder cases. Patients unable to tolerate oral agents should receive i.v. metronidazole. The combination of oral vancomycin and i.v. metronidazole is recommended in fulminant disease (80). In cases involving toxic dilatation of the colon or perforation, subtotal colectomy, diverting ileostomy, or colostomy may be required.

The safety and efficacy of probiotic agents in immunocompromised patients and patients with cancer are unknown, but it is worth noting that bacteremia has resulted occasionally from these preparations. Management of recurrences is difficult, and many different strategies have been used (repeated courses of the same antibiotic, vancomycin "pulse" therapy, and vancomycin taper) (85). Monoclonal antibodies against *C. difficile* toxins may be an option to reduce the recurrence of *C. difficile* infection (86). Prophylactic oral vancomycin when known *C. difficile* carriers are going to receive antibiotics has shown to be beneficial (87).

Anorectal Infections

Anorectal infections may be life threatening in patients who are receiving repeated courses of chemotherapy. Infection may follow the development of an anal fissure. Tiny abrasions may be a portal of entry or infection may originate in the anal crypts. Once anorectal infection is established, fascial extension to the external genitalia, pelvic floor, retroperitoneum, and peritoneal cavity may occur. Anorectal infections, with or without extensive regional spread, may lead to bacteremia. The most common pathogens in neutropenic patients are Enterobacteriaceae, anaerobes, enterococci, and *P. aeruginosa*. In most cases, the infection is polymicrobial (88).

Fever often precedes symptoms and signs suggestive of anorectal infection, and perirectal pain, often exacerbated by defecation, may initially occur in the absence of findings in the physical examination. Therefore, serial examinations of the perianal region are necessary, looking for point tenderness and poorly demarcated induration (89). Visual inspection should assess for the presence of perianal fissures, fistulas, cellulitis, and induration. Digital rectal examination should be avoided during neutropenia. A CT scan should be obtained to show the extent of perirectal involvement and drainable collections. Stool softeners and analgesics should be provided. Most cases of anorectal infections can be managed with appropriate broad-spectrum antibiotics and supportive measures without surgical intervention (88). Surgery is generally avoided or delayed until neutrophil recovery, unless the infection proves uncontrollable with medical management.

Urinary Tract Infection

Risk factors for bacterial urinary tract infection in cancer patients include the use of indwelling urethral or suprapubic catheters, ureteral stents, locally invasive neoplasias (i.e., prostatic cancer or colon cancer), and neurogenic bladder (46). *E. coli* is the most common cause of urinary tract infections. Other less common pathogens include *Klebsiella pneumoniae*, *Proteus mirabilis*, and *Enterococcus* sp. However, in patients with indwelling catheters, infections are often polymicrobial and resistant organisms are not uncommon. If feasible, adequate urine cultures prior to initiation of therapy allow tailoring of the treatment on the basis of antimicrobial susceptibility. Acceptable empiric oral therapies are TMP–SMX or oral fluoroquinolones (ciprofloxacin and levofloxacin) if local resistance is <20% (90). In ill-appearing patients, it is reasonable to start with i.v. ceftriaxone and to rule out secondary bacteremia. If the patient is known to be colonized with resistant pathogens and urosepsis is suspected, empiric therapy should include agents that target these microorganisms. In proven catheter-associated urinary tract infection, exchange of indwelling catheter can lead to improved clinical status after 72 hours and lower rates of recurrence (46,91). Ruling out obstruction is paramount. In palliative care advanced cancer patients, in whom oral agents are deemed appropriate, suppressive treatments include daily nitrofurantoin and weekly fosfomycin. Of note, asymptomatic bacteriuria should not be treated, except in neutropenic patients.

Candiduria is common among patients with indwelling catheters that receive broad-spectrum antibiotics; removal of the catheter or exchange of the catheter may be all that is needed to clear asymptomatic candiduria. Patients undergoing urologic manipulations are considered to be at risk for dissemination as well as neutropenic patients. In neutropenic patients, candiduria may be the only sign of disseminated candidiasis and antifungal treatment should be initiated (91,92). There is no evidence that treating candiduria in any other setting results in improved outcome.

Skin and Soft Tissue Infections

Skin and soft tissue infections are common among cancer and palliative care patients (35,66). Infections can be localized or be a manifestation of disseminated infections. Localized infections typically result from breaks in the skin or mucosa, usually related to physical trauma, maceration, pressure, or use of devices (i.e., around the sites of catheter insertion or ostomies). Most common localized infections are pressure ulcers and cellulitis. Sometimes skin lesions are manifestation of bacteremia (most notably ecthyma gangrenosum caused by *P. aeruginosa* and other gram-negative bacilli and also a variety of ulcers, nodules, hemorrhagic bullae, and violaceous or purpuric skin lesions), and patients that preset with fever or other signs of systemic toxicity should have blood cultures drawn before the initiation of antimicrobials. Common bacterial pathogens in cellulitis include streptococci and *S. aureus* (93). In severely immunocompromised hospitalized patients, or in neutropenic patients, gram-negative organisms (i.e., *P. aeruginosa, Aeromonas* sp., *Stenotrophomonas maltophilia*, and Enterobacteriaceae) are also common culprits and therapy should target these organisms, in addition to gram-positive cocci. It is important to consider the multiple causes of "pseudocellulitis" to avoid unnecessary use of antibiotics (94). Pressure ulcers tend to be polymicrobial. Aerobic gram-negative bacilli and gram-positive cocci are found most commonly; however, anaerobic flora is frequently isolated when deep cultures are taken. Most pressure ulcers should be treated topically and the use of systemic antibiotics reserved for evidence of cellulitis or systemic dissemination of infection.

Necrotizing infection of the skin and deeper structures (fascia and muscle) differs from the superficial skin infections in their clinical presentation and in that their outcome can be fatal. Clinical features that suggest necrosis of deeper tissues are (a) severe constant pain; (b) bullae; (c) ecchymosis that precedes skin necrosis; (d) gas, detected by palpation or imaging; (e) edema that extends beyond the area of erythema if present; (f) anesthesia; (g) systemic toxicity; and (h) rapid spread despite antibiotic therapy. These conditions are usually secondary in that they develop from an initial break in the skin due to trauma or surgery. They can be monomicrobial (usually streptococci or *Clostridium* sp.) or polymicrobial (mixed aerobic and anaerobic flora) (93). Treatment of necrotizing infections typically requires extensive surgical debridement; antimicrobial therapy for hospitalized patients or neutropenic patients should include metronidazole and cefepime or ceftazidime or monotherapy with a meropenem, imipenem, or piperacillin–tazobactam (95).

In prolonged neutropenia fungal infections are of particular concern, and skin and soft tissue lesions are usually a manifestation of disseminated disease, unless there is a clear history of trauma to the affected region. The incidence of disseminated candidiasis has substantially decreased, since the routine use of antifungal prophylaxis in HSCT and postinduction chemotherapy (9,73). About 10% of patients with invasive candidiasis develop single or multiple small (1 cm) nodular nontender erythematous skin lesions. Blood cultures are frequently positive, and skin biopsy is usually diagnostic (96).

Aspergillus spp. and *Fusarium* spp., and rarely dematiaceous molds, can spread hematogenously to the skin and subcutaneous tissue. Lesions can begin as multiple erythematous macules or subcutaneous nodules that quickly evolve to necrotic nodules. Lesions can be painful due to angioinvasion and necrosis. Mortality from these infections is high, and a diagnostic skin biopsy should be performed. Blood cultures are positive in disseminated *Fusarium* sp. infection in up to 60% of cases (57,96,97).

Herpes simplex virus (HSV) and HZ reactivations are common infections in cancer patients. HSV infection typically present as painful vesicles or ulcerations involving the nasolabial, genital or rectal skin, or mucosa. HZ reactivations present as painful papular or vesicular lesions, usually in dermatomal distribution; however, in severely immunocompromised individuals, disseminated skin lesions can appear (98). Treatment of localized HZ and HSV reactivations is with oral valaciclovir, acyclovir, or famciclovir. Treatment of disseminated disease warrants i.v. therapy. Patients with frequent reactivation could benefit from secondary prophylaxis (99,100).

COVID-19

COVID-19 stands for COronaVIrus Disease 2019. It is caused by the newly identified coronavirus SARS-CoV-2. The disease was recognized in late 2019 as a cluster of atypical cases of pneumonia in Wuhan, China, and it has become the first pandemic of the 21st century, with 18 million cases in 188 countries as of this writing (101). Although it is mainly a respiratory illness (either upper respiratory tract or pneumonia), the virus may affect other organs including nasal mucosa, GI tract, kidneys, and liver and, through thrombotic and immunopathogenic effects, almost any organ system (102,103).

After an incubation period of about 5 days (104), COVID-19 typically starts as an upper respiratory viral syndrome with cough, fever, shortness of breath, headache, and myalgias. Anosmia is a characteristic symptom. GI manifestations (diarrhea, nausea, and vomiting) may predominate in some patients. The proportion of asymptomatic cases has been estimated around 15% (105), but presymptomatic and asymptomatic cases account for a disproportionate fraction (40% to 60%) of the total transmissions. This is in part due to the fact that the highest levels of virus are found in respiratory secretions in the day preceding onset of symptoms and on the first few days of illness. In most affected individuals, the course is benign with complete resolution in 2 weeks, but at least 15% to 20% of patients develop pneumonia, typically bilateral, and require admission to the hospital for supplemental oxygen. There are several risk factors for severe disease: age, body mass index, and comorbidities like hypertension, diabetes, cardiovascular disease, chronic pulmonary disease, chronic kidney disease, and cancer.

Published data on the relationship between cancer and COVID-19 are limited by a variety of methodological problems (106). It is not yet clear whether cancer patients are at higher risk of contracting COVID-19 or not, and it is not known whether the reported increased case-fatality rates (CFR) reported by some investigators is real or artefactual (107,108). Currently, the consensus is that COVID-19 should not be considered a reason to discontinue cancer treatment (109). Guidance from national and international cancer societies is updated frequently and should be obtained (https://www.asco.org/asco-coronavirus-information/care-individuals-cancer-during-covid-19).

Of all patients with COVID-19 admitted to the hospital, 15% to 20% may need ICU care, typically for treatment of hypoxemic respiratory failure, and many of them require mechanical ventilation. The case fatality rate varies significantly with age: <1% in people younger than 50 and 20% to 30% after 70 years of age (102).

Most transmission occurs by close person to person contact, mainly by respiratory droplets, but airborne transmission is possible and has been documented mainly in poorly ventilated locales and in situations where aerosol generation is increased (110). The bulk of transmission, however, may be significantly decreased by physical distancing, use of masks, and meticulous hand hygiene.

Treatment is evolving. At the time of this writing, effective interventions include the antiviral remdesivir (111) and the anti-inflammatory dexamethasone (112). Treatment guidelines are constantly updated by the National Institutes of Health (NIH) and professional societies.

Multiple candidate vaccines are being developed (113,114), and likely more than one will be needed for different patient populations that may respond differently (e.g., elderly, immunocompromised, transplant recipients).

This section will be outdated by the time it is printed, and the reader is urged to obtain current information from the Web sites of CDC (cdc.gov, https://www.cdc.gov/coronavirus/2019-nCoV/index.html), NIH (https://www.covid19treatment-guidelines.nih.gov/), and professional societies (https://www.asco.org).

CONCLUSIONS

Infections are common in neutropenic and non-neutropenic individuals with advanced cancer. Urinary tract, respiratory tract, and bloodstream infections seem to be the most common. There is only a paucity of data on how to best manage these infections in palliative care advanced cancer patients. There is an urgent need to develop home care programs, which allow the continuity of palliative care. Studies in this population need to focus on the feasibility of administering oral regimens for certain infections and to evaluate the impact on the quality of life (Table 31.3).

TABLE 31.3 ORAL ANTIMICROBIAL THERAPY FOR SELECTED INFECTIOUS SYNDROMES IN PALLIATIVE CARE CANCER PATIENTS

Disease	Antimicrobial therapy
Neutropenic fever	*Preferred* 1. Ciprofloxacin + amox/clav[a] *Alternatives* 2. Levofloxacin 3. Ciprofloxacin + clindamycin 4. Levofloxacin + linezolid[b]
Bacterial sinusitis—non-neutropenic	*Preferred* 1. Amox/clav 2. Azithromycin 3. Cefdinir, cefprozil, or cefpodoxime
Bacterial sinusitis—neutropenic	*Preferred* 1. Levofloxacin 2. Ciprofloxacin + amox/clav *Alternatives* 3. Ciprofloxacin + clindamycin
Community-acquired pneumonia—non-neutropenic	*Preferred* 1. Levofloxacin, moxifloxacin, or gemifloxacin 2. Amox/clav and azithromycin *Alternative* 3. Doxycycline

(Continued)

TABLE 31.3 ORAL ANTIMICROBIAL THERAPY FOR SELECTED INFECTIOUS SYNDROMES IN PALLIATIVE CARE CANCER PATIENTS *(Continued)*

Disease	Antimicrobial therapy
Community-acquired pneumonia—neutropenic	*Preferred* 1. Levofloxacin
Hospital-acquired pneumonia	*Preferred* 1. Levofloxacin + linezolid
Suspected or known fungal pneumonia—neutropenic or high-dose steroids	*Preferred* 1. Voriconazole (preferred for all, except for mucormycosis) 2. Isavuconazole 3. Posaconazole
Urinary tract infection	*Preferred* 1. TMP–SMX[a] (if local resistance is <20%) 2. Ciprofloxacin, or levofloxacin (if local resistance is <20%) *Alternatives in lower UTI only* 1. Nitrofurantoin 2. Fosfomycin
Superficial skin and soft tissue infections—community-acquired and low MRSA prevalence	*Preferred* 1. Dicloxacillin 2. Cephalexin *Alternatives* 1. Doxycycline 2. TMP–SMX 3. Clindamycin
Superficial skin and soft tissue infections—community-acquired and high MRSA prevalence	*Preferred* 1. Linezolid *Alternatives* 1. TMP–SMX 2. Doxycycline 3. Clindamycin
Skin and soft tissue infections—neutropenic	*Preferred* 1. Ciprofloxacin + linezolid
Herpes simplex virus/herpes zoster	*Preferred* 1. Valaciclovir 2. Acyclovir 3. Famciclovir

These oral regimens are reasonable alternatives to the standard of care in palliative care cancer patients in whom comfort care is the main goal of therapy.

[a]Amox/clav: amoxicillin/clavulanate; TMP–SMX: trimethoprim–sulfamethoxazole.

[b]Linezolid should be considered when a catheter-related infection is suspected or when there are signs and symptoms of a skin and soft tissue infection or mucositis.

REFERENCES

1. Danai PA, Moss M, Mannino DM, Martin GS. The epidemiology of sepsis in patients with malignancy. *Chest.* 2006;129(6):1432-1440.
2. Thirumala R, Ramaswamy M, Chawla S. Diagnosis and management of infectious complications in critically ill patients with cancer. *Crit Care Clin.* 2010;26(1):59-91.
3. Wisplinghoff H, Seifert H, Wenzel RP, Edmond MB. Current trends in the epidemiology of nosocomial bloodstream infections in patients with hematological malignancies and solid neoplasms in hospitals in the United States. *Clin Infect Dis.* 2003;36(9):1103-1110.
4. Barker JN, Hough RE, van Burik JA, et al. Serious infections after unrelated donor transplantation in 136 children: impact of stem cell source. *Biol Blood Marrow Transplant.* 2005;11(5):362-370.
5. van Burik JA, Brunstein CG. Infectious complications following unrelated cord blood transplantation. *Vox Sang.* 2007;92(4):289-296.
6. Glenn J, Cotton D, Wesley R, Pizzo P. Anorectal infections in patients with malignant diseases. *Rev Infect Dis.* 1988;10(1):42-52.
7. Khardori N, Wong E, Carrasco CH, Wallace S, Patt Y, Bodey GP. Infections associated with biliary drainage procedures in patients with cancer. *Rev Infect Dis.* 1991;13(4):587-591.
8. Kalhs P, Kier P, Lechner K. Functional asplenia after bone marrow transplantation [letter]. *Ann Intern Med.* 1990;113(10):805-806.
9. Lehrnbecher T, Robinson P, Fisher B, et al. Guideline for the management of fever and neutropenia in children with cancer and hematopoietic stem-cell transplantation recipients: 2017 update. *J Clin Oncol.* 2017;35(18): 2082-2094.
10. Spielberet alger R, Stiff P, Bensinger W, et al. Palifermin for oral mucositis after intensive therapy for hematologic cancers. *N Engl J Med.* 2004;351(25):2590-2598.
11. Rosen LS, Abdi E, Davis ID, et al. Palifermin reduces the incidence of oral mucositis in patients with metastatic

colorectal cancer treated with fluorouracil-based chemotherapy. *J Clin Oncol.* 2006;24(33):5194-5200.

12. Vadhan-Raj S, Trent J, Patel S, et al. Single-dose palifermin prevents severe oral mucositis during multicycle chemotherapy in patients with cancer: a randomized trial. *Ann Intern Med.* 2010;153(6):358-367.

13. Milone G, Leotta S, Cupri A, et al. Palifermin reduces infection rate and hyperfibrinogenemia in patients treated with high-dose chemotherapy based on beam or BU-thiothepa. *Bone Marrow Transplant.* 2014;49(9): 1193-1197.

14. Tomblyn M, Chiller T, Einsele H, et al. Guidelines for preventing infectious complications among hematopoietic cell transplant recipients: a global perspective. Preface. *Bone Marrow Transplant.* 2009;44(8):453-455.

15. Fukuda T, Boeckh M, Carter RA, et al. Invasive fungal infections in recipients of allogeneic hematopoietic stem cell transplantation after nonmyeloablative conditioning: risks and outcomes. *Blood.* 2003;10:10.

16. Nichols WG, Corey L, Gooley T, Davis C, Boeckh M. High risk of death due to bacterial and fungal infection among cytomegalovirus (CMV)-seronegative recipients of stem cell transplants from seropositive donors: evidence for indirect effects of primary CMV infection. *J Infect Dis.* 2002;185(3):273-282.

17. Mackall CL, Gress RE. Pathways of T-cell regeneration in mice and humans: implications for bone marrow transplantation and immunotherapy. *Immunol Rev.* 1997;157:61-72.

18. Kulkarni S, Powles R, Treleaven J, et al. Chronic graft versus host disease is associated with long-term risk for pneumococcal infections in recipients of bone marrow transplants. *Blood.* 2000;95:3683-3686.

19. Lionakis MS, Kontoyiannis DP. Glucocorticoids and invasive fungal infections. *Lancet.* 2003;362(9398): 1828-1838.

20. Gea-Banacloche JC, Opal SM, Jorgensen J, Carcillo JA, Sepkowitz KA, Cordonnier C. Sepsis associated with immunosuppressive medications: an evidence-based review. *Crit Care Med.* 2004;32(11 suppl):S578-S590.

21. Bock SN, Lee RE, Fisher B, et al. A prospective randomized trial evaluating prophylactic antibiotics to prevent triple-lumen catheter-related sepsis in patients treated with immunotherapy. *J Clin Oncol.* 1990;8(1):161-169.

22. Martin SI, Marty FM, Fiumara K, Treon SP, Gribben JG, Baden LR. Infectious complications associated with alemtuzumab use for lymphoproliferative disorders. *Clin Infect Dis.* 2006;43(1):16-24.

23. Vidal L, Gafter-Gvili A, Leibovici L, Shpilberg O. Rituximab as maintenance therapy for patients with follicular lymphoma. *Cochrane Database Syst Rev.* 2009;(2): CD006552.

24. Gea-Banacloche JC. Rituximab-associated infections. *Semin Hematol.* 2010;47(2):187-198.

25. Pei SN, Chen CH, Lee CM, et al. Reactivation of hepatitis B virus following rituximab-based regimens: a serious complication in both HBsAg-positive and HBsAg-negative patients. *Ann Hematol.* 2009;89(3):255-262.

26. Yeo W, Chan TC, Leung NW, et al. Hepatitis B virus reactivation in lymphoma patients with prior resolved hepatitis B undergoing anticancer therapy with or without rituximab. *J Clin Oncol.* 2009;27(4):605-611.

27. Carson KR, Evens AM, Richey EA, et al. Progressive multifocal leukoencephalopathy after rituximab therapy in HIV-negative patients: a report of 57 cases from the Research on Adverse Drug Events and Reports Project. *Blood.* 2009;113(20):4834-4840.

28. Lussana F, Cattaneo M, Rambaldi A, Squizzato A. Ruxolitinib-associated infections: a systematic review and meta-analysis. *Am J Hematol.* 2018;93(3):339-347.

29. Couriel D, Saliba R, Hicks K, et al. Tumor necrosis factor-alpha blockade for the treatment of acute GVHD. *Blood.* 2004;104(3):649-654.

30. Lee DW, Gardner R, Porter DL, et al. How I treat: current concepts in the diagnosis and management of cytokine release syndrome. *Blood.* 2014;124(2):188-195.

31. Pawar A, Desai RJ, Solomon DH, et al. Risk of serious infections in tocilizumab versus other biologic drugs in patients with rheumatoid arthritis: a multidatabase cohort study. *Ann Rheum Dis.* 2019;78(4):456-464.

32. Homsi J, Walsh D, Panta R, Lagman R, Nelson KA, Longworth DL. Infectious complications of advanced cancer. *Support Care Cancer.* 2000;8(6):487-492.

33. Bauduer F, Capdupuy C, Renoux M. Characteristics of deaths in a department of oncohaematology within a general hospital. A study of 81 cases. *Support Care Cancer.* 2000;8(4):302-306.

34. Ahronheim JC, Morrison RS, Baskin SA, Morris J, Meier DE. Treatment of the dying in the acute care hospital. Advanced dementia and metastatic cancer. *Arch Intern Med.* 1996;156(18):2094-2100.

35. Nagy-Agren S, Haley H. Management of infections in palliative care patients with advanced cancer. *J Pain Symptom Manage.* 2002;24(1):64-70.

36. Pereira J, Watanabe S, Wolch G. A retrospective review of the frequency of infections and patterns of antibiotic utilization on a palliative care unit. *J Pain Symptom Manage.* 1998;16(6):374-381.

37. Girmenia C, Moleti ML, Cartoni C, et al. Management of infective complications in patients with advanced hematologic malignancies in home care. *Leukemia.* 1997;11(11):1807-1812.

38. Vitetta L, Kenner D, Sali A. Bacterial infections in terminally ill hospice patients. *J Pain Symptom Manage.* 2000;20(5):326-334.

39. Lawlor PG, Gagnon B, Mancini IL, et al. Occurrence, causes, and outcome of delirium in patients with advanced cancer: a prospective study. *Arch Intern Med.* 2000;160(6):786-794.

40. Oh DY, Kim JH, Kim DW, et al. Antibiotic use during the last days of life in cancer patients. *Eur J Cancer Care (Engl).* 2006;15(1):74-79.

41. Stiel S, Krumm N, Pestinger M, et al. Antibiotics in palliative medicine—results from a prospective epidemiological investigation from the HOPE survey. *Support Care Cancer.* 2012;20(2):325-333.

42. Enck RE. Antibiotic use in end-of-life care: a soft line? *Am J Hosp Palliat Care.* 2012;20(2):325-333.

43. Chun ED, Rodgers PE, Vitale CA, Collins CD, Malani PN. Antimicrobial use among patients receiving palliative care consultation. *Am J Hosp Palliat Care.* 2010;27(4): 261-265.

44. Macedo F, Nunes C, Ladeira K, et al. Antimicrobial therapy in palliative care: an overview. *Support Care Cancer.* 2018;26(5):1361-1367.

45. High KP, Bradley SF, Gravenstein S, et al. Clinical practice guideline for the evaluation of fever and infection in older adult residents of long-term care facilities: 2008 update by the Infectious Diseases Society of America. *Clin Infect Dis.* 2009;48(2):149-171.

46. Hooton TM, Bradley SF, Cardenas DD, et al. Diagnosis, prevention, and treatment of catheter-associated urinary tract infection in adults: 2009 International Clinical Practice Guidelines from the Infectious Diseases Society of America. *Clin Infect Dis.* 2010;50(5):625-663.

47. Klastersky J, Paesmans M, Rubenstein EB, et al. The Multinational Association for Supportive Care in Cancer risk index: a multinational scoring system for identifying low-risk febrile neutropenic cancer patients. *J Clin Oncol.* 2000;18(16):3038-3051.

48. Klastersky J, Paesmans M, Georgala A, et al. Outpatient oral antibiotics for febrile neutropenic cancer patients using a score predictive for complications. *J Clin Oncol.* 2006;24(25):4129-4134.

49. Freifeld A, Marchigiani D, Walsh T, et al. A double-blind comparison of empirical oral and intravenous antibiotic therapy for low-risk febrile patients with neutropenia during cancer chemotherapy. *N Engl J Med.* 1999;341(5):305-311.

50. Bow EJ. Fluoroquinolones, antimicrobial resistance and neutropenic cancer patients. *Curr Opin Infect Dis.* 2011;24(6):545-553.

51. Greene JN. Catheter-related complications of cancer therapy. *Infect Dis Clin North Am.* 1996;10(2):255-295.

52. Raad I, Hanna HA, Alakech B, Chatzinikolaou I, Johnson MM, Tarrand J. Differential time to positivity: a useful method for diagnosing catheter-related bloodstream infections. *Ann Intern Med.* 2004;140(1):18-25.

53. Manian FA. IDSA guidelines for the diagnosis and management of intravascular catheter-related bloodstream infection. *Clin Infect Dis.* 2009;49(11):1770-1771; author reply 1771-1772.

54. Garcia R, Raad I, Abi-Said D, et al. Nosocomial respiratory syncytial virus infections: prevention and control in bone marrow transplant patients. *Infect Control Hosp Epidemiol.* 1997;18(6):412-416.

55. Martino R, Porras RP, Rabella N, et al. Prospective study of the incidence, clinical features, and outcome of symptomatic upper and lower respiratory tract infections by respiratory viruses in adult recipients of hematopoietic stem cell transplants for hematologic malignancies. *Biol Blood Marrow Transplant.* 2005;11:781-796.

56. Walmsley S, Devi S, King S, Schneider R, Richardson S, Ford-Jones L. Invasive *Aspergillus* infections in a pediatric hospital: a ten-year review. *Pediatr Infect Dis J.* 1993;12(8):673-682.

57. Maschmeyer G, Calandra T, Singh N, Wiley J, Perfect J. Invasive mould infections: a multi-disciplinary update. *Med Mycol.* 2009;47(6):571-583.

58. De Pauw B, Walsh TJ, Donnelly JP, et al. Revised definitions of invasive fungal disease from the European Organization for Research and Treatment of Cancer/Invasive Fungal Infections Cooperative Group and the National Institute of Allergy and Infectious Diseases Mycoses Study Group (EORTC/MSG) Consensus Group. *Clin Infect Dis.* 2008;46(12):1813-1821.

59. Metlay JP, Waterer GW, Long AC, et al. Diagnosis and treatment of adults with community-acquired pneumonia. An official clinical practice guideline of the American Thoracic Society and Infectious Diseases Society of America. *Am J Respir Crit Care Med.* 2019;200(7):e45-e67.

60. Dangerfield B, Chung A, Webb B, Seville MT. Predictive value of methicillin-resistant *Staphylococcus aureus* (MRSA) nasal swab PCR assay for MRSA pneumonia. *Antimicrob Agents Chemother.* 2014;58(2):859-864.

61. Casper C, Englund J, Boeckh M. How I treat influenza in patients with hematologic malignancies. *Blood.* 2010;115(7):1331-1342.

62. Chemaly RF, Ghosh S, Bodey GP, et al. Respiratory viral infections in adults with hematologic malignancies and human stem cell transplantation recipients: a retrospective study at a major cancer center. *Medicine (Baltimore).* 2006;85(5):278-287.

63. Kalil AC, Metersky ML, Klompas M, et al. Management of adults with hospital-acquired and ventilator-associated pneumonia: 2016 clinical practice guidelines by the Infectious Diseases Society of America and the American Thoracic Society. *Clin Infect Dis.* 2016;63(5):e61-e111.

64. Ewig S. Nosocomial pneumonia: de-escalation is what matters. *Lancet Infect Dis.* 2011;11(3):155-157.

65. Evans SE, Ost DE. Pneumonia in the neutropenic cancer patient. *Curr Opin Pulm Med.* 2015;21(3):260-271.

66. Gea-Banacloche J. Pulmonary infectious complications after hematopoietic stem cell transplantation: a practical guide to clinicians. *Curr Opin Organ Transplant.* 2018;23(4):375-380.

67. Segal BH, Freifeld AG, Baden LR, et al. Prevention and treatment of cancer-related infections. *J Natl Compr Canc Netw.* 2008;6(2):122-174.

68. Symeonidis N, Jakubowski A, Pierre-Louis S, et al. Invasive adenoviral infections in T-cell-depleted allogeneic hematopoietic stem cell transplantation: high mortality in the era of cidofovir. *Transpl Infect Dis.* 2007;9(2):108-113.

69. Clark BD, Vezza PR, Copeland C, Wilder AM, Abati A. Diagnostic sensitivity of bronchoalveolar lavage versus lung fine needle aspirate. *Mod Pathol.* 2002;15(12):1259-1265.

70. Sherif R, Segal BH. Pulmonary aspergillosis: clinical presentation, diagnostic tests, management and complications. *Curr Opin Pulm Med.* 2010;16(3):242-250.

71. Meersseman W, Lagrou K, Maertens J, et al. Galactomannan in bronchoalveolar lavage fluid: a tool for diagnosing aspergillosis in intensive care unit patients. *Am J Respir Crit Care Med.* 2008;177(1):27-34.

72. Alanio A, Hauser PM, Lagrou K, et al.; 5th European Conference on Infections in Leukemia (ECIL-5), a joint venture of The European Group for Blood and Marrow Transplantation (EBMT), The European Organization for Research and Treatment of Cancer (EORTC), the Immunocompromised Host Society (ICHS) and The European LeukemiaNet (ELN). ECIL guidelines for the diagnosis of *Pneumocystis jirovecii* pneumonia in patients with haematological malignancies and stem cell transplant recipients. *J Antimicrob Chemother.* 2016;71(9):2386-2396.

73. Almyroudis NG, Segal BH. Antifungal prophylaxis and therapy in patients with hematological malignancies and hematopoietic stem cell transplant recipients. *Expert Rev Anti Infect Ther.* 2010;8(12):1451-1466.

74. Almyroudis NG, Segal BH. Prevention and treatment of invasive fungal diseases in neutropenic patients. *Curr Opin Infect Dis.* 2009;22(4):385-393.

75. Kouroussis C, Samonis G, Androulakis N, et al. Successful conservative treatment of neutropenic enterocolitis complicating taxane-based chemotherapy: a report of five cases. *Am J Clin Oncol.* 2000;23(3):309-313.

76. Ibrahim NK, Sahin AA, Dubrow RA, et al. Colitis associated with docetaxel-based chemotherapy in patients with metastatic breast cancer. *Lancet.* 2000;355(9200):281-283.

77. Kirkpatrick ID, Greenberg HM. Gastrointestinal complications in the neutropenic patient: characterization and differentiation with abdominal CT. *Radiology.* 2003;226(3):668-674.

78. Shamberger RC, Weinstein HJ, Delorey MJ, Levey RH. The medical and surgical management of typhlitis in children with acute nonlymphocytic (myelogenous) leukemia. *Cancer.* 1986;57(3):603-609.

79. Debast SB, Bauer MP, Kuijper EJ; European Society of Clinical Microbiology and Infectious Diseases. European Society of Clinical Microbiology and Infectious Diseases: update of the treatment guidance document for *Clostridium difficile* infection. *Clin Microbiol Infect.* 2014;20(suppl 2):1-26.

80. McDonald LC, Gerding DN, Johnson S, et al. Clinical practice guidelines for *Clostridium difficile* infection

in adults and children: 2017 update by the Infectious Diseases Society of America (IDSA) and Society for Healthcare Epidemiology of America (SHEA). *Clin Infect Dis.* 2018;66(7):987-994.

81. Zar FA, Bakkanagari SR, Moorthi KM, Davis MB. A comparison of vancomycin and metronidazole for the treatment of *Clostridium difficile*-associated diarrhea, stratified by disease severity. *Clin Infect Dis.* 2007;45(3): 302-307.

82. Mullane KM, Miller MA, Weiss K, et al. Efficacy of fidaxomicin versus vancomycin as therapy for *Clostridium difficile* infection in individuals taking concomitant antibiotics for other concurrent infections. *Clin Infect Dis.* 2011;53(5):440-447.

83. Herpers BL, Vlaminckx B, Burkhardt O, et al. Intravenous tigecycline as adjunctive or alternative therapy for severe refractory *Clostridium difficile* infection. *Clin Infect Dis.* 2009;48(12):1732-1735.

84. Musher DM, Logan N, Hamill RJ, et al. Nitazoxanide for the treatment of *Clostridium difficile* colitis. *Clin Infect Dis.* 2006;43:421-427.

85. Bartlett JG. Narrative review: the new epidemic of *Clostridium difficile*-associated enteric disease. *Ann Intern Med.* 2006;145(10):758-764.

86. Lowy I, Molrine DC, Leav BA, et al. Treatment with monoclonal antibodies against *Clostridium difficile* toxins. *N Engl J Med.* 2010;362(3):197-205.

87. Brown CC, Manis MM, Bohm NM, Curry SR. Oral vancomycin for secondary prophylaxis of *Clostridium difficile* infection. *Ann Pharmacother.* 2019;53(4): 396-401.

88. Lehrnbecher T, Marshall D, Gao C, Chanock SJ. A second look at anorectal infections in cancer patients in a large cancer institute: the success of early intervention with antibiotics and surgery. *Infection.* 2002;30(5): 272-276.

89. Barnes SG, Sattler FR, Ballard JO. Perirectal infections in acute leukemia. Improved survival after incision and debridement. *Ann Intern Med.* 1984;100(4):515-518.

90. Talan DA, Krishnadasan A, Abrahamian FM, Stamm WE, Moran GJ. Prevalence and risk factor analysis of trimethoprim–sulfamethoxazole- and fluoroquinolone-resistant *Escherichia coli* infection among emergency department patients with pyelonephritis. *Clin Infect Dis.* 2008;47(9):1150-1158.

91. Raz R, Schiller D, Nicolle LE. Chronic indwelling catheter replacement before antimicrobial therapy for symptomatic urinary tract infection. *J Urol.* 2000;164(4):1254-1258.

92. Pappas PG, Kauffman CA, Andes D, et al. Clinical practice guidelines for the management of candidiasis: 2009 update by the Infectious Diseases Society of America. *Clin Infect Dis.* 2009;48(5):503-535.

93. Stevens DL, Bisno AL, Chambers HF, et al. Practice guidelines for the diagnosis and management of skin and soft-tissue infections. *Clin Infect Dis.* 2005;41(10):1373-1406.

94. Strazzula L, Cotliar J, Fox LP, et al. Inpatient dermatology consultation aids diagnosis of cellulitis among hospitalized patients: a multi-institutional analysis. *J Am Acad Dermatol.* 2015;73(1):70-75.

95. Anaya DA, Dellinger EP. Necrotizing soft-tissue infection: diagnosis and management. *Clin Infect Dis.* 2007;44(5):705-710.

96. Person AK, Kontoyiannis DP, Alexander BD. Fungal infections in transplant and oncology patients. *Infect Dis Clin North Am.* 2010;24(2):439-459.

97. Nucci M, Anaissie E. Fungal infections in hematopoietic stem cell transplantation and solid-organ transplantation—focus on aspergillosis. *Clin Chest Med.* 2009;30(2):295-306, vii.

98. Meyers JD, Reed EC, Shepp DH, et al. Acyclovir for prevention of cytomegalovirus infection and disease after allogeneic marrow transplantation. *N Engl J Med.* 1988;318(2):70-75.

99. Saral R, Ambinder RF, Burns WH, et al. Acyclovir prophylaxis against herpes simplex virus infection in patients with leukemia. A randomized, double-blind, placebo-controlled study. *Ann Intern Med.* 1983;99(6): 773-776.

100. Boeckh M, Kim HW, Flowers ME, Meyers JD, Bowden RA. Long-term acyclovir for prevention of varicella zoster virus disease after allogeneic hematopoietic cell transplantation—a randomized double-blind placebo-controlled study. *Blood.* 2006;107(5):1800-1805.

101. Wu Y-C, Chen C-S, Chan Y-J. The outbreak of COVID-19: an overview. *J Chin Med Assoc.* 2020;83:217-220.

102. Wiersinga WJ, Rhodes A, Cheng AC, Peacock SJ, Prescott HC. Pathophysiology, transmission, diagnosis, and treatment of coronavirus disease 2019 (COVID-19): a review. *JAMA.* 2020. doi:10.1001/jama.2020.12839.

103. Gupta A, Madhavan MV, Sehgal K, et al. Extrapulmonary manifestations of COVID-19. *Nat Med.* 2020;26:1017-1032. doi:10.1038/s41591-020-0968-3.

104. Lauer SA, Grantz KH, Bi Q, et al. The incubation period of coronavirus disease 2019 (COVID-19) from publicly reported confirmed cases: estimation and application. *Ann Intern Med.* 2020;172:577-582. doi:10.7326/M20-0504.

105. Byambasuren O, Cardona M, Bell K, Clark J, McLaws M-L, Glasziou P. Estimating the extent of asymptomatic COVID-19 and its potential for community transmission: systematic review and meta-analysis. *medRxiv.* 2020. doi:10.1101/2020.05.10.20097543.

106. Robinson AG, Gyawali B, Evans G. COVID-19 and cancer: do we really know what we think we know? *Nat Rev Clin Oncol.* 2020;17:386-388.

107. Zhang L, Zhu F, Xie L, et al. Clinical characteristics of COVID-19-infected cancer patients: a retrospective case study in three hospitals within Wuhan, China. *Ann Oncol.* 2020;31:894-901.

108. Lee LYW, Cazier JB, Starkey T, et al.; UK Coronavirus Cancer Monitoring Project Team. COVID-19 mortality in patients with cancer on chemotherapy or other anticancer treatments: a prospective cohort study. *Lancet.* 2020;395:1919-1926.

109. Poortmans PM, Guarneri V, Cardoso M-J. Cancer and COVID-19: what do we really know? *Lancet.* 2020;395(10241):1884-1885.

110. Morawska L, Milton DK. It is time to address airborne transmission of COVID-19. *Clin Infect Dis.* 2020;ciaa939. doi:10.1093/cid/ciaa939.

111. Beigel JH, Tomashek KM, Dodd LE, et al. Remdesivir for the treatment of Covid-19—preliminary report. *N Engl J Med.* 2020. doi:10.1056/NEJMoa2007764.

112. RECOVERY Collaborative Group; Horby P, Lim WS, et al. Dexamethasone in hospitalized patients with Covid-19—preliminary report. *N Engl J Med.* 2020. doi:10.1056/NEJMoa2021436.

113. Lurie N, Saville M, Hatchett R, Halton J. Developing Covid-19 vaccines at pandemic speed. *N Engl J Med.* 2020;382:1969-1973.

114. Heaton PM. The Covid-19 vaccine-development multiverse. *N Engl J Med.* 2020. doi:10.1056/NEJMe2025111.

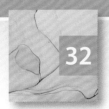

32 Management of Intracranial Metastases

Karine A. Al Feghali and Caroline Chung

INTRODUCTION

Brain metastases are the most common brain tumors in cancer patients. The incidence has been reported to range from 10% to 40% in all cancer patients and as high as 80% in patients with metastatic disease. Primary cancers that most commonly metastasize to the brain include lung cancer, breast cancer, renal cancer, colorectal cancer, and melanoma (1–4).

As advances in systemic therapies and in radiation therapy techniques continue to improve locoregional and extracranial disease control, brain metastases are having an increasing contribution to a patient's morbidity and mortality, particularly in patients who present with well-controlled systemic disease. One example is the impact of trastuzumab on HER-2 positive breast cancer patients, which has prolonged the control of extracranial disease and altered the natural progression of disease with increasing brain metastatic involvement (5). Other examples include the use of targeted therapies in EGFR-mutated or *ALK*-rearranged non–small cell lung cancer (6,7) and the use of immunotherapy such as nivolumab and ipilimumab for melanoma brain metastases (8,9).

Advances in the management of brain metastases include improvements in surgical techniques and radiotherapy delivery as well as new discoveries of systemic therapies that have effect intracranially. As a result, patients are living longer following a diagnosis of brain metastases such that the detriment of toxicity and potentially iatrogenic morbidity has become a growing concern, as patients may live much longer with deterioration in neurocognitive function and/or impairment of functional independence (10,11). Hence, it is now more important than ever to determine the appropriate goals of treatment for the individual patient before weighing the benefits and costs of the proposed treatment regimen. Largely, the goals of treatment will reflect the patient's expected overall prognosis, and there is a growing body of research aimed at improving our ability to estimate prognosis based on both patient and tumor factors.

Furthermore, with increasing use of more sensitive imaging modalities such as magnetic resonance imaging (MRI), patients are presenting with smaller, fewer and often asymptomatic brain metastases (12). There is also growing literature on the role of curative local treatment in oligometastatic disease, and it was shown to be associated with a significant progression-free survival and overall survival benefit as compared to maintenance therapy or observation (13–15). Therefore, the goals of management for patients with brain metastases have broadened to address the greater variation in goals of therapy based on the clinical presentation and overall situation at the time of brain metastasis diagnosis.

CLINICAL PRESENTATION

Historically, patients have presented with signs and symptoms of increased intracranial pressure (ICP), seizures, and/or focal neurologic symptoms due to both tumor and peritumoral edema. The specific neurological deficits are dependent on the location and size of the metastases and the extent of peritumoral edema. These can include generalized fatigue, headache, cognitive deficits and personality changes, motor or sensory deficits, balance disturbance, speech difficulties, or seizures (16–18). With increasing use of MRI, which has a higher sensitivity for the detection of brain metastases, a greater proportion of patients are presenting with radiologically detected, asymptomatic, small brain metastases (19,20). Both the presence of symptoms and the number of lesions may impact management decisions and patient outcome.

In 20% of cases, a brain metastasis is the initial presentation of malignancy with or without a known primary cancer (21). A *solitary brain metastasis* is the presence of one brain metastasis with no other sites of active metastatic disease, whereas a *single brain metastasis* is the presence of one brain metastasis with other active metastatic disease. Particularly in the setting of solitary-enhancing brain lesions, the differential diagnosis should be considered and investigations should include a metastatic workup with an aim to confirm a histologic diagnosis. If a primary malignancy cannot be found, surgical resection or biopsy of the brain lesion may be required to confirm histology.

PROGNOSIS

The prognosis of patients with brain metastases is improving. This may reflect detection of earlier, lower bulk disease in patients with better performance status at the time of diagnosis, improving systemic therapy to control intracranial and extracranial disease and more aggressive interventions to achieve durable control of brain metastases. Table 32.1 summarizes the range of reported overall survival rates following the different treatment for brain metastases. These differences in overall survival likely reflect the differences in treatment selection based on patients' prognostic factors such as disease extent and performance status. For instance, a patient with a single metastasis and well-controlled extracranial disease would likely receive more aggressive treatment than a patient with active systemic disease and multiple brain metastases.

A number of prognostic indices have been developed to help guide the appropriate goals of management and suitable care for patients with brain metastases. A key component included in most prognostic indices developed for patients with brain metastases is the Karnofsky performance status (KPS), which has been established as a reliable and valid measurement scale to guide appropriate treatment selection as well as measure treatment response in patients with brain tumors (26). KPS, however, is not specific for patients with brain metastases.

The first prognostic index specifically created for patients with brain metastases was generated from a recursive partitioning analysis (RPA) of data from 1,200 patients treated with whole brain radiotherapy (WBRT) in three randomized controlled trials of the Radiation Therapy Oncology Group (RTOG). The RPA classification system grouped patients into three prognostic classes based on patient age, status of primary tumor

TABLE 32.1 SUMMARY OF OUTCOMES FOLLOWING BRAIN METASTASIS TREATMENT (22–25)

Treatment	Overall survival (months)
Steroids alone	1
WBRT	3–6
WBRT + surgery (single metastasis)	10–15
WBRT + radiosurgery (1–4 metastases)	6–12

WBRT, whole brain radiotherapy.

control, and extent of extracranial disease (27,28). Several prognostic indices have been developed since the RPA, which incorporate various combinations of other factors including the extent of intracranial disease and the number of metastases (Table 32.2) (29–31). Despite the addition of more factors, these alternative prognostic indices do not appear to perform any better than the RPA classification in estimating the prognosis of cancer patients when tumor histology is not considered. More recently, the graded prognostic index was applied to patients with particular tumor histologies to develop a disease-specific graded prognostic assessment (DS-GPA). Retrospective multi-institutional analysis of 4,259 patients with brain metastasis, with incorporation of primary tumor histology, appeared to improve the accuracy of predicting patient prognosis beyond any of the prior prognostic indices (32). Emerging evidence suggests that the DS-GPA may best reflect prognosis in patients with brain metastases, and it has been validated in certain populations of patients with brain metastases (33–35).

In addition to the factors at presentation, other measures that reflect the pace of the disease and/

TABLE 32.2 PROGNOSTIC INDICES FOR BRAIN METASTASIS (29–31)

Prognostic index	Age	KPS	Extracranial disease status	Primary tumor control	Volume of largest metastases	Number of metastases
Golden grading system	◆	◆	◆			
Basic score for brain metastases (BS-BM)		◆	◆	◆		
Score index for radiosurgery (SIR)	◆	◆		◆	◆	◆
Graded prognostic assessment (GPA)[a]	◆	◆	◆			◆

[a]Disease-specific graded prognostic assessment, incorporating tumor histology with these prognostic factors, is currently the strongest prognostic index available (32).
KPS, Karnofsky performance status.

or response of the brain metastases to treatment over time have recently been developed as prognostic tools. Examples are brain metastasis velocity (BMV), which is the rate of development of new brain metastases (BM) after initial stereotactic radiosurgery (SRS), and initial brain metastasis velocity (iBMV) that is calculated by dividing the cumulative number of brain metastases at the time of SRS by time (years) since the initial primary cancer diagnosis (36–38). Lower BMV was shown to be associated with better overall survival, less neurologic death, and decreased rates of salvage WBRT after initial distant brain failure after SRS alone (38), and lower iBMV has been associated with better overall survival (36,37).

MANAGEMENT

Currently, the management of brain metastases may range from supportive care up to aggressive multimodal treatment with the aim of improving intracranial tumor control. The treatments that are currently used include surgery, radiosurgery, whole brain radiation, and supportive care. There are several aims for treating brain metastases, and these should reflect a patient's performance status, overall disease burden and activity, and most importantly, the patient's goals of care. In patients with limited disease burden or oligometastatic disease, the aim of the treatment may be to achieve durable intracranial tumor control or even cure utilizing a combined modality approach with surgery or radiosurgery and fractionated radiotherapy.

More recently, advances in genetic characterization of brain metastases have paved the way to new therapeutic avenues. Actionable mutations have been identified in brain metastases, which are sometimes distinct from the mutations harbored by the primary tumor (39,40). Targeted agents and immunotherapy are revolutionizing the management of brain metastases of particular tumor histologies. Tyrosine kinase inhibitors (TKIs), such as some of the *ALK*-TKIs, EGFR-TKIs, and HER2-TKIs, and other agents, such as BRAF inhibitors, have been shown to have good activity against brain metastases (41,42). Immunotherapy has shown promising change in the brain metastasis treatment landscape in recent years. Although the brain was traditionally thought of as an immune-privileged site, studies have suggested that the brain was in fact not immunologically quiescent (43). Brain metastases have been shown to contain tumor-infiltrating lymphocytes and to live in an inflammatory environment (44–46). Patients with untreated brain metastases had historically been excluded from trials exploring novel agents; however, this has recently changed and a number of clinical trials are studying the intracranial activity of different immunotherapy agents (47). Melanoma brain metastases in particular have been shown to express programmed death 1 (PD-1) and programmed death ligand 1 (PD-L1) (44). Immune checkpoint inhibitors, anticytotoxic T-lymphocyte antigen 4 (CTLA-4), and anti-PD-1 have been demonstrated to have good intracranial activity (48,49). In two recent phase II studies, the combination of ipilimumab (anti-CTLA-4) and nivolumab (anti-PD-1) had clinically meaningful intracranial activity in melanoma brain metastases, with rates of intracranial clinical benefit of 46% to 57% and intracranial complete response rates of 16% to 26% (8,50). The combination of radiation therapy and immunotherapy has also been investigated in patients with brain metastases from NSCLC, melanoma, and renal cell carcinoma with promising results (51,52), but prospective evaluation with randomized controlled trials is needed.

Surgery

Surgery has several therapeutic advantages over radiotherapy, including immediate relief of mass effect and reduced corticosteroid requirement following resection. Figure 32.1 demonstrates an example of a cerebellar metastasis that was effectively managed with surgery and postoperative radiosurgery. Additionally, surgical resection can provide histologic confirmation, particularly when the etiology of the detected brain lesion is unclear. However, surgical resection is an invasive treatment that is associated with risk of a number of potential complications, including infection, hemorrhage, thromboembolic events, and possible deterioration in neurologic function depending on the location of the tumor(s).

When surgery is used in combination with WBRT, local control and intracranial tumor control can be improved. In patients with good performance status and a single brain metastasis, this combination treatment can result in improved overall survival and greater functional independence compared with WBRT alone. Patchell et al. reported the seminal randomized controlled trial in 1990 comparing WBRT with surgical resection and WBRT alone for patients with a single brain metastasis, which demonstrated an overall survival advantage in the combined surgery and WBRT arm with a median survival of 40 weeks compared with 15 weeks for WBRT alone. In addition, the combination treatment resulted in greater functional independence of 38 weeks versus 8 weeks for the WBRT arm ($p < 0.005$) (22). A subsequent randomized study validated

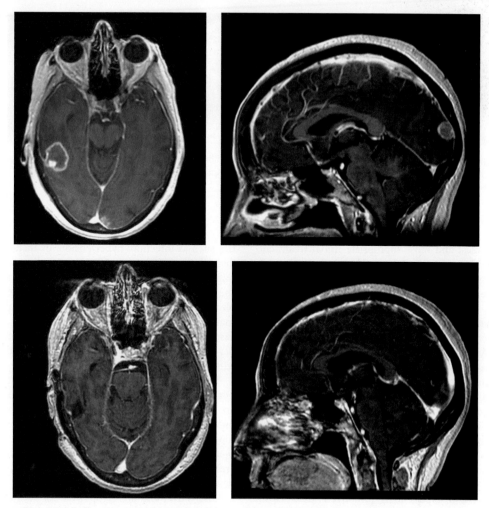

Figure 32.1 Axial (*left*) and coronal (*right*) gadolinium-enhanced T$_1$-weighted magnetic resonance images demonstrating large cystic cerebellar brain metastases (*top panel*). The *bottom panel* shows a good surgical resection with resolution of the mass effect and no evidence of recurrence 1 year after surgery and stereotactic radiotherapy to the surgical cavity.

the improvement in median overall survival with combined surgery and WBRT compared with WBRT alone, 10 months versus 6 months (53). In an attempt to minimize the treatment-related toxicity of WBRT, a multi-institutional random-ized trial of adjuvant WBRT versus stereotactic radiosurgery (NCCTG N107C/CEC.3) was per-formed, demonstrating better intracranial con-trol with postoperative WBRT, at the expense of a greater cognitive decline associated with WBRT, that persisted at the 12-month follow-up visit (54). Another trial randomized patients who had com-plete resection of one to three brain metastases to either SRS of the resection cavity (within 30 days of surgery) or observation. Two-month freedom from local recurrence was 43% in the observation group versus 72% in the SRS group (hazard ratio 0·46, $p = 0.015$) (55).

Whole Brain Radiotherapy

Whole brain radiotherapy (WBRT) has long been considered the standard of care for patients with brain metastases, either postoperatively, or as the sole treatment, especially in the setting of multiple brain metastases or leptomeningeal disease. It is an effective treatment that can provide rapid pallia-tion and tumor response in many cases. Historical studies report survival of 3 to 6 months following WBRT; however, this survival was not cause spe-cific to brain metastases (23).

Standard WBRT is typically delivered in 5 to 10 treatments to a total dose of 20 to 30 Gy with two opposed-lateral treatment fields that encom-pass the entire brain (Fig. 32.2). Alternative dos-ing schedules and higher doses of radiation have failed to show substantial benefit in patient out-come (56). Although WBRT was long considered

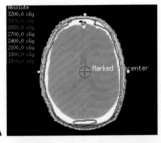
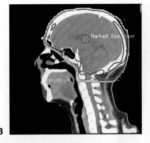
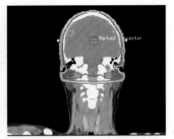

A   **B**   **C**

Figure 32.2 Example of a whole brain radiation therapy plan with a dose prescription of 30 Gray in 10 fractions. The three panels below represent cuts from the simulation computed tomography (CT) scans with isodose lines—transverse **(A)**, sagittal **(B)**, and coronal **(C)** views.

the safest and most appropriate initial treatment when lesions are not amenable to a local therapy (surgery or radiosurgery), its role in palliation for patients who are not candidate for surgical resection or radiosurgery has been challenged in the recent British QUARTZ trial, as optimal supportive care proved to be noninferior (57).

Although effective, WBRT is associated with a number of acute toxicities, including alopecia, dermatitis, headaches, nausea, otitis externa, and otitis media, as well as short-term memory and cognitive deficits (14). Despite the associated toxicities, WBRT remains the most appropriate treatment in some patients, including those with multiple diffuse brain metastases and/or leptomeningeal metastases.

As patients with brain metastases are survival longer and experiencing prolonged toxicities of WBRT, decline in neurocognitive function following WBRT has been a particular focus of research and clinical trials. A number of factors can contribute to neurocognitive decline in patients with cancer, including intracranial tumor progression, toxicity from systemic therapy, narcotic pain medications, and patient's age and existing comorbidi-

ties such as infection, hypertension, or metabolic disturbances (58–61). Genetic predisposition might also play a role in the development of neurocognitive toxicity following WBRT. For example, carrying the APOE e4 allele, the same allele that confers an increased risk to Alzheimer's disease, was shown to be a risk factor for worse memory function after treatment with WBRT (with or without memantine) (62).

Based on the hypothesis that irradiation of bilateral hippocampal regions may have the greatest impact on memory deficit (15), new treatment approaches that help avoid irradiation of the hippocampal regions have recently been investigated. This is to limit the radiation dose delivered to the neural stem cells in the hippocampal dentate gyrus, which are mitotically active and radiosensitive, and are responsible for formation of new memories (63–65). Hippocampal avoidance whole brain radiation therapy (HA-WBRT) uses conformal radiotherapy techniques including intensity-modulated radiotherapy (IMRT) or volumetric-modulated arc therapy (VMAT) to bilateral hippocampi (Fig. 32.3). This technique was tested in the phase II cooperative trial RTOG

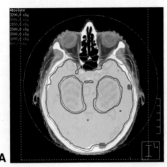
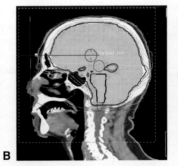
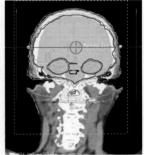

A   **B**   **C**

Figure 32.3 Example of a hippocampal avoidance whole brain radiation therapy plan using intensity-modulated radiation therapy—transverse **(A)**, sagittal **(B)**, and coronal **(C)** views.

0933, which showed significant memory preservation with hippocampal avoidance cranial irradiation, whereby relative decline in Hopkins Verbal Learning Test—Revised Delayed Recall (HVLT-R DR) at 4 months was 7% in the experimental arm, which was significantly lower than the 30% relative decline in HVLT-R DR in the prespecified historical control of patients with brain metastases treated without hippocampal avoidance (66). The promising findings of RTOG0933 motivated the trial NRG-CC001, which randomized patients with brain metastases to HA-WBRT + memantine versus conventional WBRT + memantine (67). The primary endpoint of this study was neurocognitive function failure, defined as decline using the reliable change index on HVLT-R DR, Trail Making Test, or Controlled Oral Word Association. Recently reported results demonstrated lower neurocognitive function failure risk with HA-WBRT + memantine arm as compared to conventional WBRT + memantine (hazard ratio = 0.74, p = 0.02). Age ≤61 was an independent predictor of lower neurocognitive function failure risk. There was no difference in overall survival, intracranial progression, or toxicity (67).

Another effective radiation strategy to limit radiation dose to the hippocampi is to avoid WBRT altogether and treat the known metastases using more focal radiation treatment such as stereotactic radiosurgery.

Radiosurgery

Stereotactic radiosurgery (SRS) is the delivery of a single (or very few) highly accurate treatment(s) with an ablative dose of radiation focused on a radiographically distinct target (Fig. 32.4).

Currently, radiosurgery treatment can be delivered using a linear accelerator (Linac), a CyberKnife, or Gamma Knife (68). A recent phase III trial comparing Gamma Knife and Linac-based SRS in 168 patients with 292 brain metastases revealed comparable local control and overall survival rates between these two approaches, with greater and earlier occurrences of radionecrosis in patients treated with Gamma Knife. Radiosurgery has therapeutic advantages over surgery and WBRT. Specifically, brain metastases located in eloquent cortex, such as the brainstem or motor strip, that are not amenable to surgical resection can be effectively treated with radiosurgery and/or fractionated stereotactic radiotherapy.

For patients with a limited number of brain metastases, prior randomized studies have shown that the addition of radiosurgery to the visible metastases in combination with WBRT improves local control beyond WBRT alone (23). The addition of a radiosurgery boost to WBRT also improved survival of patients with a single brain metastasis (median survival 6.5 mo SRS + WBRT vs. 4.9 mo WBRT, p = 0.0393), but a survival benefit has not been demonstrated in patients with multiple metastases, even when limited to a maximum of four metastases (24).

In a Japanese randomized trial of 132 patients with 1 to 4 brain metastases, adding WBRT to SRS was associated with significantly lower 12-month brain tumor recurrence rate (46.8% vs. 76.4%) but not with improved overall survival as compared to SRS alone (25). It is therefore important to know whether this local control benefit outweighs the possible neurocognitive side effects of adding WBRT.

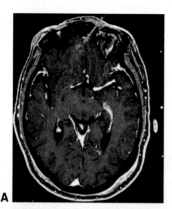
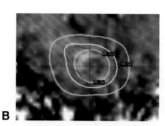
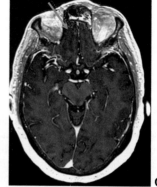

Figure 32.4 Axial T_1-weighted magnetic resonance images of a right inferior frontal brain metastasis from primary renal cell carcinoma demonstrating **(A)** baseline tumor appearance prior to radiosurgery (axial view, marked by blue arrow), **(B)** radiosurgery plan (20 Gy prescribed at the 50% isodose line) showing a very tight radiation dose targeted to the tumor with minimal dose to surrounding brain (coronal view), and **(C)** magnetic resonance images at 1 year showing a durable response with significant reduction in tumor size (axial view, marked by blue arrow).

In a randomized controlled trial of 58 patients with one to three brain metastases at MD Anderson Cancer Center, those who received WBRT plus SRS showed a significantly greater decline in HVLT-R Total Recall at 4 months than patients treated with SRS alone (52% vs. 24%, respectively), a difference which persisted at the 6-month follow-up. These patients also had greater drop in executive functioning as compared to patients randomly assigned to the SRS alone arm (69). A larger multi-institutional trial of 213 patients (N0574 trial) with one to three brain metastases also showed less cognitive deterioration at 3 months after SRS alone, although the time to intracranial failure was significantly shorter for SRS alone compared with SRS plus WBRT. Again, no difference in overall survival was noted in this trial (70).

In the postoperative setting, similar results were obtained. N107C trial is discussed in the section "surgery" of this chapter (54).

These findings suggest that even though patients treated with SRS alone (either in the definitive or adjuvant setting) had higher rates of brain recurrences as a whole, neurocognitive toxicity (learning and memory) associated with WBRT was worse than cognitive decline associated with recurrences, when close surveillance with early salvage therapy was utilized.

Nowadays and based on all the evidence, resorting to SRS monotherapy when a patient presents with a limited number of brain metastases is preferred over more aggressive upfront treatment. It is important for the patient to subsequently adhere to close clinical monitoring with high-quality neuroimaging to detect recurrences early. Systemic therapy is also sometimes needed to address microscopic disease in the brain, while SRS treats gross brain metastases. This strategy is consistent with the trend toward personalized medicine. There are, however, limited data on safety and efficacy of combining systemic therapy and SRS; more trials addressing combination treatments are therefore needed.

RECURRENT DISEASE

A growing number of patients with brain metastases are now living long enough to experience recurrences. One of the diagnostic dilemma clinicians are facing nowadays is to differentiate local recurrent brain metastasis from radiation necrosis after radiotherapy (e.g., SRS or WBRT). Conventional contrast-enhanced MRI is not always able to reliably distinguish these two entities as both can present as increasing enhancement (71), although a lesion quotient of <0.3 is suggestive of radionecrosis (lesion quotient is defined as the

proportional value of the area of the T2-weighted defined lesion over the area of the contrast-enhancing lesion on the T1-weighted post-gadolinium sequence on a comparable axial slice) (72). MR spectroscopy is also helpful in differentiating radionecrosis from recurrence, with a high choline (Cho)/normal *N*-acetylaspartate (nNAA) ratio consistent with tumor recurrence, with an 86% sensitivity and a 90% specificity (73). Chemical exchange saturation transfer (CEST) is a novel technique that is sensitive to mobile proteins and peptides and has shown early promise in identifying recurrent tumor after SRS (74). Perfusion MRI has also been found to be useful, as blood flow is expected to be different between areas of necrosis and areas of recurrent brain tumors (75,76). Positron emission tomography (PET) using amino acid tracers is also a tool that is being investigated to improve the differential diagnosis, in particular *O*-(2-[F]fluoroethyl)-L-tyrosine (FET)-PET, which when added to conventional MRI, had a specificity of 92.9% and sensitivity of 100% in primary brain tumors (77).

At the time of intracranial recurrence following prior therapy, the appropriate salvage therapy may depend on a number of factors, including location of the recurrence, the total number of recurrent lesions, and timing from previous treatment. Following prior WBRT, salvage therapy options may include repeat WBRT, radiosurgery, and surgery. Surgery is usually restricted to patients with one large metastasis in noneloquent brain associated with significant mass effect with preferably minimal or stable extracranial disease. Salvage radiosurgery is usually limited to patients with a smaller number of recurrent metastases. Some studies have shown that patients can have durable local control with salvage SRS for recurrent brain metastases, especially younger patients and those with controlled extracranial disease (78–80). A longer interval from initial RT to salvage SRS (cutoff in the study by Kurtz et al. was ≥265 days) was associated with better outcomes (78,80). Repeat WBRT is generally offered to those with a larger number of recurrent metastases that are not felt to be eligible for radiosurgery. Response to re-irradiation of recurrent disease following previous irradiation is variable and is not necessarily the same as the initial response to radiation. However, the timing of recurrence following whole brain radiation may impact radiation-related toxicity. Therefore, within 6 months of whole brain radiation, radiosurgery and surgery are favored options of salvage therapy for recurrence of a limited number of metastases. Recurrences in the region of previously resected metastases are often infiltrative and poor targets for radiosurgery, and when limited to the surgical region, it can be successfully managed with focal fractionated radiotherapy either via 3D conformal or intensity-modulated radiation therapy techniques. Other options for salvage treatment include laser interstitial thermotherapy (LITT) (81,82) and magnetic resonance high-intensity focused ultrasound (HIFU) (83).

LEPTOMENINGEAL DISEASE

Presentation

Approximately 5% to 15% of all patients with solid cancers develop leptomeningeal disease with the most common primary solid tumor histologies being breast cancer, lung cancer, and melanoma (84). Most patients presenting with leptomeningeal disease also have widely disseminated systemic cancer, and better systemic metastatic control has been associated with delayed appearance of leptomeningeal metastases (85,86). Patients can present with hydrocephalus and raised intracranial pressure or they can present with varying constellations of symptoms depending on the specific areas of leptomeningeal involvement in the cerebrum, cerebellum, cranial nerves, and/or spinal cord and roots (87).

Investigation and Diagnosis

In patients with known metastatic cancer, diagnosis of leptomeningeal brain metastases is made radiologically on a gadolinium-enhanced brain MRI. Typically, there is enhancement along the meningeal lining of the brain, classically with enhancement along the cerebellar folia (87,88). In cases where neuroimaging does not show definitive evidence of leptomeningeal disease, examination of the cerebrospinal fluid (CSF) can assist in the diagnosis of leptomeningeal metastases. Although the presence of malignant cells in the CSF is diagnostic for leptomeningeal disease, a negative CSF cytology does not reliably rule out leptomeningeal disease due to the low sensitivity of CSF cytology (89). If leptomeningeal disease is found in the brain, a gadolinium-enhanced MRI of the spine is recommended to rule out leptomeningeal disease involving the spinal cord or cauda equina.

Prognosis

The prognosis of patients with leptomeningeal disease is poor and this may be compounded when patients present with both extensive systemic disease and leptomeningeal CNS disease. The median survival of patients with leptomeningeal brain metastasis has been reported to range from 4 to 11 weeks without treatment (86,87). Median survival ranges between 4 and 6 months with cytotoxic therapy based on prior studies that include patients with varying extent of leptomeningeal

disease in the brain and/or spinal disease who were treated with radiotherapy and/or chemotherapy (84,87). A recent systematic review including patients with LMD from different histologies has demonstrated that any treatment was superior to supportive care, and that patients who received combined treatment modality (WBRT + systemic/intrathecal therapy) had the longest survival (90).

Treatment

Treatment of leptomeningeal metastasis can improve symptoms and, in some cases, prolong survival. The most common treatment for leptomeningeal brain metastasis is WBRT. Intrathecal chemotherapy or high-dose intravenous chemotherapy have been used to treat patients with leptomeningeal disease in the brain and spine (84). However, a clear survival benefit from intrathecal chemotherapy has not been demonstrated over systemic chemotherapy and/or radiotherapy (91–93). Given the uncertain benefit and the greater potential for severe complications and toxicities associated with intrathecal chemotherapy, WBRT may have a better therapeutic index for patients with radiologically visible leptomeningeal disease isolated to the brain.

SUPPORTIVE CARE

A major aim in the treatment of brain metastases is to improve symptoms and function for patients, which can include minimizing the dose and/or duration of dexamethasone required. However, most treatments are associated with toxicities and patients with limited performance status and/or extensive disease may neither tolerate nor benefit from tumor-directed treatment. In these situations, supportive care may be the most beneficial intervention, as supported by the QUARTZ trial, which enrolled patients with non–small cell lung cancer who were not candidate for surgical resection or radiosurgery (57).

STEROIDS

Most patients who present with brain metastases with symptomatic peritumoral edema benefit from corticosteroids. Dexamethasone is most commonly used as it has a long half-life, good absorption when taken orally, and minimal mineralocorticoid effect. The proposed mechanism of dexamethasone involves up-regulation of angiopoietin-1, a stabilizer of the blood–brain barrier, and down-regulation of vascular endothelial growth factor to reduce peritumoral edema (94). Evidence of reduced intracranial pressure and improvement in neurologic symptoms can be seen within hours of administration, but maximal benefit is typically seen several days after starting dexamethasone.

Recommended Dosing

There is little evidence to guide the optimal dose and tapering schedule for steroids. In general, twice daily dosing at the lowest dose that alleviates symptoms is recommended and early tapering within 1 to 2 weeks is suggested, as steroid side effects have been associated with both dose and duration of steroid use. For mild to moderately symptomatic patients, an initial dose of 4 to 8 mg/d is recommended (95,96). For patients with more severe symptoms and concerns of increased intracranial pressure, a higher dose of 16 mg/d is recommended (97).

Side Effects

Although dexamethasone can provide dramatic benefits for patients with symptomatic peritumoral edema, it is also associated with many side effects that typically worsen over longer administration, including hyperglycemia, weight gain, peripheral edema, candidiasis, myopathy, Cushing's syndrome, insomnia, hypertension, psychiatric disturbances, cataracts, and susceptibility to infection (95,98).

Diabetic Patients and Steroids

Hyperglycemia is one of the most common medical toxicities of steroid administration, either exacerbated in known diabetic patients or unmasking previously undiagnosed type 2 diabetes (99). Patients should be screened for symptoms such as polyuria and polydipsia and a random glucose with their other bloodwork may aid in early detection of hyperglycemia. Oral antidiabetic agents such as metformin are typically used. However, if hyperglycemia is severe or refractory to oral agents, insulin therapy is recommended.

Immunotherapy and Steroids

Although corticosteroids can be critical in symptom palliation in patients with brain metastases, their immunosuppressive effects can pose a problem in patients treated with immunotherapy agents, potentially diminishing their efficacy. There are several papers published on this topic (100–103), and the general accepted practice is that administration of dexamethasone 4 mg daily is allowed for most immunotherapy trials. However, the priority is to address acute neurological symptoms and deterioration associated with peritumoral edema, and the consensus is therefore to give the dose of steroids required, even if it exceeds 4 mg daily when absolutely needed.

CONCLUSION

The treatment options for patients with brain metastases have progressed with advances in surgery and radiation techniques. The aims of treatment have also evolved to reflect the changing presentation of patients due to improving systemic therapy and increasing sensitivity of brain imaging. Although the optimal management of metastases continues to be an area of active investigation, it has been recognized that the patient management should be individualized based on the patient's overall status, prognosis, tumor location, and volume, while considering the patient's goals and preferences.

REFERENCES

1. Barnholtz-Sloan JS, Sloan AE, Davis FG, et al. Incidence proportions of brain metastases in patients diagnosed (1973 to 2001) in the Metropolitan Detroit Cancer Surveillance System. *J Clin Oncol.* 2004;22:2865-2872.
2. Taillibert S, Le Rhun E. [Epidemiology of brain metastases]. *Cancer Radiother.* 2015;19:3-9.
3. Nayak L, Lee EQ, Wen PY. Epidemiology of brain metastases. *Curr Oncol Rep.* 2012;14:48-54.
4. Nussbaum ES, Djalilian HR, Cho KH, et al. Brain metastases. Histology, multiplicity, surgery, and survival. *Cancer.* 1996;78:1781-1788.
5. Lin NU, Winer EP. Brain metastases: the HER2 paradigm. *Clin Cancer Res.* 2007;13:1648-1655.
6. Zhang J, Yu J, Sun X, et al. Epidermal growth factor receptor tyrosine kinase inhibitors in the treatment of central nerve system metastases from non-small cell lung cancer. *Cancer Lett.* 2014;351:6-12.
7. Rangachari D, Yamaguchi N, VanderLaan PA, et al. Brain metastases in patients with EGFR-mutated or ALK-rearranged non-small-cell lung cancers. *Lung Cancer.* 2015;88:108-111.
8. Tawbi HA, Forsyth PA, Algazi A, et al. Combined nivolumab and ipilimumab in melanoma metastatic to the brain. *N Engl J Med.* 2018;379:722-730.
9. Tawbi HA, Boutros C, Kok D, et al. New era in the management of melanoma brain metastases. *Am Soc Clin Oncol Educ Book.* 2018;38:741-750.
10. Li J, Bentzen SM, Li J, et al. Relationship between neurocognitive function and quality of life after whole-brain radiotherapy in patients with brain metastasis. *Int J Radiat Oncol Biol Phys.* 2008;71:64-70.
11. Soussain C, Ricard D, Fike JR, et al. CNS complications of radiotherapy and chemotherapy. *Lancet.* 2009;374:1639-1651.
12. Garcia GCTE, Bockel S, Majer M, et al. Imaging of brain metastases: diagnosis and monitoring. In: Ahluwalia MS, Metellus P, Soffietti R, eds. *Central Nervous System Metastases.* 1st ed. Switzerland: Springer Nature; 2020.
13. Palma DA, Olson R, Harrow S, et al. Stereotactic ablative radiotherapy versus standard of care palliative treatment in patients with oligometastatic cancers (SABR-COMET): a randomised, phase 2, open-label trial. *Lancet.* 2019;393:2051-2058.
14. Iyengar P, Wardak Z, Gerber DE, et al. Consolidative radiotherapy for limited metastatic non-small-cell lung cancer: a phase 2 randomized clinical trial. *JAMA Oncol.* 2018;4:e173501.
15. Gomez DR, Tang C, Zhang J, et al. Local consolidative therapy vs. maintenance therapy or observation for

patients with oligometastatic non-small-cell lung cancer: long-term results of a multi-institutional, phase II, randomized study. *J Clin Oncol.* 2019;37:1558-1565.

16. Forsyth PA, Posner JB. Headaches in patients with brain tumors: a study of 111 patients. *Neurology.* 1993;43: 1678-1683.

17. Cacho-Diaz B, Lorenzana-Mendoza NA, Chavez-Hernandez JD, et al. Clinical manifestations and location of brain metastases as prognostic markers. *Curr Probl Cancer.* 2019;43:312-323.

18. Lassman AB, Deangelis LM. Brain metastases. *Neurol Clin.* 2003;21:1-23.

19. Schaefer PW, Budzik RFJ, Gonzalez RG. Imaging of cerebral metastases. *Neurosurg Clin N Am.* 1996;7: 393-423.

20. Muroff LR, Runge VM. The use of MR contrast in neoplastic disease of the brain. *Top Magn Reson Imaging.* 1995;7:137-157.

21. Gavrilovic IT, Posner JB. Brain metastases: epidemiology and pathophysiology. *J Neurooncol.* 2005;75:5-14.

22. Patchell RA, Tibbs PA, Walsh JW, et al. A randomized trial of surgery in the treatment of single metastases to the brain. *N Engl J Med.* 1990;322:494-500.

23. Tsao M, Xu W, Sahgal A. A meta-analysis evaluating stereotactic radiosurgery, whole-brain radiotherapy, or both for patients presenting with a limited number of brain metastases. *Cancer.* 2012;118:2486-2493.

24. Andrews DW, Scott CB, Sperduto PW, et al. Whole brain radiation therapy with or without stereotactic radiosurgery boost for patients with one to three brain metastases: phase III results of the RTOG 9508 randomised trial. *Lancet.* 2004;363:1665-1672.

25. Aoyama H, Shirato H, Tago M, et al. Stereotactic radiosurgery plus whole-brain radiation therapy vs stereotactic radiosurgery alone for treatment of brain metastases: a randomized controlled trial. *JAMA.* 2006;295:2483-2491.

26. Schag CC, Heinrich RL, Ganz PA. Karnofsky performance status revisited: reliability, validity, and guidelines. *J Clin Oncol.* 1984;2:187-193.

27. Gaspar L, Scott C, Rotman M, et al. Recursive Partitioning Analysis (RPA) of prognostic factors in three Radiation Therapy Oncology Group (RTOG) brain metastases trials. *Int J Radiat Oncol Biol Phys.* 1997;37: 745-751.

28. Gaspar LE, Scott C, Murray K, et al. Validation of the RTOG recursive partitioning analysis (RPA) classification for brain metastases. *Int J Radiat Oncol Biol Phys.* 2000;47:1001-1006.

29. Lorenzoni J, Devriendt D, Massager N, et al. Radiosurgery for treatment of brain metastases: estimation of patient eligibility using three stratification systems. *Int J Radiat Oncol Biol Phys.* 2004;60:218-224.

30. Viani GA, Castilho MS, Salvajoli J V, et al. Whole brain radiotherapy for brain metastases from breast cancer: estimation of survival using two stratification systems. *BMC Cancer.* 2007;7:53.

31. Golden DW, Lamborn KR, McDermott MW, et al. Prognostic factors and grading systems for overall survival in patients treated with radiosurgery for brain metastases: variation by primary site. *J Neurosurg.* 2008;109(suppl):77-86.

32. Sperduto PW, Chao ST, Sneed PK, et al. Diagnosis-specific prognostic factors, indexes, and treatment outcomes for patients with newly diagnosed brain metastases: a multi-institutional analysis of 4,259 patients. *Int J Radiat Oncol Biol Phys.* 2010;77:655-661.

33. Woody NM, Greer MD, Reddy CA, et al. Validation of the disease-specific GPA for patients with 1 to 3 synchronous brain metastases in newly diagnosed NSCLC. *Clin Lung Cancer.* 2018;19:e141-e147.

34. Nagtegaal SHJ, Claes A, Suijkerbuijk KPM, et al. Comparing survival predicted by the diagnosis-specific Graded Prognostic Assessment (DS-GPA) to actual survival in patients with 1-10 brain metastases treated with stereotactic radiosurgery. *Radiother Oncol.* 2019;138:173-179.

35. Kano H, Morales-Restrepo A, Iyer A, et al. Comparison of prognostic indices in patients who undergo melanoma brain metastasis radiosurgery. *J Neurosurg.* 2018;128:14-22.

36. Yamamoto M, Aiyama H, Koiso T, et al. Applicability and limitations of a recently-proposed prognostic grading metric, initial brain metastasis velocity, for brain metastasis patients undergoing stereotactic radiosurgery. *J Neurooncol.* 2019;143:613-621.

37. Soike MH, McTyre ER, Hughes RT, et al. Initial brain metastasis velocity: does the rate at which cancers first seed the brain affect outcomes? *J Neurooncol.* 2018;139:461-467.

38. Farris M, McTyre ER, Cramer CK, et al. Brain metastasis velocity: a novel prognostic metric predictive of overall survival and freedom from whole-brain radiation therapy after distant brain failure following upfront radiosurgery alone. *Int J Radiat Oncol Biol Phys.* 2017;98:131-141.

39. Brastianos PK, Carter SL, Santagata S, et al. Genomic characterization of brain metastases reveals branched evolution and potential therapeutic targets. *Cancer Discov.* 2015;5:1164-1177.

40. Saunus JM, Quinn MCJ, Patch A-M, et al. Integrated genomic and transcriptomic analysis of human brain metastases identifies alterations of potential clinical significance. *J Pathol.* 2015;237:363-378.

41. Lazaro T, Brastianos PK. Immunotherapy and targeted therapy in brain metastases: emerging options in precision medicine. *CNS Oncol.* 2017;6:139-151.

42. Neagu MR, Gill CM, Batchelor TT, et al. Genomic profiling of brain metastases: current knowledge and new frontiers. *Chin Clin Oncol.* 2015;4:22.

43. Dunn GP, Okada H. Principles of immunology and its nuances in the central nervous system. *Neuro Oncol.* 2015;17(suppl 7):vii3-vii8.

44. Berghoff AS, Ricken G, Widhalm G, et al. Tumour-infiltrating lymphocytes and expression of programmed death ligand 1 (PD-L1) in melanoma brain metastases. *Histopathology.* 2015;66:289-299.

45. Berghoff AS, Ricken G, Wilhelm D, et al. Tumor infiltrating lymphocytes and PD-L1 expression in brain metastases of small cell lung cancer (SCLC). *J Neurooncol.* 2016;130:19-29.

46. Berghoff AS, Fuchs E, Ricken G, et al. Density of tumor-infiltrating lymphocytes correlates with extent of brain edema and overall survival time in patients with brain metastases. *Oncoimmunology.* 2016;5:e1057388.

47. Flanigan JC, Jilaveanu LB, Faries M, et al. Melanoma brain metastasis: is it time to reassess the bias? *Curr Probl Cancer.* 2011;35:200-210.

48. Margolin K, Ernstoff MS, Hamid O, et al. Ipilimumab in patients with melanoma and brain metastases: an open-label, phase 2 trial. *Lancet Oncol.* 2012;13:459-465.

49. Goldberg SB, Gettinger SN, Mahajan A, et al. Pembrolizumab for patients with melanoma or non-small-cell lung cancer and untreated brain metastases: early analysis of a non-randomised, open-label, phase 2 trial. *Lancet Oncol.* 2016;17:976-983.

50. Long G V, Atkinson V, Lo S, et al. Combination nivolumab and ipilimumab or nivolumab alone in

melanoma brain metastases: a multicentre randomised phase 2 study. *Lancet Oncol.* 2018;19:672-681.

51. Chen L, Douglass J, Kleinberg L, et al. Concurrent immune checkpoint inhibitors and stereotactic radiosurgery for brain metastases in non-small cell lung cancer, melanoma, and renal cell carcinoma. *Int J Radiat Oncol Biol Phys.* 2018;100:916-925.

52. Pin Y, Paix A, Todeschi J, et al. Brain metastasis formation and irradiation by stereotactic radiation therapy combined with immunotherapy: a systematic review. *Crit Rev Oncol Hematol.* 2020;149:102923.

53. Patchell RA, Tibbs PA, Regine WF, et al. Postoperative radiotherapy in the treatment of single metastases to the brain: a randomized trial. *JAMA.* 1998;280:1485-1489.

54. Brown PD, Ballman KV, Cerhan JH, et al. Postoperative stereotactic radiosurgery compared with whole brain radiotherapy for resected metastatic brain disease (NCCTG N107C/CEC·3): a multicentre, randomised, controlled, phase 3 trial. *Lancet Oncol.* 2017;18:1049-1060.

55. Mahajan A, Ahmed S, McAleer MF, et al. Post-operative stereotactic radiosurgery versus observation for completely resected brain metastases: a single-centre, randomised, controlled, phase 3 trial. *Lancet Oncol.* 2017;18:1040-1048.

56. Tsao MN, Xu W, Wong RK, et al. Whole brain radiotherapy for the treatment of newly diagnosed multiple brain metastases. *Cochrane Database Syst Rev.* 2018;(1):Cd003869.

57. Mulvenna P, Nankivell M, Barton R, et al. Dexamethasone and supportive care with or without whole brain radiotherapy in treating patients with non-small cell lung cancer with brain metastases unsuitable for resection or stereotactic radiotherapy (QUARTZ): results from a phase 3, non-inferiority. *Lancet.* 2016;388:2004-2014.

58. Li J, Bentzen SM, Renschler M, et al. Regression after whole-brain radiation therapy for brain metastases correlates with survival and improved neurocognitive function. *J Clin Oncol.* 2007;25:1260-1266.

59. Giordano FA, Welzel G, Abo-Madyan Y, et al. Potential toxicities of prophylactic cranial irradiation. *Transl Lung Cancer Res.* 2012;1:254-262.

60. Wolfson AH, Bae K, Komaki R, et al. Primary analysis of a phase II randomized trial Radiation Therapy Oncology Group (RTOG) 0212: impact of different total doses and schedules of prophylactic cranial irradiation on chronic neurotoxicity and quality of life for patients with limited-disease. *Int J Radiat Oncol Biol Phys.* 2011;81:77-84.

61. Hopewell JW, Wright EA. The nature of latent cerebral irradiation damage and its modification by hypertension. *Br J Radiol.* 1970;43:161-167.

62. Wefel JS, Deshmukh S, Brown PD, et al. Impact of apolipoprotein E (APOE) genotype on neurocognitive function (NCF) in patients with brain metastasis (BM): an analysis of NRG Oncology's RTOG 0614. *J Clin Oncol.* 2018;36:2065.

63. Monje ML, Mizumatsu S, Fike JR, et al. Irradiation induces neural precursor-cell dysfunction. *Nat Med.* 2002;8:955-962.

64. Eriksson PS, Perfilieva E, Björk-Eriksson T, et al. Neurogenesis in the adult human hippocampus. *Nat Med.* 1998;4:1313-1317.

65. Gondi V, Tom WA, Mehta MP. Why avoid the hippocampus? A comprehensive review. *Radiother Oncol.* 2010;97:370-376.

66. Gondi V, Pugh SL, Tome WA, et al. Preservation of memory with conformal avoidance of the hippocampal neural stem-cell compartment during whole-brain radiotherapy for brain metastases (RTOG 0933): a phase II multi-institutional trial. *J Clin Oncol.* 2014;32:3810-3816.

67. Gondi V, Deshmukh S, Brown P, et al. NRG Oncology CC001: a phase III trial of hippocampal avoidance (HA) in addition to whole-brain radiotherapy (WBRT) plus memantine to preserve neurocognitive function (NCF) in patients with brain metastases (BM). *J Clin Oncol.* 2019;37(15 suppl):2009.

68. Mehta MP, Tsao MN, Whelan TJ, et al. The American Society for Therapeutic Radiology and Oncology (ASTRO) evidence-based review of the role of radiosurgery for brain metastases. *Int J Radiat Oncol Biol Phys.* 2005;63:37-46.

69. Chang EL, Wefel JS, Hess KR, et al. Neurocognition in patients with brain metastases treated with radiosurgery or radiosurgery plus whole-brain irradiation: a randomised controlled trial. *Lancet Oncol.* 2009;10:1037-1044.

70. Brown PD, Jaeckle K, Ballman K V, et al. Effect of radiosurgery alone vs radiosurgery with whole brain radiation therapy on cognitive function in patients with 1 to 3 brain metastases: a randomized clinical trial. *JAMA.* 2016;316:401-409.

71. Stockham AL, Tievsky AL, Koyfman SA, et al. Conventional MRI does not reliably distinguish radiation necrosis from tumor recurrence after stereotactic radiosurgery. *J Neurooncol.* 2012;109:149-158.

72. Dequesada IM, Quisling RG, Yachnis A, et al. Can standard magnetic resonance imaging reliably distinguish recurrent tumor from radiation necrosis after radiosurgery for brain metastases? A radiographic-pathological study. *Neurosurgery.* 2008;63:898-903; discussion 904.

73. Elias AE, Carlos RC, Smith EA, et al. MR spectroscopy using normalized and non-normalized metabolite ratios for differentiating recurrent brain tumor from radiation injury. *Acad Radiol.* 2011;18:1101-1108.

74. Mehrabian H, Desmond KL, Soliman H, et al. Differentiation between radiation necrosis and tumor progression using chemical exchange saturation transfer. *Clin Cancer Res.* 2017;23:3667-3675.

75. Hoefnagels FWA, Lagerwaard FJ, Sanchez E, et al. Radiological progression of cerebral metastases after radiosurgery: assessment of perfusion MRI for differentiating between necrosis and recurrence. *J Neurol.* 2009;256:878-887.

76. Barajas RF, Chang JS, Sneed PK, et al. Distinguishing recurrent intra-axial metastatic tumor from radiation necrosis following gamma knife radiosurgery using dynamic susceptibility-weighted contrast-enhanced perfusion MR imaging. *AJNR Am J Neuroradiol.* 2009;30:367-372.

77. Rachinger W, Goetz C, Popperl G, et al. Positron emission tomography with O-(2-[18F]fluoroethyl)-l-tyrosine versus magnetic resonance imaging in the diagnosis of recurrent gliomas. *Neurosurgery.* 2005;57:505-511.

78. Kurtz G, Zadeh G, Gingras-Hill G, et al. Salvage radiosurgery for brain metastases: prognostic factors to consider in patient selection. *Int J Radiat Oncol Biol Phys.* 2014;88:137-142.

79. Kelly PJ, Lin NU, Claus EB, et al. Salvage stereotactic radiosurgery for breast cancer brain metastases: outcomes and prognostic factors. *Cancer.* 2012;118:2014-2020.

80. Caballero JA, Sneed PK, Lamborn KR, et al. Prognostic factors for survival in patients treated with stereotactic radiosurgery for recurrent brain metastases after prior whole brain radiotherapy. *Int J Radiat Oncol Biol Phys.* 2012;83:303-309.

81. Bastos DCA, Rao G, Oliva ICG, et al. Predictors of local control of brain metastasis treated with laser interstitial thermal therapy. *Neurosurgery.* 2020;87(1):112-122.

82. Hong CS, Deng D, Vera A, et al. Laser-interstitial thermal therapy compared to craniotomy for treatment of radiation necrosis or recurrent tumor in brain metastases failing radiosurgery. *J Neurooncol.* 2019;142:309-317.

83. MacDonell J, Patel N, Rubino S, et al. Magnetic resonance-guided interstitial high-intensity focused ultrasound for brain tumor ablation. *Neurosurg Focus.* 2018;44:E11.

84. Chamberlain MC. Leptomeningeal metastases: a review of evaluation and treatment. *J Neurooncol.* 1998;37:271-284.

85. van Oostenbrugge RJ, Twijnstra A. Presenting features and value of diagnostic procedures in leptomeningeal metastases. *Neurology.* 1999;53:382-385.

86. Grossman SA, Krabak MJ. Leptomeningeal carcinomatosis. *Cancer Treat Rev.* 1999;25:103-119.

87. Clarke JL, Perez HR, Jacks LM, et al. Leptomeningeal metastases in the MRI era. *Neurology.* 2010;74:1449-1454.

88. Chamberlain MC, Sandy AD, Press GA. Leptomeningeal metastasis: a comparison of gadolinium-enhanced MR and contrast-enhanced CT of the brain. *Neurology.* 1990;40:435-438.

89. Wasserstrom WR, Glass JP, Posner JB. Diagnosis and treatment of leptomeningeal metastases from solid tumors: experience with 90 patients. *Cancer.* 1982;49:759-772.

90. Buszek SM, Chung C. Radiotherapy in leptomeningeal disease: a systematic review of randomized and non-randomized trials. *Front Oncol.* 2019;9:1224.

91. Bokstein F, Lossos A, Siegal T. Leptomeningeal metastases from solid tumors: a comparison of two prospective series treated with and without intra-cerebrospinal fluid chemotherapy. *Cancer.* 1998;82:1756-1763.

92. Glantz MJ, Cole BF, Recht L, et al. High-dose intravenous methotrexate for patients with nonleukemic leptomeningeal cancer: is intrathecal chemotherapy necessary? *J Clin Oncol.* 1998;16:1561-1567.

93. Boogerd W, van den Bent MJ, Koehler PJ, et al. The relevance of intraventricular chemotherapy for leptomeningeal metastasis in breast cancer: a randomised study. *Eur J Cancer.* 2004;40:2726-2733.

94. Kim H, Lee JM, Park JS, et al. Dexamethasone coordinately regulates angiopoietin-1 and VEGF: a mechanism of glucocorticoid-induced stabilization of blood-brain barrier. *Biochem Biophys Res Commun.* 2008;372:243-248.

95. Hempen C, Weiss E, Hess CF. Dexamethasone treatment in patients with brain metastases and primary brain tumors: do the benefits outweigh the side-effects?. *Support Care Cancer.* 2002;10:322-328.

96. Vecht CJ, Hovestadt A, Verbiest HB, et al. Dose-effect relationship of dexamethasone on Karnofsky performance in metastatic brain tumors: a randomized study of doses of 4, 8, and 16 mg per day. *Neurology.* 1994;44:675-680.

97. Ryken TC, Mcdermott M, Robinson PD, et al. The role of steroids in the management of brain metastases: a systematic review and evidence-based clinical practice guideline. *J Neurooncol.* 2010;96(1):103-114.

98. Roth P, Happold C, Weller M. Corticosteroid use in neuro-oncology: an update. *Neurooncol Pract.* 2015;2:6-12.

99. Lukins MB, Manninen PH. Hyperglycemia in patients administered dexamethasone for craniotomy. *Anesth Analg.* 2005;100:1129-1133.

100. Garant A, Guilbault C, Ekmekjian T, et al. Concomitant use of corticosteroids and immune checkpoint inhibitors in patients with hematologic or solid neoplasms: a systematic review. *Crit Rev Oncol Hematol.* 2017;120:86-92.

101. Jove M, Vilarino N, Nadal E. Impact of baseline steroids on efficacy of programmed cell death-1 (PD-1) and programmed death-ligand 1 (PD-L1) blockade in patients with advanced non-small cell lung cancer. *Transl Lung Cancer Res.* 2019;8:S364-S368.

102. Arbour KC, Mezquita L, Long N, et al. Impact of baseline steroids on efficacy of programmed cell death-1 and programmed death-ligand 1 blockade in patients with non-small-cell lung cancer. *J Clin Oncol.* 2018;36:2872-2878.

103. Pan EY, Merl MY, Lin K. The impact of corticosteroid use during anti-PD1 treatment. *J Oncol Pharm Pract.* 2019:1078155219872786.

Sharon M. Weinstein and Jason G. Ramirez

EPIDEMIOLOGY

The spine is the most frequent site of bony involvement in patients with metastatic malignancy (1). The major complications of spinal neoplasm are pain and neurologic injury. Compression of neural structures may be caused directly by tumor mass and/or by displacement of bony fragments into the spinal canal. Tumor of the vertebral bodies has been demonstrated in 25% to 70% of patients with metastatic cancer (2), and spinal metastases are present in 40% of patients who die of cancer (3). Metastatic lesions from other primary malignancies are three to four times as common as primary bony tumors of the spine (4).

Each year in the United States, approximately 20,000 patients with cancer are treated for malignant epidural compression (EC) of the spinal cord and/or cauda equina. It has been estimated that EC affects 5% to 10% of adult solid tumor patients and 5% of pediatric solid tumor patients (5,6). These percentages are corroborated by autopsy series (4,7). A review of over 15,000 EC cases representing over 75,000 hospitalizations revealed that patients dying of cancer in the United States have an estimated 3.4% annual incidence of EC requiring hospitalization. Inpatient management of EC varied over time and by hospital characteristics, with inpatient radiotherapy decreasing, surgical interventions increasing, and hospitalization costs increasing during the period of 1998 to 2006 (8).

It has been determined that up to 5% of patients with terminal cancer will experience EC within the last 2 years of life (9,10). With continued advances in overall cancer survival, the incidence of EC is expected to increase.

It is common for EC to be the presenting symptom of malignancy. At least a third of all patients initially presenting with EC are not known to have cancer at the time that pain or neurologic deficits begin (9–12). It is therefore important for clinicians to be familiar with the basic presentation and management algorithm for EC.

The distribution of spinal tumors reflects the prevalence of the various primary malignancies as well as the physiology of metastasis. Multiple myeloma is the most common primary bone tumor, representing 10% to 15% of malignant epidural spinal disease. Osteogenic sarcoma is the second most common primary spinal tumor, usually affecting children and adolescents. Fifty percent of chordomas affect the sacrococcygeal bones and 35% affect the base of the skull. Chondrosarcoma and Ewing's sarcoma are other bone tumors that may be primary in the vertebrae, although this is rare.

Primary tumors of the breast, lung, and prostate commonly spread to the spinal column. The spine is also a frequent site of metastasis of a nonspinal primary osteogenic sarcoma. Spinal metastases are less common in renal carcinoma, melanoma, soft tissue sarcoma, Ewing's sarcoma, germ cell tumors, neuroblastoma, and carcinomas of the head and neck, thyroid, and bladder. Rarely, malignant neoplasms of the brain, pancreas, liver, or ovary affect the bony spinal column.

Ten percent of symptomatic spinal metastases originate from unknown primary tumors (3). Some malignancies spread to the intraspinal space without directly affecting the bone. Lymphoma and neuroblastoma often invade the spinal canal through the intervertebral foramina. Ewing's sarcoma, as well as osteosarcoma, may be primary in the epidural space. Occurrence of primary epidural tumors is rare.

Considering distribution by location in the spinal column, thoracic metastases are estimated to occur twice as frequently as lumbar metastases and four times as frequently as cervical metastases (2). Almost two-thirds of metastatic spinal lesions present clinically in the thoracic region (13), although in some autopsy series, lesions of the lumbar spine have been most prevalent (3). The level of spinal involvement varies with the primary tumor type. Breast and lung tumor metastases are equally distributed throughout the spine. Prostate, renal, and gastrointestinal metastases are more often found in the lower thoracic, lumbar, and sacral levels. Tumors of the uterus and uterine cervix most commonly spread to the lower lumbar and sacral spine. Pancoast tumors of the apex of the lung extend directly into the cervicothoracic spine in 25% of cases (13), often by intraforaminal extension. Multiple noncontiguous levels of spinal tumor are present in 10% to 38% of cases (14); this pattern is relatively less common in patients with lung cancer (11).

EC is caused by the direct extension of the tumor from the vertebral body in 85% to 90% of cases (13). In pediatric patients, EC due to tumor of the posterior elements is more likely, and intraforaminal spread of tumor from paraspinal sites also occurs more frequently than in adults (14). It is noted, however, that tumor metastases in the epidural space seldom breach the dura (3,15).

The prevalence of EC varies according to the tumor type. In one series of 103 patients with lung cancer, 26% with squamous histology, 9% with adenocarcinoma, and 14% with small cell tumors had spinal cord compression (16). The prevalence of all neurologic complications in this series was approximately 40%.

Breast cancer accounts for almost one-fourth of EC diagnosed in cancer hospitals. Vertebral metastases are identified in 60% of patients with breast cancer, and multiple levels of involvement are common. EC is rarely the initial presentation or an early finding in breast cancer (17).

Approximately 7% of patients with prostate cancer develop EC. EC was noted in 12.2% of patients with poorly differentiated tumors and 2.9% of those with well-differentiated tumors (18). The average time from initial prostate cancer diagnosis to EC is 2 years, although it is shorter in stage D2. In approximately 30% of prostate cancer patients with EC, it is the initial manifestation of the cancer (19).

Renal cell carcinomas may also cause EC secondary to bony metastasis. Testicular cancer rarely metastasizes to bone, but it may grow into the spinal canal from the retroperitoneal space. Malignant melanoma may produce EC from vertebral disease, but intradural and leptomeningeal involvement are probably more common. Head and neck cancers rarely metastasize beyond the cervical lymph nodes; approximately 80% of distant metastases are detected within 2 years of initial diagnosis. Therefore, a patient with head and neck cancer presenting with EC after 2 years should be evaluated for a second primary malignancy. EC occurred at all levels of the spine in one small series of patients with head and neck cancers (20).

Esophageal cancers may rarely cause EC by direct invasion to the thoracic spinal column (21). Carcinoid tumors are associated with neurologic complications in <20% of cases; the most frequent is EC due to spinal metastases, generally a late complication.

In plasmacytoma and multiple myeloma, EC is usually due to bony collapse, occurring in >10% of patients. Hodgkin's disease and non–Hodgkin's lymphomas are associated with a 5% incidence of EC, usually in association with extranodal or extensive nodal disease. The thoracic spine is most often involved, in many cases by intraforaminal spread of tumor (22). Patients with EC due to lymphoma are at high risk for meningeal disease. Cerebrospinal fluid (CSF) examination should be considered along with spinal imaging, as concurrent meningeal lymphoma is common and affects the antineoplastic treatment regimen. Vertebral compression fracture with radicular pain is a rare presenting sign of acute leukemia (23).

EC is the presenting sign of cancer in up to 30% of pediatric cases. The time interval to presentation with EC may be twice as long in children without a known cancer compared with those already diagnosed with malignancy (24). Children without a cancer history presenting with EC are often initially misdiagnosed (6). EC is the most frequent neurologic complication of Ewing's sarcoma (25).

DIFFERENTIAL DIAGNOSIS

The differential diagnosis of back pain and neurologic dysfunction secondary to EC includes benign tumors; it is interesting to note that meningiomas occur frequently in patients with breast cancer (2). Given its high prevalence, coexisting nonmalignant disease of the spine may affect as many as 30% of patients with EC (26). Degenerative, inflammatory, and infectious processes commonly affect the spinal structures (27). Soft tissue injuries causing back pain are also very common. Trauma is the most common cause of back pain in children; other nonmalignant conditions such as Scheuermann's disease and scoliosis (28) are also present in this age group. Back pain in patients with cancer may be a secondary symptom caused by vertebral osteoporosis owing to radiation therapy or corticosteroid administration.

Spinal cord or cauda equina dysfunction may be related to direct tumor or treatment effects without EC. Leptomeningeal disease, intradural extramedullary or intramedullary spinal cord disease, paraneoplastic necrotizing myelopathy, and myelopathy induced by radiation or intrathecal chemotherapy should be considered if no compressive epidural lesion is found. Myelopathy is a late complication of radiation; epidural lipomatosis may be caused by corticosteroid therapy. Vascular events of the spinal cord may occur in association with tumor masses and hematologic dysfunctions related to cancer.

PATHOGENESIS OF NEUROLOGIC DYSFUNCTION AND PAIN

The high incidence of metastasis to the vertebrae, despite their poor blood supply, is explained by their specific physiologic features. The vertebrae have a large capillary capacity, promoting local stasis of blood. The walls of the vascular sinusoids are discontinuous, and intersinusoidal cords form cul-de-sac for tumor. Tumor products and the products of bone resorption act to stimulate tumor growth (29). Monocytes produce interleukin-1, which may promote resorption of normal bone (2). Metastases may occur more commonly in previously damaged bone (30).

Batson's plexus is a valveless system of epidural veins in which blood may flow rostrally or caudally. On Valsalva's maneuver, this system drains the viscera and may be a route of metastatic spread. Tumor also reaches the bone through the arteries and lymphatics, and by direct extension.

Epidural tumor produces dysfunction of neural structures by direct compression and by secondary demyelination, ischemia, and tissue edema. Inflammation may change vascular permeability and disrupt the blood–spinal cord barrier at the tumor site. The release of excitatory amino acids by injured neurons further promotes ischemia and injury.

In the initial stage of epidural spinal cord compression, there may be white matter edema and axonal swelling with normal blood flow. These changes are due to direct compression or venous congestion. Over time, progressive compression decreases blood flow and disturbs vascular autoregulation, leading to the development of vasogenic edema. Spinal cord infarction may result from the interruption of venous outflow or occlusion of small arteries or from the interruption of the major arterial supply to the spinal cord (including the artery of Adamkiewicz) or radicular arteries in the intervertebral foramina.

A necrotic cavity, usually located in the ventral portion of the posterior columns or dorsal horn, has been visualized on magnetic resonance imaging (MRI) (14). The effects of cord compression may also be due to coup or contrecoup injury, which is not easily predicted on the basis of the tumor location in relation to the spinal cord. Demyelination as a mechanism of neural dysfunction (5) is supported by pathologic examinations, which demonstrate greater demyelination of white matter than gray matter, a pattern that does not conform to arterial supply. Animal experiments indicate that a more rapid ischemic change produces a greater degree of irreversible neurologic injury (31,32). Similar observations have been made in the human spinal cord.

Pain due to malignancy of the spine may result from activation of afferent nociceptive neurons by mechanical distortion and inflammatory mediators (nociceptive pain) or from neural dysfunction (neuropathic pain). Nociceptors innervate the periosteum of bone, soft tissues (ligaments and muscles), facet articular cartilage, dura mater, nerve root sheaths, and blood vessels. Vertebral collapse and structural instability can give rise to mechanical pain through injury to these structures, which worsens during spine loading and weight shifting. There may be secondary myofascial pain as well. Neuropathic pain results from altered peripheral and central neural activities that may be induced by injury of the nerve roots, axonal injury, or other processes such as deafferentation (loss of primary sensory input).

PATIENT EVALUATION

Although it is widely recognized that pain is often the first symptom of spinal neoplasm, accurate assessment of back and neck pain in the patient with cancer may be challenging to even the experienced clinician. Complete history and physical examination, including a thorough neurologic examination, are essential to localize the underlying pathology. Proper clinical localization is necessary to choose diagnostic and therapeutic interventions correctly (Table 33.1). The importance of obtaining a detailed understanding of the spinal lesion(s) and elucidating the relationship of pathology to symptoms (clinicopathologic correlation) cannot be overemphasized. Inadequate evaluation increases the likelihood of otherwise preventable neurologic compromise. In a retrospective survey of patients with cancer presenting with back pain, misdiagnosis was attributed to poor history, inadequate examination, and insufficient diagnostic evaluation (33). In a review of cancer pain consultations performed by a neurology-based pain service in a cancer hospital, the comprehensive evaluation of pain led to an identification of new malignant involvement in 65% of cases (34). This underscores the importance of thorough clinical evaluation.

History

Up to 95% of adult and 80% of pediatric patients with EC present with pain (13,35). The difference in pain prevalence between adults and children may reflect greater difficulty in the pain assessment of and the underreporting of pain in children. Pain may precede other symptoms and signs of EC by 1 year (14). This interval may vary by tumor type; it is generally shorter for lung cancer than breast cancer (36). Overall, patients experience pain for an average of 4 to 5 months before presentation (3).

Pain may be local at the site of pathology or referred in a nonradicular or a radicular

TABLE 33.1 PATTERNS OF SPINAL TUMOR INVOLVEMENT

Bone
  Bone alone
    Single site
    Multiple contiguous sites
    Multiple noncontiguous sites
  Bone and paraspinal soft tissues
  Bone, paraspinal tissues, and viscera
  Bone and nerve roots
  Bone and epidural space (without thecal
    compression)
  Bone and epidural spinal cord compression
  Bone and epidural cauda equina compression

Epidural
  Intraforaminal
    Isolated
    Local extension
  Epidural and spinal cord compression
    . Single site
    Multiple contiguous sites
    Multiple noncontiguous sites
  Epidural and cauda equina compression
    Single site
    Multiple contiguous sites
    Multiple noncontiguous sites
  Diffuse

(dermatomal) distribution or have combined features. Radicular or root pain is reported in 90% of lumbosacral EC, 79% of cervical compression, and 55% of thoracic cord compression (36). Radicular pain may be bilateral in thoracic lesions and is often described as a tight band around the chest or abdomen. It is important to note that radicular pain may be experienced in only one part of a dermatome, that is, as a partial suspended sensory level. When a nerve root lesion produces chest or abdominal pain, the complaint may be mistakenly identified as referred pain of visceral origin. Radicular lesions are usually associated with segmental findings on examination. Nonradicular referred pain may be associated with vague paresthesias and tenderness at the painful site. Pain may be continuous at rest and markedly aggravated by body movements (incident pain). Although local pain from a vertebral lesion is worsened with loading due to upright posture, pain due to EC is often greatly increased by lying supine. A lesion confined to the vertebral body may also produce nonradicular referred pain. Disease at C7 may refer pain to the interscapular region, and pain due to disease at L1 may be referred to the iliac crests, hips, or sacroiliac region. Sacral disease often causes midline pain radiating to the buttocks, which is made worse with sitting. Radicular pain, in particular, may be paroxysmal, spontaneous, or provoked by movement or sensory stimulation. Valsalva's maneuver may produce or aggravate both local and radicular

pain. Pain worsened on neck flexion or straight leg raising implies dural traction. Lhermitte's sign (electric shock-like pain in the spine) is a symptom of spinal cord dysfunction. Compression of the cervical spinal cord rarely produces funicular pain, which is pain referred to the lower extremities, thorax, or abdomen as a band of paresthesias. "Pseudoclaudication" of legs may be an isolated lumbar root symptom (2).

The neurologic findings associated with EC also vary considerably. There can be extensive epidural tumor with no neurologic findings on examination. Upper motor neuron weakness may occur with lesions of the spinal cord (above the L1 vertebral body). This finding is present in 75% of patients with EC at diagnosis (13). Sensory changes occur in approximately half of patients at presentation, including paresthesias and sensory loss, which can be segmental or below the level of injury. Sensory complaint without pain is exceedingly rare. Bladder and bowel dysfunction are evident in more than half of patients on presentation with EC; constipation usually precedes urinary retention or incontinence (2).

Examination

The physical examination begins with the observation of posture, spinal curvature, symmetry of paraspinal muscles, extremities, and skin. The practitioner may appreciate tenderness of the spinous processes on palpation or percussion, although this may not correlate with the level of spinal disease. Gibbus deformity and vertebral misalignments are frequently palpable; actual crepitus of the spine is unusual. Tenderness or spasm of the paraspinal muscles may also be noted. Urinary retention may be demonstrated by bladder percussion. Laxity of the anal sphincter may be apparent on digital rectal examination. Specific areas of sacral or coccygeal tenderness may be identified by external palpation, rectal, or pelvic examination.

Spinal maneuvers to elicit pain should be performed carefully. Thoracic and abdominal radicular pain may be provoked on lateral flexion and rotation of the trunk. Increased pain on neck flexion and straight leg raise sign may be "pseudomeningeal" signs of dural traction due to epidural tumor. If neck rigidity is present, the examiner should use extreme caution with range-of-motion maneuvers. Muscle spasm may be triggered by bony instability of the cervical spine, and forced movements may dislodge bony fragments, causing acute spinal cord or brainstem injury.

The neurologic examination reveals positive findings in most patients with EC. The examination should include assessment of mental status, cranial nerves, motor function, reflexes, sensation, coordination, and gait. Proximal lower extremity weakness may be initially evident only as difficulty in rising from a chair. Although weakness due to upper motor neuron dysfunction is usually associated with increased tone and hyperreflexia, acute "spinal shock" can cause a flaccid areflexic paralysis. In the subacute phase of recovery from spinal shock, "mass reflexes" appear consisting of flexor spasms, hyperhidrosis, and piloerection due to autonomic dysfunction. Lower motor neuron weakness may be accompanied by flaccidity, atrophy, muscle fasciculations, and hyporeflexia. A cervical lesion can produce segmental hyporeflexia in the arm or arms and increased reflexes below. Lesions above the pyramidal decussation of the corticospinal tracts in the lower brainstem may be associated with the loss of contralateral abdominal reflexes; lesions below the decussation produce loss of ipsilateral abdominal reflexes. Segmental motor dysfunction due to thoracic nerve root disease may produce asymmetric abdominal muscle contraction and loss of abdominal reflexes. Beevor's sign (upward movement of the umbilicus on attempted flexion of the trunk) indicates a lesion at or near the T10 thoracic level. Lesions of the roots of the upper lumbar plexus produce hip flexion weakness and a dropped knee jerk reflex; lesions of the roots to the lower lumbar plexus may produce foot drop and diminished ankle jerk reflex. Loss of bulbocavernosus and anal reflexes may accompany spinal cord conus and cauda equina lesions (2).

Although the sensory examination may help in determining the level of epidural disease, EC results in a broad variation of sensory dysfunction, with incomplete lesions being the rule. The level of reduced sensation may be determined to be up to five segmental levels below, or one to two segments above, the level of cord compression. A sensory level on the trunk sparing the sacral dermatomes may occur in up to 20% of patients with thoracic or high lumbar compression (2). Suspended partial sensory levels or unilateral bands of sensory loss may be seen with spinal cord lesions up to the brainstem. Facial numbness may be due to upper cervical lesions. Lesions of the upper thoracic nerve roots may result in Horner syndrome, with autonomic dysfunction of the face and upper extremity. Compression of the conus of the spinal cord may produce sensory loss in the saddle area (buttocks and perineum) without lower extremity symptoms or signs.

Gait ataxia is an uncommon isolated sign of spinal cord compression. Other unusual features are signs of raised intracranial pressure; facial paresis, lower extremity fasciculations, or sciatica with cervical tumor; nystagmus with thoracic tumor; spinal myoclonus; an inverted knee jerk reflex; and "painful legs and moving toes" (14).

Diagnostic Evaluation

The selection of specific imaging tests is guided by the clinical presentation. Several imaging methods are available to confirm EC. Because the correct interpretation of symptomatic and asymptomatic lesions on diagnostic imaging studies requires a thorough knowledge of the patient's clinical presentation, it is strongly recommended that clinicoradiographic correlation be made by the examining physician. In each individual case, the "neurologic urgency" for further diagnostic tests must be modified according to the potential for treatment, the patient's condition, and overall prognosis (Fig. 33.1).

Plain radiographs confirm tumor and assess structural stability of the spinal elements. In the patient with cancer at risk for spinal metastases with neck, shoulder, or upper extremity pain, flexion and extension views of the cervical spine should not be forced. Although plain radiographs are >90% sensitive and 86% specific for demonstrating abnormalities in the patient with symptomatic spinal metastases, autopsy series suggest that up to 25% of spinal lesions are invisible on radiography (2). False negatives occur because of mild degree of pathology, because of poor visualization (e.g., the first thoracic vertebra), or because the abnormality is missed on interpretation. The false-positive rate for interpreting collapsed vertebrae as malignant may be as high as 20% (37).

It is estimated that a 30% to 50% change in bone mass is needed before plain films become abnormal (35). On anterior/posterior view, spinal radiographs may show pedicle erosion (the "winking owl" sign), increased interpeduncular distance, paraspinal widening, or paraspinal soft tissue shadow. On lateral view, vertebral collapse (wedging of the body), scalloped bodies, disk space destruction, a narrow spinal canal, hypertrophied facets, and disk calcification may be seen. Oblique views are needed to discriminate spondylotic osteophytic encroachment from tumor causing foraminal abnormality (5). Vertebral collapse and pedicle erosion >50% are especially predictive of EC. On plain radiography, multiple vertebral involvement is noted in up to 86% of patients with spinal tumor (5) and in >30% of patients with EC.

Computed tomography (CT) scan may be useful to better delineate pathology using restricted fields of view (2). CT is superior to other imaging techniques for demonstrating cortical bone architecture (4). Before the availability of MRI, CT scan in combination with myelography was considered the gold standard for demonstrating the level and extent of epidural disease. CT myelogra-

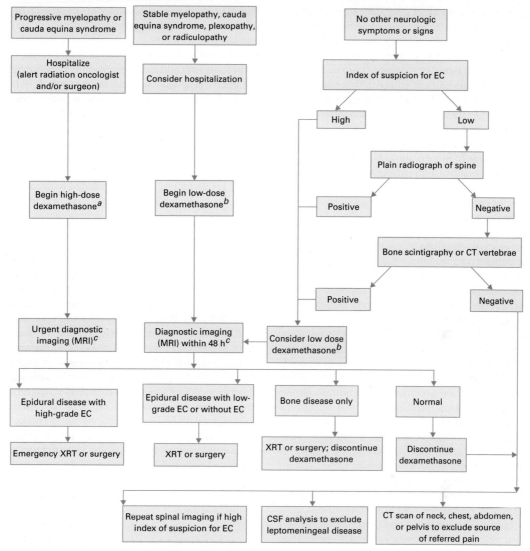

Figure 33.1 Patient with cancer and with back or neck pain—candidate for radiotherapy and/or surgery. CSF, cerebrospinal fluid; CT, computed tomography; MRI, magnetic resonance imaging; EC, epidural compression of the spinal cord and/or cauda equina; XRT, external beam radiotherapy. [a]Higher-dose dexamethasone, 100 mg followed by 24 mg q6h with taper over weeks, not generally recommended due to higher risk. [b]Lower-dose dexamethasone, 10 to 16 mg IV/PO followed by 4 to 6 mg q6h with taper over weeks after definitive therapy. [c]MRI, suggest sagittal screening of vertebral column with expanded imaging of affected areas or CT myelography (see text). (Data from Foley KM. Pain syndromes in patients with cancer. In: Portenoy RK, Kanner RM, eds. *Pain Management: Theory and Practice*. Philadelphia, PA: FA Davis Co; 1995:195; Posner, JB. *Neurological Complications of Cancer, Contemporary Neurology Series*. Vol. 45. Philadelphia, PA: FA Davis Co; 1995:112; Al-Qurainy R, Collis E. Metastatic spinal cord compression: diagnosis and management. *BMJ*. 2016;353:i2539; Kumar A, Weber MH, Gokaslan Z, et al. Metastatic spinal cord compression and steroid treatment: a systematic review. *Clin Spine Surg*. 2017;30(4):156-163; Lawton AJ, Lee KA, Cheville AL, et al. Assessment and management of patients with metastatic spinal cord compression: a multidisciplinary review. *J Clin Oncol*. 2019;37(1):61-71. doi:10.1200/JCO.2018.78.1211. with permission.)

phy may be considered if the index of suspicion for epidural disease is high, and other imaging studies are normal or if MRI cannot be interpreted or performed. Lumbar puncture should precede cervical puncture in most cases. Injection of air to supplement contrast medium may better image a CSF block. If the upper and lower extent of the block cover a long spinal segment, myelography may be repeated after treatment to determine if multiple discrete lesions are present and to better define radiotherapy portals. If repeated imaging is anticipated, oil-based contrast medium may be used to allow for follow-up radiographic imaging without repeated punctures. Another advantage of myelography over other diagnostic imaging tests is the collection of CSF for analysis. However, there is a risk of worsening neurologic function after dural puncture in the patient with partial CSF block, due to the "coning" of the spinal cord as the pressure below the block is relieved. This risk may be as high as 15% (2,14). It is therefore recommended that under these conditions, corticosteroids be administered before dural puncture.

Radionuclide bone scintigrams reveal a 5% to 10% change in bone tissue (35). Bone scintigrams are more sensitive than radiographs except in multiple myeloma (14). However, they are not as specific as radiographs in identifying the level of EC. False positives may be due to nonmalignant skeletal conditions and false negatives due to lytic lesions, for example, myeloma or solid tumors such as lung and melanoma, and prior radiation therapy. If the entire skeleton is involved by tumor, no contrast in the radionuclide uptake may be appreciated. New technology of immunoscintigraphy may prove to be more sensitive (2).

MRI is considered the imaging procedure of choice for EC. MRI without contrast enhancement may eliminate the need for other imaging studies. MRI sensitivity and specificity rival that of CT myelography and are better with contrast. In the patient with back pain and radicular symptoms but no bony tumor on plain radiograph, gadolinium-enhanced MRI is indicated to identify intraforaminal disease such as that which occurs in lymphoma and some solid tumors (35). Double-dose gadolinium-enhanced MRI may increase the accuracy. MRI with and without contrast excludes vertebral metastases, paravertebral lesions, EC, intramedullary tumor, and many leptomeningeal processes. Fat suppression and T_2 weighting, not supplemented by addition of contrast, may improve the detection of myeloma lesions (38). In previously irradiated bone, MRI signal intensity is increased and gadolinium contrast enhancement is decreased.

In the cancer patient with back pain and suspected EC, complete spine MRI is indicated when there is a high risk of noncontiguous or "skip" lesions. A full spine sagittal "screening" image to identify targets for more detailed imaging is suggested (5). Often, the cervical spine is not imaged because it adds significantly to sequencing time. Failure to identify multiple levels of EC may compromise radiotherapy if untreated lesions become symptomatic and are detected at a later time. The cost effectiveness of sagittal screening studies for identifying treatable lesions has not yet been determined. In patients with claustrophobia or severe pain in the supine position, conscious sedation or general anesthesia may be required to complete the MRI. The risk of sedation or anesthesia for MRI must be weighed against the risks of alternative imaging procedures, such as CT myelography, for each individual patient. Newer tumor imaging techniques may add to the diagnostic evaluation of patients with spinal malignancies in future. MRI is more efficient than bone scintigraphy in detecting metastases and is essential for treatment planning, but bone scintigraphy is more cost efficient for evaluating the entire skeleton (39). Cholewinski et al. (40) reported that fluorodeoxyglucose-positron emission tomography/computerized tomography (FGD-PET/CT) may be needed to precisely delineate tumor pathology. Allan et al. (41) tested a telephone hotline and a rapid referral process for cancer patients to report new symptoms of neurologic urgency that resulted in more timely diagnosis and intervention.

Scales that rate the severity of EC and spinal instability provide valid reliable instruments for clinical use and can be incorporated in a classification scheme for multicenter comparisons (42–44).

CSF examination is not required for the diagnosis of epidural tumor, and as noted in the preceding text, dural puncture may pose risk to the patient with EC and should therefore be avoided. If performed, CSF analysis may show elevated protein with normal glucose and, rarely, pleocytosis in the patient with EC.

The patient presenting with EC and an unknown primary tumor generally undergoes a battery of tests to identify the primary neoplasm. At times, biopsy of a vertebral, epidural, or paraspinal lesion is needed to determine the primary tumor histology.

MANAGEMENT OF ACUTE SPINAL CORD OR CAUDA EQUINA COMPRESSION

Metastatic EC of the spinal cord and cauda equina causes significant morbidity in patients with systemic cancer. As survival in these patients is improving with improved oncologic treatment, metastatic spine involvement is encountered increasingly often. However, the treatment for this condition remains mainly palliative. The preferred surgical management is early circumferential decompression of the spinal cord/cauda equina with concomitant spine stabilization. Advances in surgical techniques and refining approaches according to specific patient selection criteria are leading to improved clinical outcomes. Patients with radiosensitive tumors without significant neurologic deficit will likely benefit from radiotherapy. Spinal stereotactic radiosurgery and minimally invasive techniques, such as vertebroplasty and kyphoplasty, with or without radiofrequency ablation, are being used in selected patients with spinal metastases with encouraging results. There are relative contraindications to percutaneous vertebral augmentation (see below).

Pharmacologic Interventions

Corticosteroids are the mainstay of pharmacologic therapy for acute EC (45). The administration of these agents prevents lipid peroxidation of neuronal cell membranes, ischemia, and increased intracellular calcium (46). Vasogenic edema in EC has been demonstrated to be responsive to corticosteroids. Cytotoxic edema may also play a role. Typically given, dexamethasone acts by down-regulating the production of vascular endothelial growth factor and prostaglandin E2 decreasing spinal cord edema thus delaying neurologic decline. Alternative steroids and other agents to treat edema, such as mannitol, may be used.

The timing of administration and dosage of corticosteroids may affect neurologic outcome, and there is some evidence for a therapeutic window (2,46). Better analgesic effect of higher dose regimens has been demonstrated in one study (47). Many authors favored a prolonged course of high-dose corticosteroids, for example, the equivalent of a bolus of 100 mg dexamethasone followed by 96 mg/d in divided doses, tapered over a few weeks for high-grade EC, and recommended bolus of 10 to 16 mg dexamethasone followed by 16 to 24 mg/d in divided doses with a taper for low-grade EC (2,5,47). However, significant risks associated with the high-dose regimen are now thought to outweigh potential benefits for EC. High-dose corticosteroid therapy may be more analgesic, but it increases the risk of side effects (48).

Side effects depend on the duration of drug administration, cumulative dose, and regimen. In one prospective study of patients with EC treated with high-dose corticosteroids, it was noted that depressive symptoms and neuropsychiatric disorders were more common than in similar patients not receiving such treatment (49). Suppression of the hypothalamic–pituitary–adrenal axis occurs with sustained dosing; it is suggested that dosing be readministered after withdrawal in situations of severe physiologic stress. Steroid-induced osteoporosis may be reversible in the young (50). Other withdrawal symptoms, including *Pneumocystis* infection, have been reported. Corticosteroids are metabolized by the cytochrome P-450 system, which has implications for drug interactions with anticonvulsants and other medications; this potential interaction with anticonvulsants may be the least with valproate sodium (46). Clinicians should also be aware that rapid administration of steroids causes severe burning pain in the perineum;

therefore, it is preferable that doses not be given as intravenous push. Except in emergency situations, corticosteroids should be held before making the cancer diagnosis if lymphoma is suspected because of the immediate oncolytic effect, which would impede diagnosis of that condition.

Virtually all patients presenting with EC have severe pain requiring opioid analgesics. Practitioners should be prepared to initiate and rapidly titrate an opioid analgesic to effect. This may require high parenteral doses, especially in patients with neurologic involvement (51,52).

Bisphosphonates should be considered as they are effective in reducing risk of pathological fractures, relieving pain and reducing hypercalcemia associated with malignancy in neoplasms that produce osteolytic lesions. EC is considered one of the cancer pain emergencies to be immediately treated (53).

Nonpharmacologic Interventions

Radiation Therapy

Radiation therapy for EC is chosen to inhibit tumor growth, restore and preserve neurologic function, alleviate pain, and improve quality of life. The course of external beam radiotherapy (XRT) for spinal metastases and EC depends on the radiosensitivity of the tumor and its extent. XRT will be the primary treatment for some patients with EC. The treatment course may be accelerated for patients in severe pain. The spinal section routinely treated includes two vertebral segments above and below a single site of neurologic compression. Anterior/posterior portals are set to include the vertebral body, especially in low thoracic and lumbar lesions. Fields are also designed to accommodate paravertebral tumor. A single port field can be used in very ill patients affected by cachexia. As there are no known predictive factors for epidural progression with multiple sites of spinal disease, the decision to treat asymptomatic noncontiguous sites depends on clinical judgment. In addition to the clinical condition of the patient, factors to be considered include the type of tumor, presence of vertebral collapse, and anticipated future difficulty in matching radiation portals. Special techniques are required to reirradiate. XRT alone is >85% effective for EC in radiosensitive tumors (3). Motor improvement is seen in 49% and stabilization of function in another 31% of patients. However, <50% of patients regain their lost function (3). The possibility of progression to EC may be reduced by irradiating vertebral bony lesions. It is uncertain whether radiation treats micrometastases or prevents them. The response to XRT may be delayed in some cases; the factors accounting for this observation are not well understood (2).

Brachytherapy can be used for adjacent paraspinal masses and may prevent EC (54).

American Society for Radiation Oncology (ASTRO's) Evidence-Based Guideline Task Force concluded that XRT remains the mainstay of treatment for EC (55). Surgical decompression with postoperative radiotherapy is recommended for certain patients.

Loblaw et al. (56) recommended 8 Gy in single fraction is as effective as multiple fractions in patients with poor prognosis, although enrollment in clinical trials is urged. Rades et al. (57) demonstrated that long-course compared with short-course radiotherapy resulted in better progression-free survival and local disease control.

Radiosurgery of the spine was effective in a series of multiple myeloma patients, without apparent detriment to the spinal cord (58) and also in another series of patients with mixed tumor types (59). Radiosurgery following spine surgery is also being advocated to produce significantly better local disease control (60). Escalation of standard radiotherapy dose has not proven beneficial (61), but reirradiation can be considered using high-precision techniques that are now available (62). Stereotactic body radiotherapy (SBRT) has been studied (63).

Stereotactic body RT typically involves the delivery of one or a few large dose fractions of 8 to 30 Gy per fraction conformed to the shape of the tumor, under imaging guidance.

Nearly twice the amount of radiation as conventional external beam therapy can be delivered. The primary indication for SBRT pain associated with spinal metastases. The American Society for Radiation Oncology currently recommends that patients with poor performance status should not be managed with SBRT. Stereotactic radiosurgery may be considered in selected cases.

Surgery

Surgical intervention for EC may be performed for the following:

1. To establish the cancer diagnosis when it is in doubt and when tissue is required for histologic examination
2. To achieve surgical cure for a primary neoplasm
3. To treat prior irradiated radioresistant tumor with symptomatic progression of EC
4. To decompress neural structures and stabilize the spine
5. To halt a rapid clinical deterioration

The specific goals of surgery are to resect pathology, restore load-bearing capacity, decompress neural structures, achieve stability, alleviate pain, and improve quality of life. Length of survival may be extended with improvement in functional status.

Patchell et al. showed superior clinical outcomes for first-line decompressive surgery combined with postoperative radiotherapy compared with radiotherapy alone in patients with spinal cord displacement due to tumor compression. Criteria for the study entry included single-level compression, <48 hours paraplegia at the worst, prognosis of at least 3 months, and good overall condition. Patients with highly radiosensitive malignancies were excluded from participation. Study patients were treated with corticosteroids and randomized to receive 30 Gy of radiotherapy within 24 hours or surgical decompression within 24 hours followed by the same radiotherapy within 14 days of surgery. Better clinical outcomes were demonstrated for both primary end point (ability to walk) and secondary end points. The secondary end points included survival time; continence; requirement for opioid and corticosteroid medications; and function as assessed with formal functional rating scales (Frankel Functional Scale and American Spinal Injury Association Motor Score). More surgical patients retained the ability to walk ($p = 0.012$), and those able to walk at the time of enrollment retained this ability longer, having received surgery (median 153 vs. 54 days, $p = 0.024$). Continence, muscle strength, and functionality were significantly better in the surgical group ($p = 0.016$, $p = 0.001$, and $p = 0.0006$, respectively). A nonsignificant trend toward longer survival was also observed in the surgical group. Duration of hospitalization showed no difference. The results observed during the clinical trial were sufficient to meet early termination criteria, and enrollment was halted. The study supports primary surgical intervention for patients with characteristics similar to those studied (64).

For patients with more complex malignant neurologic involvement and those with a higher degree of comorbidity, individualized risk/benefit analyses may favor nonsurgical treatment (65).

Many factors affect the choice of surgical technique, including tumor location, tumor extent, integrity of adjacent vertebral segments, and general debility. In vascular tumors such as renal and thyroid, operative intervention may be preceded by vascular embolization. Tumor decompression and stabilization may be achieved through either an anterior vertebrectomy or a laminectomy. Posterior decompression through wide laminectomy is generally followed by stabilization to prevent kyphosis (2,66–68). Newer posterolateral techniques are being used for specific EC syndromes in patients with advanced cancer.

In one thorough retrospective study of 110 patients after aggressive surgical intervention for spinal metastases, 82% of patients showed improvement in pain relief and ambulatory status (69). The goals of the treatment were identified as gross total resection of tumor and spine reconstruction. Half of the patients had prior treatment and were deteriorating clinically. The "traditional" criteria for surgery, such as relapse after radiation therapy and the determination of histology, were expanded to include gross tumor resection for radioresistant or solitary lesions and for spinal stabilization. In this series, more complex surgical instrumentation was used than previously reported. Most patients received ongoing systemic therapy, partly confounding the analysis of long-term outcomes. The complication rate of 48% correlated with age older than 65, prior spinal treatment, and the presence of paraparesis. These factors also correlated with greater morbidity and poorer survival. However, in this series, nearly half of the patients were alive at 2 years, an improvement over prior studies that had compared the posterior surgical laminectomy and radiation therapy with radiation therapy alone. This improvement in survival was noted in patients with more advanced cancer and prior treatment. These authors concluded on the basis of prior reports (70,71) and the data from this series that the anterior surgical approach with stabilization may improve outcomes and suggested further definition of the subset of patients that might benefit from early anterior resection and spinal stabilization.

Early reviews of surgical outcomes have confirmed higher morbidity and mortality in patients with prior spine irradiation, age older than 70, and those with poor performance status at the time of surgery (72). In one reported series, the factors predictive of shorter survival were poorer preoperative neurologic status (leg strength grade 3/5 or weaker), anatomical site of the primary carcinoma (lung or colon cancer), and multiple vertebral body involvement. These authors consider that surgical intervention contraindicated if two or more of those factors are present (71). Several authors have suggested that a limited posterolateral approach to tumor resection be reserved for patients with expected survival <6 months (69,73). Few data are available with regard to surgical intervention for lateral epidural or intraforaminal disease. In a recent experience, a small group of patients, not considered candidates for major surgical procedures, benefited from limited resection of lateral epidural tumor. Surgery was preceded by careful correlation of symptoms with tumor mass, and good outcomes were recorded in all eight patients (73). This experience again supports careful consideration in each case until the criteria for primary surgical intervention are more fully delineated. Clearly, further refinement of surgical approaches depends on precise neuroanatomic localization of neoplastic involvement.

The complication rate for spinal surgery may be as high as 30% in patients who have undergone prior XRT (3). Coagulopathy and exogenous anticoagulants increase the risk of hematoma at the operative site. Difficult wound healing, infection, bony instability, nonfusion, displacement of implants, and other complications may occur.

There has been a steady evolution in the concepts and execution of surgical management for EC. In choosing primary surgical versus radiotherapeutic intervention, the prognosis for neurologic improvement and expected impact on functional status must be considered. In some series, radiation therapy has been shown to be equally effective to laminectomy and radiation, but with <50% neurologic improvement overall (11). De novo anterior–posterior resection with spine stabilization may result in better outcomes than laminectomy and radiation or radiation alone, as surgical complications are generally manageable, survival is improved and patients may remain ambulatory longer, although the 2-year survival rate for lung cancer may be 10% and for colorectal cancer only 17% (69). The data are as yet insufficient to draw final conclusions regarding pain and quality-of-life outcomes in all patients, but as discussed in the preceding text, there is a subset of patients presenting with single-level spinal cord displacement that will benefit from primary surgical intervention. The decision to recommend initial radiation therapy versus surgical intervention must be individualized, especially in those patients with more complex presentations. To date, the cauda equina syndrome has not been well studied. It has been suggested that without bony instability, the speed of progression of neurologic deficit and radiosensitivity of the tumor are the main factors to consider in determining primary antineoplastic treatment with either surgery or radiation. Severe deficits generally hold a poor prognosis independent of treatment.

Tancioni et al. (74) advocated a miniinvasive percutaneous approach for the poor prognostic group. Chaichana et al. (75) reported that the prognostic value of the presence of vertebral fracture with EC is independently associated with decreased postoperative ambulatory status and also that preoperative nonambulatory patients required more extensive surgery and had more postoperative complications (76). Preoperative radiotherapy decreased the likelihood of regaining ambulatory status, whereas postoperative radiotherapy and symptoms of <48 hours duration predicted positively for regaining ambulation. Putz et al. (77) found similarly and also noted individual health status to be a contributing factor to postoperative outcome. Chaichana et al. (78) also reported differences in outcomes according to primary tumor type.

Williams et al. (79) advocated aggressive surgical decompression and reconstruction for EC secondary to prostate cancer. Walcott et al. (80) and Tancioni et al. (81) reviewed their series of open spine surgeries for EC in breast cancer and concluded that aggressive therapy is warranted even in the setting of advanced and progressive systemic disease. Laufer et al. (82) suggested that reoperation in carefully selected patients can prolong ambulation and result in good functional and neurologic outcomes.

Chen et al. (83) reported good results from use of a posterolateral transpedicular approach or combined posterior anterior approaches for patients with lung cancer and also described a transpedicular partial corpectomy without anterior vertebral reconstruction in thoracic lesions (84). The posterior transpedicular approach for ventral cervical (85) and thoracic (86) spine tumors and an extended lateral parascapular approach for thoracic spine tumors (87) have been described.

Tancioni et al. (88) also reported that combined surgery and radiotherapy yielded clinical remission of pain in 91%, neurologic improvement in 72%, and 44% overall 1-year survival that was correlated with primary tumor type.

Prolonged cancer survival has led to an increase in the incidence of spinal metastases and vertebral compression fractures with associated mechanical instability, axial pain, and progressive radiculomyelopathy. Vertebral augmentation techniques, vertebroplasty and kyphoplasty, are minimally invasive techniques of percutaneous injection of bone cement (methyl methacrylate) directly into vertebral bodies. With a low complication rate, these procedures are being used more commonly in conjunction with other treatments and even as first-line approach for management of painful malignant spine fractures. Bouza et al. (89) performed an evidence-based review of balloon kyphoplasty in malignant disease and concluded that there is level III evidence for this procedure with further investigation being warranted. Dalbayrak et al. (90) reported prospectively that there is a correlation between symptom duration and restoration of vertebral body height after kyphoplasty. Positive results were reported from a randomized controlled prospective trial of kyphoplasty (91), a retrospective review of kyphoplasty

(92), and of percutaneous vertebroplasty (93,94). Zou et al. (95) suggested MRI signal localization of symptomatic myeloma lesions for targeting procedure site. Hirsch et al. (96) reported that the sequence of combined External Bean Radiation Therapy (EBRT) and Vertebral Augmentation (VA) does not affect outcomes.

Samarium 153-ethylene administered intravertebrally with kyphoplasty is a procedure to be studied further (97,98). Kyphoplasty with intraoperative radiation therapy (IORT) (99) is also being investigated. A series of patients treated with percutaneous transpedicular coblation corpectomy followed by immediate balloon kyphoplasty and subsequent radiosurgery have been reported with good outcomes (100).

In a comprehensive review, Tsoumakidou et al. (48) summarized absolute and relative contraindications to vertebral augmentation in EC as follows (modified):

Absolute contraindications:

- Asymptomatic VCFs or patient improving on medical treatment without worsening of the collapse
- Unstable spinal fracture
- Severe uncorrectable coagulopathy
- Allergy to bone cement or opacification agents

Relative contraindications:

- Radicular pain
- Tumor extension into the vertebral canal or cord compression
- Fracture of the posterior column, as there is increased risk of cement leakage and posterior displacement of loose fragment(s)
- Sclerotic metastasis, as the risk of cement leakage is high
- Diffuse metastases (>5)

Nonsurgical stabilization of the bony spine can be accomplished with a cervical collar or body bracing. The patient with cancer, neck pain, and suspected cervical spine disease should be placed in a collar, while diagnostic evaluation is being conducted.

Chemotherapy may be the sole antineoplastic therapy against EC (101), for example lymphoma, plasma cell tumors, germ cell tumors, and small cell lung cancer (9).

ONGOING CARE

Pain Management

Corticosteroid administration is the primary medical management of acute EC that confers analgesia and neuroprotection. Extended corticosteroid administration (i.e., for the duration of life in patients with EC and short prognosis) has not been well studied, but it is common in clinical practice. This practice should be discouraged unless there is an evidence of ongoing steroid-reversible neurologic deficits due to the high risk of steroid toxicities, as discussed in Section *Pharmacologic Interventions* (101).

Guidelines for the use of nonsteroidal anti-inflammatory medications, opioid analgesics, and adjuvant analgesics for neuropathic pain have been published in recent years (102–106). Chronic opioid therapy is often required for persistent pain after treatment of EC. Cases have been reported in which patients with EC required prolonged high-dose intrathecal infusion of opioid and local anesthetic to obtain adequate analgesia (107,108). Spinal instrumentation should be cautiously considered in patients with spinal tumor involvement. Radionuclides are discussed in other chapters.

Neuroablative procedures are considered when the benefit-to-risk ratio favors analgesia over the potential for further neurologic compromise. Destruction of the nervous tissue may be accomplished by anesthetic or surgical means. Chemical epidural neurolysis may be chosen to effect single or multiple nerve root interruption. Intrathecal neurolysis would be anticipated to achieve analgesia over a wider territory and may be selected when the epidural space is compromised. Both approaches entail the risk of acute neurologic deterioration, which may be irreversible (109). Neurosurgical ablation of nerve roots (rhizotomy) involves surgery and is less often indicated in very sick patients. Midline myelotomy may be indicated in patients with severe midline sacral pain and bladder or bowel compromise due to tumor of the sacrum. Spinothalamic tractotomy or cordotomy, although more easily performed as a percutaneous procedure, is not generally useful for pain in association with spine disease or EC. Hypophysectomy for diffuse painful metastatic bone disease may yield success rates as high as 90% in some endocrine-responsive tumors (110).

Integration of pharmacologic and nonpharmacologic analgesic therapies is needed for most patients with EC. A multidisciplinary approach to pain management and rehabilitation of patients with resected sacral chordoma has been reported (111).

Rehabilitation

Each patient's rehabilitation program must be individually tailored and continually reassessed and modified. For some patients, comprehensive care may be best accomplished in a formal inpatient rehabilitation setting (112). Specific rehabilitation goals are to improve ambulation, achieve weight bearing and transfers, restore bladder and bowel function, and protect the skin. The family is included in learning how to assist the patient with severely impaired mobility.

Spinal orthotics stabilize the spine and may decrease spinal pain by limiting motion. Physical therapy techniques for pain relief include ultrasound and transcutaneous electrical nerve stimulation. Evidence-based complementary integrative health modalities including massage therapy may reduce the need for medication management of cancer pain and nonpain symptoms.

Approximately, 50% of patients require urinary catheterization before and after XRT for EC (3). Sexual dysfunction may be treatable with physical and medical interventions.

A number of medical problems common to the cancer population may limit aggressive rehabilitation efforts. Organ failure due to the disease or its treatment, hemodynamic instability, poor nutrition, cancer cachexia, hematologic complications, and multiple physical and psychological symptoms may complicate rehabilitation. An active exercise program may have to be modified. Weakness due to spinal cord or nerve root compression may be complicated by concurrent peripheral neuropathy or myopathy, which are common complications of antineoplastic treatment. The skin of many patients with cancer is relatively more prone to breakdown and infection. Skin care and protection are essential, especially in the bedridden patient.

Chronic musculoskeletal problems may occur in children after spine irradiation during growth, due to the development of secondary spinal deformities. The risk of fracture in osteoporotic or tumor-laden bones should be carefully evaluated before initiating a mobility program. In patients who are paraparetic or paraplegic, prophylactic fixation of upper extremity lesions may be considered to aid mobility and weight bearing. In bedridden patients with multiple impending fractures, positioning and transfers must be undertaken with great caution.

The goals of physical medicine and rehabilitation in the patient with EC range from active programs to supportive and palliative care (113). Preventive rehabilitation therapy is directed toward achieving maximal functional restoration in patients who are cured or are in stable remission from their cancer. Continued encouragement for the effort required in aggressive rehabilitation is needed for a progressive decline in function due to advancing disease. For patients with limited prognosis, usually considered as <6 months' life expectancy, family participation receives more emphasis. The needs of the patient tend toward more dependent care as the cancer progresses. Palliative rehabilitation interventions are intended to provide comfort to the patient in the terminal stages of illness, and as noted in the preceding text, include the family.

Fattal (114,115) reviewed 38 available studies, most retrospective, to conclude that with 55% overall 12-month survival, short duration (1 to 2 month) rehabilitation stays are indicated to maximize functional benefit and patients' time with family. Improvements in ambulation, pain, and bladder/bowel function were observed.

Psychological Interventions and Palliative Care

Ongoing psychological support of the patient with metastatic spine disease is essential. Issues of loss of independence and function require careful attention. Families will often benefit from emotional support for anticipatory grieving. Professional assistance may be indicated as the burden of care increases with a patient's progressing disease. The palliative care team is able to assist with complex therapeutic decision analysis and provides essential psychosocial support in this setting.

CLINICAL OUTCOMES

The potential for the recovery of function in patients with tumor involvement of the spine and associated neurologic structures varies by tumor type (primary or metastatic), the number of vertebrae involved, the nature and degree of neurologic involvement at presentation, the oncologic status, and the general medical condition. In most series, approximately 50% of patients with metastatic spine tumors are ambulatory at presentation, 35% are paretic, and 15% are plegic (2). Up to 30% of patients with weakness become plegic within the first week of presentation (5). The prognosis for regaining ambulatory status in patients with EC who begin therapy while being ambulatory is 75%; prognosis declines to 30% to 50% for patients who begin therapy while being paretic and to 10% for those who begin therapy while being plegic (35). The duration of neurologic symptoms before treatment also affects the prognosis for neurologic recovery. If paraplegia has been present for days or if urinary retention is present for >30 hours, the likelihood of recovery is decreased (116). Rapidly progressing symptoms confer a worse prognosis.

Standardized scales have been developed to assess the degree of epidural disease and the stability of the spine (43,44). Guidelines are formulated and continually updated to assist interdisciplinary

teams in the management of these complex patients (53,117).

In a more recent meta-analysis of studies constituting almost 5,000 patients, it was confirmed that ambulatory status before treatment, interval from symptom to treatment <48 hours, and developing motor deficits in >14 days are considered as the most significant positive prognostic factors for posttreatment ambulatory status. EC is a surgical emergency and should have a higher priority with immediate intervention before patients become nonambulatory or develop irreversible neurologic deficits. Prompt identification of early symptoms and regular outpatient review might prevent poor outcomes from EC. Better ECOG-PS, KPS, and Frankel grades were noted to be positively correlated with ambulatory status, resulting in higher probability of neurologic improvement (118).

Patients who remain unable to ambulate after irradiation treatment for EC have a particularly poor prognosis for survival, owing to the complications of paresis and more advanced disease. Survival rates for patients with EC are 40% at 1 year if ambulatory before and after radiation treatment, whereas patients who are nonambulatory before and ambulatory after treatment have a survival rate of 30% at 1 year and 20% at 3 years. Prognosis falls to 7% at 1 year for patients who are nonambulatory after treatment (3).

Response to treatment for EC and survival vary with the nature of the malignancy. In patients with prostate cancer, the response to the treatment of neurologic complications depends on whether the patient has received prior hormonal therapy. Better response to hormonal manipulation correlates with longer survival. The median survival of patients with prostate cancer after diagnosis with EC is 6 months; only 34% survive at least 1 year (119). Renal cancer is poorly radioresponsive and median survival time after diagnosis with EC is <4 months (120). Hemorrhagic complications of spinal surgery for metastatic renal tumor may be avoided by preoperative embolization (121). In testicular cancer, chemotherapy is effective for untreated lesions or for responsive tumors (122), but radiation and surgery may be considered if the disease is not chemoresponsive (120). Up to 75% of patients with melanoma and EC respond to radiation therapy (123–125). Patients with carcinoid tumor and EC have a median survival of 6 months.

Ambulatory status may be preserved with radiation in up to 90% of patients with carcinoid tumors (21). In myeloma, long-term survival is common. In a series of patients with multiple myeloma, the 1-year survival rate was 100%, and the median survival 37 months after EC was diagnosed (126).

Solitary plasmacytomas are generally irradiated and surgically removed. Patients with multiple myeloma often receive radiation therapy to maximum spinal cord tolerance before surgical intervention is considered. Most lymphomas respond to chemotherapy and radiation. In pediatric patients, surgery may be preferred for radioresistant sarcomas and small cell tumors (Ewing's sarcoma, neuroblastoma, lymphoma, and germ cell tumors) presenting with rapid neurologic deterioration. A trend toward extended survival has been shown after surgical decompression in Ewing's sarcoma. Many small cell and germ cell tumors respond to chemotherapy or radiation. Grommes et al. (127). Younger age may confer greater risk of radiation complications (128). Complete resection of primary spinal extraosseous epidural Ewing's sarcoma may be difficult. The 18-month survival rate was <40% in a small series of patients with this unusual malignancy (129).

Chi et al. (130) estimated that the age at which surgery is no longer superior to radiotherapy is between 60 and 70 years and suggested that this may be a factor in selecting treatment.

In one series, overall median survival after first presentation with spinal cord compression was noted to be 2.9 months (130).

Less than half of patients treated for EC are alive after 2 months (13). EC is an indicator of poor prognosis. Definitive intervention for EC must therefore be considered in the context of the patient's overall disease status. Systemic antineoplastic therapy may at times precede or entirely supplant intervention targeted at EC. For patients with very advanced cancer, the burden of diagnostic evaluation and intervention to reverse EC often outweighs minimal potential gains in function.

A systematic review of evidence-based treatment of EC identified in 6 trials of 544 patients concluded that ambulatory patients with stable spines may be treated with radiotherapy, while surgery may be preferred for ambulatory patients with poor prognostic factors for radiotherapy and for nonambulatory patients with a single site of compression, paraplegia for <48 hours duration, radioresistant tumors, and survival prognosis of >3 months. Serious adverse effects of high-dose corticosteroids were noted (131,132).

Patients with shorter life expectancies are offered higher doses of radiation in shorter treatment courses, while those with less extensive disease are managed with lower doses over a longer period of time. Adverse effects of RT include gastrointestinal toxicity, mucositis, bone marrow suppression, and several subtypes of radiation-induced myelopathy. Acute transient radiation myelopathy is the most common subtype that presents 1 to 29 months after completion of RT is a result of demyelination of the dorsal columns. Chronic progressive radiation myelopathy occurs 9 to 15 months following RT and has been reported in 1% to 5% of patients who reach 1-year survival, presenting with ascending weakness and diminished sensation. Acute complete radiation myelopathy is related to radiation-induced vascular damage resulting in spinal cord infarction, whereas lower motor neuron disease occurs due to anterior horn cell damage (133).

Questions remain regarding the optimal treatment of EC, including defining the role of stereotactic radiotherapy to improve mobility in patients with spinal metastasis from radioresistant tumors and patients who have received prior standard radiotherapy; determining if early surgical intervention reduces the incidence of EC in those with bony disease; establishing the role of vertebral augmentation in cancer metastases; and how to refine selection criteria for specific radiotherapy treatment protocols.

Although few studies of quality of life have been conducted in this population, pain control should remain a high priority regardless of prognosis.

While we await additional scientific evidence and advances in available treatments, clinicians caring for patients with spinal neoplasm and EC are advised to work in a coordinated interdisciplinary fashion to carefully select those interventions that will achieve therapeutic goals for each individual patient. It is best for clinicians to engage with patient and family in a palliative care framework to make therapeutic decisions that are designed to alleviate pain, improve function, and enhance quality of life to the greatest extent possible.

REFERENCES

1. Loeser JD. Neurosurgical approaches in palliative care. In: Doyle D, Hanks GWC, MacDonald N, eds. *Oxford Textbook of Palliative Medicine*. Oxford, UK: Oxford University Press; 1993:221.
2. Posner JB. *Neurologic Complications of Cancer, Contemporary Neurology Series*. Vol. 45. Philadelphia, PA: FA Davis; 1995:112.
3. Perrin RG, Janjan NA, Langford LA. Spinal axis metastases. In: Levin VA, ed. *Cancer in the Nervous System*. New York, NY: Churchill Livingstone; 1996:259.
4. Byrne TN, Waxman SG. *Spinal Cord Compression: Diagnosis and Principles of Management, Contemporary Neurology Series*. Vol. 33. Philadelphia, PA: FA Davis; 1990.
5. Grant R, Papadopoulos SM, Greenberg HS. Metastatic epidural spinal cord compression. *Neurol Clin*. 1991; 9(4):825.
6. Klein SL, Sanford RA, Muhlbauer MS. Pediatric spinal epidural metastases. *J Neurosurg*. 1991;74:70.
7. Barron KD, Hirano A, Araski S, et al. Experiences with metastatic neoplasms involving the spinal cord. *Neurology*. 1959;9:91.
8. Mak KS, Lee LK, Mak RH, et al. Incidence and treatment patterns in hospitalizations for malignant spinal cord compression in the United States, 1998–2006. *Int J Radiat Oncol Biol Phys*. 2011;80(3):824-831.

9. Al-Qurainy R, Collis E. Metastatic spinal cord compression: diagnosis and management. *BMJ*. 2016;353:i2539.

10. Lawton AJ, Lee KA, Cheville AL, et al. Assessment and management of patients with metastatic spinal cord compression: a multidisciplinary review. *J Clin Oncol*. 2019;37(1):61-71. doi:10.1200/JCO.2018.78.1211.

11. Stark RJ, Henson RA, Evans SJW. Spinal metastases: a retrospective survey from a general hospital. *Brain*. 1982;105:189.

12. Boussios S, Cooke D, Hayward C, et al. Metastatic spinal cord compression: unraveling the diagnostic and therapeutic challenges. *Anticancer Res*. 2018;38:4987-4997.

13. Obbens EAMT. Neurological problems in palliative medicine. In: Doyle D, Hanks GWC, MacDonald N, eds. *Oxford Textbook of Palliative Medicine*. Oxford, UK: Oxford University Press; 1993:460.

14. Byrne TN. Spinal metastases. In: Wiley RG, ed. *Neurologic Complications of Cancer*. New York, NY: Marcel Dekker; 1995:23.

15. Harrington KD. Metastatic disease of the spine. In: Harrington KD, ed. *Orthopedic Management of Metastatic Bone Disease*. St. Louis, MO: Mosby; 1988:309.

16. Misulis KE, Wiley RG. Neurological complications of lung cancer. In: Wiley RG, ed. *Neurologic Complications of Cancer*. New York, NY: Marcel Dekker; 1995:295.

17. Anderson NE. Neurological complications of breast cancer. In: Wiley RG, ed. *Neurologic Complications of Cancer*. New York, NY: Marcel Dekker; 1995:319.

18. Kuban DA, El-Mahdi AM, Sigfred SV, et al. Characteristics of spinal cord compression in adenocarcinoma of the prostate. *Urology*. 1986;28:364.

19. Flynn DF, Shipley WU. Management of spinal cord compression secondary to metastatic prostatic carcinoma. *Urol Clin North Am*. 1991;18:145.

20. Moots PL, Wiley RG. Neurological disorders in head and neck cancers. In: Wiley RG, ed. *Neurologic Complications of Cancer*. New York, NY: Marcel Dekker; 1995:353.

21. Hagen NA. Neurological complications of gastrointestinal cancers. In: Wiley RG, ed. *Neurologic Complications of Cancer*. New York, NY: Marcel Dekker; 1995:395.

22. Friedman M, Kim TH, Panahon AM. Spinal cord compression in malignant lymphoma: treatment and results. *Cancer*. 1976;37:1485.

23. Ribeiro RC, Pui CH, Schell MJ. Vertebral compression fracture as a presenting feature of acute lymphoblastic leukemia in children. *Cancer*. 1988;61:589.

24. Jennings MT. Neurological complications of childhood cancer. In: Wiley RG, ed. *Neurologic Complications of Cancer*. New York, NY: Marcel Dekker; 1995:503.

25. Molloy PT, Phillips PC. Neurological complications of sarcomas. In: Wiley RG, ed. *Neurologic Complications of Cancer*. New York, NY: Marcel Dekker; 1995:417.

26. Galasko CSB, Sylvester BS. Back pain in patients treated for malignant tumours. *Clin Oncol*. 1978;4:273.

27. Kanner RM. Low back pain. In: Portenoy RK, Kanner RM, eds. *Pain Management: Theory and Practice, Contemporary Neurology Series*. Vol. 48. Philadelphia, PA: FA Davis; 1996:126.

28. Sty JR, Wells RG, Conway JJ. Spine pain in children. *Semin Nucl Med*. 1993;23(4):296.

29. Manishen WJ, Sivananthan K, Orr FW. Resorbing bone stimulates tumor cell growth. A role for the host microenvironment in bone metastasis. *Am J Pathol*. 1986;123:39.

30. Powell N. Metastatic carcinoma in association with Paget's disease of bone. *Br J Radiol*. 1983;56:582.

31. Tarlov IM, Klinger H. Spinal cord compression studies. II: time limits for recovery after acute compression in dogs. *Arch Neurol Psychiatry*. 1954;71:271.

32. Gledhill RF, Harrison BM, McDonald WI. Demyelination and remyelination after acute spinal cord compression. *Exp Neurol*. 1973;38:472.

33. Burger EL, Lindeque BG. Sacral and non-spinal tumors presenting as backache: a retrospective study of 17 patients. *Acta Orthop Scand*. 1994;65(3):344.

34. Gonzales GR, Elliott KJ, Portenoy RK, et al. The impact of a comprehensive evaluation in the management of cancer pain. *Pain*. 1991;47(2):141.

35. Hewitt DJ, Foley KM. Neuroimaging of pain. In: Greenberg JO, ed. *Neuroimaging*. New York, NY: McGraw-Hill; 1995:41.

36. Gilbert RW, Kim JH, Posner JB. Epidural spinal cord compression from metastatic tumor: diagnosis and treatment. *Ann Neurol*. 1978;3:40.

37. Wong DA, Fornasier VL, MacNab I. Spinal metastases: the obvious, the occult, and the imposters. *Spine*. 1990;15:1.

38. Rhamouni A, Divine M, Mathieu D, et al. Detection of multiple myeloma involving the spine: efficacy of fat-suppression and contrast-enhanced MR imaging. *AJR Am J Roentgenol*. 1993;160(5):1049.

39. Chiewvit P, Danchaivijitr N, Sirivitmaitrie K, Chiewvit S, Thephamongkhol K. Does magnetic resonance imaging give value-added than bone scintigraphy in the detection of vertebral metastasis? *J Med Assoc Thai*. 2009;92(6):818-829.

40. Cholewinski W, Castellon I, Raphael B, Heiba SI. Value of precise localization of recurrent multiple myeloma with F-18 FDG PET/CT. *Clin Nucl Med*. 2009;34(1):1-3.

41. Allan L, Baker L, Dewar J, et al. Suspected malignant cord compression—improving time to diagnosis via a "hotline": a prospective audit. *Br J Cancer*. 2009;100(12):1867-1872.

42. Bilsky MH, Laufer I, Fourney DR, et al. Reliability analysis of the epidural spinal cord compression scale. *J Neurosurg Spine*. 2010;13(3):324-328.

43. Fourney DR, Frangou EM, Ryken TC, et al. Spinal instability neoplastic score: an analysis of reliability and validity from the spine oncology study group. *J Clin Oncol*. 2011;29:3072-3077.

44. Fisher CG, DiPaola CP, Ryken TC, et al. A novel classification system for spinal instability in neoplastic disease: an evidence-based approach and expert consensus from the Spine Oncology Study Group. *Spine*. 2010;35:E1221-E1229.

45. Kumar A, Weber MH, Gokaslan Z, et al. Metastatic spinal cord compression and steroid treatment: a systematic review. *Clin Spine Surg*. 2017;30(4):156-163.

46. Vecht CJ, Verbiest HBC. Use of glucocorticoids in neuro-oncology. In: Wiley RG, ed. *Neurologic Complications of Cancer*. New York, NY: Marcel Dekker; 1995:199.

47. Greenberg HS, Kim JH, Posner JB. Epidural spinal cord compression from metastatic tumor: results with a new treatment protocol. *Ann Neurol*. 1980;8:361.

48. Tsoumakidou G, Too C, Koch G, et al. CIRSE guidelines on percutaneous vertebral augmentation. *Cardiovasc Intervent Radiol*. 2017;40:331-342.

49. Breitbart W, Stiefel F, Kornblith AB, et al. Neuropsychiatric disturbances in cancer patients with epidural spinal cord compression receiving high dose corticosteroids: a prospective comparison study. *Psychooncology*. 1993;2:233-245.

50. Pocock NA, Eisman JA, Dunstan CR, et al. Recovery from steroid induced osteoporosis. *Ann Intern Med*. 1987;107:319.

51. Yoshioka H, Tsuneto S, Kashiwagi T. Pain control with morphine for vertebral metastases and sciatica in advanced cancer patients. *J Palliat Care*. 1994;10(1):10.

52. Swarm R, Abernethy AP, Anghelescu DL, et al. NCCN adult cancer pain. *J Natl Compr Canc Netw.* 2010;8(9):1046-1086.

53. Swarm RA, Paice JA, Anghelescu DL, et al. Adult Cancer Pain, Version 3.2019, NCCN Clinical Practice Guidelines in Oncology. *JNCCN.* 2019;17(8):977-1007.

54. Armstrong JG, Fass DE, Bains M, et al. Paraspinal tumors: techniques and results of brachytherapy. *Int J Radiat Oncol Biol Phys.* 1991;20:787.

55. Lutz S, Berk L, Chang E, et al. Palliative radiotherapy for bone metastases: an ASTRO evidence-based guideline. *Int J Radiat Oncol Biol Phys.* 2011;79(4):965-976.

56. Loblaw A, Mitera G. Malignant extradural spinal cord compression in men with prostate cancer. *Curr Opin Support Palliat Care.* 2011;5(3):206-210.

57. Rades D, Lange M, Veninga T, et al. Preliminary results of spinal cord compression recurrence evaluation (score-1) study comparing short-course versus long-course radiotherapy for local control of malignant epidural spinal cord compression. *Int J Radiat Oncol Biol Phys.* 2009;73(1):228-234.

58. Jin R, Rock J, Jin JY, et al. Single fraction spine radiosurgery for myeloma epidural spinal cord compression. *J Exp Ther Oncol.* 2009;8(1):35-41.

59. Ryu S, Rock J, Jain R, et al. Radiosurgical decompression of metastatic epidural compression. *Cancer.* 2010;116(9):2250-2257.

60. Moulding HD, Elder JB, Lis E, et al. Local disease control after decompressive surgery and adjuvant high-dose single-fraction radiosurgery for spine metastases. *J Neurosurg Spine.* 2010;13(1):87-93.

61. Rades D, Freundt K, Meyners T, et al. Dose escalation for metastatic spinal cord compression in patients with relatively radioresistant tumors. *Int J Radiat Oncol Biol Phys.* 2011;80(5):1492-1497.

62. Rades D, Abrahm JL. The role of radiotherapy for metastatic epidural spinal cord compression. *Nat Rev Clin Oncol.* 2010;7(10):590-598.

63. Sahgal A, Bilsky M, Chang EL, et al. Stereotactic body radiotherapy for spinal metastases: current status, with a focus on its application in the postoperative patient. *J Neurosurg Spine.* 2011;14(2):151-166.

64. Patchell RA, Tibbs PA, Regine WF, et al. Direct decompressive surgical resection in the treatment of spinal cord compression caused by metastatic cancer: a randomised trial. *Lancet.* 2005;366:643-648.

65. Gerber DE, Grossman SA. Does decompressive surgery improve outcome in patients with metastatic epidural spinal-cord compression? *Nat Clin Pract Neurol.* 2006;2:10-11.

66. Galasko CSB. Orthopaedic principles and management. In: Doyle D, Hanks GWC, MacDonald N, eds. *Oxford Textbook of Palliative Medicine.* Oxford, UK: Oxford University Press; 1993:274.

67. Findlay GFG. Adverse effects of the management of malignant spinal cord compression. *J Neurol Neurosurg Psychiatry.* 1984;47:761.

68. McBroom R. Radiation or surgery for metastatic disease of the spine? *Soc Med Curr Med Lit—Orthop.* 1988;1:97.

69. Sundaresan N, Sachdev VP, Holland JF, et al. Surgical treatment of spinal cord compression from epidural metastasis. *J Clin Oncol.* 1995;13(9):2330.

70. Sioutos PJ, Arbit E, Meshulam BS, et al. Spinal metastases from solid tumors: analysis of factors affecting survival. *Cancer.* 1995;76(8):1453.

71. Siegal T, Siegal TZ. Surgical decompression of anterior and posterior malignant epidural tumors compressing the spinal cord: a prospective study. *Neurosurgery.* 1985;17:424-432.

72. Sundaresan N, Digiacinto GV, Hughes JEO, et al. Treatment of neoplastic spinal cord compression: results of a prospective study. *Neurosurgery.* 1991;29:645.

73. Weller SJ, Rossitch E Jr. Unilateral posterolateral decompression without stabilization for neurological palliation of symptomatic spinal metastases in debilitated patients. *J Neurosurg.* 1995;82(5):739.

74. Tancioni F, Navarria P, Pessina F, et al. Early surgical experience with minimally invasive percutaneous approach for patients with Metastatic Epidural Spinal Cord Compression (MESCC) to poor prognoses. *Ann Surg Oncol.* 2012;19(1):294-300.

75. Chaichana KL, Pendleton C, Wolinsky JP, Gokaslan ZL, Sciubba DM. Vertebral compression fractures in patients presenting with metastatic epidural spinal cord compression. *Neurosurgery.* 2009;65(2):267-274; discussion 274-275.

76. Chaichana KL, Woodworth GF, Sciubba DM, et al. Predictors of ambulatory function after decompressive surgery for metastatic epidural spinal cord compression. *Neurosurgery.* 2008;62(3):683-692; discussion 683-692.

77. Putz C, van Middendorp JJ, Pouw MH, et al. Malignant cord compression: a critical appraisal of prognostic factors predicting functional outcome after surgical treatment. *J Craniovertebr Junction Spine.* 2010;1(2): 67-73.

78. Chaichana KL, Pendleton C, Sciubba DM, Wolinsky JP, Gokaslan ZL. Outcome following decompressive surgery for different histological types of metastatic tumors causing epidural spinal cord compression. Clinical article. *J Neurosurg Spine.* 2009;11(1):56-63.

79. Williams BJ, Fox BD, Sciubba DM, et al. Surgical management of prostate cancer metastatic to the spine. *J Neurosurg Spine.* 2009;10(5):414-422.

80. Walcott BP, Cvetanovich GL, Barnard ZR, Nahed BV, Kahle KT, Curry WT. Surgical treatment and outcomes of metastatic breast cancer to the spine. *J Clin Neurosci.* 2011;18(10):1336-1339.

81. Tancioni F, Navarria P, Mancosu P, et al. Surgery followed by radiotherapy for the treatment of metastatic epidural spinal cord compression from breast cancer. *Spine (Phila Pa 1976).* 2011;36(20):E1352-E1359.

82. Laufer I, Hanover A, Lis E, Yamada Y, Bilsky M. Repeat decompression surgery for recurrent spinal metastases. *J Neurosurg Spine.* 2010;13(1):109-115.

83. Chen YJ, Chang GC, Chen HT, et al. Surgical results of metastatic spinal cord compression secondary to non-small cell lung cancer. *Spine (Phila Pa 1976).* 2007;32(15):E413-E418.

84. Chen YJ, Hsu HC, Chen KH, Li TC, Lee TS. Transpedicular partial corpectomy without anterior vertebral reconstruction in thoracic spinal metastases. *Spine (Phila Pa 1976).* 2007;32(22):E623-E626.

85. Eleraky M, Setzer M, Vrionis FD. Posterior transpedicular corpectomy for malignant cervical spine tumors. *Eur Spine J.* 2010;19(2):257-262.

86. Cho DC, Sung JK. Palliative surgery for metastatic thoracic and lumbar tumors using posterolateral transpedicular approach with posterior instrumentation. *Surg Neurol.* 2009;71(4):424-433.

87. Vecil GG, McCutcheon IE, Mendel E. Extended lateral parascapular approach for resection of a giant multicompartment thoracic schwannoma. *Acta Neurochir (Wien).* 2008;150(12):1295-1300; discussion 1300.

88. Tancioni F, Navarria P, Lorenzetti MA, et al. Multimodal approach to the management of metastatic epidural spinal cord compression (MESCC) due to solid tumors. *Int J Radiat Oncol Biol Phys.* 2010;78(5):1467-1473.

89. Bouza C, López-Cuadrado T, Cediel P, Saz-Parkinson Z, Amate JM. Balloon kyphoplasty in malignant spinal fractures: a systematic review and meta-analysis. *BMC Palliat Care*. 2009;8:12.

90. Dalbayrak S, Onen MR, Yilmaz M, Naderi S. Clinical and radiographic results of balloon kyphoplasty for treatment of vertebral body metastases and multiple myelomas. *J Clin Neurosci*. 2010;17(2):219-224.

91. Berenson J, Pflugmacher R, Jarzem P, et al. Balloon kyphoplasty versus non-surgical fracture management for treatment of painful vertebral body compression fractures in patients with cancer: a multicentre, randomised controlled trial. *Lancet Oncol*. 2011;12(3):225-235.

92. Qian Z, Sun Z, Yang H, Gu Y, Chen K, Wu G. Kyphoplasty for the treatment of malignant vertebral compression fractures caused by metastases. *J Clin Neurosci*. 2011;18(6):763-767.

93. Saliou G, Kocheida el M, Lehmann P, et al. Percutaneous vertebroplasty for pain management in malignant fractures of the spine with epidural involvement. *Radiology*. 2010;254(3):882-890.

94. Sun G, Jin P, Li M, et al. Percutaneous vertebroplasty for pain management in spinal metastasis with epidural involvement. *Technol Cancer Res Treat*. 2011;10(3):267-274.

95. Zou J, Mei X, Gan M, Yang H. Kyphoplasty for spinal fractures from multiple myeloma. *J Surg Oncol*. 2010;102(1):43-47.

96. Hirsch AE, Jha RM, Yoo AJ, et al. The use of vertebral augmentation and external beam radiation therapy in the multimodal management of malignant vertebral compression fractures. *Pain Physician*. 2011;14(5):447-458.

97. Ashamalla H, Cardoso E, Macedon M, et al. Phase I trial of Vertebral Intracavitary Cement and Samarium (VICS): novel technique for treatment of painful vertebral metastasis. *Int J Radiat Oncol Biol Phys*. 2009;75(3):836-842.

98. Gokaslan ZL, McGirt MJ. Kyphoplasty with intraspinal brachytherapy for metastatic spine tumors. *J Neurosurg Spine*. 2009;10(4):334-335; author reply 335.

99. Wenz F, Schneider F, Neumaier C, et al. Kypho-IORT—a novel approach of intraoperative radiotherapy during kyphoplasty for vertebral metastases. *Radiat Oncol*. 2010;5:11.

100. Gerszten PC, Monaco EA III. Complete percutaneous treatment of vertebral body tumors causing spinal canal compromise using a transpedicular cavitation, cement augmentation, and radiosurgical technique. *Neurosurg Focus*. 2009;27(6):E9.

101. Reid IR, King AR, Alexander CJ, et al. Prevention of steroid-induced osteoporosis with (3-amino-1-hydroxypropylidene)-1,1-bisphosphonate (APD). *Lancet*. 1988;1:143.

102. Portenoy RK. Pharmacologic management of chronic pain. In: Fields HL, ed. *Pain Syndromes in Neurologic Practice*. New York, NY: Butterworth–Heinemann; 1990:257.

103. Payne R, Weinstein SM, Hill CS. Management of cancer pain. In: Levin VL, ed. *Cancer in the Nervous System*. New York, NY: Churchill Livingstone; 1996:411.

104. World Health Organization. *Cancer Pain Relief and Palliative Care*. Geneva, Switzerland: World Health Organization; 1990.

105. Jacox A, Carr DB, Payne R, et al. *Management of Cancer Pain, Clinical Practice Guideline No. 9*. Rockville, MD: Agency for Health Care Policy and Research, U.S. Department of Health and Human Services, Public Health Services; 1994. AHCPR Publication No 94-0592.

106. American Pain Society. *Principles of Analgesic Use in the Treatment of Acute Pain and Cancer Pain*. 5th ed. Glenview, IL: American Pain Society; 2003.

107. Payne R, Cunningham M, Weinstein SM, et al. Intractable pain and suffering in a cancer patient. *Clin J Pain*. 1995;11:70.

108. Aguilar JL, Espachs P, Roca G, et al. Difficult management of pain following sacrococcygeal chordoma: thirteen months of subarachnoid infusion. *Pain*. 1994;59(2):317.

109. Morgan RJ, Steller PH. Acute paraplegias following intrathecal phenol block in the presence of occult epidural malignancy. *Anaesthesia*. 1994;49(2):142.

110. Waldman SD, Feldstein LS, Allen ML. Neuroadenolysis of the pituitary: description of a modified technique. *J Pain Symptom Manage*. 1987;2:45.

111. Watling C, Allen RR. Treatment of neuropathic pain associated with sacrectomy. In: *Proceedings of the 48th Annual Scientific Meeting of the American Academy of Neurology*; San Francisco, CA; 1996. Abstract 1996.

112. Schlicht LA, Smelz JK. Metastatic spinal cord compression. In: Garden FH, Grabois M, eds. *Cancer Rehabilitation. Physical Medicine and Rehabilitation. State of the Art Reviews*. Vol. 8(2). Philadelphia, PA: Hanley and Belfus; 1994:345.

113. Garden FH, Gillis TA. Principles of cancer rehabilitation. In: Braddom RL, ed. *Physical Medicine and Rehabilitation*. Philadelphia, PA: WB Saunders; 1996:1199.

114. Fattal C, Fabbro M, Gelis A, Bauchet L. Metastatic paraplegia and vital prognosis: perspectives and limitations for rehabilitation care. Part 1. *Arch Phys Med Rehabil*. 2011;92(1):125-133.

115. Fattal C, Fabbro M, Rouays-Mabit H, Verollet C, Bauchet L. Metastatic paraplegia and functional outcomes: perspectives and limitations for rehabilitation care. Part 2. *Arch Phys Med Rehabil*. 2011;92(1):134-145.

116. Bach F, Larsen BH, Rohde K, et al. Metastatic spinal cord compression: occurrence, symptoms, clinical presentation and progression in 398 patients with spinal cord compression. *Acta Neurochir (Wien)*. 1990;107(1-2):37-43.

117. Savage P, Sharkey R, Kua T, et al. Malignant spinal cord compression: NICE guidance, improvements and challenges. *QJM*. 2014;107:277-282.

118. Liu Y-H, Hu Y-C, Yang X-G, et al. Prognostic factors of ambulatory status for patients with metastatic spinal cord compression: a systematic review and meta-analysis. *World Neurosurg*. 2018;116:e278-e290.

119. Delattre JY, Krol G, Thaler HT, et al. Distribution of brain metastases. *Arch Neurol*. 1988;45:741.

120. Fadul CE. Neurological complications of genitourinary cancer. In: Wiley RG, ed. *Neurologic Complications of Cancer*. New York, NY: Marcel Dekker; 1995:388.

121. Sundaresan N, Choi IS, Hughes JEO, et al. Treatment of spinal metastases from kidney cancer by presurgical embolization and resection. *J Neurosurg*. 1990;73:548.

122. Cooper K, Bajorin D, Shapiro W, et al. Decompression of epidural metastases from germ cell tumors with chemotherapy. *J Neurooncol*. 1990;8:275.

123. Rate WR, Solin LJ, Turrisi AT. Palliative radiotherapy for metastatic malignant melanoma: brain metastases, bone metastases, and spinal cord compression. *Int J Radiat Oncol Biol Phys*. 1998;15:859.

124. Herbert SH, Solin LJ, Rate WR, et al. The effect of palliative radiation therapy on epidural compression due to metastatic malignant melanoma. *Cancer*. 1991;67:2472.

125. Henson JW. Neurological complications of malignant melanoma and other cutaneous malignancies. In: Wiley RG, ed. *Neurologic Complications of Cancer.* New York, NY: Marcel Dekker; 1995:333.

126. Spiess JL, Adelstein DJ, Hines DJ. Multiple myeloma presenting with spinal cord compression. *Oncology.* 1988;45:88.

127. Grommes C, Bosl GJ, DeAngelis LM. Treatment of epidural spinal cord involvement from germ cell tumors with chemotherapy. *Cancer.* 2011;117(9):1911-1916. doi: 10.1002/cncr.25693.

128. Mayfield JK, Riseborough EJ, Jaffe N, et al. Spinal deformities in children treated for neuroblastoma. *J Bone Joint Surg.* 1981;63:183.

129. Kaspars GJ, Kamphorst W, et al. Primary spinal epidural extraosseous Ewing's sarcoma. *Cancer.* 1991;68:648.

130. Chi JH, Gokaslan Z, McCormick P, Tibbs PA, Kryscio RJ, Patchell RA. Selecting treatment for patients with malignant epidural spinal cord compression—does age matter?: results from a randomized clinical trial. *Spine (Phila Pa 1976).* 2009;34(5): 431-435.

131. Loblaw DA, Laperriere NJ, Mackillop WJ. A population-based study of malignant spinal cord compression in Ontario. *Clin Oncol (R Coll Radiol).* 2003;15:211-217.

132. George R, Jeba J, Ramkumar G, Chacko AG, Leng M, Tharyan P. Interventions for the treatment of metastatic extradural spinal cord compression in adults. *Cochrane Database Syst Rev.* 2008;(4):CD006716.

133. Hammack JE. Spinal cord disease in patients with cancer. *Continuum (Minneap Minn).* 2012;18(2): 312-327.

34 Recognizing and Managing Delirium

Elizabeth L. Cobbs and Jacob W. Phillips

INTRODUCTION

Delirium is an important medical diagnosis defined as a disturbance in attention, awareness, and cognition that develops over a short period of time (usually hours to a few days), represents a change from baseline, and tends to fluctuate in severity throughout the day (1,2). Subtypes of delirium have been defined based on the presence (hyperactive) or absence (hypoactive) of psychomotor agitation, perceptual disturbances, and/or level of consciousness (3). Often both subtypes are present (mixed) (4–12).

In the context of serious illness, delirium is highly prevalent and associated with many undesirable consequences. Most physiologic disturbances can cause delirium; however, even with serious or advanced illness, causes can often be determined and reversed. Despite this, delirium is still under-recognized and undermanaged. Careful history taking, assessment of symptoms, consideration of differential diagnoses, and clear communication among the team are key to making the diagnosis. Having the diagnosis of delirium and determining prognosis, functional status, and goals of the patient/family are paramount to successful management. With this information, delirium can be conceptualized as potentially reversible or irreversible, and both workup and management strategies flow from these concepts, as well as the presence or absence of the hyperactive subtype. Both pharmacologic and nonpharmacologic interventions can be employed to improve symptoms and relieve patient and family distress.

Prevalence and Consequences

Delirium is very common in the setting of advanced illness, with reported rates of up to 56% in the hospitalized elderly (13,14), 82% to 87% in intensive care units (15–17), and 88% of patients with advanced cancer or at the end of life (8,9,18–22). It likely occurs in nearly 100% of patients who are actively dying. Disagreement about the most common subtype exists, but hypoactive is often reported as the most prevalent (9,10) and is the one most often under-recognized (8). One study of 228 end-stage cancer patients found the prevalence of delirium to be 47%, and of those, 68% were hypoactive (8).

Delirium leads to increased mortality (2,8,20,21, 23–30), decreased life expectancy (25,31,32), functional decline (24), unnecessary medical interventions, increased hospital admissions, prolonged hospitalizations (13,14,23,33), increased need for higher levels of care (23,24), and increased health care utilization and costs (14,34). Delirium and its complications account for over an estimated $38 billion in annual health care costs in the United States (35). Delirium can also impair the recognition and control of other physical and psychological symptoms, such as pain and anxiety (36–38). This all leads to a significant amount of distress for patients, families, and caregivers (39–42). One study of 101 cancer patients who recovered from delirium reported that 54% recalled the experience and that patients, spouses/caregivers, and nurses all reported moderate to severe distress from the experience, no matter the subtype (43).

Causes

The most common causes of delirium found in patients with serious and/or advanced illness are fluid and electrolyte imbalances, medications (benzodiazepines (44,45), opioids (21,45–47), steroids (45,46,48), and anticholinergics (49,50)), infections, hepatic or renal failure, hypoxia, and hematologic disturbances (21,51). A selected list of important causes to consider is presented in Table 34.1 (52).

Under-Recognition

Delirium is often unrecognized or misdiagnosed due to its complex and variable presentation, the inconsistent language used to describe it, preconceived notions about advanced illness and the dying process, and the difficulty of recognizing the hypoactive subtype. A retrospective study of 2,716 patients receiving hospice care found delirium was documented in only 17.8% of those in the homecare setting and 28.3% of those in an inpatient setting (53). Another study demonstrated that a palliative care team was only able to recognize delirium in 45% of all patients with an expert-confirmed delirium diagnosis, and in only 20% of those with hypoactive delirium (8).

TABLE 34.1 SELECTED COMMON CAUSES OF DELIRIUM

System	Causes
Brain	Stroke, seizure, head trauma, brain mass or metastases, normal pressure hydrocephalus, infection
Heart, lungs, circulation	Cardiac or pulmonary disease (anything that causes hypoxia), carotid disease, anemia, infection
Digestive, urinary	Hepatic or renal failure, peritonitis, bowel obstruction, fecal impaction, constipation, urinary retention, urinary tract infection
Endocrine	Thyroid, parathyroid, adrenal
Metabolic	Acid–base or electrolyte disturbances, abnormal glucose, dehydration
Toxicity and/or withdrawal	Drugs of abuse, opioids, steroids, benzodiazepines, anticholinergics, immunosuppressants, interferon, histamine-2 blockers (cimetidine and ranitidine)

Behaviors, Signs, and Symptoms

The diagnosis of delirium is based on a careful history that accurately captures all observed behaviors, signs, and symptoms that potentially indicate its presence, many of which are changes in mental status. To effectively communicate an evaluation, all clinicians need to know the definitions of and recognize the common behaviors, signs, and symptoms associated with delirium (Table 34.2).

ASSESSMENT

Routine screening can help identify patients at risk for delirium who can then be assessed more thoroughly. Once delirium is suspected, a careful assessment is necessary to optimally manage patients with delirium, including the following:

1. Careful description of the observed behaviors, signs, and symptoms
2. Differentiation of delirium from other related diagnoses
3. An understanding of the underlying context of the patient, that is, the primary diagnosis, associated comorbidities, functional status, and prognosis
4. The goals of care for the patient and family

Screening

Multiple tools have been developed to facilitate routine screening for delirium and tracking of

TABLE 34.2 BEHAVIORS/SYMPTOMS/SIGNS OFTEN ASSOCIATED WITH DELIRIUM

Behaviors/symptoms/signs	Definition
Acute onset	Rapid onset of symptoms over minutes to days, even if symptoms began or occurred in the past
Agitation	Unintentional, excessive, and purposeless cognitive and/or motor activity; restlessness
Altered level of consciousness	Clinically differentiable degrees of awareness and alertness, that is, hypervigilant, alert, lethargic, cloudy, stuporous, and comatose
Confusion	Not oriented to person, place, time, or situation
Delusion	A fixed and false belief or wrong judgment that opposing evidence does not change. Can be paranoid, grandiose, somatic, and persecutory
Disinhibition	Unable to control immediate impulsive response to a situation
Disorganized thinking	Thoughts are confusing, vague, and/or do not logically flow; they are loosely or not connected
Fluctuation or waxing/waning	Intensity changes rapidly; symptoms may come and go
Hallucination	Perception of an object or event that does not exist. May be visual, auditory, olfactory, gustatory, or tactile
Inattention	Inability to focus or direct thinking
Irritable	Prone to excessive impatience, annoyance, or anger to get needs met
Labile affect	Rapidly changing and out of context mood symptoms
Psychosis	Loss of contact with reality

symptom severity (52,54). The Confusion Assessment Method (CAM) is a nine-item screening tool that looks at change over time (temporal profile), attention, thought processes, and levels of consciousness (55,56). It can be easily administered by nonpsychiatrically trained personnel and has been validated in many populations, including patients with advanced illnesses (57). A shorter, four-question version of the CAM often used in intensive care units (CAM-ICU) can be administered quickly and has accuracy similar to the full nine-question version (34). It has a sensitivity of 94% to 100% and specificity of 90% to 95% (55), but this can vary by setting and the administrator's clinical discipline. Another validated delirium screening tool is the Intensive Care Delirium Screening Checklist (ICDSC), an eight-item checklist designed for patients with limited ability to communicate (34). The ICDSC assesses consciousness, orientation, hallucinations or delusions, psychomotor activity, inappropriate speech/mood, attentiveness, sleep–wake cycle disturbances, and fluctuation of symptoms (34). The ICDSC has a sensitivity of 74% and specificity of 81.9% (34). Both the CAM and CAM-ICU have higher sensitivity and specificity than the ICDSC, but all three are validated and useful screening tools in the diagnosis of delirium (34).

Gold Standard Assessment

The gold standard for assessing delirium is a thorough history, a complete mental status and physical examination, and comparison with the DSM-V criteria for delirium (1,2,58,59). As delirious patients are often not good historians, the gathering of collateral information is essential. Caregivers, including family members and support staff, can identify and describe the behaviors, signs, and symptoms they see using simple, clear, and common language (see Table 34.2). This will help make the diagnosis of delirium and differentiate it from other diagnoses with similar presentations (see Table 34.3). Each observed behavior, sign, and symptom should be described by change over time (temporal profile), severity, and response (positive or negative) to previous therapeutic interventions (60).

A careful medication history, which documents all changes in medications and dosages over recent days, weeks, or even months, especially those leading up to the mental status changes, should be included. The types and severity of all allergic and adverse reactions need to be noted and confirmed. A careful drug and alcohol history is important; of particular interest are drugs that cause withdrawal syndromes, for example, alcohol, opioids, benzodiazepines, and muscle relaxants.

Diagnostic and Severity Rating Tools

The Delirium Rating Scale Revised-98 and the Memorial Delirium Assessment Scale are diagnostic and severity rating tools that can be used to confirm the diagnosis of delirium and to monitor changes over time (61). Both tools require that the rater have familiarity with basic psychiatric concepts.

The Delirium Rating Scale Revised-98 includes 3 specific diagnostic items and a 13-item severity rating scale (61,62). When compared with expert psychiatric diagnosis with DSM criteria, it has a sensitivity of 91% to 100% and a specificity of 85% to 100%. It has been shown to differentiate delirium from disorders with similar presentations, including depression, dementia, and schizophrenia. Its predecessor, the Delirium Rating Scale, has been used to evaluate delirium in children and adolescents (63).

The Memorial Delirium Assessment Scale is another diagnostic and severity rating scale designed for serial measurements in clinical intervention trials. It is a 10-item rating scale that can be used as frequently as every 4 hours to track the course of delirium (64). It has a sensitivity of 97% and a specificity of 95%, when compared with expert psychiatric diagnosis using DSM criteria. Other tools have been designed for use in the intensive care unit (16,65–67), with children (63,66), and by nonpsychiatrically trained staff (68,69).

Several tools are often used inappropriately to screen for and assess delirium. Both the Mini-Mental State Exam and the Clock Drawing task are measures of global cognitive function, and the Mini-Mental State Exam can be used as a screen for Alzheimer's dementia. Neither of these are specific for, nor should be used to assess, delirium (70–72).

ALTERNATIVE DIAGNOSES TO CONSIDER

Many of the signs, symptoms, and behaviors associated with delirium can be associated with other

TABLE 34.3 DIFFERENTIAL DIAGNOSES

	Delirium	Dementia	Psychotic disorders	Depression	Anxiety
Onset	Hours to days	Gradual	Varies	Varies	Varies
Changes in alertness	Yes	Late	No	No	No
Frequent fluctuation	Yes	No	No	No	Varies

diagnoses. As the underlying causes and management vary greatly, it is important to differentiate delirium from dementia, depression, anxiety, bipolar disorder, psychotic disorders (e.g., schizophrenia), personality disorders, developmental disorder, and adverse effects of medications (e.g., akathisia) (2), among other things. Table 34.3 lists differences in onset, changes in alertness, and frequency of fluctuation that help clinicians to make accurate diagnoses. When in doubt, it should be assumed the patient is experiencing delirium until proven otherwise, as delirium is the most common of these related diagnoses in patients with advanced illnesses. It should not be assumed that agitation is driven by pain; careful assessment of pain and consideration of other causes of agitation are important. For complex clinical situations, mental health professionals can be consulted to quickly reduce suffering for the patient, family, and caregivers (73).

Delirium itself goes by many synonyms, including acute confusional state, ICU psychosis, encephalopathy, acute brain failure, and syndrome of cerebral insufficiency. It is important to recognize that these all refer to the same diagnosis. To ensure effective management and avoid confusion, it is best to use the term "delirium."

Underlying Diagnoses and Prognosis

Delirium in patients with advanced illnesses may or may not be reversible. To establish the potential reversibility of delirium, it is important to know each patient's goals of care, principal underlying diagnosis and comorbidities, functional status, and overall prognosis (74–78). If an underlying abnormal physiologic process is suspected, with appropriate investigation and therapies, the condition could be potentially reversible, even in the context of advanced illness, if consistent with patient/family goals.

Several studies have demonstrated the ability to find and reverse causes of delirium in the context of serious or advanced illness. One study of 213 hospice inpatients with cancer and delirium found a cause of the delirium in 93 (61%) of the 153 patients who chose to have a workup. The causes were found to be multifactorial in 52% of the cases, and a complete remission occurred in 20% (51). Another study of 104 inpatients with advanced cancer who were receiving palliative care found reversible causes in 50% of the 71 who developed delirium (21). Other studies have found reversible causes in up to 68% of cases (21,31,79).

Delirium becomes irreversible (a) if workup or attempts at reversal fail; (b) in the context of a known irreversible processes (e.g., active dying or end-stage liver failure); or (c) if workup or reversal are inconsistent with patient/family goals of care. Most patients who are actively dying (exhibiting objective signs of the dying process (74,80,81) (Table 34.4) experience either a hyperactive or a hypoactive delirium (74,80). As dying is an irreversible process of multisystem organ failure, this delirium is irreversible. Management of irreversible delirium focuses on settling and supporting the patient, the family, and caregivers.

Using the terminology of reversible versus irreversible delirium (82,83) takes into account (a) that the patient has a known medical diagnosis of delirium; (b) the potential causes of the delirium; (c) the underlying diagnoses, prognosis, and functional status of the patient; and (d) the goals of

TABLE 34.4 OBJECTIVE SIGNS OF ACTIVE DYING

Categories	Signs
Cardiac dysfunction	Tachycardia Decreased cardiac output Decreased intravascular volume Peripheral cooling Peripheral and central cyanosis Mottling of the skin (livedo reticularis) Venous pooling
Respiratory dysfunction	Tachypnea with progressive slowing and decreasing tidal volume Abnormal breathing patterns, for example, apnea, Cheyne-Stokes, agonal
Renal dysfunction	Oliguria progressing to anuria Darkening of urine
Neurologic dysfunction	Loss of swallow Loss of gag reflex Buildup of oral and tracheal secretions Loss of sphincter control Altered level of consciousness Seizures

care for the patient. With these, *prospective* workup and management decisions can be made that differ based on whether the delirium is potentially reversible or irreversible.

Goals of Care

Patients and families living with advanced illnesses have a wide range of goals for their medical care and for their lives (75–77). Some still hope for cure, many hope for prolongation of life, almost all hope for concurrent relief of the multiple issues that cause them suffering (as they define it) (78). At times they have what appear to be overlapping, and sometimes conflicting goals.

Goals of care frequently change over time as the patient's illness evolves and new information becomes available. Many patients nearing the end of their lives do not want to have aggressive or potentially life-prolonging medical therapies. They prefer to focus on care that gives them the best possible quality of life and a good death (as they define it).

If an episode of delirium is potentially reversible, the patient and family goals for medical care and goals for life should guide the diagnostic workup and management of the underlying causes. A diagnosis of delirium often causes patients living with advanced illnesses, or their surrogate decision-makers, and their families to reassess their goals for medical care. Some patients and families still find simple tests, such as blood draws and urinalysis acceptable, especially if the results might indicate an easy therapeutic intervention that could potentially reverse a hyperactive delirium, reduce distress, and improve quality of life. They choose to attempt to reverse the underlying cause of the delirium and manage any associated distressing symptoms.

Others choose to forgo a diagnostic workup and/or any treatment of the underlying cause of the delirium, thus rendering it irreversible. They may choose not to attempt to reverse the underlying cause of the delirium even when the treatment is relatively easy to do (e.g., antibiotic treatment for urinary tract infection), preferring to focus on managing distressing symptoms.

Workup of Delirium

If the patient's underlying diagnoses, prognosis, functional status, and goals for medical care are consistent with a potentially reversible delirium, after a thorough history and physical examination, obtaining a comprehensive blood count, metabolic panel, vitamin levels, and limited infection workup will often reveal the most common reversible causes of delirium. Careful thought should be given before ordering tests that are potentially more invasive or burdensome to the patient. Only tests that will lead to definitive treatment strategies should be considered.

Delirium can be caused by any physiologic disturbance. If initial investigations do not reveal an underlying cause and the goal is a comprehensive diagnostic workup, consider any medical test consistent with confirming a suspected diagnosis using a tiered approach based on the most likely causes (Table 34.5). The benefits, risks, and burdens of every investigation should be weighed.

Time-limited trials can be utilized to guide workup and/or management of underlying causes, such that clear goals and measures of success are defined over a specified period of time and unlimited workups or therapeutic trials are avoided. Should drug intoxication be suspected, a reduced dose or rotations to other medications may be considered (84,85). This is especially true for opioids (85), particularly when decreased fluid intake or urine output can lead to opioid accumulation and cause or worsen delirium.

TABLE 34.5 POTENTIAL TESTS FOR DETERMINING CAUSES OF DELIRIUM

Tier 1	Subsequent tests guided by clinical picture	
Comprehensive chemistries	PT/PTT/INR	Lumbar puncture
CBC w/differential	TSH	HIV testing
LFTs	Ammonia level	RPR testing
B_{12}/folate levels	ECG	EEG
X-rays	ABG	
Albumin	Cultures (blood, stool, etc.)	
UA and UC	CT or MRI	

PT, prothrombin time; PTT, partial thromboplastin time; INR, international normalized ratio; CBC, complete blood count; TSH, thyroid stimulating hormone; CT, computed tomography; MRI, magnetic resonance imaging; LFTs, liver function tests; HIV, human immunodeficiency virus; ECG, electrocardiogram; RPR, rapid plasma reagin; UA, urinalysis; UC, urine culture; ABG, arterial blood gas; EEG, electroencephalogram.

MANAGEMENT

If consistent with the patients' diagnoses, prognosis, functional status, and goals of care, attempt to treat the underlying cause of a potentially reversible delirium. Whether attempting to reverse or not, the associated symptoms of delirium should always be managed with nonpharmacologic interventions and, when appropriate, pharmacologic interventions. Safety for the patient, caregivers, and family is of paramount importance, as are environmental issues (2,59). Most people approaching the end of their lives want to be cared for at home in their last days to weeks, and die there (86,87). The nonpharmacologic and pharmacologic management strategies that follow can be safely administered in any setting.

Alleviating Symptoms Associated with Delirium

Nonpharmacologic Interventions

All patients can benefit from nonpharmacologic interventions, including several environmental interventions, to reduce the risk and severity of symptoms associated with delirium (31,37,88–92). These interventions can help reduce disordered thinking, disorientation, sleep disturbances, immobility, risk of falls/injury, sensory deprivation, dehydration, and other environmental factors:

- Engaging patients in mentally stimulating activities to help them with disordered thinking
- Providing orienting and familiar materials to help patients know the time and date, where they are, and which staff are working with them
- Ensuring all individuals identify themselves each time they encounter the patient, even if the encounters are minutes apart
- Minimizing the number of people interacting with the patient and the quantity of stimulation the patient receives, for example, no television or loud music
- Using family or volunteers as constant companions to help reassure and reorient a delirious patient. Encourage staff to sit with the patient while they do their documentation
- Providing adequate soft lighting so patients can see without being overstimulated by bright lights
- Managing fall risks
- Providing warm milk, massage, warm blankets, and using relaxation tapes to optimize sleep hygiene and minimize sleep disturbances
- Ensuring patients use their glasses, hearing aids, etc., to optimize orientation, decrease confusion, and promote better communication
- Ensuring patients have good nutrition and an effective bowel and bladder management strategy

- Monitoring fluid intake; rehydrate with oral fluids containing salt, for example, soups, sport drinks, red vegetable juices; when necessary, infuse fluids subcutaneously rather than intravenously (93–95)
- Avoiding physical restraints unless needed as a last resort to temporarily ensure the safety of both staff and a severely agitated and not redirectable patient (31,96), and only until less restrictive interventions are possible
- Providing education and support to help family members cope with what they are witnessing (97)

A nonpharmacologic hospital protocol targeted at delirium was developed by Inouye et al. (92) to minimize the risk of delirium in geriatric patients. Using this protocol, which supports orientation, cognitive activity, mobility, sleep, hydration, and access to sensory aids, delirium developed in only 9.9% of geriatric patients admitted to a hospital medicine service versus 15% of those receiving usual care. The intervention group also had significantly fewer and shorter episodes of delirium. A follow-up study showed that this protocol reduced the risk of developing delirium in a similar population by 89% (98).

Pharmacologic Interventions

Currently, there are

- no medications with US Food and Drug Administration (FDA)-approved indications for the management of delirium (99);
- no consensus among oncologists, geriatricians, psychiatrists, and palliative medicine specialists about how to pharmacologically treat delirium (100).

The following is an evidence-based and expert consensus approach to pharmacologically managing the symptoms associated with delirium. Pharmacologic management of delirium is guided by the presence or absence of hyperactive delirium and the potential reversibility of the delirium. Based on the delirium management decision tree presented in Figure 34.1, three approaches will be presented: (a) management of hyperactive (agitated), potentially reversible delirium; (b) management of hyperactive, irreversible delirium; and (c) management of hypoactive delirium, whether potentially reversible or irreversible.

Potentially Reversible, Hyperactive Delirium
The American Psychiatric Association (APA) guidelines for delirium management suggest the use of first-generation antipsychotics, particularly haloperidol, and the avoidance of benzodiazepines for the first-line treatment of agitation in the context of a potentially reversible delirium (NB: these

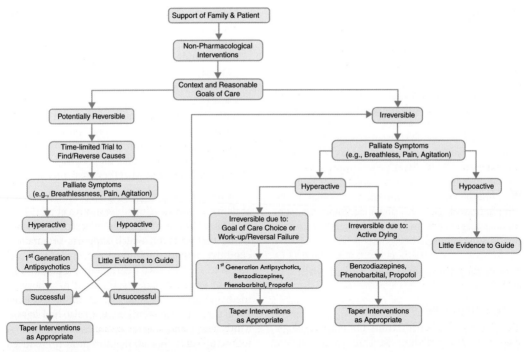

Figure 34.1 Delirium management decision tree.

guidelines do not distinguish potentially reversible from irreversible delirium, nor do they address goals of care or irreversible delirium) (2,59,101).

According to the APA guidelines, antipsychotics are the medications of choice for the management of agitation associated with potentially reversible, hyperactive delirium. However, it is important to note an October 2019 systematic review of 26 randomized controlled trials and observational studies evaluating 5,607 hospitalized adults with delirium found no difference in cognitive functioning, sedation, hospital length of stay, mortality, delirium severity, or duration between first- or second-generation antipsychotics versus placebo (99). This systematic review, published in the Annals of Internal Medicine, concluded that "current evidence does not support routine use of haloperidol or second-generation antipsychotics to treat delirium in adult inpatients" (99). Other studies have found some antipsychotics do have sedative properties (see Tables 34.6 and 34.9) (2,58,102). Furthermore, some studies posit antipsychotics may improve cognition and mental status (2,3,59,103,104).

No evidence exists for improved efficacy with atypical (second- or third-generation) antipsychotics (44,99,102,105,106). Also, they are more expensive and have limited routes of administration (103). With a few exceptions, benzodiazepines should not be used first line for managing potentially reversible delirium. They can worsen delirium, increase fall risk, create memory problems, and lead to withdrawal syndromes (2,44).

Likewise, opioids have no role in the treatment of agitation or delirium (Table 34.6). New or increased doses of opioids may worsen the symptoms of delirium. Care should be taken when titrating or tapering opioids: increase opioid doses carefully using a "catch-up" technique (75) that minimizes the risk of adverse effects (e.g., opioid-induced delirium) and reduce opioid doses carefully to avoid withdrawal syndromes.

Irreversible, Hyperactive Delirium When agitation occurs within the context of an irreversible delirium, a shift to management with benzodiazepines may be appropriate, especially if the patient is actively dying (i.e., there are associated objective signs of the dying process; Table 34.4) (21,52,80,84,107–114). This may also be appropriate when either (a) the patient's and family's goals for care are focused on symptom control without workup or management of the underlying causes or (b) the initial workup or treatment of a hyperactive, potentially reversible delirium has been refractory based on predetermined time-limited trials.

When patients are dying and experiencing an irreversible hyperactive delirium, there is significant risk of muscle tension, myoclonus, seizures, and family and caregiver distress (74,80). The goal of care is to settle the patient, relieve muscle tension, and minimize the risk of seizures. Most patients would rather not "experience" the agitated delirium associated with dying or have any "memory" of the event. Likewise, witnessing this

TABLE 34.6 ANTIPSYCHOTIC, BENZODIAZEPINE, AND OPIOID THERAPEUTIC PROPERTIES

Drug	Indication				
	Anti-agitation	Sedation	Amnesia	Muscle relaxation	Anticonvulsant
Antipsychotics	✓	✓/✗	✗	✗	–
Benzodiazepines	✓	✓	✓	✓	✓
Opioids	✗	✗	✗	✗	✗

✓, has property; ✗, does not have property; –, has opposite property.

agitation causes most caregivers and families significant distress. Benzodiazepines are ideal medications to manage and prevent these symptoms (21,52,80,84,107–114). They are sedatives, anxiolytics, skeletal muscle relaxants, amnestics, and potent antiepileptics (see Table 34.6). Only the minimum benzodiazepine dose needed to achieve the desired effect should be used.

While some clinicians worry, evidence suggests that appropriate titration of antipsychotics and benzodiazepines for the palliation of symptoms does not hasten death, and may in fact, prolong life (113–121). Doses typically needed to control these symptoms are well below FDA maximum recommended doses and far below their median lethal dosages. If a patient has an initial paradoxical reaction with more agitation, escalating the dose rapidly can overcome this reaction. If not effective, a switch to phenobarbital (122) or propofol (123,124) to control the agitation and settle the patient may be necessary.

Hypoactive Delirium Treatment of both potentially reversible and irreversible hypoactive delirium with medications is controversial. One approach is to avoid pharmacologic intervention, as medications are often the cause of delirium, and it is not clear if antipsychotics address anything besides agitation and psychotic symptoms (which are absent in hypoactive delirium). Another approach advocates for the use of antipsychotics, as they may improve cognition and other mental status changes (3,104). A third approach suggests that psychostimulants may improve cognitive performance in hypoactive delirium (125,126); however, the benefits must carefully be weighed against the risks of psychosis and worsening delirium. No evidence exists to guide the use of benzodiazepines to manage hypoactive delirium, though theoretically, their broad spectrum of therapeutic properties may be beneficial (Table 34.6) in the context of an irreversible delirium.

Pharmacologic Principles of Delirium Management

Titration of medications to control agitation or other symptoms associated with delirium should be *rapid*. All of these medications follow the same pharmacologic principles (e.g., first-order kinetics) employed when dosing medications to rapidly control other symptoms, such as pain (75).

A first dose of medication should be offered. If it does not control the symptom by the time its plasma concentration is maximum (tCmax), it will not become effective with more time. To titrate rapidly and safely to control symptoms, the medications should be dosed every tCmax until the symptom is controlled (75). Before each additional dose, the patient should be assessed for any new, undesired side effects.

Once the symptom (e.g., agitation) is controlled, the total dose used in the last 24 hours should be administered in divided, scheduled doses once every half-life (t½) over a 24-hour period. To control any breakthrough agitation or other symptoms, extra doses of the same medication should be available once every tCmax as needed.

For example, to control agitation rapidly, antipsychotics can be safely dosed intravenously (IV) once every 15 minutes, subcutaneously (SC) once every 30 minutes, or orally (PO) once every 60 minutes until the agitation is controlled or the maximum recommended dose of the medication in a 24-hour period has been reached (75). This is similar to the protocol to rapidly control agitation in emergency situations (107,125,127–129). See Tables 34.7 and 34.8 for specific dosing suggestions and sample orders.

Potential Antipsychotic Side Effects

All risks of side effects must be considered alongside the potential benefits of each medication. Table 34.9 categorizes common adverse effects for five antipsychotic medications commonly used in patients with advanced illnesses (103). These side effects correlate with a drug's affinity for the neuroreceptors most implicated in the particular side effect.

The common side effects of antipsychotics include extrapyramidal symptoms (acute dystonia, akathisia, parkinsonism, and tardive dyskinesia); anticholinergic effects (delirium, urinary retention, tachycardia, blurred vision, cognitive impairment, dry mouth, constipation, sexual dysfunction, and

TABLE 34.7 PHARMACOLOGIC PARAMETERS FOR MEDICATIONS USED TO MANAGE SYMPTOMS OF DELIRIUM

Generic and trade name	Suggested starting dosage	Breakthrough dosing based on time C_{max}	Approximate elimination $t^{1/2}$	Recommended scheduled dosing interval	Recommended maximum dosage
Haloperidol (nonsedating) aka **Haldol**	1–2 mg	p.o.: 60 min s.c./i.m.: 30 min i.v.: 15 min	21 h	Daily or twice daily	100 mg/d
Chlorpromazine (sedating) aka **Thorazine**	25–50 mg	p.o.: 60 min s.c./i.m.: 30 min i.v.: 15 min	24 h	Daily or twice daily	2,000 mg/d
Risperidone (nonsedating) aka **Risperdal**	0.25–0.5 mg	p.o.: 60 min	3 h (metabolites: 21–30 h)	Daily or twice daily	6 mg/d
Olanzapine (sedating) aka **Zyprexa**	2.5–5 mg	p.o.: 6 h (onset of action 30 min) s.c./i.m.: 30 min	30 h	Daily or twice daily	30 mg/d
Quetiapine (sedating) aka **Seroquel**	25–50 mg	p.o.: 90 min[a]	12 h	Up to three times daily	1,200 mg/d
Lorazepam aka **Ativan**	1–2 mg	p.o.: 60 min s.c./i.m.: 30 min i.v.: 15 min	12 h	Twice daily	40 mg/d[b]
Midazolam aka **Versed**	0.1–0.2 mg/kg loading dose, then 25% of the loading dose needed to control symptoms as a continuous infusion, for example, for a 50 kg person who required 0.2 mg/kg, = 10 mg to control, the continuous infusion would be 2.5 mg/h	s.c./i.m.: 30 min i.v.: 15 min	2 h	Continuous infusion	240 mg/d[b]
Phenobarbital	10–30 mg/kg loading dose, then 20–100 mg/h continuous infusion	s.c./i.m.: 2 h i.v.: 30 min	96 h	Continuous infusion	2,400 mg/d
Propofol	1 mg/kg/h starting Increase by 0.5 mg/kg until effect achieved (usually <6 mg/kg/h)	i.v.	3–12 h[c]	Continuous infusion	12 mg/kg/h

p.o., orally; PR, rectally; s.c., subcutaneously; i.v., intravenously; mg, milligram; kg, kilogram; h, hour.
[a]Caution increasing by more than 50 to 100 mg/d in ambulatory patients.
[b]Safe to use higher doses; however, management may be better with phenobarbital or propofol if symptoms are not controlled at this maximum dose.
[c]Increases with prolonged administration due to tissue distribution.

TABLE 34.8 SAMPLE ORDERS (ROUTES AND ASSOCIATED DOSING SCHEDULE MAY DIFFER)

Haloperidol

- 1 mg s.c. q30 min PRN agitation
- If three doses are not effective, call MD to reassess dose, diagnosis, or medication choice
- Do not exceed 100 mg in 24 h (wide therapeutic range)
- Schedule the total dose used in the last 24 h in divided doses administered twice daily
- Continue with same PRN schedule

Chlorpromazine

- 50 mg p.o. q60min PRN agitation
- If three doses are not effective, call MD to reassess dose, diagnosis, or medication choice
- Do not exceed 2,000 mg in 24 h
- Schedule the total dose used in the last 24 h in divided doses administered twice daily
- Continue with same PRN schedule

Risperidone

- 0.5 mg p.o. q60 min PRN agitation
- If three doses are not effective, call MD to reassess dose, diagnosis, or medication choice
- Do not exceed 6 mg in 24 h (wide therapeutic range)
- Schedule the total dose used in the last 24 h in divided doses administered twice daily
- Continue with same PRN schedule

Olanzapine

- 2.5 mg s.c. q30 min PRN agitation
- If three doses are not effective, call MD to reassess dose, diagnosis, or medication choice
- Do not exceed 30 mg in 24 h (wide therapeutic range)
- Schedule the total dose used in the last 24 h in divided doses administered twice daily
- Continue with same PRN schedule

Lorazepam

- 1 mg p.o. q60 min PRN agitation
- If three doses are not effective, call MD to reassess dose, diagnosis, or medication choice
- Do not exceed 40 mg in 24 h (wide therapeutic range)
- Schedule the total dose used in the last 24 h in three divided doses administered every 8 h
- Continue with same PRN schedule

Midazolam

- 0.2 mg/kg loading dose s.c.
- If needed give 0.1 mg/kg q30 min × 2 PRN
- Continuously infuse 25% of total dose needed for symptom control per hour
- Consider alternative if need >10 mg/h

decreased sweating); sedation; hypotension; dizziness; and orthostasis (126). Diabetes, hyperglycemia, hyperlipidemia, and weight gain may be of concern with longer term use. QTc prolongation is often cited as a concern, and some studies have shown prolongation of the QT interval with second-generation antipsychotics versus placebo or haloperidol (99).

As lower antipsychotic doses typically control agitation in medically ill patients, their side effects are less frequent in patients with advanced illnesses (44). A Cochrane review cited one study of chlorpromazine for delirium in advanced illness that found decreased cognitive function but no increase in extrapyramidal effects (130). Another Cochrane review of the efficacy and side effects of antipsychotics in delirium cited three studies, two found no significant side effects and one found that haloperidol increased the incidence of dry mouth and extrapyramidal symptoms (131).

Black Box Warnings

The FDA has issued a black box warning about the increased risk of death (3.5% with all antipsychotics vs. 2.3% with placebos) when first- or second-generation antipsychotics are used to treat *dementia-related psychosis* in elderly patients based on a number of limited studies (132–138). Other studies have not replicated this finding (139). These data do not address the risk of short-term use of these agents to manage *delirium*. In addition, no evidence for

TABLE 34.9 SIDE EFFECTS ASSOCIATED WITH ANTIPSYCHOTIC MEDICATIONS

Drug	Adverse event (receptor)				
	Anticholinergic (M_1)	Sedation (H_1)	Orthostasis (α_1)	QTc prolongation	EPS (D_2)
Haloperidol	×	✓	×	× (p.o.)	
				✓ (i.v.)	✓✓✓
Chlorpromazine	✓✓	✓✓✓	✓	✓	✓
Risperidone	×	✓	×	×	✓✓
Olanzapine	✓✓	✓✓	×	×	✓
Quetiapine	×	✓✓✓	✓	×	×

✓, relative strength of effect; ×, does not have effect; EPS, extrapyramidal side effects.

antipsychotics being the direct cause of the increased mortality in patients with dementia or delirium has yet been produced. It is not clear how long a patient must be treated with an antipsychotic before having increased risk. While the relative risk appears large (1.7 times the risk of using a placebo), the absolute risk is small (increase of 1.2%) (137,138). Similarly, the absolute increase in the risk of cerebrovascular events related to the use of newer antipsychotics in patients with *dementia* is 1% (1.9% in treated group vs. 0.9% in the placebo group) (140).

It is important to note that none of the studies of antipsychotics in dementia were designed to evaluate the risk of mortality and cerebrovascular events, and they were not stratified by risk factors for these events. They also did not account for the multiple comorbidities and medications used by the study patients. A black box warning is a sign to use caution but not a mandate to avoid the use of these medications. A recent survey found that 68% of geriatricians still use antipsychotics in geriatric patients with known vascular risk due to lack of alternatives, lack of solid evidence, and lack of clear guidelines (141). The bottom line is (a) take account of patient/family goals for care and (b) weigh the risks, benefits, burdens, and alternatives of treatment. Often, families are willing to accept these risks, if necessary, to control the severe distress everyone experiences when a patient has a delirium.

CONCLUSIONS

In patients with serious and advanced illnesses, delirium is a common diagnosis. It is associated with many negative consequences, including significant distress for patients, families, and caregivers. With a careful history, physical examination, and investigation as appropriate, the causes of delirium are often discoverable and reversible.

Delirium can be conceptualized as potentially reversible or irreversible. By knowing patient's underlying diagnoses, prognosis, functional status, and goals of care, clinicians can treat or manage the underlying cause and use nonpharmacologic and pharmacologic therapies to minimize the symptoms and reduce the distress caused by delirium. In all cases, through careful attention to the pharmacokinetics of medications, clinicians can rapidly control agitation and other symptoms associated with delirium, even in actively dying and seemingly refractory patients.

ACKNOWLEDGMENTS

We wish to acknowledge support from the staff and patients of the Geriatrics and Palliative Care departments at The George Washington University Hospital, The GW Medical Faculty Associates, the Washington DC Veterans Affairs Medical Center, and the National Institutes of Health. We also wish to acknowledge all of the brilliant minds whose research and efforts made this work possible.

The authors would like to acknowledge the contribution of Dr. Scott A. Irwin, Dr. Gary T. Buckholz, Dr. Rosene D. Pirrello, Dr. Jeremy M. Hirst, Dr. Frank D. Ferris on the previous edition.

REFERENCES

1. American Psychiatric Association. *Diagnostic and Statistical Manual of Mental Disorders.* 5th ed. Arlington, VA: American Psychiatric Association; 2013:596.
2. American Psychiatric Association. Practice guideline for the treatment of patients with delirium. *Am J Psychiatry.* 1999;156:1-20.
3. Boettger S, Breitbart W. Phenomenology of the subtypes of delirium: phenomenological differences between hyperactive and hypoactive delirium. *Palliat Support Care.* 2011;9:129-135.
4. Stagno D, Gibson C, Breitbart W. The delirium subtypes: a review of prevalence, phenomenology, pathophysiology, and treatment response. *Palliat Support Care.* 2004;2:171-179.
5. O'Keeffe ST. Clinical subtypes of delirium in the elderly. *Dement Geriatr Cogn Disord.* 1999;10:380-385.
6. Lipowski ZJ. Delirium in the elderly patient. *N Engl J Med.* 1989;320:578-582.
7. Meagher D, Moran M, Raju B, et al. A new data-based motor subtype schema for delirium. *J Neuropsychiatry Clin Neurosci.* 2008;20:185-193.
8. Fang CK, Chen HW, Liu SI, Lin CJ, Tsai LY, Lai YL. Prevalence, detection and treatment of delirium in terminal cancer inpatients: a prospective survey. *Jpn J Clin Oncol.* 2008;38:56-63.
9. Spiller JA, Keen JC. Hypoactive delirium: assessing the extent of the problem for inpatient specialist palliative care. *Palliat Med.* 2006;20:17-23.
10. Ross CA, Peyser CE, Shapiro I, Folstein MF. Delirium: phenomenologic and etiologic subtypes. *Int Psychogeriatr.* 1991;3:135-147.
11. Meagher DJ, Moran M, Raju B, et al. Motor symptoms in 100 patients with delirium versus control subjects: comparison of subtyping methods. *Psychosomatics.* 2008;49:300-308.
12. Peterson JF, Pun BT, Dittus RS, et al. Delirium and its motoric subtypes: a study of 614 critically ill patients. *J Am Geriatr Soc.* 2006;54:479-484.
13. Pompei P, Foreman M, Rudberg MA, Inouye SK, Braund V, Cassel CK. Delirium in hospitalized older persons: outcomes and predictors. *J Am Geriatr Soc.* 1994;42:809-815.
14. Inouye SK. Delirium in hospitalized older patients. *Clin Geriatr Med.* 1998;14:745-764.
15. McNicoll L, Pisani MA, Zhang Y, Ely EW, Siegel MD, Inouye SK. Delirium in the intensive care unit: occurrence and clinical course in older patients. *J Am Geriatr Soc.* 2003;51:591-598.
16. Ely EW, Margolin R, Francis J, et al. Evaluation of delirium in critically ill patients: validation of the Confusion Assessment Method for the Intensive Care Unit (CAM-ICU). *Crit Care Med.* 2001;29:1370-1379.
17. Hshieh TT, Inouye SK, Oh ES. Delirium in the elderly. *Psychiatr Clin North Am.* 2018;41:1-17. [PMID: 29412839] doi: 10.1016/j.psc.2017.10.001.
18. Massie MJ, Holland J, Glass E. Delirium in terminally ill cancer patients. *Am J Psychiatry.* 1983;140:1048-1050.

19. Breitbart W, Strout D. Delirium in the terminally ill. *Clin Geriatr Med.* 2000;16:357-372.
20. Bruera E, Miller L, McCallion J, Macmillan K, Krefting L, Hanson J. Cognitive failure in patients with terminal cancer: a prospective study. *J Pain Symptom Manage.* 1992;7:192-195.
21. Lawlor PG, Gagnon B, Mancini IL, et al. Occurrence, causes, and outcome of delirium in patients with advanced cancer: a prospective study. *Arch Intern Med.* 2000;160:786-794.
22. Gagnon P, Allard P, Masse B, DeSerres M. Delirium in terminal cancer: a prospective study using daily screening, early diagnosis, and continuous monitoring. *J Pain Symptom Manage.* 2000;19:412-426.
23. Cole MG, Primeau FJ. Prognosis of delirium in elderly hospital patients. *CMAJ.* 1993;149:41-46.
24. Inouye SK, Rushing JT, Foreman MD, Palmer RM, Pompei P. Does delirium contribute to poor hospital outcomes? A three-site epidemiologic study. *J Gen Intern Med.* 1998;13:234-242.
25. Trzepacz PT, Teague GB, Lipowski ZJ. Delirium and other organic mental disorders in a general hospital. *Gen Hosp Psychiatry.* 1985;7:101-106.
26. Inouye SK. The dilemma of delirium: clinical and research controversies regarding diagnosis and evaluation of delirium in hospitalized elderly medical patients. *Am J Med.* 1994;97:278-288.
27. Maltoni M, Amadori D. Prognosis in advanced cancer. *Hematol Oncol Clin North Am.* 2002;16:715-729.
28. Casarett DJ, Inouye SK. Diagnosis and management of delirium near the end of life. *Ann Intern Med.* 2001;135:32-40.
29. Cole MG, Ciampi A, Belzile E, Zhong L. Persistent delirium in older hospital patients: a systematic review of frequency and prognosis. *Age Ageing.* 2009;38:19-26.
30. Kiely DK, Marcantonio ER, Inouye SK, et al. Persistent delirium predicts greater mortality. *J Am Geriatr Soc.* 2009;57:55-61.
31. Fainsinger R, Bruera E. Treatment of delirium in a terminally ill patient. *J Pain Symptom Manage.* 1992;7:54-56.
32. Morita T, Tsunoda J, Inoue S, Chihara S. Survival prediction of terminally ill cancer patients by clinical symptoms: development of a simple indicator. *Jpn J Clin Oncol.* 1999;29:156-159.
33. Thomas RI, Cameron DJ, Fahs MC. A prospective study of delirium and prolonged hospital stay. Exploratory study. *Arch Gen Psychiatry.* 1988;45:937-940.
34. Gusmao-Flores D, Salluh JIF, Chalhub RÁ, Quarantini LC. The confusion assessment method for the intensive care unit (CAM-ICU) and intensive care delirium screening checklist (ICDSC) for the diagnosis of delirium: a systematic review and meta-analysis of clinical studies. *Crit Care.* 2012;16(4):R115.
35. Leslie DL, Marcantonio ER, Zhang Y, et al. One-year health care costs associated with delirium in the elderly population. *Arch Intern Med.* 2008;168:27-32. [PMID: 18195192] doi:10.1001/archinternmed.2007.4.
36. Bruera E, Fainsinger RL, Miller MJ, Kuehn N. The assessment of pain intensity in patients with cognitive failure: a preliminary report. *J Pain Symptom Manage.* 1992;7:267-270.
37. Fainsinger R, Miller MJ, Bruera E, Hanson J, Maceachern T. Symptom control during the last week of life on a palliative care unit. *J Palliat Care.* 1991;7:5-11.
38. Coyle N, Breitbart W, Weaver S, Portenoy R. Delirium as a contributing factor to "crescendo" pain: three case reports. *J Pain Symptom Manage.* 1994;9:44-47.
39. Namba M, Morita T, Imura C, Kiyohara E, Ishikawa S, Hirai K. Terminal delirium: families' experience. *Palliat Med.* 2007;21:587-594.
40. Morita T, Akechi T, Ikenaga M, et al. Terminal delirium: recommendations from bereaved families' experiences. *J Pain Symptom Manage.* 2007;34:579-589.
41. Bruera E, Bush SH, Willey J, et al. Impact of delirium and recall on the level of distress in patients with advanced cancer and their family caregivers. *Cancer.* 2009;115:2004-2012.
42. Cohen MZ, Pace EA, Kaur G, Bruera E. Delirium in advanced cancer leading to distress in patients and family caregivers. *J Palliat Care.* 2009;25:164-171.
43. Breitbart W, Gibson C, Tremblay A. The delirium experience: delirium recall and delirium-related distress in hospitalized patients with cancer, their spouses/caregivers, and their nurses. *Psychosomatics.* 2002;43:183-194.
44. Breitbart W, Marotta R, Platt MM, et al. A double-blind trial of haloperidol, chlorpromazine, and lorazepam in the treatment of delirium in hospitalized AIDS patients. *Am J Psychiatry.* 1996;153:231-237.
45. Gaudreau JD, Gagnon P, Harel F, Roy MA, Tremblay A. Psychoactive medications and risk of delirium in hospitalized cancer patients. *J Clin Oncol.* 2005;23:6712-6718.
46. Gaudreau JD, Gagnon P, Roy MA, Harel F, Tremblay A. Opioid medications and longitudinal risk of delirium in hospitalized cancer patients. *Cancer.* 2007;109:2365-2373.
47. Bruera E, Macmillan K, Hanson J, MacDonald RN. The cognitive effects of the administration of narcotic analgesics in patients with cancer pain. *Pain.* 1989;39:13-16.
48. Stiefel FC, Breitbart WS, Holland JC. Corticosteroids in cancer: neuropsychiatric complications. *Cancer Invest.* 1989;7:479-491.
49. Han L, McCusker J, Cole M, Abrahamowicz M, Primeau F, Elie M. Use of medications with anticholinergic effect predicts clinical severity of delirium symptoms in older medical inpatients. *Arch Intern Med.* 2001;161:1099-1105.
50. Ancelin ML, Artero S, Portet F, Dupuy AM, Touchon J, Ritchie K. Non-degenerative mild cognitive impairment in elderly people and use of anticholinergic drugs: longitudinal cohort study. *BMJ.* 2006;332:455-459.
51. Morita T, Tei Y, Tsunoda J, Inoue S, Chihara S. Underlying pathologies and their associations with clinical features in terminal delirium of cancer patients. *J Pain Symptom Manage.* 2001;22:997-1006.
52. Levenson JL. *Textbook of Psychosomatic Medicine.* Washington, DC: American Psychiatric Publishing; 2005:xxi, 1092 p.
53. Irwin SA, Rao S, Bower KA, et al. Psychiatric issues in palliative care: recognition of *delirium* in patients enrolled in hospice care. *Palliat Support Care.* 2008;6:159-164.
54. Schuurmans MJ, Deschamps PI, Markham SW, Shortridge-Baggett LM, Duursma SA. The measurement of delirium: review of scales. *Res Theory Nurs Pract.* 2003;17:207-224.
55. Inouye SK, van Dyck CH, Alessi CA, Balkin S, Siegal AP, Horwitz RI. Clarifying confusion: the confusion assessment method. A new method for detection of delirium. *Ann Intern Med.* 1990;113:941-948.
56. Inouye SK. *The Confusion Assessment Method (CAM): Training Manual and Coding Guide.* New Haven, CT: Yale University School of Medicine; 2003.
57. Ryan K, Leonard M, Guerin S, Donnelly S, Conroy M, Meagher D. Validation of the confusion assessment method in the palliative care setting. *Palliat Med.* 2009;23:40-45.
58. *Diagnostic and Statistical Manual of Mental Disorders: DSM-IV.* Washington, DC: American Psychiatric Association; 1994:886.
59. Cook IA. Guideline watch: practice guideline for the treatment of patients with delirium. Updated 2004.

http://psychiatryonline.org/content.aspx?bookid=28&sectionid=1681952

60. Bickley LS, Szilagyi PG, Bates B. *Bates' Guide to Physical Examination and History Taking*. Philadelphia, PA: Lippincott Williams & Wilkins; 2007.

61. Trzepacz PT, Mittal D, Torres R, Kanary K, Norton J, Jimerson N. Validation of the delirium rating scale-revised-98: comparison with the delirium rating scale and the cognitive test for delirium. *J Neuropsychiatry Clin Neurosci*. 2001;13:229-242.

62. Trzepacz PT. The Delirium Rating Scale. Its use in consultation-liaison research. *Psychosomatics*. 1999;40:193-204.

63. Turkel SB, Braslow K, Tavare CJ, Trzepacz PT. The delirium rating scale in children and adolescents. *Psychosomatics*. 2003;44:126-129.

64. Breitbart W, Rosenfeld B, Roth A, Smith MJ, Cohen K, Passik S. The memorial delirium assessment scale. *J Pain Symptom Manage*. 1997;13:128-137.

65. Ely EW, Inouye SK, Bernard GR, et al. Delirium in mechanically ventilated patients: validity and reliability of the confusion assessment method for the intensive care unit (CAM-ICU). *JAMA*. 2001;286:2703-2710.

66. Smith HA, Fuchs DC, Pandharipande PP, Barr FE, Ely EW. Delirium: an emerging frontier in the management of critically ill children. *Crit Care Clin*. 2009;25:593-614, x.

67. Truman B, Ely EW. Monitoring delirium in critically ill patients. Using the confusion assessment method for the intensive care unit. *Crit Care Nurse*. 2003;23:25-36; quiz 37-38.

68. Neelon VJ, Champagne MT, Carlson JR, Funk SG. The NEECHAM confusion scale: construction, validation, and clinical testing. *Nurs Res*. 1996;45(6):324-330.

69. Gaudreau JD, Gagnon P, Harel F, Tremblay A, Roy MA. Fast, systematic, and continuous delirium assessment in hospitalized patients: the nursing delirium screening scale. *J Pain Symptom Manage*. 2005;29:368-375.

70. Folstein MF, Folstein SE, McHugh PR. "Mini-mental state". A practical method for grading the cognitive state of patients for the clinician. *J Psychiatr Res*. 1975;12:189-198.

71. Folstein MF, Folstein SE, McHugh PR, Fanjiang G. *Mini-Mental State Examination User's Guide*. Odessa, FL: Psychological Assessment Resources; 2001.

72. Task Force for the Handbook of Psychiatric Measures. *Handbook of Psychiatric Measures*. Washington, DC: American Psychiatric Association; 2000:820.

73. Irwin SA, Ferris FD. The opportunity for psychiatry in palliative care. *Can J Psychiatry*. 2008;53:713-724.

74. Ferris FD, Danilychev M, Siegel A. Last hours of living. In: Emanuel LL, Librach SL, eds. *Palliative Care: Core Skills and Clinical Competencies*. Philadelphia, PA: Saunders Elsevier; 2007:267-293.

75. Emanuel EJ, Ferris FD, von Gunten CF, von Roenn J. *Education in Palliative and End-of-Life Care for Oncology*. Chicago, IL: The EPEC Project; 2005.

76. von Gunten CF, Sloan PA, Portenoy RK, Schonwetter RS. Physician board certification in hospice and palliative medicine. *J Palliat Med*. 2000;3:441-447.

77. Emanuel LL, Librach SL. *Palliative Care: Core Skills and Clinical Competencies*. Philadelphia, PA: Saunders/Elsevier; 2007.

78. Ferris FD, Balfour HM, Bowen K, et al. A model to guide patient and family care: based on nationally accepted principles and norms of practice. *J Pain Symptom Manage*. 2002;24:106-123.

79. Leonard M, Raju B, Conroy M, et al. Reversibility of delirium in terminally ill patients and predictors of mortality. *Palliat Med*. 2008;22:848-854.

80. Ferris FD. Last hours of living. *Clin Geriatr Med*. 2004;20:641-667.

81. Rao S, Ferris FD, Irwin SA. Ease of screening for depression and delirium in patients enrolled in inpatient hospice care. *J Palliat Med*. 2011;14:275-279.

82. Breitbart WS, Gibson C, Chochinov H. Palliative care. In: Levenson JL, ed. *Textbook of Psychosomatic Medicine*. Washington, DC: American Psychiatric Publishing; 2005:979-1007.

83. Lawlor PG, Bruera ED. Delirium in patients with advanced cancer. *Hematol Oncol Clin North Am*. 2002;16:701-714.

84. Breitbart W, Cohen K. Delirium in the terminally ill. In: Chochinov HM, Breitbart W, eds. *Handbook of Psychiatry in Palliative Medicine*. New York, NY: Oxford University Press; 2000:435.

85. de Stoutz ND, Bruera E, Suarez-Almazor M. Opioid rotation for toxicity reduction in terminal cancer patients. *J Pain Symptom Manage*. 1995;10:378-384.

86. Plonk WM Jr, Arnold RM. Terminal care: the last weeks of life. *J Palliat Med*. 2005;8:1042-1054.

87. Tang ST. Supporting cancer patients dying at home or at a hospital for Taiwanese family caregivers. *Cancer Nurs*. 2009;32:151-157.

88. Cole MG, Primeau FJ, Bailey RF, et al. Systematic intervention for elderly inpatients with delirium: a randomized trial. *CMAJ*. 1994;151:965-970.

89. Cole MG, McCusker J, Bellavance F, et al. Systematic detection and multidisciplinary care of delirium in older medical inpatients: a randomized trial. *CMAJ*. 2002;167:753-759.

90. Pitkala KH, Laurila JV, Strandberg TE, Tilvis RS. Multicomponent geriatric intervention for elderly inpatients with delirium: a randomized, controlled trial. *J Gerontol A Biol Sci Med Sci*. 2006;61:176-181.

91. Pitkala KH, Laurila JV, Strandberg TE, Kautiainen H, Sintonen H, Tilvis RS. Multicomponent geriatric intervention for elderly inpatients with delirium: effects on costs and health-related quality of life. *J Gerontol A Biol Sci Med Sci*. 2008;63:56-61.

92. Inouye SK, Bogardus ST Jr, Charpentier PA, et al. A multicomponent intervention to prevent delirium in hospitalized older patients. *N Engl J Med*. 1999;340:669-676.

93. Bruera E, Belzile M, Watanabe S, Fainsinger RL. Volume of hydration in terminal cancer patients. *Support Care Cancer*. 1996;4:147-150.

94. Dalal S, Bruera E. Dehydration in cancer patients: to treat or not to treat. *J Support Oncol*. 2004;2:467-479, 483.

95. Steiner N, Bruera E. Methods of hydration in palliative care patients. *J Palliat Care*. 1998;14:6-13.

96. Inouye SK, Zhang Y, Jones RN, Kiely DK, Yang F, Marcantonio ER. Risk factors for delirium at discharge: development and validation of a predictive model. *Arch Intern Med*. 2007;167:1406-1413.

97. Gagnon P, Charbonneau C, Allard P, Soulard C, Dumont S, Fillion L. Delirium in advanced cancer: a psychoeducational intervention for family caregivers. *J Palliat Care*. 2002;18:253-261.

98. Inouye SK, Bogardus ST Jr, Williams CS, Leo-Summers L, Agostini JV. The role of adherence on the effectiveness of nonpharmacologic interventions: evidence from the delirium prevention trial. *Arch Intern Med*. 2003;163:958-964.

99. Nikooie R, Neufeld KJ, Oh ES, et al. Antipsychotics for treating delirium in hospitalized adults: a systematic review. *Ann Intern Med*. 2019;171:485-495. doi:10.7326/M19-1860.

100. Agar M, Currow D, Plummer J, Chye R, Draper B. Differing management of people with advanced cancer and delirium by four sub-specialties. *Palliat Med*. 2008;22:633-640.

101. Rundell JR, Wise MG, Press AP. *Essentials of Consultation-Liaison Psychiatry: Based on the American Psychiatric Press Textbook of Consultation-Liaison Psychiatry.* Washington, DC: American Psychiatric Press; 1999:xxi, 671 p.

102. Sipahimalani A, Masand PS. Olanzapine in the treatment of delirium. *Psychosomatics.* 1998;39:422-430.

103. Stahl SM. *Stahl's Essential Psychopharmacology: Neuroscientific Basis and Practical Applications.* Cambridge, UK/New York, NY: Cambridge University Press; 2008:1117.

104. Boettger S, Breitbart W. An open trial of aripiprazole for the treatment of delirium in hospitalized cancer patients. *Palliat Support Care.* 2011;9:351-357.

105. Skrobik YK, Bergeron N, Dumont M, Gottfried SB. Olanzapine vs haloperidol: treating delirium in a critical care setting. *Intensive Care Med.* 2004;30:444-449.

106. Han CS, Kim YK. A double-blind trial of risperidone and haloperidol for the treatment of delirium. *Psychosomatics.* 2004;45:297-301.

107. Bottomley DM, Hanks GW. Subcutaneous midazolam infusion in palliative care. *J Pain Symptom Manage.* 1990;5:259-261.

108. Rousseau P. Palliative sedation in the management of refractory symptoms. *J Support Oncol.* 2004;2:181-186.

109. Rousseau P. Palliative sedation in the control of refractory symptoms. *J Palliat Med.* 2005;8:10-12.

110. Morita T, Tei Y, Inoue S. Agitated terminal delirium and association with partial opioid substitution and hydration. *J Palliat Med.* 2003;6:557-563.

111. Stiefel F, Fainsinger R, Bruera E. Acute confusional states in patients with advanced cancer. *J Pain Symptom Manage.* 1992;7:94-98.

112. Fainsinger RL, Waller A, Bercovici M, et al. A multicentre international study of sedation for uncontrolled symptoms in terminally ill patients. *Palliat Med.* 2000;14:257-265.

113. Rietjens JA, van Zuylen L, van Veluw H, van der Wijk L, van der Heide A, van der Rijt CC. Palliative sedation in a specialized unit for acute palliative care in a cancer hospital: comparing patients dying with and without palliative sedation. *J Pain Symptom Manage.* 2008;36:228-234.

114. Connor SR, Pyenson B, Fitch K, Spence C, Iwasaki K. Comparing hospice and nonhospice patient survival among patients who die within a three-year window. *J Pain Symptom Manage.* 2007;33:238-246.

115. Sykes N, Thorns A. Sedative use in the last week of life and the implications for end-of-life decision making. *Arch Intern Med.* 2003;163:341-344.

116. Vitetta L, Kenner D, Sali A. Sedation and analgesia-prescribing patterns in terminally ill patients at the end of life. *Am J Hosp Palliat Care.* 2005;22:465-473.

117. Morita T, Chinone Y, Ikenaga M, et al. Efficacy and safety of palliative sedation therapy: a multicenter, prospective, observational study conducted on specialized palliative care units in Japan. *J Pain Symptom Manage.* 2005;30:320-328.

118. Good PD, Ravenscroft PJ, Cavenagh J. Effects of opioids and sedatives on survival in an Australian inpatient palliative care population. *Intern Med J.* 2005;35:512-517.

119. Bercovitch M, Adunsky A. Patterns of high-dose morphine use in a home-care hospice service: should we be afraid of it? *Cancer.* 2004;101:1473-1477.

120. Bercovitch M, Waller A, Adunsky A. High dose morphine use in the hospice setting. A database survey of patient characteristics and effect on life expectancy. *Cancer.* 1999;86:871-877.

121. Portenoy RK, Sibirceva U, Smout R, et al. Opioid use and survival at the end of life: a survey of a hospice population. *J Pain Symptom Manage.* 2006;32:532-540.

122. Stirling LC, Kurowska A, Tookman A. The use of phenobarbitone in the management of agitation and seizures at the end of life. *J Pain Symptom Manage.* 1999;17:363-368.

123. Lundstrom S, Zachrisson U, Furst CJ. When nothing helps: propofol as sedative and antiemetic in palliative cancer care. *J Pain Symptom Manage.* 2005;30:570-577.

124. Lundstrom S, Twycross R, Mihalyo M, Wilcock A. Propofol. *J Pain Symptom Manage.* 2010;40:466-470.

125. Wise MG, Rundell JR. *Clinical Manual of Psychosomatic Medicine: A Guide to Consultation-Liaison Psychiatry.* Arlington, VA: American Psychiatric Publishing; 2005:xi, 338 p.

126. Richelson E. Preclinical pharmacology of neuroleptics: focus on new generation compounds. *J Clin Psychiatry.* 1996;57(suppl 11):4-11.

127. Schatzberg AF, Cole JO, DeBattista C. *Manual of Clinical Psychopharmacology.* Washington, DC: American Psychiatric Publishing; 2007:xxv, 697 p.

128. Clinical Pharmacology Online. Updated 2008. http://www.clinicalpharmacology-ipcom/defaultaspx

129. Allen MH, Currier GW, Hughes DH, Reyes-Harde M, Docherty JP. The expert consensus guideline series. Treatment of behavioral emergencies. *Postgrad Med.* 2001;1-88; quiz 89-90.

130. Jackson KC, Lipman AG. Drug therapy for delirium in terminally ill patients. *Cochrane Database Syst Rev.* 2004;(2):CD004770.

131. Lonergan E, Britton Annette M, Luxenberg J. *Antipsychotics for Delirium. Cochrane Database of Systematic Reviews.* Chichester, UK: Wiley; 2007.

132. Wang PS, Schneeweiss S, Avorn J, et al. Risk of death in elderly users of conventional vs. atypical antipsychotic medications. *N Engl J Med.* 2005;353:2335-2341.

133. Ballard C, Hanney ML, Theodoulou M, et al. The dementia antipsychotic withdrawal trial (DART-AD): long-term follow-up of a randomised placebo-controlled trial. *Lancet Neurol.* 2009;8:151-157.

134. Ray WA, Chung CP, Murray KT, Hall K, Stein CM. Atypical antipsychotic drugs and the risk of sudden cardiac death. *N Engl J Med.* 2009;360:225-235.

135. Gill SS, Bronskill SE, Normand S-LT, et al. Antipsychotic drug use and mortality in older adults with dementia. *Ann Intern Med.* 2007;146:775-786.

136. Schneeweiss S, Setoguchi S, Brookhart A, Dormuth C, Wang PS. Risk of death associated with the use of conventional versus atypical antipsychotic drugs among elderly patients. *CMAJ.* 2007;176:627-632.

137. Schneider LS, Dagerman KS, Insel P. Risk of death with atypical antipsychotic drug treatment for dementia: meta-analysis of randomized placebo-controlled trials. *JAMA.* 2005;294:1934-1943.

138. Jeste DV, Blazer D, Casey D, et al. ACNP White paper: update on use of antipsychotic drugs in elderly persons with dementia. *Neuropsychopharmacology.* 2008;33:957-970.

139. Elie D, Poirier M, Chianetta J, Durand M, Gregoire C, Grignon S. Cognitive effects of antipsychotic dosage and polypharmacy: a study with the BACS in patients with schizophrenia and schizoaffective disorder. *J Psychopharmacol.* 2010;24:1037-1044.

140. Schneider LS, Tariot PN, Dagerman KS, et al. Effectiveness of atypical antipsychotic drugs in patients with Alzheimer's disease. *N Engl J Med.* 2006;355:1525-1538.

141. Saad M, Cassagnol M, Ahmed E. The impact of FDA's warning on the use of antipsychotics in clinical practice: a survey. *Consult Pharm.* 2010;25:739-744.

35 Depression and Anxiety in Palliative Care

Paul Noufi, Haniya Raza, and Maryland Pao

"Four major existential concerns—death, meaning in life, isolation, and freedom—play a crucial role in the inner life of every human being."

—*Irvin Yalom, Love's Executioner*

EMOTIONAL RESPONSES TO ILLNESS AND DEATH

The diagnosis of medical illness is a crucial turning point for a person who is suddenly thrown into a turmoil of unknowns and uncertainties and faced with his or her vulnerability. Following onset of medical illness, spiraling stressful events with many illness-related strains may ensue. In the period of their sickness, patients may undergo frequent hospitalizations, drastic and sometimes irreversible changes in bodily functions, as well as changes in functional status (1,2). They may need to deal with pain, while still building and maintaining good relationships with multiple health care providers, and preparing for an uncertain future (1). They struggle to preserve a satisfactory body image and identity amid often unexpected and unpredictable complications of their illness and are frequently found to be fighting to maintain the social, physical, and professional homeostasis that they had previously worked to build (3). Health concerns can bring about emotional suffering, including worries about the lives of loved ones, the amount of time left to spend with them, the welfare of children, and feelings of guilt about a person's role in their disease (3). Both emotional suffering and body image impairment have been found to be highly associated with psychological stress (4).

As intuitively expected, the intensity of psychological stress and the severity of the medical illness are correlated (1). This is of particular clinical interest in the cases of patients receiving palliative care and struggling with terminal illnesses (5). Death and the influence of mortality on human existence are concepts that have preoccupied philosophers and psychologists such as Yalom, May, and Tillich for centuries, bringing about multiple reflections on the search for meaning (6–9). Human beings are the only species who can cognitively reflect on

the meaning of their mortality, but most people still manage to suppress and hide from the terrible truth of its inevitability in their daily lives, thus avoiding existential despair (10). The diagnosis of a terminal illness can shatter these unconscious defenses, exposing patients to the realization of the frailness of existence. Consequently, palliative care occurs at a time when the psyche is bombarded by overwhelming existential interrogations about the meaning of one's life and death, potentially precipitating a full mobilization and restructuring of existing psychological defenses and coping skills.

Studies have described wide interindividual variation in the responses to terminal illness (11,12). Though patterns of coping can be detected across populations, it is unrealistic to expect that all patients use the same coping strategies (13). Providers are also encouraged to keep in mind that coping is a dynamic process that changes with the specific situation and time. In other words, the subjective experience of the patient is an essential mediator of the relationship between the stress of terminal illness and the patient's affective response (Fig. 35.1). The subjective experience is shaped by multiple factors, including demographic characteristics, personality traits, previous coping styles, and illness perceptions. For example, older women living with a partner display higher rates of problem-focused coping strategies than do their younger male counterparts who are living alone (3). Heiskell and Pasnau describe a heightening of a patient's previous personality-related adaptation schemes when exposed to the stress of a medical illness that also influences their way of dealing with the stressor (14). Another factor that emerges as particularly important in the modulation of a patient's affective response is illness perception, which is the cognitive representation of the meaning of the illness to the patient, built upon previous experiences and current understanding of the medical illness (15).

Patients will experience an array of emotional responses to terminal illness, often including grief, much like the grief that accompanies the loss of a loved one (6). They may also sometimes experience anger, anxiety, sadness, and shame. Sadness is a natural emotion in the setting of illness and

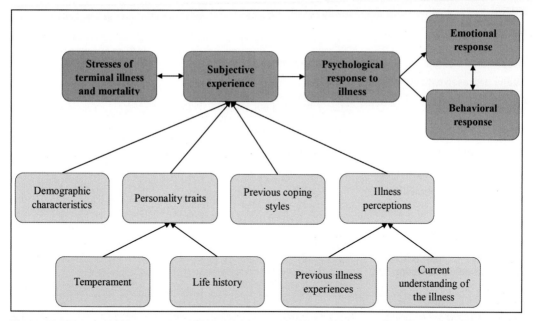

Figure 35.1 The multiple factors influencing the emotional response to illness and death. (Source: Adapted from Lazarus RS. *Stress and Emotion: A New Synthesis*. New York, NY: Springer Publishing Co.; 1999.)

particularly terminal illness, so it is not surprising to find a sick person uncomfortable, frustrated, or irritable. Though bereavement is sometimes expected to follow sequential stages, patients will often experience different emotions simultaneously. Medical providers are highly encouraged to try to understand and validate the patient's subjective experience. To avoid misinterpretation of emotional reactions as pathological or excessive, it is important to understand that patient's unique coping style given their circumstances. For example, in emergencies, patients often cope with what is most immediate while other stressors are temporarily put aside. Sometimes, emotions and fuller understanding of the personal dimension of illness are suppressed until the marathon of initial surgery, radiation treatment, and chemotherapy has been completed. Psychiatric disorders should only be diagnosed when the provider feels that the patient's presentation and symptoms are causing clinically significant distress and/or interfering with the patient's functioning or medical treatment (16).

When previous coping methods are not enough to subdue the stress of terminal illness, the patient's emotional response can become overwhelming and impairing and interfere in their care. The acute stress of medical illness initially triggers the sympathetic nervous system, releasing catecholamines that will act on different organ systems and create a generalized state of fight or flight. When they act on the central nervous system, this can lead to

cognitive and mood disturbances including anxiety and depressive disorders (17).

It is important not to overpathologize emotional responses to illness and death, but it is also crucial to recognize and diagnose mental health disorders in order to be able to offer the proper treatments.

EPIDEMIOLOGY OF DEPRESSION AND ANXIETY IN PALLIATIVE CARE PATIENTS

Major depressive disorder (MDD) is defined by the presence of low mood or anhedonia (loss of interest in daily activities) along with at least four other criteria that include appetite or sleep disturbances, difficulty concentrating, change in psychomotor activity or energy levels, hopelessness or helplessness, and suicidal thoughts. According to the DSM-5 criteria, to be able to diagnose a patient with MDD, the symptoms must be present for more than 2 consecutive weeks and need to impair the patient in daily functioning. However, though major depressive disorder is a commonly diagnosed mood disorder, it is important to remember that there are other presentations of depressive disorders that may warrant intervention and treatment. The presentations and prevalence of the different depressive disorders are presented in Table 35.1.

The reported prevalence of depressive disorders in patients receiving palliative care ranges from 1% to 88.7% across studies (18). A 2011 meta-analysis

TABLE 35.1 PRESENTATION AND PREVALENCE OF DSM-5 DEPRESSIVE DISORDERS IN THE GENERAL POPULATION

Depressive disorder	Clinical presentation	U.S. prevalence reported in the DSM-V (16)
Major depressive disorder	Persistent feeling of sadness and loss of interest, along with four other criteria including appetite and sleep disturbances, difficulty concentrating, psychomotor changes, loss of energy, feelings of worthlessness, and recurrent thoughts of death.	7%
Persistent depressive disorder	Persistent low mood for more than 2 years.	0.5%
Substance/medication-induced mood disorder	Persistent disturbance in mood that is present in the context of current or recent substance use of a substance/medication that is capable of producing this symptom.	0.26%
Depressive disorder due to another medical condition	Depressed mood that is the direct pathophysiological consequence of another medical condition.	—

of 24 studies on oncology, hematology, and palliative care patients reported a 24.5% prevalence; 16.5% of patients fulfilled the criteria for MDD (19). A recent study in India reports a 70% prevalence of MDD diagnosed using the PHQ-9 with a cutoff of 10 or more (20). Other studies led on smaller samples in Brazil and the U.S. report 88.7% and 20% prevalence, respectively (21,22).

This discrepancy in prevalence rates is thought to be due to multiple factors. First, the diagnosis of any depressive disorder can be challenging in medical patients as depression can present with neurovegetative symptoms that overlap with those of the primary medical illness. Depressive disorders can also mimic grief and sadness that often accompany terminal illness. Second, the methodologies adopted in the studies are heterogeneous. Instruments used for the screening of depression are not standardized and not always validated in medical populations; sample sizes are variable and often small due to low response rates. Additionally, the diagnosis of depression is influenced by cultural factors. For example, there may be culturally based expressions of emotional problems. Depression and other psychological distress may present as somatic symptoms. Cultures may also vary in the terms used to define and describe depression and anxiety. The differing prevalence of depression across countries may be related to variable perceptions and attitudes of providers and patients towards the nature of the illness.

Risk factors for depression are generally categorized as modifiable or not. Known nonmodifiable factors include female gender and younger age (21,23). Other factors that are difficult to modify are financial difficulties and low life satisfaction

(20,24). The latter is reported in one study to be the strongest predictor of depression. Other risk factors that are more readily modified include social support, health-related factors, and illness perception. A sense of coherence in the patient's family, a more positive attitude of the caregiver towards the illness, and a higher sense of spirituality are all protective factors against depression (23,25). Health-related risk factors include uncontrolled physical symptoms (particularly gastrointestinal symptoms), the intensity of pain, the presence of sleep or cognitive disturbances, the setting of treatment (inpatient vs. outpatient), and the illness prognosis (24,26). Finally, the patient's awareness of the prognosis influences depressive symptoms, though the direction of the association remains the subject of ongoing investigation (27,28).

Anxiety is the experience of worry, apprehension, unease, tension, or nervousness. Almost any person facing a serious illness will intermittently report some anxiety. When the emotions are brief and of low intensity, they may not be a source of significant distress and may even play the role of an adaptive function activating the person to seek treatment. However, once anxiety becomes severe or pervasive enough to cause distress or functional impairment, providers may decide that it should be the focus of clinical attention and treatment. The DSM-5 anxiety disorders are detailed in Table 35.2. Anxiety symptoms can also be present in stress-related disorders such as adjustment disorder (16).

In the palliative care setting, anxiety disorders are reported in 6.8% to 13.3% of patients, while anxiety symptoms are much more common and reported in 24% to 48% of patients (29). In a 2011

TABLE 35.2 PRESENTATION AND PREVALENCE OF DSM-5 ANXIETY DISORDERS IN THE GENERAL POPULATION

Anxiety disorder	Clinical presentation	U.S. prevalence reported in the DSM-V (16)
Generalized anxiety disorder	Excessive and uncontrollable worry about a number of events or activities, accompanied by somatic symptoms such as fatigue, restlessness, or muscle tension	2.9%
Social anxiety disorder	Anxiety triggered by specific situations where the person is exposed to unfamiliar people or to possible scrutiny by others	7%
Agoraphobia	Anxiety triggered by being in a situation where escape might be difficult or impossible, accompanied by avoidance of such situations	1.7%
Specific phobia	Excessive anxiety triggered by a specific object or situation	7%–9%
Panic disorder	Recurrent and untriggered panic attacks accompanied by significant change in behavior because of the attacks	2%–3%
Substance/medication-induced anxiety disorder	Anxiety that is present in the context of current or recent substance use of a substance/medication that is capable of producing this symptom	0.002%
Anxiety disorder due to another medical condition	Anxiety that is the direct pathophysiological consequence of another medical condition	—

meta-analysis, anxiety disorders are reported to have a prevalence of 9.8% in oncology, hematology, and palliative care patients (19). Other studies that focus on patients with advanced cancer report higher percentages of anxiety disorders ranging from 20% to 50% (30–32). Frequently, anxiety and depressive disorders are comorbid in the palliative cancer population with 10.2% of patients reporting both symptoms simultaneously (33).

Since prevalence reports are highly diverse, many studies focus instead on comorbidity of anxiety symptoms with other subjective complaints. Anxiety is found to be positively associated with physical symptoms including pain, fatigue, sleep disturbances, shortness of breath, and even cardiac arrhythmias (34–37). A study published in 2017 reports that anxiety can be predicted by sociodemographic characteristics (gender, age, performance status, assistance with activities of daily living [ADLs], organization of care, living situation), physical symptoms (pain, nausea, dyspnea, loss of appetite, tiredness), and care-related factors (use of sedatives or antidepressants). In addition, anxiety is negatively associated with the use of cardiac medications but positively associated with antibiotics (38). Finally, Kolva et al. and Thompson

et al. report a negative association between anxiety and the degree of acceptance of the illness and the belief in an afterlife (39,40).

ASSESSMENT AND DIAGNOSIS OF DEPRESSION AND ANXIETY

Clinicians should ask about mood and anxiety as these symptoms are strongly associated (41) as part of routine assessment. Patients may be more relaxed and open if depression is considered in the context of a general conversation about coping, in which they feel able to tell their story and feel heard and understood (42).

The diagnosis of depressive and anxiety disorders relies on a comprehensive interview and clinical assessment of the patient and his/her symptoms. The clinician combines the patient's subjective reports with the objective findings on the mental status exam to be able to make a final diagnosis. There is a lot to be learned about patients and their behaviors by observing and listening to them before, during, and after the psychiatric interview. It is also useful to see how the patient interacts with staff and with family or friends. A variety of adjectives are used by patients to describe a depressed or anxious mood: distraught, grieving, hopeless, overwhelmed, remorseful, sad, anxious, fearful, frightened, high-strung, nervous, on edge, overwhelmed, panicked, tense, terrified, worried, and many others. Other signs and symptoms can also be either reported by the patient or their family and/or observed by the clinician during the interview. They include changes in activity level, cognitive abilities, speech, and vegetative functions (e.g., sleep, appetite, sexual activity). An essential part of the diagnosis is also the impairment in interpersonal, social, and occupational functioning.

Diagnostic rating scales may be useful in aiding diagnosis as well as in monitoring the effects of treatment and guiding further management decisions. They help translate clinical observations or patient self-assessments into objective measures. Clinically, such tools can help screen for individuals who need treatment, evaluate the accuracy of diagnosis, determine the severity of symptoms, or gauge the effectiveness of a given intervention. Although clinician-administered instruments are generally more reliable and valid, self-completed patient instruments are less time consuming. In either case, careful consideration should be given to the clinical meanings and consequences of their results, as well as to cultural factors that could affect the tool's performance. A discussion on the challenges in the use of diagnostic instruments in the special case of palliative care patients will follow in this section.

Table 35.3 summarizes recommendations for detection, diagnosis, and assessment of depression in palliative care.

Quality of Life

The World Health Organization (WHO) defines palliative care as "an approach that improves quality of life of patients and their families by means of early identification and impeccable assessment and treatment of pain and other problems" (43). Though the definition of health-related quality of life is the subject of ongoing debate, the WHO defines it as "an individual's perception of their position in life in the context of the culture and value systems in which they live and in relation to their goals, expectations, standards, and concerns. It is a broad-ranging concept affected in a complex way by the person's physical health, psychological state, level of independence, social relationships, personal beliefs and their relationship to salient features of their environment." In this definition, psychological well-being is one of the core components of improved quality of life, and as such, the detection and treatment of psychiatric symptoms and/or disorders are a crucial component of palliative care services. Depression and anxiety can not only affect the quality of life by causing significant psychological distress but also exacerbate physical symptoms and/or their perception by the patient. Depression and anxiety may also decrease the patient's ability to care for self and to fully adhere to the recommended medical treatment. In other words, depression and anxiety impact multiple spheres of a terminal patient's life, including physical well-being, psychological well-being, and environmental health (20).

There is abundant evidence in the medical and palliative care literature for the severe negative

TABLE 35.3 DETECTION, DIAGNOSIS, AND SEVERITY ASSESSMENT: EVIDENCE AND RECOMMENDATION SUMMARY

Detection, diagnosis, and severity assessment	Quality of evidence	Strength of recommendation
Clinicians should prioritize cognitive/affective symptoms in detecting depression as physical symptoms (e.g., weight loss, fatigue) may be caused by physical disease or medical treatment.	*Moderate* Consistent evidence from nonrandomized studies	*Strong* Moderate-quality evidence; consistent with clinical opinion
Clinicians should consider screening for depression in palliative care patients. Screening tools may help clinicians detect depression, but evidence that they improve depression outcomes is lacking.	*Very low* No studies of impact on depression outcomes in palliative care	*Weak* Low-quality evidence; cost implications unclear
The psychological state of patients receiving palliative care is unstable. Clinicians should regularly review depressive symptoms to capture changes in mood.	*Moderate* Consistent evidence from nonrandomized studies	*Strong* Moderate-quality evidence; consistent with clinical opinion; low risk of harm

Source: Adapted from Rayner L, Price A, Hotopf M, Higginson IJ. Expert opinion on detecting and treating depression in palliative care: a Delphi study. *BMC Palliat Care*. 2011;10:10.

effects of psychiatric disorders on health-related quality of life. Many studies consistently report that depression and anxiety are the single strongest predictors of a decreased QoL in patients with advanced cancer (44,45). In a study published in 2019, depression was found to have a significant influence on multiple aspects of health-related QoL (physical, emotional, social, and cognitive) and global health status in patients with nonadvanced breast cancer (46). Other studies additionally report that the higher the symptoms of depression, the worse the global and functional QoL (21).

With regard to psychological well-being, depression and anxiety significantly impair the patient's mood, activity, sleep, and sexual health (46). Depressive symptoms are also associated with decreased social support (21). Hence, depression leads to decreased psychosocial functioning, alienation of the patient, and further coping difficulties with their illness (47).

In addition to direct psychological distress, depression is associated with an exacerbation of physical symptoms in the palliative care literature (44). As depressive symptoms become more severe, patients' thresholds for distress become lower, potentially leading to increased sensitivity and preoccupation with side effects of medications and physical symptoms such as pain, nausea, and vomiting (48–50). Depression can also increase fatigue that is multifactorial in palliative care patients. Consequently, psychiatric morbidity can affect willingness of patients to actively participate in their treatment and adhere to providers' recommendations, thereby reducing survival (51). In contrast, an increase in survival of patients with metastatic breast cancer after treatment of depression has been reported (52). Finally, evidence shows that the adequate treatment of depression and anxiety using antidepressants in patients with terminal illness, such as cancer, can improve both distressing symptoms and quality of life (53).

Suicide Risk Assessment

Terminal illness is highly associated with suicidal ideations and acts. In the context of palliative care, suicidality may present in different forms ranging from poor self-care to refusal of treatment and frank suicide attempts. Some authors report that half of patients diagnosed with a terminal illness express desire for hastened death (54,55). Chochinov et al. reported that 8.5% of patients admitted to palliative care services in Canada express wishes for hastened death (56). Palliative care patients are reported in some studies to have suicide prevalence

rates twice as high as the general population (55). Further, Salib et al. reported the presence of terminal illness in 5% of late-life suicides in the United Kingdom (56,57).

Physical illness thus emerges in the literature as a consistent risk factor for suicide. The association of physical illness with increased pain, a sense of loss of control, and the worry about the consequently limited lifestyle can lead to the thoughts that life is not worth living. Additionally, terminally ill patients often perceive themselves as a burden to others, which can also result in an increased desire for hastened death. In the study of the phenomenology of suicidality, some authors describe the critical role of hopelessness associated with depression and hypothesize that it is the mediator of the association between depression and suicide in the terminally ill (58).

Suicidal thoughts are the result of the complex interaction of different etiological components, and it seems oversimplistic to try and pinpoint a single unidirectional causality for this phenomenon. However, although suicide may be considered a rational decision in patients suffering from terminal illnesses with poor prognosis, it remains the ethical duty of the physician to explore the meaning and motivation underlying a refusal of life-prolonging treatment. It is also always medically indicated to investigate the presence of modifiable risk factors that could be influencing the patient's ability to cope with his or her illness. Multiple factors are found to increase the risk of suicide in the general as well as in the palliative care populations, namely male gender, marital status (divorced, widowed, or separated), and unemployment (59,60).

For a comprehensive discussion of specific suicide risk factors in patients with advanced cancer, please refer to Table 35.4. As seen in the table, the one risk factor that remains the most significant in both the general and the palliative care population is the presence of psychiatric comorbidity, and particularly of depression and/or anxiety (62). Suicidal ideation is one of the core symptoms of depression listed in the DSM-5 (16), and suicide and depression are highly correlated. As reported by the NIMH, suffering from depression or other mental disorders is one of the main risk factors for suicide (63). Furthermore, suicidal ideations can emerge even with subthreshold depressive or anxious symptoms (64). In 1986, Brown et al. found that all patients with advanced cancer in their sample who reported a desire for a rapid death met the criteria for a major depressive episode (62). This finding is not isolated; a 2000 study

TABLE 35.4 RISK FACTORS FOR SUICIDE IN CANCER PATIENTS

Sociodemographic factors
Middle or older age
Gender: male
Marital status: single, divorced, or widowed
Race: black

Psychiatric disorders
Preexisting psychopathology
Depression
Anxiety
Aggression
Family mental disorders or family history of suicide

Psychosocial factors
Poor social support
Loss of independence, feeling of being a burden

Medical factors
Pain
Advanced disease
Poor prognosis
Survival rate <5 years
Nonlocalized cancer
Short time since diagnosis disclosure
Physical symptoms
Cancer sites: head and neck, gastrointestinal, urogenital

Other factors
Previous suicide attempt
Suicidal thoughts

Source: Adapted from Spoletini I, Gianni W, Caltagirone C, Madaio R, Repetto L, Spalletta G. Suicide and cancer: where do we go from here? *Crit Rev Oncol/Hematol.* 2011;78(3):206-219. Ref. (61).

by Breitbart et al. also found that cancer patients with depression were four times more likely to request hastened death as compared to those without depression (47% vs. 12%) (65). Another study published in 2002 that investigated the association between depression and suicidal thoughts in 1,721 cancer patients reports that subjects who suffered from major depression were 1.8 times more likely to have suicidal ideations than those who did not (66). More recent studies find similar high prevalence rates of depression in late-life suicide, with percentages ranging from 23.4% to 61.4% (67). Cancer is particularly associated with increased rates of suicidal ideations, attempts, and acts (64,68). Although the risk of suicide seems to be the highest in the first month after a cancer diagnosis, some studies report persistently elevated risk up to 3 months, and sometimes even longer (68,69). However, though most studied in oncological populations, these findings are not unique to this illness, and similar reports are found in patients suffering from different types of terminal illnesses (70).

Not all patients who express suicidal ideations are necessarily suffering from a depressive disorder. However, studies have shown that suicidal ideations in the terminally ill decrease with the treatment of depression by reducing the severity of depressive symptoms. Even though this might not necessarily underline a unidirectional association between depression and suicidal ideations, it certainly adds to the argument that depression and suicidal ideations need to be screened for and treated in patients with advanced physical illnesses. For example, a 25% decrease in physician-assisted suicide requests after the use of antidepressants has been reported in the literature (71). Comparable findings are reported for patients who suffer from head and neck cancer as well as advanced AIDS, where the successful treatment of depression is found to decrease the desire for hastened death (72,73).

There are challenges in screening and diagnosis of depression in seriously medically ill patients. Given that the diagnosis of depression is clinical and relies inherently on an interpretative process on the part of the physician, clinicians' conceptualizations, attitudes, and beliefs about its diagnosis and treatment play a major role in its screening and detection. Research has identified that medical practitioners experience difficulties in reconciling the biomedical and psychosocial models of understanding depression and struggle between the different models (74,75). A spectral model spans from seeing a depressed mood as a normal reaction to stressors to the presence of several depressive symptoms and finally to a full-blown depressive disorder. The other model is dichotomous and is divided into two distinct entities: the reactive type (an understandable response to a situation) and the endogenous type (viewed as a biological illness). This debate is relevant on a clinical level as the "width" of depression conceptualization influences the readiness of clinicians to diagnose and treat depressive symptoms and disorder in a specific patient. In a study published in 2014, the authors report that clinicians who conceptualized depression in broad terms of being an illness and/or symptom, warned against adopting a narrow view of equating depression with "major depressive disorder" because of the risk of thinking that depression falling outside of such criteria was insignificant or not requiring palliation. In comparison, those with narrow concepts of depression warned against overdiagnosis and pathologizing "normal" human sadness (76).

This debate is particularly relevant in palliative care patients who are undergoing major life changes and a necessary period of grief. Attitudes towards depression are variable among different specialists: in a series of studies published between 2013 and 2015, the authors show that even though psychiatrists thought of depression in the same way in palliative and nonpalliative populations, palliative medicine specialists and palliative medicine practitioners felt that the concept of depression is different in palliative populations as, in this context, de novo depression was easier to understand because of the terminal illness (76–78). As such, depression as an emotional state was also thought of as an inevitable and unavoidable stage of the grieving process.

In the absence of purely objective and/or somatic markers for depression, the line of "normalcy" is blurred, sometimes placing depression in a gray area with indistinct boundaries with grief and other psychiatric diagnoses (79). This ongoing debate poses a challenge in the assessment and diagnosis of depression in the palliative care context.

Clinical Tools for Screening and Diagnosis of Depression and Anxiety

Given the establishment of a diagnosis of depression can be particularly challenging in medically and terminally ill patients due to the overlap of symptoms of depression with somatic symptoms secondary to the illness itself, use of clinical depression tools may be helpful. Table 35.5 compares the DSM-5 symptoms required for the diagnosis of depression to those reported in the context of

TABLE 35.5 COMPARISON OF SICKNESS SYNDROME AND MAJOR DEPRESSION

Sickness behavior	Major depression
Anhedonia	
Social isolation	
Fatigue	
Anorexia	
Weight loss	
Sleep disturbance	
Cognitive disturbance	
Decreased libido	
Psychomotor retardation	
Hyperalgesia	
	Depressed mood
	Guilt/worthlessness
	Suicidal ideation

Source: Adapted from Raison CL, Miller AH. Depression in cancer: new developments regarding diagnosis and treatment. *Biol Psychiatry*. 2003;54(3):283-294.

medical conditions including cancer and inflammatory illness (80). Neurovegetative symptoms including appetite changes, sleep disturbances, loss of concentration, and fatigue are symptoms are included in the description of depression, but they are far from being specific to the disorder.

To overcome this dilemma, various approaches have been suggested to tailor the diagnostic criteria of depression in the context of palliative care. The three most common approaches are summarized in Table 35.6. The inclusive method advocates for incorporating all depressive symptoms listed in the DSM-5 in the assessment regardless of their etiology. This strategy has evidence for a high rate of detection of depression but also an equally high rate of false positives and an overdiagnosis of depression in the medically ill (81–83). On the other hand, the substitution approach that uses the Endicott criteria advocates for the replacement of the physical symptoms of depression (disturbed sleep, poor appetite or loss of weight, poor concentration, and fatigue) with psychological symptoms that cannot be solely explained by the medical illness itself (tearfulness or depressed appearance, social withdrawal or decreased talkativeness, brooding/self-pity/pessimism, and lack of reactivity). Though these modified criteria are tailored for a more specific assessment of depression, empirical studies that provide direct data comparing the specificity of the diagnosis with and without these symptoms have unfortunately yielded inconsistent results (83–85). Finally, the exclusive approach advocates for a simplification of the depressive criteria and an altogether elimination of the somatic symptoms from the assessment. Contrary to the inclusive approach, the major disadvantage of this method is its low sensitivity, which results in an underdiagnosis and treatment of depression (81,82).

As the use of each of these approaches offers advantages and disadvantages, the clinical assessment of depression in the palliative care context remains heterogeneous among specialists. However, clinical purposes are better served by taking the inclusive approach as clinical data indicate that sickness/depressive symptoms respond to antidepressant therapy irrespective of putative etiology (86). Even in the absence of a major depressive disorder, the use of antidepressants may help in the treatment of depressive symptoms, as well as specific sickness-related symptoms, including pain and insomnia, which can also serve to prevent the development of a full-blown depressive disorder (87).

Due to these multiple approaches to depression, it is difficult to find one validated objective instrument for the screening and the measurement of depressive symptoms. Specific instruments are more useful for identifying depression either

TABLE 35.6 THE DIFFERENT APPROACHES TO THE DIAGNOSIS OF DEPRESSION IN THE PALLIATIVE CARE CONTEXT

	Inclusive	Substitutive	Exclusive
Criteria used	DSM-5 criteria for major depressive disorder	Endicott's criteria: • Low mood • Anhedonia • Feelings of guilt or worthlessness • Concentration problems • Suicidality or thoughts about death • **Tearfulness/depressed appearance** • **Social withdrawal/decreased talkativeness** • **Brooding/self-pity/pessimism** • **Lack of reactivity**	DSM-5 criteria for major depressive disorder excluding somatic symptoms
Advantages	High sensitivity	Controversial specificity	Low sensitivity
Disadvantages	Low specificity		High specificity

exclusively or inclusively, depending on the physician's approach and preference. Unlike the Beck Depression Inventory (BDI) and the Montgomery Asberg Depression Rating Scale (MAD-RS) that emphasize mood and cognitive symptoms more specific to depression, the Neurotoxicity Rating Scale assesses the full range of neurobehavioral symptoms that afflict patients with severe illnesses, including the neurovegetative symptoms shared by major depression and physical illness. The evidence base for the use of such tools in the palliative care population is very small, and most of the studies are performed in a single center and include small numbers of patients. No scale has shown superior validity, sensitivity, or specificity to become the gold-standard tool for the assessment of symptoms in palliative care patients.

The Hospital Anxiety and Depression Scale (HADS) is a 14-item scale devised in 1983 by Zigmond and Snaith for use among medical patients and is currently the most commonly used in the palliative setting (88,89). It consists of depression and anxiety subscales, with anhedonia as a major construct in the evaluation. Unfortunately, few studies have compared the HADS head-to-head with other tools (90). Validity studies also yield conflicting data concerning specificity and sensitivity, and the cutoff thresholds for both subscales are still debated. In a 2001 validity study, the sensitivity was 54% and the specificity was 74% for depression at a cutoff threshold of 11 on the depression subscale; the optimum cutoff threshold for identifying cases of depression on the anxiety subscale was 10, with a sensitivity of 59% and a specificity of 68% (91). In a meta-analysis published in 2010, sensitivity was between 71.6% and 82%, and specificity was between 77% and 82.6% for depression. For anxiety, sensitivity was between 48.7% and 83.9%, and specificity was between 69.9% and 78.7% (90). Based on these findings, Mitchell et al. recommend the use of the HADS as a screening tool, to be followed by a thorough clinical evaluation, rather than a case-finding instrument. On the other hand, acceptability studies show that, even though the 5-minute scale has a patient acceptability as high as 85% judging by the rate of full completion in clinical oncology practice, it has a staff acceptability of only 6% according to one study in cancer professionals, likely owing to the fact that it is considered too long for a routine screening tool (92–94).

The Edinburgh Postnatal Depression Screen (EPDS) is a tool initially designed to detect depression in postnatal women, excluding somatic symptoms. It consists of 10 items, each rated on a four-point scale, and includes an evaluation of guilt, thoughts of self-harm, and hopelessness. In a validity study published in 2000, the authors show a sensitivity of 81% and a specificity of 79% for the detection of depression at a cutoff value of 13 in inpatients receiving palliative care, suggesting that the EPDS may also be a useful screening instrument in palliative care patients (95).

To avoid the limitations of patient frailty and length of assessment, studies have also investigated the use of one item tool with the question "Have you felt depressed most of the day, nearly every day, for two or more weeks?." Chochinov et al. found that this screening question correctly identified the diagnosis of major depressive disorder in 197 terminally ill patients, with a sensitivity and a specificity of 100% (96). However, this result has not been replicated in all studies, and wording was found to influence the validity results. In a British study, the authors found a different single question "Are you depressed?" to have a sensitivity of 0.55 and a specificity of 0.74 (97). Payne and colleagues used a different two-item questionnaire ("Are you depressed?" and "Have you experienced loss of interest in things or activities that you would normally enjoy?") and found a sensitivity of 0.91 and a specificity of 0.68 (98). In a recent study on outpatient palliative care patients, the sensitivity and the specificity of the one-item screening tool were 0.8 and 0.85, respectively. The positive predictive value and the negative predictive value were 0.57 and 0.94, respectively (22). As such, the one-item scale, like most previously discussed scales, is mostly recommended as a screening tool to detect patients who necessitate further investigation of depression.

The Hamilton Depression Rating Scale (HDRS) is designed to measure the severity of depression and evaluate the efficacy of treatment (99). A recent study provided support for the reliability and validity of the HDRS in a large sample of terminally ill cancer patients (100). The BDI is another commonly used severity assessment scale validated in palliative care populations (101).

The literature on screening or diagnostic instruments for anxiety in the palliative care population is scarce. As mentioned above, HADS can also be used as a screening tool for anxiety in the palliative population. Generalized Anxiety Disorder-7 Screener (GAD-7) may be useful among cancer patients (102). According to the American Society of Clinical Oncology (ASCO), a GAD-7 score of >10, for example, indicates moderate to severe levels of anxiety (103). The Hamilton Anxiety Scale (HAM-A) is a valid measure for anxiety in the medically ill (104).

Somatic versus Psychological Causes of Anxiety

Much like depression, the symptom of anxiety is not specific to anxiety disorders and can be secondary to different medical issues. In the palliative care setting, it may be particularly challenging to differentiate between the somatic and the psychological causes of anxiety and to fully understand the complex bidirectional relationship of anxiety with other symptoms. Although findings are not entirely consistent across studies, symptoms such as pain, dyspnea, fatigue, nausea, and insomnia are known to be associated with increased anxiety in clinical practice (49,105). Other somatic etiologies that may be associated with anxiety symptoms include sepsis, bleeding, pulmonary embolus, hypercalcemia, nutritional failure, myocardial infarction, and substance intoxication and/or withdrawal.

A patient who is having acute suboptimally controlled pain may present with restlessness, perspiration, and agitation—symptoms highly suggestive of a panic attack. In a study published in 2019, patients reported pain and dyspnea as a frequent cause of anxiety, but also noted that the thought of future exacerbation was an important source of apprehension as well (31). It was also noted that patients who experience breakthrough pain (episodes of severe or excruciating pain superimposed on relatively stable, well-controlled baseline pain) also clinically report significantly more anxiety than do patients who do not report these episodes.

Though the exact pathophysiological mechanisms that underline the association between anxiety and dyspnea are not fully understood to date, potential pathways are postulated (Fig. 35.2). Acute hyperventilation due to any breathing disorder is thought to significantly decrease the level of carbon dioxide in the blood, which reduces blood flow to the brain and triggers emotional symptoms, including anxiety. Additionally, hyperventilation may worsen breathlessness, which also provokes

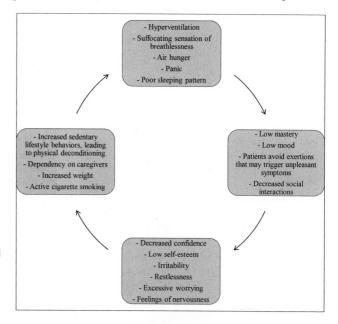

Figure 35.2 A cognitive–behavioral conceptualization of the "Dyspnea–Anxiety cycle." (Source: Adapted from Yohannes AM, Junkes-Cunha M, Smith J, Vestbo J. Management of dyspnea and anxiety in chronic obstructive pulmonary disease: a critical review. *J Am Med Direct Assoc.* 2017;18(12):1096.e1091-1096.e1017.)

the exacerbation of anxiety through inappropriately aligned cognitive perceptions of the increased work of breathing (106).

On the other hand, a change in metabolic state or an impending medical catastrophe such as a pulmonary embolus, a myocardial infarction, or a stroke may also sometimes be heralded by symptoms of anxiety and a feeling of "jumping out of my skin" (107). Anxiety can also be a frequent epileptic symptom, especially in the context of temporal lobe epilepsy (108).

Finally, substance withdrawal from alcohol, opioids, and benzodiazepines needs to be considered as an etiological and/or a concomitant contributor to the presentation of anxiety and agitation. Patients in the palliative care setting are frequently prescribed shorter-acting benzodiazepines and may experience rebound anxiety between doses (107).

Substance-Induced Symptoms

Medications can cause activation of immune-inflammatory responses, impacting central nervous system functions and consequently sleep–wake cycles, brain activity, and behaviors. Some medications can also result in medical complications such as anemia or thyroid dysfunction that can present with mood symptoms, akathisia, or anxiety. Palliative care patients are often simultaneously prescribed multiple medications and procedures for symptom relief. Often, patients will present with a combination of a primary psychiatric disorder along with substance-induced psychiatric symptoms (17). Though the investigation of a specific etiology for mood symptoms does not always necessarily change a provider's management plan, it makes the evaluation of psychiatric symptoms more challenging as substance-induced mood symptoms often have an atypical presentation. Psychotropic medications are useful to treat psychiatric side effects of these medical therapies that are often necessary in the management of the patient.

Depression represents approximately 1% of reported adverse drug reactions (109). The main medications related to substance-induced mood disturbances are presented in Table 35.7. Treatment categories that commonly induce psychiatric symptoms are discussed below.

Steroids

Corticosteroids, particularly dexamethasone and prednisone, are frequently used in chemotherapy protocols to treat central nervous system edema, inflammation, and acute and delayed chemotherapy-related nausea and for prevention of hypersensitivity to taxanes. The hypothalamic–pituitary axis (HPA) plays an essential role in the regulation

TABLE 35.7 DRUGS ASSOCIATED WITH DEPRESSION AND/OR DEPRESSIVE SYMPTOMS

Drugs causing the syndrome of major depression	None
Drugs causing depressive symptoms	Corticosteroids, contraceptive implants, GnRHA, interferon-alpha, interleukin-2, mefloquine
Drugs causing side effects informally labeled as depression	Propranolol, sotalol

Source: Adapted from Patten SB, Barbui C. Drug-induced depression: a systematic review to inform clinical practice. *Psychother Psychosom.* 2004;73(4):207-215.

of mood and the sleep–wake cycle. A disruption in the glucocorticoid function through a change in secretion or a change in receptor function can thus result in mood disturbances as well as anxiety symptoms.

Corticosteroids are frequently implicated in causing or precipitating psychiatric presentations. A small study published in 1994 reports a 75% incidence of mood disturbances after a 5-day challenge with 80 mg of oral prednisone. These symptoms include depression, tearfulness, irritability, anger, insomnia, talkativeness, giddiness, increased appetite, mood elevation, increased energy, confusion, racing thoughts, and depersonalization (110). More specifically, Naber et al. report a 10% incidence of depression after a 5- to 8-day high-dose steroid treatment (111). Most studies describe a positive correlation between the severity of the symptoms and the treatment dosage with uncommon reports of depression and anxiety with doses <40 mg/d but increasing to 18.4% at doses above 80 mg/d (112). However, more recent studies show an equally high incidence of psychiatric symptoms with long-term therapy at lower doses. A 2003 study by Bolanos reported that 60% of patients receiving long-term steroids at lower doses met diagnostic criteria for a prednisone-induced mood disorder (113). These results are reproduced more recently with a 2012 study that reports an increased hazard ratio for suicide, depression, and panic disorder in patients receiving glucocorticoids (114).

Interferon

Interferon alfa is frequently used at high dosages for the treatment of infectious illnesses, neoplastic diseases, and chronic hepatitis B or C. In 2002, interferon alfa treatment received a U.S. FDA black box warning for causing or aggravating fatal or life-threatening neuropsychiatric disorders. Among these, the most frequently reported adverse events associated with interferon are depression and irritability (115–117). One recent study reported that approximately one-third of nondepressed subjects treated for hepatitis C with interferon developed major depression (118).

On the other hand, interferon causes symptoms that mimic depression without necessarily causing a full-blown depressive disorder. Multifactorial fatigue secondary to endocrine, autoimmune, and neuropsychiatric etiologies is a common side effect of treatment, reported in up to 70% to 100% of patients (119). Anorexia, weight loss, early satiety as well as anhedonia, impaired concentration, and sleep disturbances are also commonly reported with interferon treatment (120). These depressive symptoms develop insidiously over weeks to months. Finally, interferon treatment is also associated with suicidal ideations and attempts (121).

Chemotherapy

Chemotherapeutic medications have been shown to contribute to depressive symptoms. Agents such as vincristine, vinblastine, vinorelbine, procarbazine, asparaginase, paclitaxel, and docetaxel are reported to cause neurotoxicity as well as a decrease of emotional functioning (122–125). One case–control study published in 2008 shows that breast cancer patients who received taxanes had higher emotional distress and worse mental quality of life throughout adjuvant chemotherapy, and took longer to recover emotionally than did patients in the nontaxane group (126).

Radiation Therapy

Radiation therapy is reported to contribute to depressive symptomatology in palliative patients. As radiation therapy increases the release of inflammatory cytokines, this activation may extend beyond the cancer area to peripheral tissues and ultimately contribute to behavioral morbidities such as depression (127,128). Multiple studies agree that depressive symptoms tend to reach their highest peak at the end of radiation treatment, leading to the maximal deterioration of the quality of life at that time, even in patients with no previous diagnosis of depression (129–131). Behavioral side effects are particularly amplified when radiation therapy and chemotherapy are combined, possibly due to an even more significant activation of the neuroinflammatory system (127).

Depression due to Concomitant Medications

Though the current medical literature does not confirm the direct implication of some medications in developing depression and anxiety, several medication categories are still reported in smaller studies to cause psychiatric symptoms.

Some beta-blockers, most notably propranolol, are associated with reports of depression in clinical trial adverse event reports (132,133). Even when beta-blockers cause neuropsychiatric side effects, the clinical presentation is unlikely to resemble a classical depressive syndrome, and there is no evidence that beta-blockers are associated with any DSM-5 defined depressive disorder (123).

Notably, tamoxifen and aromatase inhibitors are reported to be associated with depressive symptoms in smaller studies, mainly by inducing antiestrogenic states that cause hot flashes, insomnia, and dysphoria (134–136). Providers should also be cautious about drug–drug interactions that emerge with the combination of antidepressants and tamoxifen as paroxetine, fluoxetine, and bupropion can cause CYP2D6 inhibition. It would be prudent to use an alternate agent such as venlafaxine or citalopram due to their minimal interaction with CYP2D6 (137).

Other Diagnostic Challenges

Negative attitudes of society and a patient towards depression and anxiety combined with the stigma that may surround such diagnoses might prevent practitioners from addressing these issues (76). Patients and clinicians often avoid further investigation of psychiatric symptoms for fear that such exploration will cause further distress (138). On the other hand, depression and anxiety can be considered a normal part of dying in some cultures and lead to minimizing available treatments for psychological suffering. In others, the stigma that surrounds a psychiatric diagnosis might prevent these disorders from being expressed in usual psychological terms; patients might instead present with atypical features, including somatic and/or neurovegetative symptoms, that are out of proportion to the physical findings at the time of the exam. These atypical presentations might be confusing to the physician who is not alert to the cultural variability of psychiatric symptoms, thus preventing adequate diagnosis and treatment of depression and anxiety.

The attitudes and beliefs of practitioners towards psychiatric disorders can additionally influence the diagnoses of depression and anxiety. For example, therapeutic nihilism is defined as the phenomenon when physicians are reluctant to prescribe medications due to concerns about additional adverse effects without significant benefit (139,140). Due to therapeutic nihilism, physicians may hesitate to diagnose a condition that they do not feel they can treat successfully. Moreover, the physicians' limited experience in the assessment and treatment of depression and anxiety are also challenges preventing these disorders from getting adequate attention, evaluation, and treatment (141).

DIFFERENTIAL DIAGNOSES

Delirium

A 2019 systematic review reported a 35% pooled point prevalence of delirium on admission to inpatient palliative care units, a 9% to 57% prevalence across hospital palliative care services, a 6% to 74% prevalence in inpatient palliative care units, and a 42% to 88% prevalence of delirium before death in palliative care contexts (142). Despite the high prevalence of this disorder in medically ill patients, delirium is often mistaken for depression and anxiety by clinicians. Studies show a consistent misdiagnosis of delirium postoperatively in medical and geriatric units even in the setting of palliative care services (143–145). Fang et al. report that oncology teams misdiagnose delirium in more than one-third of cases (146) and a study published in 2009 reported that oncologists miss a diagnosis of delirium in 36.7% of patients with advanced cancer (147). Primary providers are similarly found to misdiagnose delirium in up to 61% of cases. When delirium presents with the hypoactive symptoms of psychomotor retardation and lethargy, 63% of cases go unrecognized by the patient's primary team (148). Though palliative care specialists seem to be overall more familiar with the diagnosis, they are still reported to recognize hypoactive delirium in only 20.5% of terminally ill patients (146).

In its hypoactive subtype, delirium can present with tearfulness, anhedonia, psychomotor retardation, decreased appetite, and feelings of hopelessness or helplessness that could initially be suggestive of a depressive disorder. In the hyperactive form, psychomotor agitation and perceptual disturbances predominate and are often accompanied by feelings of anxiety and angst, frequently assumed to be symptoms of an anxiety disorder. However, unlike depression and anxiety, delirium is part of the neurocognitive disorders of the DSM-5 and is an acute-onset disturbance that often accompanies or is the consequence of a medical illness or substance. Though delirium can manifest with clinical pictures that mimic other psychiatric disorders, one core finding that helps distinguish it is the alteration of attention and awareness over time. Contrary to depression and anxiety, delirium is also characterized by symptoms that are specific to the disorder: acute onset, fluctuating course, and accompanying rapid cognitive decline.

Demoralization

The concept of demoralization has been recognized and described in different fields throughout human history as people may question the meaning of life when faced with existential crises. When a person lacks the resources to cope with such inner conflict, the person will feel trapped and unable to control or modify his or her predicament. This, in turn, can lead to feelings of hopelessness, helplessness, isolation, and despair. This state is generally known as demoralization (149).

The concept of demoralization was initially coined in the context of philosophical and literary thought, with various terms emerging to describe similar or comparable notions. Acedia or "spiritual torpor" is a term that originates from the Christian culture and refers to an amotivational state seen in monks who had lost their spirituality and hence their main drive to seek meaning in life (150). Other terms such as "giving-up given-up complex" and "the social breakdown syndrome" were also previously used to describe similar affective states characterized by a feeling of reaching a "dead end" with regards to the meaning of existence (151). The famous concept of "learned helplessness" similarly describes the condition when a person gives up on trying to change or control their situation after multiple unsuccessful attempts (152).

A more formal discussion of the demoralization syndrome was only initiated over the past half-century when the existence of demoralization was suggested in the psychotherapeutic and psychiatric settings. In the face of a terminal illness, some patients were found to deduce that their behavior no longer influenced the outcomes and consequently they fall into a state of poor self-care and help-seeking. Studies focusing on patients coping with a terminal illness in the palliative care context gave way to further discussion of the clinical presentation and psychotherapy with a focus on the human condition, the "will to meaning," and the meaning-based coping strategies emerged with therapists such as Yalom, Frankl, and Folkman (9,153,154).

Kissane et al. presented the most modern conceptualization of demoralization in 2001 and argued for including the disorder as a distinct entity in the DSM-5. Demoralization is presented as a medical psychiatric syndrome that describes an abnormal response to illness with the core features of hopelessness and loss of purpose. In its extreme form, the disorder may lead to a rational decision of suicide. To diagnose demoralization, the following criteria need to persist for at least 2 weeks, in the absence of a primary diagnosis of MDD:

- Affective symptoms of existential distress, including hopelessness or loss of meaning and purpose in life
- Cognitive attitudes of pessimism, helplessness, sense of being trapped, personal failure, or lack of a worthwhile future
- Conative absence of drive or motivation to cope differently
- Associated features of social alienation and lack of support (155)

A major paradigm shift from the DSM-4 to the DSM-5 was the understanding of psychiatric disorders in a dimensional rather than a categorical approach. Demoralization is also reported to lie on a spectrum of coping with a terminal illness that extends from disheartenment through despondency and despair to complete demoralization that might warrant medical intervention (155). The presentation of the syndrome can thus be clinically challenging to distinguish from MDD. However, one key difference is the experience of pleasure: while anhedonia is one of the core symptoms of depression and a patient suffering from MDD typically presents with a generalized and persistent loss of pleasure, a terminally ill patient with demoralization might still be reactive to pleasurable stimuli while feeling hopeless and not motivated to seek it out (156). In a study by de Figueiredo on the phenomenological differences between the two syndromes, depression is reported to be associated with a prominent loss of motivation to pursue a pleasurable activity whereas demoralization is perceived as a feeling of helplessness in front of choices that all seem futile (157).

Despite this similarity in presentation, it is important to clinically distinguish between depression and demoralization as the treatment options differ. While treatment of depression and anxiety respond to different pharmacological and psychosocial interventions discussed later in this chapter, the treatment of demoralization relies more heavily on meaning-based psychotherapeutic interventions (70). The strategies for approaching the subject of demoralization with patients and the premises of the treatment for demoralization are presented in Tables 35.8 and 35.9.

Grief

Palliative care patients cope with multiple losses including the loss of health, autonomy, role, and the future loss of relationships, all of which may be sources of grief. The debate concerning the fine line that distinguishes grief from depression has a long history in both psychology and psychiatry, dating back to Freud's differentiation between mourning (grief in the modern literature) and melancholia (depression in the modern literature) (159).

TABLE 35.8 THE PREMISES OF THE TREATMENT OF DEMORALIZATION SYNDROME
Proactively manage physical symptoms
Explore attitudes towards meaning of life while instilling hope
Encourage the search for the meaning of the illness and of life
Provide spiritual support as needed
Break the cycle of isolation by encouraging social involvement and involvement of family and friends
Regularly review goals of care with patient in multidisciplinary meetings

Source: Adapted from Kissane DW, Clarke DM, Street AF. Demoralization syndrome—a relevant psychiatric diagnosis for palliative care. *J Palliat Care.* 2001;17(1):12-21.

While depressive disorders are pathological, grief is considered an expected and universal adaptive reaction to loss. It is a time-limited response that usually does not impact a person's functioning. Providers are hence encouraged to refrain from treating grief as a disorder. Most patients benefit instead from education about the symptoms of normal grief as well as the support of a health care professional who actively listens and accepts the feelings of grief associated with loss (160).

Prolonged or complicated grief is a syndrome that is currently a topic of great interest but is not yet an acknowledged DSM-5 diagnosis. The symptoms of complicated grief include an intense yearning for the loss, preoccupation with thoughts of the loss, anger and bitterness, and intrusive thoughts related to the loss (161). The definition of complicated grief varies among authors; the duration (symptoms lasting for more than 6 months) and degree of functional impairment are variables that distinguish it from normal grief but are still the subject of ongoing debate. Nevertheless, in bereaved family members of cancer patients, recent studies report that prolonged grief and major depressive disorder have distinct clinical presentations, though they frequently are comorbid (162). It is clinically important to distinguish complicated grief from MDD as psychotherapy designed specifically for prolonged grief disorder demonstrates specific efficacy for this entity (163).

EVIDENCE-BASED TREATMENT APPROACHES

There is strong evidence for the management of depression and anxiety in palliative care settings using a collaborative care model that combines primary care and mental health providers (164).

TABLE 35.9 STRATEGIES AND QUESTIONS THAT HELP WITH APPROACHING THE SUBJECT OF DEMORALIZATION WITH PATIENTS

Coherence vs. Confusion

How do you make sense of what you are going through?

When you are uncertain how to make sense of it, how do you deal with feeling confused?

To whom do you turn for help when you feel confused?

(For a religious patient) Do you have a sense that God has a way of making sense of it? Do you sense that God sees meaning in your suffering?

Communion vs. Isolation

Who really understands your situation?

When you have difficult days, with whom do you talk?

In whose presence do you feel a bodily sense of peace?

(For religious patients) Do you feel the presence of God? How? What does God know about your experience that other people may not understand?

Hope vs. Despair

From what sources do you draw hope?

On difficult days, what keeps you from giving up?

Who have you known in your life who would not be surprised to see you stay hopeful amid adversity? What did this person know about you that other people may not have known?

Purpose vs. Meaninglessness

What keeps you going on difficult days?

For whom, or for what, does it matter that you continue to live?

(For terminally ill patients) What do you hope to contribute in the time you have remaining?

(For religious patients) What does God hope you will do with your life in days to come?

Agency vs. Helplessness

What is your prioritized list of concerns/what concerns you most? What next most?

What most helps you to stand strong against the challenges of this illness?

What should I know about you as a person that lies beyond your illness?

How have you kept this illness from taking charge of your entire life?

Courage vs. Cowardice

Have there been moments when you felt tempted to give up but didn't?

How did you make a decision to persevere?

If you were to see someone else taking such a step even though feeling afraid, would you consider that an act of courage? If so, can you imagine viewing yourself as a courageous person? Is that a description of yourself that you would desire?

Can you imagine that others who witness how you cope with this illness might describe you as a courageous person?

Gratitude vs. Resentment

For what are you most deeply grateful?

Are there moments when you can still feel joy despite the sorrow you have been through?

If you could look back on this illness from some future time, what would you say that you took from the experience that added to your life?

Source: Adapted from Griffith JL, Gaby L. Brief psychotherapy at the bedside: countering demoralization from medical illness. *Psychosomatics.* 2005;46(2):109-116. Ref. (158).

In this model, primary care providers deliver systematic screening, initial management, and brief counseling for mental health disorders and then make referrals to specialists as needed. It allows primary care providers to work conjointly with mental health providers and concomitantly treat distressing physical symptoms that could be causing or exacerbating depressive or anxiety symptoms (165). When referral is made for specialized psychiatric care, a combination of pharmacotherapy, psychotherapy, and psychoeducation is the mainstay of treatment.

DEPRESSION

Pharmacotherapy

General Principles

The general principles for the prescription of medications for the treatment of depression in the palliative care setting are summarized in Tables 35.10 and 35.11. The treatment of depression in this context follows the same principles as in the general population. For mild depressive symptoms, clinicians are recommended to begin with nonpharmacological therapies and

TABLE 35.10 THE GENERAL PRINCIPLES FOR THE PRESCRIPTION OF MEDICATIONS FOR THE TREATMENT OF DEPRESSION IN THE PALLIATIVE CARE SETTING

Follow same principles as in general population.
- Start with nonpharmacological therapies for mild depressive symptoms.
- Consider pharmacotherapy for moderate to severe depressive symptoms and/or if behavioral therapy is not effective or available.
- All antidepressants are equally effective though every patient can respond differently to different antidepressants.
- A trial of antidepressant is considered adequate after 8–12 weeks at therapeutic dose.

Take into consideration the prognosis of the patient.
- For patients with a prognosis of weeks, consider the use of psychostimulants.

Be mindful of drug–drug interactions.
- Psychotropic medications impact cytochrome P450 enzymes, which metabolize various drugs, including antiepileptics, antibiotics, and antiretrovirals.
- When polypharmacy is present, consider eitalopram, escitalopram, or mirtazapine.

Attempt to target as many symptoms with as few medications as possible.

Take into consideration the other comorbid symptoms.
- When neuropathic pain is present, consider duloxetine or venlafaxine.
- When insomnia, nausea, or anorexia is present, consider mirtazapine.
- When fatigue/lethargy is present, consider stimulants or bupropion.

Closely monitor patients initiated on an antidepressant for emergence of adverse events.
- Risk of delirium due to anticholinergic effect.
- Common initial side effects of serotoninergic agents include anxiety, agitation, restlessness, insomnia, drowsiness, nausea, diarrhea, emesis, anorexia, dizziness, tremor, sweats, headaches, cognitive fogginess, emotional blunting, and sexual dysfunction.
- More serious side effects of serotoninergic agents include bleeding, bruising, interference with platelet adhesion, hyponatremia due to SIADH, and serotonin syndrome.
- Side effects of TCAs include anticholinergic (dry mouth, constipation, urinary retention, cognitive impairment), antinoradrenergic (orthostasis, fainting, falling), antihistaminergic (sedation, weight gain), cardiac (slow conduction, atrioventricular block with bundle branch block).

Take into consideration the patient's past responses to specific agents.

If the patient has a history of good response to a specific agent, consider restarting it.

Take into consideration hepatic and renal impairment when dosing medications.

Consider alternate routes of administration when oral medication administration is not possible.
- Most SSRIs are available in liquid formulation (fluoxetine, sertraline, and paroxetine most readily available in the United States of America).
- Mirtazapine is available as orally disintegrating tablet.
- Methylphenidate is available in transdermal patches and liquid extended release.
- Ketamine is available in intravenous or intranasal formulations.
- Trazodone is available in liquid form.
- Amitriptyline and imipramine are available in liquid form.
- Dextroamphetamine is available in liquid form.

Involve social worker and/or spiritual support services if depression is related to social or spiritual factors.

Refer to a mental health specialist for treatment-refractory symptoms, comorbid psychiatric illnesses, and psychiatric polypharmacy.

Refer to a mental health clinician or to the emergency department if patient presents with suicidal ideations.

only consider adding medication treatment when symptoms are more severe or refractory (42,166). There is significant evidence that all antidepressants are equally effective; therefore, the choice of agent should be based on an evaluation of the specific patient profile and can be aimed at targeting concomitant symptoms that are frequently comorbid in palliative patients (neuropathic pain, insomnia, anorexia, and fatigue) (167,168). Table 35.12 gives specific suggestions for the choice of antidepressant agents in a symptom-targeted approach.

Clinicians should also consider a patient's previous response to specific agents and favor medications with a history of a good response or remission of symptoms. In the choice of

TABLE 35.11 THE GENERAL GUIDELINES FOR THE TREATMENT OF DEPRESSION IN THE PALLIATIVE CARE SETTING

Mild depression *Characterized by a small number of symptoms with limited impact on the patient's everyday life*	**First-line treatment:** • Assess quality of relationships with significant others; facilitate communication. • Consider a guided self-help program. • Consider a brief psychological intervention (e.g., problem-solving therapy, brief CBT). **If symptoms persist:** • Consider using an antidepressant. • Reassess and possibly revise the diagnosis.
Moderate depression *Characterized by a larger number of symptoms that make it difficult for the patient to function as they would normally*	**First-line treatment:** • Do all recommended for mild depression. • Initiate antidepressant medication and/or psychological therapy. **If symptoms persist:** • Assess compliance to treatment. • Consider combining antidepressant treatment and psychological therapy. • After 4 weeks of antidepressant treatment, consider raising the dose of antidepressant or switching to a different drug.
Severe depression *Characterized by a large number of symptoms that make it very difficult for the patient to carry out everyday activities. There may be psychotic symptoms, food and/or fluid refusal, or severe and persistent suicidal ideation*	**First-line treatment:** • Do all recommended for mild depression. • Initiate antidepressants and psychological therapy. • Consider using a hypnotic or sedative in sleep-disturbed or very distressed patients. **If symptoms persist:** • Refer to a mental health specialist. • Lithium augmentation, electroconvulsive therapy, and antipsychotic drugs may be considered (under supervision of a mental health specialist).

Source: Adapted from Rayner L, Price A, Hotopf M, Higginson IJ. Expert opinion on detecting and treating depression in palliative care: a Delphi study. *BMC Palliat Care.* 2011;10:10.

the agent, clinicians should also be mindful of drug–drug interactions as psychotropic medications impact cytochrome p450 enzymes, which also metabolize various drugs, including antiepileptics, antibiotics, and antiretrovirals. Among antidepressants, citalopram, escitalopram, duloxetine, and mirtazapine are the least implicated in drug–drug interactions (169). When the decision for initiation of medications is made, clinicians are recommended to consider hepatic and renal functions with regards to dosing and need subsequent close monitoring for the emergence of adverse effects. Medications

should typically be started at a low dose and then titrated to the minimum effective dose to minimize adverse effects (169).

Patients in the palliative care context may have comorbidities that prevent them from taking oral medications, including swallowing difficulties, mucositis, esophageal lesions, and GI obstruction, among others. It is recommended that clinicians become familiar with alternate routes of administration of common agents used for the treatment of depression (see Table 35.10). Since a trial of an antidepressant is considered adequate only after 8 to 12 weeks of treatment at an appropriate dose, it is also recommended that the prognosis of the patient be taken into consideration when determining the treatment strategy (139). For patients with a prognosis of months, antidepressants are the first-line agents for treatment. However, for patients that are only expected to have a prognosis of days to weeks, the use of antidepressants is not highly recommended, and faster-acting agents such as psychostimulants or ketamine should be considered (169).

When depressive symptoms are refractory to treatment with a first-line agent prescribed by a primary physician or by a palliative specialist, the patient should be referred to a mental health

TABLE 35.12 SYMPTOM-TARGETED APPROACH TO ANTIDEPRESSANT CHOICE

Depression with insomnia	Mirtazapine
Depression with poor appetite	Mirtazapine Paroxetine
Depression with pain	High dose Venlafaxine Duloxetine TCAs
Depression with prominent fatigue	Bupropion Fluoxetine

specialist. Also, when the patient is receiving multiple psychiatric medications for other psychiatric comorbidities, consider a psychiatric consultation. Finally, if a patient presents with an acute psychiatric emergency such as suicidal ideation, clinicians are recommended to urgently refer them to a mental health practitioner or the emergency department.

Antidepressants

There is evidence that antidepressants are effective for the treatment of depression in the physically ill. Specifically, despite no formal FDA approval, studies have also shown that antidepressants are effective for the treatment of depression in life-threatening illness. A meta-analysis published in 2011 reported significantly higher effect of tricyclic antidepressants (TCAs) and selective serotonin reuptake inhibitors (SSRIs) as compared to placebo at 6 to 8 weeks of treatment, with a subsequent significant improvement in measures of quality of life. In addition, in this study, antidepressants were reported to be generally well tolerated with a number needed to harm (NNH) of approximately 6, which reflects a low incidence of adverse events (170).

Selective Serotonin Reuptake Inhibitors (SSRIs)—SSRIs are the most commonly prescribed and first-line antidepressants for the treatment of depressive disorders. SSRIs block 5HT reuptake, increasing serotonin in the synapse. To minimize common side effects, including QTc prolongation, initial anxiety and agitation, insomnia, and gastrointestinal side effects (nausea, diarrhea, emesis, anorexia), SSRIs should be started at a low dose and then titrated up to the minimum effective dose. Fluoxetine can be used in patients presenting with prominent psychomotor retardation because of its activating effect, but clinicians should also monitor for worsening of anxiety. Paroxetine can be sedating because of its anticholinergic effects and can lead to withdrawal with missed doses because of its short half-life. Because sertraline, citalopram, and escitalopram have lower side effect profiles and are neither activating nor sedating, they may be better choices for palliative care patients (171). SSRIs also have a slight risk of increased bleeding secondary to platelet dysfunction (172).

Serotonin Norepinephrine Reuptake Inhibitors (SNRIs)—In addition to serotonin, SNRIs also inhibit reuptake of norepinephrine at the synapse level. Because of this additional molecular effect, SNRIs may be used for the treatment of depression in the context of neuropathic pain, vasomotor instability, and depressive disorders with prominent anxiety features. SNRIs may prolong bleeding times and therefore may not be safe in patients with active bleeding or intracranial metastases. To increase the norepinephrine effect, venlafaxine needs to be prescribed at higher doses. This medication can cause discontinuation symptoms with missed doses and requires monitoring of hypertension. Duloxetine is an SNRI even at lower doses. It has been associated with hepatic insufficiency and a worsening of acute angle glaucoma (169).

Mirtazapine—Mirtazapine is one of the most commonly used antidepressant agents in patients with advanced cancer because of its antihistaminergic effects causing increased appetite and sedation. These side effects of the medication can be used to an advantage in palliative care patients who are suffering from anorexia and sleep disturbances. In addition, the 5-HT3 receptor blocking properties of mirtazapine have led some palliative care clinicians to recommend it as first-line treatment for nausea (173). Mirtazapine tends to cause more sedation and increased appetite at lower doses, but this becomes less significant with higher doses. Major side effects include hypertension, orthostatic hypotension, dizziness, and constipation.

Tricyclic Antidepressants (TCAs)—TCAs are an older class of antidepressants that are nonselective inhibitors of norepinephrine reuptake and usually recommended as second-line treatment for depressive disorders in the general population. Even though TCAs have proven good efficacy in the treatment of depression in palliative care patients (170), their use is limited by the wide array of side effects: QTc prolongation, anticholinergic effects (dry mouth, constipation, cognitive impairment, delirium), antinoradrenergic effects (tachycardia, orthostasis, dizziness), and antihistaminergic effects (sedation, weight gain). TCAs can also be lethal in overdose and should be used with caution in patients at risk of medication overdose. Even though TCAs are not recommended as first-line treatment in palliative care patients, they can still be useful in heart-healthy young patients with comorbid neuropathic pain and/or insomnia.

Monoamine Oxidase Inhibitors (MAOIs)—MAOIs are also an older generation of antidepressants that inhibit monoamine oxidase enzymes. Due to their high side effect profile, need for dietary restriction, potential for drug–drug interactions, and the risk of serotonin syndrome, MAOIs are rarely used in palliative care patients.

Bupropion—Bupropion is a norepinephrine and dopamine reuptake inhibitor antidepressant. It is thought to be less sedating and have a lower incidence of sexual side effects. It can thus be effective if the core symptoms of the presentation include amotivation, poor attention, low energy, or fatigue.

However, this medication is associated with a risk of seizure; therefore, it is recommended to avoid its use in patients with a history of a seizure disorder (especially if uncontrolled), electrolyte imbalances, and in patients at risk of benzodiazepine and/or alcohol withdrawal.

Psychostimulants

Except for modafinil and caffeine, psychostimulants directly increase synaptic activity of the monoamine neurotransmitters (dopamine, noradrenaline, and serotonin) and have an indirect agonist effect by increasing neurotransmitter function/release. All psychostimulants produce a similar increase in monoamine activity. Due to this direct agonist effect of psychostimulants on a molecular level, they appear to clinically act quickly by relieving targeted symptoms of depression, which differentiates them from typical antidepressant agents. In several studies, psychostimulants are reported to start showing clinical benefit as early as 2 to 3 days after initiation (174). The U.S. National Cancer Institute guidelines on cancer-related fatigue recommend the use of psychostimulants for the symptomatic treatment of fatigue (175). However, evidence for effectiveness of this treatment is lacking (176).

Similarly, there is mixed evidence for the use of psychostimulants for the treatment of depressive symptoms, particularly in palliative care patients. Unfortunately, randomized controlled trials have yielded mixed results with regards to this outcome (174,177). A 2009 Cochrane review underscores these conflicting results and concludes that, even though results from three small trials of psychostimulants involving a total of 62 participants indicated a short-term significant reduction in depressive symptoms when compared with placebo, the overall quality of the trials was poor, limiting confidence in the findings (178). It is also unclear if the effect of psychostimulants on depression is only mediated by its effect on fatigue, which is a major component of the presentation of depression in palliative care (174). Certain trials report an improvement in anorexia, a reduction in sedation secondary to opiates, and even an adjuvant analgesic effect of these medications (178,179). Therefore, despite the lack of overwhelming evidence, dextroamphetamine, methylphenidate, methylamphetamine, and pemoline may still be clinically valid options for palliation of depressive symptoms in terminally ill patients in whom the concern for abuse is clinically not relevant. Psychostimulants can also sometimes be used in conjunction with antidepressants to palliate symptoms while treatment takes full effect.

Other Agents

Ketamine—There is a growing interest in the use of ketamine, which is thought to have a rapid therapeutic effect on depression. Ketamine is most commonly used as an anesthetic agent and as an adjuvant treatment of cancer pain in subanesthetic doses, mainly because of its μ, κ, and δ opioid–like effects. It is unclear what exact molecular mechanisms of action contribute to its antidepressant effect, but it is thought to be due to the N-methyl-D-aspartate (NMDA) receptor antagonism as well as to the interactions with other calcium and sodium channels, cholinergic transmission, noradrenergic and serotonergic reuptake inhibition, glutamate transmission, and synapse formation. Notably, anesthesia dosing is significantly higher than analgesia and depression dosing (180).

Studies investigating the use of ketamine in depressed palliative patients are scarce, have small sample sizes, and only report short-term effects of the medication; no randomized controlled trials are available. Despite this lack of evidence, recent open-label trials and retrospective chart reviews have yielded positive preliminary results for the early improvement of depressive symptoms (180,181). In a 2013 open-label study, 100% of patients had a significant improvement of depression starting day 14, independent of improvement of pain. However, no change in quality of life using standardized measures was noted, though the authors report a subjective clinical improvement in the patient (180). In the 2015 retrospective chart review of 31 patients receiving hospice care, ketamine was reported to be therapeutically effective through the first week postdosing, with the first response most significant on days 0 to 1 of initiation. In both studies, patients did not experience clinically significant side effects, though authors do caution against the risk of delirium (181).

Antipsychotics—Aripiprazole has been discussed as a possible treatment for depression in the palliative care context, as monotherapy or as an augmentation medication with antidepressants (182). However, no formal evidence exists for its use. Though quetiapine is used as an adjunctive treatment for major depression in the general population, there is scant evidence for its use in the palliative care population. Olanzapine is also sometimes used off-label as an adjunct treatment of depression in patients presenting with nausea (173). However, it is recommended to use these agents with caution, carefully weighing the risk-to-benefit ratio.

Psychotherapies

As mentioned previously, psychotherapy is indicated at all levels of depression severity, alone or in conjunction with pharmacotherapy. Although not all studies that investigate the effect of psychotherapy on depression in palliative patients show positive results, recent reviews and meta-analyses highlight significant effect of any psychotherapeutic intervention on the reduction of depression in palliative care patients (167,183–185). In a 2008 Cochrane review, the combined data from six randomized controlled trials showed that psychotherapy had a significant effect on the treatment of depressive symptoms among participants with advanced cancer, with a subsequent significant effect on general psychological distress (184). These findings suggest that the effects of psychotherapy are almost comparable to those obtained in antidepressant pharmacotherapy in general psychiatry settings (186). A more recent meta-analysis published in 2018 investigated the effect of any type of psychotherapy on depression among adults with any condition appropriate for palliative care. This study also reported a large treatment effect of psychotherapy on depressive symptoms with a subsequent significant though small effect on quality of life. More specifically, this study found a larger effect for interventions with a greater number of short treatment sessions in younger patients, and for psychotherapy administered by mental health professionals rather than by other types of providers. The authors conclude with a recommendation to integrate mental health providers into palliative care teams (183).

Cognitive–Behavioral Therapy

Cognitive–behavioral therapy (CBT) is a short-term structured psychotherapeutic approach that uses active collaboration between patient and therapist to resolve the patient's active current problems. It is usually conducted on an individual basis, although group methods are also available. Underlying the practice of CBT is the theory that cognitions, emotions, and behaviors are interrelated. The intervention aims to make patients aware of their cognitive distortions, thereby improving their affective state and behavioral patterns.

In the specific context of palliative care, CBT has shown good results in the management of depression, and review articles have concluded that CBT is generally an effective nonpharmacological treatment for depression in the terminally ill (183,187). However, evidence also shows that the effects of CBT can be transient and that benefits tend to decrease when the patient is no longer in treatment (183,188). This could highlight that the stresses and worries of the final phase of life possibly go unaddressed by CBT. As such, in a 2012 review study, the authors suggest that CBT might be more useful for patients in the earlier stages of advanced disease rather than for those in the final weeks of life (187).

Existential Therapies

Therapies that target existential distress, life meaning, and spiritual well-being have newly emerged as possible nonpharmacological interventions for the treatment of depression in the terminally ill. Multiple modalities have been suggested, including dignity therapy, short-term life reviews, meaning-centered therapy, narrative therapy, and Managing Cancer and Living Meaningfully (CALM) therapy (189–193). Evidence is scant regarding the efficacy of these strategies for the treatment of clinically diagnosed depressive disorders, and few RCTs have been done to investigate their effects on illness severity. However, it is thought that these strategies can still impact spiritual suffering, death-related distress, and other outcomes that may not be reflected in measures of psychological distress but are targets of palliative care interventions (70,183,187,192,193).

Dignity therapy—Dignity therapy is a short-term therapy consisting of 3 to 4 sessions, originally designed and studied by Chochinov et al. The aim of the sessions is to go over the achievements that the patient takes most pride of during the lifetime, and to define the legacy that the patient wants to pass down to the generations that follow. The result of this therapy is a "generativity document" that records these accomplishments and expresses unsaid things to loved ones. The final session is a ceremony to pass down the document to a family member (189).

Short-term life reviews—In this therapy, patients review their lives with the therapist in the first session, and the review is recorded and edited. In the second session, the patient and the therapist view the album made by the therapist and confirm the contents. This therapy posits the healing power of memories by allowing a "progressive return to consciousness of prior experience, which can be reevaluated with the intention of resolving and integrating past conflict, thereby giving new significance to one's life" (194,195).

Meaning-centered therapy—This therapy was initially designed for patients with advanced cancer, based on the works of Frankl, Yalom, and Kissane (9,153,196) on existential themes in psychotherapy. The focus of this therapy by Breitbart et al. is to find meaning and purpose in life in the face of medical illnesses with limited prognoses (197).

Narrative therapy—Narrative therapy offers patients a safe space where they can freely express in a narrative form their personal experience with their illness. This strategy has been promoted as a way to provide holistic support to the dying patients and their families, in order to decrease emotional distress and establish meaning (198).

CALM therapy—Based on the relational and existential theories, CALM therapy provides an intervention focused on four domains: symptom management and communication with health care providers, changes in self and relations with close others, spiritual well-being and the sense of meaning and purpose, and mortality and future-oriented concerns (125).

ANXIETY

Ongoing monitoring and close assessment of patients is very important in treating palliative care patients with anxiety. While anxiety symptoms are common and expected to a degree in patients with serious medical illness, they may increase and create great distress and suffering for certain patients. A close and supportive relationship between the patient and treatment team lends itself to improved communication, clinicians being more attuned to changes in patients' anxious distress levels, and ultimately addressing anxiety symptoms expeditiously and accurately. Clinical assessment tools should be utilized regularly to track symptoms so that more aggressive treatments can be implemented once it is established that the patient meets criteria for an anxiety disorder. In cases where anxiety symptoms do not remit or continue to worsen despite treatment interventions, or in situations in which persistent anxiety interferes with treatment of the underlying illness/disease, referral for psychiatric evaluation and management should be considered.

Pharmacotherapy

There is a lack of good evidence for the use of pharmacotherapy specifically in the treatment of anxiety in terminally ill patients. In a Cochrane review published in 2017, the authors did not find any RCT that investigated the role of drug therapy for the treatment of symptoms of anxiety in adult palliative care patients (199). Thus, clinical guidelines in cancer therapy and palliative care recommend minimizing the use of medications and, instead, favoring nonpharmacological treatments such as psychological support and therapies except in the last days of life (200). When medications are used, it is recommended to cautiously weigh the risk-to-benefit ratio as many of these treatments can cause an exacerbation of preexisting medical problems. In addition, any medication that is used for the treatment of anxiety should preferably be started at a lower dose than in the general population due to potential for side effects and interactions with other drugs (199).

SSRIs and Buspirone—Buspirone is an antianxiety medication that has a high affinity for serotonin 5-HT$_{1A}$ and 5-HT$_2$ receptors, without affecting GABA receptors like benzodiazepines. Like SSRIs, buspirone requires multiple weeks to achieve therapeutic effect. The use of SSRIs and buspirone is limited due to this prolonged clinical onset of action, and the evidence for their use in the palliative care population is limited as compared to the general population. If SSRIs are used, sedating agents like mirtazapine or trazodone are likely preferred to help with anxiety.

Benzodiazepines—Benzodiazepines are the most frequently used agents for the management of anxiety in terminally ill patients even though this strategy lacks the support of high-quality evidence (199). Because benzodiazepines can worsen respiratory depression and delirium in palliative patients, it is appropriate to favor short-acting agents like lorazepam or midazolam to symptomatically treat severe anxiety. For patients with severe hepatic dysfunction, it is preferable to use lorazepam, oxazepam, and temazepam, and in patients who cannot take oral medications, providers may use diazepam in its rectal form for the management of severe anxiety, with dosages equivalent to those used in oral regimens (201).

Antihistamines—Though low doses of antihistamines can be useful for breakthrough anxiety, they should be used cautiously in terminally patients as they can exacerbate confusion and delirium because of their anticholinergic effect.

Antipsychotics—Just as in depression, no high-quality data exist to justify the use of any antipsychotic for the management of anxiety in the palliative care population. In practice, if a patient presents with anxiety in the context of hyperactive delirium, off-label use of antipsychotics may target symptoms of agitation, insomnia, and anxiety (202).

Opioids—As mentioned previously, anxiety can be triggered and/or maintained by dyspnea and pain. As opioids are effective for the management of both symptoms, they can also consequently be effective for the symptomatic treatment of anxiety on a short-term basis only. It is however recommended to be careful with the prescription of opiate medications as they can cause central respiratory depression and lead to tolerance and dependence. In a prospective nonrandomized study published in 2011, the authors reported that the concomitant use of opioids and anxiolytics is a safe and effective method for the management of dyspnea and anxiety in a small palliative care population (203).

Psychotherapies

A targeted approach to treating anxiety should be considered when symptoms interfere with the individual's functioning, indicating moderate to severe levels. Therapy strategies may include a variety of treatment approaches beyond pharmacotherapy, such as psychotherapy, and other supportive treatments. Complementary and alternative approaches may also be useful.

Psychotherapy can be useful in exploring factors that may be driving patients' anxiety, including fears about medical interventions, social impacts of illness, worries about being a burden on others, spiritual factors, feelings of grief and loss, and issues related to end of life and death. Modalities include individual, couple, or family therapy. A variety of therapy approaches could be utilized to treat anxiety, including brief individualized approaches, Cognitive-behavioral therapy (CBT), supportive therapy in the group setting, dignity therapy, and meaning-centered therapy (204).

Effective therapeutic approaches involve an individualized and patient-tailored approach. In choosing the therapeutic strategy, consideration should be given to individual factors, such as diagnosis and prognosis, comorbid conditions, and physical status. Patients' needs regarding their anxiety treatment should be assessed. In a qualitative study of palliative cancer care in a hospice setting, patients' six main needs included honest information, a sense of feeling in control, feeling safe and not alone (with physical proximity to others), adequate physical symptom management (of pain, nausea, and insomnia for example), and respect for their own coping strategies (31).

In addition, the psychological status of the patient is important in that the process of psychotherapy has the potential to ease and improve the patient's anxiety or, on the other hand, possibly cause further emotional distress and discomfort. In seriously ill patients, more frequent shorter sessions may be preferable than fewer lengthy sessions of any psychotherapeutic modality (183). Indeed, some individuals may not have the psychological reserves to tolerate the work of a more intensive psychotherapy, and therefore a brief individual supportive intervention may be more helpful than a more detailed CBT approach in these patients.

Some clinical scenarios may be more suited to using a CBT intervention. For example, patients expressing distorted cognitions about their medical status and treatment, patients who seem to benefit from distraction and activation, patients who catastrophize, patient with panic symptoms, patients who are stuck and helpless, and patients who are overly inhibited may specifically benefit from CBT (205).

Overall, psychotherapy for the palliative patient population with serious medical illness can be beneficial and improve symptoms of anxiety and quality of life according to a recent meta-analysis (183). Findings suggest that the clinical care of palliative care patients with anxiety (and depression) can improve when specific therapies, including CBT and other therapies (such as mindfulness and acceptance therapy) are provided by mental health clinicians (183).

Other Interventions

In addition to psychotherapy, there are numerous complementary and alternative methods (CAM) that may ease anxiety of individuals with serious medical illness and those receiving palliative care. These include hypnotherapy, music therapy, relaxation training, acupuncture, mindfulness meditation, aromatherapy, massage, and art therapy. Evidence suggests that CAM may result in a modest short-term benefit in palliative care patients (206). There is limited evidence supporting statistically significant benefits of CAM; however, many studies report CAM may result in clinical improvement of distressing symptoms (both physical and psychological) and of quality of life. Music therapy may have short-term benefit in reducing anxiety in palliative care patients. There are also limited data to support the use of meditation, relaxation training, and mindfulness exercises for longer-term improvement in anxiety, if patients learn strategies and use them consistently over time (207,208). It is suggested that CAM methods be provided by individuals who have expertise in the specific type modality being provided to ensure that high-quality and sound treatment is being delivered.

Other lifestyle modifications may offer low-cost and relatively simple strategies to improve anxiety. For example, exercise, even in seriously medically ill patients, may reduce anxiety, worry, and stress. Further, exercise, even simple movement repetitions in a hospital bed, may improve a patient's well-being, provide control, and create a sense of accomplishment thus improving anxiety symptoms. Improved sleep hygiene can help with insomnia and unrestful sleep, which may be driving an individual's anxiety. Assessment of daily and caffeine and/or alcohol intake and modifying these could also potentially improve anxiety symptoms.

CONCLUSION

Depressive and anxiety symptoms are common throughout the course of a person's serious medical illness and may heighten at the end of life. Palliative approaches suggest addressing these emotional and psychological symptoms early and comprehensively improves patients' quality of life. Depending on the severity and degree of impairment caused by these symptoms, psychiatric disorders may become apparent and warrant treatment to mitigate the patient's suffering and improve the care of the whole patient.

ACKNOWLEDGEMENT OF NIMH SUPPORT

This research was supported (in part) by the Intramural Research Program of the NIMH and includes the relevant Annual Report number ZIAMH002922.

REFERENCES

1. Bishop GD. *Health Psychology: Integrating Mind and Body*. Needham Heights, MA: Allyn & Bacon; 1994.
2. Zachariades FK. Coping with health-related problems and psychological distress amongst older adult hospital patients; 2000 [thesis].
3. Garg R, Chauhan V, Sabreen B. Coping styles and life satisfaction in palliative care. *Indian J Palliat Care*. 2018;24(4):491-495.
4. Diaz-Frutos D, Baca-Garcia E, Garcia-Foncillas J, Lopez-Castroman J. Predictors of psychological distress in advanced cancer patients under palliative treatments. *Eur J Cancer Care*. 2016;25(4):608-615.
5. Lazarus RS. *Stress and Emotion: A New Synthesis*. New York, NY: Springer Publishing Co.; 1999.
6. Sand L, Olsson M, Strang P. Coping strategies in the presence of one's own impending death from cancer. *J Pain Symptom Manage*. 2009;37(1):13-22.
7. Tillich P. *The Courage To Be*. New Haven, CT: Yale University Press; 1952.
8. May R. *The Meaning of Anxiety*. W.W Norton & Company; 1996.
9. Yalom ID. *Existential Psychotherapy*. Basic Books; 1980.
10. Becker E. *The Denial of Death*. New York, NY: Free Press; 1973.
11. Heim E, Augustiny KF, Schaffner L, Valach L. Coping with breast cancer over time and situation. *J Psychosom Res*. 1993;37(5):523-542.
12. Silver RL, Wortman CB. *Coping with Undesirable Life Events*. New York, NY: Academic Press; 1980.
13. Nipp RD, El-Jawahri A, Fishbein JN, et al. The relationship between coping strategies, quality of life, and mood in patients with incurable cancer. *Cancer*. 2016;122(13):2110-2116.
14. Heiskell LE, Pasnau RO. Psychological reaction to hospitalization and illness in the emergency department. *Emerg Med Clin North Am*. 1991;9(1):207-218.
15. Krok D, Telka E, Zarzycka B. Illness perception and affective symptoms in gastrointestinal cancer patients: a moderated mediation analysis of meaning in life and coping. *Psychooncology*. 2019;28(8):1728-1734.
16. *Diagnostic and Statistical Manual of Mental Disorders: DSM-5*. 5th ed. Arlington, VA: American Psychiatric Association; 2013.
17. Miller AH, Ancoli-Israel S, Bower JE, Capuron L, Irwin MR. Neuroendocrine-immune mechanisms of behavioral comorbidities in patients with cancer. *J Clin Oncol*. 2008;26(6):971-982.
18. Hotopf M, Chidgey J, Addington-Hall J, Ly KL. Depression in advanced disease: a systematic review. Part 1. Prevalence and case finding. *Palliat Med*. 2002;16(2): 81-97.
19. Mitchell AJ, Chan M, Bhatti H, et al. Prevalence of depression, anxiety, and adjustment disorder in oncological, haematological, and palliative-care settings: a meta-analysis of 94 interview-based studies. *Lancet Oncol*. 2011;12(2):160-174.
20. Sudarisan SSP, Abraham B, George C. Prevalence, correlates of depression, and its impact on quality of life of cancer patients attending a palliative care setting in South India. *Psychooncology*. 2019;28(6):1308-1313.
21. Azevedo C, Pessalacia JDR, Mata L, Zoboli E, Pereira MDG. Interface between social support, quality of life and depression in users eligible for palliative care. *Rev Esc Enferm USP*. 2017;51:e03245.
22. Taylor L, Lovell N, Ward J, Wood F, Hosker C. Diagnosis of depression in patients receiving specialist community palliative care: does using a single screening question identify depression otherwise diagnosed by clinical interview? *J Palliat Med*. 2013;16(9):1140-1142.
23. Mollerberg ML, Arestedt K, Swahnberg K, Benzein E, Sandgren A. Family sense of coherence and its associations with hope, anxiety and symptoms of depression in persons with cancer in palliative phase and their family members: a cross-sectional study. *Palliat Med*. 2019:269216319866653.
24. Fisher KA, Seow H, Brazil K, Freeman S, Smith TF, Guthrie DM. Prevalence and risk factors of depressive symptoms in a Canadian palliative home care population: a cross-sectional study. *BMC Palliat Care*. 2014;13(1):10.
25. Soldato M, Liperoti R, Landi F, Carpenter IG, Bernabei R, Onder G. Patient depression and caregiver attitudes: results from The AgeD in HOme Care study. *J Affect Disord*. 2008;106(1-2):107-115.
26. Walsh D, Rybicki L. Symptom clustering in advanced cancer. *Support Care Cancer*. 2006;14(8):831-836.
27. Chochinov HM, Tataryn DJ, Wilson KG, Ennis M, Lander S. Prognostic awareness and the terminally ill. *Psychosomatics*. 2000;41(6):500-504.
28. Ray A, Block SD, Friedlander RJ, Zhang B, Maciejewski PK, Prigerson HG. Peaceful awareness in patients with advanced cancer. *J Palliat Med*. 2006;9(6):1359-1368.
29. Atkin N, Vickerstaff V, Candy B. 'Worried to death': the assessment and management of anxiety in patients with advanced life-limiting disease, a national survey of palliative medicine physicians. *BMC Palliat Care*. 2017;16(1):69.
30. Pidgeon T, Johnson CE, Currow D, et al. A survey of patients' experience of pain and other symptoms while receiving care from palliative care services. *BMJ Support Palliat Care*. 2016;6(3):315-322.
31. Zweers D, de Graeff A, Duijn J, de Graaf E, Witteveen PO, Teunissen S. Patients' needs regarding anxiety management in palliative cancer care: a qualitative study in a hospice setting. *Am J Hosp Palliat Care*. 2019;36(11):947-954.
32. American Cancer Society. *Cancer Facts & Figures*. Atlanta, GA: American Cancer Society; 2013.
33. Wilson KG, Chochinov HM, Skirko MG, et al. Depression and anxiety disorders in palliative cancer care. *J Pain Symptom Manage*. 2007;33(2):118-129.
34. Jehn CF, Flath B, Strux A, et al. Influence of age, performance status, cancer activity, and IL-6 on anxiety and depression in patients with metastatic breast cancer. *Breast Cancer Res Treat*. 2012;136(3):789-794.
35. Barlow DH. *Anxiety and its Disorders: The Nature and Treatment of Anxiety and Panic*. 2nd ed. New York, NY: Guilford Press; 2002.
36. Brintzenhofe-Szoc KM, Levin TT, Li Y, Kissane DW, Zabora JR. Mixed anxiety/depression symptoms in a

large cancer cohort: prevalence by cancer type. *Psychosomatics.* 2009;50(4):383-391.

37. Thielking PD. Cancer pain and anxiety. *Curr Pain Headache Rep.* 2003;7(4):249-261.

38. Hofmann S, Hess S, Klein C, Lindena G, Radbruch L, Ostgathe C. Patients in palliative care—development of a predictive model for anxiety using routine data. *PLoS One.* 2017;12(8):e0179415.

39. Kolva E, Rosenfeld B, Pessin H, Breitbart W, Brescia R. Anxiety in terminally ill cancer patients. *J Pain Symptom Manage.* 2011;42(5):691-701.

40. Thompson GN, Chochinov HM, Wilson KG, et al. Prognostic acceptance and the well-being of patients receiving palliative care for cancer. *J Clin Oncol.* 2009;27(34): 5757-5762.

41. Block SD. Perspectives on care at the close of life. Psychological considerations, growth, and transcendence at the end of life: the art of the possible. *JAMA.* 2001;285(22):2898-2905.

42. Rayner L, Price A, Hotopf M, Higginson IJ. Expert opinion on detecting and treating depression in palliative care: a Delphi study. *BMC Palliat Care.* 2011;10:10.

43. World Health Organization. WHO definition of palliative care; 2016. http://www.who.int/cancer/palliative/definition/en/

44. Grotmol KS, Lie HC, Hjermstad MJ, et al. Depression—a major contributor to poor quality of life in patients with advanced cancer. *J Pain Symptom Manage.* 2017;54(6):889-897.

45. Choi S, Ryu E. Effects of symptom clusters and depression on the quality of life in patients with advanced lung cancer. *Eur J Cancer Care.* 2018;27(1).

46. Calderon C, Carmona-Bayonas A, Hernandez R, et al. Effects of pessimism, depression, fatigue, and pain on functional health-related quality of life in patients with resected non-advanced breast cancer. *Breast.* 2019;44:108-112.

47. Rajmohan V, Kumar SK. Psychiatric morbidity, pain perception, and functional status of chronic pain patients in palliative care. *Indian J Palliat Care.* 2013;19(3): 146-151.

48. Mystakidou K, Parpa E, Katsouda E, Galanos A, Vlahos L. Influence of pain and quality of life on desire for hastened death in patients with advanced cancer. *Int J Palliat Nurs.* 2004;10(10):476-483.

49. Delgado-Guay M, Parsons HA, Li Z, Palmer JL, Bruera E. Symptom distress in advanced cancer patients with anxiety and depression in the palliative care setting. *Support Care Cancer.* 2009;17(5):573-579.

50. Girgis A, Currow D, Waller A, et al. *Palliative Care Needs Assessment Guidelines Summary.* Australian Government Department of Health and Ageing; 2006.

51. Somerset W, Stout SC, Miller AH, Musselman D. Breast cancer and depression. *Oncology (Williston Park).* 2004;18(8):1021-1034; discussion 1035-1036, 1047-1048.

52. Giese-Davis J, Collie K, Rancourt KM, Neri E, Kraemer HC, Spiegel D. Decrease in depression symptoms is associated with longer survival in patients with metastatic breast cancer: a secondary analysis. *J Clin Oncol.* 2011;29(4):413-420.

53. Yu ES, Shim EJ, Kim HK, Hahm BJ, Park JH, Kim JH. Development of guidelines for distress management in Korean cancer patients. *Psychooncology.* 2012;21(5):541-549.

54. Cheung G, Douwes G, Sundram F. Late-life suicide in terminal cancer: a rational act or underdiagnosed depression? *J Pain Symptom Manage.* 2017;54(6):835-842.

55. Misono S, Weiss NS, Fann JR, Redman M, Yueh B. Incidence of suicide in persons with cancer. *J Clin Oncol.* 2008;26(29):4731-4738.

56. Chochinov HM, Wilson KG, Enns M, et al. Desire for death in the terminally ill. *Am J Psychiatry.* 1995;152(8): 1185-1191.

57. Salib E, Rahim S, El-Nimr G, Habeeb B. Elderly suicide: an analysis of coroner's inquests into two hundred cases in Cheshire 1989–2001. *Med Sci Law.* 2005;45(1):71-80.

58. Chochinov HM, Wilson KG, Enns M, Lander S. Depression, hopelessness, and suicidal ideation in the terminally ill. *Psychosomatics.* 1998;39(4):366-370.

59. Hirschfeld RM, Russell JM. Assessment and treatment of suicidal patients. *N Engl J Med.* 1997;337(13): 910-915.

60. Llorente MD, Burke M, Gregory GR, et al. Prostate cancer: a significant risk factor for late-life suicide. *Am J Geriatr Psychiatry.* 2005;13(3):195-201.

61. Spoletini I, Gianni W, Caltagirone C, Madaio R, Repetto L, Spalletta G. Suicide and cancer: where do we go from here? *Crit Rev Oncol/Hematol.* 2011;78(3):206-219.

62. Brown JH, Henteleff P, Barakat S, Rowe CJ. Is it normal for terminally ill patients to desire death? *Am J Psychiatry.* 1986;143(2):208-211.

63. NIMH. *Suicide Prevention.* National Institute of Mental Health Web site. Bethesda, MD; 2019. https://www.nimh.nih.gov/health/topics/suicide-prevention/index.shtml. Accessed February 14, 2020.

64. Druss B, Pincus H. Suicidal ideation and suicide attempts in general medical illnesses. *Arch Intern Med.* 2000;160(10):1522-1526.

65. Breitbart W, Rosenfeld B, Pessin H, et al. Depression, hopelessness, and desire for hastened death in terminally ill patients with cancer. *JAMA.* 2000;284(22):2907-2911.

66. Akechi T, Okamura H, Nishiwaki Y, Uchitomi Y. Predictive factors for suicidal ideation in patients with unresectable lung carcinoma. *Cancer.* 2002;95(5):1085-1093.

67. Cheung G, Merry S, Sundram F. Medical examiner and coroner reports: uses and limitations in the epidemiology and prevention of late-life suicide. *Int J Geriatr Psychiatry.* 2015;30(8):781-792.

68. Yousaf U, Christensen ML, Engholm G, Storm HH. Suicides among Danish cancer patients 1971-1999. *Br J Cancer.* 2005;92(6):995-1000.

69. Hem E, Loge JH, Haldorsen T, Ekeberg O. Suicide risk in cancer patients from 1960 to 1999. *J Clin Oncol.* 2004;22(20):4209-4216.

70. Breitbart W, Rosenfeld B, Gibson C, et al. Meaning-centered group psychotherapy for patients with advanced cancer: a pilot randomized controlled trial. *Psychooncology.* 2010;19(1):21-28.

71. Meier DE, Emmons CA, Wallenstein S, Quill T, Morrison RS, Cassel CK. A national survey of physician-assisted suicide and euthanasia in the United States. *N Engl J Med.* 1998;338(17):1193-1201.

72. Lydiatt WM, Denman D, McNeilly DP, Puumula SE, Burke WJ. A randomized, placebo-controlled trial of citalopram for the prevention of major depression during treatment for head and neck cancer. *Arch Otolaryngol Head Neck Surg.* 2008;134(5):528-535.

73. Breitbart W, Rosenfeld B, Gibson C, et al. Impact of treatment for depression on desire for hastened death in patients with advanced AIDS. *Psychosomatics.* 2010;51(2): 98-105.

74. Thomas-MacLean R, Stoppard JM. Physicians' constructions of depression: inside/outside the boundaries of medicalization. *Health.* 2004;8(3):275-293.

75. Schumann I, Schneider A, Kantert C, Lowe B, Linde K. Physicians' attitudes, diagnostic process and barriers regarding depression diagnosis in primary care: a

systematic review of qualitative studies. *Fam Pract.* 2012;29(3):255-263.

76. Ng F, Crawford GB, Chur-Hansen A. Depression means different things: a qualitative study of psychiatrists' conceptualization of depression in the palliative care setting. *Palliat Support Care.* 2015;13(5):1223-1230.

77. Ng F, Crawford GB, Chur-Hansen A. How do palliative medicine specialists conceptualize depression? Findings from a qualitative in-depth interview study. *J Palliat Med.* 2014;17(3):318-324.

78. Ng F, Crawford GB, Chur-Hansen A. Palliative medicine practitioners' views on the concept of depression in the palliative care setting. *J Palliat Med.* 2013;16(8): 922-928.

79. Wasteson E, Brenne E, Higginson IJ, et al. Depression assessment and classification in palliative cancer patients: a systematic literature review. *Palliat Med.* 2009;23(8):739-753.

80. Raison CL, Miller AH. Depression in cancer: new developments regarding diagnosis and treatment. *Biol Psychiatry.* 2003;54(3):283-294.

81. Trask PC. Assessment of depression in cancer patients. *J Natl Cancer Inst Monogr.* 2004(32):80-92.

82. Akechi T, Ietsugu T, Sukigara M, et al. Symptom indicator of severity of depression in cancer patients: a comparison of the DSM-IV criteria with alternative diagnostic criteria. *Gen Hosp Psychiatry.* 2009;31(3): 225-232.

83. Kathol RG, Mutgi A, Williams J, Clamon G, Noyes R Jr. Diagnosis of major depression in cancer patients according to four sets of criteria. *Am J Psychiatry.* 1990;147(8):1021-1024.

84. Chochinov HM, Wilson KG, Enns M, Lander S. Prevalence of depression in the terminally ill: effects of diagnostic criteria and symptom threshold judgments. *Am J Psychiatry.* 1994;151(4):537-540.

85. Ciaramella A, Poli P. Assessment of depression among cancer patients: the role of pain, cancer type and treatment. *Psychooncology.* 2001;10(2):156-165.

86. Yirmiya R, Weidenfeld J, Pollak Y, et al. Cytokines, "depression due to a general medical condition," and antidepressant drugs. *Adv Exp Med Biol.* 1999;461: 283-316.

87. Breslau N, Roth T, Rosenthal L, Andreski P. Sleep disturbance and psychiatric disorders: a longitudinal epidemiological study of young adults. *Biol Psychiatry.* 1996;39(6):411-418.

88. Zigmond AS, Snaith RP. The hospital anxiety and depression scale. *Acta Psychiatr Scand.* 1983;67(6): 361-370.

89. Lawrie I, Lloyd-Williams M, Taylor F. How do palliative medicine physicians assess and manage depression. *Palliat Med.* 2004;18(3):234-238.

90. Mitchell AJ, Meader N, Symonds P. Diagnostic validity of the Hospital Anxiety and Depression Scale (HADS) in cancer and palliative settings: a meta-analysis. *J Affect Disord.* 2010;126(3):335-348.

91. Lloyd-Williams M, Friedman T, Rudd N. An analysis of the validity of the Hospital Anxiety and Depression scale as a screening tool in patients with advanced metastatic cancer. *J Pain Symptom Manage.* 2001;22(6): 990-996.

92. Snaith RP. The Hospital Anxiety and Depression Scale. *Health Qual Life Outcomes.* 2003;1:29.

93. Sellick SM, Edwardson AD. Screening new cancer patients for psychological distress using the hospital anxiety and depression scale. *Psychooncology.* 2007;16(6):534-542.

94. Mitchell AJ, Kaar S, Coggan C, Herdman J. Acceptability of common screening methods used to detect distress and related mood disorders—preferences of cancer specialists and non-specialists. *Psychooncology.* 2008;17(3):226-236.

95. Lloyd-Williams M, Friedman T, Rudd N. Criterion validation of the Edinburgh postnatal depression scale as a screening tool for depression in patients with advanced metastatic cancer. *J Pain Symptom Manage.* 2000;20(4):259-265.

96. Chochinov HM, Wilson KG, Enns M, Lander S. "Are you depressed?" Screening for depression in the terminally ill. *Am J Psychiatry.* 1997;154(5):674-676.

97. Lloyd-Williams M, Dennis M, Taylor F, Baker I. Is asking patients in palliative care, "are you depressed?" Appropriate? Prospective study. *BMJ.* 2003;327(7411): 372-373.

98. Payne A, Barry S, Creedon B, et al. Sensitivity and specificity of a two-question screening tool for depression in a specialist palliative care unit. *Palliat Med.* 2007;21(3):193-198.

99. Hamilton M. A rating scale for depression. *J Neurol Neurosurg Psychiatry.* 1960;23:56-62.

100. Olden M, Rosenfeld B, Pessin H, Breitbart W. Measuring depression at the end of life: is the Hamilton Depression Rating Scale a valid instrument? *Assessment.* 2009;16(1):43-54.

101. Loosman WL, Siegert CE, Korzec A, Honig A. Validity of the Hospital Anxiety and Depression Scale and the Beck Depression Inventory for use in end-stage renal disease patients. *Br J Clin Psychol.* 2010;49(Pt 4): 507-516.

102. Esser P, Hartung TJ, Friedrich M, et al. The Generalized Anxiety Disorder Screener (GAD-7) and the anxiety module of the Hospital and Depression Scale (HADS-A) as screening tools for generalized anxiety disorder among cancer patients. *Psychooncology.* 2018;27(6):1509-1516.

103. Andersen BL, DeRubeis RJ, Berman BS, et al. Screening, assessment, and care of anxiety and depressive symptoms in adults with cancer: an American Society of Clinical Oncology Guideline Adaptation. *J Clin Oncol.* 2014;32(15):1605-1619.

104. Bech P. Mood and anxiety in the medically ill. *Adv Psychosom Med.* 2012;32:118-132.

105. Zweers D, de Graaf E, de Graeff A, Stellato RK, Witteveen PO, Teunissen S. The predictive value of symptoms for anxiety in hospice inpatients with advanced cancer. *Palliat Support Care.* 2018;16(5):602-607.

106. Yohannes AM, Junkes-Cunha M, Smith J, Vestbo J. Management of dyspnea and anxiety in chronic obstructive pulmonary disease: a critical review. *J Am Med Direct Assoc.* 2017;18(12):1096.e1091-1096.e1017.

107. Roth AJ, Massie MJ. Anxiety and its management in advanced cancer. *Curr Opin Support Palliat Care.* 2007;1(1):50-56.

108. Boulogne S, Catenoix H, Ryvlin P, Rheims S. Long-lasting seizure-related anxiety in patients with temporal lobe epilepsy and comorbid psychiatric disorders. *Epileptic Disord.* 2015;17(3):340-344.

109. Freemantle SN, Pears GL, Wilton LV, Mac Kay FJ, Mann RD. The incidence of the most commonly reported events with 40 newly marketed drugs—a study by prescription-event monitoring. *Pharmacoepidemiol Drug Saf.* 1997:1–62.

110. Wolkowitz OM. Prospective controlled studies of the behavioral and biological effects of exogenous corticosteroids. *Psychoneuroendocrinology.* 1994;19(3):233-255.

111. Naber D, Sand P, Heigl B. Psychopathological and neuropsychological effects of 8-days' corticosteroid treatment. A prospective study. *Psychoneuroendocrinology.* 1996;21(1):25-31.

112. Acute adverse reactions to prednisone in relation to dosage. *Clin Pharmacol Ther.* 1972;13(5):694-698.

113. Bolanos SH, Khan DA, Hanczyc M, Bauer MS, Dhanani N, Brown ES. Assessment of mood states in patients receiving long-term corticosteroid therapy and in controls with patient-rated and clinician-rated scales. *Ann Allergy Asthma Immunol.* 2004;92(5):500-505.

114. Fardet L, Petersen I, Nazareth I. Suicidal behavior and severe neuropsychiatric disorders following glucocorticoid therapy in primary care. *Am J Psychiatry.* 2012;169(5):491-497.

115. Trask PC, Paterson AG, Esper P, Pau J, Redman B. Longitudinal course of depression, fatigue, and quality of life in patients with high risk melanoma receiving adjuvant interferon. *Psychooncology.* 2004;13(8):526-536.

116. Hauser P. Neuropsychiatric side effects of HCV therapy and their treatment: focus on IFN alpha-induced depression. *Gastroenterol Clin North Am.* 2004; 33(1 suppl):S35-S50.

117. Malek-Ahmadi P. Mood disorders associated with interferon treatment: theoretical and practical considerations. *Ann Pharmacother.* 2001;35(4):489-495.

118. Hauser P, Khosla J, Aurora H, et al. A prospective study of the incidence and open-label treatment of interferon-induced major depressive disorder in patients with hepatitis C. *Mol Psychiatry.* 2002;7(9):942-947.

119. Hauschild A, Gogas H, Tarhini A, et al. Practical guidelines for the management of interferon-alpha-2b side effects in patients receiving adjuvant treatment for melanoma: expert opinion. *Cancer.* 2008;112(5):982-994.

120. Musselman DL, Lawson DH, Gumnick JF, et al. Paroxetine for the prevention of depression induced by high-dose interferon alfa. *N Engl J Med.* 2001;344(13): 961-966.

121. Janssen HL, Brouwer JT, van der Mast RC, Schalm SW. Suicide associated with alfa-interferon therapy for chronic viral hepatitis. *J Hepatol.* 1994;21(2):241-243.

122. Holland J, Fasanello S, Onuma T. Psychiatric symptoms associated with L-asparaginase administration. *J Psychiatr Res.* 1974;10(2):105-113.

123. Patten SB, Barbui C. Drug-induced depression: a systematic review to inform clinical practice. *Psychother Psychosom.* 2004;73(4):207-215.

124. Denicoff KD, Rubinow DR, Papa MZ, et al. The neuropsychiatric effects of treatment with interleukin-2 and lymphokine-activated killer cells. *Ann Intern Med.* 1987;107(3):293-300.

125. Holland JC. *Psycho-oncology.* Oxford University Press. Oxford, United Kingdom; 2015.

126. Thornton LM, Carson WE III, Shapiro CL, Farrar WB, Andersen BL. Delayed emotional recovery after taxane-based chemotherapy. *Cancer.* 2008;113(3): 638-647.

127. Torres MA, Pace TW, Liu T, et al. Predictors of depression in breast cancer patients treated with radiation: role of prior chemotherapy and nuclear factor kappa B. *Cancer.* 2013;119(11):1951-1959.

128. Braunstein S, Formenti SC, Schneider RJ. Acquisition of stable inducible up-regulation of nuclear factor-kappaB by tumor necrosis factor confers increased radiation resistance without increased transformation in breast cancer cells. *Mol Cancer Res.* 2008;6(1):78-88.

129. Hammerlid E, Silander E, Hornestam L, Sullivan M. Health-related quality of life three years after diagnosis of head and neck cancer—a longitudinal study. *Head Neck.* 2001;23(2):113-125.

130. Kelly C, Paleri V, Downs C, Shah R. Deterioration in quality of life and depressive symptoms during radiation therapy for head and neck cancer. *Otolaryngol Head Neck Surg.* 2007;136(1):108-111.

131. Sehlen S, Lenk M, Herschbach P, et al. Depressive symptoms during and after radiotherapy for head and neck cancer. *Head Neck.* 2003;25(12):1004-1018.

132. Head A, Kendall MJ, Ferner R, Eagles C. Acute effects of beta blockade and exercise on mood and anxiety. *Br J Sports Med.* 1996;30(3):238-242.

133. Conant J, Engler R, Janowsky D, Maisel A, Gilpin E, LeWinter M. Central nervous system side effects of beta-adrenergic blocking agents with high and low lipid solubility. *J Cardiovasc Pharmacol.* 1989;13(4):656-661.

134. Shariff S, Cumming CE, Lees A, Handman M, Cumming DC. Mood disorder in women with early breast cancer taking tamoxifen, an estradiol receptor antagonist. An expected or unexpected effect? *Ann N Y Acad Sci.* 1995;761:365-368.

135. Breuer B, Anderson R. The relationship of tamoxifen with dementia, depression, and dependence in activities of daily living in elderly nursing home residents. *Women Health.* 2000;31(1):71-85.

136. Cella D, Fallowfield L, Barker P, Cuzick J, Locker G, Howell A. Quality of life of postmenopausal women in the ATAC ("Arimidex", tamoxifen, alone or in combination) trial after completion of 5 years' adjuvant treatment for early breast cancer. *Breast Cancer Res Treat.* 2006;100(3):273-284.

137. Desmarais JE, Looper KJ. Interactions between tamoxifen and antidepressants via cytochrome P450 2D6. *J Clin Psychiatry.* 2009;70(12):1688-1697.

138. Maguire P. The recognition and treatment of affective disorder in cancer patients. *Appl Psychol.* 2008;33: 479-491.

139. Block SD. Assessing and managing depression in the terminally ill patient. ACP-ASIM End-of-Life Care Consensus Panel. American College of Physicians—American Society of Internal Medicine. *Ann Intern Med.* 2000;132(3):209-218.

140. Block SD, Billings JA. Patient requests to hasten death. Evaluation and management in terminal care. *Arch Intern Med.* 1994;154(18):2039-2047.

141. Noorani NH, Montagnini M. Recognizing depression in palliative care patients. *J Palliat Med.* 2007;10(2): 458-464.

142. Watt CL, Momoli F, Ansari MT, et al. The incidence and prevalence of delirium across palliative care settings: a systematic review. *Palliat Med.* 2019;33(8):865-877.

143. Irwin SA, Rao S, Bower KA, et al. Psychiatric issues in palliative care: recognition of delirium in patients enrolled in hospice care. *Palliat Support Care.* 2008;6(2): 159-164.

144. Inouye SK, Westendorp RG, Saczynski JS. Delirium in elderly people. *Lancet.* 2014;383(9920):911-922.

145. Mittal D, Majithia D, Kennedy R, Rhudy J. Differences in characteristics and outcome of delirium as based on referral patterns. *Psychosomatics.* 2006;47(5):367-375.

146. Fang CK, Chen HW, Liu SI, Lin CJ, Tsai LY, Lai YL. Prevalence, detection and treatment of delirium in terminal cancer inpatients: a prospective survey. *Jpn J Clin Oncol.* 2008;38(1):56-63.

147. Wada T, Wada M, Wada M, Onishi H. Characteristics, interventions, and outcomes of misdiagnosed delirium in cancer patients. *Palliat Support Care.* 2010;8(2): 125-131.

148. de la Cruz M, Fan J, Yennu S, et al. The frequency of missed delirium in patients referred to palliative care in a comprehensive cancer center. *Support Care Cancer.* 2015;23(8):2427-2433.

149. Robinson S, Kissane DW, Brooker J, Burney S. A review of the construct of demoralization: history, definitions, and future directions for palliative care. *Am J Hosp Palliat Care.* 2016;33(1):93-101.

150. Finlay-Jones R. Disgust with life in general. *Aust N Z J Psychiatry.* 1983;17(2):149-152.

151. Engel GL. A psychological setting of somatic disease: the 'giving up–given up' complex. *Proc R Soc Med.* 1967;60(6):553-555.

152. Maier SF, Seligman ME. Learned helplessness: theory and evidence. *J Exp Psychol Gen.* 1976;105(1):3-46.

153. Frankl VE. *Man's search for meaning.* Pocket Books; 1985.

154. Folkman S. Positive psychological states and coping with severe stress. *Soc Sci Med.* 1997;45(8):1207-1221.

155. Kissane DW, Clarke DM, Street AF. Demoralization syndrome—a relevant psychiatric diagnosis for palliative care. *J Palliat Care.* 2001;17(1):12-21.

156. Robinson S, Kissane DW, Brooker J, Burney S. A systematic review of the demoralization syndrome in individuals with progressive disease and cancer: a decade of research. *J Pain Symptom Manage.* 2015;49(3):595-610.

157. de Figueiredo JM. Depression and demoralization: phenomenologic differences and research perspectives. *Compr Psychiatry.* 1993;34(5):308-311.

158. Griffith JL, Gaby L. Brief psychotherapy at the bedside: countering demoralization from medical illness. *Psychosomatics.* 2005;46(2):109-116.

159. Freud S. Mourning and melancholia. *SE.* 1917;14.

160. Widera EW, Block SD. Managing grief and depression at the end of life. *Am Fam Physician.* 2012;86(3):259-264.

161. Zisook S, Shear K. Grief and bereavement: what psychiatrists need to know. *World Psychiatry.* 2009;8(2):67-74.

162. Aoyama M, Sakaguchi Y, Morita T, et al. Factors associated with possible complicated grief and major depressive disorders. *Psychooncology.* 2018;27(3):915-921.

163. Boelen PA, de Keijser J, van den Hout MA, van den Bout J. Treatment of complicated grief: a comparison between cognitive-behavioral therapy and supportive counseling. *J Consult Clin Psychol.* 2007;75(2):277-284.

164. Miovic M, Block S. Psychiatric disorders in advanced cancer. *Cancer.* 2007;110(8):1665-1676.

165. Potash M, Breitbart W. Affective disorders in advanced cancer. *Hematol/Oncol Clin North Am.* 2002;16(3):671-700.

166. Excellence. NIfHaC. Depression in adults: recognition and management. Clinical guideline 90; 2009. Last updated April 2016.

167. Fujisawa D. Depression in cancer care. *Keio J Med.* 2018;67(3):37-44.

168. Janberidze E, Hjermstad MJ, Brunelli C, et al. The use of antidepressants in patients with advanced cancer—results from an international multicentre study. *Psychooncology.* 2014;23(10):1096-1102.

169. Rosenberg L, deLima Thomas J. Pharmacologic Management of Depression in Advanced Illness #309. *J Palliat Med.* 2016;19(7):783-784.

170. Rayner L, Price A, Evans A, Valsraj K, Hotopf M, Higginson IJ. Antidepressants for the treatment of depression in palliative care: systematic review and meta-analysis. *Palliat Med.* 2011;25(1):36-51.

171. Lloyd-Williams M, Friedman T, Rudd N. A survey of antidepressant prescribing in the terminally ill. *Palliat Med.* 1999;13(3):243-248.

172. de Abajo FJ, Garcia-Rodriguez LA. Risk of upper gastrointestinal tract bleeding associated with selective serotonin reuptake inhibitors and venlafaxine therapy: interaction with nonsteroidal anti-inflammatory drugs and effect of acid-suppressing agents. *Arch Gen Psychiatry.* 2008;65(7):795-803.

173. Kast RE, Foley KF. Cancer chemotherapy and cachexia: mirtazapine and olanzapine are 5-HT3 antagonists with good antinausea effects. *Eur J Cancer Care.* 2007;16(4):351-354.

174. Kerr CW, Drake J, Milch RA, et al. Effects of methylphenidate on fatigue and depression: a randomized, double-blind, placebo-controlled trial. *J Pain Symptom Manage.* 2012;43(1):68-77.

175. Mock V, Atkinson A, Barsevick A, et al. NCCN practice guidelines for cancer-related fatigue. *Oncology (Williston Park).* 2000;14(11a):151-161.

176. Mücke M, Mochamat, Cuhls H, et al. Pharmacological treatments for fatigue associated with palliative care. *Cochrane Database Syst Rev.* 2015;(5).

177. Sullivan DR, Mongoue-Tchokote S, Mori M, Goy E, Ganzini L. Randomized, double-blind, placebo-controlled study of methylphenidate for the treatment of depression in SSRI-treated cancer patients receiving palliative care. *Psychooncology.* 2017;26(11):1763-1769.

178. Candy M, Jones L, Williams R, Tookman A, King M. Psychostimulants for depression. *Cochrane Database Syst Rev.* 2008;(2):CD006722.

179. Bruera E, Fainsinger R, MacEachern T, Hanson J. The use of methylphenidate in patients with incident cancer pain requiring regular opiates. A preliminary report. *Pain.* 1992;50(1):75-77.

180. Irwin SA, Iglewicz A, Nelesen RA, et al. Daily oral ketamine for the treatment of depression and anxiety in patients receiving hospice care: a 28-day open-label proof-of-concept trial. *J Palliat Med.* 2013;16(8):958-965.

181. Iglewicz A, Morrison K, Nelesen RA, et al. Ketamine for the treatment of depression in patients receiving hospice care: a retrospective medical record review of thirty-one cases. *Psychosomatics.* 2015;56(4):329-337.

182. Meyer-Junco LE. Aripiprazole for the treatment of depression in palliative care. *J Palliat Med.* 2015;18(4):316.

183. Fulton JJ, Newins AR, Porter LS, Ramos K. Psychotherapy targeting depression and anxiety for use in palliative care: a meta-analysis. *J Palliat Med.* 2018;21(7):1024-1037.

184. Akechi T, Okuyama T, Onishi J, Morita T, Furukawa TA. Psychotherapy for depression among incurable cancer patients. *Cochrane Database Syst Rev.* 2008;(2):Cd005537.

185. Okuyama T, Akechi T, Mackenzie L, Furukawa TA. Psychotherapy for depression among advanced, incurable cancer patients: a systematic review and meta-analysis. *Cancer Treat Rev.* 2017;56:16-27.

186. Bech P, Cialdella P, Haugh MC, et al. Meta-analysis of randomised controlled trials of fluoxetine v. placebo and tricyclic antidepressants in the short-term treatment of major depression. *Br J Psychiatry.* 2000;176:421-428.

187. Stagg EK, Lazenby M. Best practices for the nonpharmacological treatment of depression at the end of life. *Am J Hosp Palliat Care.* 2012;29(3):183-194.

188. Edelman S, Bell DR, Kidman AD. A group cognitive behaviour therapy programme with metastatic breast cancer patients. *Psychooncology.* 1999;8(4):295-305.

189. Chochinov HM, Kristjanson LJ, Breitbart W, et al. Effect of dignity therapy on distress and end-of-life experience in terminally ill patients: a randomised controlled trial. *Lancet Oncol.* 2011;12(8):753-762.

190. Noble A, Jones C. Benefits of narrative therapy: holistic interventions at the end of life. *Br J Nurs.* 2005;14(6):330-333.

191. Ando M, Morita T, Akechi T, Okamoto T. Efficacy of short-term life-review interviews on the spiritual well-being of terminally ill cancer patients. *J Pain Symptom Manage*. 2010;39(6):993-1002.

192. Breitbart W, Poppito S, Rosenfeld B, et al. Pilot randomized controlled trial of individual meaning-centered psychotherapy for patients with advanced cancer. *J Clin Oncol*. 2012;30(12):1304-1309.

193. Rodin G, Lo C, Rydall A, et al. Managing cancer and living meaningfully (CALM): a randomized controlled trial of a psychological intervention for patients with advanced cancer. *J Clin Oncol*. 2018;36(23):2422-2432.

194. Ando M, Morita T, Okamoto T, Ninosaka Y. One-week short-term life review interview can improve spiritual well-being of terminally ill cancer patients. *Psychooncology*. 2008;17(9):885-890.

195. Butler RN. Succesful aging and the role of the life review. *J Am Geriatr Soc*. 1974;22(12):529-535.

196. Kissane DW, Bloch S, Smith GC, et al. Cognitive-existential group psychotherapy for women with primary breast cancer: a randomised controlled trial. *Psychooncology*. 2003;12(6):532-546.

197. Breitbart W, Poppito HR. *Meaning-Centered Group Psychotherapy for Patients with Advanced Cancer: A Treatment Manual*. Oxford University Press; 2015.

198. Lloyd-Williams M, Shiels C, Ellis J, et al. Pilot randomised controlled trial of focused narrative intervention for moderate to severe depression in palliative care patients: DISCERN trial. *Palliat Med*. 2018;32(1):206-215.

199. Salt S, Mulvaney CA, Preston NJ. Drug therapy for symptoms associated with anxiety in adult palliative care patients. *Cochrane Database Syst Rev*. 2017;(5):CD004596.

200. National Clinical Guideline Centre. National Institute for Health and Care Excellence: clinical guidelines. In: *Care of Dying Adults in the Last Days of Life*. London, UK: National Institute for Health and Care Excellence (UK) Copyright (c) 2015 National Clinical Guideline Centre; 2015.

201. Levenson JL. *The American Psychiatric Association Publishing Textbook of Psychosomatic Medicine and Consultation-Liaison Psychiatry*. 3rd ed. American Psychiatric Association Publishing. Washington, DC; 2018.

202. Meagher DJ, McLoughlin L, Leonard M, Hannon N, Dunne C, O'Regan N. What do we really know about the treatment of delirium with antipsychotics? Ten key issues for delirium pharmacotherapy. *Am J Geriatr Psychiatry*. 2013;21(12):1223-1238.

203. Clemens KE, Klaschik E. Dyspnoea associated with anxiety—symptomatic therapy with opioids in combination with lorazepam and its effect on ventilation in palliative care patients. *Support Care Cancer*. 2011;19(12):2027-2033.

204. Breitbart W, Holland JC. *Psychiatric Aspects of Symptom Management in Cancer Patients*. American Psychiatric Press. Washington, DC; 1993.

205. Levin TT, White CA, Bialer P, Charlson RW, Kissane DW. A review of cognitive therapy in acute medical settings. Part II: strategies and complexities. *Palliat Support Care*. 2013;11(3):253-266.

206. Zeng YS, Wang C, Ward KE, Hume AL. Complementary and alternative medicine in hospice and palliative care: a systematic review. *J Pain Symptom Manage*. 2018;56(5):781-794.e784.

207. Williams JW Jr, Gierisch JM, McDuffie J, Strauss JL, Nagi A. VA evidence-based synthesis program reports. In: *An Overview of Complementary and Alternative Medicine Therapies for Anxiety and Depressive Disorders: Supplement to Efficacy of Complementary and Alternative Medicine Therapies for Posttraumatic Stress Disorder*. Washington, DC: Department of Veterans Affairs (US); 2011.

208. Poletti S, Razzini G, Ferrari R, et al. Mindfulness-based stress reduction in early palliative care for people with metastatic cancer: a mixed-method study. *Complement Ther Med*. 2019;47:102218.

Cognitive Decline Following Cancer Treatment

Elizabeth Ryan, Alexandra M. Gaynor, Katrazyna McNeal, Tim A. Ahles, and James C. Root

INTRODUCTION

Cognitive decline following cancer diagnosis and treatment is an important clinical problem for cancer survivors that may have far-reaching consequences in home life, educational attainment, and occupational success. Increasingly, cognitive decline has been identified in individuals treated for non-CNS cancers, in which no primary neurological etiology can be identified. Patient- and physician-reported cognitive decline in breast and other cancers following treatment led to investigation of various treatment modalities and their potential effect on cognition in these groups. While earlier reports generally focused on the effects of chemotherapy exposure ("chemobrain"), other factors and treatment modalities are recognized as potential contributors to cognitive dysfunction. In addition to chemotherapy exposure, hormone treatment, stem cell transplant, pain medications, genetic susceptibilities, immune system dysfunction, and the psychological and physical stress of diagnosis and treatment may all potentially affect self-report and objective findings of cognitive dysfunction. For this reason, we mainly discuss posttreatment difficulties in cognition with a focus on chemotherapy exposure, mainly derived from studies in women with breast cancer, but with the caveat that several other factors may also contribute to reported and observed dysfunction. Studies utilizing neuropsychological measures have defined the objective cognitive effects following treatment and have been extended through the use of structural and functional neuroimaging to better understand potential pathology underlying cognitive dysfunction. In addition, while still in the early stages of investigation, mechanisms by which cancer treatments might influence cognitive abilities and brain function have been proposed that might help to explain resulting cognitive dysfunction.

In this chapter, we describe a typical case of cognitive dysfunction putatively associated with cancer treatment to provide the reader a better understanding of how this syndrome presents in a routine clinical setting. We then review research literature documenting the self-report of individuals

posttreatment in regard to their most prominent cognitive symptoms and how these affect day-to-day functioning. Research documenting formal, objective measurement of cognitive abilities in this group is then reviewed and contrasted. Contributions of structural and functional imaging, which may help to clarify the underlying changes in brain structure and function following treatment, are then discussed, followed by potential mechanisms by which treatment may exert an effect on the brain and cognition. We then close with a review of the emerging literature on cognitive rehabilitation and pharmacologic interventions that have been developed for the treatment of cognitive changes following non-CNS cancer.

CASE SUMMARY

Ms. C., a 25-year-old woman diagnosed with non-Hodgkin's lymphoma approximately 2 years before, was referred to our service with reports of forgetfulness, poor concentration, and difficulties in understanding instructions and learning new tasks. Ms. C. had undergone chemotherapy treatment consisting of four rounds: rituximab, cyclophosphamide, doxorubicin, vincristine, and prednisone (R-CHOP), and two rounds: ifosfamide, carboplatin, and etoposide (ICE) after her diagnosis, resulting in no evidence of disease. While she had had no difficulties performing her work in office administration before treatment, she found herself making increasing errors on routine assignments, felt more easily distracted, and experienced problems with new tasks. These difficulties only increased when she took a new position with similar responsibilities in a different, faster-paced environment with new coworkers. She found herself making significant errors on a daily basis and increasingly relying on her coworkers for additional help, both of which led to reprimands from her supervisors. Ms. C. expressed considerable anxiety about her situation, fearing that her many mistakes were putting her job in jeopardy.

Ms. C. was administered a standard neuropsychological test battery, which included measures of processing speed, attention, language functioning, verbal and visuospatial reasoning, learning and memory, as well as executive functioning; emotional factors that may have been contributing to the reported issues were also assessed by self-report. Our assessment found mildly impaired cognitive and motor slowing across all timed tasks in which speed and efficiency are prerequisites, as well as difficulties in recollection of previously learned information. Complicating the clinical picture, Ms. C.'s profile was also notable for considerable anxiety, manifested by rumination, tension, and constant worry. These difficulties were discussed with Ms. C., who found the objective results broadly overlapping with the symptoms she had identified at work and at home; specifically, she identified feelings of being forgetful, being "slower," being "less efficient," difficulties in real-time, pressured situations, and constant anxiety that appeared in reaction to mistakes as well as distracted her from tasks at hand. Cognitive rehabilitation, tailored to her specific tasks and difficulties at work, was recommended, as well as regular psychotherapy for treatment of the attendant anxiety in relation to her diagnosis and current difficulties.

SELF-REPORTED COGNITIVE DECLINE FOLLOWING TREATMENT

The kinds of difficulties described above are widely cited in literature studying self-reported cognitive issues following treatment. Slowing, inattention, distraction, forgetfulness, difficulties in multitasking, and word finding problems are all implicated in patients' self-report to varying degrees. Early research on self-reported cognitive difficulties in mixed etiology cancer patients found that roughly half of patients reported difficulties in memory or concentration at some point in their treatment (1). Follow-up by this group in a sample of 91 lymphoma patients 6 or more months posttreatment found 30% of patients reported difficulties in concentration, with significant forgetfulness being reported by 52% of patients (2). That these self-reported cognitive difficulties persisted for longer interims posttreatment was confirmed by Schagen et al. (3), who found persistent reported cognitive difficulties, including poor concentration (31%) and forgetfulness (21%) in breast cancer survivors treated with cyclophosphamide, methotrexate, and fluorouracil 5FU (CMF) compared with surgery and radiation treatment alone. Similarly, Ahles et al. (4) found persistent reports of difficulties in concentration and complex attention up to 10 years posttreatment in individuals who received systemic chemotherapy for breast cancer and lymphoma. Several other studies, including patients with different cancers at various time points during and after completion of treatment, have found similar increased incidence of reported cognitive difficulties putatively associated with chemotherapy and hormone exposure (5–13).

OBJECTIVE MEASUREMENT OF COGNITION FOLLOWING TREATMENT

The first studies that investigated objective differences in cognition of individuals posttreatment were cross-sectional, contrasting individuals posttreatment with healthy controls or cancer-diagnosed controls undergoing a different treatment. Initial cross-sectional studies of breast cancer survivors found that 17% to 75% of patients experienced cognitive difficulties anywhere between 6 months and 10 years posttreatment. A meta-analysis that included mainly cross-sectional studies (5,6,14) found small to moderate effect sizes across motor function, executive function, learning and memory, spatial reasoning, and language function; these results square with reports of cancer survivors and their clinicians, which document difficulties including forgetfulness, difficulties in attention and multitasking, cognitive slowing, and difficulties in word finding (15,16). Ahles et al. (4) documented that a subset of cognitive difficulties appear even at longer intervals posttreatment, with chemotherapy-exposed individuals exhibiting significantly worse performance overall and lower performance specifically in verbal ability and psychomotor speed 10 years posttreatment.

The cross-sectional design of these studies, which do not include pretreatment baseline assessments, qualifies the interpretation of their results. Cancer patients may present with pretreatment, baseline cognitive dysfunction, with these difficulties persisting through treatment and posttreatment testing (17,18). Wefel et al. (18) found that 35% of women pre–chemotherapy treatment exhibited cognitive impairment. Ahles et al. (17) investigated pretreatment cognitive ability in healthy controls and patients diagnosed with invasive (stages I to III) and noninvasive (stage 0) breast cancer and found significantly slowed reaction time in the invasive group compared with healthy controls, and lower overall performance in the invasive group compared with the healthy and noninvasive patient groups. While pretreatment/baseline differences remain poorly understood in regard to mechanism or etiology, the fact that differences are present between groups prior to treatment requires that longitudinal assessments be conducted.

More recent longitudinal studies that can control for these pretreatment differences have contrasted cancer-diagnosed individuals undergoing different treatment regimens with each other and with healthy, non–cancer diagnosed individuals. Results of these longitudinal studies suggest more specific and more subtle cognitive decline associated with chemotherapy treatment than previous cross-sectional studies indicated. A subset of these studies find no observable cognitive effect of chemotherapy exposure (19), observable decline in only a subset of patients treated with a specific regimen of chemotherapy (CTC vs. FEC) (20), or declines in only a subset of cognitive abilities with no overall decline in neuropsychological performance (21). Positive studies generally suggest that declines in performance following chemotherapy exposure will be in specific cognitive abilities and that these declines will only be exhibited in a subset of individuals. Quesnel et al. (22) compared chemotherapy-exposed and radiotherapy-treated patients pretreatment and at 3 months posttreatment and found that verbal memory was affected in both groups regardless of treatment, but with a specific effect on verbal fluency in the chemotherapy-exposed group.

Recent work complicates the interpretation that chemotherapy, in isolation, is responsible for cognitive decline posttreatment and reinforces the argument that effects posttreatment are likely multifactorial. In addition to chemotherapy treatment, longitudinal studies that included patients not exposed to chemotherapy and healthy controls revealed that the no-chemotherapy group frequently performed as poorly as the chemotherapy group or at an intermediate level between the chemotherapy-exposed group and the healthy controls. This pattern of results raised the question of whether endocrine therapy could impact cognitive functioning. Initial examination of this issue produced mixed results; however, most studies were not powered to adequately examine the independent effects of endocrine therapy. A longitudinal study examining patients not treated with chemotherapy who were randomized to tamoxifen or exemestane revealed that patients treated with tamoxifen, but not with exemestane, experienced cognitive problems compared with healthy controls (23). Even though investigators assumed that they were studying the effects of chemotherapy, in reality, most breast cancer patients receive multimodality treatment including surgery with exposure to general anesthesia, radiation therapy, and endocrine therapy in addition to chemotherapy. This, in combination with the evidence for pretreatment cognitive issues, led Hurria and colleagues to propose the phrase "cancer and cancer treatment–associated cognitive change" as a more accurate descriptor of the phenomenon (24).

The research cited above confirms the presence of objective cognitive difficulties in a subset of cancer patients posttreatment, and these difficulties have been linked specifically to chemotherapy treatment as well as to several other variables, including endocrine therapies and more recently, immunotherapy (25), where 37.5% of leukemia and non-Hodgkin's lymphoma patients reported cognitive difficulties after CAR T-cell therapy.

SUBJECTIVE VERSUS OBJECTIVE MEASUREMENT OF COGNITION FOLLOWING TREATMENT

Similar to findings in other disorders, subjective cognitive reports exhibit poor agreement with results of objective testing at the level of the individual. Depending on the study, this discrepancy appears to be due either to a tendency to overestimate cognitive difficulties by self-report where objective measures find no significant issue or a failure to report cognitive dysfunction where objective measures would suggest significant difficulties. Importantly, most studies do find increased objective cognitive difficulties in individuals posttreatment but report little overlap with subjective reports.

As an example, following on their observation of patient reports of cognitive difficulties described above, Cull et al. (2) found no significant difference in performance on objective memory or concentration tasks between those reporting cognitive difficulties and those reporting no issues. Similarly, Schagen et al. (3) found no relationship between the cognitive reports and objective cognitive performance of breast cancer survivors treated with CMF, despite a higher rate of objective cognitive difficulties in the CMF-exposed group. This same inconsistency between self-report and objective measures is found across several later studies and in those described above, with studies finding either no relationship between subjective and objective measures or that subjective reports were better accounted for by other variables.

While objective findings of cognitive dysfunction have been documented in previous studies, it is important to note that use of these objective measures either clinically or in research applications may tend to underestimate cognitive dysfunction. To what extent these measures are actually predictive of day-to-day functioning, that is, their ecological validity, is unclear; to what extent neuropsychological measures are adequately sensitive to what are likely subtle deficits is questionable. Additionally, formal assessments typically take place in a somewhat rarefied environment that includes no distractions and no competing demands in a quiet, generally predictable setting, all important factors for individuals who complain of attentional difficulties and distractibility. In the research context, in addition to being subject to all of the caveats described in the clinical setting, prior research has excluded individuals who may be at most risk for cognitive dysfunction because of a history of neurological, medical, or psychological difficulties that may in fact act as risk factors to treatment-related effects. As Pullens et al. (25) note, several factors may be in play: (a) the sensitivity of objective measures may be questioned in their ability to identify what may be subtle cognitive deficits; (b) objective measures may fail to measure the kinds of difficulties that most affect patients posttreatment; (c) patients may be describing their worst functioning over a period of months versus a one-time, cross-sectional objective measurement; (d) increasing patient exposure and knowledge of "chemobrain" may lead to increased reporting; (e) subjective reports may reflect poor self-evaluation as a result of distress. Emotional factors have been found to be associated with increased reporting of cognitive decline posttreatment in the absence of objective decline. Van Dam et al. (13) found a higher incidence of objective cognitive difficulties in high versus low dose and healthy control patients as well as a higher incidence of reported cognitive difficulties between chemotherapy-treated patients and healthy control participants. Significantly, while objective performance and subjective reports were not associated, subjective reports were associated with elevated anxiety and depression scores with similar findings in a subset of other studies (3,7,12,26,27). Subjective expectation of cognitive difficulties may also affect increased self-reporting as a result of increasing awareness of treatment-related effects. This is suggested by Schagen et al. (28) who found that, similar to other schema induction research, individuals who had preexisting knowledge of potential treatment effects reported more cognitive difficulties.

Additionally, it has been suggested that one reason for the discordance between self-reported cognitive impairment in traditional neuropsychological tasks may be due to limitations of traditional statistical methods used to assess this relationship. Researchers typically rely on correlation-based statistical approaches to assess the relationship between ratings of cognitive difficulties on self-report measures and total or domain scores on neuropsychological assessments, which do not take into account the frequency or pattern of endorsement of specific items on self-report. Past research has shown that latent regression Rasch modeling, in which individual item-level

responses on self-report measures of cognitive function are directly modeled such that endorsement of rare symptoms is weighted more heavily than commonly reported symptoms, results in better concordance between subjective and objective measures of cognitive performance. For example, a recent study of breast cancer patients showed that while traditional correlational analyses resulted in no relationship between self-report and objective cognitive test performance, latent regression Rasch models showed that changes in neuropsychological test performance from pre- to posttreatment significantly predicted self-reported cognitive problems, suggesting discrepancies between self-report and neuropsychological performance found in past research may in part be due to limitations of traditional statistical approaches (29). Furthermore, this work raises the possibility that discrepancies between subjective and objective measures of performance may be due to survivors misattributing attention problems to memory problems. This hypothesis is further supported by research showing that breast cancer survivors demonstrate deficits in attention and initial learning, but normal performance on delayed memory tests (30,31), suggesting that survivors' perception that they do not remember information is correct, but the problem stems from a failure during initial learning of new material rather than retrieval or memory decay (i.e., "forgetting"). Therefore, in addition to limitations of traditional statistical approaches, the discordance between self-reported cognitive difficulties and neuropsychological test performance may also be due to the relative insensitivity of traditional memory assessments to detect attentional failures during initial learning as compared to retrieval or forgetting problems, given that subjects compensate for initial learning failures over the course of multiple trials.

RISK FACTORS AND MODERATORS OF COGNITIVE CHANGE FOLLOWING TREATMENT

In light of previous research finding pretreatment differences in a subset of cancer-diagnosed individuals together with the more recent research that suggests only a subset of individuals experience cognitive decline following treatment, a next logical step is to examine risk factors that increase vulnerability to cognitive change and factors that may compensate for, or confer resilience to, these changes. Cognitive changes may be understood as the product of intrinsic factors—age-appropriate and pathological changes in structural and functional integrity in the brain—together with what may be broadly characterized as environmental exposures, either currently or by history, that may either be protective or represent a risk factor to cognitive functioning. Work on the concept of brain reserve, that is, the theory that structural integrity or burden in the brain can influence the course of cognitive function in the face of new-onset insults, has realized increasing attention in studies of dementing conditions and traumatic brain insult (32). This work has mainly focused on resilience to cognitive deterioration in conditions in which progressive decline is a natural course (Alzheimer's disease, frontotemporal dementia, Lewy body disease) (33) (for review, see Ref. 34). The concept of cognitive reserve, that is, innate and developed cognitive capacity that is influenced by various factors including genetics, education, occupational attainment, and lifestyle, is related to brain reserve but is defined as a more active, compensatory process (34). Age, premorbid cognitive ability, and genetic inheritance have all been identified as significant factors that may moderate or mediate cognitive difficulties following treatment. Age is a well-established risk factor for cognitive decline in other disorders; researchers have speculated that older adults may be more vulnerable to a variety of insults partly as a result of decreased brain reserve mediated by brain pathology and the accumulated effects of age-appropriate changes in brain structure (35). Individuals with lesser cognitive abilities pretreatment, which may be indicative of lesser cognitive reserve, may also be at greater risk for posttreatment cognitive changes. Research has demonstrated that people with low cognitive reserve are more vulnerable to the development of neurocognitive disorders (Alzheimer's disease)

and to cognitive decline following a variety of insults to the brain. Further, research has demonstrated poorer cognitive outcomes secondary to neurotoxic exposures (e.g., lead) in people with low cognitive reserve (36). Based on the concepts of brain and cognitive reserve, one would predict that older patients with lower than expected cognitive performance at pretreatment would demonstrate poorer cognitive performance posttreatment. Ahles and colleagues found support for an interaction of age, cognitive reserve, and exposure to chemotherapy as risk factors for cognitive decline. In the context of a longitudinal study, they demonstrated that older patients who had lower levels of estimated premorbid function demonstrated significantly reduced performance on posttreatment measures of processing speed (see Fig. 36.1) (37).

Genetic factors have also been examined as potential risk factors for cognitive decline. Apolipoprotein E (ApoE) is a complex glycolipoprotein that facilitates the uptake, transport, and distribution of lipids. It appears to play an important role in neuronal repair and plasticity after injury. A four-exon gene codes for ApoE on chromosome 19 in humans. There are three major alleles: E2, E3, and E4. These alleles differ in amino acids at positions 112 and 158: E2 (cysteine/cysteine), E3 (cysteine/arginine), and E4 (arginine/arginine). Animal models suggest a link between the E4 allele and increased mortality, extent of damage, and poor repair following trauma (38). The human E4 allele has been associated with a variety of disorders with prominent cognitive dysfunction including healthy individuals with memory difficulties,

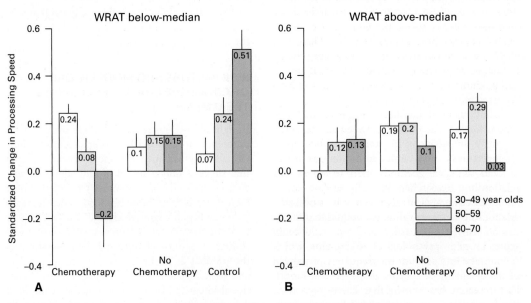

Figure 36.1 Effect of age and premorbid cognitive ability on the speed of processing.

Alzheimer's disease, and poor outcomes in stroke and traumatic brain injury. Ahles et al. (39) evaluated the relationship between the ApoE genotype and neuropsychological performance in long-term cancer survivors treated with standard-dose chemotherapy. The results demonstrated that survivors with at least one E4 allele scored significantly lower in the visual memory and spatial ability domains, with a trend to score lower in the psychomotor domain, compared with survivors who did not carry an E4 allele. A recent longitudinal study of breast cancer patients in survivors showed that survivors with the E4 allele had short-term decreases in learning and memory performance following hormone treatment, and worse performance on attention, processing speed, and executive function tasks at 24 months following chemotherapy, as compared to controls (40). Another longitudinal study showed that APOE4 status was associated with climbing processing speed and working memory pre- to posttreatment, but only for survivors without a history of smoking, suggesting that a smoking history may moderate the degree to which carrying the E4 allele increases the risk of cognitive decline following treatment (37).

Small et al. (41) studied catechol-O-methyltransferase (COMT), which influences the metabolic breakdown of catecholamines through the methylation of dopamine (DA). The valine version (val allele) is almost four times as active as the methionine version of the gene (met allele). Thus individuals homozygous for the val allele presumably metabolize DA much more rapidly than do those with the met allele. COMT becomes a major modulator of dopaminergic tone in the frontal cortex, accounting for approximately 60% of the metabolic degradation of DA. These researchers found that breast cancer patients who had the COMT-Val allele and were treated with chemotherapy performed more poorly on tests of attention, verbal fluency, and motor speed compared with COMT-Met homozygotes.

Other genetic factors that have been suggested as potential candidates for increasing risk for chemotherapy-induced cognitive change include genes that regulate DNA repair (e.g., x-ray repair cross complementing protein 1, XRCC1; Meiotic recombination 11 homolog A, MRE11A), cytokine regulation (e.g., Interleukin 1, IL1; IL6; tumor necrosis factor alpha, TNF-alpha), neurotransmitter activity (e.g., BDNF), and blood–brain barrier efficiency (e.g., multidrug resistance 1, MDR1; organic anion transporting polypeptide, OATP). However, no studies have directly examined the relationship between these genes and chemotherapy-induced cognitive function (4).

STRUCTURAL AND FUNCTIONAL MRI FINDINGS

A crucial, intermediate step in understanding potential mechanisms of chemotherapy-induced cognitive decline will utilize structural brain imaging techniques that enable measurement of changes in regional cerebral volume and cortical thickness. A handful of relatively recent investigations utilizing various methodologies have studied this issue, with a focus on changes in gray matter volumes in individuals postchemotherapy. These studies utilize voxel-based morphometry (VBM), which estimates gray matter volume after segmentation of MRI-derived structural images. In a cross-sectional study, which incorporated data collection points at 1 and 3 year post–chemotherapy treatment in a cohort of breast cancer survivors, brain structure and neuropsychological performance were compared between a chemotherapy and healthy control group (42). Results suggested significantly decreased gray matter volume in prefrontal cortex, precuneus, cingulate cortex, and parahippocampal gyri relative to healthy controls initially, with no difference observed at a 3-year follow-up. A more recent cross-sectional study utilized diffusion tensor imaging (DTI) to examine white matter tract integrity in breast cancer survivors treated with chemotherapy and unaffected controls (43). While complementary to VBM analysis, DTI relies on measures of regional diffusion to estimate white matter tract integrity and efficiency. Significantly, results suggest decreased white matter tract integrity indicated by increased fractional anisotropy and mean diffusion measures in chemotherapy-treated individuals relative to controls. Focal deficits were exhibited in frontal and temporal white matter tracts, consistent with VBM gray matter findings described above, and correlated with neuropsychological measures of processing speed and attention.

While suggestive, interpretation of the results from the above studies is qualified given the relatively small patient groups, the absence of control groups of cancer survivors with no chemotherapy treatment, and the use of cross-sectional designs that prevent interpretation of interval changes from pretreatment baseline. As noted above, pretreatment baseline structural measurement is an important element in any investigation because of pretreatment differences in cognition in individuals prior to adjuvant chemotherapy treatment (17). Results from Ahles et al.'s study also underscore the importance of the inclusion of cancer-diagnosed individuals who are not treated with chemotherapy to delineate the effects of chemotherapy treatment versus cancer diagnosis alone on cognition. More recently, Menning et al. (44) found that breast cancer patients had greater prefrontal activation during a working memory task and decreased white matter integrity prior to chemotherapy. These results suggest that brain structural and functional changes may be present before starting adjuvant chemotherapy, consistent with the findings of neuropsychological deficits pretreatment, and can be further disrupted with chemotherapy treatment. In the first longitudinal study of structural changes associated with chemotherapy treatment, pretreatment baseline scans were collected in breast cancer survivors treated with (CTx+) and without (CTx−) chemotherapy and healthy controls and compared with structural scans at 1 month and 1 year posttreatment in the same individuals. VBM analysis found decreases in frontotemporal cortex and cerebellum at 1 month relative to baseline in the chemotherapy-treated group, with partial recovery of volume at 1 year. While the CTx- group exhibited gray matter reduction in cerebellum at 1 month, the CTx+ group exhibited more widely distributed gray matter reductions across frontal and temporal cortical regions as well as cerebellum and thalamus. Partial recovery of volume in these same regions was exhibited in the CTx+ group at 1 year posttreatment, but reduced volume remained relative to pretreatment baseline (45). The course of recovery of gray matter volume described in this study parallels the finding that individuals' neuropsychological deficits are most pronounced immediately following treatment, with subsequent, partial recovery of function over time (26,46).

Studies utilizing functional imaging methods such as functional magnetic resonance imaging (fMRI), positron emission tomography (PET), or single proton emission computed tomography are relatively sparse in the literature at this point. In a cross-sectional study comparing verbal memory performance between 14 women post–chemotherapy treatment and 14 healthy controls (47), patients exhibited increased prefrontal cortex recruitment during the recall task. The areas of increased recruitment were described as atypical for the declarative memory task based on previous findings associated with this task, and interpreted, again, as compensatory for more typical cortical sites recruited in this paradigm; behavioral performance and accuracy did not significantly differ between groups. A recent, prospective longitudinal fMRI study of memory function in breast cancer survivors showed that survivors demonstrated altered hippocampal conductivity that was associated with poorer objective memory performance and greater subjective complaints about memory function. Furthermore, authors reported increased

activity of prefrontal regions during memory tasks in survivors, suggesting compensatory activation in the face of memory weaknesses (48). Two fMRI studies investigated functional activation in chemotherapy-exposed individuals at longer intervals posttreatment. In a PET study, Silverman et al. (49) investigated differences in regional recruitment between women who had been treated with chemotherapy 5 to 10 years earlier and control subjects who had not been exposed to chemotherapy while performing a memory task. While task performance was equivalent between groups, increased inferior frontal gyrus recruitment was exhibited in the chemotherapy-exposed group during task completion, suggesting that increased prefrontal activity may be compensatory. The suggestion that the chemotherapy group employed compensatory strategies for task completion is further supported by the fact that this inferior frontal gyrus recruitment was not found in the control group, in whom parietal and occipital cortex recruitment was more typical. De Ruiter et al. (50) studied 19 women approximately 10 years post–chemotherapy treatment compared with 15 women previously diagnosed with breast cancer but not treated with chemotherapy on a task of executive functioning and planning (Tower of London) and on a paired associate memory task. In contrast to the previously described studies, the chemotherapy-exposed group exhibited decreased recruitment in dorsolateral prefrontal cortex on the executive functioning task, as well as decreased recruitment in parahippocampal gyri on the paired associates task, with corresponding poorer performance on each task in the chemotherapy group. Similar to previous research in objective neurocognitive assessment of cancer-diagnosed patients, an fMRI study (51) compared 10 cancer-diagnosed women prior to chemotherapy with nine healthy controls on a working memory task. Consistent with findings of pretreatment cognitive issues in cancer-diagnosed individuals, the patient group was less accurate on the working memory task in the context of wider and more diffuse recruitment of prefrontal cortex, and specifically inferior frontal gyrus. This study, similar to studies using objective neuropsychological testing that found pretreatment differences in cognition in cancer-diagnosed individuals, underscores the need for longitudinal design in fMRI studies that would account for pretreatment differences.

Collectively, functional imaging studies suggest that in tasks in which performance is essentially equivalent between groups, the affected group generally employs compensatory prefrontal mechanisms for task completion; there is also evidence that in the subset of studies in which performance was decreased in the affected group, typical brain regions that would otherwise be recruited exhibit reduced recruitment. Still unclear are the precise mechanisms by which treatment may influence brain structure and function.

MECHANISMS

As treatment-related cognitive changes have been increasingly supported in previous studies, central to understanding the etiology of these changes will be the investigation of how prescribed treatments affect underlying brain structure and function. While a number of mechanisms have been proposed to explain cognitive dysfunction associated with cancer treatments, still little is known regarding biological risk factors or mechanisms of damage (52).

The most intuitive explanation for the effects of treatment, and specifically chemotherapy, on brain structure and function is the direct effect of chemotherapy agents on the brain (e.g., neurotoxic or inflammatory mechanisms). Chemotherapy agents exhibit different profiles in their ability to cross the blood–brain barrier, although in rare cases, most agents can cause CNS disorders, suggesting that some permeability of the blood–brain barrier is common to these drugs under certain conditions. Research utilizing PET, a neuroimaging technique that radio-labels chemotherapy agents, has shown that cisplatin, BCNU, and paclitaxel, are detectable in the CNS postadministration (53–55). Furthermore, some animal studies have shown that higher levels of chemotherapy reach the brain than was previously thought, and even low doses can result in increased cell death and decreased cell division in the hippocampus and corpus callosum (56,57). It is clear, however, that the absolute levels of chemotherapy reaching the CNS are much lower than outside the CNS, as evidenced by the poor efficacy of systemic chemotherapy treatment on CNS tumors. This may suggest that, while chemotherapy permeability of the blood–brain barrier is relatively low, little drug is necessary to have an effect on the brain. Evidence of this is found in nonhuman animal studies that find cell death and decreased cell division in hippocampal, parahippocampal, and corpus callosum regions following systemic chemotherapy treatment in mice (56). Differences in blood–brain barrier permeability between individuals may also be an important factor in the extent of chemotherapy exposure in the CNS. The gene multidrug resistance 1 (MDR1) has been found to play a role in blood–brain barrier functioning through its role in encoding the protein P-glycoprotein (P-gp), which is implicated in transporting toxic substances out of the cell.

Select MDR1 polymorphisms may be associated with P-gp function, which may in turn alter the efficiency with which toxic agents, including chemotherapy, are transported from the blood–brain barrier (58).

DNA damage as a result of oxidative stress has also been proposed as a potential intermediate mechanism to CNS damage. One mechanism through which chemotherapy agents affect tumor cell growth is through DNA damage to tumor cells. Importantly, chemotherapy treatment also leads to DNA damage in nontumor cells and is associated with increased levels of non–protein-bound iron, free radicals, and reduced antioxidant capacity, leading to increased oxidative stress more generally. Evidence of an association between increased oxidative DNA damage and cognitive dysfunction has been found in previous studies of neurocognitive disorders, including Alzheimer's disease, and mild cognitive impairment (59). At this point, it is not clear how DNA damage might affect the CNS. The production of defective proteins leading to neuronal apoptosis, deficient DNA repair mechanisms, as well as the loss of essential gene products as a result of DNA damage have all been considered (60,61). Finally, chemotherapy treatment may have a direct effect on telomere length (62–64). With each DNA replication, telomeres become shorter, and past a given threshold, this shortening leads to cell death or cell senescence. Chemotherapy treatment therefore may essentially accelerate the aging process through either direct effect on telomere length in the CNS or the more general effect on genomic stability and biological systems.

Cytokines, cell-signaling proteins that play an important role in immune system functioning as well as in the nervous system, have also been identified as one potential mechanism in CNS damage related to treatment. Cytokines have been found to modulate neuronal and glial cell functioning, neural repair, as well as the action of the neurotransmitters dopamine and serotonin, and cytokine dysregulation has been associated with neural cell death and degenerative neurological disorders associated with aging. In cancer patients, the role of cytokines in cognitive functioning is most clear in patients undergoing IL2 or IFN-α treatment, which are associated with increased fatigue, depression, and cognitive difficulties (65). Importantly, chemotherapy treatment has been associated with increased cytokine levels in the acute phase of treatment (66–68). Chemotherapy-exposed individuals with significant and chronic fatigue at longer intervals posttreatment exhibit elevated levels of cytokines (69,70), and several recent animal studies have demonstrated that chemotherapy elevates probably inflammatory cytokines and decreases anti-inflammatory cytokines, and that these changes are associated with decreased hippocampal activity and poor performance on cognitive tasks, suggesting that impaired cognition following chemotherapy may result from disruptions in cytokine regulation (71–73).

Research has been initiated and continues in our lab and others that seek to better understand and locate mechanistic explanations for treatment-related cognitive dysfunction. Regardless of how such changes come about, an important clinical issue is how best to measure and define these difficulties such that treatment recommendations can be made with an aim toward ameliorating difficulties in cognition.

CLINICAL NEUROPSYCHOLOGICAL TESTING OF POSTTREATMENT COGNITIVE DYSFUNCTION

Neuropsychology is a subspecialty of psychology with a primary interest in understanding brain–behavior relationships, with a particular focus on higher level cognitive processes and their dysfunction in clinical syndromes. Given the disagreement between subjective reports and objective cognitive measures, neuropsychological testing remains the most direct and accurate way in which to measure cognitive effects post-cancer treatment. Even given this disagreement, the most typical reason for referral is generally subjective complaint of difficulties or caregiver/family observation of cognitive difficulties in the patient.

Depending on the setting, referrals may be made by the primary oncologist involved in the patient's care, by rehabilitation medicine, by psychiatry, by a general practitioner, or, most often in older patients, by the primary geriatrician. There are many questions to consider when contemplating referral for assessment of postcancer treatment, and more generally, in any medically ill population: Are the patients at their "new" baseline? Are they currently on an active treatment regimen that may have acute effects not predictive of longer term adjustment (current chemotherapy treatment, intracranial irradiation, etc.)? Will their medical care change dramatically in the near future and would this alteration be expected to affect cognition (initiation of chemotherapy regimen, initiation of intracranial irradiation)? Is there a significant psychiatric issue that may affect cognition (uncontrolled depression, anxiety, adjustment reaction)? Is there significant fatigue, pain, or physical discomfort that may influence cognitive testing? These considerations are meant to ensure that the results of the assessment will be indicative and predictive of long-term, future cognitive function and will not be overwhelmed by state-like transient factors or subject to change because of a change in treatment, physical condition, or emotional/psychological status.

Once a referral is made, a typical neuropsychological consultation begins with a full diagnostic interview, which gathers information on the chief cognitive difficulties, cancer, medical, neurological, psychiatric, psychosocial, substance use, and educational/vocational history, all of which will help to contextualize the results of the neuropsychological assessment. If a neuropsychological assessment is considered appropriate, formal testing is recommended, which will vary in terms of time and measures administered depending on patient characteristics and referral question; time for an assessment may range from as little as 30 minutes to an hour, to several hours. Older patients, patients with significant fatigue, or patients with significant pain who cannot tolerate a full evaluation may be given briefer screening measures or stand-alone batteries.

A flexible approach to test selection will allow tailoring of the assessment to the specific referral question; while most practitioners will employ a somewhat standard, "core" battery of measures, additional measures may be administered for specific issues or difficulties (multitasking, attention/concentration issues over longer periods of time). Neuropsychological and psychological measures are generally in a paper and pencil as well as interview and computer administered formats, and should have acceptable validity and reliability. Most assessments will attempt to sample cognitive ability in multiple domains, including attention and concentration, psychomotor speed, verbal functioning, visuospatial reasoning, praxis and construction, verbal and visual learning and recall, and executive functioning (abstraction, reasoning, cognitive flexibility, problem solving, planning and organization) (see Table 36.1 for a list of typical measures used in our Neuropsychological Evaluation Service). Depending on the patient's presentation, stand-alone measures of personality, emotional, and psychological functioning may also be administered either by course or when there is suspicion that a significant psychiatric issue may be affecting cognition.

Once testing is complete, patient performance on individual measures is compared with normative groups defined by age, or, increasingly, age, education, gender, and ethnicity to ensure the most exact matching of patients to their respective cohorts. In contrast to a "deficit testing" model of assessment, in which performance is categorized as either normal or aberrant, comparison of patients' performance with that of normative groups, and

TABLE 36.1 LIST OF COMMONLY USED NEUROPSYCHOLOGICAL MEASURES IN ASSESSMENT OF POSTTREATMENT COGNITIVE DYSFUNCTION

Measure	Function
Premorbid intelligence	
Wide Range Achievement Test 5th Edition-Reading subtest (WRAT5)	A measure estimating premorbid cognitive abilities, highly correlated with general intellectual abilities
Verbal ability	
FAS-Controlled Oral Word Association Test	A timed measure of phonemic fluency
Animal Naming Test	A timed measure of semantic fluency
Boston Naming Test	A measure of confrontation naming (word finding)
Learning and memory	
California Verbal Learning Test II (CVLT-III)	A measure of verbal list learning and recall
Logical Memory I and II (WMS-IV)	A measure of verbal story learning and recall
Rey-Osterreith Complex Figure	A measure of visual figure learning and memory
Attention	
Digit Span (WAIS-IV)	A measure of brief span of attention
Arithmetic (WAIS-IV)	A measure of brief span of attention and working memory
Connors Continuous Performance Test 3rd Edition (CPT3)	A measure of sustained attention
Processing speed	
The Trail Making Test (Part A)	A measure of visual scanning and graphomotor speed
The Trail Making Test (Part B)	A measure of visual scanning, graphomotor speed and set-shifting
Digit Symbol—Coding (WAIS-IV)	A speeded graphomotor measure
Symbol Search (WAIS-IV)	A speeded measure of visual scanning and attention
Visual reasoning/construction	
Rey-Osterreith Complex Figure	A measure of visual construction
Judgment of Line Orientation	A measure of visuospatial judgment and reasoning
Block Design (WAIS-IV)	A timed measure of visual construction and reasoning
Executive functioning	
Wisconsin Card Sorting Task (WCST)	A measure of abstract reasoning and problem solving
Stroop	A measure of speeded word reading, color naming, and inhibition
Psychological/emotional	
Personality Assessment Inventory (PAI)	A self-report measure of psychological functioning
Beck Depression Inventory Fast Screen for Medical Patients (BDI-Fast Screen)	A self-report measure of affective depressive symptomatology
Generalized Anxiety Disorder-7 (GAD-7)	A self-report measure of affective anxiety symptomatology

with their own premorbid functioning, allows for finer gradations of interpretation; test results can indicate how well, or how poorly, an individual patient performs on a given task and also allows for detection not only of absolute deficits but also of deficits that are relative to the patient's normative cohort or to the patient's own premorbid functioning.

Results are then integrated and contextualized with the patient's report of difficulty as well as with the patient's medical and other history. Differential diagnosis is a particularly important aspect of neuropsychological assessment in cancer survivors. Because the incidence of a subset of cancers increases with age, referrals for neuropsychological assessment in a cancer center typically skew to older patients. Since older patients may present with several possible etiologies or, at the very least, contributors to cognitive dysfunction, a detailed assessment and analysis of the pattern of strengths and weaknesses is especially necessary. While some etiologies or syndromes may express a typical pattern of neuropsychological performance, few exhibit pathognomonic signs, and it is more likely that a combination of a given pattern of performance together with an association of history of treatment and onset of difficulties will guide interpretation. Once the pattern of neuropsychological performance is analyzed and interpreted, recommendations for further treatment, evaluations, and rehabilitation can be made. These can include referrals for neurological evaluation and neuroimaging studies, psychiatric evaluation, and cognitive rehabilitation.

TREATMENT OPTIONS

Treatment options following cancer therapy will depend on the nature of the cognitive impairment, the presence of additional potential etiologies, and patient preference. The two discussed here are cognitive rehabilitation and pharmacologic intervention. Follow-up treatment by psychiatry, neurology, and physical therapy are also potential directions in the event that the patient has a significant psychological or emotional component, there is suspicion of a primary neurological disorder that better explains results of neuropsychological testing, or there is a significant impact of physical limitations.

Cognitive Rehabilitation

In traditional rehabilitation settings, cognitive rehabilitation has been employed to assist individuals in learning, or in most cases relearning, ways to concentrate, remember, and solve problems after an illness or injury affecting the brain. Cognitive rehabilitation involves a structured set of therapeutic activities designed to retrain an individual's ability to think, use judgment, and make decisions. The focus is on improving deficits in memory, attention, perception, learning, planning, and judgment through both restoration and compensatory strategies (74). The desired outcome of cognitive rehabilitation is an improved quality of life or an improved ability to function in home and community life. Cognitive rehabilitation has been generally characterized as either restorative, which focuses on retraining basic cognitive skills, or compensatory, which focuses on developing skills and strategies that work around the presenting cognitive issue. Often, interventions may consist of a mixture of both strategies in treating cognitive symptoms.

Research on the efficacy of cognitive rehabilitation has been mixed in other neurological disorders (minimal cognitive impairment, traumatic brain injury), as well as in posttreatment issues. Ferguson and colleagues (75) conducted a single-arm pilot study utilizing a cognitive behavioral treatment approach to aid breast cancer survivors in managing deficits with attention and memory following treatment with adjuvant chemotherapy. In brief, 29 adult women who received adjuvant chemotherapy for stage I or II breast cancer underwent Memory and Attention Adaptation Training (MAAT) at least 3 years posttreatment (mean years postchemotherapy was 8.20, SD = 4.40). Inclusion criteria included complaint of memory and attention problems postchemotherapy but not a deficit on neuropsychological testing. The program consisted of seven contact sessions: four individual, in-person monthly sessions and three phone contacts. Participants were given a workbook that reviewed knowledge of chemotherapy-associated memory deficits, introduced self-awareness training, gave instruction on self-regulation including relaxation training and activity scheduling, and supplied compensatory strategies and tailored recommendations. Participants demonstrated significant improvements in verbal memory and executive functions and reported improvement in overall cognitive functioning and quality of life. While MAAT demonstrated efficacy, there was no control group and treatment was participant specific, thus limiting generalization. Given these limitations, Ferguson and colleagues (76) conducted a randomized clinical trial to further evaluate the efficacy of MAAT. Forty adult women who received adjuvant chemotherapy for stage I or II breast cancer were enrolled in the study; 19 were randomized to the treatment condition (MAAT) and 21 were randomized to the waitlist control condition. Inclusion criteria were a memory or attention complaint, but an actual cognitive deficit was not a prerequisite. Participants in the treatment condition underwent MAAT training as described above. Results indicated that MAAT participants demonstrated a significant improvement in verbal memory and spiritual well-being compared with controls. This randomized clinical trial did not replicate the previous finding of improved executive functioning or improvement in self-reported cognitive functioning or quality of life.

In a randomized controlled trial comparing the effects of memory training and speed of processing training on cognitive function in 82 breast cancer survivors, it was found that memory training improved performance on neuropsychological tests of memory at 2-month follow-up posttraining, while speed of processing training increased scores on objective tests of processing speed immediately follow training and at a 2-month follow-up. This suggests both types of training were effective in improving targeted cognitive domains, but speed of processing training resulted in both immediate and lasting changes in performance (77). A pilot study testing the effects of a 12-week compensatory cognitive training intervention in 54 breast cancer patients receiving chemotherapy also found improvement in performance on standard neuropsychological tests of immediate memory, delayed memory, and verbal fluency in the intervention group as compared to waitlisted controls (77). In addition to at-home and clinic-based interventions, there is some evidence that web-based cognitive training may also be effective in improving cognitive function in cancer survivors. One recent pilot study tested the effects of a 4-week online cognitive training program on survivors of non-CNS cancers and found that the intervention improved attention and executive function for both the cancer and noncancer intervention groups as compared to a noncancer waitlisted control group (78). As a follow-up to the in-person MAAT training described above, a randomized controlled trial to determine the efficacy of videoconference-delivered MAAT to improve cognitive function in 35 breast cancer survivors was conducted, and results found that participants assigned to the MAAT condition ($n = 22$) had significant improvements in processing speed compared to supportive therapy controls. Taken together, these results suggest that the use of web-based and videoconference-delivered therapies may serve as an effective means by which to improve cognitive function in cancer survivors, while limiting the need for clinic visits and thereby, participant and clinician burden.

In contrast to the positive findings of cognitive interventions in this population, Poppelreuter and colleagues (79) failed to find a specific cognitive intervention effect in their study. They investigated two forms of cognitive rehabilitation training: a Neuropsychological Training Group (NTG), which consisted of functional training groups in which participants practiced compensatory strategies and techniques to improve attention and memory as they relate to everyday activities, and an individualized, computer-based training software package (PC) under direct supervision also targeted at improving attention and memory. These intervention groups were compared with a control group of participants that received no training. Participants had received high-dose chemotherapy and hematopoietic stem cell transplantation for systemic cancer; median time since therapy conclusion was 3 months. At the time of the study, they were undergoing inpatient rehabilitation following their

oncological therapy, which is standard care for individuals in Germany. Participants had to have demonstrated a cognitive deficit in order to be in the study. Subtests from the Test Battery for Attentional Performance were used, and participants had to score in the lowest quartile of the normative sample in at least two of the five parameters (61.1% of participants screened had a cognitive deficit). Eligible participants were randomly assigned to either one of the two treatment groups (NTG: $n = 21$; PC: $n = 26$) or a control group ($n = 28$). Training was implemented four times per week for 1 hour a day over the course of their inpatient stay. They found significant improvements across all cognitive domains among the three study groups concluding no specific intervention effect. This study was replicated in stage I or II breast cancer patients. Participants had to have demonstrated a cognitive deficit in order to be in the study. Subtests from the Test Battery for Attentional Performance were used, and participants had to score in the lowest quartile of the normative sample in at least two of the five parameters (47.1% of participants screened had a cognitive deficit). They found similar results as with the hematopoietic stem cell transplantation study in that there were no specific intervention effects (80).

Emerging research suggests that noninvasive brain stimulation, which has been shown to improve cognitive deficits and other populations (81), also improves attention performance in cancer survivors, with one recent pilot study showing that transcranial direct current stimulation (tDCS) improved breast cancer survivors' sustained attention performance on a continuous performance test (81). These promising findings suggest a utility for tDCS to enhance the effects of cognitive training to improve functioning cancer survivors, but further research is needed to determine whether stimulation can produce long-lasting changes in brain structure and function to resultant fall and lasting remediation of cancer-related cognitive dysfunction.

As can be seen from the above studies, current research on the efficacy of cognitive rehabilitation for posttreatment cognitive difficulties is mixed, and this may reflect research findings on cognitive rehabilitation more generally. One complicating issue is whether restorative or compensatory therapy is prescribed and the manner in which postrehabilitation abilities are measured. A restorative model would predict that objective performance should improve since training is focused on the underlying ability and this should generalize to other tasks in which that ability is a prerequisite. In contrast, compensatory rehabilitation, with its focus on developing strategies and managing the environment in which cognitive tasks are performed, would likely not lead to changes in objective measures since at least a subset of alternate strategies most likely cannot be used (e.g., patients could not keep a list of memory items). At this point, given the paucity of literature in this area, more research needs to be conducted to measure the efficacy of various treatment approaches.

Pharmacologic Interventions

Pharmacologic interventions have generally taken the form of stimulant treatment with more recent research in the efficacy of modafinil. Dexmethylphenidate (Focalin) has been approved for the treatment of attentional symptoms in attention deficit disorder through its action as a psychostimulant. To test for more generalized effects of dexmethylphenidate on attention in other etiologies, its effect on cognition and fatigue was studied in women undergoing adjuvant chemotherapy (82). During chemotherapy for breast cancer, women were randomized to D-methylphenidate ($n = 29$) or placebo ($n = 28$) to see if it improved cognitive functioning, QOL, or fatigue. In the D-MPH group, the percentage of patients classified as having moderate to severe cognitive dysfunction by the High Sensitivity Cognitive Screen, a test of six major neuropsychological domains, decreased from 3.6% at baseline to 0% at the end of chemotherapy. Rate of impairment was stable at 11% in the placebo group. However, a correction factor applied for practice effects at the follow-up assessments led to 11% with moderate to severe impairment in the D-MPH group and 22% in the placebo group with no statistically significant difference in cognitive outcomes between groups. In a randomized placebo-controlled trial of D-methylphenidate as a treatment for cognitive dysfunction and fatigue in 250 nonanemic breast and ovarian cancer patients, patients (76% breast cancer and 13.6% ovarian cancer) were randomized to placebo ($n = 75$) or D-methylphenidate ($n = 77$). Significant improvement in memory and fatigue was observed in the D-methylphenidate group (83). Similarly, Escalante et al. (2014) conducted a double-blind randomized controlled crossover trial to test the effects of 4 weeks of methylphenidate on cognitive performance in 33 breast cancer patients, and found that methylphenidate treatment significantly improved verbal learning, memory, and processing speed relative to placebo. Patients were able to work significantly more hours following treatment with 58% of patients wanting to continue treatment following the 4-week intervention (84).

Modafinil (Provigil) has been approved for the treatment of narcolepsy and shift-work disorder and, as such, has been considered in the treatment of attentional and fatigue symptoms in several other disorders. Kohli and colleagues (85) examined the effects of modafinil on cognitive functioning in patients with breast cancer. Sixty-eight participants with breast cancer who had completed treatment with chemotherapy and/or radiation more than 1 month prior to commencement of the study completed both the open-label phase of the study (phase 1) and the randomization phase to continue treatment with modafinil or placebo (phase 2). Results indicated that 200 mg/d of modafinil during phase 1 significantly increased participants' ability to store, retain, and retrieve verbal and nonverbal information and that they were more accurate in doing so. These results were also found at the end of phase 2 for individuals receiving continued treatment with modafinil. Further, increased attention was also found at the end of phase 2 for individuals receiving modafinil. Lundorff and colleagues (86) also examined the effects of modafinil on cancer-related cognitive dysfunction. They conducted a double-blind, randomized, crossover, single-dose trial of modafinil in an advanced cancer patient population. Twenty-eight patients with advanced cancer (breast, genitourinary, gastrointestinal, head/neck, hematologic, lung, other) were randomly assigned to receive a single dose of 200 mg modafinil or placebo on day 1 and were crossed over to the alternative treatment on day 4. Attention and psychomotor speed were assessed with the Finger Tapping Test (FTT) and Trail Making Test B (TMT-B), which were administered before tablet intake on each day and again 4.5 hours after tablet intake. Statistically significant improvements were found in both FTT with the dominant hand and TMT-B after treatment with modafinil compared with placebo. Taken together, these studies demonstrate that modafinil is effective in improving cancer-related cognitive dysfunction.

CONCLUSIONS

Since the early studies documenting patients' report of cognitive difficulties putatively associated with treatment, significant progress has been made in better defining these issues objectively and understanding potential mechanisms. We have discussed the nature of subjective reports and objective cognitive performance posttreatment, as well as potential reasons for their disagreement. Changes in cortical thickness and subcortical volumes from pre- to posttreatment were also discussed together with their association with changes in brain function following treatment. Potential risk factors and mediators of cognitive dysfunction were identified that may explain individual outcome differences posttreatment. The role of neuropsychological assessment was discussed in clarifying cognitive dysfunction posttreatment, together with identification of specific cognitive issues that may be a focus of treatment through rehabilitation or pharmacologic intervention. Some qualifications and caveats are suggested given what we now know in regard to cancer therapies and cognitive issues. Cognitive decline is most likely associated with broader treatment variables and chemotherapy treatment alone does not fully explain cognitive dysfunction. Cognitive changes following treatment are far from uniform; subsets of individuals, as a result of age, premorbid cognitive reserve, brain reserve, or genetic variants, may be more likely or more severely affected by treatment. Cognitive differences are also exhibited in cancer-diagnosed individuals pretreatment, underscoring the necessity of longitudinal studies; this observation also suggests that cancer diagnosis and pretreatment cognitive differences may be related by an as yet undetermined factor. The exact mechanism of treatment variables' effect on brain structure and function is not clear; research studying oxidative stress, DNA repair mechanisms, and cytokine deregulation in response to treatment is ongoing.

REFERENCES

1. Cull A, Stewart M, Altman DG. Assessment of and intervention for psychosocial problems in routine oncology practice. *Br J Cancer.* 1995;72(1):229-235. doi: 10.1038/bjc.1995.308.
2. Cull A, Hay C, Love SB, Mackie M, Smets E, Stewart M. What do cancer patients mean when they complain of concentration and memory problems? *Br J Cancer.* 1996;74(10):1674-1679.
3. Schagen SB, van Dam FS, Muller MJ, Boogerd W, Lindeboom J, Bruning PF. Cognitive deficits after postoperative adjuvant chemotherapy for breast carcinoma. *Cancer.* 1999;85(3):640-650. doi: 10.1002/(SICI)1097-0142(19990201)85:3<640::AID-CNCR14>3.0.CO;2-G [pii].
4. Ahles TA, Saykin AJ, Furstenberg CT, et al. Neuropsychologic impact of standard-dose systemic chemotherapy in long-term survivors of breast cancer and lymphoma. *J Clin Oncol.* 2002;20(2):485-493.
5. Castellon SA, Ganz PA, Bower JE, Petersen L, Abraham L, Greendale GA. Neurocognitive performance in breast cancer survivors exposed to adjuvant chemotherapy and tamoxifen. *J Clin Exp Neuropsychol.* 2004;26(7):955-969.
6. Downie FP, Mar Fan HG, Houede-Tchen N, Yi Q, Tannock IF. Cognitive function, fatigue, and menopausal symptoms in breast cancer patients receiving adjuvant chemotherapy: evaluation with patient interview after formal assessment. *Psychooncology.* 2006;15(10):921-930. doi: 10.1002/pon.1035.
7. Hermelink K, Untch M, Lux MP, et al. Cognitive function during neoadjuvant chemotherapy for breast cancer: results of a prospective, multicenter, longitudinal study. *Cancer.* 2007;109(9):1905-1913. doi: 10.1002/cncr.22610.
8. Jansen CE, Dodd MJ, Miaskowski CA, Dowling GA, Kramer J. Preliminary results of a longitudinal study of changes in cognitive function in breast cancer patients undergoing chemotherapy with doxorubicin and cyclophosphamide. *Psychooncology.* 2008;17(12):1189-1195. doi: 10.1002/pon.1342.
9. Mehnert A, Scherwath A, Schirmer L, et al. The association between neuropsychological impairment, self-perceived cognitive deficits, fatigue and health related quality of life in breast cancer survivors following standard adjuvant versus high-dose chemotherapy. *Patient Educ Couns.* 2007;66(1):108-118. doi: 10.1016/j.pec.2006.11.005.
10. Poppelreuter M, Weis J, Kulz AK, Tucha O, Lange KW, Bartsch HH. Cognitive dysfunction and subjective complaints of cancer patients. A cross-sectional study in a cancer rehabilitation centre. *Eur J Cancer.* 2004;40(1):43-49.
11. Schagen SB, Boogerd W, Muller MJ, et al. Cognitive complaints and cognitive impairment following BEP chemotherapy in patients with testicular cancer. *Acta Oncol.* 2008;47(1):63-70. doi: 10.1080/02841860701518058.
12. Shilling V, Jenkins V. Self-reported cognitive problems in women receiving adjuvant therapy for breast cancer. *Eur J Oncol Nurs.* 2007;11(1):6-15. doi: 10.1016/j.ejon.2006.02.005.
13. Van Dam FS, Schagen SB, Muller MJ, et al. Impairment of cognitive function in women receiving adjuvant treatment for high-risk breast cancer: high-dose versus standard-dose chemotherapy. *J Natl Cancer Inst.* 1998;90(3):210-218.
14. Falleti MG, Sanfilippo A, Maruff P, Weih L, Phillips KA. The nature and severity of cognitive impairment associated with adjuvant chemotherapy in women with breast cancer: a meta-analysis of the current literature. *Brain Cogn.* 2005;59(1):60-70.
15. Berglund G, Bolund C, Fornander T, Rutqvist LE, Sjoden PO. Late effects of adjuvant chemotherapy and postoperative radiotherapy on quality of life among breast cancer patients. *Eur J Cancer.* 1991;27(9):1075-1081.
16. Phillips KA, Bernhard J. Adjuvant breast cancer treatment and cognitive function: current knowledge and research directions. *J Natl Cancer Inst.* 2003;95(3):190-197.
17. Ahles TA, Saykin AJ, McDonald BC, et al. Cognitive function in breast cancer patients prior to adjuvant treatment. *Breast Cancer Res Treat.* 2008;110(1):143-152.
18. Wefel JS, Lenzi R, Theriault R, Buzdar AU, Cruickshank S, Meyers CA. "Chemobrain" in breast carcinoma?: a prologue. *Cancer.* 2004;101(3):466-475. doi: 10.1002/cncr.20393.
19. Jenkins V, Shilling V, Deutsch G, et al. A 3-year prospective study of the effects of adjuvant treatments on cognition in women with early stage breast cancer. *Br J Cancer.* 2006;94(6):828-834. doi: 10.1038/sj.bjc.6603029.
20. Schagen SB, Muller MJ, Boogerd W, Mellenbergh GJ, van Dam FS. Change in cognitive function after chemotherapy: a prospective longitudinal study in breast cancer patients. *J Natl Cancer Inst.* 2006;98(23):1742-1745. doi: 10.1093/jnci/djj470. 98/23/1742 [pii].
21. Wefel JS, Lenzi R, Theriault RL, Davis RN, Meyers CA. The cognitive sequelae of standard-dose adjuvant chemotherapy in women with breast carcinoma: results of a prospective, randomized, longitudinal trial. *Cancer.* 2004;100(11):2292-2299. doi: 10.1002/cncr.20272.
22. Quesnel C, Savard J, Ivers H. Cognitive impairments associated with breast cancer treatments: results from a longitudinal study. *Breast Cancer Res Treat.* 2009;116(1):113-123. doi: 10.1007/s10549-008-0114-2.
23. Schilder CM, Seynaeve C, Beex LV, et al. Effects of tamoxifen and exemestane on cognitive functioning of postmenopausal patients with breast cancer: results from the neuropsychological side study of the tamoxifen and exemestane adjuvant multinational trial. *J Clin Oncol.* 2010;28(8):1294-1300. doi: 10.1200/JCO.2008.21.3553.

24. Hurria A, Somlo G, Ahles T. Renaming "chemo-brain." *Cancer Invest* 2007;25(6):373-377. doi: 10.1080/07357900701506672.

25. Pullens MJ, De Vries J, Roukema JA. Subjective cognitive dysfunction in breast cancer patients: a systematic review. *Psychooncology*. 2010;19(11):1127-1138. doi: 10.1002/pon.1673.

26. Weis J, Poppelreuter M, Bartsch HH. Cognitive deficits as long-term side-effects of adjuvant therapy in breast cancer patients: "subjective" complaints and "objective" neuropsychological test results. *Psychooncology*. 2009;18(7):775-782. doi: 10.1002/pon.1472.

27. Tannock IF, Ahles TA, Ganz PA, Van Dam FS. Cognitive impairment associated with chemotherapy for cancer: report of a workshop. *J Clin Oncol*. 2004;22(11):2233-2239. doi: 10.1200/JCO.2004.08.094.

28. Schagen SB, Das E, van Dam FS. The influence of priming and pre-existing knowledge of chemotherapy-associated cognitive complaints on the reporting of such complaints in breast cancer patients. *Psychooncology*. 2009;18(6):674-678. doi: 10.1002/pon.1454.

29. Li Y, Root JC, Atkinson TM, Ahles TA. Examining the association between patient-reported symptoms of attention and memory dysfunction with objective cognitive performance: a latent regression rasch model approach. *Arch Clin Neuropsychol*. 2016;31(4):365-377. doi: 10.1093/arclin/acw017.

30. Root JC, Ryan E, Barnett G, Andreotti C, Bolutayo K, Ahles T. Learning and memory performance in a cohort of clinically referred breast cancer survivors: the role of attention versus forgetting in patient-reported memory complaints: Memory performance in breast cancer survivors. *Psychooncology*. 2015;24(5):548-555. doi: 10.1002/pon.3615.

31. Root JC, Andreotti C, Tsu L, Ellmore TM, Ahles TA. Learning and memory performance in breast cancer survivors 2 to 6 years post-treatment: the role of encoding versus forgetting. *J Cancer Surviv*. 2016;10(3):593-599. doi: 10.1007/s11764-015-0505-4.

32. Sole-Padulles C, Bartres-Faz D, Junque C, et al. Brain structure and function related to cognitive reserve variables in normal aging, mild cognitive impairment and Alzheimer's disease. *Neurobiol Aging*. 2009;30(7):1114-1124.

33. Mortimer JA, Borenstein AR, Gosche KM, Snowdon DA. Very early detection of Alzheimer neuropathology and the role of brain reserve in modifying its clinical expression. *J Geriatr Psychiatry Neurol*. 2005;18(4):218-223.

34. Stern Y. What is cognitive reserve? Theory and research application of the reserve concept. *J Int Neuropsychol Soc*. 2002;8(3):448-460.

35. Bartres-Faz D, Arenaza-Urquijo EM. Structural and functional imaging correlates of cognitive and brain reserve hypotheses in healthy and pathological aging. *Brain Topogr*. 2011;24(3-4):340-357. doi: 10.1007/s10548-011-0195-9.

36. Bleecker ML, Ford DP, Celio MA, Vaughan CG, Lindgren KN. Impact of cognitive reserve on the relationship of lead exposure and neurobehavioral performance. *Neurology*. 2007;69(5):470-476. doi: 10.1212/01.wnl.0000266628.43760.8c.

37. Ahles TA, Saykin AJ, McDonald BC, et al. Longitudinal assessment of cognitive changes associated with adjuvant treatment for breast cancer: impact of age and cognitive reserve. *J Clin Oncol*. 2010;28(29):4434-4440. doi: 10.1200/JCO.2009.27.0827.

38. Bookheimer S, Burggren A. APOE-4 genotype and neurophysiological vulnerability to Alzheimer's and cognitive aging. *Annu Rev Clin Psychol*. 2009;5:343-362. doi: 10.1146/annurev.clinpsy.032408.153625.

39. Ahles TA, Saykin AJ, Noll WW, et al. The relationship of APOE genotype to neuropsychological performance in long-term cancer survivors treated with standard dose chemotherapy. *Psychooncology*. 2003;12(6):612-619. doi: 10.1002/pon.742.

40. Mandelblatt JS, Small BJ, Luta G, et al. Cancer-related cognitive outcomes among older breast cancer survivors in the thinking and living with cancer study. *J Clin Oncol*. 2018;36(32):3211-3222. doi: 10.1200/JCO.18.00140.

41. Small BJ, Rawson KS, Walsh E, et al. Catechol-O-methyltransferase genotype modulates cancer treatment-related cognitive deficits in breast cancer survivors. *Cancer*. 2011;117(7):1369-1376. doi: 10.1002/cncr.25685.

42. Inagaki M, Yoshikawa E, Matsuoka Y, et al. Smaller regional volumes of brain gray and white matter demonstrated in breast cancer survivors exposed to adjuvant chemotherapy. *Cancer*. 2007;109(1):146-156.

43. Deprez S, Amant F, Yigit R, et al. Chemotherapy-induced structural changes in cerebral white matter and its correlation with impaired cognitive functioning in breast cancer patients. *Hum Brain Mapp*. 2010;32(3):480-493. doi: 10.1002/hbm.21033.

44. Menning S, de Ruiter MB, Veltman DJ, et al. Multi-modal MRI and cognitive function in patients with breast cancer prior to adjuvant treatment—the role of fatigue. *Neuroimage Clin*. 2015;7:547-554. doi: 10.1016/j.nicl.2015.02.005.

45. McDonald BC, Conroy SK, Ahles TA, West JD, Saykin AJ. Gray matter reduction associated with systemic chemotherapy for breast cancer: a prospective MRI study. *Breast Cancer Res Treat*. 2010;123(3):819-828.

46. Yamada TH, Denburg NL, Beglinger LJ, Schultz SK. Neuropsychological outcomes of older breast cancer survivors: cognitive features ten or more years after chemotherapy. *J Neuropsychiatry Clin Neurosci*. 2010;22(1):48-54.

47. Kesler SR, Bennett FC, Mahaffey ML, Spiegel D. Regional brain activation during verbal declarative memory in metastatic breast cancer. *Clin Cancer Res*. 2009;15(21):6665-6673. doi: 10.1158/1078-0432.CCR-09-1227.

48. Pergolizzi D, Root JC, Pan H, et al. Episodic memory for visual scenes suggests compensatory brain activity in breast cancer patients: a prospective longitudinal fMRI study. *Brain Imaging Behav*. 2019;13(6):1674-1688. doi: 10.1007/s11682-019-00038-2.

49. Silverman DH, Dy CJ, Castellon SA, et al. Altered frontocortical, cerebellar, and basal ganglia activity in adjuvant-treated breast cancer survivors 5-10 years after chemotherapy. *Breast Cancer Res Treat*. 2007;103(3):303-311. doi: 10.1007/s10549-006-9380-z.

50. de Ruiter MB, Reneman L, Boogerd W, et al. Cerebral hyporesponsiveness and cognitive impairment 10 years after chemotherapy for breast cancer. *Hum Brain Mapp*. 2011;32(8):1206-1219. doi: 10.1002/hbm.21102.

51. Cimprich B, Reuter-Lorenz P, Nelson J, et al. Prechemotherapy alterations in brain function in women with breast cancer. *J Clin Exp Neuropsychol*. 2010;32(3):324-331. doi: 10.1080/13803390903032537.

52. Ahles TA, Saykin AJ. Candidate mechanisms for chemotherapy-induced cognitive changes. *Nat Rev Cancer*. 2007;7(3):192-201.

53. Ginos JZ, Cooper AJ, Dhawan V, et al. [13N]cisplatin PET to assess pharmacokinetics of intra-arterial versus intravenous chemotherapy for malignant brain tumors. *J Nucl Med*. 1987;28(12):1844-1852.

54. Mitsuki S, Diksic M, Conway T, Yamamoto YL, Villemure JG, Feindel W. Pharmacokinetics of 11C-labelled BCNU and SarCNU in gliomas studied by PET. *J Neurooncol*. 1991;10(1):47-55.

55. Gangloff A, Hsueh WA, Kesner AL, et al. Estimation of paclitaxel biodistribution and uptake in human-derived xenografts in vivo with (18)F-fluoropaclitaxel. *J Nucl Med.* 2005;46(11):1866-1871.

56. Dietrich J, Han R, Yang Y, Mayer-Proschel M, Noble M. CNS progenitor cells and oligodendrocytes are targets of chemotherapeutic agents in vitro and in vivo. *J Biol.* 2006;5(7):22. doi: 10.1186/jbiol50.

57. Seigers R, Fardell JE. Neurobiological basis of chemo-therapy-induced cognitive impairment: a review of rodent research. *Neurosci Biobehav Rev.* 2011;35(3):729-741. doi: 10.1016/j.neubiorev.2010.09.006.

58. Muramatsu T, Johnson DR, Finch RA, et al. Age-related differences in vincristine toxicity and biodistribution in wild-type and transporter-deficient mice. *Oncol Res.* 2004;14(7-8):331-343.

59. Mariani E, Polidori MC, Cherubini A, Mecocci P. Oxidative stress in brain aging, neurodegenerative and vascular diseases: an overview. *J Chromatogr B Anal Technol Biomed Life Sci.* 2005;827(1):65-75. doi: 10.1016/j.jchromb.2005.04.023.

60. Caldecott KW. DNA single-strand breaks and neurode-generation. *DNA Repair (Amst).* 2004;3(8-9):875-882. doi: 10.1016/j.dnarep.2004.04.011.

61. Harrison JF, Hollensworth SB, Spitz DR, Copeland WC, Wilson GL, LeDoux SP. Oxidative stress-induced apop-tosis in neurons correlates with mitochondrial DNA base excision repair pathway imbalance. *Nucleic Acids Res.* 2005;33(14):4660-4671. doi: 10.1093/nar/gki759.

62. Schroder CP, Wisman GB, de Jong S, et al. Telomere length in breast cancer patients before and after chemotherapy with or without stem cell transplantation. *Br J Cancer.* 2001;84(10):1348-1353. doi: 10.1054/bjoc.2001.1803.

63. Lahav M, Uziel O, Kestenbaum M, et al. Nonmyeloabla-tive conditioning does not prevent telomere shortening after allogeneic stem cell transplantation. *Transplanta-tion.* 2005;80(7):969-976.

64. Maccormick RE. Possible acceleration of aging by adjuvant chemotherapy: a cause of early onset frailty? *Med Hypotheses.* 2006;67(2):212-215. doi: 10.1016/j.mehy.2006.01.045.

65. Trask PC, Esper P, Riba M, Redman B. Psychiat-ric side effects of interferon therapy: prevalence, pro-posed mechanisms, and future directions. *J Clin Oncol.* 2000;18(11):2316-2326.

66. Penson RT, Kronish K, Duan Z, et al. Cytokines IL-1beta, IL-2, IL-6, IL-8, MCP-1, GM-CSF and TNFalpha in patients with epithelial ovarian cancer and their rela-tionship to treatment with paclitaxel. *Int J Gynecol Can-cer.* 2000;10(1):33-41.

67. Tsavaris N, Kosmas C, Vadiaka M, Kanelopoulos P, Boulamatsis D. Immune changes in patients with advanced breast cancer undergoing chemotherapy with taxanes. *Br J Cancer.* 2002;87(1):21-27. doi: 10.1038/sj.bjc.6600347.

68. Pusztai L, Mendoza TR, Reuben JM, et al. Changes in plasma levels of inflammatory cytokines in response to paclitaxel chemotherapy. *Cytokine.* 2004;25(3):94-102.

69. Bower JE, Ganz PA, Aziz N, Fahey JL. Fatigue and proinflammatory cytokine activity in breast cancer sur-vivors. *Psychosom Med.* 2002;64(4):604-611.

70. Collado-Hidalgo A, Bower JE, Ganz PA, Cole SW, Irwin MR. Inflammatory biomarkers for persistent fatigue in breast cancer survivors. *Clin Cancer Res.* 2006;12(9):2759-2766. doi: 10.1158/1078-0432.CCR-05-2398.

71. Bagnall-Moreau C, Chaudhry S, Salas-Ramirez K, Ahles T, Hubbard K. Chemotherapy-induced cognitive impair-ment is associated with increased inflammation and oxidative damage in the hippocampus. *Mol Neurobiol.* 2019;56(10):7159-7172. doi: 10.1007/s12035-019-1589-z.

72. Salas-Ramirez KY, Bagnall C, Frias L, Abdali SA, Ahles TA, Hubbard K. Doxorubicin and cyclophospha-mide induce cognitive dysfunction and activate the ERK and AKT signaling pathways. *Behav Brain Res.* 2015;292:133-141. doi: 10.1016/j.bbr.2015.06.028.

73. Shi D-D, Huang Y-H, Lai CSW, et al. Chemotherapy-induced cognitive impairment is associated with cyto-kine dysregulation and disruptions in neuroplasticity. *Mol Neurobiol.* 2019;56(3):2234-2243. doi: 10.1007/s12035-018-1224-4.

74. Lustig C, Shah P, Seidler R, Reuter-Lorenz PA. Aging, training, and the brain: a review and future directions. *Neuropsychol Rev.* 2009;19(4):504-522. doi: 10.1007/s11065-009-9119-9.

75. Ferguson RJ, Ahles TA, Saykin AJ, et al. Cognitive-behavioral management of chemotherapy-related cog-nitive change. *Psychooncology.* 2007;16(8):772-777. doi: 10.1002/pon.1133.

76. Ferguson RJ, McDonald BC, Rocque MA, et al. Devel-opment of CBT for chemotherapy-related cognitive change: results of a waitlist control trial. *Psychooncol-ogy.* 2012;21(2):176-186. doi: 10.1002/pon.1878.

77. Park J-H, Jung YS, Kim KS, Bae SH. Effects of compen-satory cognitive training intervention for breast cancer patients undergoing chemotherapy: a pilot study. *Sup-port Care Cancer.* 2017;25(6):1887-1896. doi: 10.1007/s00520-017-3589-8.

78. Mihuta ME, Green HJ, Shum DHK. Efficacy of a web-based cognitive rehabilitation intervention for adult cancer survivors: a pilot study. *Eur J Cancer Care.* 2018;27(2):e12805. doi: 10.1111/ecc.12805.

79. Poppelreuter M, Weis J, Mumm A, Orth HB, Bartsch HH. Rehabilitation of therapy-related cognitive defi-cits in patients after hematopoietic stem cell transplan-tation. *Bone Marrow Transpl.* 2008;41(1):79-90. doi: 10.1038/sj.bmt.1705884.

80. Poppelreuter M, Weis J, Bartsch HH. Effects of specific neuropsychological training programs for breast cancer patients after adjuvant chemotherapy. *J Psychosoc Oncol.* 2009;27(2):274-296. doi: 10.1080/07347330902776044.

81. Gaynor AM, Pergolizzi D, Alici Y, et al. Impact of transcranial direct current stimulation on sustained attention in breast cancer survivors: evidence for fea-sibility, tolerability, and initial efficacy. *Brain Stimul.* 2020;13(4):1108-1116. doi: 10.1016/j.brs.2020.04.013.

82. Mar Fan HG, Clemons M, Xu W, et al. A randomised, placebo-controlled, double-blind trial of the effects of d-methylphenidate on fatigue and cognitive dysfunc-tion in women undergoing adjuvant chemotherapy for breast cancer. *Support Care Cancer.* 2008;16(6):577-583. doi: 10.1007/s00520-007-0341-9.

83. Lower E, Fleishman S, Cooper A, Zeldis J, Faleck H, Manning D. A phase III, randomized placebo-con-trolled trial of the safety and efficacy of d-MPH as new treatment of fatigue and "chemobrain" in adult cancer patients. *J Clin Oncol.* 2005;23(16_suppl):8000. doi: 10.1200/jco.2005.23.16_suppl.8000.

84. Escalante CP, Meyers C, Reuben JM, et al. A random-ized, double-blind, 2-period, placebo-controlled cross-over trial of a sustained-release methylphenidate in the treatment of fatigue in cancer patients. *Cancer J.* 2014;20(1):8-14. doi: 10.1097/PPO.0000000000000018.

85. Kohli S, Fisher SG, Tra Y, et al. The effect of modafinil on cognitive function in breast cancer survivors. *Can-cer.* 2009;115(12):2605-2616. doi: 10.1002/cncr.24287.

86. Lundorff LE, Jonsson BH, Sjogren P. Modafinil for attentional and psychomotor dysfunction in advanced cancer: a double-blind, randomised, cross-over trial. *Palliat Med.* 2009;23(8):731-738. doi: 10.1177/0269216309106872.

37 Substance Use Disorders and Palliative Care

Karen Blackstone

INTRODUCTION

Substance use disorders in patients with advanced illness pose complex clinical challenges. Particularly alarming is the recent sharp increase in controlled prescription drug abuse (also referred to as nonmedical opioid use or diversion) in the United States (1). Physicians and other health care providers need to be continually mindful of the potential for substance use disorders in the palliative care setting. The severity of substance-related problems varies significantly. Some patients exhibit minor risky behaviors, such as escalating drug dosages without informing their physicians or using analgesics to treat symptoms other than those intended. At the other end of the continuum, some patients present to the palliative care team with a known history of or current substance use disorder that requires immediate action by the treatment team. Proper identification, assessment, and clinical management of the entire spectrum of substance-related behaviors are critically important for optimal treatment of patients in palliative care settings.

Clinicians must balance the obligation to be thorough in assessing potential opioid abuse or diversion with the duty to ensure that patients' pain is not undertreated. Regulatory pressures only add to this burden, leading some physicians to believe that they must avoid being duped by those abusing prescription pain medications at all costs. Although it is tempting to reduce the clinical implications of patient behavior to dichotomous labels of "addiction" or "not addiction," this oversimplification is not in the patient's best interests. In fact, pain management can be adapted to address the multiple possibilities that might be behind the problematic behaviors noted in an assessment. Physicians can assert control over prescriptions without necessarily ceasing to prescribe controlled substances entirely. Although these situations invariably defy simple solutions, knowledgeable clinicians can implement strategies to simultaneously address the need for compassionate care, symptom relief, and substance use disorder risk reduction.

Safe and effective palliative symptom management demands attention to the risks of prescribed controlled substances and the potential biological, societal, ethical, and legal consequences of substance use disorders. When opiates, benzodiazepines, and other controlled substances are indicated, palliative care providers may reduce risks of injury or death through interdisciplinary teamwork, comprehensive patient risk assessment, risk minimization strategies, coordinated monitoring for substance use disorders, and ongoing treatment plan review and revision. Substance use disorders are common and result in high morbidity and mortality. The U.S. Department of Health and Human Services has declared an opioid crisis in the United States and a public health emergency. In 2018, 2 million U.S. adults were diagnosed with an opioid use disorder, more than 130 people died every day from opioid drug overdoses, and 40% of these deaths involved a prescription opioid (2). Recently increased opioid prescription practice is one factor that contributes to the current widespread misuse of both prescription and nonprescription opioids.

In addition to opioids, the American Psychiatric Association recognizes substance use disorders resulting from alcohol, cannabis, hallucinogens, inhalants, sedatives, hypnotics, anxiolytics, stimulants, tobacco, and other or unknown substances (3). Substance use disorders are characterized by cognitive, physiological, and behavioral symptoms indicating that an individual continues to use one of these substances despite significant substance use–related problems. The Diagnostic and Statistical Manual of Mental Disorders (DSM-5) defines substance use disorder by the presence of behaviors of impaired control, social impairment, risky use, and pharmacological criteria. Substance use disorder severity can be categorized as mild (2 to 3 symptom behaviors), moderate (4 to 5 symptom behaviors), severe (6 or more symptom behaviors) (3).

Impaired control behaviors

- Take the substance in larger amounts or for longer than originally intended
- Express a persistent desire to cut down or regulate substance use and report multiple unsuccessful efforts to decrease or discontinue use

- Spend a great deal of time obtaining, using, or recovering from the effects of the substance
- Experience cravings and urges to use the substance

Social impairment behaviors

- Failure to fulfill major role obligations at work, school, or home
- Continue substance use despite persistent or recurrent social or interpersonal problems cause or exacerbated by the effects of the substance
- Give up or reduce important social, occupational, or recreational activities because of substance use

Risky use behaviors

- Recurrent substance use in situations in which it is physically hazardous
- Continued substance use despite knowledge of having a persistent or recurrent physical or psychological problem that is likely to have been cause or exacerbated by the substance

Pharmacologic criteria

- Tolerance: requiring a markedly increased dose of the substance to achieve the desired effect or a markedly reduced effect when the usual dose is consumed.
- Withdrawal: a syndrome that occurs when blood or tissue concentration of a substance decline in an individual who had maintained prolonged heavy use of the substance. After developing withdrawal symptoms, the individual is likely to consume the substance to relieve the symptoms. Withdrawal symptoms vary across the classes of substances.

PREVALENCE OF SUBSTANCE USE DISORDERS AMONG SERIOUSLY ILL PATIENTS

Substance use disorders are common in the U.S. general population and may be more prevalent than previously reported among patients with advanced illnesses. Approximately half the individuals aged 15 to 54 in the United States reported illegal drug use at some point in their lives and 6% to 15% reported a current or past substance use disorder of some type (4–10). Substance use disorders coexist with several life-threatening diseases (acquired immunodeficiency syndrome, cirrhosis, and some cancers) commonly treated in palliative care settings (11–14). Alcohol-related substance use disorder is common in the general population and has been identified in more than 25% of patients admitted to a palliative care unit (15). Adults with medical illness (including

chronic obstructive pulmonary disease, heart disease, kidney disease, and cancer) reported marijuana use more often than those without medical conditions (16).

The rapid rise in controlled prescription drug abuse is of particular concern for the palliative care team. When misused, prescription opioids and central nervous system depressants and stimulants can be deadly. In 2002, controlled prescription drugs were implicated in 30% of drug-related emergency room deaths and in at least 23% of emergency department admissions (1). Contrary to past data suggesting that most controlled prescription drug abusers were regular or experienced users, approximately one-third of abusers in 2000 were new users of controlled prescriptions according to the data from the National Center of Addiction and Substance Abuse (1). Between the years 1992 and 2003, there was 225% increase in new opioid abuse, 150% increase in new tranquilizer abuse, 127% increase in new sedative abuse, and 171% increase in new stimulant abuse (1). Particular regions of the United States, most notably the south and west, have been disproportionately affected.

The growing rates of nonmedical prescription drug use and diversion raise questions about the prevalence of substance use disorders in patient populations with cancer and how palliative care physicians can best address the needs of their patients. Despite its prevalence in the general population, substance abuse appears to be very uncommon within the tertiary care population with cancer. In a 6-month period, in 2005, fewer than 1% of inpatient and outpatient consultations performed by the psychiatry service at Memorial Sloan-Kettering Cancer Center (MSKCC) were requested for substance abuse–related issues and only 3% of patients who were referred to the psychiatry department were subsequently diagnosed with a substance abuse disorder of any type (15). This prevalence is much lower than the frequency of substance abuse disorders in society at large, in general medical populations, and in emergency medical departments (4,8,17–19). A 1983 study of the Psychiatric Collaborative Oncology Group, which assessed psychiatric diagnoses in ambulatory patients with cancer from several tertiary care hospitals also found a low prevalence of substance-related disorders with fewer than 5% of 215 patients with cancer meeting the American Psychiatric Association definition (18,20).

The relatively low prevalence of substance abuse among patients with cancer treated in tertiary care hospitals may reflect institutional biases or a tendency for patients to underreport in these settings. Many patients with substance use disorders are poor, feel alienated from the health care system, may not seek care in tertiary centers, and may be reluctant to acknowledge the stigmatizing history of drug use. For these reasons, the low prevalence of substance use disorders in cancer centers may not be representative of the true prevalence in the cancer population overall. In support of this conclusion, the findings of a 1995 survey of patients admitted to a palliative care unit indicate alcohol abuse in more than 25% of patients (21). Additional studies are needed to clarify the current epidemiology of substance use disorders in patients with cancer and others with progressive medical diseases.

COMMON LANGUAGE

Both epidemiologic studies and clinical management depend on an accepted, valid nomenclature for terms associated with substance use disorder. Adding to confusion and complexity, some have advocated for different standards to diagnose substance use disorders among people with concurrent medical illness. Clear terminology is an essential step in improving the diagnosis, prevention, and management of substance use disorders in palliative care settings (Table 37.1).

Tolerance

Tolerance is a pharmacologic property defined by the need for increasing doses to maintain effects (22–24). An extensive clinical experience with opioid drugs in the medical context has not confirmed that tolerance causes substantial problems (25,26). Although tolerance to a variety of opioid effects, including analgesia, can be reliably observed in animal models and tolerance to nonanalgesic effects, such as respiratory depression and cognitive impairment, occurs routinely in the clinical setting, analgesic tolerance seldom interferes with the clinical efficacy of opioid drugs (25,26). Indeed, most patients attain stable doses associated with a favorable balance between analgesia and side effects for prolonged periods; dose escalation, when it is required, usually heralds the appearance of a progressive painful lesion (27–34). Unlike

TABLE 37.1 SUBSTANCE ABUSE DEFINITIONS IN THE MEDICALLY ILL

Tolerance	The need for increasing doses to maintain analgesic effects
Addiction	Continuing and compulsive use despite physical, psychological, or social harm
Physical dependence	Presence of withdrawal following abrupt dose reduction

tolerance to the side effects of opioids, clinically meaningful analgesic tolerance, which would yield the need for dose escalation to maintain analgesia in the absence of progressive disease, appears to be a rare phenomenon. Clinical observation also fails to support the conclusion that analgesic tolerance is a substantial contributor to the development of substance dependence.

Physical Dependence

Physical dependence is defined solely by the occurrence of an abstinence syndrome (withdrawal) following abrupt dose reduction or administration of an antagonist (22–24,35). There is great confusion among clinicians about the differences between physical dependence and true substance dependence. Physical dependence, like tolerance, has been suggested to be a component of substance dependence, and the avoidance of withdrawal has been postulated to create behavioral contingencies that reinforce drug-seeking behavior (35). These speculations, however, are not supported by experience acquired during opioid therapy for chronic pain. Physical dependence does not preclude the uncomplicated discontinuation of opioids during multidisciplinary pain management of nonmalignant pain (36), and opioid therapy is routinely stopped without difficulty in the patients with cancer whose pain disappears following effective antineoplastic therapy. Indirect evidence for a fundamental distinction between physical dependence and substance dependence is even provided by animal models of opioid self-administration, which have demonstrated that persistent drug-taking behavior can be maintained in the absence of physical dependence (37).

Addiction

The terms addiction and addict are particularly troublesome. These labels are often inappropriately applied to describe both aberrant drug use (reminiscent of the behaviors that characterize active abusers of illicit drugs) and phenomena related to tolerance or physical dependence. The labels "addict" and "addiction" should never be used to describe patients who are only perceived to have the capacity for an abstinence syndrome. These patients must be labeled "physically dependent." Use of the word "dependent" *alone* also should be discouraged, because it fosters confusion between physical dependence and psychological dependence, a component of substance dependence. For the same reason, the term habituation should not be used.

Identification of substance use disorder and nonmedical prescription drug use or diversion must be based on the identification of behaviors that are outside of cultural or societal norms. The ability to categorize questionable behaviors (e.g., consuming a few extra doses of a prescribed opioid, particularly if this behavior was not specifically prescribed by the clinician, or using an opioid drug prescribed for pain as a nighttime hypnotic) as nonnormative presupposes that there is certainty about the parameters of normative behavior. In fact, even experienced pain clinicians disagree on the interpretation of varied drug-taking patterns. In a recent survey, pain clinicians expressed significant individual differences in the perception of which behaviors were the most problematic when asked to rank order a list of aberrant drug-taking behaviors (38). In general, physicians rated illegal behaviors as the most aberrant, followed by alteration of the route of delivery and self-escalation of dose.

There are few empirical data in medically ill populations that define the meaning of specific drug-related behaviors in relation to substance use disorders; as a result, the boundaries of normative behavior remain ill defined. The confusing nature of normative prescription drug use was highlighted in a pilot survey performed in 2000 at MSKCC, which revealed that inpatients with cancer harbor attitudes supporting misuse of drugs in the face of symptom management problems and that women with human immunodeficiency virus (at MSKCC for palliative care) engage in such behaviors commonly (39). The prevalence of such behaviors and attitudes among the medically ill raises concern about their predictive validity as a marker of any diagnosis related to substance abuse. Clearly, there is a need for empirical data that illuminate the prevalence of drug-taking attitudes and behaviors in different populations of medically ill patients.

The core concepts used to define substance dependence also may be problematic as a result of changes induced by a progressive disease. Deterioration in physical or psychosocial functioning caused by the disease and its treatment may be difficult to separate from the morbidity associated with drug abuse. This may particularly complicate efforts to evaluate the concept of "use despite harm," which is critical to the diagnosis of substance abuse or dependence. For example, the nature of questionable drug-related behaviors can be difficult to discern in the patient who develops social withdrawal or cognitive changes following brain irradiation for metastases. Even if impaired cognition is clearly related to the drugs used to treat symptoms, this outcome might only reflect a narrow therapeutic window, rather than a desire on the patient's part for these psychic effects.

Definitions of Substance Dependence in the Medically Ill

Previous definitions that include phenomena related to physical dependence or tolerance cannot be the model terminology for medically ill populations who receive potentially abusable drugs for legitimate medical purposes. A more appropriate definition of substance dependence notes that it is a chronic disorder characterized by "the compulsive use of a substance resulting in physical, psychological, or social harm to the user and continued use despite that harm" (40). Although this definition was developed from experience in substance-abusing populations without medical illness, it appropriately emphasizes that substance dependence is, fundamentally, a psychological and behavioral syndrome. Any appropriate definition of substance abuse or dependence must include the concepts of loss of control over drug use, compulsive drug use, and continued use despite harm.

Even appropriate definitions of substance dependence will have limited utility, however, unless operationalized for a clinical setting. The concept of "aberrant drug-related behavior" is a useful first step in operationalizing the definitions of substance abuse and dependence and recognizes the broad range of behaviors that may be considered problematic by prescribers. Although the assessment and interpretation of these behaviors can be challenging, as discussed previously, the occurrence of aberrant behaviors signals the need to reevaluate and manage drug taking, even in the context of an appropriate medical indication for a drug.

If drug-taking behavior in a medical patient can be characterized as aberrant, a "differential diagnosis" for this behavior can be explored. That a patient has a true substance use disorder is only one of several possible explanations. The challenging diagnosis of pseudoaddiction must be considered if the patient is reporting distress associated with unrelieved symptoms. In the case of pseudoaddiction, behaviors such as aggressively complaining about the need for higher doses and occasional unilateral drug escalations indicate desperation caused by pain and disappear if pain management improves.

Alternatively, impulsive drug use may indicate the existence of another psychiatric disorder, the diagnosis of which may have therapeutic implications. Patients with borderline personality disorder can express fear and rage through aberrant drug taking and behave impulsively and self-destructively during pain therapy. Passik and Hay (41) reported a case in which one of the more worrisome aberrant drug-related behaviors, forging of a prescription for a controlled substance, was an impulsive expression of fears of abandonment, having little to do with true substance abuse in a borderline patient. Such patients are challenging and often require firm limit-setting and careful monitoring to avoid impulsive drug taking.

Similarly, patients who self-medicate for anxiety, panic, depression, or even periodic dysphoria and loneliness can present as aberrant drug takers. In such instances, careful diagnosis and treatment of these problems can at times obviate the need for such self-medication. Occasionally, aberrant drug-related behavior appears to be causally related to a delirium, with confusion about the appropriate therapeutic regimen. This may be a concern in the treatment of the elderly patient. Rarely, problematic behaviors indicate criminal intent, such as when patients report pain but intend to sell or divert medications.

These diagnoses are not mutually exclusive. A thorough psychiatric assessment is critically important, both in the population without a prior history of substance abuse and the population of known abusers, who have a high prevalence of psychiatric comorbidity (42,43).

In assessing the differential diagnosis for drug-related behavior, it is useful to consider the degree of aberrancy (Table 37.2). The less aberrant behaviors (such as aggressively complaining about the need for medications) are more likely to reflect untreated distress of some type, rather than substance dependence–related concerns. Conversely, the more aberrant behaviors (such as injection of an oral formulation) are more likely to reflect true substance use disorder. Although empirical studies are needed to validate this conceptualization, it may be a useful model when evaluating aberrant behaviors.

TABLE 37.2 DEGREES OF ABERRANCE IN DRUG-TAKING BEHAVIOR

Mildly aberrant	Requests for specific pain medication Aggressive complaints about the need for medication Using drugs prescribed for a friend or family member Frequent prescription losses Hoarding drugs
More highly aberrant	Forging prescriptions Obtaining drugs from nonmedical source Sale of prescription drugs Crushing sustained-release tablets for snorting or injecting

From Passik SD, Kirsh KL, Whitcomb L, et al. Pain clinicians' rankings of aberrant drug-taking behaviors. *J Pain Palliat Care Pharmacother*. 2002;16:39-49.

EMPIRICAL STUDIES USING THE ABERRANT DRUG-TAKING CONCEPT

Several studies have investigated the usefulness of considering aberrant drug taking as occurring on a continuum. Although the studies performed to date all involve small samples, they have shown that conceptualizing aberrant drug taking in this way has important implications for clinicians. The first study examined the relationship between aberrant drug-taking behaviors and compliance-related outcomes in patients with a history of substance abuse receiving chronic opioid therapy for nonmalignant pain. Dunbar and Katz (44) examined outcomes and drug taking in 20 patients with diverse histories of drug abuse who underwent a year of chronic opioid therapy. During the year of therapy, 11 patients were adherent with the drug regimen and 9 were not. The authors examined patient characteristics and aberrant drug-taking behaviors that differentiated the two groups. The patients who did not abuse the therapy were abusers of solely alcohol (or had remote histories of polysubstance abuse), were participating in 12-step programs, and had good social support. The patients who abused the therapy were polysubstance abusers, were not participating in 12-step programs, and had poor social support. The specific behaviors that were recorded more frequently by those who abused the therapy were unscheduled visits and multiple phone calls to the clinic, unsanctioned dose escalations, and acquisition of opioids from more than one source.

A second study examined the relationship between aberrant drug taking and the presence or absence of a psychiatric diagnosis of substance use disorder in pain patients. Compton et al. (45) studied 56 patients seeking pain treatment in a multidisciplinary pain program who were referred for "problematic drug taking." The patients all underwent structured psychiatric interviews, and the sample was divided between those qualifying and those not qualifying for psychiatric diagnoses of substance use disorders. The authors then examined the subjects' reports of aberrant drug-taking behaviors on a structured interview assessment. The patients who qualified for a substance use disorder diagnosis were more likely to have engaged in unsanctioned dose escalations, received opioids from multiple sources, and reported a subjective impression of loss of control of their prescribed medications.

Passik and researchers at a major cancer center (40) examined the self-reports of aberrant drug-taking attitudes and behaviors in samples of patients with cancer ($N = 52$) and patients with AIDS ($N = 111$) on a questionnaire designed for the purposes of the study. Reports of past drug use and abuse were more frequent than the present reports in both groups. Current aberrant drug-related behaviors were seldom reported, but attitude items revealed that patients would consider engaging in aberrant behaviors or would possibly excuse them in others, if pain or symptom management were inadequate. It was found that aberrant behaviors and attitudes were endorsed more frequently by the women with AIDS than by male and female patients with cancer. Overall, patients greatly overestimated the risk of substance dependence during pain treatment. Experience with this questionnaire suggests that patients both with cancer and AIDS respond in a forthcoming fashion to drug-taking behavior questions and describe attitudes and behaviors that may be highly relevant to the diagnosis and management of substance use disorders.

These studies help clarify the meanings ascribed by clinicians to the various behaviors that occur during long-term administration of a potentially abusable drug. Ultimately, such studies may define the true "red flags" in a given population.

Far too often, anecdotal accounts shape the way clinicians view drug-related behaviors. Some behaviors are regarded almost universally as aberrant despite limited systematic data to suggest that this is the case. Consider, for example, the patient who requests a specific pain medication or a specific route or dose. Although this behavior may reflect a patient who is knowledgeable and assertive—favorable characteristics in other contexts—it is often greeted with suspicion on the part of practitioners. Other behaviors may be common in medically ill non–substance-abusing populations, and although aberrant, they may have little predictive value for true substance dependence. For example, the finding that many non–substance-abusing patients with cancer use anxiolytic medications prescribed for a friend or others (39) more than likely reflects the undertreatment and underreporting of anxiety in patients with cancer than true substance abuse.

CLINICAL MANAGEMENT

When opioid and other controlled prescription medications are indicated for symptom management, palliative care providers may adapt evidence-based and consensus-developed risk mitigation guidelines. The 2016 Centers for Disease Control and Prevention Guideline for Prescribing Opioids for Chronic Pain advises clinicians to establish treatment goals with patients and consider how opioids will be discontinued if benefits do not outweigh risks. This report recommends clinicians prescribe the lowest effective opioid dosage,

carefully reassess benefits and risks when considering increasing dosage to 50 morphine milligram equivalents or more per day, and avoid concurrent opioids and benzodiazepines whenever possible, with reassessment of risks and benefits with patients every 3 months or more frequently and review prescription drug monitoring program data, when available, for high-risk combinations or dosages (46). The American Society for Clinical Oncology similarly recommends universal precautions when considering controlled prescription medications to treat symptoms of cancer, including screening risk for all patients, discussing risks, benefits, adverse effects and alternative therapies, providing education on safe use, storage, and disposal, and use of prescription drug monitoring programs (PDMPs), urine testing, patient provider agreements, and close observation of behaviors to help ensure treatment adherence, detect substance use disorder symptoms, and shared therapeutic decision-making (47).

Interdisciplinary Approach

Substance use disorders among patient with symptoms from advanced illness (with or without a prior history of substance use disorder) are serious and complex clinical occurrences. An interdisciplinary team approach can promote patient safety while optimizing symptom management and addressing health care provider stress. Palliative care teams may enhance their expertise (physician, nurse, social worker, chaplain, pharmacist) and collaborate with mental health professionals with specialization in substance use disorders. The palliative care team can communicate concerns, review and revise the comprehensive care plan, and support each other through regular meetings. Teams may create universal risk mitigation policies and implement procedures based on individual patient risks and goals (Table 37.3).

Risk Assessment

Palliative care providers may implement a graduated interview style developed for use with chronic pain patients, beginning with broad questions about the role of substances such as nicotine and caffeine have in the patient's life and gradually becoming more specific with questions about controlled medication and illicit drug use. Such an approach is helpful in reducing denial and resistance. This interviewing style may also assist in the detection of coexisting psychiatric disorders. Comorbid psychiatric disorders can significantly contribute to aberrant drug-taking behavior. Studies suggest that 37% to 62% of people with alcohol use disorder have one or more coexisting psychiatric disorders, and the patient's drug history may

TABLE 37.3 RISK MITIGATION PROCEDURES

Universal Risk Assessment

Use graduated interview approach beginning with broad questions about substances such as nicotine or caffeine and becoming more specific
Assess for comorbid psychiatric disorders, such as anxiety, personality disorders, and mood disorders
Use screening tools (e.g., RIOSORD, SOAPP-R, ORT)

Treatment Risk Reduction Strategies

General	Listen and accept patient's report of distress
	Develop shared treatment goals
	Educate patients about risks of controlled medications
	Use behavioral and nonopioid interventions for pain when possible
	Consider drugs with slower onset and longer duration (e.g., transdermal fentanyl and modified-release opioids). Note that higher doses may be needed for adequate pain control in patients with a history of abuse or dependence
	Frequently assess adequacy of symptom and pain control
	Use monitoring tools (PDMP, urine toxicology, pill counting)
Outpatients	Develop patient/provider agreement
	Limit amount of drug dispensed per prescription
	Make refills contingent on clinic attendance
	Consider urine toxicology screenings to assess usage
	Involve family members and friends in the treatment plan
Inpatients	Assess and treat withdrawal symptoms (delirium tremens)
	Consider close observation (a private room, near the nurses' station)
	Consider daily urine toxicology testing

be a clue to comorbid psychiatric disorders (e.g., drinking to quell panic symptoms). Anxiety, personality disorders, and mood disorders are those most commonly encountered (9,43,48). The Centers for Disease Control and Prevention have promulgated alcohol screening tools than have been validated for general use (49). The assessment and treatment of comorbid psychiatric disorders can greatly enhance management strategies and reduce the risk of relapse.

Universal Screening

Although many substance use disorder risk assessment screening tools are available, few are specific for patients with symptoms from advanced or progressive illnesses. Palliative care providers may use general screening tools such as the Risk Index for Serious Opioid-Induced Respiratory Depression (RIOSORD) to identify patients with factors that might increase the risk for opioid overdose, such as sleep-disordered breathing, end-organ dysfunction leading to impaired medication clearance, pulmonary disease, and concomitant use of sedating medications (50). Palliative care providers may also use screening tools developed for patients with chronic pain to estimate the likelihood of substance use disorder development during treatment. The Screener and Opioid Assessment for Patients with Pain (SOAPP-R) tool is a 24-item self-administered survey initially studied among patients with chronic noncancer pain (51). A retrospective analysis including 69 patients with cancer

pain who needed an opioid prescription demonstrated the SOAPP-R's sensitivity (0.75) and specificity (0.80) to predict substance use disorders. Although not specific for palliative care patients, the Opioid Risk Tool (ORT), with 5 items addressing personal and family history of substance use disorders, age, history of preadolescent sexual abuse, and certain psychological conditions, may sensitively and specifically identify patients prescribed opioids for chronic pain to determine who may develop opioid-related aberrant behaviors (52). When an active substance use disorder is suspected, palliative care providers can explore further with validated tools such as the Rapid Opioid Dependency Screen (53).

Most recent research has focused on tools that can aid prescreening patients to determine the level of risk when considering opioids as part of the treatment regimen. While mislabeling patients as either a good or bad risk can have negative consequence, safe opioid prescribing relies on proper risk stratification and the accommodation of that risk into a treatment plan. In addition, providers must always keep in mind that a spectrum of nonadherence exists and that this spectrum is distinct for pain patients versus those who use controlled substances for nonmedical purposes (54) (Fig. 37.1). Nonmedical opioid users can be seen as self-treating personal issues, purely as recreational users, or as having a more severe and consistent substance use disorder. On the other hand, pain patients are more complex and their behaviors

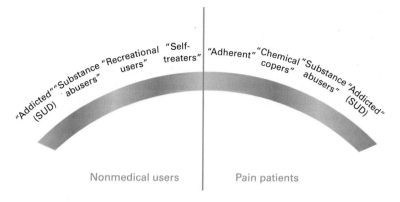

SUD, substance use disorder.

Figure 37.1 The spectrum of adherence for pain patients versus the spectrum of illicit use by nonmedical users. (From Kirsh KL, Passik SD. The interface between pain and drug abuse and the evolution of strategies to optimize pain management while minimizing drug abuse. *Exp Clin Psychopharmacol*. 2008;16(5):400-404.)

might range from strict adherence to chemically coping to a frank addiction. Thus, scores indicating increased risk on the screening tools may not necessarily indicate substance use disorder but might be uncovering some of the gray areas of opioid noncompliance.

Monitoring Strategies

Palliative care providers may follow opioid risk reduction monitoring strategies developed for chronic pain patients. One checklist tool describes "Four A's" domains to be monitored, including

analgesia, activities of daily living, adverse side effects, and aberrant drug-taking behaviors (55,56). The monitoring of these outcomes over time should inform therapeutic decision-making and provide a framework for documentation (Table 37.4).

Development of a Treatment Plan— General Considerations

Clear treatment goals are essential in managing aberrant drug-related behaviors. Depending on the history, a complete remission of the patient's substance use disorder may not be a reasonable

TABLE 37.4 FOUR A'S FOR ONGOING MONITORING

Analgesia	Document and monitor patient's pain, using scales such as a 0–10 pain rating scale. Although listed as the first "A," analgesia is not necessarily to be considered the most important outcome of pain management. An alternate view is how much relief it takes for a patient to feel that their life is meaningfully changed so they can work toward the attainment of their own goals.
Activities of daily living	Monitor patient's typical level of daily activities and psychosocial functioning to observe increases over time. The second "A" concerning activities of daily living refers to quality of life issues and functionality. It is necessary that patients understand that they must comply with all of their recommended treatment options so that they are better able to return to work, avocation, and social activities.
Adverse effects	Strive for highest analgesia with most benign side effect profile. Patients must also be made aware of the adverse side effects inherent in the treatment of their pain condition with opioids and other medications. Side effects must be aggressively managed so that sedation and other side effects do not overshadow the potential benefits of drug therapy. The most common side effects of opioid analgesics include constipation, sedation, nausea and vomiting, dry mouth, respiratory depression, confusion, urinary retention, and itching.
Aberrant behaviors	Be aware of aberrant behaviors suggestive of drug use, such as multiple "lost" prescriptions or unauthorized dose escalations. Patients must be educated through agreements, or other means, about the parameters of acceptable drug taking. Even an overall good outcome in every other domain might not constitute satisfactory treatment if the patient is not compliant with the contract in worrisome ways. Dispensing pain medicine in a highly structured fashion may become necessary for some patients who are in violation or constantly on the fringes of appropriate drug taking.

goal. The distress of coping with a life-threatening illness and the availability of prescription drugs for symptom control can undermine efforts to maintain control over comorbid substance abuse or dependence (56). For some patients, "harm reduction" may be a better model. It aims to enhance social support, maximize treatment compliance, and contain harm done through episodic relapse. Several elements are key in this approach. First, clinicians must establish a relationship based on empathic listening and accept the patient's report of distress. Second, it is important to use nonopioid and behavioral interventions for pain when possible but not as substitutes for appropriate pharmacologic management. Third, specific aspects of drug selection and dosing should be informed by a history of problematic drug use. For example, a history of active opioid abuse usually means that higher doses may be needed more rapidly than commonly observed in patients who are opioid-naive. Underdosing may lead to a degree of persistent pain that drives the patient's attempts to self-medicate. Finally, the team should make plans to frequently reassess the adequacy of pain and symptom control.

Prescription Drug Monitoring Programs

Prescription drug monitoring programs allow review of a patient's controlled prescription history. A patient-specific query is required before opioid initiation in several U.S. states. Although patients in hospice care may be exempt from PDMP requirements in some locations, palliative care providers can use PDMP resources to identify multiple prescribers of controlled medications, concomitant opioid and benzodiazepine prescriptions, and evidence of an undisclosed opioid use disorder by previous prescriptions for buprenorphine (57).

Controlled Substance Agreements

Previously known as "pain contracts," controlled substance agreements may promote patient adherence, safety, trust, and shared decision-making with prescribers. Palliative care providers may adapt and personalize agreement checklists created for use in chronic pain management. Common controlled substance agreement elements include goals of medication therapy, risks and benefits, prescribing policies of the practice, patient and provider responsibilities, and patient's informed consent (58).

Urine Toxicology Screening

Urine toxicology screening has the potential to be a useful tool to the practicing clinician for both diagnosing potential concerns and monitoring active substance use disorders. Although generally considered important, providers do not consistently request urine toxicology, and when ordered, providers do not completely document reasons for ordering or follow-up recommendations. A 2000 tertiary care center chart review found that nearly 40% of the charts surveyed listed no reason for obtaining the urine toxicology screen and the ordering physician could not be identified nearly 30% of the time (59). Staff education efforts can help to address this problem.

One might wonder how good clinicians are at detecting adherence and misuse in their patients. Bronstein et al. (60) addressed this question by asking clinicians to identify patients who they thought were at risk for medication misuse and those who were not based on risk assessment methods used in their practice. Urine drug testing results were then compared with these assessments. A total of 755 samples were received from 62 clinicians in 50 practices. Patients who were thought to potentially be misusing their medications ($N = 226$) had urine drug tests (UDTs) showing illicits, missing prescribed medication, unprescribed medication present, and/or results above or below the range using Rx Guardian methodology 79% of the time. In patients who clinicians thought were not at risk for misuse of medications ($N = 297$), 72% had UDTs showing illicits, missing prescribed medication, unprescribed medication present, and/or results above or below the range using Rx Guardian methodology. The third group (random with no risk assessment identified, $N = 232$) showed 71% of samples had illicits, missing prescribed medication, unprescribed medication present, and/or results above or below the range using Rx Guardian methodology. Bronstein et al. went on to relax the criteria for labeling a test abnormal to see if that lead to improved clinician's accuracy. For this data cut, tests were considered abnormal only if illicits were present and/or prescribed drug was not found. This resulted in a data set of 549 samples. In group A ($N = 204$, those patients not suspected of medication misuse), 60% still had abnormal results; in group B ($N = 173$, those suspected of medication misuse), 72% had abnormal results; and the random group C ($N = 172$) had 61% abnormal tests.

As demonstrated by Bronstein et al. (60), it is difficult to predict which patients are likely to be misusing opioids or taking an illicit drug. Clinicians were better able to predict medication misuse in patients where they thought there might be an issue based on whatever risk assessments they used in the clinic. Thus, if clinicians only test patients suspected of likely misusing medications, they are missing a significant group of patients, up to 72% in the large data set and 60%

in the narrower data set that were likely misusing their medications without any identifiable risk behaviors.

Patients with Advanced Disease and Substance Use Disorders

Symptom management for patients with both advanced medical illness and substance use disorders may be particularly challenging. Although clinicians may be tempted to overlook a patient's use of illicit substances or alcohol, viewing these behaviors as a last source of pleasure for the patient, drug use that is out of control may have a highly deleterious impact on palliative care efforts. Aberrant drug-related behaviors may be associated with poor symptom control, distress, increased stress for family members, family concern over the misuse of medication, poor compliance with the treatment regimen, and diminished quality of life. Complete abstinence from drugs of abuse may not be a realistic outcome, but reduction in use can certainly have positive effects for the patient (61).

Management of risk is a "package deal." It comprises a suite of assessment, monitoring, and treatment tools that need to be considered for each patient and individualized as clinically indicated (62) (Table 37.5). Screening tools are available to help in the assessment of known risk factors for opioid abuse, including smoking, psychiatric disorders, and personal or family history of substance abuse. When available, prescription monitoring programs can provide physicians with valuable information about prescription compliance (63). Patients determined to be at minimal risk can receive minimal structure, whereas those determined to be at greater risk can receive more structure, such as more frequent visits, fewer pills per prescription, specialist-level care (e.g., an addiction specialist or psychotherapist), and urine toxicology testing. Patients must be made aware of the responsibility of safeguarding these medications against diversion by friends, family, or visitors who may have access to medications left out or in unlocked locations. Up to 50% or more of prescription opioids diverted for nonmedical use are obtained from friends and family (63). Finally, opioid formulations that incorporate barriers to common forms of manipulation are an emerging component of risk management. Novel subclasses of opioid formulations, incorporating pharmacological strategies and physical barriers, are designed to deter or resist misuse and abuse by making it difficult to obtain euphoric effects from opioid use.

Outpatient Management Strategies

There are a number of additional strategies for promoting treatment adherence in an outpatient setting. A controlled substance agreement between the team and patient helps provide structure to the treatment plan, establishes clear expectations of the roles played by both parties, and outlines the consequences of aberrant substance use behaviors. The inclusion of spot urine toxicology screens in the agreement can be useful in maximizing treatment compliance. Expectations regarding follow-up visits and management of drug supply also should be stated. For example, clinicians may wish to limit the amount of medication dispensed per prescription and make refills contingent upon clinic attendance. The clinician may consider the requirement for joint management by a specialist in substance abuse or required attendance at a 12-step program. Attention to the spiritual and social-based recovery process of 12-step programs can help support healthy coping practices, particularly in times of distress for people with serious illness. Palliative care providers may help to serve those living with addiction disorders better by assessing not only patient histories of substance use/abuse and other addictive behaviors but by facilitating their ongoing support recovery efforts (64). With the patient's consent, the clinician may wish to contact the patient's sponsor and make him or her aware that the patient is being treated for a chronic illness that requires medications (e.g., opioids). This action will reduce the potential for stigmatization of the patient as being noncompliant with the ideals of the 12-step program. Finally, clinicians and patients may involve family members and friends in the treatment to help bolster social support and functioning.

Inpatient Management Strategies

The management of patients with active substance use disorders who have been admitted to the hospital for treatment of a life-threatening illness is based on the guidelines discussed in the preceding text for outpatient settings. These guidelines aim

TABLE 37.5 RISK MANAGEMENT PACKAGE FOR PATIENTS UNDERGOING OPIOID THERAPY

Screening and risk stratification
Use of prescription monitoring program data
Compliance monitoring
Urine drug testing
Pill or patch counts
Education about drug storage and sharing
Psychotherapy and highly structured approaches
Abuse-deterrent or abuse-resistant strategies in opioid formulation

From Kirsh KL, Passik SD. The interface between pain and drug abuse and the evolution of strategies to optimize pain management while minimizing drug abuse. *Exp Clin Psychopharmacol*. 2008;16(5):400-404.

to promote the safety of patients and staff, contain manipulative behaviors by patients, enhance the appropriate use of medication for pain and symptom management, and communicate an understanding of pain and substance abuse management. First, the patient's drug use needs to be discussed in an open manner. It may be necessary to reassure the patient that steps will be taken to avoid adverse events such as drug or alcohol withdrawal. In some challenging cases, it would be best to admit a patient several days in advance of a planned procedure for stabilization of the drug regimen. While addressing pain and other symptoms, inpatient health care providers may implement facility-specific policies and procedures to reduce risks of patient elopement and trafficking of illicit substances between patients and visitors (such as admitting to a private room, close nursing observation, search of belongings, screening or limiting visitors). Inpatient providers may order frequent or daily urine toxicology screens.

Management approaches should be tailored to reflect the clinician's assessment of the severity of drug abuse. Open and honest communication between the clinician and the patient throughout the admission reassures the patient that these guidelines were established in their best interest.

In some cases, these guidelines fail to curtail aberrant drug use despite repeated interventions by staff. At that point, the patient should be considered for discharge. This appears to be necessary only in the most recalcitrant of cases. The clinician should involve members of the staff and administration for discussion about the ethical and legal implications of such a decision.

Methadone

Oral methadone can be used safely and effectively as an analgesic for patients with cancer (65–69). Hospice and palliative care experts published consensus guidelines in 2018 on appropriate candidates for methadone, detail in dosing, titration, and monitoring of patients' response to methadone therapy (69). This guideline advises that health care providers be informed about the unique pharmacokinetic and pharmacodynamic properties of methadone and risks of interacting medications (those that prolong QTc or are metabolized by cytochrome P-450 enzymes) prior to prescribing and carefully consider appropriate candidates for methadone with attention to detail in dosing and monitoring the patient's response to therapy. Methadone is especially of interest for the treatment of seriously ill people because of its long duration of action, availability of multiple dosage formulas (tablet, oral solution, intravenous), high

bioavailability, low cost, lack of pharmacologically active metabolites, and perceived enhanced effectiveness in difficult pain syndromes. Precautions and contraindications to methadone therapy include impaired liver function, active illicit drug use or misuse, congenital QTc syndrome (patient or family), structural heart disease, electrolyte abnormalities, disordered breathing syndromes, and paralytic ileus. The consensus group recommends a very low dose of methadone, such as 1 mg by mouth twice daily, as a starting dose. The consensus group cautions that the long and unpredictable half-life of methadone elimination requires allowing 5 to 7 days before adjusting the does for most patients. Others have reported that once-daily methadone as used for substance use disorder treatment is rarely useful as an analgesic, and patients receiving maintenance methadone for opioid dependence cannot obtain pain relief merely by increasing their dose (70,71).

Alcohol Withdrawal and Serious Illness

Patients with life-threatening illness who are dependent on alcohol require careful assessment and management. When these patients are not identified and are admitted to the hospital, alcohol withdrawal can be an unexpected complication. Patients at the end of life can also inadvertently experience withdrawal symptoms if they decrease their alcohol intake as their physical condition declines. Withdrawal symptoms may be mistaken for general anxiety when the full extent of the patient's use of alcohol is not known (72). The first symptoms of withdrawal usually manifest a few hours following the cessation of alcohol intake and often consist of tremors, agitation, and insomnia. In mild to moderate cases, these symptoms lessen within 2 days. Patients with advanced illness are more likely than the physically healthy to progress from these milder symptoms to a state of delirium characterized by autonomic hyperactivity, hallucinations, incoherence, and disorientation (73). Delirium tremens (DTs) occur in approximately 5% to 15% of patients in alcohol withdrawal (72), typically within the first 72 to 96 hours of withdrawal. Severe DTs is a medical emergency and requires prompt treatment.

In surgical settings, alcohol withdrawal can cause up to a threefold increase in postoperative mortality when unrecognized and not addressed (74–76). Patients with cancer who abuse alcohol are at high risk for delirium postoperatively due to poor nutrition, prior head trauma, and other causes of brain injury.

The extreme vulnerability of patients who are terminally ill necessitates that potential alcohol withdrawal symptoms be managed aggressively and prevented whenever possible (76). To date, no research exists to determine the best approach to treat acute alcohol withdrawal in the palliative care setting; in its absence, basic management steps, such as the use of hydration, benzodiazepines, and in some cases, neuroleptics, should be taken to manage alcohol withdrawal syndrome (72). The administration of a vitamin–mineral solution is indicated, including parenteral thiamine 100 g for 3 days before switching to oral administration to prevent the development of Korsakoff's syndrome. A daily dose of folate 1 mg should also be given throughout treatment (72).

Patients in Substance Use Recovery

Symptom management with advanced illness patients in substance use recovery presents a unique challenge. Depending on the structure of the recovery program (e.g., alcoholics anonymous, 12 steps, and interdisciplinary methadone maintenance programs), a patient may fear ostracism from the program's members or have intense fear regarding susceptibility to relapsing into substance use disorder behaviors. Nonopioid therapies should be optimized, which may require referral to a pain center or other specialists (70). If opioids or other controlled substances are required, therapy should be structured based on a thorough assessment, the goals of care, and the life expectancy of the patient. In some cases, it is necessary to use controlled substance agreements, random urine toxicology screens, and pill counts. If possible, attempts should be made to include the patient's recovery program sponsor in order to garner their cooperation and support of the patient.

CONCLUSION

Safe and effective symptom management of patients with advanced illness necessitates a comprehensive approach that recognizes the biological, chemical, social, and psychiatric aspects of substance use disorders and provides practical means to manage risk, treat symptoms, and assure patient safety. Palliative care providers may follow or adapt guidelines for risk assessment, mitigation, and safe practice developed for the general population and by specialty pain, oncology, and palliative care expert consensus groups. More research is needed to clarify the prevalence and risks of substance use disorder among seriously ill patients and develop and test specialized assessment tools, monitoring programs, and treatment guidelines. More research may lead to improved symptom management and patient safety through knowledge, new models of care, and policy changes.

ACKNOWLEDGMENT

The authors would like to acknowledge the contribution of Dr. Julie R. Hamrick, Dr. Steven D. Passik, Dr. Kenneth L. Kirsh on the previous edition.

REFERENCES

1. National Center on Addiction and Substance Abuse of Columbia University. Paper presented at: Under the Counter: The Diversion and Abuse of Controlled Prescription Drugs in the U.S.; July 2005; New York, NY.
2. US Department of Health and Human Services. What is the opioid crisis? https://www.hhs.gov/opioids/about-the-epidemic/. Content last reviewed on September 4, 2019. Accessed December 17, 2019.
3. American Psychiatric Association. *Diagnostic and Statistical Manual of Mental Disorders.* 5th ed. Washington, DC: American Psychiatric Association; 2013.
4. Colliver JD, Kopstein AN. Trends in cocaine abuse reflected in emergency room episodes reported to DAWN. *Public Health Rep.* 1991;106:59-68.
5. Warner LA, Kessler RC, Hughes M, et al. Prevalence and correlates of drug use and dependence in the United States. Results from the National Comorbidity Survey. *Arch Gen Psychiatry.* 1995;52:219-229.
6. Kessler RC, Chui WT, Demler O, et al. Prevalence, severity, and comorbidity of 12-month DSM-IV disorders in the National comorbidity survey replication. *Arch Gen Psychiatry.* 2005;62:617-627.
7. Kessler RC, Berglund P, Demler O, et al. Lifetime prevalence and age-of-onset distributions of DSM-IV disorders in the National comorbidity survey replication. *Arch Gen Psychiatry.* 2005;62:593-602.
8. Groerer J, Brodsky M. The incidence of illicit drug use in the United States, 1962–1989. *Br J Addict.* 1992;87:1345.
9. Regier DA, Farmer ME, Rae DS, et al. Comorbidity of mental disorders with alcohol and other drug abuse. *J Am Med Assoc.* 1990;264:2511-2518.
10. Wells KB, Golding JM, Burnam MA. Chronic medical conditions in a sample of the general population with anxiety, affective, and substance use disorders. *Am J Psychiatry.* 1989;146:1440.
11. Smith-Warner SA, Spiegelman D, Yaun S, et al. Alcohol and breast cancer in women: a pooled analysis of cohort studies. *J Am Med Assoc.* 1998;279:535-540.
12. Blot WJ. Alcohol and cancer. *Cancer Res.* 1992;52: S2119-S2123.
13. Thun MJ, Peto R, Lopez AD, et al. Alcohol consumption and mortality among middle-aged and elderly U.S. adults. *N Engl J Med.* 1997;337:1705-1714.
14. Room R, Babor T, Rehm J. Alcohol and public health. *Lancet.* 2005;365:519-530.
15. Yu DK. Review of Memorial Sloan-Kettering Counselling Center Database (Unpublished) 2005.
16. Dai H, Richter KP. A national survey of marijuana use among US adults with medical conditions, 2016–2017. *JAMA Netw Open.* 2019;2(9):e1911936.
17. Burton RW, Lyons JS, Devens M, et al. Psychiatric consults for psychoactive substance disorders in the general hospital. *Gen Hosp Psychiatry.* 1991;13:83.
18. Derogatis LR, Morrow GR, Fetting J, et al. The prevalence of psychiatric disorders among cancer patients. *J Am Med Assoc.* 1983;249:751.
19. Regier DA, Meyers JK, Dramer M, et al. The NIMH epidemiologic catchment area program. *Arch Gen Psychiatry.* 1984;41:934.

20. American Psychiatric Association. *Diagnostic and Statistical Manual for Mental Disorders*. 3rd ed. Washington, DC: American Psychiatric Association; 1983.

21. Bruera E, Moyano J, Seifert L, et al. The frequency of alcoholism among patients with pain due to terminal cancer. *J Pain Symptom Manage*. 1995;10(8):599.

22. Dole VP. Narcotic addiction, physical dependence and relapse. *N Engl J Med*. 1972;286:988.

23. Martin WR, Jasinski DR. Physiological parameters of morphine dependence in man-tolerance, early abstinence, protracted abstinence. *J Psychiatr Res*. 1969;7:9.

24. Portenoy RK. Opioid tolerance and efficacy: basic research and clinical observations. In: Gebhardt G, Hammond D, Jensen T, eds. *Proceedings of the VII World Congress on Pain, Progress in Pain Research and Management*. Vol. 2. Seattle, WA: IASP Press; 1994:595.

25. Foley KM. Clinical tolerance to opioids. In: Basbaum AI, Besson J-M, eds. *Towards a New Pharmacotherapy of Pain*. Chichester: Wiley; 1991:181.

26. Ling GSF, Paul D, Simantov R, et al. Differential development of acute tolerance to analgesia, respiratory depression, gastrointestinal transit and hormone release in a morphine infusion model. *Life Sci*. 1989;45:1627.

27. Bruera E, Macmillan K, Hanson JA, et al. The cognitive effects of the administration of narcotic analgesics in patients with cancer pain. *Pain*. 1989;39:13.

28. Twycross RG. Clinical experience with diamorphine in advanced malignant disease. *Int J Clin Pharmacol Ther Toxicol*. 1974;9:184.

29. Kanner RM, Foley KM. Patterns of narcotic drug use in a cancer pain clinic. *Ann N Y Acad Sci*. 1981;362:161.

30. Chapman CR, Hill HF. Prolonged morphine self-administration and addiction liability: evaluation of two theories in a bone marrow transplant unit. *Cancer*. 1989;63:1636.

31. Meuser T, Pietruck C, Radruch L, et al. Symptoms during cancer pain treatment following WHO guidelines: a longitudinal follow-up study of symptom prevalence, severity, and etiology. *Pain*. 2001;93:247-257.

32. McCarberg BH, Barkin RC. Long-acting opioids for chronic pain: pharmacotherapeutic opportunities to enhance compliance, quality of life, and analgesia. *Am J Ther*. 2001;8:181-186.

33. Aronoff GM. Opioids in chronic pain management: is there a significant risk of addiction? *Curr Rev Pain*. 2000;4:112-121.

34. Zenz M, Strumpf M, Tryba M. Long-term opioid therapy in patients with chronic nonmalignant pain. *J Pain Symptom Manage*. 1992;7:69.

35. Redmond DE, Krystal JH. Multiple mechanisms of withdrawal from opioid drugs. *Annu Rev Neurosci*. 1984;7:443-478.

36. Wikler A. *Opioid Dependence: Mechanisms and Treatment*. New York, NY: Plenum Press; 1980.

37. Halpern LM, Robinson J. Prescribing practices for pain in drug dependence: a lesson in ignorance. *Adv Alcohol Subst Abuse*. 1985;5:184.

38. Dai S, Corrigal WA, Coen KM, et al. Heroin self—administration by rats: influence of dose and physical dependence. *Pharmacol Biochem Behav*. 1989;32:1009.

39. Passik SD, Kirsh KL, Whitcomb L, et al. Pain clinicians' rankings of aberrant drug- behaviors. *J Pain Palliat Care Pharmacother*. 2002;16:39-49.

40. Passik S, Kirsh KL, McDonald M, et al. A pilot survey of aberrant drug-taking attitudes and behaviors in samples of cancer and AIDS patients. *J Pain Symptom Manage*. 2000;19:274-286.

41. Hay J, Passik SD. The cancer patient with borderline personality disorder: suggestions for symptom-focused management in the medical setting. *Psychooncology*. 2000;9:91-100.

42. Khantzian EJ, Treece C. DSM-III psychiatric diagnosis of narcotic addicts. *Arch Gen Psychiatry*. 1985;42:1067.

43. Grant BF, Stinson FS, Dawson DA, et al. Prevalence and co-occurrence of substance use disorders and independent mood and anxiety disorders. *Arch Gen Psychiatry*. 2004;61:807-816.

44. Dunbar SA, Katz NP. Chronic opioid therapy for nonmalignant pain in patients with a history of substance abuse: report of 20 cases. *J Pain Symptom Manage*. 1996;11:163.

45. Compton P, Darakjian J, Miotto K. Screening for addiction in patients with chronic pain with "problematic" substance use: evaluation of a pilot assessment tool. *J Pain Symptom Manage*. 1998;16:355-363.

46. Dowell D, Haegrerich TM, Chou R. CDC Guideline for prescribing opioids for chronic pain—United States, 2016. *JAMA*. 2016;315(15):1624-1645.

47. Dalal S, Bruera E. Pain management for patients with advanced cancer in the opioid epidemic era. *Am Soc Clin Oncol Educ Book*. 2019;39:24-35.

48. Penick E, Powell B, Nickel E, et al. Comorbidity of lifetime psychiatric disorders among male alcoholics. *Alcohol Clin Exp Res*. 1994;18:1289-1293.

49. https://www.cdc.gov/ncbddd/fasd/alcohol-screening.html. Accessed May 18, 2020.

50. Zedler B, et al. Development of a risk index for serious prescription opioid-induced respiratory depression or overdose in Veterans' Health Administration patients. *Pain Med*. 2015;16:1566-1579.

51. Butler SF. Validation of the revised screener and opioid assessment for patients with pain (SOAPP-R). *J Pain*. 2008;9(4):360-372.

52. Webster LR, Webster RM. Predicting aberrant behaviors in opioid-treated patients: preliminary validation of the opioid risk tool. *Pain Med*. 2005;6(6):432-442.

53. Wickersham JA, et al. Validation of a brief measure of opioid dependence: the rapid opioid dependence screen (RODS). *J Correct Health Care*. 2015;21(1):12-26.

54. Passik SD, Weinreb HJ. Managing chronic nonmalignant pain: overcoming obstacles to the use of opioids. *Adv Ther*. 2000;17:70-80.

55. Passik SD, Kirsh KL, Whitcomb LA, et al. A new tool to assess and document pain outcomes in chronic pain patients receiving opioid therapy. *Clin Ther*. 2004;26:552-561.

56. Passik SD, Portenoy RK, Ricketts PL. Substance abuse issues in cancer patients: part 2: evaluation and treatment. *Oncology (Huntingt)*. 1998;12:729-734.

57. Centers for Disease Control and Prevention, National Center for Injury Prevention and Control. What healthcare providers need to know about PDMP. https://www.cdc.gov/drugoverdose/pdmp/providers.html. Last reviewed July 12, 2019. Accessed December 17, 2019.

58. Tobin DG, Keogh FK, Johnson MS. Breaking the pain contract: a better controlled-substance agreement for patients on chronic opioid therapy. *Cleve Clin J Med*. 2016;83(11):827-835.

59. Passik S, Schreiber J, Kirsh KL, et al. A chart review of the ordering and documentation of urine toxicology screens in a cancer center: do they influence patient management? *J Pain Symptom Manage*. 2000;19:40-44.

60. Bronstein K, Passik S, Munitz L, et al. Can clinicians accurately predict which patients are misusing their medications? Poster presentation at: The 30th Annual Scientific Meeting of the American Pain Society; May 2011; Austin, TX.

61. Passik S, Theobald D. Managing addiction in advanced cancer patients: why bother? *J Pain Symptom Manage*. 2000;19:229-234.

62. Kirsh KL, Passik SD. The interface between pain and drug abuse the evolution of strategies to optimize pain management while minimizing drug abuse. *Exp Clin Psychopharmacol.* 2008;16(5):400-404.

63. Passik SD. Issues in long-term opioid therapy: unmet needs, risks, and solutions. *Mayo Clin Proc.* 2009;84(7):593-601.

64. Groninger H, Knapik M. Twelve-step programs and spiritual support at the end of life. *Am J Hosp Palliat Care.* 2019;36(9):807-811.

65. Ripamonti C, Groff L, Brunelli D, et al. Switching from morphine to oral methadone in treating cancer pain: what is the equianalgesic dose ratio? *J Clin Oncol.* 1998;16:3216-3221.

66. Mercadante S, Sapio R, Serretta M, et al. Patient-controlled analgesia with oral methadone in cancer pain: preliminary report. *Ann Oncol.* 1996;7:613-617.

67. Carrol E, Fine E, Ruff R, et al. A four-drug pain regimen for head and neck cancers. *Laryngoscope.* 1994;104:694-700.

68. Lawlor P, Turner K, Hanson J, et al. Dose ratio between morphine and methadone in patients with cancer pain: a retrospective study. *Cancer.* 1998;82:1167-1173.

69. McPherson ML, et al. Safe and appropriate use of methadone in hospice and palliative care: expert consensus white paper. *J Pain Symptom Manage.* 2019;57:635-645.

70. Parrino M. *State Methadone Treatment Guidelines, Treatment Improvement Protocol (TIP)—Series 1.* Rockville, MD: Center for Substance Abuse Treatment; 1993. DHHS publication no. (SMA) 93–1991.

71. Zweben JE, Payte JT. Methadone maintenance in the treatment of opioid dependence: a current perspective. *West J Med.* 1990;152:588-599.

72. Myrick H, Anton RF. Treatment of alcohol withdrawal. *Alcohol Health Res World.* 1998;22:38-43.

73. Lundberg JC, Passik SD. Alcohol and cancer: a review for psycho-oncologists. *Psychooncology.* 1997;6:253-266.

74. Sonne NM, Tonnesen H. The influence of alcoholism on outcome after evacuation of subdural haematoma. *Br J Neurosurg.* 1992;6:125-130.

75. Maxmen JS, Ward NG. Substance-related disorders. In: Hamrick J, ed. *Essential Psychopathology and Its Treatment.* New York, NY: W.W. Norton and Company; 1995:132-172.

76. Spies CD, Nordmann A, Brummer G, et al. Intensive care unit stay is prolonged in chronic alcoholic men following tumor resection of the upper digestive tract. *Acta Anaesthesiol Scand.* 1996;40:649-656.

Issues in Palliative Care

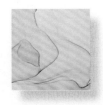 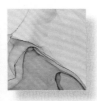 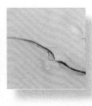 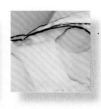 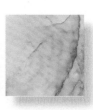

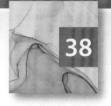

38 Hospice

Martha L. Twaddle and Laura Patel

END-OF-LIFE CARE

If medicine takes aim at death prevention, rather than at health and relief of suffering, if it regards every death as premature, as a failure of today's medicine—but avoidable by tomorrow's—then it is tacitly asserting that its true goal is bodily immortality. Physicians should try to keep their eyes on the main business, restoring and correcting what can be corrected and restored, always acknowledging that death will and must come, that health is a mortal good, and that as embodied beings, we are fragile beings that must stop sooner or later, medicine or no medicine (1).

National data reports tell us that over 80% of those who die in the United States do so after a lengthy, progressively debilitating illness (2). In essence, over 80% of the time, the outcome of the disease is predictable, but the timing of the outcome is not. In oncology, the trajectory of the illness has changed over the recent decades to increasingly be one of a chronic progressively debilitating illness, punctuated by acute exacerbations with temporary recoveries. Like nonmalignant illness, oncology patients may likely experience more frequent exacerbations in their final months and years, these crises coming closer and closer together with less and less time or capacity for an interval sustained recovery. These frequent exacerbations may be related directly to the malignant illness or are often caused by treatment-related morbidities or infections. This pattern of closely occurring crises focuses the health care teams on deeply ingrained "rescue" behaviors and may obscure the clinicians' perspectives on the overall pattern of decline, which, in far advanced malignant disease, is most often predictable and is characterized by a precipitous decline in functional status associated with nutritional and cognitive deterioration (3–5).

PATIENT AND FAMILY GOALS MAY LACK SYNERGY WITH MODERN HEALTH CARE

When faced with approaching death, modern Americans prefer to maximize the time with those activities that are meaningful to them and support the integrity of their individual well-being

(6–12). Unfortunately, with advancing illness, the time spent in organizing resources, navigating the complexity of health care systems, and receiving procedures, tests, and other interventions at hospitals and other institutions often overwhelm the energies of patients and families. Given the choice, most patients likely would not elect to focus their last days and energies on interactions with health care systems. But the operative phrase within that statement is "when given the choice." Often, however, such choice is not offered. Although informed consent regarding procedures is the standard of care in health care, advanced care planning discussions that might provide opportunity for patients and families to modify or decline further disease-focused interventions without the risk of abandonment, real or perceived, are not yet routine practice in all settings of care (13–16).

Goals of the disease management model are to eradicate disease and prolong life. Resources are directed to these ends. The physician, nurse, and others laboring in this model work as "warriors" tend to see death as failure and often view the lessening or absence of disease-interventional treatments as "doing nothing." It is normative, for example, for a physician who has exhausted all protocols in fighting a malignancy to say "I have nothing left to offer you" when in fact, an armamentarium of beneficial supportive care modalities may be available.

The warrior perspective often does not create an atmosphere that allows for the kind of questions and sharing of information that could lead to choices for comfort-oriented care and acceptance of decline and death. This may not be for any lack of empathy or compassion on the part of doctors and other health care agents. Rather, it attests to the emphasis of contemporary training and practice and the prioritization of finely honed intervention skills within the highly technologic, science-based environment of health care centers.

PALLIATIVE CARE COMPLEMENTS TREATMENTS

Palliative care by definition and practice is not *alternative* care. It is rather *complementary* to traditional medical care and is, simply put, the very foundation of good medical care (17). The palliative approach views the patient as a whole person in the context of his or her family and community and seeks to understand and mitigate the cultural, social, spiritual, and psychological elements that contribute to suffering and which, if addressed, can improve quality of life, even if life is short.

Palliative care starts with clarification of the goals of care in the light of how the individual defines quality of life and its meaning. With the goals defined and documented, care ideally moves from crisis intervention to crisis avoidance, resources for support and advocacy are defined earlier in the illness, and discussions of the burden and benefit of interventions are revisited regularly. Palliative care is thus a continuum of supportive care that ideally begins at the time of a potentially life-limiting diagnosis and actively supports the patient and family throughout the course of illness, however long that journey may be (Fig. 38.1) (18–20).

HOSPICE CULMINATES THE CONTINUUM

Within this continuum of palliative care is hospice—a place where the most intensive form of palliative care, typically supported by defined insurance coverage, is practiced. As such, hospice

is also a philosophy of care that recognizes that the disease is not curable, that time is limited, and that symptom control and quality of life are preeminent goals. In this paradigm, *all* interventions and therapies must have immediate, tangible benefit to the patient and family, consistent with their personally defined goals. Hospice views death as an expected outcome within a discrete time frame. It offers a support system to patients, families, and professionals that affirms the outcome of death not as failure, but its heralded approach as opportunity to maximize quality so that the patient might live well until death. Recognizing the time limitations of life allows patients and families to prioritize the activities and interactions that have meaning, to seek closure personally and practically, and to have an opportunity to "leave a legacy," if so desired, or to have some focused intent as to how or even in what manner one will be remembered after death.

ROOTS OF HOSPICE CARE

The term "hospice" has a long history: Originally, hospices were places of safety for travelers on pilgrimage throughout the ancient Middle East (c. AD 400). These centers of "hospitality" evolved into the first hospitals of Europe, often operated and staffed by religious orders. Dame Cicely Saunders of Great Britain is credited with launching the

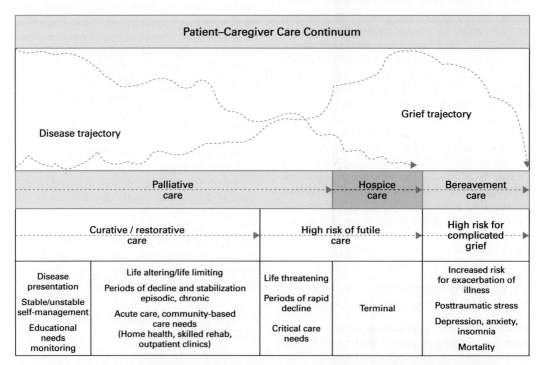

Figure 38.1 Diagram of the continuum of palliative care through hospice. (AsceraCare Hospice, used with permission. Created by Bob Parker, RN, MSN/ED; Angie Hollis-Sells, RN CHPN; Martha L. Twaddle, MD, FACP, FAAHPM; and David B. Friend, MD, MBA.)

modern concept of hospice care (Fig. 38.2) (21). Dame Saunders initially practiced as a nurse during the World War II, but a back injury forced her to redirect her career to medical social work. In this context, she cared for and befriended a young man, David Tasma, a 40-year-old dying of inoperable cancer. Visiting him frequently in hospital, she witnessed how his symptoms were controlled by the administration of morphine and noted particularly how, when free of pain, he "had time to sort out who he was dying at the age of 40, and coming from the Warsaw ghetto. Of course, leaving nobody behind and feeling he had made no impression on the world for ever having lived in it. But as we were talking, he said he would leave me something in his will, he had insurance, and he said, 'I'll be a window in your home.' And the idea of openness to everybody who might come, openness to every future challenge, really stems from that gift, which was, I think, the founding gift of the whole hospice movement, made by David Tasma, who thought his name would never mean anything to anybody" (22).

THE EXPANSION OF THE BRITISH MODEL OF HOSPICE

The original concept of hospice in England, sparked into being by Dame Saunders and David Tasma's gift, was care for those with advanced cancer provided in an institutional setting, in essence, a specialty hospital. St. Christopher's hospice opened in 1967, and in this setting, Dame Saunders pioneered the application of the scientific approach to the care of the dying, establishing many of the current best practices of palliative medicine, in particular, the around-the-clock administration of analgesic therapy to control pain symptoms. Dame Saunder's trainees further developed hospice in the world.

- Dr. Robert Twycross established the World Health Organization's Collaborating Center for Hospice/Palliative Care at the Sir Michael Sobell House in Oxford. A prolific writer and erudite teacher, he has written and published extensively on pharmacologic interventions in pain and symptom management.

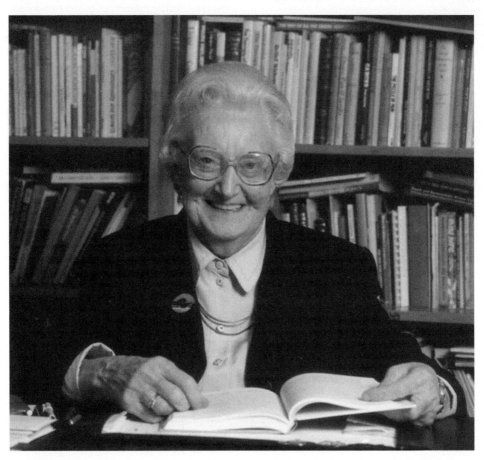

Figure 38.2 Dame Cicely Saunders of Great Britain is credited as launching the modern concept of hospice care.

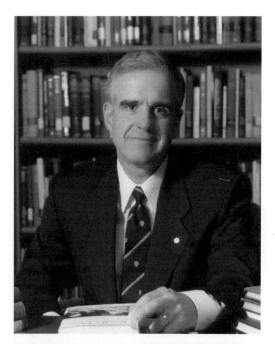

Figure 38.3 Dr. Balfour Mount is credited for having coined the term "palliative medicine" to describe the medical discipline of hospice care.

- Dr. Balfour Mount (Fig. 38.3), a urologic surgeon at McGill University, is credited with having coined the term "palliative medicine" to describe the medical discipline of hospice care. His work at the Royal Victoria Hospital in Montreal helped moved forward the integration of this care model throughout North America and, along with Dr. Josefina Magno, contributed substantially to the formation in 1988 of the Academy of Hospice Physicians which later evolved to the American Academy of Hospice and Palliative Medicine (AAHPM) (23).
- Florence Wald, PhD, Dean of the Graduate School of Nursing at Yale University, opened the New Haven Connecticut Hospice in 1974. This was a sentinel event for hospice, the introduction of the hospice care model into the United States, and the form of hospice care being delivered in the home setting, a model that is most common within the United States to this day. Early models of inpatient hospice care were established at Calvary Hospital and St. Luke's-Roosevelt Hospital in New York City; however, the model that has grown prolifically in the United States has been home care (24).

GROWTH WITHIN THE UNITED STATES

The growth of hospice in the United States found fertile soil in the work of Dr. Elisabeth Kübler-Ross, who raised the awareness of death and the recognition of the patient's coping mechanisms through her observational studies published in *Death and Dying* in 1969 (25). In keeping with the grassroots psychology of the American, hospice programs were established at the community level, often by professional volunteers, to provide an alternative to institutional-based dying. The early pioneers of hospice in the United States were vocal in their condemnation of "modern" health care's inattention to the needs of dying patients and their families and sought to establish health care systems that existed outside of the mainstream in reaction to this deficit. Within the United States, terminally ill patients with diagnoses other than cancer were increasingly served by hospice programs: By 2017, over 70% of patients were admitted with noncancer diagnoses, with the most common being end-stage heart disease and dementia (26). The New Haven program brought together hospice leaders and advocates in the late 1970s to establish guidelines for the operations of hospice programs in the United States. This led to the development of the National Hospice Organization, now the National Hospice and Palliative Care Organization (NHPCO). The mission of this membership organization that represents the nation's hospice programs is "to lead and mobilize social change for improved care at the end of life" (27).

Through the involvement and advocacy of such leaders, the United States Congress authorized the Medicare Hospice Benefit (MHB) in 1982. This entitlement benefit addresses the types of services provided within hospice care, the persons eligible to elect the benefit, and the payment system that supports the care. Hospice programs throughout the United States moved to become Medicare certified by adhering to these federal regulations. Medicaid and commercial insurance developed similar guidelines, and hospice programs thereby could bill and receive insurance dollars to support care. The Hospice Medicare benefit is divided into periods, the initial being two 90-day periods with an unlimited number of 60-day increments to follow. Each benefit period requires physician recertification around prognosis and goals of care (28).

The regulations for Medicare-certified hospice providers were published in the Federal Register as the *Hospice Conditions of Participation* in 1983 and updated further in 2008. The 2008 update reflects the Centers for Medicare and Medicaid Services' (CMS) increased emphasis on both patient-centered care and the development of quality and performance measures to monitor hospice care and its outcomes. The stated goal of CMS is to ensure access to high-quality end-of-life care for Medicare beneficiaries electing the benefit and the agency contracted for the development of quality measurement tools. Currently, hospices have two reporting requirements: the Hospice Item Set (HIS) and the Hospice Consumer Assessment of Healthcare Providers and Systems (CAHPS) survey. HIS and Hospice CAHPS data are used to calculate performance on quality measures (29). National Hospice CAHPS survey data is publicly reported on the Hospice Compare website (30).

In addition, CMS' requirements for the determination of *continued* hospice eligibility have become more accountable with the enactment of the face-to-face visit requirement (Federal Register May 9, 2010). As of January 2011, the hospice physician or hospice nurse practitioner is required to have a face-to-face encounter with the Medicare beneficiary within 30 days of the start of the third and each subsequent benefit period. The goal of this increased clinician involvement is to improve the documentation of the patient's medical condition and clinical justification that supports the prognosis of a life expectancy of 6 months or less. As such, it is part of the overall effort to administer health care resources to guarantee affordable, quality health care for all Americans, as outlined in the Patient Protection and Affordable Care Act in March 2010.

THE BUSINESS OF HOSPICE CARE

As is typical with any philosophical approach that moves to a business model, hospice care in America has been challenged by the tension between its philosophy and what is economically feasible to support. In truth, the MHB was one of the first capitated insurance programs and also one of the most successful. Until 2016, the MHB payment model provided a flat per diem rate for routine level hospice care. In 2016, the payment model changed to a two-tiered rate, with higher payments in the first 60 days and lower payment after 60 days, as well as additional payment (service intensity add-on) for visits provided in the last 7 days of life. Under this payment structure, the hospice program is responsible to provide the professional care of nurses, social workers, chaplains, and therapists in an interdisciplinary team structure. The per diem also covers all the medications, therapies, and procedures related to the hospice diagnosis and any durable medical equipment necessary to care for the patient. The MHB also specifically calls for the involvement of volunteers to provide support to the patient and family. The benefit requires the participation of a hospice medical director to oversee the medical management and, along with the primary attending physician, to certify the patient has a life expectancy of 6 months or less if the disease follows its normal course. Clinical care provided by a physician in the domain of either primary care or palliative medicine is not part of the per diem and is reimbursed through established billing protocols that cover physician services. The benefit also requires a minimum of 12 months of bereavement support for the survivors of the deceased; the per diem payment does not continue through that time period (Table 38.1).

The MHB also requires and covers three other levels of care. The general inpatient (GIP) level of care was established to address the short-term needs of hospice patients when an acute condition precluded the safe delivery of care in any other setting. Under this portion of the benefit, the hospice patient could be hospitalized for acute symptom exacerbations or physical, psychological, or existential issues around dying that could not be safely or effectively managed in another setting. The goal of GIP is to stabilize or resolve the issue(s) that led to inpatient care and return the patient to a less acute setting. No more than 20% of the hospice's overall patient days can be at the GIP level of care. Continuous care is available to address high-acuity situations in the home setting that require additional care in a low-tech environment for a finite period of time. By definition, the hospice team is providing continuous care to the patient; the majority must be nursing care. The MHB also provides respite care, a 5-day provision that is allowed within each benefit period to ease care giving strain. Under this provision, the patient is typically transferred from a home to a nursing home or other inpatient facility for a finite period of time, and a small per diem rate goes for room and board as well as to cover all medications and equipment related to the hospice diagnosis supplied within the facility. Most commercial insurance programs mimic the MHB but with variations that require hospice programs to negotiate and clarify the scope of coverage.

The MHB is a capitated reimbursement program. The CMS determines the adjusted cap amount and works through Medicare Administrative Contractors (MACs) to distribute the funds for hospice services. The MAC is responsible for calculating each hospice's cap amount by multiplying the adjusted cap by the number of Medicare beneficiaries who elected to receive hospice care from each hospice during a 12-month period ending with September 30 of each year. If in excess of the cap, each hospice must refund Medicare payments in excess of this aggregated cap amount (31).

TABLE 38.1 COMPARISON OF HOME HEALTH AND HOSPICE REQUIREMENTS AND SERVICES

	Home health	Hospice
Eligibility	Any diagnosis Need to have a skilled need (this can be nursing or therapy) Need to be homebound	Any diagnosis No such requirement No such requirement
Site of care delivery	Can only be provided in the home or assisted living (not skilled, LTCF, or hospital)	Many sites of care: home, LTCF, ALF, hospital, adult day care, etc.
Certification	Only one medical director certifies Certification periods are 60 d Face-to-face encounter and attestation by eligible health care provider required 90 d prior or 30 d after initiation of benefit	Need two physicians to certify Certification periods are two 90 d and then 60 d Face-to-face encounter and attestation by eligible health care provider within 30 d of the third and all subsequent benefit periods. Certification for continued eligibility within 15 d of the benefit periods
Care management	Physician directed; prescriptive	Interdisciplinary team directed
Services covered	Payment does not include meds or DME Includes supplies related to admitting diagnosis Can only be provided in the home or assisted living (not skilled, LTCF, or hospital)	Includes meds and DME Includes supplies related to admitting diagnosis plus general care (diapers, skin care, etc.) Many sites of care: home, LTCF, ALF, hospital, adult day care, etc.
Levels of care	N/A	Four different levels of care: routine home care, inpatient respite, continuous care, and general inpatient
Hours of coverage	Varies from agency to agency. Most will direct patient to ER after hours	24 h on call support
Physician reimbursement	*Attending Physician* may bill for accumulation of 30-min increments of "oversight" care. *Medical director* is salaried if has no medical practice	*Attending Physician* bills insurance with a GW or GV modifier if not employed by hospice. *Consulting physicians* bill hospice program. *Hospice medical director* receives administrative salary or stipend

LTCF, long-term care facility; ALF, assisted living facility; DME, durable medical equipment; N/A, not applicable; ER, emergency room.

CHALLENGES AND LIMITATIONS TO ACCESS

The challenges of fully utilizing hospice care exist more in its business model than philosophy. Given the regulatory issues and cost constraints, many hospice programs accept patients who have made the decision to forego further disease-related treatments and disease-modifying therapies, consistent with the Medicare regulations. The advent of immunotherapy and changing treatment landscape can make timely referral challenging, particularly with the potential of delayed response to therapy. Hospice is often unable to provide concurrent coverage of costly treatments, while oncologists and patients may want additional attempts at immunotherapy or even chemotherapy or have uncertainty around prognosis. In a study of referral patterns, those patients referred by oncologists typically have the shortest length of stay in hospice care, as opposed to patients referred from primary care practitioners (32). Despite the steady growth in the utilization of hospice services in the United States, increasing from 340,000 in 1994 to 885,000 in 2002 and 1.49 million in 2017, the median length of stay in hospice programs in 2017 was only 24 days, with 27% of hospice patients dying within 7 days or less of accessing hospice support (26). Patients with hematologic malignancies are often referred late or never to hospice care with an average of only 2% of these patients using hospice for an average length of stay of <9 days (33). For patients with cancer, initiation of early multidisciplinary hospice care is associated with better pain relief, quality of life, reduced cost, and less aggressive care at the EOL as well as less psychiatric morbidity for caregivers (34).

INCREASING ACCESS—THE NATIONAL AGENDA

Despite the financial and regulatory limitations of hospice care, larger hospice programs in the United States have sought ways to increase access and provide the fullness of support to patients who are grappling with the decisions of foregoing further disease-modifying treatment. The NHPCO and the National Association of Home Care and Hospice (NAHC) have focused many resources on improving access to care, particularly for underserved patients. More common now are hospice programs that accept patients who are still receiving disease-modifying treatments with palliative intent, who have not yet established a "Do Not Attempt Resuscitation Order" or who do not have a caregiver living with them. Hospice programs will more typically underwrite such therapies as palliative radiation or blood transfusions if the goals of care are clearly for enhanced quality of life and symptom management, and if the treatments have little, if any, associated morbidity. The developments within the field of oncology of improved supportive therapies that may slow the progression of the disease with little, if any, dose-limiting side effects have fueled the discussions further regarding continuing such therapies in the setting of hospice. Although great variations exist in the field of hospice as to eligibility around admissions, the overarching theme is to enhance access and stretch the model of care beyond confines that limit its utilization (35). This desire to increase access to support is reflected in the development of a new model called Medicare Care Choices Model developed through the Center for Medicare and Medicaid Innovation. This model is testing a new payment approach for hospice eligible Medicare patients who are still seeking disease directed treatments, allowing people to still receive chemotherapy while also receiving support from a home-based hospice team. Eighty-five hospice programs have participated in this 5-year pilot which ends in 2021 (36).

PEDIATRIC HOSPICE CARE

The pediatric population benefits significantly from this enhanced access model. Pediatric palliative and/or hospice care (PP/HC) is a philosophical and organized method to provide competent, compassionate, and consistent care to children with chronic, complex, and/or life-threatening conditions and their families. PP/HC differs significantly from the models of hospice care provided to adults because of the wide age and developmental ranges of the patients, the inherent differences in the pediatric trajectories of illness, clinical models of care delivery, funding support for care, communication strategies with patients and their families, staffing models and ratios, symptom management interventions, and the ethical concerns that can arise during care (37).

In the United States, cancer is the second most common cause of death for children aged 1 to 14. More than 16 out of 100,000 children are diagnosed with cancer; 3 out of 100,000 die. Over the past 25 years, the 5-year survival rate for all major childhood cancers has improved significantly, and a large percentage of children may survive childhood cancer. Pediatric palliative care and hospice service programs may serve patients and their families with chronic complex illness over a much longer period of time. While most chronic conditions do not lead to death in childhood, the death rate is more than twice that of age-matched unaffected populations, and death can occur suddenly for the affected children (38).

The Institute of Medicine's *When Children Die; Improving Palliative and End-of-Life Care for Children and their Families* reinforced that the best model to approach the care for seriously ill children is palliative care (39). The cessation of supportive modalities such as fluids and many medications is typically not feasible for a child; palliative care allows continued active physical support with intensive psychosocial spiritual care for the child and their parents. Bereavement care for parents following the death of a child is critically important. Morbidity and mortality increase in this circumstance, particularly for the mother who has experience the death of her child and for surviving siblings (39,40).

DOES HOSPICE MEAN GIVING UP?

The philosophical barriers regarding access to hospice care are matters of ongoing debate. Physicians and patients will argue that accepting hospice support is "giving up." There is, however, a substantive difference in acceptance of a terminal diagnosis and resignation to the illness. Acceptance confers that the reality is acknowledged, and plans, attitudes, and priorities are adjusted given this reality. Patients live within this new reality—with new limitations. Resignation confers passivity, an inactive waiting. Although some individuals may live their lives and their last days in this manner, it is not the imposed paradigm for those receiving a terminal diagnosis or choosing the support of hospice care. Many in hospice care speak of hope and would likely define that as trust and reliance in the people and process of support as opposed to hope as an expectation of fulfillment (cure) (41). In hospice, these individuals and families are *hopeful* in living well despite advanced disease, seeking active supportive care to enhance their living in the time they have left. There are, in addition, a percentage of patients who survive hospice care, discharged after a period in hospice with stabilization of their disease process, if not improvement in their condition. These patients are most often those with noncancer diagnoses and a higher functional status (42).

HOSPICE OUTCOMES ARE POSITIVE

The reported satisfaction ratings of hospice care are extremely high, and the testimonials of individuals who access hospice support further fuel the passion of its advocates (43,44). The data also suggest that the well-being and survival of the survivors themselves is directly impacted by hospice support. A 2003 retrospective cohort study by Dr. Nicholas Christakis matched over 30,000 couples who used hospice care with an equal number who did not. The results suggested strongly that hospice care might attenuate the ordinarily increased mortality following the death of a spouse, particularly so for women (45).

Along with high satisfaction ratings of hospice care are significant cost savings. The cost of provisioning care to patients choosing palliative care or hospice support services is significantly less compared with those expenditures for patients who pursue a disease-intervention model until death (46). This is particularly significant because Medicare recipients tend to consume the highest percentage of their health care dollars in the weeks and months just prior to death, in large part due to the utilization of intensive care services. Of concern is the trend toward the increasingly aggressive treatment of cancer patients in the weeks just before death, which is reflected in higher utilization of emergency rooms and intensive care units (47–49). In a study of over 8,700 Medicare patients, mean and median costs were lower for patients enrolled in hospice care. The data also show that the maximum reduction in Medicare expenditures per user occurred when a decedent with a primary diagnosis of cancer used hospice care for their last 58 to 103 days of life (50). Lower costs, however, were not associated with a shorter time frame until death; in fact, the patients in hospice care tended to live longer than matched controls that did not elect hospice care (51).

THE GROWTH OF MEDICAL PROFESSIONALISM IN HOSPICE CARE

A significant and ongoing reintegration of hospice into the mainstream of health care began gradually throughout the 1990s. This process has many routes:

President Clinton's health care reform proposals of 1993 recognized hospice care as an accepted part of the health care continuum. Hospital systems have increasingly recognized the benefits in terms of clinical outcomes, patient satisfaction, and cost savings achieved through the integration of palliative and hospice services (52). The MHB GIP level of care allows patients to activate their hospice benefit while still hospitalized: In essence, discharging them from the acute care admission and readmitting them to hospice care with a series of medical orders, as opposed to any physical changes in setting. Hospices and hospitals often have partnered in these arrangements to facilitate hospice patients receiving inpatient hospice care and also accessing a revenue stream that can help support the care (53,54). These integrative models have been further developed on the national level through the encouragement and mentoring of NHPCO, NAHC, and the Center for Advancement of Palliative Care (CAPC) (55). CAPC has taught and mentored several different models for the integration of palliative care and hospice into the hospital/institution settings through its national meetings and training sites. Leaders from NHPCO, CAPC, AAHPM, and the Hospice and Palliative Nursing Association along with the prior consumer group, the Last Acts Project, collaborated to create the inaugural *National Consensus Project in Quality Palliative Care*, which was published in April 2004 and revised for the fourth time in 2018, providing institutions and agencies with best practice guidelines in palliative care (17). Intrinsic to these guidelines is the idea of the continuum of palliative and hospice care and the defining presence of the interdisciplinary team. Domain 7, caring for patients nearing the end of life asserts: "The interdisciplinary model of hospice care is recognized conceptually and philosophically as the best care for patients nearing the end of life. Discussion regarding hospice as an option for support should be introduced early so that patients and families can understand eligibility, and the benefits and limitations of accessing this care model. Early access to hospice support should be facilitated whenever possible to optimize care outcomes for the patient and the family. Palliative care teams, hospice providers and other health care organizations must work together to find innovative, sustainable supportive care solutions for all patients and families in their final months of life" (17).

CONCLUSION

Hospice is a vital support system for the end-of-life care for patients and families and has steadily integrated into traditional health care, particularly in the continuum with palliative care. The medical community and the public have become increasingly aware of the benefits of hospice, yet the utilization of hospice support for patients with cancer continues to remain limited and measured in days to weeks, not months. The utilization of the palliative care continuum, the emphasis on access to care, and the expansion of insurance and regulatory guidelines allow more patients and families who face life-limiting illnesses to experience the fullness of hospice support. Hospice care clearly promotes the concept of "live until you die" by actively supporting patients and families with attention to the physical, psychological, social, cultural, and spiritual aspects of care. Patients who elect hospice care may live longer than those who forego this support, and yet their health care costs are significantly less. Ongoing support for families in bereavement promotes wellness and opportunities for healing and positively protects against the raised mortality risk of the bereaved.

REFERENCES

1. Kass LR. Ethical dilemmas in the care of the III: II. What is the patient's good? *JAMA*. 1980;244(17):1946-1949.
2. Heron M. Deaths: leading causes for 2017. *Natl Vital Stat Rep*. 2019;68(6):1-77.
3. Murray SA, Kendall M, Boyd K, Sheikh A. Illness trajectories and palliative care. *BMJ*. 2005;330(7498):1007-1011. doi:10.1136/bmj.330.7498.1007.
4. Teno JM, Weitzen S, Fennell ML, et al. Dying trajectory in the last year of life: does cancer trajectory fit other diseases? *J Palliat Med*. 2001;4:457-464.
5. Constantini M, Beccaro M, Higginson IJ. Cancer trajectories at the end of life: is there an effect of age and gender? *BMC Cancer*. 2008;8:127-131.
6. McSkimming S, London M, Lieberman C, et al. Improving response to life-threatening illness. *Health Prog*. 2004;1:26-56.
7. Steinhauser KD, Clipp EC, McNeilly M, et al. In search of a good death: observations of patients, families, and providers. *Ann Intern Med*. 2000;132:825-832.
8. Teno JM, Clarridge BR, Casey V, et al. Family perspectives on end-of-life care at the last place of care. *JAMA*. 2004;291:88-93.
9. Steinhauser KE, Christakis NA, Clipp EC, et al. Preparing for the end of life: preferences of patients, families, physicians, and other care providers. *J Pain Symptom Manage*. 2001;22:727-737.
10. Steinhauser KE, Christakis NA, Clipp EC, et al. Factors considered important at the end of life by patients, family, physicians and other care providers. *JAMA*. 2000;284:2476-2482.
11. Dunn A, Litrivis E. Aligning patient preferences and patient care at the end of life. *J Gen Intern Med*. 2011;26(7):681-682. doi:10.1007/s11606-011-1738-1.
12. Winter L. Patient values and preferences for end-of-life treatments: are values better predictors than a living will? *J Palliat Med*. 2013;16(4):362-368.
13. Lamont EB, Christakis NA. Prognostic disclosure to patients with cancer near the end of life. *Ann Intern Med*. 2001;134:1096-1105.
14. Casarett D, Crowley R, Stevenson C, et al. Making difficult decisions about hospice enrollment: what do patients and families want to know? *J Am Geriatr Soc*. 2005;53:249-254.
15. The SUPPORT Principle Investigators. A controlled trial to improve care for seriously ill hospitalized patients. The study to understand prognoses and preferences for outcomes and risks of treatments (SUPPORT). *JAMA*. 1995;274:1591-1598.
16. Baker R, Wu AW, Teno JM, et al. Family satisfaction with end-of-life care in seriously ill hospitalized adults. *J Am Geriatr Soc*. 2000;48(5 suppl):S61-S69.
17. Ferrell BR, Twaddle ML, Melnick A, Meier DE. National consensus project clinical practice guidelines for quality palliative care guidelines, 4th edition. *J Palliat Med*. 2018;21(12):1684-1689.
18. Hui D, Hannon B, Zimmerman C, Bruera E. Improving patient and caregiver outcomes in oncology: team-based, timely, and targeted palliative care. *CA Cancer J Clin*. 2018;68(5):356-376. doi:10.3322/caac.21490.
19. Meyers FJ, Linder J. Simultaneous care: disease treatment and palliative care throughout illness. *J Clin Oncol*. 2003;21:1412-1415.
20. Nickolich MD, El-Jawahri A, Temel JS, LeBlanc TW. Discussing the evidence for upstream palliative care in improving outcomes in advanced cancer. *Am Soc Clin Oncol Educ Book*. 2016;35:e534-e538. doi:10.14694/EDBK_159224.
21. Clark D. *Cicely Saunders—Founder of the Hospice Movement*. Oxford, England: Oxford University Press; 2002.
22. Curriculum Emanuel LL, von Gunten CF, Ferris FD, eds. *The Education in Palliative and End-of-Life Care (EPEC) Curriculum: © The EPEC Project*. Chicago, IL: Northwestern University, Feinberg School of Medicine; 2003.
23. Holman GH, Forman WB. On the 10th anniversary of the organization of the American Academy of Hospice and Palliative Medicine (AAHPM): the first 10 years. *Am J Hosp Palliat Care*. 2001;18:275-278.
24. Buck J. Home hospice versus home health. *Nurs Hist Rev*. 2004;12:25-46.
25. Kubler-Ross E. *On Death and Dying*. New York, NY: Macmillan; 1969.
26. *Hospice Facts and Figures*. NHPCO. https://www.nhpco.org/wp-content/uploads/2019/07/2018_NHPCO_Facts_Figures.pdf. Accessed November 13, 2019.
27. *Mission and Vision*. NHPCO. http://my.nhpco.org/aboutourcommunity/aboutnhpco/nhpcomissionvision/. Accessed October 7, 2019.
28. *Conditions for Coverage (CfC) & Conditions of Participation (COPs); Hospice*. 42 CFR 418.3, 418.52-116. https://www.cms.gov/CFCsAndCoPs/05_Hospice.asp. Accessed November 21, 2019.
29. *Hospice Quality Reporting Program*. https://www.cms.gov/Medicare/Quality-Initiatives-Patient-Assessment-Instruments/Hospice-Quality-Reporting/Current-Measures. Accessed November 21, 2019.
30. *Hospice Compare Datasets*. https://data.medicare.gov/data/hospice-compare. Accessed November 21, 2019.
31. *Medicare Benefit Policy Manual. Chapter 9. Coverage of Hospice Services Under Hospital Insurance*. 2018. https://www.cms.gov/media/125141. Accessed January 12, 2020.
32. Lamont EB, Christakis NA. Physician factors in the timing of cancer patient referral to hospice palliative care. *Cancer*. 2002;94:2733-2737.
33. Sexauer A, Cheng MJ, Knight L, et al. Patterns of hospice use in patients dying from hematologic malignancies. *J Palliat Med*. 2014;17:195-199.
34. Amano K, Morita T, Tatara R, Katayama H, Uno T, Takagi I. Association between early palliative care referrals, inpatient hospice utilization, and aggressiveness of care at the end of life. *J Palliat Med*. 2015;18(3):270-273.

35. Jennings B, Ryndes T, D'Onofrio C, et al. Access to hospice care: expanding boundaries, overcoming barriers. *Hastings Cent Rep.* 2003;2:S3-S9, S9-S13, S15-S21.

36. ABT Associates. *Evaluation of the Medicare Care Choices Model: Annual Report #1.* https://innovation.cms.gov/Files/reports/mccm-firstannrpt.pdf. Accessed November 19, 2019.

37. Friebert S. *NHPCO Facts and Figures: Pediatric Palliative and Hospice Care in America.* 2009. http://www.nhpco.org/files/public/quality/Pediatric_Facts-Figures.pdf. Accessed October 7, 2011.

38. Institute of Medicine Board on Health Science Policy. *When Children Die: Improving Palliative and End-of-Life Care for Children and Their Families.* 2003. https://www.nap.edu/catalog/10390/when-children-die-improving-palliative-and-end-of-life-care. Accessed January 12, 2020.

39. Li J, Precht DH, Mortensen PB, et al. Mortality in parents after death of a child in Denmark: a nationwide follow-up study. *Lancet.* 2003;361(9355):363-367.

40. Yu Y, Liew Z, Cnattingius S, et al. Association of mortality with the death of a sibling in childhood. *JAMA Pediatr.* 2017;171(6):538-545. doi:10.1001/jamapediatrics.2017.0197.

41. Tulsky J. Hope and hubris. *J Palliat Med.* 2002;5:339-341.

42. Kutner JS, Blake M, Meyer SA. Predictors of live hospice discharge: data from the National Home and Hospice Care Survey (NHHCS). *Am J Hosp Palliat Care.* 2002;19:331-337.

43. Casarett DJ, Hirschman KB, Crowley R, et al. Caregivers' satisfaction with hospice care in the last 24 hours of life. *Am J Hosp Palliat Care.* 2003;20:205-210.

44. Miceli PJ, Mylod DE. Satisfaction of families using end-of-life care: current successes and challenges in the hospice industry. *Am J Hosp Palliat Care.* 2003;20:360-370.

45. Christakis NA, Iwashyna TJ. The health impact of health care on families: a matched cohort study of hospice use by decedents and mortality outcomes in surviving, widowed spouses. *Soc Sci Med.* 2003;57:465-475.

46. Elsayem A, Swint K, Fisch M, et al. Palliative care inpatient service in a comprehensive cancer center: clinical and financial outcomes. *Clin Oncol.* 2004;22:2008-2014.

47. Campbell ML, Frank RR. Experience with an end-of-life practice at a university hospital. *Crit Care Med.* 1997; 25:197-202.

48. Harrison JP, Ford D, Wilson K. The impact of hospice programs on US hospitals. *Nurs Econ.* 2005; 23:78-84.

49. Earle CC, Neville BA, Landrum MB, et al. Trends in the aggressiveness of cancer care near the end of life. *J Clin Oncol.* 2004;22:315-321.

50. Taylor DH, Osterman J, Van Houtven CH, Tulsky J, Steinhauser K. What length of hospice use maximizes reduction in medical expenditures near death in the US Medicare program? *Soc Sci Med.* 2007;65: 1466-1478.

51. Pyenson B, Connor S, Fitch K, et al. Medicare cost in matched hospice and non-hospice cohorts. *J Pain Symptom Manage.* 2004;28:200-210.

52. Higginson IJ, Finlay IG, Goodwin DM, et al. Do hospital-based palliative teams improve care for patients or families at the end of life? *J Pain Symptom Manage.* 2002;23:96-106.

53. Dunlop RJ, Hockey JM. *Hospital-Based Palliative Care Teams: The Hospital-Hospice Interface.* New York, NY: Oxford University Press; 1998.

54. Meier DE. When pain and suffering do not require a prognosis: working toward meaningful hospital-hospice partnership. *J Palliat Med.* 2003;6:109-115.

55. *Center for Advancement of Palliative Care.* http://www.capc.org/. Accessed January 12, 2020.

WEB-BASED RESOURCES

56. American Academy of Hospice and Palliative Medicine (AAHPM). http://www.aahpm.org

57. Center for Advancement of Palliative Care (CAPC). http://www.capc.org

58. National Association of Homecare (NAHC). http://www.nahc.org

59. *Clinical Practice Guidelines for Quality Palliative Care, 4th Edition.* https://www.nationalcoalitionhpc.org/ncp/. Accessed November 19, 2019.

60. National Hospice and Palliative Care Organization. http://www.nhpco.org

61. Pediatric Palliative Care. https://pediatrics.aappublications.org/content/106/2/351

62. https://www.uptodate.com/contents/pediatric-palliative-care

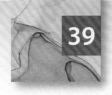

39 Cultural Issues in Palliatives and Supportive Oncology

Joseph F. O'Neill, Margaret M. Mahon, and Gregory Pappas

INTRODUCTION

"Analogous to the 3 physical states of water, which can exist as a solid, a liquid, or a gas, and still be constituted of the same fundamental substances...persons experiencing illness exist in 3 interrelated states or identities. Attention to the multiplicity of perspectives of individuals rendered vulnerable by illness is at the heart of providing competent and humane medical care. Recognizing that every person is "like all others" identifies the notion of a shared common humanity and universal needs when facing serious and life-threatening illness. Recognizing that every person is "like some others" acknowledges that we share commonalities with certain tribal and cultural groups and not with others. Finally, affirming that every person is "like no others" speaks to the very important need to individualize care and to assess the specific circumstances of illness and the particular needs of individuals with unique preferences and personal values."

Richard Payne, MD (1)

The challenge of addressing all these states of personhood is never trivial, especially when providing support and palliative care to someone living with, or dying from, cancer. Often the humanity that is shared by patient and provider ("like all others") allows a relationship to form that feels natural and easy and that allows the provider to imagine and comprehend the patient's perspective despite differences in language, experience, or education. Similarly, understanding the unique aspects of a particular person's disease, psychology, or other needs ("like no others") can also be, if not straightforward, at least easier for health care providers to understand than the "like some others"—the cultural—aspects of personhood.

CULTURE

The Cambridge English Dictionary defines "culture" as "the way of life, especially the general customs and beliefs, of a particular group of people at a particular time" (2). This definition can be useful in the clinical setting only insofar as it is understood that, ultimately, the "particular group" is the patient and family being treated, and the particular time is the immediate clinical situation you and your patient face. To draw broader generalizations risks stereotyping the patient; this can harm, sometimes seriously, the doctor–patient relationship.

All of us, patient and provider alike, live and work in complex and dynamic cultural contexts that influence how illness is viewed, understood, treated, and discussed. These cultural contexts have an impact on every aspect of life: language, dress, interpersonal interactions, traditions, definitions of family, styles of communication, decision making processes, perspectives, beliefs, attitudes, understanding of history, and individual expressions of thoughts and emotions. Culture is part of what makes us individuals. It influences how we connect with others, including those we care for and those who care for us.

Cultural beliefs and practices are often fundamental guideposts on the search to find meaning in life and, hence, are especially important when facing care transitions, suffering, and death. Culture is an integral dimension of each person. Therefore, respect for the individual person, a fundamental ethical principle of contemporary bioethics, must encompass understanding of, and respect for, each patient's cultures.

MEDICAL CULTURE

Medicine itself can be understood as a culture, with shared experience, goals, and rites of passage. The Editors of the JAMA Journal of Ethics noted in an editorial (3) *"The culture of medicine is an elusive concept; it can at once evoke images of benevolent men and women offering themselves in service of the sick and vulnerable and images of a patriarchal institution marred by elitism and the abuse of power. A complex interplay among the people in medicine, the institutions that train them, and the society within which both function contributes to these incongruous images. The culture of medicine is influenced by its rich history and the most recent trends in medical attitudes and practices. In order to portray adequately the discourse and norms surrounding the profession, we must take all of these elements into account. Perhaps one reason defining and discussing culture can be so challenging is that so much of what forms and sustains it is implicit. The culture of medicine is not only defined by what doctors do, say, feel, and think, but also by what they do not do, say, feel, or think. What one is expected to read between the lines, or to "pick up on," without being explicitly told is very much a part of medical—indeed any— culture; the norms and expectations that lie just beneath the surface can be as influential as anything codified. Thus, there can be a disconnect between what the medical field purports to do and what actually happens on the wards or in the classroom."*

This shared culture borne of common experiences and beliefs, despite the heterogeneity of those who are physicians, can itself lead to different life and death experiences. For example, at end of life, physicians are less likely to have care in an emergency department, but more likely to have hospital care and intensive care. Similarly, physicians with cancer were more likely to receive chemotherapy at end of life. Physicians were also more likely to receive opioids, and to have them for a longer period of time (4). In this case, it is unclear if differences were due to physician choices or physicians writing orders differently for colleagues, but it does seem apparent that the culture of medicine led to differences in care.

It is important, therefore, for physicians who are caring for cancer patients to understand that, just as a patient's views, beliefs and attitudes are influenced by culture, so too are their own. One's professional education plays no small part in this.

Medical Education and Culture

Individuals grow up in the context of not only their ethnicity but in the environment of their neighborhood, religion (or lack thereof), school and more. Medicine adds to this its own culture, as do disciplines of medical specialties and subspecialties: Surgeons can be said to have a different culture, for example, than psychiatrists, and, in turn, biomedically oriented psychiatrists may differ from psychoanalysts in cultural and professional norms.

Medical education itself is affected by ethnicity and other dimensions of culture. Nameni and Dowlatabadi (5) studied multiple dimensions of intercultural sensitivity (IS) and intercultural communicative competence (ICC) by studying, and finding variability between, four ethnic groups of Iranian medical students. Health care providers unfamiliar with the complexities of Iranian society might think of there being a single culture in Iran and be surprised to learn that even between Iranian medical students, people differed in awareness, knowledge, and skills. Foong and colleagues (6) also found difference between cultural subgroups (i.e., Chinese). Such differences may affect attitudes about communication skills and even educational success. This points to the complexity of culture and the challenges medical educators

face in developing young physicians' intercultural skills.

In a study of the educational experiences of nonwhite students in medicine and biomedical sciences in the United Kingdom (7), ethnicity or race was perceived by both students and faculty as having significant effects across educational experiences. These differences in experiences were posited to lead to attainment gap. Minority students had smaller social networks that were divided by race/ethnicity. Faculty believed that minority students might therefore have fewer resources, because of informal transmission of knowledge that occurs within social networks. The authors also suggested that faculty bias might affect students' experiences, further leading to the attainment gap. As a result, even Black students, Asian students, or students from other minorities who have been accepted to medical or biomedical education might be less likely to progress to graduation.

Health Disparities

No discussion of cultural aspects of palliative and supportive oncology in the United States (and many other countries) can ignore the reality of racial/ethnic health disparities and the roles that the majority society and medicine have historically played, and can still play, in their etiology.

A systematic review (8) of end of life care for patients with cancer showed, for example, that African Americans typically perceived a need for hospice care. Nonetheless, respondents frequently had poor knowledge of hospice care, preferred aggressive treatments, less often had documented care plans, and used hospice care less frequently than did white Americans. Similarly, systematic reviews of pain and ethnicity (9) and palliative care and ethnic disparities (10) found that minority patients were more likely to have less access to pain management, were more likely to have their pain underestimated by providers, and were less likely to have their pain treated than whites.

It is particularly important to note that many patients may have a personal, family, or community history of discrimination or poor health care. These personal experiences of discrimination may, if not addressed, undermine trust, and complicate efforts to palliate symptoms and to provide supportive care.

Cultural Health Practices: Beliefs and Healing

One of the rich and rewarding aspects of medical practice is the opportunity it affords to engage with, and learn from, patients with cultural backgrounds and beliefs different from one's own. Setting aside for the moment, cultural or religious practices that are, from western medicine's perspective, deleterious to health, (e.g., refusal of blood products), many healing practices can complement, and some may even augment, the oncologist's skills. An NIH consensus statement (11), for example, found some promising results for acupuncture in management of chemotherapy-associated nausea. Similarly, acupuncture has been found to relieve dyspnea in patients with severe disease (12).

Healing, a concept here defined broadly as the transcendence of suffering (i.e., not just pain or symptom management or management of disease), can occur even when medical therapies prove to be inadequate to achieve hoped-for goals. Such healing can be heavily reliant on psychosocial and spiritual practices that, in turn, are often founded in cultural beliefs and practices. Identifying, understanding, and respecting rituals, beliefs, notions, patterns of decision making, practices, and even the use of certain objects can therefore be very helpful in care and support of oncology patients.

Approach to the Patient

The U.S. Department of Health and Human Services Office of Minority Health established its Center for Linguistic and Cultural Competence in Health Care in 1995 and in 2000 promulgated National Standards in this regard. Since then a range of activities and trainings designed to assist health practitioners improve cultural competency have been made available, including specific guides and training for physicians (13).

Cultural competence training is believed to be an important means to decrease disparities in access to health care (14). A 2014 Cochrane review (15) of cultural competence education for health professionals found five studies that assessed the impact of cultural competence training on patient-related outcomes. They found positive but low-quality evidence for improvement in involvement of culturally and linguistically diverse (CALD) patients in their care but concluded that "uncertainty exists about the best and most effective way to educate health professionals in cultural competence that leads to improved health outcomes for CALD populations."

Kleinman and Benson (16) note that the Cultural Competency approach: (a) "...suggests that culture can be reduced to a technical skill for which clinicians can be trained"; (b) "...cultural factors are not always central to a case"; (c) the culture of the clinician is often not factored into the analysis; (d) "attention to cultural difference can be interpreted by patients and families intrusive, and might even contribute to a sense of being singled out and stigmatized"; and (e) "overemphasis on cultural difference can lead to the mistaken idea that if we can only identify the cultural root of the problem, it can be resolved." These authors prefer an "ethnographic" approach to the patient and family that is intended to better see the illness experience through the their eyes. The ethnographic approach emphasizes frank conversation to understand the patient's and family's view of their ethnicity and how important it is to their sense of self; what is at stake as they face illness; how they understand and explain their illness, its cause, and its treatment; what they fear; what psychosocial stressors and supports they have; and, finally how culture (theirs and yours) might impact on the ongoing physician–patient relationship.

Ethnography to improve cultural competence in medicine has been attempted in several venues. Dao and colleagues have used ethnography to improve care via a cultural consultation service. They acknowledge its limitations, however, writing, "while clinical ethnographic interviewing skills can be successfully taught and learned, the 'real-world' context of medical practice may impose barriers to such patient-centered interviewing" (17).

Another means of assessing culture in the clinical setting has been suggested by Kagawa-Singer as a means of avoiding stereotyping and improving communication (see Fig. 39.1) (18).

All of these approaches are intended to assist the development of an effective relationship between health care provider and patient during a stressful time of illness while avoiding stigmatization and stereotyping. The easiest way to do this is to simply talk to the patient (or appropriate family member or friend) exploring the issues identified by Kleinman, Benson, Kawaga-Singer, and Blackhall, and to be open to the education that will ensue. This requires both curiosity and humility but, in the long run, can greatly benefit the clinical relationship.

ETIQUETTE

Following basic rules of etiquette when interacting with a patient, family, or loved one, especially one where cultural difference between the provider and patient could increase the chance of misunderstandings, can be helpful. Additionally, as Judith Martin (Miss Manners) pointed out, etiquette is important because it "makes you feel at ease, helps you exude confidence, and contributes to overall confidence." It can have the same impact on patients if, for no other reason, it helps to avoid making a bad first impression—something that can be all too easy to do if there are cultural differences at play. Showing interest in a patient's culture and how they view health and illness, on the other hand, almost always helps.

While, for example, it may be permissible, or even desirable, for a physician working in a college health center to address a patient by first name, an

Issue	Possible Consequences of Ignoring the Issue	Techniques and Strategies to Address the Issue
Responses to inequities in care.	Lack of trust Increased desire for futile aggressive care at the end of life Lack of collaboration with patient and with the family Dissatisfaction with care by all parties involved	Address directly: "I wonder whether it's hard for you to trust a physician who is not____[of your same background]?" Make explicit that you and the patient and their family will work together in achieving the best care possible Work to improve access and reduce inequities Understand and accommodate desires for more aggressive care, and use respectful negotiation when this is contraindicated or medically futile
Communication/language barriers	Bidirectional misunderstanding Unnecessary physical, emotional, and spiritual suffering	Take time to: Avoid medical or complex jargon Check for understanding: "So I can make sure I'm explaining this well for you, please tell me what your understanding is about your illness and the treatment we're considering" Hire bilingual, bicultural staff and train in medical translation to be bridges across cultures. Translators are preferable in person, but use AT&T language line or similar services, if trained staff unavailable Avoid use of family as translators, especially minors
Religion and spirituality	Lack of faith in the physician Lack of adherence to the treatment regimen	"Spiritual or religious strength sustains many people in times of distress. What is important for us to know about your faith or spiritual needs?" "How can we support your needs and practices?" "Where do you find your strength to make sense of this experience?"
Truth telling	Anger, mistrust, or even removal of patient from health care system if team insists on informing the patient against the wishes of the family Hopelessness in the patient if he or she misunderstands your reason for telling him or her directly	Informed refusal: "Some patients want to know everything about their condition, others prefer that the doctors mainly talk to their families. How would you prefer to get this information?" Use a hypothetical case, eg, "Others who have conditions similar to yours have found it helpful to consider several options for care, such as nutrition, to keep them feeling as well as possible" Be cognizant of nonverbal or indirect communication when discussing serious information
Family involvement in decision-making	Disagreement and conflict between family and medical staff when the family, rather than the patient, insists on making decisions	Ascertain the key members of the family and ensure that all are included in discussions as desired by the patient: "Is there anyone else that I should talk to about your condition?" Talk with whomever accompanies the patient and ask the patient about this individual's involvement in receiving information and decision-making
Hospice care	Reduced use of hospice services, leading to decreased quality of end-of-life care	Emphasize hospice as an adjunct or assistance to the family but not as a replacement: "When the family is taking care of the patient at home, hospice can help them do that"

Figure 39.1 Techniques for negotiating issues influenced by culture that are important in end of life care.

older patient, especially one from a culture where formality is normative, may be offended. Similarly, a male physician placing a stethoscope on the chest of an adult male without first formally asking permission to conduct a physical examination would raise few eyebrows. Doing the same thing to a woman recently arrived in the United States from Saudi Arabia could be experienced as a serious violation of cultural norms.

The point of establishing one's own etiquette habits is, then, to ensure, as far as possible, that one does not unknowingly offend a patient. Short of developing an encyclopedic base of knowledge about every culture on the planet, behaving in ways that minimize the risk of error, etiquette, is good practice.

Some basic rules of medical etiquette include the following:

- Sit, facing the patient directly. If you are using a language interpreter make sure you address the patient, not the interpreter.
- Introduce yourself.
- Unless faced with an emergency situation do not touch the patient without first asking permission.
- Ask the patient how he or she wishes to be addressed.
- Maintain a professional appearance.
- Start your interview with a little "small talk." Important information (e.g., "Do you have children? Where are they?") can be asked before diving directly into disease or symptom-oriented questions and will, thereby, communicate your interest in, and openness to, understanding psychosocial and spiritual aspects of their lives.

CONCLUSION

Culture is most often understood as relating to race and heritage. Customs, practices, and beliefs may, however, arise from shared life experiences and identities, such as neighborhood, profession, religion, school, professional union, sports team, or other factors. These many variables that the physician and the patient bring to the clinical interaction affect both content and process. Culture, then, is not just complex, but the *experience* of culture can also be complex and result in even the most open-minded, aware, knowledgeable, and skilled physician or nurse struggling to have an interaction with a patient and family unimpeded by cultural stereotypes or unconscious bias.

Self-awareness, a basic set of etiquette skills and a good faith, and open and humble willingness to learn from patients what their culture means to them and how best to work across cultural differences will go a long way to minimize these difficulties and foster the kind of therapeutic and supportive relationship that cancer patients seek.

REFERENCES

1. Payne R. Culturally relevant palliative care. *Clin Geriatr Med.* 2015;31:271-279.
2. Culture. In *Cambridge English Dictionary*. https://dictionary.cambridge.org/dictionary/english/culture. Accessed April 10, 2020.
3. Michalska-Smith M. Describing a Culture from Within. *AMA J Ethics.* 2015;17(2):108-110. https://journalofethics.ama-assn.org/sites/journalofethics.ama-assn.org/files/2018-06/vm-1502.pdf
4. Wunsch H, Scales D, Gershengorn HB, et al. End-of-life care received by physicians compared with non-physicians. *JAMA Netw Open.* 2019;2(7):e197650. doi: 10.1001/jamanetworkopen.2019.7650.
5. Nameni A, Dowlatabadi H. A study of the level of intercultural communicative competence and intercultural sensitivity of Iranian medical students based on ethnicity. *J Intercult Commun Res.* 2019;48(1):21-34. doi: 10.1080/17475759.2018.1549586 2 Ibid, p. 5.
6. Foong ALS, Sow CG, Ramasamy S, Yap PS. Pre-tertiary education, ethnicity, and attitudes of Asian medical undergraduates towards communication skills. *Int J Med Educ.* 2019;10:1-8. doi: 10.5116/ijme.5c30.988d. p. 5.
7. Claridge H, Stone K, Ussher M. The ethnicity attainment gap among medical and biomedical science students: a qualitative study. *BMC Med Educ.* 2018;18:325. doi: 10.1186/s12909-018-1426-5.
8. LoPresti MA, Dement F, Gold HT. End-of-life care for people with cancer from ethnic minority groups: a systematic review. *Am J Hosp Palliat Care.* 2016;33(3): 291-305.
9. Cintron A, Morrison RS. Pain and ethnicity in the United States: A systematic review. *J Palliat Med.* 2006;9(6):1454-1473.
10. Johnson KS. Racial and ethnic disparities in palliative care. *J Palliat Med.* 2013;16(11):1329-1334.
11. NIH Consensus Conference. Acupuncture. *JAMA.* 1998;280(17):1518-1524. https://www.ncbi.nlm.nih.gov/pubmed/9809733
12. von Trott P, Oei SL, Ramsenthaler C. Acupuncture for breathlessness in advanced diseases: a systematic review and meta-analysis. *J Pain Symptom Manage.* 2020;59(2):327-338.
13. US Department of Health & Human Services. *A Physician's Practical Guide to Culturally Competent Care. Think Cultural Health website.* Accessed December 1, 2020. https://cccm.thinkculturalhealth.hhs.gov/
14. Sorensen J, Norredam M, Dogra N, Essink-Bot ML, Suurmond J, Krasnik A. Enhancing cultural competence in medical education. *Int J Med Educ.* 2017;8:28-30. doi: 10.5116/ijme.587a.0333.
15. Horvat L, Horey D, Romios P, Kis-Rigo J. Cultural competence education for health professionals. *Cochrane Database Syst Rev.* 2014;(5):CD009405. doi: 10.1002/14651858.CD009405.pub2.
16. Kleinman A, Benson P. Anthropology in the clinic: the problem of cultural competency and how to fix it. *PLoS Med.* 2006;3(10):e294.
17. Dominicé Dao M, Inglin S, Vilpert S, et al. The relevance of clinical ethnography: reflections on 10 years of a cultural consultation service. *BMC Health Serv Res.* 2018;18:19. doi: 10.1186/s12913-017-2823.
18. Kagawa-Singer M, Blackhall LJ. Negotiating cross-cultural issues at the end of life: "You got to go where he lives". *JAMA.* 2001;286(23):2993-3001.

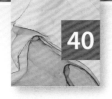

40 Communication During Transitions of Care

Anne M. Kelemen, Clara Van Gerven, and Terry Altilio

INTRODUCTION

There was no sudden, striking, and emotional transition. Like the warming of a room or the coming of daylight. When you first observe them, they have already been going on for some time (1).

This C.S. Lewis quote from his book *A Grief Observed* captures the nature of some of the transitions that an oncology patient may experience as they move from health through illness to possible remission, cure, or death. Some transitions are subtle and occur quietly over time with impact and significance felt only after the fog lifts and the landscape emerges. A pesky symptom that ceases to go away may be accommodated unobserved until a family member or friend comments on a pained facial expression, a limp, or change in mood. Other transitions may occur dramatically and elicit immediate attention like the results of a diagnostic study that dashes hope for a cure and raises the specter of life with a chronic illness or the anticipation of death.

Transitions can be a time of loss and adaptation, celebration, threat, or crises when equilibrium, often barely reestablished, may be disrupted by challenges to one's sense of self and the anticipated future. They may also elicit a process of defining what brings meaning to life and identifying strengths, supports, and values that sustain the patient and family for what comes next.

Clinicians, patients, and families experience many transitions from diagnosis to death. Many oncology specialists engage with patients and families over time and through periods of adjustment, adaptation, and moments of profound meaning (Nancy Bourque, M.S.W., email communication, September 30, 2019) such as:

- The surgeon who has to tell a patient that a surgical procedure revealed an inoperable cancer, leaving a visible scar, a permanent and constant reminder of a foreshortened life (Eugene Choi, MD, private communication, December 12, 2019).
- The oncologist who shares diagnostic findings that may warrant radiation therapy thereby asking patient and family to forge new relationships and build trust at a time of increased vulnerability.

- The cancer patient whose therapy has been successful and transitions to "survivorship" which may come with its own set of expectations, complex emotions, and fears as they separate from treatment teams that have become important as an integral part of their illness experience.
- The pediatric patient, their family, and caregivers who prepare for transition to "adult" practice and face thoughts and feelings that color this transition. For some it is a cause for celebration, for others a time of anticipatory anxiety and profound loss, and for many a combination of both.

Transitions occur within the course of active treatment and after treatments have ended. Patients may transition to different settings such as extended care or subacute rehabilitation facilities or be asked to consider accepting help in their homes—events that often require adaptation and effort to maintain a coherent sense of self in the face of increased physical dependence and potential loss of privacy. During these transitions, the words used to communicate, the information shared, the silence to be honored, and the patience practiced impact the emotional and cognitive response of the patient, their family, or fictive kin to what is said (and what is not said).

Conversations that mark transitions are not just about sharing serious information. Because they occur within relationships, they are also an opportunity for an empathic exchange that can explore the patient's unique narrative and discover their feelings, fears and hopes, strengths, and supports that bring meaning and direction to a plan of care.

Communication in health care has been enhanced through the creation of learning tools focused on skill training often directed toward the delivery of important news and the recognition of emotion in the responses of patients, families, and clinicians (2). Finally, communication technology has progressed and has the potential both to create and support connection or to distance and thereby enhance or impede relationship and care. Thus, the integration of technology often requires education as well as a shared understanding of the potential benefits for patient and family and clinician.

This chapter intends to:

1. Review recent literature concerning health care clinician communication about transitions in care and between clinicians across settings.
2. Identify transitions that may serve as opportunities to enhance adaptation and reframe meaning as illness evolves.
3. Provide guidance in recognizing and intervening with common topics that arise when caring for patients with serious illness—sharing important news, discussing advance care planning (ACP), changing goals of care, and mediating prognostic awareness.

HEALTH CARE CLINICIANS' COMMUNICATION

Communication between health care clinicians and seriously ill patients is fundamental to good care. How this occurs, however, can vary—sometimes greatly. Importantly, in addition to the unique training and communication skills of individuals, effective communication is often most productive when it is an interdisciplinary team (IDT) effort where different disciplines collaborate and utilize their expertise to the best effect (3).

How health care teams balance organizational expectations while maintaining professional and personal standards can change the nature of any single team member's labor. The effect of team versus solo communication is especially notable. Team communication in safe practice environments enhances "deep acting" where clinicians identify, regulate, and modify emotion to match expressed affect (4). In a theme that will recur throughout this chapter, the quality of communication between those providing care sets the stage for conversations with patients, families, and colleagues and provides support to all involved when it is effective.

How information is delivered matters. Training clinicians in communication can reduce patient anxiety and enhance trust (5). In practice, however, communication is often hindered by lack of both training and self-awareness. Clinicians can miss opportunities to elicit patients' concerns and, when they do elicit them, will often interrupt the patient and, in doing so, abort chances to enhance empathy and better understand and validate the unique narrative of their experience of illness (6). How communication around transitions in care is handled, for better or worse, has significant impacts on patients' quality of life (7). The shared discovery of values, feelings, hopes, and concerns informs critical thinking that guides clinicians to effectively bridge transitions.

While communication skills are essential to each professional discipline, the unique role of physicians makes the impact of their choice of words (or decision to remain silent) especially important. For those who accompany and guide patients through illness and difficult transitions, being able to communicate well is a critically important tool, yet it is not often high on the list of skills prioritized during formal medical training.

Poor communication, while common, is not inevitable. Fortunately, as the emphasis on patient-centered, family-focused care has grown, so too have the tools available to improve clinicians' communication skills (8–12). Communication training for clinicians is expanding rapidly and is still building its evidence base (13–15). In this evolving area, it is important to rely on proven approaches where they are available and to follow current developments in this specialty area of practice.

WHAT MAKES FOR GOOD COMMUNICATION?

The skills honed by communication training, including the ability to express empathy, are linked to improved outcomes (16). While a primary focus of medical conversations during transitions is often on information to be delivered and plans to be made, this can leave little room for pauses—the silences that allow those present to process what has been conveyed—and to consider their responses. The ability to sit with silence, listen, and maintain a calm body language is a clinician's ally in building trust and facilitating a two-way conversation with patients and their families. Both verbal and nonverbal communications contribute to the level of rapport that develops and, in turn, to patient outcomes (16,17).

How clinicians manage their own emotions in the context of their roles and institutional pressures has consequences for patient care especially when working with patients who are expected to die (18). The mandate to lessen mortality rates in hospital settings is an example of these institutional pressures. The nature of these emotional responses is often discipline specific. For the physician, a range feeling such as failure, guilt, sadness, or impotence can surface. These may be acknowledged and valued, yet not necessarily experienced in the same way, by team members who do not have responsibility for the medical treatment of cancer. Although medical education has historically de-emphasized this component, it is essential to recognize that clinicians are active participants in clinical communication encounters. As discussed below, recognizing and addressing both the patient's and the clinician's emotions is an important aspect of good communication that builds trust (19). Attending to one's own emotional reactions to caring for patients requires a consciousness of the words or behaviors that reflect these emotions and influence the process of communication. This dynamic will be explored more fully following an overview of basic communication skills.

COMMUNICATION SKILLS

Explaining the implications of a chronic disease, the need for rehabilitation, or talking about a terminal illness or end-of-life care all requires basic communication skills. The primary difference between these communications is the emotional significance the clinician may place on the conversation and the anticipation of its meaning to patients and families. Recognizing one's feelings of sadness, worry, or vulnerability is often an indication that the conversation is likely needed and preparation might begin with the clinician processing, privately or with team members, their own emotions about the patient and family—the questions and emotions they anticipate. It is helpful to remember that patients often have an intuitive sense and understanding when things are not going well and if given time and opportunity will share these perceptions. Thus the conversation may not necessarily be a surprise. Clinicians who allow for open communication starting from diagnosis create relationships that may make the transition of care conversations a natural part of shared care planning as the disease progresses.

Basic communication etiquette includes sitting at eye level, turning pagers or cell phone off, and striving to avoid other interruptions. While the pressures of documentation and productivity are real, attending to a computer screen rather than maintaining eye contact creates distance and impairs the process of observing nonverbal and behavioral cues. This, in turn, disrupts the interpersonal connection with the patient and family that is so important to successful communication. Consider abandoning the computer, pen and paper, and other distractions, and focus your attention on the reactions and responses of patients and their families.

Differences in culture impact communication and may influence verbal and behavioral response of patient and their family. The chapter on culture in this volume provides further information on this topic. Critically, it is important for the clinician to practice empathic inquiry rather than making assumptions about patients' and families' preferences, decision-making process, who is part of their family, how they function and provide care. For patients or families for whom English is not their first language or who are deaf, engage a trained interpreter unless you are fluent. It is not appropriate to utilize hospital staff unless they have been trained as interpreters. Using family members can place an unnecessary burden on family who may agree to the role, unaware of the information they will be asked to interpret (20). In addition, engaging family to interpret creates a circumstance and a risk as clinicians do not know if their words have been interpreted correctly.

A serious conversation with a patient or family can be no less risky than an invasive procedure. Both require thoughtful preparation including an understanding of who the patient chooses to be present. If the patient is able, they can tell you. Advance directives and living wills provide direction when the patient is unable to provide this guidance. It is best, whenever possible, to meet in person, but using various communication technologies can be helpful if face-to-face meetings are not possible. Additionally, with careful planning these technologies allow participation of family or clinicians who may be geographically very distant.

It is helpful for the involved teams to meet prior to discussions with patient and family to decide which clinicians from the IDT are essential to the conversation. Often the participation of nurses, chaplains, or social workers in family meetings enriches the process by bringing in different perspectives, information, and communication skills. Equally important is a sharing across teams of the information to be shared, acknowledging where disagreement may exist, and deciding how that disagreement will be handled within the meeting. Anticipating questions and concerns can serve to mitigate clinician anxiety. While medical and nursing jargon is appropriate and comfortable within teams, it can confuse and distance patients and families and when used requires clear explanation by clinicians. Pause frequently to invite questions, check for understanding, allow words to settle, and acknowledge emotion or nonverbal behavior.

Ask open-ended questions which invite answers beyond a brief response or a "yes" or "no." Focus on patient and family affects as well as their concerns. Open-ended questions invite dialogue and are an antidote to the tendency of physicians to do most of the talking in family meetings (21).

There are a variety of algorithms that exist to guide clinicians and to invite the naming and exploration of emotions. These include SPIKES (Table 40.1) which provides a protocol and structure for family meetings and NURSE, which guides clinicians in addressing emotions (22–25).

Below is a sample script which uses SPIKES to help guide the discussion. Prior to the start of this conversation, the clinician has invited the patient

TABLE 40.1 THE SPIKES PROTOCOL

SPIKES	
S	**Setting** up the Interview: Be comfortable with the history: who participates, when, and where
P	Assessing the Patient's **Perception**: Beyond knowledge to what is seen and realized
I	Obtaining the Patient's **Invitation**: How do they wish to receive information and plan
K	Giving **Knowledge** and Information: In clear language, reflecting awareness of illness history
E	Addressing the Patient's **Emotions**: After listening and allowing for silence
S	**Strategy or Summary**: After insuring all have expressed feelings, thoughts, and questions

Baile W, Buckaman R, Lenzi R, Glober G, Beale E, Kudelka A. SPIKES—a six-step protocol for delivering bad news: application to the patient with cancer. *Oncologist.* 2000;5:302-311.

to engage necessary family members, sets up a quiet room to meet, had enough chairs and tissues available, and coordinated the use of SKYPE or conference calls to engage distant family. Start with introductions and a request for others to raise questions and concerns to create a shared agenda.

Doctor: I'm wondering if you can share what you have been told about your cancer, what you are seeing day to day and how you've been feeling?

Patient: I know there are multiple tumors and the cancer has spread beyond my breast. We are talking today because you have some results of my latest scans. I feel a bit weaker, but my pain is manageable and my appetite okay.

Doctor: That is correct. Good to hear that your pain is managed, and we can talk a bit later about your tiredness. Have you other things that you would want us to talk about today?

Silence while waiting for an answer.

Doctor: How would you like me to share information today? I know that in the past, you have wanted to hear everything. Is that how you feel today, or would you prefer I share with your family?

Patient: Yes. I would prefer you speak with me and my family.

Family members agree so the meeting can continue.

Doctor: So the scans did not show what we had been hoping for; the cancer has now spread to your liver and lungs.

Patient: I've been worried about this. I mean I can feel my body changing.

Doctor: I wish that things were different.

Patient: It's not (starts to cry…allow for some silence).

Doctor: Can you talk a bit about how you feel your body is changing?

Patient: The weakness and I know I am losing weight.

Doctor: It is difficult to experience changes in your body (silence).

Doctor: Is it okay if I ask your family to share their thoughts, feelings, or questions?

Patient: No, I do not want to hear anymore.

Doctor: Okay. We talked about important things today, and we need to think about planning for your care and where we go from here. Do you want to do that now or when I see you next week?

Patient: I think maybe next week.

Doctor: Do you want to talk a bit about your tiredness?

Patient: No that can wait.

Doctor: Okay, I want to give you my direct number again if you think of anything when you leave. I'm also going to call you in a few days to check in and make sure your pain and other symptoms are controlled.

Patient: That sounds good. Thank you.

COMMUNICATING OVER THE TRANSITION

Implicit in all transitions, regardless of intent or significance, is change, and change makes demands on the patient, the family, and the clinicians involved in care. Transition to a subacute rehabilitation facility with the intent of improved function and continued treatment creates a very different set of responses and communication challenges than referral, for example, for a home hospice plan of care.

It is never safe to assume the meaning and impact of any transition. Every situation, patient, and family are unique. Placement in a facility even for a short time, for some, means separation from family and imposition of an undesired structure and set of rules. For others it may mean a welcome respite. A family with resources and good insurance may experience no financial consequences, whereas families with limited resources or physical limitations might have to travel long distances and endure financial and physical hardship simply to visit the patient.

A discussion about transition to home care might elicit varied, and even mixed, responses—a feeling of relief, a loss of privacy, intrusion or fear that this implies disease progression, or a judgment that family cannot provide care. Placement of a semielectric bed in the home with the intent of easing care and enhancing comfort may also symbolize the loss of comfort and the intimacy that comes from sharing a bed with partners.

All clinicians can be sensitized to the potential impacts and meaning of changes in care. Social work can play a central role in responding to the psychosocial and cultural meanings which may be implicit in some transitions while also attending to logistical concerns. Times of transition and changes in care plans create opportunity to better understand how patients, families, and care partners are adapting and to join with them in discovering meaning and sources of support and solving problems.

The meaning attributed to transitions may differ between team members. Such variation may be a function of role, relationship with the patient and family, and professional as well as personal expectations. A physician, for example, whose focus has been on extending life may struggle with feelings of failure, sadness, abandonment, and even despair when a hospice referral is warranted. On the other hand, they may feel relief and satisfaction that they did all that could be done and had done it well. Likewise, the same situation may elicit varied emotional responses from members of other disciplines whose role does not include decisions about disease management and the responsibility for communicating difficult information.

Perhaps the most important goal of any communication with patients or family is to understand the important and enduring values and beliefs that support and sustain them beyond the medical setting and illness experience. These sustaining forces weave through the past, inform the present, and frame the imagining of the future. By placing a current transition in this context, we demonstrate respect for continuity of life and relationships and perhaps identify strengths to face current challenges.

These questions and statements invite sharing of values and may help to place a current transition into the larger context of a life, a future, and treatment relationships:

- We know that many patients and families have managed difficult circumstances in their lives. I wanted to start by understanding a bit about how you and your family have managed troubles in the past?
- Have you had illness and deaths in your family? Current? Past?
- What helps you make sense of the current situation?
- Have you had religious or spiritual practice that has grounded you over the years?

- Do you feel a sense of control in your situation? Are there others who might have some control over your situation?

THE POWER OF LANGUAGE; RAISING WORD CHOICE TO CONSCIOUSNESS

"Words not only convey something, but are something; that words have color, depth, texture of their own, & the power to evoke vastly more than they mean; that words can be used not merely to make things clear, make things vivid, make things interesting; but to make things happen inside the one who hears them." (26)

The language of health care abounds with unconscious use of jargon, idioms, and metaphors which have become second nature for many. While these words and phrases may enhance professional communication between peers, they can cloud conversation with patients and family members the intent of which is to be understood, build trust, engage, and support their participation in decision-making and discover what brings meaning to their lives (27).

Oncology conversations are often replete with war and sports metaphors. Terms like "winning," "losing," "victory," "defeat," or "failure" are woven through the media, public discourse, and the messages of oncology advocacy groups. The inferences of winning and losing, victory or defeat, and victim or survivor for some may be energizing and for others project an expectation that bears no relationship to their sense of self or the experience of illness (28). The following spontaneous hallway exchange links clinician and patient in a unique and poignant example of the conscious and unconscious thoughts and feelings that infuse relationships and drive word choice.

Oncology Physician Fellow referring a patient to palliative care: She has failed chemotherapy.
Palliative Social Worker: Patients don't fail chemotherapy.
Oncology Fellow: If she did not fail then I did.
Palliative Social Worker: There is no place for failure if all did the best they could with the tools available to them.

The above exchange captures the potential of varied disciplines who hear differently to create an opportunity to notice and challenge the dynamics that underlie word choice toward the goal of increasing insight and perhaps mitigating distress related to transitions that portend end of life. Consider the implications of the following statement.

"If you go to rehab we can see if you get stronger and then perhaps give you more chemotherapy."

At times these well-intended words reflect an authentic possibility, and at other times, they can confuse, set unreal expectation, and delay difficult conversation about evolving disease and end of life. Rather than place a burden on patient and family to pursue an elusive possibility, it is often more appropriate to focus on a transition that involves increased awareness and invites preparation for end of life.

Language used during transitions has the potential to link the past, present, and future in clear and understandable ways—to build and join rather than negate and distance. Consider the difference between the words "but" and "and" and the words "wish" and "hope" in the following exchange with a daughter struggling to integrate the meaning of mother's responsiveness (29,30).

"I hear your **hope** that your mother is responding **but** the doctors indicate this is not purposeful."
"I hear your **hope** that your mother is responding **and** we **wish** her responses were purposeful."

The uncertainty inherent in clinical care, along with time pressures, conflicting agendas and other factors inherent in contemporary health care can disrupt relationships and the sense of shared humanity between patient and provider that could, if allowed to flourish, transcend disease and enrich therapeutic interventions. Consider, for example, how acknowledgement of a patient's history joins family and provider to enhance a conversation about present decisions and planning for the future.

"As we talked about this past Monday, we continued ventilator support to see if the antibiotics might improve Mr. J's lungs so he could breathe on his own. The antibiotics have not created the outcome we had hoped for."

This introduction to discussion might simply be followed by silence allowing time for thoughts and feelings before introducing options that might integrate advance directives with the medical circumstances. By using "Mr. J," we honor the patient as a person and avoid making assumptions implicit in descriptors such as "loved one" which presumes a knowledge of the patient and their relationships that may be grounded in hope rather than reality. The following statement joins with family and invites their feelings and thoughts.

"We can only imagine how difficult it is to come to the ICU every day and not see the changes we had hoped for."

Explicit attention to care and treatments that could be provided no matter the decision about Mr. J's ventilator support replaces clinician passivity with expertise and shared thoughtfulness. This, in turn, mitigates any message that might be interpreted as helplessness and abandonment (27).

TABLE 40.2 WORD CHOICE PROMPTS

Common statement	Reframe with focus on word choice
There is nothing more I can do for you	The chemotherapy has ceased to be effective; we need to think together about what is possible and most important to you …
We need to put mom in a subacute rehab	Mom needs specialized and daily rehab and the best way for her to receive that every day is …
You need to go to hospice	We hear you hope to be cared for at home and the program that can best do that is called hospice. Have you heard of hospice?
We need to stop "life-sustaining therapies"	We have learned over the past days that the ventilator and medications are keeping their lungs working; we cannot recover his living in the way he did before. We might think about a new antibiotic—a time-limited trial as in the next 2–5 days, we would all know if it were working
If you get stronger, we can talk about more chemotherapy	I worry that your body is so weak to tolerate more chemotherapy. I would love to be wrong about this, and if I am, we can revisit this.

Another example of problematic language is choosing to describe a plan of care as "comfort care." While this may have specific meaning for clinicians, it often is confusing for lay people and does not provide clarity as to what specifically will and will not be done. It may also be interpreted to mean that comfort was not maximized over previous hours and days—a confusing and inaccurate message about both the care provided and the colleagues who provided that care. Table 40.2 identifies words and phrases that can be problematic during clinical transitions.

COMMUNICATION AT THE END OF LIFE

Principles and practice of communication outlined above are relevant to end-of-life discussions: honesty, pacing and the timing of revealing serious news, awareness of emotional and cognitive capacity, and familiarity with cultural religious and spiritual mores are especially important. Cancer patients often have the most trusting relationship with the oncologist who has cared for them over time and may want that physician to initiate end-of-life care discussions (31) and to give prognostic information. These conversations require a focus on care that will continue as well as acknowledgment of those treatments which are no longer effective (32). Using language of patient "failure" can be particularly distressing at this juncture. Yet it is authentic to state that therapy is no longer working (e.g., the chemotherapy is no longer effective in treating the cancer) (33). Concurrently, it is essential to reassure patients they won't be abandoned and to listen and respond to their emotions (31,34). Below is a narrative example of a discussion focused on a transition to end-of-life care.

Case Example: Ms. Jones is a 40-year-old female with pancreatic cancer. You have been her primary oncologist for the last 18 months, and she is nearing the end of her life. She is coming to clinic today, and you hope to discuss hospice care at this visit. You estimate her prognosis to be weeks to maybe a month.

Doctor: Hi. Ms. Jones. It's good to see you today. I was hoping we could discuss a few things regarding your care. First, I wanted to see how you are doing. How are you feeling today?

Ms. Jones: Not good, I feel weak all of the time. I don't have an appetite and my pain is worse.

Doctor: I'm sorry to hear that. I want to help with your pain. Can you tell me a little more about the pain?

Ms. Jones: It's just there all the time and I'm just wondering if this will get any better. I'm scared.

Doctor: Tell me more about what frightens you.

Ms. Jones: I just worry that I'm not going to get better…ever.

Doctor: I worry about that too.

Ms. Jones: Do you think I'm dying?

Doctor: Yes, I do think that is what's happening to your body (allow silence), and I wish things were different.

Ms. Jones: What can we do now?

Doctor: Well, there is a lot we can do to help manage your symptoms, and I have some ideas on how we can get you more help at home when needed. Would you like to talk about that now?

Ms. Jones: Yes.

Doctor: There are services that you can get at home at the end of your life. It's called hospice care. What do you know about hospice?

Ms. Jones: That's just a place you go to die. I don't want that.

Doctor: Well, that is often what people think when we talk about hospice care. Yes, there are hospice places where patients can receive care. However, most hospice care takes place at home.

Ms. Jones: Well, I would like to be at home. How long do you think I have?

Doctor: That's a good question. I worry that your time is short; it's hard to predict exactly and I think you likely have a few weeks to maybe a couple of months (allow for silence).

Ms. Jones: Okay. (Getting emotional.)

Doctor: Does that surprise you how short your time might be?

Ms. Jones: Yes, a little.

Doctor: I wish things were different. I know this is not what you were hoping for. I wanted to make sure you understand that our team is still here to help care for you. Is there anything we can do today—for you or your family—in addition to helping with your pain?

Ms. Jones: I'll try and talk with my family but if they have questions. I might ask for your help in explaining some of this to them.

Doctor: Sure. I would be happy to help.

In the above script, the doctor gives honest information while providing space for Ms. Jones to ask questions. The reference to family is an invitation for Ms. Jones to share thoughts or worries about family as she leaves the office with knowledge that she is coming to the end of life. The following sections will address how to respond to emotions and affect of patients, families, and clinician.

THE ROLE OF EMOTION

Recognizing and identifying emotion can enhance the effectiveness of conversations just as a lack of recognition can sabotage the goals of well-intended clinicians. A family member upset about a mixup in their mother's care is not likely to respond well to efforts to force the clinician's agenda until that anger has been heard. A patient who has just learned that their life expectancy is much shorter than they thought may not comprehend much of a care plan being offered if the feelings and thoughts related to the prognosis are ignored. The complex and stressful nature of many health care interactions, especially those occurring in an inpatient setting (35), can mean that patients and their families are often anxious before the physician even walks into the room. Minimal acknowledgement of emotion improves recall of information after interactions (36). Thus, recognition of emotion allows both patients and caregivers to more effectively process cognitive and other aspects of transition conversations.

Working with the Patient's Emotions

Some clinicians are skilled and comfortable in addressing feelings and eliciting the key concerns of the cancer patient while, for others, it can be a daunting task. Effectively accompanying patients and families through transitions is, however, an important undertaking which taps into the shared humanity between clinician, patients, and their families. It can make a vulnerable time easier and, using very simple strategies, can benefit the patient greatly.

It is important to approach a patient's emotions with curiosity and empathy which allows the patient to expand upon their feelings in an open and nonjudgmental way. This kind of sharing and connection can help clinicians to understand the patient's point of view, check their understanding, and validate their insights. Empathy, expressed verbally or nonverbally, is associated with positive outcomes, including greater enablement defined as the ability to cope and manage illness (37–39). Robert Smith has created a useful mnemonic delineating four basic techniques to use when exploring patient emotions: NURS (*Name*, *Understand*, *Respect*, and *Support*) with a final "E" added in this discussion to include *Explore* (40).

- **Naming** the emotion serves to acknowledge feeling and to demonstrate that it is a legitimate area for discussion. Naming is often best done in a quizzical fashion that does not presuppose the emotion: "Many people would feel angry if that happened to them. I wonder if you ever feel that way."
- Expressing a sense of **understanding** normalizes emotion and conveys empathy. At the same time, clinicians cannot ever assume full understanding of the patient's experience. This is especially true in the presence of cross-cultural communications where cultural inquiry and humility are essential to begin exploring the many aspects of history and personhood that are brought to an illness experience (41–43).
- **Respect** acknowledges and builds upon family strength, affirms resilience, and demonstrates attention to supports beyond those offered by the health care system. A statement as simple as "I hear how you have advocated for your friend and made sure we know their needs" can affirm strengths and relationships in a stressful situation.
- **Support** outlines the follow-up a patient can expect which may help decrease a sense of isolation or abandonment as the focus of treatment or place of care changes. Acknowledging community, spiritual, and family supports beyond health care affirms the world of the patient that sustains no matter the outcome of disease.

Finally, exploring patient's reactions and resources can provide vital information about their emotions, values and beliefs, needs, and preferences. When a patient or family member, for example, says "I'm afraid of what happens when I go home," a simple follow-up question such as "what are you most worried about?" can provide important insight about social supports, existential distress, safety concerns, barriers to medication adherence, and other anxieties.

There are a number of simple strategies that enhance the effectiveness of clinical responses to patient emotion. Checking assumptions at the door, asking open-ended questions, reflecting back and paraphrasing statements, openly acknowledging emotion, and staying attuned to patient and family behavioral cues and one's own reactions contribute to creating a safe and responsive environment for patient and family. These approaches also enrich both the relationship and the information needed to evolve a shared plan of care.

Working with the Clinician's Emotions

Clinician affect can directly impact the patient and appropriate training can mitigate some of the anxiety and distress that often accompanies the sharing of serious news with patients and families (5). Managing clinician emotion in the clinical setting is an important skill which requires insight and acknowledgment of those emotions.

The physician's resilience provides some protection from the effects of distress (44). Death anxiety, on the other hand, may be a significant contributing factor to burnout in palliative care and oncology physicians and nurses (45,46). No professional is exempt from the emotional impact of difficult conversations, yet those emotions are not always the same for each. Here too curiosity without judgment is an asset. A clinician's attention to their own emotional reactions can prompt empathic inquiry and benefit both patient and clinician. There is evidence that such engagement may reduce burnout risk (47).

The concept of countertransference for the purpose of this chapter is defined as the reaction to the patient's condition or words emanating from the clinician's own emotions and experiences. This is a useful way to conceptualize and address the reaction of the professionals to the patient. One way to mitigate the impact countertransference is to debrief with colleagues or other trusted individuals. The IDT where trust and safety are prioritized can be a good venue for this and can meet the need identified by primary palliative care practitioners for individual and coworker support, shared education, and collaborative feedback (48,49).

There are some promising interventions for reducing burnout and countertransference risks on teams including various forms of mindfulness practice (50,51). Mindfulness-based stress reduction

(MBSR), for example, is a well-studied intervention for burnout and depression across a variety of health care disciplines (52).

HOPE IN THE CONTEXT OF TRANSITIONS

While hope can be a resource and source of strength, clinicians can become concerned when they believe that specific hopes, in the face of uncertainty, are incongruous with medical realities. Hope is a fluid concept. It can be influenced by age, gender, religious, spiritual, and cultural beliefs. Creating environments of care that include presence, inquiry, and patience allow the emotional and cognitive space for reframing of hopes over time.

Stuart et al. (53) propose two phases of hope in advanced illness: "focused hope" and "intrinsic hope." Focused hope is outer-directed, supports the desire for cure or relief from disease, and depends on external and tangible goals. Thus, it is reactive to events such as the results of a CT scan or blood test. Intrinsic hope is described as inborn, centering on the subjective and personal, within the self, families, and relationships and such and thus can emerge concurrently with diagnosis or over time as outcomes of treatments evolve (53).

While clinicians may initially rely on focused hope to support patients as they receive therapies, over time the evolution of disease invites increased presence of "intrinsic hope." Hope for cure, for example, may be replaced by hope for remission, hope for a peaceful death, or the enhancement of legacy. Thus, clinicians and patients shift from "doing" to "being" underscoring that relationships and life, however modified, continue even as treatment options wane (54,55). As both forms of hope are explored, therapeutic benefit can be achieved even as transitions inherent in serious illness unfold. Good symptom management, presence, honesty, cultural awareness, and openness to spirituality and spiritual expression are important to sustain hope (56).

A clinician who listens for hope or messages of hopelessness may engage with patients and families as they reframe the focus of hope or invite the expression of grief over loss. The following sample questions may be used to explore hope:

- Hope is important in many people's lives; can you help me understand how you think about hope?
- Over your life, what or who has been a source of hope?
- How does your illness influence your hope?
- What are you hoping for now for you and those you care about?
- For the future, tomorrow, next week, or next month?

ADVANCE CARE PLANNING

Advance care planning is the shared decision-making process between health care professionals, patients, and families (57). ACP can include addressing treatment preferences, appointment of a health care agent, and education (58,59). This is ideally done over multiple sessions, to allow patients time to think, review advance directives, and discuss their preferences with family. It's often most helpful to focus on values and goals of the patient rather than specific outcomes or interventions such as code status or artificial nutrition (60). One's own perception of the value of ACP can greatly influence the process of ACP. For example, having experienced the impact of a patient's documented wishes on any feelings of guilt on the part of their friends or family can be a motivator to help facilitate ACP. As with other conversations, it is important for one to be aware of their own thoughts, feelings, and judgments prior to meeting with the patient (61). General resources on ACP can be found in Table 40.3.

MOLST forms—medical orders for life-sustaining treatments for persons with serious advancing illness—or POLST, physician orders for

TABLE 40.3 ADVANCE CARE PLANNING RESOURCES

Advance care planning resources	Web site	When to use
Prepare for your Care	www.prepareforyourcare.org	Easy to read advance directive. Has been translated in different languages. Includes pictures to enhance understanding.
The Conversation Project	www.theconversationproject.org	Can be used by clinicians and patients. Includes videos and materials to guide the conversation.
My Directives	https://mydirectives.com/	A place for a patient to upload an advance directive online
Five Wishes	www.fivewishes.org	Ability to order five wishes

scope of treatment, now exist in most states. For many patients leaving the hospital, MOLST forms are helpful to ensure good transitions of care. For patients at end of life, a MOLST can help guide discussion and ensure specific interventions (CPR, intubation, etc.) will or will not be attempted. Oregon has led the initiative with their POLST (Portable Orders for Life-Sustaining Treatment) since 1995 (62). Below are some suggestions to begin and continue the ACP conversations throughout disease progression.

A Start to ACP: Normalizing the Conversation

Julie is a 30-year-old female with a new diagnosis of metastatic lung cancer. As her primary oncologist, you recognize her prognosis is likely a year. When she comes to a clinic appointment prior to starting her next round of chemotherapy, you want to initiate a conversation around ACP. You hope to discuss identifying a health care agent and broaching the topic of an advance directive. Below is a sample dialogue for how to approach this topic:

Doctor: It's good to see you. How are you doing?

Julie: I'm okay, anxious to start the next round of treatment.

Doctor: Yes, I want to talk with you about that. I want to be sure I was clear when we discussed your care and treatment at the last appointment. It would be helpful for me if you explained a bit about what we discussed and your thoughts about it. Is that okay?

Julie: Yes, well you talked about how the first round of chemotherapy didn't do as much as you hoped. I mean I know my cancer can't go away, but you're hoping you can control it.

Doctor: Yes, that is correct. As we discussed previously, the treatments we have can't cure your cancer, and the goal for the chemotherapy is to see if we can stabilize the tumors and prevent future growth.

Julie: Yes. I understand that.

Doctor: One thing I wanted to think about today is who in your life is aware of your medical condition and might be helpful if something happens during the treatments and you become sicker. While we will continue to talk with you about treatments and decisions, sometimes patients choose to share decision-making with trusted persons in their lives, and sometimes things happen that prevent patients from being able to make decisions. Who would help make medical decisions if you were unable to?

Julie: My sister, Barbara.

Doctor: Can you share a bit about how much she understands about your care?

Julie: I have not told her a lot. I do not want her to worry.

Doctor: In order to ensure that Barbara is the person we might talk with if necessary, we would need to help you to complete an advance directive—a path for you to appoint her as your health care decision-maker. It sounds as if we might start with asking Barbara to come with you for your next appointment to begin to help her understand your illness. She knows that you have cancer and come here for treatments so that is a beginning. I heard that you do not want Barbara to worry—can you share a bit more about your concern? Or what seems like a wish to protect her?

Julie: Sure, I don't want to be a burden to Barbara with all that. Why would I not be able to make decisions?

Doctor: Sometimes with the treatments and the cancer, you can get very sick. We want to make sure we know how you think about your life and what is important to you so we can honor your wishes and have someone who knows you to help guide us in decision-making.

Julie: Okay. I will ask if she can come with me next time.

There are a number of online resources that can be shared with patients to help initiate the conversation on their own with family.

ACP Continued: Eliciting Preferences

When Julie returns for her next visit with her oncologist, she arrives with her sister, Barbara, who has seen the changes in her and understands the seriousness of her diagnosis. She agrees to accept the role of surrogate decision-maker, and the following questions begin a dialogue about Julie's values in preparation for completing an advance directive.

- Tell me a little about yourself as a person.
- What brings you joy?
- What makes life worth living for you?
- In addition to Barbara, if you got sicker who else could you rely on for support?
- Can you share what might make life intolerable for you?

IDEAS FOR RESPONDING TO COMMON REACTIONS

Finally, it is useful to consider some examples of questions or comments that come up when there are transitions in care. Drawing upon the communication strategies discussed in this chapter, it is important to remain curious, avoid assumption, check your understanding, and acknowledge the emotion it expresses. Table 40.4 has some

TABLE 40.4 COMMON QUESTIONS AND ANSWERS

Common Questions	Common Answers
How long do I have to live?	Provide ranges: hours to days, days to weeks, or weeks to months.
Does this mean you're giving up on me?	The treatments are no longer effective for your body, and you are more than your body. We will make sure that you and your family continue to get care.
Are you telling me that I am going to die?	I wish that were not the case.
Are there any other treatment options?	There are no options to further manage the disease; there are many options to manage symptoms and to care for you and your family.
This is in God's hands.	It sounds like your faith is really important to you.
I'm hoping for a miracle.	Help me understand what a miracle might look like to you.
I want you to do everything.	Can you tell me more so I can understand what everything means to you and to your family? (30)

questions and comments that may seem challenging with suggested responses.

MITIGATING CONFLICT

Patients, families, and clinicians are often brought together not by choice but by an untoward event involving a threat to health and often to life itself. Regardless of setting, patients and their families can be abruptly faced with crises exacerbated by confusing health care hierarchies, unfamiliar language, new environments, and their own thoughts, feelings, and fears—sometimes expressed, sometimes not. Often decisions need to be made in situations of high stress and time pressures—a setting where distress and perhaps conflict might reasonably be expected. Additionally, there may be racial and cultural history or prior experience with health care that impact trust in clinicians and in the beneficent intent of the health care system. Demands on time and decision-making pressures coupled with clinician's own perspectives and responses to conflict can exacerbate rather than mitigate conflict both within families and between patient, families, and care teams.

Transitions that involve the discontinuing of life-extending treatments or interventions such as ventilator support often foreshadow death.

While clinicians might have carefully weighed the balance of harm and benefit and arrived at an opinion on continuing these treatments, family members and decision-makers may see the situation very differently. Their perspective on the meaning of suffering, the importance of quality of life versus sanctity of life, and confidence in the health care systems are among the many variables that engender potential conflict between the care team and family and within the family itself.

The following suggestions may be helpful both to build relationships and organize family meetings that might prevent conflict and then to mitigate harm if it occurs:

- Engage interdisciplinary colleagues who may enhance communication, listening, and support.
- Understand the history of illness, so patient and family hear both knowledge of and respect for the care they have received and the illness experience they have lived.
- Prepare patient and family, when possible, so they can collaborate on the choice of time and arrange for significant persons to participate.
- Start on time.

When the need is to share important information:

- Create a shared agenda accepting that patient and family's is primary; "what would you like to discuss; anything you are particularly worried about?"
- Ask patient and/or family what they observe or understand about the illness—inviting cognitive feedback as well as their observations and interpretations of what they see.
- Frame information as "important" or "serious"—bad news assumes that clinicians know the meaning of information to unique patients and families.
- Prepare patient and family by saying "I have some important news to share."
- Share information succinctly and clearly without euphemism and medical jargon, acknowledging previous hopes, expectations, treatments, and outcomes.
- Allow silence, observe physical and affective responses of self and others, and take some focused breaths to contain anxiety and internal pressures to fill silence or react defensively.
- When conflict arises, imagine what the source might be. Consider that anger or challenge may be response to terror, fear of dependence, situational mistrust, coming to the end of one's life, or being pressured before emotionally ready to receive and accept life-altering information.
- Acknowledge areas of disagreement or conflict and concurrent emotion; contain assumptions

and judgment creating an open environment which allows for authentic response.

- Resist interrupting, defending, or responding in anger. Listen much more than you speak (34).

Cohering around plan of care:

- Describe care and treatments that may continue and may be added and those that have not had the expected or hoped for outcome; offer suggestions for care moving forward as differences are further explored or resolved.
- Listen for consensus, misunderstanding, discrepancy, disagreement, fears, feelings of hopelessness, abandonment, anger, etc.
- Clarify where necessary; contain the impulse to respond with more data or information.
- Acknowledge the differences in feelings, opinions, and values being expressed.
- When appropriate give voice to fears, anger, or accusations related to bias; wait to be corrected or to be affirmed in your understanding.
- Provide a time frame for further conversation, being explicit about the current plans, including treatments that can continue and those that might be added to serve as negotiated trial for shared observation of outcome.
- Affirm the uncertainty and complexity of caring for persons with serious illness.
- Respect the "tincture of time and patience" as therapeutic forces that at times are the most important and immeasurable factors in resolution of conflict (63).
- Ask for help from colleagues and engage other experts, including ethics consultants.

The compassion and competence of the clinicians, in the presence or absence of conflict, often influences how that illness is integrated into the family legacy—a dynamic especially poignant and meaningful when the transition is to end of life.

BEREAVEMENT

Death, to the clinician, often affords little time to acknowledge the loss it represents to the patient's family, friends, and even to the clinicians themselves. Good care, however, extends beyond the patient's end of life into the ways the illness and death become a part of family legacy. It also involves attention to the emotional, spiritual, and socioeconomic impacts of a person's death on friends and family members. It is, for example, necessary to anticipate when there may be risk of complicated grief. While most grief allows for readjustment after a death, complicated grief, which occurs in about 7% of people after a major loss, has a more severe course (64). Those who are at risk may benefit from screening by a team social worker or chaplain and, if necessary, referral to treatment. Risk factors for complicated grief include the following:

- Preloss dependency
- Female gender
- Death of a spouse OR child
- Low social support
- High developmental burden to caregiver (i.e., loss of expected activities)
- Multiple losses (64–67)

Additional risk factors are listed at https://www.mayoclinic.org/diseases-conditions/complicated-grief/symptoms-causes/syc-20360374.

The clinician's knowledge of and relationship with the patient's family system are the most useful tool in providing or arranging appropriate care in bereavement (68). Many resources can assist individuals who have lost a friend or relative, including the grief counseling services available through hospice and other organizations—https://www.nhpco.org/is a good starting point.

Those professionals who care for dying patients often grieve quietly and in isolation from colleagues. In many settings where patient death is routine and expected, rituals have been developed to honor those deaths. Finding a time and place for remembrances can provide an invitation and a useful framework for recognizing clinician grief and facilitating varied forms of grief work (69).

CONCLUSION

Transitions are a vulnerable time for patients and their support systems and can expose them to a great deal of stress. Acknowledging and working with patient and clinician emotion can forge an alliance that brings meaning to the shared experience of transitions, including the transition to end of life. The discovery of values and supports that sustain and foster resilience validates the patient family narrative beyond the illness experience. The clinician who merges empathy with good communication skills has the potential to minimize the impacts of transitions along the continuum of illness—a gift to patients and families that may also fuel the resilience of the clinicians themselves. Continuity, collaboration across teams and disciplines, consensus around a clear plan of care, and, most of all, attention to patient priorities can help adapt the patient's goals to the changed situation, create a plan for the future, and tailor the plan of care to their needs and values.

REFERENCES

1. Lewis CS. *A Grief Observed*. New York, NY: Harper Collins; 1961.
2. Tulsky JA, Arnold RM. Communication during transitions of care. In: Berger AM, Schuster JL, VonRoenn JH, eds. *Principles and Practices of Palliative Care and Supportive Oncology*. 4th ed. Philadelphia, PA: Lippincott Williams & Wilkins; 2013:624-635.
3. Nedjat-Haiem F, Carrion I, Gonzalez K, Ell K, Thompson B, Mishra S. Exploring health care clinicians' views about initiating end-of-life care communication. *Am J Hosp Palliat Med*. 2016;34(4):308-317. doi:10.1177/1049909115627773.
4. Drach-Zahavy A, Yagil D, Cohen I. Social model of emotional labour and client satisfaction: exploring inter- and intrapersonal characteristics of the client–clinician encounter. *Work Stress*. 2017;31(2):182-208. doi:10.1080/02678373.2017.1303550.
5. Zwingmann J, Baile WF, Schmier JW, Bernhard J, Keller M. Effects of patient-centered communication on anxiety, negative affect, and trust in the physician in delivering a cancer diagnosis: a randomized, experimental study. *Cancer*. 2017;123(16):3167-3175. doi:10.1002/cncr.30694.
6. Ospina NS, Phillips KA, Rodriguez-Gutierrez R, et al. Eliciting the patient's agenda—Secondary analysis of recorded clinical encounters. *J Gen Intern Med*. 2018;34(1):36-40. doi:10.1007/s11606-018-4540-5.
7. Fröjd C, Lampic C, Larsson G, Essen L. Is satisfaction with doctors' care related to health-related quality of life, anxiety and depression among patients with carcinoid tumours? A longitudinal report. *Scand J Caring Sci*. 2009;23(1):107-116. doi:10.1111/j.1471-6712.2008.00596.x.
8. King S, Exley J, Parks S, et al. The use and impact of quality of life assessment tools in clinical care settings for cancer patients, with a particular emphasis on brain cancer: insights from a systematic review and stakeholder consultations. *Qual Life Res*. 2016;25(9):2245-2256. doi:10.1007/s11136-016-1278-6.
9. Boissy A, Windover AK, Bokar D, et al. Communication skills training for physicians improves patient satisfaction. *J Gen Intern Med*. 2016;31:755. doi:10.1007/s11606-016-3597-2.
10. Ferrell B, Buller H, Paice J, Anderson W, Donesky D. End-of-life nursing and education consortium communication curriculum for interdisciplinary palliative care teams. *J Palliat Med*. 2019;22:1082-1091.
11. Rucker B, Browning DM. Practicing end-of-life conversations: physician communication training program in palliative care. *J Soc Work End Life Palliat Care*. 2015;11(2):132-146.
12. National Coalition for Hospice and Palliative Care; National Consensus Project for Quality Palliative Care. Clinical Practice Guidelines for Quality Palliative Care, 4th ed. Published 2018. https://www.nationalcoalitionhpc.org/ncp. Accessed November 29, 2019.
13. Brighton LJ, Koffman J, Hawkins A, et al. A systematic review of end-of-life care communication skills training for generalist palliative care clinicians: research quality and reporting guidance. *J Pain Symptom Manage*. 2017;54(3):417-425.
14. Fischer F, Helmer S, Rogge A, et al. Outcomes and outcome measures used in evaluation of communication training in oncology—a systematic literature review, an expert workshop, and recommendations for future research. *BMC Cancer*. 2019;19(1):808. doi:10.1186/s12885-019-6022-5.
15. Back AL, Arnold RM, Baile WF, et al. Efficacy of communication skills training for giving bad news and discussing transitions to palliative care. *Arch Intern Med*. 2007;167(5):453-460.
16. De Vries AMM, Roten Y, Meystre C, Passchier J, Despland J-N, Stiefel F. Clinician characteristics, communication, and patient outcome in oncology: a systematic review. *Psychooncology*. 2014;23(4):375-381. doi:10.1002/pon.3445.
17. Davis DL. Simple but not always easy: improving doctor-patient communication. *J Commun Healthc*. 2010;3(3/4):240-245. doi:10.1179/175380710X12870623776397.
18. Draper EJ, Hillen MA, Moors M, Ket JC, van Laarhoven HW, Henselmans I. Relationship between physicians' death anxiety and medical communication and decision-making: a systematic review. *Patient Educ Couns*. 2019;102(2):266-274.
19. Adams K, Cimino JE, Arnold RM, Anderson WG. Why should I talk about emotion? Communication patterns associated with physician discussion of patient expressions of negative emotion in hospital admission encounters. *Patient Educ Couns*. 2012;89(1):44-50.
20. Schenker Y, Lo B, Ettinger KM, Fernandez A. Navigating language barriers under difficult circumstances. *Ann Intern Med*. 2008;149(4):264-269.
21. Walter JK, Sach E, Schall TE, et al. Interprofessional teamwork during family meetings in the pediatric cardiac intensive care unit. *J Pain Symptom Manage*. 2019;57(6):1089-1098.
22. Baile W, Buckaman R, Lenzi R, Glober G, Beale E, Kudelka A. SPIKES—A six-step protocol for delivering bad news: application to the patient with cancer. *Oncologist*. 2000;5:302-311. doi:10.1634/theoncologist.5-4-302.
23. Fischer GS, Tulsky JA, Arnold RM. Communicating a poor prognosis. In: Portenoy RK, Bruera E, eds. *Topics in Palliative Care*. Vol. 4. New York, NY: Oxford University Press; 2000.
24. Maguire P, Faulkner A, Booth K, et al. Helping cancer patients disclose their concerns. *Eur J Cancer*. 1996;32A(1):78-81.
25. Fogarty LA, Curbow BA, Wingard JR, et al. Can 40 seconds of compassion reduce patient anxiety? *J Clin Oncol*. 1999;17(1):371-379.
26. Buechner F. *The Sacred Journey: A Memoir of Early Days*. San Francisco, CA: Harper Collins Publishers; 1982.
27. Bibler TM. Why I no longer say "withdrawal of care" or "life-sustaining technology". *J Palliat Med*. 2013;16(9):1146-1147.
28. Dvorak A. I am not a fighter because I survived cancer at 19. *Washington Post*. August 29, 2019. https://www.washingtonpost.com/outlook/2019/08/21/i-am-not-fighter-because-i-survived-cancer-nineteen/. Accessed November 29, 2019.
29. Margaritis P. The difference between "But" & "And". Published April 5, 2016. http://petermargaritis.com/the-difference-between-but-and. Accessed November 29, 2019.
30. Quill TE, Arnold RM, Platt F. "I wish things were different": expressing wishes in response to loss, futility, and unrealistic hopes. *Ann Intern Med*. 2001;135(7):551-555.
31. Balaban R. A physician's guide to talking about end-of-life-care. *J Gen Intern Med*. 2000;15(3):195-200. doi:10.1046/j.1525-1497.2000.07228.x.
32. Clayton JM, Butow PN, Arnold RM, et al. Fostering coping and nurturing hope when discussing the future with terminally ill cancer patients and their caregivers. *Cancer*. 2005;103(9):1965-1975.
33. Kelemen A, Groninger H. Therapy first, not the patient? *J Soc Work End Life Palliat Care*. 2017;13(1):9-12. doi:10.1080/15524256.2017.1282918.
34. McDonagh JR, Elliott TB, Engelberg RA, et al. Family satisfaction with family conferences about end-of-life care in the intensive care unit: increased proportion of

family speech is associated with increased satisfaction. *Crit Care Med.* 2004;32(7):1484-1488.

35. Chang BP. Can hospitalization be hazardous to your health? A nosocomial based stress model for hospitalization. *Gen Hosp Psychiatry.* 2019;60:83-89.

36. Jansen J, van Weert JC, de Groot J, van Dulmen S, Heeren TJ, Bensing JM. Emotional and informational patient cues: the impact of nurses' responses on recall. *Patient Educ Couns.* 2010;79(2):218-224.

37. Derksen F, Bensing J, Lagro-Janssen A. Effectiveness of empathy in general practice: a systematic review. *Br J Gen Pract.* 2013;63(606):e76-e84.

38. Mercer SW, Neumann M, Wirtz M, Fitzpatrick B, Vojt G. General practitioner empathy, patient enablement, and patient-reported outcomes in primary care in an area of high socio-economic deprivation in Scotland—a pilot prospective study using structural equation modeling. *Patient Educ Couns.* 2008;73(2):240-245.

39. Derksen F, Hartman TC, van Dijk A, Plouvier A, Bensing J, Lagro-Janssen A. Consequences of the presence and absence of empathy during consultations in primary care: a focus group study with patients. *Patient Educ Couns.* 2017;100(5):987-993.

40. Smith RC, Hoppe RB. The patient's story: integrating the patient- and physician-centered approaches to interviewing. *Ann Intern Med.* 1991;115(6):470-477.

41. Lorié Á, Reinero DA, Phillips M, Zhang L, Riess H. Culture and nonverbal expressions of empathy in clinical settings: a systematic review. *Patient Educ Couns.* 2017;100(3):411-424.

42. Fleming BD, Thomas SE, Shaw D, Burnham WS, Charles LT. Improving Ethnocultural Empathy in Healthcare Students through a Targeted Intervention. *J Cult Divers.* 2015;22(2):59-63.

43. Fisher-Borne M, Cain JM, Martin SL. From mastery to accountability: cultural humility as an alternative to cultural competence. *Social Work Educ.* 2015;34(2):165-181. doi:10.1080/02615479.2014.977244.

44. McFarland DC, Roth A. Resilience of internal medicine house staff and its association with distress and empathy in an oncology setting. *Psychooncology.* 2017;26(10):1519-1525. doi:10.1002/pon.4165.

45. Samson T, Shvartzman P. Association between level of exposure to death and dying and professional quality of life among palliative care workers. *Palliat Support Care.* 2018;16(4):442-451.

46. Granek L, Ben-David M, Nakash O, et al. Oncologists' negative attitudes towards expressing emotion over patient death and burnout. *Support Care Cancer.* 2017;25(5):1607-1614.

47. Lamothe M, Rondeau É, Malboeuf-Hurtubise C, Duval M, Sultan S. Outcomes of MBSR or MBSR-based interventions in health care clinicians: a systematic review with a focus on empathy and emotional competencies. *Complement Ther Med.* 2016;24:19-28.

48. Brighton LJ, Selman LE, Bristowe K, Edwards B, Koffman J, Evans CJ. Emotional labour in palliative and end-of-life care communication: a qualitative study with generalist palliative care clinicians. *Patient Educ Couns.* 2019;102(3):494-502.

49. Grandey A, Foo SC, Groth M, Goodwin RE. Free to be you and me: a climate of authenticity alleviates burnout from emotional labor. *J Occup Health Psychol.* 2012;17(1):1-14. doi:10.1037/a0025102.

50. Sansó N, Galiana L, Oliver A, Cuesta P, Sánchez C, Benito E. Evaluación de una intervención mindfulness en equipos de cuidados paliativos. *Psychosoc Interv.* 2018;27(2):81-88.

51. Hayes JA, Gelso CJ, Goldberg S, Kivlighan DM. Countertransference management and effective psycho-therapy: meta-analytic findings. *Psychotherapy (Chic).* 2018;55(4):496-507. doi:10.1037/pst0000189.

52. Goodman MJ, Schorling JB. A mindfulness course decreases burnout and improves well-being among healthcare clinicians. *Int J Psychiatry Med.* 2012;43(2):119-128.

53. Stuart B, Begoun A, Berry L. The dual nature of hope at the end of life. *The BMJ Opinion.* Published April 13, 2017. https://blogs.bmj.com/bmj/2017/04/13/the-dual-nature-of-hope-at-the-end-of-life/. Accessed November 29, 2019.

54. Ofri D. When doing nothing is the best medicine. *New York Times.* October 20, 2011. https://well.blogs.nytimes.com/2011/10/20/when-doing-nothing-is-the-best-medicine/. Accessed November 29, 2019.

55. Herth KA, Cutcliffe JR. The concept of hope in nursing 3: hope and palliative care nursing. *Br J Nurs.* 2002;11(14):977-983. doi:10.12968/bjon.2002.11.14.10470.

56. Duggleby W, Hicks D, Nekolaichuk C, et al. Hope, older adults, and chronic illness: a metasynthesis of qualitative research. *J Adv Nurs.* 2012;68(6):1211-1223. doi:10.1111/j.1365-2648.2011.05919.

57. Gjerberg E, Lillemoen L, Forde R, Pedersen R. End-of-life care communications and shared decision-making in Norwegian nursing homes—experiences and perspectives of patients and relatives. *BMC Geriatr.* 2015;15(103):1-13. doi:10.1186/s12877-015-0096-y.

58. Singer PA, Martin DK, Lavery JV, et al. Reconceptualizing advance care planning from the patient's perspective. *Arch Intern Med.* 1998;158:879-884.

59. Stewart F, Goddard C, Schiff R, Hall S. Advanced care planning in care homes for older people: a qualitative study of the views of care staff and families. *Age Ageing.* 2011;40(3):330-335. doi: 10.1093/ageing/afr006.

60. Mullick A, Martin J, Sallnow L. An introduction to advance care planning in practice. *BMJ.* 2013;21:60-64. doi:https://doi.org/10.1136/bmj.f6064.

61. Nortje N, Stepan K. Advance care planning conversations in the oncology setting: tips from the experts. *J Cancer Educ.* 2019. doi:10.1007/s13187-019-01631-1.

62. Tolle SW, Teno JM. Lessons from Oregon in embracing complexity in end-of-life care. *N Engl J Med.* 2017;376(11):1078-1082.

63. Masters P. The power of the tincture of time. KevinMD Blog. Published December 6, 2018. www.kevinmd.com/blog/2018/12/the-power-of-the-tincture-of-time.html. Accessed November 29, 2019.

64. Kersting A, Brähler E, Glaesmer H, Wagner B. Prevalence of complicated grief in a representative population-based sample. *J Affect Disord.* 2011;131(1-3):339-343.

65. Lai C, Luciani M, Morelli E, et al. Predictive role of different dimensions of burden for risk of complicated grief in caregivers of terminally ill patients. *Am J Hosp Palliat Med.* 2014;31(2):189-193.

66. Bonanno GA, Wortman CB, Lehman DR, et al. Resilience to loss and chronic grief: a prospective study from preloss to 18-months postloss. *J Pers Soc Psychol.* 2002;83(5):1150-1164. doi:10.1037/0022-3514.83.5.1150.

67. Shear MK, Ghesquiere A, Glickman K. Bereavement and complicated grief. *Curr Psychiatry Rep.* 2013;15(11):406. doi:10.1007/s11920-013-0406-z.

68. Nielsen MK, Neergaard MA, Jensen AB, Vedsted P, Bro F, Guldin MB. Predictors of complicated grief and depression in bereaved caregivers: a nationwide prospective cohort study. *J Pain Symptom Manage.* 2017;53(3):540-550.

69. Morris SE, Kearns JP, Moment A, Lee KA, deLima Thomas J. "Remembrance": a self-care tool for clinicians. *J Palliat Med.* 2019;22(3):316-318.

41 The Family Meeting

Sumi K. Misra and Mohana B. Karlekar

INTRODUCTION

Palliative care specialists excel in communication. The goal of excellent palliative care is to collaboratively meet the needs of the patients, families, and treatment teams during times of transition in the context of life-limiting and serious illness (1). Excellent communication between medical clinicians and families of seriously ill patients is recognized as a key factor in successful shared decision-making and family perception of quality care (2–4).

Formal family meetings have increasingly been seen as an effective tool to facilitate this dialogue (5,6). Through this communication method, not only do families improve their understanding of the patient's diagnosis, therapeutic options, and prognosis, but additionally, clinicians better recognize the emotional weight and the personal meaning of the patient's illness. Through family meetings, clinicians and families build honest relationships based on each other's desire to provide the best care for the patient (7). Family meetings should allow for families to identify patient's goals and patient's views of quality of life, which allows clinicians to provide medical recommendations based on those identified goals. This process results in a shared decision plan (8,9).

This chapter is designed to:

1. Review recent literature relevant to optimal communication during family meetings.
2. Outline the anatomy of a family meeting, including setting, population targeted, planning, execution, pitfalls, and documentation of the event.
3. Highlight the family meeting as a tool for enhanced shared decision-making.

THE ROLE OF THE FAMILY MEETING

Communication occurs best, face to face. Given that over 50% of communication is nonverbal, not paying attention to nonverbal cues puts clinicians at a disadvantage creating a missed opportunity for clarity and connection with patients and families at a time of confusion, potential conflict, and critical decision-making (10). While most patients and family members want to receive support and hope from clinicians, they also desire honest information about the patient's medical condition and prognosis (11,12). Yet, studies reveal that up to a third of families of critically ill patients are dissatisfied with the lack of communication or conflicting information from different clinicians (13,14).

Even when clinicians spend time communicating the patient's medical diagnosis, treatment, and prognosis with the family, only half of families actually comprehend what was said despite both clinicians' and families' perception of understanding (15). This disconnect is alarming since clinical decisions are made based upon these misunderstandings.

Physicians rarely effectively communicate with their seriously ill patients about their goals, values, or basic treatment decisions. When physicians communicate effectively they are more apt to understand and address the issues that are important for the patient or the patient–family unit. Consequently, patients are better able to understand their medical situation in the context of their psychosocial situation. This could affect their understanding of their medical issues and treatment options more concretely (16). In addition, effective communication improves patient satisfaction and reduces anxiety and distress (17,18). Even brief expressions of empathy may reduce patient anxiety (19).

Optimal communication has been identified by patients and their families as one of the more important aspects of medical care at a time of serious illness and at the end of life (20–22). The family meeting is a useful format for clarification ensuring that everyone involved is on the same page regarding the patient's condition.

WHEN SHOULD A FAMILY MEETING BE CONSIDERED?

A family meeting should be considered in any of the following clinical situations (9):

1. Complicated decision-making about current or future care particularly when multiple teams are involved in a patient's care.
2. Medical updates are indicated to ensure delivery of complex medical information to patients and families.

3. Communication of a significant change in condition and/or functional status.
4. Communication of a poor prognosis and or medical futility.
5. If there is report or evidence of conflict, tension, or lack of trust between treatment teams involved and patient or family.

Family meetings provide an opportunity to clarify treatment goals, advocate for the patient, and ensure that all parties involved in care (both medical and nonmedical) understand treatment decisions and prognosis (23). Family meetings are an invaluable part of all levels of hospital-based care and are an important step in providing the best care to patients and their loved ones. Meetings are recommended during transitions in care and critical decision-making points in a patient's disease trajectory. For the cancer patient, a proactive meeting soon after the initial diagnosis may help the patient and family ask questions and begin to think about quality-of-life issues as they make treatment decisions. Consider follow-up family meetings when there is progression of cancer despite current therapy, when there are complications from therapy, and when patients are eligible for hospice.

Currently, the majority of family meetings happen in the hospital in situations where the patient is not able to make decisions for himself/herself due to sedation, intubation, delirium, or confusion due to underlying medical condition. However, we anticipate that there will be an increase in outpatient family meetings conducted in the community based palliative care continues to grow (24,25). The majority of literature detailing the timing of family meetings comes from the ICU literature and recommends that meetings should take place upon admission to the ICU, if a patient's condition changes, if there is conflict within the family, or if there is conflict between family and clinicians (10,26).

Lilly et al. (2) instituted early family meetings for critically ill patients, which identified patient's goals sooner and paved the road for follow-up family meetings when the clinical course became incompatible with either the patient's goals or restoring life, which subsequently permitted earlier withdrawal of life-sustaining therapy (2). Family members were more satisfied about the quality of a patient's death in the ICU if a family meeting was held to discuss patient's goals (27).

The data on the pediatric population mirror the adult side. Many parents believed they shared the same beliefs as the physicians on prognosis of their children's illness; however, 70% of parents were more optimistic than their physicians regarding prognosis, again highlighting the clear chasm between clinicians and families in areas of optimism and hope (28). In the pediatric ICU, a single formal meeting results in increased shared decision-making (29,30).

THE FAMILY MEETING SETUP (THE PRE-MEETING)

Planning is an essential component to the success of any conference, and family meetings are no different. It is important that a "pre-meeting" occurs prior to the actual designated meeting with family to prevent common pitfalls (31) (Table 41.2). It is an important step to help identify the stakeholders from the medical staff who are going to be involved in the meeting. Physicians, nurses, social workers, and chaplains should be included in this step if they plan to participate in the meeting. This allows time for the medical team to discuss potential family dynamics (e.g., siblings that do not get along or distrust of medical staff) (32).

The medical staff should jointly discuss the patient's current medical condition and hospital course to date and come to a consensus regarding prognosis and treatment course. This is an opportunity to discuss with any other consultants their medical opinions and ensure that a cohesive plan is being presented to the family. Proposed treatments should be reviewed and consensus reached about what will be recommended to the family.

TABLE 41.1 REASONS TO CONDUCT A PRE-MEETING

Identify and gather key stakeholders
Review medical issues and advance directives
Identify and address areas of potential conflict
Discuss and reach consensus
Designate the "leader"
Identify key additional "presenters"
Emphasize role of empathetic active listening

TABLE 41.2 PATIENT AND FAMILY CENTERED REASONS TO CONDUCT A FAMILY MEETING

To provide a sense of autonomy and control
To understand their illness, disease trajectory, and treatment options
To present and understand their illness in their unique psychosocial context
To have a preference and value-based discussion for goals of care
To gain realistic expectations aligned with their goals
To actively participate in the care plan
To provide a coping mechanism and plan and prioritize for the future
To provide a platform to reframe "hope"

During the pre-meeting, the person that will lead the meeting should be designated. Each member involved should be informed of any information they will be asked to give in the meeting (update on medical condition, discuss current "brain function," etc.). By telling each participant what they will be expected to present, they can begin to prepare what they wish to communicate to the family prior to the actual meeting (23,31). Attempts should be made to minimize "surprise revelations and opinions" during the actual family meeting.

The medical participants should review any pertinent advance directives and ensure that they understand them and are proposing a treatment plan in alignment with those directives. Careful attention should be paid to review if the patient has identified a surrogate decision maker or made any explicit statements about treatment options (e.g., feeding tubes).

By attempting to do the above prior to a family meeting, all the providers can enter the meeting adequately prepared and, more importantly, with an understanding of their role in the meeting. Each step in this pre-meeting is a potential pitfall, where things can go wrong in the family meeting. If a leader is not designated, medical provider roles are not clear, or communication regarding prognosis is not consistent, then it will be challenging to establish trust with the family and reach any conclusive shared patient-centered decisions (33–35).

THE ANATOMY OF THE FAMILY MEETING

Most of the evidence discussing the family meeting originates from the ICU and medical oncology literature. Though there are many different well-established methods on how to conduct a family meeting, the fundamental principles remain

TABLE 41.3 THE 12-STEP PROCESS FOR AN EFFECTIVE FAMILY MEETING

Step 1: The pre-meeting
Step 2: Meeting logistics and physical setup
Step 3: Introductions, setting expectations, and a framework
Step 4: Eliciting patient and family position, perspectives, and concerns
Step 5: Establishing boundaries (if any) on information sharing
Step 6: Communication of relevant medical fact
Step 7: Responding to emotions and managing conflict
Step 8: Eliciting patient-centered goals of care
Step 9: Establishing and summarizing mutually acceptable plans of care
Step 10: Outlining the "next steps"
Step 11: Expressing appreciation for involvement and attendance
Step 12: Communicating, debriefing, and documenting, in written form, a summary of the interaction

constant. As discussed above, much of the work for the family meeting is done before the actual meeting. Von Gunten et al. (32) divided the actual family meeting into a seven-step process (32). We recommend a 12-step process (Table 41.3).

Step 1: *Conduct the pre-meeting* (Tables 41.1 and 41.2). Here the clinician must ascertain the following: What is the purpose of the meeting? Which individuals in the family need to attend? Who are the relevant medical team members from both the primary team and consulting team? The clinicians chosen to participate in the family meeting should meet prior to the meeting and determine who will lead the discussion. Each participant should know what the other will communicate.

Step 2: *Agree upon a convenient time to meet.* A mutually acceptable time needs to be agreed upon with enough prior notice to all, in order to maximize attendance (9). To better prepare the family prior to the meeting, Nelson et al. (36) discussed giving family members a written checklist of what they should consider prior to the meeting. A decisional patient can be asked who he or she wants to participate from his or her family and community, including faith leaders. In general, it is wise not to set any arbitrary limits on the number of attendees. The medical care team should likewise decide whom they want to participate. It is wise to not overwhelm a family with too many health professionals. On the other hand, a physician from the primary team as well as a nurse and social worker should attend when possible; these individuals can help ensure the consistency of information as well as help deal with complicated dynamics. If the patient has a long-time treating physician whom he or she trusts, this person should ideally be present (26,31,33,37,38).

The ideal setting is private and quiet, with chairs arranged in a circle or around a table. Everyone should be able to sit down if they wish. All pagers and cellular telephones should be turned off.

Step 3: *Make introductions.* At the start of the meeting, the clinician leading the meeting should initiate introductions and have each individual present to explain his or her role in the patient's care. Family should be asked to introduce themselves. Ground rules should be established, emphasizing that everyone interested in speaking will have an opportunity to do so.

Phrases that may be helpful: "We are here to discuss the next steps in the care of Mrs. X."

If you do not know the patient or family well, take a moment to build relationships. Ask a non-medical question such as "I am just getting to know you. I had a chance to look at your chart and learn about your medical condition, but it does not say much about your life before you got sick. Can you tell us about the things you liked to do before you got sick?" Similarly, if the patient is not able to participate in the meeting, ask family to describe the patient prior to his or her becoming ill: "As we get started, can you describe what Mrs. X was like before she became ill?" (39).

Step 4: *Determine what the family understands.* Prior to imparting information, it is recommended that the team actively listen to the patient and family and elicit their full list of concerns (16). Physicians cannot assume that patients will volunteer all their concerns spontaneously. It is important to ask the family what they know about the patient's condition, treatment options, and prognosis using open-ended questions. The extent to which the patient's concerns have been disclosed and resolved directly correlate with lower levels of depression and anxiety. When a holistic and thoughtful approach is taken to establish a safe space for the patient and family to discuss the issues, they feel more satisfied and may comply better with the offered advice (40–42).

Phrases that may be helpful:

- "What is your understanding of what is going on with Mrs. X?"
- "What has been most difficult about this illness for you?"
- "As you think about your illness, what is the best and worst that can happen?"

Step 5: *Communicate the medical facts.* Multiple factors determine how much information is to be shared (Table 41.4). This will be a function of both the family's ability to process information and how much they would like to know. The majority of English-speaking people in North America who have a serious illness prefer to be fully informed about a variety of topics related to their health, including diagnosis, prognosis, and treatment options (43–45). However, not all patients want very extensive information about their illness and prognosis (46). It is noted that patients' information needs may be strongly influenced by their unique culture, by country of origin, or by subculture within a country. Some patients may want minimal information

TABLE 41.4 FACTORS THAT COULD INFLUENCE INFORMATION DISCLOSURE TO PATIENTS

Culture

Country of origin

Disease progression and life expectancy

Age

Sex

Socioeconomic background

Level of education

Relationship with health care team

or nondisclosure when their life expectancy is very short (47). The evidence is inconclusive in non-Western countries, but the overall trend has been more disclosure based on insightful understanding of where the patient and family are in their journey of experiencing the serious illness. Patients from some cultural backgrounds may prefer disclosure negotiated through the family when the prognosis is poor (47). Higher levels of information are often sought by younger patients (44,48,49), females (44), individuals in a middle socioeconomic class (50), and those who have a higher level of education (48).

Phrases that may be helpful:

- "Is there anything you are particularly concerned about, that would help us understand your/your loved one's illness better?"
- "How have you adapted to difficult circumstances in the past?"
- "Would it help to have someone with you as we discuss this further?"

Step 6: *Communicate the relevant medical facts.* The information delivered should be done so with clarity without the use of medical jargon or excessive and complex physiology. Some patients and surrogates are comfortable using numbers when talking about probabilities, whereas others could be quantitatively challenged (51,52). Information should be presented based on elicited patient preferences, and many patients will leave decisions to the judgment of the medical team, based on the team's best interpretation of wide-ranging medical data.

Phrases that may be helpful:

- "I would like to update everyone here about Mrs. X's condition."
- "Mrs. X has been in the ICU for 27 days. She has had many people involved in her medical care and has had many test and procedures. I would like to summarize these for you."

Step 7: *Acknowledge, validate, and respond to emotions.* It is important to tolerate and allow silence. Although conflict is often avoided by clinicians and patients, conflict managed well can be productive. Denial of conflict and nonrevelation of "hidden agendas" and unexplored strong negative emotions can derail honest communication and exacerbate indecision in goal setting. Back and Arnold (53) have described a seven-step approach to conflict management and resolution that takes into account active listening, empathizing, reframing, explaining, self-disclosure, and trying to reach a "middle ground."

Phrases that may be helpful:

- "Although I have never shared your experience, I do understand that this is a really difficult time for you."

- "Many people would feel angry/sad/overwhelmed if this happened to them. I wonder if you ever feel that way."

Step 8: *Elicit patient-centered goals of care.* Establish treatment plans based on the patient's wishes, values, goals, and treatment priorities. Discussions based on vague terms such as "quality of life" should be avoided; instead, it is more important to identify how a patient or their surrogates identify a good quality of life. Identifying what conditions the patient would find unacceptable can also help clarify a patient's preferences. A useful question is "Can you imagine any situations in which life would not be worth living?" (54). This question can be followed by asking what the patient would want in the current context of illness and treatment plans. Emphasize to family members that they should be communicating the wishes of their loved one, not their own. The literature clearly demonstrates poor concordance between patient preferences and surrogate perceptions of those preferences. It is recommended that it be stressed that the patient communicates his or her preference with the proxy decision maker as well as communicates how much leeway the proxy should have in the decision-making (55,56).

Phrases that may be helpful:

- "What makes life worth living for you?"
- "What do you think Mrs. X would say if she were at this table and listening to this question/discussion?"
- "We realize it is sometimes very difficult to take our own emotions and feelings out of a decision regarding a loved one, knowing that we could face a life without them."

Step 9: *Summarize the salient points of the meeting to the group.*

Review and establish the plan of care and communicate this concisely to the group at the conclusion of the meeting.

Phrases that may be helpful:

- "I appreciate everybody's input into Mrs. X's plan to help us jointly make some decisions. We can now agree to move forward with…."
- "I believe, after this very helpful discussion, that you would prefer…."

Step 10: *Outline the next steps.* Patients may have specific questions about further tests, treatment options, and interventions. A succinct short-term plan as well as a general clear overview of the next immediate few hours to days can go a long way in allowing the patient and family to reframe and reconceptualize their future. It could provide a "safe haven" during the current period of turmoil

and transition. This is an opportunity to schedule the next family meeting if appropriate.

Phrases that may be helpful:

- "We have covered a lot of ground today; let's go over some of the things we have discussed and see what we will be doing over the next few hours/days."
- "I will keep you updated about his breathing over the next few hours, as well as his x-ray results while you think about your decision regarding the breathing machine."
- "There is a lot that we can do. Let's talk about what goals are most important for your loved one."

Step 11: *Express appreciation for involvement and attendance*: One cannot always achieve a happy ending or make the participants happy in a family meeting, given the circumstance under which most meetings are held. Instead, a closing statement that focuses on appreciation of the attendees' support of and dedication to the patient's best interests is recommended. Emphasize that the meeting is an important step in a series of communications that may occur in the care and caring of the patient.

Phrases that may be helpful:

- "Thank you for being here today. Your presence and involvement were very helpful in coming to these important decisions."
- "Mrs. X is so very fortunate to have you keeping her best interests in mind at a time like this. Thank you for being there for her and us."

Step 12: *Communication, debriefing, and documentation of the meeting.* It is critically important to communicate all relevant information to the health care team both verbally and in the medical record immediately following the family meeting. Family meetings are often billed using time as the factor in determining the appropriate E/M code (57).

SKILL SETS AND COMMUNICATION TOOLS TO CONDUCT THE FAMILY MEETING

All clinicians should strive to improve their communication strategies in the family meeting setting. A good physician–patient relationship is the cornerstone of effective communication in the scenario of advancing chronic as well as sudden illnesses (58,59). Unfortunately, most physicians have received little to no training regarding effective communication. For many, this skill set has been learned by trial and error. Clinicians are often very uncomfortable when they must discuss prognosis and treatment options with the patient if the information is unfavorable. Based on our own observations and those of others (60–66), we believe that the discomfort is based on a number of concerns that physicians experience. These include uncertainty about the patient's expectations, fear of destroying the patient's hope, fear of their own inadequacy in the face of uncontrollable disease, not feeling prepared to manage the patient's anticipated emotional reactions, and sometimes embarrassment at having previously painted too optimistic a picture for the patient.

Communication Skills

In general, it is recommended that the health care team create a holistic patient-centered climate where the patient is treated as a "whole person" and it clearly communicates that the physician is interested, is attuned, and is sensitive to their medical needs as well as their psychosocial needs and emotions of the patient (16). Over the last decade, communication tools have been developed to help clinicians become more adept at family meetings. The SPIKES protocol is a commonly used practical protocol for disclosing unfavorable information— "breaking bad news"—to cancer patients about their illness. The protocol (SPIKES) consists of six steps (67) (Table 41.5).

The goal is to enable the clinician fulfill the four most important objectives of the interview disclosing bad news: gathering information from the patient, transmitting the medical information, providing support to the patient, and eliciting the patient's collaboration in developing a strategy or treatment plan for the future. Oncologists, oncology trainees, and medical students who have been taught the protocol have reported increased confidence in their ability to disclose unfavorable medical information to patients. Another such tool is an acronym VALUE that incorporates the following techniques (68):

- Value and appreciate what families communicate.
- Acknowledge emotions with reflective summary statements.
- Listen carefully.
- Understand who the patient is as a person by asking open-ended questions.
- Elicit questions from families.

Leadership Skills

A cornerstone skill in palliative medicine is leadership of family meetings to establish goals of care, typically completed at a time of patient change in status, where the value of current treatments needs to be reevaluated. Leading a family meeting requires considerable flexibility to ensure that all relevant participants have the opportunity to have their points of view expressed. Although it is useful to have one person designated as the main orchestrator and coordinator of the meeting, the essential skills for making a family meeting successful can come from more than one participant. These skills include group facilitation skills, counseling skills, knowledge of medical and prognostic information, and a willingness to provide leadership and guidance in decision-making (31).

Conflict Management and Resolution Skills

Conflicts about medical care occur frequently at the end of life. These conflicts threaten therapeutic relationships and lead to patient, health care provider, and family dissatisfaction. Conflict between the patient/family and physician may arise from simple factual misunderstandings about medical care. Frequently, however, conflict is driven by a patient's or family's emotions such as feeling unheard or ignored, as well as having goals that conflict with those of the medical team. In these instances, attempting to convince a patient or family with additional medical information will not work (Table 41.6).

Information gaps can arise when there is an inaccurate understanding of the patient's medical condition. Inconsistent information that varies between providers or confusing information that is embedded in medical jargon and presented in an illogical and nonsequential manner can create informational gaps, leading to conflict. Additionally, information in excess of what needs to be communicated at a certain time or information that is presented at times of genuine uncertainty such as immediate post cerebrovascular accident and brain injury in children as well as in adults can cause information disconnects. All the above can be exacerbated if additional issues of language and cultural barriers exist.

TABLE 41.5 THE SPIKES PROTOCOL FOR BREAKING BAD NEWS

Setting up
Perception
Invitation
Knowledge
Emotions/empathy
Strategy and summary

TABLE 41.6 POTENTIAL CAUSES FOR CONFLICT DURING A FAMILY MEETING

Information gaps
Treatment goal confusion
Emotions
Family/team dynamics
Relationship between the clinician and the patient/surrogate

Treatment goal confusion arises from a disparity between the perception of the treating team and the patient–family dynamics. This includes lack of clarity about short-term and long-term goals when multiple issues need to be addressed and inconsistent and illogical treatment plans that are driven on emotion rather than logic. This can also arise when phrases and terms such as "comfort care" and "do everything" are used, which can mean different things to different people unless clarified explicitly (69).

Humans are intensely emotional beings and the combination of uncertainty in the context of serious, life-limiting, and sometimes sudden illness can give rise to situations fraught with conflict. Emotions such as grief, fear, anxiety, guilt, anger, hope, and despair can all cause conflict situations and should be recognized in context and addressed directly and with empathy if possible.

Family dynamics can often cause conflict between family members and between the family and health care team or between the family and patient. Issues pertinent are families and surrogates confusing patients' best interests and wishes with their own needs, poor coping and decision-making capacity of surrogate decision makers, and unrecognized history/presence of psychiatric illness in family that impedes rational decision-making.

Health care team dynamics, such as disagreement with regard to prognosis, approach to treatment plan, and level of disclosure, when not recognized and addressed appropriately in a timely fashion can unfairly and unfortunately jeopardize the family meeting, putting the patient/family in the middle of the dispute.

The relationship between the clinician and the patient/surrogate has a potential to play a significant role in conflict development, management, and resolution during times of crisis. Lack of trust in the health care team/health care system, past experiences where the patient has had a better outcome than predicted by the health care team, and genuine value differences in the arena of cultural/religious values concerning life, dying, and death can all play an important role in how issues could be addressed and resolved (38,53,70–72).

Addressing the underlying roots of conflict will have considerable impact. The following method emphasizes resolving conflict through mutual trust and shared goals between physicians, patients, and families. Weissman's approach to conflict resolution is based on understanding a patient's or a family's story, attending to their emotions, and establishing shared decision-making (35).

Principled negotiation is an approach to resolving conflict that avoids power struggles and unwanted compromises (Table 41.7) (34,71). The

TABLE 41.7 STRATEGIES FOR CONFLICT MANAGEMENT AND RESOLUTION

Learn the patient's and family's story

Attend to emotions

Establish shared goals for treatment

Separate people from the problem

Focus on interests

Invent solutions

Outline objective criteria

Establish shared goals for treatment

process recommends that one identify the fundamental problem, separating this from the individual's judgment on both sides. It next involves listening to requests and demands but making an attempt to look into underlying interests, for all parties concerned. This would include a clear expression of the intentions and goals of the medical team. It is recommended that one avoid contrasting different philosophies of medical care. Instead, it would be prudent to propose a plan of care that meets a family's expectations without detracting from good medical care. Provision of objective information to substantiate medical recommendations rather than anecdotes is also recommended in this approach.

Empathetic Truth-Telling Skills

Health care providers are often afraid that by telling someone the truth about his/her diagnosis, they would be responsible for taking away hope. The conflict, between truth telling and fear of destroying hope, is commonly noted by patients and families who feel that "the doctor is not really telling me everything," a feeling that is highly corrosive to the doctor–patient relationship (73).

Brody (74) writes, "Hope means different things to different people, and different things to the same person as he/she moves through stages of illness." The physician can play a valuable role in helping the individual patient define his/her hopes and fears. When close to death, hope often becomes refocused away from long-term goals and toward short-term or spiritual goals. Hope may mean a pain-free day, a sense of security, love and nonabandonment, or a wedding to attend in the near future. Factors that often increase hope in the terminally ill include feeling valued, maintaining meaningful relationships, reminiscence, humor, realistic goals, and optimal symptom relief. Factors that often decrease hope include feeling devalued or abandoned, lack of direction and goals, and unrelieved pain and discomfort (75).

Strategic Use of a Therapeutic Silence

When communicating distressing information, it is important to allow for silence. In the authors' experience, no matter what one might imagine the response from the patient or family will be to any information being communicated, particularly information in the setting of a life-threatening or life-limiting illness, one really cannot predict their expressed as well as repressed emotional reaction (e.g., relief, anxiety, anger, regret, and fear). The ensuing silence can be uncomfortable. It is important to resist the urge to fill it with more facts as they will likely not be heard. Not all patients and families express emotions at this point and instead respond practically. It is still recommended that one wait, silently, to see what response the patient or family demonstrates. Curtis et al. (76,77) demonstrated that when clinicians spend a greater proportion of their time during family conferences listening rather than speaking, family members report increased satisfaction with the communication.

POPULATIONS, SITUATIONS, AND CIRCUMSTANCES THAT REQUIRE A SPECIAL MENTION

Pediatrics

Caring for the seriously ill and dying children is a stressful job. Insufficient training and competence in communication skills may exacerbate staff members' stress and affect the quality of care (78). This stress affects not only the physicians and nurses who work closely with children and families in the palliative phases of treatment but also a host of other hospital staff members. The staff members and family members often experience anguish at watching children suffer and a sense of helplessness with respect to alleviating the pain (78–80). Staff members also conveyed concerns about their lack of preparation and their feelings of inadequacy in pain management. In addition, they described instances of disagreements among attending physicians and refusal to consult with the pain management team (78,80). The expanding literature and experiences of families and staff members emphasize the continuing need for improvements in communication (81) and caring at the end of life for the pediatric population. An abundance of adequate and timely support is necessary for staff members as well as families (78,82). Although children are typically allowed to assent, rather than consent to plans regarding their care, parents and health care providers must recognize the subjective personal nature of suffering and respect the child's autonomy and capacity to make decisions, particularly for emancipated and mature minors.

Surgical Patients

Navigating family meetings within the surgical population poses distinct challenges as compared to patients with medical illnesses. Surgical patients who benefit from palliative care typically are diagnosed with either a subacute or chronic condition that is worsening or a sudden event like a trauma or burn injury. There are several unique characteristics of trauma patients that make family meetings imperative (83). First, there is a 10% to 20% mortality incidence in trauma ICUs. A significant minority of these patients are young, healthy patients who become critically ill in a matter of seconds. Second, the illness course is usually either brief (patient succumbing to devastating neurologic injury in the first 72 hours) or long and drawn out (patient who initially survives trauma injury but has complications from multiple organ failure and sepsis) (83). The prognostication tools for these patients are of limited value at the individual patient level (84). Surgical patients with more subacute or chronic disease have often been followed by their surgeon for years. As a result, the physician patient bond in these patients is strong, and patients generally defer to their treating surgeons for all major medical decisions. In these situations, it is paramount to have buy-in and ideally direct involvement from the primary surgeon before embarking on a family meeting (85). It is equally important that information communicated to patients and families is consistent amongst all providers to minimize the miscommunication. Often, communication about the end-of-life decisions is not done until the last hours of a patient's life. Measures to hold a family meeting early on to address prognosis or prognostic uncertainty and goals of care have improved communication in the surgical setting including both trauma ICUs and surgical ICUs (86).

Chronic Progressive Illness

As a result of advances in medicine, patients are able to live longer despite having an incurable and or progressive illness. Access to these novel therapies has extended life, but quality of life and functionality can vary considerably between patients and disease. It is imperative therefore that clinicians familiarize themselves with the different disease trajectories for chronic progressive illness, as this will allow them to identify the key points in time when a family meeting is indicated (87–89).

Withdrawal of Life-Sustaining Measures

It is important not to directly ask the family to make a decision about withdrawal of life support but to rather make a shared decision based on your medical knowledge and the family's input about patient's goals or wishes. Do not use language that causes fear of abandonment such as "There's nothing more we can do" or "I've done all I can." Instead, empathetic phrases such as "I wish your dad's liver could be fixed. Unfortunately, it can't be fixed. Based on what you've told me about your dad's wishes, I recommend focusing on your dad's comfort." Discussing what the patient would want rather than what the family desires also relieves family guilt (90). Giving concrete information about what withdrawal of life support looks like, including anticipated time of death, reassurance that the patient will be continued to be cared for, and common terminal symptoms, decreases caregivers' depression and anxiety (91).

Language Barrier

During times of emotional stress and during conversations that are ripe with emotion, vulnerability, and those that touch the very sense and core of the inner soul, it is most comforting and safe for patients and families to describe feelings and thoughts in their primary language. Although using family members as interpreters may seem convenient, and tempting, it is fraught with problems. There is no assurance they will have the necessary language skills to convey medical information, and the patient may not feel comfortable expressing his or her feelings through family members. Family members may misinterpret medical phrases, censor sensitive/taboo topics, or summarize discussions rather than translating them completely (92). Family members may have strong emotions that affect their objectivity and impartiality. In addition, being the bearer of bad news or discussing contentious information may have negative implications for a family member following the encounter.

When communicating to patients and families with limited English proficiency, one should utilize a medical interpreter who has acquired the specific training and meet the national standards/ethics of practice (National Council on Interpreting in Healthcare) (93). The need to use an interpreter implies that significant cultural differences exist between the practitioner and the patient/family. Professional interpreters can help one to provide effective and efficient communication that is culturally sensitive and factually accurate upon translation. Accomplished and qualified uses of translators prevent the "lost in translation" phenomenon, which can cause conflict and misunderstandings in communications (94).

Cultural Beliefs

The cultural backgrounds of not only patients and families but also of health care teams profoundly influence their preferences and needs regarding

---

TABLE 41.8 A FRAMEWORK FOR A CULTURALLY SENSITIVE INTERACTION

Communication
Unique cultural values
Locus of decision-making
Translators
Understanding the patient's needs
Ritualized practice and restrictions
Environment at home

From Lum H, Arnold R. Asking about cultural beliefs in palliative care. Fast Facts and Concepts #216. June 2009.

---

discussing bad news, decision-making, and the dying experience (Table 41.8).

It is important to identify the patient's preferences regarding how and with whom medical information is shared. For those who request that the physician discuss their condition with family members, identify the main contacts to give information to, about the patient's condition. Use respectful, curious, and open-ended questions about a patient's cultural heritage to identify their values (95).

For some patients, medical decision-making is communally driven rather than individualistic. Multiple family members or a community elder or leader may need to be involved, often without prior official documentation because it is assumed or understood from the patient's perspective. As discussed in a previous section, language barriers are extremely challenging, especially during times of severe illness. Utilize medical interpreters frequently and effectively.

Reassess what is being heard, understood, and agreed upon frequently, from both the patient's and clinician's standpoint. Specifically confirm that the patient understands (96). This is particularly important if a medical translator is involved, as miscommunication is common even when using trained medical interpreters. Determine if there are specific customs the patient desires to be followed. These must be communicated to other health care providers, especially in the hospital setting. It may be necessary to advocate for the patient and negotiate with health care facility administrators to find an agreeable way to honor a patient's wishes. Given that a majority of hospice care happens in the patient's home environment, respectfully explore whether there are any needs that can be met by the health care system, and how open the patient, family, or community is to receiving care at home. Even if a trusting, collaborative relationship has developed between a patient/family and clinicians in the hospital, this may not immediately translate into the home setting. With the patient's permission, expectations about cultural-specific aspects of a patient's care should be explicitly communicated to care providers outside the hospital (97–100).

WHAT CAN GO WRONG IN EVEN WELL-PLANNED FAMILY MEETINGS?

The family meeting can be the most effective tool for clinicians when handled well. However, when conducted poorly, it can be catastrophic. What can go wrong? Often there is insufficient preparation that is done prior to the meeting. Clinicians may not agree on treatment decisions. This gets reflected in the meetings causing confusion among the family members, ultimately making it difficult to delineate a cohesive plan (26). Physicians often talk too much. McDonagh et al. noted that typically in the ICU settings, physicians spent about 70% of the time talking during family meetings while families spent only 30%. Further, they found that when families had a greater opportunity to speak more during these meetings, satisfaction increased (77). Finally, clinicians often use too much medical jargon when communicating, decreasing the ability of the families to truly understand an already complicated situation (6). Following a clear structure as outlined in Tables 41.1 to 41.3 when conducting a meeting is often helpful in avoiding some of the anticipated pitfalls.

CONCLUSION

Good communication and organizational skills are critical to delivering effective and timely care to all patients, particularly those with serious illnesses. Using a stepwise approach to family meetings provides a framework to optimize shared decision-making. A family meeting and other patient–physician interactions when executed well have correlated with improved health outcomes, patient satisfactions, and emotional well-being and should be considered (8,101–103).

REFERENCES

1. Joshi R. Family meetings: an essential component of comprehensive palliative care. *Can Fam Physician.* 2013;59: 637-639.
2. Lilly CM, De Meo DL, Sonna LA, et al. An intensive communication intervention for the critically ill. *Am J Med.* 2000;109(6):469-475.
3. Lautrette A, Darmaon M, Megarbane B, et al. A communication strategy and brochure for relatives of patients dying in the ICU. *N Engl J Med.* 2007;356(5):469-478.
4. Stapleton RD, Engelberg RA, Wenrich MD, Goss CH, Curtis JR. Clinician statements and family satisfaction with family conferences in the intensive care unit. *Crit Care Med.* 2006;34(6):1679-1685.
5. Mularski RA, Curtis JR, Billings JA, et al. Proposed quality measures for palliative care in the critically ill: a consensus from the Robert Wood Johnson Foundation

6. Critical Care Workgroup. *Crit Care Med.* 2006;34(11): S404-S411.
6. Curtis JR, Patrick DL, Shannon SE, Treece PD, Engelberg RA, Rubenfeld GD. The family conference as a focus to improve communication about end-of-life care in the intensive care unit: opportunities for improvement. *Crit Care Med.* 2001;29(2):N26-N33.
7. Billings JA. The end-of-life family meeting in intensive care part I: indications, outcomes, and family needs. *J Palliat Med.* 2011;14(9):1042-1050.
8. Billings JA. The end-of-life family meeting in intensive care part II: family-centered decision making. *J Palliat Med.* 2011;14(9):1051-1057.
9. Hudson P, Quinn K, O'Hanlon B, Aranda S. Family meetings in palliative care: multidisciplinary clinical practice guidelines. *BMC Palliat Care.* 2008;7:12.
10. Breen CM, Abernethy AP, Abbott KH, Tulsky JA. Conflict associated with decisions to limit life-sustaining treatment in intensive care units. *J Gen Intern Med.* 2001;16(5): 283-289.
11. Hofmann JC, Wenger NS, Davis RB, et al. Patient preferences for communication with physicians about end-of-life decisions. SUPPORT Investigators. Study to understand prognoses and preference for outcomes and risks of treatment. *Ann Intern Med.* 1997;127(1):1-12.
12. Clarke EB, Curtis JR, Lucw JM, et al. Quality indicators for end-of-life care in the intensive care unit. *Crit Care Med.* 2003;31(9):2255-2262.
13. Abbott KH, Sago JG, Breen CM, Abernethy AP, Tulsky JA. Families looking back: one year after discussion of withdrawal or withholding of life-sustaining support. *Crit Care Med.* 2001;29(1):197-201.
14. Baker R, Wu AW, Teno JM, et al. Family satisfaction with end-of-life care in seriously ill hospitalized adults. *J Am Geriatr Soc.* 2000;48(5):S61-S69.
15. Azoulay E, Chevret S, Leleu G, et al. Half the families of intensive care unit patients experience inadequate communication with physicians. *Crit Care Med.* 2000;28(8):3044-3049.
16. Maguire P, Pitceathly C. Key communication skills and how to acquire them. *BMJ (Clin Res Ed).* 2002;325(7366): 697-700.
17. Roberts CS, Cox CE, Reintgen DS, Baile WF, Gibertini M. Influence of physician communication on newly diagnosed breast patients' psychologic adjustment and decision-making. *Cancer.* 1994;74(1):336-341.
18. Kaplan SH, Ware JE. The patients role in healthcare and quality assessment. In: Goldfield N, Nash DB, eds. *Providing Quality Care: Future Challenges.* Chicago, IL: Health Administration Press; 1995:26-27.
19. Fogarty LA, Curbow BA, Wingard JR, McDonnell K, Somerfield MR. Can 40 seconds of compassion reduce patient anxiety? *J Clin Oncol.* 1999;17(1):371-379.
20. Curtis JR, Wenrich MD, Carline JD, Shannon SE, Ambrozy DM, Ramsey PG. Understanding physicians' skills at providing end-of-life care perspectives of patients, families, and health care workers. *J Gen Intern Med.* 2001;16(1):41-49.
21. Steinhauser KE, Clipp EC, McNeilly M, Christakis NA, McIntyre LM, Tulsky JA. In search of a good death: observations of patients, families, and providers. *Ann Intern Med.* 2000;132(10):825-832.
22. Wenrich MD, Curtis JR, Shannon SE, Carline JD, Ambrozy DM, Ramsey PG. Communicating with dying patients within the spectrum of medical care from terminal diagnosis to death. *Arch Intern Med.* 2001;161(6):868-874.
23. Weissman DE, Quill TE, Arnold RM. The family meeting: end-of-life goal setting and future planning #227. *J Palliat Med.* 2010;13(4):462-463.

24. Meyer DL, Gershman K, Broberg L, Craigie FC Jr, Antonucci J. Conducting family meetings in nursing homes: resident, nurse, and family perceptions. *Fam Med.* 1991;23:36-39.

25. Gritti P. The family meetings in oncology: some practical guidelines. *Front Psychol.* 2014;5:1552.

26. Lautrette A, Ciroldi M, Ksibi H, Azoulay E. End-of-life family conferences: rooted in the evidence. *Crit Care Med.* 2006;34(11):S364-S372.

27. Lilly CM, Sonna LA, Haley KJ, Massaro AF. Intensive communication: four-year follow-up from a clinical practice study. *Crit Care Med.* 2003;31(5):S394-S399.

28. Mack JW, Cook EF, Wolfe J, Grier HE, Cleary PD, Weeks JC. Understanding of prognosis among parents of children with cancer: parental optimism and the parent-physician interaction. *J Clin Oncol.* 2007;25(11): 1357-1362.

29. Garros D, Rosychuk RJ, Cox PN. Circumstances surrounding end of life in a pediatric intensive care unit. *Pediatrics.* 2003;112(5):e371.

30. Walter JK, Sachs E, Schall TE, et al. Interprofessional teamwork during family meetings in the Pediatric Cardiac Intensive Care Unit. *J Pain Symptom Manage.* 2019;57:1089-1098.

31. Weissman DE, Quill TE, Arnold RM. Preparing for the family meeting #222. *J Palliat Med.* 2010;13(2):203-204.

32. von Gunten CF, Ferris FD, Emanuel LL. The patient-physician relationship. Ensuring competency in end-of-life care: communication and relational skills. *JAMA.* 2000;284(23):3051-3057.

33. Curtis JR, Engelberg RA, Wenrich MD, Shannon SE, Treece PD, Rubenfeld GD. Missed opportunities during family conferences about end-of-life care in the intensive care unit. *Am J Respir Crit Care Med.* 2005;171(8):844-849.

34. King DA, Quill T. Working with families in palliative care: one size does not fit all. *J Palliat Med.* 2006; 9(3):704-715.

35. Weissman DE, Quill TE, Arnold RM. The family meeting: causes of conflict #225. *J Palliat Med.* 2010;13(3): 328-329.

36. Nelson JE, Walker AS, Luhrs CA, Cortez TB, Pronovost PJ. Family meetings made simpler: a toolkit for the intensive care unit. *J Crit Care.* 2009;24(4):626.e7-626.e14.

37. Tobin B, Lobb E, Roper E, Ingham J. Is the patient's voice under-heard in family conferences in palliative care? A question from Sydney, Australia. *J Pain Symptom Manage.* 2011;41(2):e3-e6.

38. Back A. *Mastering Communication with Seriously Ill Patients: Balancing Honesty with Empathy and Hope.* Cambridge, UK/New York, NY: Cambridge University Press; 2009.

39. Weissman DE, Quill TE, Arnold RM. The family meeting: starting the conversation #223. *J Palliat Med.* 2010;13(2):204-205.

40. Radwany S, Albanese T, Clough L, Sims L, Mason H, Jahangiri S. End-of-life decision making and emotional burden: placing family meetings in context. *Am J Hosp Palliat Care.* 2009;26(5):376-383.

41. Parle M, Jones B, Maguire P. Maladaptive coping and affective disorders among cancer patients. *Psychol Med.* 1996;26(4):735-744.

42. Maguire P. Improving communication with cancer patients. *Eur J Cancer.* 1999;35(14):2058-2065.

43. Butow PN, Maclean M, Dunn SM, Tattersall MH, Boyer MJ. The dynamics of change: cancer patients' preferences for information, involvement and support. *Ann Oncol.* 1997;8(9):857-863.

44. Jenkins V, Fallowfield L, Saul J. Information needs of patients with cancer: results from a large study in UK cancer centres. *Br J Cancer.* 2001;84(1):48-51.

45. Kutner JS, Steiner JF, Corbett KK, Jahnigen DW, Barton PL. Information needs in terminal illness. *Soc Sci Med (1982).* 1999;48(10):1341-1352.

46. Leydon GM, Boulton M, Moynihan C, et al. Cancer patients' information needs and information seeking behaviour: in depth interview study. *BMJ (Clin Res Ed).* 2000;320(7239):909-913.

47. Goldstein D, Thewes B, Butow P. Communicating in a multicultural society. II: Greek community attitudes towards cancer in Australia. *Intern Med J.* 2002;32(7): 289-296.

48. Cassileth BR, Zupkis RV, Sutton-Smith K, March V. Information and participation preferences among cancer patients. *Ann Intern Med.* 1980;92(6):832-836.

49. Blanchard CG, Labrecque MS, Ruckdeschel JC, Blanchard EB. Information and decision-making preferences of hospitalized adult cancer patients. *Soc Sci Med (1982).* 1988;27(11):1139-1145.

50. Jones R, Pearson J, McGregor S, et al. Cross sectional survey of patients' satisfaction with information about cancer. *BMJ (Clin Res Ed).* 1999;319(7219): 1247-1248.

51. Mazur DJ, Hickam DH. Patients' interpretations of probability terms. *J Gen Intern Med.* 1991;6(3): 237-240.

52. Woloshin KK, Ruffin MT IV, Gorenflo DW. Patients' interpretation of qualitative probability statements. *Arch Fam Med.* 1994;3(11):961-966.

53. Back AL, Arnold RM. Dealing with conflict in caring for the seriously ill: 'it was just out of the question'. *JAMA.* 2005;293(11):1374-1381.

54. Pearlman RA, Cain KC, Patrick DL, et al. Insights pertaining to patient assessments of states worse than death. *J Clin Ethics.* 1993;4(1):33-41.

55. Seckler AB, Meier DE, Mulvihill M, Paris BE. Substituted judgment: how accurate are proxy predictions? *Ann Intern Med.* 1991;115(2):92-98.

56. Sehgal A, Galbraith A, Chesney M, Schoenfeld P, Charles G, Lo B. How strictly do dialysis patients want their advance directives followed? *JAMA.* 1992; 267(1):59-63.

57. von Gunten CF, Ferris FD, Kirschner C, Emanuel LL. Coding and reimbursement mechanisms for physician services in hospice and palliative care. *J Palliat Med.* 2000;3(2):157-164.

58. Wenrich MD, Curtis JR, Ambrozy DA, Carline JD, Shannon SE, Ramsey PG. Dying patients' need for emotional support and personalized care from physicians: perspectives of patients with terminal illness, families, and health care providers. *J Pain Symptom Manage.* 2003;25(3):236-246.

59. Steinhauser KE, Christakis NA, Clipp EC, McNeilly M, McIntyre L, Tulsky JA. Factors considered important at the end of life by patients, family, physicians, and other care providers. *JAMA.* 2000;284(19):2476-2482.

60. Oken D. What to tell cancer patients. A study of medical attitudes. *JAMA.* 1961;175:1120-1128.

61. Taylor KM. 'Telling bad news': physicians and the disclosure of undesirable information. *Soc Health Illn.* 1988;10(2):109-132.

62. Miyaji NT. The power of compassion: truth-telling among American doctors in the care of dying patients. *Soc Sci Med (1982).* 1993;36(3): 249-264.

63. Siminoff LA, Fetting JH, Abeloff MD. Doctor-patient communication about breast cancer adjuvant therapy. *J Clin Oncol.* 1989;7(9):1192-1200.

64. Maguire P. Barriers to psychological care of the dying. *BMJ (Clin Res Ed).* 1985;291(6510):1711-1713.

65. Buckman R. Breaking bad news: why is it still so difficult? *BMJ (Clin Res Ed).* 1984;288(6430):1597-1599.

66. Del vecchio Good MJ, Good BJ, Schaffer C, Lind SE. American oncology and the discourse on hope. *Cult Med Psychiatry*. 1990;14(1):59-79.

67. Baile WF, Buckman R, Lenzi R, Glober G, Beale EA, Kudelka AP. SPIKES—a six-step protocol for delivering bad news: application to the patient with cancer. *Oncologist*. 2000;5(4):302-311.

68. Curtis JR, White DB. Practical guidance for evidence-based ICU family conferences. *Chest*. 2008;134(4):835-843.

69. Quill TE, Arnold R, Back AL. Discussing treatment preferences with patients who want 'everything'. *Ann Intern Med*. 2009;151(5):345-349.

70. Lazare A, Eisenthal S, Frank A. Clinician/patient relations II: conflict and negotiation. In: *Outpatient Psychiatry*. Baltimore, MD: Lippincott Williams & Wilkins; 1989:137-157.

71. Fisher R. *Getting to Yes: Negotiating Agreement Without Giving In*. 2nd ed. Boston, MA: Houghton Mifflin; 1991.

72. Quill TE. Recognizing and adjusting to barriers in doctor-patient communication. *Ann Intern Med*. 1989;111(1):51-57.

73. Tywcross R, Lichter I. The terminal phase. In: Doyle D, Hanks, G, MacDonald N, eds. *Oxford Textbook of Palliative Medicine*. 2nd ed. New York, NY: Oxford University Press; 1998:977-978.

74. Brody H. Hope. *JAMA*. 1981;246(13):1411-1412.

75. Ambuel B, Weissman DE. Discussing spiritual issues and maintaining hope. In: Weissman DE, Ambuel B, eds. *Improving End-of-Life Care: A Resource Guide for Physician Education*. 2nd ed. Milwaukee, WI: Medical College of Wisconsin; 1999:113-121.

76. Curtis JR, Engelberg RA, Wenrich MD, et al. Studying communication about end-of-life care during the ICU family conference: development of a framework. *J Crit Care*. 2002;17(3):147-160.

77. McDonagh JR, Elliott TB, Engelberg RA, et al. Family satisfaction with family conferences about end-of-life care in the intensive care unit: increased proportion of family speech is associated with increased satisfaction. *Crit Care Med*. 2004;32(7):1484-1488.

78. Hilden JM, Emanuel EJ, Fairclough DL, et al. Attitudes and practices among pediatric oncologists regarding end-of-life care: results of the 1998 American Society of Clinical Oncology survey. *J Clin Oncol*. 2001;19(1):205-212.

79. Contro NA, Larson J, Scofield S, Sourkes B, Cohen HJ. Hospital staff and family perspectives regarding quality of pediatric palliative care. *Pediatrics*. 2004;114(5):1248-1252.

80. Contro N, Larson J, Scofield S, Sourkes B, Cohen H. Family perspectives on the quality of pediatric palliative care. *Arch Pediatr Adolesc Med*. 2002;156(1):14-19.

81. Khaneja S, Milrod B. Educational needs among pediatricians regarding caring for terminally ill children. *Arch Pediatr Adolesc Med*. 1998;152(9):909-914.

82. Vachon ML. Staff stress in hospice/palliative care: a review. *Palliat Med*. 1995;9(2):91-122.

83. Mosenthal AC, Murphy PA, Barker LK, Lavery R, Retano A, Livingston DH. Changing the culture around end-of-life care in the trauma intensive care unit. *J Trauma*. 2008;64(6):1587-1593.

84. Sinuff T, Adhikari NK, Cook DJ, et al. Mortality predictions in the intensive care unit: comparing physicians with scoring systems. *Crit Care Med*. 2006;34(3):878-885.

85. Schwarze ML, Bradley CT, Brasel KJ. Surgical "buy-in": the contractual relationship between surgeons and patients that influences decisions regarding life-supporting therapy. *Crit Care Med*. 2010;38:843-848.

86. Mosenthal AC, Murphy PA. Interdisciplinary model for palliative care in the trauma and surgical intensive care unit: Robert Wood Johnson Foundation Demonstration Project for Improving Palliative Care in the Intensive Care Unit. *Crit Care Med*. 2006;34(11):S399-S403.

87. Seow H, O'Leary E, Perez R, Tanuseputro P. Access to palliative care by disease trajectory: a population-based cohort of Ontario decedents. *BMJ Open*. 2018;8:e021147.

88. Mizuno A, Yoshida S, Hayashi K. Not illness trajectory but Bayesian-estimated rate model should be appropriately explained when discussing palliative care in heart disease. *J Palliat Med*. 2017;20:580-581.

89. Beernaert K, Pardon K, Van den Block L, et al. Palliative care needs at different phases in the illness trajectory: a survey study in patients with cancer. *Eur J Cancer Care (Engl)*. 2016;25:534-543.

90. Way J, Back AL, Curtis JR. Withdrawing life support and resolution of conflict with families. *BMJ (Clin Res Ed)*. 2002;325(7376):1342-1345.

91. Kirchhoff KT, Palzkill J, Kowalkowski J, Mork A, Gretarsdottir E. Preparing families of intensive care patients for withdrawal of life support: a pilot study. *Am J Crit Care*. 2008;17(2):113-121; quiz 122.

92. Haffner L. Translation is not enough. Interpreting in a medical setting. *West J Med*. 1992;157(3):255-259.

93. Howard S. Use of interpreters in palliative care. Fast facts and concepts #154. April 2006.

94. Haffner L. Guide to interpreter positioning in health care settings. *The National Council on Interpreting in Health Care Working Paper Series*; 2003. http://www.ncihc.org/mc/page.do?sitePageId=57022&orgId=ncihc

95. Lum H, Arnold R. Asking about cultural beliefs in palliative care. Fast facts and concepts #216. June 2009.

96. Maugans TA. The SPIRITual history. *Arch Fam Med*. 1996;5(1):11-16.

97. Pham K, Thornton JD, Engelberg RA, Jackson JC, Curtis JR. Alterations during medical interpretation of ICU family conferences that interfere with or enhance communication. *Chest*. 2008;134(1):109-116.

98. Searight HR, Gafford J. Cultural diversity at the end of life: issues and guidelines for family physicians. *Am Fam Physician*. 2005;71(3):515-522.

99. Crawley LM, Marshall PA, Lo B, Koenig BA. Strategies for culturally effective end-of-life care. *Ann Intern Med*. 2002;136(9):673-679.

100. Arnold R. Palliative care case of the month: the family says not to tell. *University of Pittsburgh Institute to Enhance Palliative Care*; 2006. http://www.dom.pitt.edu/dgim/IEPC/case-of-the-month.html

101. Hallenbeck J, Arnold R. A request for nondisclosure: don't tell mother. *J Clin Oncol*. 2007;25(31):5030-5034.

102. Bertakis KD, Roter D, Putnam SM. The relationship of physician medical interview style to patient satisfaction. *J Fam Pract*. 1991;32(2):175-181.

103. Roter DL, Hall JA, Kern DE, Barker LR, Cole KA, Roca RP. Improving physicians' interviewing skills and reducing patients' emotional distress. A randomized clinical trial. *Arch Intern Med*. 1995;155(17):1877-1884.

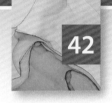

42 Psychosocial Consequences of Advanced Cancer

James R. Zabora and Matthew J. Loscalzo

When a cancer patient is confronted by advanced disease, how should clinical providers describe upcoming changes in their cancer care? Is it supportive care? Or, is the patient offered palliative care? Following the keynote panel at the American Society of Clinical Oncology's (ASCO) first palliative care conference in 2014, a robust discussion erupted that centered on this significant transition in care. The questions above dominated the remainder of the opening plenary session. Finally, an audience participant stepped to the microphone and said,

> "In Canada, if the intent of treatment is curative, we deliver supportive care. If curative treatment is not feasible, then palliative care is offered. In both instances, psychosocial interventions are highly integrated."

Following this interaction, the respondent was asked for the name of his department, and he responded, "The Department of Supportive and Palliative Care." Since 2014, cancer centers have slowly evolved in the consolidation of resources into a more continuous care model that allows patients and families to easily move from one program to another. Excellent examples are the City of Hope's Department of Supportive Care Medicine (Duarte, CA) and the Life With Cancer Program within the Inova Health System (Fairfax, VA).

All psychosocial care is palliative in nature. Attention must be directed to the realities of one's life within their unique social context in order to maximize internal resources, activate external support systems, and focus on the dignity and quality of life (QOL) for each patient and family member. Psychosocial care within supportive and palliative care programs deliver ongoing evidence-based interventions that deliver measurable benefit to patients, family caregivers, and the health care system. Supportive and palliative care are provided by interdisciplinary teams of compassionate experts, but if there is no team in place, true whole-patient–centered care is not possible (1). The debate of supportive versus palliative care in hospitals has dramatically increased over the past 5 years (2); however, the integration of clearly defined programs within standard cancer care is still far less than is desirable.

Psychosocial concerns and dilemmas based on context and predisposition continue to be at the core of the cancer experience. Life-limiting illness and related stressors generate ongoing challenges. However, there are opportunities to learn how to manage demands in order to achieve meaningful experiences during care for advanced disease. In the absence of moderate to severe distress caused by physical symptoms, such as pain, nausea, and difficulty in breathing, the psychosocial and spiritual aspects of a person's identity and life become paramount. The psychosocial aspects of a person's life are what give them a sense as vital human beings within a social context of living with a life-threatening illness. In this context, the possibility for emotional growth and transcendence becomes obtainable.

Despite significant progress in research and treatments, the diagnosis of cancer creates fear and turmoil in the lives of every patient and family. In many respects, cancer generates a greater sense of dread than other life-threatening illnesses with similar prognoses (3). Some studies have found that patients with cancer are sicker and have more symptoms than patients without cancer in the year before death, and most often, it is easier to predict the course of the illness (4). Yabroff and Youngmee (5) documented that many noxious physical and psychological symptoms are prevalent in the year after diagnosis, after disease-directed treatments have ceased, regardless of prognosis. Consequently, supportive and palliative approaches must be offered and provided based on psychosocial needs of each patient and family.

Frequently, the greatest concern of patients with cancer is not death, pain, or physical symptoms but rather the impact of the disease on their families (6). People see themselves as imbedded in a larger social construct that gives them a sense of place and meaning. For most cancer patients, it is the family that is at the most basic core of that identity. According to the World Health Organization (7), family refers to those individuals who are either relatives or other significant people as defined by the patient. Health care professionals must acknowledge the role of the family to maximize treatment outcomes. If the family is actively incorporated into patient care, the health care team gains valuable allies and resources. Families are the primary source of support and also fill in the caregiving roles for persons with cancer. Of note, men are taking a greater responsibility for the care of seriously ill spouses, but women still comprise most of the individuals who serve in these caregiving roles (8,9). However, families vary widely in their ability to provide this necessary care and support.

Although access to ongoing supportive and palliative care could potentially provide support for both patient and family, financial resources to fully support these two related approaches to care remain limited in many cancer centers and hospital systems. In the United States, most palliative care is still perceived as being associated with hospice programs, but the median length of service for hospice patients continues at 3 weeks or less (10,11). Furthermore, a discussion concerning a referral to palliative care or hospice can seem quite sudden, and the patient and family can experience this transition as rejection. Despite the sobering survival statistics for many cancers, relatively few hospitals have truly developed a continuum of cancer care, which clearly informs patients and families that most antineoplastic therapy in advanced disease is palliative and not curative. In particular, this is true for patients with cancer who enroll in phase I and II clinical trials (12). This is significant given that most patients with cancer overestimate the probability of long-term survival (13). At present, patients and family members enter hospice care, which is the primary resource for comprehensive palliative care services, and attempt to accept that prolongation of life is no longer the goal of care. In addition to the shift in the focus from cure to care, the patient and family experience the loss of the health care team with whom trust has been imbued over months and sometimes many years. The loss occurs simultaneously at multiple levels. Although palliative care at the end of life should be a time of refocusing and resolution, the hospice referral process may cause an iatrogenic crisis rather than comfort. But even when patients are not transferred to an external setting trauma is common. This is especially true of patients who are admitted to ICUs where the caregivers of deceased patients all too frequently report symptoms (up to 20%) of posttraumatic distress disorder from the experience many years after the death (14). Consequently, the focus of care for patients with advanced disease needs to be the early identification of vulnerability, such as significantly elevated distress, that is followed by evidence-based psychosocial interventions.

PSYCHOLOGICAL RESPONSES TO ADVANCED CANCER

The psychological impact of advanced cancer and its management is directly influenced by the interactions among the degree of physical disability, the severity of symptoms, the internal resources of the patient, the level of social support, the intensity of the treatment, side effects and other adverse reactions, and the relationship with the health care team. The degree of physical distress placed on any individual and the inevitable drive to give meaning to the experience is the core from which the psychosocial concerns arise. At present, active support for these aspects of supportive and palliative care is still lacking in many nonacademic medical settings (15).

Adaptation to advancing disease begins with an appraisal of the extent of perceived harm, loss, threat, and challenge that this experience generates. In many respects, this appraisal is linked to the intensity and quality of the patient's emotional response. Emotional regulation is at the core of coping and "problem solving" and has significant implications for maintaining a sense of direction and control. Overall, this primary appraisal, efficiency of emotional regulation, and definition of the meaning of advanced cancer result in an assessment of the potential harm and threat as well as a secondary appraisal. In this secondary level, patients must assess their personal (internal) and social (external) resources necessary to begin to address the demands and problems associated with advanced cancer. This process can be significantly influenced by the patient's ability to maintain emotional regulation (16).

In addition, two salient continuums related to patient and family adaptation must also be considered. The level of psychological distress forms the first continuum and the second consists of the predictable and transitional phases of the disease process. Patients with a preexisting high level of psychological distress can experience significant difficulty with any attempt to adapt to the stressors associated with a cancer diagnosis and related treatments. Although most patients experience significant distress at the time of their diagnosis, most patients gradually adjust during the following 6 months (17). Evidence indicates that the best predictor of positive adaptation is the psychological state of the patient with cancer before the initiation of any therapeutic regimens (18). Although clinical experience would clearly indicate that the health system can influence the ability of patients and their families to adapt, literature to support this premise empirically continues to be unavailable. Clinically, it is quite evident that hospitals still

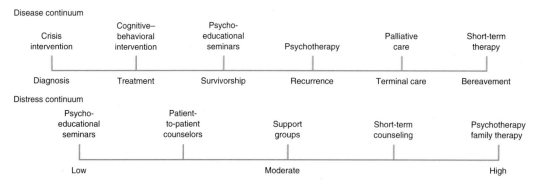

Figure 42.1 Continuum of care for patients with cancer and their families.

experience difficulty with critical transition points in the care of seriously ill patients. But, there are now strong data that indicate supportive and palliative care for specific groups of cancer patients with advancing disease can extend both QOL and length of life (19).

Figure 42.1 details evidence-based psychosocial interventions along the disease and distress continuums. The level of psychological vulnerability also falls along a continuum from low to high distress and should guide this selection of interventions (20). In addition, "a problem-solving intervention" has been demonstrated to reduce distress among patients with cancer as well as among family members (21,22). Prevalence studies demonstrate that one of every three newly diagnosed patients (regardless of prognosis) needs psychosocial or psychiatric intervention (23–26). As disease advances, a positive relationship exists between the increase in the occurrence and severity of physiologic symptoms and the patient's level of emotional distress and overall QOL. For example, a study of 268 patients with cancer having recurrent disease observed that patients with higher symptomatology, greater financial concerns, and a pessimistic outlook experience higher levels of psychological distress and lower levels of general well-being (27).

In 2011, the National Comprehensive Cancer Network (NCCN) initiated an effort to establish the early identification of patients at high risk for poor adaptation. NCCN developed and published guidelines for the management of psychological distress among cancer patients across the disease continuum. The NCCN described distress in a manner consistent with the focus and goals of supportive and palliative care, as an experience that can be psychological, social, or spiritual, which interferes with one's ability to manage or problem-solve in relation to the diagnosis, treatment, side effects, and symptoms associated with cancer (28). These guidelines provided a framework for the development and implementation of psychosocial

interventions based on the perspectives of social work, psychiatry, psychology, nursing, and pastoral care. Psychosocial distress screening served as the mechanism to identify patients at higher levels of risk in order to provide interventions at a much earlier point in time. The current guidelines can be accessed at www.nccs.org.

If distress levels can be identified through techniques such as psychosocial screening, patients can then be introduced into supportive care systems earlier in the treatment or at the beginning of the palliative care process. In fact, nationally and internationally, a number of investigators have successfully implemented robust biopsychosocial screening initiatives as part of the standard of clinical care in cancer setting (e.g., J. Zabora, M. Loscalzo, B. Bultz, and A. Mitchell). All of these screening programs use instruments that include psychological and physical symptoms, as well as social, spiritual, and practical concerns (28). Some of these programs use automated referrals or triages, provide educational information, and send clinical summary alerts to the physician and team during the clinical encounter (29). Of significant importance, the influential Institute of Medicine report in 2007, Cancer Care for the Whole Patient: Meeting Psychosocial Health Needs, has endorsed biopsychosocial screening as the minimum standard of quality cancer care (30). Subsequently in 2016, the American College of Surgeons (ACoS) has established a new standard that requires screening for distress in ACoS accredited programs. In Canada, distress has been endorsed as the sixth vital sign (31).

Accordingly, any attempt to identify vulnerable patients and families in a prospective manner is worthwhile. Screening techniques are available through the use of standardized instruments that are able to prospectively identify patients and families that may be more vulnerable to the cancer experience (32,33). Preexisting psychosocial resources are critical in any predictive or screening

TABLE 42.1 VARIABLES ASSOCIATED WITH PSYCHOSOCIAL ADAPTATION

Social support	History	Current concerns	Other variables
Marital status	Substance abuse	Health	Education
Living arrangements	Depression	Religion	Employment
Number of family members and relatives in vicinity	Mental health	Work-finance	Physical symptoms
Church attendance	Major illness	Family	Anatomic staging
	Past regrets	Friends	
	Optimism vs. pessimism	Existential	
		Self-appraisal	

From Weisman AD, Worden JW, Sobel HJ. *Psychosocial Screening and Interventions with Patients with Cancer: A Research Report*. Boston, MA: Harvard Medical School and Massachusetts Hospital; 1980, with permission.

process. In one approach, Weisman et al. (34) delineated key psychosocial variables in the format of a structured interview accompanied by a self-report measure (Table. 42.1). However, in hospitals, clinics, or community agencies, which provide care to a high volume of patients and family members, a structured interview by a psychosocial provider is seldom feasible or even warranted. Consequently, brief and rapid methods of screening are necessary. Brief screening techniques that examine components of distress, such as anxiety or depression, can be incorporated into the routine clinical care of the patient. But only screening for psychiatric symptoms is not adequate. Just as cancer patients should not have to be dying to receive the full suite of palliative care services, patients and their families should not have to manifest psychiatric symptoms to receive psychosocial support. Early psychosocial interventions may be less stigmatizing to the patient and more readily accepted by patients, families, and staff if screening identifies the management of distress as one component of comprehensive care (35). Screening is also a cost-effective technique for case identification in comparison to an assessment of all new patients (36). Although screening for distress and disease-related problems have received much attention, there are relatively few extensive screening and intervention programs in place, including some comprehensive cancer centers (37). The City of Hope National Medical Center and NCI-designated Comprehensive Cancer Center in Duarte, California, is one of the few cancer programs that is screening patients with cancer for common problems and related distress. A fully automated touchscreen system (*SupportScreen*) has been in place since 2009 and has been licensed to a number of hospitals (29). *SupportScreen* provides an opportunity for the patients (and in some clinics family caregivers) to input their own information

(in English and Spanish) relating to immediate psychological and physical symptoms as well as social, spiritual, and practical concerns. Patients are able to indicate the degree of distress they are experiencing as well as the kind of assistance they are seeking from the health care team. Personalized educational sheets and resources are also provided, all in real time during the actual clinical encounter. The physician and health care team also automatically receive paper and electronic clinical alerts right before they meet with the patient. This technology has been very well received by physicians and staff, patients (of all adult ages), and family members. The experience at the City of Hope and other hospitals has demonstrated that patients prefer touchscreen technology to either paper or pencil and to personal interviews and provide more personal information in this medium (38). The items on the screening instrument have also been tailored for individual clinics by medical specialty. The implications for the integration of palliative care into the standard of clinical care are of major importance. Many of the domains that relate to serious illness are emotionally laden and many physicians and health care providers lack the time, training, or inclination to open conversations that are essential to the psychological well-being of patients and their concerned family members. In this instance, it is quite evident that this technology and biopsychosocial content have the potential to transform the clinical encounter and the relationship between patients and their health care providers.

For each of the problems listed, a triage plan is in place and can be accessed during the clinical visit by the physician, nurse, or social worker. The social worker assesses the potential need for referrals to psychology and psychiatry. Not surprisingly, the 10 most common problems in rank order manifested by the first 300 patients with cancer at the City of Hope were fatigue (feeling tired), fear and worry about the future, finances, pain, feeling down, depressed or blue, being dependent on others, understanding my treatment options, sleeping, managing my emotions, and solving problems due to my illness. Of particular note, although pain was not the most frequently endorsed problem, it was the most emotionally distressing.

Standardized measures of psychological distress can differentiate patients into low, moderate, or high degrees of vulnerability. Patients with a low or moderate level of distress may benefit from a psychoeducational program, which can enhance adaptive capabilities and problem-solving skills; high distress patients possess more complex psychosocial needs that require brief therapy or family therapy along with psychotropic drug therapy for the patient. For some patients, ongoing mental health services are essential, whereas other patients may require assistance only at critical transition points. Clinical practice suggests that virtually all patients could benefit from some type of psychosocial intervention at some point along the disease continuum, especially at the end of life. Psychosocial interventions include educational programs, support groups, cognitive–behavioral techniques, problem-solving therapy or education, and psychotherapy (39). To further facilitate the process of screening, the brief standardized instruments have been developed to create greater ease of administration and scoring and to develop gender-based norms (40,41). Finally, Zabora and BrintzenhofeSzoc developed the Chronic Illness Distress Scale (CIDS) that has been in use at Life With Cancer in the Inova Health System in northern, Virginia, and acceptable levels of sensitivity and specificity have been established. The CIDS has been administered to over 8,000 new cancer patients at 5 Inova cancer clinics via Epic and handheld tablets. Patient and staff satisfaction has been high, and manuscripts that describe this process are in process.

The second continuum relates to the predictable phases of the disease process. This disease continuum extends from the point of diagnosis to cancer therapies and beyond. Across this continuum, patients acquire experiences, knowledge, and skills that enable them to respond to the demands of their disease. The needs of a newly diagnosed patient with intractable symptoms differ significantly from a patient who has advanced disease and no further options for curative treatments.

The patient and family may be supported throughout the illness process and the family requires continuing support following the death of the patient. At times families are overwhelmed by the illness and as a result are unable to effectively respond. For some families, a death may represent a major loss of the family's identity and may paralyze the family's coping and problem-solving responses. Failure to respond and solve problems leads to a lack of control and may generate a significant potential for a chronic grief reaction (42). Although the disease continuum consists of specific points, Table 42.2 identifies a series of predictable and relevant crisis events and psychosocial challenges that occur as patients and families confront advanced disease.

FAMILY ADAPTABILITY AND COHESION

The circumplex model of family functioning, as developed by Olson et al. (43), categorizes families in a manner that explains the variation in their behavior. Although not specifically developed for cancer, this model conceptualizes families' responses to stressful events based on two constructs: adaptability and cohesion. End of life care simultaneously generates significant stressors for both patients and families, especially in issues related to power, structure, and role assignments. Adaptability reflects the capability of a family to reorganize internal roles, rules, and power structure in response to a significant stressor. Given the impact of advancing cancer on the total family unit, families must frequently reassign roles, alter rules for daily living, and revise long-held methods for problem solving. Dysfunction in the family can relate to either low adaptability (rigidity) or excessively high adaptability (chaotic). A family characterized as rigid in its adaptability persists in the use of coping behaviors, such as frequent manifestations of anger, even when they are ineffective. Those that exhibit high adaptability create a chaotic response within the power structure, roles, and rules of the family; such families lack structure in their responses and attempt different coping strategies with every new stress. Although most families are in the more functional category of "structured adaptability," 30% are rigid or chaotic. These latter families are likely to exhibit problematic behaviors such as excessive demands of staff time or interference with the delivery of medical care that the health care team may find difficult to manage (44).

The second construct of Olson et al.—cohesion—is indicative of the family's ability to provide adequate support (43). Cohesion is the level of emotional bonding that exists among family members and is also conceptualized on a continuum from low to high. Low cohesion (disengagement) suggests little or no connectedness among family members. A commitment to care for other family members is not evident, and, as a result, these

TABLE 42.2 ADVANCING DISEASE AND PSYCHOSOCIAL TREATMENT

Crisis event	Personal meaning	Manifestation	Coping tasks	Survivor goals	Professional interventions
Recurrence/new primary	What did I do wrong? Was it my negative attitude? Was I foolish to hope this was over forever? God has failed me I beat this last time, I will beat it again	Anger Fear Depression Anxiety Shock Loss of hope Denial Guilt	Reestablish hope Accept the uncertainty about the future Understand information about new situation Regain a life focus and time perspective appropriate to the changed prognosis	Integrate reality with family functioning, maintain self-worth	Information Support Education Cognitive/behavioral skills training Physical availability Supportive psychotherapy Resource provision/referral
	Nothing ever works out good for me They said I was okay but I am not Do I have to start all over again?	Loss of trust Feelings of alienation Increased vulnerability Loss of control Confronting mortality Search for meaning	Communicate new status to others Make decisions about the new treatment course Integrate reality of ongoing nature of disease to probable death from cancer Tolerate changes in routine and roles again Adjust to increased dependency again Reinvest in treatment		
Advanced disease	I am out of control Will they offer new treatment? What am I doing wrong? Will it be as bad as the last time? Will I go broke?	Depression Anxiety Demoralization Fear Denial Anger Fear of intimacy	Maintain hope and direction Tolerate medical care Enhance coping skills Maintain open communication with family, friends, and health care professionals Assess treatment and care options Maintain relationships with medical team	Dignity Direction Role in work, family, and community	Support Cognitive/behavioral skills training Supportive psychotherapy Physical availability Resource provision/referral Information Education

(Continued)

TABLE 42.2 ADVANCING DISEASE AND PSYCHOSOCIAL TREATMENT (*Continued*)

Crisis event	Personal meaning	Manifestation	Coping tasks	Survivor goals	Professional interventions
Terminal	When am I going to die? Does dying hurt? What happens after you die? Why me? Why now? What did I do to deserve this? What will happen to my family? Will I be remembered by my family and friends? What if I start to die and I am all alone? Can't the doctors do something else, are they holding back on me, have they given up on me?	Depression Fear Anxiety Denial Demoralization Self-destructive behavior Loss of control Guilt Anger Fear of abandonment Fear of isolation Increased dependency Acceptance Withdrawal Search for meaning in past as well as present Pain/suffering Need to discuss afterlife	Maintain a meaningful quality of life Adjust to physical deterioration Plan for surviving family members Accept reality of prognosis Mourn actual losses Mourn the death of dreams Get things in order Maintain and end significant relationships Say good-bye to family and friends Accept impending death Confront the relevant existential and spiritual issues Talk about feelings Review one's life	Dignity Family support and bereavement	Physical availability Support Cognitive/behavioral skills training Therapeutic rituals Coordination of services Advocacy Information

From Mitchell SL, Teno JM, Miller SC, Mor V. A national study of the location of death for older persons with dementia. *J Am Geriatr Soc.* 2005;53(2):299-305.

families are frequently unavailable to the medical staff for support of the patient or for participation in the decision-making process. At the other extreme, high cohesion (enmeshment) blurs the boundaries among family members. This results in the perception by health care providers that some family members seem to be just as affected by the diagnosis or treatment or by each symptom, as the patient. Enmeshed families may demand excessive amounts of time from the health care team and be incapable of following simple medical directives. These families are not able to objectively receive and comprehend information that may be in the best interest of the patient. Also these families may assume a highly overprotective position in relation to the patient and may speak for the patient even when the patient's self-expression could be encouraged.

When engaging families, it is necessary to gain an appreciation for the rules and regulations within each particular family. Each family has its own rules, regulations, and communication styles. In gaining an understanding of the role of the patient in the family, it is helpful to ask the patient to describe the specific responsibilities he or she performs in the family, especially during a crisis. Generalities are less informative than descriptions of the specific experiences and duties of each family member during a crisis. These queries enable the patient to openly communicate and objectively evaluate his or her role and importance in the family system and provide a clinical opportunity to assess ongoing progress or deterioration. Patients and families can usually tolerate even the worst news or the most dire prognosis as long as it is framed within a context in which the patient and family know how they are expected to respond and that the health care team will not abandon them.

IMPACT OF PHYSICAL AND PSYCHOLOGICAL SYMPTOMS

Patients with advanced illness experience pain, delirium, dyspnea, fatigue, nausea, anxiety, depression, sleeplessness, and many other symptoms that impair QOL. These noxious symptoms also compromise cognition, concentration, and memory (45) and may override the underlying mental schema of patients. For the person in pain or acute physical distress, perception is confined to only the most immediate and essential elements of his or her sensory experience, and there is only a distant remnant of a past or future. The immediate need and goal is to stop or minimize the noxious experience. In some sense, pain and other symptoms absorb the limited psychic energy of the patient, and valuable energy can only be made available if physical distress is effectively managed. The psychic life is subservient and dependent to the bodily experience. This is an important point for health care providers. Therefore, psychosocial interventions must simultaneously focus on physical symptoms in order to be effective. Furthermore, interventions that do not address the physical concerns of the patient may be unethical. The essence of psychosocial care is to raise the "bar" of what humanistic medical care means so that all concerns and needs of patients are effectively addressed and resolved. Unless physical and psychosocial distress are managed simultaneously, psychosocial interventions are less likely to be effective.

Moderate to severe pain is reported by 30% to 45% of patients undergoing (34) cancer treatments and 75% to 90% of patients with advanced disease (46). Pain seems to stand alone in its ability to gain the active attention of others although dramatically demonstrating a sense of being alone and vulnerable. This is especially true of patients with advanced disease and their families. Although a patient is experiencing pain, another person only inches away is incapable of truly understanding what is so central and undeniable to the patient. This invisible and almost palpable boundary between the person in pain and his or her caregivers has significant implications for the quality and effectiveness of the therapeutic relationship (47,48). Of note, a significant problem has been documented where minority populations such as African Americans may be consistently undertreated for cancer pain (49,50), and this disparity must be addressed.

Given that cancer pain can be adequately managed in almost all circumstances, its deleterious and at times life-threatening impact on the physical, psychological, and spiritual resources of both the patient and family are not only unnecessary but also evil. There is no known benefit to ongoing unrelieved pain. There are many known negative consequences. For example, O'Mahony et al. (49) found that the desire for death was correlated with ratings of pain and low family support but most significantly with depression. Given the relationship between pain and depression, the importance of adequate pain management can hardly be overstated. Cobb et al. (50), in their comprehensive review of the delirium literature, found that poor pain control was identified as the number one cause or contributor for delirium. Given the obvious importance and prevalence of delirium as an indicator of QOL at the end of life, this is very critical information.

Serlin et al. (51) were able to demonstrate that there is a positive correlation between pain intensity and function. As expected, low levels of pain intensity cause low levels of interference with life, whereas moderate to high levels of pain make it virtually impossible to have meaningful interactions with others and to feel part of a larger whole. Clinical experience consistently demonstrates that people with physical illness accompanied by high levels of pain intensity experience acute isolation, are unable to advocate for themselves, and are at very high risk to be badly cared for even in the best medical centers. Family and health care providers can be sensitive, caring, supportive, and concerned, but if pain is not adequately managed, the person confronting death has little possibility to think clearly, express his or her concerns, make a contribution, and have anything resembling a peaceful death.

It is generally accepted that pain is poorly managed despite the availability of effective therapies (52–54). Of particular note, effective pain management may also be influenced by the race and ethnicity of the patient, but socioeconomic disadvantage is the more important predictor of disabling pain (55). Patients, families, and professional staff may share a reluctance to use opioid analgesics even when life expectancy is quite limited. Dysfunctional processes continue to exist, which enable patients to accept suffering and to allow the health care team to permit unnecessary pain. This type of response represents an adaptive but "dark side" of professional care. Although most patients with cancer are psychologically healthy (23,56), inadequately managed cancer pain and other symptoms can produce a variety of "pseudopsychiatric" syndromes, which are anxiety provoking and confusing to patients, families, and clinicians. Patients with cancer and pain are also more likely to develop psychiatric disorders than patients with cancer without significant pain (54). In the short term, pain provokes anxiety; over the long term, it generates depression and demoralization. Misguided priorities in the health care system frequently result in needless pain and suffering in patients, and long-term guilt in family members and permanent mistrust of the intentions of health care providers.

The differences between depression and demoralization as clinical constructs have yet to be empirically explored. Depression is significantly related to higher levels of cancer pain and pain is likely to play a causal role related to depression. Overall depression rates for cancer patients are 20% to 25% (57), and estimates as high as 50% to 70% have been applied to populations with advanced disease (58). Patients who are demoralized are disheartened or discouraged by their circumstances but not in a pathologic sense. There is a significant correlation between affective disorders and pain and among the negative emotional states associated with pain (dysphoria, hopelessness, guilt, suicidal ideation, etc.). Anecdotal clinical experience consistently demonstrates that once pain and related distressing physical symptoms are relieved, and suffering, anxiety, depression, demoralization, and suicidal ideation are ameliorated, the impact on the family is equally significant (59).

Patients who are depressed distort reality and grossly minimize their perceived abilities in managing the demands of the illness and its treatment. Furthermore, patients with cancer who are depressed and have inadequately controlled pain are at increased risk for suicide (49,60). For the patient who is depressed, acute sensitivity to physical sensations may lead to or exaggerate preexisting morbid or catastrophizing thoughts. The complex and interactive associations among physical sensations (neutral or noxious sensations), mentation (personal meaning given to the sensations), and behaviors (attempts to minimize threat and regain control) are all negatively influenced by depression. The destructive synergy of unrelieved pain and depression may lead to overwhelming suffering in patients and families and to a shared sense of helplessness and hopelessness (61). Consequently, a patient or family may develop the faulty perception that suicide is their only remaining vestige of control. From this perspective, the value of a multimodality approach that combines pharmacology, supportive psychotherapy, and cognitive–behavioral skills training is clear (62). From a psychological perspective, promotion of compliance with medical regimens; correction of distorted cognitive perceptions; acquisition of coping skills to manage physical tension, stress, and pain; and the effective use of valuable physical energy to maximize engagement of life become the focus of care.

SOCIOCULTURAL INFLUENCES ON PATIENT AND FAMILY ADAPTATION

Perceptions of illness and death can be conceptualized as experiences with both conscious and unconscious associations. These perceptions include concerns and fears that are beyond the limits of objective knowledge. Sociocultural beliefs may soothe anxiety or fear by providing comfort when a vacuum exists due to a lack of experience in the management of a chronic illness. Sociocultural attitudes also exert considerable influence as patients approach the end of their lives (63,64). These beliefs and attitudes are evident in direct observations of how the family cares for the patient, views of an afterlife, and rituals related to how the corpse is to be managed.

Koenig and Gates-Williams (65) offer a framework to assess cultural responses relevant to palliative care. This framework, which is consistent with a comprehensive psychosocial assessment, posits that "culture is only meaningful when interpreted in the context of a patient's unique history, family constellation, and socioeconomic status." Dangers exist in creating negative stereotypes—in simply supplying clinicians with an atlas or map of "cultural traits common among particular ethnic groups."

Patients and their families can simply not be adequately understood without knowledge of their sociocultural backgrounds (66). Patients and families vary according to interests, beliefs, values, and attitudes. Individuals learn attitudes or values through family interactions and these patterns influence how patients respond to the health care team. Although the health care team represents expertise, safety, and authority, it is also an external and foreign force, which only through necessity has gained influence and power within the family system. In stressful situations, the patient and family may project their own perceptions about themselves onto the health care team.

Although cultural characteristics are important, these influences often diminish over time as families are assimilated into the predominant culture. Second-generation families are more similar to the host country than the country of origin. First-generation immigrants may possess old-world attitudes and values about authority and illness, whereas the perspectives of their offspring will be more consistent with the health care team.

Given the many and complex demands already made on health care professionals and the rapidly increasing diversity of institutions, is it reasonable to expect that staff be informed about the myriad cultures represented in such a pluralistic environment? For example, it is estimated that there are over 150 different languages spoken among the Native Americans, with each tribe having its own rituals around the end of life (67). One can only imagine trying to provide bereavement services to a group that demands that the name of the deceased never be mentioned again. Or that believes that even mentioning the word death will cause the event to happen. These barriers to effective and open communication, so respected by health care professionals in the United States, are not unique to Native Americans (68). Furthermore, evidence exists that African Americans are far less likely to discuss the end of life issues due to a belief that these discussions may result in less care being delivered (69). Consequently, ineffective communication about terminal care creates a significant potential for disparities in how these patients receive support at the end of life.

Although there is no formula to making a connection with another person when he or she is ill, there are some areas that can be explored together that can be mutually enriching. The health care provider needs to specifically ask the patient and family about them as a system, patient, family, tribe, group, and so on. Some examples are as follows:

- Because everyone is different, can you teach me how to help you get the information you need about your illness?
- How would you like me to share information with you about your illness?
- How much information, if any, would you like me to share with your family and others?
- Is there a particular person you would like me to include when you and I talk about serious matters?
- Would you like me to give you an overview of what is happening to you each time we meet, or would you like me to simply answer your specific questions?
- What is your understanding of your health right now?
- What kinds of information would you like me to tell you?
- You have a very serious illness. Some people want to know what they have to prepare for in the near future. Is there anything that you would like to know now?
- Is there anything you think we need to share with your family and others that may be helpful to them and you?
- Is there anything we can do together to make this time meaningful for you and your family?
- Would you feel comfortable contacting me if you have any questions?

Ultimately, a relationship is always between two people at a time. Opening up one's self to be taught by the patient and family about who they are and how they want to manage the illness is the perfect counterpoint to the awesome power held by health care professionals.

PRINCIPLES OF EFFECTIVE PATIENT AND FAMILY MANAGEMENT

The family, as defined by the patient, is virtually always the primary supportive structure for the patient. The family serves as a supportive environment, which provides instrumental assistance, psychological support, and consistent encouragement, so that the patient seeks and acquires the best available medical care. Early in the diagnostic and treatment planning phases, a family's primary functions are to instill hope and facilitate communication. For the patient whose disease is beyond life-prolonging therapy, caregiving becomes the primary focus for the family. In the latter situation, families must prepare psychologically and financially for the experience of life without the patient (anticipatory grief). Cancer and its treatments are always a crisis and an assault on the family system. As an uninvited intruder, cancer challenges the viability of the family structure to tolerate and integrate a harsh and threatening reality, which cannot be overcome by force, denial, or even joint action. Joint action can be successful in terms of adaptation, and if the goals are clearly defined, there is an ongoing plan that promotes the optimal opportunity for successful goal attainment of support for the patient.

The health care team can guide the family in developing a problem-solving approach to the demands of the illness. Problem-solving therapy conceived by D'Zurilla, Nezu, and others defines problem solving as a series of tasks rather than a single skill. According to the theoretical model, successful problem solving requires five component processes, each of which contributes directly to effective problem resolution (70,71). The five components are as follows:

1. Problem orientation, definition, and formulation
2. Generation of alternatives
3. Decision-making
4. Solution implementation
5. Verification

Problem orientation involves a motivational process; the other components consist of specific skills and abilities that enable a person to effectively solve a particular problem. Because problem solving is a set of skills, this approach has also been provided as an educational format.

The basic notion underlying the relevance of problem solving for cancer patients lies in the moderating role of coping through problem solving serves in the general stress–distress relationship (72). The more effective people are in resolving or coping with stressful problems, the more probable it is that they will experience a higher QOL as compared with those persons facing similar problems who have difficulty in coping. Families also require guidance and support in managing the multiple problems associated with cancer, related treatments, adverse reactions, and rehabilitation. Following the diagnosis of cancer, families need to have honest, intelligible, and timely information whereas being reassured that competent health care professionals are genuinely caring for their family member.

Previous research indicates that problem-solving education for family caregivers improves their ability to manage care better and cope more effectively with the stressors generated by caregiving. D'Zurilla, Nezu, and others (73,74) have developed conceptual frameworks for problem-solving therapy and have conducted research that demonstrates that counseling caregivers, who are under stress, reduces their distress while increasing their problem-solving competence. This conceptual model has been applied successfully with a number of diverse health-related problems, including cancer (75). Toseland et al. (76) have shown that problem-solving counseling of family caregivers lessened caregiver distress and reduced long-term depression in the patients. Finally, Bevans et al. has applied problem-solving education to a specific treatment, that is, bone marrow transplantation and demonstrated clear value and benefit to bone marrow recipients and their family caregivers (77,78).

A therapeutic treatment plans must always be clearly communicated because it delineates each individual's responsibility so that the potential for goal attainment is maximized. For many families with histories of effective functioning, the cancer experience represents the first time that their joint action may not overcome an external threat. Consequently, the cancer experience must be reframed into more realistic terms so that the threat can be perceived as manageable rather than destructive. If this is not achieved, the family can manifest anger, avoidance, displacement, or other forms of regressive behavior. For the family with a history of multiple defeats and failures, the cancer experience may be perceived as more evidence that they are incapable of managing the demands of an overwhelming world. The cancer experience temporarily alters the family structure, but it also has the potential to inflict permanent change. The health care team can significantly influence how these changes are interpreted and integrated into family life.

Patients often identify the effect on the family as the most upsetting repercussion of the cancer (5). Therefore, any effective intervention must include the patient, family, and other social support networks. When patients consider their families, they may experience guilt, shame, anger, frustration, and fear of abandonment. Family members may experience anger, fear, powerlessness, survivor guilt, and confusion as they attempt to care for the patient. Family members may demonstrate the defense mechanism of displacement, transferring emotion from one person or situation to another and potentially confusing health care professionals. This confusion can create tension for family members and providers at a time when clarity and effective interactions are essential.

With little exception, assessment of the primary members in the family system is a rather straightforward process. The patient can be asked the following directly:

- Who do you rely on most to assist you in relation to the practical needs of your illness (e.g., transportation and insurance company negotiations)?
- With whom do you share your emotional concerns? (e.g., the kind of thoughts you have if you wake up in the middle of the night and experience fears about dying)?
- When you get scared or confused, with whom in your family are you most able to talk?
- Who in your family most concerns you?
- Is anyone in your family overwhelmed with your ongoing medical and practical needs?
- Who in your family is coping least well with your illness?
- Is anyone in your family openly angry with you because of your illness?
- Are you particularly worried about how a specific person in your family is coping?
- Who is most dependent on you in your family?
- For what are they dependent on you?
- What would happen to your family if you were unable to maintain your present level of functioning?
- Are you ever concerned that the demands of your illness will be too much for your family?

The answers to these questions communicate to the patient and family that it is appropriate and necessary to gauge the impact of the cancer and its treatment on their lives and also provide the groundwork for the coordination of patient and family functions. In addition, role modeling of open communication provides an environment of emotional support, flexibility in roles, trust, and the implied and spoken promise never to abandon each other. This cannot be achieved unless the patient and family accept that some treatment effects and life events are beyond their control and there are limits to what is possible. The medical team has the responsibility to manage the physical aspects of the disease, whereas the patient and family actively strive to integrate change, maintain normalcy, and accept the reality of the illness. The course of the illness—including death—must be identified as one of the potentially uncontrollable issues so the patient and family can focus on areas that are amenable to their influence.

Financial resources are virtually always a major concern of patients and families. When discussions of money and resources occur within the family system, shame and guilt are common. These emotions are frequently alluded to but not openly discussed. This can be a barrier to open communication and can lead to patient's fears and fantasies of abandonment. This is especially true for patients with advancing disease. Simultaneously, the family may have concerns about life goals after the patient's acute need is past or death occurs. The expected range of emotional reactions within the family includes anger, fear, guilt, anxiety, frustration, powerlessness, and confusion. Cancer confronts people with the reality of limitations.

In addition to the increasing costs of health insurance and home care, there is a wide variety of nonreimbursable, illness-related costs that can be financially devastating to patients and families. Transportation, nutritional supplements, temporary housing, child care, and lost work days are but a few examples of costs borne almost totally by patients and families for which there is seldom any form of reimbursement (77). Schulz et al. (27) found that respondents spent more than $200 per month on health-related expenses and reported significant negative effects on the amount of time worked. Other studies have confirmed the negative financial impact of advanced cancer (78,79).

Money is almost always a metaphor for value, control, and power (80). How patients and family members communicate about money can be an indication of their perceptions of whether treatment is progressing or not. Therefore, interchanges about financial matters can actively represent latent communications about the perceived but unexpressed value of care and its potential outcome. For example, the patient and family may at the beginning of treatment state that money is no object and all resources must be expended so that the patient survives. When treatment becomes prolonged, however, a much more sober and realistic view concerning valuable and vanishing resources may become evident, and a greater discussion of investment and return may ensue. At this point in time, both patient and family may be actually talking about their ability to persevere. Concerns about money may then be an expression of exhaustion, diminishing hope, or anger. It is important that this metaphorical communication be seen as inadequate for open and direct communication. A metaphor is a signal and cue that indicate the need for open discussion. Openness is essential for the patient and family to discuss both their common and increasingly diverging needs. Patients and families must discuss their physical and spiritual fatigue, as well as specific financial concerns related to diminishing resources as a result of their struggle with cancer. The following clinical example illustrates a number of these points.

A 54-year-old married woman with three adolescent daughters expressed concern to the medical team about the ongoing cost of care for her terminally ill husband. The team felt that she was selfish and that it was unethical for them to consider the financial impact on the family in caring for the patient. Sensing their resistance to her plight, she felt rejected and became irate. A meeting with the patient, family, and relevant staff was organized by the social worker to openly address her financial concerns. The family had existing financial debts due to past medical treatments and consequently had ample reason for its concern related to the additional costs of care. Once this meeting resolved concerns over additional unneeded expenditures, the focus shifted to the much more emotionally laden issues related to the slow deterioration of the patient and the family's intense grief over the impending loss. It became evident that money for the family represented the loss of "everything."

In some cases, the family may begin to perceive the dying patient as already being deceased. Anticipatory grief and premature emotional withdrawal from the dying patient creates confusion and a sense of terror in the patient. As a result, the family experiences guilt and shame because they are prepared for the loss, but the patient is still alive. If this final process is prolonged, a great deal of anger can be manifested by family members.

SPECIFIC PROBLEMATIC PATIENT AND FAMILY BEHAVIORS

Physicians almost always identify "difficult families" as one of the most challenging tasks as a medical provider. Within the context of the family milieu, conflicts with staff may be unavoidable. It is the management of these conflicts that will determine the quality of the relationship between the patient, family, and professional staff. Conflicts may result if a family cannot follow simple guidelines or is intolerant of any physical discomfort that the patient may experience. Families that frequently criticize staff may be held to more rigid standards of behavior. Unit guidelines become laws, and the struggle for control results in fear and mistrust. Conversely, patients and families who endear themselves to staff through verbal praise of the quality of care often receive warmth and flexibility, and, as a result, unit guidelines, such as visiting hours or number of visitors, may be relaxed.

The professional staff must be flexible in their communication styles or they may be perceived as violating family boundaries. This type of interaction can devolve into a battle for power and control. Conflicts that remain at the level of power and control make it virtually impossible to work with the patient and family to develop action-oriented, problem-solving strategies, which unite all in a common set of values and goals. Effective symptom management is essential to engage the patient, family, and the staff toward a common goal. Poor management can lead to estrangement and abandonment (81). Open communication can establish goals within the context of the family and significantly reduce the strain. However, health care providers must accept that at times any approach may be ineffective because the family structure cannot tolerate the influence of external forces. When this occurs, continued attempts at open communication is the only alternative that can achieve some sense of mutual understanding and trust.

Families can exhibit a range of behaviors that the health care team defines as problematic and can potentially interfere with the delivery of medical care. Families can delay or prevent the completion of a procedure, verbally abuse the staff, or divide the team. Families may demand excessive amounts of staff time, repeatedly demanding sessions to review the same information. Confusion may reflect intense anxiety and the overwhelming nature of this experience for caregivers. Some families have unrealistic expectations and compare the responses of staff members searching for inconsistencies. Others fail to follow unit guidelines, consistently arriving well before visiting hours or delaying their departure from the hospital at the end of the day. Families may encourage patients to refuse medical recommendations or directives. Family members at times may speak for the patient and encourage the patient to withdraw and regress. Families may also possess unrealistic expectations of staff. Family members may perceive the staff as their own medical providers and seek personal care from the team (44).

Family functions include facilitation of medical decision-making, reduction of stress, initiation of effective problem solving, and provision of comfort to the patient. If the family cannot provide these functions or is unavailable to the patient and staff, the staff may need to assume and fulfill these roles. At times, the staff may be resentful when families are unavailable or withdraw from participation. The burden on staff to care for these patients can be dramatically increased.

SPECIAL PATIENT AND FAMILY ISSUES

Children in the Home

Children of adult patients with cancer may be an unseen and forgotten population. In acute care settings, children are not observed due to the patients' daytime appointments or policies that prohibit visits to inpatient units. Within the palliative setting, however, children and grandchildren are often present and may play an active role in the caregiving process.

Although salient developmental differences exist among children of different ages, those 3 years or older are able to verbally communicate their concerns so that an ongoing dialogue can occur. Highly sensitive to emotional and physical changes, children benefit most from an environment where they are continually given information in a manner that they can understand and are then encouraged to ask questions. Adults should be prepared for questions to be rather concrete and egocentric, centered around the immediate needs of the child and any potential change in the immediate family. Children are specifically concerned about the continued presence of parents and their own safety. Questions from children usually come one or two at a time. Children often need time to interpret and integrate the adult responses before returning for additional information, which may occur days or weeks later.

Methods to deliver medical information or relieve distress must vary according to each child's developmental stage. Children have fantasies about the etiology, meaning, and duration of a parent's illness. Young children need consistent information about the chronic nature of the disease so that they can anticipate changes and incorporate an understanding of these medical events into their world. Young children cannot fully appreciate the concept of permanence. The permanence of death or abstract terms, such as "forever," are beyond their ability to integrate on a cognitive level. Children need consistent support, measured doses of information, and an environment that can respond to their questions.

Developmentally, adolescence is the time for resolution of conflicts with parents as well as a quickened pace to individuation from the family. These processes can be delayed or significantly complicated by the family's focus on a loved one who is slowly deteriorating and dying. Competitiveness, sexuality, aggression, and peer relationships may compound and confuse attempts to cope with a loss and the end of a specific relationship.

Familial roles can be disrupted or confused during a parent's illness, and, as a result, adolescents may be required to assume adult responsibilities. There is a danger in treating an adolescent as an adult. The demands of adolescence under normal circumstances generate numerous stressors for the family, and a chronic illness at this point in the life cycle can significantly exacerbate the family's level of distress. Of particular concern, adolescents may be "parentified." Physical maturity should not be equated with emotional, intellectual, or spiritual development. Adolescents can easily be overwhelmed with guilt and shame when their normal sense of power and grandiosity cannot control symptoms or death. This may have a long-term negative effect on the ability to tolerate emotional relationships. If the death of a parent or grandparent is to occur in the home, children must be carefully assessed, and appropriate interventions and support should be offered.

Psychiatric Illness

Histories of psychiatric disorders present further challenges in the effective management of patients and families. Psychiatric symptoms must be assessed and appropriately managed if the patient is to truly benefit from supportive care interventions. For example, symptoms, such as severe depression, may dramatically influence a patient's perception of pain and the ability of the health care team to control it. Furthermore, psychiatric symptoms of a family member can also cause a significant concern given the health care team's expectations concerning caregiving in the home by family members. Frequently, expectations of family members as caregivers are relatively uniform despite the significant variation that exists in each family's level of functioning. Families must be assessed not only for their availability but also for their ability to provide adequate supportive care.

Patients or family members with a history of physical or sexual abuse may exhibit significant difficulty in the ability to develop a trusting relationship with the health care team and may require psychiatric management. Families with a history of abuse may try to withhold information related to the abuse and any attempt to assess the patient or family as an intrusion. Trust can only be developed over time as the health care team consistently verbalizes their concern for patient and family as well as their availability for support and intervention. Families with severe dysfunction isolate and protect themselves from the outside world with rigid outer boundaries. Health care providers may define such a family as problematic when initial offers of assistance are refused. The team may experience frustration and rejection, which is inevitably communicated directly to the patient and family. Consequently, the family is lost as an ally and resource and, as a result, their isolation is increased. Although few in number, timely psychiatric referrals for these patients and family members are essential.

Addictions

A current or past history of substance abuse or an active addiction within the patient or the family creates a sense of alarm within the health care team. For example, the patient with a history of substance abuse may simply not be trusted by health care providers. The patient's behavior may be viewed as manipulative and if pain is a problem, there may be reticence to prescribe higher opioid doses if the patient is in pain or even when dying.

Patients should not needlessly suffer as a result of a prior history of substance abuse or their current treatment in a methadone clinic. Patients with a history of substance addiction that is remote or has been effectively managed in a drug treatment program are at much greater risk for the undertreatment of cancer pain. Consultation with a drug treatment facility may be necessary to plan effective management strategies.

Family members of a substance abuser can negatively influence or reinforce the patient's drug-seeking behavior. These families frequently possess an extremely high level of cohesion, which can be characterized as enmeshment. Within this type of family, boundaries between family members are nebulous, and, as a result, family members may appear to be equally affected by the status of the patient. The care provided to the patient may be sporadic or inconsistent because the family may be overwhelmed by the severity of the illness. Careful medical and psychosocial coordination between patient, family, staff, and, when appropriate, a drug treatment center is necessary to maximize cooperation and maintain quality care. Despite the level of frustration associated with this group of patients, dignified care is possible and attainable.

Intimacy and Sexuality

Advanced disease always affects sexuality and sexual functioning. Notwithstanding, the lack of libido and impaired sexual functioning are frequently overlooked or ignored as a concern of the patient. Open discussion of intimacy and sexuality with the team can actually result in enhancement of emotional vitality. In fact, an increase in intimacy can evolve as closeness is redefined and openly discussed. Patients' needs for intimacy and sexual activity must be examined and supported. A couple's expression of intimacy, even during terminal care, can create a sense of normalcy and relief in the midst of a highly traumatic course of medical events. As patients enter the terminal phase, these discussions require a high level of sensitivity. Most patients long to be touched and held, and it is not uncommon for spouses or children to lie in bed with a dying patient to provide comfort and experience closeness or intimacy. Models for assessment of these issues with effective interventions are available (82).

Dying at Home

Although many patients and families describe a preference for death to occur in the comfort of their homes, this goal is not always attainable. While the majority of patient deaths continue to occur in medical institutions, the return to home, nursing homes, or hospices as the chosen places of death continues to increase, primarily as a result of the Medicare Hospice Benefit (83,84) and physician availability for home visits (85,86). A number of key psychosocial variables (Table 42.2) may inhibit or prevent the occurrence of death in the home even with the highest level of supportive care or hospice services. Families must be carefully assessed and prepared for the death event. Key family members can be specifically questioned concerning their level of comfort or toleration for stressful events within the home. Preparations, including advance directives, wills, and do-not-resuscitate orders, should begin as early as possible to resolve all questions and informational needs that the family may have. Typically, hospice services are only available in the home for a fraction of each day. Consequently, the patient's death will probably occur when the family is alone (87).

A family that wants to maintain a dying member at home despite complex needs may suddenly request that the patient die in the hospital. Reasons for rapid changes may be obvious and practical or may be irrational and unconscious. Either way, the resources and limitations of the family must be assessed and supported. Many patients who are terminally ill possess acute care needs (e.g., pain control and mental status changes), and admission may be warranted to provide brief respite for the family or to actually manage the death event.

When the Patient Dies

The final hours of the patient's life have significant meaning for the family and offer an opportunity for closure (88,89). The ritualistic need to be present at the exact moment of death can be very powerful for family members. The desire to be present for the death event is common, and for family members who are absent, significant regrets may result (90,91). Unexpected deaths occur in approximately 30% of patients; attempts to notify the family of the impending event is possible in 70% of cases (92).

Family members may require objective information concerning the cause of death, especially if the death was unexpected. Despite the terminal prognosis, many families need to understand why the patient died when he or she did. This information can mitigate a high level of mistrust and resulting distress and address any irrational concerns and fears associated with the death as it is happening.

Interactions with staff that occur immediately following the death can have a long-term effect. Emotional reactions of family members are expected, and crying, sobbing, and wailing are common. The therapeutic demands associated with the provision of terminal care challenges the health care professional to communicate with empathy while facilitating the initiation of essential tasks such as removal of the body and funeral arrangements. Families vary in their ability to receive information and emotional support during this time. The relationship between the family and the health care team influences how much of these preparations can be made prior to the death event and how much clinical intervention the family requires and can tolerate. Generally, families elect a spokesperson to provide and receive information but care must also be taken to assess other members of the family. A follow-up meeting with the family by a social worker or nurse in the home can be very helpful to identify any family member who may be at risk for an abnormal grief response (42,90).

CONCLUSIONS

All patients and families possess a personal meaning of disease, prolonged illness, and death. These meanings are influenced over time by numerous factors. A clear understanding of these meanings, associated emotions, and their antecedents enhances the health care team's ability to provide care and anticipate potential problems. Information and education must be consistently available as the patient and family move across the disease continuum toward and post the death event (90).

In essence, a model of care is proposed that promotes active engagement in therapies for the treatment of advanced cancers while engaging the individual patient and their family caregivers. This treatment approach must be evidence based in terms of distress screening tools, comprehensive psychosocial assessments, and, most importantly, established interventions and measurement of effectiveness that clinicians can apply to this population. Furthermore, "simultaneous care" provided to alleviate symptoms and side effects might be incorporated earlier on in the disease continuum than much later when palliative care is introduced (91). As previously stated, a cancer such as multiple myeloma presents numerous complex problems for patients and their family caregivers, and the focus should be on ensuring that these patients possess the most effective resources with which to manage this difficult disease (92). This model may

also benefit patients and family who grapple with other advanced cancers (93).

Variables, such as family cohesion, describe the quality and intensity of relationships within the family. High cohesion or enmeshed families lose more than a family member when the patient dies. For these families, part of their identity is also lost. Given their extreme level of dependence on one another, these families may experience the death as catastrophic, which prevents the effective resolution of the loss. Chronic grief can exacerbate current psychological symptoms and influence health care practices. Bereavement follow-up among high-risk families is essential as a means to develop psychosocial prevention programs. The psychosocial obligation to the family does not end with the patient's death, and some families may require follow-up beyond the customary 1-year period as the bereaved experience salient dates such as a birthday or anniversary for the first time without the loved one who has died (94). Most often, bereaved family members must experience the "four seasons of the year" as they attempt to celebrate holidays or experience a vacation following the death of their loved one (95). Given the intensity of the loss and the family's level of risk, grief must be monitored and resolved.

As with palliative care, despite data supporting effectiveness and benefits to patients, their caregivers, and to the system, psychosocial services have been actively supported and increasingly demanded by consumers of these services. In addition, numerous professional organizations have created clinical standards that support the importance of whole-patient–centered care. To its detriment, the health system has for too long resisted a wider view of the patient experience. Paradoxically, just as professional groups and the public are demanding a more comprehensive model of cancer care that minimally includes a full biopsychosocial (and sometimes spiritual) approach to care and caring, given international demographics relating to aging, population growth, the ongoing obesity epidemic, and increasingly sedentary lifestyles palliative care is being recognized as an essential element to health care systems. Recent empirical support for the value of palliative care will only accelerate this process.

Palliative care has actively promoted the importance of psychosocial services and has created an opportunity to give a strong voice to the humanistic agenda, where respect, dignity, and identifying personal and social strengths are synergized into a health caring system where the needs of people are more wisely and appropriately balanced with the inquisitiveness and natural desire to defy the limits of what humans can presently accomplish while still maintaining our humanity.

Ultimately, the role of the health care team and the compassionate expertise they provide is to create an environment with exquisite symptom management and honest and open communication (96). If these components are present, the opportunity exists to provide meaning to the death event. If this occurs, a sense of growth is possible for patients who are dying, their surviving family members, their health care providers, and society at large.

ACKNOWLEDGMENTS

The authors thank Sheri and Les Biller for their generous and ongoing support of the Sheri & Les Biller Patient and Family Resource Center and for City of Hope administrative leadership who had the audacity and vision to create the integrated interdisciplinary Department of Supportive Care Medicine.

REFERENCES

1. Loscalzo MJ. Palliative care: an historical perspective. *Hematology Am Soc Hematol Educ Program*. 2008;2008:465.
2. National Hospice and Palliative Care Organization. *Facts and Figures: Hospice Care in America*. Alexandria, VA: NHPCO; September 2010.
3. Mishel MH. Reconceptualization of the uncertainty in illness theory. *Image J Nurs Sch*. 1990;22:256.
4. Seale C, Cartwright A. *The Year before Death*. Brookfield, WI: Ashgate Publishing Company; 1994.
5. Yabroff CR, Youngmee K. Time costs associated with informal caregiving for cancer survivors. *Cancer*. 2009;115(suppl 18):4362-4373.
6. Levin DN, Cleeland CS, Dar R. Public attitudes toward cancer pain. *Cancer*. 1985;56:2337.
7. World Health Organization. Cancer pain and palliative care. *Technical Report 804*. Geneva: World Health Organization; 1990.
8. Zarit SH, Todd PA, Zarit JM. Subjective burdens of husbands and wives as caregivers: a longitudinal study. *Gerontologist*. 1986;26:260.
9. Brody EM. Women in the middle and family help to older people. *Gerontologist*. 1981;21:471.
10. Iwashyna TJ, Christakis NA. Attitude and self-reported practice regarding hospice referral in a national sample. *J Palliat Med*. 1998;1(3):241.
11. Bomba PA. Enabling the transition to hospice through effective palliative care. *Case Manager*. 2005;16(1):48.
12. Zwerding T, Hamann K, Meyers F. Extending palliative care: is there a role for preventive medicine? *J Palliat Med*. 2005;8(3):486.
13. Weeks JC, Cook EF, O'Day SJ, et al. Relationship between cancer patients' predictions of prognosis and their treatment preferences. *JAMA*. 1998;279:1709.
14. Azoulay E, Pochard F, Kentish-Barnes N, et al. Risk of post-traumatic stress symptoms in family members of intensive care unit patients. *Am J Respir Crit Care Med*. 2005;171:987-994.
15. Gott M, Ingleton C, Bennett MI, Gardiner C. Transitions to palliative care in acute hospitals in England: qualitative study. *BMJ*. 2011;342:d1773.
16. Lazarus RS. *Emotion and Adaptation*. New York, NY: Oxford University Press; 1991.

17. Weisman AD, Worden JW. The existential plight in cancer: significance of the first 100 days. *Int J Psychiatry Med*. 1976–1977;7:1.
18. Carlsson M, Mamrin E. Psychological and psychosocial aspects of breast cancer treatments. *Cancer Nurs*. 1994;17:418.
19. Ternel JS, Greer JA, Muzinkansky A, et al. Early palliative care for patients with metastatic non-small-cell lung cancer. *N Engl J Med*. 2010;363(8):733–742.
20. Zabora JR, Loscalzo MJ, Weber J. Managing complications in cancer: identifying and responding to the patient's perspective. *Semin Oncol Nurs*. 2003;19(4 suppl 2):1.
21. Houts PS, Nezu AM, Nezu CM, et al. A problem-solving model of family care giving for cancer patients. *Patient Educ Couns*. 1996;27:63.
22. Bucher J, Loscalzo MJ, Zabora JR, et al. Problem-solving cancer care education for patients and caregivers. *Cancer Pract*. 2001;9(2):66.
23. Derogatis LR, Morrow GR, Fetting J. The prevalence of psychiatric disorders among cancer patients. *JAMA*. 1983;249(6):751.
24. Farber JM, Weinerman BH, Kuypers JA. Psychosocial distress in oncology outpatients. *J Psychosoc Oncol*. 1984;2:109.
25. Stefanek M, Derogatis L, Shaw A. Psychological distress among oncology outpatients. *Psychosomatics*. 1987;28:530.
26. Zabora J, BrintzenhofeSzoc K, Curbow B, et al. The prevalence of psychological distress by cancer site. *Psychooncology*. 2001;10:19.
27. Schulz R, Williamson GM, Knapp JE, et al. The psychological, social, and economic impact of illness among patients with recurrent cancer. *J Psychosoc Oncol*. 1995;13(3):21.
28. National Comprehensive Cancer Network. *The NCCN Distress Practice Guidelines in Oncology*. Vol 1.2011. Fort Washington, PA: NCCN; 2011:2.
29. Clark K, Bardwell WA, Arsenault T, DeTeresa D, Loscalzo M. Implementing touch-screen technology to enhance recognition of distress. *Psycho-Oncology*. 2009;18(8):822-830.
30. Institute of Medicine. *Cancer Care for the Whole Patient: Meeting Psychosocial Health Needs*. Washington, DC: Institute of Medicine; 2007.
31. Bultz BD, Johansen C. Screening for distress, the 6th vital sign: where are we, and where are we going? *Psycho-Oncology*. 2011;20(6):569-571.
32. Zabora JR. Pragmatic approaches in the psychosocial screening of cancer patients. In: Holland J, Breitbart P, Loscalzo M, eds. *Handbook of Psychooncology*. 2nd ed. London: Oxford Press; 1998.
33. Jacobsen PB, Donovan KA, Trask PC, et al. Screening for distress in ambulatory cancer patients. *Cancer*. 2005;103(7):1494.
34. Weisman AD, Worden JW, Sobel HJ. *Psychosocial Screening and Interventions with Cancer Patients: A Research Report*. Boston, MA: Harvard Medical School and Massachusetts Hospital; 1980.
35. Fawzy FI, Fawzy NW, Arndt LA, et al. Critical review of psychosocial interventions in cancer care. *Arch Gen Psychiatry*. 1995;52:100.
36. Zabora JR, Smith-Wilson R, Fetting JH, et al. An efficient method for the psychosocial screening of cancer patients. *Psychosomatics*. 1990;31(2):192.
37. Jacobsen PB, Ransom S. Implementation of NCCN Distress Management Guidelines by Member Institutions. *J Natl Compr Canc Netw*. 2007;5(1):99-103.
38. Velikova G, Booth L, Smith AB, et al. Measuring quality of life in routine oncology practice improves communi-

cation and patient well-being: a randomized controlled trial. *J Clin Oncol*. 2004;22(4):714-724.

39. Zabora JR, Loscalzo MJ, Smith ED. Psychosocial rehabilitation. In: Abeloff MD, Armitage JO, Lichter AS, et al., eds. *Clinical Oncology*. New York, NY: Churchill Livingstone; 2002.

40. Derogatis LR. *BSI-18: Administration, Scoring and Procedures Manual*. Minneapolis, MN: National Computer Systems; 2000.

41. Zabora J, BrintzenhofeSzoc K, Jacobsen P, et al. Development of a new psychosocial screening instrument for use with cancer patients. *Psychosomatics*. 2001; 42(3):19.

42. BrintzenhofeSzoc K, Smith E, Zabora J. Development of a screening approach to predict complicated grief in surviving spouses of cancer patients. *Cancer Pract*. 1999;7(5):233.

43. Olson DH, McCubbin HI, Barnes HL, et al. Predicting conflict with staff among families of cancer patients during prolonged hospitalizations. *J Psychosoc Oncol*. 1989;7(3):103.

44. Zabora JR, Fetting JH, Shaley VB, et al. Predicting conflict with staff among families of cancer patients during prolonged hospitalization. *J Psychosoc Oncol*. 1989;7(3):103.

45. Jamison RN, Sbrocco T, Parris W. The influence of problems in concentration and memory on emotional distress and daily activities in chronic pain patients. *Int J Psychiatry Med*. 1988;18:183.

46. Daut RL, Cleeland CS. The prevalence and severity of pain in cancer. *Cancer*. 1982;50(9):1913.

47. Bond MR, Pearson IB. Psychological aspects of pain in women with advanced cancer of the cervix. *J Psychosom Res*. 1969;13:13.

48. Cleeland CS. The impact of pain on the patient with cancer. *Cancer*. 1984;54:2635.

49. O'Mahony S, Goulet J, Kornblith A, et al. Desire for hastened death, cancer pain and depression: report of a longitudinal observational study. *J Pain Symptom Manage*. 2005;29(5):446.

50. Cobb JL, Glantz MJ, Martin EW, et al. Delirium in patients with cancer at the end of life. *Cancer Pract*. 2000;8(4):172.

51. Serlin RC, Mendoza TR, Nakamura Y, et al. When is cancer pain mild, moderate or severe? *Pain*. 1995;61(2):277.

52. Von Roemn JH, Cleeland CS, Gonin R, et al. Physician attitudes and practice in cancer pain management. *Ann Intern Med*. 1993;119:121.

53. Cleeland CS, Gonin R, Hatfield AK, et al. Pain and its treatment in outpatients with metastatic cancer. *N Engl J Med*. 1994;330(9):592.

54. Grossman SA, Sheidler VR, Sweeden K, et al. Correlation of patient and caregiver ratings of cancer pain. *J Pain Symptom Manage*. 1991;692:53.

55. Portenoy RK, Ugarte C, Fuller I, et al. Population-based survey of pain in the United States: differences among white, African American, and Hispanic subjects. *J Pain*. 2004;5(6):317.

56. Spiegel D, Sands SS, Koopman C. Pain and depression in patients with cancer. *Cancer*. 1994;74:2579.

57. Razavi D, Delvaux N, Farvacques C, et al. Screening for adjustment disorders and major depressive disorders in cancer inpatients. *Br J Psychiatry*. 1990;156:79.

58. Shacham S, Reinhart LC, Raubertas RF, et al. Emotional states and pain: intraindividual and interindividual measures of association. *J Behav Med*. 1983;6:405.

59. Bucher JA, Trostle GB, Moore M. Family reports of cancer pain, pain relief, and prescription access. *Cancer Pract*. 1999;792:71.

60. Bolund C. Suicide and cancer II: medical and care factors in suicide by cancer patients in Sweden, 1973–1976. *J Psychosoc Oncol*. 1985;3:17.

61. Breitbart W, Rosenfeld B, Pessin H, et al. Depression, hopelessness, and desire for hastened death in terminally ill patients with cancer. *JAMA*. 2000;284(22):2907.

62. Massie MJ, Holland JC. Depression and the cancer patient. *J Clin Psychiatry*. 1990;51(suppl 7):12.

63. Kagawa-Singer M. Diverse cultural beliefs and practices about death and dying in the elderly. In: Wieland D, ed. *Cultural Diversity and Geriatric Care: Challenges to the Health Professions*. New York, NY: Haworth Press; 1994.

64. Hellman C. *Culture, Health and Illness*. 3rd ed. Newton, MA: Butterworth–Heinemann; 1995.

65. Koenig BA, Gates-Williams J. Understanding cultural difference in caring for dying patients. Caring for patients at the end of life. *West J Med*. 1995;163(3):244.

66. Power PW, Dell Orto AE. Understanding the family. In: Power PW, Dell Orto AE, eds *Role of the Family in the Rehabilitation of the Physically Disabled*. Baltimore, MD: University Park Press; 1980.

67. Van Winkle NM. End of life decision making in American Indian and Alaska Native cultures. In: *Cultural Issues in End-of-Life Decision Making*. Thousand Oaks, CA: Sage Publications Inc; 2000.

68. Parker SG. The challenge of bringing hospice to the Zuni Tribe. *Last Acts*. 2001;10.

69. Hopp F, Duffy SA. Racial variations in end-of-life care. *J Am Geriatr Soc*. 2000;48(6):658.

70. Nezu AM, Nezu CM, Friedman SH, et al. *Helping Cancer Patients Cope*. Washington, DC: American Psychological Associates; 1998.

71. Meyers FJ, Carducci M, Loscalzo MJ, et al. Effects of a problem-solving intervention (COPE) on quality of life for patients with advanced cancer on clinical trials and their caregivers: simultaneous care educational intervention (SCEI): linking palliation and clinical trials. *J Palliat Med*. 2011;14(4):465-473.

72. Nezu AM, Nezu CM, Perri MG. *Problem-Solving Therapy for Depression: Theory, Research, and Clinical Guidelines*. New York, NY: Wiley; 1989.

73. D'Zurilla TJ, Nezu AM. Social problem-solving in adults. In: Kendall P, ed. *Cognitive-Behavioral Research and Therapy*. New York, NY: Academic Press; 1982.

74. Nezu AM, Nezu CM, Houts PS, et al. Relevance of problem-solving therapy to psychosocial oncology. *J Psychosoc Oncol*. 1999;16(3-4):5-26.

75. Nezu AM, D'Zurilla TJ. Social problem-solving and negative affective states. In: Kendall P, Watson D, eds. *Anxiety and Depression: Distinctive and Overlapping Features*. New York, NY: Academic Press; 1989.

76. Toseland RW, Blanchard CG, McCallion P. A problem solving intervention for caregivers of cancer patients. *Soc Sci Med*. 1995;40(4):517.

77. Bevans M, Wehrlen L, Prachenko O, Soeken K, Zabora J, Wallen G. Distress screening in allogeneic hematopoietic stem cell (HSCT) caregivers and patients. *Psycho-Oncology*. 2011;20(6):615.

78. Bevans M, Wehrlen L, Castro K, et al. A problem-solving education intervention in caregivers and patients during allogeneic hematopoietic stem cell transplantation. *J Health Psychology*. 2014;19(5):602.

79. Lansky SB, Cairns N, Lowman J, et al. Childhood cancer: non-medical costs of the illness. *Cancer*. 1979;43(1):403.

80. Houts PS, Lipton A, Harvey HA, et al. Nonmedical costs to patients and their families associated with outpatient chemotherapy. *Cancer*. 1984;53:2388.

81. Mor V, Guadagnoli E, Wool M. An examination of the concrete service needs of advanced cancer patients. *J Psychosoc Oncol*. 1987;5(1):1.

82. Farkas C, Loscalzo M. Death without indignity. In: Kutscher AH, Carr AC, Kutscher LG, eds. *Principles of Thanatology.* New York, NY: Columbia University Press; 1987:133.

83. Loscalzo M, Amendola J. Psychosocial and behavioral management of cancer pain: the social work contribution. In: Foley KM, Bonica JJ, Ventafridda V, eds. *Advances in Pain Research and Therapy.* Vol 16. New York, NY: Raven Press; 1990:429.

84. Cagle JG, Bolte S. Sexuality and life-threatening illness: implications for social work and palliative care. *Health Soc Work.* 34(3):223-233.

85. Jordhoy MS, Saltvedt I, Fayers P, et al. Which cancer patients die in nursing homes? Quality of life, medical and sociodemographic characteristics. *Palliat Med.* 2003;17(5):433.

86. Bruera E, Sweeney C, Russell N, et al. Place of death of Houston area residents with cancer over a two-year period. *J Pain Symptom Manage.* 2003;26(1):637.

87. Sager M, Easterling D, Kindig D, et al. Changes in the location of death after passage of Medicare's prospective payment system. A national study. *N Engl J Med.* 1989;320:433.

88. McMullan A, Mentnech R, Lubitz J, et al. Trends and patterns in place of death for medicare enrollees. *Health Care Financ Rev.* 1990;12:1.

89. Leff B, Kaffenbarger KP, Remsburg RN. Prevalence, effectiveness, and predictors of planning the place of death among older persons followed in community-based long term care. *J Am Geriatr Soc.* 2000;48(8):943.

90. Tolle SW, Bascom PB, Hickam DA, et al. Communication between physicians and surviving spouses following patient death. *J Gen Intern Med.* 1986;1:309.

91. Tolle SW, Girard DW. The physician's role in the events surrounding patient death. *Arch Intern Med.* 1982;143:1447.

92. Zabora J, Buzaglo J, Kennedy V, et al. Clinical perspective: linking psychosocial care to the disease continuum in patients with multiple myeloma. *J Palliat Support Care.* 2014(June 24):1.

93. Myers FJ, Linder J. Simultaneous care: disease treatment and palliative care throughout illness. *J Clin Oncol.* 2003;21(7):1412.

94. Abbott KH, Sago JG, Breen CM, et al. Looking back: one year after discussion of withdrawal or withholding of life-sustaining support. *Crit Care Med.* 2001;25(1):197.

95. Worden JW. *Grief Counseling and Grief Therapy: A Handbook for the Mental Health Practitioner.* 2nd ed. New York, NY: Springer Publishing Company; 1991.

96. Steinhauser KE, Christakis NA, Clipp EC, et al. Factors considered important at the end of life by patients, families, physicians, and other care providers. *JAMA.* 2000;284(19):2476.

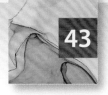

43 Disorders of Sexuality and Reproduction

Mary K. Hughes

INTRODUCTION

While the goal of palliative and supportive care is to support the ideal life of cancer patients and their partners, it often overlooks sexuality (1). Guidelines recommend providers assess the impact of illness on intimacy and sexuality (2). Most societies have a taboo around illness, sexuality, and dying (3). Hordern and Street (4) found that clinicians medicalized patient's sexuality and intimacy by discussing fertility, contraception, and erectile or menopause status rather than intimacy issues. According to Leiblum et al. (5), all patients regardless of age, sexual orientation, marital status, or life circumstances should have the opportunity to discuss sexual matters with their health care professional.

According to Gilley (6), in the context of palliative care sexuality is defined as "the capacity of the individual to link emotional needs with physical intimacy" within the limits of their ability. One of the goals of palliative care is intense symptom management, and many unmanaged symptoms affect sexuality (7). By the time one is referred to palliative care, they may have barely functional sexual lives (3). Sexual changes after treatment are not routinely addressed or only barely touched on despite patients having significant needs for education, support, and practical help with managing them (8). Lemieux et al. (9) found that the emotional connection to another at the end of life may be more important that the physical connection of sexuality. Maslow (10) described sexual activity to be a basic need on his hierarchy of needs while love and connection to others were at a higher level. Everyone has a lifelong need for touch and emotional connection to others regardless of current relationship status (11). Touching changes with cancer. Often the partner becomes the caregiver, changing dressings, and managing drains and wounds, and intimate touching decreases and becomes treatment related. Sexual intercourse is not the defining characteristic of a person's sexuality. A sexual relationship includes the need to be touched and held along with closeness and tenderness (12,13).

SEXUALITY

In order for providers to begin assessing sexuality in people with cancer, they must first understand what sexuality encompasses. It is a broad term including social, emotional, and physical components. It is not just genitals or gender but includes body image, love of self and others, relating to others, and pleasure (14). It is genetically endowed, phenotypically embodied, and hormonally nurtured; is not age related; but is matured by experience and cannot be destroyed despite what is done to a person (15,16). Sexuality includes affection, sexual orientation, sexual activity, eroticism, reproduction, intimacy, and gender roles and encompasses feelings of trust (17,18).

Gregoire (19) reports that men are more attracted to visual sexual stimuli, whereas women are more attracted to auditory and written material, particularly stimuli associated within the context of a loving and positive relationship. Women are not linear in their sexual response, but more circular (20) and may experience sexual excitement before they have a desire for sexual activity. Sexual excitement is the phase where the penis becomes rigid enough to use and in the female, the vagina lubricates and enlarges in depth and width, and the clitoris enlarges (21–23). Erection is the male counterpart to vaginal lubrication from the sexual physiology perspective (24). Orgasm is the height of sexual pleasure and the release of sexual tension. The penis emits semen through muscular spasms, there are rhythmic contractions of the vagina, and the cervix lifts up out of the vaginal vault. The last phase of the cycle is the resolution phase where the genitals return to their normal, nonexcited state. During this phase, there is an evaluation of the sexual experience as well as relaxation and contentment (25,26). The refractory period, where the genitals are resistant to sexual stimulation, happens during this stage. In males, this period can be a matter of minutes in youth but can take days in older men or with certain medications or medical conditions like cancer.

Sexual expression is influenced by cultural norms, past experiences, and the developmental stage of the individual. A medically underserved and diverse population is the lesbian, gay, bisexual, transgender, and queer/questioning (LGBTQ) community also referred to as sexual and gender minorities (SGMs) (27). National Institutes of Health designated them as a minority population in 2016 (28).

645

There have been limited efforts to address cancer disparities by sexual orientation and gender identity (SOGI), but these questions are not a part of most research studies (29–32). Expressions of sexuality include style of dress, values and attitudes, as well as hugging, touching, kissing, acting out scenarios/fantasies, sex toys, masturbation, sexual intercourse, and oral genital stimulation, either alone or with another (19,33). Sexual behaviors may involve oral, vaginal, and/or anal penetration (34). Sexual behavior is influenced by religious beliefs, age, education, level of comfort with one's body and physical functioning, experiences of sexual abuse and trauma, their partner's wishes, and comfort level with one's own SOGI (34). Jabson and Bowen (35) found that heterosexual breast cancer survivors perceived less stress than LGBTQ breast cancer survivors.

LGBTQ population have lower access to health care and increased cancer risks, resulting in a higher incidence of cancer that is diagnosed at a later stage (36,37). Schabath et al. (38) found that oncologists were interested in receiving education on the unique health needs of LGBTQ patients. Unfortunately, there is little literature to guide the oncologist in caring for SGM patients (39). Most cancer centers do not have institutional policies, guidelines, or practices that focus on patient-centered care for SGM patients (40).

SEXUAL DYSFUNCTION

Sexual dysfunction is failure of any aspect of the sexual response cycle to function properly (41). Goldstein et al. (42) report that 90% of sexual dysfunction cases have a psychological component and 75% have clear physiologic sources, so there is a significant overlap. But when a person with cancer has sexual dysfunction, it is mostly physiological. Causes of sexual dysfunction include psychosocial/interpersonal stressors, medical illness, depressive illness, medication, and sexual disorders (DSM-V) (43). According to Gregoire (19), a sexual problem includes physiological dysfunction, altered experiences, one's own perceptions and beliefs, partner's perceptions and expectations, altered circumstances, and past experiences. Causes of sexual dysfunction in a person with cancer are often treatment related due to the changes in physiological, psychological, and social dimensions of sexuality and disruption in one or more phases of the sexual response cycle (11,44). Radiation and surgery can have long-lasting effects on sexuality due to chronic pain, scarring, and body image issues. Besides chemotherapy, biologic agents, immunotherapy, and hormones, there are numerous medications that can have sexual side effects that range from decreased desire to difficulty reaching orgasm. Many of these medications are used in palliative care (19,45,46) and include the following:

- Neurotransmitters
- Stimulants
- Hallucinogens
- Sedatives
- Narcotics
- Anxiolytics
- Anticholinergics
- Antipsychotics
- Lipid-lowering drugs
- H$_2$ antagonists
- Many antidepressants
- Phenothiazines
- Antihypertensives
- Recreational drugs
- Alcohol
- Herbals and vitamins
- Serotonin reuptake inhibitors
- Anticonvulsants

Table 43.1 provides a list of menopausal symptoms and sexual side effects (42,47–52).

Menopausal symptoms can be very distressing to women and interfere with sexuality because of the changes on her body (53). These changes happen gradually in women without cancer, and they have time to adjust and enjoy sexual activity 5 to 10 years longer with fewer sexual problems than women with cancer who rapidly experience menopause (54,55). One should note that while dyspareunia assumes pain with penile–vaginal intercourse, it may be a source of distress as well for women with same-sexed partners, where touch and/or finger or object penetration is uncomfortable (56). Katz (57) found that physical appearance was important in gay culture and having a partner show acceptance of treatment- or disease-related physical changes was comforting. Table 43.2 describes types of sexual dysfunction as defined by the DSM-V (19,43,45,58–67).

It should be remembered that sexual dysfunctions are not all-or-nothing phenomena, but occur on a continuum in terms of frequency and severity. Comorbidity of sexual dysfunctions is common. Gregoire (19) reports that almost half the men with low libido also have another sexual dysfunction, and 20% of men with erectile dysfunction have low libido. The patient's partner and their relationship probably have a more profound effect on sexual health than on any other aspect of health. Sexual dysfunction in men is not as complicated as that in women and is usually associated with age and illness. Table 43.3 describes sexual dysfunctions and possible causes (19,51,52,55,58,60–64,66–72).

Reese et al. found that women with colorectal cancer had poor body image and that men

TABLE 43.1 MENOPAUSAL SYMPTOMS (42,47–52)

Menopausal symptoms	Sexual effects
Vaginal dryness and atrophy	Painful intercourse
Decreased vaginal ridges	Decreased friction on the vagina
Labia minora and vulvar atrophy	Painful intercourse
Hot flashes	Decreased libido and arousal and difficulty having an orgasm, hard to remain physically close
Change in body aroma	Decreased libido and arousal
Decreased clitoral sensation	Decreased arousal and longer time to achieve orgasm
Insomnia	Fatigue
Joint pain and decreased muscle mass	Harder to engage in sexual activities due to pain
Irritability; mood swings	Lower libido and arousal; partner doesn't know what to expect
Decreased bone density	Fear of fractures with sexual activity
Skin and hair changes	Poor body image, decreased libido, altered sense of sexual self
Migraine headaches	Decreased libido
Stature loss	Poor body image
Decreased sexual hair	Poor body image, less cushioning during sex, altered sense of sexual self
Increased urinary tract infections	Painful intercourse
Vaginal itching	Painful intercourse
Loss of tissue elasticity	Painful intercourse, bleeding
Infertility	Change in body image
Urogenital atrophy	Dyspareunia, vaginal dryness, decreased libido

TABLE 43.2 SEXUAL DYSFUNCTION ACCORDING TO DSM V (19,43,45,58–67)

Type of sexual dysfunction	Description
Persistent or recurrent disorders of interest/desire (hypoactive sexual desire disorder)	An absence of sexual fantasies or thoughts, desire, or receptivity to sexual activity at anytime during the sexual experience designates disorder
Disorders of subjective and genital arousal	If subjective, no response to any type of sexual stimulation but may have genital arousal If genital arousal disorder, subjective arousal to nongenital stimulation (usually postmenopausal women), but impaired or absent genital sexual arousal. Inability to attain or maintain adequate lubrication or swelling response during sexual activity Combined: Absence or very diminished feelings of sexual arousal from any type of sexual stimulation as well as absent genital sexual arousal
Persistent sexual arousal disorder	In the absence of sexual interest and desire, spontaneous, intrusive, unwanted genital throbbing unrelieved by orgasm
Male erectile disorder	Episodic or continuous inability to obtain and/or maintain an erection during sexual activity
Orgasmic disorder (female orgasmic disorder) Retrograde ejaculation Anejaculation	Lack of, markedly diminished, or delay of orgasms despite sexual arousal regardless of stimulation Ejaculation disorders—hard to collect sperm Body image, relationship satisfaction, and self-esteem may affect the ability of women to orgasm
Vaginismus	Reflexive tightening around the vagina when vaginal entry is attempted despite woman's desire for penetration. No physical abnormalities present. Often associated with fear, anticipation, or pain
Dyspareunia	Recurrent genital pain with attempted vaginal penetration or penile thrusting
Orgasmic disorder	Episodic, continuous, or complete absence of orgasm following excitement phase
Sexual dysfunction secondary to a general medical condition or substance induced	Medications, chronic or acute illnesses, fatigue, pain

TABLE 43.3 CAUSES OF SEXUAL DYSFUNCTION (19,51,52,55,58,60–64,66–72)

Sexual dysfunction	Causes
Low libido	Chemotherapy, androgen deprivation therapy, fatigue, pain, dementia, delirium, depression, boredom, benzodiazepines, antipsychotics, neuroleptics, sedatives, opioids, diuretics, brain tumors, low testosterone, histamine-2 antagonists, nicotine, alcohol
Erectile dysfunction/female arousal	Antihypertensives, chemotherapy, androgen deprivation therapy, surgery, loss of a willing partner, opportunity, privacy, decreased frequency of activity, decreased tactile sensation, increased refractory period after orgasm, peripheral vascular disease, diabetic neuropathy, nicotine, diuretics, alcohol, opioids, neuroleptics, brain and spine tumors, anxiety, antihistamines, histamine-2 antagonists, high body mass, St. John's wort, cocaine, marijuana, lipid-lowering agents, genital vasodilation, urogenital atrophy
Ejaculation problems: retrograde, dry, premature, delayed	SSRIs, surgery, radiation, opioids, antipsychotics, neuroleptics
Orgasmic disorder	Antidepressants, antihypertensives, diuretics, neuroleptics, antipsychotics, anxiety, neuropathy, radiation, SSRIs, serotonin reuptake inhibitors, bowel and bladder problems

had poorer sexual function (72). If an SMM participates in insertive anal sex, his penis needs to be very rigid to be successful. If he is receptive, rigidity is not as important. Some studies show that partners of patients with cancer experience more psychological distress than do their cancer-affected mates (73).

Body image is a key aspect of sexuality and includes one's feelings and attitudes about one's body (17,74). Body image changes can profoundly alter feelings of attractiveness, an important aspect of sexuality. External changes that are visible to others as well as internal changes affect body image (17,75). Temporary body changes include the following:

- Alopecia
- Change in facial hair growth
- Skin changes (color and texture)
- Ostomies and stomas
- Placement of drains and venous access lines
- Weight changes
- Incontinence of bowel and/or bladder
- Gynecomastia
- Penile/testicular atrophy
- Change in shape of breasts
- Rashes, acne, peeling of palms, and soles of feet
- Fertility
- Neuropathies

Permanent body changes may have been temporary, but became permanent and affect body image and include the following:

- Alopecia from radiation
- Change in facial hair growth
- Scarring
- Dry mouth, unable to move tongue
- Ostomies and stomas
- Pain control pumps

- Skin changes
- Amputations
- Incontinence of bowel and/or bladder
- Thinning hair
- Penile/testicular atrophy
- Change in shape of breasts
- Pelvic exenteration
- Hemipelvectomy
- Vaginal stenosis
- Fertility
- Neuropathies

Mitchell et al. (76) assert that mood can affect sexual functioning in a negative or positive way. Psychological issues that can alter sexual functioning include the following:

- Frustration
- Stigma
- Embarrassment
- Anxiety
- Anger
- Irritability
- Depression
- Loneliness
- Despair
- Grief
- Interference of age-appropriate goals (education, marriage, child bearing, and retirement)
- Performance anxiety
- Changes in personality
- Mood swings
- Misinformation
- Guilt and shame
- Disappointment
- Fear of
  - Death
  - Rejection
  - Never feeling better
  - Abandonment
  - How cancer will affect others

○ Social role change
○ How attractiveness changes
○ Never finishing treatment
○ Pain—major obstacle to enjoying sex
○ Recurrence with sexual activity
○ Cancer spread with sexual activity
○ Loss of control
○ Dependency (47,53,74,77,78)

FERTILITY

Treatment decisions made at the time of diagnosis impact interpersonal relationships, sexuality, and reproductive capacity of all survivors (79). Those diagnosed with cancer during their reproductive years hope to have children after treatment (80,81). Reproductive concerns may also affect their treatment decisions (82,83). There is a significant reduction in mortality thanks to modern treatments, but there are increased unwanted side effects such as reduced fertility (84).The ability to preserve fertility depends on these variables: age, type of cancer, history of prior infertility treatments and comorbidities, and types of treatment (85).

Ovarian-stimulating drugs with standard treatment protocols can be used without increasing the risk of developing breast cancer (86). A study (87) showed that breast cancer patients who became pregnant after treatment had a 41% reduced risk of death compared with those who didn't become pregnant. The ideal interval to wait between completing treatment and conception is unclear. Two main intervals are considered: wait until the chemotherapy is out of the patient's system or until the patient is at lower risk for recurrence (88). The timing should be personalized.

The American Society of Clinical Oncologists and the American Society of Reproductive Medicine recommends that:

- Oncologists address the possibility of infertility with all patients, including LGBTQ, in their reproductive years
- Fertility preservation should be considered as early as possible during treatment
- Standard fertility preservation practice is
  - Sperm cryopreservation for men (successful in most postpubertal cancer patients)
  - Embryo/oocyte cryopreservation for women
  - Other methods considered investigational (89)
  - Ovarian suppression with LHRHa during chemotherapy (90)
  - Ovarian transposition (oophoropexy) (91,92)

Fertility preservation takes time, is expensive, and can delay treatment and many cancers need to be treated promptly (86). Barriers to undergoing fertility preservation include cost, lack of

TABLE 43.4 REPRODUCTIVE OPTIONS (94,95)

Option	Challenge
Adoption	Limited availability of infants Emotional and financial constraints Discrimination
Third-party reproduction Assisted reproduction technologies (ART)	Society often considers this a less favorable option Some major religions forbid this Expensive

knowledge about options, and feeling too overwhelmed at the time of diagnosis (93). Psychological responses to infertility include a variety of emotions such as grief, anger, depression, sadness, loss of femininity/masculinity, and/or changes in self-image (9).

Traditional reproductive options are seen in Table 43.4 (94,95).

Psychosocial issues surrounding infertility are complicated. Postpubertal minor children before cancer treatment can undergo semen cryopreservation and oocyte freezing with patient assent and parental consent (89). Oncofertility describes an integrated network of clinical resources that focus on sparing or restoring reproductive function in people diagnosed with cancer (96).

There are emotional aspects of losing one's fertility that can include the whole spectrum of grieving. The patient may have fear of undergoing additional treatment as well as fear of abandonment by the partner. There are numerous financial issues related to pursuing treatment for infertility. How does one tell the family, friends, and significant others? Often it makes the patient feel like a failure. The couple has to address issues of child-free living.

SEXUAL ASSESSMENT AND TREATMENT

According to Bober (97), most practitioners do not have experience discussing sexuality and intimacy in a frank, authentic, and direct manner. In most published studies, patients have stated that they would like more information about sex than they received from their physician. The patient usually does not voluntarily ask sex-related questions, so it is up to the health care provider to integrate sexuality into the routine care of all oncology patients (98). Davis and Taylor's (99) Extended PLISSIT model can provide a framework for doing a sexual assessment. It stresses the importance of *explicit* permission-giving, which validates the importance of the intimate relationship. It has four components: P, permission; LI, limited information; SS, specific suggestions; and IT, intensive therapy.

The practitioner gives the patient permission (P) to think about cancer and sexuality at the same time by asking, "What sexuality changes have you noticed since your cancer?" which lets them know that they are not the only ones to experience sexuality changes. By asking open-ended questions, the health care provider is better able to get a thoughtful response from the patient (76). Giving them the time to answer is important. Try to remain relaxed with good eye contact to let them know that you are interested in this area of their lives. Addressing sexuality and developing supportive interventions early on in the assessment and treatment of the patient allows the practitioner to open up a line of communication with the patient across the spectrum of cancer care (100). Giving them LI about side effects from treatments by saying, "Sometimes people notice sexuality changes when they get this treatment," lets them know that you are comfortable talking about sexuality issues. Ways to incorporate assessment of sexuality concerns into clinical practice include addressing sexuality through patients' perceptions of their body image, family roles and functions, relationships, and sexual function (101). Describing SS such as books to read, or positions to use, can offer them help with the problem.

Some patients are in difficult relationships, which only get worse with cancer treatment and need IT from a marital or a sex therapist. Having a list of those resources in the community can be helpful to the patient specialist. Giving referrals depends on what specialized assistance would benefit the patient.

The culture in which the person grew up as well as the culture in which the person currently lives not only will affect how one copes with cancer but influences one's sexuality (53). After cancer treatment gay men are concerned about erectile problems or libido, which may lead to feelings of exclusion from sexual communities (102). Often the health care practitioner does not know the sexual orientation or gender identity of his or her patients. Dibble et al. (33) state that because of heterosexism, those who do not share a heterosexual orientation may have difficult lives especially when they are ill. Heterosexism is the belief that heterosexuality is the only "normal" option for relationships (33). People in isolated, rural areas may feel a lack of support and resources to address sexuality changes. Someone with cancer may mistakenly feel they are contagious. Partners of women with cancer often are fearful of inflicting pain, causing fractures, or infecting them because of lack of information or misinformation from the practitioner about resuming sexual activity (48,103). Cancer is expensive to treat and often financial

and insurance concerns interfere with sexuality because of the patient being distracted. The stress of cancer and its treatments can exacerbate underlying marital tension and likewise affect the sexual relationship (54). There are many socioeconomic factors that can affect sexuality, and these include marital status, race, education, attitude toward cancer/treatment, gender preference, family traditions, religion, lack of partner, significance of body part, role change, job loss/pressures, end of life issues, and relationship inequalities (4,47,48,98).

Sexual morbidities after breast cancer diagnosis include an immediate reduction in sexual activity, interest, responsiveness, and pleasure (104,105). Andersen (106) found that women diagnosed with breast cancer recurrence initially were less sexually active but increased their activity to pre-recurrence rates unless they had distance metastases. Even when patients are dealing with end-of-life issues, it is important to be aware of their sexuality concerns and address these (77). Interventions for sexual dysfunction resulting from cancer treatment can be limited because of the hormone status of the tumor. Women with estrogen receptive positive breast cancer are often unable to use any estrogen products, while some oncologists give them the go-ahead to use an estrogen vaginal ring, vaginal creams, or tablets. A study reported that the use of vaginal estradiol tablet was associated with a rise in systemic estradiol levels, which reverses estrogen suppression achieved by aromatase inhibitors and should be avoided (46). Onujiogu et al. (107) report that 90% of patients with gynecologic cancer report sexual dysfunction that impacts their psychosocial adjustment and quality of life. Most of the symptoms of sexual dysfunction in patients with breast cancer are related to estrogen deprivation due to premature menopause caused by chemotherapy and antiestrogen hormonal therapy. There are some oncologists that will approve the use of off-label androgen gel for those women to improve libido. Studies have shown that testosterone has positive effects on women's sexuality and higher doses show greater effects (108). It is controversial and should be left to the discretion of the medical oncologist. Women with other types of cancer can use oral estrogen replacement if they are comfortable with this and their oncologist gives them the approval. Maintenance of vaginal health through hormonal and nonhormonal methods is important not only for the overall well-being in the postmenopausal female but also for the elimination of sexual dysfunctions that occur because of urogenital atrophy (95).

Levine (109) reports that sexual activity serves as a rebonding mechanism by serving as an eraser for ordinary annoyances, preventing hostility

TABLE 43.5 TREATMENT OF SEXUAL DYSFUNCTION (4,24,48,53,115–125)

Treatment	Example
Vaginal dilator (use with lubricant)	Different sizes to find comfortable fit with partner or to be able to tolerate gynecological examination. Silicone ones can be heated or cooled
Erotica	Videos, magazines, books, music, Web sites
Water-soluble or silicone personal lubricants and moisturizers, natural oils	K-Y, Astroglide, or other lubricants for sexual activity, Replens, or other vaginal moisturizers for vaginal health and comfort; olive or coconut oil
Videos	Better Sex Videos, an inexpensive, tastefully done option
Contraceptive options	Oral contraceptives may not be option, use barrier protection (female or male condoms and diaphragm)
Planning for sexual activity	Take medications to control symptoms 30 minutes before encounter Schedule encounters when energy is highest
Communicating more openly about sexual needs	Tell partner what feels good, when sexual desire is highest
Exploring one's own body	Finding out new erogenous zones, pleasuring self to improve blood flow into the genitals
Safer sexual practices	If not in committed relationship, use barrier protection (condoms)
Different means of sexual expression	Oral–genital, anal activity, manual stimulation, different sexual positions, vibrators
Better symptom control	Take medications for pain, nausea, fatigue, diarrhea as needed. Bowel and bladder training
Using erotic devices	Vibrators can enhance sexual activity and improve blood flow in the vagina and to the penis
Sensate focus	Focuses on receiver's pleasure, no genital activity, uses all of the senses
PDE-5 inhibitors	Tadafil, vardenafil, sildenafil Best if taken on an empty stomach 30 minutes prior to sexual activity. Needs sexual stimulation to be effective
Penile implants	Genitourinary specialist referral
Penile injections	Alprostadil, Caverject Needs prescription
Penile bands	Over the counter; improve sustainability of erection
OhNut	Provides a spacer on the penis when the vagina has shortened
Vacuum erection device	Need prescription
Fertility specialists	Both male and female, oncofertilitist consult
EROS-CT for women	Vacuum device for female (need prescription)
Physical therapist for pelvic floor exercises	P.T. must have specialized training
Reconstructive surgery	Plastic surgeon, dentists, wound ostomy nurses
Breast implants	Plastic surgeon
Acupuncture	Improve erectile dysfunction, decrease menopause symptoms, pain
Vaginal laser	Improve vaginal atrophy, gynecology consult
L-Arginine	Reportedly improves genital blood flow to improve arousal. Does not stimulate estrogen
Hormone therapy	Endocrinology; improves libido and erections
Psychosexual therapy	Sexual therapist
Lidocaine	For dyspareunia

between partners, decreasing extramarital temptations, and providing psychological intimacy. According to Boa and Grenman (110), cancer is a "relationship disease" that affects not only the sexual relationship but other intimate relationships as well. Sexuality is important to many people's self-concept and personal integrity (111). It can improve sleep quality and may be sedating (112,113), comforts, and relaxes (114). A study found that American women masturbate to fall asleep and also for pain relief (115,116). Treatment options for female and male sexual dysfunction are shown in Table 43.5 (4,24,48,53,115–126).

Men with prostate cancer do not have the option to take testosterone replacements for low libido for fear of stimulating the tumor. However, men with other types of cancer can take testosterone replacements without fear of increasing their risk of prostate cancer (127). Asking about desire includes inquiring about sexual fantasies and dreams which are dependent on testosterone levels.

Many people have adopted a pattern of sexual behavior before their diagnosis and attempt to return to it after treatment. If they experience discomfort or failure to function as before, they will stop trying and feel they cannot enjoy sexual activity (106). Some couples who are cancer survivors and are in a stressful relationship with an unsupportive partner tend to have more distress, which can lead to avoidant coping behaviors (128). They avoid talking about difficult issues, including sexuality. Conversely, during the time of treatment, the cancer experience encourages a more intimate and intense interpersonal relationship. There are few studies that have attempted any type of psychosocial intervention to assist survivors in integrating the cancer experience into their personal life. Whether one is partnered or not, a large portion of cancer survivors remain sexually active, which makes it important to address sexual issues soon after their diagnosis. Ussher et al. (100) found it important to address sexual and body image issues in patients with nonreproductive cancers as well. If one is not partnered, there is the question of when to reveal one's cancer history: at the beginning of a relationship or wait until the relationship develops, but that is up to the person with cancer. There is no right or wrong answer.

CONCLUSION

The Institute of Medicine report, *From Cancer Patient to Survivor: Lost in Transition*, recommends intervention for consequences of cancer and its treatment including sexual side effects (129). Palliative care can address these side effects as they treat other side effects the patient

experiences. Both patients and their partners value pretreatment preparation for sexual recovery and support after treatment for sexual recovery (130). According to the Institute of Medicine report, *The health of lesbian, gay, bisexual, and transgender people: building a foundation for better understanding,* (131) there are numerous factors contributing to SGM health care disparities even in the palliative care setting. According to Davis and Taylor (99), sexual well-being includes participation in sexual activity, satisfaction with sexual experiences, and sexual function. When a serious illness occurs patient intimacy is critically threatened and most patients want to talk about sexuality and intimacy issues with palliative care providers (2). Recognizing the importance of patient-centered care helps them feel safe in disclosing sexual issues. The patient will realize that the practitioner is holistic and focused not just on physical concerns, but the patient's quality of life.

REFERENCES

1. Kusakabe A, Hirano K, Mawatari H, et al. Are the medical staff ready to respond to the suffering from sexuality of terminal cancer patients (article in Japanese). *Gan To Kagaku Ryoho.* 2019;46(suppl 1):57-59.
2. Kelemen A, Cagle J, Chung J, Groninger H. Assessing the impact of serious illness on patient intimacy and sexuality in palliative care. *J Pain Symptom Manage.* 2019;58(2):282-288.
3. Releman MJ. Is there a place for sexuality in the holistic care of patients in the palliative care phase of life? *Am J Hosp Palliat Care.* 2008;25(5):366-371.
4. Hordern AJ, Street AF. Let's talk about sex: risky business for cancer and palliative care clinicians. *Contemp Nurse.* 2007;27(1):49-60.
5. Leiblum SR, Baume RM, Croog SH. The sexual functioning of elderly hypertensive women. *J Sex Marital Ther.* 1994;20:259-270.
6. Gilley J. Intimacy and terminal care. *J R Coll Gen Pract.* 1988;38:121-122.
7. Leung MW, Goldfarb S, Dizon DS. Communication about sexuality in advanced illness aligns with a palliative care approach to patient-centered care. *Curr Oncol Rep.* 2016;18:11.
8. Tomlinson JM. Talking a sexual history. In: Tomlinson JM, ed. *ABC of Sexual Health.* Malden, MA: Blackwell Publishing, Inc.; 2005:13-16.
9. Lemieux L, Kaiser S, Pereira J, Meadows LM. Sexuality in palliative care: patient perspectives. *Palliat Med.* 2004;18:630-637.
10. Maslow A. A theory of human motivation. *Psychol Rev.* 1943;50:370-396.
11. Matzo M, Hijjazi K. If you don't ask me…don't expect me to tell. A pilot study of the sexual health of hospice patients. *J Hosp Palliat Nurs.* 2009;11:271-281.
12. Kelemen AM, Cagle JG, Groninger H. Screening for intimacy concerns in a palliative care population: findings from a pilot study. *J Palliat Med.* 2016;19:1102-1105.
13. Masters WH, Johnson VE. *Human Sexual Response.* 1st ed. Boston, MA: Little Brown; 1966.
14. Southard NZ, Keller J. The importance of assessing sexuality: a patient perspective. *Clin J Oncol Nurs.* 2009;13:213-217.

15. Smith DB. Sexuality and the patient with cancer: what nurses need to know. *Oncol Patient Care Pract Guidel Special Nurse.* 1994;4:1-3.

16. Winze JP, Carey MP. *Sexual Dysfunction: A Guide for Assessment and Treatment.* New York, NY: Guilford Press; 1991.

17. Krebs L. What should I say? Talking with patients about sexuality issues. *Clin J Oncol Nurs.* 2006;10:313-315.

18. Wilmoth MC. Life after cancer: what does sexuality have to do with it? 2006 Mara Mogensen Flaherty Memorial Lectureship. *Oncol Nurs Forum.* 2006;33:905-910.

19. Gregoire A. Male sexual problems. In: Tomlinson JM, ed. *ABC of Sexual Health.* 2nd ed. Malden, MA: Blackwell Publishing, Inc.; 2005:37-39.

20. Basson R. Human sex-response cycles. *J Sex Marital Ther.* 2001;27:33-43.

21. Kandeel FR, Koussa VK, Swerdloff RS. Male sexual function and its disorders: physiology, pathophysiology, clinical investigation, and treatment. *Endocr Rev.* 2001;22:342-388.

22. Katz A. *Breaking the Silence on Cancer and Sexuality.* Pittsburgh, PA: Oncology Nursing Society; 2007.

23. Schiavi RC, Segraves RT. The biology of sexual function. *Psychiatr Clin North Am.* 1995;18:7-23.

24. Sarrel P. Genital blood flow and ovarian secretions. *J Clin Pract Sex.* 1990;14-15.

25. Zilbergeld B, Ellison C. Desire discrepancies and arousal problems in sex therapy. In: Leiblum S, Pervin L, eds. *Principles and Practice of Sex Therapy.* New York, NY: Guilford Press; 1980:65-104.

26. Gallo-Silver L. The sexual rehabilitation of persons with cancer. *Cancer Pract.* 2000;8,10-15.

27. Quinn GO, Sanchez JA, Sutton SK, et al. Cancer and lesbian, gay, bisexual, transgender/transsexual, and queer/questioning (LGBTQ) populations. *CA Cancer J Clin.* 2015;65:384-400.

28. National Cancer Institute. Cancer disparities. Updated October 21, 2016. https://www.cancer.gov/about-cancer/understandingdisparities. Accessed March 3, 2020.

29. Fredriksen-Goldsen KI, Kim HJ, Barkan SE, et al. Health disparities among lesbian, gay, and bisexual older adults: results from a population-based study. *Am J Public Health.* 2013;103:1802-1809.

30. Lisy K, Peters MDJ, Schofield P, et al. Experiences and unmet needs of lesbian, gay, and bisexual people with cancer care: a systematic review and metasynthesis. *Psychooncology.* 2018;27:1480-1489.

31. Matthews AK, Breen E, Kittieerasack P. Social determinants of LBT cancer health inequities. *Semin Oncol Nurs.* 2018;34:12-20.

32. Simoni JM, Smith L, Oosl KM, et al. Disparities in physical health conditions among lesbian and bisexual women: a systematic review of population-based studies. *J Homosex.* 2017;64:32-44.

33. Dibble S, Eliason MJ, Dejoseph JF, Chinn P. Sexual issues in special populations: lesbian and gay individuals. *Semin Oncol Nurs.* 2008;24:127-130.

34. Dibble SL, Eliason MJ, Christiansen MA. Chronic illness care for lesbian, gay, bisexual individuals. *Nurs Clin North Am.* 2007;42:655-674; viii.

35. Jabson JM, Bowen DJ. Perceived stress and sexual orientation among breast cancer survivors. *J Homosex.* 2014;61:889-898.

36. Cochran SD, Maya VM, Bowen D, et al. Cancer-related risk indicators and preventive screening behaviors among lesbians and bisexual women. *Am J Public Health.* 2001;91:591-597.

37. Roberts JR, Siekas LL, Kaz AM. Anal intraepithelial neoplasia: a review of diagnosis and management. *World J Gastrointest Oncol.* 2017;9:50-61.

38. Schabath MB, Blackburn CA, Sutter ME, et al. National survey of oncologists at National Cancer Institute-designated comprehensive cancer centers: attitudes, knowledge, and practice behaviors about LGBTQ patients with cancer. *J Clin Oncol.* 2019;37(7):547-560.

39. Cathcart-Rake EJ. Cancer in sexual and gender minority patients: are we addressing their needs? *Curr Oncol Rep.* 2018;20:85.

40. Wheldon CW, Schabatth MB, Sudson J, et al. Culturally competent care for sexual and gender minority patients at National Cancer Institute-designated comprehensive cancer centers. *LGBT Health.* 2018;5(3):203-211.

41. Montejo-Gonzalez AL, Llorca G, Izquierdo JA, et al. SSRI-induced sexual dysfunction: fluoxetine, paroxetine, sertraline, and fluvoxamine in a prospective, multicenter, and descriptive clinical study of 344 patients. *J Sex Marital Ther.* 1997;23:176-194.

42. Goldstein I, Meston CM, Traish AM, et al. Future directions. In: *Women's Sexual Function and Dysfunction: Study, Diagnosis, and Treatment.* London: Taylor & Francis; 2007:745-748.

43. American Psychiatric Association. *Diagnostic and Statistical Manual of Mental Disorders: DSM-V.* Washington, DC: Author; 2013.

44. Schover L. Reproductive complications and sexual dysfunction in cancer survivors. In: Ganz PA, ed. *Cancer Survivorship; Today and Tomorrow.* New York, NY: Springer; 2007:251-271.

45. Crenshaw TL, Goldberg JP, eds. *Sexual Pharmacology: Drugs that Effect Sexual Functioning.* New York, NY: WW Norton; 1996.

46. Sadock V. Psychotropic drugs and sexual dysfunction. *Prim Psychiatry.* 1995;4:16-17.

47. Hughes MK. Gynecological cancer. In: Holland JC Golant M, Greenberg DM, et al., eds. *Psycho-Oncology: A Quick Reference on the Psychosocial Dimensions of Cancer Symptom Management.* 2nd ed. New York, NY: Oxford University Press; 2015:171-178.

48. Hughes MK. Sexual dysfunction. In: Holland JC, Golant M, Greenbert DM, et al., eds. *Psycho-Oncology: A Quick Reference on the Psychosocial Dimensions of Cancer Symptom Management.* 2nd ed. New York, NY: Oxford University Press; 2015:115-119.

49. Stein KD, Jacobsen PB, Hann DM, Greenberg H, Lyman G. Impact of hot flashes on quality of life among postmenopausal women being treated for breast cancer. *J Pain Symptom Manage.* 2000;19:436-445.

50. Gupta P, Sturdee DW, Palin SL, et al. Menopausal symptoms in women treated for breast cancer: the prevalence and severity of symptoms and their perceived effects on quality of life. *Climacteric.* 2006;9(1):49-58.

51. Santoro N. The menopause transition. *Am J Med.* 2005;118(12B):85-135.

52. Ganz PA, Desmond KA, Belin TR, Meyerowitz BE, Rowland JH. Predictors of sexual health in women after a breast cancer diagnosis. *J Clin Oncol.* 1999;17(8):2371-2380.

53. Hughes MK. Alterations of sexual function in women with cancer. *Semin Oncol Nurs.* 2008;24:91-101.

54. Conde DM, Pinto-Neto AM, Cabello C, Sa DS, Costa-Paiva L, Martinez EZ. Menopause symptoms and quality of life in women aged 45 to 65 years with and without breast cancer. *Menopause.* 2005;12:436-443.

55. Fobair P, Stewart SL, Chang S, D'Onofrio C, Banks PJ, Bloom JR. Body image and sexual problems in young women with breast cancer. *Psychooncology.* 2006;15:579-594.

56. Rosenbaum TY. Managing postmenopausal dyspareunia: beyond hormone therapy. *Fem Patient.* 2006;31:1–5.

57. Katz A. Gay and lesbian patients with cancer. *Oncol Nurs Forum.* 2009;36:203-207.

58. Carter J, Stabile C, Gunn A, Sonoda Y. The physical consequences of gynecologic cancer surgery and their impact on sexual, emotional, and quality of life issues. *J Sex Med.* 2013;10(suppl 1):21-34.

59. Kupelian V, Shabsigh R, Araujo AB, O'Donnell AB, McKinlay JB. Erectile dysfunction as a predictor of the metabolic syndrome in aging men: results from the Massachusetts Male Aging Study. *J Urol.* 2006;176: 222-226.

60. Krychman ML, Carter J, Aghajanian CA, Dizon DS, Castiel M. Chemotherapy induced dyspareunia: a case study of vaginal mucositis and pegylated liposomal doxorubicin injection in advanced stage ovarian carcinoma. *Gynecol Oncol.* 2004;93:561-563.

61. Taylor MJ, Rudkin L, Hawton K. Strategies for managing antidepressant-induced sexual dysfunction: systematic review of randomized controlled trials. *J Affect Disord.* 2005;88:241-254.

62. Zemishlany Z, Weizman A. The impact of mental illness on sexual dysfunction. *Adv Psychosom Med.* 2008; 29:89-106.

63. Basson R, Schultz WW. Sexual sequelae of general medical disorders. *Lancet.* 2007;369:409-424.

64. Hitiris N, Barrett JA, Brodie JJ. Erectile dysfunction associated with pregablin add-on treatment in patients with partial seizures: five case reports. *Epilepsy Behav.* 2006;8:418-421.

65. Hypericum Depression Trial Study Group. Effect of *Hypericum perforatum* (St. John's wort) in major depressive disorder. A randomized controlled trial. *JAMA.* 2002;287:1807-1814.

66. Lue T. Physiology of penile erection and pathophysiology of erectile dysfunction and priaprism. In: Walsh C, ed. *Campbell's Urology.* 8th ed. Philadelphia, PA: W.B. Saunders; 2002:1591-1618.

67. Do C, Huyghe E, Lapeyre-Mestre M, Montastruc JI, Bagheri H. Statins and erectile dysfunction: results of a case/noncase study using the French Pharmocovigilance System Database. *Drug Saf.* 2009;32:591-597.

68. Basson R, Leiblum S, Brotto L, et al. Revised definitions of women's sexual dysfunction. *J Sex Med.* 2004;1:40-48.

69. Basson R. Women's sexual dysfunction: revised and expanded definitions. *CMAJ.* 2005;172:1327-1333.

70. Clayton AH. Sexual function and dysfunction in women. *Psychiatr Clin North Am.* 2003;26:673-682.

71. Basson R, Althof S, Davis S, et al. Summary of the recommendations on sexual dysfunctions in women. *J Sex Med.* 2004;1:24-34.

72. Reese JB, Handorf E, Haythornthwaite JA. Sexual quality of life, body image distress, and psychosocial outcomes in colorectal cancer: a longitudinal study. *Support Care Cancer.* 2018;26(10):3431-3440.

73. Harden J. Developmental life stage and couples' experiences with prostate cancer: a review of the literature. *Cancer Nurs.* 2005;28:85-98.

74. DeFrank JT, Mehta CC, Stein KD, Baker F. Body image dissatisfaction in cancer survivors. *Oncol Nurs Forum.* 2007;34:E36-E41.

75. Brotto LA, et al. Women's sexual desire and arousal disorders. *J Sex Med.* 2010;1(Pt 2):586-614.

76. Mitchell WB, DiBartolo PM, Brown TA, Barlow DH. Effects of positive and negative mood on sexual arousal in sexually functional males. *Arch Sex Behav.* 1998;27:197-207.

77. Shell JA, Carolan M, Zhang Y, Meneses KD. The longitudinal effects of cancer treatment on sexuality in individuals with lung cancer. *Oncol Nurs Forum.* 2008;35:73-79.

78. Gevirtz C. How chronic pain affects sexuality. *Nursing.* 2008;38:17.

79. Schover LR. Sexuality and fertility after cancer. *Hematol Am Soc Hematol Educ Program.* 2005;523:7.

80. Kirkman M, Stern C, Neil S, et al. Fertility management after breast cancer diagnosis: a qualitative investigation of women's experiences of and recommendations for professional care. *Health Care Women Int.* 2013;34:50-67.

81. Schmidt R, Richter D, Sender A, Geue K. Motivations for having children after cancer—a systematic review of the literature. *Eur J Cancer Care.* 2014;25:6-17.

82. Ruddy KJ, Gelber SI, Tamimi RM, et al. Prospective study of fertility concerns and preservation strategies in young women with breast cancer. *J Clin Oncol.* 2014;32(11):1151-1156.

83. Senkus E, Gomez H, Dirix L, et al. Attitudes of young patients with breast cancer toward fertility loss related to adjuvant systemic therapies. EoRTC study 10002 BIG 3-98. *Psychooncology.* 2014;23(2):173-182.

84. Johnson J-A, Tough S. Delayed childbearing. *J Obstet Gynaecol Can.* 2012;34(1):80-93.

85. Wallace WHB, Smith AG, Kelsey TW, Edgar AE, Anderson RA. Fertility preservation for girls and young women with cancer: population-based validation of criteria for ovarian tissue cryopreservation. *Lancet Oncol.* 2014;15(19):1129-1136.

86. Practice Committee of the American Society for Reproductive Medicine. Fertility preservation in patients undergoing gonadotoxic therapy or gonadectomy: a committee opinion. *Fertil Steril.* 2019;112:1022-1033.

87. Azim HA Jr, Santoro L, Pavlidis N, et al. Safety of pregnancy following breast cancer diagnosis: a meta-analysis of 14 studies. *Eur J Cancer.* 2011;47(1):74-83.

88. Peccatori FA, Azim HA Jr, Orecchia R, et al. Cancer, pregnancy and fertility: ESMO Clinical Practice guidelines for diagnosis treatment and follow-up. *Ann Oncol.* 2013;24(suppl 6):160-170.

89. Loren AW, Mangu PB, Beck LN, et al. Fertility preservation for patients with cancer: American Society of Clinical Oncology Clinical Practice Guideline update. *J Clin Oncol.* 2013;31(19):2500-2510.

90. Coates AS, Winer EP, Goldhirsch A, et al. Tailoring therapies-improving the management of early breast cancer: St Gallen International Expert Consensus on the Primary Therapy of Early Breast Cancer 2015. *Ann Oncol.* 2015;26(8):1533-1546.

91. Oktay K, Harvey BE, Partridge AH, et al. Fertility preservation in patients with cancer: ASCO Clinical Practice Guideline update. *J Clin Oncol.* 2018;36: 1994-2001.

92. Bisharah M, Tulandi T. Laparoscopic preservation of ovarian function: an underused procedure. *Am J Obstet Gynecol.* 2003;188:367-370.

93. Benedict C, Thom B, Friedman F, et al. Young adult female cancer survivors' unmet information needs and reproductive concerns contribute to decisional conflict regarding posttreatment fertility preservation. *Cancer.* 2016;122:2101-2109.

94. Carr SV. Surrogacy and ethics in women with cancer. *Best Pract Res Clin Obstet Gynaecol.* 2019;55:117-127.

95. Lester JL, Bernhard LA. Urogenital atrophy in breast cancer survivors. *Oncol Nurs Forum.* 2009;36(6):693-698.

96. Woodruff TK. The oncofertility consortium—addressing fertility in young people with cancer. *Nat Rev Clin Oncol.* 2010;7(8):466-475.

97. Bober SL, From the guest editor. Out in the open: addressing sexual health after cancer. *Cancer J.* 2009;15:13-14.

98. Hughes MK. Sexuality and the cancer survivor: a silent coexistence. *Cancer Nurs.* 2000;23:477-482.

99. Davis S, Taylor B. From PLISSIT to EX-PLISSIT. In: Davis S, ed. *Rehabilitation: The Use of Theories and Models in Practice.* Oxford, UK: Elsevier LTD.; 2006: 101-129.

100. Ussher JM, Perz J, Gilbert E; the Australian Cancer and Sexuality Study Team. Perceived causes and consequences of sexual changes after cancer for women and men: a mixed method study. *BMC Cancer.* 2015;15: 268-286.

101. Mick JM. Sexuality assessment: 10 strategies for improvement. *Clin J Oncol Nurs.* 2007;11:671-675.

102. Ussher JM, Perz J, Rose D, et al. Threat of sexual disqualification: the consequences of erectile dysfunction and other sexual changes for gay and bisexual men with prostate cancer. *Arch Sex Behav.* 2017;46: 2043-2057.

103. Kwan KSH, Roberts LJ, Swalm DM. Sexual dysfunction and chronic pain: the role of psychological variables and impact on quality of life. *Eur J Pain.* 2005;9: 643-652.

104. Kedde H, et al. Sexual dysfunction in young women with breast cancer. *Support Care Cancer.* 2013;21(1):271-280.

105. Ussher JM, Perz J, Gilbert E. Changes to sexual well-being and intimacy after breast cancer. *Cancer Nurs.* 2012;35(6):456-465.

106. Andersen BL. In sickness and in health: maintaining intimacy after breast cancer recurrence. *Cancer J.* 2009;15:70-73.

107. Onujiogu N, et al. Survivors of endometrial cancer: who is at risk for sexual dysfunction? *Gynecol Oncol.* 2011;123(2):356-359.

108. Heiman JR. Treating low sexual desire—new findings for testosterone in women. *N Engl J Med.* 2008;359: 2047-2949.

109. Levine SB. What patients mean by love, intimacy, and sexual desire. In: Levine SB, Risen CB, Althof SE, eds. *Handbook of Clinical Sexuality for Mental Health Professionals.* 2nd ed. New York, NY: Routledge; 2010:19-34.

110. Boa R, Grenman S. Psychosexual health in gynecologic cancer. *Int J Gynecol Obstet.* 2018;143(suppl 2): 147-152.

111. Masters WH, Johnson VE, Kolodny RC. *Human Sexuality.* New York, NY: Harper Collins; 1992.

112. Weeks D, James J. *Secrets of the Superyoung.* New York, NY: Villard; 1999.

113. Odent M. *The Scientification of Love.* London, UK: Free Assoc Books; 1999.

114. Weeks DJ. Sex for the mature adult: health, self-esteem and countering ageist stereotypes. *Sex Relat Ther.* 2002;17: 231-240.

115. Komisaruk Br, Whipple B. The suppression of pain by genital stimulation in females. *Annu Rev Sex Res.* 1995;6: 151-186.

116. Juraskova I, Jarvis S, Mok K, et al. The acceptability, feasibility, and efficacy (phase/I/II study) of the OVER-come (Olive oil, Vaginal Exercise, and MoisturizeR)

117. Rahn DD, Carberry C, Sanses TV, et al. Vaginal estrogen for genitourinary syndrome of menopause: a systemic review. *Obstet Gynecol.* 2014;124(6):1147-1156.

118. ohnut.co/products/ohnut-set. Accessed March 13, 2020.

119. Lemke EA, Madsen LT, Dains JE. Vaginal testosterone for management of aromatase inhibitor-related sexual dysfunction: an integrative review. *Oncol Nurs Forum.* 2018;44(3):296-301.

120. Campbel G, Thomas TH, Hand L, et al. Caring for survivors of gynecologic cancer: assessment and management of long-term and late effects. *Semin Oncol Nurs.* 2019;35:192-201.

121. Bond CB, Jensen PT, Groenvold M, Johnsen AT. Prevalence and possible predictors of sexual dysfunction and self-reported needs related to the sexual life of advanced cancer patients. *Acta Oncol.* 2019;12:1-7.

122. Pagano I, Gieri S, Nocera F, et al. Evaluation of the CO_2 laser therapy on vulvo-vaginal atrophy (VV) in oncological patients: preliminary results. *J Cancer Ther.* 2017;8: 452-463.

123. Katz A, Dizon DS. Sexuality after cancer: a model for male survivors. *J Sex Med.* 2016;12:70-78.

124. Albaugh JA. Intracavernosal injection algorithm. *Urol Nurs.* 2006;26:449-453.

125. Guirguis WR. Oral treatment of erectile dysfunction: from herbal remedies to designer drugs. *J Sex Marital Ther.* 1998;24:69-73.

126. White A, Hayhoe S, Hart A, Ernst E; Volunteers from BMAS and AACP. Adverse events following acupuncture (SAFA): a prospective survey of 32,000 consultations. *Acupunct Med.* 2001;19:84-92.

127. Slater S, Oliver RT. Testosterone: its role in development of prostate cancer and potential risk from use as hormone replacement therapy. *Drugs Aging.* 2000;17: 431-439.

128. Manne SL, Ostroff J, Winkel G, Grana G, Fox K. Partner unsupportive responses, avoidant coping, and distress among women with early stage breast cancer: patient and partner perspectives. *Health Psychol.* 2005;24: 635-641.

129. Institute of Medicine. *From Cancer Patient to Cancer Survivor: Lost in Transition.* Washington, DC: National Academies Press; 2005.

130. Mehta A, Pollack CE, Gillespie TW, et al. What patient and partners want in intervention that support sexual recovery after prostate cancer treatment: an exploratory convergent mixed methods study. *Sex Med.* 2019;7(2): 184-191.

131. Institute of Medicine. *The Health of Lesbian, Gay, Bisexual, and Transgender People Building a Foundation for Better Understanding.* Washington, DC: National Academy of Science; 2011.

intervention to improve dyspareunia and alleviate sexual problems in women with breast cancer. *J Sex Med.* 2013;10:2549-2558.

44 Caregiving in the Home

Betty Ferrell and Pierce DiMauro

CAREGIVING

Background

The United States is experiencing a dramatic shift toward becoming an older society. With the aging population have come increased health care costs and an increased use of overall health care services. In its essence, growing older is expensive. Chronic illness begins to impair older adults' physical and cognitive abilities, and by doing so, dramatically increases the necessity for health care services. Yet, as more people have grown older, Medicare has undergone marked changes and policy reformations ranging from service coverage and reimbursement to, most dramatically, reductions for home health care (HHC). Over the years, health care professionals and policy makers have been challenged with the following question: *How do we balance quality, cost, and access to health care, particularly at home* (1)?

Prior to the 1980s, most HHC was provided by informal (family/unpaid) caregivers. At-home care consisted largely of noncomplex interventions, such as administering oral medication or changing simple dressings. Patients in need of more complex care remained as hospital inpatients. In the mid-1980s, however, with the expansion of Medicare access and usage, there was a dramatic shift to formal HHC, wherein discharged patients were treated by formal, paid caregivers. During this time, large incentives were in place to make HHC the fastest growing U.S. medical service (2). At home, formal and informal caregivers worked as a team to address patients' needs. Often home health nurses performed home visits prior to discharge. This practice allowed the nurse to meet the family, introduce the care plan, and address any issues within the home environment that could present challenges for the patient once home. Meeting a nurse and becoming familiar with the treatment plan lessened the family's worry, particularly on how to address their loved one's special needs. Before the patient came home, the nurse could have all necessary medications, supplies, and medical equipment in place. The nurse–family caregiver team could then be sufficiently prepared to care for the family member at home.

The Balanced Budget Act in 1997 (3) greatly impacted HHC provided by Medicare by instituting some of the largest Medicare reductions since 1981. Prior to the Act's passage, HHC was paid for by Medicare on a retrospective cost basis; this reimbursement model provided financial incentives to HHC agencies to provide more, and longer services. By October 2000, however, HHC was paid for on a prospective basis; a predetermined rate schedule limits patients to 60 days of HHC (2). Additionally, the eligibility parameters were narrowed and more frequent, complex documentation complicated patient access (3). The Balanced Budget Act sparked a significant shift back to informal caregiving at home. Today, formal caregiving is most often paid for out of pocket, with some care provided by long-term private health insurance or community-based services (4).

New technologies, innovative surgical techniques, and advances in medication modalities are changing how and where cancer care is delivered. The majority of cancer treatments may now occur in outpatient clinics in their entirety; while decrease in the need for inpatient treatment is positive, health care systems have not adequately adjusted to accommodate the growing needs of care provided in the home setting (5–7).

Complex Care in the Home Setting

Family caregivers provide much of the necessary care that enables chronically ill patients to live at home (8). The quality of home care provided is influenced by several factors, especially the delivery of palliative care. Heavy reliance on family caregivers, access to diagnostic facilities, and pharmacy services available all influence the effectiveness of pain and symptom management at home and all aspects of patient care (9).

Often health care professionals, family members, and patients voice strong preference for care in the home setting, viewing it as preferential to institutional care. The assumption is that comfort will be maximized while at home. Family members, however, encounter several barriers when implementing care. Pain management has been found to be a particularly difficult task for caregivers, and 71%

of patients with advanced cancer experience pain. Caregivers are expected to administer analgesics, including opioids, to provide relief (8).

Research has revealed that at home, caregivers are impeded by a lack of knowledge and adequate assessment skills. Additionally, caregivers cope with fears regarding side effects, addiction, and concerns about tolerance to pain medications (10,11). When planning cancer home care, consideration must be given to the accessibility of services and to family caregivers' knowledge, values, and abilities. If potential home care issues have not been identified, not only can patient comfort level be compromised, but such issues can evoke a sense of inadequacy and despair in family caregivers. Challenges in managing pain have become even more important in recent years with the opioid crisis often impacting availability of medications and fears associated with their use.

At home, caregivers may dramatically lack the resources that are available to health care providers within inpatient settings. For patients with complex problems, inpatient care may include a variety of aggressive or invasive strategies for diagnosis and definitive treatment of the underlying conditions. With immediate access to specialists and high-tech equipment in the inpatient setting, an appropriate plan can be determined and initiated immediately. Conversely, at-home caregivers must rely on low-tech care methodologies, and attention must be paid most to symptom management. The dynamic nature of cancer and its treatment side effects make effective symptom management especially challenging for home care patients and family caregivers. A change in symptoms may indicate disease progression or treatment-related side effects. Support for caregivers when preparing to provide at-home care is needed. Research is also needed to further understand how health care professionals can provide this support (8,10,11).

Cancer as a Family Experience

A cancer diagnosis places a burden not only on the patient but also on familial relatives, friends, and caregivers (12–15). Care that was once provided by intensive care units (ICUs), delivered by specially trained health care providers, is now thrust upon families to be provided in the home. Often family members have little or no preparation for the physical and emotional demands of such a role (16,17). Although the patient may be the sole member affected physically by illness, chronic disease can inflict challenges on every family member. Conflicts can arise from different needs and/or different coping strategies. For instance, spouses often experience more burden and depression than do other family members. Spousal well-being and self-efficacy have been found to decrease when a partner is diagnosed with a chronic illness (6,18). Spouses are also the most likely to provide the highest degree of care among family caregivers, and are the least likely to seek professional caregiving assistance. For many, marriage is the most significant relationship in their life; as such, spousal caregivers are often the most vulnerable to distress from their caregiving role (18). Research has indicated that partner caregivers experience the highest rate of caregiver depression, while they try to balance providing care and coping with the distress of a prognosis, disease progression, and end-of-life preparation. Partner depression rates may, in fact, surpass patient depression in some couples (15).

Patients note that relational difficulties are often more challenging to navigate than the cancer treatment itself (12). Family members of patients undergoing serious surgeries can have heightened physical and psychological distress, which can result in reduced participation in family activities and changes in familial relationship dynamics (19). Caregivers and relatives are faced with the patient's increased need for assistance, heightening their personal stress (12). When one family member performs the majority of caregiving duties, resentment toward other family members may occur. Saritas and colleagues, in an analysis of family caregivers, found that as perceived burden reported by caregivers increased, correspondingly the perceived social support from their family lessened (20).

Family members are integral to making treatment decisions and developing care plans. Patients, caregivers, and extended family members can have different, subjective understandings and theories of illness and health care. This can cause conflict among the parties, stemming from disagreement on the cause of disease or the medical treatment benefits the family can expect (12). Thus, it is important for family members and patients to establish effective communication. The National Consensus Project for Quality Palliative Care (NCP) emphasizes the importance of family communication (21). A family's openness toward discussing topics related to a patient's chronic illness may change and evolve over time. So, too, changes in familial roles, interactions, and relationship interdependence can occur. Health care professionals must understand how family communication patterns vary and that improved communication can promote the well-being of the patient and family members throughout illness progression (13).

Case Study

To further illustrate cancer as a family experience and the long-term consequences, a case study is included.

Six-year-old Trevor was diagnosed with acute lymphoblastic leukemia 3 months ago. He has two older sisters, 8 and 10 years old. His parents, Amy and Sam, both teach in an inner city high school 45 minutes from their home. For the first 6 weeks, Sam took time off to be with Trevor while he was an inpatient receiving high-dose chemotherapy. He has no more paid time off. Trevor's mother is worried about taking time off now, in case he gets "really sick from the chemo" and has to return to the hospital. He has 2 more years of outpatient chemotherapy.

On discharge, Trevor's parents were given 35 medications and a 2-page list of instructions on diet, activity, infection prevention, and signs of infection, such as redness, tenderness, or pus at his Port-a-Cath site. If Trevor's temperature reached 38.3°C or higher, they were instructed to rush him to the hospital immediately. He started his outpatient chemotherapy a month ago. Since then he has been to the emergency room twice and admitted to the hospital once for 4 days.

Fortunately, Trevor's family lives in a closely knit neighborhood that has reached out to support the family. Transportation for the sisters' school and activities has been organized by their neighbors who have also ensured that food is well supplied and their dog is cared for. Amy's parents live nearby and spend the day with Trevor while the rest of the family is away at work and school.

Amy no longer allows the girls to have friends over, fearing they may bring germs into the house. She disinfects the whole house twice a day and has established "Trevor only" items such as keyboards, toys, and furniture. Upon their return from work and school, everyone in the family has to shower before they are allowed in the same room with Trevor. Other than work and school, the family has stopped outside activities, including church. Even the dog, which has always slept in the girls' room, is no longer allowed in the house.

Sam is anxious to keep Trevor "normal" during his 2-year treatment period. He feels like Amy is overreacting and is making the girls feel as if they don't matter. When Sam tries to discuss this with Amy, she gets defensive telling him he doesn't care about his son. She says it's just for 2 years and that he and the girls will just have to adjust.

THE FAMILY CAREGIVER

Demographics

"In 2013, about 40 million family caregivers in the United States provided an estimated 37 billion hours of care to adults with limitations in daily activities. The estimated economic value of their unpaid contributions was approximately $470 billion in 2013, up from an estimated $450 billion in 2009" (22). Without at-home family caregivers, the costs of long term HHC would rise drastically.

In 2015, an estimated 43.5 million adults in the United States provided unpaid care to an adult or child; this equates to a prevalence of caregiving of 16.6%. Ninety percent of dependent patients living in communities with acute and chronic illness are looked after by family caregivers (23). Today, the majority of caregivers are female at 60%, while 40% are male. Sixty percent of all caregivers have less than a college degree (24). The average caregiver is 49 years old, with 8 out of every 10 taking care of just one person. Eighty-five percent care for a relative, while one in every 10 cares for a spouse (22,25). Cancer caregivers provide, on average, 32.9 hours per week of care, with 32% providing 41 or more hours of weekly care; family caregiving is truly a full-time job for most (24). Caregivers are composed of many different demographic backgrounds.

Elderly

Approximately 1 in every 10 family caregivers is 75 years old or older (25). The proportion of the elderly in the global society will increase over the next few decades; by 2050, the global population of elderly adults (defined as 60 years or older) will triple, reaching 1.6 billion individuals (26,27). Further, 80% of these elderly adults will be living in developing nations, and the majority of their care will be provided by family caregivers (26). This is also true for developed nations, including the United States.

Elderly caregivers are predominantly female and often live in the same household as the elderly family member for whom they provide care (26). The responsibility of caring for an older family member may also fall upon adult children. Among older caregivers, a concurrent increase in the prevalence of comorbidities is observed (26,28). Providing care for a geriatric oncology patient is particularly burdensome. Older spousal caregivers have been found to provide more extensive and comprehensive care while also remaining in the caregiving role longer. This results in more interruptions to daily life and is correlated with a greater reported struggle than that observed in younger caregivers (28). Older caregivers are observed to experience increased disability, decreased physical mobility, and limited financial resources (29). Certain familial arrangements may find older caregivers dually providing care to an older spouse while concurrently providing care to grandchildren. These multiple caring responsibilities, in addition to the presence of comorbidities, predispose elderly caregivers to higher levels of stress.

Inadvertently, this heightened stress can exacerbate comorbidities and cause other health declines (28,30). The unique needs of elderly caregivers must be explored further, and their risk for requiring concomitant care while caregiving should be considered (29).

Children

Caregivers of pediatric patients face immense challenges and stresses. For children under 14 years of age, cancer remains the leading cause of death due to disease (31). Parents and other caregivers of children with chronic, life-threatening illness are tasked with providing care while simultaneously coping with the possibility of a future loss of their child (32). However, with medical advancements, pediatric cancer patients are experiencing improved outcomes. The 5-year survival rate for pediatric cancers has reached 83% in developed nations (31,33). These improvements also mean that children are increasingly cared for at home for longer periods of time. Parents must provide not only routine childcare but also comprehensive care regimens consisting of emotional, technical, and nursing tasks (32). During cancer treatment, children experience symptoms such as fatigue, pain, nausea, and vomiting. Although children can reliably report their symptoms, the treatment of pediatric illnesses involves the oversight and additional reporting of symptoms from guardians. Family caregivers often act as proxy reporters, and when doing so can add their own perceptions and responses to the child's symptoms (34).

Pediatric cancers can present significantly stressful experiences; an elevated risk of depression in parents of children undergoing intensive procedures, such as hematopoietic stem cell transplants, has been observed (35). For caregivers, chronic illness in children is additionally correlated with increased stress, heightened anxiety, increased fatigue, and poorer overall health (31,32,36). Providing care to an ill child leaves caregivers exhausted, with a reported below-average quality of life (QOL). The impending mortality of a child with cancer is overwhelming for many parents. Parents must continue to perform their parental duties in order to ensure the delivery of the best care possible. At the same time, parents must process their situation and deal with the intense emotional challenges of preparing for the loss of their child (32). Despite the progress in managing pediatric oncology, effective ways to address caregiver needs still are greatly lacking (32,33). Recognizing the needs and special concerns of caregivers of pediatric patients is important and can affect the child's well-being and further influence adherence to medication, disclosure of information, and overall survival (33).

Gender

From a global perspective, the majority of family caregivers remain predominantly female. In the United States, however, approximately 40% of caregivers today are now male (18), up from 25% in 1987 (37). Caregivers' need to care for a relative is often driven out of necessity for both male and female caregivers, rather than caregivers' voluntarily accepting the role. The commitments associated with the caregiving role can change the dynamics of the household, including gender roles, functions of family members, work outside of the home, and social activities.

Research has found observable differences in caring patterns and responses to caregiving between men and women. Learned, societal and cultural gender roles can influence approaches and interpretations of the caregiving role. Women may be more likely to feel a sense of obligation to caregiving. Women often perceive caregiving as a part of their other household and parental roles. Further, they are more likely to feel judgment when deciding against providing caregiving services and respond more often with feelings of guilt (38). The typical gender role for women is often associated with a nurturing nature, and for many women, caregiving can feel almost like an innate role. Female caregivers are often reported to be more emotionally connected to the patient, more willing to sacrifice their social life, and less likely to ask for assistance (39). Gender can, however, affect caregiver outcomes. Women, while taking on the caregiving role more often, rate their health lower, and experience higher levels of depression while reporting lower levels of social support and maintaining lower levels of physical activity in the caregiving role (29).

The influence of gender roles for men differs; male caregivers may interpret the role of caregiving as "work to be done," which can translate as a means to uphold one's masculinity. Society at large still values the maintenance of masculinity among male caregivers, even during the most distressful times of the role. The "work" of caregiving can present itself as difficult problems in need of solving, and when solved, can instill feelings of proudness and accomplishment. The influence of masculinity often delegates male caregivers to focusing more on the immediate aspects of caregiving at hand, such as daily medication administration and appointment scheduling, with little of their focus spent processing the emotional strains that the caregiving role imposes (18). The influence of gender roles on caregiver outcomes and approaches to care still requires more research, and is rarely factored in by health care professionals.

Distance and New Technologies

Today, more than 7 million people are long-distance caregivers. In fact, an estimated one-third of all informal caregiving occurs from a distance (40,41). Long-distance caregivers organize and orchestrate care for loved ones over physical separation. Although more proximal caregivers may carry out the majority of physical care responsibilities, long-distance caregivers often take on the burden of coordinating care demands (41). Caregiving is very much a team effort and involves a network of family and friends. Yet, due to the physical separation, long-distance caregivers often do not consider themselves caregivers since they do not provide direct-contact care. Feelings of guilt, sadness, and disconnect can all contribute to a feeling of being "out of the loop" regarding a loved one's care (40).

As personal technologies have advanced, their applicability to assist in caregiver preparedness and through connecting long-distance caregivers has just begun to be explored. Long distance caregivers often report a lack of access to information (42). In this new "tech-enabled" era of caregiving, several smartphone apps have been developed to allow long-distance caregivers to organize gatherings, share a guestbook for visitation tracking, and update a patient's condition among friends (42,43). Caregivers can also utilize new resources such as Roobrik, which offers various online support services on navigating complex care decisions including driving cessation and for the possible future selection of residential care facilities. Another tool, Everplans, is a cloud-based communication system focused on end-of-life directives; it can serve as a digital archive for the end-of-life wishes of a patient (43).

Aside from distance from their loved one, long-distance caregivers, particularly in rural areas, can be distant from caregiver support services. Blusi and colleagues found that rural caregivers using Internet-based support services experienced a reduction in their feelings of isolation (44). This is especially pertinent, as rural populations are consistently found to be underserved regarding palliative care, from a national and international perspective (45). Much of this software is designed to be responsive and sensitive to the individual needs of each caregiver. Further, many caregivers are unaware of these new and ever-developing technologies available to them, and nurses in particular can advocate for their use (43,44).

Minority Patients and Caregivers

Inequalities among racial and ethnic minorities are consistently documented in literature, and include access to care, the quality of care received, insurance coverage, and health outcomes. Cancer mortality rates have remained disproportionately high among racial and ethnic minorities, and for those from disadvantaged socioeconomic backgrounds (46). Cultural competency must be factored in when addressing minority caregivers. For instance, minority caregivers and patients are less likely than non-Hispanic, Caucasian patients to hire and trust health care professionals and to have confidence in their competence. Minority patients further demonstrate lower improvements in mobility than do Caucasian patients while under home care (47). Minority caregivers, on average, have lower incomes, yet provide higher levels of care and report more unmet care needs than do Whites. When considering this, in comparison to Whites, minority caregivers still report a lower burden of stress, higher levels of personal meaningfulness, and additional informal support with caregiving duties (48).

For many patients from a racial/ethnic minority group, family is at the core of the caregiving experience. Knight and colleagues found that familism is valued most by Koreans and Hispanics, less so by African Americans, and has the least regard among Whites (49). Iranian and Turkish familial culture also have been found to foster strong family bonds, wherein families provide the patient with the highest level of care possible. Conversely, these families are found to be less likely to express their caregiving problems and needs (50,51). Trends in caregiver demographics thus vary among ethnic/racial groups. Among Koreans, the majority of caregivers have been found to be daughters-in-law, while among Korean Americans and Caucasians, the majority are daughters or spouses. Other studies have found the majority of African American caregivers to be adult sons, with African American samples having a higher prominence of nonfamilial caregivers (49).

As to QOL, different cultures can incorporate variant metrics and values. In Latino populations for instance, decision making is often done as a family and is a major determinant of QOL (52). This relevance of familism on QOL is also found in Asian societies (53). In Singapore, when asking determinants of QOL, the nonresponse rate regarding sexual health is far higher than in Europe or the United States, suggesting that the level of comfort with and relevance of certain QOL parameters varies from culture to culture (53). When it comes to educating, and supporting the burden of family caregivers, cultural competence is of utmost importance, and much work is still needed toward its implementation into clinical practice (49,52).

LGBT+ Patients and Caregivers

As social rights for LGBT+ patients have expanded over the last decade, the cultural relevance and demand to address their specific needs are more pertinent than ever. Individuals from the LGBT+ community face unique challenges regarding family caregivers. Older LGBT+ adults often lack a robust informal social care network when compared to their heterosexual counterparts; while only 40% of LGBT+ adults have a permanent spouse or partner, only 20% to 25% report having a living child. Care for many can then rely on the "family of choice," who may be more limited for providing care particularly over a long period of time (54). Capistrant and colleagues found that among gay/bisexual men with prostate cancer, specific care considerations are different, particularly with regard to referrals to gay-friendly health care providers. In addition, emotional support is unique, and providers should address the manner in which their prostate cancer limits their capacity for male to male sexual intimacy (56). Overall, LGBT+ adults have been found to underutilize health and social services, in particular, caregiver support resources (54).

LGBT+ individuals, who may experience the same "kin-related" life experiences such as marriage, parenting, and bereavement as the general population, have distinct experiences nonetheless due to their historical social exclusion. With the onset of federal recognition for same-sex marriages, and the advancement of workplace protections in many states, it is likely more LGBT+ individuals in the future will be taken care of by a family caregiver when faced with a chronic illness. As palliative care clinicians, it is important to bear in mind the historical traumas that LGBT+ individuals have faced within health care, perhaps most markedly the AIDS epidemic. More research is thus necessary on the needs of older LGBT+ adults and the composition of their caregiving networks (55,56). There also remains vast room for improvement in considering the supportive care needs of LGBT+ patients, especially within the palliative care setting.

Caregiver Roles and Responsibilities

Family caregivers navigate a range of multifaceted roles and responsibilities; they are often demanding and affect all aspects of QOL, including psychological, physical, emotional, spiritual, and financial stresses (57). Without any proper training or compensation, family caregivers perform daily tasks such as meal preparation, transportation, and feeding, to medical care and pain management. Caregivers often provide wound care, and the management, dosing, and injections of medication. They additionally provide and coordinate social support, communicating with friends and family, and often are expected to provide reassurance regarding the patient's well-being. Family caregivers are burdened with the role of protection

and advocacy, wherein they must advocate for their loved one's needs when interacting with health care providers and insurance companies. Family caregivers can spend upwards of 8 hours per day performing their various duties (17,57,58).

The administration of medication is a primary task for many family caregivers. It is enlightening to realize that health care professionals assume similar responsibilities in inpatient and other settings only after formal courses in pharmacology and with direct access to and support available from professional colleagues such as pharmacists. Family caregivers at home navigate these responsibilities without such resources, and often are challenged with administering medications on an as-needed basis or administering around-the-clock dosages, such as the titration of analgesics.

Family caregivers of cancer patients experience a higher reported level of burden than do caregivers of older adults and those of patients with dementia (59). Cancer caregivers deal with the devastating initial diagnosis of cancer in ones they love. They first undergo primary appraisals, the initial evaluation of the significance of the patient's cancer. Caregivers are then tasked with secondary appraisals, serving as an assessment of their ability to manage the needs of the patient's illness and fulfill the now necessary caregiving role. They can remain in the role for extended periods of time, with many cancer patients living at least 5 years past their diagnosis (60,61).

Most cancer treatments and interventions are provided for in outpatient settings (59). As the condition of the patient declines, nurses and health care providers rely more and more on the caregiver to report the status of symptoms, with unrelieved symptoms tending to increase near the end of life (62). Providing proper pain management is immensely challenging for caregivers. Although analgesics have improved, pain often persists among patients (51). Further, reluctance toward using analgesics can stem from erroneous understandings of pain management (63).

Caregivers are also tasked with complex choices regarding the patient's care plan. The discussion of terminating disease management, when and if it occurs at all, is made under the context of "looming death" and is influenced by the deteriorating condition of the patient and the emotions and interactions of family members present. Caregivers and patients indeed traverse the health care system together (64); they form an interdependent "unit of care," the patient and caregiver experiencing health care services in tandem (65–67). Effective palliative care must continue to acknowledge the role of the family caregiver and the central role he or she plays in patient care.

Case Study

To further illustrate the impact cancer has on the caregiver's roles and responsibilities, this case study is included.

Chen, a 45-year-old Chinese American woman, works 7 days a week with her husband, Hui, in their small grocery store. In addition to shop keeping, she is responsible for their household, which includes a teenage son and Hui's non–English-speaking aging parents. The son does not drive and is involved in many after-school activities. Hui is the leader of the family.

Several months ago, Hui began experiencing nausea, vomiting, and gastric pain. After many doctor visits, tests, and treatment regimens, he was diagnosed with stage III gastric cancer. He is scheduled for surgery, which will be followed by chemotherapy. Although the surgery will be inpatient, the 6 months of chemotherapy will be outpatient at the same site, 15 miles away. The chemotherapy will require a minimum of three visits per week.

Neither Hui's parents nor the son has been told of his cancer diagnosis. His obvious illness has been explained as a passing virus. Chen is a reluctant driver but has been able to transport Hui to his medical appointments and take their son to his frequent after-school activities. She is feeling overwhelmed as she struggles to keep the grocery store (their only income) open, to transport/support their son at school, to protect her in-laws and son from any knowledge of the diagnosis, and to take care of all of Hui's needs. Hui's only brother, who lives in China, has been told about the cancer diagnosis; he is unable to leave his job to come to help. He agrees that his parents should not be told about the cancer diagnosis. At this point, the surgery is only 1 week away. Chen is bravely trying to embrace her new role as the quasi–family leader while shouldering all her new responsibilities.

Family Caregiver Needs

Like cancer patients, family caregivers have diverse, specific needs and health concerns. Cancer presents specific challenges for caregivers. With the shift toward at-home care, caregivers of cancer patients experience new burdens and interruptions to their lives (68). Family caregiver needs are wide, variant, and dependent on several factors, including, but not limited to, age, gender, culture, gender, education, socioeconomic, and geographic setting (16,68). The needs of family caregivers range from informational, personal, and household to care issues that, when not acknowledged by health care providers, may impact adherence and decision making regarding medical care (68).

Informal caregiving can cause a massive financial burden. Many families report losing a significant amount of their savings when serving in the caregiving role; as many as 40% of families report someone having to quit current employment. Often the duration of care needed for a family member far surpasses the time-off allotted in the Family Medical Leave Act (FMLA) for the caregiver and/or patient (65).

Caregivers are often thrust into the role suddenly and under extreme circumstances (67). Family caregivers consistently express a desire to be more adequately prepared on how to help their loved one deal with the diagnosis of a chronic disease. This can include learning how to watch for infections while managing side effects, especially when providing care post-op (5). Throughout the treatment process, caregivers have a substantial amount of interaction with health care professionals. Contemporary perspectives in health care have long placed an emphasis on patient autonomy and confidentiality, but are slowly incorporating the need for family-centered approaches to care delivery, wherein caregivers are included in consultations and treatment plans (23). Still, health care systems often fail to meet caregivers' needs for information, with communication being described as suboptimal. Caregivers express the need to have their contributions acknowledged during consultations with providers and to have the value of their role emphasized (16,23). The need for improved communication among health care systems and caregivers prevails (68).

Caregiver QOL encompasses the domains of physical, psychological, social, and spiritual well-being (SWB) (68–71). Caregiver burden can be defined as the extent to which caregivers feel their QOL determinants have declined as a result of providing informal care (69). Anxiety and depressive symptoms have been found to be correlated to the degree of reported caregiver burden (72). Caregivers typically prioritize the needs of their family members first, leaving little room for self-care (50). Older caregivers face the prevalence of multimorbidities, with their own symptoms warranting attention, particularly for predispositions to diseases like diabetes, chronic heart disease, and arthritis (27,61).

The demands and burdens of caregiving can change over disease progression (64–66,68). As oncological survival rates improve, caregiving duties have been extended longer than ever before (65,73). These improvements in mortality correspond to increased rates of ambulatory and home care (15). In the initial phases of cancer treatment, on average, caregivers attend to 80% of needs; near the end of life, caregivers address roughly

60% (72). The caregiving burden can increase if and when a metastatic stage is reached, and fluctuates temporally from the time of diagnosis, during treatment, and the transition out of treatment (59,66). Cognitive impairment, particularly in patients with brain cancers, is markedly challenging for caregivers to navigate. Making end of life decisions for patients who are cognitively impaired can be the most distressing responsibility during the caregiving experience and increasingly put caregivers at risk for feelings of guilt and bereavement (68,72).

There has been little research into how caregiver needs vary among cancer type (74). For instance, caregivers of glioma patients present a particularly higher adjusted mortality; this is likely due in part to the fact that these caregivers are dealing with dual oncological and neurological challenges (75). Additionally, there is a lack of caregiver support services to aid in making such stressful decisions; such services are often neither standardized nor systemized. For caregivers, it remains a matter of chance whether their health care system has proper support resources and makes them accessible (67).

Caregiver Burden Assessment

The degree of burden that caregiving places upon an individual is of growing interest among health care professionals. The needs, satisfaction, and QOL of caregivers are not systematically monitored nor regulated in clinical settings. In a literature review, Tanco and colleagues identified 59 assessment tools developed and utilized by health care professionals to address burden, satisfaction with health care, and QOL of family caregivers (76). Very few have been incorporated into regular clinical practice and this paucity highlights the need for comparative clinical assessments of caregiver assessment instruments (76). One such tool, the Edmonton Symptom Assessment System (ESAS), is a 10-item scale that addresses physical and psychosocial burdens in caregivers. An updated version, ESAS-FS, includes items for financial and spiritual distress. One study concluded that ESAS was a feasible tool in identifying caregiver burden symptoms, and out of the sample studied, the majority of caregivers found that the tool was useful for expressing their burden (77). More research is needed on the effectiveness, and further implementation of universal assessment tools for caregiver burden.

Self-Care

Caregiver burden can often be lessened by internal coping factors and external social support. Caregivers more often report the negative effects

of caregiving than the positive ones (78). Among caregivers, insomnia and poor sleep are widespread issues. Sleep disturbances stem from actual and perceived difficulties with sleep and can impair the caregiver's well-being (79). Sleep disturbance correlates with the advancement of stages of cancer diagnosis and disease progression. Additionally, disruptions from care demands, hypervigilance, and worry can contribute to and perpetuate sleep disturbances; even after being relieved of caregiving responsibilities, some family caregivers still report them (79).

The need to implement health-promoting behaviors in caregivers is of growing interest. Health behaviors are habits or actions implemented or avoided for the purpose of preventing, detecting, and managing illness (80). Many patients after surviving a cancer diagnosis are inspired to incorporate healthier lifestyle habits into their lives, most often centered around smoking cessation, nutrition, and exercise (79). More research is needed to determine how self-care and healthier lifestyle habits in caregivers can improve both patient and caregiver outcomes. Some studies have found that cancer caregiving is associated with inadequate exercise, poor nutrition habits, smoking, and overconsumption of alcohol (81). However, there are studies to the contrary. For example, Han Lo found that caregivers, when compared to noncaregivers in Taiwan, practice health-promoting behaviors significantly more, and that health-promoting behaviors may more prominently affect QOL in caregivers (82). Thus, the influence or lack thereof of health-promoting behaviors in caregivers requires more study.

Quality of Life

Health-related QOL is a person's self-concept of well-being, affected, and defined by disease or a treatment regimen (83). Cancer negatively affects both the patient's and family caregiver's QOL (83,84). The essential goal of palliative care is to improve QOL across the four domains that define QOL: physical, psychological, social, and SWB (85,86). According to the World Health Organization, these goals are not limited to just patients; QOL improvements must include family members as well (87). Patient and caregiver QOL innately affect and influence one another. As so, it is necessary to address concerns regarding QOL in the patient and family caregiver concurrently (85). To date, the majority of psychosocial interventions focused on improving QOL address the patient and caregiver separately. Family-based interventions that address both are in demand and may offer benefits to improving QOL throughout disease progression (88).

Physical Well-Being. The physical demands of caregiving are diverse, widespread, and highly variant depending on the health concerns of the patient (89). In general, the physical detriments of caregiving are less intensive than the psychological burdens (90). The physical demands are related to the care needs of the patients (16,17). Factors that determine the degree of care necessary include behavioral problems, cognitive impairment, functional disabilities, the duration, and amount of care provided, as well as the amount of vigilance paid (90). In the Evercare study, caregivers indicated that for some, their health had gotten "a lot" worse as a result of their experienced burden. Overall, health was found to decline among caregivers, with participants indicating their health as fair to poor (91).

Psychological Well-Being. Stress, one of the most impactful detriments to psychological well-being, has been found to be the most common negative consequence of duties reported by caregivers (57). The role and perspectives of the patient and caregiver are distinct, with each experiencing different challenges. Mosher et al. found that processing emotions around diagnosis, fear of recurrence, coping with continual uncertainty, and observing the patient suffer and decline were some of the largest detriments to QOL regarding psychological well-being in family caregivers (92). Caregiving produces intense emotional stressors including depression, sadness, anger, and hopelessness. Correspondingly, the prevalence of depression in caregivers is estimated between 10% and 53% (93). Caregivers also may experience a lack of self-identity, lowered self-esteem, uncertainty, lowered self-acceptance, a lost sense of control, and feelings of ineffectiveness (78,94). Additionally, coping strategies are found to be lower in caregivers (95). Frustration can arise with the feeling of being a "prisoner in their own home" (78), wherein caregivers feel no escape from the constant attendance of their loved one's needs. Fear of cancer recurrence is also one of the most frequently reported and unmet needs of both patients and caregivers. It is negatively associated with QOL and positively associated with psychological distress in both patients and caregivers (96).

Assessing declines in caregiver QOL factors is often subjective, and the need for standardized parameters remains, particularly with regard to psychological well-being (65).

Social Well-Being. The social demands of caregiving are affected by relationships, financial burdens, and disruptions in daily activities. When assessing family caregivers' social well-being, factors to consider include (a) patient/family caregiver communication and relationships, for example, marital quality, marital tension, emotional and physical intimacy, and role adaptation; (b) family members' way of interrelating, for example, family cohesions, conflict, communication, interpersonal support, and relationship quality with patient; and (c) parenting behavior and parenting quality. Social well-being studies have examined the interpersonal effect of cancer on patients and their family caregivers, mostly with a focus on couples. Among couples with a wife dealing with breast cancer, Lewis and colleagues found that spousal caregivers receiving educational intervention sessions experienced significant improvements in their measures of QOL. Wives in the study significantly improved their marital communication ratings and positive perceptions of their spouse's interpersonal support as well (97). Keesing and colleagues found that among couples dealing with a breast cancer diagnosis, concerns of communication, intimacy, and sexuality are widely shared. Using thematic analysis, it was found that couples first experience a disconnection within their relationship, wherein the survivor prioritized her own needs, sometimes at the expense of the spouse. Reformulation of the relationship followed, wherein couples navigated these new relational dynamics. Lastly, support to negotiate the relationship occurs, wherein couples focus on the need to utilize external resources like therapy and caregiver support groups, for the maintenance of their relationship during early survivorship (98).

Family communication is especially important during cancer treatment. *The Clinical Practice Guidelines for Quality Palliative Care* established by the NCP recommends that routine patient and family meetings be conducted with the interdisciplinary team to facilitate communication and develop an individualized plan of care (21). The family meeting can affirm the work done by caregivers and address caregiver concerns and unmet needs.

Spiritual Well-Being. Among palliative care providers, there is a growing awareness of the necessity to address spirituality as a pertinent determinant of QOL (99,100). Most studies concur that spirituality has positive effects on patient well-being, with distressing influences limited to negative religious coping and spiritual struggles (99). The onset of a cancer diagnosis can spark increased spiritual or religious beliefs that can improve coping strategies, with resultant improvements in QOL (101). Most importantly, cancer patients and family caregivers can derive spiritual meaning from their treatment process (99,102). Meaningfulness can result in positive coping mechanisms for a cancer diagnosis and the improved management of stress (102). Vespa and colleagues found that oncology caregivers with self-expressed high SWB have significant differences in reported bodily pain, vitality, social activities, and mental health subscale ratings (100). Shim and colleagues found that a caregiver's discovery of new meanings through spirituality is correlated with expressing positive emotions toward the patient, having faith in a "higher power," incorporating altruism, and inferring strength from persevering through previously stressful life events (103). Aside from focusing on the burdens of caregiving, clinicians can emphasize the importance of personal spirituality when addressing caregiver needs (101).

Case Study

The case of Renee, a distance caregiver for her mother, illustrates how communication issues fostered feelings of distress and impacted Renee's overall QOL.

Renee is an African American woman born in Washington, DC where she was raised by her single parent mother, Dorothy. Dorothy was the sole provider for their household and worked as an appointment clerk in a downtown hospital. Her priority was to provide a good education for Renee so "she can do whatever she wants to do." Although the rent has doubled, Dorothy still lives in the same rented row house. After graduating from law school a year ago, Renee moved 100 miles away to Richmond, VA, where she works for the state of Virginia. Although the job requires her to work a 80-hour week, she loves it.

At the age of 53, Dorothy was diagnosed with breast cancer and retired from her hospital job. Renee begged her mother to come to Richmond for her surgery and treatment, but Dorothy wanted to be close to her Baptist Church and go to "her" hospital.

Dorothy's surgery was on a Friday in "her" hospital, which enabled Renee to be with her for the overnight inpatient stay and at her home through the weekend. Dorothy's church friends promised to care for her and assured Renee they would call her if her mother needed anything. Nevertheless, when Renee left on Sunday to return to Richmond, she was overcome with feelings of guilt. "My mother gave up her life for me; now I can't even be with her when she needs me the most."

Since the surgery, there have been issues with lymphedema and pain. Renee's long-distance attempts to talk to the oncologist or surgeon have been unsuccessful. Even though she travels to be with her mother every weekend, Renee has been unable to meet with her mother's health care providers or to establish a communication plan.

Her mother is scheduled to start her chemotherapy within the next 2 weeks. Renee has become depressed and is unable to concentrate at work.

SUPPORTING THE FAMILY CAREGIVER

Caregiver Bill of Rights

Caregivers often struggle to find a balance between the needs of their loved one and the need to take care of themselves. The Caregiver's Bill (104) of Rights is helpful in providing a guideline for caregivers to appreciate their responsibilities and their limitations as they partner with their loved ones in the cancer experience.

Case Study

In this case, Ellen and Joe, long-married and dependent on each other, illustrate the need for early intervention to support patients and families throughout the cancer experience.

Ellen and Joe have been married for 65 years. Joe retired from his bus driver job 20 years ago; now he spends most of his time watching sports on television. He is diabetic and arthritic and has congestive heart failure. Ellen was a homemaker and stay-at-home mother and had many close friends. She says most of them have died, "I miss them; I don't have anyone to talk to anymore." She has been healthy, "just a little arthritis," but recently she has lost weight and has fallen several times. They have lived in their two-bedroom two-level condo in a run-down area of Los Angles for the past 10 years. Most of their neighbors are new, and they do not know them. They have two children (one married and one divorced) who live within 45 miles, but with LA traffic taking at least 2 hours, they get to their house only every few months. Ellen's and Joe's three adult grandchildren rarely visit as they are busy taking care of their own grandchildren.

When Ellen started having difficulty breathing, she attributed it to age. The problem progressively worsened and she was too fatigued to leave the house. Ellen was ultimately diagnosed with stage IV lung cancer and referred to her local oncologist. Joe was devastated by the diagnosis. He insisted she have every treatment available. The children and grandchildren agreed to help Joe with the caregiving responsibilities. Even though Ellen wanted to talk about advance directives, her family refused, saying that was giving up. She started her chemotherapy 3 days after her diagnosis. The first day Joe and Ellen arrived at the clinic at 7:00 AM for blood tests, x-rays, doctors' visits, and then 4 hours of chemotherapy. They did not eat breakfast, as Ellen was too nervous to cook or eat. By midday, Joe was in a wheelchair needing medical assistance for his low blood sugar. By the end of the 12-hour day, they had to call their son to pick them up; Joe could not drive home.

As the chemotherapy treatment continued, Ellen became weaker and weaker. She was constantly nauseated, had diarrhea, and could not eat. Joe's health deteriorated faster than Ellen's. She no longer could administer his insulin or make his meals. They did not want to burden their children/grandchildren with their caregiving needs. Joe discouraged the children's and grandchildren's offers of help.

CONCLUSION

With resultant changes in health care delivery systems and HHC accessibility, the majority of oncological patient care occurs in the home setting today, tended to most often by (family/unpaid) caregivers. Although the home setting is rich with benefits to enhance patient comfort, it also provides challenges in providing optimum physical, psychological, social, and spiritual care. The existing literature emphasizes a need to recognize the immense role that family caregivers play, and further, to have health care providers adequately prepare and educate family members for the caregiving role.

There is a tremendous need for continuity of care as patients are increasingly cared for across many settings. It is essential that issues of care in the home are communicated to those involved, including the health care professionals, patients, and family caregivers. Quality care for patients at home, similar to all aspects of palliative care, begins with a thorough assessment of the patients' and the family caregivers' needs. Organized care based on a comprehensive perspective, which recognizes the needs for physical, psychological, social, and SWB during the cancer experience, is best accomplished by empowering family caregivers to provide excellent care for their loved ones and to care for themselves.

REFERENCES

1. Sullivan-Marx E. Looking ahead after 50 years of Medicare. *J Gerontol Nurs.* 2015;41(9):15-18.
2. Huai CE, Greener HT. Medicare home health care patient case mix before and after the balanced act of 1997: effect on dual eligible beneficiaries. *Home Health Care Serv Q.* 2014;33(1):58-76.
3. Schneider A. *Overview of Medicaid Provisions in the Balanced Budget Act of 1997, P.L. 105-33.* Washington, DC: Center on Budget and Policy Priorities; 1997.
4. Long CO. The spiritual self: pathways to inner strength for caregivers. *J Am Geriatr Soc.* 2016;22(2):14-18.
5. Chen SC, Lai YH, Liao CT, et al. Unmet supportive care needs and characteristics of family caregivers of patients with oral cancer after surgery. *Psychooncology.* 2014;23:569-577.
6. Gröpper S, van DM, Landes T, Bucher H, Stickel A, Goerling U. Assessing cancer-related distress in

cancer patients and caregivers receiving outpatient psycho-oncological counseling. *Support Care Cancer.* 2016;24(5):2351-2357.
7. van Ryn M, Sanders S, Kahn K, et al. Objective burden, resources, and other stressors among informal cancer caregivers: a hidden quality issue? *Psychooncology.* 2011;20:44-52.
8. Latter S, Hopkinson JB, Richardson A, Hughes JA, Lowson E, Edwards D. How can we help family carers manage pain medicines for patients with advanced cancer? A systematic review of intervention studies. *BMJ Support Palliat Care.* 2016;6(3):263-275.
9. Meeker MA, Finnell D, Othman AK. Family caregivers and cancer pain management: a review. *J Fam Nurs.* 2011;17(1):29-60.
10. Chi NC, Demiris G, Pike KC, Washington K, Oliver DP. Pain management concerns from the hospice family caregivers' perspective. *Am J Hosp Palliat Care.* 2018;35(4):601-611.
11. McPherson CJ, Hadjistavropoulos T, Devereaux A, Lobchuk MM. A qualitative investigation of the roles and perspectives of older patients with advanced cancer and their family caregivers in managing pain in the home. *BMC Palliat Care.* 2014;13:39.
12. Preisler M, Heuse S, Riemer M, Kendel F, Letsch A. Early integration of palliative cancer care: patients' and caregivers' challenges, treatment preferences, and knowledge of illness and treatment throughout the cancer trajectory. *Support Care Cancer.* 2018;26(3):921-931.
13. Goldsmith J, Wittenberg E, Small PC, Iannarino NT, Reno J. Family caregiver communication in oncology: advancing a typology. *Psychooncology.* 2015;25:463-470.
14. Wittenberg E, Kravits K, Goldsmith J, Ferrell B, Fujinami R. Validation of a model of family caregiver communication types and related caregiver outcomes. *Palliat Support Care.* 2017;15(1):3-11.
15. Masterson MP, Hurley KE, Zaider T, Kissane DW. Toward a model of continuous care: a necessity for caregiving partners. *Palliat Support Care.* 2015;13(5):1459-1467.
16. Lund L, Ross L, Petersen MA, Groenvold M. The interaction between informal cancer caregivers and health care professionals: a survey of caregivers' experiences of problems and unmet needs. *Support Care Cancer.* 2015;23(6):1719-1733.
17. Lambert SD, Lydia OB, Morrison M. Priorities for caregiver research in cancer care: an international delphi survey of caregivers, clinicians, managers, and researchers. *Support Care Cancer.* 2019;27(3):805-817.
18. Friedemann ML, Buckwalter KC. Family caregiver role and burden related to gender and family relationships. *J Fam Nurs.* 2014;20(3):313-336.
19. Sun V, Kim JY, Raz DJ. Preparing cancer patients and family caregivers for lung surgery: development of a multimedia self-management intervention. *J Cancer Educ.* 2018;33(3):557-563.
20. Saritas SC, Kavak F, Aksoy, Asude A, Saritas S. Examination of the care burden of caregivers of oncology patients and the perceived social support from family. *Int J Caring Sci.* 2017;10(1):448-455.
21. National Consensus Project for Quality Palliative Care. *Clinical Practice Guidelines for Quality Palliative Care.* 4th ed. Richmond, VA: National Coalition for Hospice and Palliative Care; 2018.
22. Reinhard S, Feinberg L, Choula R, Houser A. *Valuing the Invaluable: 2015 Update—Undeniable Progress, but Big Gaps Remain.* Washington, DC: AARP Public Policy Institute; 2015.
23. Mitnick S, Leffler C, Hood VL; American College of Physicians Ethics, Professionalism and Human Rights

Committee. Family caregivers, patients and physicians: ethical guidance to optimize relationships. *J Gen Intern Med*. 2010;25(3):255-260.

24. National Alliance for Caregiving. *Cancer Caregiving in the U.S.: An Intense, Episodic and Challenging Care Experience*; 2016. https://www.caregiving.org/wp-content/uploads/2016/06/CancerCaregivingReport_FINAL_June-17-2016.pdf. Accessed July 22, 2019.

25. National Alliance for Caregiving. *Caregiving in the U.S.*; 2015. https://www.caregiving.org/research/caregivingusa.pdf. Accessed July 22, 2019.

26. Luchesi BM, Alexandre TS, de Oliveira NA, et al. Factors associated with attitudes toward the elderly in a sample of elderly caregivers. *Int Psychogeriatr*. 2016;28(12):2079-2089.

27. Naganthan G, Kuluski K, Gill A, Jaakkimanen L, Upshur R, Wodchis WP. Perceived value of support for older adults coping with multi-morbidity: patient, informal care-giver and family physician perspectives. *Ageing Soc*. 2016;36(9):1891-1914.

28. Wittenberg-Lyles E, Demiris G, Oliver DP, Burchett M. Exploring aging-related stress among older spousal caregivers. *J Gerontol Nurs*. 2014;40(8):13-16.

29. Cuthbert CA, King-Shier K, Tapp D, Ruether D, Culos-Reed S. Exploring gender differences in self-reported physical activity and health among older caregivers. *Oncol Nurs Forum*. 2017;44(4):435-445.

30. de Oliveira NA, Souza ÉN, Luchesi BM, Inouye K, Iost Pavarini SC. Stress and optimism of elderlies who are caregivers for elderlies and live with children. *Rev Bras Enferm*. 2017;70(4):697-703.

31. Crane S, Haase JE, Hickman SE. Well-being of child and family participants in phase 1 pediatric oncology clinical trials. *Oncol Nurs Forum*. 2018;45(5):E67-E97.

32. Verberne LM, Kars MC, Schouten-van Meeteren AN, et al. Parental experiences and coping strategies when caring for a child receiving paediatric palliative care: a qualitative study. *Eur J Pediatr*. 2019;178(7):1075-1085.

33. El Malla HE. Having a child diagnosed with cancer: raising the challenges encountered by the caregivers at the pediatric oncology ward in Egypt. *Diseases*. 2017;5(4):36.

34. Cheng L, Wang L, Mengxue H, Feng S, Zhu Y, Rodgers C. Perspectives of children, family caregivers, and health professionals about pediatric oncology symptoms: a systematic review. *Support Care Cancer*. 2018;26(9):2957-2971.

35. Devine KA, Manne SL, Mee L, et al. Barriers to psychological care among primary caregivers of children undergoing hematopoietic stem cell transplantation. *Support Care Cancer*. 2016;24(5):2235-2242.

36. Daniel LC, Walsh CM, Meltzer LJ, Barakat LP, Kloss JD. The relationship between child and caregiver sleep in acute lymphoblastic leukemia maintenance. *Support Care Cancer*. 2018;26(4):1123-1132.

37. Kim Y, Mitchell HR, Ting A. Application of psychological theories on the role of gender in caregiving to pyscho-oncology research. *Psychooncology*. 2019;28:228-254.

38. Robinson C, Bottorff J, Pesut B, Oliffe J, Tomlinson J. The male face of caregiving: a scoping review of men caring for a person with dementia. *Am J Mens Health*. 2014;8(5):409-426.

39. Brank EM, Wylie LE. Differing perspectives on older adult caregiving. *J Appl Gerontol*. 2014;35(7):698-720.

40. O'Brien C. Supporting the Cancer Patient's Long Distance Caregiver, *Oncol Nurs Advis*. 2015. https://www.oncologynurseadvisor.com/home/departments/from-cancercare/supporting-the-cancer-patients-long-distance-caregiver/

41. Cagle JG, Munn JC. Long-distance caregiving: a systematic review of the literature. *J Gerontol Soc Work*. 2012;55(8):682-707.

42. Piraino E, Byrne K, Heckman, GA, Stolee P. Caring in the information age: personal online networks to improve caregiver support. *Can J Geriatr*. 2017;20(2):85-93.

43. Andruszkiewicz G, Fike K. Emerging technology trends and products: how tech innovations are easing the burden of family caregiving. *Generations*. 2016;39(4):64-68.

44. Blusi M, Kristiansen L, Jong M. Exploring the influence of internet-based caregiver support on experiences of isolation for older spouse caregivers in rural areas: a qualitative interview study. *Int J Older People Nurs*. 2015;10(3):211-220.

45. Dionne-Odom JN, Taylor R, Rocque G, et al. Adapting an early palliative care intervention to family caregivers of persons with advanced cancer in the rural deep south: a qualitative formative evaluation. *J Pain Symptom Manage*. 2018;55(6):1519-1530.

46. Patel M, Nevedal A, Bhattacharya J, Coker TR. A community-partnered, evidence-based approach to improving cancer care delivery for low-income and minority patients with cancer. *J Community Health*. 2019;44(5):1-9.

47. Davitt JK, Bourjolly J, Frasso R. Understanding inequities in home health care outcomes: staff views on agency and system factors. *Res Gerontol Nurs*. 2015;8(3): 119-129.

48. Sawchuk CN, Van Dyke E, Omidpanah A, Russo JE, Tsosie U, Buchwald D. Caregiving among American Indians and Alaska natives with cancer. *Support Care Cancer*. 2015;23(6):1607-1614.

49. Knight BC, Robinson CS, Flynn Longmire CV, Chun M, Nakao K, Kim J. Cross cultural issues in caregiving for dementia: do familism values reduce burden and distress? *Ageing Int*. 2002;27:70-93.

50. Hashemi M, Irajpour A, Taleghani F. Caregivers needing care: the unmet needs of the family caregivers of end of life cancer patients. *Support Care Cancer*. 2018;26(3):759-766.

51. Ovayolu Ö, Ovayolu N, Aytaç S, Serçe S, Sevinc A. Pain in cancer patients: pain assessment by patients and family caregivers and problems experienced by caregivers. *Support Care Cancer*. 2015;23(7):1857-1864.

52. Juarez G, Branin JJ, Rosales M. Perceptions of QOL among caregivers of Mexican ancestry of adults with advanced cancer. *Qual Life Res*. 2015;24(7):1729-1740.

53. Lee GL, Ow MYL, Akhileswaran R, et al. Quality of life domains important and relevant to family caregivers of advanced cancer patients in an Asian population: a qualitative study. *Qual Life Res*. 2015;24(4):817-828.

54. Brennan-Ing M, Seidel L, Larson B, Karpiak SE. Social care networks and older LGBT adults: challenges for the future. *J Homosex*. 2014;61(1):21-52.

55. Fredriksen-Goldsen KI, Bryan AE, Jen S, Goldsen J, Kim HJ, Muraco A. The unfolding of LGBT lives: key events associated with health and well-being in later life. *Gerontologist*. 2017;57(1):15-29.

56. Capistrant B, Torres B, Merengwa E, West W, Mitteldorf D, Rossser S. Caregiving and social support for gay and bisexual men with prostate cancer. *Psychooncology*. 2016;25:1329-1336.

57. Lund L, Ross L, Petersen MA, Groenvold M. Cancer caregiving tasks and consequences and their associations with caregiver status and the caregiver's relationship to the patient: a survey. *BMC Cancer*. 2014;14:541.

58. Al-Daken L, Ahmad MM. Predictors of burden and quality of sleep among family caregivers of patients with cancer. *Support Care Cancer*. 2018;26(11):3967-3973.

59. Finley J. Caregiver café: providing education and support to family caregivers of patients with cancer. *Clin J Oncol Nurs*. 2018;22(1):91-96.

60. Hendrix CC, Bailey DE, Steinhauser KE, et al. Effects of enhanced caregiver training program on cancer caregiver's self-efficacy, preparedness, and psychological well-being. *Support Care Cancer*. 2016;24(1):327-336.

61. Ellis KR, Janevic MR, Kershaw T, Caldwell CH, Janz NK, Northouse L. The influence of dyadic symptom distress on threat appraisals and self-efficacy in advanced cancer and caregiving. *Support Care Cancer*. 2017;25(1):185-194.

62. Ezenwa MO, Fischer DJ, Epstein J, Johnson J, Yao Y, Wilkie DJ. Caregivers' perspectives on oral health problems of end-of-life cancer patients. *Support Care Cancer*. 2016;24(11):4769-4777.

63. Valeberg BT, Miaskowski C, Steven P, Rustoen T. Comparison of oncology patients' and their family caregivers' attitudes and concerns toward pain and pain management. *Cancer Nurs*. 2016;39(4):328-334.

64. Norton SA, Wittink MN, Duberstein PR, Prigerson HG, Stanek S, Epstein RM. Family caregiver descriptions of stopping chemotherapy and end-of-life transitions. *Support Care Cancer*. 2019;27(2):669.

65. Merrigi F, Federica A, Premi V, et al. Assessing cancer caregivers' needs for an early targeted psychosocial support project: the experience of the oncology department at the Poliambulanza Foundation. *Palliat Support Care*. 2015;13(4):865-873.

66. Tolbert E, Bowie J, Snyder C, Bantug E, Smith K. A qualitative exploration of the experiences, needs, and roles of caregivers during and after cancer treatment: "That's what I say. I'm a relative survivor". *J Cancer Surv*. 2018;12(1):134-144.

67. Preisler M, Rohrmoser A, Goerling U, et al. Early palliative care for those who care: a qualitative exploration of cancer caregivers' information needs during hospital stays. *Eur J Cancer*. 2019;28(2):e12990.

68. Ferrell B, Hanson J, Grant M. An overview and evaluation of the oncology family caregiver project: improving quality of life and quality of care for oncology family caregivers. *Psychooncology*. 2013;22(7):1645-1652.

69. Naoki Y, Matsuda Y, Maeda I, et al. Association between family satisfaction and caregiver burden in cancer patients receiving outreach palliative care at home. *Palliat Support Care*. 2018;16(3):260-268.

70. Rohrmoser A, Preisler M, Bär K, Letsch A, Goerling U. Early integration of palliative/supportive cancer care—healthcare professionals' perspectives on the support needs of cancer patients and their caregivers across the cancer treatment trajectory. *Support Care Cancer*. 2017;25(5):1621-1627.

71. Jolliffe R, Collaco N, Seers H, Farrell C, Sawkins MJ, Polley MJ. Development of measure yourself concerns and wellbeing for informal caregivers of people with cancer—a multicentred study. *Support Care Cancer*. 2019;27(5):1901-1909.

72. Saria MG, Courchesne N, Evangelista L, et al. Cognitive dysfunction in patients with brain metastases: influences on caregiver resilience and coping. *Support Care Cancer*. 2017;25(4):1247-1256.

73. Seven M, Yilmaz S, Sahin E, Akyüz A. Evaluation of the quality of life of caregivers in gynecological cancer patients. *J Cancer Educ*. 2014;29(2):325-332.

74. Seekatz B, Lukasczik M, Löhr M, et al. Screening for symptom burden and supportive needs of patients with glioblastoma and brain metastases and their caregivers in relation to their use of specialized palliative care. *Support Care Cancer*. 2017;25(9):2761-2770.

75. Ramirez C, Christophe V, Dassonneville C, Grynberg D. Caregivers' quality of life and psychological health in response to functional, cognitive, neuropsychiatric and social deficits of patients with brain tumours: protocol for a cross-sectional study. *BMJ Open*. 2017;7(10): e016308.

76. Tanco K, Park JC, Cerana A, Sisson A, Sobti N, Bruera E. A systematic review of instruments assessing dimensions of distress among caregivers of adult and pediatric cancer patients. *Palliat Support Care*. 2017;15(1): 110-124.

77. Tanco K, Vidal M, Arthur J, et al. Testing the feasibility of using the Edmonton symptom assessment system (ESAS) to assess caregiver symptom burden. *Palliat Support Care*. 2018;16(1):14-22.

78. Goldzweig G, Schapira L, Baider L, Jacobs JM, Andritsch E, Rottenberg Y. Who will care for the caregiver? Distress and depression among spousal caregivers of older patients undergoing treatment for cancer. *Support Care Cancer*. 2019;27(11):4221-4227.

79. Mazanec SR, Flocke SA, Daly BJ. Health behaviors in family members of patients completing cancer treatment. *Oncol Nurs Forum*. 2015;42(1):54-62.

80. Ross A, Sundaramurthi T, Bevans M. A labor of love: the influence of cancer caregiving on health behaviors. *Cancer Nurs*. 2013;36(6):474-483.

81. Litzelman K, Kent EE, Rowland JH. Interrelationships between health behaviors and coping strategies among informal caregivers of cancer survivors. *Health Educ Behav*. 2018;45(1):90-100.

82. Lo MH. Health-promoting behavior and quality of life among caregivers and non-caregivers in Taiwan: a comparative study. *J Adv Nurs*. 2009;65:1695-1704.

83. Almutairi KM, Alodhayani AA, Alonazi WB, Vinluan JM. Assessment of health-related quality of life among caregivers of patients with cancer diagnosis: a cross-sectional study in Saudi Arabia. *J Relig Health*. 2017;56(1):226-237.

84. Fujinami R, Sun V, Zachariah F, Uman G, Grant M, Ferrell B. Family caregivers' distress levels related to quality of life, burden, and preparedness. *Psychooncology*. 2015;24(1):54-62.

85. Lee YJ, Kim JE, Choi YS, et al. Quality of life discordance between terminal cancer patients and family caregivers: a multicenter study. *Support Care Cancer*. 2016;24(7):2853-2860.

86. Ferrell BR, Ferrell FB, Rhiner M, Grant M. Family factors influencing cancer pain management. *Postgrad Med J*. 1991;67:S64-S69.

87. World Health Organization. *National Cancer Control Programmes: Policies and Managerial Guidelines*. 2nd ed. Geneva, Switzerland: WHO; 2002.

88. Badr H. Psychosocial interventions for patients with advanced cancer and their families. *Am J Lifestyle Med*. 2014;10(1):53-63.

89. *European Association Working for Carers: Reconciling Work and the Need to Support Informal Carers*. Brussels, BE: Eurocarers; 2017.

90. Schulz R, Sherwood PR. Physical and mental health effects of family caregiving. *Am J Nurs*. 2008;108(9):23-27.

91. National Alliance for Caregiving and Evercare. *Evercare® Study of Caregivers in Decline: A Close-Up Look at the Health Risks of Caring for a Loved One*. Bethesda, MD/Minnetonka, MN: National Alliance for Caregiving and Evercare; 2006.

92. Mosher CE, Adams RN, Helft PR, et al. Family caregiving challenges in advanced colorectal cancer: patient and caregiver perspectives. *Support Care Cancer*. 2016;24(5):2017-2024.

93. Mitchell AM, Pössel P. Repetitive negative thinking: the link between caregiver burden and depressive symptoms. *Oncol Nurs Forum*. 2017;44(2):210-216.

94. Marcotte J, Tremblay D, Turcotte A, Michaud C. Needs-focused interventions for family caregivers of older adults with cancer: a descriptive interpretive study. *Support Care Cancer*. 2019;27(8):2771-2781.

95. Tokem Y, Ozcelik H, Cicik A. Examination of the relationship between hopelessness levels and coping strategies among the family caregivers of patients with cancer. *Cancer Nurs*. 2015;38(4):E28-E34.

96. Leske S, Allan BS, Lambert SD, Girgis A. A protocol for an updated and expanded systematic mixed studies review of fear of cancer recurrence in families and caregivers of adults diagnosed with cancer. *Syst Rev*. 2018;7(1):134.

97. Lewis FM, Griffith KA, Alzawad Z, Dawson PL, Zahlis EH, Shands ME. Helping her heal: randomized clinical trial to enhance dyadic outcomes in couples. *Psychooncology*. 2019;28:430-438.

98. Keesing S, Rosenwax L, McNamara B. A dyadic approach to understanding the impact of breast cancer on relationships between partners during early survivorship. *BMC Womens Health*. 2016;16(1):57.

99. Tan SJY, Lim HA, Kuek NMY, et al. Caring for the caregiver while caring for the patient: exploring the dyadic relationship between patient spirituality and caregiver quality of life. *Support Care Cancer*. 2015;23(12):3403-3406.

100. Vespa A, Spatuzzi R, Merico F, et al. Spiritual well-being associated with personality traits and quality of life in family caregivers of cancer patients. *Support Care Cancer*. 2018;26(8):2633-2640.

101. Damianakis T, Wilson K, Marziali E. Family caregiver support groups: spiritual reflections' impact on stress management. *Aging Ment Health*. 2018;22(1):70-76.

102. Adelstein KE, Anderson JG, Taylor AG. Importance of meaning-making for patients undergoing hematopoietic stem cell transplantation. *Oncol Nurs Forum*. 2014;41(2):E172-E184.

103. Shim B, Barroso J, Gilliss CL, Davis LL. Finding meaning in caring for a spouse with dementia. *Appl Nurs Res*. 2013;26:121-126.

104. Horne J. *Caregiving: Helping an Aging Loved One*. Washington, DC: American Association of Retired Persons Books; 1985.

45 Management of Symptoms in the Actively Dying Patient

Teresa Khoo and Christopher J. Pietras

INTRODUCTION

The obligation of physicians to relieve suffering is universal, particularly when death is imminent and the indignities of illness consume patients' final days and hours of life. This honored duty is fundamental to a death free of unyielding symptoms and a satisfactory bereavement for surviving family members (1). Unfortunately, the dying process can be a time of untold loss and suffering, and unrelieved physical suffering can detract the attention from important spiritual and psychosocial issues at the end of life. Accordingly, therapy during this time should be supportive and focus on symptom control and, in so doing, maintain patient dignity and familial equanimity (2). Just as every stage is marked by its own challenges, so too is the management of the actively dying patient (3).

The actively dying phase is defined as "the hours or days preceding imminent death during which time the patient's physiologic functions wane" but can last as long as weeks in some circumstances (4). For this chapter, the management will be focused on the last few hours to days of life. Prospectively recognizing that a patient has entered this actively dying stage is important not only to be able to appropriately manage the patient's symptoms but also to maintain the patient's autonomy and dignity (5).

During the last days of life, there are characteristic signs and symptoms that commonly occur, which include (6)

- Weight loss
- Fatigue with prolonged periods of drowsiness
- Decreasing need for food and drink
- Difficulty swallowing
- Difficulty breathing and changes in breathing patterns
- Cool extremities, sometimes with mottling
- Decreased response to touch or sound
- Decreased urine output
- Pain
- Increased restlessness and confusion

In addition, there are seven signs associated with a high likelihood of death within 3 days (7):

- Decreased response to visual stimuli
- Hyperextension of the neck
- Drooping of nasolabial fold
- Nonreactive pupil
- Decreased response to verbal stimuli
- Grunting of vocal cords
- Inability to close eyelids.
- Kennedy ulcer development (discuss)

We must note the inherent challenge of differentiating symptoms from signs in the nonverbal patient. Although such signs and symptoms are often multifactorial in etiology, treatment is usually empiric and symptom directed. Diagnostic evaluation is limited in recognition of short life expectancy and impending death. Nevertheless, empiric treatment strategies do not suggest or encourage clinical indifference but rather mandate ongoing clinical assessment of therapeutic interventions in a continual effort to allay suffering. During this period of time, it is imperative that only essential medications be given by the least invasive route to provide adequate relief from suffering. Likewise, any medication or medical investigations that do not contribute to comfort should be discontinued. From time to time, terminal symptoms are refractory and unresponsive to aggressive and exhaustive interventions. In such cases, palliative sedation (PS) is an ethically and morally appropriate option that may be utilized to afford a more peaceful and tranquil death for the patient and a satisfactory grieving.

PAIN

Definition

Pain is as "an unpleasant sensory and emotional experience associated with actual or potential tissue damage" (8).

Epidemiology

At the end of life, pain is one of the most common symptoms, with a prevalence of 45% to 60% (9–13).

Etiology

Pain at the end of life can be multifactorial—from progression of a patient's disease process to iatrogenic causes (i.e., turning, aggressive suctioning, presence of endotracheal tube, and wound care) (14). Minimizing iatrogenic causes of pain should be done as part of pain management. Other causes of pain include mucositis, bone pain, malignant bowel obstruction, nerve pain, or wound pain.

Diagnosis

Assessment of pain requires asking the patient about pain intensity on a numerical pain scale from 0 to 10 (0 being no pain and 10 being the worst pain). The levels of pain intensity are then divided into three different levels of pain intensity: mild pain (1 to 3), moderate pain (4 to 7), and severe pain (8 to 10) (15). However, in the final days or hours of life, assessment of pain may become difficult as patients may not be able to verbalize their discomfort. In such cases, use of validated pain tools like Pain Assessment like the Pain Assessment in Advanced Dementia (PAIN-AD) or the Critical-Care Pain Observation Tool (CPOT) may be useful (Table 45.1) (16,17). It is recommended to treat for pain above a score of 2 on either the PAINAD or CPOT at the end of life (18). However, no tools are yet validated specifically for the actively dying patient. During this time, it is important to look for nonverbal signs of pain, including tension across the forehead, furrowing of the eyebrows, or facial grimacing (19–21). Patients may appear to show signs of pain when turned or repositioned, even when unconscious. Such pain may be due to an underlying medical disorder or due to joint stiffness secondary to bed rest and minimal body movement (22). Conversely, moaning and groaning are not uncommon in actively dying patients and may be interpreted as pain by family members. However, it is rare for uncontrolled pain to develop during the last hours of life. In such patients, it is helpful to look for nonverbal signs, which further support that the moaning and groaning are secondary to pain (23).

Treatment

Opioids are the mainstay of treatment. Morphine, hydromorphone, and fentanyl are the typical medications used (24,25). Typically, short-acting formulations are emphasized given that long-acting formulations may accumulate excessively. Long-acting opioid doses should be guided by the short-acting requirement. In the final hours of life, patients may be unable to swallow, and intravenous, subcutaneous, or rectal administration of analgesics may be necessary (26). Because patients may be unable to ask for medications, it is important that prescriptions be written "as needed for specific symptoms" or scheduled for symptom management with the ability for patients to refuse. It is also important to consider side effects, including nausea and constipation, and treat them appropriately. For instance, in patients who are placed on increasing doses of opioids, their bowel regimens should be titrated accordingly.

General Approach

1. In an opioid-naïve patient, start morphine at 2 to 4 mg i.v. every 15 minutes or 5 to 10 mg p.o. every 30 to 60 minutes until patient is comfortable (27).

TABLE 45.1 PAIN ASSESSMENT IN ADVANCED DEMENTIA (PAINAD)

Category	Scoring		
	0	**1**	**2**
Breathing	Normal	Occasional labored breathing. Short period of hyperventilation.	Noisy labored breathing. Long period of hyperventilation. Cheyne-Stokes respirations.
Negative vocalization	None	Occasional moan or groan. Low-level speech with a negative or disapproving quality.	Repeated trouble calling out. Loud moaning or groaning. Crying.
Facial expressions	Smiling or inexpressive	Sad. Frightened. Frown.	Facial grimacing.
Body language	Relaxed	Tense. Distressed pacing. Fidgeting.	Rigid. Fists clenched, knees pulled up. Pulling or pushing away. Striking out.
Consolability	No need to console	Reassured by occasional touching, hugging, or being talked to. Distractible.	Unable to console, distract, reassure.
Total	___	PAINAD >2: Treatment recommended.	

2. In an opioid-tolerant patient, for i.v./s.c., bolus every 15 to 30 minutes approximately 5% of the morphine equivalent daily dose (MEDD). Or, if p.o./s.l., then bolus every 60 minutes 10% to 20% of the MEDD.
3. In patients with uncontrolled pain, repeat and increase the bolus up to 50% to 100% every 15 to 30 minutes (i.v./s.c.) or every 60 minutes (p.o./s.l.).
4. For significant persistent pain, a continuous infusion or scheduled p.o./s.l. liquid may be administered to equal the last 24 hours of opioids required.
5. Remember to adjust bowel regimen as opioids are titrated up.

DYSPNEA

Definition

Dyspnea is defined as "a subjective experience of breathing discomfort that consists of qualitatively distinct sensations that vary in intensity" (28).

Epidemiology

Dyspnea occurs in 25% to 95% of terminally ill patients and is one of the most common severe symptoms as death approaches (10,11,28–31).

Etiology

Dyspnea in terminally ill patients derives from five primary causes, namely:

1. Existing disease (i.e., chronic obstructive pulmonary disease [COPD] and congestive heart failure)
2. Acute superimposed illness (i.e., pneumonia and pulmonary embolus)
3. Cancer-related complications (i.e., pleural effusion, lymphangitic carcinomatosis, tumor-induced bronchial obstruction, and ascites)
4. Effects of cancer therapy (i.e., radiation and chemotherapy-induced pulmonary fibrosis)
5. Miscellaneous causes (i.e., anemia, uremia, and anxiety) (29,32–34)

Diagnosis

Dyspnea is often very distressing for patients. And, it must be emphasized that dyspnea can only be perceived by the person experiencing it. Like pain, dyspnea is a symptom and must be distinguished from signs that the health care team may cite as evidence of respiratory distress—tachypnea, intercostal retractions, the use of accessory muscles. There is no validated assessment tool to assess for dyspnea. Patients will describe feeling air hunger, breathlessness, increased work of breathing, and even suffocation (35). They may also note an inability to catch their breath or complete an inhalation.

Treatment

The main priority is to help reduce the distress it causes. As with any symptom, the treatment of dyspnea should address any easily and rapidly correctable underlying cause, all the while recognizing and considering the limited life expectancy of the imminently dying patient and the invasiveness and discomfort of the proposed therapeutic interventions.

Opioids are the treatment of choice for dyspnea at the end of life (36). Opioids purportedly relieve dyspnea by altering the perception of breathlessness, decreasing ventilatory response to hypoxia and hypercapnia, and reducing oxygen consumption at rest and with exercise. Numerous studies on "opioids for the palliation of refractory dyspnea in adults with advanced disease and terminal illness" included in a recent *Cochrane Review* showed that the use of oral or parenteral opioids demonstrated a reduction in dyspnea (32). There was no evidence to support the use of nebulized opioids (37). Although morphine preparations are generally utilized, any opioid should potentially alleviate dyspnea (38). Opioids can be administered orally, rectally, sublingually, subcutaneously, and intravenously, but during the final hours of life when the ability to swallow declines and consciousness wanes, rectal, subcutaneous, and intravenous routes are more commonly used (Table 45.2).

Benzodiazepines may be helpful in treating dyspnea. Anxiety can be a result of dyspnea or, in some cases, the contributing cause. Benzodiazepines can alter the perception and reduce the patient's response to dyspnea. In a recent *Cochrane Review*, studies on various populations demonstrated no benefit of benzodiazepines for the relief of dyspnea (39). Nevertheless, benzodiazepines are frequently beneficial in reducing dyspnea, particularly during the final days of life. In one study, concurrent treatment with benzodiazepines and opioids was associated with a lower rate of admission seen in patients with WHO statuses 3 and 4 (40). Lorazepam when used as an adjuvant to opioids showed significant benefit in the relief of dyspnea when compared with opioids as a single agent without further risk of respiratory depression or change in gas exchange (41–43). This study shows the relationship between dyspnea and anxiety and how the use of opioid and anxiolytic together may well be suited to actively dying patients where the benefits clearly outweigh the risk.

Corticosteroids are frequently used for symptom management in treatment of patients with terminal illnesses. Corticosteroids reduce airway inflammation and edema, However, the evidence supporting their use is weak, except in cases of severe airway or parenchymal lung disease, and

TABLE 45.2 PHARMACOLOGIC TREATMENT OF DYSPNEA

Drug	Dose
Opioids	
Morphine	*Opioid naïve*—1–4 mg i.v./s.c. q15–30min or 5–10 mg p.o./s.l. q1h *Opioid tolerant*—increase opioid dose by 50%–100% until symptoms improve.
Oxycodone	5–10 mg p.o./s.l./p.r. q1–4h
Hydromorphone	0.2–1 mg i.v./s.c. q15–30min or 2–4 mg p.o. q60min
Corticosteroids	
Dexamethasone	4–8 mg p.o./s.l./i.v./s.c./p.r. daily
Prednisone	20–40 mg p.o./s.l. daily
Benzodiazepines	
Lorazepam	0.25–2 mg p.o./s.l./i.v./s.c. q1–4h
Diazepam	5–10 mg p.o./s.l./i.v./p.r. q1–4h

should be used judiciously and with caution (32). Corticosteroids can be administered orally, rectally, subcutaneously, intravenously, and by inhalation. Although side effects are of concern during chronic use, such concerns are negated by short-term use in actively dying patients.

Other medications are also available to attenuate dyspnea in the dying patient. These include diuretics, bronchodilators, and inhaled anesthetics. Oral and intravenous diuretics are useful when pulmonary edema and ascites contribute to dyspnea. The use of nebulized diuretics is not recommended. Although bronchodilators are best utilized in patients with a bronchospastic component to dyspnea (i.e., asthma and COPD with reactive airways), these drugs are frequently used when there is little-to-no evidence of bronchospasm and appear to provide subjective reduction of dyspnea in many patients. The use of adrenergic agonist bronchodilators should be tempered by the possibility of resultant agitation, tremor, and heightened anxiety, potentially aggravating terminal dyspnea (29).

Nonpharmacologic interventions that are useful for terminal dyspnea include oxygen, a bedside fan, thoracentesis for pleural effusion, and paracentesis for ascites (44). The role of oxygen therapy in reducing dyspnea in patients near the end of life is somewhat controversial (45). In hypoxemic patients with disorders such as COPD, congestive heart failure, or pulmonary fibrosis, most studies suggest that there is a significant symptomatic improvement. In patients without hypoxemia, however, its use is not advantageous.

A bedside fan may also be useful in alleviating dyspnea by reportedly stimulating thermal and mechanical receptors of the trigeminal nerve (V2 branch) in the cheek and nasopharynx, altering the central perception of breathlessness

(29,44,46). The fan should be placed at the bedside, set on a low speed, and directed at the patient's face (46).

General Approach

1. In a patient who is opioid naïve, start morphine at 1 to 4 mg i.v./s.c. every 15 to 30 minutes or 5 mg p.o./s.l. every 60 minutes as needed for shortness of breath until patient is comfortable without adverse effects.
   a. For a patient who is already on opioids, consider increasing opioid by 50% to 100% until patient is comfortable without adverse effects.
2. If a patient's dyspnea is persistent, either add a schedule oral opioid or add a continuous infusion with continued as needed bolus dosing every 15 minutes (i.v.) or 30 minutes (p.o./s.l.) for breakthrough dyspnea.
3. If the patient is experiencing anxiety with the dyspnea, start Lorazepam 0.25 to 1 mg p.o., s.c., or i.v. every 1 hour as needed.

DEATH RATTLE

In the last 24 to 48 hours of life, most patients retain secretions in the back of the throat that produces a gurgling type of respiration frequently referred to as the death rattle (29,47). The presence of these enhanced secretions is felt to predict death within 48 hours in over 75% of patients (48). Fortunately, the patient is usually unaware of the noise. Oropharyngeal suctioning is often provided, but gagging and coughing may generate patient discomfort. Instead, treatment with anticholinergic drugs is recommended to desiccate bronchial secretions and abolish the need for suctioning. Suggested medications include atropine, glycopyrrolate, scopolamine, and hyoscyamine (Table 45.3)

TABLE 45.3 PHARMACOLOGIC TREATMENT OF THE DEATH RATTLE

Drug	Dose
Scopolamine	1.5 mg patch TD q72h
Hyoscyamine	0.125–0.250 mg p.o./s.l. q2–4h
Glycopyrrolate	0.2–0.4 mg s.c./i.v. q4h
Atropine	0.1–0.4 mg s.c./i.v q4h or 1% solution 1–2 GTT s.l. q2h

(29,49). In one study, scopolamine patch was more immediately efficacious when compared with subcutaneous glycopyrrolate; however, glycopyrrolate has a longer duration of action (6,50). Nevertheless, most anticholinergic medications may provide relief and are widely used in clinical practice, although the overall efficacy has been challenged by a recent *Cochrane Review* (51). These antisialagogues do not dry up secretions that are already present, and they should therefore be used at the first sign of noisy respirations (52). In addition, placing patients in a lateral recumbent position with the head slightly elevated may help reduce the pooling of secretions and diminish noisy respirations, as may discontinuing parenteral and enteral infusions whenever possible (53).

ANXIETY, RESTLESSNESS, AND DELIRIUM

Anxiety

Definition

Anxiety is a condition characterized by excessive worry or nervousness and changes how a patient emotionally copes and functions. It also may make symptoms more difficult to treat (54).

Epidemiology

Anxiety is one of the most common psychological problems in terminally ill patients and like most symptoms can have numerous etiologies. The prevalence of anxiety can range from 2% to 14%, while significant symptoms can range from 25% to 48% (55–57). Increased rates of anxiety can be seen in women, unmarried patients, and those with poor functional status (54,56).

Etiology

Anxiety can be a component of a preexisting anxiety disorder or, more commonly in actively dying patients, accompany medical disorders and complications of illness and medications (55). Medical disorders that can cause anxiety include hyperthyroidism, pheochromocytoma, and primary and metastatic brain tumors. Medical complications and medications that can precipitate anxiety include hypoxia, sepsis, unrelieved pain, dyspnea, and medications such as corticosteroids, bronchodilators, and antiemetics that cause akathisia (58–60). In addition, withdrawal states from benzodiazepines and opioids can result in anxiety and may occur inadvertently when medications are suddenly discontinued after admission to a hospital or a long-term care facility (59). Anxiety can also occur in patients with poorly controlled symptoms, loss of independence, and social isolation.

Diagnosis

The symptoms of anxiety can present as agitation, restlessness, sweating, tachycardia, hyperventilation, panic attack, worry, or tension (61). There are many different assessments for anxiety; however the hospital anxiety and depression scale (HADS) has been validated with high reliability in a variety of medically ill populations (55,62,63). It is a 14-component self-reported measure that includes 7 anxiety items and 7 depression items, but does not include symptoms that may confound the diagnosis of anxiety or depression (63).

Treatment

The treatment of anxiety in the terminally ill often depends on etiology, but it generally involves nondrug maneuvers, specific interventions, and pharmacotherapy. Nondrug mainstays of treatment for anxiety earlier in the life trajectory, including meditation, biofeedback, progressive relaxation, and psychotherapy, are of little value in the actively dying patient (59). In some cases, specific interventions can be of benefit and include such measures as oxygen and opioids for dyspnea and opioids and other analgesics for pain, and discontinuing medications that cause akathisia, a movement disorder precipitated by neuroleptic medications (i.e., haloperidol, chlorpromazine, and prochlorperazine) and characterized by motor restlessness, compulsive moving, and anxiety.

The principal therapy for anxiety includes the judicious use of benzodiazepines and neuroleptics (58–60). Benzodiazepines are the mainstay of treatment in the terminally ill patient, with the shorter-acting agents, such as lorazepam preferred in the patient with advanced disease (Table 45.4) (64). These drugs are metabolized by conjugation in the liver and are the safest when hepatic disease is present (58–60). This is in contrast to alprazolam and other benzodiazepines, which are metabolized through oxidative pathways and may accumulate in debilitated patients. Midazolam, a water-soluble benzodiazepine, may be infused intravenously or subcutaneously and is very useful in controlling anxiety in the terminal phase of illness (65).

TABLE 45.4 PHARMACOLOGIC TREATMENT OF ANXIETY/DELIRIUM

Drug	Dose
Benzodiazepines	
Lorazepam	0.25–2 mg p.o./s.l./i.v./s.c. q1–2h
Midazolam	0.5–5 mg i.v./s.c. q1–2h
Diazepam	5–10 mg p.o./s.l./i.v./p.r. q1–4h
Neuroleptics	
Haloperidol	0.5–1 mg p.o./i.v./i.m./s.c. q1h
Olanzapine	2.5–5 mg p.o. q4h

The cost of midazolam may limit its use, particularly in managed care and capitated health systems, although a generic version is now available. Diazepam, an older but efficacious benzodiazepine, may be used rectally when no other route is available and the cost is of concern, with recommended dosages equivalent to oral regimens.

Other nonbenzodiazepine medications that are useful for anxiety include the neuroleptics chlorpromazine, thioridazine, and haloperidol. Neuroleptics may be used when benzodiazepines fail to relieve anxiety, when psychotic symptoms accompany anxiety, or when there is concern regarding the respiratory depressant effects of benzodiazepines. In one case report, gabapentin is useful in treating generalized anxiety (66). Trazodone has been shown to be effective in patients with anxiety, depression, and insomnia (67).

Restlessness

Restlessness is commonly observed during the last hours of life. Although it has multiple causes (and may overlap with delirium), specific treatment may not be possible (52). Restless patients may have diverse symptoms, including impaired consciousness, intermittent sleepiness, tossing and turning, moaning, grunting, crying out, and agitation, and muscle spasms or twitching (52). Restlessness may be caused by spiritual conflicts; by physical discomfort, such as a distended urinary bladder or bladder spasms, fecal impaction, unrelieved pain, and pressure ulcers; or by nausea, dyspnea, pruritus, hypoxia, extreme weakness, corticosteroids, and sudden withdrawal from benzodiazepines. Treatment involves identifying and managing the underlying cause or, if that is not possible, providing spiritual support, verbal, and tactile reassurance and utilizing a benzodiazepine such as midazolam or a neuroleptic such as chlorpromazine (68,69).

Delirium

Definition

According to the *Diagnostic and Statistical Manual of the American Psychiatric Association* (70), delirium is characterized by

- Disturbance of consciousness (reduced awareness of the environment), with reduced ability to focus, sustain, or shift attention
- Change in cognition (memory deficit, disorientation, and perceptual disturbances such as hallucinations, illusions, and delusions) that is not related to a preexisting dementia
- Development over a short period of time, with usual fluctuation throughout the day
- Evidence from the history, physical examination, or laboratory tests of a general medical condition judged to be etiologically related to the causation of delirium

In contrast to dementia, delirium is considered a reversible disorder with rapid onset; in the last 24 to 48 hours of life; however, it is often irreversible.

Epidemiology

Delirium is a nonspecific global disorder of cognition and attention that occurs in 8% to 75% of hospitalized patients with cancer (59,60,71) and in 62% to 83% of patients just before death (71,72).

Etiology

It is a significant sign of physiologic disturbance and, analogous to anxiety, may be secondary to multiple etiologies, including primary or metastatic brain tumors, infection, organ failure, metabolic disturbances, vascular complications, nutritional deficiencies, medication side effects, radiotherapy, and paraneoplastic syndromes (73). At the end of life, delirium can result from end-stage organ failure confounded by other irreversible causes.

Diagnosis

The assessment of delirium must take into consideration the life expectancy of the patient and the patient's goals for care. Most palliative care clinicians would undertake a diagnostic workup only when a clinically suspected cause can be easily identified and treated effectively with simple interventions that carry a minimal burden or risk of causing further distress (i.e., hypodermoclysis for dehydration). Most often, the cause of delirium in the actively dying patient is multifactorial and irreversible, and treatment is usually empiric (73). Similar to anxiety, nondrug supportive measures are of limited value (other than the presence of family members, a well-lit room, and familiar sounds and music). Consequently, pharmacologic interventions are the primary methods for treating hyperactive or agitated delirium in patients near death.

Treatment

Recent studies suggest that in patients near the end of life (but not specifically those actively dying), neuroleptics may worsen delirium symptoms when used for mild to moderate symptoms at lower doses (74). However, these studies do not utilize the aggressive q1h frequency and rapid dose titrations implemented by most hospice and palliative medicine providers. Unfortunately, this leaves providers in a place of uncertainty, where they should remain cautious in the use of neuroleptics. Often, neuroleptics are utilized when preserving consciousness is a goal while treating hyperactive delirium but are avoided in hypoactive or with mild to moderate delirium that can be managed with nonpharmacologic measures when possible. Until further evidence is available, benzodiazepines are generally preferred as the first-line medication for hyperactive delirium when not contraindicated.

When using neuroleptics, Haldol is the preferred pharmacologic agent (Table 45.4) (74). However, Haldol should be used with caution, and if it is ineffective, it should be stopped or changed out with another medication. The sedative effects at higher doses are likely still helpful for select patients. Haldol still has not been studied in patients who are actively dying with prognosis of days and who often require rapid titration to cause an effect. For patients that are expected to live longer (weeks and longer), providers should be particularly cautious about use of neuroleptics (75). The atypical neuroleptics such as olanzapine, risperidone, and quetiapine can also be considered in management of delirium with lower extrapyramidal but more metabolic side effects.

A short-acting benzodiazepine can be added if the patient is overly agitated, although benzodiazepines alone are not indicated in the treatment of delirium earlier in the life trajectory (50). In fact, benzodiazepines may actually exacerbate the delirious state, and if no improvement at initial dosing, they should either be uptitrated to maximize the sedative and amnesic effect or discontinued if delirium worsens and further sedation is not in line with goals of care. When delirium is difficult to control in the last days of life, PS with a goal of deep continuous sedation to alleviate intractable suffering may be required (76,77). In such situations a benzodiazepine, such as lorazepam or midazolam, is the drug of choice, either alone or in conjunction with a neuroleptic. If the goal of deep continuous sedation is not achieved by increased doses of benzodiazepines, then phenobarbital is next option. If a patient is in the ICU and hyperactive delirium has required propofol for effective management, the patient may alternatively continue on this regimen.

In addition to pharmacological treatment of delirium, it is important to consider an integrated approach to include modification of clinical factors that may precipitate delirium (74). There are multiple behavioral and educational interventions that should be considered as part of management through minimizing interruptions at night, bringing in familiar objects and pictures, returning eyeglasses and hearing aids, and reorienting the patient.

General Approach

1. Explore possible causes of anxiety and delirium. If restlessness or agitation is seen in isolation, unrelieved symptoms should be investigated—for example, unrelieved pain, constipation, or full bladder.
2. Consider nonpharmacological management of anxiety, restlessness, and delirium at the end of life.
3. Treat any reversible causes of anxiety, restlessness, and delirium.
4. For management of anxiety or agitation, start lorazepam at 0.25 to 2 mg p.o., s.l., s.c., or i.v. every 1 to 2 hours as needed.
5. For management of delirium, consider starting lorazepam 1 mg p.o. or i.v. every 1 hour as needed or Haldol 0.5 to 1 mg p.o. or i.v. every 1 hour as needed.

NAUSEA AND VOMITING

Definition

Nausea is an entirely subjective experience for the patient defined by the sensation of the need to vomit. In contrast, vomiting is a physical event as evidenced by forceful expulsion of gastric contents (78).

Epidemiology

Among patients with advanced cancer, AIDS, heart disease, COPD, and renal disease, symptom prevalence of nausea and vomiting (NV) was reported at 16% to 68% (79). Similarly, in a systematic review of symptoms during the last 2 weeks of life, the prevalence of NV was 19.4%, with a range of 8.4% to 71% (11). Risk factors are age <65, female gender, patients with specific types of tumors (breast, gynecological, stomach, and esophageal), presence of metastases to the lung, pleura, or peritoneum, opioid medication, and gastrointestinal obstruction.

Etiology

The etiology of NV in terminal illness varies and is frequently multifactorial (29), particularly as death approaches. At the end of life, common causes of nausea include constipation, opioids, malignant bowel obstruction, and chemotherapy (80). Although diagnostic evaluation can be done in the actively dying patient, treatment usually involves the empiric use of nonpharmacologic measures and antiemetics.

Diagnosis

The history of NV is imperative to determining its etiology. The history should detail duration, frequency, and severity of the NV in addition to the characteristics and associated symptoms. Associated symptoms such as reflux or constipation should be ruled out.

Treatment

An integrative approach should be used when treating NV. Nonpharmacologic measures used to treat NV include dietary manipulations, elimination of emetogenic medications (i.e., nonsteroidal anti-inflammatories, digoxin, and iron), and the limited use of nasogastric suctioning, particularly for high gastrointestinal bowel obstruction (81). Nasogastric tubes can be uncomfortable and difficult to place, especially in the home environment, but intermittent use may be considered for severe and intractable vomiting refractory to antiemetic therapy. A percutaneous venting gastrostomy is useful if placed prior to the active dying process. However, its placement in the patient near death is usually not practical.

There are two different pharmacologic approaches to treating NV: empirical and mechanistic. The empirical approach uses a variety of antiemetics to cover a range of emetic pathways and neurotransmitter or any medication that is well tolerated with proven efficacy regardless of underlying cause (52). The mechanistic approach utilizes understanding of the emetic pathway and neurotransmitters involved to select an antiemetic agent. These pathways use one or more of the following neurotransmitters, including dopamine, serotonin types 2-4, histamine type 1, acetylcholine, neurokinin, and cannabinoid. As such, treatment aimed at these neurotransmitters is utilized in the treatment of terminal NV: dopamine antagonists, anticholinergics, antihistamines, corticosteroids, serotonin antagonists, octreotide, cannabinoids, and benzodiazepines (Table 45.5) (27,29,68,81). While the mechanistic approach is based on understanding of the underlying pathway, etiology of NV is often multifactorial or unidentifiable, especially at

TABLE 45.5 PHARMACOLOGIC TREATMENT OF NAUSEA AND VOMITING

Drug	Dose
Dopamine antagonists	
Haloperidol	0.5–2 mg p.o./i.m./i.v./s.c. q1–2h
Prochlorperazine	5–20 mg p.o./i.m./i.v. q4–6h or 25 mg p.r. q4h
Promethazine	25 mg p.o./p.r. q4–6h or 12.5–25 mg i.v. q4–6h
Metoclopramide	5–10 mg p.o./i.v./s.c./i.m. q6h
Anticholinergics	
Scopolamine	1.5-mg transdermal patches q72h
Hyoscyamine	0.125–0.25 mg p.o./s.l. q4h; 0.25–0.5 mg s.c. q4–6h
Antihistamines	
Meclizine	25–50 mg p.o. q4–6h
Diphenhydramine	25–50 mg p.o./i.m./i.v. q4–6h
Corticosteroids	
Dexamethasone	4–8 mg p.o./i.v./s.c. q24h
Serotonin antagonists	
Ondansetron	4–8 mg p.o./i.v./s.c. q4–8h
Granisetron	0.5–1 mg p.o./i.v./s.c. q12h
Somatostatin analog	
Octreotide	100–600 µg i.v./s.c. q8h
Cannabinoid	
Dronabinol	2.5–7.5 mg p.o. b.i.d. or t.i.d.
Benzodiazepines	
Lorazepam	0.5–2 mg p.o./s.l./i.v./s.q. q1–4h

the end of life. Thus, an empiric approach is more commonly used.

Dopamine antagonists include haloperidol and prochlorperazine and are the usual first-line antiemetics chosen by most clinicians. Haloperidol is an excellent antiemetic and is particularly useful in delirious patients with NV because the symptoms may be improved with a single medication, although a recent *Cochrane Review* cited insufficient evidence to support its usefulness (82). As mentioned earlier (see Section "Delirium"), parenteral doses are twice as potent as oral doses, and there is a reported ceiling effect at approximately 30 mg a day. Prochlorperazine is also efficacious, has a rectal formulation, and is preferred by many clinicians, and while promethazine and chlorpromazine are also prescribed, there is probably little advantage in using them over prochlorperazine, except in the treatment of NV as an effect of increased intracranial pressure for which promethazine is preferred (78,81,83). Although combination therapy for NV is common in the terminally ill, two or more dopamine antagonists should not be prescribed concurrently as the potential for adverse extrapyramidal reactions is increased without additional antiemetic benefit.

Metoclopramide is both a dopamine antagonist and a serotonin (5-HT4) agonist, but at doses >120 mg a day, it becomes a serotonin (5-HT3) antagonist (27,81). It is very useful as an antiemetic and a prokinetic agent for gastroparesis-induced vomiting, but caution must be exercised with older patients as it may cause extrapyramidal reactions that may not be dose dependent (81).

Anticholinergic medications are most efficacious in NV related to colic and mechanical bowel obstruction (81,84). They include scopolamine, hyoscyamine, and glycopyrrolate. Antihistamines are effective in motion sickness, mechanical bowel obstruction, and increased intracranial pressure. These drugs comprise meclizine and diphenhydramine.

Corticosteroids have a synergistic effect with metoclopramide and the serotonin antagonists, but they are rarely useful as single agents (however, they may reduce peritumor edema of gastrointestinal malignancies and brain metastases and, in so doing, lessen emetic episodes) (81). Dexamethasone is the favored agent due to the small pill size, minimal mineralocorticoid activity, and availability of intravenous and subcutaneous administration.

Serotonin antagonists are frequently utilized in dying patients and are reportedly effective in reducing emesis, particularly NV associated with radiation, bowel obstruction, and renal failure (68,78,83,84). Depending on formulation, they can be relatively expensive. Although quite useful in chemotherapy-induced and radiation-induced emesis, their value in terminal NV is not completely studied.

Octreotide is a somatostatin analog that is useful in reducing NV associated with intestinal obstruction. This drug decreases gastrointestinal secretions, stimulates absorption of water and electrolytes, and inhibits intestinal peristalsis (85,86).

Dronabinol is a tetrahydrocannabinol (THC) that can be helpful in refractory forms of NV. It is rarely used in terminal NV. It exhibits antikinetic properties in the stomach and small bowel and may be most useful in emesis related to small bowel obstruction (81). It may, however, potentially worsen gastroparetic conditions.

The benzodiazepines have little role as singular antiemetics in the actively dying patient unless anxiety is a dominant component. They are best utilized as adjuncts to other antiemetics through their amnesic, anxiolytic, and sedative properties.

Olanzapine is an antipsychotic agent with significant binding affinity for dopamine, serotonin, histamine, and muscarinic cholinergic receptors (87). In the actively dying patient, it is most often utilized for nausea that has been resistant to other antiemetics.

Many hospice programs utilize compounding pharmacists to prepare diverse and innovative medications and delivery systems for symptom control in dying patients. A compounding pharmacist can prepare a topical gel and/or suppository variously known as *ABHR*, *ABHRD*, or *ABHRDC* that contain commercially available antiemetics, including Ativan (lorazepam), Benadryl or Dramamine (diphenhydramine), Haldol (haloperidol), Reglan (metoclopramide), Decadron (dexamethasone), or Cogentin (benztropine). These drugs are combined in various dosages (i.e., Ativan, 1.0 mg; Benadryl, 12.5 to 25 mg, or Dramamine, 25 to 50 mg; Haldol, 0.5 to 1 mg; Reglan, 5 to 10 mg; Decadron, 10 mg; and Cogentin, 1 mg). The suppositories have been quite useful in refractory NV and may be very effective in patients near death. Although there have been no studies that support the use of varied combinations, they appear to benefit some patients because of both antiemetic and sedative effects.

General Approach

1. Determine causes and emetic pathways involved in order to help identify reversible causes of NV and/or select an antiemetic treatment.
   a. If possible, reverse any underlying cause when possible.
2. If patient does not have a bowel obstruction, start with ondansetron 4 to 8 mg p.o., s.c., or i.v. q6h or metoclopramide 10 mg p.o, s.c., or i.v. q4h as needed for NV.
   a. If symptoms persist despite utilizing the as needed medications above, consider scheduling the antiemetics.
3. Consider adding anticholinergic medications, for example, meclizine or scopolamine, especially if there is a vestibular component to the nausea.
4. Corticosteroids, neuroleptics (e.g., olanzapine), benzodiazepines (e.g., lorazepam), and synthetic cannabinoids (e.g., dronabinol) can be added for refractory nausea.

PALLIATIVE SEDATION

The National Hospice and Palliative Care Organization (NHPCO) defines PS as "the lowering of patient consciousness using medications for the express purpose of limiting patient awareness of suffering that is intractable and intolerable. For the limited number of imminently dying patients who have pain and suffering that is (a) unresponsive to other palliative interventions and (b) intolerable to the patient, NHPCO believes that PS is an important option" (88).

The prevalence of PS varies from 3.1% to 51% (89). This variation is attributable to diverse definitions of PS, the retrospective nature of studies, and cultural and ethnic diversities.

A refractory symptom is a severe clinical symptom—for example, pain, dyspnea, delirium, agitation, nausea/vomiting—that is uncontrollable with the usual medications. It is at times subjective and nonspecific and includes physical as well as psychological symptoms (90). Cherny and Portenoy clarify the boundaries of a refractory symptom by offering three criteria that suggest a symptom is refractory:

1. It cannot be controlled adequately despite aggressive efforts to identify a tolerable therapy that does not compromise consciousness.
2. Additional invasive and noninvasive interventions are incapable of providing adequate relief.
3. The therapy directed at the symptom is associated with excessive and intolerable acute or chronic morbidity and is unlikely to provide relief within a tolerable time frame (91).

The ethical validity of PS derives from the doctrine of double effect, a doctrine that is applied to situations in which it is impossible for a person to avoid all harmful actions, and the precept of informed consent. The traditional formulations of the doctrine of double effect involve four basic conditions:

1. The nature of the act must be good or morally neutral and not in a category that is absolutely prohibited and intrinsically wrong.
2. The intent of the clinician must be good, and the good effect, not the bad effect, must be intended.
3. The demarcation between the means and effects must be acceptable, in other words, the bad effect must not be the means to the good effect.
4. Proportionality, whereby the good effect must exceed or balance the bad effect (92).

Contentious issues regarding PS revolve around artificial nutrition and hydration. Decisions regarding whether to continue or begin artificial nutrition and hydration should be discussed with family before PS begins. This decision should be made independent from a decision to proceed with PS. Whether or not artificial nutrition and

TABLE 45.6 GUIDELINES FOR PALLIATIVE SEDATION

Presence of a terminal illness with refractory symptom(s)

A do-not-resuscitate order

Exhaustion of all palliative treatments, including treatment for depression, delirium, anxiety, and familial discord

Consideration of ethical and psychiatric consultations

Consideration of assessment for spiritual issues by a skilled clinician or clergy member

Discussion regarding the discontinuation of parenteral or enteral nutrition or hydration

Obtaining informed consent

Consideration of respite sedation, particularly in patients with refractory existential distress

hydration relieves or exacerbates symptoms should be thoroughly discussed.

It is important to also distinguish PS from euthanasia and physician-assisted dying. Euthanasia is *intentionally* ending the life of another person by administration of a lethal agent with the goal of alleviating suffering. Physician-assisted dying is when a physician facilitates a patient's death by providing the means. PS involves giving sedative medications to reduce a patient's consciousness to make their suffering more tolerable (93). When PS is utilized for patients who are actively dying, the length of life is no different than when PS is not used (94).

If PS is employed in a dying patient, guidelines should be followed, including obtaining informed consent, as it is intimately integrated with autonomy and self-determination, and allowing a reasonable person or surrogate to make independent and noncoerced treatment decisions (Table 45.6) (95). The reason for PS should be documented, as should the people present during the discussion, and if required by institutional or corporate policy, a completed consent form should be placed in the patient's chart. All involved providers and staff should have an opportunity to voice concerns and discuss their role prior to initiation of PS. The choice of medications for PS is practitioner dependent; clinicians should choose the drugs they are most familiar with, considering efficacy, cost, and clinical circumstance. Drugs frequently used for PS include benzodiazepines, barbiturates, neuroleptics, and propofol.

ACKNOWLEDGMENTS

We would like to acknowledge and thank Drs. Paul Rousseau and Leigh Vaughan for their prior contributions to this chapter, upon which this work is built.

REFERENCES

1. Rousseau P. The losses and suffering of terminal illness. *Mayo Clin Proc.* 2000;75:197-198. doi:10.4065/75.2.197.
2. Svenaeus F. To die well: the phenomenology of suffering and end of life ethics. *Med Health Care Philos.* 2019;23:335-342. doi: 10.1007/s11019-019-09914-6.
3. Lamont EB. A demographic and prognostic approach to defining the end of life. *J Palliat Med.* 2005;8(suppl 1):S12-S21.
4. Hui D, Nooruddin Z, Didwaniya N, et al. Concepts and definitions for "actively dying," "end of life," "terminally ill," "terminal care," and "transition of care": a systematic review. *J Pain Symptom Manage.* 2014;47(1):77-89.
5. Meier EA, Gallegos JV, Montross-Thomas LP, Depp CA, Irwin SA, Jeste DV. Defining a good death (successful dying): literature review and a call for research and public dialogue. *Am J Geriatr Psychiatry.* 2016;24(4):261-271. doi:10.1016/j.jagp.2016.01.135.
6. Pitorak EF. Care at the time of death. *Home Healthc Nurse.* 2005;23(5):318-327.
7. Hui D, Dos Santos R, Chisholm G, Bansal S, Crovador CS, Bruera E. Bedside clinical signs associated with impending death in patients with advanced cancer: preliminary findings of a prospective, longitudinal cohort study. *Cancer.* 2015;121(6):960-967. doi:10.1002/cncr.29048.
8. Merskey H, Bogduk N. *Classification of Chronic Pain.* 2nd ed. Seattle: IASP Task Force on Taxonomy, IASP Press; 1994.
9. Singer AE, Meeker D, Teno JM, Lynn J, Lunney JR, Lorenz KA. Symptom trends in the last year of life from 1998 to 2010: a cohort study. *Ann Intern Med.* 2015;162(3):175-183. doi:10.7326/M13-1609.
10. Kobewka D, Ronksley P, McIsaac D, Mulpuru S, Forster A. Prevalence of symptoms at the end of life in an acute care hospital: a retrospective cohort study. *CMAJ Open.* 2017;5(1):E222-E228. doi:10.9778/cmajo.20160123.
11. Kehl KA, Kowalkowski JA. A systematic review of the prevalence of signs of impending death and symptoms in the last 2 weeks of life. *Am J Hosp Palliat Med.* 2013;30(6):601-616. doi:10.1177/1049909112468222.
12. Clark K, Connolly A, Clapham S, Quinsey K, Eagar K, Currow DC. Physical symptoms at the time of dying was diagnosed: a consecutive cohort study to describe the prevalence and intensity of problems experienced by imminently dying palliative care patients by diagnosis and place of care. *J Palliat Med.* 2016;19(12):1288-1295. doi:10.1089/jpm.2016.0219.
13. McCarthy EP, Phillips RS, Zhong Z, Drews RE, Lynn J. Dying with cancer: patients' function, symptoms, and care preferences as death approaches. *J Am Geriatr Soc.* 2000;48(S1):S110-S121. doi:10.1111/j.1532-5415.2000.tb03120.x.
14. Truog RD, Campbell ML, Curtis JR, et al. Recommendations for end-of-life care in the intensive care unit: a consensus statement by the American College of Critical Care Medicine. *Crit Care Med.* 2008;36(3):953-963. doi:10.1097/CCM.0B013E3181659096.
15. Swarm RA, Paice JA, Anghelescu DL, et al. Adult cancer pain, version 3.2019, NCCN Clinical Practice Guidelines in Oncology. *J Natl Compr Cancer Netw.* 2019;1(9):1046-1086. doi:10.6004/jnccn.2019.0038.
16. Groninger H, Vijayan J. Pharmacologic management of pain at the end of life. *Am Fam Physician.* 2014;90(1):26-32.
17. Gélinas C, Harel F, Fillion L, Puntillo KA, Johnston CC. Sensitivity and specificity of the critical-care pain observation tool for the detection of pain in intubated adults after cardiac surgery. *J Pain Symptom Manage.* 2009;37:58-67. doi:10.1016/j.jpainsymman.2007.12.022.
18. Goebel JR, Ferolito M, Gorman N. Pain screening in the older adult with delirium. *Pain Manag Nurs.* 2019;20:519-525. doi:10.1016/j.pmn.2019.07.003.
19. Ferris FD, Von Gunten CF, Emanuel LL. Competency in end-of-life care: last hours of life. *J Palliat Med.* 2003;6:605-613. doi:10.1089/109662103768253713.
20. Ferris FD. Last hours of living. *Clin Geriatr Med.* 2004;20:641-667. doi:10.1016/j.cger.2004.07.011.
21. Mularski RA. Pain management in the intensive care unit. *Crit Care Clin.* 2004;20(3):381-401. doi:10.1016/j.ccc.2004.03.010.
22. Saunders C, Platt M. Pain and impending death. In: Melzack R, Wall PD, eds. *Handbook of Pain Management: A Clinical Companion to Textbook of Pain.* 1st ed. Edinburgh: Churchill Livingstone; 2003.
23. Warden V, Hurley AC, Volicer L. Development and psychometric evaluation of the pain assessment in advanced dementia (PAINAD) scale. *J Am Med Dir Assoc.* 2003;4(1):9-15. doi:10.1097/01.JAM.0000043422.31640.F7.
24. Durán-crane A, Laserna A, López-olivo MA, et al. Clinical practice guidelines and consensus statements about pain management in critically ill end-of-life patients: a systematic review. *Crit Care Med.* 2019;47:1619-1626. doi:10.1097/CCM.0000000000003975.
25. Portenoy RK, Ahmed E. Principles of opioid use in cancer pain. *J Clin Oncol.* 2014;32(16):1662-1670. doi:10.1200/JCO.2013.52.5188.
26. Parsons HA, Shukkoor A, Quan H, et al. Intermittent subcutaneous opioids for the management of cancer pain. *J Palliat Med.* 2008;11(10):1319-1324. doi:10.1089/jpm.2008.0155.
27. Blinderman CD, Billings JA. Comfort care for patients dying in the hospital. *N Engl J Med.* 2015;373(26):2549-2561. doi:10.1056/NEJMra1411746.
28. Parshall MB, Schwartzstein RM, Adams L, et al. An official American Thoracic Society Statement: update on the mechanisms, assessment, and management of dyspnea. *Am J Respir Crit Care Med.* 2012;185(4):435-452. doi:10.1164/rccm.201111-2042ST.
29. Rousseau P. Nonpain symptom management in the dying patient. *Hosp Physician.* 2002;38(2):51-56.
30. Campbell ML, Kiernan JM, Strandmark J, Yarandi HN. Trajectory of dyspnea and respiratory distress among patients in the last month of life. *J Palliat Med.* 2018;21(2):194-199. doi:10.1089/jpm.2017.0265.
31. Lau C, Stilos K, Nowell A, Lau F, Moore J, Wynnychuk L. The comfort measures order set at a tertiary care academic hospital: is there a comparable difference in end-of-life care between patients dying in acute care when CMOS is utilized? *Am J Hosp Palliat Med.* 2018;35(4):652-663. doi:10.1177/1049909117734228.
32. Pisani L, Hill NS, Maria A, Pacilli G, Polastri M, Nava S. Management of dyspnea in the terminally ill. *Chest.* 2018;154(4):925-934. doi:10.1016/j.chest.2018.04.003.
33. Farncombe M. Dyspnea: assessment and treatment. *Support Care Cancer.* 1997;5:94-99.
34. Lok CW. Management of breathlessness in patients with advanced cancer: a narrative review. *Am J Hosp Palliat Care.* 2016;33(3):286-290. doi:10.1177/1049909114554796.
35. Shoemaker LK, Estfan B, Induru R, Walsh TD. Symptom management: an important part of cancer care. *Cleve Clin J Med.* 2011;78(1):25-34. doi:10.3949/ccjm.78a.10053.
36. Marciniuk DD, Goodridge D, Hernandez P, et al. Managing dyspnea in patients with advanced chronic obstructive pulmonary disease: a Canadian Thoracic Society clinical practice guideline. *Can Respir J.* 2011;18(2):69-78. doi:10.1155/2011/745047.

37. Vargas-bermúdez A, Cardenal F, Porta-sales J, Cardenal F, Porta-sales J. Opioids for the management of dyspnea in cancer patients: evidence of the last 15 years—a systematic review. *J Pain Palliat Care Pharmacother.* 2015;29:341-352. doi:10.3109/15360288.2015.1082005.

38. Qaseem A, Snow V, Shekelle P, Casey DE, Cross JT, Owens DK. Evidence-based interventions to improve the palliative care of pain, dyspnea, and depression at the end of life: a clinical practice guideline from the American College of Physicians. *Ann Intern Med.* 2008;148(2):141-146.   doi:10.7326/0003-4819-148-2-200801150-00009.

39. Simon ST, Higginson IJ, Booth S, Harding R, Weingärtner V, Bausewein C. Benzodiazepines for the relief of breathlessness in advanced malignant and non-malignant diseases in adults. *Cochrane Database Syst Rev* 2016;(10):CD007354. doi:10.1002/14651858.CD007354. pub3.

40. Ekström MP, Abernethy AP, Currow DC. The management of chronic breathlessness in patients with advanced and terminal illness. *BMJ.* 2015;349(January): 1-7. doi:10.1136/bmj.g7617.

41. Clemens KE, Klaschik E. Dyspnoea associated with anxiety-symptomatic therapy with opioids in combination with lorazepam and its effect on ventilation in palliative care patients. *Support Care Cancer.* 2011;19:2027-2033. doi:10.1007/s00520-010-1058-8.

42. Ekström MP, Abernethy AP, Currow DC. Safety of benzodiazepines and opioids in very severe respiratory disease: national prospective study. *BMJ.* 2014;348:g445. doi:10.1136/bmj.g445.

43. Morita T, Tsunoda J, Inoue S, Chihara S. Effects of high dose opioids and sedatives on survival in terminally ill cancer patients. *J Pain Symptom Manage.* 2001;21(4): 282-289. doi:10.1016/S0885-3924(01)00258-5.

44. Bausewein C, Booth S, Gysels M, Ij H. Non-pharmacological interventions for breathlessness in advanced stages of malignant and non-malignant diseases. *Cochrane Database Syst Rev.* 2008;(2):CD005623.

45. Elkington H, White P, Addington-Hall J, Higgs R, Edmonds P. The healthcare needs of Chronic obstructive pulmonary disease patients in the last year of life. *Palliat Med.* 2005;19(6):485-491. doi:10.1191/02692163 05pm1056oa.

46. Galbraith S, Fagan P, Dip G, et al. Does the use of a handheld fan improve chronic dyspnea ? A randomized, controlled, crossover trial. *J Pain Symptom Manage.* 2010;39(5):831-838. doi:10.1016/j.jpainsymman.2009.09.024.

47. Sorenson HM, Manning HL, Fins JJ, Rubenfeld GD, Curtis JR, Viles L. Managing secretions in dying patients. *Respir Care.* 2000;45:1355-1364.

48. Kompanje EJO. "The death rattle" in the intensive care unit after withdrawal of mechanical ventilation in neurological patients. *Neurocrit Care.* 2005;3:107-110. doi:10.1385/NCC:3:2:107.

49. Wildiers H, Dhaenekint C, Demeulenaere P, et al. Atropine, hyoscine butylbromide, or scopolamine are equally effective for the treatment of death rattle in terminal care. *J Pain Symptom Manage.* 2009;38:124-133. doi:10.1016/j.jpainsymman.2008.07.007.

50. Plonk WM, Arnold RM. Terminal care: the last weeks of life. *J Palliat Med.* 2005;8:1042-1054. doi:10.1089/jpm. 2005.8.1042.

51. Wee B, Hillier R. Interventions for noisy breathing in patients near to death. *Cochrane Database Syst Rev.* 2008;(1):CD005177. doi:10.1002/14651858.CD005177. pub2.

52. Cherny N, Fallon M, Kaasa S, Portenoy RK, Currow DC. *Oxford Textbook of Palliative Medicine.* 5th ed. Oxford: Oxford University Press; 2015.

53. Von Roenn JH, Paice JA. Control of common, non-pain cancer symptoms. *Semin Oncol.* 2005;32:200-210. doi:10.1053/j.seminoncol.2004.11.019.

54. Spencer R, Nilsson M, Wright A, Pirl W, Prigerson H. Anxiety disorders in advanced cancer patients: correlates and predictors of end-of-life outcomes. *Cancer.* 2010;116:1810-1819. doi:10.1002/cncr.24954.

55. Atkin N, Vickerstaff V, Candy B. 'Worried to death': the assessment and management of anxiety in patients with advanced life-limiting disease, a national survey of palliative medicine physicians. *BMC Palliat Care.* 2017;16:69. doi:10.1186/s12904-017-0245-5.

56. Kolva E, Rosenfeld B, Pessin H, Breitbart W, Brescia R. Anxiety in terminally ill cancer patients. *J Pain Symptom Manage.* 2011;42(5):691-701. doi:10.1016/j.jpainsymman.2011.01.013.Anxiety.

57. Kozlov E, Phongtankuel V, Prigerson H, et al. Prevalence, severity, and correlates of symptoms of anxiety and depression at the very end of life. *J Pain Symptom Manage.* 2019;58(1):80-85. doi:10.1016/j.jpainsymman.2019.04.012.Prevalence.

58. Breitbart W, Jacobsen PB. Psychiatric symptom management in terminal care. *Clin Geriatr Med.* 1996;12:329-347. doi:10.1016/s0749-0690(18)30230-1.

59. Roth AJ, Breitbart W. Psychiatric emergencies in terminally ill cancer patients. *Hematol Oncol Clin North Am.* 1996;10:235-259. doi:10.1016/S0889-8588(05) 70337-3.

60. Breitbart W. Psycho-oncology: Depression, anxiety, delirium. *Semin Oncol.* 1994;21:754-769.

61. Fine RL. Depression, anxiety, and delirium in the terminally ill patient. *Proc (Bayl Univ Med Cent).* 2001;14:130-133.

62. Brennan C, Worrall-davies A, Mcmillan D, Gilbody S, House A. The hospital anxiety and depression scale: a diagnostic meta-analysis of case-finding ability. *J Psychosom Res.* 2010;69(4):371-378. doi:10.1016/j.jpsychores.2010.04.006.

63. Bjelland I, Dahl AA, Tangen T, Neckelmann D. The validity of the hospital anxiety and depression scale an updated literature review. *J Psychosom Res.* 2002;52: 69-77.

64. Roth AJ, Massie MJ. Anxiety and its management in advanced cancer. *Curr Opin Support Palliat Care.* 2007;1:50-56. doi:10.1097/spc.0b013e32813aeb23.

65. Sandvik RK, Selbaek G, Bergh S, Aarsland D, Husebo BS. Signs of imminent dying and change in symptom intensity during pharmacological treatment in dying nursing home patients: a prospective trajectory study. *J Am Med Dir Assoc.* 2016;17:821-827. doi:10.1016/j. jamda.2016.05.006.

66. Markota M, Morgan RJ. Treatment of generalized anxiety disorder with gabapentin. *Case Rep Psychiatry.* 2017;2017:1-4. doi:10.1155/2017/6045017.

67. Arriaga F, Cavaglia F, Pires AM, Lara E, Paiva T. Effects of trazodone on insomnia and anxiety in depressed patients: a clinical and sleep EEG study. *Int J Psychiatry Clin Pract.* 1997;1(4):281-286. doi:10.3109/13651509709024740.

68. Lindqvist O, Lundquist G, Dickman A, et al. Four essential drugs needed for quality care of the dying: a Delphi-study based international expert consensus opinion. *J Palliat Med.* 2013;16(1):38-43. doi:10.1089/ jpm.2012.0205.

69. Gambles M, McGlinchey T, Latten R, Dickman A, Lowe D, Ellershaw JE. How is agitation and restlessness managed in the last 24 h of life in patients whose care is supported by the Liverpool care pathway for the dying patient? *BMJ Support Palliat Care.* 2011;1:329-333. doi:10.1136/bmjspcare-2011-000075.

70. American Psychiatric Association. *Diagnostic and Statistical Manual of Mental Disorders.* 5th ed. Arlington, TX: American Psychiatric Association; 2013.

71. Massie MJ, Holland J, Glass E. Delirium in terminally ill cancer patients. *Am J Psychiatry.* 1983;140:1048-1050. doi:10.1176/ajp.140.8.1048.

72. Casarett DJ, Inouye SK, Snyder L. Diagnosis and management of delirium near the end of life. *Ann Intern Med.* 2001;135:32-40. doi:10.7326/0003-4819-135-1-200107030-00011.

73. Breitbart W, Strout D. Delirium in the terminally ill. *Clin Geriatr Med.* 2000;16:357-372. doi:10.1016/S0749-0690(05)70061-6.

74. Grassi L, Caraceni A, Mitchell AJ, et al. Management of delirium in palliative care: a review. *Curr Psychiatry Rep.* 2015;17:550. doi:10.1007/s11920-015-0550-8.

75. Agar MR, Lawlor PG, Quinn S, et al. Efficacy of oral risperidone, haloperidol, or placebo for symptoms of delirium among patients in palliative care: a randomized clinical trial. *JAMA Intern Med.* 2017;177:34-42. doi:10.1001/jamainternmed.2016.7491.

76. Bush SH, Leonard MM, Agar M, et al. End-of-life delirium: issues regarding recognition, optimal management, and the role of sedation in the dying phase. *J Pain Symptom Manage.* 2014;48(2):215-230. doi:10.1016/j.jpainsymman.2014.05.009.

77. Jackson KC, Lipman AG. Drug therapy for delirium in terminally ill adult patients. *Cochrane Database Syst Rev.* 2004;(2):CD004770. doi:10.1002/14651858.CD004770.

78. Glare P, Miller J, Nikolova T, Tickoo R. Treating nausea and vomiting in palliative care: a review. *Clin Interv Aging.* 2011;6:243-259. doi:10.2147/CIA.S13109.

79. Solano JP, Gomes B, Higginson IJ. A comparison of symptom prevalence in far advanced cancer, AIDS, heart disease, chronic obstructive pulmonary disease and renal disease. *J Pain Symptom Manage.* 2006;31:58-69. doi:10.1016/j.jpainsymman.2005.06.007.

80. Kreher M. Symptom control at the end of life. *Med Clin North Am.* 2016;100(5):1111-1122. doi:10.1016/j.mcna.2016.04.020.

81. Davis MP, Walsh D. Treatment of nausea and vomiting in advanced cancer. *Support Care Cancer.* 2000;8:444-452. doi:10.1007/s005200000151.

82. Murray-Brown F, Dorman S. Haloperidol for the treatment of nausea and vomiting in palliative care patients. *Cochrane Database Syst Rev.* 2015;2015:CD006271. doi:10.1002/14651858.CD006271.pub3.

83. Glare PA, Dunwoodie D, Clark K, et al. Treatment of nausea and vomiting in terminally ill cancer patients. *Drugs.* 2008;68:2575-2590. doi:10.2165/0003495-200868180-00004.

84. Wood GJ, Shega JW, Lynch B, Von Roenn JH. Management of intractable nausea and vomiting in patients at the end of life. *JAMA.* 2007;298(10):1196-1207.

85. Mercadante S, Porzio G. Octreotide for malignant bowel obstruction: twenty years after. *Crit Rev Oncol Hematol.* 2012;83:388-392. doi:10.1016/j.critrevonc.2011.12.006.

86. Hisanaga T, Shinjo T, Morita T, et al. Multicenter prospective study on efficacy and safety of octreotide for inoperable malignant bowel obstruction. *Jpn J Clin Oncol.* 2010;40:739-745. doi:10.1093/jjco/hyq048.

87. Harder S, Groenvold M, Isaksen J, Sigaard J, Frandsen KB. Antiemetic use of olanzapine in patients with advanced cancer: results from an open-label multicenter study. *Support Care Cancer.* 2019;27:2849-2856.

88. Kirk TW, Mahon MM. National Hospice and Palliative Care Organization (NHPCO) position statement and commentary on the use of palliative sedation in imminently dying terminally ill patients. *J Pain Symptom Manage.* 2010;39(5):914-923. doi:10.1016/j.jpainsymman.2010.01.009.

89. Claessens P, Menten J, Schotsmans P. Palliative sedation: a review of the research literature. *J Pain Symptom Manage.* 2008;36(3):310-333. doi:10.1016/j.jpainsymman.2007.10.004.

90. Rousseau P. The ethical validity and clinical experience of palliative sedation. *Mayo Clin Proc.* 2000;75:1064-1069. doi:10.4065/75.10.1064.

91. Cherny NI, Portenoy RK. Sedation in the management of refractory symptoms: guidelines for evaluation and treatment. *J Palliat Care.* 1994;10:31-38. doi:10.1177/082585979401000207.

92. Quill TE, Dresser R, Brock DW. The rule of double effect—A critique of its role in end-of-life decision making. *N Engl J Med.* 1997;337:1768-1771. doi:10.1056/NEJM199712113372413.

93. Have H, Welie JVM. Palliative sedation versus euthanasia: an ethical assessment. *J Pain Symptom Manage.* 2014;47(1):123-136. doi:10.1016/j.jpainsymman.2013.03.008.

94. Maltoni M, Scarpi E, Rosati M, et al. Palliative sedation in end-of-life care and survival: a systematic review. *J Clin Oncol.* 2012;30(12):1378-1383. doi:10.1200/JCO.2011.37.3795.

95. Rousseau P. Palliative sedation in the management of refractory symptoms. *J Support Oncol.* 2004;2:181-186.

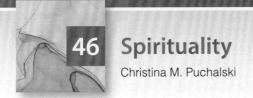

46 Spirituality

Christina M. Puchalski

Palliative care is a specialty based in the whole person care model. Thus, care of the patient and family includes addressing psychosocial and spiritual needs as well as the physical needs. In a whole person–centered model, preservation of human dignity is considered an important part of quality of life. Spiritual care is based in honoring the dignity of each person. In doing so, spiritual care supports the whole person and recognizes that a goal of care is helping each patient find a sense of wholeness and integrity in the midst of suffering and illness. This is especially important in caring for seriously ill and dying patients.

When my mother was hospitalized a few years before she died, she was interviewed by a neurologist. He fired questions at her trying to assess her mental status. He never asked about her story, where she was from. All he wanted was to obtain a number for her MMSE. Her dignity was not honored, her story was not heard. In the middle of the rapid-fire questions, she said to me in her native language, Polish, "I feel so stupid. What are all these questions about?" Later, after he left and she calmed down, she told me that her whole sense of who she was in that moment was torn away from her. What she needed was reassurance, connection, respect, and compassion—she needed good spiritual care.

Illness can strip away one's meaning and purpose and one's important relationships in life; illness can call into question patients' beliefs and values thus triggering profound questions of deep meaning purpose and what is most important to a person. It can be an opportunity for deep reflection and growth. Health care professionals can hinder that opportunity by not providing attention and space for patients to address these deeper questions in their lives. Illness can also cause deep suffering. Addressing only the physical pain does not address the spiritual and existential suffering seriously ill and dying patients experience. How the health care professionals interact with patients in the midst of their illness can have profound effects on how that person will understand their illness, cope with it, find a will to live and persevere, or the strength to let go and die peacefully when it is time. This process, that is, the patients'

confronting their illness and the health care system working with the patients to treat that illness, is a spiritual one. Spiritual care is the act of partnering with patients to help them find meaning, wholeness, and healing. Spirituality and spiritual care are the fabrics that underlie the process of honoring the dignity of each person.

THE BIOPSYCHOSOCIAL–SPIRITUAL MODEL

The basic tenets of whole person, patient-centered care are rooted in the biopsychosocial–spiritual model: attention to all the dimensions of a patient—physical, emotional, social, and spiritual (Table 46.1) (1).

The biopsychosocial care model developed by Engel (2) and White et al. (3) forms another theoretical framework for spiritual care by recognizing that each person is a "being-in-relationship." In support of extending the biopsychosocial care model to encompass the spiritual, Jonas said, "Life is essentially a relationship; and relation as such implies 'transcendence,' a going-beyond-itself on the part of that which entertains the relation" (4). Sulmasy took the association a step farther by describing disease as a disturbance in the right relationships that constitute the unity and integrity of what we know to be a human being (see Fig. 46.1) (5,6).

Spiritual care recognizes that a person's relationships—from those inside the physical body that define health to external or transcendent relationships that give a person's life meaning—are disrupted by illness and, thus, all relationships must be attended to in the treatment or care plan to enhance quality of life.

According to the biopsychosocial–spiritual model, everyone has a spiritual history. For many people, this spiritual history unfolds within the context of an explicit religious tradition; for others, it unfolds as a set of philosophical principles or significant experiences. Regardless, this spiritual history helps shape who each patient is as a whole person. An illness experience is unique to each individual in his or her totality (7). This totality includes not only simply the biologic,

TABLE 46.1 DIMENSIONS OF THE DYING EXPERIENCE

Physical	Pain and other symptom management
Psychological	Anxiety and depression
Social	Social isolation and economic issues
Spiritual	Purpose and meaning, relationships with the transcendent, search for ultimate meaning, hope, reconciliation, and despair

psychological, and social aspects of the person (8) but also the spiritual aspects as well (9,10). The biologic, psychological, social, and spiritual are distinct dimensions of each person. No one aspect can be disaggregated from the whole. Each aspect can be affected differently by a person's history and illness and each aspect can interact and affect other aspects of the person (6).

Based on this model, one can reframe the standard assessment and plan to include all dimensions of the person, not just the physical. This radically changes how we approach the patient as person. By attending to the whole person, spiritual care embraces the definition of health as not just absence of disease, but as a state of well-being that includes a sense that life has purpose and meaning (11) as stated in the Pew-Fetzer definition of health: "We are coming to understand health not as the absence of disease, but rather as the process by which individuals maintain their sense of coherence (i.e., sense that life is comprehensible,

manageable and meaningful) and ability to function in the face of changes in themselves and their relationship with the environment."

MEANING AND PURPOSE

Illness and the prospect of dying can call into question the very meaning and purpose of a person's life. Illness can also cause people to suffer deeply. Victor Frankl wrote that man is not destroyed by suffering; he is destroyed by suffering without meaning (12). Writing about concentration camp victims, he noted that survival itself might depend on seeking and finding meaning. Harold Kushner also noted that pain may be the reason, and out of pain and suffering may come the answer (13). In my own clinical experience, I have found that people may cope with their suffering by finding meaning in it. Illness can present people with the opportunity to find new meaning in their lives. Many patients say that out of their despair, they were able to realize an entirely new and more fulfilling meaning in their lives. Rabbi Cohen wrote,

> When my mother died, I inherited her needlepoint tapestries. "When I was a little boy, I used to sit at her feet as she worked on them. Have you ever seen needlepoint from underneath? All I could see was chaos; strands of thread all over with no seeming purpose. As I grew, I was able to see her work from above. I came to appreciate the patterns, the need for the dark threads as well as the light and gaily colored ones. Life is like that. From our human perspective, we cannot see the whole picture, but we should not despair or feel that there is no purpose. There is meaning and purpose even for the dark threads, but we cannot see that right away" (14).

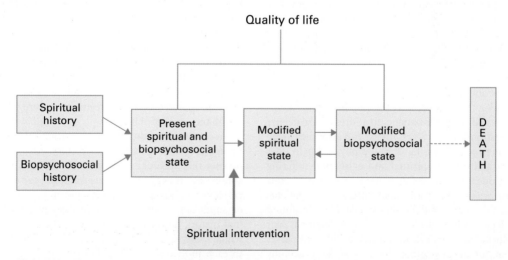

Figure 46.1 The biopsychosocial–spiritual model of care. (From Sulmasy DP. A biopsychosocial–spiritual model for the care of patients at the end of life. *Gerontologist*. 2002;42(spec 3):24-33. Used with permission.)

Spirituality helps people find hope in the midst of despair. As caregivers, we need to engage our patients on that spiritual level. This is where spirituality plays such a critical role—the relationship with a transcendent being or concept can give meaning and purpose to people's lives, to their joys, and to their sufferings. Spirituality is concerned with a transcendental or existential way to live one's life at a deeper level, "with the person as human being" (15). All people seek meaning and purpose in life; this search may be intensified when someone is facing serious illness, the possibility of death or dying.

There are many different ways people can derive meaning from their lives:

- Work
- Relationships
- Hobbies
- Art, music, and dance
- Reflective writing
- Sports
- Relationship with God/sacred/Divine
- Religious, spiritual, philosophical, or existential beliefs
- Religious, spiritual, or cultural rituals

Some of these activities or practices provide an important but perhaps transient meaning (meaning with a small m); others provide a more transcendent and spiritual meaning (meaning with a large M). For example, work may provide an immense amount of meaning to a person. But when that person is ill or dying and unable to work, what then will provide meaning? Therefore, there are activities, relationships, and values that are meaningful but do not define the ultimate purpose of one's life. Illness, aging, and dying strip away all those things that were meaningful but that do not ultimately sustain us. When we confront ourselves in the nakedness of our dying, it is then that we have the opportunity to find deep and transcendent meaning, that is, values, beliefs, practices, relationships, expressions that lead one to the awareness of transcendence/God/Divine and to a sense of ultimate value and purpose in life. Everyone's sense of meaning evolves over their life in response to experiences and life in general. People can fluctuate between "meaning" and "Meaning."

Downey defined spirituality as "an awareness that there are levels of reality not immediately apparent and that there is a quest for personal integration in the face of forces of fragmentation and depersonalization" (16). Spirituality is that aspect of human beings that seeks to heal or be whole. Foglio and Brody wrote,

> For many people religion [spirituality] forms a basis of meaning and purpose in life. The profoundly disturbing effects of illness can call into question

a person's purpose in life and work; responsibilities to spouse, children, and parents ... Healing, the restoration of wholeness (as opposed to merely technical healing) requires answers to these questions (17).

Healing, then, is not synonymous with recovery. Indeed, healing may occur at any time, independent of recovery from illness. In dying, for example, restoration of wholeness may be manifested by a transcendent set of meaningful experiences while very ill. Eric Cassell has noted that "Transcendence is probably the most powerful way in which one is restored to wholeness after an injury to personhood. When experienced, transcendence locates the person in a far larger landscape" (18). It may be reflected by a peaceful death. In chronic illness, healing may be experienced as the acceptance of limitations (15). A person may look to medical care to alleviate his or her suffering, and when the medical system fails to do so, begin to look toward spirituality for meaning, purpose, and understanding. As people are faced with serious illness or the prospect of dying, questions often arise:

- Why did this happen to me?
- What will happen to me after I die?
- Why would God allow me to suffer this way?
- Will I be remembered?
- Will I be missed?

These questions can cause people to undergo a life review whereby they analyze their lives, accomplishments, relationships, and perceived failings (19). This questioning can result in fears, anxieties, and unresolved feelings, which in turn can result in despair and suffering as people face themselves and their eventual mortality. Cassell wrote, "Since in suffering, disruption of the whole person is the dominant theme, we know of the losses and their meaning by what we know of others out of compassion for their suffering" (20). Compassion is essential in the care of all patients, particularly those who are dealing with chronic and serious illnesses and are dying. Two Latin words form the root of the word compassion: "cum," meaning "with," and "passio," meaning "suffering with" (21). What compassionate care asks us to do is to suffer with our patients, that is, to be present to them fully as they suffer and to partner with them in the midst of their pain.

SPIRITUALITY IN CLINICAL PRACTICE PROFESSIONAL GUIDELINES

Guidelines from several organizations, including the American College of Physicians (ACP) and The Joint Commission on Healthcare Accreditation,

American Association of Nursing, and National Association of Social Workers, recognize the need for spiritual care. In a recent ACP consensus conference on end of life, it was concluded that physicians have the obligation to address all dimensions of suffering, including spiritual, religious, and existential suffering (22). It also developed guidelines for communicating with patients about spiritual and religious matters (23). JCAHO (Joint Commission on Accreditation of Healthcare Organizations) requires that spiritual care be available to patients in hospital settings (24). In 1978, the first nursing diagnosis related to spirituality, spiritual distress, was established in the North American Nursing Diagnosis Association (NANDA). Spiritual distress is the "impaired ability to experience and integrate meaning and purpose in life through a person's connectedness with self, others, art, music, literature, nature, or a power greater than oneself" (25). The Code of Ethics for professional nurses in the United States recognizes the importance of spirituality and health, illustrated by Provision 1 of the code, which states, "The nurse, in all professional relationships, practices with compassion and respect for the inherent dignity, worth, and uniqueness of each individual, unrestricted by considerations of social and economic status, personal attributes, or the nature of health problems" (26). The National Association of Social Workers' Code of Ethics declares that a social worker must include spirituality when completing an assessment (27).

The National Quality Forum identified spiritual care as one of eight domains of the Clinical Practice Guidelines developed by the National Consensus Project for Quality Palliative Care (NCP) (28). The NCP is a coalition of the leading palliative care organizations in the United States. The NCP recommendations for spiritual care emphasize regular and ongoing assessment and response to patients' spiritual and existential issues and concerns. They emphasize the use of a spiritual assessment to identify religious or spiritual/existential preferences, beliefs, rituals, and practices of the patient and family. These guidelines also recognize the need for inclusion of pastoral care in the interdisciplinary care team.

DATA DEMONSTRATING PATIENT NEED

Studies, as well as theoretical and philosophical literature, demonstrate the impact of religious and spiritual beliefs on people's moral decision-making, way of life, ability to transcend suffering, dealing with life's challenges, interactions with others, and life choices. Spiritual and religious beliefs have been shown to have an impact on how people cope

with serious illness, aging, and life stresses. Spiritual practices can foster coping resources (29,30), promote health-related behavior (31), enhance a sense of well-being and improve quality of life (32), provide social support (33), and generate feelings of love and forgiveness (34). Spiritual beliefs can also impact health care decision-making (35). Spiritual/religious beliefs, however, can also be harmful (36). Thus, spirituality may be a critical dynamic of how patients understand their illness and cope with it either positively or negatively.

Research also indicates that patients would like their spiritual beliefs addressed by physicians and other health care professionals in a variety of health care circumstances (37). One study shows that patients feel increased trust in their clinicians if a spiritual history is obtained. They also note that they experience an increased sense of being listened to (37). Interestingly, a study by Balboni et al. showed that 75% of dying cancer patients did not have their spiritual needs met even when 95% of them said spirituality was important to them (38). These data indicate the importance of developing guidelines and resources for patients and clinicians.

RELATIONSHIP BETWEEN SPIRITUALITY AND COPING

The beneficial effects of spirituality in helping people cope with serious illness and dying are well documented (39). Furthermore, researchers have noted that most patients with cancer in a palliative care setting experience spiritual pain, which is expressed as an internal conflict, a loss or interpersonal conflict, or in relation to God/Divine. Fitchett et al. have shown that spiritual struggles are associated with poor physical outcome and higher rates of morbidity (40). Spiritual pain is also related to psychological distress so that patients presenting with depression or anxiety may actually be suffering from spiritual conflict (41).

Quality of life instruments used in end-of-life care try to measure an existential domain, which addresses purpose, meaning in life, and capacity for self-transcendence. In studies of one such instrument, three items have been found to correlate with good quality of life for patients with advanced disease: if the patient's personal existence is meaningful; if the patient finds fulfillment in achieving life goals; and if life to this point has been meaningful (42). This supports the importance of addressing meaning and purpose in a dying person's life. Spirituality and nonorganized religion have also been associated positively with the will to live in patients with acquired immunodeficiency syndrome (HIV) (43).

The observations noted in patient stories (15) and in the writings of Foglio and Brody (17)—that illness can cause people to question their lives, their identities, and what gives their life meaning—are supported by research. For example, in a study of 108 women undergoing treatment for gynecologic cancer, 49% noted becoming more spiritual after their diagnosis (30). In a study of parents with a child who had died of cancer, 40% of those parents reported a strengthening of their own spiritual commitment over the course of the year before their child's death (44). Illness, facing one's mortality, is an opportunity for new experience, self-awareness, and meaning in life.

Religion and religious beliefs can play an important role in how patients understand their illness. In a study asking older adults about God's role in health and illness, many respondents saw health and illness as being partly attributable to God and, to some extent, God's interventions (45). Pargament et al. have studied both positive and negative coping and have found that religious experiences and practices, such as seeking God's help or having a vision of God, extend the individual's coping resources and are associated with improvement in health care outcomes (46). Patients showed less psychological distress if they sought control through a partnership with God or a higher power in a problem-solving way, if they asked God's forgiveness or were able to forgive others, if they reported finding strength and comfort from their spiritual beliefs, and if they found support in a spiritual community. Patients had more depression, poorer quality of life, and callousness toward others if they saw the crisis as a punishment from God, if they had excessive guilt, or if they had an absolute belief in prayer and cure and an inability to resolve their anger if cure did not occur. Pargament et al. have also noted that sometimes patients refuse medical treatment based on religious beliefs (36).

There are a number of studies on meditation as well as other spiritual and religious practices that demonstrate a positive physical response, especially in relation to levels of stress hormones and modulation of the stress response (47). Although more solid evidence is needed, there appears to be an association between meditation and some spiritual or religious practices and certain physiologic processes, including cardiovascular, neuroendocrine, and immune function.

SPIRITUAL COPING

How does spirituality work to help people cope with their dying (Table 46.2)? One mechanism might be through hope. Hope is a powerful inner strength that helps one transcend the present situation and helps foster a positive belief or outlook.

TABLE 46.2 SPIRITUAL COPING

Hope: for a cure, for healing, for finishing important goals, and for a peaceful death

Sense of control

Acceptance of the situation

Strength to deal with the situation

Meaning and purpose: in life and in midst of suffering

Spirituality and religion offer people hope and help people find hope in the midst of the despair that often occurs in the course of serious illness and dying. Hope can change during a course of an illness. Early on, the person may hope for a cure; later, when a cure becomes unlikely, the person may hope for time to finish important projects or goals, travel, make peace with loved ones or with God, and have a peaceful death. This can result in a healing, which can be manifested as a restoration of one's relationships or sense of self. Often our society thinks in terms of cures. Whereas cures may not always be possible, healing—the restoration of wholeness—may be possible to the very end of life. Hope has also been shown to be an effective coping mechanism. Patients who are more hopeful tend to be less depressed.

Religious beliefs offer a sense of hope. For example, in Catholicism, hope in Jesus' promise of victory over death through resurrection and salvation gives Catholics hope in a life beyond death. In the funeral rites, it is stated, "I believe in the resurrection of the dead and the life of the world to come" (48). In the Protestant view, the concept of salvation in death gives hope. Jesus' dying and rising from the dead means that those who participate in His death no longer participate in the sinful human nature (49). In Eastern traditions such as Buddhism and Hinduism, the hope of rebirth and a belief in karma offer people hope in the face of mortality (50). In Judaism, there are many diverse ways of viewing death. For some, hope is found in living on through one's children. In the orthodox and conservative views, there is a belief in a resurrection in which the body arises to be united with the soul (51). For patients with and without specific religious beliefs, there is a need to transcend death, which may also be manifested through living on through one's relationships or one's accomplishments and deeds (52). Irion suggests that humans may create abstractions by portraying a life after death (53). For the religious, this may take the form of concepts found in their religious traditions. For others, life after death might be in terms of one's descendants. For some, it might be being immortalized in the memory of others or in the contributions one makes in life. Cultural beliefs and traditions can also contribute to how people find meaning and hope in the midst of despair (54).

Finding meaning in the midst of suffering and uncertainty is critical to effective coping. Spiritual beliefs in general and religious, in particular, can help people find this meaning and purpose. Religion provides a system of beliefs, ritual, and community that can help people find meaning in the context of their illness and dying (55). One very powerful intervention that addresses meaning with patients with advanced cancer has had positive outcomes in these patients. It involved a brief meaning-centered group psychotherapy intervention that is centered on helping patients find meaning in the midst of their suffering (56).

Spirituality can offer people a sense of control. Illness can disrupt life completely. Some people find a sense of control by turning worries or a situation over to a higher power or to God (57). Similarly, people can use their beliefs to help them accept their illness and find strength to deal with their situation (58). Reconciliation may be an important aspect of a dying person's spiritual journey. Often people seek to forgive others or themselves as they review their lives and their relationships.

SPIRITUAL ISSUES: DIAGNOSIS AND RESOURCES OF STRENGTH

The diagnosis of chronic or life-threatening illness or other adverse life events can lead to spiritual struggles for patients. The turmoil may be short for some patients and protracted for others as individuals attempt to integrate the reality of their diagnosis with their spiritual beliefs. The journey may result in growth and transformation for some people and to distress and despair for others (59).

Studies have found that patients with spiritual or religious struggles had poorer physical health, worse quality of life, and greater depression (60); those with chronic spiritual or religious struggles also had increased disability (59) and higher indices of pain and fatigue and more difficulties with daily physical functioning (61). Religious struggle has also been found to be a significant predictor of increased mortality, even when controlling for demographic, physical health, and mental health factors (62). Poorer quality of life and greater emotional distress were found among patients with diabetes and congestive heart failure who experience religious struggle (41).

Spirituality may also present as a source of strength for patients. The act of seeking forgiveness or the willingness to forgive may be a spiritual strength. The Joint Commission notes that adult and older adult strengths may include "cultural/ spiritual/religious and community involvement" (63). Another example of spiritual strength may be a patient's connection to God or the sacred. Spiritual strengths may help patients cope, find hope in the midst of suffering, find joy in life, and/or find the ability to be grateful (64).

The clinical aspect of spirituality that is critical especially in patients with serious and chronic illness is spiritual distress seen as a symptom that must be managed with the same intensity as physical pain. The NCCN defined spiritual distress symptoms (cite) and in the 2009 consensus conference a list of those diagnosis and others were defined as spiritual distress diagnosis.

These are described in the table below.

SPIRITUAL DISTRESS OR CONCERNS (6)

Diagnoses (primary)	Key feature from history	Example statements
Existential	Lack of meaning/Questions meaning about one's own existence/Concern about afterlife/ Questions the meaning of suffering/Seeks spiritual assistance	"My life is meaningless" "I feel useless"
Abandonment God or others	Lack of love, loneliness/Not being remembered/No Sense of Relatedness	"God has abandoned me" "No one comes by anymore"
Anger at God or others	Displaces anger toward religious representatives/Inability to Forgive	"Why would God take my child... its not fair"
Concerns about relationship with deity	Closeness to God, deepening relationship	"I want to have a deeper relationship with God"
Conflicted or challenged belief systems	Verbalizes inner conflicts or questions about beliefs or faith Conflicts between religious beliefs and recommended treatments/Questions moral or ethical implications of therapeutic regimen/Express concern with life/death and/or belief system	"I am not sure if God is with me anymore"

Personal and professional caregivers also have similar spiritual issues, as well as spiritual issues that relate to the caregiving role.

In addition to identifying and addressing the spiritual issues discussed in the preceding section, it is important to assess the spiritual resources of strength for patients—hope, sense of meaning and purpose, ability to transcend suffering, as well as support from spiritual or religious community, family, or friends.

Communities, such as churches, temples, mosques, spiritual, or other support groups or a group of like-minded friends, can serve as strong support systems for some patients. The absence of these resources could impact in an adverse way on how patients cope with illness and/or dying.

SPIRITUAL CARE: FRAMEWORK OF CARE

An approach to the care of a patient is to recognize that spirituality is an essential part of being human. It is the part of a person that seeks transcendent meaning and purpose in life. It is that part of each individual from which each person can heal by becoming whole again in the midst of suffering, loss, and stress. Therefore, in caring for patients, health care professionals must not only attend to the physical, emotional, and social domains of a patient's life as is supported by the biopsychosocial model of care but also the spiritual domain, therefore a biopsychosocial–spiritual model of care. In a recent Ethics Conference with the George Washington Institute of Spirituality and Health, as well as the AAMC, spiritual care was described as an essential element of health care and not an amenity (65).

During the time a person experiences illness, suffering, loss, or stress, he or she will engage actively in the health care system. Health care professionals will often meet people during profoundly difficult times in their patients' lives. During these times, patients are vulnerable and often afraid, lonely, and confused. Spiritual care offers a framework for health care professionals to connect with their patients, listen to their fears, dreams, and pain, collaborate with their patients as partners in their care, and provide through the therapeutic relationship an opportunity for healing. Healing is distinguished from cure in this context. It refers to the ability of a person to find solace, comfort, connection, meaning, and purpose in the midst of suffering, disarray, and pain. The care the clinician provides is rooted in spirituality through compassion, hopefulness, and the recognition that although a person's life may be limited or no longer socially productive, it remains full of possibility (66).

There are studies that document the importance of the doctor–patient relationship (67). Dr. Francis Peabody wrote in his 1927 medical classic, *The Care of the Patient*, "One of the essential qualities of the clinician is interest in humanity, for the secret care of the patient is in caring for the patient" (68). This relationship can have potential positive impact on health care outcomes, compliance, and patient satisfaction (67). Because healing springs from the therapeutic relationship, spiritual care is grounded in relationship-centered care. Spiritual care begins from the moment the health care professional enters the patient's room.

SPIRITUAL CARE: PRACTICE WITH INTENTION

The health care practitioner intentionally opens himself or herself to the possibility of openness, connection, and mystery. Intention to openness refers to the willingness to listen to the patient without a preconceived agenda, with full respect of the patient as an individual with a unique story (cultural, personal, and spiritual), and a commitment to be fully present in the encounter with the patient. Intention to connection refers to the willingness and ability to actively and appropriately form a connection with the patient on a spiritual and emotional level thereby affording the patient the opportunity to experience a sense of belonging, care, and love. By relating from our humanness, we can help to form deeper and more meaningful connections with our patients. Intention to mystery refers to the acceptance that none of us controls another, life, outcome, or ourselves. Life is full of mysteries—being open to mystery allows the health care practitioner to let go of a need to be in control and fully responsible for outcome. It implies a humbleness as one accepts that both the health care practitioner and the patient are walking a journey together, which may have many unplanned and unexpected turns. This reframes the commitment from fixing or solving to a commitment of presence, persistence, partnership, and a willingness to walk with the unknown and handle situations as they arise together. It removes the illusion of expert and client and offers the reality of spiritually equal partners.

In order to be able to engage in spiritual care, health care professionals need training on how to be intentionally open, willing, and accepting of mystery. This means that the clinician brings his or her whole being to the encounter and places full attention on the patient, not allowing distractions to interfere with that attention. Integral to this is the ability to listen and to be attentive to all dimensions of patients' and their family's lives.

Some clinicians suggest that current medical practices do not allow enough time for this. However, being wholly present to the patient is not time dependent. It simply requires the intention on the part of the physician to be fully present for their patients. One becomes fully present when one approaches the patient with deep respect, respect stemming from a commitment to honoring of the whole person. Mohamad Reaz Abdullah of the Asian Institute for Development Communication (AidCom) said, "When we say 'I respect you,' what exactly are we saying? We are really respecting a quality that has been expressed by the person, and we are forming a symbiotic relationship with a quality that we admire. However, when the divinity in the individual that is common to all beings is respected, then the meaning of respect is taken on golden wings to a new height." This is the essence of a spiritually based relationship with others.

Relationship-centered care is intense and personal as it opens up to the possibility of emotional and spiritual reaction on the part of both patient and health care professional. Both patients and health care professionals can be transformed as a result of their interaction in clinical environments. This requires an awareness of the clinician's own values, beliefs, and attitudes, particularly toward their own mortality. By confronting one's own mortality, one can better understand what the patient is facing. Many clinicians speak of their own spiritual practices and how those practices help them in their ability to deliver good spiritual care and, in fact, good medical care (15,69). Therefore, in order to practice spiritual care effectively, the health care professional needs to be aware of, and supported in, their spiritual needs and journey. It is also critical to train and support the health care professional on how to practice relationship-centered care in a way that respects the power differential of the contextual relationship—doctor–patient, nurse–patient, and so on.

INTRINSIC AND EXTRINSIC SPIRITUAL CARE

All medical care has intrinsic (the behavior, attitudes, and values the health care professionals bring to the encounter) and extrinsic aspects (the knowledge and skills applied in the encounter). The relationship-centered aspect of medical care is the intrinsic essential aspect of all care from which extrinsic care emanates, including physical, emotional, and social care. That is, spiritual intrinsic care refers to the intention of presence; physical extrinsic care refers to taking vital signs, for example, and spiritual extrinsic care refers to the ability to reorganize spiritual issues and problems

as they present in relationship to the presenting health care problem or situation. It also refers to recognizing patients' inner resources of strength or a lack of those resources. Once these are recognized, clinicians then incorporate patients' spirituality into the care plan if appropriate to the clinical situation. Everyone on the interdisciplinary health care team practices spiritual care, but the specifics of how the spiritual care is delivered is dependent on the context, which it is given. A chaplain provides spiritual care in the context of his or her training as a spiritual counselor in health care setting, a clergy provides spiritual care in the context of a religious setting, and a nurse and physician practice spiritual care in the context of caring for patients in a spiritual health care situation (hospital, clinic, patient visits, and education). Although the relationship-centered caring aspects are similar in how each profession deals with the patient, how patient's spiritual issues and problems are dealt with depend on the health care professional's level of training and context. Chaplains and clergy work primarily with spiritual issues and spiritual problems in-depth and not necessarily in relation to health and illness. They may be secondarily aware of and interface with social, emotional, and physical issues but deal with them more in a supportive way. Nurses and doctors are trained primarily to address the physical issues with which patients present. However, emotional, social, and spiritual issues may affect or be related to the physical issue. Therefore, nurses and doctors recognize, support, and/or triage those spiritual issues appropriately to the spiritual care professionals (Table 46.3).

TABLE 46.3 SPIRITUAL CARE

Compassionate presence
Intention to openness
Intention to connection
Intention to mystery

Relationship-centered care
Partnership
Not agenda driven
Listening to patients' fears, hopes, dreams, and meaning

Spirituality of health care professional
Awareness of one's own spirituality
Awareness of one's own mortality
Having a spiritual practice

Extrinsic spiritual care
Taking a spiritual history
Recognizing patients' spiritual issues
Recognizing patients' spiritual problems or spiritual pain
Recognizing patients' resources of inner strength or lack of resources
Incorporating patients' spirituality into treatment or care plans (presence, referral, rituals, meditation, etc.)

A CONSENSUS-BASED INTERPROFESSIONAL MODEL OF SPIRITUAL CARE

In 2009, 40 interdisciplinary experts in palliative care participated in the 2009 National Consensus Conference for Spiritual Care in Palliative Care (NCC) to develop recommendations for improving spiritual care in palliative care settings, with palliative care broadly defined as care for patients with chronic or life-threatening illness (6). Conference participants produced a consensus-based definition of spirituality for clinical settings that recognizes that each person's spirituality is unique and may or may not include religious beliefs and/or cultural practices:

> Spirituality is the aspect of humanity that refers to the way individuals seek and express meaning and purpose, and the way they experience their connectedness to the moment, to self, to others, to nature, and to the significant or sacred. Building on this meeting a global consensus conference developed a definition of spirituality that included many different cultural perspectives: "Spirituality is a dynamic and intrinsic aspect of humanity through which persons seek ultimate meaning, purpose, and transcendence, and experience relationship to self, family, others, community, society, nature, and the significant or sacred. Spirituality is expressed through beliefs, values, traditions, and practices" (70).

The practice of spiritual care is based on a generalist-specialist model of care called the Interprofessional Spiritual Care Model. Spiritual care involves the assessment and treatment of spiritual distress, support for spiritual resources of strength and in-depth spiritual counseling when appropriate (71). Clinicians address spiritual concerns, do spiritual screening or histories to assess for spiritual distress and work with spiritual care specialists such as chaplains, pastoral counselors, or spiritual directors in treating and attending to spiritual distress. Health care chaplains have the skill and expertise to assess and address the spiritual and existential issues frequently faced by pediatric and adult patients with acute or chronic pain or receiving palliative care and their families would be available to address these needs. Chaplains play a strong role as professional members of the health care team. Spiritual care is best provided in an interdisciplinary, team-based care environment with strong ties to the communities they serve (70). In the community setting, the spiritual care expert may be clergy, pastoral counselors, or spiritual directors.

Spiritual care refers to many different aspects of care ranging from the intrinsic (presence to patients' suffering, honoring dignity of patients, recognition of the concept of healing, and the role of spirituality in the healing process) to extrinsic (doing a spiritual history, integration of spirituality into the treatment plan, and follow-up on spiritual issues as appropriate). As cited in many guidelines, it is the obligation of all clinicians, to attend to all dimensions of the suffering of the patient and the patient's family; second to elicit the patient's spiritual needs; and third, to respect those beliefs and struggles. But, nonchaplain clinicians need to recognize the limits of their expertise (64) and should not engage in significant spiritual counseling. The separation of responsibilities between clinicians and chaplains and/or the patient's personal clergy recognizes both specific expertise and ethical concerns—patients may tell physicians things they would not tell clergy and vice versa.

Thus, the physician, nurse, and social worker should engage in the spiritual aspects of illness by being present to all patients, honoring their dignity, and taking a spiritual history or a screening to identify patients' spiritual issues. For simple issues, as discussed below, medical clinicians may work with patients to address those needs. For more complex issues or if the simple issues are not resolved, then patients should be referred to board-certified or board-eligible chaplains. All issues, whether simple or complex, should be documented in the patient's chart appropriately and shared with the health care team.

The NCC also described the concept of spiritual distress as a diagnosis, which should be treated with the same intensity as physical pain. An algorithm was developed whereby clinicians would evaluate patient distress in the biopsychosocial–spiritual framework. This framework recognized that pain not only may be physical but also may have psychosocial or spiritual aspects as well, that is, suffering. Spiritual screening would identify if a patient is in spiritual distress and should therefore need an urgent chaplain referral. Spiritual history, a more complete assessment done by clinicians doing a treatment or care plan, would further identify more about types of spiritual issues that cause the distress as well as identify spiritual resources of strength. Clinicians would then refer to chaplains for a more complete spiritual assessment as well as treatment of spiritual distress. Ideally, the treatment or care plan is developed by the interdisciplinary team, which should also include a chaplain.

The NCC produced guidelines, for taking a spiritual history and for the formulation of spiritual treatment or care plans, which include the following:

- All health care professionals should be trained in doing a spiritual screening or history as part of their routine history and evaluation.
- Spiritual screenings, histories, and assessments should be communicated and documented in patient records (e.g., charts and computerized

databases shared with the interprofessional health care team).

- Follow-up spiritual histories or assessments should be conducted for all patients whose medical, psychosocial, or spiritual condition changes and as part of routine follow-up in a medical history.
- A spiritual issue becomes a diagnosis if the following criteria are met: (a) the spiritual issue leads to distress or suffering (e.g., lack of meaning, conflicted religious beliefs, and inability to forgive); (b) the spiritual issue is the cause of a psychological or physical diagnosis such as depression, anxiety, or acute or chronic pain (e.g., severe meaninglessness that leads to depression or suicidality and guilt that leads to chronic physical pain); and (c) the spiritual issue is a secondary cause or affects the presenting psychological or physical diagnosis (e.g., hypertension is difficult to control because the patient refuses to take medications because of his or her religious beliefs).
- Treatment or care plans should include but not be limited to referral to chaplains, spiritual directors, pastoral counselors, and other spiritual care providers, including clergy or faith-community healers for spiritual counseling; development of spiritual goals; meaning-oriented therapy; mind–body interventions; rituals, spiritual practices; and contemplative interventions.
- Spiritual diagnosis, resources of strength, as well as the spiritual treatment plan should be documented in the chart.

Obtaining a spiritual history is one way of listening to what is deeply important to the patient (72). When one gets involved in a discussion with a patient about his or her spirituality, one enters the domain of what gives the person meaning and purpose in life and how that person copes with stress, illness, and dying. The spiritual history affords the patient the space and opportunity to address his or her suffering and hopes. A spiritual history validates the importance of a patient's spirituality and gives the patient permission to discuss their spirituality, if they desire to. Having the physician or other clinician inquire about the patient's spiritual beliefs gives the patient an opening and an invitation to discuss spiritual beliefs, if that is what the patient would like to do. It also enables the physician to connect with the patient on a deep, caring level. In fact, many physicians who obtain spiritual histories remark that the nature of the doctor–patient relationship changes. As soon as they bring up these questions, they feel that it establishes a level of intimacy and an understanding of who the person is at a much deeper level than is typical. The relationship feels less superficial (72).

Patients note that they feel more trusting of a physician who addresses and respects their spiritual beliefs. In one survey, 65% of patients in a pulmonary outpatient clinic noted that a physician's inquiry about spiritual beliefs would strengthen their trust in the physician (73).

TREATMENT OF CARE PLAN

Once the clinician identifies the spiritual distress or spiritual resources of strength or resources for coping, the clinician should then integrate that into the patient treatment or care plan and document this in the chart. Spiritual distress needs to be attended with the same urgency as any other distress. Thus, patients with moderate or severe spiritual distress or with religious-specific needs should be referred to the board-certified chaplain. Some types of spiritual distress, which one might classify as minimal or mild, might be able to be attended to by other clinicians on the team. In the NCC, these would be classified as simple spiritual issues. An example might be patient not clear about meaning and purpose but is not particularly distressed by this. Talking about this to the clinician might be helpful as just telling of one's story can sometimes be enough for the patient to find an answer for themselves. Or other providers, such as art therapists, might be a helpful resource. The patient might also share spiritual practices that are important to the patient. These might be prayer, meditation, listening to certain music, enjoying solitude, writing poetry, or journeying. The clinician can then incorporate these practices as appropriate. However, if the patient is in significant spiritual distress, this would be a complex spiritual issue, and therefore, a referral to the chaplain would be recommended. If the clinician initially thought the spiritual issue was simple, but the initial interventions did not work, then a referral should be made to the board-certified chaplain.

Possible options for a spiritual care plan, then, are as follows:

- Referrals to:
  - Appropriate spiritual care professionals, such as chaplains, pastoral counselors, and spiritual directors—especially with complex spiritual issues
  - A meaning-centered psychotherapy group
  - Music thanatologists
  - Art therapy
  - Meditation
  - Yoga and tai chi
  - Specific spiritual support groups
  - Religious or sacred spiritual reading or rituals (based on what the patient has identified as appropriate for them)

- Incorporating spiritual practices or rituals as appropriate
- Presence to patient as he or she works on spiritual issues with the health care professional

SPIRITUAL HISTORY

The main elements of a spiritual history, which have been developed for physicians and other health care providers, can be recalled by using the acronym "FICA" (Table 46.4) (72). This acronym helps clinicians to structure questions that help elicit patients' spiritual beliefs and values. This tool was developed with a focus group of primary care physicians. The goal was to identify the basic information clinicians need to know in order to determine how a patient's spirituality might impact their care. The tool is primarily used as a way to invite the patient to share their spiritual beliefs and values with their clinician, if they would like to. Anecdotal evidence suggests that patients experienced increased trust in their clinician once these conversations are initiated. Patients also express feeling respected and that the clinician is interested in who they are as people. Clinicians also find that the information obtained from the spiritual history allows the clinician to come up with a more comprehensive treatment plan.

The initial question of FICA affords the patient the opportunity to talk about spiritual matters. These spiritual issues can be religious, spiritual, or other sources of deep meaning and purpose in life. In this first question, it is important to assess what the patient's belief system is and also if that belief system or something else gives meaning to the person's life. The second question allows the clinician to determine if these belief systems are important to the patient. For some people, identified spiritual beliefs may not be important to them but there may be other philosophies or activities that give deeper meaning or purpose. This is also the place where patients might reveal if they have any spiritual issues that need attending to. For example, patients might reveal spiritual distress, such as meaninglessness or guilt. It is also important to know if there is anything else about the belief system that might impact health care decision-making. This is particularly important with advanced directives: wishes for how a patient would like to be treated and who should be involved in the decision-making process. Many patients would like their clergy or culturally based healers involved. The fourth question has to do with the extrinsic aspect of the patient's belief system—is there a community that the patient identifies as their spiritual or main support community. This could be church, temple, or mosque or could be like-minded friends, family, or other spiritual support group (e.g., a cancer support group could be thought of by some as a spiritual support group). Finally, the "A" (assessment or action) section is not a specific question one has to ask, but rather it is one to be considered in terms of what specific aspects of the treatment plan might be affected. So, if the patient is in spiritual distress, a referral to a chaplain might be appropriate. Or if a patient would like to learn to meditate, then a referral to a teacher or class might be beneficial.

FICA is not meant to be used as a checklist, but rather as a guide as to how to start the spiritual history and what to listen for as the patient talks about his or her beliefs. Mostly, FICA is a tool to help physicians and other health care providers know how to open a conversation to spiritual issues and issues of meaning and value. In the context of the spiritual history, patients may relate those fears, dreams, and hopes to their care provider. The spiritual history can be done in the context of a routine history or at any time in the patient interview, usually as a part of the social history. In addition to religious or spiritual beliefs and values and other aspects of the spiritual history, the social history should address lifestyle, home situation, and primary relationships; other important relationships and social environment; work situation and employment; social interests/avocation; life stresses; and lifestyle risk factors (e.g., tobacco, alcohol, or illicit drugs).

The spiritual history is patient centered. One should always respect patients' wishes and understand appropriate boundaries. Physicians and other health care providers must respect patients' privacy regarding matters of spirituality and religion and should avoid imposing their own beliefs on the patient (74).

The following case illustrates how FICA can be used. A patient who died of metastatic malignant melanoma was an Episcopalian. Her religious beliefs were central to her life and, in fact, were the means through which she came to be at peace with dying. During her last hospitalization, the house officers caring for her were apprehensive about discussing advance directives and dying. However, during the spiritual history, the patient told them how her religious beliefs helped her come to terms with dying and how she was ready to die naturally. She handed them her living will. She also asked that her church members be allowed to visit her often. She later told me that being asked about her beliefs helped her feel respected and valued by the physicians and that she felt that she could trust them more. The physicians stated that once they asked a spiritual history, the nature of the interaction between themselves and this patient changed. It felt "more natural, more comfortable, warmer, and more honest."

TABLE 46.4 FICA

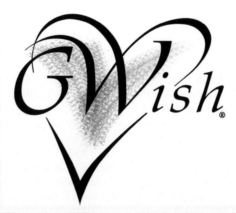

FICA Spiritual History Tool©*

Spiritual histories are taken as part of the regular history during an annual examination or new patient visit, but they also can be taken as part of follow-up visits, as appropriate. The acronym FICA not only can help to structure questions for health care professionals who are taking a spiritual history to learn more about a patient's spirituality and meaning but also may help identify spiritual distress and resources of strength. The FICA Spiritual History Tool© is not a checklist, but rather serves as a guide for conversations in clinical settings.

F—Faith, Belief, Meaning

"Do you consider yourself to be spiritual?" or "Is spirituality something important to you?"
"Do you have spiritual beliefs, practices, or values that help you to cope with stress, difficult times, or what you are going through right now?" *(Contextualize question to reason for visit if it is not the routine history.)*

"What gives your life meaning?" *(The question of meaning should be asked regardless of whether the patient answered "yes" or "no" about spirituality. Sometimes patients respond to the meaning question with answers involving family, career, or nature.)*

I—Importance and Influence

"What importance does spirituality have in your life?" *(For people not identifying with spiritual ask about the importance of their sources of meaning)*

"Has your spirituality (*or sources of meaning*) influenced how you take care of yourself, particularly regarding your health?" "Does your spirituality affect your health care decision-making? *(Answers to these questions may provide insight regarding treatment plans, advance directives, etc.)*

C—Community

"Are you part of a spiritual community?"
"Is your community of support to you and how?" For people who don't identify with a community consider asking "Is there a group of people you really love or who are important to you?"
(Communities such as churches, temples, mosques, family, groups of like-minded friends, or yoga or similar groups can serve as strong support systems for some patients.)

A—Address/Action in Care

"How would you like me, as your health care provider, to address spiritual issues in your health care?" *(With newer models, including the diagnosis of spiritual distress, "A" also refers to the "Assessment and Plan" for patient spiritual distress, needs and/or resources within a treatment or care plan.)*

© Copyright Christina Puchalski, MD, and The George Washington University 1996 (updated 2021). All rights reserved.
*Adapted from Puchalski, C, Romer, AL. Taking a spiritual history allows clinicians to understand patients more fully. *J Palliat Med.* 2000;3(1):129-137.

Another case illustrates the variability encountered in practice. When asked "if you have any spiritual beliefs that help you with stress," a patient undergoing a routine examination answered that she found meaning and purpose while sitting in the woods near her house—that nature brought her peace. This was very important to her, as she noted that on days when she did not meditate there in the morning, she would become scattered and tense. Her community consisted of a group of like-minded friends who shared her beliefs. She asked that her medical record indicate that when she became seriously ill or dying, she wanted a room in her hospice overlooking the trees. She also asked to learn basic meditation techniques. In a subsequent visit many months later, she reported that she had stopped meditating, with negative results; resuming meditation helped her cope better with her stress.

ETHICAL ISSUES: ROLE OF SPIRITUALITY IN THE CLINICAL SETTING

It is critical for physicians and other health care providers to address spiritual issues with their patients because spirituality affects patients' clinical care in a direct manner. Spiritual issues can impact clinical care in various ways, which are illustrated by the following cases.

Case 1

Spiritual beliefs may be a dynamic in patients' understanding of their illness. Julie was a 28-year-old woman whose husband left her recently. She learned through the family grapevine that he has HIV. She came into a clinic and saw a physician for the first time to get tested for HIV. When she returned to the clinic for her test results, she found out that she was HIV positive. The physician attempted to present an optimistic picture by relaying all the newest information on treatment for HIV. The patient, however, continued to cry out about "God doing this to me." The physician persisted in discussion of the medical and technical aspects of the diagnosis, while the patient continued to make references to God. After some time, the physician asked the patient why she thought her illness was coming from God. She told the physician that she was raped as a teenager, got pregnant, and had an abortion. She said, "I have been waiting for the punishment for 15 years, and this is it." The patient refused all medications and treatment.

Patients come to understand their health, illness, and dying through their beliefs, cultural backgrounds, past experience, and values. In this case, Julie had been carrying guilt for an event that happened many years before. The temptation for the physician was to alleviate this guilt by talking about how understandable the abortion was in the context of the rape. However, this is not what the patient felt, and by trying to erase her guilt, it actually precluded the patient from talking about her feelings. The physician instead listened to the patient and did not force the issue of medications and preventive care. The physician continued to see the patient regularly, listening to her issues around the diagnosis. She also referred Julie to a chaplain who worked further with Julie on these

issues. It took approximately a year before Julie was able to see God as forgiving and was able to forgive herself. It was then that she could focus on the treatment of her HIV disease. Issues like these can be complicated. What part of Julie's beliefs came from strongly held religious dogma and what part from low self-esteem or depression? Chaplains are trained to understand the difference in the roots of these beliefs, and they are trained to help patients resolve these types of conflicts. In addition, physicians can be helpful by listening to patients, giving patients the time to resolve conflicts, and respecting patients' rights to their own beliefs.

Case 2

Religious convictions/beliefs may affect health care decision-making. Frank was an 88-year-old man dying of pancreatic cancer in the intensive care unit. He was on pressors and a ventilator. The team approached the family about withdrawing support. The family was very religious and believed that their father's life was in God's hands; they believed that there would be a miracle and that their father would survive.

These types of cases are very common and are often handled poorly. Physicians and intensive care unit teams get frustrated that patients' families cannot see that their loved one is dying, and the family feels hurt and angry that the medical teams do not understand their beliefs. The discussion often gets polarized and difficult to resolve. It is critical that the medical teams, even if they do not agree with the family, respect family beliefs. Often, simply listening to the family about what they mean by a "miracle" can open up the conversation to many feelings that the family is experiencing. For example, the physician could simply say, "I can understand that a miracle would be wonderful," and then wait to see what the family says. Or the physician could ask, "What does a miracle mean to you?" If families feel respected, they are not as likely to feel threatened and that the medical team opposes them. The medical team, in turn, can get to know the values and beliefs of the family. Referral to a chaplain would be critical in this case. The chaplain, someone who is not perceived as being a part of the medical team per se, can explore the issues of miracles in a very nonthreatening way.

In Frank's case, the chaplain worked with the family. Over time, they began to see the possibility of a miracle independent of whether their father was on a ventilator. The family was then at peace with withdrawing ventilator support. The family was invited to bring their minister in during the whole process, and there were prayers and rituals at the bedside. Their father lived for several days and then died at peace.

Case 3

Spirituality may be a patient need. Rebecca was a 60-year-old woman who had a stroke and had had diabetes and hypertension for many years. She was very debilitated, being wheelchair bound with a speech impediment. Her major coping strategy was prayer. She was Catholic. Her church group and family were her major social supports. It was very important for her to discuss her spiritual beliefs with her physician.

Rebecca's faith was central to her life and was the basis of all her decisions. It was the way she coped with the effects of her chronic illnesses and with her dying. It was important for her to talk about her faith at every visit. She had an inner strength that was rooted in her religious beliefs and enabled her to withstand numerous physical and emotional challenges. In the end, it was her faith that probably gave her the will to live beyond what medical statistics would have predicted for someone as ill as she was. Daily prayer was so important to her that it also became an indicator for her well-being. At one point in her illness, she became very depressed. Although she denied symptoms of depression, she related that she was too tired to pray. She was then able to recognize symptoms of depression. Her church group was also a strong support. In fact, they were so present to her that they were clearly part of her extended family.

Case 4

Spirituality may be important in patient coping. Ronda was a 54-year-old woman with advanced ovarian cancer. Her husband, who was her major support, died unexpectedly. Ronda, who was Jewish, dealt with her suffering and depression through her faith in God. She also joined Jewish Healing Services for support and guidance.

Ronda was raised Jewish but was not observant throughout her adult life. She described herself as an optimist and saw that attitude as an inner strength. Her will to live was strong, and her fight to survive her cancer in the face of dismal odds gave her meaning in life. She spoke of her cancer as a gift in that it gave her a new perspective of life. She came to understand her life in a different, deeper way. She expressed a sense of gratitude for being alive each moment of the day and did not take anything, or anyone, for granted. During times of stress and loss, she relied on her inner strength as a resource. She reached out to support networks, such as the Jewish Healing Services. When her cancer metastasized, she looked at her religious roots for an understanding of death and of suffering. It was important for her to talk with her physicians about these issues and for her to be respected. For a physician to dismiss her will to live and try new therapies simply because of a statistical understanding of her disease would be to dismiss who she is as a person, a "statistic of one," as she said. It was important for her to be able to talk with her physician about her will to live and also about her search for meaning in the midst of suffering. She made a "dream list" as to what was important for her to accomplish before her death. Therapy was adjusted around her ability to complete her dream list.

Case 5

Spirituality may be integral to whole patient care. Joe was a 42-year-old man with irritable bowel syndrome. He had major stressors in his life, including a failed marriage and dissatisfaction at work. He had signs of depression, including insomnia, excessive worrying, decreased appetite, and anhedonia. Overall, he felt that he had no meaning and purpose in life.

Joe did not respond to medication and diet changes alone. However, with the addition of meditation and counseling, Joe improved. In this case, the physical, emotional, social, and spiritual issues all interplayed and affected how he coped with illness.

ETHICAL ISSUES: PROFESSIONAL AND PERSONAL BOUNDARIES

Performing a spiritual history has been included in coursework on spirituality and medicine (50). The spiritual history emphasizes the practice of compassion with one's patients and helps the clinician learn to integrate patients' spiritual concerns into the therapeutic plans. Given the data suggesting that spirituality may be beneficial for patients who are coping with illness, health care institutions should have written policies stating that the patient has a right to express his or her spirituality and religiosity in a respectful and supportive clinical environment.

Physicians should strive to discuss patients' spiritual concerns in a respectful manner and as directed by the patient. The spiritual history is patient centered, not physician centered (Table 46.5). A physician should always respect patients' privacy regarding matters of spirituality and religion and must be vigilant in avoiding imposing his or her beliefs on the patients. The relationship between physician and patient is not an equal one. There is an intimacy in the relationship, but it is intimacy with formality. The patient comes to the physician in a vulnerable time of his or her life, often looking to the physician as a person of authority. The physician should not abuse that authority by imposing his or her own beliefs, or lack of beliefs, onto patients. A vulnerable patient may adopt a physician's belief simply

TABLE 46.5 ETHICAL AND PROFESSIONAL BOUNDARIES

Spiritual history: patient centered

Recognition of pastoral care professionals as experts

Proselytizing is not acceptable in professional settings

More in-depth spiritual counseling should be under the direction of chaplains and other spiritual leaders

Praying with patients:
    Not initiated by physicians unless there is no pastoral care available and the patient requests it
    Physician can stand in silence as patient prays in his or her tradition
    Referral to pastoral care for chaplain-led prayer

because the patient is fearful and assumes the physician knows more. In terms of spiritual intervention, physicians can recommend a variety of interventions, such as chaplain referral, meditation, yoga, prayer, or other spiritual practice. But the decision to recommend these comes from the patient. For example, physicians could recommend religious and spiritual practices to a patient if these practices are already part of that patient's belief system. However, an agnostic patient should not be told to engage in worship any more than a highly religious patient should be criticized for frequent church attendance. Therefore, if a patient states that prayer helps with stress, the physician could suggest that prayer might help in dealing with a serious diagnosis. Or, if a patient finds meaning and purpose in nature, a physician might suggest meditation techniques focused on nature.

Patients sometimes ask their physician about the physician's beliefs. Given the unequal relationship between patient and physician, it is important that the question be handled carefully and with the same guidelines that are used when addressing other sensitive issues such as sexual history or domestic violence. Patients sometimes ask personal questions of their physicians to take the attention off themselves. Sometimes, it is to see if they can connect with the physician by reassuring themselves that the physician has the same beliefs as they. In general, if asked about his or her own beliefs, the physician could ask the patient why it is important for him or her to know that information. The physician can reassure the patient that the focus of the encounter is on the patient's needs and issues, not the doctor's. In some cases, patients still feel the need to know. A patient of a certain religious belief may want to work only with a doctor of that same religion. In some cases, it may not be possible to accommodate the patient, but at least the physician can explore with the patient the rea-

sons for the request. Some patients want to know that their beliefs will not be ridiculed. A response from the physician that he or she respects and supports a patient's beliefs might serve to reassure the patient. In general, it is best to avoid sharing one's personal beliefs unless one already knows the patient and is comfortable that this sharing would not coerce the patient into adopting the physician's beliefs or intimidate the patient from sharing more about his or her own beliefs. A physician should not do anything that violates his or her own comfort level as well. Many physicians prefer to keep their private lives private in the professional context of the doctor–patient relationship.

Patients often ask physicians to pray with them. A physician need not worry that it is somehow inappropriate to allow a moment of silence or a prayer if the patient requests this. In fact, walking away and not showing respect for the request may leave the patient with a sense of abandonment by the physician. If the physician feels conflicted about praying with patients, he or she needs to only stand by quietly as the patient prays in his or her own tradition. Alternatively, the physician could suggest calling in the chaplain or the patient's clergyperson to lead a prayer. Physician-led prayer is generally not recommended, as that is usually the role of the clergy or chaplain. In addition, having the physician lead a prayer opens the possibility of having the prayer be of the physician's belief, not of the patient's. Furthermore, clergy and chaplains are trained specifically in techniques of leading prayer in ecumenical and health care contexts.

Appropriate referrals to chaplains are important to good health care practice and are as appropriate as referrals to other specialists. Chaplains are clergy or laypersons certified in a pastoral training program designed to train them as chaplains. Chaplains work in hospital settings, outpatient clinics, businesses, schools, and prisons. They are trained to be spiritual care providers working with people to explore meaning in life, cope with suffering, and use their beliefs to help them cope with illness or stress. Chaplains work with people of all faiths, as well as with nonreligious people. Clergy are trained to provide religious care usually only to people of their specific denomination.

Where are the boundaries between what chaplains do and what physicians do? Some would argue that discussions with patients about spiritual matters should be initiated solely by chaplains (75). Physicians can use spiritual histories as a screening tool. By inquiring about a patient's beliefs, the physician can evaluate whether the beliefs are helpful or harmful to the patient's health and medical care. If a patient has beliefs that support him or her and give meaning and peace of mind, the physician can encourage those beliefs. In cases in which spiritual beliefs interfere with a patient's getting needed therapy, for example, a patient who thinks an illness is a punishment caused by God and therefore refuses medicine or treatment because of a feeling that the punishment is deserved, a referral to a chaplain would be very helpful. Patients have the right to refuse medical treatment. However, it is important that the choice be made with full informed consent. Therefore, if a patient refuses treatment based on a religious or spiritual belief, it may be appropriate to refer the patient to a chaplain so that the chaplain can explore these beliefs with the patient.

Sometimes, refusal of treatment is based on accepted religious tenets. Other times, the patient may attribute the reasons for refusal to religious beliefs when it actually stems from other concerns, such as lack of self-esteem or depression. The chaplain is trained to explore the beliefs with the patient further and help the patient differentiate between the two. The physician should be respectful of the patient's beliefs, but still explain the consequences of refusal of treatment without being coercive. This way the patient can have enough medical and spiritual information to make a fully informed decision. Physicians in general are not trained to explore the theological aspects of belief, although they can listen and learn about belief from patients. However, physicians can listen to and support patients as they make decisions for themselves. Sometimes, simply listening to a patient in a nonjudgmental fashion and asking a few open-ended questions, such as "tell me more about your belief," can help patients resolve issues of belief and treatment for themselves.

Although many studies suggest that spirituality can be helpful, there are also circumstances in which spirituality can have a negative effect on health. It is important for health care providers to recognize this dynamic. For example, a person who interprets his or her illness as a punishment from God might attempt to refuse treatment. In such a scenario, a chaplain or other religious advisor could perhaps work with the patient's beliefs to help him or her work through the guilt issues. The patient might accept treatment or refuse it, but at least the decision would not be motivated solely by guilt and would be more of an informed decision. Some people who feel guilt in their relationships with God might also relate to others in their lives in a similar way. Counseling may also be helpful. Some religious beliefs forbid certain medical practices, such as Jehovah's Witnesses' refusal to accept blood transfusions. It is important to recognize the difference between refusing treatment based on an established religious principle versus

refusal of treatment stemming from depression, unwarranted guilt, or a misperceived sense of punishment from God. Some patients may have complicated ethical and spiritual issues. Physicians need not feel that they must solve these dilemmas on their own. Chaplains, members of ethics committees, and counselors often work with physicians in the care of patients.

It is important to recognize that spirituality in the health care setting is not in any one person's domain. Physicians, nurses, social workers, and chaplains all can deal with patient's spirituality. It also is true, however, that most physicians are not trained to deal with complex spiritual crises and conflicts but chaplains and other spiritual caregivers are. Therefore, it is important that physicians obtain a spiritual history as a way of inquiry about spiritual issues that might impact a patient but that physicians also recognize when to make a referral to these specialists.

CARING FOR OUR PATIENTS

Beyond the data, writings, and courses are personal stories from physicians and their patients. In the experience of many physicians who care for patients with chronic and terminal illnesses, there is a feeling of being privileged and honored to care for people who are facing death. Their strength and courage in the midst of suffering is inspiring. Our patients are greater teachers to us and to our students on the meaning of life than any philosophical text. The stories they share are ones of personal transcendence, courage, and dignity. Our patients continually live with dying and, in the midst of that, are often able to face their losses, their fears, and their pain, and transcend to a place where they see their lives as rich and fulfilling. They reprioritize and thereby are able to find a place of deep meaning and purpose in their lives. It is often humbling for us to recognize that what we now place importance on in life may have little or no importance in the end when facing our own mortality. Annoyance at rush hour traffic when late or our emphasis on academic success pale in comparison to our patients' descriptions of a glowing sunrise or the deep love they feel for another. We would encourage all students reading this text to look on your patients as teachers and to approach dying patients not with trepidation and fear but with openness to all the joy and wisdom you can experience with them.

We should have systems of care that allow for people to die in peace, to die the way they want to, and to be able to engage in those activities that bring peace to them: prayer, meditation, listening to music, art, journaling, sacred ritual, and relationships with others. Our systems of care should be interdisciplinary, with physicians, nurses, social workers, chaplains, and other spiritual care providers all working together to provide spiritual and holistic care for our patients. It is then that health care systems will become caring communities rather than impersonal, technologically driven ones.

Our culture and our profession as a whole must look at dying very differently from the way it currently does. We need to see dying not as a medical problem but as a natural part of life that can be meaningful and peaceful. We can broaden and perhaps even enhance our lives now by knowing that one day we will die. By thinking about our mortality early in life, we will not be caught off guard and pressured by the dilemmas of choices at the end of life. We will have had a chance to think about some of those choices sooner and to come to peace with our mortality. This is where religious organizations can be particularly helpful. They can facilitate our discussions of dying and what that means to us. They can educate their members about the importance of preparing themselves for the choices, both spiritual and medical that need to be made near the end of life. We, the interdisciplinary care team, can jointly assist the dying person come to peace in life's last moments.

All of us, whether actively dying or helping care for the dying, have one thing in common: we all will die. The personal transformation that is often seen in patients as they face death can occur in all of our lives. By facing our inevitable dying, we can ask ourselves the same questions that dying patients face—what gives meaning and purpose to our lives, who are we at our deepest core, and what are the important things we want to do in our lives. By attending to the spiritual dimensions of our personal and professional lives, however, we express that, we can better provide care to our patients (76).

> Wayne Muller has written that "There are times in all of our lives when we are forced to reach deep into ourselves to feel the truth of our real nature. For each of us, there comes a moment when we can no longer live our lives by accident. Life throws us into questions that some of us refuse to ask until we are confronted by death or some tragedy in our lives. What do I know to be most deeply true? What do I love, and have I loved well? Who do I believe myself to be and what have I placed on the center of the altar of my life? Where do I belong? What will people find in the ashes of my incarnation when it is over? How shall I live my life knowing that I will die? And what is my gift to the family of earth?" (77).

Of all life's difficult yet important experiences, dying may be the most difficult one we will ever have. The moment of death, and the dying that precedes it, brings to a close the journey that each one of us has been on. We are the privileged persons who attend people while they are dying, be they our patients or our loved ones and friends. We are the persons who can bring hope and comfort to dying patients as they complete their lives. We need to ensure that our society and our systems of care preserve and enhance the dignity of all people, especially when they are made vulnerable by illness and suffering. We need to listen to the dying and to all our patients, and be with them, for them. The process of dying can be a meaningful one, one that we can all embrace and celebrate rather than fear and dread.

How might the assessment and plan look for an 87-year-old female with a history of dementia and hypertension now hospitalized for pneumonia?

Physical:

- Pneumonia, oxygen saturation 98%, on Zithromax, blood and urine culture pending
- Dementia: stable, continue Aricept
- Hypertension: stable continue Vasotec

Psychological: No evidence of depression; some anxiety about being in the hospital.

- Reassurance, private room, family to stay with her, consider massage and music
  Social: strong family support
- Plan to discharge home with home physical therapy (PT)
- Offer additional resource education to family

Spiritual: faith important to patient and family. Patient appears peaceful and accepting of her situation.

- Faith important to patient, gets comfort from prayer and the Eucharist. Will contact chaplain as well as patients' family priest.
- Staff to offer continued presence and compassion to patient and family.
- Encourage husband to sing to patient in hospital to bring her comfort and connection.

COMMUNICATING WITH PATIENTS ABOUT SPIRITUAL ISSUES

A key component of spiritual care is the spiritual assessment. Every person on the interdisciplinary team has a role in assessing patients' spiritual issues, as well as the physical, emotional, and social issues. Every person on the team also has a different area of expertise. Thus, physical issues may be dealt with in depth by the nurse or physician; social issues by the social worker; emotional issues by the psychologist; and spiritual by the chaplain. The chaplain will identify and discuss physical pain, for example, with the patient. The chaplain will then refer to the physician for more specialized handling of the pain issues. The physician will identify and discuss spiritual issues with patient but will also refer to the chaplain for more in-depth counseling on these issues. All health care professionals ideally should communicate with each other and develop a treatment plan together so that the practice of the biopsychosocial–spiritual model of care is seamless and fully integrated.

The spiritual assessment that nonchaplain health care professionals do is, therefore, more of a history and a screening than the full assessment chaplains do. The spiritual history can be done as part of the social history in an intake or initial visit and then be brought up at follow-up visits as appropriate. The goal of the spiritual history is to offer the patient and their family the opportunity to discuss issues that relate to meaning, purpose, hope, suffering, transcendence, as well as values and beliefs that may affect health care decision-making. The spiritual history invites people to share their experiences of the sacred in their lives or of hope, joy, or sadness. It is listening to their inmost stories. There are several spiritual history tools that have been developed. These include SPIRIT (78), FICA (72), and HOPE (79). FICA is described in Table 46.4.

Anecdotal evidence from health care professionals who use the FICA tool suggests that the act of taking the spiritual history is transformative to the clinical encounter. One medical student noted, "The whole feeling of the interview changed. My patient became more open, more comfortable. There was less tension and more trust, it seemed, in me. I also felt more human. It felt like we moved from the purely technical visit to a human encounter." The patient said, "I really felt she (the medical student) cared deeply for me, was interested in me, … in who I really am and what I really feel." Spirituality is an essential element of what makes a person human. Talking about spirituality reaches the human being, not just the patient. The spiritual history gives the health care professional the opportunity to be compassionate and to know of their patient's suffering through the act of being present to that suffering, being open to caring, and being committed to honoring the dignity of that patient.

CONCLUSION

Two weeks before my mother died, she was in the hospital again. The nurse was tender and caring, making sure my mother and I were comfortable and that my mother's needs were attended to. She bathed her with the utmost tenderness, respecting her privacy and dignity. This time, her physician was open, warm, and honored her for who she was. He asked her how she felt and responded to her nonverbal answer in her facial expression. He asked her about her family. He knew her faith was important to her and asked us if she would like to see the chaplain. He reassured her with his touch. He told her that he saw in her a strong yet tender woman, a loving mother and wife. My mother was so happy with her visit with him that even with the difficulty she had with speech, she was able to tell him "you are so nice" and then offer him part of the banana she was eating. When the chaplain came, she offered my mother and me communion. In her prayer, she honored my mother's life, her strength, and her holiness in her suffering with dementia. The health care team created an atmosphere of trust and peace in which my mother was happy and I was able to come to a deep sense of acceptance that my mother would die soon. Most importantly, she was honored for who she was as a person. Her illness was obscured by the enormity of her life, her passions, and her love. Spirituality is the expression of all that is meaningful in one's life, it is the foundation of the dignity and worth of a person, and it is essential to healing and wholeness.

REFERENCES

1. Sulmasy DP. A biopsychosocial–spiritual model for the care of patients at the end of life. *Gerontologist.* 2002;42:24-33.
2. Engel GL. The need for a new medical model: a challenge for biomedicine. *Science.* 1977;196:129-136.
3. White KL, Williams TF, Greenberg BG. The ecology of medical care. *Acad Med.* 1996;73:187-205.
4. Jonas H. *The Phenomenon of Life: Towards a Philosophical Biology.* Evanston, IL: Northwestern University Press; 2001.
5. Sulmasy DP. *The Rebirth of the Clinic: An Introduction to Spirituality in Health Care.* Washington, DC: Georgetown University Press; 2006.
6. Puchalski CM, Ferrell B, Virani R, et al. Improving the quality of spiritual care as a dimension of palliative care: the report of the Consensus Conference. *J Palliat Med.* 2009;12(10):885-904.
7. Ramsey P. *The Patient as Person.* New Haven, CT: Yale University Press; 1970.
8. Engel GL. How much longer must medicine's science be bound by a seventeenth century world view? *Psychother Psychosom.* 1992;57(1-2):3-16.
9. King DE. *Faith, Spirituality and Medicine: Toward the Making of a Healing Practitioner.* Binghamton, NY: Haworth Pastoral Press; 2000.
10. McKee DD, Chappel JN. Spirituality and medical practice. *J Fam Pract.* 1992;5:201, 205-208.
11. Medical School Objectives Project (MSOP). *Report III: Contemporary Issues in Medicine: Communication in Medicine.* Washington, DC: AAMC; 1999:21.
12. Frankl V. *Man's Search for Meaning.* New York, NY: Simon & Schuster; 1984.
13. Kushner HS. *When Bad Things Happen to Good People.* New York, NY: Schocken Books; 1981.

14. Cohen KL. Good Grief. rabbicohen.com. http://www.rabbicohen.com/good-grief.html. Accessed November 22 2020.

15. Doka KJ, Morgan JD, eds. *Death and Spirituality*. Amityville, NY: Baywood Publishing; 1993.

16. Downey M. *Understanding Christian Spirituality*. New York, NY: Paulist Press; 1997.

17. Foglio JP, Brody H. Religion, faith and family medicine. *J Fam Pract*. 1988;27:473-474.

18. Cassell EJ. The nature of suffering and the goals of medicine. *Loss Grief Care*. 1998;8(1-2):129-142.

19. Kubler-Ross E. *On Death and Dying*. New York, NY: Collier Books/Macmillan; 1997.

20. Cassell EJ. *The Nature of Suffering and Goals of Medicine*. New York, NY: Oxford University Press; 1991.

21. *Webster's 7th New Collegiate Dictionary*. Springfield, MA: Merriam-Webster; 1965.

22. Lo B, Quill T, Tulsky J. Discussing palliative care with patients. ACP-ASIM End-of-Life Care Consensus Panel. *Ann Intern Med*. 1999;130:744-749.

23. Karlawish J, Quill T, Meier D. A consensus-based approach to providing palliative care to patients who lack decision-making capacity. ACP-ASIM End-of-Life Care Consensus Panel. *Ann Intern Med*. 1999;130:835-840.

24. Joint Commission for Accreditation of Healthcare Organizations (JCAHO). Spiritual assessment; 2004. http://www.jointcommission.org/AccreditationPrograms/Home Care/Standards/FAQs/Provision+of+Care/Assessment/Spiritual_Assessment.htm. Accessed November 15, 2007.

25. Burkhart, L. Documenting spiritual care. *J Christian Nurses*. 2005;22(1):6-12.

26. American Nursing Association. *Nursing's Social Policy Statement*. 2nd ed. Washington, DC: ANA; 2003.

27. National Association of Social Workers. Code of ethics, 1996 (revised 1999). http://www.socialworkers.org/pubs/code/code.asp. Accessed August 2007.

28. National Consensus Guidelines for Quality Palliative Care. *American Academy of Palliative Care*; 2004. www.nationalconsensusproject.org/guideline.pdf. Accessed June 29, 2008.

29. Keonig HG, McCullough ME, Larson DB. *Handbook of Religion and Health*. New York, NY: Oxford University Press; 2001.

30. Roberts JA, Brown D, Elkins T, Larson DB. Factors influencing views of patients with gynecologic cancer about end-of-life decisions. *Am J Obstet Gynecol*. 1997;176(1):166-172.

31. Powell LH, Shabbi L, Thoreson CE. Religion and spirituality linkages to physical health. *Am Psychol*. 2003;58:36-52.

32. Cohen SR, Mount BM, Tomas JJ, Mount LF. Existential well-being is an important determinant of quality of life. Evidence from the McGill Quality of Life Questionnaire. *Cancer*. 1996;77:576-586.

33. Burgener SC. Predicting quality of life in caregivers of Alzheimer's patients: the role of support from and involvement with the religious community. *J Pastoral Care*. 1999;53:443-446.

34. Worthington E. *Five Steps to Forgiveness: The Art and Science of Forgiveness*. New York, NY: Crown Publishers; 2001.

35. Silvestri GA, Knittig S, Zoller JS, Nietert PJ. Importance of faith on medical decisions regarding cancer care. *J Clin Oncol*. 2003;21:1379-1382.

36. Pargament KI, Smith BW, Koenig HG, Perez L. Patterns of positive and negative religious coping with major life stresses. *J Sci Study Relig*. 1998;37(4):710-724.

37. McCord G, Gilchrist V, Grossman S, et al. Discussing spirituality with patients: a rational and ethical approach. *Ann Fam Med*. 2004;2(4):356-361.

38. Balboni TA, Vanderwerker LC, Block SD, et al. Religiousness and spiritual support among advanced cancer patients and associations with end-of-life treatment preferences and quality of life. *J Clin Oncol*. 2007;25(5):555-560.

39. Cohen SR, Boston P, Mount BM, et al. Changes in quality of life following admission to palliative care units. *Palliat Med*. 2001;15(5):363-371.

40. Fitchett G, Rybarczyk BD, DeMarco GA, et al. The role of religion in medical rehabilitation outcomes: a longitudinal study. *Rehabil Psychol*. 1999;44(4):333-353.

41. Fitchett G, Murphy PE, Kim J, Gibbons JL, Cameron JR, Davis JA. Religious struggle: prevalence, correlates and mental health risks in diabetic, congestive heart failure, and oncology patients. *Int J Psychiatry Med*. 2004;34(2):179-196.

42. Cohen SR, Mount BM, Strobel MG, et al. The McGill Quality of Life Questionnaire: a measure of quality of life appropriate for people with advanced disease. A preliminary study of validity and acceptability. *Palliat Med*. 1995;9:207-219.

43. Cotton S, Puchalski, CM, Sherman SN, et al. Spirituality and religion in patients with HIV/AIDS. *J Gen Intern Med*. 2006;21:S5-S13.

44. Cook JA, Wimberly DW. If I should die before I wake: religious commitment and adjustment to death of a child. *J Sci Study Relig*. 1983;22:222-238.

45. Bearon LB, Koenig RG. Religious cognitions and use of prayer in health and illness. *Gerontologist*. 1990;30: 249-253.

46. Pargament KI, David SE, Kathryn F, et al. God help me: I, religious coping efforts as predictors of the outcomes to significant negative life events. *Am J Community Psychol*. 1990;18:793-824.

47. Seeman TE, Aubin LF, Seema M. Religiosity/spirituality and health: a critical review of the evidence for biological pathways. *Am Psychol*. 2003;58(1):53-63.

48. Rutherford R. *The Death of a Christian: The Rite of Funerals*. New York, NY: Pueblo; 1980.

49. Klass D. Spirituality, protestantism and death. In: Doka KJ, Morgan JD, eds. *Death and Spirituality*. Amityville, NY: Baywood Publishing; 1993:61.

50. Ryan D. Death: eastern perspectives. In: Doka KJ, Morgan JD, eds. *Death and Spirituality*. Amityville, NY: Baywood Publishing; 1993:81.

51. Grollman EA. Death in Jewish thought. In: Doka KJ, Morgan JD, eds. *Death and Spirituality*. Amityville, NY: Baywood Publishing; 1993:25-27.

52. VandeCreek L, Nye C. Trying to live forever: correlates to the belief in life after death. *J Pastoral Care*. 1994;48(3):273-280.

53. Irion PE. Spiritual issues in death and dying for those who do not have conventional religious beliefs. In: Doka KJ, Morgan JD, eds. *Death and Spirituality*. Amityville, NY: Baywood Publishing; 1993.

54. Meagher D, Bell CP. Perspectives on death in the African American community. In: Doka KJ, Morgan JD, eds. *Death and Spirituality*. Amityville, NY: Baywood Publishing; 1993:113-130.

55. Puchalski CM, O'Donnell E. Religious and spiritual beliefs in end-of-life care: how major religions view death and dying. *Tech Reg Anesth Pain Manag*. 2005;9(3):114-121.

56. Breithart W. Spirituality and meaning in supportive care. Spirituality and meaning-centered group psychotherapy interventions in advanced cancer. *Support Care Center*. 2002;10:272-280.

57. 44 Questions: Questions and Answers About Alcoholics Anonymous. General Service Office of Great Britain: AA World Services; 1952.

58. Strachan JG. *Alcoholism, Treatable Illness: An Honorable Approach to Man's Alcoholism Problem*. Center City, MN: Hazelden; 1982.

59. Pargament KI, Koenig HG, Tarakeshwar N, Hahn J. Religious coping methods as predictors of psychological, physical and spiritual outcomes among medically ill elderly patients: a two-year longitudinal study. *J Health Psychol*. 2004;9(6):713-730.

60. Koenig HG, Pargament KI, Nelson J. Religious coping and health status in medically ill hospitalized older adults. *J Nerv Ment Dis*. 1998;186(9):513-521.

61. Sherman AC, Simonton S, Latif U, Spohn R, Tricot G. Religious struggle and religious comfort in response to illness: health outcomes among stem cell transplant patients. *J Behav Med*. 2005;28(4):359-367.

62. Pargament KI, Koenig HG, Tarakeshwar N, Hahn J. Religious struggle as a predictor of mortality among medically ill elderly patients: a two-year longitudinal study. *Arch Intern Med*. 2001;161(15):1881-1885.

63. Joint Commission. *Specifications Manual for Joint Commission National Quality Core Measures*; 2010. http://manual.jointcommission.org/releases/TJC2010A2/rsrc/Manual/TableOfContentsTJC/HBIPS_2010A2.pdf

64. Puchalski CM, Ferrell B. *Making Health Care Whole: Integrating Spirituality into Patient Care*. West Conshohocken, PA: Templeton Press; 2010.

65. Puchalski CM, Anderson BM, Lo B, et al. *Ethical Guidelines for Spiritual Care*. Washington, DC: AAMC Report; 2006.

66. O'Connor P. The role of spiritual care in hospice. Are we meeting patients' needs? *Am J Hosp Care*. 1988;5:31-37.

67. DiBlasi Z, Harkness E, Ernst E, et al. Influence of context effects on health outcomes: a systematic review. *Lancet*. 2001;357(9258):757-762.

68. Peabody FW. *The Care of the Patient*. Cambridge, MA: Harvard University Press; 1927.

69. Sulmasy DP. *The Healer's Calling: A Spirituality for Physicians and Other Health Care Professionals*. New York, NY: Paulist Press; 1997.

70. Puchalski CM, Vitillo R, Hull SK, Reller N. Improving the spiritual dimension of whole person care: reaching national and international consensus. *J Palliat Med*. 2014;17(6):642-656.

71. Puchalski CM, Sbrana A, Ferrell B, et al. Interprofessional spiritual care in oncology: a literature review. *ESMO Open*. 2019;4(1):e000465.

72. © Copyright Christina Puchalski, MD, and The George Washington University 1996 (updated 2021). All rights reserved. Adapted from Puchalski C, Romer AL. Taking a spiritual history allows clinicians to understand patients more fully. *J Palliat Med*. 2000;3(1):129-137.

73. Ehman JW, Ott BB, Short TH, et al. Do patients want physicians to inquire about their spiritual or religious beliefs if they become gravely ill? *Arch Intern Med*. 1999;159:1803-1806.

74. Post SG, Puchalski CM, Larson DB. Physicians and patient spirituality: professional boundaries, competency, and ethics. *Ann Intern Med*. 2000;132(7):578-583.

75. Sloan RP, Bagiella E, VandeCreek L, et al. Should physicians prescribe religious activities? *N Engl J Med*. 2000;342(25):1913-1916.

76. Newman LF, Epstein L. Doctor–patient relationships: know thy patient, know thyself. *Med Health R I*. 1996;79(8):308-310.

77. Muller W. *Touching the Divine: Teachings, Meditations and Contemplations to Awaken Your True Nature [Audiocassettes]*. Louisville, CO: Sounds True; 1994.

78. Maugans TA. The SPIRITual history. *Arch Fam Med*. 1996;5(1):11-16.

79. Anandarajah G, Hight E. Spirituality and medical practice: using HOPE questions as a practical tool for spiritual assessment. *Am Fam Physician*. 2001;63(1):81-89.

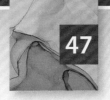

47 Grief and Bereavement

Carol Kummet and Susan E. Merel

MY GRIEF AFFAIR (1)

I met Grief at your funeral. He was wearing a T-shirt,
jeans, and flip-flops in January, smoking a joint
in the corner; he put it out just as the funeral
director rushed over. Goddamn, Grief was sexy,
brooding in that corner, not crying, just being himself
without apology. I knew he would be in my bed that night.
We got drunk and stayed up late crying, reminiscing
about you, fucking, laughing, holding each other's hair back
while we puked. We slept for a while, fucked some more,
smoked cigarettes on the porch, and ate leftover pizza.
I thought it would be a one-night stand, but now Grief
knew where I lived. He started showing up at my door in the evenings,
and sometimes first thing in the morning, too. He begged me
to stay home from work. He wanted us to scream from a rooftop,
cry together in public, break bottles in the street. We drank
all the whiskey in Portland, yelled at no one in particular,
made out with strangers, tripped and fell countless times on the way
home. Once, we lost my keys inside the lining of my jacket
and had to sleep on the front doorstep. We would
lie in bed for days, eating tiramisu and watching movies.
My friends weren't crazy about him. A few told me he would
eventually have to leave. We fought a lot. I got tired
of his constant presence, always right next to me,
even when I peed. Sometimes I would ignore him for days,
but he was patient, sitting in the corner, reading *The New Yorker*,
waving whenever I looked in his direction.

— *Jennifer Foreman*

GRIEF REACTIONS, ANTICIPATORY GRIEF, BEREAVEMENT, AND MOURNING

Patients experience loss, change, and challenges when they are ill and consequently often present to clinicians with grief reactions. Grief will also be common in the family members of your seriously ill patients. In this chapter, we will outline important modern grief theories and discuss simple interventions that clinicians can use with adults and children experiencing grief and loss.

Jennifer Foreman's poem highlights some important concepts about grief. Grief is a constant, insistence, and important presence in the lives of many people (hence grief is depicted as "patient, sitting in the corner, reading *The New Yorker*"). The bereaved may have periods of time when they think less about their deceased loved one, but having an ongoing relationship with the deceased is normal and not a pathological grief response. The poem also depicts grief changing the behavior of the bereaved, and this is also common and expected.

Grief is the human response to a loss, change, challenge, or death. *Bereavement* is an Old English word meaning "to be robbed" and describes the state of experiencing loss. *Mourning* is the process by which people adapt to a loss (2). An individual's mourning process is shaped not only by their individual grief reactions but also by social rules, cultural customs, and cultural or religious rituals. When caring for patients from a culture different from our own, it is appropriate to ask about mourning rituals so that they can be respected (2).

Grief reactions manifest in many ways (3). We list common grief reactions in Table 47.1. All of these are more or less common responses to grief and you may encounter them in patients

TABLE 47.1 COMMON GRIEF MANIFESTATIONS

Domain	Common manifestations	
Psychological	Shock	Anxiety
	Numbness	Emotional lability
	Sadness	Irritability
	Disbelief	Guilt
	Fear	Helplessness
	Relief	Impaired concentration
	Denial	Impaired memory
	Anger	Impaired decision-making
Physical	Anorexia	Temperature changes
	Weight changes	Chest pain
	Sleep changes	Headache
	Fatigue	Hair loss
	Palpitations	Gastrointestinal distress
Behavioral	Restlessness	
	Crying	
	Social withdrawal, sensitivity in social situations	
	Experiencing symptoms of the loved one's illness	
	Seeing, hearing or feeling the presence of the deceased	
	Speaking aloud to the deceased	
Social	Any or all of the following in relationships with friends and relatives: desire for support from and connection with from others, withdrawal from others, increased dependency on others, increased conflict including marital difficulties	
	Increased sensitivity in conversations to topics of loss (e.g., airplane crashes, auto accidents)	
Spiritual	Searching for meaning	
	Questioning priorities and values	
	Increased or decreased spiritual or religious practice	

who have recently experienced a loss. When the bereaved report new physical symptoms, they should be medically evaluated as usual, but the clinician should also consider whether grief could be contributing.

Anticipatory grief is a particularly important concept for clinicians caring for people with serious illness. Anticipatory grief is experienced by patients and loved ones during the course of a life-threatening illness. Patients are adapting to their uncertain future, may be undergoing internal life review or questioning choices made in their life or health care in the past, and may be trying to come to terms with leaving their loved ones (2). Table 47.2 outlines important characteristics of anticipatory grief and suggested brief interventions.

You may read elsewhere about the distinction between complicated and uncomplicated grief or

TABLE 47.2 COMMON MANIFESTATIONS OF ANTICIPATORY GRIEF IN SERIOUSLY ILL PATIENTS AND THEIR FAMILIES

Family member experiencing loss	Anticipatory grief response	Suggested interventions
Seriously ill patient	Worries about comfort and support of family	Family can reinforce and support his or her unique role within the family; clinicians can reinforce that family will be cared for and supported after death.
Seriously ill patient	Concerned about unfinished business (e.g., financial business, legacy work)	Counseling can help discover areas of unfinished business and help make a plan to complete. Social workers, counselors, and clinicians can provide opportunities for legacy work.
Caregiver	Social isolation	Clinicians, social workers, and counselors can help family ask for help from others.
Caregiver and patient	Relationships strained, communication not optimal between them	Clinicians can lead family meetings, facilitate information exchange within the family, acknowledge role changes within the family.
Caregiver and patient	Fear and uncertainty	Clinicians can assess family's coping skills and provide support; provide supportive listening about fear and uncertainty; provide prognostic information if desired.

about the DSM-5 proposed criteria set of persistent complex bereavement disorder (PCBD); a similar set of diagnostic criteria for prolonged grief disorder will be included in ICD-11 (4–6). However, many experts do not use the term "complicated grief," and the DSM-5 category was intended as a criteria set for further study but not yet for clinical use. Some experts in the field feel strongly that specific grief symptoms lasting >6 months (for PGD, the ICD-11 criteria) or 12 months (for PCBD, the DSM-5 criteria) constitute a subset of patients that should be identified and treated in a particular way, and there is some evidence that a particular protocol for grief treatment based on exposure therapy for PTSD might be more efficacious than interpersonal psychotherapy for those fitting research criteria for complicated grief (6,7). However, the DSM-5 and ICD-11 criteria correlate poorly with each other and with other diagnostic criteria for complicated grief used to test the currently available specific psychotherapeutic interventions, and experts warn of the risk of unnecessarily pathologizing grief reactions with currently available diagnostic criteria (8).

We feel that terms like complicated grief, PGD, and PCBD can pathologize common and expected grief reactions, including grief reactions lasting longer than 6 months, and potentially distract clinicians from diagnosing other conditions such as major depression. Rather than making these specific diagnoses, we recommend that clinicians consider whether some grieving patients and bereaved family members are depressed or have other psychiatric conditions underlying their symptoms; Table 47.3 outlines some important distinctions between grief and clinical depression. Many patients experiencing grief would benefit from grief counseling from a professional, whether they fit criteria for a complicated grief disorder or not.

MODERN GRIEF THEORIES

For many years, the dominant theory of grief was Elisabeth Kübler-Ross's 5 Stages of Grief (9). This theory, while still frequently encountered and appreciated for stimulating discussion of grief, dying, and death at a time when these topics were not commonly openly discussed, has in recent years been supplanted by others. Key flaws in the Kübler-Ross theory are that it describes a linear process of grieving, describes only emotional grief reactions and assumes that humans come to closure with their relationship with the deceased (10,11).

Clinicians working with grieving patients and families should be familiar with three modern grief theories: Kenneth Doka's description of the two dominant styles of grieving, William Worden's four tasks of mourning, and the continuing bonds theory (12–14). We outline all three here, with a special focus on how cancer patients themselves may experience grief related to their illness.

Doka's Two Dominant Styles of Grieving

Two dominant styles of grieving have been identified by Kenneth Doka: intuitive and instrumental grieving (12). While the intuitive style, characterized by outward displays of emotion, will be more familiar to many, both are common, normal, and experienced by both men and women. Assessing a patient or family member's grieving style is important in understanding their experience and offering targeted support. An intuitive or emotional griever expresses, experiences, and adapts to grief on an emotional level. The intuitive griever talks about grief as waves of sorrow, which are expressed through emotions such as crying, anger, depression, relief, or irritability. Clinicians can support intuitive grievers by giving them time to talk, tell

TABLE 47.3 CHARACTERISTICS OF GRIEF AND CLINICAL DEPRESSION

Grief	Clinical depression
Can still experience moments of joy and lightness	Often with significant anhedonia, without moments of joy and lightness
Feelings of emptiness and loss often predominate	Depressed mood and anhedonia predominate; depressed mood is persistent and not tied to specific thoughts or preoccupations
Preoccupation with thoughts and memories of the deceased	Self-critical or pessimistic ruminations
If has related somatic symptoms, these are transient	Somatic symptoms of depression are more often persistent
Often openly angry	Less often openly angry; more often irritable
Expresses guilt over a specific aspect of illness, loss or change	Expresses a more general feeling of guilt
Milder loss of self-esteem	Deep loss of self-esteem

their story, and express their emotions and then by helping intuitive grievers connect with counselors, oncology social workers, chaplains, and/or support groups to give them more opportunities to express emotions. Cues from your patient that they are an intuitive griever might include comments such as, "I just need to tell you this" or "I was telling my neighbor about how tired I am after treatment and they just couldn't listen. I had to learn who I can share things with or talk to" or "I am just so weepy all the time" or "I suddenly got so angry with the grocery clerk and wanted to shout 'I have cancer?'" or "I really need to talk about all that has been going on since my diagnosis" or "When I need to talk my sister won't let me and just tells me all of her problems."

An instrumental griever expresses, experiences, and adapts to grief in active or cognitive ways. The instrumental griever might experience grief through difficult memories, lack of concentration, physical complaints, appetite changes, sleep pattern changes, or changes in behaviors. These grieving individuals may find reading information about grief from books, websites, handouts, and blogs more helpful than intuitive grievers. They often find exercise helpful as well as "doing" something like participating in a walk against cancer or a run to raise money for research. It is particularly important to identify an instrumental griever as some ask multiple questions and have a detail-oriented approach to care that can cause them to be labeled as a "difficult patient" or "difficult family member." Understanding that this behavior is part of the patient or family member's grief response can be helpful to clinicians. Cues from your patient that they are an instrumental griever might include comments such as, "I found a great website about what to eat when you feel nauseated" or "My wife wants me to talk about how I feel. I just don't want to talk about it" or "I'm not really a support group kind of person" or "Is there something I can do to sleep better?" or "When I

am done with treatments I'm going to volunteer at the reception desk."

Most grieving patients and family members will use one style predominantly but show characteristics of both (e.g., an instrumental griever may certainly still cry). Different grieving styles within a family can sometimes contribute to conflict. In stressful times, grieving patients often want their family members to react the same way, with the same intensity, at the same time as they do. Clinicians can help patients and family members when they identify and discuss the different styles of grieving within a family.

Worden's Four Tasks of Mourning

Oncology clinicians are often the first people to offer support to a patient who is grieving their diagnosis and the accompanying losses, changes, and challenges. Knowing grief and loss theories will build the clinicians' skill set so that they can provide compassionate medical care to grieving cancer patients. Meeting with a clinician who acknowledges grief and can address it helps a patient face grief rather than suppressing it which can have negative repercussions. J. William Worden's Four Tasks of Mourning are a very helpful framework for clinicians working with patients experiencing either grief related to a death or anticipatory/expected grief during an illness (13). His original four tasks described for an individual grieving a death are described in Table 47.4, and we present a framework based on Worden's four tasks for brief grief counseling with patients with cancer or other serious illness in the section below. Of note, the four tasks are not linear. Grieving patients will at times be working on two or more tasks at one time, while still other times they will toggle between two tasks or not be open to or able to work on any task. Although these tasks are written for grieving a death, they also work for grieving nondeath losses, as we discuss in the next section.

TABLE 47.4 J. WILLIAM WORDEN'S FOUR TASKS OF MOURNING

Task	Important elements of the task
1. Accept the reality of the loss	Acknowledges all the additional losses brought about by the death including roles, finances, future dreams, etc. Gives the bereaved perspective on what they are grieving and offers some self-compassion about why grief might take longer than expected.
2. Experience the pain of the grief	Processing grief involves experiencing uncomfortable reactions. Numbing sorrow does not help the bereaved.
3. Adjust to the environment in which the deceased is missing.	Learn to cope and function in the world without the deceased.
4. Find an enduring connection to the deceased while embarking on a new life.	Stay connected or in relationship with the deceased while forming new relationships and a new life.

Continuing Bonds Theory

Many of us were taught the appropriate approach to the death of someone we cared about was to come to closure with that relationship and move on without them. This kind of detachment is no longer thought of as healthy grieving. The continuing bonds theory, described by Klass, Silverman, and Nickman, encourages a different or new relationship in the present with the deceased (14). The theory can be summarized by a quote from Robert Anderson's play *I Never Sang for my Father*, "Death ends a life, but it does not end a relationship (15)." The continuing bonds approach is seen in the Oban Ceremony in Japan, the Dia de los Muertos (Day of the Dead) Celebration in Mexico, the Qingming or Grave Sweeping Day in China, and the Celtic festival of Samhain. All these cultural celebrations are times to remember deceased loved ones, tell stories about their lives, and grieve as a community.

SUPPORTING GRIEVING PATIENTS AND FAMILIES

Patients with cancer will experience multiple losses, changes, and challenges throughout their disease course whether the outcome is a return to health, a remission, or their death. Clinicians who can identify grief in their patients and address it during their treatment will improve patient care. To identify grief in your patients, listen for statements such as, "So many things have changed since I was diagnosed" or "I really miss being able to bike to work" or "I always just took walking to the bus stop for granted" or "I had to put school on hold" or "It is a lot to ask my family to drive me to appointments." These are openings for clinicians to acknowledge how the patient's life has changed and ask about other losses. Clinicians can gently suggest to their patients that they might be grieving. "Things really have changed in your life, do you think you are grieving?" or "With all those losses you might be feeling some grief." Once grief is identified, it is appropriate to refer grieving patients to oncology or palliative care social workers, grief counselors, or other community resources for ongoing grief counseling during their treatment. A meta-analysis of randomized controlled trials of psychological interventions for grief in adults found a statistically significant pooled effect on grief symptoms, with greater effect sizes in studies of one-one-one counseling (16). However, patients also expect support from their clinicians; those who have basic knowledge of the skills of grief counseling can offer limited grief support in just a few minutes during appointment times. Below we offer a framework based on Worden's four tasks of mourning for brief grief counseling during a routine office visit for a grieving patient with cancer or another serious illness.

Task 1: Acknowledge the Loss

Patients going through cancer treatment experience losses, changes, and challenges each day as they live with their diagnosis, manage symptoms from treatment, and often face their own death.

Your Intervention

In 1 to 2 minutes, clinicians can support the grieving patient by acknowledging losses and encouraging the patient to share some of the most challenging ones. Identifying grief helps to normalize the patient's reactions to the diagnosis or symptoms associated with cancer or treatment. Acknowledging the patient's losses, changes, and challenges builds rapport between the provider and patient. Note this is a time to listen to the patient, not to solve a problem.

Suggested Language

- "Since your diagnosis, you have really faced a lot of changes in your life. Would you tell me about some of the most challenging changes you have faced?"
- "You mentioned that you love being outdoors yet while you are immunosuppressed, you haven't had the opportunity to get fresh air as often as before. What other losses are you experiencing?"

Task 2: Experience the Pain of the Loss

Patients may have grief reactions while discussing the changes in their life or may report symptoms in a clinic visit that you can identify as grief reactions. The reactions might be emotional, physical, social, spiritual, cognitive, or behavioral (Table 47.1).

Your Intervention

Be knowledgeable about the varying manifestations of grief so that you do not pathologize a common or expected manifestation. Support the grieving patient by being a compassionate presence to their pain. Do not try to take the pain away. It is helpful to the patient to be able to express sorrow in the presence of a kind witness. Don't offer judgments, opinions, or suggestions right away. This does not need to take a lot of time during the patient's appointment. A pause of just 15 seconds while the patient is tearful shows the patient that their grief is worthy of attention. Having tissues available within reach of the patient gives the patient the power to choose to reach for one or not. This avoids the patient misinterpreting a clinician's offer of a tissue as a sign that they should stop crying.

Suggested Language

- Use silence rather than language—sit with the person in their grief. Allow them time to speak if they wish.
- "I'm sorry you are going through this grief."
- "Some people feel grief in their body, while others have trouble concentrating and still others have changes in how they interact with friends and family. Many different reactions can be common."
- If the patient begins to cry, you might say "Please take your time," or "It is okay to let your tears fall."
- If the patient expresses anger, you might say one of the following:
  - "You have the right to be upset about this happening."
  - "How do you get your anger out at home?"
  - "Anger at the situation is understandable. If you are angry at our clinic I'd like to address it, with your permission."

Task 3: Adjust to the Losses, Changes, and Challenges of Serious Illness

This task is about adjusting, coping, learning to live with changes, and fully engaging with life even with a cancer diagnosis.

Your Interventions

Task 3 is the counterpart to Task 2. Help the patient identify where they are doing well, succeeding in their commitment to health, coping with their symptoms, and addressing their challenges by adjusting their attitude or adapting though the support of family, friends, counselors, or community resources. Grieving patients need to both express their grief and adjust to living with the new challenges. Here, the clinician's task is to highlight the patient's steps toward adjustment.

Suggested Language

- "I am glad you saw the social worker. Sometimes patients don't use all the resources available to them."
- "I am glad you tried deep breathing and yoga. I'm sorry they did not work for you. Have you found something else that does address your anxiety?"

Task 4: Identify Lessons the Patient Will Take Forward Into Their Life

This task complements the continuing bonds approach to grief work introduced above. While Worden's original fourth task speaks to staying connected to deceased loved ones, it also can serve grieving patients who will regain their health, returning to their lives cured or in remission from their illness.

Your Interventions

Without sentimentality, clinicians can encourage the grieving patient to reflect on ways in which all the losses, changes, and challenges have impacted them. Here it's best to reserve judgment and to simply acknowledge the ways they are now different since the diagnosis. For patients who are dying and are ready to discuss their death, legacy work is part of this task. See Box 47.1 for suggested

---

Box 47.1 How to Encourage Patients to Complete Legacy Work

Here's one way of explaining legacy work to a seriously ill patient:

"Have you written or recorded your legacy for your family? Your legacy might be stories from your life that pass on your beliefs and values or it might be a retelling of a child's birth and how you loved them from first sight. Your legacy might be a video in which you express your love for family members, or it might be a video of your worst and/ or dirtiest jokes so that they will remember your sense of humor. It might be a heartfelt statement of your hopes for future generations. Maybe it is your family's genealogy tree or secret lasagna recipe."

Here are some specific questions patients can use to think about their legacy. These questions can be used for private reflection, writing, video or audio recording or in conversation with family.

- What are your most strongly held beliefs? Did any of your beliefs change as you aged?
- What are your hopes for yourself and others?
- What are your concerns for yourself and others?
- Where did you get inspiration in life? What motivated you?
- Who influenced you or was there an event that shaped you?
- What did you struggle with in life?
- What did you desire most on in life?
- Why did you marry? Why did you not get married?
- How many children did you have? Did you choose not to have children?
- How did you choose your profession?
- How did you choose your hobbies?
- Did you ever change your view on life?
- Do you have a memory from childhood that you still think about or relive?
- Are there life lessons you know now but wished you knew when you were younger?
- What matters the most to you right now?
- What do you enjoy most right now?
- How do you define a successful life?
- What do you hope to accomplish in your life?
- What are your hopes for your loved ones?
- What would you like to be remembered for after you die?

Box 47.2 Template for a Letter That
Seriously Ill Patients Can Consider
Writing to Loved Ones

The following is a template that can be shared with seriously ill patients who are considering writing letters to loved ones as part of their legacy work.

Dear …

I am writing to you because I love and care for you very much. I want you to know how I feel about you and I want you to know what is important to me. I want to give you what I learned as gifts for your life.

Of your many traits I especially love your…

You have given me strength in many ways including…

My hope for you is that you will always…

Don't be afraid to…

I think it is important for you to take time to enjoy…

You may have tough times in your life, but I want to encourage you to…

Some of the best times with you include…

Something I learned is to never take for granted…

The beliefs I hold dear are…

A family story I want you to know and remember is…

I hope your life will be full of…

I will always love you. You are precious to me. Thank you for being in my life.

Love,

prompts to open conversations about legacy work with patients and Box 47.2, "A Love Letter," which patients can modify and use with loved ones.

Examples

- "What have you noticed you are now grateful for that perhaps you took for granted before your diagnosis?"
- "What changes happened that you are actually okay with now?"
- If the patient is dying:
  - "What is the most important thing or story you want your family to know about you?"
  - "Have you said all you need to your family? Your words connect them to you long after your death and give them comfort in their grief."

Knowledge of your health care system's grief and loss resources allows you to make timely and appropriate referrals. Most health care systems have social workers and/or chaplains who offer supportive grief counseling. Some health care systems have a dedicated grief counselor available to the patient during treatment and the family/friends after a death. Often the social workers, chaplains, and grief counselors serve the staff as well as the patients and their families in processing the grief of caring for seriously ill patients. Currently, a minority of US intensive care units have any bereavement follow-up services (17). While there is a need for bereavement services within health systems, bereavement services are part of the Medicare hospice benefit for all patients receiving hospice care and are sometimes available to those in the larger community as well. There is increasing recognition of the importance of institutional support for bereavement within hospitals and health systems, and this is an area for quality improvement and further study.

SUPPORTING GRIEVING CHILDREN AND THEIR FAMILIES

Clinicians encounter grieving children either when caring for the child (e.g., a grieving child who presents for medical care in clinic) or when caring for a patient facing death who has children or grandchildren. Children do not grieve in the same manner as adults. For example, children often have intense quick bursts of reactions and then just as quickly return to playing as though nothing is wrong. Clinicians should be familiar with common grief responses for children of different ages and be able to briefly counsel families about reactions to expect and how adults can best help grieving children in a particular age group (Table 47.5). Younger children who may not be familiar with the concept of death need concrete, simple explanations that reinforce the permanence of death, such as "When a person dies, his or her body stops working. The heart stops beating and the body stops moving, eating, and breathing." (11) It is important to avoid euphemisms like "went to sleep," "passed away," or "we lost him" as these can be confusing or even frightening for children.

The common messages for bereaved children of all ages are "it is not your fault" and "you will be safe"; these messages are delivered differently depending on the age of the child. When children ask questions about illness and death, parents and clinicians should answer these simply but honestly, avoiding overexplanation. Clinicians may be asked if children should be brought to the bedside of a dying loved one—this is a decision that each family should make for themselves, but families should be encouraged to take the child's lead and facilitate this if the child desires the visit. Child life specialists and/or social workers in hospitals can help

TABLE 47.5 COMMON GRIEF RESPONSES IN CHILDREN AND RECOMMENDED CAREGIVER INTERVENTIONS

Age	Common reactions	How an adult can best help
Birth to 3 years old	Affected most by mood of caregiver. Toddlers may demand more attention.	Maintain routines. Provide attention and reassurance.
3–6 years old	May not see death as permanent. May worry about the deceased. May use imaginative play to process the information. May regress in behavior.	Maintain routines. Answer all questions concretely. Allow expression of feelings through play.
6–9 years old	May feel responsible for death. May want to talk about the death over and over. May express a range of emotions from none to sorrow to distress. May fear other deaths or abandonment.	Tell the child it was not their fault. Answer questions honestly. If leaving, tell the child when you will return and how to contact you. Listen to their thoughts and feelings without judgment.
9–12 years old	Understands that death is permanent. May show anger, guilt or relief. May have physical reactions as well as emotional ones.	Provide time to talk. Encourage child to express their grief reactions and be honest about your own feelings. Reassure the child that they will be cared for.

support families and children during these visits. Box 47.3 provides a summary of the main points clinicians might cover when offering brief counseling to families about how to support a grieving child.

Many communities have organizations that support bereaved children and/or children living with a parent with serious illness. Pediatric hospice provides important concurrent care to children with advance illness, and hospices providing care for adults also often provide special bereavement services for children. The Sesame Street Workshop has produced an excellent online toolkit offering advice for families and excellent videos for children and families to watch (18). Many families may wish to use children's literature in their home to help them open conversations with their children about illness and death; a recent systematic review provides brief summaries of children's books about death and dying, including separate lists of books about a child's dying experience and books featuring African, African American, Asian, Hispanic, and Native cultures (19).

HOW CLINICIANS GRIEVE

Physicians and other clinicians grieve for their patients; it is important to identify grief over the loss of a patient and distinguish it from depression and burnout. Qualitative studies of oncologists' responses to patient loss suggest they grieve when a patient receives a poor prognosis or at any time

Box 47.3 Counseling Families of Bereaved Children

Information to offer to families with grieving children of any age:

- Tell the child their loved one's disease is not the child's fault. Children of all ages make incorrect assumptions: "I did not make my bed so mom got sick." Children often believe that their misbehaving caused the illness.
- Keep the child's routine the same as much as possible.
- Children are good "lie detectors." Tell the truth and tell it often. Give the child honest information at a level they will understand. If you do not share information the child will arrive at their own conclusions which will cause them emotional harm.
- The child might ask very direct questions such as "Will Mom die?" Give honest answers that are as optimistic as the situation allows. Give no more information than what the child is asking. Do not over-explain.
- Ask the child what they understand is happening. Ask the child what they want to know. Correct misunderstandings.
- Tell the child's teacher what is happening.
- Allow the child to have a wide range of reactions including emotional responses and physical responses. Some children regress in their behaviors.
- Help the child find a way to remember the deceased.

after the patient's death. Oncologists in the studies reported typical grief symptoms including sadness, anxiety, helplessness, and physical symptoms including chest pain, fatigue, insomnia, and general physical discomfort (20). Oncologists reported coping with grief by compartmentalization and distancing themselves from patients. Some also reported a positive impact of grief; while they sometimes brought grief home with them, they also felt it helped them develop a better perspective on life (21). Trainees may be particularly susceptible to grief and may be more likely to feel personally responsible for a loss (22).

Self-reflection, informal discussions with colleagues, and structured small group discussions can all be helpful for clinicians needing to process grief. We provide some prompts for written or quiet personal reflection about grief in Box 47.4. At our institution, we provide several opportunities for reflection and discussion of the emotional impact of caring for seriously ill patients including "Death Rounds" with multiple groups of trainees. In one study of this intervention, a majority of intern participants in "Death Rounds" found it helpful, and 98% of respondents thought that having an opportunity to discuss the emotional aspects of patient death should be included in their training (23).

Some providers have found an effective tool for processing their grief after the death of patient is to write a condolence card to the surviving family or friends. Writing a personal note of sympathy is a way of acknowledging the death (Worden Task 1), taking time to feel whatever emotion or response you have over the death of the particular patient (Worden Task 2), have perspective on, and adjust to your work in which many patients survive and go on to live long lives while others die (Worden Task 3), and if you offer the family/friends a story

---

Box 47.5 Elements to Include in a Condolence Card or Letter

- A condolence card or letter can be handwritten or typed.
- It can be quite short (just a few sentences are appropriate).
- Consider including the following:
  - Acknowledge the patient's death, using their name.
  - Share a brief personal memory of the deceased.
  - If applicable, share a reflection on the relationship between the deceased and the bereaved (e.g., "it was always clear to me how much she cared about you.")
- Conclude the letter simply.

---

or a thought about the uniqueness of the patient who died, you are adding to that deceased patient's legacy (Worden Task 4). Box 47.5 provides a suggested framework for a clinician's condolence letter.

REFERENCES

1. Foreman J. My Grief Affair. Reprinted with permission from both the author and the publisher of the site on which the poem initially appeared. The Sun Magazine, October 2015. https://www.thesunmagazine.org/issues/478/my-grief-affair. Accessed October 31, 2019.
2. Grief and Bereavement. In: Quill TE, Bower KA, Holloway RG, et al. *Primer of Palliative Care.* 6th ed. Chicago, IL: American Academy of Hospice and Palliative Medicine; 2014.
3. Cassarett D, Kutner JS, Abrahm J. Life after death: a practical approach to grief and bereavement. *Ann Intern Med.* 2001;134(3):208-215.
4. Shear MK. Complicated grief. *N Engl J Med.* 2015;372:153-160.
5. American Psychiatric Association. *Diagnostic and Statistic Manual of Mental Disorders.* 5th ed. Arlington, VA: American Psychiatric Association; 2013. https://dsm-psychiatryonlineorg.offcampus.lib.washington.edu/doi/full/10.5555/appi.books.9780890425596.ConditionsforFurtherStudy. Accessed online February 16, 2020.
6. Simon NM, et al. Commentary on evidence in support of a grief-related condition as DSM diagnosis. *Depress Anxiety.* 2020;37(1):9-16.
7. Shear K, et al. Treatment of complicated grief: a randomized controlled trial. *JAMA.* 2005;293:2601-2608.
8. Lenferink LIM, et al. The importance of harmonizing diagnostic sets for pathological grief. *Br J Psychiatry.* 2019:1-4.
9. Kubler-Ross E. *On Death and Dying.* New York, NY: MacMillan; 1969.
10. McVean A. *It's Time to Let the Five Stages of Grief Die.* McGill Office for Science and Society Newsletter. Montreal, CA; 2019. https://www.mcgill.ca/oss/article/health-history/its-time-let-five-stages-grief-die. Accessed February 16, 2020.
11. Rosenbaum R. *Dead Like Her: How Elisabeth Kübler-Ross Went Around The Bend.* Slate. New York, NY; 2004. https://slate.com/culture/2004/09/the-treacly-legacy-of-kubler-ross.html. Accessed February 16, 2020.

Box 47.4 A Professional's Grief Self-Assessment

The following prompts are meant to be used by health care professionals for self-reflection. This could be done alone or in a small trusted group with the understanding that reflections will be confidential.

The family rules about grieving I grew up with are (e.g., "be strong," "don't cry"):

The family rules about grieving I now follow are:

I know I'm grieving when I:

These are some ways I'll grieve my personal and professional losses:

When I'm overwhelmed by grief it helps to:

12. Doka K, Martin TL. *Grieving Beyond Gender: Understanding the Ways Men and Women Mourn*. Revised Edition. New York, NY: Routledge; 2010. https://ebookcentral.proquest.com/lib/washington/reader.action?docID=646557. Accessed November 5, 2019.

13. Worden JW. *Grief Counseling and Grief Therapy: A Handbook for the Mental Health Practitioner*. 5th ed. New York, NY: Springer; 2018.

14. Klass D, Silverman P, Nickman, S. *Continuing Bonds, New Understanding of Grief*. Washington, DC: Taylor and Francis; 1996.

15. Anderson R. *I Never Sang For My Father*. New York, NY: Random House; 1968:3.

16. Johannsen M, Damholdt MF, Zachariae R, et al. Psychological interventions for grief in adults: a systematic review and meta-analysis of randomized controlled trials. *J Affect Disord*. 2019;253:69-86.

17. McAdam JL, Erikson A. Bereavement services offered in adult intensive care units in the United States. *Am J Crit Care*. 2016:25(2):110-117.

18. Sesame Workshop. Grief Toolkit. https://www.sesamestreet.org/toolkits/grief/. Accessed October 15, 2019.

19. Aruda-Colli MNF, Weaver MS, Weiner L. Communication about dying, death and bereavement: a systematic review of children's literature. *J Palliat Med*. 2017;20(5):548-559.

20. Granek L, Ben-David M, Shapira S, Bar-Sela G, Ariad S. Grief symptoms and difficult patient loss for oncologists in response to patient death. *Psychooncology*. 2017;26:960-966.

21. Granek L, Tozer R, Mazzota P, Ramjuan A, Krzyzanowska M. Nature and impact of grief over patient loss on oncologists/personal and professional lives. *Arch Intern Med*. 2012;172(12):964-965.

22. Vallurupalli M. Mourning on morning rounds. *N Engl J Med*. 2013;369(5):404-405.

23. Smith L, Hough CL. Using death rounds to improve end-of-life education for internal medicine residents. *J Palliat Med*. 2011;14(1):55-58.

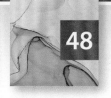

48 Staff Stress and Burnout

Laura D. Johnson, Alvin L. Reaves III, and Hunter Groninger

INTRODUCTION

In this ever-changing world of health care reform, limited resources, reduced reimbursement, and increased demands for quality performance measures, clinicians are experiencing less autonomy in their scope of practice (1–10). Health care providers increasingly report job-related stressors, including employee dissatisfaction, mental exhaustion, and documentation time (11–13), as the availability of their personal resources (e.g., time and emotion/empathy) diminishes in the face of increased patient demands and complexity and severity of illness grows (14,15). The concept of "burnout" (defined below) is a common means of capturing the cumulative deleterious impact of these stressors. Currently, over half of all nurses report burnout (16). A 2017 study of American physicians reveals that just over 40% report burnout and they have a greater risk for burnout compared to the rest of the workforce (10).

Definition Box

According to the WHO's ICD-11, burnout is defined as: "a syndrome conceptualized as resulting from chronic workplace stress that has not been successfully managed. It is characterized by three dimensions: (a) feelings of energy depletion or exhaustion; (b) increased mental distance from one's job, or feelings of negativism or cynicism related to one's job; and (c) reduced professional efficacy. Burn-out refers specifically to phenomena in the occupational context and should not be applied to describe experiences in other areas of life."
World Health Organization. Burn-out an "occupational phenomenon": International Classification of Diseases. May 28, 2019. https://www.who.int/mental_health/evidence/burn-out/en/. Accessed October 1, 2019.
Compassion fatigue is when "the ongoing exposure to and empathetic concern for the suffering of others leads to deep physical, emotional, and spiritual exhaustion, hopelessness, disconnection from others, and decreased capacity for and interest in empathetic attunement with clients."

This quote is from Pelon SB. Compassion fatigue and compassion satisfaction in hospice social work. *J Soc Work End Life Palliat Care.* 2017;13(2-3):134-150. The author is summarizing a definition based off work by Radey M, Figley CR. The social psychology of compassion. *Clin Soc Work J.* 2007;35:207-214.

This is particularly true in the disciplines of oncology and palliative care, examples of subspecialties in which clinicians care for individuals with chronic, progressive, and often life-limiting diseases, with whom they develop deep, meaningful provider–patient relationships. The well-being and job satisfaction of these clinicians should be tantamount to the wellness that they expect from the delivery of their services to their patients (1). After all, it has been noted that the wellness of a care provider has direct negative effects on important outcomes, including quality of patient care, efficiency, and productivity, as well as increased resource utilization (17,18). Work-related stressors may lead to problems with substance abuse and psychiatric and/or medical illnesses. They can affect interpersonal relationships, resulting in compassion fatigue before culminating later in burnout or even early retirement (1,6,9–11,19–29). This rippling effect has the potential to decrease clinical workforce substantially, creating gaps in the ability to provide expert care (1,15).

With physicians at increased risk for burnout (10) and over half of nurses reporting burnout (16), health care professionals' well-being has received a significant amount of attention, causing organizations to invest in efforts to improve upon reducing stress, burnout, and compassion fatigue. The National Academy of Medicine report *Taking Action Against Burnout: A Systems Approach to Professional Well-Being* released in October 2019 highlights the complexity of addressing burnout and calls for urgent responses tailored to each organization (15). Results from a 2015 American Hospital Association Study indicate that 87% of hospitals surveyed have an employee wellness program (30). Nevertheless, reviews of interventions geared toward reducing physician burnout indicate that they provide only "small, significant reductions in burnout" (31). One review found that efforts led by organizations have greater effects than those only led by physicians, suggesting the imperative for making changes on a system level (31). Another study concluded that both intervention types can provide "clinically meaningful reductions in burnout," and these initiatives decreased physician overall burnout scores by 10% (32). With work hours being a strong indicator for burnout (27), the Accreditation Counsel on Graduate Medical Education's work hour restrictions have significantly reduced resident physician burnout (33). Without a "one size fits all" intervention to mitigate burnout, organizations are encouraged to scrutinize and address triggers specific to their system and report their findings (15). Therefore, it is also imperative that workers in the human service industry incorporate measures into their daily routine to effectuate professional sustainability and find tenable ways to ensure adequate and frequent maintenance of their mind, body, and soul so that delivery of quality care may persist (15,17,34–37).

The aims of this chapter are to describe work-related stressors in the fields of oncology and palliative care and to delineate their impact on burnout and compassion fatigue. Given the proliferation of literature focused on mitigating burnout and compassion fatigue over the last decades, we will provide a recent and selective review of the literature. We will then provide an overview of strategies for sustained self-care.

BURNOUT DEFINITION AND PREVALENCE

Much attention has been given to the concept of *burnout* or *burnout syndrome* over the last 50 years, more so from an organizational business model, but of late from a health care perspective (15,31,32,38–42). Much of the literature historically focused on physician job satisfaction (19,43–47). *Burnout* is a term first described in the 1970s by psychologist and psychoanalyst Herbert Freudenberger (6,48–50) and expanded upon two decades later by Christina Maslach. Burnout is described to be a "stress-induced occupational disease" affecting many health care professionals (51–54). While 'burnout' is not a DSM-5 diagnosis, many of the sequelae of burnout are.

The Maslach Burnout Inventory-Human Services Survey (MBI-HSS) is now considered the gold standard measurement of burnout syndrome, in which the domain metrics are *emotional exhaustion* (feelings of being overextended with loss of emotional and physical resources and reserve), *depersonalization* ("negative, callous, or excessively detached responses" to work), and *personal accomplishment* (inversely proportional to burnout, refers to the feelings of incompetence and underachievement at work) (6,31–33,51,53–57). The MBI consists of a 22-item questionnaire assessing the frequency with which clinicians experience certain feelings related to their jobs in the three aforementioned subscales where scores are rated low, moderate, and high (Table. 48.1) (53). One is said to have burnout when emotional exhaustion or depersonalization scores are high (10,15,58).

Researching burnout in oncology and palliative care has yielded mixed, but striking, statistics. In a 2014 study of oncologists using the MBI, nearly 45% exhibited burnout, scoring high in the emotional exhaustion (38%) and depersonalization (25%) domains. More time spent directly with patients was "the dominant professional predictor of burnout for oncologists" (27). Other studies show prevalence hovering at about 30%, including oncology physician assistants (29,59–61).

Globally, prevalence of burnout in oncologists is high, with about half of oncologists exhibiting burnout in New Zealand and Australia (48.5%) as well as Lebanon (47%), and more than half in China (51%), Belgium (51.2%), and Brazil (58.1%) (62–66). Strikingly, two-thirds of oncologists aged 40 or younger across Europe meet criteria for burnout (67). Among trainees, more than half of U.S. oncology fellows exhibit burnout, as do one-third of radiation oncology residents, with that number higher among radiation oncology residents in France and New Zealand (68–71).

TABLE 48.1 MASLACH BURNOUT INVENTORY SCALE

Depersonalization	I feel I treat some patients as if they were impersonal objects.
	I do not really care what happens to some patients.
Emotional exhaustion	I still feel tired when I wake up on the workday mornings.
Personal accomplishment	I deal effectively with my patient's problems.
	I can easily create a relaxed atmosphere for my patients.
	I feel exhilarated after working closely with my patients.

Excerpts from modified Maslach Burnout Inventory (MBI). MBI consists of a 22-item questionnaire consisting of three domains: depersonalization, emotional exhaustion, and personal accomplishment. The frequency with which one experiences these feelings is scored on a seven-point Likert scale and rated low, moderate, and high. The hallmark of burnout is high emotional exhaustion (48,51,105).
Adapted from Maslach C, Schaufeli WB, Leiter MP. Job burnout. *Ann Rev Psychol*. 2001;52:397-422.

Comparatively, 38.7% of U.S. palliative care clinicians (physicians, nurses, social workers, and chaplains) surveyed in 2016 showed at least one symptom of burnout, either high emotional exhaustion or high depersonalization (28,72). A recent survey of palliative care chaplains found two-thirds exhibited work-related distress (73). A 2017 review of literature that included palliative care physicians, nurses, and social workers revealed overall burnout prevalence at 17.3%, with social workers exhibiting the highest prevalence at 27% (74).

In the 11th Revision of the International Classification of Diseases, the World Health Organization classifies burnout as an occupational phenomenon "resulting from chronic workplace stress that has not been successfully managed," characterized by: exhaustion, mental distancing or cynicism, and decreased efficacy (54). In other words, one may be more prone to experiencing feelings of "being burned out," if one's work conditions do not align with one's work goals. Maslach noted that burnout occurs when there is a mismatch of the person and the job, as it relates to workload or resources, control, reward, community, fairness, and values (15,50,75,76). This is not to say that one will find perfection in each of the aforementioned domains—rather that there will be acceptable or substantial levels of satisfaction in them such that one remains satisfied and committed to his/her job. This commitment or job engagement may help mitigate job burnout.

For all intents and purposes, these domains reflect organizational, often modifiable elements, more so than personal, perhaps less modifiable traits. Therefore, burnout, in its deconstruction, seems to stem from external influences that are beyond the care provider's own locus of control. Potter cites Gentry and Baranowsky who describe burnout as "the chronic psychological syndrome of perceived demands from work outweighing perceived resources in the work environment" (11). Thus, this imbalance produces a stress reaction in the individual; if such stress persists unaddressed, it manifests fertile conditions for burnout (15,31).

COMPASSION FATIGUE DEFINITION AND PREVALENCE

By contrast, where burnout relates to extrinsic issues of the workplace environment, the basis of compassion fatigue seems due to internal qualities of the care provider. Summarized by Pelon (77), compassion fatigue is when "the ongoing exposure to and empathetic concern for the suffering of others leads to deep physical, emotional, and spiritual exhaustion, hopelessness, disconnection from others, and decreased capacity for and interest in empathetic attunement with clients" (77–82). Joinson initially described the phenomenon of compassion fatigue in 1992, a concept derived from research on burnout in emergency department nurses suggesting that compassion fatigue was "a unique form of burnout that affects people in care giving profession" (11,78,83). She noted particular behaviors characteristic of compassion fatigue in "cancer care providers," which included the following: chronic fatigue, irritability, dread going to work, aggravation of physical ailments, and a lack of joy in life (78).

Some investigators purport that the "cost of caring" (84) for patients with cancer and other chronic life-limiting diseases in which deep emotional, empathic investment is made undergirds the concept of compassion fatigue (81,82). They suggest that repeated exposure to highly emotional care, often with frequent losses, is akin to posttraumatic stress disorder (PTSD). Compassion fatigue has also been described as *secondary trauma* or *vicarious trauma*—a consequence of trauma of another rather than trauma to oneself (55,80,84–86). It is characterized by classic symptomatology of PTSD, including recurring and intrusive thoughts, avoidance, and emotional hyperarousal. Compassion fatigue can lead to burnout (55,80–82,85).

Orlovsky helped to differentiate compassion fatigue from job dissatisfaction or frustration with the organizational mechanics of the workplace (78,87). Compassion fatigue may be considered a loss of the continued "ability to nurture" (83) as it relates to loss of empathic restoration due to repeated encounters with those dying from their chronic diseases. Although one may be unable to nurture anymore and is suffering from compassion fatigue or perhaps is even burned out, there can still exist a degree of compassion satisfaction. *Compassion satisfaction* is defined as positive benefits that helping professionals derive from working with traumatized or suffering persons and the degree to which they feel successful in their jobs (88). Research on hospice workers reveals compassion satisfaction is negatively associated with compassion fatigue and burnout, suggesting its protective power (77,89). In a small study of American palliative care interdisciplinary clinicians, more years of experience correlated with higher compassion satisfaction and lower burnout (81).

Reviewing the growing body of literature on compassion fatigue has yielded many descriptions of the caregiver's experience, including discontentment, depression, and loss of self-worth, in addition to feelings of mental and physical exhaustion (11,51,55,82,90). For a clinician, periodic physical or mental exhaustion can be normal.

TABLE 48.2 INTERVENTIONS TO PROMOTE WORK–LIFE BALANCE

Supportive work community

Appropriate recognition and reward

Training in communication skills

Practice of self-care activities

Development of self-awareness skills

Promotion of feelings of choice and control

Sustainable workload

Adapted from Kearney MK, Weininger RB, Vachon MLS, Harrison RL, Balfour MM. Self-care of physicians caring for patients at the end of life: being connected…a key to my survival. *JAMA*. 2009;301:1155-1164.

However, it is the loss of the caregiver's ability to be an empathic witness for one's patients and their families that constitutes compassion fatigue—colloquially, "when the well runs dry" (78). Here, we consider compassion fatigue to be a unique form of burnout that occurs earlier on the "trajectory" of job burnout where there is the loss of "ability to nurture" (83). It is a phenomenon where timely and upstream intervention can ameliorate its vastly devastating effects. Interventions are listed in Table. 48.2.

ETIOLOGIES/MANIFESTATIONS OF BURNOUT AND COMPASSION FATIGUE

Given the high prevalence of burnout in the medical world, and in particular oncology and palliative care, there is an imperative to understand and mitigate its influencing factors (28,29,72). Research has demonstrated that young physicians are more prone to burnout than their older counterparts, the sentiments of which are speculated to start as early as residency (1,28,33,58,67,72,91,92). Nearly one-quarter of medical residents surveyed would like to change career paths, due to long work hours, heavy workload, and little autonomy and control (1,93). Additional risk factors for burnout found in this demographic included single relationship status, poor self-esteem, situations in which the clinician feels a lack of control, high student loan debt, and personality traits of perfectionism, workaholism, and/or type A personality (1,6,27,92,94,95).

Compassion fatigue and burnout are also associated with negative clinical adverse events such as increased medical errors and suboptimal patient care. A large 2018 systematic review and meta-analysis found that "burnout is associated with twofold increased odds for unsafe care, unprofessional behaviors, and low patient satisfaction" (17). Physicians with higher depersonalization have three times increased reports of unprofessional behaviors (17). A study examining the effects of workload on physicians' quality of care found that 57% of those studied purported that exhaustion, fatigue, or sleep deprivation resulted in suboptimal patient care (1,96). Additional studies further highlight the dangers of fatigue, tiredness, and sleep deprivation in health care professionals as sleep deprivation was noted to be more incapacitating than a high blood alcohol concentration (1,97).

Professionally, burned out health care providers have experienced increased absenteeism, decreased productivity, and increased job turnover (6,15,18,22,25,52,98–100). Among gynecologic oncologists, burnout significantly decreased RVUs and academic publications, especially with female physicians experiencing burnout (18). Such loss of physician workforce is financially costly to organizations, about $4.6 billion a year (101). Ultimately, the consumer (patient and family member) suffers the greatest from clinician compassion fatigue and burnout. Patients who trust and have confidence in their physicians because of the physician's job satisfaction are more likely to comply with the prescribed regimen of care (19,42,102).

As noted previously, physicians are noted to have greater job stress and emotional distress than the general population (10). It is not surprising that clinicians in oncology and palliative care are more vulnerable to burnout due to the intensity and frequency of losses in the field (11,29,103). With respect to oncology nursing burnout, the following stress factors have been identified: the nature of the cancer, complex treatments, death, a personal sense of failure and futility, intense involvement with patients and families, ethical issues in treatment, surrogate decision-making, and palliative care issues (79,104). In palliative care, clinicians noted similar stressors, along with the feeling of being understaffed (28,73). These issues are applicable to the entire interdisciplinary team caring for the individual patient (87).

Physicians were also found to work longer hours per week (50 to 60 hours per week) even when not on call (1,105). Over the last decade, ACGME work hour restrictions for house officers appear to reduce resident physician burnout as well as medical errors (33). More interestingly, researchers investigating the negative impact of stress upon one's physical being found abnormal biological markers, including ketonuria and cardiac arrhythmias on examination of subjects (106). A study of the association between workload and burnout in intensive care unit physicians correlated such physiologic changes with more intense workloads and were factors suggestive of future burnout (107). Palliative care clinicians with higher burnout scores have significantly higher cortisol secretions (108). With this objective evidence, one might be better able to conceptualize that burnout is not merely a subjective phenomenon, but it gives merit to stress serving as the forerunner to disease.

Occupational injuries such as percutaneous needle sticks increase with fatigue and lack of attentiveness (1,109). For individuals working 16 consecutive hours or more, a rise in medical errors occurred due to lack of attentiveness (1,17,110). These factors are also likely culprits in the increased motor vehicle accidents noted within the profession. Additionally, while the electronic health record (EHR) is meant to increase the quality of care provided, it is instead increasing clinician burnout and frustration. Clinicians are spending more time on clerical work that typically has an inefficient workflow and using time afterhours to finish notes (13,15).

Finally, clinicians' personal lives are also impacted by such rigorous work hours and demanding workloads. Researchers have found that substance abuse and increased alcohol use are often evident in the lives of those providers who have a difficult time with the person–job fit due to factors, both intrinsic and extrinsic (2–5,9,17,20,21,29,55,59). Such negative coping mechanisms of avoidance and denial underscore how this type of self-medication can be a slippery slope, as often there are real underlying psychiatric disorders (depression, anxiety) that should be professionally addressed (1,29,59,70,111–114). Several studies suggest that greater burnout puts a clinician at higher risk for suicidal ideation and suicide (15,115). Further, interpersonal relations, those that are considered beneficial in protecting one from burnout, often suffer as a result of unrecognized and untreated compassion fatigue and burnout (2–5).

SELF-CARE

Characterizing compassion fatigue and burnout helps delineate where things can go wrong. For more sustainable professional development—including within the fields of oncology and palliative medicine—one must routinely incorporate principles of self-care. These deliberate practices help to ensure self-preservation and daily restoration of the care provider; they function to keep work–life balance at greater equilibrium, lessening the effects of compassion fatigue that can lead to burnout (34,78,87,116).

Perhaps one might conceptualize stress as a multidimensional entity that has repercussions expressed in many modalities. In the palliative care

world, Dame Cicely Saunders, who put extensive efforts in the development of modern hospice care, theorized a model for total pain. She postulated that pain, in its finer analysis, is a constellation of physical, social, psychological, and spiritual pain elements, coexisting in one individual, with dynamic interplay on the other. Using this paradigm of total pain as an example, one might consider an analogous model of *total stress*. Total stress is then influenced by physical, social, psychological, and spiritual factors (Fig. 48.1). The interplay of these components can either ameliorate or exacerbate one's stress response.

Implementation of self-care practices into one's routine can be challenging. As busy health care professionals with seemingly limited time resources and other constraints, self-care is often neglected. However, although discrete data are lacking, daily participation in self-care practices that address all domains of "total stress" is likely beneficial in preventing or combating compassion fatigue and burnout (Table 48.3) (28,72,116,117). Clinical literature reinforces anecdotal findings that physicians often work when sick, self-medicate their ailments, and are less likely to be open about physical or mental illness, for fear these are signs of provider weakness and/or incompetence (1,118). Although literature is lacking, it is possible to assume that these behaviors are not physician-only but occur across other health disciplines. This underscores the importance of obtaining preventative medical care, appropriate screening tests, and routine dental care as integral parts of self-care practices (119). However, as we have already discussed, not disclosing or recognizing one's limitations has profound negative influences on the care provider, the patient/families, and the organization.

Self-care research findings consistently show important trends. Physical activity, particularly exercise, is a key component to self-care and is consistently noted in the literature (90,113,119). Intuitively, exercise likely promotes overall general cardiovascular health in this population. As it has been suggested that the cardiovascular mortality in physicians is "higher than average," one might speculate that this is one intervention to help reduce stress and promote vigor and vitality (1). In addition to exercise, health care providers are encouraged to take vacations, engage in personal passions and hobbies, and read nonmedical literature (28,72,120).

In order to be an effective care provider, one has to be not only physically but also emotionally well to function at a high and sustainable level of service. One study of palliative care clinicians in Spain found that practices of self-care related to one's "inner life" including focusing on and being aware of one's own

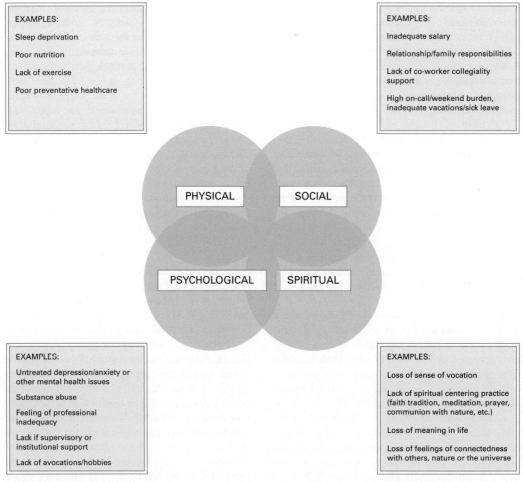

Figure 48.1 Conceptual model of total stress and examples.

emotions, as well as having a healthy social life, fostered healthier coping with patients' deaths and less burnout (34). Furthermore, psychotherapy or mental health counseling provides opportunities for clinicians to process these emotionally intense situations, develop greater self-awareness, and develop skills for coping. More than 90% of hospitals have Employee Assistance Programs or mental health services for employees, which signals an attempt to provide these resources (30).

TABLE 48.3 TABLE OF SELF-CARE INTERVENTIONS

Do	Don't
Honor yourself	Blame others
Recharge, renew daily: regular exercise program, mediation, a walk	Ignore the problem
Have a meaningful conversation each day; value time with family, friends	Complain to coworkers or look for a new job (make rash decisions)
Get enough sleep and rest	Self-medicate
Identify your own personal goals	Neglect your own needs, interests, and desires
Take some time off	Work harder and longer

Adapted from Showalter SE. Compassion fatigue: what is it? Why does it matter? Recognizing the symptoms, acknowledging the impact, developing the tools to prevent compassion fatigue, and strengthen the professional already suffering from the effects. *Am J Hosp Palliat Care*. 2010;27:239-242.

Further, fostering interpersonal relationships (professionally with colleagues and personally with family members) is one protective mechanism against burnout, including peer support groups (6,34,78,121–124). The culture of medicine suggests that physicians are reluctant to talk about their own health issues or distress or even those problems affecting their colleagues. This "conspiracy of silence" often fosters feelings of isolation without access to supportive resources (1,125).

Though the hospice interdisciplinary care team was developed by Saunders to facilitate best care for the dying patient, the interconnectedness of the various members of the team may help to balance the caregiving investment of any one provider. Saunders expressed that

> The care of the dying patient should not be an individual work but one that is shared. Shared with the relative with all the various members of the staff, spiritual, medical, and lay; and, as far as we can, with the patient himself. Where this is so we are left with the sense of completion and fulfillment which makes this such a rewarding branch of medical and nursing care (126).

In the late 1950s, British psychoanalyst Michael Balint understood the dynamics of the doctor–patient relationship realizing that it can evoke considerable stress in the physician (78,121). Hosting forums for physicians to meet and discuss challenging patients helped to stave off internal turmoil and stresses generated by such patients. In later years, continued emphasis has been placed on the importance of this type of group intervention for health care providers in an effort to further combat compassion fatigue and burnout (78,122,123,127,128). The presence of other colleagues lends support as empathic/sympathetic witnesses when one has encountered a difficult family member or a dying child, had to deliver bad news, or make a difficult decision to withdraw or forgo care in someone who has experienced an unexpected trauma. Challenges even occur when discussing any of the above clinical scenarios with interdisciplinary staff caring for the patient/family who themselves are experiencing a difficult time with the clinical situation, from executing orders to grappling with their own morals and beliefs regarding difficult decisions, particularly at end of life.

Recent research examining burnout in intensive care unit physicians demonstrated that the quality of collegial relationships and the support derived from them are protective against compassion fatigue (106). Interdisciplinary clinical frameworks and organizational support of self-care may also be protective (55,129–131). This again underscores the importance of communication and sharing the caregiver burden as it helps to increase compassion

satisfaction, lessen compassion fatigue and hopefully, to prevent later burnout.

Still, communication can also be the source of great conflict, particularly in oncology and palliative care. Ramirez et al. noted that oncologists and other clinicians working with cancer patients were more susceptible to burning out if they felt poorly equipped to handle the emotional needs of this patient population (129). This ineffective doctor–patient communication dyad causes distress in the workplace. As part of this perpetuating cycle, oncologists with low job satisfaction and greater secondary traumatic stress are "less likely to communicate prognosis with their patients" (132,133). Continued efforts must be invested into the implementation of communication and interpersonal skills early on in medical education, as research has proven it beneficial in building therapeutic alliance with patients, particularly those with cancer (78,129,134,135).

Spirituality remains an important, often overlooked area in holistic support of the patient and caregiver. Spirituality is often used interchangeably with religiosity and faith. However, spirituality more so pertains to what gives meaning to one's life or experiences. As caregivers in oncology and palliative care repeatedly, often daily, encounter death and dying, they are witness to meaning-making experiences of their patients. Naturally, these interactions can and do bring pause to the health professional allowing for introspection and reflection regarding one's own significance and mortality. Several investigators have postulated that a clinician's spirituality or spiritual well-being is protective against burnout and is inversely related to burnout (35,136–138).

Engaging in "personally meaningful rituals" following a patient's death mitigates burnout and compassion fatigue in hospice workers. Examples of rituals provided in one study include inward reflection, journaling, walking, lighting candles, attending funerals, and calling bereaved family members (35). Another palliative care team creates "Bereavement Rounds" to commemorate those who have died and provide an opportunity to share and debrief (36). Rituals of this kind provide an opportunity for clinicians to grieve and reflect on the people they serve and thus create meaning out of their work. Without an opportunity to grieve and acknowledge their emotions and the connection they share with patients, clinicians are at risk for burnout (35–37,139).

Personal accomplishment, one of the three domains of burnout that was discussed earlier, also seems to be a protective factor in preventing burnout. In those physician and nursing populations where the risk of burnout was deemed to be the highest, personal accomplishment was found to be protective (6–8,59,140–142). Literature has demonstrated that high personal accomplishment may be protective against emotional exhaustion and depersonalization, avoiding burnout syndrome (59). This is perhaps due to the influence of spirituality; how a caregiver's work gives meaning to another's life including their own (137).

From an institutional perspective, it may behoove the global medical profession to borrow from organizational management strategies researched and developed by Kaiser Permanente Medical Group over the last several years in their thrust to enhance physicians' professional satisfaction and job retention (143). They have recognized that in order to quell the severity of the experience of compassion fatigue, subsequent burnout, and eventual loss of their physician work pool, they must be more attentive to the needs of their physicians. Anticipating their needs prior to their official start times with the company, during the early affiliation/working for the organization, and throughout the tenure of their employment with the company is one of the ways that the organization has tried to achieve this. Striving to find and maintain a work–life balance is dynamic force changing from day to day, so are the needs of physicians/employees. King and Speckart concluded that there exist 10 evidence-based practices that are needed for successful physician retention (143) (Table 48.4).

Organizations have become increasingly creative in mitigating burnout for their associates. The Stanford Emergency Department engaged in

a "time banking" study, in which physicians who picked up a colleague's shift, served on a committee, or mentored students could then "bank" this time for assistance for both their careers (assistance in grant-writing or preparing presentations) and personal lives (various meal and housecleaning services). Through this, the team members were more willing to both cover for each other and ask for help, reported greater job satisfaction, and all positions were retained (144,145).

Therefore, as noted previously, organizations, such as hospitals, health maintenance organizations, or physician practices, should reasonably attend to those institutional factors that will enhance job satisfaction and promote job engagement as much as possible. This is facilitated by prioritizing health providers' needs in the organizational hierarchy such that there is a greater sense of control and autonomy in shaping the work environment with the aim of maintaining as ideal a person–job fit as possible (Table 48.4). The effort toward fostering clinician wellness impacts the quality of care patients and families receive.

SUMMARY

As an empathic witness to a patient's stress and distress, caregivers must be able to respond to the emotional needs of the patient. This is best enhanced through effective communication skills (78,129). By corollary, health care providers in oncology and palliative care must practice recognizing their own limitations, when they feel "stressed out" or unable to find the appropriate words to effectively mediate difficult patient/family situations. There must be an impetus to move from tacit isolation to finding a voice to let others know that one needs help and to recognizing when colleagues are displaying signs of burnout and are in need of help. Relationship building, rapport, and teamwork, where effective communication is timely and frequent, along with daily, multidimensional self-care interventions, are perhaps the most effective tools against compassion fatigue and subsequent burnout.

Traditionally, the medical education curriculum, however, has not met the needs of young clinicians in this regard. With more research and clarity on burnout and compassion fatigue, perhaps this awareness will trickle down to young trainees in the profession (15). Future research endeavors might focus on the field of palliative care, as it is a relatively new and growing discipline, to assess how self-care interventions affect rates of attrition and retention of its workforce.

Work–life balance is crucial to self-preservation and diminishing, if not preventing, compassion fatigue. One must set appropriate boundaries

TABLE 48.4 PRACTICE STRATEGIES FOR PHYSICIAN RETENTION

Realistic job preview and behavioral interviewing
Essential startup resources and administrative processes planned and in place
Practical, timely, comprehensive orientation programs delivered in multiple ways
Physician enculturation, socialization, and fostering feelings of belonging
Mentoring program
Perceived control over the practice environment
Accurate, effective, and timely feedback
Recognition, rewards, and opportunities for advancement/career development
Open and trustworthy communication; belief that management listens and acts on suggestions
Reduction of stress in the workplace

Adapted from King H, Speckart C. Ten evidence-based practices for successful physician retention. *Perm J.* 2002;6:52-54.

and expectations and recognize limitations so that the empathic presence required to help others is not emotionally depleted. If depleted, the caregiver may certainly become less productive or efficacious. Attention must be given to foster a sense of well-being and wholeness in health care professionals to thwart the infectious and destructive pattern of burnout that permeates and threatens to undermine the future of medicine. If physicians, nurses, pharmacists, social workers, and chaplains are enduring more stress, feeling less supported, and more overworked, they then are less likely to encourage subsequent generations to pursue careers in the profession, thus jeopardizing the quality of our health care system (19).

REFERENCES

1. Wallace JE, Lemaire JB, Ghali WA. Physician wellness: a missing quality indicator. *Lancet*. 2009;374:1714-1721.
2. Sargent MC, Sotile W, Sotile MO, Rubash H, Barrack RL. Stress and coping among orthopaedic surgery residents and faculty. *J Bone Joint Surg Am*. 2004;86:1579-1586.
3. Firth-Cozens J. Individual and organizational predictors of depression in general practitioners. *Br J Gen Pract*. 1998;48:1647-1651.
4. Frank E, Dingle AD. Self-reported depression and suicide attempts among U.S. women physicians. *Am J Psychiatry*. 1999;156:1887-1894.
5. Graham J, Albery IP, Ramirez AJ, Richards MA. How hospital consultants cope with stress at work: implications for their mental health. *Stress Health*. 2001;17:85-89.
6. Hyman SA, Michaels DR, Berry JM, Schildcrout JS, Mercaldo ND, Weinger MB. Risk of burnout in perioperative clinicians: a survey study and literature review. *Anesthesiology*. 2011;114:194-204.
7. Gabbe SG, Melville J, Mandel L, Walker E. Burnout in chairs of obstetrics and gynecology: diagnosis, treatment and prevention. *Am J Obstet Gynecol*. 2002;186:601-612.
8. Ramirez AJ, Graham J, Richards MA, Cull A, Gregory WM. Mental health of hospital consultants: the effects of stress and satisfaction at work. *Lancet*. 1996;347:724-728.
9. Spickard A Jr, Gabbe SG, Christensen JF. Mid-career burnout in generalist and specialist physicians. *JAMA*. 2002;288:1447-1450.
10. Shanafelt TD, West CP, Sinsky C, et al. Changes in burnout and satisfaction with work-life integration in physicians and the general US working population between 2011 and 2017. *Mayo Clin Proc*. 2019;94(9):1681-1694.
11. Potter P, Deshields T, Divanbeigi J, et al. Compassion fatigue and burnout: prevalence among oncology nurses. *Clin J Oncol Nurs*. 2010;14:e56-e62.
12. Ferrans C. Quality of life: conceptual issues. *Semin Oncol Nurs*. 1990;6:248-254.
13. Shanafelt TD, Dyrbye LN, Sinsky C, et al. Relationship between clerical burden and characteristics of the electronic environment with physician burnout and professional satisfaction. *Mayo Clin Proc*. 2016;91:836-848.
14. Saint S, Zemencuk JK, Hayward RA, et al. What effect does increasing inpatient time have on outpatient-oriented internist satisfaction? *J Gen Intern Med*. 2003;18:725-729.
15. National Academies of Sciences, Engineering, and Medicine. *Taking action against clinician burnout: A systems approach to professional well-being*. Washington, DC: The National Academies Press; 2019. https://doi.org/10.17226/25521.
16. Zhang H-Y, Han W-L, Qin W, et al. Extent of compassion satisfaction, compassion fatigue, and burnout in nursing: a meta-analysis. *J Nurs Manag*. 2018;26:810-819.
17. Panagioti M, Geraghty K, Johnson J, et al. Association between physician burnout and patient safety, professionalism, and patient satisfaction. *JAMA Intern Med*. 2018;178(10):1317-1330.
18. Turner TB, Dilley SE, Smith HJ, et al. The impact of physician burnout on clinical and academic productivity of gynecologic oncologists: a decision analysis. *Gynecol Oncol*. 2017;146(3):642-646.
19. Scheurer D, McKean S, Miller J, Wetterneck T. U.S. physician satisfaction: a systematic review. *J Hosp Med*. 2009;4:560-568.
20. Brooke D, Edwards G, Taylor C. Addiction as an occupational hazard: 144 doctors with drug and alcohol problems. *Br J Addict*. 1991;86:1011-1016.
21. Juntunen J, Asp S, Olkinuora M, Aarimaa M, Strid L, Kauttu K. Doctors' drinking habits and consumption of alcohol. *BMJ*. 1988;297:951-954.
22. Ahola K, Kivimaki M, Honkonen T, et al. Occupational burnout and medically certified sickness absence: a population-based study of Finnish employees. *J Psychosom Res*. 2008;64:185-193.
23. Gardulf A, Soderstrom IL, Orton ML, Ericksson LE, Arnetz B, Nordstrom G. Why do nurses at a university hospital want to quit their jobs? *J Nurs Manag*. 2005;13:329-337.
24. Sharma A, Sharp DM, Walker LG, Monson JR. Stress and burnout among colorectal surgeons and colorectal nurse specialists working in the National Health Service. *Colorectal Dis*. 2008;10:397-406.
25. Borritz M, Rugulies R, Christensen KB, Villadsen E, Kristensen TS. Burnout as a predictor of self-reported sickness absence among human service workers: prospective findings from three year follow up of the PUMA study. *Occup Environ Med*. 2006;63:98-106.
26. Garelick AI, Gross SR, Richardson I, von der Tann M, Bland J, Hale R. Which doctors and with what problems contact a specialist service for doctors? *BMC Med*. 2007;5:26.
27. Shanafelt TD, Gradishar WJ, Kosty M, et al. Burnout and career satisfaction among US oncologists. *J Clin Oncol*. 2014;32(7):678-686.
28. Kamal AH, Bull JH, Wolf SP, et al. Prevalence and predictors of burnout among hospice and palliative care clinicians in the U.S [retracted in: *J Pain Symptom Management*. 2020;59(5):965]. *J Pain Symptom Manage*. 2016;51(4):690-696.
29. Medisauskaite A, Kamau C. Prevalence of oncologists in distress: systematic review and meta-analysis. *Psychooncology*. 2017;26(11):1732-1740.
30. Health Research & Educational Trust. *Health and Wellness Programs for Hospital Employees: Results from a 2015 American Hospital Association survey*. Chicago, IL: Health Research & Educational Trust; 2016, October. Accessed at www.hope.org
31. Panagioti M, Panagopoulou E, Bower P, et al. Controlled interventions to reduce burnout in physicians: a systematic review and meta-analysis. *JAMA Intern Med*. 2017;177(2):195-205.
32. West CP, Dyrbye LN, Erwin PJ, Shanafelt TD. Interventions to prevent and reduce physician burnout: a

systematic review and meta-analysis. *Lancet*. 2016; 388(10057):2272-2281.

33. Busireddy KR, Miller JA, Ellison K, Ren V, Qayyum R, Panda M. Efficacy of interventions to reduce resident physician burnout: a systematic review. *J Grad Med Educ*. 2017;9(3):294-301.

34. Sanso N, Galiana L, Oliver A, Pascual A, Sinclair S, Benito E. Palliative care professionals' inner life: exploring the relationships among awareness, self-care, and compassion satisfaction and fatigue, burnout, and coping with death. *J Pain Symptom Manage*. 2015;50(2):200-207.

35. Montross-Thomas LP, Scheiber C, Meier EA, Irwin SA. Personally meaningful rituals: a way to increase compassion and decrease burnout among hospice staff and volunteers. *J Palliat Med*. 2016;19(10):1043-1050.

36. Morris SE, Kearns JP, Moment A, Lee KA, deLima Thomas J. "Remembrance": a self-care tool for clinicians. *J Palliat Med*. 2019;2(3):316-318.

37. Kapoor S, Morgan CK, Siddique MA, Guntupalli KK. "Sacred Pause" in the ICU: evaluation of a ritual and intervention to lower distress and burnout. *Am J Hosp Palliat Med*. 2018;35(10):1337-1341.

38. Rochester SR, Vachon MLS, Lyall WAL. Immediacy in language: a channel to care of the dying patient. *J Comp Psychol*. 1974;2:75-76.

39. Lyall WAL, Vachon MLS, Rogers J. A study of the degree of stress experienced by professionals caring for dying patients. In: Ajemian I, Mount BM, eds. *The RVH Manual on Hospice/Palliative Care*. New York, NY: ARNO Press; 1980: 498-508.

40. Grunfeld, E, Whelan TJ, Zitzelsberger L, et al. Cancer care workers in Ontario: prevalence of burnout, job stress and job satisfaction. *Can Med Assoc J*. 2000;163:166-169.

41. Grunfeld E, Zitzelsberger L, Coristine M, et al. Job stress and job satisfaction of cancer care workers. *Psychooncology*. 2005;14:61-69.

42. Shanafelt T, Goh J, Sinsky C. The business case for investing in physician well-being. *JAMA Intern Med*. 2017;177(12):1826-1832.

43. Keeton, K, Fenner DE, Johnson TRB, Hayward RA. Predictors of physician career satisfaction, work–life balance, and burnout. *Obstet Gynecol*. 2007;109: 949-955.

44. Doan-Wiggins L, Zun L, Cooper MA, Meyers DL, Chen EH. Practice satisfaction, occupational stress, and attrition of emergency physicians. Wellness Task Force, Illinois College of Emergency Physicians. *Acad Emerg Med*. 1995;2:556-563.

45. Freeobrn DK. Satisfaction, commitment, and psychological well-being among HMO physicians. *West J Med*. 2001;174:13-18.

46. Gallery ME, Whitley TW, Klonic LK, Anzinger RK, Revicki, DA. A study of occupational stress and depression among emergency physicians. *Ann Emerg Med*. 1992;21:58-64.

47. Linzer M, Visser MR, Oort FJ, et al. Predicting and preventing physician burnout: results from the United States and Netherlands. *Am J Med*. 2001;111:170-175.

48. Freudenberger HJ. The staff burn-out syndrome in alternative institutions. *Psychother Theory, Res Pract*. 1971;12:73-82.

49. Freudenberger HJ. Burn-out: occupational hazard of the child care worker. *Child Care Q*. 1977;6:90-99.

50. Maslach C, Schaufeli WB, Leiter MP. Job burnout. *Annu Rev Psychol*. 2001;52:397-422.

51. Trufelli DC, Bensi CG, Garcia JB, et al. Burnout in cancer professionals: a systematic review and meta-analysis. *Eur J Cancer Care*. 2008;17:524-531.

52. Felton JS. Burnout as a clinical entity—its importance in health care workers. *Occup Med*. 1998;48:237-250.

53. Maslach C, Jackson S, Leiter MP. *Maslach Burnout Inventory Manual*. Palo Alto, CA: Consulting Psychologists Press; 1996.

54. World Health Organization. Burn-out an "occupational phenomenon": International Classification of Diseases. May 28, 2019. https://www.who.int/mental_health/evidence/burn-out/en/. Accessed October 1, 2019.

55. Kearney MK, Weininger RB, Vachon MLS, Harrison RL, Balfour MM. Self-care of physicians caring for patients at the end of life: being connected … a key to my survival. *JAMA*. 2009;301:1155-1164.

56. Maslach C, Leiter MP. Early predictors of job burnout and engagement. *J Appl Psychol*. 2008;93:498-512.

57. Maslach C. Job burnout: new directions in research and intervention. *Curr Dir Psychol Sci*. 2003;12:189-192.

58. Shanafelt TD, Bradley KA, Wipf JW, Back AL. Burnout and self-reported patient care in an internal medicine residency program. *Ann Intern Med*. 2002;136: 358-367.

59. Rath KS, Huffman LB, Phillips GS, Carpenter KM, Fowler JM. Burnout and associated factors among members of the Society of Gynecologic Oncology. *Am J Obstet Gynecol*. 2015;213(6):824.e1-824.e9.

60. Balch CM, Shanafelt TD, Sloan J, Satele DV, Kuerer HM. Burnout and career satisfaction among surgical oncologists compared with other surgical specialties. *Ann Surg Oncol*. 2011;18(1):16-25.

61. Tetzlaff ED, Hylton HM, DeMora L, Ruth K, Wong YN. National study of burnout and career satisfaction among physician assistants in oncology: Implications for team-based care. *J Oncol Pract*. 2018;14(1):e11-e22.

62. Leung J, Rioseco P, Munro P. Stress, satisfaction and burnout amongst Australian and New Zealand radiation oncologists. *J Med Imaging Radiat Oncol*. 2015;59(1):115-124.

63. Salem R, Akel R, Fakhri G, Tfayli A. Burnout among Lebanese oncologists: prevalence and risk factors. *Asian Pac J Cancer Prev*. 2018;19(8):2135-2139.

64. Ma S, Huang Y, Yang Y, et al. Prevalence of burnout and career satisfaction among oncologists in China: A National Survey. *Oncologist*. 2019;24(7):e480-e489.

65. Eelen S, Bauwens S, Baillon C, Distelmans W, Jacobs E, Verzelen A. The prevalence of burnout among oncology professionals: oncologists are at risk of developing burnout. *Psychooncology*. 2014;23(12):1415-1422.

66. Paiva CE, Martins BP, Paiva BSR. Doctor, are you healthy? A cross-sectional investigation of oncologist burnout, depression, and anxiety and an investigation of their associated factors. *BMC Cancer*. 2018;18(1):1044.

67. Banerjee S, Califano R, Corral J, et al. Professional burnout in European young oncologists: results of the European Society for Medical Oncology (ESMO) Young Oncologists Committee Burnout Survey. *Ann Oncol*. 2017;28(7):1590-1596.

68. Mougalian S, Lessen D, Levine R, et al. Palliative care training and associations with burnout in oncology fellows. *J Support Oncol*. 2013;11(2):95-102.

69. Ramey SJ, Ahmed AA, Takita C, Wilson LD, Thomas CR Jr, Yechieli R. Burnout evaluation of radiation residents nationwide: results of a survey of United States residents. *Int J Radiat Oncol Biol Phys*. 2017; 99(3):530-538.

70. Lazarescu I, Dubray B, Joulakian MB, et al. Prevalence of burnout, depression and job satisfaction among French senior and resident radiation oncologists. *Cancer Radiother*. 2018;22(8):784-789.

71. Leung J, Rioseco P. Burnout, stress and satisfaction among Australian and New Zealand radiation oncology trainees. *J Med Imaging Radiat Oncol*. 2017;61(1):146-155.

72. Kamal AH, Bull JH, Wolf SP, et al. Retraction of "Prevalence and predictors of burnout among hospice and palliative care professionals from 2016 Apr;51(4):690-6". *J Pain Symptom Manage.* 2020;59(5):965.

73. White KB, Murphy PE, Jeuland J, Fitchett G. Distress and self-care among chaplains working in palliative care. *Palliat Support Care.* 2019;17(5):542-549.

74. Parola V, Coelho A, Cardoso D, Sandgren A, Apostolo J. Prevalence of burnout in health professionals working in palliative care: a systematic review. *JBI Database System Rev Implement Rep.* 2017;15(7):1905-1933.

75. Vachon MLS, Sherwood C. Staff stress and burnout. In: Berger AM, Shuster DL Jr, Von Roenn JH, eds. *Principles and Practice of Palliative Oncology and Supportive Oncology.* Philadelphia, PA: Lippincott Williams and Wilkins; 2007:667-683.

76. French JRP, Rodgers W, Cobb S. Adjustment as person–environment fit. In: Coelho GV, Hamburg DA, Adams E, eds. *Coping and Adaptation.* New York, NY: Basic Books; 1974: 316-333.

77. Pelon SB. Compassion fatigue and compassion satisfaction in hospice social work. *J Soc Work End Life Palliat Care.* 2017;13(2-3):134-150.

78. Najjar N, Davis LW, Beck-Coon K, Doebbeling CC. Compassion fatigue: a review of the research to date and relevance to cancer-care providers. *J Health Psychol.* 2009;14:267-277.

79. McHolm F. Rx for compassion fatigue. *J Christ Nurs.* 2006;23:12-19; quiz 20-21.

80. O'Mahony S, Gerhart JI, Grosse J, Abrams I, Levy MM. Posttraumatic stress symptoms in palliative care professionals seeking mindfulness training: prevalence and vulnerability. *Palliat Med.* 2016;30(2):189-192.

81. O'Mahony S, Ziadni M, Hoerger M, Levine S, Baron A, Gerhart J. Compassion fatigue among palliative care clinicians: findings on personality factors and years of service. *Am J Hosp Palliat Care.* 2018;35(2):343-347.

82. Barnett MD, Ruiz IA. Psychological distress and compassion fatigue among hospice nurses: The mediating role of self-esteem and negative affect. *J Palliat Med.* 2018;21(10):1504-1506.

83. Joinson C. Coping with compassion fatigue. *Nursing.* 1992;22:116-121.

84. Figley CR, ed. *Compassion Fatigue: Coping with Secondary Traumatic Stress Disorder in Those Who Treat the Traumatized.* New York, NY: Brunner/Mazel; 1995:7-12.

85. Figley CR, ed. *Treating Compassion Fatigue.* New York, NY: Brunner-Routledge; 2002.

86. Breen LJ, O'Connor M, Hewitt LY, Lobb EA. The "specter" of cancer: exploring secondary trauma for health professionals providing cancer support and counseling. *Psychol Serv.* 2014;11(1):60-67.

87. Orlovsky C. Compassion fatigue. *Prairie Rose.* 2006;75:13.

88. Stamm B. Measuring compassion fatigue as well as fatigue: developmental history of the compassion satisfaction and fatigue testing. In: Figley C, ed. *Treating Compassion Fatigue.* New York, NY: Brunner-Routledge; 2002.

89. Slocum-Gori S, Hemsworth D, Chan WW, Carson A, Kazanjian A. Understanding compassion satisfaction, compassion fatigue and burnout: a survey of the hospice palliative care workforce. *Palliat Med.* 2013;27(2):172-178.

90. Showalter SE. Compassion fatigue: what is it? Why does it matter? Recognizing the symptoms, acknowledging the impact, developing the tools to prevent compassion fatigue, and strengthen the professional already suffering from the effects. *Am J Hosp Palliat Care* 2010;27:239-242.

91. Tang. L, Pang Y, He Y, Chen Z, Leng J. Burnout among early-career oncology professionals and the risk factors. *Psychooncology.* 2018;27(10)2436-2441.

92. Ramondetta LM, Urbauer D, Brown AJ, et al. Work related stress among gynecologic oncologists. *Gynecol Oncol.* 2011;123(2):365-369.

93. Cohen JS, Patten S. Well being in residency training: a survey examining resident physician satisfaction both within and outside of residency training and mental health in Alberta. *BMC Med Educ.* 2005;5:21.

94. Firth-Cozens J, King J. Are psychological factors linked to performance? In: Firth-Cozens J, King J, Hutchinson A, McAvoy P, eds. *Understanding Doctors' Performance.* Oxford, UK: Radcliffe Publishing; 2006.

95. Vetter MH, Vetter MK, Fowler J. Resilience, hope and flourishing are inversely associated with burnout among members of the Society for Gynecologic Oncology. *Gynecol Oncol Rep.* 2018;(25):52-55.

96. Firth-Cozens J, Greenhalgh J. Doctors' perceptions of the links between stress and lowered clinical care. *Soc Sci Med.* 1997;44:1017-1022.

97. Williamson AM, Feyer AM. Moderate sleep deprivation produces impairments in cognitive and motor performance equivalent to legally prescribed levels of alcohol intoxication. *Occup Environ Med.* 2000;57:649-655.

98. Middaugh DJ. Presenteeism: sick and tired at work. *Dermatol Nurs.* 2007;19:172-173, 185.

99. Pilette PC. Presenteeism in nursing: a clear and present danger to productivity. *J Nurs Adm.* 2005;35: 300-303.

100. Toppinen-Tanner S, Ojajarvi A, Vaananen A, Kalimo R, Japinen P. Burnout as a predictor of medically certified sick-leave absences and their diagnosed causes. *Behav Med.* 2005;31:18-27.

101. Han S, Shanafelt TD, Sinsky CA, et al. Estimating the attributable cost of physician burnout in the United States. *Ann Intern Med.* 2019;170(11):784-790.

102. DiMatteo MR, Sherbourne CD, Hays RD, et al. Physicians' characteristics influence patients' adherence to medical treatment: results from the Medical Outcomes Study. *Health Psychol.* 1993;12: 93-102.

103. Lewis AE. Reducing burnout: development of an oncology staff bereavement program. *Oncol Nurs Forum.* 1999;26:1065-1069.

104. Kash K, Breitbart W. The stress of caring for cancer patients. In: Breitbart W, Holland JC, eds. *Psychiatric Aspects of Symptom Management in Cancer Patients.* Washington, DC: American Psychiatric Press; 1993: 243-260.

105. Williams ES, Rondeau KV, Xiao Q, Francescutti LH. Heavy physician workloads: impact on physician attitudes and outcomes. *Health Serv Manage Res.* 2007;20:261-269.

106. Embriaco N, Papazian L, Kentish-Barnes N, Pochard F, Azoulay E. Burnout syndrome among critical care healthcare workers. *Curr Opin Crit Care.* 2007;13: 482-488.

107. Parshuram C, Dhanni S, Kirsch J, Cox P. Fellowship training, workload, fatigue and physical stress: a prospective observational study. *CMAJ.* 2004;170: 965-970.

108. Fernández-Sánchez JC, Pérez-Mármol JM, Blásquez A, Santos-Ruiz AM, Peralta-Ramírez MI. Association between burnout and cortisol secretion, perceived stress, and psychopathology in palliative care unit health professionals. *Palliat Support Care.* 2017;16(3):286-297.

109. Ayas NT, Barger LK, Cade BE, et al. Extended work duration and the risk of self-reported percutaneous injuries in interns. *JAMA.* 2006;296:1055-1062.

110. Lockley SW, Cronin JW, Evans EE, et al.; for the Harvard Work Hours, Health and Safety Group. Effect of reducing interns' weekly work hours on sleep and attentional failures. *N Engl J Med.* 2004;351:1829-1837.

111. Baldisseri MR. Impaired healthcare professional. *Crit Care Med.* 2007;35(suppl):S106-S116.

112. Firth-Cozens J. Interventions to improve physicians' well being and patient care. *Soc Sci Med.* 2001;52:215-222.

113. Whitebird RR, Asche SE, Thompson GL, Rossom R, Heinrich R. Stress, burnout, compassion fatigue, and mental health in hospice workers in Minnesota. *J Palliat Med.* 2013;16(12):1534-1539.

114. Shanafelt TD, Boone S, Tan L, et al. Burnout and satisfaction with work-life balance among US physicians relative to the general US population. *Arch Intern Med.* 2012;172(18):1377-1385.

115. Shanafelt TD, Balch CM, Dyrbye L, et al. Special report: Suicidal ideation among American surgeons. *Arch Surg.* 2011;146(1):54-62.

116. Hotchkiss JT. Mindful self-care and secondary traumatic stress mediate a relationship between compassion satisfaction and burnout risk among hospice care professionals. *Am J Hosp Palliat Med.* 2018;35(8):1099-1108.

117. Gillman L, Adams J, Kovac R, Kilcullen A, House A, Doyle C. Strategies to promote coping and resilience in oncology and palliative care nurses caring for adult patients with malignancy: a comprehensive systematic review. *JBI Database System Rev Implement Rep.* 2015;13(5):131-204.

118. Thompson WT, Cupples ME, Sibbett CH, Skan DI, Bradley T. Challenges of Culture, Conscience, and Contract to General Practitioners' 2008; 63 care of their own health: qualitative study. *BMJ.* 2001;323:728-731.

119. Chittenden EH, Ritchie CS. Work–life balancing: challenges and strategies. *J Palliat Med.* 2011;14:870-874.

120. Marchalik D, Rodriguez A, Namath A, et al. The impact of non-medical reading on clinician burnout: a national survey of palliative care providers. *Ann Palliat Med.* 2019;8(4):428-435.

121. Balint M. *The Doctor, His Patient and the Illness.* New York, NY: International University Press; 1957.

122. Benson J, Magraith K. Compassion fatigue and burnout. *Aust Fam Physician.* 2005;34:497-498.

123. Lyckholm L. Dealing with stress, burnout, and grief in the practice of oncology. *Lancet Oncol.* 2001;2:750-755.

124. Peterson U, Bergstrom G, Samuelsson M, Asberg M, Nygren A. Reflecting peer-support groups in the prevention of stress and burnout: randomized controlled trail. *J Adv Nurs.* 2008;63:506-516.

125. Arnetz BB. Psychological challenges facing physicians of today. *Soc Sci Med.* 2001;52:203-213.

126. Saunders C. The last achievement. *Nurs Times.* 1976;72:1247-1249.

127. Stojanovic-Tasic M, Latas M, Milosevic N, et al. Is Balint training associated with the reduced burnout among primary health care doctors? *Libyan J Med.* 2018;13(1):1440123.

128. Popa-Velea O, Trutescu CI, Diaconescu LV. The impact of Balint work on alexithymia, perceived stress, perceived social support and burnout among physicians working in palliative care: a longitudinal study. *Int J Occup Med Environ Health.* 2019;32(1):53-63.

129. Ramirez A, Graham J, Richards M, et al. Burnout and psychiatric disorder among cancer clinicians. *Br J Cancer.* 1995;71:1263-1269.

130. Vachon MLS. Staff stress in hospice/palliative care: a review. *Palliat Med.* 1995;9:91-122.

131. Edmonds C, Lockwood GM, Bezjak A, Nyhof-Young J. Alleviating emotional exhaustion in oncology nurses: an evaluation of Wellspring's "Care for the Professional Caregiver Program". *J Cancer Educ.* 2012;27(1):27-36.

132. Raphael MJ, Fundytus A, Hopman WM, et al. Medical oncology job satisfaction: results of a global survey. *Semin Oncol.* 2019;46(1):73-82.

133. Granek L, Nakash O, Cohen M, Ben-David M, Ariad S. Oncologists' communication about end of life: The relationship among secondary traumatic stress, compassion satisfaction, and approach and avoidance communication. *Psychooncology.* 2017;26(11):1980-1986.

134. Gysels M, Richardson A, Higginson IJ. Communication training for health professionals who care for patients with cancer: a systematic review of effectiveness. *Support Care Cancer.* 2004;12:692-700.

135. Fellowes D, Wikinson S, Moore P. Communication skills training for health care professionals working with cancer patients, their families and/or carers. *Cochrane Database Syst Rev.* 2004;(2):CD003751.

136. Harrison RL, Westwood MJ. Preventing vicarious traumatization of mental health therapists: identifying protective practices. *Psychotherapy (Chic).* 2009;46(2):203-219.

137. Boston PH, Mount BM. The caregiver's perspective on existential and spiritual distress in palliative care. *J Pain Symptom Manage.* 2006;32:13-26.

138. Huggard PK. *Managing Compassion Fatigue: Implications for Medical Education [dissertation].* Auckland, New Zealand: University of Aukland; 2008.

139. Granek L, Krzyzanowska MK, Nakash O, et al. Gender differences in the effect of grief reactions and burnout on emotional distress among clinical oncologists. *Cancer.* 2016;122(23):3705-3715.

140. Johns MM III, Ossoff RH. Burnout in academic chairs of otolaryngology: head and neck surgery. *Laryngoscope.* 2005;115:2056-2061.

141. Bertges YW, Eshelman A, Raoufi M, Abouljoud MS. A national study of burnout among American transplant surgeons. *Transplant Proc.* 2005;37:1399-1401.

142. Guntupalli KK, Fromm RE Jr. Burnout in the internist–intensivist. *Intensive Care Med.* 1996;22(7):625-630.

143. King H, Speckart C. Ten evidence-based practices for successful physician retention. *Perm J.* 2002;6:52-54.

144. Fassiotto M, Simard C, Sandborg C, Valantine H, Raymond J. An integrated career coaching and time-banking system promoting flexibility, wellness, and success. *Acad Med.* 2018;93(6):881-887.

145. Schulte, B. Time in the bank: a Stanford plan to save doctors from burnout. *The Washington Post.* August 20, 2015.

Ethical Considerations in Palliative Care

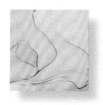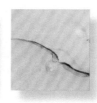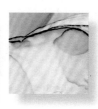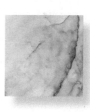

49 Advance Care Planning, Advance Directives, and Withholding and Withdrawing Treatment[1]

Hae Lin Cho and Christine Grady

Patients should make their own medical decisions whenever possible. However, some patients, especially those with serious illnesses or near the end of life, may be too sick or incapacitated to make decisions for themselves. One study found that about 30% of elderly Americans at the end of life required decision-making but lacked decision-making capacity (1), and other studies have shown that most critically ill patients are unable to participate in end-of-life treatment decisions (2). Around 25% of Americans die in the hospital, although most say they want to die at home (3,4); and more than half a million Americans die of cancer annually, often supported by technology in the impersonal and isolated environment of an intensive care unit (5). Publically debated cases, such as those of Nancy Cruzan and Terry Schiavo, brought attention to the complexity of making treatment and end-of-life care decisions, especially in the face of uncertainty about individuals' previously expressed wishes (6,7). Advance directives (AD) and advance care planning (ACP) evolved as a response to most people's desire to retain some control over their future medical care. AD and ACP provide patients with the opportunity to process and document their values and goals for treatment and specify them in writing, so that others can make decisions consistent with their wishes when they are no longer capable of making their own.

COMPLETING ADVANCE DIRECTIVES AND ENGAGING IN ADVANCE CARE PLANNING

Advance Directives

There are two general types of AD: the instructional directive and designation of a proxy. An instructional directive allows a person to express her preferences for or give instructions about future medical care for such a time when she is no longer able to make decisions herself. The living will,

a well-known instructional directive, allows people to document their desire to accept or refuse particular interventions used in serious illness or to sustain life, including mechanical ventilation, cardiopulmonary resuscitation (CPR), dialysis, and pain control.

The other advance directive option is designating a proxy or substitute to make decisions at such time a person cannot make them for herself. A designated proxy is referred to by several names, including Durable Power of Attorney for Health Care or DPA, Health Care Agent, Health Care Proxy, or medical power of attorney, often depending on state laws. Importantly, a DPA or medical power of attorney is distinct from a traditional power of attorney, which is a legal designation that grants another person jurisdiction over one's financial and personal matters.

Patients may be well served by both designating a DPA and providing instructions about future medical care, as these types of directives are complementary. Assigning a DPA is helpful because one cannot anticipate all possible future health care situations and decisions. Specific instructions related to patient preferences, in turn, can provide welcome guidance for the DPA and medical team when making decisions. Most available forms developed at the state level or by specialty organizations allow both. An example of an advance directive form that provides the option for both kinds of advance directive is included here (Fig. 49.1).

All Medicare participating health care facilities are required by the U.S. Patient Self-Determination Act of 1990 to provide patients with information about their rights to make health care decisions, ask patients at admission about AD, and provide further information or assistance if desired (8). All 50 U.S. states and the District of Columbia have statutes that support AD and permit physicians to follow them without fear of liability. Although state statutes differ in some ways, many states honor documents completed in accordance with other state laws, and any written advance directive, as well as oral statements previously made by patients, can help guide treatment decisions (9).

---

[1]Disclaimer: The views expressed are those of the authors and do not necessarily reflect those of the NIH or the U.S. Department of Health and Human Services.

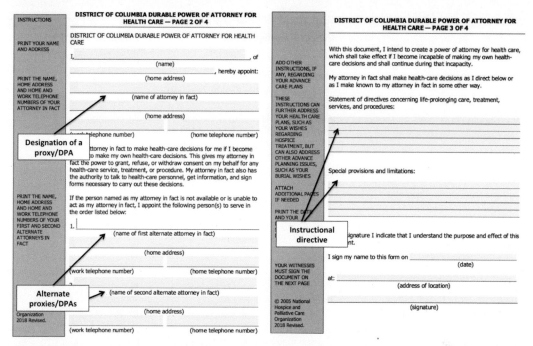

Figure 49.1 Example of an advance directive form with both an instructional directive and designation of a proxy option.

Specific advance directive forms and instructions for each of the 50 states are available online, as well as from state or municipal Departments of Health, hospitals, and some physicians' offices (10). These forms are often available in languages besides English (e.g., available language forms for all states can be found online through PREPARE for Your Care) (11). Some state initiatives allow people to complete an advance directive online and store it in a registry (12). Advance Directive/Living Will Registries are public or proprietary databases that electronically store AD and make them available to patients and providers when needed.

In addition to state forms, other initiatives aim to improve or supplement the traditional advance directive process, and expand patients' options for specifying values and preferences about their future medical care. Selected examples include Five Wishes, Let Me Decide, Respecting Choices, and Physicians or Medical Orders for Life-Sustaining Treatment (POLST/MOLST) paradigm.

- "Five Wishes" is an advance directive document that includes appointment of a proxy and documentation of a range of issues that people might care about, but are not usually included in a traditional advance directive, including emotional, spiritual, and personal needs (13).

- "Let Me Decide" is an advance directive document developed in Canada that offers patients and families an opportunity to specify choices about levels of care, nutrition, CPR, and treatment of life-threatening illness, as well as to assign a proxy (14).

- "Respecting Choices" is an ACP program that uses a staged approach; emphasizes training of physicians, health care providers, and ACP facilitators; and encourages the use of hospice and palliative care services. This program began as a community-wide planning system in Lacrosse, Wisconsin, through the Gundersen Lutheran Hospital system, which has since experienced a reduced number of hospital days at the end of life and lowered Medicare spending compared to other centers (15).

- Medical Orders for Life-Sustaining Treatment (POLST or MOLST) forms (referred to as the POLST paradigm) are portable medical orders that travel with a patient. A doctor, nurse practitioner, or other authorized health care provider completes and signs POLST/MOLST order forms after discussions with the patient about her values and preferences, diagnosis, treatment options, and likely course of disease. A POLST or MOLST is not the same as an advance directive but can complement one. The chart below describes the differences (Table 49.1) (16).

TABLE 49.1 COMPARISON OF POLST AND ADVANCE DIRECTIVES

	POLST Paradigm Form	Advance Directive
Type of Document	Medical Order	Legal Document
Who Completes the Document	Health care professional (which health care professional can sign varies by state)	Individual
Who Should Have One	Any seriously ill or frail individual (regardless of age) whose health care professional wouldn't be surprised if he/she died in the year	All competent adults
What Document Communicates	Specific medical orders	General treatment wishes
Can this Document Appoint a Surrogate Decision-Maker?	No	Yes
Surrogate Decision-Maker Role	Can engage in discussion and update or void form if patient lacks capacity	Cannot complete
Can Emergency Personnel Follow this Document?	Yes	No
Ease In Locating/Portability	Patient has original; a copy is in patient's medical record. A copy may be in a state registry (if state has one).	No set location. Individuals must make sure surrogates have most recent version.
Periodic Review	Health care professional responsible for reviewing with patient or surrogate	Patient is responsible for periodically reviewing.

Reproduced from polst.org with permission.

Advance Care Planning

ACP is a process that involves discussion, deliberation, and communication about clinical circumstances, prognosis, and goals, and the development of plans and preferences for future care to approximate those goals (Fig. 49.2) (17). ACP is a more iterative and interactive process than simply filling out an advance directive and should precede and surround the completion of a written advance directive. The ACP process often starts with health care providers giving patients information about their current clinical circumstances, likely trajectory, and available treatment options. Discussion of the patient's values and goals can help guide clinicians and surrogate decision makers when called upon later to make decisions. One study showed that giving patients question prompts that lay out potential points of discussion prior to ACP significantly increased the number of questions patients asked, as well the length of ACP consultations (18).

As shown in Figure 49.2, decisions made through the ACP process should be documented in written AD that can specify who and how decisions will be made for patients in the future. Even patients who already have AD should partake in ACP. Studies have found that ACP can increase alignment with patient preferences and palliative care use, decrease the rate of patients dying in hospitals and receiving life-sustaining treatment, and provide emotional support to patients' loved ones (19). These same studies also found that written AD are more useful in guiding decision-making when complemented by discussions with proxies, family members, physicians, and others who might be involved in later decisions (19).

ACP can be beneficial for patients at various stages of illness, and is not synonymous with end-of-life discussions, although end-of-life care planning can certainly be a part of ACP. Determining when to initiate ACP is critical and can be challenging. Although providers worry about the psychological effects of ACP on patients, studies suggest that these concerns are unsubstantiated, and most patients wait for their physicians to initiate ACP and/or end-of-life discussions (20–22). Currently, the American Society of Clinical Oncology (ASCO) recommends that end-of-life discussions occur within a month of diagnosis in patients with incurable cancer (23), although qualitative studies suggest that some patients prefer to postpone such discussions until further disease progression (21). Whenever a clinician initiates ACP, it may be helpful to reassure the patient that ACP does not necessarily mean that she has poor prognosis.

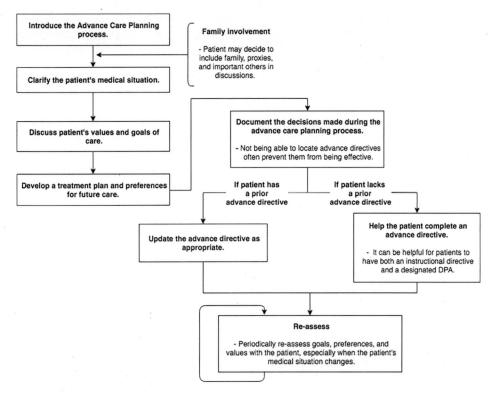

Figure 49.2 Advance care planning process.

Plans and decisions made during ACP should be revisited whenever the patient's clinical or social situation changes or when a patient wishes to re-examine her goals or directives. For patients with cancer, ASCO lays out specific sentinel events that trigger renewed ACP discussions, such as cancer progression, decline in functional status, or consideration of high-risk procedures such as surgery (23).

Completing Instructional Directives

Patients should document their preferences and instructions in writing whenever possible. Two general formats are available for instructional directives: predrafted and open-ended. Patients who want to make and document specific decisions regarding certain interventions might find the use of validated and predrafted instruments helpful; for example, the medical directive describes a number of situations and presents choices for the patient to make (24). Here is one example:

"If I am in a coma or a persistent vegetative state and, in the opinion of my physician and two consultants, have no known hope of regaining awareness and higher mental functions no matter what is done, then my goals and specific wishes—if medically reasonable—for this and any additional illness would be:

- Prolong life; treat everything
- Attempt to cure, but reevaluate often
- Limit to less invasive and less burdensome interventions
- Provide comfort care only
- Other (please specify)"

Other patients may prefer open-ended formats: discussing general parameters and using them as guides to their wishes rather than making a series of specific treatment decisions. With either format, patients often need information about interventions used in serious illness or to sustain life: what they are, when they are used, and the advantages or disadvantages of choosing them under certain circumstances. Health care providers can offer patients realistic and accessible information about these and other interventions and provide opportunities for discussion and questions. It is also helpful to inform patients that it is very difficult to imagine all the possible interventions or scenarios that may need to be decided upon.

Patients may already have strong preferences for or against certain interventions based on previous experience with a friend or relative, or exposure to the issue through a news story, movie, or other experience. These strong preferences should be explored to ensure they are based on a realistic understanding of the interventions involved.

Assigning a Health Care Proxy or DPA

Health care providers should help patients understand important aspects of selecting a health care proxy or DPA. For example, providers should reassure a patient that a DPA will only be asked to make decisions when it is found that the patient is unable to make decisions for herself. Both patient and DPA should be informed that at such a time, the DPA will have the authority to make all treatment and care decisions that the patient would be asked to make if she were able. These might include choosing a doctor, a caregiver, or a place of care; accepting or refusing medical treatments including life-sustaining treatments; making discharge or transfer decisions; and authorizing the release of medical information, among others.

When possible, a DPA makes decisions based on the patient's previously expressed wishes. However, in situations where previously expressed wishes do not provide sufficient guidance, the DPA might be asked to make a decision using "substituted judgment," or what they imagine the patient would have wanted based on their knowledge of the patient. Substituted judgment is a complex concept and can be hard to implement, especially when the patient is in a situation that neither she nor the DPA had previously considered or discussed. When substituted judgment is not feasible, the DPA makes decisions based on the patient's best interests. Some patients authorize their DPA to have more discretion or instruct the DPA to consult with other family members or loved ones when making health-related decisions. Data suggest that surrogates often do rely on other factors including their own best interests or mutual interests that they share with the patient (25).

Growing evidence shows that surrogates, even or especially those who are close to the patient, are not very good at accurately guessing what the patient would have wanted, and often choose more aggressive care than the patient would have chosen (26). Although there is limited evidence, more specific and frequent ACP discussions, especially about medical circumstances or types of treatments that the patient cares strongly about, could be helpful. Making decisions for a loved one can be emotionally difficult for the DPA, as well as other family and close friends. Surrogates sometimes feel stress, guilt, and doubt—especially when making end-of-life decisions and letting go of loved ones—but knowing that the treatment selected was consistent with the patient's preferences appears to reduce the negative effect on surrogates (26).

Patients may want some assistance from their health care provider in deliberating and choosing a DPA or health care agent. For legal and practical reasons, the designated DPA should be an adult (usually 18 years or older), someone that the patient trusts, and someone who knows the patient well, understands her values and beliefs, and is willing and available to speak on her behalf. The designated DPA should also be comfortable asking questions of the health care team and advocating for the patient even at emotionally difficult times, and be willing to make decisions that represent the patient's wishes and values. Sometimes, a patient's choice of DPA is not the most obvious choice; for example, a patient might designate her sister as DPA instead of her spouse, or a friend instead of a parent. Although there may be very good reasons for these choices, patients may need support in making this decision and communicating it to their loved ones.

The name and contact information of the designated DPA should be documented on an advance directive form, and copies given to the patient, DPA, and primary physician, and placed in the medical record when appropriate. Many advance directive forms ask patients to designate an alternate DPA, which is useful in the event that the primary DPA is unavailable or no longer willing or able to serve in this role. The patient should be encouraged to talk with the designated and any alternate DPAs about treatment preferences and values that are important to her and that will help the DPAs make health-related decisions on her behalf. These discussions should occur periodically, especially when there are important health or life changes.

AD do not automatically expire, but a capacitated patient can change or revoke an advance directive at any time. For either type of directive, patients may want to periodically revisit their choices and any specific parameters that they set. Once a patient loses capacity, the advance directive will be activated.

IMPLEMENTING ADVANCE DIRECTIVES

Assessing Decision-Making Capacity

The DPA or surrogate will become the legal decision maker for health-related decisions only when a patient loses decision-making capacity. However, deciding when a patient is unable to make decisions for herself is rarely straightforward. Sometimes a patient's capacity waxes and wanes, and decision-making capacity is task specific, meaning a patient may have the capacity to make some decisions but not others. In most cases, the patient's physician will make the determination that the patient does or does not have the capacity to make the decision at hand, often with the help of other members of the health care team (Fig. 49.3).

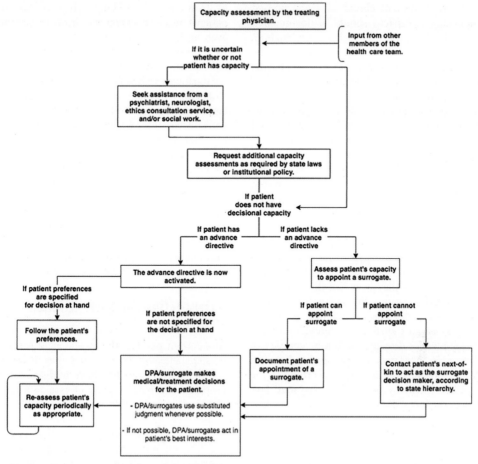

Figure 49.3 Assessing decision-making capacity.

A patient with decision-making capacity is able to take in information, evaluate and deliberate about the information, and make and communicate a preference or choice. Capacity to make a specific treatment or care decision requires (a) a basic understanding of the medical situation, (b) an understanding of the nature of the decision, including the risks and benefits of treatments being considered and any alternatives, and (c) the ability to communicate a decision that is logical and consistent with the patient's values. Some decisions are more complex than others, and some treatment choices are likely to expose the patient to higher risk. For example, information is more complex and there is more at stake when deciding about bone marrow transplantation for a serious illness than about antibiotics for an infection. The capacity to make the former decision requires a higher threshold of understanding and ability to deliberate and make a choice.

Several instruments are available to assist health care providers in determining decision-making capacity. A review evaluating 19 instruments identified three as easy to use and useful: the Aid to Capacity Evaluation, The Hopkins Competency Assessment Test, and the Understanding Treatment Disclosure (27). The authors note that the Aid to Capacity Evaluation was validated in the largest cohort, and is available for free online (28). When the treating physician is uncertain about a patient's capacity, consultation from a psychiatrist, neurologist, ethics consultant or committee, or social services can be helpful.

Physicians and other health care providers should minimize the influence of any possible barriers to understanding, such as language, timing, sedating medications, etc. When assessing capacity, they should also assure that the patient has received the information she would need to make an informed decision. When the patient communicates a decision, it should make sense within the context of her values and history and be reasonably consistent and free of influence from other people.

A determination of absent or compromised decision-making capacity should be documented in the medical record. After such a determination, the DPA will be asked to make decisions on the patient's behalf. The patient, however, should be kept involved in treatment decisions to the extent possible. If the patient is capable of receiving such information, she should be informed about treatment and care decisions made by her proxy, and allowed to assent or dissent. When appropriate, there should be regular repeat assessment of a patient's capacity to make decisions, as patients may have the capacity to make some decisions but not others, or may regain the ability to make decisions.

Some patients with uncertain or absent capacity do not have a previous instructional directive or a designated proxy. Recent research has shown that some patients retain the capacity to assign a surrogate even if they have lost the capacity to make medical decisions themselves (29). However, if a patient does not herself have either the capacity to assign a surrogate or provide instructions, an advance directive cannot be completed. In these cases, a relative can be asked in lieu of a DPA to make medical decisions according to the next-of-kin hierarchy as specified by state law. Although the hierarchy varies by state, the list usually includes spouses, adult children, parents, siblings, and others in that or a similar order.

Honoring Advance Directives

State laws, professional ethics, and respect for persons underlie an obligation to honor a patient's wishes as expressed in a valid advance directive. Unfortunately, having an advance directive does not always ensure that expressed wishes are followed. One critical barrier to effectively using AD is that they are often unavailable when needed. In order to follow an advance directive, the treating physician and health care team need physical access to it, as well as understanding of what it expresses and how to apply it to the situation at hand. In a summary of studies supported by the U.S. Agency for Healthcare Research and Quality, fewer than 50% of the severely or terminally ill patients studied had an advance directive available in their medical record, and almost 75% of physicians whose patient did have an advance directive were not aware that it existed (30). AD are also difficult to follow when they are vague, unclear, or too general (e.g., statements like "don't keep me alive if I am a vegetable") or when the designated proxy feels unprepared, unwilling, or too anxious to make decisions.

Early findings from the "Study to understand prognoses and preferences for outcomes and risks of treatment" (SUPPORT) showed that many patients received aggressive, invasive treatments even against their previously stated wishes (31). In contrast, more recent studies have found that AD substantially improve the correlation between what patients want and the care they receive at the end of life. For example, Silveira et al. found strong agreement between stated preferences on a living will and care received, and say that their data indicate that "living wills have an important effect on care received and that a durable power of attorney for health care is necessary to account for unforeseen factors" at least in elderly patients (p. 1217) (1). Other studies have shown that AD were associated with fewer hospital deaths (1, 32–34), less use of certain procedures such as feeding tubes or respirators (33), more use of hospice (34), and lower health care costs in regions characterized by high baseline levels of Medicare spending (34).

WITHHOLDING AND WITHDRAWING TREATMENT

At a certain point in the trajectory of serious illness, patients or their proxies may decide that continued aggressive treatment of disease is inappropriate and reorder goals of care so that comfort and palliation of symptoms are primary. Sometimes this reordering raises questions about withholding or withdrawing treatment, including life-sustaining treatment. Despite common misconceptions about the ethical appropriateness of limiting life-sustaining treatment, when the burdens of a treatment outweigh the benefits as determined by the patient's goals of care, withholding, changing, or withdrawing the treatment may be the most appropriate course of action, even when that course anticipates the patient's death (Table 49.2). There are several reasons a physician might agree to withhold or withdraw life-sustaining treatment from a patient: (a) to comply with an adult patient's competent wishes or wishes expressed through an authorized proxy or a previously completed advance directive; (b) because the treatment cannot achieve care goals; and (c) because the therapy has failed and is simply prolonging the dying process (35).

When a patient makes an informed, clear, consistent, and well-considered request, treatment can be withheld or stopped, even if it results in the patient's death. If a patient lacks the capacity to make decisions about starting or stopping a treatment, her DPA or, in the absence of a DPA, her next-of-kin can also act to make such decisions. Respecting an informed and considered choice of the patient or her DPA to refuse or withdraw a treatment is consistent with respect for patient

TABLE 49.2 COMMON MISPERCEPTIONS

Question	Misperceptions	Realities
Does an advance directive have to be on a particular form or in a particular format to be valid?	Health care providers will only follow an advance directive if it is on the approved state form.	Written advance directives are useful in guiding decision-making by proxies and health care providers even if all the legal formalities are not met. Oral expressions of a patient's wishes can also be useful and valid guides for decision makers.
When the DPA is asked to make decisions for a patient, will he or she make all future health-related decisions?	Once the DPA is activated, the patient cannot make any more decisions.	A person's capacity can wax and wane, and capacity is task specific. Even if a patient is determined to not have capacity for a certain medical decision, she may have capacity to make other medical decisions. The patient's decision-making capacity should be reassessed as appropriate and the patient involved in decisions to the extent possible.
When should advance care planning be initiated?	Some worry that initiating advance care planning or bringing up advance directives implies a poor prognosis.	Advance care planning is appropriate at any time to explore a person's values and medical care preferences for a possible future time when she cannot make these decisions. Advance care planning is not a one-time event, and should coincide with clinical or life changes to reflect the patient's wishes.
If a patient or surrogate decides to limit a life-sustaining intervention, will other care provided to the patient change?	Patients, families, and some health care providers fear that limiting a life-sustaining intervention means limiting care.	Patients, proxies, and the health care team should agree on the goals of care. Treatment should be consistent with those goals and an analysis of the benefits and burdens. Symptoms will be treated regardless of other treatment choices throughout a person's life.
Is it ethically or legally better to withhold treatment than to withdraw it?	Once a treatment is begun, it is more ethically problematic to stop it.	Patients or their proxies can accept or refuse the initiation of treatment, as well as the continuation of treatment they no longer want. Although withdrawing treatment is ethically and legally similar to withholding treatment, health care providers and families often find withdrawal emotionally challenging.
Can a physician withdraw life-sustaining treatment?	When withdrawing a treatment leads to a patient's death, it could be seen as murder or euthanasia.	Termination of life support at the request of the patient or family is honoring their right to make treatment decisions. Death is understood as a result of the patient's underlying disease. Current law supports the termination of life support that is consistent with the patient's wishes or best interests.

Adapted from Meisel A, Snyder L, Quill T, et al. Seven legal barriers to end-of-life care: myths, realities, and grains of truth. *JAMA.* 2000;284:2495-2501; Ackermann R. Chapter 32. In: Berger A, Shuster J, Von Roenn J, eds. *Principles and Practice of Palliative Care and Supportive Oncology.* 3rd ed. Philadelphia, PA: Lippincott Williams & Wilkins; 2007(36).

autonomy, or the right of a competent adult to accept or refuse treatments and interventions. Some states limit what a proxy decision maker can refuse, or have additional safeguards specifically related to decisions about discontinuing life-sustaining treatments (37).

Withdrawing treatment often creates more controversy and psychological distress for the family and health care team than not starting a treatment to begin with. However, in certain cases it may be preferable to start a treatment with the option of later stopping it than not starting it at all, especially if there is uncertainty about the burdens and benefits of treatment or about the patient's wishes. Despite some consensus that both withholding and withdrawing treatment are morally and legally comparable and acceptable, health care providers do not always agree and practices vary (38, 39). Hospital ethics committees, legal counsel, and professional society guidelines can provide helpful advice and assist health care teams with decisions about withholding or withdrawing care (39).

Decisions about withholding or withdrawing treatment are stressful for all involved, including the DPA, family members, and health care providers, especially those who have been caring for a patient over an extended period of time. Health care providers can help facilitate decision-making about withholding or withdrawing treatment, and possibly relieve some stress through frank and regular communication that allows the patient, DPA, and/or family to discuss the patient's medical situation as well as her cultural, spiritual, and other values and preferences. Patients and their DPA may also need assistance in deciphering complex medical and prognostic information. The Society for Critical Care Medicine has online reader-friendly descriptions of many interventions used in the intensive care unit. Patients and their families may also have different decision-making preferences; some will prefer recommendations from the physician while others may prefer a more shared decision-making process. Multidisciplinary patient care conferences as well as family conferences provide useful opportunities to review care goals, decipher complex medical and prognostic information, update everyone about the patient's clinical course, and discuss options. The Medical College of Wisconsin's Palliative Care Network publishes a comprehensive and useful set of Fast Facts and Concepts for Clinicians, including one entitled Moderating an End-of-Life Family Conference (41). Effective communication between a patient and/or DPA and health care providers helps ensure that decisions are sound and based on an understanding of the medical condition, prognosis, benefits and burdens of the life-sustaining treatment, and the goals of care.

Symptom management and palliation are important management goals at every stage of illness, even when a decision has been made to withhold or withdraw aggressive treatment. Physicians and health care providers should reassure the patient and family that the patient will continue to receive appropriate care, and that symptoms will be managed to make the patient as comfortable as possible. Some patients and their families worry that if they opt for palliative or comfort care, the patient will not receive good medical care and die sooner. Yet studies have shown that patients with various cancers, including lung and gastrointestinal cancers, who received early palliative care had better quality of life and mood than did those who continued to receive standard aggressive care (42,43). Patients with metastatic non–small cell lung cancers who received early palliative care also lived on average a few months longer (44). Nonetheless, despite the availability of palliative care, cancer patients in some places received more aggressive care at the end of life in 2008 than in 2002 (33,44).

CONCLUSION

AD and ACP, although somewhat underutilized and imperfect in realizing their original goals, are helpful tools that facilitate deliberation and discussion and help health care providers and loved ones understand patients' preferences and values. Thoughtful and respectful consideration of patients' wishes—expressed presently or previously—and of the difficult and emotional challenges facing surrogate decision makers and other loved ones can help guide health care providers in providing quality care for all patients.

REFERENCES

1. Silveira MJ, Kim SYH, Langa KM. Advance directives and outcomes of surrogate decision making before death. *N Engl J Med.* 2010;362:1211-1218.
2. White DB, Braddock CH III, Bereknyei S, et al. Toward shared decision making at the end of life in intensive care units: opportunities for improvement. *Arch Intern Med.* 2007;167:461-467.
3. Teno JM, Gozalo PL, Bynum JPW, et al. Change in end-of-life care for Medicare beneficiaries: site of death, place of care, and health care transitions in 2000, 2005, and 2009. *JAMA.* 2013;309:470-477.
4. Hamel L, Wu B, Brodie M. *Views and Experiences with End-of-Life Medical Care in the U.S.* The Henry J. Kaiser Family Foundation; 2017. https://www.kff.org/report-section/views-and-experiences-with-end-of-life-medi-cal-care-in-the-us-findings/. Accessed March 27, 2019.
5. *Cancer Statistics.* National Cancer Institute; 2015. https://www.cancer.gov/about-cancer/understanding/statistics. Accessed March 22, 2019.
6. Annas GJ. "Culture of life" politics at the bedside—the case of Terri Schiavo. *N Engl J Med.* 2005;352: 1710-1715.

7. Quill TE. Terri Schiavo—a tragedy compounded. *N Engl J Med.* 2005;352:1630-1633.

8. Patient Self-Determination Act. 42 C.F.R. § 489.102.

9. Meisel A, Snyder L, Quill T, et al. Seven legal barriers to end-of-life care: myths, realities, and grains of truth. *JAMA.* 2000;284:2495-2501.

10. See for example, National Hospice and Palliative Care Organization, Caring Connections. http://www.caringinfo.org/i4a/pages/index.cfm?pageid=3289. Accessed March 25, 2019.

11. *PREPARE Advance Directive: All States and Languages.* PREPARE for Your Care. https://prepareforyourcare.org/advance-directive-library. Accessed April 23, 2019.

12. Holmes P. Commission on Law & Aging Research: a tour of state advance directive registries. *Bifocal.* 2016;37:122-127.

13. *Aging with Dignity.* Five Wishes Online. https://agingwithdignity.org/. Accessed March 25, 2019.

14. Molloy DW, Russo R, Stiller A, et al. How to implement the "Let Me Decide" advance health and personal care directive program. 7:7. *J Coop Organ Manage.* 2000;7(9):41-47.

15. Respecting Choices. *Respecting Choices.* https://respectingchoices.org. Accessed March 27, 2019.

16. *Chart: POLST & Advance Directives.* National POLST Paradigm. https://polst.org/polst-and-advance-directives/.

17. Emanuel LL, Danis M, Pearlman RA, et al. Advance care planning as a process: structuring the discussions in practice. *J Am Geriatr Soc.* 1995;43:440-446.

18. Bestvina CM, Polite BN. Implementation of advance care planning in oncology: a review of the literature. *J Oncol Pract.* 2017;13:657-662.

19. Brinkman-Stoppelenburg A, Rietjens JAC, van der Heide A. The effects of advance care planning on end-of-life care: a systematic review. *Palliat Med.* 2014;28:1000-1025.

20. Balaban RB. A physician's guide to talking about end-of-life care. *J Gen Intern Med.* 2000;15:195-200.

21. Barnes KA, Barlow CA, Harrington J, et al. Advance care planning discussions in advanced cancer: analysis of dialogues between patients and care planning mediators. *Palliat Support Care.* 2011;9:73-79.

22. Gesme DH, Wiseman M. Advance care planning with your patients. *J Oncol Pract.* 2011;7:e42-e44.

23. Gilligan T, Coyle N, Frankel RM, et al. Patient-Clinician Communication: American Society of Clinical Oncology Consensus Guideline. *J Curr Oncol.* 2017;35:3618-3632.

24. Medical Directives LLC. http://www.medicaldirectives.net/index.html. Accessed March 27, 2019.

25. Vig EK, Taylor JS, Starks H, et al. Beyond substituted judgment: how surrogates navigate end-of-life decision-making. *J Am Geriatr Soc.* 2006;54:1688-1693.

26. Shalowitz DI, Garrett-Mayer E, Wendler D. The accuracy of surrogate decision makers: a systematic review. *Arch Intern Med.* 2006;166:493-497.

27. Sessums LL, Zembrzuska H, Jackson JL. Does this patient have medical decision-making capacity? *JAMA.* 2011;306:420-427.

28. Scott D. *Toolkit for Primary Care: Capacity Assessment*; 2008. https://admin.rgpc.ca/uploads/documents/1%20capacity%20assessment%20toolkit%20overview.pdf.

29. Kim SYH, Karlawish JH, Kim HM, et al. Preservation of the capacity to appoint a proxy decision maker: implications for dementia research. *Arch Gen Psychiatry.* 2011;68:214-220.

30. Kass-Bartelmes B, Hughes R, Rutherford M. *Advance Care Planning: Preferences for Care at the End of Life.* Issue #12. AHRQ Pub No. 03-0018. Rockville, MD: Agency for Healthcare Research and Quality; 2003. http://www.scribd.com/fullscreen/47966710

31. The SUPPORT Investigators. A controlled trial to improve care for seriously ill hospitalized patients. The study to understand prognoses and preferences for outcomes and risks of treatments (SUPPORT). *JAMA.* 1995;274:1591-1598.

32. Degenholtz HB, Rhee Y, Arnold RM. Brief communication: the relationship between having a living will and dying in place. *Ann Intern Med.* 2004;141:113-117.

33. Teno JM, Gruneir A, Schwartz Z, et al. Association between advance directives and quality of end-of-life care: a national study. *J Am Geriatr Soc.* 2007;55:189-194.

34. Nicholas LH, Langa KM, Iwashyna TJ, et al. Regional variation in the association between advance directives and end-of-life Medicare expenditures. *JAMA.* 2011;306:1447-1453.

35. Prendergast TJ, Puntillo KA. Withdrawal of life support: intensive caring at the end of life. *JAMA.* 2002;288:2732-2740.

36. Ackermann R. Chapter 32. In: Berger A, Shuster J, Von Roenn J, eds. *Principles and Practice of Palliative Care and Supportive Oncology.* 3rd ed. Philadelphia, PA: Lippincott Williams & Wilkins; 2007.

37. Wynn S. Decisions by surrogates: an overview of surrogate consent laws in the United States managing someone else's money. *Bifocal.* 2014;36:10-14.

38. Dickenson DL. Are medical ethicists out of touch? Practitioner attitudes in the US and UK towards decisions at the end of life. *J Med Ethics.* 2000;26:254-260.

39. Glick S. Withholding versus withdrawal of life support: is there an ethical difference? *BMJ.* 2011;342:d728.

40. American Medical Association. *Withholding or Withdrawing Life-Sustaining Treatment.* American Medical Association. https://www.ama-assn.org/delivering-care/ethics/withholding-or-withdrawing-life-sustaining-treatment. Accessed April 22, 2019.

41. Ambuel B, Weissman DE. *Moderating An End-of-Life Family Conference. Fast Facts and Concepts*; 2015. https://www.mypcnow.org/blank-qy84d. Accessed April 23, 2019.

42. Temel JS, El-Jawahri A, Greer JA, et al. Randomized trial of early integrated palliative and oncology care. *J Curr Oncol.* 2016;34:10003-10003.

43. Temel JS, Greer JA, Muzikansky A, et al. Early palliative care for patients with metastatic non–small-cell lung cancer. *N Engl J Med.* 2010;363:733-742.

44. Gonsalves W, Tashi T, Davies T, et al. Aggressiveness of end-of-life care before and after the utilization of a palliative care service. *J Curr Oncol.* 2011;29:9135-9135.

50 Palliative Care: Ethics and the Law[1]

Ryan R. Nash and Nicole Shirilla

INTRODUCTION TO ETHICS

Ethics is the study of right and wrong, good and evil. Ethics assumes that such categories exist, although these categories are not always dichotomous. Ethics does not always deal with absolutes; instead, it entails trying to find the better option on the moral gradient. The ultimate determination of right and wrong, or the meta-ethical claim, is based on how one knows truth and how one values or orders life. Therefore, the ultimate ethical determination is based on epistemology. Epistemologies are diverse. Various philosophical theories and religions have made claim to define the good, the evil, virtue, and vice. However, they often do not agree. One may place the highest value on self-determination and freedom, another on equal opportunity for all, and yet another on self-sacrifice and love of another. When there is no agreement on where humankind comes from, where it is going, and what in life is most valuable and good, then agreement on what is ethical is all but impossible. Even if two persons from competing epistemologies find that they agree on an ethical claim, they may do so for very different reasons. Thus, making a claim that something is ethical or unethical begs the question, "According to whose ethics? and why?" In a pluralistic society such as that of the United States, it is expected that two may meet as moral strangers (1), not having an agreed-upon epistemology or understanding of right and wrong. In such as anticipated scenario, how are we to "do ethics" and determine the best path forward? We strive to come to an agreement of mutual consent, a modus vivendi (way of life), and to work toward the best ethic possible within the reality of moral pluralism. This is not a claim that we are agreeing on the ultimate ethic, nor is it saying that all of ethics is personal and relative. The claim is that we come to an agreed-upon operation that allows for variation on points of disagreement. Mistakenly many in health care use the phrase ethical or unethical as an ultimate truth

claim and pretend, perhaps unknowingly, that all ethics is agreed upon. Much in ethics is not agreed upon. Thus, how we "do ethics" in health care is more procedural, based on agreements and precedence over time. Though consensus statements exist (2,3), we fail to give ethics and ultimate truth claims their due if we think our laws, procedures, or professional statements are the ultimate source of right and wrong, good and evil. This chapter will not focus on the ultimate meta-ethical claims or differing epistemological approaches to finding the good but on the practical approach of doing bedside clinical medical ethics, describing the usual modus vivendi and shared wisdom of those that have wrestled with what to do in the past. It will not attempt to solve the legion of disagreements that do and will exist.

DIVERSE FOUNDATIONS

Many ethical systems or approaches have been promoted. Some of these are summarized in Table 50.1. However, these ethical systems are often an attempt to identify or at least define the ultimate ethical nature of an action. As previously mentioned, all attempts to reach the ultimate ethical judgment depend on presuppositions of how life is valued or ordered. These systems do give focus for reflection and are helpful in ethical discourse by giving a shared vocabulary. However, at the bedside they too often fail to give sufficient clarity and direction. For instance, using the principle-based approach, how does one decide which ethical principle takes priority if differing ethical principles conflict? Should autonomy or beneficence receive greater ethical weight?

PALLIATIVE CARE TERMS

To establish a common ground of meaning, palliative care terms are defined in Table 50.2. These terms reflect hospice and palliative medicine's emphasis on improving quality of life for patients with serious disease through management of pain and other distressing symptoms. Misunderstanding of these terms often leads to needless ethical conflicts or false dilemmas.

---

[1]This material is also covered with modification and greater depth in Nash RR, Nelson LJ. *UNIPAC 6: Ethical and Legal Dimensions of Care*. 4th ed. AAHPM; 2012.

TABLE 50.1 SELECTED ETHICAL FRAMEWORKS AND FOUNDATIONS

Principle based

Focuses on the following ethical principles:

- Beneficence—promote patient well-being
- Autonomy—respect patient self-determination
- Nonmaleficence—do no harm
- Justice—protect vulnerable populations and provide fair allocation of resources

Professionalism

Professionalism involves the qualities that make a good professional or a good physician. The ways in which a practitioner is true to a standard when honoring established principles, oaths, or examples determines his or her level of professionalism.

Virtue based

Virtues defining the character of a good physician include the following:

- Fidelity to trust and promise—honoring the ineradicable trust of the patient–physician relationship
- Effacement of self-interest—protecting the patient from exploitation and refraining from using the patient as a means to advance power, prestige, profit, or pleasure
- Compassion and caring—exhibiting concern, empathy, and consideration for the patient's plight
- Intellectual honesty—knowing when to say "I do not know"
- Prudence—deliberating and discerning alternatives in situations of uncertainty and stress

Caring based

The ethics of caring assumes that connections to others are central to what it means to be human. Caring requires empathy and compassion for patients, assuming responsibility for patients by performing actions that meet their needs, and creating an educational environment that fosters caring.

Consequentialism

"Consequentialism" is a general theory of morality in which the moral worth of an action can be determined by looking at its consequences. A prominent form of consequentialism is utilitarianism, which states that what one ought to do in any given situation is to take the action that brings about the most amount of collective well-being and minimizes the most amount of collective suffering.

Deontology

Deontological frameworks judge the moral worth of an action on the basis of whether or not the action is compatible with a certain set of ethical rules. A prominent form of deontology is Immanuel Kant's moral philosophy, which is based upon categorial imperatives that he described as commands of action that are derived from reason and held unconditionally.

Respect for personhood

Respect for personhood proposes the following:

- Treatment of patients must reflect the inherent dignity of every person regardless of age, debility, dependence, race, color, or creed.
- Actions must reflect the patient's current needs.
- Decisions must value the person and accept human mortality and medical finitude.

Humanities

Uses literature, history, the arts, and narrative to arrive at principles or sentiment of the right and wrong

Religious and cultural

Application of deep and rich contextual understandings of the good or ways of life. Such considerations may or may not be able to be reduced into philosophical categories or language. The truth claims are at times exclusive to the group.

RESPONSIBILITY AND OBLIGATIONS OF PALLIATIVE CARE

Related to the definition of palliative care are its responsibilities. It has been proclaimed that the role of medicine is to restore health or to fight disease and death. More realistic views have emphasized the sentiment attributed to a number of famous physicians including Sir William Osler and Edward Trudeau, "to cure sometimes, to relieve often, to comfort (or to care) always" (4,5). Palliative care professionals have understood this latter call and have championed it. However, some have taken the call for comfort and relief of all suffering as a responsibility and an obligation. Although

TABLE 50.2 DEFINITIONS ASSOCIATED WITH HOSPICE AND PALLIATIVE CARE

Hospice care

Patients who are terminally ill can elect to receive hospice care, which focuses on comforting the patient and managing symptoms rather than curing the terminal illness. In general, terminal illness is defined for hospice eligibility as having a prognosis with a life expectancy of 6 months or less if the illness runs its normal course. Hospice care is generally provided where the patient resides, and services are provided by a team including nursing, physician, social work, chaplaincy, and bereavement services to help meet physical, psychosocial, and spiritual needs of the patient and their family.

Palliative care is patient- and family-centered care that anticipates, prevents, and treats burdens of disease. Palliative care throughout the continuum of illness involves addressing physical, intellectual, emotional, social, and spiritual needs and facilitating patient access to information and choice. Palliative care is ideally delivered by an interprofessional team including a physician, nurse, social worker, chaplain, counselor, and others. (Modified from 73 FR 32204, June 5, 2008, Medicare—Final Rule.) **Palliative care deals with the burden of disease regardless of the stage of disease and attempts to encourage effective and desired interventions delivered in the right place and at the right time.**

Palliative treatments are treatments and interventions that enhance comfort and improve the quality of a patient's life. No specific therapy is excluded from consideration. The decision to intervene with a palliative treatment is based on the treatment's ability to meet the stated goals rather than on its effect on the underlying disease. The treatments are explored and evaluated within the context of the patient's values, symptoms, and clinical circumstances.

What palliative care is not

Palliative care is **not only end-of-life care**. Palliative care deals with the burden of disease regardless of the stage of disease. It includes treating patients with serious, but not necessarily life-limiting, illnesses as well as those who likely are dying.

Palliative care is **not** an attempt to **contain medical costs or ration care**. Palliative care attempts to encourage effective and desired interventions in the right place and at the right time. Palliative care has been shown to be a good steward of medical resources and sometimes is associated with cost savings, but controlling costs is not its primary aim.

Palliative care does **not hasten death**. In fact, many patients receiving palliative care may live longer and have opportunity to pursue additional "aggressive" or curative interventions due to enhanced symptom management, communication, and coordination of care. Appropriate pain and symptom management and addressing other burdens of disease have not been shown to hasten death.

Palliative care is **not** a dichotomy of care between **"do everything" vs. "do nothing"** or aggressive care vs. comfort care only. Palliative care helps involved parties navigate the complex range of medical choices and make the best possible medical decisions under difficult circumstances.

Palliative care is **not** always a **choice**. Most patients receiving palliative care will have a goal to live longer and have a better quality life. Many would choose life-prolonging, curative therapies if they were available and could be effective for them, but often they are not. For those with incurable disease, palliative care is an essential part of their treatment plan alongside the disease-directed therapies they continue to try.

Palliative care is **not** an attempt to force one definition of **"the good death"** upon all patients.

relief of suffering is a worthy goal and should be attempted with great effort and skill, the hospice and palliative medicine specialist's responsibility is not to perfectly relieve all suffering but to use the best of one's knowledge, skill, and abilities to provide the best possible care (6). Palliative care teams also must appreciate the finitude of medicine. Not only is medicine not the source of eternal life but it often fails at being the source of perfect relief of suffering or "a good death." Attempts to "totalize" the dying experience with medicine in the name of compassion can lead to actions held by many to be wrong or evil in the name of compassion (7). Ironically, palliative care providers often must be reminded of the original hospice movement goals of not medicinalizing, institutionalizing, or trying to hide death.

Ethics, Law, and Practice

In giving clinical ethics advice, it is common for a clinical ethicist to address three perspectives: the legal, the professional, and the consultant's judgment or opinion on the case. This chapter provides a suggested framework to practically address clinical ethical decision making, describes key legal considerations and gives an overview of ethical issues important in palliative care. Hospice and palliative medicine, unlike many other specialties, has less univocity regarding many ethical issues. Thus, the chapter will not emphasize professional standards. The American Academy of Hospice and Palliative Medicine (AAHPM) has ethical statements readily available, which are frequently updated and sometimes changed (www.aahpm.org).

The Law

The law and ethics are not synonyms. We hope that our laws are ethical but history has shown that such is not guaranteed. At least theoretically, if a law were ethically wrong then one may willfully disobey the law. Further, some may suggest that we may have duty to try to change unethical laws. However, the laws we currently have throughout the United States are an attempt for a modus vivendi (mentioned in the Introduction). Laws vary from state to state and a description of each is beyond the scope of this chapter. Needless to say, it behooves all health care professionals to know the laws of their land (8,9), as many myths and misconceptions exist (10–12). Failure to correct these misconceptions may result in physicians stepping outside of accepted standards of medical practice (13). Most state laws are a reaction to landmark court cases around the country that became precedence. These cases, at times, had misinformation or needless court involvement, but nevertheless have defined the current legal terrain. Upon review of state laws and landmark cases, one may be surprised how often the well-intended laws are impractical and often not followed in clinical settings.

RIGHT TO REFUSE AND RIGHT TO DIE

Two distinct but related movements occurred in end-of-life law during the recent technological age of medicine and were in part a reaction against the perception of a paternalistic medicine. The *right to refuse* is the belief that medical care is optional for adults with decisional capacity (or determined by their appropriate proxy decision maker). This negative or forbearance right has become accepted in clinical care and ethical discourse and is legal precedence. Further, it is constitutive of palliative care.

The *right to die* movement agrees that medical care is optional and can be refused, but adds a claim or positive right for a person to choose the method, manner, and timing of death. Some advocates argue for the right to demand help in causing death from health care professionals and systems. The right to die movement advocates assisted suicide and some types of euthanasia. The right to die has not been broadly accepted legally, ethically, or clinically. As opposed to the right to refuse, the right to die is not constitutive of palliative care.

Finally, another positive or claim right, the *right to demand medical care*, movement has come to the fore, as seen in several court cases (14). This right to demand a particular treatment is similar to the right to die (which is a type of demand) in that they are both positive or claim rights. Currently, the right to demand is mainly being considered in the context of reproductive technologies and chronic treatments such as hemodialysis. Currently, a right to demand a particular treatment is not broadly accepted in law or medical ethics.

LANDMARK CASES ON THE RIGHT TO REFUSE

The Quinlan Case[2]

In April 1975, at age 21 years, Karen Ann Quinlan suffered severe anoxic brain injury. Karen Ann was eventually diagnosed to be in a persistent vegetative state and remained on a mechanical ventilator. Her father requested guardianship and requested the mechanical ventilator be removed. Mr. Quinlan's requests were opposed by the treating physicians, the hospital, the local prosecutor, the State of New Jersey, and Karen's guardian ad litem. The Supreme Court of New Jersey authorized the withdrawal of mechanical ventilation and the appointment of Mr. Quinlan as guardian for that purpose if it was concluded, after appropriate consultation with a hospital ethics committee, that there was no reasonable possibility of Karen ever emerging from a persistent vegetative state. The court also noted that this decision was consistent with Karen Ann's and Mr. Quinlan's Roman Catholic faith (the decision had been endorsed by their bishop).

The Supreme Court of New Jersey found that the right of Karen Ann Quinlan to refuse medical treatment, even if exercised by her surrogate or proxy, was protected by a right of privacy. The court noted that the claimed interests of the state were to preserve life and protect the right of physicians to administer treatment in accordance with their best judgment, but these interests were outweighed by the poor prognosis of the patient and great bodily invasion involved in sustaining her life. The court endorsed the use of a substituted judgment standard (i.e., allowing her guardian and family "to render their best judgment" regarding whether she would refuse the continuation of treatment if she could wake up for a few minutes and tell her family what she would want them to do before returning to her vegetative state). The court also endorsed the use of hospital ethics committees in reviewing decisions to withdraw life-sustaining treatment as preferable to court proceedings. After this decision, mechanical ventilation was removed, but Karen Ann Quinlan was able to breathe on her own (as predicted by only one expert witness). She lived for several years being fed by artificial nutrition and hydration (ANH) and in 1985 died from an overwhelming infection (15). Despite the expanded role for ethics committees envisioned in the *Quinlan* decision, few hospitals created such committees (16).

---

[2]*In re Quinlan*, 355 A2d 647 (NJ 1976).

The failure of hospitals to adopt ethics committees was attributed to a "reluctance to disturb the status quo, together with a sense of confusion over what an ethics committee could accomplish" (16).

The Cruzan Case[3]

In January 1983, Nancy Cruzan, a 25-year-old Missourian, was seriously injured in an automobile accident. When she was found lying facedown, there was no detectable heartbeat or respiration, but these functions were restored at the scene by paramedics. She was taken to a hospital where she remained unconscious. Physicians implanted a gastrostomy tube with permission. Her condition subsequently was diagnosed as a persistent vegetative state. Eventually, Cruzan's parents asked hospital employees to stop ANH administration, but hospital employees refused to accede without a court order. The trial court recognized a constitutional right to refuse life-sustaining treatment and authorized withdrawal of ANH based upon its finding that before her injury Cruzan had told a friend that if she were seriously injured she would not want to live unless she could live "halfway normally." The Missouri Supreme Court reversed the decision of the trial court. Although the court recognized a right to refuse treatment under the common law doctrine of informed consent, it refused to recognize a constitutional right and found strong state interest in preservation of life as expressed in the Missouri Living Will Statute. On that basis, the court found that treatment could not be terminated in the absence of a valid living will unless it could be shown by "clear and convincing evidence" that the patient would have wanted it terminated and found that the statements relied on by the trial court were unreliable and did not meet the clear and convincing evidence standard. The US Supreme Court affirmed the decision of the Supreme Court of Missouri, holding that the state could require clear and convincing evidence of a person's expressed wishes made while competent. While the majority opinion upheld the constitutionality of the State of Missouri's requirement of clear and convincing evidence, it also acknowledged that "a constitutionally protected liberty interest in refusing unwanted medical treatment may be inferred from our prior decisions." The court stated, however, that because incompetent patients need certain protection given they cannot exercise this right of refusal, it was appropriate for the State of Missouri to impose additional safeguards in the form of the clear and convincing evidence standard in light of its interest in preserving life. After the Supreme Court's decision,

the Cruzans petitioned the trial court in Missouri, again requesting discontinuation of tube feedings. Her coworkers testified that Cruzan stated she would not like to live "like a vegetable." Cruzan's treating physician and court-appointed guardian also supported discontinuation of ANH. As a result, the Missouri court authorized the discontinuation of feeding, and Cruzan died shortly thereafter. The publicity surrounding this case fostered interest in advance directives and health care proxy appointments. It also generated support for the federal Patient Self-Determination Act passed in 1991 (17), which requires some health facilities to present patients with information on advance health care directives.

The Schiavo Case

On February 25, 1990, Theresa Schiavo suffered anoxic brain injury following a cardiac arrest as the result of a potassium imbalance. She never regained consciousness, and eventually her condition was diagnosed as a persistent vegetative state. A feeding tube was inserted and ANH started, but in 1998 her husband asked a Florida state trial court for permission to remove the feeding tube. The court granted permission after determining this was what she would have wanted. At the time feeding tube removal was sought, it was clear that with ANH Terri Schiavo could continue to live for many years, but, if withdrawn, she would die in a few days. The Florida trial court authorized the withdrawal of ANH. The trial court decision was affirmed by the Florida District Court of Appeals, holding that the trial judge had properly found under the clear and convincing evidence standard that Theresa would have wanted the feeding discontinued.[4] The Florida courts—applying a substituted judgment standard—authorized the withdrawal of ANH based on the assumption that she, if competent to make the decision, would have wanted it withdrawn. Schiavo and her family were Roman Catholic, so Catholic teaching was an issue in the case, bearing on the question of what she would have wanted. In the original proceedings before the trial court, a Catholic priest from the Diocese of St. Petersburg, FL, testified regarding Church teaching on the withdrawal of ANH from patients in a persistent vegetative state. Schiavo's husband's attorney asked the priest whether removal of ANH would be consistent with the teaching of the Catholic Church. He further asked the priest to assume, for purposes of this question, that Theresa Schiavo had told her husband she would not want to live "if she was dependent on the care of others" and further that she

[3]*Cruzan v Director, Missouri Department of Health,* 497 US 261 (1990).

[4]*In re Guardianship of Schiavo,* 780 So2d 176, 180 (FL App. Ct. 2001).

"mentioned to her husband and to her brother and sister-in-law that she would not want to be kept alive artificially." The priest answered: "After all that has transpired, I believe, yes, it would be consistent with the teaching of the Catholic Church." On cross-examination, Fr. Murphy was asked if he was familiar with Directive 58 in the 1994 Ethical and Religious Directives for Catholic Health Care Services, which states there should be a presumption in favor of providing ANH. He stated that he was familiar with Directive 58, but characterized it as providing an ideal standard; further, "You have to go back and evaluate the proportion" (18). The appellate court sided with the husband, permitting him to order the withdrawal of treatment. After this decision came several years of additional legal wrangling in both state and federal courts between her parents, who opposed removal of the feeding tube, and her husband, who sought its removal. The parents continued to contend that Theresa was in a minimally conscious state rather than in a persistent vegetative state and that in light of her Catholic faith she would want the feeding continued. On October 15, 2003, Theresa's feeding tube was removed. Six days later, the Florida legislature passed a law allowing Governor Jeb Bush to order that the feeding be resumed. The feeding tube was reinserted, but this law subsequently was declared unconstitutional by the Florida Supreme Court.[5]

Theresa Schiavo died on March 31, 2005, approximately 2 weeks after the removal of her feeding tube pursuant to a court order (19).

The Schiavo case focused attention on Catholic teaching on withdrawal of ANH from patients in a persistent vegetative state and eventually resulted in a revision of Directive 58 of the Ethical and Religious Directives for Catholic Health Care Services (see box below).

Catholic Health Care Directives

The 2009 version of Ethical and Religious Directives for Health Care Services, 5th edition (20) (the norms adopted by Catholic bishops in the United States that apply to Catholic hospitals) states

56. A person has a moral obligation to use ordinary or proportionate means of preserving his or her life. Proportionate means are those that in the judgment of the patient offer a reasonable hope of benefit and do not entail an excessive burden or impose excessive expense on the family or the community.

57. A person may forgo extraordinary or disproportionate means of preserving life. Disproportionate means are those that in the patient's judgment do not offer a reasonable hope of benefit or entail an excessive burden, or impose excessive expense on the family or the community.

58. In principle, there is an obligation to provide patients with food and water, including medically assisted nutrition and hydration for those who cannot take food orally. This obligation extends to patients in chronic and presumably irreversible conditions (e.g., the "persistent vegetative state") who can reasonably be expected to live indefinitely if given such care. Medically assisted nutrition and hydration become morally optional when they cannot reasonably be expected to prolong life or when they would be "excessively burdensome for the patient or [would] cause significant physical discomfort, for example resulting from complications in the use of the means employed." For instance, as a patient draws close to inevitable death from an underlying progressive and fatal condition, certain measures to provide nutrition and hydration may become excessively burdensome and therefore not obligatory in light of their very limited ability to prolong life or provide comfort.

59. The free and informed judgment made by a competent adult patient concerning the use or withdrawal of life-sustaining procedures should always be respected and normally complied with, unless it is contrary to Catholic moral teaching.

Other noteworthy cases include the following.

The Barber Case[6]

In 1983, two physicians were found not guilty of murder and conspiracy to commit murder when they withdrew ANH from a patient in a persistent vegetative state at the request of the patient's family and the patient died. The ruling held that ANH should be viewed as medical treatment, that it was permissible to withdraw ANH without appointment of a legal guardian, and that the patient's wife and children could act as surrogate decision makers. The panel noted that surrogate decision makers should apply a substituted judgment standard (what the patient would want), but, even in the absence of evidence of the patient's wishes, ANH could be withdrawn under a best interests standard

---

[5]*Bush v Schiavo*, 885 So2d 321 (FL 2004).

[6]*Barber v Superior Court*, 147 CA Rptr 484 (Ct App 1983).

(what seems to be the best for the patient) when its burdens exceeded its benefits.

Vacco v Quill[7]

In this case, the US Supreme Court upheld state laws prohibiting physician-assisted death, rejecting an argument that the ban irrationally distinguished between physician-assisted suicide or euthanasia and palliative sedation (21). The US Supreme Court also has recognized that the withdrawal of life-sustaining treatment is not equivalent to physician-assisted death. The right to die was not recognized though the right to refuse was again affirmed.

Ethical Decision Making

The decisions made by terminally ill patients and their physicians can profoundly affect the life of the patient and his or her family. When physicians and patients face ethical decisions about emotionally charged issues, such as withholding or withdrawing life-sustaining treatment, the palliative medicine model of care recognizes the importance of shared communication and respect for the multiple and sometimes conflicting needs of physicians, patients and family members, and interdisciplinary team members. Palliative medicine also acknowledges the intellectual, emotional, and spiritual challenges accompanying ethical decision making for everyone involved in the process—patients, family members, physicians, and other health care professionals. To arrive at the best decision for a patient and to minimize unnecessary decision-making burden while honoring patient self-determination, an informed consent process using shared decision making should be used.

The shared decision-making process is a response to past medical paternalism, when physicians decided for patients and often acted without adequate communication or opportunity for refusal. Medical paternalism assumed that the physician knew what was best for the patient. Shared decision-making models reflect the fact that physicians and patients have differing spheres of expertise: the physician has knowledge of diseases and their treatments, while the patient has a lifetime of personal experiences and knowledge about his or her own values and priorities. The goal of a shared decision-making or informed consent process is to give an opportunity for *informed refusal* (protecting the patient from unwanted treatments or advice from health care professionals) and to have the best plan for a patient. Thus, shared decision making helps to align patient goals and values with available treatments. Patients should be given the opportunity to accept or refuse potentially effective treatments. However, physicians are not ethically obligated to provide any and all treatments that a patient or family member may demand.

THE PHYSICIAN IN DECISION MAKING

The physician plays a key role as facilitator of the decision-making process. In an understandable reaction against paternalism, many physicians may be reluctant to share their recommendations with patients for fear of overly influencing them and diminishing patient autonomy; however, this reluctance may deprive patients and families of the physician's expertise and guidance. Physicians should make recommendations based on their medical knowledge and what they have learned about the patient's values and priorities.

In hospice and palliative care settings, the physician is responsible for decisions about medical care and recommending courses of action with input from members of the interdisciplinary team. Nonphysician team members must advise the patient's physician about changes in the patient's condition and include the physician in treatment-related decisions. The hospice and palliative care physician also is an integral member of the interdisciplinary team. When difficult decisions must be made, other team members can and should help with the decision and help communicate with and educate patients and families. However, it is not ethically appropriate for professionals to work outside of their scope of practice and competency. It is vital that physicians take a leadership role in assisting patients in making these decisions.

It is the responsibility of the care provider to gather all relevant information about the decision to be made. A number of potentially important questions are included in the 4-Box Model (22) (Table 50.3). Practical procedural approaches such as the 4-Box Model may not address the ultimate ethical nature of an action, but they provide a practical construct or approach to attempting to reach ethical decisions in given circumstances. An approach such as the 4-Box Model can help with the vast majority of ethical dilemmas in clinical practice.

The 4-Box Model is organized with a hierarchy in mind; clinical and biographical facts that focus on what makes sense medically and respect patient wishes are given more weight than quality of life or cultural considerations This hierarchy does not suggest that the questions in the bottom two boxes are insignificant but rather is more attuned to the avoidance of unnecessary conflicts or dilemmas through emphasis on first clarifying the relevant medical information and understanding options that make sense medically. If the patient prefers a plan of care that makes practical medical sense to

---

[7]*Vacco v Quill*, 521 US 793, 807 (1997).

TABLE 50.3 THE 4-BOX MODEL

I. Medical information	**II. Patient and professional preferences**
What is the patient's diagnosis and prognosis? How has the patient's condition changed? Are symptoms adequately treated? What is the proposed intervention? How effective is the intervention likely to be for this patient? What is the intention of the proposed intervention? What are possible alternatives?	What is known about the patient's wishes and values? What is known about the wishes of surrogates, family members, and other involved parties? Does the patient have the capacity to make decisions about medical treatments? Who is involved in making the decision and what is his or her involvement? What is the recommendation of the physician and interdisciplinary team?
III. Benefits and burdens	**IV. Contextual features**
What are the potential benefits and burdens/risks of the treatment in question? How does the patient describe his or her quality of life or burden of life? What brings meaning or sustains the patient? How has the patient made treatment decisions in the past? What types of treatments would provide a satisfactory outcome for this patient's life? What is achievable with regard to the patient's preferences?	Who is this patient? What are the patient's life story and primary values? What is the patient's relationship with family members and significant others? What are the patient's cultural, religious, and spiritual beliefs and values? What are the potential benefits and burdens of each alternative for the patient and family, including financial and emotional costs? What are the legal considerations? How will the decision affect the patient and family physically, emotionally, spiritually, socially, and economically?

Adapted with modification from Jonsen AR, Siegler M, Winslade WJ. *Clinical Ethics: A Practical Approach to Ethical Decisions in Clinical Medicine.* 7th ed. New York, NY: McGraw-Hill; 2010:8. Copyright © 2010 by McGraw-Hill.

the physician and team, there is a reduced likelihood of conflict.

Of note, the 4-Box Model shared in this chapter differs from that referenced in that we chose to focus on the benefits and burdens of treatments instead of quality of life in Box III. The palliative physician (as well as the clinical ethicist) is encouraged to ask whether a treatment is worth giving (in the context of the patient with predicted benefits and burdens) instead of the more troubling—is a life worth living.

THE PATIENT IN DECISION MAKING

Hospice and palliative medicine recognizes the patient and family as the unit of care. When possible the patient is the key decision maker, with authority to give consent or refuse treatment.

Decision-Making Capacity

It is important to confirm decision-making capacity to ensure that the patient has the ability to execute an informed refusal or to give informed consent (23). In medical settings, it is the physician's responsibility to determine decisional capacity. Capacity may change depending on the patient's condition and the complexity of the decision in question. Decision-making capacity is decision specific. The same patient may be able to express a simple value judgment (e.g., "I want my son to make decisions for me because I trust him") but not be able to understand the risks, benefits, and alternatives of a complex treatment (e.g.,

aortic valve replacement with lifelong warfarin therapy). To have capacity to make a specific decision, a patient needs to be able to (22)

- ***express insight*** (express sufficient understanding of relevant information and the implications of various treatment choices)
- make an ***internally rational*** choice (a decision that is in accordance with personal values and goals); external rationality standards usually equate to whether a person agrees with a decision
- demonstrate that he or she is ***not delusional*** as a consequence of delirium or other psychiatric diseases (capacity evaluation in the latter may necessitate a psychiatrist)
- express a ***static preference*** (not change his or her mind rapidly based on cognitive difficulties)

SURROGATE DECISION MAKERS

If a patient becomes incapacitated, treatment decisions may be made by a proxy or surrogate decision maker (i.e., a third person who has the authority to make medical decisions). Most states have adopted laws permitting a legally competent individual to execute a document authorizing a proxy to make health care decisions on behalf of a patient if he or she loses decision-making capacity. Sometimes, these documents are referred to as *durable powers of attorney for health care.* It is becoming more common to combine a proxy appointment with an instructive advance directive (e.g., Five Wishes document) or advance physician orders (e.g., POLST). While some states by statute specifically authorize proxies to make decisions to withhold or withdraw life-sustaining treatment, other states by statute limit the authority of a proxy, setting standards of evidence required for certain decisions in that regard (24). Even if there is an advance directive, its instructions often will not be sufficient to cover the current situation. Thus, designation of a surrogate should always be recommended. A proxy appointment is important particularly in certain circumstances, such as when a patient desires to name someone other than a legal spouse to act as his or her surrogate. A proxy also is important when disagreements among family members cannot be resolved or when family members are unavailable or nonexistent.

When a patient is incapacitated and there is no proxy or guardian with authority to make a medical decision, many states have statutes designating the patient's spouse, then adult children, and then parents or siblings to act as the patient's surrogate decision maker. Even in the absence of such a statute, it may be appropriate to presume that close family members who know the patient well have decision-making authority (24).

In the case of an incapacitated patient with no proxy, no guardian with authority to make medical decisions, and no family, court designation of a surrogate may be necessary. Sometimes a patient may have indicated that a friend should act as a surrogate when he or she becomes incapacitated. It may be appropriate in some cases for the physician to accept this designation. Neither the patient's physician nor members of an interdisciplinary care team should serve as a patient's surrogate decision maker.

Decisions by Surrogates

The essential role of the surrogate is to make decisions in accordance with the "substituted judgment" standard that attempts to mirror the decisions the patient would make under the same circumstances. If unknown or uncertain, it is appropriate for a surrogate to apply the best interest standard. Although ethicists and clinicians expect surrogates to use substituted judgment or patients' best interests when making decisions, data indicate that many surrogates rely on other factors such as their own best interests or mutual interests of themselves and the patient (25).

The term *substituted interests*, coined in a 2010 *Journal of the American Medical Association* article, describes a practical approach employed by many experienced physicians. This approach includes physician leadership in listening to the values and wishes of patients, contextualizing medical recommendations appropriately for patients, and offering guidance to surrogates in decision making, but not in such a way that reverts to paternalism (Table 50.4) (26).

TABLE 50.4 THE SUBSTITUTED INTERESTS MODEL OF SURROGATE DECISION MAKING

Step	Sample conversation starters and points
Empathy and connection: acknowledge stresses of the situation and difficulty of the task and attend to needs of the surrogate	"It must be very difficult to see your loved one so sick."
Authentic values: understand the patient as a person *Values*: interpersonal, moral, religious, familial, psychological *Directives*: substantive treatment preferences and process considerations, such as who should decide and how	"Tell us about your loved one." "Has anyone else in the family ever experienced a situation like this?"
Clinical data: share understanding of the patient's clinical circumstances and prognosis	"All of that is important for us to know as we face the current situation." "Here is what is wrong …" "This is what is likely to happen …"
Substituted interests: determine what the patient's real interests are, given the patient's values and these circumstances	"Knowing your loved one, what do you think would be the most important for him/her right now? Avoiding pain? Having family members here?"
Clinical judgment: share understanding of the options and offer recommendation based on clinical experience, tailored to the particular patient's real interests	"Here's what could be done." "This is what we would recommend, based on what we know and what you've told us about your loved one."
Best judgment for the patient: best path to promote the good of this patient as a unique person, in the context of his or her relationships, authentic values, known wishes, and real interests, given the circumstances and options	"Knowing your loved one, does our recommendation seem right for him or her? Do you think another plan would be better, given his or her values, preferences, relationships?"

Adapted from Sulmasy DP, Snyder L. Substituted interests and best judgments: an integrated model of surrogate decision making. *JAMA*. 2010;304(17):1946-1947. Copyright © 2010 by the American Medical Association.

SELECTED ETHICAL ISSUES

Proportionate Pain and Symptom Management

Some physicians fail to prescribe adequate amounts of pain medication because they fear the required dosages may inadvertently shorten a patient's life. They tend to grossly overestimate the toxicity of carefully titrated dosages of opioids.

Although advocates of effective pain management may invoke the principle of double effect (see box below) to encourage adequate pain control, in most cases the principle is irrelevant. Carefully titrated opioid dosages are not likely to shorten a patient's life (27). The principle of double effect may be more applicable in treating severe terminal dyspnea; however, this is an unproven speculation. In fact, many hospice and palliative care physicians have observed that prescribing dosages of an opioid sufficient to relieve pain and dyspnea can improve activity levels, quality of life (28), and perhaps even survival (29). Formal informed consent processes and drug agreements can be used to enhance understanding and shared expectations for symptom treatment (these should not be viewed as "drug contracts" (30)).

Principle of Double Effect

Although it has been criticized in recent years, the principle of double effect has had a significant role in secular and religious bioethics and also has influenced criminal law (31).

It validates the use of treatments that are honestly intended to relieve suffering or restore health even if the intervention has potential untoward effects. The four elements of the doctrine are as follows:

1. The good effect has to be intended (e.g., relieving pain or dyspnea).
2. The bad effect can be foreseen but not intended (could possibly shorten life, but not the intent).
3. The bad effect cannot be the means to the good effect (cannot end the patient's life to relieve the pain).
4. The symptom must be severe enough to warrant taking risks; this is known as proportionality.

Medical Futility

The concept of futility has been controversial, and attempts to implement it to limit treatment despite the wishes of the patient's family have led to serious disagreements (32). Texas, alone, has enacted legislation giving physicians the authority, upon approval of a hospital ethics committee, to remove life-sustaining medical treatment without consent of the patient or family under circumstances deemed medically futile (33,34). The Texas law remains very controversial.

Difficulties regarding medical futility are partly attributable to varying definitions. Medical futility can be defined on quantitative and qualitative grounds (35). If an intervention has a theoretical chance of providing benefit but has failed to do so in the last 100 cases, it is *quantitatively medically futile*. A treatment is *qualitatively futile* when it is perceived that the burdens outweigh the benefits of the treatment in the context of a certain patient. Qualitative futility often is considered if a technology is perceived as merely maintaining a patient in a state of permanent unconsciousness or in a state that continues to require management in an ICU with no hope of benefit other than maintenance. Consent from the patient or family to forgo (withhold or withdraw) quantitatively futile treatments may not be required, but qualitatively futile treatments generally require at least assent prior to forgoing or withdrawing them. The Texas law does not distinguish between the two types of futility.

When physicians use the term *futile* to describe a treatment, they often are reacting to a profound sense that it would be "wrong" to provide the treatment for a particular patient in a specific situation (36). The challenge is to honor the physician's sense of wrongdoing by exploring relevant issues with the patient instead of implying the existence of objective and dispassionate standards of medical futility that do not exist. When a patient or family demands treatment the physician believes is medically futile, full disclosure and compassionate communication usually result in medically appropriate decisions without resorting to the legal system. When treatment issues cannot be resolved, the case should be referred to an ethics consultant. Throughout this process, it is important for the treatment team to remember that in most cases family members are struggling with how to love their loved one.

Organ Donation

Although organ procurement and transplantation generally are not the domain of palliative care, it is important to realize that it is a potential source for concern, comfort, or both for patients and their families (37). If a patient or family is interested in organ donation, it is the responsibility of the health care team to contact the appropriate organ procurement organization (OPO). Early contact with the OPO staff gives the patient and family time to discuss their concerns about organ donation such as logistics, cost, and time. The OPO staff is trained at effectively discussing these issues with families and providing appropriate psychosocial support (38–40). Increasingly, palliative care teams may be asked to participate in certain types of organ procurement called donation after circulatory death. Palliative care teams should become familiar with the protocols used at their institution, as they vary. Controversially, the determination of death after circulatory death no longer has a verification time requirement. Participation in organ procurement without verification of death over several minutes may violate the ethical standards of some health care workers and patients (41).

Health Care Provider Conscientious Refusal

Federal laws known as the Church Amendments, established in 1973 a few weeks following the legalization of elective abortion, support the rights of health care providers to conscientiously refuse to participate in any "program or activity that would be contrary to his religious beliefs or moral convictions."[8] Since 1994, three additional United States federal statutes have been passed that provide increased conscience protections for health care providers including the Public Health Service Act, the Weldon Amendment, and the Affordable Care Act. The Affordable Care Act includes specific conscience protections regarding the intentional hastening of death.[9] Violations of these laws are to be reported to the U.S. Department of Health and Human Services Office for Civil Rights (42). Those invoking conscience protection may not be doing so only to protect themselves from being involved in an action they believe to be morally wrong. They may be attempting to protect the patient from an action they believe may be harmful.

Withdrawing ANH

ANH is a medical procedure that involves placing a tube or needle into the alimentary tract, in a vein, or under the skin to deliver fluids and nutrients. It does not refer to assisted oral feeding. Physicians must consider the withdrawal of ANH within an ethical framework, using all of the medical data available. As with other medical interventions, ANH should have a clearly defined therapeutic goal. The treatment can be discontinued when the patient's condition or appropriate time-limited trials indicate that the therapeutic goal is not achievable, when the intervention has become more burdensome than beneficial, or when it no longer serves the patient's goals (43).

The decision to withdraw ANH is complicated by many issues. There is debate and uncertainty among the general public and some care providers whether this is a basic need or a medical intervention. The fear of death by starvation and dehydration remains an emotionally charged subject.

A judicial and increasingly an ethical consensus has emerged that ANH is a medical treatment and may be refused under the same standards as other medical treatment, and in general it is accepted that adult patients with decision-making capacity can refuse ANH (24). In the aftermath of the Cruzan case, discussed in this chapter, many states revised their advance directive and proxy appointment statutes to permit refusal of ANH. However, sometimes the instructions in an advance directive may not adequately cover the situation and some states by statute limit the right of proxies to refuse ANH (44).

Palliative Sedation

Palliative sedation at the end of life refers to the use of high-dose sedatives to relieve extreme suffering as a last resort (45,46). The intent of the sedation is to provide relief from the distressing symptom and not to hasten death (47). Some physicians believe sedation at the end of life offers a humane alternative to suicide and assisted suicide. Others fear a "slippery slope" to euthanasia. *The intent of sedation is to provide relief and not to hasten death* (47).

The nomenclature for palliative sedation has changed and remains of poor consistency. Some will refer to palliative sedation as a situation in which a person dies sleepy from disease or drug. This is inaccurate. Some will include in the term *palliative sedation* the following: ordinary sedation (sedation as a side effect of regular symptom management), intermittent sedation (intentional sedation for a limited time period), and sedation to decreased awareness but not to unconsciousness, but these are not particularly ethically controversial issues. *Palliative sedation to unconsciousness* and continued until death is the controversial form, and this usually is referred to as palliative sedation. Before instituting palliative sedation to unconsciousness, the following conditions should be met (48):

- The patient is diagnosed with a terminal illness with a very short prognosis.
- All palliative treatment has been exhausted and profound symptoms persist.
- A psychological assessment has been made.
- A spiritual assessment has been made.
- There is a DNAR order (Do Not Attempt Resuscitation).
- There is informed consent.
- ANH was discussed before sedation.
- A policy and procedure should be in place and followed.

---

[8]Sterilization or Abortion Act, 42 USC, §300a-7 (1973).
[9]Affordable Care Act, § 42-1553 (2010).

- Appropriate documentation is assured.
- Complicated bereavement follow-up for family is available.

In the past, sedation at the end of life was referred to as "terminal sedation." However, use of this phrase often is discouraged because it may be misinterpreted to imply an intent to "terminate" a patient's life (49). It may be prudent to further modify our nomenclature to refer only to sedation to unconsciousness until death as palliative sedation. If we did so, "ordinary sedation" and palliative sedation that is not to unconsciousness or intermittent sedation would not potentially fall under the same heading. In the meantime, this nomenclature has yet to be agreed upon.

The debate regarding palliative sedation is that for the wrong patient or if inappropriately applied it can be a form of "slow euthanasia" (50); however, this is possibly not true if reserved for the rare case described here when palliative sedation has a legitimate and ethically defensible place in end-of-life-care as a measure of last resort in certain extreme cases when necessary to palliate severe symptoms for a person who is imminently dying. In general, the proximal cause of death ought to be the underlying disease, and not an intervention prescribed by a physician. Medically controlled sedation ought not to hasten or be the proximal cause of a person's death, including preventing a person from eating and drinking who would otherwise be able if not in state of medically controlled sedation (51). In general, for a person who is imminently dying, natural or medically assisted nutrition and hydration cease for physiologic reasons related to the irreversible progression of the disease, but this still ought to be carefully considered prior to initiation of any medically controlled sedation that will lessen the ability to eat and increase the risk of aspiration. As with all symptom management, the lowest effective doses should be utilized for the goal of the acceptable palliative of the symptom, after informed consent and thorough discussion of the expected benefits and risks (52).

Another issue of debate is that some centers seem to use palliative sedation to unconsciousness quite frequently, while other top centers use it rarely, if at all. Such variation is difficult to explain based on patient characteristics and values. Further, many world religions and cultures value awareness at the end of life and are opposed to intentional sedation at that time, even if symptoms are not optimally managed. Most experienced palliative care clinicians believe that palliative sedation to unconsciousness should be needed quite rarely, and only after other rigorous attempts have been made to relieve the patient's suffering.

Physician-Assisted Death

AAHPM defines *physician-assisted death* "as a physician providing, at the patient's request, a lethal medication that the patient can take by his own hand to end otherwise intolerable suffering" (53). *Euthanasia* is when a physician personally ends a patient's life (54). The US Supreme Court has rejected arguments that there is a constitutional right to physician-assisted death, and it is illegal in most states.[10,11] Eight states including California,[12] Colorado,[13] Hawaii,[14] Maine,[15] New Jersey,[16] Oregon,[17] Vermont,[18] and Washington[19] and the District of Columbia[20] now have laws permitting physician-assisted death. The Montana Supreme Court has ruled that patients with terminal illness have a right to physician-assisted death.[21] The protection offered by this court ruling is questionable. Other states are free to legalize physician-assisted death. No state at this time has legalized euthanasia.

Each state and the District of Columbia with laws permitting physician assisted suicide contain exemption clauses for health care providers who conscientiously object to participation in physician-assisted death. Under the Affordable Care Act, federal and state governments and health care providers receiving federal financial assistance may not discriminate against individuals and institutions for refusing to offer physician-assisted death, euthanasia, or mercy killing.[22]

The Debate

Thoughtful and compassionate people have compelling arguments for both prohibiting physician-assisted death and allowing it under carefully

---

[10]*Vacco v Quill,* 521 US 793, 807 (1997).

[11]*Washington v Glucksberg,* 521 US 702 (1997).

[12]California End of Life Options Act, Cal Health & Safety Code § 443 (2016).

[13]Colorado End-of-Life Options Act, Colo. Rev. Stat. § 25-48 (2017).

[14]Our Care, Our Choice Act, Hawaii Rev Stat § 327L (2019).

[15]Maine Death with Dignity Act, Maine Revised Stat Title 22 § 2140.

[16]New Jersey Aid in Dying for the Terminally Ill Act, N.J. Stat § 26:16 (2019).

[17]Oregon Death with Dignity Act, Or Rev Stat, §127.800 (2003).

[18]Patient Choice at End of Life Act, Vt. Stat.Ann. tit.18, § § 5281 (2016).

[19]Washington Death with Dignity Act, Wash Rev Code, §70.245 (2008).

[20]Death with Dignity Act, D.C. Code § 7-661 (2017).

[21]*Baxter v State,* 224 P3d 1211 (2009).

[22]Patient Protection and Affordable Care Act, Pub L No. 111-48, 124 Stat 119, §1553 (2010).

defined circumstances (55). Proponents of physician-assisted death base their arguments on autonomy and compassion (56). Proponents view physician-assisted death—in compelling cases and with adequate safeguards—as a humane way to end a life characterized by intense suffering resulting from uncontrollable physical, psychosocial, or spiritual pain. They also point out that such practices have historical and cultural precedence. When a patient's life has become intolerable, some proponents view a refusal to participate in assisted death as contrary to the principle of patient autonomy, which, they argue, includes the patient's right to determine when and how life ends. Some believe assisted death is compatible with a physician's professional integrity, but only when it is used as a last resort to relieve intractable physical suffering (57). Those supporting physician-assisted death tend to believe society is systematically diverging from what is right by forcing dying patients to endure unwanted days of meaningless suffering (58).

Opponents of physician-assisted death and euthanasia often base their arguments on moral codes or religious traditions that assert the wrongness or evil of intentionally killing innocents even at their request. Physicians, opponents believe, have a professional obligation to avoid harming a patient. They will point to a history of medical professionalism opposed to such practices. They will point out that most physicians, hospice groups, and physician societies oppose physician-assisted dying. Opponents also voice concerns about the dangers of social policies that condone killing; the initiation of a "slippery slope" that could be used to justify the elimination of disabled or expensive patients; and subtle family, societal, or financial pressures on patients to choose assisted death. Many believe in the likelihood that pain and suffering can be alleviated with skillful palliative interventions that will help patients view life as worth living until death occurs, and that the nature of requests for assisted death, which generally are withdrawn when pain and depression effectively are treated, are temporary. Further, people may believe that suicide may be harmful to bereaved families or even harmful transcendentally to the patient after death. Opponents often express fears that societal trust toward medicine (and particularly hospice and palliative care) will wane if medicine becomes an instrument of death. They often want to respect autonomy, but they embrace the long-held view that suicide presents a limit to respecting self-determination (59). Finally, they often lament the societal denigration of all that is not youth, beauty, sexuality, independence, and productivity (54,60,61).

Common Ground

Proponents and opponents of physician-assisted death should share an ethic of compassion and must agree that abandonment is not a viable alternative to assisted death. Further, universal agreement should exist that suffering among dying patients remains all too prevalent, and lack of access to expert hospice and palliative care contributes to the suffering. Although this chapter *about* ethics cannot offer an universally accepted answer (though the author believes one exists) for physicians grappling with the issue of physician-assisted death, it does offer unequivocal recognition of the need to support improved access to expert palliative care.

REFERENCES

1. Engelhardt HT. *Foundations of Bioethics.* 2nd ed. London, UK: Oxford University Press; 1996.
2. Meisel A. The legal consensus about foregoing life sustaining treatment: its status and its prospects. *Kennedy Inst Ethics J.* 1992;2(4):309-345.
3. Snyder L. *Ethics Manual.* 6th ed. Philadelphia, PA: American College of Physicians; 2012.
4. Stoneberg JN, von Gunten CF. Assessment of palliative care needs. *Anesthesiol Clin.* 2006;24(1):1-17.
5. Cayley WE Jr. Our most important role as a physician is being a comforter to the sick. *Fam Pract Manag.* 2006;13(9):74.
6. Daneault S, Lussier V, Mongeau S, et al. The nature of suffering and its relief in the terminally ill: a qualitative study. *J Palliat Care.* 2004;20(1):7-11.
7. Bishop, J. *The Anticipatory Corpse: Medicine, Power, and the Care of the Dying.* Notre Dame, IN: Notre Dame Press; 2011 (theme of the book). www.aahpm.org
8. Koppel A, Sullivan SM. Legal considerations in end-of-life decision making in Louisiana. *Ochsner J.* 2011;11(4):330-333.
9. Schuklenk U, van Delden JJ, Downie J, McLean SA, Upshur R, Weinstock D. End-of-life decision making in Canada: the report by the Royal Society of Canada expert panel on end-of-life decision making. *Bioethics.* 2011;25(suppl 1):1-73.
10. Sato K, Miyashita M, Morita T, Suzuki M. The long-term effect of a population-based educational intervention focusing on end-of-life home care, life-prolongation treatment, and knowledge about palliative care. *J Palliat Care.* 2009;25(3):206-212.
11. Feltman DM, Du H, Leuthner SR. Survey of neonatologists' attitudes toward limiting life-sustaining treatments in the neonatal intensive care unit. *J Perinatol.* 2012;32(11):886-892.
12. Solomon MZ, O'Donnell L, Jennings B, et al. Decisions near the end of life: professional views on life-sustaining treatments. *Am J Public Health.* 1993;83(1):14-23.
13. Meisel A, Snyder L, Quill T. Seven legal barriers to end-of-life care: myths, realities, and grains of truth. *JAMA.* 2000;284(19):2495-2501.
14. Bradley A. Positive rights, negative rights and health care. *J Med Ethics.* 2010;36(12):838-841.
15. Kinney HC, Korein J, Panigrahy A, Dikkes P, Goode R. Neuropathological findings in the brain of Karen Ann Quinlan. The role of the thalamus in the persistent vegetative state. *N Engl J Med.* 1994;330(21):1469-1475.

16. Cranford RE, Doudera AE. The emergence of institutional ethics committees. *Law Med Health Care*. 1984;12(1):13-20.
17. Lewin T. Nancy Cruzan dies, outlived by a debate over the right to die. *New York Times*; December 27, 1990.
18. University of Miami Ethics Programs, Shepard Broad Law Center at Nova Southeastern University. Key events in the case of Theresa Marie Schiavo. http://www6.miami.edu/ethics/schiavo/timeline.htm. Accessed January 12, 2012.
19. Goodnough A. The Schiavo case: the overview. *New York Times*; April 1, 2005:A1.
20. United States Conference of Catholic Bishops. *Ethical and Religious Directives for Catholic Health Care Services*. 5th ed. http://www.ncbcenter.org/document.doc?id=147. Accessed January 11, 2012.
21. Burt RA. The Supreme Court speaks—not assisted suicide but a constitutional right to palliative care. *N Engl J Med*. 1997;337(17):1234-1236.
22. Jonsen AR, Siegler M, Winslade WJ. *Clinical Ethics: A Practical Approach to Ethical Decisions in Clinical Medicine*. 7th ed. New York, NY: McGraw-Hill; 2010.
23. Miller SS, Marin DB. Assessing capacity. *Emerg Med Clin North Am*. 2000;18(2):233-242.
24. Meisel A, Cerminara KL. *Right to Die: The Law of End-of-Life Decision Making*. 3rd ed. Riverwoods, IL: Aspen Publishers; 2011.
25. Vig EK, Taylor JS, Starks H, Hopley EK, Fryer-Edwards K. Beyond substituted judgment: how surrogates navigate end-of-life decision-making. *J Am Geriatr Soc*. 2006;54(11):1688-1693.
26. Sulmasy DP, Snyder L. Substituted interests and best judgments: an integrated model of surrogate decision making. *JAMA*. 2010;304(17):1946-1947. © 2010 by the American Medical Association.
27. Brown DJ. Palliation of breathlessness. *Clin Med*. 2006;6(2):133-136.
28. El-Jawahri A, Greer JA, Temel JS. Does palliative care improve outcomes for patients with incurable illness? A review of the evidence. *J Support Oncol*. 2011;9(3):87-94.
29. Temel JS, Greer JA, Muzikansky A, et al. Early palliative care for patients with metastatic non-small-cell lung cancer. *N Engl J Med*. 2010;363(8):733-742.
30. Payne R, Anderson E, Arnold R, et al. A rose by any other name: pain contracts/agreements. *Am J Bioeth*. 2010;10(11):5-12.
31. Quill TE, Dresser R, Brock DW. The rule of double effect—a critique of its role in end-of-life decision making. *N Engl J Med*. 1997;337(24):1768-1771.
32. Bernat JL. Medical futility: definition, determination, and disputes in critical care. *Neurocrit Care*. 2005;2(2):198-205.
33. Procedure if Not Effectuating a Directive or Treatment Decision, Texas Health & Safety Code, §166.046 (2003).
34. Burge CR. Texas Advance Directives Act versus "state-created danger" theory: a prima facie analysis. *Am J Trial Advoc*. 2009;32:552.
35. Schneiderman LJ, Jecker NS, Jonsen AR. Medical futility: its meaning and ethical implications. *Ann Intern Med*. 1990;112(12):949-954.
36. Alpers A, Lo B. When is CPR futile? *JAMA*. 1995;273(2):156-158.
37. Nelson JL. Internal organs, integral selves, and good communities: opt-out organ procurement policies and the 'separateness of persons'. *Theor Med Bioeth*. 2011;32(5):289-300.
38. Arnold RM. Fast facts and concepts #79: discussing organ donation with families; 2006. www.aahpm.org/cgi-bin/wkcgi/view?status=A%20&search=155&id=390&offset=0&limit=258. Accessed August 3, 2007.
39. Arnold RM, Siminoff LA, Frader JE. Ethical issues in organ procurement: a review for intensivists. *Crit Care Clin*. 1996;12(1):29-48.
40. Siminoff LA, Arnold RM, Caplan AL, Virnig BA, Seltzer DL. Public policy governing organ and tissue procurement in the United States. Results from the National Organ and Tissue Procurement Study. *Ann Intern Med*. 1995;123(1):10-17.
41. Stein R. Changes in controversial organ donation method stir fears. *Washington Post*; September 19, 2011.
42. Public Welfare: Definitions. To be codified at 45 CFR §88.2. *Fed Regist*. 2008;73:414-415.
43. Fuhrman MP, Herrmann VM. Bridging the continuum: nutrition support in palliative and hospice care. *Nutr Clin Pract*. 2006;21(2):134-141.
44. Gillick MR. The use of advance care planning to guide decisions about artificial nutrition and hydration. *Nutr Clin Pract*. 2006;21(2):126-133.
45. Quill TE, Lo B, Brock DW, Meisel A. Last-resort options for palliative sedation. *Ann Intern Med*. 2009;151(6):421-424.
46. Quill TE, Byock IR. Responding to intractable terminal suffering. *Ann Intern Med*. 2000;133(7):561-562.
47. Lo B, Rubenfeld G. Palliative sedation in dying patients: "we turn to it when everything else hasn't worked." *JAMA*. 2005;294(14):1810-1816.
48. Rousseau P. Palliative sedation in the management of refractory symptoms. *J Support Oncol*. 2004;2(2):181-186.
49. Krakauer EL, Penson RT, Truog RD, King LA, Chabner BA, Lynch TJ Jr. Sedation for intractable distress of a dying patient: acute palliative care and the principle of double effect. *Oncologist*. 2000;5(1):53-62.
50. Billings JA, Block SD. Slow euthanasia. *J Palliat Care*. 1996;12(4):21-30.
51. American Academy of Hospice and Palliative Medicine Statement on Palliative Sedation. Approved by the AAHPM Board of Directors on December 5, 2014. http://aahpm.org/positions/palliative-sedation. Accessed March 10, 2020.
52. Olsen ML, Swetz KM, Mueller PS. Ethical decision making with end-of-life care: palliative sedation and withholding or withdrawing life-sustaining treatments. *Mayo Clin Proc*. 2010;85(10):949-954.
53. American Academy of Hospice and Palliative Medicine. *AAHPM Statement on Physician-Assisted Suicide*. www.aahpm.org/positions/default/suicide.html. Accessed December 15, 2011.
54. Moulin DE, Latimer EJ, Macdonald N, et al. Statement on euthanasia and physician-assisted suicide. *J Palliat Care*. 1994;10(2):80-81.
55. Foley KM. Competent care for the dying instead of physician-assisted suicide. *N Engl J Med*. 1997;336(1):54-58.
56. Battin MP. *Ethical Issues in Suicide*. 2nd ed. Englewood Cliffs, NJ: Prentice-Hall; 1995.
57. Emanuel EJ, Fairclough D, Clarridge BC, et al. Attitudes and practices of U.S. oncologists regarding euthanasia and physician-assisted suicide. *Ann Intern Med*. 2000;133(7):527-532.
58. Warnock M. *Easeful Death: Is There a Case for Assisted Dying?* New York, NY: Oxford University Press; 2009.
59. Foley KM, Hendin H, eds. *The Case Against Assisted Suicide: For the Right to End-of-Life Care*. Baltimore, MD: Johns Hopkins University Press; 2004.
60. Hendin H. Selling death and dignity. *Hastings Cent Rep*. 1995;25(3):19-23.
61. Cherny NI, Coyle N, Foley KM. The treatment of suffering when patients request elective death. *J Palliat Care*. 1994;10(2):71-79.

51 Assisted Suicide or Understanding and Responding to Requests for Hastened Death

Margaret M. Mahon

[T]he problem of coping with death unites people of all times

Spronk, 2004, p. 987

(If you are looking for concrete suggestions or practical advice, see page, 12, "When the request comes.")

INTRODUCTION

Among the oldest of human constructions are tombs. This should not be surprising, for among the oldest of human preoccupations is an understanding of human mortality, that human life is finite. This paradox, that human life culminates in its own extinction, has been a foundational issue of philosophy, religion, and literature, transcending time and culture. To confront this paradox, our ancestors built tombs, perhaps to demonstrate that a meaningful life did not end in meaninglessness. For our ancestors, the good death, a death that was not meaningless, was in part a matter of proper memorialization. Today, however, the good death is not nearly as passive. Unlike our ancestors, in much of today's Western culture, medical intervention has become integral to the good death. While medical knowledge and skills have increased dramatically, traditional notions of the good death have not been explored at the same pace. Understanding the role of medical interventions in the context of traditional notions of the good death is a challenge unique to our time.

Assisted suicide and euthanasia are not constructs of the late 20th century. Rather, they have been contemplated for millennia. In this chapter, perspectives on dying well and on suffering are described. Notions about a good life, a good death, and the role of suffering can inform health caregivers' responses when facing a request for or questions about hastened death.

ANCIENT HISTORY

In ancient times, as exemplified in the Hebrew Bible,[1] a good death comprised long life, being at peace at the time of death, living in the context of family (including one's forebears and progeny), and being buried near home (1). In Greco-Roman times (approximately 332 BC to 395 AD), death in battle was a reason to be glorified (2). The Roman emperor Augustus (63 BC to 14 AD) wished for euthanasia, which, at the time, meant a good death, one that was quick and painless (2). In ancient millennia, the dimensions of a good death were often congruent with the core elements of living well.

A bad death included, in part, the absence of the dimensions of a good life. What people believed constituted a bad death varied, but included violence, death alone, death far from home, or death from suicide (3).

The role of the physician was to recognize when death was near, but not to intervene. "In the medical texts, no mention is made of the doctor's task to relieve the suffering of those who are fatally ill" (2, p. 980). Sophocles, the tragedian of the fifth century BCE, believed that no role existed for hastening of death; life was given by the gods and therefore was of the highest good (4). Euripides, also fifth century BCE, wrote that physicians should not usually hasten death, though he described acceptable conditions for hastening death at least twice (4). Plato (427? to 347 BCE) suggested severe punishment for any physician who caused a person's death with a medication. Plato did recognize the right of a person living with severe pain to commit suicide, though opposed it in other circumstances (4).

THE 19TH CENTURY: FOUNDATIONS OF PALLIATIVE CARE

Looking forward two millennia, the discussion remained largely the same, though knowledge about illness and some factors about how people died

---

[1]The Hebrew Bible was written over centuries, at least as early as 1000 BCE (From Drummond J. What is the oldest Hebrew Bible? Bible History Daily Web site. Published 2016.

Updated December 16, 2016. Accessed December 18, 2019; Faigenbaum-Golovin S, Shaus A, Sober B, et al. Algorithmic handwriting analysis of Judah's military correspondence sheds light on composition of biblical texts. *Proc Natl Acad Sci U S A*. 2016;113(17):4664-4669; and Ngo R. When was the Hebrew Bible written? Bible History Daily Web site. Published 2016. Updated May 10, 2017. Accessed December 18, 2019).

were changing. Starting in the 1840s, more deaths occurred outside of the home, as institutions who cared for people at the end of life developed in Europe (France, Ireland, England), Australia, and the United States (5). Contemporaneously, physicians and nurses published information about how to provide care to the dying (5). These authors also developed nascent ideas that could form a philosophy of care of the dying (5), revealing an evolution of thought about end of life care, as well as points of disagreement that continue two centuries later.

Though discussions about how people live and how people die were similar millennia apart, the foundation for the discussion was rapidly evolving. Scientific advancements of the 19th century formed the foundation of modern health care. Germ theory was described. The fields of microbiology and bacteriology burgeoned, and physiology evolved past its Galenic assumptions. These discoveries led to current practices of antisepsis and of anesthesia in surgery. Vaccines were developed, including for rabies, cholera, typhoid, and others, though use was quite limited. These advances in knowledge provided a foundation for reflections on the role of physiology in scientific medicine.

William Munk (1816–1898), a recognized expert physician in London, was a staunch advocate for the use of opioids and other analgesics for pain management for those with serious illness (6). Though not often touted as such, Munk was, in many ways, an early champion of what we now call palliative care.

After more than 40 years practicing medicine, in 1887, Munk published *Euthanasia: Or, Medical treatment in aid of an easy death* (7). He used "euthanasia" in the way of his century, as conveyed in his subtitle. The word is from the Greek, εάθανασία, in which εὐ, eu means "good" and θάνατος, thanatos means "death." Munk was the first modern physician to use this term to describe the amelioration of suffering[2] associated with dying.

Munk sought to educate people about dying and about death. He provided multiple examples of good deaths. For example, he described the death of William Hunter, an anatomist. "He retained his consciousness to the last, and just before he died he whispered to his friend, Dr. Combe, 'If I had strength enough to hold a pen, I would write about how easy and pleasant a thing it is to die'" (7, p. 10). He wrote about near drowning, deaths following surgery, and deaths from illness. He recognized that being around the dying was uncomfortable for some, but expressed, "… *"the physical process of death loses much of its horror on a near view."*

---

[2]Suffering comes from Latin, *suffere*, from *sub* (from below) + *ferrer* (to bear). The word "patient" comes from the Latin verb *pati* (to suffer). Patient, then, means, the one who suffers.

Physicians, the clergy, and intelligent nurses—all, indeed, who are practically conversant with the dying testify to the truth of this statement" (7, p. 8, 9). Munk recognized that some deaths were not easy. Furthermore, the ministrations or interference of health care providers could impede what otherwise might be an "easy death." "In the intelligent trained nurses of the present day, we have the best security against such barbarity" (7, p. 96).

Munk described symptoms that typically occur with dying, including waning levels of consciousness, delirium, altered sensorium, circulatory changes, restlessness, fatigue, dyspnea, changes in appearance, and other aspects of dying. Munk wrote about the decreased need for food as death approaches. "Food is given too frequently, and in quantities too large. The dying person is induced by the wearisome importunity of his attendants to take food or stimulants, against which nature and his stomach revolt" (7, p. 66).

How many times do we have this same discussion in the 21st century? Let the patient eat what she wants, be guided by her own appetites. Munk also advocated respect for patient preferences in this area. "The wishes of the patient himself, when he has reached the stage of existence here contemplated, may generally be taken as a correct indication in all that relates to the administration of food and stimulants" (7, p. 67). He espoused doing what is necessary and no more. "The fewer the drugs and the less of medicine we can do with in the treatment of the dying, the better" (7, p. 85).

Finally, Munk wrote about the use of medications or other substances to enhance the dying person's comfort. He included "wine or spirit" ("Of wines, sherry is perhaps the most useful") (7, p. 70). Munk described the benefits of small quantities of water and ice in providing comfort. He strongly endorsed the use of opium. "Opium is here worth all the rest of the material medica. Its object and action must however be clearly understood" (7, p. 73).

It is in Munk's discussion of the optimal use of opium that we see that a reemergence of the points made by Euripides and Plato millennia earlier, and the harbinger of consideration of providers' roles in patients' dying and deaths in the 21st century. "Opium should rarely be administered to the dying as a mere hypnotic, or with a view to enforce sleep. To do so would be to risk throwing the patient into a sleep from which he may not awake. But opium often induces sleep indirectly, and in the kindest way, by the relief of pain, or sinking that had hitherto rendered sleep impossible" (7, p. 73, 74). Munk challenges providers to be cognizant of their motives. He clearly demarcated an intervention meant to cause death from those intended to manage symptoms, avoiding harmful side effects when possible.

Most physicians in England and the United States in the late 19th century believed that intentional killing was wrong, even if a person were dying. Furthermore, hastening death was construed as dangerous not only to individuals but also to society as a whole (5). At the same time, though, a debate began outside of the circles of professional medicine. In 1872, schoolteacher Samuel Williams presented a paper to the Birmingham Philosophical Society in which he strongly supported voluntary euthanasia (5,8). Despite many publications supporting Williams' ideas, the idea of hastening death had little impact on the medical community until almost the 20th century (8).

Munk's view of death was straightforward, almost simple. The dying person should be relatively unencumbered, except by that that would increase comfort. Although Munk's framework for care of the dying was novel, his writings reflected the cultural notions prevailing in the England of his time, as well as the technical and scientific realities of his day.

Munk could not foresee the current technological abilities to extend human life long past its "natural" end. Exploring the roles of potentially life-extending technologies has led to a need to reframe the notion of the good death. Unlike Munk's contemporaries, we contend with the possibility that our ministrations may prolong dying as well as extend life. We may even increase suffering. Further, as a disciple of Enlightenment rationalism and living in a time of unfettered belief in human progress, Munk's saw all suffering as needless, meaningless, an absolute evil. This view of suffering as something to be avoided is common in discussions about hastening death today. This view does not, however, allow for the idea that in some cultures and for some individuals, suffering has redemptive purpose, itself necessary for a good death.

SUFFERING AT END OF LIFE

The role of suffering at the end of life has received increased attention in the 20th and 21st centuries. Beliefs about the role of suffering in dying are wide ranging. Many answers have been proposed to the question, "Why do people suffer?" Some people perceive suffering as just punishment for sins; for some, suffering is inevitable (9). Suffering may be construed as an inevitable part of the human condition, or suffering may be understood as a means to be closer to God. (I had a patient, an elderly woman with a great deal of physical pain. She was close to death and had benefitted from low dose opioids. She started to refuse them, because "When I'm in pain, I am closer to God. When I'm in pain, I share his suffering.") For each of these hypotheses, however, Foley described *some* meaning (9).

Suffering may be the most difficult or challenging when it is perceived to be devoid of meaning.

Viktor Frankl, MD, PhD was an Austrian, psychiatrist and neurologist who was a prisoner at four concentration camps during the Holocaust. Based on his work prior to imprisonment, as well as his experiences at the camps, in 1946, Frankl published one of the most meaningful publications of the 20th century, *Man's Search for Meaning* (10). Frankl wrote this book to "try to answer this question: How was everyday life in a concentration camp reflected in the mind of the average prisoner" (10, p. 3). Frankl wrote, "Man's search for meaning is the primary motivation in his life and not a 'secondary rationalization' of instinctual drives. The meaning is unique and specific in that it must and can be fulfilled by him alone; only then does it achieve a significance which will satisfy his own *will* to meaning" (10, p. 99). Based on what he witnessed in the camps, the suffering, the cruelty, the despair, the compassion, and the choices, Frank recognized the unavoidability of suffering and concluded that meaning can be found in *any* situation.

Frankl specifically addressed suffering while dying, and the opportunity to find meaning even then. "Those things which seem to take meaning away from human life include not only suffering but dying as well" (10, p. 120). Meaning can decrease or evolve with suffering, including at end of life. "[T]he transitoriness of our existence in no way makes it meaningless" (10, p. 120). Finding meaning in the face of suffering is work. Frankl developed *logotherapy*, which "focuses on the meaning of human existence as well as on man's search for such a meaning. According to this logotherapy, this striving to find a meaning in one's life is the primary motivational force in man" (10, p. 98, 99). For Frankl, then, finding meaning in suffering is a choice, it is active. A patient at the end of life is often suffering. One dimension for the clinician to consider is whether the person who is dying ascribes any meaning to this point in living. In addition, does the clinician find meaning in this stage in the patient's life?

Suffering in Literature

Comfort with dying is integral to palliative care and is increasingly recognized as important to other medical specialties. Tolstoy's *The Death of Ivan Ilyich* (11), and Margaret Edson's play, *W;t* (12) (Wit) each provide intimate descriptions not only of death but of living at the end of life. Both portray suffering at the end of life. Both provide glimpses of what the protagonists believe are a good life and a good death, even though the good death might not be achieved. In understanding these two examples, dimensions of the debate about assisted suicide come into focus.

Suffering in "The Death of Ivan Ilyich"

In Tolstoy's novella, Ivan Ilyich Golovan is dying from an illness that his physician cannot identify. Ivan Ilyich is wracked with pain, and eventually becomes bedridden. "There was no deceiving himself: something new and dreadful was happening to him, something of such vast importance that nothing in his life could compare with it. And he alone was aware of this. Those about him either did not understand or did not wish to understand and thought that nothing in the world had changed" (11, p. 80). Isolation was a predominant component of Ivan Ilyich's suffering from the first.

As he contemplated his living and his dying, Ivan Ilyich also struggled with the notion of what is right, what is fair. "'What does it all mean? Why has it happened? It's inconceivable, inconceivable that life was so senseless and disgusting. And if it really was so disgusting and senseless, why should I have to die, and die in agony? Something must be wrong. Perhaps I did not live as I should have,' it suddenly occurred to him. 'But how can that be when I did everything one is supposed to?'…" (11, p. 120). The relatively short time of his disease upended the previously settled and assured beliefs about his life he held until he became ill.

Ivan Ilyich believed he had lived right, done right, and done well, so he did not deserve to suffer. Even more, he deserved *not* to suffer. And yet, physically, he did suffer. "Morning or night, Friday or Sunday, made no difference, everything was the same: the gnawing, excruciating, incessant pain; that awareness of life irrevocably passing but not yet gone; that dreadful, loathsome death, the only reality, relentlessly closing in on him; and that same endless lie. What did days, weeks, or hours matter?" Increasing physical agony was surpassed by the mounting agony of isolation. Physical isolation expanded to encompass the interpersonal, psychological, and spiritual. "[W]hat tormented Ivan Ilyich most was that no one gave him the kind of compassion he craved. There were moments after long suffering when what he wanted most of all (shameful as it might be for him to admit) was to be pitied like a sick child. He wanted to be caressed, kissed, cried over, as sick children are caressed and comforted" (11, p. 104).

Ivan Ilyich does receive, and eventually accept the intimacy of care and presence, when, not his wife, nor his children, nor his friends, but his servant, Gerasim provided the care and compassion that Ivan Ilyich both needed and craved. Gerasim not only took care of Ivan Ilyich's physical needs, he stayed. Not because he had to, but because he chose to. "Once, as Ivan Ilyich was sending him away, he came right out and said: 'We all have to die someday, so why shouldn't I help you?'" (11, p. 104).

In his severe illness, in his dying, Ivan Ilyich perceived himself as powerless, taken over by his disease. Strandmark described powerlessness as consisting "of a self-image of worthlessness, feeling imprisoned by one's situation and emotional suffering" (13, p. 138). She continued, "Powerlessness implies vulnerability" (13, p. 138). As Gerasim gave to Ivan Ilyich, compassionate contact can alleviate powerlessness and suffering. In understanding suffering, and sometimes in understanding requests for hastened death, we have to understand if we can meet a patient's needs. These needs might take the form of substantive conversation, of talking about football, of contact with one's pet, or of a shared cup of tea. This presence can be compassion. This presence does not alleviate the terminal illness, but it may decrease suffering. It may validate that one is more than one's illness.

When people talk with palliative care providers (or with a nurse, oncologist, cardiologist, gerontologist, or others) about hastening death, it is essential to understand the nature of the individual's suffering. Is the patient or family requesting death *or* are they requesting an end to suffering? Are those notions separable? Is the family able or ill prepared to sit with dying? It is sometimes surprising how many adults, even senior health care providers, have never seen death up close. We must be like Gerasim and be willing to learn *this* patient's perspective, to witness what the suffering actually is for *this* person, in *this* minute.

Suffering in "W;t"

W;t is a one-act play written by Margaret Edson. Edson's writings were informed, in part, by her work in a hospital. The protagonist, Vivian Bearing, is an English professor, specializing in the works of the poet and Anglican cleric John Donne (1572–1631).[3] Dr. Bearing had always been singularly focused on her work and, as a result, chose to lead a somewhat isolated existence. The play portrays the last hours of Dr. Bearing's life, with frequent flashbacks that provide greater understanding of the professor. When diagnosed with stage IV ovarian cancer, Dr. Bearing accepts the opportunity, the challenge proffered by her oncologist, Dr. Kelekian: eight cycles of an experimental regimen … at full dosage. Dr. Bearing perceives a link between her own scholastic rigor and taking the most difficult treatment regimen. She likened her choice to become a rigorous scholar to her choice about participating in research "Simple

---

[3]Of Donne's work, one of Dr. Bearing's favorite subjects was Sonnet X, Death Be Not Proud, which includes the lines, And soonest our best men with thee do go, Rest of their bones, and soul's delivery.

human truth, uncompromising scholarly standards? …. All right, significant contribution to knowledge. Eight cycles of chemotherapy. Give me the full dose, the full dose every time" (12, p. 15). When she realizes that she is being treated as a research subject rather than a patient (the one who suffers), she recognizes the parallel with her own background as an educator and researcher: focusing on learning, on knowledge, more than on people. "The attention was flattering. For the first five minutes. Now I know how poems feel" (12, p. 15). She sees both sides. "I always want to know more things. I'm a scholar. Or I was when I had shoes, when I had eyebrows" (12, p. 54).

In the isolation of her medical treatments and her dying, Dr. Bearing realizes she would appreciate kindness. (It feels much akin to Ivan Ilyich's search for compassion.) The most meaningful discussion of the play comes with someone Dr. Bearing barely knows, Susie Monahan, Dr. Bearing's primary nurse. Ms. Monahan laughs and shares a popsicle with Dr. Bearing, and, then, she asks the professor about code status. Dr. Bearing chooses not to have resuscitation attempted. Reflecting on her conversation with Ms. Monahan, Dr. Bearing recognizes the gift of the simple. "Now is not the time for verbal swordplay, for unlikely flights of imagination and wildly shifting perspectives, for metaphysical conceit, for wit. […] Now is a time for simplicity. Now is a time for, dare I say it, kindness. I thought being extremely smart would take care of it. But I see that I have been found out" (12, p. 55, 56).

Dr. Bearing dies alone, much as she had lived. She chose to be alone in her living, throughout her illness, and in her dying. The reader (or viewer) gets the impression that isolation allowed Dr. Bearing to interact primarily on the intellectual plane she so valued. It was only in her dying that isolation became a source of suffering. She came to recognize the difference that being known, perhaps being loved might add to her life.

Common Messages

Despite being vastly different portrayals, the parallels in the lives of Ivan Ilyich and Dr. Bearing are notable. Both lived life as they had chosen; both were successful in their chosen fields and took pride in that. That success, their achievements, was an important component of their self-identity.

For both Ivan Ilyich and Dr. Bearing, the value of what was important changed as death became a proximal reality. Both were suffering, and mostly suffered alone. Both recognized the desire for different types of relationships as death approached. Both Ivan Ilyich and Dr. Bearing had a single

person who saw past the disease, the physical suffering, and the existential suffering, and who chose to step into the difficult, the intimate[4] place. It is the choice of Garasim and of Ms. Monahan to become intimate, to *know*, to be present with the suffering of the dying person.

SUFFERING AND REQUESTS FOR HASTENED DEATH

A request for hastened death typically comes from a place of suffering, perhaps physical, but more often interpersonal, psychological, or spiritual. Suffering may have a component of fear of future suffering. Twenty-first century health care is very much focused on doing, on intervening, and on being active. There is sometimes greater value in being still. Both Gerasim and Ms. Monahan evidenced the value of presence, of understanding, and of acceptance. Their most helpful, treasured interventions were that they stayed in the room, acknowledged discomfort (physical and otherwise), and listened. In discussions about assisted suicide, caregivers are challenged to be present with the pain, the burdens of the person requesting hastened death.

People often suffer at the end of their lives,[5] but it is rarely only the patient who suffers. Family members and loved ones suffer. Ferrand and colleagues (14) found that, in France, where assisted suicide is not legal, 60.8% of requests for hastened death came from patients, 32.9% came from family or others in a "close circle" (p. 6), and 6.3% came from nurses.

Physicians, nurses, social workers, chaplains, and others involved in the care of the dying may be uncomfortable when the patient no longer is receiving disease-directed therapies. Some perceive this as a time of "doing nothing." If death is not near-immediate, some perceive a vast expanse of inactivity until death (though the time might be minutes or hours or days). This perceived inactivity may be difficult for some; it might be a time of clinicians' suffering. Some physicians and other professionals perceive a patient's death as personal failure. This is the time at which some clinicians might start a continuous opioid infusion, though perhaps the IV is not warranted by the patient's symptoms. For some providers, when they realize that they cannot cure, that they do not have any further disease- or injury-focused therapies to offer. This action to shorten the period of

---

[4]Intimate comes from the Latin, *intimare*, to make familiar.

[5]Suffering comes from Latin, *pati,*patient, suffering. Patient, then, means, the one who suffers.

a patient's dying may allow providers to separate themselves more rapidly from a patient's dying and death. They feel less confronted with the inability to "do something."

In *W;t*, Dr. Bearing develops acute pain, and her suffering is stark. "Oh, God, it is so painful. So painful. So much pain. So much pain" (12, p. 56). Ms. Monahan requests a PCA, but she is forcefully overruled. Dr. Kelekian, the attending physician, says, "I want a morphine drip." He acknowledged that a PCA might be the right choice in other circumstances. "Ordinarily, yes. But in her case, no." He continues, "She's earned a rest. (*To* [the fellow].) Morphine, ten push now, then start at ten an hour" (12, p. 57). If the patient were sedated, then neither the attending nor Dr. Bearing would have to witness the suffering. Dr. Kelekian's goal was not to manage the pain, it was to sedate (at least) the patient. The intimation was that it was easier for the physician (and likely also for the nurses in Ferrand's and colleagues' study who requested hastened death for a patient) if the patient were not conscious. Both Ms. Monahan and Dr. Kelekian wanted to intervene to decrease (avoid?) to avoid Dr. Bearing's suffering. Each perceived different responsibilities in the face of impending death.

DEFINITIONS

Several terms are commonly used to describe clinicians' interventions to hasten a patient's death. Professionals vary in the terms that they choose. A common understanding of terms, or reasons for specific vocabulary, might allow for open discussion apart from personal judgments about differing points of view.

The term **euthanasia**, "good death," formerly referred to interventions focused on providing comfort during the time until natural death. The term has evolved from Munk's time. Rather than allowing death, however, euthanasia now refers to someone other than the patient (e.g., physician, another provider, or a nonmedical person) completing the act that causes a person's death. The European Association for Palliative Care (EAPC) defined euthanasia as, "a physician (or other person) intentionally killing a person by the administration of drugs, at that person's voluntary and competent request" (15, p. 108). The EAPC emphasizes the voluntary dimension of euthanasia. "Medicalized killing of a person without the person's consent…is not euthanasia: it is murder" (15, p. 108). A clinicians' administration of more medication, typically an opioid, than is warranted by the patient's symptoms is euthanasia oft borne of provider discomfort.

Emanuel and colleagues clarified different definitions of euthanasia, specifically **involuntary euthanasia**, "when the patient is mentally competent but did not request euthanasia" or **nonvoluntary euthanasia**, "when the patient is not mentally competent and could not request euthanasia" (16, p. 80). In some countries, these cases of medically causing a patient's death without the patient's consent is called, "**termination of life without the patient's explicit request**" (16, p. 80).

Involuntary and nonvoluntary euthanasia are not legal in the United States but are legal in the Netherlands, Belgium, Columbia, Luxembourg, and Canada (16). In some of these countries, the consent of the patient is not always required, differentiating it from the EAPC definition, in which voluntariness is central.

"**Passive euthanasia**" is used by some to indicate withdrawing or withholding a potentially life-prolonging therapy (16,17). This language does not fit with the EAPC definition of euthanasia, in which the intent of administrating the medication is to cause death. Withdrawing or withholding a life-prolonging therapy is not done to cause death. Rather, medical intervention is refused or discontinued because the burdens outweigh the benefits, or because the therapy is not providing the intended benefit. Withdrawing or withholding is "ethically distinct from PAS/Euthanasia because of critical differences in intention, causation, and other factors" (18, p. 5). Discontinuing a nonbeneficial or burdensome therapy is not assisted death. Death, if it occurs, is not caused, but allowed. Distinguishing withdrawing or withholding a life-prolonging therapy from euthanasia is essential; some physicians refuse to withdraw nonbeneficial interventions, because they do not want any perception that they are hastening dying (19). This distinction between *causing* and *allowing* is often an important point in family meetings about end of life care.

The EAPC defined **assisted suicide** as, "a person intentionally helping another person to terminate his or her life, at that person's voluntary and competent request" (15, p. 108). Again, the focus is on relief of suffering (20–22). Rather than a provider completing the act intended to cause death, a person who is terminally ill ingests substances intended to cause death. The means to complete this act may be medication obtained from a licensed provider, but some use nonmedically obtained substances. The terminally ill person is both the requestor and the actor.

According to the EAPC, **physician assisted suicide** (PAS) is "a physician intentionally helping a person to terminate his or her life by providing drugs for self-administration, at that person's voluntary and competent request" (15, p. 109). That is, the physician provides the means of death, but the medications are used by the patient to complete suicide.

The American Academy of Hospice and Palliative Medicine (AAHPM) uses the phrase **physician assisted dying (PAD)** to refer to what EAPC calls physician assisted suicide (23). That is, the physician provides "at the patient's request, a prescription for a lethal dose of medication that the patient can self-administer by ingestion, with the explicit intention of ending life" (23). We have chosen *not* to use the term physician-assisted dying, because, at its best, palliative care also assist patients to die well by providing excellent symptom management, including management of both physical and non-physical symptoms, as well as provide family support. The distinction is that, with PAD (as defined by AAHPM), the goal is to hasten death, while with palliative care, the goal is to allow death. Both have the goal of patient comfort and decreased suffering.

Similarly, the term **aid in dying** is sometimes used to describe hastening death. For every dying person, however, excellent care acknowledges the fact of dying and provides the opportunity for interventions to decrease suffering, to aid in comfortable dying, without hastening death.

LEGISLATION REGARDING ASSISTED SUICIDE IN THE UNITED STATES

The phrase "**Death with Dignity**" has many meanings in the discussion about end of life care. It refers to an organization, is the title of multiple legislative efforts, and is the phrase used by some to refer to PAS or hastened death.

In 1993, "Oregon Right to Die," a political action committee, was founded to develop legislation to legalize assisted suicide at the state and the national level. In 1994, Oregon voters passed legislation to legalize the right of people who are terminally ill to hasten their own dying, with the involvement of a medical provider (24).

During this same time, efforts to choose to allow the hastening of dying were happening around the United States and around the world. In the United States, it was previously illegal for a medical provider intentionally to be involved in hastening a person's death. In 1997, in the case *Washington v Glucksberg,* the United States Supreme Court ruled that medical assistance in dying is *not* a fundamental right, therefore, it is *not* protected by the due process clause of the Constitution (in the 14th Amendment). Though the Court rejected the notion of a Constitutional right to die, to medical assistance in hastening death, the justices returned the issues to the states. Each state, therefore, has

the right to determine the legality of medical assistance in hastening death within its boundaries (25).

Over ensuing years, several organizations and individuals worked locally and nationally to legalize physician assisted suicide, or **medical aid in dying** (deathwithdignity.org) in many states. As of this writing, medical assistance in dying is legal in Oregon (1997), Washington (2008), Vermont (2013), California (2016), Colorado (2016), District of Columbia (2017), Hawai'i (2018), Maine (2019), and New Jersey (2019). Other states have legislation pending.

ON LANGUAGE

As with many other subjects that explore how we live and how we die, there are sometimes harsh divides. Unfortunately, this may take the form of value judgments about those with different views. In any discussion of hastening death, the words chosen are crucial. Too often, words are used to divide, to establish an *us vs them* framework. We can presume that almost everyone is providing care considering the best interest of the patient. Much of our differences come in varying understandings of "best interest." Understanding why and how words are used, choosing words that accept another's viewpoint may facilitate conversation, ultimately improving the patient's care.

The term "death with dignity" is often used to entitle legislation to legalize hastened death, as well as to frame discussions about assisted suicide. Implicit in this title are two assumptions. The first, which is true enough, is that certain manners of dying rob patients of their dignity. The second, which is not necessarily true, is that a hastened death will restore that dignity. No thought is given to the notion that a hastened death may be as undignified as any other.

The term **assisted suicide** is sometimes labeled as a pejorative term (26). The term **hastened death** may be less objectionable for some. "Hastened death" does not overlap with the definition of palliative care (27) that intends the relief of suffering without hastening death.

It is still not uncommon for language to be divisive. For example, Canetto wrote, "In the pro physician-assisted-suicide discourse, medical aid in dying is the modern and rational way to death. It is about being informed and logical; clear headed, lucid, and matter-of-fact; pragmatic; free thinking, and sophisticated; sane and sensible; enlightened and progressive; noble and brave" (28, p. 44). The implication being that those who oppose are uninformed, illogical, muddled headed, etc. Cannetto posited a juxtaposition, "By contrast, opposition to physician-assisted suicide is viewed as a sign of irrationality, ignorance, and superstition" (28, p. 44). Some have suggested that it is only opponents who use the phrase PAS, while others choose more "neutral" phrases: physician aid in dying, physician assisted death, hastening death, or medical assistance in dying (26).

Those who oppose any form of hastening death may use the word "killing." For some, "The very nature of terms like 'physician-assisted' ... or 'death with dignity'... make tacit and possibly misleading assertions that function to legitimize the practice, or to legally distance suicide in terminal disease from other chronic disorders such as addiction or depression" (29, p. 1072). Kussmaul wrote, "'euthanasia' and 'medical assistance in dying' do what euphemisms are supposed to do: make a distasteful subject palatable or at least discussable" (30, p. 595).

Those who support and those who oppose using medicine to hasten death both want to do right and want to do good. Respect for the presumption of good intent may facilitate at least collegial relations between those with disparate views.

CONSCIENTIOUS OBJECTION

Conscientious objection (CO) occurs when "a health care professional refuses to participate in health care service provision for moral or religious reasons" (31, p. 1). The foundation is that clinicians have a right to refuse to participate in medical procedures to which they object, including PAS. To address the rightness of CO in the setting of considerations of hastened death, two fundamental questions are juxtaposed. If hastening death is legal, as it is in several jurisdictions in the United States, do clinicians have an obligation to provide hastened death? If PAS is legal, do individuals have a right to receive it?

The American Thoracic Society (ATS) developed a policy statement on managing conscientious objections in the ICU (32). The ATS described reasons to accommodate CO, including "to protect clinicians' moral integrity," "[t]o respect clinicians' autonomy," "to improve the quality of medical care," and "to identify needed changes in professional norms and practices" (32, p. 220, 221). Reasons *not* to accommodate COs included "to honor professional commitments," "to protect vulnerable patients," "to prevent undue excessive hardships on other clinicians or the institution," and "to avoid invidious discrimination" (32, p. 221, 222). The ATS policy does a thorough job of balancing the rights and responsibilities of individuals and organizations, with an overarching theme of continuous, high-quality patient care.

Schuklenk and Smalling asserted that professionals have *no* right to CO. Because societal norms and values are changing, and "assisted dying" is increasingly legal, if clinicians are permitted CO, then there might not be enough providers to provide the services to which patients are legally entitled (33). The right to conscientious objection is expected in the United States; however, in Sweden, Finland, and Iceland, physicians are not permitted CO for abortion (32,33). The authors argue that one should not enter a profession without recognizing that change might occur within the profession. Some accommodation might be made for those for whom PAS was not legal when they entered the profession; they allow, however, that if one pursues a career in health knowing that PAS is legal, then one does not have a right to CO.

Others disagree. Goligher and colleagues, a group convened to explore a range of opinions regarding hastening death, wrote, "We unanimously agree that accommodation for the matter of conscience is necessary. Patients should respect the fact that PAS/[euthanasia] is an ethically controversial topic, and they should expect many physicians to be unwilling to provide it upon request" (18, p. 7).

The ATS proposed several recommendations to help the patient, the provider, and the institution in addressing the question of CO, including institutional guidelines, ways to accommodate CO without burdening other providers, the CO does not apply to potentially inappropriate or futile medical services, and that discussions about CO exist within a context of respect (32, p. 220). Is essence, the establishment of guidelines *a priori* can minimize the interruption of patient care while recognizing personal values and respecting the autonomy of clinicians.

In some U.S. jurisdictions, health care organizations prohibit any form of hastening death in their facilities. Section 1553 of the Affordable Care Act mandated that any organization that receives federal funds may not discriminate against any person or organization who refuses to provide assisted suicide, euthanasia, or mercy killing (34). In May, 2019, the U.S. Office of Civil Rights (OCR) acted to enforce 25 different laws intended to protect those who object to certain medical procedures on moral or religious grounds (35).

The Colorado End-of-Life Options Act was to go into effect in 2020, though is delayed because of expected legal appeals. The act was intended to make legal the actions of individuals who chose to participate in hastening a patient's death, even if it were against their organizations policies (36). A similar discussion (and legal battle) is ongoing in California (37). As these cases work their ways through the courts, discussions continue to balance the right to CO against a patient's right to pursue care without too much difficultly in the process.

WHO REQUESTS ASSISTED SUICIDE

There is rarely a single reason someone requests hastened dying. Reasons are complex and multidimensional (15). Reasons involve facts, and reasons involve fears.

When Oregonians passed their Right to Die legislation (passed in 1994, implemented in 1997), they also established a range of supportive interventions. They established mechanisms for excellent end of life care, so that people would not perceive assisted suicide as the sole means to avoid suffering at end of life. In addition, the Oregon Health Authority has published detailed records about who requests and who completes PAS, and their reasons for doing so. These data allow a more complete understanding of the reality of PAS (38).

Not everyone who receives medications to hasten death uses them. In the 21 years that PAS has been legal in Oregon, rates of completion ranged from 47.4% in 2001 to 81.8% in 1999. The mean rate of completion over 21 years was 65.8%. The wider range of numbers reflects the smaller numbers of requests and completions. In 2001, there were 44 requests and 21 completions (47.7%); in 1999, there were 33 requests and 27 completions (81.8%). Since 2011, there have been more than 100 requests for medications to hasten death each year; since 2014, there have been more than 100 completions per year (38).

In Oregon, from 1998 to 2018, 1,459 people died following ingestion of a lethal dose of medication prescribed by a physician; 168 of those people died in 2018. In 2018, 249 prescriptions were written; 168 completed their dying using these medications, though 11 people had received their prescriptions during the previous year (67.5%) (38).

Over the time this law has been in effect, 22,016 people have received prescriptions under the Oregon law; 1,459 (65.8%) have hasted their death with these medications. Data from 2019 (capturing 2018 deaths) were similar to those of earlier years. Most people who chose hastened death were older; 79.2% were 65 years or older, and the median age was 74 years. Slightly more than half were male (51.8%). Less than half were married or had a domestic partner (43.4%) (38).

The data about race are striking. In 2018, 97% of those who completed PAS were white. From 1998 to 2018, only 1 African American completed PAS (0.1%), as did 15 Hispanics (1%), 3 American Indians (0.2%), 21 Asians (1.4%), 1 Pacific Islander (0.1%), 7 people of two or more races (0.5%).

Nirappil wrote, "the law has been enacted in a handful of states with mostly white population." Many blacks fear that discrimination in health care will continue at end of life, with hastened death being one tool of this. A Boston minister, the Reverend Eugen Rivers called legislation for PAS "back end eugenics" (39).

In 2018, 47.3% of those who completed PAS in Oregon had a bachelor's degree or higher; since the inception of the law, 42.8% of participants had at least a bachelor's degree. Over 90% of patients were enrolled in hospice at the time of their death (38).

In Oregon, and most other places in the United States, and around the world, people who request hastened death must have a terminal illness (see Table 51.1 for causes of death). The most common cause of death for hastened deaths is cancer, both nationally and internationally (14,16).

Someone considering PAS is almost certainly suffering or anticipates the possibility of future suffering. Data collected in Oregon included questions about why people requested PAS, which allows greater understanding of their suffering. Understanding others' suffering provides guidance for interactions with our own patients and their families.

Healthy people, anticipating what they would want at the time of their dying, typically project that they would seek hastened death because of physical symptoms, especially of pain (41). In one study, 49% of physician respondents believed that main reason a person would request PAS would be pain (40). As described in *Ivan Ilyich* and *W;t*,

TABLE 51.1 TERMINAL ILLNESSES OF PEOPLE COMPLETING HASTENED DEATH IN OREGON

Cause of death	1998–2018 n (%) n = 1,459	2018 n (%) n = 168
Cancer	1,107 (75.9)	105 (62.5)
Neurological disease	161 (11.0)	25 (14.9)
Respiratory disease	75 (5.1)	13 (7.7)
Heart/circulatory disease	66 (4.5)	16 (9.5)
Infectious disease	0 (0)	13 (0.9)
Gastrointestinal disease	9 (0.6)	9 (0.6)
Endocrine/ metabolic disease	11 (0.8)	2 (1.2)
Other illnesses	17 (1.2)	6 (3.6)

Oregon Public Health Division CfHS. *Oregon Death with Dignity Act.* Oregon Health Authority. 2019. Updated April 25, 2019. Accessed December 31, 2019.

physical pain is a sometimes prominent dimension of suffering. Suffering, however, typically is much more encompassing. In Oregon, one-quarter of respondents reported that one of the reasons they sought PAS was a physical symptom, or concern that one would develop. Most people sought PAS for reasons related to loss of control. Loss of autonomy and decreased ability to engage in enjoyable activities were a concern for more than 90% of those who completed PAS in Oregon in 2018. Though these data are from Oregon, the findings are similar to those reported by others: that people who request hastened death do so due to loss of control, loss of dignity, or the presence of a desire to avoid suffering (18,41,42).

In the 21st century, in part because of the increased medicalization of illness, and hence, of death, fewer people are familiar with, or have witnessed death. Misconceptions might prevail (Hudson & Hudson) affecting actions, interactions, and choices. That which used to occur at home is now typically geographically separate, spoken of euphemistically, and kept from children (43). What people have witnessed of death often come from media portrayals that, though typically rather unrealistic, influence people's expectations, both good and bad (3,19). Misinformation or misunderstandings affect expectations. For example, people have been told that aggressive pain management will hasten death (44), despite knowledge that opioids, when managed well, will not hasten death.

Social media also affects people's expectations. Many patients reported that they value the support and understanding of others in a social media group with the same disease or injury. A challenge with social media is that what is posted is a snapshot, not the whole story. A patient's family member recently said, "Social media is good for increasing your contacts, but not your reality. It's contrived."

Other Factors Affecting Decision-Making

Beliefs about dying and beliefs about suffering affect decision-making regarding one's end of life in many situations, including considerations of hastened death. Perhaps the core question regarding access to hastened death is whether causing death is "morally acceptable" (18). Those who support hastening death might say, "There is a significant possibility that this patient will develop a terminal event that would cause suffering. We can see no reason why that patient should not be allowed to die at a time of their own choosing, rather than being obliged to wait for the unpredictable terminal event with a possibility of suffering despite adequate/maximal palliative care" (18, p. 6). Autonomy is an oft-cited reason for why

people should have access to, or why they choose to pursue hastened dying. Compassion & Choices advocate that allowing PAS places "control back in the hands of people" (45, p. 5). One must consider, though, whether the terminal illness represents the ultimate loss of control. Choosing to control the timing of one's dying is seen by some as a means to garner autonomy (Table 51.2) (45, p. 5).

A serious illness may be portrayed as transformative (3). For those supporting PAS, the question becomes whether one has an obligation to look for transformation. Goliger and colleagues wrote, "the dying process can also be a time of existential and spiritual healing through growth in personal and relational wholeness as well as individual learning for patients, their loved ones, and those caring for them (18, p. 4). Considering Frankl's logotherapy, though one *might* find meaning in the suffering at the end of life, it does not follow that one is obligated to search for meaning at end of life. Decades later, Frankl wrote, "More people today have the means to live, but no meaning to live for" (46, p. 21, 22).

For those who support hastening death, moral acceptability comes with a goal of decreasing suffering by increasing control. For those who oppose hastening death, the morally acceptable care is excellent palliative care of the whole person, recognizing and allowing death, but never hastening it. Those who are opposed to hastening death cite the "incalculable value and intrinsic worth" of a human life (18, p. 6). They might state that no one has a right, much less an obligation to shorten that life.

TABLE 51.2 REF: REASONS FOR COMPLETING PAS IN OREGON

End of life concerns	1998–2018 n (%) (n = 1,459)	2018 n (%) (n = 168)
Losing autonomy	1,322 (90.6)	154 (91.7)
Less able to engage in activities making life enjoyable	1,300 (89.1)	152 (90.5)
Loss of dignity	989 (74.4)	112 (66.7)
Losing control of bodily functions	647 (44.3)	62 (36.9)
Burden on family, friends/caregivers	654 (44.8)	91 (54.2)
Inadequate pain control, or concern about it	375 (25.7)	43 (25.6)
Financial implications of treatment	57 (3.9)	9 (5.4)

Oregon Public Health Division CfHS. *Oregon Death with Dignity Act.* Oregon Health Authority. 2019. Updated April 25, 2019. Accessed December 31, 2019.

Depression Screening

Screening for depression is an essential component of requests for hastened death in almost every jurisdiction where it is legal. Physical symptoms are a rare cause for hastening death; psychological, interpersonal, and spiritual reasons are common. For unclear reasons, however, few physicians who are helping people pursue hastened death require further psychological screening (41). In Oregon, in 2018, only three people (1.8%) were referred for psychiatric evaluation. Over the 21 years of the program, 65 people (4.5%) have been referred (38). The clinician is challenged to consider whether hastening death is appropriate for someone with the possibility of mental illness (20). Involvement of a psychiatrist or other mental health worker does not preclude hastening death, but it assures that the person's decision is not shaded by mental health concerns. Olié & Courtet have suggested that a psychiatrist should be involved in every case in which a patient is considering hastening death (20).

The Role of Religion in Requests for Hastened Death

For many people, religious beliefs are central to their beliefs and philosophies, including their support or opposition for hastening death. Magelssen and colleagues found that people whose beliefs are more secular are more likely to support assisted dying and oppose the right to conscientious objection, where people who are more religious are less likely to support assisted dying and more likely to support conscientious objection (31). Among older adults, those who describe religious values as important in their daily lives are less likely to believe that PAS is an option for them (47).

As with most faith and cultures, there is rarely homogeneity of beliefs within any group. Understanding common teaching of major religions can facilitate discussions with patients and families making decisions about how to live at end of life. It shouldn't be presumed that someone comes from a particular spiritual tradition that one will adhere to the tenets of that tradition. What unifies all these beliefs is that our life is not our possessions; that life is a gift from the God of Abraham, who is commonly revered by these four faith traditions.

In **Judaism**, "Human life is the paramount ethical value" (48, p. 437). This single statement provides guidance for many actions and choices in a Jew's life. Scholars acknowledge that the balancing of expectations and responsibilities is sometimes difficult (48). Jews believe that all life is sacred, because all human life is in the image of God. Most Judaic scholars oppose hastened death in every circumstance (48–50). Some Reform scholars support

euthanasia (49,50). Even while dying, the person is "a living person in every respect and, being even in the last moments of his life, he has to be treated according to this living status" (50, p. 783). At the same time, "Judaism is extremely concerned about pain and suffering" (49, p. 567). Efforts for comfort and the alleviation of suffering in multiple dimensions should be implemented. Clinicians "may use all measures to alleviate pain and suffering that will not actually cause the patient to die" (48, p. 443).

There is some variation in Jews' beliefs about withdrawing and withholding care at the end of life. "Distinguishing between actions that cross over into the realm of active euthanasia from those that only reach the level of 'removal of an impediment' can be difficult, particularly in the modern age, where technology can permit the survival of the patients in conditions not considered by the original theorists" (48, p. 447). Consulting a rabbi, especially one who is familiar with health care decision-making can be most helpful for patients and families.

A fundamental teaching of the **Roman Catholic** Church is, "that human life is sacred and that the dignity of the human person is the foundation of a moral vision for society" (51). Church leaders have written specifically about interventions to end life, "As a gift from God, every human life is sacred from conception to natural death" (51). They also prohibit individuals and institutions from participating in euthanasia or hastened death. "Catholic health care intuitions may never condone or participate in euthanasia or assisted suicide in any way. Dying patients who request euthanasia should receiving loving care, psychological and spiritual support, and appropriate remedies for pain and other symptoms so that they can live with dignity until the time of natural death" (53, p. 60).

While no active means can be taken to cause death, Catholic teaching allows refusal of treatments that "involve too grave a burden" (54, p. 2). Excessive burden includes "excessive expense on the family or the community" (55). The Roman church acknowledge that suffering is a part of many aspects of human life that can lead one to question the meaning life and God's intent. Much as the woman described earlier who refused opioids to allow herself pain (and suffering), the Church believes in a "redemptive nature of suffering" (56). One's suffering on this earth can help redeem the world.

Protestantism constitutes a broad spectrum of beliefs and practices within the Christian tradition, comprising at least 10 denominations. Within each denomination members have a range of beliefs. A core belief in Protestantism is that its members are redeemed by Christ's sacrifice and the acceptance of God's grace, and therefore their lives belong to Him. Attainment of the afterlife is assured by faith alone. There is not one position statement of Protestant beliefs, including about whether or not hastened death is supported. Some denominations do have specific statements against hastening death. Most Protestant religions encourage their members to study scripture and to use scripture to inform a reasoned decision. Individuals' beliefs and practices are respected. At the same time, people are encouraged to use the expertise in their community, including palliative care, casting the net broadly. Discernment about the choices one makes at end of is strongly encouraged. This consideration is a process.

The community is encouraged to care for the suffering, including at end of life. Someone who is dying remains a member of the community, though some will be truly challenged to allow others to provide care to them. Care might be visiting, driving someone to appointments, cooking a meal, and doing laundry. To accept care allows others the grace of caring.

Some Protestant denominations have a more formal administration and rule structure (e.g., Seventh Day Adventists). Within and between Protestant denominations, those that are more conservative are less likely to support access to hastened death.

Islam means "to surrender oneself" (57, p. 25). Core beliefs of Islam are those that were identified by the Prophet Muhammad (PBUH), the messenger of Islam. There is, however, not one Islamic authority (58). Though there is a range of beliefs within Islam, there is general agreement on the core beliefs. One core belief is that human life, the soul is a gift from God and belongs to God (57). Therefore, life cannot be taken; death cannot be hastened (59). "[M]ercy killing is ethically wrong and it comes under the broader guidelines of the Quran and *Sunnah* which are against killing innocent beings and against participating or collaborating in committing sin (*ithm*)" (59, p. 5). "God is the giver and the taker of life" (58, p. 2). Physicians are instructed not to participate in hastening death (58). At the same time, physicians also have a responsibility to diminish suffering whenever possible, including the aggressive use of medications and other tools. Hospice is encouraged. The distinction between allowing death without hastening death is crucial.

Suffering is believed to have value; forbearance is important (Pew Research Center). One is encouraged to be patient, tolerant of a disease. "The Prophet said: 'There is no disease that Allah has created, except that He has also created its treatment'" (59, p. 8). Endurance in suffering is a way to closeness with God. The Ṣaḥīḥ al-Bukhārī contain *hadith* or statements providing moral guidance about how to live as a Muslim. Book 68 of the Ṣaḥīḥ al-Bukhārī is the Book of Patients; Chapter One is, "The saying that sickness is expiation for sins." Forebearance is rewarded. Hadith number 1958 begins, "None of you should wish for death." The words are reiterated in Hadith 1960. Only God chooses the time of dying.

Understanding a person's religious or spiritual perspective does not definitely indicate a person's beliefs or choices. Being confronted with a terminal illness might lead someone toward or away from previously held beliefs. Serious illness may change the perspectives of an individual or a family. Being able to consider religious perspectives in discussions with patients and families can increase the comfort of patients and families.

WHEN THE REQUEST COMES

It will happen. Mr. Washington, a 78-year-old with COPD might say to you, "I just don't want to do this anymore. Can't you just give me something so I can get it over with?"

Ms. Adams, a 50-year-old undergoing treatment for gastric cancer will say, "I'm okay now, but I don't want to suffer at the end. When the time comes, will you help me find someone who will just end it peacefully?"

Mr. Jefferson, the adult son of a man who has had a very large stroke, was recently extubated, and isn't expected to recover, says, angrily, "This shouldn't be taking so long! Why do we have to wait? Just end it now."

Before you continue reading, pause. Is your first thought to promise that you will do whatever the patient and family want? Is your instinct to say, "I don't believe in that. I'm sorry. I can't help you." Your response will depend on what you believe, on how you choose to practice. You should know the laws in your jurisdiction, as well as the policies of your institution. Some health care systems, especially religious institutions, prohibit acts that hasten death, including the prescription of medications that are part of the process of PAS. What are your professional obligations, and your professional limitations?

Responding to questions or concerns of patients or families about hastening death is one of the most difficult interactions a provider can have (16,19). The clinician is likely to be challenged both professionally and personally (60). No clinician should have to address these concerns alone. Hopefully before you ever are in the situation of receiving a request for hastened death, you are sure you would not be responding to the request in isolation. Know your partners. Know who will support you, regardless of what you believe and choose to do. What colleagues can help you, and in so doing, help this patient and family? Consider psychiatry, pastoral care, social workers; which nurses or physicians will work this through with you?

Okay. You have just been confronted with a perhaps unwelcome and disconcerting request. Your first instinct might be to say, "Sorry. That's my cellphone. I have to get this. We'll talk later," and exit stage left. Instead, pause. Take a breath. Search for calm. Know your strength. The best thing you can do for your patient is to stay. You do not have to have all the answers. The first, best thing to do is to be present, to witness these statements of suffering or, as is true with Ms. Adams, anticipated suffering. Ask, "Do you mind if I sit down?" Pull up a chair.

When you get back to the conversation, do not forget to breathe. As with any interaction that is fraught, listen well. Clarify. "Mr. Washington, you sound very upset. I want to help you, but I want to make sure I understand what you are saying. Can you tell me more?"

"Ms. Adams, I'm glad you're doing well with your cancer treatments. I share the goal of wanting you not to suffer. Do you have concerns about anything in particular?" (In this particular discussion, Ms. Adams was very clear about requesting hastened death. She wanted to get right into who, what, where, when, and how she could hasten her own dying when the time comes.) "Mr. Jefferson, your father is so fortunate to have you here for him. I know you are concerned about your father. What is your greatest concern?"

Explore people's symptoms and their fears (60). Everyone has a unique story. Listen. Hear the story. Sometimes it is tempting to provide guidance or direction early in the discussion. Rather, if you have to, count to 10 your head to make sure the patient has the time to gather and express thoughts. Ask questions. Ask what they think will happen? What have they seen? What do they know? At this point, there may be a balance of hearing the story, considering hyperbole, and suggesting considerations that might help the patient and her family discuss options.

It is also important to ask who is helping the person living with the serious illness. In Oregon in 2018, about 6% of people did not inform their families about their decision to hasten death (38). If someone says, "No one know. I'm doing this by myself," ask more questions. This solitariness, isolation in choosing to hasten one's death is a red flag.

If the request come from family, rather than the patient, the need to understand that person's suffering is no less important. It is also no less time consuming. Sometimes, requests from family come, despite the lack of patient suffering. At that time, show the patient what you see. "Mr. Jefferson, I know this is difficult for you. Your father is so fortunate to have you at his bedside; you have seen that not everyone has that." Explore what it is like for the family members. Very often they haven't slept, they haven't eaten, they haven't had a decent shower. Hear the story. Then focus on the patient. "Mr. Jefferson, I hear that you are suffering; you have been through a lot. Let me tell you what I see with your father. He looks comfortable to me. If he were uncomfortable, I would expect to see a furrowed brow, tightened muscles, or other signs of discomfort. I don't see that. You know your father far better than I. Do you see anything that I am missing?" It is also necessary to specify *your* professional limits. This is another difficult conversation. "I will do everything I can to keep your father comfortable, but I will not to anything to hasten his dying." Allow silence. Reassure the son of the gift of his presence to his father. Involve pastoral care, social work, or others who can be present and provide support. Keep checking in; demonstrate that not providing high tech interventions does *not* mean that his father is not continuing to receive care.

There is an extensive body of literature on communication in palliative care (see Chapters 40 and 62) and workshops. Perhaps not only because of increased technology in health care but also because of the expectation of charting *during* a patient encounter, clinician–patient communication has become less personal, perhaps with less interpersonal connection. Although previously the core of medicine, improving physician–patient relationships has garnered a lot of attention recently. Zulman and colleagues identified specific skills to help build connections between provider and patient and family (61). Many of the suggestions are for nonverbal actions: sit, lean forward, and attend to the emotional content of the message as much of the words. Before the visit, prepare yourself to focus on this interaction at this time. Listen without interrupting. Hear the patient's concerns and priorities. Let the patient know you understand their verbal and emotional messages. Listen to learn and understand before you give your message.

CONCLUSION

Regardless of an individual's beliefs or practices regarding hastening death, the responsibility for excellence in end of life care remains (41). Palliative care or hospice is often the means to this end. Advocate for a palliative care consult (18) or a hospice referral. We cannot promise that palliative care will alleviate all suffering. We can promise to remain present, to remain persistent, and to involve the best interdisciplinary team.

Those unfamiliar or inexperienced with the complexities of providing end of life care, that always includes symptom management and the existential dimensions of care, may more quickly consider hastened death as the way to relieve suffering (18). Identifying and having a relationship with colleagues who can support the patient and family, as well as the clinician, allows focus on the patient's concerns. Do not handle these discussions without support.

These discussions are difficult. Perhaps they always should be difficult, be somewhat uncomfortable. You will be helping a person explore whether to end her life.

REFERENCES

1. Spronk K. Good death and bad death in ancient Israel according to biblical lore. *Soc Sci Med*. 2004;58(5): 987-995.
2. Van Hooff AJL. Ancient euthanasia: 'good death' and the doctor in the graeco-Roman world. *Soc Sci Med*. 2004;58(5):975-985.
3. Seale C, van der Geest S. Good and bad death: introduction. *Soc Sci Med*. 2004;58(5):883-885.
4. Papadimitriou JD, Skiadas P, Mavrantonis CS, Polimeropoulos V, Papadimitriou DJ, Papacostas KJ. Euthanasia and suicide in antiquity: viewpoint of the dramatists and philosophers. *J R Soc Med*. 2007;100(1):25-28.
5. Hughes N, Clark D. "A thoughtful and experienced physician": William Munk and the care of the dying in late Victorian England. *J Palliat Med*. 2004;7(5): 703-710.
6. Brown GH. William Munk. Royal College of Physicians; Inspiring physicians. Updated December 21, 1898. https://history.rcplondon.ac.uk/inspiring-physicians/william-munk. Accessed December 19, 2019.
7. Munk W. *Euthanasia: Or, Medical Treatment in Aid of An Easy Death*. London: Longmans, Green, and Co.; 1887.
8. Clark D. *To Comfort Always: A History of Palliative Medicine Since the Nineteenth Century*. Oxford, UK: Oxford University Press; 2016.
9. Foley DP. Eleven interpretations of personal suffering. *J Relig Health*. 1988;27(4):321-328.
10. Frankl VE. *Man's Search for Meaning*. Boston, MA: Beacon Press; 2006.
11. Tolstoy L. *The Death of Ivan Ilyich*. New York, NY: Bantam Books; 1981.
12. Edson M. *Wit (W;t)*. New York, NY: Dramatists Play Service Inc.; 1993.
13. Margaretha Strandmark K. Ill health is powerlessness: a phenomenological study about worthlessness, limitations and suffering. *Scand J Caring Sci*. 2004;18(2): 135-144.
14. Ferrand E, Dreyfus J-F, Chastrusse M, Ellien F, Lemaire F, Fischler M. Evolution of requests to hasten death among patients managed by palliative care teams in France: A multicentre cross-sectional survey (DemandE). *Eur J Cancer*. 2012;48(3):368-376.
15. Radbruch L, Leget C, Bahr P, et al. Euthanasia and physician-assisted suicide: A white paper from the European Association for Palliative Care. *Palliat Med*. 2015;30(2):104-116.
16. Emanuel EJ, Onwuteaka-Philipsen BD, Urwin JW, Cohen J. Attitudes and Practices of Euthanasia and Physician-Assisted Suicide in the United States, Canada, and Europe. *JAMA*. 2016;316(1):79-90.
17. Legal Information Institute. n.d. Right to die. https://www.law.cornell.edu/constitution-conan/amendment-14/section-1/right-to-die
18. Goligher EC, Ely EW, Sulmasy DP, et al. Physician-assisted suicide and euthanasia in the intensive care unit: a dialogue on core ethical issues. *Crit Care Med*. 2017;45(2):149-155.
19. Hudson P, Hudson R, Philip J, Boughey M, Kelly B, Hertogh C. Legalizing physician-assisted suicide and/or euthanasia: pragmatic implications. *Palliat Support Care*. 2015;13(5):1399-1409.
20. Olié E, Courtet P. The controversial issue of euthanasia in patients with psychiatric illness. *JAMA*. 2016;316(6):656-657.
21. Hamric AB, Schwarz JK, Cohen L, Mahon M. Assisted suicide/aid in dying: what is the nurse's role? *Am J Nurs*. 2018;118(5):50-59.
22. Sulmasy DP. An open letter to norman cantor regarding dementia and physician-assisted suicide. *Hastings Cent Rep*. 2018;48(4):28-30.
23. American Academy of Hospice & Palliative Physicians. Statement on Physician-Assisted Dying. 2019. http://aahpm.org/positions/pad Last updated June 24, 2016. Accessed June 15, 2019.
24. Death with Dignity National Center Death with dignity. n.d. https://www.deathwithdignity.org/
25. Gostin LO. Deciding life and death in the courtroom: from Quinlan to Cruzan, Glucksberg, and Vacco—a brief history and analysis of constitutional protection of the 'right to die'. *JAMA*. 1997;278(18):1523-1528.
26. Derse AR, Moskop JC, McGrath NA, et al. Physician-assisted death: ethical implications for emergency physicians. *Acad Emerg Med*. 2019;26(2):250-255.
27. World Health Organization. *WHO Definition of Palliative Care*. n.d. Accessed January 6, 2020.
28. Canetto SS. If physician-assisted suicide is the modern woman's last powerful choice, why are White women its leading advocates and main users? *Prof Psychol Res Pract*. 2019;50(1):39-50.
29. Katz J, Mitsumoto H. ALS and physician-assisted suicide. *Neurology*. 2016;87(11):1072-1073.
30. Kussmaul WG, III. The slippery slope of legalization of physician-assisted suicide. *Ann Intern Med*. 2017;167(8):595-596.
31. Magelssen M, Le NQ, Supphellen M. Secularity, abortion, assisted dying and the future of conscientious objection: modelling the relationship between attitudes. *BMC Med Ethics*. 2019;20(1):65.
32. Lewis-Newby M, Wicclair M, Pope T, et al. An official American Thoracic Society Policy Statement: managing conscientious objections in intensive care medicine. *Am J Respir Crit Care Med*. 2015;191(2):219-227.
33. Schuklenk U, Smalling R. Why medical professionals have no moral claim to conscientious objection accommodation in liberal democracies. *J Med Ethics*. 2017;43(4):234.
34. Department of Health and Human Services. *Section 1553 of the Affordable Care Act*. n.d. HHS.gov. Accessed January 15, 2020.
35. Keith K. Trump administration finalizes broad religious and moral exemptions for health care workers. In. *Health Affairs Blog. Following the ACA*. Vol 2020. Health Affairs; 2019. https://www.healthaffairs.org/do/10.1377/hblog20190503.960127/full/
36. Wynia M. Colorado end-of-life options act: a clash of organizational and individual conscience. *JAMA*. 2019;322(20):1953-1954.
37. Cain CL, Koenig BA, Starks H, et al. Hospital and health system policies concerning the california end of life option act. *J Palliat Med*. 2019;23(1):60-66.

38. Oregon Health Authority, Public Health Division. Oregon's Death with Dignity Act (DWDA). 2018 Data Summary. Published n.d. https://www.oregon.gov/oha/PH/PROVIDERPARTNERRESOURCES/EVALUATIONRESEARCH/DEATHWITHDIGNITYACT/Pages/faqs.aspx. Accessed December 31, 2019.9.

39. Nirappil F. Right-to-die law faces skepticism in nation's capital: 'It's really aimed at old black people'. In: *Washington Post*. D.C. Politics; 2016.

40. Hetzler PT III, Nie J, Zhou A, Dugdale LS. A report of physicians' beliefs about physician-assisted suicide: a national study. *Yale J Biol Med*. 2019;92(4):575-585.

41. Emanuel EJ. Euthanasia and physician-assisted suicide: focus on the data. *Med J Aust*. 2017;206(8):339-340.

42. Quill TE, Arnold RM, Youngner SJ. Physician-assisted suicide: finding a path forward in a changing legal environment. *Ann Intern Med*. 2017;167(8):597-598.

43. Amir D. Love, death, and other forgotten traditions. In: *Nautilus*. 2017:54. http://nautil.us/issue/54/the-unspoken/love-death-and-other-forgotten-traditions

44. Ball H. Physician assisted death in America: ethics, law, and policy conflicts. Cato Institute. In: *The last choice: Death and dignity in the United States Web site*. 2012. Accessed December 31, 2019.

45. Compassion and Choices. *Our mission. Our work*. 2019. compassionandchoices.org/wp-content/uploads/Our-Mission-Our-Work-FINAL-2-19-19.pdf. Updated February 10, 2019. Accessed November 29, 2019.

46. Frankl V. *The Unheard Cry for Meaning*. New York, NY: Simon & Schuster; 1978.

47. Lapierre S, Castelli Dransart DA, St-Amant K, et al. Religiosity and the wish of older adults for physician-assisted suicide. *Religions*. 2018;9(3):66.

48. Bentley PJ. The shattered vessel: the dying person in Jewish law and ethics. *Loyola Univ Chicago Law J*. 2006;37(2):433-454.

49. Kinzbrunner BM. Jewish medical ethics and end-of-life care. *J Palliat Med*. 2004;7(4):558-573.

50. Baeke G, Wils J-P, Broeckaert B. 'There is a time to be born and a time to die' (Ecclesiastes 3:2a): Jewish perspectives on euthanasia. *J Relig Health*. 2011;50(4):778-795.

51. United States Conference of Catholic Bishops. *Seven Themes of Catholic Social Teaching*. n.d. USCCB. What we believe. Web site. Accessed January 16, 2020.

52. United States Conference of Catholic Bishops. *Human Life and Dignity*. n.d. USCCB. Issues and action. Web site. Accessed January 16, 2020.

53. United States Conference of Catholic Bishops. *Ethical and Religious Directives for Catholic Health Care Services*, 5th ed. United States Conference of Catholic Bishops; 2009. www.usccbpublishing.org

54. Activities NCoCBCfP-L. Statement on uniform rights of the terminally ill act. In: *Committee for Pro-Life Activities*. Washington, DC: NCCB; 1986:8.

55. National Catholic Bioethics Center. *End-of-Life Care*. National Catholic Bioethics Center; 2013. https://www.ncbcenter.org/resources/position-papers-ncbc/

56. National Catholic Bioethics Center. A Catholic guide to end-of-life decisions. In: *An Explanation of Church Teaching on Advance Directives, Euthanasia, and Physician Assisted Suicide*. National Catholic Bioethics Center; 2011. Accessed December 24, 2019.

57. Choudry M, Latif A, Warburton KG. An overview of the spiritual importances of end-of-life care among the five major faiths of the United Kingdom. *Clin Med (Lond)*. 2018;18(1):23-31.

58. Ahaddour C, Van den Branden S, Broeckaert B. "God is the giver and taker of life": Muslim beliefs and attitudes regarding assisted suicide and euthanasia. *AJOB Empir Bioeth* 2018;9(1):1-11.

59. Ayuba MA. Euthanasia: a muslim's perspective. *Scriptura*. 2016;115:1-13.

60. Quill TE, Back AL, Block SD. Responding to patients requesting physician-assisted death: physician involvement at the very end of life. *JAMA*. 2016;315(3):245-246.

61. Zulman DM, Haverfield MC, Shaw JG, et al. Practices to foster physician presence and connection with patients in the clinical encounter. *JAMA*. 2020;323(1):70-81.

Special Interventions in Supportive and Palliative Care

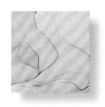 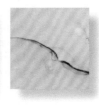 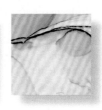 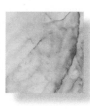 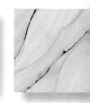

52 Hematologic Support of the Cancer Patient

Vanessa Wookey and Lee Schwartzberg

INTRODUCTION

The bone marrow, site of origin for blood cells, is the organ most at risk for collateral damage from the modalities of modern cancer therapy. Each of the constituent components of blood—granulocytes, erythrocytes, and platelets—is at risk for compromise. Reduction in quantity and/or function in any component can lead to profound consequences for the patient. Moreover, the bone marrow itself is a frequent site of metastases for many solid tumors and the primary site of many hematologic malignancies, rendering it particularly vulnerable to insult. Indeed, neutropenia, anemia, and thrombocytopenia are the most common complications of cancer and its treatment. Physicians caring for cancer patients must be fully versed in the consequences of cytopenias.

In the early decades of oncology, the armamentarium for hematologic support was limited to transfusions, antibiotics, and the passage of time. The development of growth factors was a technologic tour de force, which profoundly transformed hematologic supportive care. However, growth factors are expensive and are associated with real and theoretical complications. Clinicians should recognize the reasons to consider hematologic support for patients and carefully evaluate the risk–benefit ratio of growth factors, and other available measures to maximize patient outcomes. By utilizing appropriate supportive care cancer patients can undergo more effective therapy with reduced morbidity and mortality.

ANEMIA

Anemia is defined as a reduction in the number of circulating red blood cells (RBCs) or by the hemoglobin (Hb) level and the hematocrit (Hct), all reported on a complete blood count. It is the most common hematologic abnormality in patients with cancer. Depending on the tumor type, between 32% and 49% of patients are anemic at the time of cancer diagnosis (1) and approximately 50% of all patients will develop anemia at some time during their treatment. Anemia is graded as mild, moderate, severe, or life threatening (Table 52.1).

When oxygen delivery to tissue is impaired by anemia, subtle or profound organ dysfunction occurs depending on the rapidity of the fall of RBCs, availability of compensatory mechanisms, absolute RBC levels, baseline functional state, and comorbid conditions. Signs of anemia include pallor in mucous membranes, conjunctiva, and nail beds, tachycardia, and increased respiratory rate and may progress to hypoxemia and orthostatic hypotension in patients with acute blood loss and hypovolemia. A widened pulse pressure, hyperdynamic precordium, and systolic flow murmur can be ascertained along with, in decompensated states, signs of high output cardiac failure, peripheral edema, S_3 and S_4 gallops, and pulmonary rales.

Symptoms of anemia can be insidious and include early decrease in exercise tolerance, shortness of breath on exertion, and fatigue that does not resolve with rest. Some patients describe muscle cramps, irritability, and other signs of neuropsychiatric dysfunction, including depression and confusion. Strain on the cardiovascular system is manifested by breathlessness and rapid heartbeat and can precipitate angina. While cancer-related fatigue itself has many etiologic causes, anemia is a common and contributing factor (2–4).

Anemia can have a direct impact on cancer responsiveness to radiation therapy and may impact the ability to deliver full doses of curative chemotherapy on schedule (5). Cancer-associated anemia is an independent risk factor for survival regardless of tumor type (6).

Etiologies of Anemia in Cancer Patients

There are a myriad of possible etiologies for anemia in cancer patients. The particular type of cancer, patient comorbidities, and the treatment itself may all act independently or together to result in anemia (7). Non–cancer-related causes include preexisting nutritional deficiencies, renal dysfunction, bleeding, hemolysis, hemoglobinopathies, and infection (8). Malignancy itself can promote the development of anemia (anemia of cancer [AOC]), and anemia frequently develops as a consequence of cancer treatment (chemotherapy-induced anemia [CIA]).

TABLE 52.1 ANEMIA GRADE

Grade	Scale (Hb g/dL)
1 (mild)	10 to lower limit of normal
2 (moderate)	8 to <10
3 (severe)	<8
4 (life threatening)	Urgent intervention indicated
5 (death)	Death

Adapted from the Common Terminology Criteria for Adverse Events. https://ctep.cancer.gov/protocoldevelopment/electronic_applications/docs/CTCAE_v5_Quick_Reference_5x7.pdf

Due to the numerous potential etiologies of anemia in patients with cancer, the evaluation may be complex. Thus, knowledge of the pathophysiology behind cancer and chemotherapy resulting in anemia is essential. The most common anemias in the world are nutritional, particularly those resulting from iron deficiency, as well as deficiency of folate and vitamin B_{12} (9). These are more often seen in noncancer populations but should always be considered in patients with cancer. In a study of anemic cancer patients receiving chemotherapy, 17% had ferritin levels <100 mg/L, 6% had low vitamin B_{12} levels, and 2% had high creatinine levels (10).

A useful framework for the assessment of anemia arises from evaluating three factors: the degree of RBC proliferation, the size of the RBCs, and the quality of hemoglobinization. Proliferation is estimated by the reticulocyte production index (RPI), which is calculated by multiplying the reticulocyte count by the actual Hct divided by the normal expected Hct and corrected for the longer life span of prematurely released reticulocytes (11). The RBC size is determined by the mean corpuscular volume (MCV) and can be normal (normocytic), small (microcytic), or large (macrocytic). The degree of hemoglobinization is derived from the mean corpuscular hemoglobin concentration (MCHC). RBCs may have normal levels of Hb (normochromic), low amounts of Hb (hypochromic), or high amounts of Hb (hyperchromic). These simple tests, along with serum iron, total iron-binding capacity, ferritin, vitamin B_{12}, folate, and creatinine levels, and a visual examination of the peripheral blood smear can help diagnose the majority of anemias quickly.

Iron deficiency leads to a microcytic, hypochromic anemia. Conversely, vitamin B_{12} or folate deficiencies typically lead to macrocytic and normochromic anemias. In the absence of therapy, anemia associated with myelodysplastic syndrome

(MDS) will be normocytic to macrocytic and is often associated with other cytopenias. The RPI will be low in nutritional anemias, but it will be high in the setting of acute or chronic hemolysis and may also be high in occult or acute blood loss. A careful history is always a cost-effective tool in determining if there is a hereditary component to anemia such as hemoglobinopathy or a prior GI surgical procedure that could lead to nutritional deficiency. Endocrine and metabolic deficiencies should be ruled out as well, as anemia is a frequent consequence.

Anemia of Cancer

RBCs developed from primitive bone marrow progenitor cells that are functionally defined as burst forming units-erythroid. These red cell precursors are simulated to proliferate and differentiate largely as a result of the actions of erythropoietin, a growth factor hormone synthesized and secreted by the kidney in response to sensing tissue hypoxemia. There is an inverse relationship between the Hb and Hct and erythropoietin levels, which begin to rise above normal when the Hb is <10 g/dL, and/or the Hct is <30% (12). Erythropoietin production can be impaired in multiple ways and is frequently compromised in individuals with reduced renal function from any cause, including nephrotoxic chemotherapy, diabetes, and aging.

Many cancer patients experience activation of the immune system. At its most extreme, autoantibodies can destroy RBCs leading to autoimmune hemolytic anemia or even profound suppression of RBC production (RBC aplasia). More commonly, there appears to be a less-specific activation of the immune system in the bone marrow leading to increased cytokine production of interferon gamma, interleukin-1 (IL-1), interleukin-6 (IL-6), and tumor necrosis factor, each of which can suppress erythropoietin production (13,14). These cytokines may also interact synergistically and perpetuate each other's production leading to a chronically elevated cytokine state and reduction in erythropoietin (Fig. 52.1) (15,16).

Iron metabolism is intrinsically linked to RBC production as iron is incorporated into the functioning Hb molecule through a complex physiology. Abnormalities of iron metabolism play a significant role in etiology of AOC. Hepcidin, a small peptide, serves a critical regulatory role in the transfer of iron to RBC precursors. Hepcidin is up-regulated by IL-6, acts principally to decrease both iron absorption in the GI tract and macrophage iron release, and decreases erythropoietin levels (17) with a net effect of decreased iron available for erythropoiesis (18).

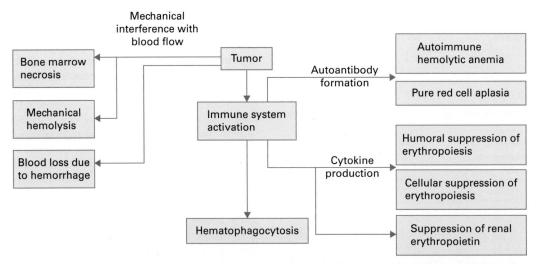

Figure 52.1 Causes of anemia of cancer. Solid tumors can cause anemia by a range of mechanisms. Immune system activation with direct and indirect inhibition of red blood cell (RBC) production is most common, but other factors as described are also operant. Hematopoietic tumors involve similar mechanisms with the addition of intrinsic genetic abnormalities in the erythroid progenitor cells as the most common cause of reduced RBCs.

RBC life span, typically around 90 days in normal individuals, is reduced by cytokines, and shortened survival cannot be overcome by compensatory increase in production. Finally, AOC can occur due to myelophthisis, which is replacement of the marrow-forming elements by cancer, a situation frequently seen in prostate cancer, breast cancer, and small cell lung cancer.

The clinical manifestations of AOC are a hypoproliferative state with normocytic to microcytic RBCs, normal to mildly reduced MCHC, and a low reticulocyte count. Serum ferritin levels are typically normal to increased, while both serum iron and serum transferrin may be low. These studies help to differentiate AOC from iron deficiency anemia. Severe AOC with an Hb <8 g/dL is rare. Other etiologies should be entertained in this circumstance.

Chemotherapy-Induced Anemia

Myelosuppressive effects of cytotoxic chemotherapy on erythropoiesis are generally cumulative in nature, and up to 50% of patients with cancer may develop CIA over the course of treatment (19). A steady increase in the rate of anemia occurs with additional cycles of chemotherapy as demonstrated by the European Cancer Anemia Survey (ECAS), which followed 15,367 patients in 24 countries (20). This study showed that the rate of anemia, defined as an Hb <12 g/dL, increased from 19.5% in cycle 1 to 46.7% by cycle 5. The percentage of patients with more severe, grade 2/3 anemia also increased with greater number of chemotherapy cycles.

A separate analysis of ECAS data in patients who were not anemic (Hb > 12 g/dL) prior to initiating chemotherapy revealed that 62% of patients experienced an Hb decline of 1.5 g/dL within a median time of 6.1 to 7.2 weeks and 51% experienced an Hb reduction of ≥2 g/dL within a median time of 7.3 to 8.9 weeks (21).

A retrospective observational study of US community-based oncology practices defined anemia as an Hb <11 g/dL at any time during chemotherapy. At baseline, 20.9% of the 42,923 patients evaluated were anemic. The highest prevalences of anemia were ovarian cancer at 56.3%, breast cancer at 53.3% and non–small cell lung cancer at 50.9% (22).

Type of chemotherapy and the length and intensity of treatment can affect the prevalence of anemia. The commonly used platinum-based agents can cause anemia through a variety of mechanisms, including direct effect on renal function as well as occasionally causing hemolytic anemia (23). Patients who received gemcitabine-based regimens (59%), platinum-based regimens (50.7%), and anthracycline-based regimens (50.8%) were the most likely to develop anemia (22).

Additionally, in the era of biologic agents, there may be a greater risk for the development of anemia with the newer drugs. For example, imatinib therapy for GI stromal tumors resulted in almost 90% of patients developing anemia, with 10% developing grade 3 or 4 anemia (24). Patients with metastatic renal cell carcinoma receiving temsirolimus as monotherapy experienced an increased rate of clinically significant anemia compared with patients receiving sunitinib or sorafenib (25–27).

Erythropoiesis-Stimulating Agents to Treat Anemia

The discovery of erythropoietin as the hormone responsible for RBC production led to the purification, cloning, and manufacture of recombinant human erythropoietin (rHuEPO) in quantities useful as a therapeutic agent. First approved to treat anemia associated with chronic renal disease, in 1993 rHuEPO was approved to treat CIA. Several varieties of rHuEPO are available commercially including epoetin alfa (Procrit, Ortho Biotech) and darbepoetin alfa (Aranesp, Amgen) in North America and epoetin beta (NeoRecormon, Roche) in Europe. Together, they are termed erythropoiesis-stimulating agents (ESAs). Rising costs of cancer and supportive care therapeutics have stimulated the recent development of biosimilar drugs, including biosimilar ESAs that are now widely available.

The use of ESAs rapidly increased through the 1990s and early 2000s, based on randomized trials that demonstrated improvement in Hb levels, reduction in the need for blood transfusions, and improvement in quality of life (28–30). In the mid-2000s, safety concerns were raised with ESA use, leading to a series of US Food and Drug Administration (FDA) advisory boards examining the issue and ultimately to several FDA label changes and a black box warning. As a result, ESA usage dropped very substantially in patients with CIA.

Large community-based prospective trials of rHuEPO were completed and reported in the late 1990s. The first trial evaluating 10,000 units (U) of epoetin alfa subcutaneously (SQ) every 3 weeks enrolled 2,370 patients with a variety of nonmyeloid malignancies with Hb levels <11 g/dL (31). Sixty-three percent of patients had a >1 g/dL rise in Hb after 4 weeks, and after 16 weeks, 61% had a 2 g/dL rise or Hb >12 g/dL and a mean rise of Hb of 2 g/dL. A weekly fixed dosing schedule of 40,000 U (32) demonstrated an Hb response of 68%, mean Hb rise of 1.8 g/dL, and reduction in transfusion requirements. Given the convenience of weekly compared with thrice-weekly dosing, 40,000 U weekly of epoetin alfa quickly became the community standard dosage.

Darbepoetin alfa is a modified recombinant form of erythropoietin with a slightly different amino acid structure that adds additional glycosylation to the native glycoprotein (33). Thus, darbepoetin alfa has a prolonged half-life and altered receptor affinity and was FDA approved for treatment of CIA in 2002. Randomized clinical trials (RCTs) showed a reduction in transfusion requirements, an increase in Hb levels, and improvement in quality of life in patients with solid tumors and nonmyeloid hematologic malignancies (27,34,35).

A 2012 Cochrane systemic review of 91 randomized trials examining treatment with epoetin or darbepoetin demonstrated a reduction in transfusion rate by 35% compared to untreated or placebo-treated patients (relative risk [RR] 0.65, 95% CI 0.62 to 0.68) (36). A subanalysis of 46 trials demonstrated that patients receiving epoetin or darbepoetin were more likely to have a hematologic response, defined as a risk in Hb of at least 2 g/dL or a rise in Hct by at least 6 percentage points (RR 3.39; 95% CI 3.10 to 3.71). Subsequent RCTs and systemic reviews have reinforced the value of ESAs reduction in transfusion requirements (37).

Several clinical trials have compared weekly epoetin alfa with darbepoetin alfa given less frequently (every 2 to 3 weeks) and have demonstrated similar efficacy endpoints (38,39). Therefore, the decision of the agent to be used should be based on scheduling and economic considerations. Darbepoetin alfa was initially FDA approved on a weight-based weekly dosage. More recent trials have demonstrated that a fixed dosage given as infrequently as every 3 weeks retains efficacy with far greater patient convenience (40–42). The American Society of Clinical Oncology (ASCO) and the American Society of Hematology (ASH) 2019 guidelines state that epoetin alfa, darbepoetin alfa, and ESA biosimilars are therapeutically equivalent with regard to both efficacy and safety (37).

Risks of ESAs

Initial studies with ESAs suggested a potential survival advantage for patients treated for CIA. There was rationale for the signal; anemic patients in many different settings including cancer have an inferior survival over nonanemic matched controls, and hypoxia can potentially reduce the effectiveness of radiotherapy and even chemotherapy. This hypothesis led to the conduct of several trials in nonanemic patients designed either to prevent significant anemia from occurring or to increase Hb levels to supranormal values. However, a trial in nonanemic head and neck cancer patients receiving radiation therapy and a study in metastatic breast cancer patients receiving first-line chemotherapy showed higher mortality rates with this strategy (43,44).

Overall, inferior outcomes were demonstrated in 8 of 59 controlled phase III trials of ESAs in a variety of cancers. Only four of these eight trials included patients with CIA, the FDA-labeled indications for ESAs, and all four targeted higher than normal Hb levels as the endpoint for stopping the ESA. A cervical cancer trial was terminated early in 2003 before the primary endpoint could be assessed (45). In another breast cancer trial with intent of ESA to increase Hb in nonanemic patients, the event-free survival and overall survival were unplanned analyses (46). No difference in survival was detected in a more mature analysis (47).

An individual patient-level data meta-analysis was published in 2009 (48). This involved 53 studies with 13,933 cancer patients receiving ESAs and included both concurrently chemotherapy-treated patients and those not receiving chemotherapy while on study with the ESA. A significantly increased RR for mortality on study Hazard Ratio (HR) (1.17, $p = 0.003$) and for overall survival duration (HR 1.06, $p = 0.005$) was noted. When analysis was restricted to 10,441 patients receiving chemotherapy, there was a nonsignificant increase in on-study mortality (HR 1.10, $p = 0.26$). Other meta-analyses published subsequently have reached conflicting conclusions (49). Based on these results, the consensus of expert opinion concurs that ESAs should not be administered to patients with AOC not receiving chemotherapy.

There is substantial evidence that ESAs are associated with an increased risk of thrombovascular events in cancer patients. Venous thromboembolism (VTE) is a frequent complication of cancer in the absence of ESA therapy. Multiple risk factors for VTE in cancer patients include cancer type, stage, chemotherapy regimen, comorbidities, and immobilization (50).

Several meta-analyses have evaluated the risk of VTE in patients receiving ESAs with chemotherapy, radiotherapy, or without additional treatment, and each showed a significant increase in the RR for VTE events. The Agency for Healthcare Research and Quality (AHRQ) comparative effectiveness review of 30 RCTs published in 2006 revealed an RR of 1.69 (95% CI 1.36 to 2.10, $p < 0.001$) (51). The event rates for VTE was 7% (range 0% to 30%) in patients treated with epoetin alfa versus 4% in controls (range 1% to 23%) and 5% in patients treated with darbepoetin alfa versus 3% in controls. A pooled analysis of individual patient-level data from RCTs comparing darbepoetin with placebo showed an increased risk for VTE (HR 1.5, 95% CI 1.10 to 2.26) (52). No increase was observed in mortality in progression-free survival (HR 0.93, 95% CI 0.84 to 1.04) or disease progression. A meta-analysis of long-term follow-up in 18 RCTs utilizing ESAs in CIA demonstrated an odds ratio of 1.47 and 95% CI of 1.24 to 1.74 for VTE (49).

The relative rate for VTE appears to be dependent on target Hb, increasing as Hb rises to ≥13 g/dL. The actual dose or schedule of ESAs utilized does not seem to play a role in the RR of VTEs. None of the trials evaluated specific factors that might impact VTE risk. It is reasonable to weigh the risks and benefits of ESAs carefully in patients judged to be at an increased risk for VTE based on history or clinical findings.

ESA Dosing

Epoetin alfa can be initiated at doses of 150 U/kg SQ 3 times per week (t.i.w.) or 40,000 U weekly in patients with CIA as per the FDA label. The dose should be increased to 300 U/kg t.i.w. or 60,000 U weekly, respectively, if no response in Hb or no reduction in transfusion requirement is noted after 4 to 6 weeks of therapy. Doses can be reduced or held once target Hb levels are obtained with careful monitoring, reinitiating when Hb levels begin to drop toward a level where transfusion might be contemplated. Extended dosing with epoetin alfa at 80,000 U every 2 weeks or 120,000 U every 3 weeks has also been evaluated (53,54).

Darbepoetin alfa can be initiated at 2.25 μg/kg SQ weekly or 500 μg every 3 weeks as per the FDA-approved dose. In addition, randomized trials support starting doses of darbepoetin at 200 μg every 3 weeks or 300 μg every 3 weeks (39,55). The weekly dose of darbepoetin should be doubled to 4.5 μg/kg, the biweekly dose increased to 300 μg, and a starting dose of 300 μg every 3 weeks can be escalated to 500 μg if inadequate response by week 6. There is no evidence to support doses of darbepoetin >500 μg every 3 weeks.

ESA should be discontinued following completion of chemotherapy or if there is no response after 8 to 9 weeks of therapy as measured by Hb levels or continued need for transfusions. Overall, approximately 50% to 70% of patients will achieve an Hb response, and unfortunately no pretreatment factors predictive of response or nonresponsiveness have yet been identified (56). Current labels for ESAs include a black box warning against usage in patients with curative malignancies given the potential risk from harm from ESAs (57).

Attempts to improve the response to ESAs have focused on providing additional iron, given the functional iron deficiency that occurs in both AOC and CIA. Nine prospective RCTs of intravenous (IV) iron supplementation to oral iron or no iron in CIA patients receiving ESAs have been conducted (58). Eight of these trials showed benefit from the addition of IV iron as measured by Hb response, decrease in blood transfusions, or less ESA requirement (59–62). Patients had ferritin levels from 160 to 460 mg/L and transferrin saturations from 19% to 36%. Given the weight of the data, all patients initiating ESA therapy should be screened for iron deficiency and functional iron deficiency. Concurrent IV iron should be strongly considered for those with evidence of functional iron deficiency.

Transfusion to Treat Cancer-Associated Anemia

Modern day blood banks typically fractionate whole blood collections into packed red blood cells (PRBCs), fresh frozen plasma, and platelet concentrates. In general, use of blood products is more appropriate than administering whole blood except in the rare instance of severe hypovolemia from large-volume acute blood loss. In cancer patients, anemia is generally treated with PRBC units. One 300-mL unit typically raises the recipient's Hb by approximately 1 g/dL and the Hct by 3% to 4%.

Indications for a transfusion in anemia associated with cancer are not clearly defined. The US Department of Health and Human Services suggests that transfusion should be used for "treatment of symptomatic deficit oxygen-carrying capacity" and should not be used "to treat anemias that could be corrected with specific medications should as iron, vitamin B12, folic acid, or erythropoietin" (58).

Many clinicians utilize an Hb of ≤7 g/dL or Hct of ≤21 to initiate transfusions in relatively asymptomatic patients, but there is little evidence base around this recommendation in ambulatory patients. Symptomatic patients and in those where anemia develops rapidly may require PRBCs at a higher Hb level. The availability of PRBCs varies by season, blood type, and other local and regional factors. Considerable resource utilization occurs with blood transfusions, requiring several hours to perform and crossmatch followed by several hours to deliver the transfusion, typically in an outpatient setting, but occasionally as an inpatient at significantly higher costs.

Transfusion Risks

Blood transfusions are generally safe but not without consequence. Transfusion-related mortality remains a reality. The annual number of transfusion-related deaths in 2015 was 37 (63), with nearly 12 million transfusions in the United States in 2015 (64). Hemolytic transfusion reactions occur infrequently but lead to 16% of transfusion-related deaths in 2015. Transfusion-related circulatory overload is also associated with morbidity and mortality (63).

Alloimmunization is the most frequent complication of transfusions with estimates of rates ranging from 7% to 31%. A retrospective analysis of patients with myeloproliferative or lymphoproliferative disorders found an overall immunization rate in 9% of patients receiving long-term transfusion support with the risk of immunization approximately 0.5% for each unit of PRBCS transfused (65). Acute reactions to blood transfusions range from an allergic skin reaction with urticaria to life-threatening hemolysis and multi-organ dysfunction. Modern molecular techniques of crossmatching have reduced acute hemolytic reactions to rare events, <1/200 U transfused (66).

As a biologic product, blood transfusions carry the risk of transmitting infection. Remarkable progress has been made over the years in reducing the approximate chance of infection from hepatitis C to 1:1.1 million and 1:1.5 million for HIV (67). However, there remains the possibility of infection from other transmissible agents, including bacteria, parasites, and other viruses, including West Nile and Zika viruses (68,69), and there are other viruses and infectious agents, such as prions, capable of causing hepatitis, which are not currently screenable. Bacterial infection is rare, but it can occur as an outgrowth of contaminated blood products (70).

The most common cause of treatment-related deaths from transfusion occurs from transfusion-related acute long injury (TRALI). TRALI develops during or within 6 hours of a transfusion and is characterized by rapid onset of dyspnea, tachypnea, cyanosis, and hypoxemia. Radiographic studies reveal diffuse fluffy infiltrates consistent with noncardiogenic pulmonary edema. Treatment consists of supplemental oxygen and mechanical ventilation. Milder forms of disease have also been reported (71). TRALI is thought to originate from granulocyte-mediated lung tissue injury. Mortality from TRALI may be as high as 6% to 10%. Transfusion of blood products from female donors is associated with increased risk of TRALI, and the incidence decreased from 1:4,000 units to 1:12,000 units when predominantly male plasma donors were used (72).

Cytomegalovirus (CMV) is worthy of mention because of the high seroprevalence in the United States (35% to 80% by region). There is a risk of acute infection in immunosuppressed hosts, particularly bone marrow/stem cell transplant patients. CMV is a leukocyte-associated virus. Therefore, any blood products containing white blood cells is capable of transmitting infection. With the widespread use of leukodepleted blood products, the risk of CMV infection is lessened. However, in the absence of prospective trials comparing leukocyte depleted with seronegative CMV products, CMV-negative donors are still the standard of care for severely immunocompromised CMV-seronegative recipients (73).

Irradiated blood products should be given to cancer patients at increased risk for graft versus host disease. Such groups would include allergenic and autologous bone marrow/stem cell transplant patients and patients who are severely immunocompromised including Hodgkin's disease and other lymphomas (74).

NEUTROPENIA

Neutrophils are the immune system's first line of defense against bacterial and fungal infection. Patients with severe neutropenia (SN), defined as absolute neutrophil counts (ANCs) <500 cells/µL are at substantial risk for blood-borne infection, especially if ANC <100 cells/µL. Fever associated with neutropenia, or febrile neutropenia (FN), is defined as a temperature of >38.3°C orally or >38.0°C for 1 hour with an ANC of <1,000 cells/µL. A broad range of symptomology is associated with FN, from none to severe sepsis. Because in the early stages of FN the outcome cannot be predicted, all patients with an FN should be carefully evaluated and presumed to be infected (75). It should be kept in mind that the absence of neutrophils markedly reduces the inflammatory response characteristically seen with infections, for example, pulmonary infiltrates in the setting of pneumonia. Signs and symptoms of infection may therefore be lacking. As a result, broad-spectrum antibiotics should be initiated immediately after a careful search for localizing sources of infection and pan culturing.

There is significant morbidity and mortality risk for FN, which represents 5.2% of hospitalizations related to cancer (76). Hospitalization for FN is associated with substantial resource utilization, including a mean length of stay of 9.6 days and mean cost of $24,770 per hospitalization based on 2012 U.S. data (76). A scoring system can help predict the risk of complications in patients with FN (77,78).

Patients presenting with FN can be characterized into low-risk groups who could be treated as outpatients with oral antibiotics, and high-risk groups requiring IV antibiotics and prolonged hospitalizations (79,80). Low-risk patients tend to have solid tumors under control, are without serious comorbidities, and expect relatively shorter duration of SN/FN. At least two prediction models are validated and are useful to make decisions or hospitalizations for patient to present with FN (81,82). Given the expense of hospitalization for FN and the ability to reliably identify low-risk patients (83), utilizing risk stratification in FN is cost-effective.

The use of antibiotic prophylaxis to prevent FN is not well established for solid tumors, although often utilized along with colony-stimulating factor (CSF) support in hematologic malignancy when long periods of neutropenia are expected. Evidence is too limited to routinely recommend prophylactic antibiotics in patients with solid tumors receiving myelosuppressive chemotherapy (84–86).

Determination of Risk of Neutropenia

The likelihood of FN/SN with chemotherapy is dependent mainly on the intrinsic myelosuppression of the regimen utilized, but patient and disease factors should also be considered. Many clinical trials, which determine the efficacy of a particular chemotherapy regimen, did not formally establish the risk of FN as a component of the trial. Therefore, there is still a knowledge gap for many established combination chemotherapy programs. However, the National Comprehensive Cancer Network (NCCN) guidelines has grouped regimens into a moderate risk of FN, defined as 10% to 20%, or high-risk, >20% chance of FN.

Patient factors should also be taken into consideration when determining the risk of SN/FN (Table 52.2) (87,88). The most important patient risk factor is age, with patients >65 years old at highest risk for any given chemotherapy regimen (89,90). Other important factors include previous exposure to chemotherapy or radiation therapy, prior chemotherapy-induced neutropenia, bone marrow involvement with tumor, poor performance status, poor renal function, liver dysfunction, and preexisting conditions including neutropenia, infection, or recent surgery (91,92).

Several risk models have been developed to integrate patient related factors into a useful tool to predict SN/FN, particularly when regimens

TABLE 52.2 PATIENT-RELATED PREDICTIVE FACTORS FOR FEBRILE NEUTROPENIA

Older age (>65)
Poor performance status
Female sex
Multiple comorbidities
No G-CSF use
Advanced disease
Abnormal liver function tests
Low body mass index/body surface area
Prior chemotherapy with three or more agents
Baseline neutrophils <1.5
Anemia
Cardiovascular disease
Renal disease
High-intensity chemotherapy
Lack of antibiotic prophylaxis
Baseline albumin <3.5 g/dL

G-CSF, granulocyte colony-stimulating factor.
Adapted from Lyman GH, Abella E, Pettengell R. Risk factors for febrile neutropenia among patients with cancer receiving chemotherapy: a systemic review. *Crit Rev Oncol Hematol.* 2014;90(3):190-199.

with intermediate intrinsic risk are utilized (93). Lyman et al. developed a predictive model that was retrospectively validated with a dataset of over 3,760 patients (87). Cycle 1 neutropenic events were predicted in 34% of high-risk and 4% of low-risk patients with a sensitivity of 90% and specificity of 59%. Another model utilizes a validated web-based tool for predicting the severity of hematologic toxicity in lymphoma patients receiving cyclophosphamide, doxorubicin, vincristine, and prednisone (CHOP)-like regimens (94) and another for non-Hodgkin's lymphoma (NHL) showed high sensitivity of 81% and specificity of 80% for predicting cycle 1 FN with 28% positive and 98% negative predictive value (95). All of the models to date suffer from a lack of prospective validation, but they can still serve as a useful adjunct to decision-making for primary prophylaxis with growth factors.

Growth Factor Use for Prevention of FN

Granulocyte colony-stimulating factor (G-CSF) is a lineage-specific myeloid growth factor that hastens maturation and release of the committed progenitor pool, prolongs circulation of released granulocytes, and stimulates the margination of neutrophils in the vascular pool. It also enhances neutrophil function through increases in chemotaxis and phagocytosis, and primes granulocytes for respiratory burst. The normal proliferation and maturation of neutrophils from progenitors in the bone marrow is markedly enhanced by the addition of pharmacologic doses of recombinant human G-CSF (filgrastim [Neupogen], Amgen), such that the normal 5-day maturation process may occur within a single day. Normal volunteers receiving filgrastim experience a dose-dependent increase in ANC (96).

Pegfilgrastim (Neulasta, Amgen) is a modified version of recombinant G-CSF with a 20-kDa polyethylene glycol molecule attached to the N-terminus of the standard molecule. Due to this modification, pegfilgrastim is not cleared by the kidneys and has a prolonged serum half-life, while maintaining all other biologic effects of G-CSF. When patients receive myelosuppressive chemotherapy, pegfilgrastim given afterward remains at high circulating concentrations until stimulation of accelerated recovery of the neutrophil compartment, which then binds the pegfilgrastim and clears it internally (97). This mode of metabolism is termed as self-regulation and explains why a single dose of pegfilgrastim per cycle of chemotherapy can be clinically effective in reducing duration and depth of neutropenia.

Granulocyte–macrophage colony-stimulating factor (GM-CSF) is a lineage-nonspecific factor, which acts synergistically with other cytokines to enhance myeloid, macrophage, and erythrocyte lineage expansion and maturation with resulting broader hematologic effects. Recombinant human GM-CSF is available commercially (sargramostim [Leukine], Genzyme). Clinically, GM-CSF can increase the neutrophil and monocyte counts and modestly affect the erythroid compartment; immunologic enhancement is also seen. GM-CSF is not FDA approved for the treatment of chemotherapy-induced neutropenia.

Initial RCTs testing G-CSF as primary prophylaxis after myelotoxic chemotherapy with an expected risk of FN of >40% demonstrated a 50% reduction in FN rate with daily growth factor administration until neutrophil recovery (98,99). Subsequent trials examined less myelosuppressive regimens and showed reduction in FN rate with G-CSF prophylaxis. Pegfilgrastim compared with daily filgrastim showed equal or better efficacy with the benefit of administration of only one dose per cycle compared with an average of 10 daily doses of filgrastim for equivalent effects (100,101). A trial examining the use of primary prophylaxis with pegfilgrastim versus placebo in patients receiving myelosuppressive doses of docetaxel in breast cancer demonstrated a dramatic reduction in the rate of FN from 17% to 1% (102).

A systemic analysis of RCTs including 3,493 patients utilizing G-CSF as primary prophylaxis against FN showed a risk reduction of 46% (RR 0.54, 95% CI 0.43 to 0.67, $p < 0.001$) for the incidence of FN (103). Moreover, the relative dose intensity (RDI) of chemotherapy delivered was improved by 8.4%, $p = 0.001$. Notably, this meta-analysis demonstrated a reduction in infection-related mortality (RR 0.05, 95% CI 0.33 to 0.90, $p = 0.018$) and also for early mortality during chemotherapy (RR 0.60, 95% CI 0.43 to 0.83, $p = 0.002$). A more recent systemic review of 25 randomized trials involving 12,000 patients showed an RR of 0.897 for all-cause mortality with the use of prophylactic growth factor, translating into a 3.4% absolute reduction and mortality (104).

Growth Factor Indications and Dosing

G-CSF prophylaxis is recommended for patients receiving myelotoxic chemotherapy with an expected FN rate of around 20% or higher (Table 52.3). NCCN (1), ASCO (105), and European Organization for Research and Treatment of Cancer (EORTC) guidelines (106) are concordant on this recommendation. For patients receiving curative intent therapy, or in the setting of life-prolonging treatments where delivered dose intensity may be extremely important, growth factor support is considered for regimens with a 10% to 20% risk of FN. Alternatively, for patients receiving purely palliative chemotherapy it may be more appropriate to

TABLE 52.3 DISEASE SETTINGS AND CHEMOTHERAPY REGIMENS WITH A HIGH RISK OF FEBRILE NEUTROPENIA (>20%)

Acute Lymphoblastic Leukemia (ALL)
- Select ALL Regimens as directed by treatment protocol.

Bladder Cancer
- Dose-dense MVAC (methotrexate, vinblastine, doxorubicin, cisplatin)

Bone Cancer
- VAI (vincristine, doxorubicin, ifosfamide)
- VDC-IE (vincristine, doxorubicin, cyclophosphamide alternating with ifosfamide and etoposide)
- VIDE (vincristine, ifosfamide, doxorubicin, etoposide)

Breast cancer
- Dose-dense AC -> T (doxorubicin, cyclophosphamide, paclitaxel)
- TAC (docetaxel, doxorubicin, cyclophosphamide)
- TC (docetaxel, cyclophosphamide)
- TCH (docetaxel, carboplatin, trastuzumab)

Head and Neck Squamous Cell Carcinoma
- TPF (docetaxel, cisplatin, 5-fluorouracil)

Hodgkin's Lymphoma
- Brentuximab vedotin + ACD (doxorubicin, vinblastine, dacarbazine)
- Escalated BEACOPP (bleomycin, etoposide, doxorubicin, cyclophosphamide, vincristine, procarbazine, prednisone)

Kidney Cancer
- Doxorubicin/gemcitabine

Non-Hodgkin's Lymphoma
- Dose-adjusted EPOCH (etoposide, prednisone, vincristine, cyclophosphamide, doxorubicin)
- ICE (ifosfamide, carboplatin, etoposide)
- Dose-dense CHOP-14 (cyclophosphamide, doxorubicin, vincristine, prednisone)
- MINE (mesna, ifosfamide, mitoxantrone, etoposide)
- DHAP (dexamethasone, cisplatin, cytarabine)
- ESHAP (etoposide, methylprednisone, cisplatin, cytarabine)
- HyperCVAD (cyclophosphamide, vincristine, doxorubicin, dexamethasone)

Melanoma
- Dacarbazine-based combination with IL-2, interferon alfa (dacarbazine, cisplatin, vinblastine, IL-2, interferon alfa)

Multiple Myeloma
- DT PACE (dexamethasone, thalidomide, cisplatin, doxorubicin, cyclophosphamide, etoposide ± bortezomib (VTD-PACE)

Ovarian Cancer
- Topotecan
- Docetaxel

Soft Tissue Sarcoma
- MAID (mesna, doxorubicin, ifosfamide, dacarbazine)
- Doxorubicin
- Ifosfamide/doxorubicin

Small Cell Lung Cancer
- Topotecan

Testicular Cancer
- VeIP (vinblastine, ifosfamide, cisplatin)
- VIP (etoposide, ifosfamide, cisplatin)
- TIP (paclitaxel, ifosfamide, cisplatin)

From The NCCN Clinical Practice Guidelines in Oncology. Hematopoietic growth factors. Version 2.2019. https://www.nccn.org/professionals/physician_gls/pdf/growthfactors.pdf. Accessed July 25, 2019.

reduce doses of chemotherapy when the risk of FN is high or after a prior episode of FN to a particular treatment regimen. Prophylactic G-CSF is recommended for any patient considered to be at high risk for FN regardless of the intent of therapy. Moreover, patients receiving a lower risk regimen should be considered for growth factor support when there is a high chance for serious morbidity or mortality.

Growth factor support allows for the delivery of full doses of chemotherapy on schedule. Reduction in RDI of even modest amounts has been associated with inferior outcomes in curative disease settings such as NHL treated with CHOP and adjuvant chemotherapy in early-stage breast cancer (107,108). Neutropenia remains the major dose-limiting toxicity of adjuvant chemotherapy for early-stage breast cancer (109). A meta-analysis of 10 studies that reported RDI and compared prophylaxis with growth factors versus none showed an increase in RDI to 95.1% of anticipated in patients who received G-CSF compared with 86.7% in those without growth factor support (103).

Filgrastim and pegfilgrastim should be administered 1 to 3 days after completion of chemotherapy to achieve optimal effects and reduce potential complications. Filgrastim is dosed at 5 µg/kg SQ daily, adjusted to the closest vial size available, until neutrophil recovery. Pegfilgrastim is given at a single fixed dose of 6 mg SQ to adults, with chemotherapy occurring every 2 weeks or greater. Studies examining alternative or shorter programs of growth factor support have generally demonstrated inferior results (110,111). Trials examining growth factors on the same day as chemotherapy have also been shown to be less effective than beginning at least 1 day after chemotherapy, and same-day administration is not recommended (112,113).

The first cycle of a myelosuppressive regimen is associated with the highest risk of FN (114). Indeed, in many prospective and retrospective analyses the first cycle constitutes up to 50% of the risk of FN for the entire chemotherapy program (102,115). Therefore, primary prophylaxis beginning with the first cycle of chemotherapy and continuing with each cycle represents the most effective way to reduce the chance of FN with appropriately myelotoxic chemotherapy. A patient who develops FN after chemotherapy not supported by prophylactic growth factors should be strongly considered for subsequent cycle prevention with CSF.

Patients who develop FN without growth factors can be treated with filgrastim at the time of neutropenia until the ANC recovers. Studies have not demonstrated a robust effect for treatment of established FN, although neutrophil recovery maybe hastened by 1 to 2 days (116). Nonetheless, older patients and those with comorbidities or complications like pneumonia or sepsis should be strongly considered for treatment with growth factors during FN (1). A patient who receives pegfilgrastim following myelosuppressive chemotherapy and still develops SN or FN should not receive further filgrastim as circulating levels of G-CSF will be high and there is no benefit of additional growth factor in this situation.

Toxicity of Growth Factors

Filgrastim and pegfilgrastim are generally considered safe. Occasional skin and other allergic reactions have been reported. The most common adverse reaction is mild to moderate bone pain and myalgias, probably secondary to the marrow stimulation. Typical onset is 2 to 5 days after growth factor administration. Pretreatment patient education and early intervention with nonsteroidal anti-inflammatory drugs or other nonopioid analgesics work well to alleviate the symptoms (117). Incidentally, long-acting H_2-blockers have been reported to reduce bone pain, but no formal prospective evaluations of this strategy have been conducted (118). Evaluation of RCTs has demonstrated no evidence that pegfilgrastim is more likely to cause bone pain compared with daily filgrastim (119). Myeloid growth factors should be used with caution, if at all, in patients with sickle cell disease due to the chance of precipitating a crisis (120).

There is a small increased risk of secondary malignancies, notably acute myeloid leukemia and MDS, in patients receiving growth factors with chemotherapy (104). Some of the increase may well be due to dose escalation of chemotherapy, which was the strategy attempted to improve the efficacy of the regimen, usually without benefit. It is difficult to distinguish the growth factor affects from the high-dose chemotherapy effect. The benefits of growth factor in preventing FN, hospitalization, and potential early mortality outweigh the small risk.

THROMBOCYTOPENIA

Thrombocytopenia is common in patients with cancer. Causes include chemotherapy, radiation therapy, bone marrow infiltration by tumor, nutritional deficiencies, and tumor-associated immune effects, including autoimmune thrombocytopenic purpura. Thrombocytopenia is particularly prevalent in patients with hematologic malignancies, including MDS and acute and chronic leukemia. Patients with solid tumors increasingly experience thrombocytopenia with the chronicity of sequential multi-agent chemotherapy, as well as newer biologic agents, which exacerbate hematologic toxicity and may also independently increase bleeding. Complications from thrombocytopenia vary from asymptomatic to mild bleeding characterized by ecchymoses and petechiae through disruptive epistaxis and gingival bleeding to life-threatening GI or intracranial hemorrhage.

The treatment of thrombocytopenia largely remains prophylactic platelet transfusions for asymptomatic patients with severe thrombocytopenia and therapeutic platelet transfusions in the setting of active bleeding. Platelets for transfusion are either collected as a fraction of whole blood, which is then pooled with 4 to 6 donors, or collected from a single donor by apheresis to constitute an adequate transfusion dose. The quality of apheresis platelets is similar to that of pooled random donor platelet concentrates (121,122), and therefore, these two products can be used interchangeably based on availability and cost considerations (123).

Prophylactic platelet transfusions should be initiated when a platelet count declines to 10,000/µL as per most recent ASCO guidelines (124). Several randomized studies have demonstrated no difference in bleeding events when a trigger of 10,000/µL is utilized versus a higher trigger of 20,000/µL (125,126).

Therapeutic platelet transfusions are generally initiated when there is an evidence of active bleeding due to platelet dysfunction or thrombocytopenia. For chronic thrombocytopenia, evidence of gross bleeding with or without the need for PRBC transfusions usually triggers platelet transfusions. Some other factors like anatomical abnormalities, quantitative platelet dysfunction, coagulation factor deficiencies, and others contribute to bleeding. It is not surprising that therapeutic platelet transfusions are only modestly effective in controlling bleeding in clinical trials (127). For major surgical procedures, a platelet count of at least 50,000/µL should be established. Because the count itself is not the only indication of hemostatic function, patients undergoing neurosurgical procedures should have platelet counts closer to 100,000/µL.

Platelet Refractoriness

Cancer patients who require frequent platelet transfusions often show inadequate rise in platelet count afterward, termed refractoriness to transfusions. Both immune and nonimmune mechanisms play a role in this inadequate response. However, alloimmunization against major histocompatibility antigens is the major determinant of refractoriness. Providing ABO compatible platelets achieves the highest posttransfusion platelet count and reduces the incidence of alloimmunization.

A large trial in leukemia patients demonstrated the value of leukoreduced platelets (and PRBC) compared with standard blood products to prevent the development of human leukocyte antigen (HLA) antibodies (128). Leukodepleted transfusions are also less likely to cause transfusion reactions, which is thought to be mediated by cytokines from leukocytes. Many institutes have instituted universal leukoreduction of the blood supply (129).

Strategies for dealing with alloimmunized recipients include selecting HLA-matched donors from an HLA-typed registry of apheresis donors, identifying HLA-antibody specificities, and selecting antigen-compatible apheresis donors or performing platelet crossmatch tests to select compatible donors (130). Even with these techniques, up to one-third of the patients will remain refractory likely due to nonalloimmunization factors like splenomegaly, concurrent heparin use, disseminated intravascular coagulation, sepsis, and immune thrombocytopenia (ITP). Persistently, refractory patients with ongoing bleeding may derive some benefit from immunoglobulin G (IgG) infusions, fibrinolytic inhibitors, or recombinant factor VIIa (130).

Thrombopoietic Agents

Platelet transfusions are costly, at times ineffective, and place the recipient at risk for transfusion reactions and infectious exposure. Given the proven benefit of utilizing pharmacologic doses of erythroid and myeloid growth factors, there has been considerable interest in developing a biologic treatment for thrombocytopenia. Analogous to G-CSF and erythropoietin, thrombopoietin (TPO) is the endogenous ligand for the TPO receptor expressed on the surface of megakaryocytes, platelet precursors, and platelets. First-generation recombinant human TPO and its derivatives were ineffective and led to prolonged thrombocytopenia and autoantibodies in some patients (131). Clinical development of these agents was therefore abandoned.

rHIL-11, also known as oprelvekin (Neumega, Wyeth), was initially approved as a thrombopoietic agent based on a 30% reduction in platelet transfusions in patients with breast cancer (132). IL-11 promotes megakaryocytopoeisis and increases platelet production, in vivo. However, side effects of IL-11 are substantial and include edema, fatigue, myalgias, and cardiovascular events, and oprelvekin now has only orphan drug designation by the FDA.

Second-generation thrombopoiesis-stimulation agents, including romiplostim (Nplate, Amgen), an IV peptide-antibody construct, and eltrombopag (Promacta, GlaxoSmithKline) and avatrombopag (Doptelet, Dova), which are oral small molecules, are commercially available. These drugs carry an FDA label for treating chronic ITP, a condition occasionally encountered in cancer patients, particularly those with lymphoma, who have had an incomplete response to a prior ITP treatment. These agents carry an increased risk of thrombus formation and are contraindicated in MDS due to increased risk of transformation to acute myeloid leukemia (133). Eltrombopag also carries an FDA black box warning for hepatotoxicity (134).

In 2018, fostamatinib (Tavalisse, Rigel), an oral small molecule spleen tyrosine kinase inhibitor that reduces antibody-mediated platelet destruction, was approved for refractory chronic ITP. Two parallel phase 3 RCTs reported an overall response, defined as >1 platelet count > 50,000/μL in the first 12 weeks of treatment, in 43% of patients treated with fostamatinib compared to 14% on placebo ($p = 0.0006$). The most common side effects included diarrhea (31% vs. 15% in placebo arm) and hypertension (28% vs. 13% in placebo arm) (135). Other less common but potential adverse effects included nausea, neutropenia, and hepatotoxicity (135,136).

Hematologic Consequences of Immune Checkpoint Inhibitors

The development of immune checkpoint inhibitors (ICI) in recent years has drastically altered the treatment for many cancer types and is accompanied by a unique profile of immune-related adverse effects (irAEs) on many organ systems due to T-cell hyperactivation (137,138). Though the overall frequency of hematologic irAEs is low and ranged from 1% to 3.6% (137,139), they can be fatal with a reported mortality rate of 14% and require a high index of suspicion (139). Hematologic irAEs typically occur early in treatment, with a median onset of 10 weeks, but can occur at any time with a range of 1 to 84 weeks (139), and may require permanent discontinuation of immune therapy (140).

There are a variety of possible hematologic irAE, but hemolytic anemias and ITP are the most common (137–139). The overall prevalence of all grades of anemia was reported to be 5%, with a slightly increased frequency of all grades of anemia with combination immunotherapy versus monotherapy; however, there was no difference for high-grade anemias (138). Autoimmune hemolytic anemia (AIHA) can be life threatening and requires prompt identification and treatment. Cold AIHA represented 33% of cases (141), and glucocorticoids typically have poor efficacy in these patients (139). Grades 2 to 4 AIHA require glucocorticoids, with a long taper over, and grades 3 to 4 require permanent discontinuation of ICI and may need further immunosuppressants (139,140).

ITP is the most common irAE affecting platelets (137,141), though acquired thrombotic thrombocytopenic purpura can also occur (140), and treatment options are similar to classic ITP. For grades 2 to 4 glucocorticoids should be promptly initiated, and IVIG or other second-line ITP treatments may be required if bleeding risk is high (139,140). ITP typically responds to steroids, and it may be reasonable to resume ICI after shared decision-making in select patients (139).

Isolated neutropenia is rare, though the true prevalence is difficult to identify due to confounders and comorbidities (137,142). However, immune-related neutropenia is typically severe and prolonged and typically requires GCSF and glucocorticoids, though there is a lack of clear guidelines for treatment (139).

Acquired hemophilia can also occur with ICIs but is rare (139,140). Severe hemophilia A (<1% factor VIII) is classified as a grade 3 to 4 adverse event and requires permanent discontinuation of ICI, though it may be possible to resume ICI with shared decision-making with the patient after resolution of grade 1 (mild hemophilia) or grade 2 (moderate hemophilia) (139,140) Ultimately, treatment of all irAEs differs by grade and specific adverse event and guidelines are available (140), but glucocorticoids remain the backbone for treatment (137,140). Table 52.4 summarizes management of several ICI-related irAEs.

BIOSIMILARS

The rising costs of cancer care, and biologics in particular, in the United States over recent years has stimulated the development of biosimilar drugs in the hopes of lowering costs (143). A biosimilar is highly similar to an FDA-approved biologic agent with "no clinically meaningful differences in terms of safety, purity, and potency" and is designated by the FDA by a 4-letter suffix added to the originator drug name. Once biosimilarity has been shown for one indication of the reference product, existing data can be used to justify approval of the biosimilar product for other indications of the reference, known as extrapolation, which can decrease time to approval and development costs (144).

The implementation of biosimilars is relatively new in the United States. However, the European Medicines Agency (EMA) approved the first ESA biosimilar (epoetin alfa [Binocrit, Sandoz]) in 2007, and the first GCSF biosimilar (filgrastim [Zarxio, Sandoz]) in 2009, which provides a decade of clinical experience and postmarketing surveillance for biosimilars in treating CIA and neutropenia. Multiple European studies have demonstrated similar efficacy and safety profile of ESA (145–147) and GSCF biosimilars (148,149). A European analysis of the cost-effectiveness of biosimilar epoetin alfa demonstrated a 13.8% reduction in cost compared to epoetin alfa and 44.2% compared to darbepoetin alfa (150).

Filgrastim-sndz (Zarxio, Sandoz) was the first biosimilar approved by the FDA in March 2015 based on the PIONEER study, a phase III RCT in breast cancer patients receiving myelosuppressive chemotherapy that demonstrated noninferiority of filgrastim-sndz compared to filgrastim (151). Other subsequent real-world studies have further supported the safety and efficacy of filgrastim-sndz (152,153) and other GSCF biosimilars (154).

Since the approval of filgrastim-sndz, further biosimilars of filgrastim have been FDA approved, as well as an ESA biosimilar, epoetin alfa-epbx (Retacrit, Pfizer), which was FDA approved in May 2018 and pegfilgrastim biosimilars, pegfilgrastim-jmdb (Fulphila, Mylan) and pegfilgrastim-cbqv (Udenyca, Coherus) (155). Recent meta-analyses have continued to demonstrate no significant differences in efficacy or safety profile (154,156). However, widespread adoption of existing biosimilars in the United States has yet to be seen. Postmarket surveillance is important to ensure continued safety of biosimilars as the FDA approval process relies largely on extrapolation of pharmacologic data for approval of other approved indications of the reference drug, after the initial FDA approval. Extrapolation facilitates the potential for decreased costs and improved access, the magnitude of which will be seen in the coming years (157).

CONCLUSION

Cancer patients remain highly susceptible to hematologic complications, which impact every aspect of oncologic care. The clinical complications of neutropenia, anemia, and thrombocytopenia are now well characterized and range from minimal to life threatening. The discovery of hematopoietic growth factors and their introduction into clinical practice dramatically changed our treatment approach to hematologic support of cancer patients. Over the last decades, better

TABLE 52.4 HEMATOLOGIC ADVERSE EVENTS ASSOCIATED WITH IMMUNE CHECKPOINT INHIBITORS (ICI)

Grade	Management
Autoimmune hemolytic anemia	
Grade 1: Hb 10 g/dL—LLN	Continue ICI
Grade 2: Hb 8–10 g/dL	Hold and strongly consider permanent discontinuation
	Prednisone 0.5–1.0 mg/kg/d
Grade 3: Hb < 8 g/dL	Permanently discontinue ICI
	Prednisone 1–2 mg/kg/d
	Consider RBC transfusion to relieve symptoms
Grade 4: Life Threatening	Permanently dissolve ICI
	Admit Patient
	IV Prednisone 1–2 mg/kg/d
	Consider IVIG, rituximab, other immunosuppressive drugs
Immune thrombocytopenia	
Grade 1: Platelets < 100 µL	Continue ICI
Grade 2: Platelets < 75 µL	Hold ICI until resolves to G1
	Administer prednisone 0.5–2 mg/kg/d
	Consider IVIG 1 g/kg
Grades 3–4: Platelets <50 µL	Hold ICI until resolves to G1
	Prednisone 1–2 mg/kg/d PO or IV
	IVIG 1 g/kg
Aplastic anemia	
Grade 1: ANC > 500 µL Hypocellular marrow; platelet >20/µL Reticulocyte count >20,000	Hold ICI and provide growth factor support and supportive transfusions
Grade 2: Severe hypocellular marrow < 25% and two of the following: ANC < 500/µL and reticulocyte count < 20,000	Hold ICI and provide growth factor support and supportive transitions ATG + cyclosporine, HLA typing. All blood products should be irradiated and filtered
Grade 3–4: Very severe: UNC <500/µL, Platelet <20/µL Reticulocyte count <20,000	Hold ICI until resolves to G1 Horse ATG + cyclosporine, HLA typing. All blood products should be irradiated and filtered If no response, repeat immunosuppression with rabbit ATG and cyclosporine and cyclophosphamide Consider eltrombopag
Acquired TTP (thrombotic thrombocytopenia purpura)	
Grade 1: Evidence of RBC destruction w/o anemia, renal insufficiency or thrombocytopenia	Hold ICI, discuss restart after resolution
Grade 2: Evidence of RBC destruction with grade 2 anemia/thrombocytopenia	Prednisone 0.5–1 mg/kg/d Hold ICI Discuss restart after resolution
Grade 3: Grade 3 thrombocytopenia, anemia, renal insufficiency OR	Discontinue ICI
Grade 4: Life threatening	Initiate plasma exchange, methylprednisone IG or IV daily × 3 days May offer rituximab

Adapted from Brahmer J, Lacchetti C, Schneider B, et al. Management of immune-related adverse events in patients treated with immune checkpoint inhibitor therapy: American Society of Clinical Oncology Clinical Practice Guidelines. *J Clin Oncol.* 2018;36(17):1714-1768.

understanding of the risks and benefits of hemato-poietic growth factors has been defined. The recent adoption of hematopoietic growth factor biosim-ilars may reduce supportive care costs of cancer patients.

Advances in blood product transfusions have improved safe delivery of blood components, but better pharmacologic approaches to hematologic support remains the preferred approach. In this dynamic supportive care environment, readers are encouraged to fold the results of ongoing RCTs, as well as frequent updates of evidence-based clini-cal practice guidelines to best incorporate use of hematopoietic growth factors, transfusion sup-port, and antibiotics in the clinical care of their patients. ICIs produce hematologic toxicity at a delayed time point, and clinicians must be vigilant to screen for them. Modulation of the immune response is the most effective strategy for these toxicities.

REFERENCES

1. The NCCN Clinical Practice Guidelines in Oncol-ogy. Hematopoietic growth factors. Version 2.2019. https://www.nccn.org/professionals/physician_gls/pdf/growthfactors.pdf. Accessed July 25, 2019.
2. Berger AM, Abernathy AP, Atkinson A, et al. Cancer-related fatigue. *J Natl Compr Canc Netw.* 2010;8(8):904-931.
3. Balducci L. Anemia, fatigue and aging. *Transfus Clin Biol.* 2010;17(5-6):375-381.
4. Wagner, LI, Cella D. Fatigue and cancer: causes, prevalence and treatment approaches. *Br J Cancer.* 2004;91(5):822-828.
5. Glaser CM, Millesi W, Kornek GV, et al. Impact of hemoglobin level and use of recombinant erythropoietin on efficacy of preoperative chemoradiation therapy for squamous cell carcinoma of the oral cavity and orophar-ynx. *Int J Radiat Oncol Biol Phys.* 2001;50(3):705-715.
6. Caro JJ, Salas M, Ward A, Goss G. Anemia as an inde-pendent prognostic factor for survival in patients with cancer: a systemic quantitative review. *Cancer.* 2001;91(12):2214-2221.
7. Birgegard G, Aapro MS, Bokemeyer G, et al. Cancer-related anemia: pathogenesis, prevalence and treat-ment. *Oncology.* 2005;68(suppl 1):3-11.
8. Marks P. *Hematologic Manifestations of Systemic Disease: Infection, Chronic Inflammation, and Cancer.* 5th ed. Philadelphia, PA: Churchill Livingstone Elsevier; 2009.
9. Kaushansky K, Tipps TJ. *Hematopoietic Agents: Growth Factors, Minerals, and Vitamins.* 13th ed. New York, NY: McGraw-Hill; 2018.
10. Henry D. Iron or vitamin B_{12} deficiency in anemic can-cer patients prior to erythropoiesis-stimulating agent therapy. *Community Oncol.* 2007;4(2):95-101.
11. Hillman RS, Finch CA. Erythropoiesis: normal and abnormal. *Semin Hematol.* 1967;4(4):327-336.
12. Spivak JL. The anaemia of cancer: death by all thousand cuts. *Nat Rev Cancer.* 2005;5(7):543-555.
13. Maccio A, Madeddu C, Massa D, et al. Hemoglobin levels correlate with interleukin-6 levels in patients with advanced untreated epithelial ovarian cancer: role of inflammation in cancer-related anemia. *Blood.* 2005;106(1):362-367.
14. Faquin WC, Schneider TJ, Goldberg MA. Effect of inflammatory cytokines on hypoxia-induced erythro-poietic production. *Blood.* 1992;79(8):1987-1994.
15. Hellwig-Burgel T, Rutkowski K, Metzen E, Fandrey J, Jelkmann W. Interleukin-1 beta and tumor necrosis fac-tor-alpha stimulate DNA binding of hypoxia-inducible factor-1. *Blood.* 1999;94(5):1561-1567.
16. Herrmann F, Gebauer G, Lindemann A, Brach M, Mertelsmann R. Interleukin-2 and interferon-gamma recruit different subsets of human peripheral blood monocytes to secrete interleukin-1 beta and tumor necro-sis factor-alpha. *Clin Exp Immunol.* 1989;77(1):97-100.
17. Nicolas G, Chauvet C, Viatte L, et al. The gene encod-ing the iron regulatory peptide hepcidin is regulated by anemia, hypoxia, and inflammation. *J Clin Invest.* 2002;110(7):1037-1044.
18. Weiss G, Goodnough LT. Anemia of chronic disease. *N Engl J Med.* 2005;352(10):1011-1023.
19. Groopman JE, Itri LM. Chemotherapy-induced anemia in adults: incidence and treatment. *J Natl Cancer Inst.* 1999;91(19):1616-1634.
20. Ludwig H, Van Belle S, Barrett-Lee P, et al. The Euro-pean Cancer Anaemia Survey (ECAS): a large, multi-national, prospective survey defining the prevalence, incidence, and treatment of anaemia in cancer patients. *Eur J Cancer.* 2004;40(15):2293-2306.
21. Barrett-Lee PJ, Ludwig H, Birgegard G, et al. Indepen-dent risk factors for anemia in cancer patients receiv-ing chemotherapy: results from the European Cancer Anaemia Survey. *Oncology.* 2006;70(1):34-48.
22. Wu Y, Aravind S, Ranganathan G, Martin A, Nalysnyk L. Anemia and thrombocytopenia in patients undergo-ing chemotherapy for solid tumors: a descriptive study of a large outpatient oncology practice database, 2000-2007. *Clin Ther.* 2009;31(pt 2):2416-2432.
23. Wood PA, Hrushesky WJ. Cisplatin-associated anemia: an erythropoietin deficiency syndrome. *J Clin Invest.* 1995;95(4):1650-1659.
24. Duffaud F, Lecesne A, Ray-Coquard I. Erythropoietin for anemia treatment of patients with GIST receiving imatinib. *J Clin Oncol.* 2004;22(14):9046.
25. Hutson TE, Figlin RA, Kuhn JG, Motzer RJ. Targeted therapies for metastatic renal cell carcinoma: an over-view of toxicity and dosing strategies. *Oncologist.* 2018;13(10):1084-1096.
26. Sher A, Wu S. Anti-vascular endothelial growth fac-tor antibody bevacizumab reduced the risk of anemia associated with chemotherapy—a meta-analysis. *Acta Oncol.* 2011;50(7):997-1005.
27. Glaspy JA, Jadeja JS, Justice G, et al. Darbepoetin alfa given every 1 or 2 weeks alleviates anaemia associated with cancer chemotherapy. *Br J Cancer.* 2002;87(3):268-276.
28. Littlewood TJ, Bajetta E, Nortier JW, Vercammen E, Rapoport B. Effects of epoetin alfa on hematologic parameters and quality of life in cancer patients receiv-ing nonplatinum chemotherapy: results of a random-ized, double-blind, placebo-controlled trial. *J Clin Oncol.* 2001;19(11):2865-2874.
29. Lyman GH, Glaspy J. Are there clinical benefits with early erythropoietic intervention for chemother-apy-induced anemia? A systematic review. *Cancer.* 2006;106(1):223-233.
30. Crawford J, Cella D, Cleeland CS, et al. Relationship between changes in hemoglobin level and quality of life during chemotherapy in anemic cancer patients receiv-ing epoetin alfa therapy. *Cancer.* 2002;95(4):888-895.
31. Demetri GD, Kris M, Wade J, Degos L, Cella D. Qual-ity-of-life benefit in chemotherapy patients treated

with epoetin alfa is independent of disease response or tumor type: results from a prospective community oncology study. Procrit Study Group. *J Clin Oncol.* 1998;16(10):3412-3425.

32. Gabrilove JL, Cleeland CS, Livingston RB, Sarokhan B, Winer E, Einhorn LH. Clinical evaluation of once-weekly dosing of epoetin alfa in chemotherapy patients: improvements in hemoglobin and quality of Life are similar to three-times-weekly dosing. *J Clin Oncol.* 2001;19(11):2875-2882.

33. Macdougall IC, Gray SJ, Elston O, et al. Pharmacokinetics of novel erythropoiesis stimulating protein compared with epoetin alfa in dialysis patients. *J Am Soc Nephrol.* 1999;10(11):2392-2395.

34. Vansteenkiste J, Pirker R, Massuti B, et al. Double-blind, placebo-controlled, randomized phase III trial of darbepoetin alfa in lung cancer patients receiving chemotherapy. *J Natl Cancer Inst.* 2002;94(16):1211-1220.

35. Glaspy JA, Jadeja JS, Justice G, Fleishman A, Rossi G, Colowick AB. A randomized, active-control, pilot trial of front-loaded dosing regimens of darbepoetin-alfa for the treatment of patients with anemia during chemotherapy for malignant disease. *Cancer.* 2003;97(5):1312-1320.

36. Tonia T, Mettler A, Robert N, et al. Erythropoietin or darbepoetin for patients with cancer. *Cochrane Database Syst Rev.* 2012;(12):CD003407.

37. Bohlius J, Bohlke K, Castelli R, et al. Management of cancer-associated anemia with erythropoiesis-stimulating agents: American Society of Clinical Oncology/American Society of Hematology clinical practice guideline update. *Blood Adv.* 2019;3:1197-1210.

38. Schwartzberg LS, Yee LK, Senecal FM, et al. A randomized week darbepoetin alfa and weekly epoetin alfa for the treatment of chemotherapy-induced anemia in patients with breast, lung, or gynecologic cancer. *Oncologist.* 2004;9(6):696-707.

39. Glaspy J, Vadhan-Raj S, Patel R, et al. Randomized comparison of every-2-week darbepoetin alfa and weekly epoetin alfa for the treatment of chemotherapy-induced anemia: the 20030125 Study Group Trial. *J Clin Oncol.* 2006;24(15):2290-2297.

40. Schwartzberg L, Burkes R, Mirtsching B, et al. Comparison of darbepoetin alfa dosed weekly (QW) vs. extended dosing schedule (EDS) in the treatment of anemia in patients receiving multicycle chemotherapy in a randomized, phase 2, open-label trial. *BMC Cancer.* 2010;10:581.

41. Muller RJ, Baribeault D. Extended-dosage-interval regimens of erythropoietic agents in chemotherapy-induced anemia. *Am J Health Syst Pharm.* 2007;64(24): 2547-2556.

42. Canon JL, Vansteenkiste J, Bodoky G, et al. Randomized, double-blind, active-controlled trial of darbepoetin alfa for the treatment of chemotherapy-induced anemia. *J Natl Cancer Inst.* 2006;98(4):273-284.

43. Henke M, Laszig R, Rube C, et al. Erythropoietin to treat head and neck cancer patients with anaemia undergoing radiotherapy: randomized, double-blind, placebo-controlled trial. *Lancet.* 2003;362(9392): 1255-1260.

44. Leyland-Jones B, Semiglazov V, Pawlicki M, et al. Maintaining normal hemoglobin levels with epoetin alfa in mainly non-anemic patients with metastatic breast cancer receiving first-line chemotherapy: a survival study. *J Clin Oncol.* 2005;23(25):5960-5972.

45. Thomas G, Ali S, Hoebers FJ, et al. Phase III trial to evaluate the efficacy of maintaining hemoglobin levels above 12.0 g/dL with erythropoietin vs above 10.0 g/dL without erythropoietin in anemic patients receiving

concurrent radiation and cisplatin for cervical cancer. *Gynecol Oncol.* 2008;108(2):317-325.

46. Untch M, Fasching P, Bauerfeind I, et al. PREPARE trial: a randomized phase III trial comparing preoperative, dose-dense, dose-intensified chemotherapy with epirubicin, paclitaxel and CMF with a standard dosed epirubicin/cyclophosphamide followed by paclitaxel (+/−) darbepoetin alfa in primary breast cancer: a preplanned interim analysis of efficacy at surgery. *J Clin Oncol.* 2008;26(15):517.

47. Untch M, von Minckwitz G, Konecny GE, et al. PREPARE trial: a randomized phase III trial comparing preoperative, dose-dense, dose-intensified chemotherapy with epirubicin, paclitaxel and CMF with a standard dosed epirubicin/cyclophosphamide followed by paclitaxel with or without darbepoetin alfa in primary breast cancer—outcome on prognosis. *Ann Oncol.* 2011;22(9):1999-2006.

48. Bohlius J, Schmidlin K, Brillant C, et al. Erythropoietin or darbepoetin for patients with cancer—meta-analysis based on individual patient data. *Cochrane Database Syst Rev.* 2009;(3):CD007303.

49. Glaspy J, Crawford J, Vansteenkiste J, et al. Erythropoiesis-stimulating agents in oncology: a study-level meta-analysis of survival and other safety outcomes. *Br J Cancer.* 2010;102(2):301-315.

50. Khorana AA, Connolly GC. Assessing risk of venous thromboembolism in the patient with cancer. *J Clin Oncol.* 2009;27(29):4839-4847.

51. Seidenfeld J, Piper M, Bohlius J, et al. *Comparative Effectiveness of Epoetin and Darbepoetin for Managing Anemia in Patients Undergoing Cancer Treatment.* Rockville, MD: Agency for Healthcare Research and Quality (US); 2006.

52. Ludwig H, Crawford J, Osterbr A, et al. Pooled analysis of individual patient-level data from all randomized, double-blind, placebo-controlled trials of darbepoetin alfa in the treatment of patients with chemotherapy-induced anemia. *J Clin Oncol.* 2009;27(17):2838-2847.

53. Glaspy JA, Charu V, Luo D, Moyo V, Kamin M, Wilhelm FE. Initiation of epoetin-alpha therapy at a starting dose of 120,000 units once every 3 weeks in patients with cancer receiving chemotherapy: an open-label, multicenter study with randomized and nonrandomized treatment arms. *Cancer.* 2009;115(5):1121-1131.

54. Henry DH, Gordan LN, Charu V, et al. Randomized, open-labed comparison of epoetin alfa extended dosing (80 000 U Q2W) vs weekly dosing (40 000 U QW) in patients with chemotherapy induced anemia. *Curr Med Res Opin.* 2006;22(7):1403-1413.

55. Boccia R, Malik IA, Raja V, et al. Darbepoetin alfa administered every three weeks is effective for the treatment of chemotherapy-induced anemia. *Oncologist.* 2006;11(4):409-417.

56. Littlewood TJ, Zagari M, Pallister C, Perkins A. Baseline and early treatment factors are not clinically useful for predicting individual response to erythropoietin in anemic cancer patients. *Oncologist.* 2003;8(1):99-107.

57. US Food and Drug Administration. FDA Alert. Information for Healthcare Professionals: Erythropoiesis Stimulating Agents (ESA) [Aranesp (Darbepoetin), Epogen (Epoetin Alfa), and Procrit (Epoetin Alfa)]. https://wayback.archive-it.org/7993/20170723113601/; https://www.fda.gov/Drugs/DrugSafety/PostmarketDrugSafetyInformationforPatientsandProviders/ucm126481.htm. Accessed November 13, 2019.

58. Henry DH. Parental iron therapy in cancer-associated anemia. *Hematology Am Soc Hematol Educ Program.* 2010;2010:351-356.

59. Auerbach M, Ballard H, Trout JR, et al. Intravenous iron optimizes the response to recombinant human erythropoietin in cancer patients with chemotherapy-related anemia: a multicenter, open-label, randomized trial. *J Clin Oncol.* 2004;22(7):1301-1307.

60. Hedenus M, Birgegard G, Nasman P, et al. Addition of intravenous iron to epoetin dose requirement in anemic patients with lymphoproliferative malignancies: a randomized multicenter study. *Leukemia.* 2007;21(4): 627-632.

61. Bastit L, Vandebroek A, Altintas S, et al. Randomized, multicenter, controlled trial comparing the efficacy and safely of darbepoetin alpha administered ever 3 weeks with or without intravenous iron in patients with chemotherapy-induced anemia. *J Clin Oncol.* 2008;26(10):1611-1618.

62. Pedrazzoli P, Farris A, Del Prete S, et al. Randomized trial of intravenous iron supplementation in patients with chemotherapy-related anemia without iron deficiency treated with darbepoetin alpha. *J Clin Oncol.* 2008;26(10):1619-1625.

63. Steensma DP, Sloan JA, Dakhil SR, et al. Phase III, randomized study of the effects of parental iron, oral iron, or no iron supplementation on the erythropoietic response to darbepoetin alfa for patients with chemotherapy-associated anemia. *J Clin Oncol.* 2011;29(1):97-105.

64. Food and Drug Administration. Fatalities reported to FDA following blood collection and transfusion annual summary for fiscal year 2015. http://wayback.archive-it.org/7993/20171114162532/https://www.fda.gov/downloads/BiologicsBloodVaccines/SafetyAvailability/ReportaProblem/TransfusionDonationFatalities/UCM518148.pdf. Accessed November 12, 2019.

65. Schonewille H, Haak HL, van Zijl AM. Alloimmunization after blood transfusion in patients with hematologic and oncologic diseases. *Transfusion.* 1999;39(7): 763-771.

66. Goodnough LT, Brecher ME, Kanter MH, AuBuchon JP. Transfusion medicine. First of two parts—blood transfusion. *N Engl J Med.* 1999;340(6):438-447.

67. Zou S, Dorsey KA, Notari EP, et al. Prevalence, incidence, and residual risk of human immunodeficiency virus and hepatitis C virus infections among United States blood donors since the introduction of nucleic acid testing. *Transfusion.* 2010;50(7):1495-1504.

68. Pealer LN, Marfin AA, Petersen LR, et al. Transmission of West Nile virus through blood transfusion in the United States in 2002. *N Engl J Med.* 2003;349(13):1236-1245.

69. Magnus MM, Espósito DLA, Costa VAD, et al. Risk of Zika virus transmission by blood donations in Brazil. *Hematol Transfus Cell Ther.* 2018;40(3):250–254.

70. Brecher ME, Hay SN. Bacterial contamination of blood components. *Clin Microbiol Rev.* 2005;18(1):195-204.

71. Cherry T, Steciuk M, Reddy VV, Marques MB. Transfusion-related acute lung injury: past, present, and future. *Am J Clin Pathol.* 2008;129(2):287-297.

72. Toy P, Gajic O, Bacchetti P, et al. Transfusion-related acute lung injury: incidence and risk factors. *Blood.* 2012;119(7):1757-1767.

73. Vamvakas EC. Is white blood cell reduction equivalent to antibody screening and preventing transmission of cytomegalovirus by transfusion? A review of the literature and meta-analysis. *Transfus Med Rev.* 2005;19(3):181-199.

74. Ruhl H, Bein G, Sachs UJ. Transfusion-associated graft-versus-host disease. *Transfus Med Rev.* 2009;23(1):62-71.

75. Taplitz RA, Kennedy EB, Bow EJ, et al. Antimicrobial prophylaxis for adult patients with cancer-related immunosuppression: ASCO and IDSA clinical practice guideline update. *J Clin Oncol.* 2018;36(30):3043-3054.

76. Tai E, Guy JP, Dunbar A, Richardson LC. Cost of cancer-related neutropenia for fever hospitalizations, United States, 2012. *J Oncol Pract.* 2017;13(6):e552-e561.

77. Klastersky J, Paesmans M, Rubenstein EB, et al. The Multinational Association for Supportive Care in Cancer risk index: a multinational scoring system for identifying low-risk febrile neutropenic cancer patients. *J Clin Oncol.* 2000;18(16):3038-3051.

78. de Souza Viana L, Serufo JC, da Costa Rocha MO, Costa RN, Duarte RC. Performance of a modified MASCC index score for identifying low-risk sub brown neutropenic cancer patients. *Support Care Cancer.* 2008;16(7):841-846.

79. Talcott JA, Whalen A, Clark J, Rieker PP, Finberg R. Home antibiotic therapy for low-risk cancer patient with fever and neutropenia: a pilot study of 30 patients based on a validated prediction rule. *J Clin Oncol.* 1994;12(1):107-114.

80. Raber-Durlacher JE, Epstein JB, Raber J, et al. Peridontal infection in cancer patients treated with high-dose chemotherapy. *Support Care Cancer.* 2002;10(6):466-473.

81. Talcott JA, Yeap BY, Clark JA, et al. Safety of early discharge for low-risk patients with febrile neutropenia: a multicenter randomized controlled trial. *J Clin Oncol.* 2011;29(30):3977-3983.

82. Klastersky J, Paesmans M, Georgala A, et al. Outpatient oral antibiotics for febrile neutropenic cancer patients using a score predictive for complications. *J Clin Oncol.* 2006;24(25):4129-4134.

83. Carstensen M, Sorensen JB. Outpatient management of febrile neutropenia: time to revise the present treatment strategy. *J Support Oncol.* 2008;6(5):199-208.

84. Gafter-Gvili A, Fraser A, Paul M, Leibovici L. Meta-analysis: antibiotic prophylaxis reduces mortality in neutropenic patients. *Ann Intern Med.* 2005;142(12 pt 1):979-995.

85. Herbst C, Naumann F, Kruse EB, et al. Prophylactic antibiotics or G-CSF for the prevention of infections and improvement of survival in cancer patients undergoing chemotherapy. *Cochrane Database Syst Rev.* 2009;(1):CD007107.

86. van de Wetering MD, de Witte MA, Kremer LC, Offringa M, Scholten RJ, Caron HN. Efficacy of oral prophylactic antibiotics in neutropenic afebrile oncology patients: a systemic review of randomised controlled trials. *Eur J Cancer.* 2005;41(10):1373-1382.

87. Lyman GH, Kuderer NM, Crawford J, et al. Predicting individual risk of neutropenic complications in patients receiving cancer chemotherapy. *Cancer.* 2011;117(9):1917-1927.

88. Lyman GH, Abella E, Pettengell R. Risk factors for febrile neutropenia among patients with cancer receiving chemotherapy: a systemic review. *Crit Rev Oncol Hematol.* 2014;90(3):190-199.

89. Dees EC, O'Reilly S, Goodman SN, et al. A prospective pharmacologic evaluation of age-related toxicity of adjuvant chemotherapy in women with breast cancer. *Cancer Invest.* 2000;18(6):521-529.

90. Lyman GH, Morrison VA, Dale DC, Crawford J, Delgado DJ, Fridman M. Risk of febrile neutropenia among patients with intermediate-grade non-Hodgkin's lymphoma receiving CHOP chemotherapy. *Leuk Lymphoma.* 2003;44(12):2069-2076.

91. Jenkins P, Freeman S. Pretreatment haematological laboratory values predict for excessive myelosuppression in patients receiving adjuvant FEC chemotherapy for breast cancer. *Ann Oncol.* 2009;20(1):34-40.

92. Matter-Walstra KW, Dedes KJ, Schwenkglenks M, Brauchli P, Szucs TD, Pestalozzi BC. Trastuzumab beyond progression: a cost-utility analysis. *Ann Oncol.* 2010;21(11):2161-2168.

93. Aapro M, Crawford J, Kamioner D. Prophylaxis of che-motherapy-introduced febrile neutropenia with gran-ulocyte colony-stimulating factors: where are we now? *Support Care Cancer.* 2010;18(5):529-541.

94. Ziepert M, Schmits R, Trumper L, Pfreundschuh M, Loeffler M. Prognostic factors for hematotoxicity of chemotherapy in aggressive non-Hodgkin's lym-phoma. *Ann Oncol.* 2008;19(4):752-762.

95. Pettengell R, Bosly A, Szucs TD, et al. Multivariate analysis of febrile neutropenia occurrence in patients with non-Hodgkin lymphoma: data from the INC-EU Prospective Observational European Neutropenia Study. *Br J Haematol.* 2009;144(5):677-685.

96. Bensinger WI, Price TH, Dale DC, et al. The effects of daily recombinant human granulocyte colony-stimulating factor administration on normal gran-ulocyte donors undergoing leukapheresis. *Blood.* 1993;81(7):1883-1888.

97. Holmes FA, Jones SE, O'Shaughnessy J, et al. Com-parable efficacy and safety profiles once-per-cycle pegfilgrastim and daily injection filgrastim in che-motherapy-induced neutropenia: a multicenter dose-finding study in women with breast cancer. *Ann Oncol.* 2002;13(6):903-909.

98. Crawford J, Ozer H, Stoller R, et al. Reduction by gran-ulocyte colony-stimulating factor of fever and neu-tropenia induced by chemotherapy and patients with small-cell lung cancer. *N Engl J Med.* 1991;325(3):164-170.

99. Trillet-Lenoir V, Arpin D, Brune J. Optimal deliv-ery of dose in cancer chemotherapy with the sup-port of haematopoietic growth factors. *Eur J Cancer.* 1993;29A(suppl 5):S14-S16.

100. Holmes FA, O'Shaughnessy JA, Vukelja S, et al. Blinded, randomized, multicenter study to evaluate single administration pegfilgrastim once per cycle ver-sus daily filgrastim as an adjunct to chemotherapy in patients with high-risk stage II or stage III/IV breast cancer. *J Clin Oncol.* 2002;20(3):727-731.

101. Green MD, Koelbl H, Baselga J, et al. A randomized double-blind multicenter phase III study of fixed-dose single administration pegfilgrastim versus daily fil-grastim in patients receiving myelosuppressive che-motherapy. *Ann Oncol.* 2003;14(1):29-35.

102. Vogel CL, Wojtukiewicz MZ, Carroll RR, et al. First and subsequent cycle use of pegfilgrastim prevents febrile neutropenia in patients with breast cancer: a multicenter, double-blind, placebo-controlled phase III study. *J Clin Oncol.* 2005;23(6):1178-1184.

103. Kuderer NM, Dale DC, Crawford J, Lyman GH. Impact of primary prophylaxis with granulocyte colony-stim-ulating factor on febrile neutropenia and mortality in adult cancer patients receiving chemotherapy: a sys-temic review. *J Clin Oncol.* 2007;25(21):3158-3167.

104. Lyman GH, Dale DC, Wolff DA, et al. Acute myeloid leukemia or myelodysplastic syndrome in random-ized controlled clinical trials of cancer chemotherapy with granulocyte colony-stimulating factor: a systemic review. *J Clin Oncol.* 2010;28(17):2914-2924.

105. Smith TJ, Bohlke K, Lyman GH, et al. Recommenda-tions for the use of WBC growth factors: American Society of Clinical Oncology clinical practice guide-lines update. *J Clin Oncol.* 2015;33(28):3199-3212.

106. Aapro MS, Bohlius J, Cameron DA, et al. 2010 update of EORTC guidelines for the use of granulocytes-colony stimulating factor to reduce the incidence of chemotherapy-induced febrile neutropenia in adult patients with lymphoproliferative disorders and solid tumours. *Eur J Cancer.* 2011;47(1):8-32.

107. Kwak LW, Halpern J, Olshen RA, Horning SJ. Prognos-tic significance of actual dose intensity in diffuse large-cell lymphoma: results of a tree-structured survival analysis. *J Clin Oncol.* 1990;8(6):963-977.

108. Budman DR, Berry DA, Cirrincione CT, et al. Dose and dose intensity as determinants of outcome in the adjuvant treatment of breast cancer. The Cancer and Leukemia Group B. *J Natl Cancer Inst.* 1998;90(16):1205-1211.

109. Link BK, Budd GT, Scott S, et al. Delivering adju-vant chemotherapy to women with early-stage breast carcinoma: current patterns of care. *Cancer.* 2001;92(6):1354-1367.

110. Papaldo P, Lopez M, Marolla P, et al. Impact of five pro-phylactic filgrastim schedules on hematologic toxicity in early breast cancer patients treated with epirubi-cin and cyclophosphamide. *J Clin Oncol.* 2005;23(28):6908-6918.

111. Nabholtz JM, Cantin J, Chang J, et al. Phase III trial comparing granulocyte colony-stimulating factor to leridistim in the prevention of neutropenic complica-tions in breast cancer patients treated with docetaxel/doxorubicin/cyclophosphamide: results of the BCIRG 004 trial. *Clin Breast Cancer.* 2002;3(4):268-275.

112. Burris HA, Belani CP, Kaufman PA, et al. Pegfilgrastim on the same day versus next day of chemotherapy in patients with breast cancer, non-small-cell lung cancer, ovarian cancer, and non-Hodgkin's lymphoma: results of four multicenter, double-blind randomized phase II studies. *J Oncol Pract.* 2010;6(3):133-140.

113. Skarlos DV, Timotheadou E, Galani E, et al. Pegfilgras-tim administered on the same day with dose-dense adjuvant chemotherapy for breast cancer is associated with a higher incidence of febrile neutropenia as com-pared to conventional growth factor support: match case-control study of the Hellenic Cooperative Oncol-ogy Group. *Oncology.* 2009;77(2):107-112.

114. Dale DC. Advances in the treatment of neutropenia. *Curr Opin Support Palliat Care.* 2009;3(3):207-212.

115. Crawford J, Dale DC, Kuderer NM, et al. Risk and timing of neutropenic events in adult cancer patients receiving chemotherapy: the results of a prospective nationwide study of oncology practice. *J Natl Compr Canc Netw.* 2008;6(2):109-118.

116. Garcia-Carbonero R, Mayordomo JI, Tornamira MV, et al. Granulocyte colony-stimulating factor in the treatment of high-risk febrile neutropenia: a multi-center randomized trial. *J Natl Cancer Inst.* 2001;93(1):31-38.

117. Moore DC, Pellegrino AE. Pegfilgrastim-induced bone pain: a review on incidence, risk factors, and evidence-based management. *Ann Pharmacother.* 2017;51(9):797-803.

118. Gavoli E, Abrams M. Prevention of granulocyte-col-ony stimulating factor (G-CSF) induced bone pain using double histamine blockade. *Support Care Can-cer.* 2017;25(3):817-822.

119. Pinto L, Liu Z, Doan Q, Bernal M, Dubois R, Lyman G. Comparison of pegfilgrastim with filgrastim on febrile neutropenia grade IV neutropenia and bone pain: a meta-analysis of randomized controlled trials. *Curr Med Res Opin.* 2007;23(9):2283-2295.

120. Fitzhugh CD, Hsieh MM, Bolan CD, Saenz C, Tisdale JF. Granulocyte colony-stimulating factor (G-CSF) administration in individuals with sickle cell dis-ease: time for moratorium? *Cryotherapy.* 2009;11(4):464-471.

121. Keegan T, Heaton A, Holme S, Owens M, Nelson E, Carmen R. Paired comparison of platelet concentrates

prepared from platelet-rich plasma and buffy coats using a new technique with ^{111}IN and ^{51}Cr. *Transfusion.* 1992;32(3):113-120.

122. Cardigan R, Williamson LM. The quality of platelets after storage for 7 days. *Transfus Med.* 2003;13(4):173-187.

123. Chambers LA, Herman JH. Considerations in the selection of a platelet component: apheresis versus whole blood-derived. *Transfus Med Rev.* 1999;13(4):311-322.

124. Schiffer CA, Bohlke K, Delaney M, et al. Platelet transfusion for patients with cancer: American Society of clinical oncology clinical practice guidelines update. *J Clin Oncol.* 2018;36(3):283-299.

125. Wandt H, Frank M, Ehninger G, et al. Safety and cost-effectiveness of a 10 × 10(9)/L trigger for prophylactic platelet transfusions compared with the traditional 20 × 10(9)/L trigger: a prospective comparative trial in 105 patients with acute myeloid leukemia. *Blood.* 1998;91(10):3601-3606.

126. Rebulla P, Finazzi G, Marangoni F, et al. The threshold for prophylactic platelet transfusions in adults with acute myeloid leukemia. Gruppo Italiano Malattie Ematologiche Maligne dell'Adulto. *N Engl J Med.* 1997;337(26):1870-1875.

127. Heddle NM, Cook RJ, Sigouin C, Slichter SJ, Murphy M, Rebulla P. A descriptive analysis of international transfusion practice and bleeding outcomes in patients with acute leukemia. *Transfusion.* 2006;46(6):903-911.

128. Leukocyte reduction and ultraviolet B irradiation of platelets to prevent alloimmunization and refractoriness to platelet transfusions. The Trial to Reduce Alloimmunization to Platelets Study Group. *N Engl J Med.* 1997;337(26):1861-1869.

129. Slichter SJ. Evidence-based platelet transfusion guidelines. *Hematology Am Soc Hematol Educ Program.* 2007;172-178.

130. Delaflor-Weiss E, Mintz PD. The evaluation and management of platelet refractoriness and alloimmunization. *Transfus Med Rev.* 2002;14(2):180-196.

131. Vadhan-Raj S. Management of chemotherapy-induced thrombocytopenia: current status of thrombopoietic agents. *Semin Hematol.* 2009;46(1 suppl 2):S26-S32.

132. Tepler I, Elias L, Smith JW II, et al. A randomized placebo-controlled trial of recombinant human interleukin-11 in cancer patients with severe thrombocytopenia due to chemotherapy. *Blood.* 1996;87(9):3607-3614.

133. Al-Samkari H, Kuter D. Optimal use of thrombopoietin receptor agonists in immune thrombocytopenia. *Ther Adv Hematol.* 2019;10:1-13.

134. GlaxoSmithKline. Promacta (eltrombopag) [package insert]. U.S. Food and Drug Administration website. https://www.accessdata.fda.gov/drugsatfda_docs/label/2011/022291s006lbl.pdf. Revised December 2011. Accessed November 11, 2019.

135. Bussel J, Arnold D, Grossbard E, et al. Fostamatinib for the treatment of adult persistent and chronic immune thrombocytopenia: results of two phase 3, randomized placebo-controlled trials. *Am J Hematol.* 2018;93(7):921-930.

136. Rigel Pharmaceuticals, Inc. Tavalisse (fostamatinib) [package insert]. U.S. Food and Drug Administration website; 2018. https://www.accessdata.fda.gov/drugsatfda_docs/label/2018/209299lbl.pdf. Accessed November 11, 2019.

137. Davis E, Salem J, Young A, et al. Hematologic complications of immune checkpoint inhibitors. *Oncologist.* 2019;24(5):584-588.

138. Sui J, Wang Y, Wan Y, Wu Y. Risk of hematological toxicities with programmed cell death-1 inhibitors in cancer patients: a meta-analysis of current studies. *Drug Des Devel Ther.* 2018;12:1645-1657.

139. Michot J, Lazarovici J, Tieu A, et al. Haematological immune-related adverse events with immune checkpoint inhibitors, how to manage? *Eur J Cancer.* 2019;122:72-90.

140. Brahmer J, Lacchetti C, Schneider B, et al. Management of immune-related adverse events in patients treated with immune checkpoint inhibitor therapy: American Society of Clinical Oncology Clinical Practice Guidelines. *J Clin Oncol.* 2018;36(17):1714-1768.

141. Delanoy N, Michot JM, Comont T, et al. Haematological immune-related adverse events induced by anti-PD-1 or anti-PD-L1 immunotherapy: a descriptive observational study. *Lancet Haematol.* 2019;6(1):e48-e57.

142. Naqash A, Ebenezer A, Yang L, et al. Isolated neutropenia as a rare but serious adverse event secondary to immune checkpoint inhibition. *J Immunother Cancer.* 2019;7:169. doi: 10.1186/s40425-019-0648-3.

143. Prasad V, De Jesús K, Mailankody S. The high price of anticancer drugs: origins, implications, barriers, solutions. *Nat Rev Clin Oncol.* 2017;14:381-390.

144. US Food and Drug Administration. Biosimilar product regulatory review and approval. https://www.fda.gov/media/108621/download. Accessed August 8, 2019.

145. Kerkhofs L, Boschetti G, Lugini A, Stanculeanu D, Paloma A. Use of biosimilar epoetin to increase hemoglobin levels in patients with chemotherapy-induced anemia: real-life experience. *Future Oncol.* 2012;8(6):751-756.

146. Michallet M, Luporsi E, Soubeyran P, et al. BiOsimilars in the management of anaemia secondary to chemotherapy in HaEmatology and Oncology: results of the ORHEO observational study. *BMC Cancer.* 2014;14(1):503.

147. Aapro M, Krendyukov A, Schiestl M, Gascon P. Epoetin biosimilars in the treatment of chemotherapy-induced anemia: 10 years' experience gained. *BioDrugs.* 2018;32(2):129-135.

148. Gascón P, Krendyukov A, Mathieson N, Natek M, Aapro M. Extrapolation in practice: lessons from 10 years with biosimilar filgrastim. *BioDrugs.* 2019;33(6):635-645. doi: 10.1007/s40259-019-00373-2.

149. Harbeck N, Gascón P, Krendyukov A, Hoebel N, Gattu S, Blackwell K. Safety profile of biosimilar filgrastim (Zarzio/Zarxio): a combined analysis of phase III studies. *Oncologist.* 2018;23(4):403-409.

150. Aapro M, Comes P, Sun D, Abraham I. Comparative cost efficiency across the European G5 countries of originators and a biosimilar erythropoiesis-stimulating agent to manage chemotherapy-induced anemia in patients with cancer. *Ther Adv Med Oncol.* 2012;4(3):95-105.

151. Blackwell K, Gascón P, Krendyukov A, et al. Safety and efficacy of alternating treatment with EP2006, a filgrastim biosimilar, and reference filgrastim: a phase 3, randomised, double-blind clinical study in the prevention of severe neutropenia in patients with breast cancer receiving myelosuppressive chemotherapy. *Ann Oncol.* 2018;29(1):244-249.

152. Gascón P, Aapro M, Ludwig H, et al. Treatment patterns and outcomes in the prophylaxis of chemotherapy-induced (febrile) neutropenia with biosimilar filgrastim (the MONITOR-GCSF study). *Support Care Cancer.* 2016;24(2):911–925.

153. Schwartzberg L, Lal L, Balu S, et al. Clinical outcomes of treatment with filgrastim versus a filgrastim biosimilar and febrile neutropenia-associated costs among patients with nonmyeloid cancer undergoing chemotherapy. *J Manag Care Spec Pharm.* 2018;24(10):976-984.

154. Botteri E, Krendyukov A, Curigliano G. Comparing granulocyte colony-stimulating factor filgrastim and pegfilgrastim to its biosimilars in terms of efficacy and safety: a meta-analysis of randomised clinical trials in breast cancer patients. *Eur J Cancer*. 2018;89:49-55.

155. US Food and Drug Administration. Biosimilar product information. https://www.fda.gov/drugs/biosimilars/biosimilar-product-information. Accessed August 8, 2019.

156. Yang J, Yu S, Yang Z, et al. Efficacy and safety of supportive care biosimilars among cancer patients: a systemic review and meta-analysis. *BioDrugs*. 2019;33(4):373-389.

157. Lyman G, Balaban E, Diaz M, et al. American Society of Clinical Oncology statement: biosimilars in oncology. *J Clin Oncol*. 2018;36(12):1260-1265.

53 Issues in Nutrition and Hydration

Elizabeth Kvale and Christine S. Ritchie

The issues surrounding artificial nutrition and hydration (ANH) pose challenges for clinicians, patients, families, and society. Legal precedent and ethical principles guide medical practice; yet with regard to critical questions in this area, our scientific base for establishing benefit or harm is inadequate to provide guidance that is fully evidence based. Two recent *Cochrane Reviews* evaluated the use of ANH in palliative populations, including the terminal and dying phases of illness. It concluded that the evidence base is insufficient to make any recommendation for practice with regard to the use of ANH in patients receiving palliative care (1,2). Decisions regarding the use of hydration and nutrition in palliative care often boil down to an honest if imperfect discussion of the potential harm and benefit of nutrition and hydration in a particular setting, filtered through the values of each patient and their family. This chapter reviews some of the elements to consider in such a discussion, including the historic context of artificial hydration and nutrition, the legal and ethical framework for decision-making, and a review of the evidence base related to the benefits and potential harms of ANH.

WHAT IS NUTRITION AND HYDRATION?

Definitions

Artificial hydration is the provision of water or electrolyte solutions through any nonoral route. *Artificial nutrition* includes total parenteral nutrition (TPN) and enteral nutrition (EN) by nasogastric tube (NGT), percutaneous endoscopic gastrostomy (PEG) tube, percutaneous endoscopic gastrostomy jejunostomy (PEG-J) tube, gastrostomy tube, or gastrojejunostomy tube.

History

In the 1920s, continuous infusion of IV glucose was introduced in humans. It was not until the 1960s that parenteral nutrition was used, first in seriously ill adult surgical patients and then in children and adults with short bowel syndrome (3). These children, who before these therapies died of starvation, were able to live for years, sustained

with artificial nutrition. Parenteral nutrition use then expanded to many other patient populations, often without clear or well-established indications. Only in the last decade has some light been shed in critical care settings as to when TPN is beneficial and when it may be more harmful (4,5).

In the late 1970s, gastrostomies began to be performed and were often used for swallowing problems in children (6). Their use became widely generalized to adults such that EN is now commonly used among patients with stroke, neurologic disease, and cancer (7). Between 1988 and 1995, the number of tubes placed in the United States doubled; in 2000, more than 216,000 tubes were placed. Recent data from Veterans Administration (VA) and Medicare database reviews suggest a stabilization of this trend in some settings (Fig. 53.1).

Whereas IV hydration is a well-established part of medical practice, its role in end-of-life care remains less clear. Intravenous hydration is often used for the treatment of terminal delirium and agitation. Whether it is beneficial, and if so, for what outcomes and at what rate of infusion, remains an area of controversy.

ETHICAL AND LEGAL FRAMEWORK

Nutrition and hydration decisions may be more difficult for some families than ventilator support or cardiac resuscitation. Families may equate foregoing of artificial nutrition with starvation. The potential harms associated with artificial nutrition (such as restraint use, immobility, and decreased social contact) are often not considered. Because of the dearth of good scientific data to assist clinicians in addressing whether or not artificial nutrition has meaningful benefit, it is often difficult to provide guidance to patients' families.

In medicine, ethical principles guide how a patient should be treated or how a treatment dilemma should be handled. The ethical principle of *autonomy* states that a person should have the ability to govern oneself. This principle was applied in the court decisions of Barber in 1983, Bouvia in 1986, and Cruzan in 1990, all of which stated that competent adults should be the final arbiters of

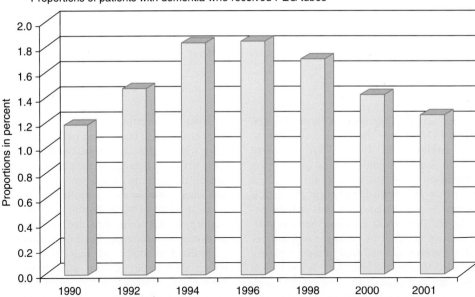

Figure 53.1 Time trends in the use of percutaneous endoscopic gastrostomy (PEG) tube feeding: proportion of demented patients in the administrative database of the Veterans Health Administration shown as percentage of total number of demented patients. A decreasing trend since 1996 is identified.

decisions regarding their own health care. If nutritional support is unwanted, then providing artificial nutrition does not adhere to the principle of *autonomy* and lessens patient dignity. *Beneficence* is the ethical principle that states that physicians should always provide care that benefits the patient. In the case of artificial nutrition, the physician needs to ask if the artificial nutrition is actually "doing good" for their patient. The principle of *nonmaleficence* addresses the complimentary principle that one should "do no harm"—primum non nocere. In the case of ANH, physicians must weigh the potential for this medical treatment to harm their patient in any way. If ANH were contributing to more harm than benefit, then the principle of *nonmaleficence* would support its discontinuation (Fig. 53.2).

The argument for the discontinuation of nutritional support states that ANH are indistinguishable from other medical treatments. In the 1990 Cruzan decision, the US Supreme Court stated that "the law does not distinguish artificial feeding from other forms of medical treatment" (8). The right of patients to refuse this treatment is supported, and within this framework, artificial nutrition is considered medical intervention and not basic care. Withdrawing artificial nutritional support and allowing a patient to die is *not* considered equivalent to euthanasia. In the former instance, the goal of discontinuing therapy is to remove burdensome

interventions; in the latter, the intended result is the death of the patient. Nevertheless, as demonstrated by the Schiavo case, public acceptance of these distinguishing features in nutritional support varies greatly. Furthermore, some faith communities take issue with the distinction between artificial and basic nutrition (proposition 52).

In addition, much legal confusion persists because advance directive statutes may make it more difficult for a person capable of making decisions to prospectively forego ANH and many state statutes are poorly written and confusing (9).

INDICATIONS

No clear palliative indications exist for artificial nutrition. The American Gastroenterological Association (AGA) endorses PEG tube placement for prolonged tube feeding (specifically more than 30 days) and nasogastric feeding when enteral feeding is required for shorter periods (Table 53.1). In practice, PEG tubes are placed for a variety of different clinical conditions, including dysphagia, prolonged illness, anorexia, neurologic/psychiatric disorders, oropharyngeal or esophageal disorders or cancers, or increased nutritional needs that the patient is unable to meet with oral intake. Studies show that neurologic illnesses (e.g., dysphagia following stroke and dementia), cancer (obstruction secondary to tumor, postradiation, postchemotherapy, or postresection),

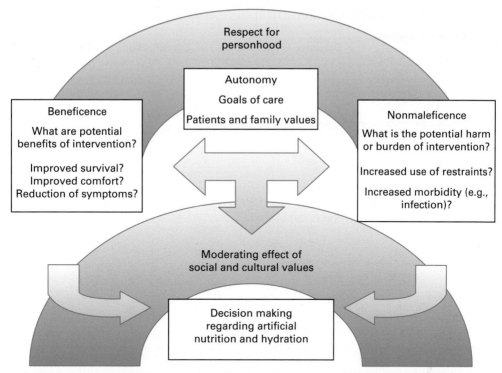

Figure 53.2 Integration of ethical principles into decision-making regarding artificial nutrition and hydration.

and the prevention of aspiration account for most placements (10–12).

Indications for artificial hydration are relatively straightforward in critical care settings or when an otherwise healthy patient presents with volume depletion. Indications for hydration at the end of life have not been established. In the acute care setting, parenteral hydration is routinely given. In the hospice setting, parenteral hydration is not routine but may be considered in instances where the patient is experiencing neuropsychiatric symptoms such as delirium, myoclonus, and agitation.

With regard to ANH, the scientific literature lacks high-quality randomized trials that might yield clear indications to guide practice. Benefits and harms are often gleaned from imperfect evidence from heterogeneous populations.

TABLE 53.1 AMERICAN GASTROENTEROLOGICAL ASSOCIATION GUIDELINES ON ENTERAL FEEDING

- The patient cannot or will not eat
- The gut is functional
- The patient can tolerate the placement of the device[a]

[a]From American Gastroenterological Association. American Gastroenterological Association medical position statement: guidelines for the use of enteral nutrition. *Gastroenterology.* 1995;108:1280-1301.

POTENTIAL BENEFIT OF ARTIFICIAL NUTRITION

Common rationale for use of artificial nutrition includes improved survival, comfort, reduction or healing in pressure ulcers, and reduction in aspiration. Although most of the studies performed to date are compromised by substantial methodological problems, none have consistently demonstrated improved outcomes in these arenas with the exceptions of improved survival for short bowel syndrome, decreased hepatic encephalopathy in alcoholic cirrhosis, decreased length of hospital stay in hip fracture patients, and decreased postoperative complications of patients with gastric cancer given artificial nutrition preoperatively (13,14). Although no controlled trials exist, follow-up studies suggest increased survival of patients in persistent vegetative state who are likely to die within weeks without artificial nutrition, but they may live for many years with artificial nutrition (15). There is also moderately strong evidence that artificial nutrition can prolong life when it is used in short-term critical care (16). A summary of the levels of evidence for benefit from artificial nutrition is given in Tables 53.2 and 53.3.

Survival

A number of retrospective studies and a few prospective studies have been performed in patients to

TABLE 53.2 LEVELS OF EVIDENCE FOR ARTIFICIAL NUTRITION

Population/type of artificial nutrition	Outcome	Classification	Level of evidence
Stroke			
PEG vs. NG tube	Improved albumin/weight	IIa	B1
PEG vs. NG tube/oral feeding	Survival	IIb	B1
Acquired immunodeficiency syndrome			
TPN in advanced disease	Increased weight	IIa	B1
TPN in advanced disease	Survival	IIb	B1
Cancer			
TPN	During chemotherapy	III	B1
Prophylactic enteral nutrition[a] before treatment in head and neck cancer	Weight stabilization	IIa	B2
Enteral nutrition before surgery	Gastrointestinal cancer	IIa	A
Dementia			
Enteral nutrition	Survival	III	B2
Enteral nutrition	Aspiration	III	B2
Enteral nutrition	Pressure sores	IIb	C

[a]Enteral nutrition includes NG, gastrostomy, and PEG tube feeding.
PEG, percutaneous endoscopic gastrostomy; NG, nasogastric; TPN, total parenteral nutrition.

ascertain survival benefit in patients receiving artificial nutrition. The largest study to date was a retrospective review by Grant et al. of 81,105 Medicare beneficiaries who received gastrostomies in 1991. No comparison group was identified for this study. Cerebrovascular disease, neoplasms, fluid and electrolyte disorders, and aspiration pneumonia were the most common primary diagnoses. The mortality

TABLE 53.3 RECOMMENDATION CLASSIFICATIONS AND LEVELS OF EVIDENCE

Classification

Class I: Intervention is useful and effective

Class IIa: Weight of evidence/opinion is in favor of usefulness/efficacy

Class IIb: Usefulness/efficacy less well established by evidence/opinion

Class III: Intervention is not useful/effective and may be harmful

Level of evidence

A: Sufficient evidence from multiple randomized trials

B: Limited evidence from

  1. Single, randomized trial or

  2. Other nonrandomized studies

C: Based on expert opinion, case studies, or standard of care

rate at 1 and 3 years was 63.0% to 81.3%. The median survival was 28.9 weeks for women and 17.6 weeks for men. At 30 days, primary diagnoses of malnutrition and fluid and electrolyte disorders and secondary diagnoses of swallowing disorders, dementia, or cerebrovascular disease were characterized by the *lowest* mortality rates. Thirty-day mortality rates were *highest* among those with primary diagnoses of nonaspiration pneumonia or influenza and secondary diagnoses of congestive heart failure or any neoplasm (12). Rabeneck et al. studied 7,369 patients receiving PEG tubes at VA facilities between 1990 and 1992. In this retrospective cohort study, 23.5% died during their index hospitalization. The median survival of the full cohort was 7.5 months from the time of tube placement. The overall mortality rates at 1, 2, and 3 years were 59%, 71%, and 77%, respectively. The highest mortality rates were observed for patients with lung or pleural cancer (46.4%), followed by esophageal cancer (20.8%) and head and neck cancer (18.8%) (17). Survival decreased with increasing age. The median survival across clinical diagnostic categories was 13.9 months for cerebrovascular disease, 13.4 months for other organic neurologic diseases, 9.6 months for nutritional deficiency, 8.0 months for head and neck cancer, and 4 or fewer months for all other cancers. Among 674 older (age > 50 years) adults referred to a community gastroenterology group for PEG insertion over a 10-year period, mortality rates at 1, 2, and 3 years were 54.3%, 73.2%, and 84.5%, respectively. Like Rabeneck's study, the overall median survival was between 6 months and 1 year; however, those receiving tube feeding in this cohort were much more likely to be patients with stroke or other neurologic conditions. Very few of the PEGs were placed in patients with cancer. Risk factors for mortality in this cohort were being male, having feeding difficulty, having diabetes, being referred from a hospital, and being 80 years of age or greater (18). Similar to Grant's cohort, dementia was *not* an independent risk factor for decreased survival. Because these studies used large databases, identification of truly comparable control groups would have been challenging. Nevertheless, because there was no comparable control group, the impact of gastrostomies on survival could not be ascertained.

Comfort

The small body of literature evaluating the patient symptoms at the end of life suggests a relatively low prevalence of hunger (19). In McCann's study of 32 patients in a comfort care unit, 63% denied hunger entirely, while 34% reported hunger during the first quarter of their course in the unit. In all patients reporting either hunger or thirst, these symptoms were consistently and completely relieved by oral care or the ingestion of small amounts of food and fluid. In a case study of a patient refusing nutrition and hydration, the patient experienced no discomfort and died peacefully (19). A survey of Oregon hospice nurses found that among those who had cared for patients who declined nutrition and hydration, the majority reported the ensuing death to be peaceful (20).

Studies of healthy volunteers engaged in fasting report resolution of hunger in 24 hours. The resulting ketosis is associated with the relief of hunger and a mild euphoria. Animal studies suggest that ketosis may also have a mild analgesic effect. When ketosis is minimized by small feedings, hunger may persist (21).

Reduction in Pressure Ulcers

There is some evidence that malnutrition is positively correlated with pressure ulcer incidence and severity (22,23). However, only two nutrition intervention studies for pressure ulcer prevention or treatment included artificial nutrition. Hartgrink et al. performed a randomized controlled trial (RCT) of 140 patients with fracture of the hip and an increased pressure ulcer risk. The intervention group was treated with a standard hospital diet and an additional NGT feeding administered overnight. The comparison group received the standard hospital diet alone (24). No significant difference was found between the groups. Ohura

et al. utilized artificial nutrition in a trial that enrolled 60 tube-fed patients. The treatment comparison, however, was protein and micronutrient intake, not tube feeding (25). Thus, while it is not possible to draw any firm conclusions on the effect of enteral and parenteral nutrition on the prevention and treatment of pressure ulcers, there is growing evidence that disease-specific nutrition support may offer benefit with regard to pressure ulcer incidence and healing (26).

Reduction in Aspiration Rates

In prospective studies of EN, aspiration pneumonia is not demonstrably decreased. Progression of aspiration to pneumonia is difficult to predict and is influenced by a number of factors, including decreased level of alertness, prolonged supine position, and colonization of the oropharynx (27). Tube feeding is a risk factor for the development of aspiration pneumonia among nursing home residents (odds ratio 3.0) (28). A recent meta-analysis suggests that small bowel feeding reduces the frequency of aspiration pneumonia compared with intragastric feeding in critical care settings (29).

POTENTIAL HARM

Complications

Complications from nasal intubation can include pharyngeal or esophageal perforation and accidental bronchial insertion. Approximately 25% of NGTs "fall out" or are pulled out by patients soon after insertion; fine bore tubes can be displaced by coughing or vomiting. Immediate complications of percutaneous gastrostomy and jejunostomy tubes include abdominal wall or intraperitoneal bleeding and bowel perforation (30). Significant surgical intervention is needed in fewer than 5% of cases. Postinsertion tube–related complications from percutaneous gastrostomy and jejunostomy tubes include infection at the insertion site, peristomal leaks, accidental tube removal, peritonitis, sepsis, and necrotizing fasciitis.

Restraints

Families are often unaware that patients with PEG tubes may require restraints (31). In Peck's study of nursing home residents with dementia, those receiving EN were more likely to be restrained (71%) than those who were not (56%) (32). When a select cohort of nursing home residents were asked, a third stated that they would prefer tube feeds if they were unable to eat. But 25% then declined when they were informed that restraints are sometimes applied during the feeding process.

Social Isolation

Patients fed enterally may be given fewer opportunities to taste food or experience the social interaction that can occur at mealtimes. They may experience sensory deprivation and social isolation if feeding comprises simply hanging a bag of nutrients on a pole for delivery through a tube. Hand-feeding, though more labor intensive than EN, enhances the dietary impact of feeding through touch, social engagement, and nurturing interactions.

CONDITIONS FOR WHICH ARTIFICIAL NUTRITION IS OFTEN CONSIDERED

Stroke

Two randomized studies of stroke patients with dysphagia who received PEG tube feeds showed improvement in albumin and weight gain at 6 weeks follow-up (33,34). Norton et al. performed a prospective randomized comparison of PEG versus NGT feeding after acute dysphagic stroke (33). Thirty patients with persisting dysphagia 14 days after acute stroke were randomly assigned to PEG (16 patients) versus NGT feeding (14 patients). Mortality at 6 weeks was significantly lower in the PEG group, with two deaths compared with eight deaths in the NGT group. Patients with PEG were more likely to have received the total amount of prescribed feeding and showed statistically greater improvement in nutritional state as well as discharge rate at 6 weeks. The comparison groups for both of these studies were patients receiving NGT feeding, not oral feeding. A meta-analysis of the three completed trials comparing PEG and NGTs estimated that the odds ratio for death is 0.88 (95% confidence interval [CI], 0.59-1.33) in favor of PEG. This value is not significant; CIs were wide and included the possibility of a large advantage or disadvantage with respect to survival for PEG over nasogastric feeding.

More recently, Iizuka and Reding performed a case-matched control of PEG versus no-PEG for 193 PEG patients. Controls were matched to the greatest extent possible on (from highest to lowest priority):

1. Sex
2. Duration from onset to stroke unit admission (interval poststroke)
3. Functional status on admission
4. Age
5. Diagnosis (ischemic vs. hemorrhagic)
6. Year of admission

No significant differences were found between the two groups except for functional status, which was significantly lower for the PEG group. There

was a 4.7-fold greater frequency of death in the PEG group. Medical complications (pneumonia, cardiac events, and stroke progression) were also greater in this group. Both groups, however, showed a similar frequency of home discharge for survivors (35).

The largest controlled trials in stroke patients are the Feed or Ordinary Diet (FOOD) trials, which consisted of two trials for dysphagic stroke patients. In one trial, patients enrolled within 7 days of admission were randomly allocated to early enteral tube feeding or no tube feeding for more than 7 days (early vs. avoid). In the other, patients were assigned to PEG or nasogastric feeding. In the early versus avoid trial, early tube feeding was associated with a nonsignificant reduction in absolute risk of death of 5.8% (95% CI, 0.8-12.5; $p = 0.09$). There was no increase in pneumonia associated with early tube feeding; however, the improved survival was offset by a 4.7% excess of survivors with a poor outcome, with a worse quality of life. Thus, early feeding might have kept patients alive in a severely disabled state when they would otherwise have died. This finding is reinforced by a study utilizing data from the Centers for Medicare and Medicaid Services that evaluated outcomes related to PEG tube placement among 31,301 patients discharged with acute ischemic stroke. This study identified no association between PEG placement and mortality at 30 days; however, at 1 year, PEG patients had a 2.59-fold greater mortality hazard (95% CI, 2.38-2.82) (36). In the PEG versus nasogastric trial, PEG feeding was associated with a nonsignificant increase in the absolute risk of death of 1.0% (37).

End-Stage Acquired Immunodeficiency Syndrome

Retrospective and prospective observational studies have reported conflicting results regarding the impact of TPN or EN on body weight and body composition in patients with human immunodeficiency virus infections. In a 2-month RCT of 31 malnourished and severely immunodepressed acquired immunodeficiency syndrome patients, subjects were assigned to receive either dietary counseling ($n = 15$) or home TPN ($n = 16$). Body-weight increased by 8 kg in the TPN group and decreased by 3 kg in the control group ($p < 0.0006$). Lean body mass increased in the TPN group and decreased in the control group ($p < 0.004$). However, no difference in survival rate was noted. Quality of life in this trial was measured with a self-assessed "subjective health feeling" that demonstrated improvement in 83% of participants in the intervention arm, while 91% of participants in the control group reported feeling worse. Karnofsky scores stabilized in the intervention group and decreased in the control group (−12%), though this change was only statistically significant at one-time point (38). Other studies of TPN have also demonstrated increases in lean body mass and body weight, but only in patients who do not have a systemic infection (39).

Cancer

TPN and EN cancer–randomized studies in patients with a variety of tumors and therapies have generated inconsistent results. In a meta-analysis of 28 prospective RCTs evaluating the use of TPN in patients with cancer, TPN was found to be possibly useful when used preoperatively in patients with gastrointestinal tract cancer. It appeared to be beneficial in reducing major surgical complications and operative mortality, but it increased risk of infection. No statistically significant benefit from TPN could be demonstrated in survival, treatment tolerance, treatment toxicity, or tumor response in patients receiving chemotherapy or radiotherapy (40). A meta-analysis of patients receiving TPN during chemotherapy failed to demonstrate any clinical benefit (41). The poor outcomes observed in these trials culminated in a consensus statement from the American College of Physicians. This statement advised that the routine use of parenteral nutrition should be discouraged in patients undergoing chemotherapy and that when it is used in patients with cancer with malnutrition, physicians should consider the possibility of increased risk (42). This statement and the clinical trials that led to its issuance have curbed the use of TPN in the United States in patients with metastatic, incurable disease. However, subsequent studies evaluating TPN and EN remain mixed. In other countries, TPN continues to be used regularly for patients with advanced cancer.

Like TPN, EN in patients with cancer has not been shown to improve survival, improve tumor response, decrease toxicity, or decrease surgical complications. The only exception is in patients with cancer in head and neck and esophagus (43). In a retrospective case–control study of 88 patients treated for locally advanced head and neck cancer with accelerated radiation or concurrent chemoradiotherapy, prophylactic gastrostomy tubes (PGTs) were associated with half of the weight loss compared with the control group. There were significantly fewer hospitalizations for nutritional or dehydration issues in those with PGTs than in the control group; the use of PGTs had no influence on overall survival or local control. Although in animal studies nutritional support has been shown to increase rates of tumor growth, this has not been demonstrated consistently in humans (44).

Both TPN and EN have been able to improve some nutritional indices, such as body weight, fat mass, nitrogen balance, and whole body potassium. Thyroxine-binding prealbumin and retinol-binding protein levels increase only with TPN, whereas some immune response indices (complement factors and lymphocyte number) improve only with EN. EN appears to be more available for use in protein synthesis than TPN (45). The results of randomized studies comparing TPN and EN have been conflicting but demonstrated a potential marginal advantage to TPN with regard to weight gain and nitrogen balance (46,47). Taken as a whole, TPN and EN both appear able to prevent further deterioration of the nutritional state and sometimes improve some metabolic indices in patients with cancer. However, no real demonstrable benefit has been shown on quality of life, and no large randomized trials have been performed in patients with advanced cancer.

Dementia

Dementia is a progressive disease that worsens in recognizable stages. In the Functional Assessment Staging System (FAST), one system used to follow the course of Alzheimer's disease; it is at the final stage seven when Alzheimer's disease patients may stop eating spontaneously. At stage seven, patients usually die within a year. They lose the ability to speak, ambulate, eat, control their muscles, and smile. When patients reach this stage, it is very difficult to maintain nutrition because encouragement to eat becomes less successful. In this instance, difficulty eating is a marker for the terminal phase of Alzheimer's dementia.

The same is not true in other forms of dementia. For example, patients with Parkinson's disease often lose the ability to maintain adequate caloric intake at an earlier stage of their disease; in this setting, a feeding tube may be required. Weight loss is characteristic of Parkinson's disease even in the early phases of the illness, thus some authors speculate that the role of dysphagia as a mediator of weight loss is limited (48). PEG tube placement does not prevent aspiration; aspiration rates may continue to range between 25% and 40% (49). PEG tubes in patients with advanced dementia do not prevent aspiration pneumonia, reduce the risk of infection or pressure sores, or improve function. Based on Rimon's findings and those of others not showing dementia to be a risk factor for increased mortality, the impact of EN on survival remains unclear (18).

Amyotrophic Lateral Sclerosis

Some studies suggest that the benefits of a PEG in amyotrophic lateral sclerosis are adequate nutritional intake and weight stabilization (50–52). Studies indicate lower survival in malnourished patients. Whether PEG increases survival time remains unclear (53). One study indicates that PEG tube placement is associated with greater survival than NGT placement. This study was retrospective, however, and the indications for treatment and nutritional indices differed between groups (54). PEG placement may be associated with increased pulmonary risks and shorter survival time when done in patients with reduced vital capacity, defined as forced vital capacity 50% of predicted. Recent studies, however, call this into question (55,56).

POTENTIAL BENEFIT FROM ARTIFICIAL HYDRATION

Comfort

A common argument for providing artificial hydration in palliative care is to alleviate thirst. Healthy volunteers who undergo experimentally induced dehydration often report thirst, yet this sensation is relieved by ad lib sips of fluid in cumulative volumes insufficient to restore physiologic fluid balance. The few studies evaluating patient symptoms at the end of life suggest a high prevalence of dry mouth and thirst that is not correlated with hydration status, but it can be alleviated with ice chips and sips of water (19). In several studies of palliative care patients, no statistically significant association was found between thirst and fluid intake, serum sodium, urea, or osmolality (57,58).

Reduction of Delirium or Opioid Toxicity

Retrospective studies have suggested that hydration might be able to reduce neuropsychiatric symptoms such as sedation, hallucinations, myoclonus, and agitation. In the first RCT of hydration versus placebo in patients with cancer, Bruera et al. compared the effects of hydration with either 1,000 or 100 mL of normal saline on target symptoms of sedation, fatigue, hallucinations, and myoclonus (59). Although the study did not meet its accrual goals, 53 (73%) of 73 target symptoms experienced by the treatment group improved compared with 33 (49%) of 67 target symptoms in the placebo group ($p = 0.006$), suggesting a potential benefit of hydration in this population. This study was underpowered and characterized by many subjective measures and was not performed in hospice patients. Nevertheless, it highlights the importance of further study in this controversial area.

POTENTIAL HARM FROM ARTIFICIAL HYDRATION

Commonly cited side effects of artificial hydration in palliative care include fluid overload and increased respiratory secretions. Because no controlled trials exist, the association between these adverse effects and artificial hydration is hard to measure.

Fluid Overload

Concerns regarding hydration often center on the potential impact such hydration might have on edema, ascites, and respiratory distress. A comparison of two different health care settings (a palliative care unit and an acute care unit) demonstrated marked differences in volume of hydration ordered. The acute care group ordered higher volumes of hydration, but it also prescribed a higher number of diuretics, suggesting that increased hydration could be associated with greater likelihood for fluid overload (60). Morita's study of terminally ill patients also noted an association between hydration and symptom scores for edema, ascites, and pleural effusion (61).

Increased Respiratory Secretions

Many palliative care providers believe that hydration may worsen retained respiratory secretions at the very end of life. However, the effect of hydration on respiratory secretions at the end of life is unclear. Neither Ellershaw nor Morita found a correlation between hydration status and bronchial secretions.

METHODOLOGICAL ISSUES IN EVALUATING EFFECTIVENESS OF NUTRITION INTERVENTIONS

In reviewing the current ANH literature, one is struck by the dearth of methodologically rigorous studies available to inform practice. With the exception of several large retrospective cohort studies, most studies had small sample sizes and heterogeneous patient populations. These cohort studies did not include meaningful comparison groups, so evaluating the true impact of ANH is problematic.

Very little attention has been given to the nature of the nutritional intervention being provided through artificial nutrition. PEG placement or tube feeding might or might not lead to adequate caloric intake. Evaluating differences in outcome between those receiving adequate nutrients and those that did not would elucidate whether or not outcomes varied by actual caloric intake. In most studies, the composition of the nutrition or fluid formulations in these studies was rarely addressed or identified.

In almost all instances, RCTs either do not exist or are underpowered to evaluate the main outcomes. Most studies had difficulty with recruitment and high dropout rates. Furthermore, the follow-up time was often very short (days to weeks). Hence, these trials are not likely to detect true effects of the intervention.

For the preponderance of observational studies influencing this field, confounding is not adequately addressed. For example, in observational studies of patients with dementia receiving EN, it is possible that tubes are placed primarily in a subgroup of patients whose oral intake has become insufficient to sustain life, thus prolonging their survival from 0 to 1 month to 6 to 7 months (confounding by indication). On the other hand, it is likely that tubes were not placed in the subgroup of patients who retained some capacity to eat; those patients also survived a median of roughly 6 to 7 months. The ability to eat could then be a confounding factor that explains the similar survival between groups receiving and not receiving artificial nutrition. Measuring the ability to eat and controlling for this risk factor in the analysis could help to ascertain the true association between tube placement and survival. Because many patients have multiple conditions, the nature and severity of these conditions (especially in Medicare databases) may be difficult to capture and therefore adequately control for in analyses.

Many of the outcomes chosen in these studies provide inadequate information for clinicians to guide patients. Most studies have evaluated survival and nutritional or medical indicators. Most have not addressed quality-of-life outcomes or quality-adjusted life years.

WHAT ARE CULTURAL AND RELIGIOUS DIMENSIONS TO THESE FORMS OF TREATMENT?

Ethnicity

Among nursing home residents with severe cognitive impairment, African Americans were almost four times more likely than Whites to have a feeding tube (62). Despite a recent trend toward decreased PEG tube placement in dementia patients, racial discrepancies persist. In a review of the Veterans Health Administration database, Braun et al. found that although only 18.4% of dementia patients were African Americans, they accounted for 28.8% of all PEG tube recipients with dementia (63). Reasons cited for this discrepancy include mistrust of the health care system, a greater desire for more aggressive medical treatment near the end of life, and differences in underlying religious beliefs and values. The possibility remains that African Americans are receiving a different standard of care with regard to ANH at end of life.

Religious Background

Jewish, Islamic, and Catholic traditions place a priority on "sanctity of life," often preferring greater life-sustaining treatments over "quality of life." Jewish and Islamic traditions do not distinguish tube feeding from other forms of basic nutrition (64). According to most Jewish religious authorities, "nutrition in any form is a basic human need and should be provided to all patients" (65). How cognitively impaired the patient is, is not relevant, because human life of any quality is of supreme value. Jewish tradition, however, does not argue for *any* treatment that is not of benefit to the patient and relies on scientific evidence in making an ethical judgment on a particular treatment modality.

GUIDELINES FOR ENTERAL/PARENTERAL NUTRITION IN PALLIATIVE CARE

Improve the Scientific Literature Base

Because all the current data regarding ANH have significant methodological weaknesses, providers should be circumspect about the true benefits and harm of nutrition support, especially in the enteral form. Improvements in the overall quality could be made by

1. Collaboration with epidemiologists/biostatisticians from the beginning stages of the study
2. Agreement on appropriate outcome measures
3. Use of the highest quality design for the clinical question at hand

More rigorous studies are needed to increase the confidence that current clinical practice is based on the higher levels of evidence.

Improve the Assessment Process

Before initiating artificial nutrition, it is worth asking the following questions:

1. Is the patient able to swallow properly? If so, oral nutrition is preferable and safer than tube feeding.
2. If the patient can swallow properly, is the patient maintaining adequate nutritional intake to meet nutritional needs? If not, dietary supplementation is preferable and safer than tube feeding.
3. If the patient can swallow but cannot maintain adequate nutritional intake, is it due to a specific modifiable cause? If so, addressing the underlying cause is preferable and safer than tube feeding. For example:
   - Does the patient have a psychological condition such as depression that affects nutritional intake?
   - Does the patient have mouth pain, poorly fitted dentures, or loss of teeth?
   - Is the food or the eating environment unappealing?
   - Does the patient have the physical dexterity needed to eat without assistance?

- Does the patient need to be reminded how to chew and swallow?
- Is the patient receiving the help he or she needs to eat?
- Are language barriers, ethnic or cultural dietary restrictions, or religious beliefs keeping the patient from taking an adequate amount of nutrition?

4. If the patient is unable to eat or does not have adequate nutritional intake, address the following questions before considering tube feeding:

- Does the clinical decision to employ tube feeding respect the autonomy of the patient and family to decline the intervention?
- Is conservative treatment a better option? Has it been tried? If not, why?
- Is there scientific evidence that supports tube feeding as a better option than oral intake in this situation?
- Are there any contraindications to artificial feeding in this patient?
- When and how will the effectiveness of and continued need for tube feeding be reassessed (i.e., reaching a specific therapeutic goal or a prespecified time period)?

Improve the Informed Consent Process

The current quality of informed consent for EN and, in particular, placement of gastrostomy tubes is poor. In a review of 154 consecutive hospitalized adults undergoing placement of gastrostomy tubes, only 1 medical record documented a procedure-specific discussion of benefits and burdens of and alternatives to tube feeding (66).

Specific Information that Should Be Provided

The informed consent process should include discussion of median, 1-year, and 3-year survival rates. It should also identify both physical (restraints) and potential psychosocial (social isolation and sensory deprivation) adverse effects associated with artificial nutrition. In patients who are not imminently dying, alternatives such as carefully monitored hand-feeding should be discussed, including the observation that there is no difference in survival for PEG tubes versus hand-feeding for demented and nondemented patients (67). In patients who are in the terminal phase of their illness, findings regarding the common lack of hunger experienced by patients should be communicated to patients' families to allay concerns regarding potential patient distress associated with minimal oral intake.

Poor prognostic factors consistently noted in the literature should be described, including increased age (>80 years), chewing and swallowing disorders, and the presence of underlying malignancies (68).

GUIDELINES FOR HYDRATION IN PALLIATIVE CARE

Hydration may be of benefit in patients with potential opioid toxicity, confusion, or nausea. Patients and families should be informed regarding the lack of correlation between hydration and thirst and the finding that sips of water, ice chips, lip moisteners, salivary substitutes, mouth swabs, hard candy, and routine mouth care are more effective at addressing the sense of dry mouth and thirst than is artificial hydration.

CONCLUSION

Evidence regarding the potential benefit or harm associated with ANH in palliative care continues to be limited by underpowered or poorly designed studies. Decisions regarding ANH should be informed by treatment goals and patient preference (autonomy) and the application of the principles of nonmaleficence and beneficence where potential harm or benefits can be determined. While case law regards artificial nutrition as medical treatment, in the absence of a developed literature to provide a scientific basis for decision-making, social values may continue to guide decisions in some instances. Many religious traditions do not distinguish artificial nutrition from basic food and water, a point that renders moot discussion of harm and benefits for some decision makers. Physicians should inform the patient or their family as fully as possible regarding the potential benefit and harm associated with ANH and assist them to make the best decision possible based on the patient's values and available information about risks and benefits.

REFERENCES

1. Good P, Cavenagh J, Mather M, Ravenscroft P. Medically assisted nutrition for palliative care in adult patients. *Cochrane Database Syst Rev.* 2008;(4):CD006274.
2. Good P, Cavenagh J, Mather M, Ravenscroft P. Medically assisted hydration for palliative care patients. *Cochrane Database Syst Rev.* 2008;(2):CD006273.
3. Dudrick SJ. Rhoads Lecture: a 45-year obsession and passionate pursuit of optimal nutrition support: puppies, pediatrics, surgery, geriatrics, home TPN, A.S.P.E.N., et cetera. *JPEN J Parenter Enteral Nutr.* 2005;29(4):272-287.
4. Heyland DK, Montalvo M, MacDonald S, Keefe L, Su XY, Drover JW. Total parenteral nutrition in the surgical patient: a meta-analysis. *Can J Surg.* 2001;44(2):102-111.
5. Heyland DK, MacDonald S, Keefe L, Drover JW. Total parenteral nutrition in the critically ill patient: a meta-analysis. *JAMA.* 1998;280(23):2013-2019.
6. Gauderer MW. Percutaneous endoscopic gastrostomy-20 years later: a historical perspective. *J Pediatr Surg.* 2001;36(1):217-219.
7. Callahan CM, Haag KM, Buchanan NN, Nisi R. Decision-making for percutaneous endoscopic gastrostomy

among older adults in a community setting. *J Am Geriatr Soc.* 1999;47(9):1105-1109.

8. Cruzan v. Director, Missouri Department of Public Health. In: 110 S. Court; 1990; 2841.

9. Kapp MB. Regulating the foregoing of artificial nutrition and hydration: first, do some harm. *J Am Geriatr Soc.* 2002;50(3):586-588.

10. Taylor CA, Larson DE, Ballard DJ, et al. Predictors of outcome after percutaneous endoscopic gastrostomy: a community-based study. *Mayo Clin Proc.* 1992;67(11):1042-1049.

11. Light VL, Slezak FA, Porter JA, Gerson LW, McCord G. Predictive factors for early mortality after percutaneous endoscopic gastrostomy. *Gastrointest Endosc.* 1995;42(4):330-335.

12. Grant MD, Rudberg MA, Brody JA. Gastrostomy placement and mortality among hospitalized Medicare beneficiaries. *JAMA.* 1998;279(24):1973-1976.

13. Wasa M, Takagi Y, Sando K, Harada T, Okada A. Long-term outcome of short bowel syndrome in adult and pediatric patients. *JPEN J Parenter Enteral Nutr.* 1999;23(5 suppl):S110-S112.

14. Klein S, Kinney J, Jeejeebhoy K, et al. Nutrition support in clinical practice: review of published data and recommendations for future research directions. *Clin Nutr.* 1997;16(4):193-218.

15. Tresch DD, Sims FH, Duthie EH, Goldstein MD, Lane PS. Clinical characteristics of patients in the persistent vegetative state. *Arch Intern Med.* 1991;151(5):930-932.

16. Heyland DK, Dhaliwal R, Drover JW, Gramlich L, Dodek P. Canadian clinical practice guidelines for nutrition support in mechanically ventilated, critically ill adult patients. *JPEN J Parenter Enteral Nutr.* 2003;27(5):355-373.

17. Rabeneck L, Wray NP, Petersen NJ. Long-term outcomes of patients receiving percutaneous endoscopic gastrostomy tubes. *J Gen Intern Med.* 1996;11(5):287-293.

18. Rimon E, Kagansky N, Levy S. Percutaneous endoscopic gastrostomy: evidence of different prognosis in various patient subgroups. *Age Ageing.* 2005;34(4):353-357.

19. McCann RM, Hall WJ, Groth-Juncker A. Comfort care for terminally ill patients. The appropriate use of nutrition and hydration. *JAMA.* 1994;272(16):1263-1266.

20. Ganzini L, Goy ER, Miller LL, Harvath TA, Jackson A, Delorit MA. Nurses' experiences with hospice patients who refuse food and fluids to hasten death. *N Engl J Med.* 2003;349(4):359-365.

21. Byock I. Patient refusal of nutrition and hydration: walking the ever-finer line. *Am J Hosp Palliat Care.* 1995;12(2):8, 9-13.

22. Berlowitz DR, Wilking SV. Risk factors for pressure sores. A comparison of cross-sectional and cohort-derived data. *J Am Geriatr Soc.* 1989;37(11):1043-1050.

23. Bergstrom N, Braden B. A prospective study of pressure sore risk among institutionalized elderly. *J Am Geriatr Soc.* 1992;40(8):747-758.

24. Hartgrink HH, Wille J, Konig P, Hermans J, Breslau PJ. Pressure sores and tube feeding in patients with a fracture of the hip: a randomized clinical trial. *Clin Nutr.* 1998;17(6):287-292.

25. Ohura T, Nakajo T, Okada S, Omura K, Adachi K. Evaluation of effects of nutrition intervention on healing of pressure ulcers and nutritional states (randomized controlled trial). *Wound Repair Regen.* 2011;19(3):330-336.

26. Stratton RJ, Ek AC, Engfer M, et al. Enteral nutritional support in prevention and treatment of pressure ulcers: a systematic review and meta-analysis. *Ageing Res Rev.* 2005;4(3):422-450.

27. McClave SA, DeMeo MT, DeLegge MH, et al. North American Summit on Aspiration in the critically ill

patient: consensus statement. *JPEN J Parenter Enteral Nutr.* 2002;26(6 suppl):S80-S85.

28. Langmore SE, Terpenning MS, Schork A, et al. Predictors of aspiration pneumonia: how important is dysphagia? *Dysphagia.* 1998;13(2):69-81.

29. Heyland DK, Drover JW, MacDonald S, Novak F, Lam M. Effect of postpyloric feeding on gastroesophageal regurgitation and pulmonary microaspiration: results of a randomized controlled trial. *Crit Care Med.* 2001;29(8):1495-1501.

30. Stroud M, Duncan H, Nightingale J. Guidelines for enteral feeding in adult hospital patients. *Gut.* 2003;52(suppl 7):vii1-vii12.

31. Sullivan-Marx EM, Strumpf NE, Evans LK, Baumgarten M, Maislin G. Predictors of continued physical restraint use in nursing home residents following restraint reduction efforts. *J Am Geriatr Soc.* 1999;47(3):342-348.

32. Peck A, Cohen CE, Mulvihill MN. Long-term enteral feeding of aged demented nursing home patients. *J Am Geriatr Soc.* 1990;38(11):1195-1198.

33. Norton B, Homer-Ward M, Donnelly MT, Long RG, Holmes GK. A randomised prospective comparison of percutaneous endoscopic gastrostomy and nasogastric tube feeding after acute dysphagic stroke. *BMJ.* 1996;312(7022):13-16.

34. Park RH, Allison MC, Lang J, et al. Randomised comparison of percutaneous endoscopic gastrostomy and nasogastric tube feeding in patients with persisting neurological dysphagia. *BMJ.* 1992;304(6839):1406-1409.

35. Iizuka M, Reding M. Use of percutaneous endoscopic gastrostomy feeding tubes and functional recovery in stroke rehabilitation: a case-matched controlled study. *Arch Phys Med Rehabil.* 2005;86(5):1049-1052.

36. Golestanian E, Liou JI, Smith MA. Long-term survival in older critically ill patients with acute ischemic stroke. *Crit Care Med.* 2009;37(12):3107-3113.

37. Dennis MS, Lewis SC, Warlow C. Effect of timing and method of enteral tube feeding for dysphagic stroke patients (FOOD): a multicentre randomised controlled trial. *Lancet.* 2005;365(9461):764-772.

38. Melchior JC, Chastang C, Gelas P, et al. Efficacy of 2-month total parenteral nutrition in AIDS patients: a controlled randomized prospective trial. The French Multicenter Total Parenteral Nutrition Cooperative Group Study. *AIDS.* 1996;10(4):379-384.

39. Klein S, Kinney J, Jeejeebhoy K, et al. Nutrition support in clinical practice: review of published data and recommendations for future research directions. Summary of a conference sponsored by the National Institutes of Health, American Society for Parenteral and Enteral Nutrition, and American Society for Clinical Nutrition. *Am J Clin Nutr.* 1997;66(3):683-706.

40. Klein S, Simes J, Blackburn GL. Total parenteral nutrition and cancer clinical trials. *Cancer.* 1986;58(6):1378-1386.

41. McGeer AJ, Detsky AS, O'Rourke K. Parenteral nutrition in cancer patients undergoing chemotherapy: a meta-analysis. *Nutrition.* 1990;6(3):233-240.

42. Parenteral nutrition in patients receiving cancer chemotherapy. American College of Physicians. *Ann Intern Med.* 1989;110(9):734-736.

43. Lee JH, Machtay M, Unger LD, et al. Prophylactic gastrostomy tubes in patients undergoing intensive irradiation for cancer of the head and neck. *Arch Otolaryngol Head Neck Surg.* 1998;124(8):871-875.

44. Bozzetti F, Gavazzi C, Mariani L, Crippa F. Artificial nutrition in cancer patients: which route, what composition? *World J Surg.* 1999;23(6):577-583.

45. Dresler CM, Jeevanandam M, Brennan MF. Metabolic efficacy of enteral feeding in malnourished cancer and noncancer patients. *Metabolism.* 1987;36(1):82-88.

46. Burt ME, Gorschboth CM, Brennan MF. A controlled, prospective, randomized trial evaluating the metabolic effects of enteral and parenteral nutrition in the cancer patient. *Cancer.* 1982;49(6):1092-1105.

47. Lim ST, Choa RG, Lam KH, Wong J, Ong GB. Total parenteral nutrition versus gastrostomy in the preoperative preparation of patients with carcinoma of the oesophagus. *Br J Surg.* 1981;68(2):69-72.

48. Barichella M, Cereda E, Pezzoli G. Major nutritional issues in the management of Parkinson's disease. *Mov Disord.* 2009;24(13):1881-1892.

49. McClave SA, Chang WK. Complications of enteral access. *Gastrointest Endosc.* 2003;58(5):739-751.

50. Klor BM, Milianti FJ. Rehabilitation of neurogenic dysphagia with percutaneous endoscopic gastrostomy. *Dysphagia.* 1999;14(3):162-164.

51. Mazzini L, Corra T, Zaccala M, Mora G, Del Piano M, Galante M. Percutaneous endoscopic gastrostomy and enteral nutrition in amyotrophic lateral sclerosis. *J Neurol.* 1995;242(10):695-698.

52. Kasarskis EJ, Scarlata D, Hill R, Fuller C, Stambler N, Cedarbaum JM. A retrospective study of percutaneous endoscopic gastrostomy in ALS patients during the BDNF and CNTF trials. *J Neurol Sci.* 1999;169(1-2):118-125.

53. Desport JC, Preux PM, Truong CT, Courat L, Vallat JM, Couratier P. Nutritional assessment and survival in ALS patients. *Amyotroph Lateral Scler Other Motor Neuron Disord.* 2000;1(2):91-96.

54. Rio A, Ellis C, Shaw C, et al. Nutritional factors associated with survival following enteral tube feeding in patients with motor neurone disease. *J Hum Nutr Diet.* 2010;23(4):408-415.

55. Gregory S, Siderowf A, Golaszewski AL, McCluskey L. Gastrostomy insertion in ALS patients with low vital capacity: respiratory support and survival. *Neurology.* 2002;58(3):485-487.

56. Boitano LJ, Jordan T, Benditt JO. Noninvasive ventilation allows gastrostomy tube placement in patients with advanced ALS. *Neurology.* 2001;56(3):413-414.

57. Ellershaw JE, Sutcliffe JM, Saunders CM. Dehydration and the dying patient. *J Pain Symptom Manage.* 1995;10(3):192-197.

58. Burge FI. Dehydration symptoms of palliative care cancer patients. *J Pain Symptom Manage.* 1993;8(7):454-464.

59. Bruera E, Franco JJ, Maltoni M, Watanabe S, Suarez-Almazor M. Changing pattern of agitated impaired mental status in patients with advanced cancer: association with cognitive monitoring, hydration, and opioid rotation. *J Pain Symptom Manage.* 1995;10(4):287-291.

60. Lanuke K, Fainsinger RL, DeMoissac D. Hydration management at the end of life. *J Palliat Med.* 2004;7(2):257-263.

61. Morita T, Hyodo I, Yoshimi T, et al. Association between hydration volume and symptoms in terminally ill cancer patients with abdominal malignancies. *Ann Oncol.* 2005;16(4):640-647.

62. Gessert CE, Curry NM, Robinson A. Ethnicity and end-of-life care: the use of feeding tubes. *Ethn Dis.* 2001;11(1):97-106.

63. Braun UK, Rabeneck L, McCullough LB, et al. Decreasing use of percutaneous endoscopic gastrostomy tube feeding for veterans with dementia-racial differences remain. *J Am Geriatr Soc.* 2005;53(2):242-248.

64. Gordon M, Alibhai SH. Ethics of PEG tubes—Jewish and Islamic perspectives. *Am J Gastroenterol.* 2004;99(6):1194.

65. Jotkowitz AB, Clarfield AM, Glick S. The care of patients with dementia: a modern Jewish ethical perspective. *J Am Geriatr Soc.* 2005;53(5):881-884.

66. Brett AS, Rosenberg JC. The adequacy of informed consent for placement of gastrostomy tubes. *Arch Intern Med.* 2001;161(5):745-748.

67. Franzoni S, Frisoni GB, Boffelli S, Rozzini R, Trabucchi M. Good nutritional oral intake is associated with equal survival in demented and nondemented very old patients. *J Am Geriatr Soc.* 1996;44(11):1366-1370.

68. Mitchell SL, Buchanan JL, Littlehale S, Hamel MB. Tube-feeding versus hand-feeding nursing home residents with advanced dementia: a cost comparison. *J Am Med Dir Assoc.* 2003;4(1):27-33.

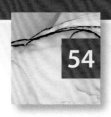

54 Complementary and Integrative Therapies in Oncology

Maleeha Ruhi, Karen Baker, and M. Jennifer Cheng

Complementary and integrative medicine encompasses a group of diverse medical and health care systems, practices, and products that are distinct from conventional medical modalities and used in conjunction (complementary) with standard biomedical management (Table 54.1) (1,2). The use of complementary and integrative medicine in the United States has substantially increased. In the 2012 National Health Interview Survey (NHIS), 33.2% of US adults used complementary health approaches. This is similar to the percentages in 2007 (35.5%) and 2002 (32.3%). The most commonly used complementary approach was natural products and herbs, and the most predominant symptom to be addressed by the use of complementary modalities was pain (Table 54.2 Figure 54.1 (3,4). According to the 2012 National Health Interview Survey, the total out-of-pocket spending on complementary medicine was 30.2$ billion a year; with total or partial insurance coverage, most insurance coverage was for chiropractic care (60%) followed by acupuncture (25%) and massage (15%) (1).

Patients often do not reveal their use of complementary health approaches to their providers, so it is wise to proactively query patients in a nonjudgmental tone ("Tell me what else do you do or take to treat your symptoms or this disease.") (5). Some complementary modalities are supported by more robust clinical trial data than others. These include acupuncture, yoga, tai chi, massage therapy, and relaxation techniques (6). In 2009, the Society for Integrative Oncology issued evidence-based clinical practice guidelines for health care providers to consider complementary health approaches to control symptoms and enhance patients' well-being (1).

DEFINITIONS: While used in the same acronym, a distinction must be made between complementary and alternative therapies.

- **Alternative therapies:** They are used *in place* of mainstream treatments. There has not been convincing evidence to date of the effectiveness of alternative cancer treatments.

- **Complementary therapies:** They are used *together with* mainstream oncologic treatments, and there is growing research addressing their safety and efficacy.
- Patients are increasingly seeking holistic cancer care that is tailored to the unique needs of the individual. (Greek word Holos means "all or entire." **Holistic approach** in medicine means treatment targeting toward patient's mental, physical, emotional, functional, spiritual, social, and community aspects and treating the whole person rather than, e.g., one organ system).

This trend has fueled the establishment of the field of integrative oncology in 2000, which interweaves conventional and evidence-based complementary therapies in oncology (7). Complementary therapies usually serve as adjuncts to mainstream cancer treatments to enhance well-being and self-empowerment, manage cancer and cancer treatment symptoms, and provide survivor care (8–11). There is limited evidence that complementary and integrative medicine therapies might modulate immune system function (12); however, there is no evidence for improved survival from this effect.

This chapter will review various modalities of complementary therapies in integrative oncology: mind–body interventions (hypnosis, relaxation therapies, meditation/mindfulness-based stress reduction [MBSR], biofeedback, yoga, and creative therapy), energy therapies (Reiki, healing/therapeutic touch), manipulative and body-based methods (chiropractic, massage therapy, exercise, Qigong, and tai chi chuan), acupuncture, and biologically based therapies (herbs and vitamins). The biologically based therapies section also examines specific phytochemicals and vitamins that are under investigation for cancer prevention and enhance cancer treatment and symptom management. Multiple complementary interventions can be concurrently utilized, and some care should be taken to make sure that integrative therapies do not conflict with other treatments (e.g., thrombocytopenia, neutropenia, and acupuncture).

TABLE 54.1 MODALITIES OF COMPLEMENTARY THERAPIES IN INTEGRATIVE ONCOLOGY

Mind–body interventions

Relaxation
Meditation
Hypnosis
Biofeedback
Guided imagery
Prayer
Labyrinth
Humor
Art
Yoga

Manipulative/body-based interventions

Feldenkrais
Massage
Reflexology
Music
Exercise
Chiropractic

Energy therapies

Magnetics
Acupuncture
Qi Gong
Reiki
Light/phototherapy

Biological/plant based

Herbs
Aromatherapy
Vitamins
Phytochemical
Cannabis

This chapter is not intended to be an exhaustive description of all types of complementary or integrative therapies. It will, rather, address some of the most common approaches and those that have the benefit of some degree of research analysis behind them.

MIND–BODY INTERVENTIONS

Mind–body interventions utilize the interactions among the brain, mind, body, and behavior and are defined by the National Center for Complemen-

TABLE 54.2 COMPLEMENTARY MODALITY APPS

Herb List (National Library of Medicine at NIH)
Breathe2Relax
Headspace: Meditation & Sleep
Insight Timer—Free Meditation App
Calm—Meditate, Sleep, Relax
Smiling Mind (pediatrics)
Ten Percent Happier

tary and Integrative Health as "a variety of techniques designed to enhance the mind's capacity to affect bodily function and symptoms" (1,13–15).

Hypnosis

In 1985, Kihlstrom defined hypnosis as "a social interaction in which one person, designated the subject, responds to suggestions offered by another person, designated the hypnotist, for experiences involving alterations in perception, memory, and voluntary action" (16). Hypnosis allows for a highly relaxed state in which the patient purposefully altered state of consciousness is open to intentional, therapeutic suggestions.

Hypnosis has been well researched in randomized clinical studies as treatment interventions for outcomes in controlling chronic pain including modulating cancer-related pain (17–21); improving acute and procedural pain in adults and children including procedures such as bone marrow aspiration, lumpectomy/core needle breast biopsy/breast cancer surgery, and vascular access procedures (22–24); alleviating stress, anxiety, and depression in breast cancer surgery patients and terminally ill cancer patients (13,25); improving anticipatory nausea and vomiting in children and adults receiving chemotherapy use (26–28); and reducing frequency and intensity of hot flashes among breast cancer survivors (29) without significantly increasing procedure time or cost (22). Some studies support the use of self-hypnosis in the medical setting, where brief training sessions that build self-hypnosis skills result in improved clinical outcomes, coupled with increased sense of mastery and self-control (30,31).

Self-hypnosis has also been utilized in conjunction with other complementary therapies. In a 1989 prospective study by Spiegel et al. published in *The Lancet*, women with metastatic breast cancer are randomly assigned to the intervention or control groups. Intervention includes 1 year of group therapy led by a psychiatrist or social worker with a therapist and self-hypnosis training for pain control. At 10-year follow-up, there was significantly improved survival in the intervention group, with a mean survival of 36.6 months compared with 18.9 months in the control group (32). However, subsequent multicenter randomized clinical trials (RCTs) did not replicate the survival benefit found by Spiegel et al. This may be due to the innovations in breast cancer treatment subsequent to Spiegel's publication, including selective estrogen receptor modulators and earlier detection of breast cancer through routine cancer screening. However, all of these studies demonstrate improvements in quality of life and reductions in distress and pain among women utilizing self-hypnosis and group support strategies (33). The responsiveness to suggestion

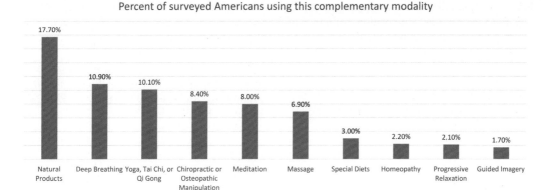

Figure 54.1 Top 10 complementary modalities among U.S. adults in 2012. (Source: Clarke TC, Black LI, Stussman BJ, Barnes PM, Nahin RL. Trends in the use of complementary health approaches among adults: United States, 2002-2012. *Natl Health Stat Report*. 2015;(79):1-16.)

with the ability to dissociate can effectively change perceptions modulating symptoms and curbing anticipatory distress.

Relaxation Therapies

Beginning in the early 1900s with Jacobson's progressive muscle relaxation technique (34), many relaxation techniques have evolved, such as visualization, centering, meditation, and abdominal breathing that aim to engender a state free of mental and/or physical tension (14).

A literature review by Kwekkeboom et al. found six studies where relaxation was implemented as the key intervention in treating two or more symptoms in the pain–fatigue–sleep disturbance cancer symptom cluster. Pain benefit was demonstrated in three of the four studies in which it was the key outcome. Other cancer-related symptoms mitigated by relaxation intervention include physical tension and sleep (35). Results of the 2017 U.S. National Health Interview Survey showed 59.2% of surveyed cancer survivors reported sleep problems, and a considerable number of cancer survivors with sleep problems use mind–body modalities (36). Other populations studied include hospitalized patients with cancer pain, outpatients with chronic cancer pain, and women with early-stage breast cancer. While symptoms generally improved compared with no treatment group, results have not been consistent (37).

Guided Imagery

Guided imagery engages the imagination in creating a sensory experience to achieve a specific clinical outcome (38). Imagery is often combined with other mind–body techniques such as relaxation techniques and music therapy.

The National Comprehensive Cancer Network recommends guided imagery for the treatment of anticipatory nausea and vomiting (39). In one study, guided imagery with music therapy was found to improve the quality of life and mood disturbance in cancer survivors (40). Mood and quality of life improved significantly in the guided imagery group as well as the progressive muscle relaxation group compared with usual care in an RCT of 56 participants with advanced cancer receiving palliative care at home (41). While studies evaluating the use of guided imagery in participants receiving chemotherapy showed mixed response in improvements in nausea and vomiting prior to and hours to days after chemotherapy, there have generally been significant improvements in emotional response and anxiety during chemotherapy treatment associated with the use of guided imagery (42–45).

Few RCTs compared imagery alone with a treatment or another active intervention group. In general, imagery alone is more effective than no treatment in improving symptoms of depression, anxiety, pain, and quality of life. Its effects are generally comparable to other mind–body techniques such as hypnosis or relaxation (38,40). However, more stringently designed clinical trials are needed, as current studies lack explicit descriptions of the intervention procedures, duration, and outcome measures. Therapist-directed guided imagery can assist patients in diversion and distraction during procedures. This modality is also convenient and quickly accessible through various electronic media (phone, computer, etc.)

Meditation/Mindfulness-Based Stress Reduction

Meditation is a family of techniques with the goal of training the mind to focus on a single target perception to realize an ultimate benefit. While purported to have its origin from Eastern traditions, many religious and spiritual traditions have developed their own meditative practices. The most well-studied meditation technique is the mindfulness-based stress reduction (MBSR), a secular meditation technique developed by Jon Kabat-Zinn and colleagues with its roots in Buddhist Vipassana and Zen practices (46). The primary goal of mindfulness meditation is to complete engagement in the present moment experience with a nonjudgmental attitude of acceptance and patience—without ruminations about prior or future experience. Through this training, one develops a nonreactive awareness even during stressful situations (47).

MBSR is a well-defined patient-focused intervention typically offered in 7 to 10 weekly group sessions, each lasting for 1 to 1.5 hours. While the oncology populations most evaluated in MBSR study interventions are those with breast and prostate cancer, the literature is growing on its impact on other oncology populations. Most interventions generally demonstrate improvements in mood and stress (48), quality of life (49), cytokine production (49), sleep quality (50), coping styles, decreases in helplessness–hopelessness (51), and pain. Speca's prospective, randomized, treatment controlled trial demonstrated significant decreases in overall symptoms of stress, depression, anxiety, anger, and confusion following a mindfulness meditation-based stress reduction program in cancer outpatients with various stages of disease. A study by Carlson et al. demonstrated improvements at 1 year following MBSR interventions in quality of life and stress symptoms. This study also found clinical and lab evidence consistent with reductions in the stress response, including hormonal, immunological, and vascular parameters (49,52). In a systematic review article by Duong et al., there is evidence of mindfulness and relaxation's effectiveness at reducing fatigue severity in patients with cancer and HSCT recipients (53).

One controlled study showed that brain MRI of adults who meditate have more gyri than adults who don't meditate; it also affects the amygdala even when the person is not doing meditation (54). Similarly, other studies have shown that meditation may slow, stall, or even reverse normal aging of the brain. While meditation can provide cost-effective benefit, providers need to be aware that it could also cause or worsens some psychiatric symptoms like anxiety or depression (55).

Overall, meta-analyses demonstrate that MBSR is effective in oncology populations for psychological stressors, with more modest effect sizes for physiological measurements and physical health measures. Mindfulness-based practices are increasingly being explored in various aspects of cancer patient care and symptom management (56).

Yoga

The practice of yoga originates from Eastern traditions. The word *yoga* is derived from the Sanskrit root *yuj*, meaning to bind, join, and yoke. The goal of yoga is to strengthen the union between mind, body, and spirit through ethical disciplines, physical postures, and spiritual practices (14,57). Listed in Table 54.3 are various styles of yoga and corresponding clinical studies assessing its effectiveness in symptom management among cancer patients (14,57,68).

Overall, there has been preliminary positive evidence supporting the use of yoga through single-arm pilot trials and small-scale RCTs largely focused on breast cancer population (69). Data suggest improved overall quality of life, emotional well-being, mood, hot flashes, spiritual well-being, and sleep (Table 54.3). The first nationwide, multisite, phase II/III RCT led by Mustian et al. using a standardized, 4-week, yoga intervention demonstrated that it can significantly improves cancer-related fatigue. In this study, cancer patients who participated in yoga as compared to patients who received standard survivorship care alone felt reduced daytime fatigue/dysfunction and had improved sleep quality which contributed to more daytime energy and reduction in cancer-related fatigue (67).

The emphasis of its use in cancer population is on controlled movements and deep breathing, increasing the patient's body awareness, flexibility, and balance. Of course, thought must be given to the patient's overall physical stamina and ability to participate in yoga, especially if they are a novice. It is wise, in addition, to caution against hot yoga or other intensive variants in oncology patients. Other less strenuous and taxing forms of yoga such as modified bed yoga have been clinically well accepted by hospitalized patients and should be considered.

Biofeedback

Biofeedback enables an individual to learn how to change physiologic functions by measuring these activities and providing real-time "feedback" to patients in order to facilitate changes in behavior, emotions, and cognition. Physiologic measures can include brainwaves, heart function, breathing, muscle activity, and skin temperature. The goal is for the physiologic changes to persist without the need for an instrument (70). Biofeedback can be helpful in cancer-related pain, fatigue, and cognitive impairments (71). There are studies showing effectiveness of biofeedback therapy in improving anal function in rectal cancer patients with anterior resection syndrome after sphincter-saving surgery (72).

TABLE 54.3 VARIOUS STYLES OF YOGA WITH CORRESPONDING CLINICAL STUDIES IN SYMPTOM MANAGEMENT AMONG CANCER PATIENTS

		Selected studies	Design	Result
Hatha yoga	Focuses on postures (asanas) and breathing exercises (pranayama)	Moadel et al. (58)	RCT 128 patients (stages I–III) breast cancer. ECOG performance status of <3 recruited from urban cancer center to a 12-wk yoga intervention or a 12-wk waitlist control group	Improved overall QOL ($p < 0.008$), emotional well-being ($p < 0.015$), social well-being ($p < 0.004$), spiritual well-being ($p < 0.009$), and distressed mood ($p < 0.031$)
Iyengar yoga	Focuses on body alignment, precision, and sequencing of poses; uses props such as blankets and blocks	Blank et al. (59)	RCT Pilot study of 18 women diagnosed with stage I–III breast cancer and receiving antiestrogen or aromatase inhibitor hormonal therapy. Yoga classes were conducted two times per week for 8 wk	More than 60% experienced less anxiety and improved mood
		Duncan et al. (60)	Single-arm pilot trial 24 postmenopausal women with stage I–III breast cancer who reported aromatase inhibitor–associated arthralgia were enrolled in a single-arm pilot trial. A yoga program was provided twice a week for 8 wk	Improvement in patient-reported QOL, spiritual well-being, and mood
		Speed-Andrews et al. (61)	Single-arm pilot trial 24 breast cancer survivors participated in 12-wk classes in Iyengar yoga and completed a questionnaire measuring generic and disease-specific QOL and psychosocial function before and after the intervention	Improvement in mental health (mean change, +4.2; $p = 0.045$), vitality (mean change, +4.9; $p = 0.033$), role-emotional (mean change, +6.4; $p = 0.010$), and bodily pain (mean change, +4.4; $p = 0.024$)
Restorative yoga	"Gentle type" of yoga. Traditional poses performed with props (e.g., an exercise ball) to support the body	Danhauer et al. (62)	Single-arm pilot trial 51 women with ovarian ($n = 37$) or breast cancer ($n = 14$). The majority (61%) were actively undergoing cancer treatment. All study participants participated in 10 weekly classes	Significant improvements in depression, negative affect, state anxiety, mental health, and quality of life
		Danhauer et al. (63)	RCT 44 women with breast cancer enrolled, 34% were actively undergoing cancer treatment. Study participants were randomized to the intervention (10 weekly 75-min classes) or a waitlist control group	Improved mental health, depression, fatigue, positive affect, and spirituality

(Continued)

TABLE 54.3 VARIOUS STYLES OF YOGA WITH CORRESPONDING CLINICAL STUDIES IN SYMPTOM MANAGEMENT AMONG CANCER PATIENTS *(Continued)*

	Selected studies	Design	Result
	Cohen et al. (64)	Single-arm pilot trial A pilot trial in 14 postmenopausal women experiencing ≥4 moderate to severe hot flushes per day or ≥30 moderate to severe hot flushes per week. Eight restorative yoga poses taught in a 3-h introductory session and eight weekly 90-min sessions	Mean number of hot flushes per week decreased by 30.8% (95% CI 15.6%–45.9%) and mean hot-flash score decreased 34.2% (95% CI 16.0%–52.5%) from baseline to week 8
Yoga of awareness program	Carson et al. (65)	RCT 37 breast cancer disease-free women experiencing hot flashes were randomized to the 8-wk yoga of awareness program (gentle yoga poses, meditation, and breathing exercises) or to waitlist control	Improvements in hot-flash frequency, severity, and total scores and in levels of joint pain, fatigue, sleep disturbance, symptom-related bother, and vigor
8-wk protocol involving gentle yoga postures, breathing exercises, meditation, didactic, and group exchanges	Peppone et al. (66)	Nationwide, multisite, phase II/III RCT in breast cancer survivors (*n* = 167) were randomized into 2 groups: 1. Standard care monitoring (*n* = 92) 2. Standard care plus the 4-wk yoga intervention (two times per week; 75 min/session) (*n* = 75)	Yoga participants had reductions in total body aches (*p* = 0.02; OR = 2.19) The brief community-based YOCAS intervention significantly reduced general pain, muscle aches, and physical discomfort
The effect of yoga for musculoskeletal symptoms among breast cancer survivors on hormonal therapy	Mustian et al. (67)	RCT; nationwide, multisite, phase II/III study 410 early-stage cancer survivors randomized to usual care or 75-min yoga class twice a week for 4 wk	Treatment group reported 22% improvement in sleep quality compared with a 12% improvement in control group. Treatment group reduced the use of sleep medication by 12% compared with 5% increase in sleep medication in the control. Treatment group with 42% reduction in fatigue compared with the 12% in control group
UR yoga for cancer survivors (YOCAS)		Mindfulness exercises that covered breathing, meditation, visualization, and 18 poses	

RCT, randomized clinical trial; QOL, quality of life; ECOG, Eastern Cooperative Oncology Group.

A small randomized control study in advanced cancer patients demonstrates reduction in cancer-related pain using electromyography biofeedback-assisted relaxation over a 4-week period. The mechanism of action is thought to be associated with attenuation of physiologic arousal (73).

The study of audiovisual feedback in respiratory-gated radiotherapy for lung cancer patients by George et al. assesses the effect of five weekly breath-training sessions with a goal of improved compliance during radiotherapy. Within each session the patients initially breathed without any instruction (free breathing), then with audio instructions, and finally with audiovisual biofeedback. Audiovisual biofeedback significantly reduces residual motion compared with free breathing and audio instruction (74–76). Biofeedback has also been explored in liver cancer stereotactic body radiotherapy (77). However, results in biofeedback have not been consistent. Bladder ultrasound biofeedback training did not produce a reproducible increase in bladder filling in prostate cancer patients during pelvic tumor irradiation (78). Additional area explored includes the impact of biofeedback therapy on anorectal function after the reversal of temporary stoma in rectal cancer patients with sphincter-saving surgery (79).

Biofeedback is often used in conjunction with other integrative techniques. For example, a model for social work teaches cancer patients and their relatives ways of coping through a combination of cognitive behavioral intervention, relaxation methods with guided imagery, and biofeedback (80). It has also been studied for preprocedural distress in children with cancer (81). However, clinician should be aware that biofeedback can sometimes exacerbate existing symptoms transiently, which usually resolves after a few sessions (82).

Creative Therapies

Creative therapies are a group of creative processes that aim to enhance individuals' physical, mental, and emotional well-being. This category includes visual arts, music therapy, creative writing, and mixed-modality programs. Music therapy is one of the best studied creative therapies in the literature.

Music therapy in its strictest definition is provided by professional musicians trained at the university level whose training includes music theory, psychology, supervision, and personal psychotherapy (83). In recent years, the definition has broadened to include listening to prerecorded music offered by medical staff.

In a descriptive review written by Gallagher from the Cleveland Clinic Arts and Medicine Institute, music therapy can be used throughout the spectrum of the cancer care process, including palliation, hospice, the active dying process, and bereavement. Common interventions include instrument playing, lyric analysis, musical entrainment, music-assisted relaxation, musical life review, music listening (live or recorded), participation (i.e., clapping, humming, and tapping foot), planning funeral music, singing, song writing, and verbal processing (84–86).

A Cochrane review by Bradt et al. examines the effects of music intervention on physical and psychological outcomes in cancer patients. The review includes all randomized controlled trials and quasi-randomized trials—52 trials with a total of 3,731 participants are included. The results suggest that music interventions may have beneficial effects in people with cancer, including quality of life and symptoms such as anxiety, pain, fatigue, and quality of life. Music therapy may have a small effect on heart rate, respiratory rate, and blood pressure. No strong evidence is found for improvements in fatigue, physical status, or depression. The authors conclude that the systematic review suggests beneficial effects of music therapy in the aforementioned outcome, but caution that these trials are at high risk for bias (87). Toning is one aspect of music therapy. It is the elongation of a note/tone from the voice, aimed at specific body part or symptom—for example, toning the abdomen for treating constipation. Music therapy also can be utilized as an energy modality. Each chakra (concentrated energy centers of the body) is assigned a music note, which when played can assist in balancing that chakra.

Art therapy, including Mandala therapy which allows for meditation and self-exploration, is another creative therapy modality commonly utilized by that enables the oncology patient to emotionally express through nonverbal means. A literature review by Geue et al. identifies 17 papers evaluating the effectiveness of using painting/drawing intervention for adult cancer patients. Nine out of the 17 papers are quantitative papers with two studies using randomization; the rest are qualitative studies. The sample sizes range from 7 and 70 participants with considerable variation in the structure and content of interventions. The results are generally positive, revealing decreases in anxiety and depression, increases in quality of life, and positive effects on personal growth, coping, and social interactions (88).

Acupuncture

Acupuncture is considered to be a part of mind–body medicine, but it is also considered a component of energy medicine, manipulative and body-based practices, and traditional Chinese medicine (1). Acupuncture involves the insertion of fine needles into predefined meridian acupuncture points to relieve symptoms and improve disease processes through energy flow. Acupuncture needles are FDA-approved medical device since 1996 (89). The Australian Acupuncture and Chinese Medicine Association published a comprehensive literature review on available evidence on acupuncture and identified eight conditions with strong evidence supporting its effectiveness, including chemotherapy-induced nausea and vomiting (with antiemetics), chronic low back pain, headache (tension-type and chronic), knee osteoarthritis, migraine prophylaxis, postoperative nausea and vomiting, postoperative pain, and allergic rhinitis. Several of the listed indications are commonly experienced by cancer patients (90). Additionally, the World Health Organization reports 31 diseases, symptoms, and conditions for which evidence from controlled trials suggests benefit from acupuncture (91).

Review of the evidence supports the use of acupuncture in oncologic settings for pain, xerostomia, and fatigue (Table 54.4) (108,109). There is also evidence for acupuncture use in peripheral neuropathy, postsurgical pain and dysfunction, joint pain from aromatase inhibitors, cancer-related fatigue, and hyperemesis associated with chemotherapy (1,110–114).

Acupressure is similar to acupuncture, but instead of needles, applies pressure with fingertips to the meridian points. This technique can be used with patients who are unable to or unwilling to receive needles.

The strength of the evidence supporting acupuncture use varies, with randomized controlled trials available for postoperative pain in head and neck cancer patients (96), fatigue (102,103), hyperemesis (115), xerostomia (98), and aromatase inhibitor–induced arthralgias (92).

Lu and Rosenthal discuss safety considerations in acupuncture use and recommend against acupuncture use in the following conditions: absolute neutrophil count <500/µL, platelet count <25,000/µL, altered mental state, clinically significant cardiac arrhythmias, and other unstable medical conditions evaluated on a case-by-case basis (116). Acupuncturist should be very careful about using sterile needles in cancer patient with decreased immunity from chemotherapy and radiation therapy to prevent any infection (1).

ENERGY HEALING

Energy healing techniques include a group of therapies where the caregiver transfers and/or conducts energy through their hands to the patient. Among the more commonly used energy practices are Reiki, therapeutic touch, and healing touch.

Reiki was developed in Japan and is widely practiced in the United States. Reiki is a Japanese word for "universal life force energy" and is conveyed through noninvasive, nonmanipulative progression of hand placement on or near the recipient's body. The benefits from Reiki and other touch therapies are proposed to derive from improved flow of life energy (chi) that is associated with achieving and maintaining good health; the tenant is based on that the body wants to heal itself. The theory of chi flow is that it may activate the parasympathetic system. The Reiki master has gone through an attunement process to better open the patient's energy channels. There is also a shared *intention*: what to focus on during the session between the care giver and receiver of Reiki, such as pain reduction.

The touch interventions are easy to implement; the patient remains clothed and can be carried out with the patient sitting in a chair or bed. They are readily embraced by pediatrics, geriatric, and the medically fragile due to its passive style. The most common symptoms treated with energy techniques are depression, fear, anxiety, support of overall well-being, and relaxation.

A systematic review by Agdal et al. of the use of energy healing in cancer patients identifies a total of six quantitative and two qualitative studies in which practitioners explicitly intend to direct energy to the cancer patient for therapeutic purpose without the use of other technical devices, remedies, or massage (117). Studies utilizing prayer or ritual healing interventions are not included in this review, although there is acknowledged similarity between these modalities and energy healing.

Positive marginal to moderate effects of energy healing are found on pain, fatigue, well-being, and quality of life. There are mixed results concerning anxiety, physical indicators, and medication use for symptom management. A recent literature review done on the effect of therapeutic touch in cancer patients showed the benefit of therapeutic touch for nausea, fatigue, depressed mood, severe pain, and improved sleep quality in cancer patients (118). Additional study has evaluated the role of energy healing in children with cancer (119).

Methodological weaknesses such as lack of or inadequately described blinding process, modest sample size, self-selection, and sparse descriptions on the interaction between the practitioner and patient limit the interpretation of many studies in energy healing. Lack of documented working mechanisms makes it a challenge to design sham treatments that do not activate the same working mechanism as the intervention. Thus far, the differences between intervention and sham

TABLE 54.4 CLINICAL TRIALS OF ACUPUNCTURE USE IN CANCER-RELATED SYMPTOMS

	Source	Intervention	Design	No. of participants	Setting	Outcomes	Results
Aromatase inhibitor–induced arthralgia	Crew et al. (92)	Full body/auricular acupuncture and joint-specific point prescriptions vs. sham acupuncture of superficial needle insertion at nonacupoint locations	RCT[a]; blinded study	51	Women with breast cancer treated with aromatase inhibitors with joint symptoms	Difference in mean Brief Pain Inventory-Short Form worst pain scores at 6 wk	Lower pain score for intervention group compared with sham acupuncture (3.0 vs. 5.5; $p < 0.001$)
	Mao et al. (93,94)	Based on Chinese medicine diagnosis of "Bi" syndrome with electrostimulation of needles around the painful joint(s)	Single-arm feasibility trial	12	Postmenopausal women with stage I–III breast cancer who reported aromatase inhibitor–related arthralgia	Pain severity of the modified Brief Pain Inventory was used as the primary outcome	Patients reported reduction in pain severity (from 5.3 to 1.9), stiffness (from 6.9 to 2.4), and joint symptom interference (from 4.7 to 0.8), all $p < 0.001$
Metastatic and advanced cancer pain	Dean-Clower et al. (95)	Manual acupuncture with a standardized acupuncture point protocol	Single-arm prospective pilot	40	Women with advanced ovarian or breast cancer at an outpatient academic oncology center (Karnofsky performance scale >60)	Symptom severity and quality of life questionnaires over 8 wk of treatment	There was improvement in anxiety ($p = 0.001$), fatigue ($p = 0.0002$), pain ($p = 0.0002$), and depression ($p = 0.003$) as well as general quality of life relief
Postsurgical cancer pain	Pfister et al. (96)	Manual acupuncture once a week. Acupuncture needles were placed at both standard and customized anatomic points	RCT; acupuncture once a week for 4 wk vs. usual care	58	Patients at a tertiary cancer center with chronic pain or dysfunction attributed to neck dissection	The Constant-Murley score, a composite measure of pain, function, and activities of daily living, was the primary outcome measure. Xerostomia, a secondary end point, was assessed using the Xerostomia Inventory	Constant-Murley scores improved more in the acupuncture group (adjusted difference between groups = 11.2; 95% CI, 3.0–19.3; $p = 0.008$). No significant difference in medication use. Acupuncture produced greater improvement in reported xerostomia (adjusted difference in Xerostomia Inventory = −5.8; 95% CI, −0.9 to −10.7; $p = 0.02$)
	Deng et al. (97)	Preoperative implantation of small intradermal needles that were retained for 4 wk	RCT; acupuncture vs. preoperative placement of sham needles at the same schedule	162	Patients with cancer undergoing thoracotomy	Comparison of Brief Pain Inventory pain intensity scores at the 30-d follow-up	A special acupuncture technique did not reduce pain or use of pain medication after thoracotomy more than a sham technique

(Continued)

TABLE 54.4 CLINICAL TRIALS OF ACUPUNCTURE USE IN CANCER-RELATED SYMPTOMS *(Continued)*

	Source	Intervention	Design	No. of participants	Setting	Outcomes	Results
Xerostomia	Deng et al. (98)	Unilateral manual acupuncture stimulation at LI-2, a point commonly used in clinical practice to treat xerostomia	RCT; sham acupuncture controlled	20	Healthy volunteers	Cortical regions that were activated or deactivated during the interventions were evaluated by functional magnetic resonance imaging. Saliva production was also measured	Acupuncture at LI-2 was associated with neuronal activations absent during sham acupuncture stimulation. True acupuncture induced more saliva production than sham acupuncture
	Wong et al. (99)	ALTENS[b] daily with radiotherapy for radiation-induced xerostomia	RCT	56	Head and neck cancer patients	Stimulated and basal unstimulated WSP[c] plus RIXVAS[d] were assessed at specific time points	There was no significant difference in mean WSP and RIXVAS between the two groups, so ALTENS is not recommended as a prophylactic intervention
	Simcock et al. (100)	Each received eight weekly sessions of acupuncture using four bilateral acupuncture points (Salivary Gland 2; Modified Point Zero; Shen Men and one point in the distal radial aspect of each index finger [LI1])	Single-arm study	12	Men with established radiation-induced xerostomia	Sialometry and quality of life assessments were performed at baseline and at the end of treatment	There were objective increases in the amounts of saliva produced for 6/12 patients post intervention and the majority also reported subjective improvements. Mean quality of life scores for domains related to salivation and xerostomia also showed improvement
	Simcock et al. (101)	Weekly acupuncture as compared to oral care for treatment of radiation-induced xerostomia	RCT	145 patients divided into two groups: 1. Oral care (*n* = 75) 2. 8 weeks acupuncture (one time per week) (*n* = 70)	chronic radiation-induced xerostomia	Acupuncture compared with oral care, produced significant reductions in patient with severe dry mouth	Acupuncture group reported improvement of severe dry mouth (OR = 2.01, *p* = 0.031) sticky saliva (OR = 1.67, *p* = 0.048), needing to sip fluids to swallow food (OR = 2.08, *p* = 0.011) and in waking up at night to drink (OR = 1.71, *p* = 0.013)

TABLE 54.4 CLINICAL TRIALS OF ACUPUNCTURE USE IN CANCER-RELATED SYMPTOMS (Continued)

	Source	Intervention	Design	No. of participants	Setting	Outcomes	Results
Cancer fatigue cancer	Mao et al. (94)	Manual acupuncture. Patients received up to 12 treatments of acupuncture over the entire course of their RT[e]	Cross-sectional survey study and a single-arm acupuncture clinical trial	16	Patients undergoing radiation therapy	The LFS[f] was administered at baseline, in the middle of RT, and at the end of RT, along with the PGIC[g]	Among the 16 trial participants, average fatigue and energy domains of the LFS remained stable during and after RT, without any expected statistical decline owing to RT. Based on the PGIC at the end of RT, 2 subjects (13%) reported their fatigue as worse, 8 (50%) as stable, and 6 (37%) as better
	Balk et al. (102)	Manual acupuncture once to twice per week during the 6-wk course of radiation therapy	RCT; modified double blind	27	Cancer patients receiving external radiation therapy	Fatigue, fatigue distress, quality of life, and depression	Both true and sham acupuncture groups had improved fatigue, fatigue distress, quality of life, and depression from baseline to 10 wk, but the differences between the groups were not statistically significant
	Molassiotis et al. (103)	Manual acupuncture vs. acupressure vs. sham acupressure group	RCT	47	Patients with cancer who experienced moderate to severe fatigue after chemotherapy	Patients completed the Multidimensional Fatigue Inventory before randomization, at the end of the 2-wk intervention and again about 2 wk after the end of the intervention	Significant improvements were found with regard to general fatigue ($p < 0.001$), physical fatigue ($p = 0.016$), activity ($p = 0.004$), and motivation ($p = 0.024$). At the end of the intervention, there was a 36% improvement in fatigue levels in the acupuncture group, while the acupressure group improved by 19% and the sham acupressure by 0.6%
Chemotherapy-induced neuropathy	Wong et al. (104)	Manual acupuncture	Prospective case series	5	Patients with advanced gynecological cancers requiring chemotherapy with carboplatin and paclitaxel and developed severe paresthesia	Patient self-reported pain score (0–10), analgesic dosage	Average pain score was reduced to 3 out of 10 (range 1–5). All patients had a reduction in analgesic dosage

(Continued)

TABLE 54.4 CLINICAL TRIALS OF ACUPUNCTURE USE IN CANCER-RELATED SYMPTOMS *(Continued)*

	Source	Intervention	Design	No. of participants	Setting	Outcomes	Results
Vasomotor symptoms in breast and prostate cancers	Walker et al. (105)	12 wk of manual acupuncture or venlafaxine treatment (37.5 mg orally at night for 1 wk, then 75 mg at night for the remaining 11 wk)	RCT	50	Women with stage 0–III pre- or postmenopausal breast cancer patients on hormone therapy with tamoxifen or Arimidex with ≥14 hot flashes per week; must be within 5 yr after treatment; Karnofsky performance status >70	The primary end point was hot-flash frequency via the Hot Flash Diary; the MenQOL[h] Questionnaire; the SF-12[i] Survey; the BDI-PC[j]; and the National Cancer Institute Common Toxicity Criteria scale. Patients were observed for 1-yr posttreatment	Both groups exhibited significant decreases in hot flashes, depressive symptoms, and other quality of life symptoms, indicating that acupuncture was as effective as venlafaxine. The acupuncture group experienced no negative adverse effects
	Ashamalla et al. (106)	Electroacupuncture twice a week for 4 wk	Single-arm prospective study	14	Men with hot flashes and history of androgen ablation therapy for prostate cancer	An HFS[k] was used to measure daily hot flashes. The composite daily score was calculated as the product of frequency x severity	The mean initial HFS was 28.3; it dropped to 10.3 (*p* = 0.0001) at 2 wk posttreatment, 7.5 (*p* = 0.0001) at 6 wk, and 7.0 (*p* = 0.001) at 8 mo
	Beer et al. (107)	Acupuncture with electrostimulation biweekly for 4 wk, then weekly for 6 wk	Single-arm prospective study	22	Men who had a hot-flash score >4 who were receiving androgen deprivation therapy for prostate cancer	The primary end point was a 50% reduction in the hot-flash score after 4 wk of therapy, calculated from the patients' daily hot-flash diaries	Of the 22 patients, 41% had responded by week 4 and 55% had a >50% reduction in the hot-flash score at any point during the therapy course

RCT, randomized clinical trial.

[a]Acupuncture-like transcutaneous electrical nerve stimulation.
[b]Whole saliva production.
[c]RIX symptoms visual analog score.
[d]Radiation treatment.
[e]Lee Fatigue Scale.
[f]Patient Global Impression of Change.
[g]Menopause-Specific Quality of Life.
[h]Short Form 12-Item.
[i]Beck Depression Inventory-Primary Care.
[j]Hot-flash score.

treatments are small, and patient expectation may be a large factor influencing outcome (120). Psychosocial processes should be taken into account and explored, rather than dismissed. Additional validated spiritual healing outcome tools will hopefully improve the reliable measurement of efficacy in energy healing techniques (121).

MANIPULATIVE AND BODY-BASED THERAPIES

Exercise Therapy

The benefit of regular exercise has been well recognized in chronic illnesses such as coronary artery disease and chronic obstructive pulmonary disease. More recently, the American Cancer Society (ACS) recommends regular exercise to reduce the risk of colon, breast, renal, and other cancers (122). The field of exercise oncology began with the first studies exploring the effect of exercise training on fatigue and nausea associated with chemotherapy and radiation and loss of fitness found in breast cancer patients (123–125). Since then, the number of studies in this field has increased steadily, covering the spectrum of cancer survivorship—from cancer diagnosis through palliation (126).

The beneficial effects of regular exercise on cancer-specific and all-cause mortality in breast cancer was first demonstrated in a study by Holmes et al. in 2005 (127). Jones et al. demonstrate that peak oxygen consumption ($Vo_{2\,peak}$) is a strong independent predictor of long-term overall survival in non–small cell lung cancer (NSCLC) (128). In a single-arm intervention study, NSCLC patients undergoing lung resection engaged in presurgical daily exercise training at intensities varying from 60% to 100% of baseline peak oxygen consumption $Vo_{2\,peak}$. This training was associated with significant $Vo_{2\,peak}$ increases of 2.4 mL/kg/min that did not decrease below baseline values following surgery (129). Available literature also suggests that higher preoperative physical activity in patients undergoing cancer surgery may be associated with better postoperative outcomes, including better quality of life and shorter lengths of stay (130).

Current studies provide promising evidence that structured exercise training during and after adjuvant cancer therapy is a well-tolerated adjunct therapy for mitigating common treatment-related side effects. Improvements in cancer-related fatigue, anxiety, cardiopulmonary fitness, and enhanced activities of daily living have been demonstrated with exercise training programs. The majority of studies utilize aerobic training alone, resistance training alone, or the combination of both in accordance with the traditional exercise **prescription

guidelines (3 to 5 days per week at 50% to 75% of baseline $Vo_{2\,peak}$ for 12 to 15 weeks) (131). Further studies clarifying the optimal frequency, intensity, type, and duration of exercise intervention, tailored for different types and/or stages of cancer, are needed (131–135).

Finally, a systematic review by Lowe et al. identifies six studies that evaluated the effect of exercise on quality of life, fatigue, or physical function in patients with advanced cancer (136,137). While findings are generally positive, more rigorously designed studies are needed before exercise therapies should be routinely recommended as effective for this population.

The aforementioned exercise intervention mainly consists of aerobic, resistance training, or a combination of both. In recent years, alternative forms of exercise, such as tai chi chuan and qigong, had gained increasing popularity in the Western Hemisphere. Both forms of exercise originated from China, and their popularity has spread extensively throughout the world and is increasing, being used and studied in cancer care. Available literature suggests clinically meaningful benefit in fatigue and sleep quality, with positive trends observed for anxiety, stress, depressive symptoms, and overall quality of life (138,139).

Labyrinth walking is another form of body-based therapy that is considered kinesthetic meditation, combining exercise and spiritual reflection to promote overall well-being. They are often found outdoors in public gardens, but portable, indoor labyrinth canvases are also available in hospital settings.

Generally, a multimodal approach of exercise plus other nonpharmaceutical interventions is more beneficial than the use of one complementary treatment option. For example, a systematic review found that there is moderate to large effect sizes benefit for using combination of CBT, massage, relaxation, and yoga along with aerobic and resistance training to reduce CRF during or after cancer treatment (140).

Massage Therapy

Massage therapy focuses on manual manipulation of soft tissue of whole body areas using pressure and traction (141,142). It is one of the oldest forms of therapeutic interventions, and various cultures have developed their unique styles of massage. It is a complementary modality familiar to cancer survivors for symptom relief and/or relaxation (143). Systematic review and meta-analysis of impact of massage therapy on cancer pain showed potential benefit of massage therapy for the treatment of pain, fatigue, and anxiety (142).

Classical massage, described as manual treatment, using effleurage (long, light strokes), friction (small circular strokes), percussion (chopping motion), and petrissage (kneading action) has been demonstrated in several RCTs to alleviate pain, nausea, depression, anxiety, stress, and fatigue. However, the effect sizes in most trials are small to moderate, with a paucity of high-quality studies (141). Similarly, reflexology is another popular form of massage in which manual pressure is applied to the feet or hands, under the premise that internal organs can be stimulated by pressing particular areas of the extremity. Deep pressure massage should be avoided especially in areas directly over the tumor or radiation therapy affected skin (1). Currently, there is no convincing evidence of efficacy for reflexology in cancer care, but studies are ongoing (144,145). In clinical practice, massage can be helpful with lymphedema and to lessen the feeling of isolation through positive tactile stimulation.

Chiropractic

Chiropractic comes from the Greek words *cheir* (hands) and *praktikos* (efficient) and is defined by the ACS as "a health care system that focuses on the relationship between the body's skeletal and muscular structure and its functions. Treatment often involves manipulating (moving) the bones of the spine to correct medical problems." In addition to chiropractic adjustments, techniques such as massage, stretching, electrical stimulation of the muscles, traction, heat, and ice can be employed (1). While studies suggest chiropractic is effective in some forms of acute lower back pain (146), there is no strong evidence for efficacy in chronic lower back pain. Currently, the nature of the chiropractic clinical encounter and its reported benefits remain to be fully investigated for cancer-related symptoms (147). More research is encouraged in this field as chiropractic services remain well utilized among cancer patients (148).

BIOLOGICALLY BASED THERAPIES

Biologically based therapies, such as phytochemicals and vitamins, are consistently polled to be the most frequently utilized complementary and alternative therapy by cancer patients. For some cancer patients, using botanicals and vitamins may provide an increased sense of control and participation in their health care. For others, these supplements may be viewed as natural complementary therapies that help with cancer- and therapy-related side effects. For still others, herbs and vitamins may represent an alternative to cancer treatment, especially if conventional therapies have failed

(149). Despite the frequent use of phytochemicals and vitamins, many health care providers are not aware of the use of supplements by their patients (150,151). There is the common assumption that "natural" means safe, when many biologically based therapies may interact with cancer treatments (152,153). Furthermore, patients are commonly unaware that dietary supplements are not regulated by the Food and Drug Administration, and preparations of herbs and supplements may vary from manufacturer to manufacturer (154). It is therefore important for clinicians to encourage open discussions of complementary and integrative therapies that patients may be using.

Phytochemicals

Phytochemicals consist of bioactive compounds found in plants. It is estimated that approximately 50% of drugs used in the last few decades are either derived directly from plants or chemically similar to naturally occurring compounds (155,156). In the field of cancer treatment, there is currently an abundance of cancer research invested in finding other phytochemicals that may have anticancer properties like paclitaxel (derived from the Pacific yew). Table 54.5 lists some of the botanically based therapies currently under investigation for cancer treatment or as adjunctive therapy for symptom alleviation as described by Ulbricht and Chao (154). Coffee is a rich source of bioactive compounds that have potential anticarcinogenic effects. However, it remains unclear whether coffee drinking is associated with colorectal cancer. One study done in Japan showed a lower risk of colon cancer among female drinkers of >3 cups coffee/day, no such association in men. Coffee drinking was not associated with risk of rectal cancer in men or women. Results were virtually the same among never smokers except for an increased risk of rectal cancer associated with frequent coffee consumption (176).

Similarly, one study done in Italy evaluated the role of Mediterranean diet which is rich in antioxidant fibers, phytochemicals, and unsaturated fatty acids which may have favorable effect on endometrial cancer (177).

Vitamins (Nutrition and Hydration Are Discussed in Chapter 54)

Vitamins are organic compounds that organisms are required to ingest as nutrients as it cannot be synthesized in sufficient quantities by the organism and must be taken in through diet or the environment. Vitamins have a variety of functions, including hormone-like properties (vitamin D), regulation of cell and tissue growth and differentiation (vitamin A), and act as antioxidants

TABLE 54.5 PHYTOCHEMICALS AND THEIR PROPERTIES, IN CANCER-RELATED STUDIES, AND SAFETY CONSIDERATIONS

Phytochemicals	Properties	Study findings	Safety considerations	General comment/other
Ginger (*Zingiber officinale*)	The rhizome (underground stem) can be used fresh, dried, and powdered, or as a juice or oil	Mixed results for use of ginger for chemotherapy-induced nausea when compared with standard antiemetics though overall more effective than placebo (157,158)	May inhibit platelet function with increased risk of bleeding, gastrointestinal upset, bloating May have estrogenic modulating effect based on in vitro evidence (159)	Special consideration should be taken in estrogen receptor–positive patients and those at increased risk for bleeding
Ginkgo biloba	Extract from the leaves of the *Ginkgo* tree	Mostly in vitro and animal studies on the effects of gingko extract on ovarian and colon cancer cells	May inhibit platelet function Common side effects include headache and gastrointestinal discomfort	Insufficient data to recommend its use for cancer-related symptoms Avoid use with NSAID and anticoagulants
Ginseng (*Panax* spp. and American)	The root is used to make medicine. It is a common ingredient in traditional Chinese medicine	Trials using American ginseng to treat cancer-related fatigue showed nonsignificant trends toward benefit (160,161)	Headache, insomnia, gastrointestinal toxicities, increased risk of bleeding American ginseng preparations that contain chemicals called ginsenosides might act like estrogen	Further clinical trials are needed for the use of ginseng in cancer patients and its effect on cancer treatment Caution when used with medications metabolized by cytochrome P-450 2D6 and in estrogen receptor–positive patients
Green tea (*Camellia sinensis*)	A product made from the *Camellia sinensis* plant. Can be prepared as a beverage or an extract from the leaves	Decreased occurrence of prostate cancer treated with green tea extract vs. placebo with high-grade prostate intraepithelial neoplasia (162) Green tea ingestion associated with improved prognosis in stage I and II breast cancer among Japanese women (163)	Interfere with the action of boronic acid–based proteasome inhibitors	Additional human research is needed in the use of green tea in prevention and treatment of cancer Avoid use in combination with boronic acid–based chemotherapy agents
Milk thistle (*Silybum marianum*)	The aboveground parts and seeds of this plant are used	In vitro and animal model studies show that silibinin, the flavonoid found in the milk thistle, may have antitumorigenesis properties. For example, silibinin has been shown to inhibit mouse lung tumorigenesis (164), induce a loss of cell viability and apoptotic cell death in MCF-7 human breast cancer cells (165), and inhibit the growth of colorectal cancer (166)	Oral milk thistle has generally been well tolerated for up to 6 yr (167). Some side effects include mild gastrointestinal symptoms, urticaria, eczema, and headache. Case reports of anaphylactic reactions Inhibition of cytochrome P-450 3A4 and 2C9	Preliminary studies are promising for silibinin's potential anticancer effects, but more studies are needed before it can be recommended as an anticancer treatment (168) Extracts from milk thistle plant might have estrogen-like properties. Milk thistle seed extracts do not seem to act like estrogen

(Continued)

TABLE 54.5 PHYTOCHEMICALS AND THEIR PROPERTIES, IN CANCER-RELATED STUDIES, AND SAFETY CONSIDERATIONS *(Continued)*

Phytochemicals	Properties	Study findings	Safety considerations	General comment/ other
Mistletoe (*Viscum album*)	Mistletoe is a semiparasitic plant that grows on several species of trees native to Great Britain, Europe, and western Asia. The plant's leaves and twigs are used in herbal remedies; the berries are not used. Mistletoe injections are one of the most widely used unconventional cancer treatment in Europe (154)	While numerous studies have evaluated the effect of mistletoe in survival and quality of life and suggest positive effects among cancer patients, most were of poor methodological quality with publication bias. Further well-designed randomized controlled trials are needed (169)	Contraindicated in patients with protein hypersensitivity or chronic progressive infections Most common reactions are erythema and hyperemia (170,171)	The mistletoe plant should not be eaten because all parts of it are poisonous Patients generally tolerate the intervention well and may have quality of life benefit when used as an adjunct therapy in cancer treatment (172,173). Until more high-quality studies are available, cannot recommend its use as alternative cancer treatment
Turmeric (*Curcuma longa*)	Used as the main spice in curry. The root of the turmeric plant is used to make medicine Curcumin is the hydrophobic polyphenol derived from turmeric and is the active ingredient studied in cancer research	Multiple clinical trials are underway to evaluate the use of turmeric in treatment of cancer In vitro and in vivo research has shown various activities, such as anti-inflammatory, cytokines release, antioxidant, immunomodulatory, enhancing of the apoptotic process, and antiangiogenic properties (174,175)	The most common side effect is epigastric burning, dyspepsia, nausea, and diarrhea. Phase I trial found limited toxicity with doses as high as 8 g daily (154). Can induce liver transaminase abnormalities (in rats) Increased bleeding risk with high doses of curcumin	Use in caution with hepatotoxic agents and those at increased risk of bleeding

NSAIDs, nonsteroidal anti-inflammatory drugs.

(vitamins E and C) and enzyme cofactors (vitamin B complex) (178). The majority of data in the cancer literature regarding vitamins focuses on cancer prevention and investigates potential anticancer properties of vitamin supplements.

β-Carotene is a group of carotenoids that can be found in fruits, vegetables, and whole grains and provide vitamin A. Two large RCTs demonstrate no efficacy from β-carotene supplementation in the prevention of lung cancer (Alpha-Tocopherol and Beta-Carotene Cancer Prevention Trial [ATBC] and Beta-Carotene and Retinol Efficacy Trial); in fact, ATBC study demonstrates an increase in the incidence of lung cancer for those who received β-carotene. In people who smoke, β-carotene supplements might increase the risk of lung and prostate cancer (179). β-Carotene intake is currently recommended through food sources rather than nutritional supplements. Two large-scale studies found that β-carotene increases the risk of lung cancer in tobacco smokers (180).

Vitamin B complex includes thiamine (B1), riboflavin (B2), niacin (B3), pantothenic acid (B5), pyridoxine (B6), biotin (B7), folic acid (B9), and cobalamin (B12). Folic acid is one of the more well-studied B vitamins. Through the years, there have been conflicting results on how folic acid may affect cancer risk. The Nurses' Health Study which followed nurses from 1980 to 1994 reports that the women receiving more than 400 µg of folic acid per day are much less likely to develop colon cancer than those with <200 µg intake (181). However, the large European Prospective Investigation into Cancer and Nutrition (EPIC) study in Europe reports no significant link between folic acid levels in the blood and colon or rectal cancer risk

(182). A similarly mixed result is seen in breast cancer risk and folic acid intake (183). Until more is known, the ACS recommends eating a variety of healthful foods—with most of them coming from plant sources—rather than relying on supplements. As high doses of folic acid may interfere with the actions of methotrexate and other similar class of agents, the use of over-the-counter supplements and vitamins should routinely be investigated in the cancer patient.

Vitamin C is a water-soluble vitamin found in abundance in citrus fruits and in green leafy vegetables. Many studies demonstrate a connection between eating foods rich in vitamin C and a reduced risk of cancer. However, clinical trials of high doses of vitamin C as a treatment for cancer show no benefit (184–186). This suggests that the beneficial effects may be the combination of vitamin C and other phytochemicals found in food products, rather than vitamin C alone. Most oncologists recommend that people with cancer avoid large doses of vitamin C during treatment due to its potential antioxidant effects (187).

Observational epidemiologic studies suggest that higher levels of vitamin D in the body might be linked to lower cancer risk. In a study of more than 3,000 adults who had colonoscopies between 1994 and 1997, those with the highest vitamin D intake are less likely to have advanced cancer than those with low intake. In randomized control trials, the Women's Health Initiative study randomly divides 36,000 menopausal women into the intervention group of vitamin D with calcium and placebo (sham pill) group. After 7 years, the cancer risk is not significantly different between the two groups. Criticisms of this study cite the low dose of vitamin D given (400 IU/d) and the allowance of supplemental vitamin D and calcium possibly diluting the effect of intervention (188,189). Subsequent studies with long-term follow-up did not find evidence to suggest vitamin D supplementation alone reduces the incidences of cancer or cancer mortality (190,191).

Lappe's randomized control trial, including calcium, calcium plus vitamin D3, and placebo arms, demonstrates a reduction in cancer risk conferred to women receiving supplemental calcium and vitamin D (192). However, it is difficult to tease out the effect of calcium from vitamin D in many of these studies, and more studies are needed to confirm this finding.

There are several pilot studies evaluating the use of vitamin D in prostate cancer treatment and its use in combination with chemotherapy agents (Taxotere). More studies are likely to follow, and further investigations are needed before conclusions can be made (193,194).

Vitamin E represents a group of fat-soluble substances that function as antioxidants in the body. The Woman Health Study showed that vitamin E has no effect on lung, breast, and colorectal cancers. The Selenium and Vitamin E Cancer Prevention Trial (SELECT) showed that vitamin E alone or in combination with selenium did not prevent prostate cancer. Vitamin E supplement taken alone in higher dose increases the risk of prostate cancer in men but no increase in prostate cancer risk when vitamin E and selenium were taken together (195). It is unclear how the antioxidant effect of vitamin E interacts with radiation therapy and some chemotherapy agents—whether reducing or potentiating the treatments' effectiveness (196). Patients taking Vitamin E supplements should be aware of its increased risk of hemorrhagic stroke.

Finally, small clinical studies on the effect of menatetrenone, a vitamin K2 analog, on liver cancer development and recurrence show promising results. More research is needed to demonstrate the strength of this effect (197).

In general, one should be aware of the following when considering the use of natural product while receiving cancer treatment (198):

- Natural products with antioxidant properties that may interfere with radiation and/or chemotherapy efficacy.
- Natural products with anticoagulant properties, especially in setting of thrombocytopenia.
- Phytoestrogenic herbs may interfere with hormone therapies or affect hormone sensitive cancers.
- Immunostimulant herbs may affect immunosuppressive therapies.
- Renal and hepatic toxicities have been associated with natural products.
- Quality control of natural product varies.

Pediatric

Pediatric integrative medicine is increasingly found in academic settings where it has institutional support, funding, and trained clinicians. Outpatient practices are readily available in larger communities but often require to pay for service out of pocket.

Children undergoing oncological treatments are agreeable to trying and accepting complementary therapies for symptom relief, often, simply because they are not medications. In the midst of "high-tech" care, massage and Reiki are perceived as nicer, gentle touch. Utilization of biofeedback and guided imagery parallels in their understanding through the similarity to gaming. Breathing techniques, hypnosis, and music therapy are easier to teach to children in that they have less blocks to disassociating then adults. Acupuncture is embraced by adolescents, in younger patients it is suggested to describe acupuncture as getting "taps" versus needles inserted. Yoga designed for kids is an effective method for exercise in those who are deconditioned or neutropenic.

When introducing a novel, complementary therapy, ask if the parents or sibling can participate with the patient or have the parent go first in the case of acupuncture application. The best strategy for success and adaption into the plan of care is to keep sessions short, 10 to 15 minutes each.

Examples of Breathing Techniques

1. Balloon breathing: Pretend there is a balloon in your tummy. Watch your tummy expand while you breathe in and then deflate the balloon in your stomach as you exhale.
2. Bumble bee breathing: Plug your ears with your fingers, breathe in your mouth making a buzzing/humming noise, and breath out your nose making a buzzing/humming noise.
3. Beach breathing: As you inhale imagine the waves coming up on the beach; when exhaling imagine the wave receding back to the ocean.

Practical Considerations in Implementing Complementary Modalities

1. Initiate one modality at a time as you would introduce a new medication.
2. Periodically reassess its effectiveness in treating your target symptom(s).
3. Therapies can be combined for synergy—for example, combining Reiki and hypnosis for anxiety.
4. It is unlikely that one treatment session of any complementary modalities will resolve the target symptom. Most require a series of the intervention to determine effectiveness.

FUTURE DIRECTIONS

In this chapter, we reviewed the indications and evidence for mind–body interventions, energy therapies, manipulative and body-based methods, and biologically based therapies in integrative oncologic care. While integrative oncology is a relatively young field, preliminary results from some clinical trials and bench research are promising, and certain complementary interventions have shown to significantly affect a person's well-being during conventional cancer treatment and cancer survivorship.

The trend in oncologic care over the past decades has been toward a multidisciplinary as well as a multidimensional approach to patient care. There is a growing recognition of cancer patients' needs beyond conventional cancer treatment, and the importance of an interdisciplinary team that includes nurse, social worker, chaplain, physical therapist, occupational therapist, recreational therapist, and physician to address problems and concerns that arise through cancer diagnosis, management, remission, and end-of-life care. Similarly, the goal of integrative oncology is to assess the needs of the whole person and to utilize safe, effective, and well-tolerated complementary interventions to manage symptoms, be they physical, psychological, or spiritual.

Future research should focus on standardizing definition of various complementary therapies and performing studies with larger sample sizes and more stringent study designs. Ongoing research is also underway in the field of phytochemicals and vitamins, exploring their roles in cancer risk and cancer treatment. Finally, increasing awareness of complementary therapies throughout the professional and public communities will promote evidence-based recommendations, encourage open dialogue between patients and physicians regarding complementary and integrative medicine use, and encourage critical appraisal of inadequately studied and regulated products and therapies. It is likely that the field of integrative oncology will continue to evolve and increasingly inform and influence the care of cancer patients.

USEFUL WEB SITES

Society for Integrative Oncology: https://integrativeonc.org/

MD Anderson Cancer Center Integrative Medicine Program: https://www.mdanderson.org/research/departments-labs-institutes/programs-centers/integrative-medicine-program.html

Memorial Sloan Kettering Cancer Center Integrative Medicine Service: https://www.mskcc.org/integrativemedicine

Consumer Lab: http://cms.herbalgram.org/herbstream/mdanderson/homePage/ (subscription)

Natural Medicines Comprehensive Database: https://naturalmedicines.therapeuticresearch.com/ (subscription)_

National Cancer Institute Office of Cancer Complementary and Alternative Medicine: https://cam.cancer.gov/

Office of Dietary Supplements: https://ods.od.nih.gov/

National Center for Complementary and Integrative Health: https://nccih.nih.gov/

University of Arizona Center for Integrative Medicine: https://integrativemedicine.arizona.edu/

REFERENCES

1. National Center for Complementary and Integrative Health. https://nccih.nih.gov/health/integrative-health. Accessed November 9, 2019.
2. Verhoef MJ, Mulkins A, Carlson LE, Hilsden RJ, Kania A. Assessing the role of evidence in patients' evaluation of complementary therapies: a quality study. *Integr Cancer Ther.* 2007;6(4):345-353.
3. Clarke TC, Black LI, Stussman BJ, Barnes PM, Nahin RL. Trends in the use of complementary health approaches among adults: United States, 2002-2012. *Natl Health Stat Rep.* 2015;(79):1-16.
4. Clarke TC. The use of complementary health approaches among U.S. adults with a recent cancer diagnosis. *J Altern Complement Med.* 2018;24(2):139-145.
5. Sanford NN, Sher DJ, Ahn C, Aizer AA, Mahal BA. Prevalence and nondisclosure of complementary and alternative medicine use in patients with cancer and cancer survivors in the United States. *JAMA Oncol.* 2019;5(5):735-737.
6. Nahin RL, Boineau R, Khalsa PS, Stussman BJ, Weber WJ. Evidence-based evaluation of complementary health approaches for pain management in the United States. *Mayo Clin Proc.* 2016;91(9):1292-1306.
7. Geffen JR. Integrative oncology for the whole person: a multidimensional approach to cancer care. *Integr Cancer Ther.* 2010;9(1):105-121.
8. Menendez-Aponte YGRM, Turcott Chaparro JG, De la Piedra Gomez A, et al. Effect of complementary Integrative Oncology on anxiety, depression and quality of life in thoracic cancer patients: a pilot study. *Complement Ther Clin Pract.* 2019;36:56-63.
9. Frenkel M, Balneaves LG. Integrative oncology: an essential feature of high-quality cancer care. *J Altern Complement Med.* 2018;24(9-10):855-858.
10. Lopez G, McQuade J, Cohen L, et al. Integrative oncology physician consultations at a comprehensive cancer center: analysis of demographic, clinical and patient reported outcomes. *J Cancer.* 2017;8(3):395-402.
11. John GM, Hershman DL, Falci L, Shi Z, Tsai WY, Greenlee H. Complementary and alternative medicine use among US cancer survivors. *J Cancer Surviv.* 2016;10(5):850-864.
12. Ding SS, Hong SH, Wang C, Guo Y, Wang ZK, Xu Y. Acupuncture modulates the neuro-endocrine-immune network. *QJM.* 2014;107(5):341-345.
13. Neron S, Stephenson R. Effectiveness of hypnotherapy with cancer patients' trajectory: emesis, acute pain, and analgesia and anxiolysis in procedures. *Int J Clin Exp Hypn.* 2007;55(3):336-354.
14. Elkins G, Fisher W, Johnson A. Mind-body therapies in integrative oncology. *Curr Treat Options Oncol.* 2010;11(3-4):128-140.
15. Carlson LE. Distress management through mind-body therapies in oncology. *J Natl Cancer Inst Monogr.* 2017;2017(52).
16. Kihlstrom JF. Hypnosis. *Annu Rev Psychol.* 1985;36:385-418.
17. Elkins G, Jensen MP, Patterson DR. Hypnotherapy for the management of chronic pain. *Int J Clin Exp Hypn.* 2007;55(3):275-287.
18. Integration of behavioral and relaxation approaches into the treatment of chronic pain and insomnia. NIH Technology Assessment Panel on Integration of Behavioral and Relaxation Approaches into the Treatment of Chronic Pain and Insomnia. *JAMA.* 1996;276(4):313-318.
19. Juel J, Abrahamsen R, Olesen SS, Drewes AM. A pilot-study of hypnotherapy as complementary treatment for pain in chronic pancreatitis. *J Complement Integr Med.* 2018;15(4).
20. Brugnoli MP, Pesce G, Pasin E, Basile MF, Tamburin S, Polati E. The role of clinical hypnosis and self-hypnosis to relief pain and anxiety in severe chronic diseases in palliative care: a 2-year long-term follow-up of treatment in a nonrandomized clinical trial. *Ann Palliat Med.* 2018;7(1):17-31.
21. Willmarth EK. Clinical hypnosis in pain therapy and palliative care: a handbook of techniques for improving the patient's physical and psychological well-being by Brugnoli, Maria Paola. *Am J Clin Hypn.* 2017;59(3):318-320.
22. Lang EV, Berbaum KS, Faintuch S, et al. Adjunctive self-hypnotic relaxation for outpatient medical procedures: a prospective randomized trial with women undergoing large core breast biopsy. *Pain.* 2006;126(1-3):155-164.
23. Liossi C, White P, Hatira P. Randomized clinical trial of local anesthetic versus a combination of local anesthetic with self-hypnosis in the management of pediatric procedure-related pain. *Health Psychol.* 2006;25(3):307-315.
24. Stoelb BL, Molton IR, Jensen MP, Patterson DR. The efficacy of hypnotic analgesia in adults: a review of the literature. *Contemp Hypn.* 2009;26(1):24-39.
25. Rajasekaran M, Edmonds PM, Higginson IL. Systematic review of hypnotherapy for treating symptoms in terminally ill adult cancer patients. *Palliat Med.* 2005;19(5):418-426.
26. Zeltzer LK, Dolgin MJ, LeBaron S, LeBaron C. A randomized, controlled study of behavioral intervention for chemotherapy distress in children with cancer. *Pediatrics.* 1991;88(1):34-42.
27. Jacknow DS, Tschann JM, Link MP, Boyce WT. Hypnosis in the prevention of chemotherapy-related nausea and vomiting in children: a prospective study. *J Dev Behav Pediatr.* 1994;15(4):258-264.
28. Syrjala KL, Cummings C, Donaldson GW. Hypnosis or cognitive behavioral training for the reduction of pain and nausea during cancer treatment: a controlled clinical trial. *Pain.* 1992;48(2):137-146.
29. Elkins G, Marcus J, Stearns V, et al. Randomized trial of a hypnosis intervention for treatment of hot flashes among breast cancer survivors. *J Clin Oncol.* 2008;26(31):5022-5026.
30. Liossi C, Hatira P. Clinical hypnosis in the alleviation of procedure-related pain in pediatric oncology patients. *Int J Clin Exp Hypn.* 2003;51(1):4-28.
31. Lang EV, Benotsch EG, Fick LJ, et al. Adjunctive non-pharmacological analgesia for invasive medical procedures: a randomised trial. *Lancet.* 2000;355(9214):1486-1490.
32. Spiegel D, Bloom JR, Kraemer HC, Gottheil E. Effect of psychosocial treatment on survival of patients with metastatic breast cancer. *Lancet.* 1989;2(8668):888-891.
33. Spiegel D, Cordova M. Supportive-expressive group therapy and life extension of breast cancer patients: Spiegel et al. (1989). *Adv Mind Body Med.* 2001;17(1):38-41.
34. Jacobson E. *Progressive Relaxation.* Chicago, IL: University of Chicago Press; 1929.
35. Cannici J, Malcolm R, Peek LA. Treatment of insomnia in cancer patients using muscle relaxation training. *J Behav Ther Exp Psychiatry.* 1983;14(3):251-256.
36. Voiss P, Hoxtermann MD, Dobos G, Cramer H. Cancer, sleep problems, and mind-body medicine use: results of the 2017 National Health Interview Survey. *Cancer.* 2019;125(24):4490-4497.
37. Kwekkeboom KL, Cherwin CH, Lee JW, Wanta B. Mind-body treatments for the pain-fatigue-sleep disturbance

symptom cluster in persons with cancer. *J Pain Symptom Manage.* 2010;39(1):126-138.

38. Carlson LE, Zelinski E, Toivonen K, et al. Mind-body therapies in cancer: what is the latest evidence? *Curr Oncol Rep.* 2017;19(10):67.

39. NCC Network. NCCN guidelines for patients nausea and vomiting. *Supportive Care Book Series 2016.* Accessed March 3, 2020.

40. Roffe L, Schmidt K, Ernst E. A systematic review of guided imagery as an adjuvant cancer therapy. *Psychooncology.* 2005;14(8):607-617.

41. Sloman R. Relaxation and imagery for anxiety and depression control in community patients with advanced cancer. *Cancer Nurs.* 2002;25(6):432-435.

42. Feldman CS, Salzberg HC. The role of imagery in the hypnotic treatment of adverse reactions to cancer therapy. *J S C Med Assoc.* 1990;86(5):303-306.

43. Troesch LM, Rodehaver CB, Delaney EA, Yanes B. The influence of guided imagery on chemotherapy-related nausea and vomiting. *Oncol Nurs Forum.* 1993;20(8):1179-1185.

44. Kapogiannis A, Tsoli S, Chrousos G. Investigating the effects of the progressive muscle relaxation-guided imagery combination on patients with cancer receiving chemotherapy treatment: a systematic review of randomized controlled trials. *Explore (NY).* 2018;14(2):137-143.

45. Hosseini M, Tirgari B, Forouzi MA, Jahani Y. Guided imagery effects on chemotherapy induced nausea and vomiting in Iranian breast cancer patients. *Complement Ther Clin Pract.* 2016;25:8-12.

46. Kabat-Zinn J. *Full Catastrophe Living: Using the Power of Your Body and Mind to Face Stress, Pain, and Illness.* Delta Trade Paperbacks. New York, NY: Bantam Books Trade Paperbacks; 1991.

47. Ott MJ, Norris RL, Bauer-Wu SM. Mindfulness meditation for oncology patients: a discussion and critical review. *Integr Cancer Ther.* 2006;5(2):98-108.

48. Brown KW, Ryan RM. The benefits of being present: mindfulness and its role in psychological well-being. *J Pers Soc Psychol.* 2003;84(4):822-848.

49. Carlson LE, Speca M, Patel KD, Goodey E. Mindfulness-based stress reduction in relation to quality of life, mood, symptoms of stress, and immune parameters in breast and prostate cancer outpatients. *Psychosom Med.* 2003;65(4):571-581.

50. Shapiro SL, Bootzin RR, Figueredo AJ, Lopez AM, Schwartz GE. The efficacy of mindfulness-based stress reduction in the treatment of sleep disturbance in women with breast cancer: an exploratory study. *J Psychosom Res.* 2003;54(1):85-91.

51. Tacón AM, Caldera YM, Ronaghan C. Mindfulness-Based Stress Reduction in Women with Breast Cancer. *Fam Syst Health.* 2004;22(2):193-203.

52. Carlson LE, Speca M, Patel KD, Goodey E. Mindfulness-based stress reduction in relation to quality of life, mood, symptoms of stress and levels of cortisol, dehydroepiandrosterone sulfate (DHEAS) and melatonin in breast and prostate cancer outpatients. *Psychoneuroendocrinology.* 2004;29(4):448-474.

53. Duong N, Davis H, Robinson PD, et al. Mind and body practices for fatigue reduction in patients with cancer and hematopoietic stem cell transplant recipients: a systematic review and meta-analysis. *Crit Rev Oncol Hematol.* 2017;120:210-216.

54. Holzel BK, Carmody J, Vangel M, et al. Mindfulness practice leads to increases in regional brain gray matter density. *Psychiatry Res.* 2011;191(1):36-43.

55. Luders E, Kurth F, Mayer EA, Toga AW, Narr KL, Gaser C. The unique brain anatomy of meditation practitioners: alterations in cortical gyrification. *Front Hum Neurosci.* 2012;6:34.

56. Mehta R, Sharma K, Potters L, Wernicke AG, Parashar B. Evidence for the role of mindfulness in cancer: benefits and techniques. *Cureus.* 2019;11(5):e4629.

57. DiStasio SA. Integrating yoga into cancer care. *Clin J Oncol Nurs.* 2008;12(1):125-130.

58. Moadel AB, Shah C, Wylie-Rosett J, et al. Randomized controlled trial of yoga among a multiethnic sample of breast cancer patients: effects on quality of life. *J Clin Oncol.* 2007;25(28):4387-4395.

59. Blank S, Kittel J, Haberman M. Active practice of Iyengar yoga as an intervention for breast cancer survivors. *Int J Yoga Therap.* 2005;15(1):51-59.

60. Duncan MD, Leis A, Taylor-Brown JW. Impact and outcomes of an Iyengar yoga program in a cancer centre. *Curr Oncol.* 2008;15(Suppl 2):s109.es72-s109.es108.

61. Speed-Andrews AE, Stevinson C, Belanger LJ, Mirus JJ, Courneya KS. Pilot evaluation of an Iyengar yoga program for breast cancer survivors. *Cancer Nurs.* 2010; 33(5):369-381.

62. Danhauer SC, Tooze JA, Farmer DF, et al. Restorative yoga for women with ovarian or breast cancer: findings from a pilot study. *J Soc Integr Oncol.* 2008;6(2):47-58.

63. Danhauer SC, Mihalko SL, Russell GB, et al. Restorative yoga for women with breast cancer: findings from a randomized pilot study. *Psychooncology.* 2009;18(4): 360-368.

64. Cohen BE, Kanaya AM, Macer JL, Shen H, Chang AA, Grady D. Feasibility and acceptability of restorative yoga for treatment of hot flushes: a pilot trial. *Maturitas.* 2007;56(2):198-204.

65. Carson JW, Carson KM, Porter LS, Keefe FJ, Seewaldt VL. Yoga of Awareness program for menopausal symptoms in breast cancer survivors: results from a randomized trial. *Support Care Cancer.* 2009;17(10): 1301-1309.

66. Peppone LJ, Janelsins MC, Kamen C, et al. The effect of YOCAS(c)(R) yoga for musculoskeletal symptoms among breast cancer survivors on hormonal therapy. *Breast Cancer Res Treat.* 2015;150(3):597-604.

67. Mustian KM, Palesh O, Sprod L, et al. Effect of YOCAS yoga on sleep, fatigue, and quality of life: a URCC CCOP randomized, controlled clinical trial among 410 cancer survivors. *J Clin Oncol.* 2010;28(15 suppl):9013.

68. Hede K. Supportive care: large studies ease yoga, exercise into mainstream oncology. *J Natl Cancer Inst.* 2011;103(1):11-12.

69. El-Hashimi D, Gorey KM. Yoga-specific enhancement of quality of life among women with breast cancer: systematic review and exploratory meta-analysis of randomized controlled trials. *J Evid Based Integr Med.* 2019;24:2515690X19828325.

70. Applied psychophysiology and biofeedback. https:// www.aapb.org/i4a/pages/index.cfm?pageid=1. Accessed November 15, 2019.

71. Hetkamp M, Bender J, Rheindorf N, et al. A systematic review of the effect of neurofeedback in cancer patients. *Integr Cancer Ther.* 2019;18:1534735419832361.

72. Liang Z, Ding W, Chen W, Wang Z, Du P, Cui L. Therapeutic evaluation of biofeedback therapy in the treatment of anterior resection syndrome after sphincter-saving surgery for rectal cancer. *Clin Colorectal Cancer.* 2016;15(3):e101-e107.

73. Tsai PS, Chen PL, Lai YL, Lee MB, Lin CC. Effects of electromyography biofeedback-assisted relaxation on pain in patients with advanced cancer in a palliative care unit. *Cancer Nurs.* 2007;30(5):347-353.

74. George R, Chung TD, Vedam SS, et al. Audio-visual biofeedback for respiratory-gated radiotherapy: impact of audio instruction and audio-visual biofeedback on respiratory-gated radiotherapy. *Int J Radiat Oncol Biol Phys.* 2006;65(3):924-933.

75. Pollock S, O'Brien R, Makhija K, et al. Audiovisual bio-feedback breathing guidance for lung cancer patients receiving radiotherapy: a multi-institutional phase II randomised clinical trial. *BMC Cancer.* 2015;15:526.

76. Katz JE, Chinea FM, Patel VN, et al. Disparities in Hispanic/Latino and non-Hispanic Black men with low-risk prostate cancer and eligible for active surveillance: a population-based study. *Prostate Cancer Prostatic Dis.* 2018;21(4):533-538.

77. Pollock S, Tse R, Martin D, et al. Impact of audiovisual biofeedback on interfraction respiratory motion reproducibility in liver cancer stereotactic body radiotherapy. *J Med Imaging Radiat Oncol.* 2018;62(1):133-139.

78. Stam MR, van Lin EN, van der Vight LP, Kaanders JH, Visser AG. Bladder filling variation during radiation treatment of prostate cancer: can the use of a bladder ultrasound scanner and biofeedback optimize bladder filling? *Int J Radiat Oncol Biol Phys.* 2006;65(2):371-377.

79. Kye BH, Kim HJ, Kim G, Yoo RN, Cho HM. The effect of biofeedback therapy on anorectal function after the reversal of temporary stoma when administered during the temporary stoma period in rectal cancer patients with sphincter-saving surgery: the interim report of a prospective randomized controlled trial. *Medicine (Baltimore).* 2016;95(18):e3611.

80. Cohen M. A model of group cognitive behavioral intervention combined with bio-feedback in oncology settings. *Soc Work Health Care.* 2010;49(2):149-164.

81. Shockey DP, Menzies V, Glick DF, Taylor AG, Boitnott A, Rovnyak V. Preprocedural distress in children with cancer: an intervention using biofeedback and relaxation. *J Pediatr Oncol Nurs.* 2013;30(3):129-138.

82. Luctkar-Flude M, Groll D. A systematic review of the safety and effect of neurofeedback on fatigue and cognition. *Integr Cancer Ther.* 2015;14(4):318-340.

83. Olofsson A, Fossum B. Perspectives on music therapy in adult cancer care: a hermeneutic study. *Oncol Nurs Forum.* 2009;36(4):E223-E231.

84. Gallagher LM, Lagman R, Rybicki L. Outcomes of music therapy interventions on symptom management in palliative medicine patients. *Am J Hosp Palliat Care.* 2018;35(2):250-257.

85. Gallagher LM. The role of music therapy in palliative medicine and supportive care. *Semin Oncol.* 2011;38(3):403-406.

86. Gallagher LM, Lagman R, Bates D, et al. Perceptions of family members of palliative medicine and hospice patients who experienced music therapy. *Support Care Cancer.* 2017;25(6):1769-1778.

87. Bradt J, Dileo C, Magill L, Teague A. Music interventions for improving psychological and physical outcomes in cancer patients. *Cochrane Database Syst Rev.* 2016;(8):CD006911.

88. Geue K, Goetze H, Buttstaedt M, Kleinert E, Richter D, Singer S. An overview of art therapy interventions for cancer patients and the results of research. *Complement Ther Med.* 2010;18(3-4):160-170.

89. Kemper KJ, Sarah R, Silver-Highfield E, Xiarhos E, Barnes L, Berde C. On pins and needles? Pediatric pain patients' experience with acupuncture. *Pediatrics.* 2000;105(4 Pt 2):941-947.

90. McDonald J, Janz S. *The Acupuncture Evidence Project: A Comparative Literature Review (Revised Edition).* Brisbane: Australian Acupuncture and Chinese Medicine Association Ltd; 2017. http://www.acupuncture.org.au/. Accessed November 10, 2019.

91. World Health Organization. *Acupuncture: Review and Analysis of Reports on Controlled Clinical Trial.* 2002.

http://apps.who.int/bookorders/anglais/detart1.jsp?codlan=1&codcol=93&codcch=196. Accessed November 15, 2019.

92. Crew KD, Capodice JL, Greenlee H, et al. Randomized, blinded, sham-controlled trial of acupuncture for the management of aromatase inhibitor-associated joint symptoms in women with early-stage breast cancer. *J Clin Oncol.* 2010;28(7):1154-1160.

93. Mao JJ, Bruner DW, Stricker C, et al. Feasibility trial of electroacupuncture for aromatase inhibitor—related arthralgia in breast cancer survivors. *Integr Cancer Ther.* 2009;8(2):123-129.

94. Mao JJ, Styles T, Cheville A, Wolf J, Fernandes S, Farrar JT. Acupuncture for nonpalliative radiation therapy-related fatigue: feasibility study. *J Soc Integr Oncol.* 2009;7(2):52-58.

95. Dean-Clower E, Doherty-Gilman AM, Keshaviah A, et al. Acupuncture as palliative therapy for physical symptoms and quality of life for advanced cancer patients. *Integr Cancer Ther.* 2010;9(2):158-167.

96. Pfister DG, Cassileth BR, Deng GE, et al. Acupuncture for pain and dysfunction after neck dissection: results of a randomized controlled trial. *J Clin Oncol.* 2010;28(15):2565-2570.

97. Deng G, Rusch V, Vickers A, et al. Randomized controlled trial of a special acupuncture technique for pain after thoracotomy. *J Thorac Cardiovasc Surg.* 2008;136(6):1464-1469.

98. Deng G, Hou BL, Holodny AI, Cassileth BR. Functional magnetic resonance imaging (fMRI) changes and saliva production associated with acupuncture at LI-2 acupuncture point: a randomized controlled study. *BMC Complement Altern Med.* 2008;8:37.

99. Wong RK, Sagar SM, Chen BJ, Yi GY, Cook R. Phase II randomized trial of acupuncture-like transcutaneous electrical nerve stimulation to prevent radiation-induced xerostomia in head and neck cancer patients. *J Soc Integr Oncol.* 2010;8(2):35-42.

100. Simcock R, Fallowfield L, Jenkins V. Group acupuncture to relieve radiation induced xerostomia: a feasibility study. *Acupunct Med.* 2009;27(3):109-113.

101. Simcock R, Fallowfield L, Monson K, et al. ARIX: a randomised trial of acupuncture versus oral care sessions in patients with chronic xerostomia following treatment of head and neck cancer. *Ann Oncol.* 2013;24(3):776-783.

102. Balk J, Day R, Rosenzweig M, Beriwal S. Pilot, randomized, modified, double-blind, placebo-controlled trial of acupuncture for cancer-related fatigue. *J Soc Integr Oncol.* 2009;7(1):4-11.

103. Molassiotis A, Sylt P, Diggins H. The management of cancer-related fatigue after chemotherapy with acupuncture and acupressure: a randomised controlled trial. *Complement Ther Med.* 2007;15(4):228-237.

104. Wong R, Sagar S. Acupuncture treatment for chemotherapy-induced peripheral neuropathy—a case series. *Acupunct Med.* 2006;24(2):87-91.

105. Walker EM, Rodriguez AI, Kohn B, et al. Acupuncture versus venlafaxine for the management of vasomotor symptoms in patients with hormone receptor-positive breast cancer: a randomized controlled trial. *J Clin Oncol.* 2010;28(4):634-640.

106. Ashamalla H, Jiang ML, Guirguis A, Peluso F, Ashamalla M. Acupuncture for the alleviation of hot flashes in men treated with androgen ablation therapy. *Int J Radiat Oncol Biol Phys.* 2011;79(5):1358-1363.

107. Beer TM, Benavides M, Emmons SL, et al. Acupuncture for hot flashes in patients with prostate cancer. *Urology.* 2010;76(5):1182-1188.

108. Capodice JL. Acupuncture in the oncology setting: clinical trial update. *Curr Treat Options Oncol.* 2010;11(3-4): 87-94.

109. Birch S, Lee MS, Alraek T, Kim TH. Evidence, safety and recommendations for when to use acupuncture for treating cancer related symptoms: a narrative review. *Integr Med Res.* 2019;8(3):160-166.

110. Chen L, Lin CC, Huang TW, et al. Effect of acupuncture on aromatase inhibitor-induced arthralgia in patients with breast cancer: a meta-analysis of randomized controlled trials. *Breast.* 2017;33:132-138.

111. Lau CH, Wu X, Chung VC, et al. Acupuncture and related therapies for symptom management in palliative cancer care: systematic review and meta-analysis. *Medicine (Baltimore).* 2016;95(9):e2901.

112. Assy Z, Brand HS. A systematic review of the effects of acupuncture on xerostomia and hyposalivation. *BMC Complement Altern Med.* 2018;18(1):57.

113. Zhang Y, Lin L, Li H, Hu Y, Tian L. Effects of acupuncture on cancer-related fatigue: a meta-analysis. *Support Care Cancer.* 2018;26(2):415-425.

114. Li K, Giustini D, Seely D. A systematic review of acupuncture for chemotherapy-induced peripheral neuropathy. *Curr Oncol.* 2019;26(2):e147-e154.

115. Shen J, Wenger N, Glaspy J, et al. Electroacupuncture for control of myeloablative chemotherapy-induced emesis: a randomized controlled trial. *JAMA.* 2000;284(21):2755-2761.

116. Lu W, Rosenthal DS. Recent advances in oncology acupuncture and safety considerations in practice. *Curr Treat Options Oncol.* 2010;11(3-4):141-146.

117. Agdal R, von B Hjelmborg J, Johannessen H. Energy healing for cancer: a critical review. *Forsch Komplementmed.* 2011;18(3):146-154.

118. Tabatabaee A, Tafreshi MZ, Rassouli M, Aledavood SA, AlaviMajd H, Farahmand SK. Effect of therapeutic touch in patients with cancer: a literature review. *Med Arch.* 2016;70(2):142-147.

119. Zucchetti G, Candela F, Bottigelli C, et al. The power of reiki: feasibility and efficacy of reducing pain in children with cancer undergoing hematopoietic stem cell transplantation. *J Pediatr Oncol Nurs.* 2019;36(5):361-368.

120. Pohl G, Seemann H, Zojer N, et al. "Laying on of hands" improves well-being in patients with advanced cancer. *Support Care Cancer.* 2007;15(2):143-151.

121. Bishop FL, Barlow F, Walker J, McDermott C, Lewith GT. The development and validation of an outcome measure for spiritual healing: a mixed methods study. *Psychother Psychosom.* 2010;79(6):350-362.

122. Kushi LH, Doyle C, McCullough M, et al. American Cancer Society Guidelines on nutrition and physical activity for cancer prevention: reducing the risk of cancer with healthy food choices and physical activity. *CA Cancer J Clin.* 2012;62(1):30-67.

123. Doyle C, Kushi LH, Byers T, et al. Nutrition and physical activity during and after cancer treatment: an American Cancer Society guide for informed choices. *CA Cancer J Clin.* 2006;56(6):323-353.

124. Winningham ML, MacVicar MG. The effect of aerobic exercise on patient reports of nausea. *Oncol Nurs Forum.* 1988;15(4):447-450.

125. Gianni L, Dombernowsky P, Sledge G, et al. Cardiac function following combination therapy with paclitaxel and doxorubicin: an analysis of 657 women with advanced breast cancer. *Ann Oncol.* 2001;12(8): 1067-1073.

126. Jones LW, Peppercorn J, Scott JM, Battaglini C. Erratum to: Exercise therapy in the management of solid tumors. *Curr Treat Options Oncol.* 2010;11(3-4):73-86.

127. Holmes MD, Chen WY, Feskanich D, Kroenke CH, Colditz GA. Physical activity and survival after breast cancer diagnosis. *JAMA.* 2005;293(20):2479-2486.

128. Jones LW, Watson D, Herndon JE II, et al. Peak oxygen consumption and long-term all-cause mortality in nonsmall cell lung cancer. *Cancer.* 2010;116(20): 4825-4832.

129. Jones LW, Peddle CJ, Eves ND, et al. Effects of presurgical exercise training on cardiorespiratory fitness among patients undergoing thoracic surgery for malignant lung lesions. *Cancer.* 2007;110(3):590-598.

130. Steffens D, Beckenkamp PR, Young J, Solomon M, da Silva TM, Hancock MJ. Is preoperative physical activity level of patients undergoing cancer surgery associated with postoperative outcomes? A systematic review and meta-analysis. *Eur J Surg Oncol.* 2019;45(4):510-518.

131. Speck RM, Courneya KS, Masse LC, Duval S, Schmitz KH. An update of controlled physical activity trials in cancer survivors: a systematic review and meta-analysis. *J Cancer Surviv.* 2010;4(2):87-100.

132. Segal R, Evans W, Johnson D, et al. Structured exercise improves physical functioning in women with stages I and II breast cancer: results of a randomized controlled trial. *J Clin Oncol.* 2001;19(3):657-665.

133. Courneya KS, Segal RJ, Mackey JR, et al. Effects of aerobic and resistance exercise in breast cancer patients receiving adjuvant chemotherapy: a multicenter randomized controlled trial. *J Clin Oncol.* 2007;25(28):4396-4404.

134. Furmaniak AC, Menig M, Markes MH. Exercise for women receiving adjuvant therapy for breast cancer. *Cochrane Database Syst Rev.* 2016;9:CD005001.

135. Cramp F, Byron-Daniel J. Exercise for the management of cancer-related fatigue in adults. *Cochrane Database Syst Rev.* 2012;11:CD006145.

136. Lowe SS, Watanabe SM, Baracos VE, Courneya KS. Physical activity interests and preferences in palliative cancer patients. *Support Care Cancer.* 2010;18(11): 1469-1475.

137. Lowe SS, Watanabe SM, Courneya KS. Physical activity as a supportive care intervention in palliative cancer patients: a systematic review. *J Support Oncol.* 2009;7(1):27-34.

138. Pan Y, Yang K, Shi X, Liang H, Zhang F, Lv Q. Tai chi chuan exercise for patients with breast cancer: a systematic review and meta-analysis. *Evid Based Complement Alternat Med.* 2015;2015:535237.

139. Zeng Y, Xie X, Cheng ASK. Qigong or Tai Chi in cancer care: an updated systematic review and meta-analysis. *Curr Oncol Rep.* 2019;21(6):48.

140. Hilfiker R, Meichtry A, Eicher M, et al. Exercise and other non-pharmaceutical interventions for cancer-related fatigue in patients during or after cancer treatment: a systematic review incorporating an indirect-comparisons meta-analysis. *Br J Sports Med.* 2018;52(10):651-658.

141. Ernst E. Massage therapy for cancer palliation and supportive care: a systematic review of randomised clinical trials. *Support Care Cancer.* 2009;17(4):333-337.

142. Boyd C, Crawford C, Paat CF, et al. The impact of massage therapy on function in pain populations—a systematic review and meta-analysis of randomized controlled trials: part ii, cancer pain populations. *Pain Med.* 2016;17(8):1553-1568.

143. Gansler T, Kaw C, Crammer C, Smith T. A population-based study of prevalence of complementary methods use by cancer survivors: a report from the American Cancer Society's studies of cancer survivors. *Cancer.* 2008;113(5):1048-1057.

144. Kim JI, Lee MS, Kang JW, Choi DY, Ernst E. Reflexology for the symptomatic treatment of breast cancer: a systematic review. *Integr Cancer Ther.* 2010;9(4): 326-330.

145. Ernst E, Posadzki P, Lee MS. Reflexology: an update of a systematic review of randomised clinical trials. *Maturitas.* 2011;68(2):116-120.

146. Lawrence DJ, Meeker W, Branson R, et al. Chiropractic management of low back pain and low back-related leg complaints: a literature synthesis. *J Manipulative Physiol Ther.* 2008;31(9):659-674.

147. Alcantara J, Alcantara JD, Alcantara J. The chiropractic care of patients with cancer: a systematic review of the literature. *Integr Cancer Ther.* 2012;11(4):304-312.

148. Evans RC, Rosner AL. Alternatives in cancer pain treatment: the application of chiropractic care. *Semin Oncol Nurs.* 2005;21(3):184-189.

149. Chang KH, Brodie R, Choong MA, Sweeney KJ, Kerin MJ. Complementary and alternative medicine use in oncology: a questionnaire survey of patients and health care professionals. *BMC Cancer.* 2011;11:196.

150. Frenkel M, Ben-Arye E, Baldwin CD, Sierpina V. Approach to communicating with patients about the use of nutritional supplements in cancer care. *South Med J.* 2005;98(3):289-294.

151. Frenkel M. Is there a role for nutritional supplements in cancer care? Challenges and solutions. *Future Oncol.* 2015;11(6):901-904.

152. Ulbricht C, Chao W, Costa D, Rusie-Seamon E, Weissner W, Woods J. Clinical evidence of herb-drug interactions: a systematic review by the natural standard research collaboration. *Curr Drug Metab.* 2008;9(10):1063-1120.

153. Alsanad SM, Williamson EM, Howard RL. Cancer patients at risk of herb/food supplement-drug interactions: a systematic review. *Phytother Res.* 2014;28(12): 1749-1755.

154. Ulbricht CE, Chao W. Phytochemicals in the oncology setting. *Curr Treat Options Oncol.* 2010;11(3-4): 95-106.

155. Amin A, Gali-Muhtasib H, Ocker M, Schneider-Stock R. Overview of major classes of plant-derived anticancer drugs. *Int J Biomed Sci.* 2009;5(1):1-11.

156. Kotecha R, Takami A, Espinoza JL. Dietary phytochemicals and cancer chemoprevention: a review of the clinical evidence. *Oncotarget.* 2016;7(32):52517-52529.

157. Ernst E, Pittler MH. Efficacy of ginger for nausea and vomiting: a systematic review of randomized clinical trials. *Br J Anaesth.* 2000;84(3):367-371.

158. Saneei Totmaj A, Emamat H, Jarrahi F, Zarrati M. The effect of ginger (*Zingiber officinale*) on chemotherapy-induced nausea and vomiting in breast cancer patients: a systematic literature review of randomized controlled trials. *Phytother Res.* 2019;33(8):1957-1965.

159. Kang SC, Lee CM, Choi H, et al. Evaluation of oriental medicinal herbs for estrogenic and antiproliferative activities. *Phytother Res.* 2006;20(11):1017-1019.

160. Barton DL, Liu H, Dakhil SR, et al. Wisconsin Ginseng (*Panax quinquefolius*) to improve cancer-related fatigue: a randomized, double-blind trial, N07C2. *J Natl Cancer Inst.* 2013;105(16):1230-1238.

161. Yennurajalingam S, Tannir NM, Williams JL, et al. A double-blind, randomized, placebo-controlled trial of panax ginseng for cancer-related fatigue in patients with advanced cancer. *J Natl Compr Canc Netw.* 2017;15(9):1111-1120.

162. McLarty J, Bigelow RL, Smith M, Elmajian D, Ankem M, Cardelli JA. Tea polyphenols decrease serum levels of prostate-specific antigen, hepatocyte growth factor, and vascular endothelial growth factor in prostate cancer patients and inhibit production of hepatocyte growth factor and vascular endothelial growth factor in vitro. *Cancer Prev Res (Phila).* 2009;2(7):673-682.

163. Nakachi K, Suemasu K, Suga K, Takeo T, Imai K, Higashi Y. Influence of drinking green tea on breast cancer malignancy among Japanese patients. *Jpn J Cancer Res.* 1998;89(3):254-261.

164. Tyagi A, Agarwal C, Dwyer-Nield LD, Singh RP, Malkinson AM, Agarwal R. Silibinin modulates TNF-alpha and IFN-gamma mediated signaling to regulate COX2 and iNOS expression in tumorigenic mouse lung epithelial LM2 cells. *Mol Carcinog.* 2012;51(10):832-842.

165. Noh EM, Yi MS, Youn HJ, et al. Silibinin enhances ultraviolet B-induced apoptosis in mcf-7 human breast cancer cells. *J Breast Cancer.* 2011;14(1):8-13.

166. Kauntz H, Bousserouel S, Gosse F, Raul F. Silibinin triggers apoptotic signaling pathways and autophagic survival response in human colon adenocarcinoma cells and their derived metastatic cells. *Apoptosis.* 2011;16(10):1042-1053.

167. Cheung CW, Gibbons N, Johnson DW, Nicol DL. Silibinin—a promising new treatment for cancer. *Anticancer Agents Med Chem.* 2010;10(3):186-195.

168. Li J, Li B, Xu WW, et al. Role of AMPK signaling in mediating the anticancer effects of silibinin in esophageal squamous cell carcinoma. *Expert Opin Ther Targets.* 2016;20(1):7-18.

169. Bussing A, Raak C, Ostermann T. Quality of life and related dimensions in cancer patients treated with mistletoe extract (iscador): a meta-analysis. *Evid Based Complement Alternat Med.* 2012;2012:219402.

170. Kleijnen J, Knipschild P. Mistletoe treatment for cancer review of controlled trials in humans. *Phytomedicine.* 1994;1(3):255-260.

171. Huber R, Schlodder D, Effertz C, Rieger S, Troger W. Safety of intravenously applied mistletoe extract—results from a phase I dose escalation study in patients with advanced cancer. *BMC Complement Altern Med.* 2017;17(1):465.

172. Eisenbraun J, Scheer R, Kroz M, Schad F, Huber R. Quality of life in breast cancer patients during chemotherapy and concurrent therapy with a mistletoe extract. *Phytomedicine.* 2011;18(2-3):151-157.

173. Brandenberger M, Simoes-Wust AP, Rostock M, Rist L, Saller R. An exploratory study on the quality of life and individual coping of cancer patients during mistletoe therapy. *Integr Cancer Ther.* 2012;11(2):90-100.

174. Shakeri A, Ward N, Panahi Y, Sahebkar A. Anti-angiogenic activity of curcumin in cancer therapy: a narrative review. *Curr Vasc Pharmacol.* 2019;17(3):262-269.

175. Bar-Sela G, Epelbaum R, Schaffer M. Curcumin as an anti-cancer agent: review of the gap between basic and clinical applications. *Curr Med Chem.* 2010;17(3): 190-197.

176. Kashino I, Akter S, Mizoue T, et al. Coffee drinking and colorectal cancer and its subsites: a pooled analysis of 8 cohort studies in Japan. *Int J Cancer.* 2018;143(2):307-316.

177. Filomeno M, Bosetti C, Bidoli E, et al. Mediterranean diet and risk of endometrial cancer: a pooled analysis of three Italian case-control studies. *Br J Cancer.* 2015;112(11):1816-1821.

178. National Institute on Aging. Vitamins and minerals. https://www.nia.nih.gov/health/vitamins-and-minerals. Accessed November 15, 2019.

179. Lawson KA, Wright ME, Subar A, et al. Multivitamin use and risk of prostate cancer in the National Institutes of Health-AARP Diet and Health Study. *J Natl Cancer Inst.* 2007;99(10):754-764.

180. Park SJ, Myung SK, Lee Y, Lee YJ. Effects of vitamin and antioxidant supplements in prevention of bladder cancer: a meta-analysis of randomized controlled trials. *J Korean Med Sci.* 2017;32(4):628-635.

181. Giovannucci E, Stampfer MJ, Colditz GA, et al. Multivitamin use, folate, and colon cancer in women in the Nurses' Health Study. *Ann Intern Med.* 1998;129(7):517-524.

182. Eussen SJ, Vollset SE, Igland J, et al. Plasma folate, related genetic variants, and colorectal cancer risk in EPIC. *Cancer Epidemiol Biomarkers Prev.* 2010;19(5):1328-1340.

183. Feigelson HS, Jonas CR, Robertson AS, McCullough ML, Thun MJ, Calle EE. Alcohol, folate, methionine, and risk of incident breast cancer in the American Cancer Society Cancer Prevention Study II Nutrition Cohort. *Cancer Epidemiol Biomarkers Prev.* 2003;12(2):161-164.

184. Moertel CG, Fleming TR, Creagan ET, Rubin J, O'Connell MJ, Ames MM. High-dose vitamin C versus placebo in the treatment of patients with advanced cancer who have had no prior chemotherapy. A randomized double-blind comparison. *N Engl J Med.* 1985;312(3):137-141.

185. Bjelakovic G, Nikolova D, Gluud LL, Simonetti RG, Gluud C. Mortality in randomized trials of antioxidant supplements for primary and secondary prevention: systematic review and meta-analysis. *JAMA.* 2007;297(8):842-857.

186. van Gorkom GNY, Lookermans EL, Van Elssen C, Bos GMJ. The effect of vitamin C (ascorbic acid) in the treatment of patients with cancer: a systematic review. *Nutrients.* 2019;11(5):977.

187. Labriola D, Livingston R. Possible interactions between dietary antioxidants and chemotherapy. *Oncology (Williston Park).* 1999;13(7):1003-1008; discussion 1008, 1011-1012.

188. Jackson RD, LaCroix AZ, Gass M, et al. Calcium plus vitamin D supplementation and the risk of fractures. *N Engl J Med.* 2006;354(7):669-683.

189. LaCroix AZ, Kotchen J, Anderson G, et al. Calcium plus vitamin D supplementation and mortality in postmenopausal women: the Women's Health Initiative calcium-vitamin D randomized controlled trial. *J Gerontol A Biol Sci Med Sci.* 2009;64(5):559-567.

190. Hossain S, Beydoun MA, Beydoun HA, Chen X, Zonderman AB, Wood RJ. Vitamin D and breast cancer: a systematic review and meta-analysis of observational studies. *Clin Nutr ESPEN.* 2019;30:170-184.

191. Goulao B, Stewart F, Ford JA, MacLennan G, Avenell A. Cancer and vitamin D supplementation: a systematic review and meta-analysis. *Am J Clin Nutr.* 2018;107(4):652-663.

192. Lappe JM, Travers-Gustafson D, Davies KM, Recker RR, Heaney RP. Vitamin D and calcium supplementation reduces cancer risk: results of a randomized trial. *Am J Clin Nutr.* 2007;85(6):1586-1591.

193. Attia S, Eickhoff J, Wilding G, et al. Randomized, double-blinded phase II evaluation of docetaxel with or without doxercalciferol in patients with metastatic, androgen-independent prostate cancer. *Clin Cancer Res.* 2008;14(8):2437-2443.

194. Beer TM, Lemmon D, Lowe BA, Henner WD. High-dose weekly oral calcitriol in patients with a rising PSA after prostatectomy or radiation for prostate carcinoma. *Cancer.* 2003;97(5):1217-1224.

195. Nicastro HL, Dunn BK. Selenium and prostate cancer prevention: insights from the selenium and vitamin E cancer prevention trial (SELECT). *Nutrients.* 2013;5(4):1122-1148.

196. Lawenda BD, Kelly KM, Ladas EJ, Sagar SM, Vickers A, Blumberg JB. Should supplemental antioxidant administration be avoided during chemotherapy and radiation therapy? *J Natl Cancer Inst.* 2008;100(11):773-783.

197. Miyazawa S, Moriya S, Kokuba H, Hino H, Takano N, Miyazawa K. Vitamin K2 induces non-apoptotic cell death along with autophagosome formation in breast cancer cell lines. *Breast Cancer.* 2020;27(2):225-235.

198. Latte-Naor S, Mao JJ. Putting integrative oncology into practice: concepts and approaches. *J Oncol Pract.* 2019;15(1):7-14.

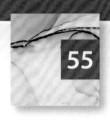

55 Cannabinoids

Sonia Malani, Mary Brown, Jessica Streufert, and Sunil Kumar Aggarwal

INTRODUCTION

For centuries, botanical therapies have been utilized for the treatment of various ailments. These therapies often provide clinical improvement but lack both standardization and evidence-based dosing protocols. As a result, they often are considered anecdotal therapies versus standards of care. The growing patient demand, along with convincing evidence, suggests that the medical community reevaluates the role of one important botanical, cannabis, as a therapeutic. Initially authorized for the treatment of nausea in 1985, then FDA approved for cachexia in 1992, cannabinoids have earned their place in palliative medicine (1). Preclinical and early clinical data suggest that cannabinoids might also have a place in onco-therapeutics for their documented anti-inflammatory and antiproliferative actions. It is becoming widely accepted that cannabinoids have an array of therapeutic potential that spans beyond palliative care. While the safety of the individual cannabis constituents remain under investigation, reported serious adverse effects are rare. Cannabis therapeutics are beginning to spur international interest and are projected to be a multibillion dollar industry. Due to the scheduled status of this drug, this movement also reveals the inevitable intersection of health care and politics. This chapter will provide an overview of the history and botany as well as discuss the pharmacodynamics, pharmacokinetics, drug interactions, and contraindications of cannabinoid as a therapeutic in palliative medicine and supportive oncology.

HISTORICAL SIGNIFICANCE

Cannabis sativa L. is considered one of the 50 traditional Chinese herbs. The first use of cannabis in medicinal applications is traceable as far back as 2737 BC to Chinese emperor Shen-Nung who is credited with using the hemp plant (*Ma*) for constipation, gout, and rheumatism. Dating back to the earliest recorded references, cannabis has been revered as an entheogen, which translates to "becoming divine within," in writings spanning across India to West Africa (2). Perhaps the most influential maven was Irish physician William Brooke O'Shaughnessy, who is credited with introducing the therapeutic use of cannabis to Western medicine. Documenting careful *in vivo* case studies in the 1830s, his experiments involved both animal models as well as human subjects of all ages (3). His findings provided the foundation for medicinal cannabis in modern times. From the mid 19th century to the 1930s, American physicians prescribed cannabis for a variety of indications, until the federal government imposed restrictions on its use in 1937. In 1964, Raphael Mechoulam, an Israeli chemist, discovered the structure of Δ9-tetrahydrocannabinol (THC), thus reintroducing cannabinoids into the global pharmacopoeia. Despite these scientific achievements, the U.S. Congress ultimately classified cannabis as a Schedule I substance in 1970 (4). In 1992, Allyn Howlett and William Devane determined a primary mechanism of action of THC and anandamide as well as other endogenous cannabinoids in central and peripheral organs, further supporting Mechoulam's work and the discovery of the human endocannabinoid system (ECS) (5). The findings and commitments of these scientists were instrumental to the role *Cannabis sativa L.* has in modern medicine.

BOTANY

Cannabis sativa L. is a mostly dioecious, annual plant. *Cannabis* is part of the Cannabaceae family, which is also sometimes known as Cannabiaceae. With access to abundant light, nutrients, and water, the plant can grow up to 6 m in height with roots reaching approximately 2.5 m underground (6). Characteristics of the leaf are dictated by the plant's genetics; however, commonalities include a palmate structure, serrated edges, and deep green hue dotted with brown resin. Female and male plants are grossly indistinguishable until they begin flowering. Once mature, male plants tend to be taller and have fewer branches than their female counterparts. When the female flower is pollinated, the ovule bears an achene or single-seeded fruit. The fruit shares the shape of an ellipsoid and can germinate in 3 to 7 days. Cannabis seeds are known to contain both essential fatty acids (EFAs) and all dietary essential amino acids (7). Seeds are usually planted in the spring; however, *Cannabis* prefers to flower in late summer, when the days grow shorter and there is <12 to 14 hours of sunlight.

Human intervention and climate influences have resulted in a wide variety of chemical compositions of the plant. Breeding techniques have been finessed to customize the concentration and potency of the plant's constituents. The variations of these constituents in the plant phenotype have a direct influence on the mammalian ECS.

Endocannabinoid System

The ECS is comprised of the endogenous cannabinoid receptors located in the mammalian brain and throughout the central and peripheral nervous system. This system contains three principal elements: endocannabinoid receptors, specialized modulators (endocannabinoids) that interact with those receptors, and enzymes that either metabolize or synthesize the endocannabinoids (8). This lipid signaling system has shown to be vital in maintaining homeostasis in organisms. Unlike most neurotransmitters, endocannabinoids are produced in an on-demand fashion (9). In neural tissue, cannabinoids transmit an inhibitory or excitatory response from cells at any given time. Endocannabinoids modulate neurotransmitter activity rather than signaling the brain to action (10).

According to Pacher and Kunos, the ECS regulates, modulates, and plays a role in every major biological function of the human body. This includes, but is not limited to, immune function, newborn suckling, appetite reward, temperature regulation, memory, inflammation regulation, and neuroprotection (9). A 2013 Health Canada summary adds digestion, bone development, bone density, synaptic plasticity, learning, pain, memory, circadian rhythm, and regulation of stress and emotional health to this list (11).

CANNABINOID RECEPTORS

The most well-studied receptors are cannabinoid type-1 (CB1) receptor and cannabinoid type-2 (CB2) receptor. CB1 and CB2 are seven-transmembrane G-protein–coupled receptors that affect cyclic-AMP. CB1 is abundant in the central nervous system (CNS) and spinal cord and is found in particularly high levels in the neocortex, hippocampus, basal ganglia, and cerebellum (12). CB1 receptors can also be found in the peripheral nervous system; synergistic activity between the peripheral and central cannabinoid receptors has been demonstrated (13). CB1 receptors have key roles in the regulation of pain, pruritus, and

muscle tone but also modulate the propulsion and secretory aspects of digestion. The CB1 receptor binds to Δ9-THC and mediates THC's effects in the CNS (14). CB1 receptors are minimally found in the brainstem, which explains why respiratory depression is an unlikely side effect of cannabinoid use (15).

CB2, unlike CB1, is a nonpsychoactive receptor commonly referred to as the peripheral receptor. Research has shown the CB2 receptors to predominantly be found on immune cells, notably B-lymphocytes, T-lymphocytes, monocytes, and NK cells. They can also be found on peripheral dorsal root ganglia cells and in the enteric nervous system. CB2 expression has been shown to be up-regulated in the setting of traumatic brain injury or certain neurodegenerative diseases (10).

There is evidence that a third receptor, transient receptor potential vanilloid-one (TRPV1), is also part of the ECS. TRPV1 is associated with pain transmission and is specifically activated by a temperature >109°F/43°C (16). It is proposed to be an actionable target for treating certain kinds of neuropathic pain via *N*-arachidonoyl ethanolamine (AEA) and cannabidiol (CBD), but not THC.

Cannabinoid interaction has been postulated to extend far beyond just CB1 and CB2 receptors to other CB-type receptors and related ion channels. Termed "orphan CB receptors," GPR55, GPR18, GPR19, and the peroxisome proliferator-activated nuclear receptors (PPAR-alpha and -gamma) regulate important metabolic functions involving fatty acid storage, glucose metabolism, immune function, and proliferation of malignancies (17).

CANNABINOIDS

Cannabinoids can be divided into three categories: endogenous cannabinoids, phytocannabinoids, and pharmaceutical cannabinoids. In this section, we will expand upon endogenous and phytocannabinoids, while pharmaceutical cannabinoids will be addressed later in the chapter. Endogenous cannabinoids are produced in the body. There are two primary endogenous cannabinoids, otherwise known as arachidonoyl ethanolamide (AEA) and 2-arachidonoyl glycerol (2-AG). First discovered in 1992, AEA was the first endocannabinoid discovered to activate CB1. In 1995, 2-arachidonoyl glycerol (2-AG) was discovered in the gut tissue of a canine by one of Mechoulam's doctoral students, Shimon Ben-Shabat (simultaneously discovered by the Japanese team of Sugiura, T., et al). Both AEA and 2-AG are neuromodulators that act as retrograde messengers on G-protein–coupled receptors are synthesized on demand and are particularly active at glutamatergic and GABAergic synapses (18).

These endocannabinoids are derived from EFAs and have the ability to perform separate functions on the same organ, system, or cell (19). AEA is important in pain pathways, while 2-AG is more important to brain injury (10). Fatty acid amide hydrolase (FAAH) is responsible for the breakdown of AEA while 2-AG is degraded by monoacylglycerol lipase (MAGL), which also breaks down FAAH. Two enzymes, phospholipase C (PLC) and diacylglycerol lipase (DAGL), mediate the synthesis of 2-AG. The body synthesizes AEA from N-arachidonoyl phosphatidylethanolamine (NAPE) using multiple pathways employing enzymes phospholipase A2, PLC, and NAPE-PLD (20).

Phytocannabinoids are plant-derived natural terpenophenolic compounds produced by the cannabis plant (21). There are more than 700 chemical constituents produced by the cannabis plant of which phytocannabinoids are included. Phytocannabinoids resemble endogenous cannabinoids by interacting directly with the ECS. Phytocannabinoids are produced by the cannabis plant in the form of carboxylic acids; when they undergo decarboxylation most commonly by heating, they become neutral. More than 100 phytocannabinoids have been isolated, characterized, and divided into 11 chemical classes. The most abundant phytocannabinoids are Δ-9 tetrahydrocannabinolic acid (THCA) and THC. Fibre-type plants are known to contain mainly cannabinoid acids, such as cannabidiolic acid (CBDA) and cannabigerolic acid (CBGA). When decarboxylated, these acids become CBD and cannabigerol (CBG). Other minor cannabinoids include cannabichromenic acid (CBCA), cannabichromene (CBC), cannabinolic acid (CBNA), and cannabinol (CBN); the latter two are the oxidative degradation products of THCA and THC, respectively (22–25).

While most phytocannabinoids have not been approved by federal health regulators, it is important to note that the U.S. Department of Health and Human Services, which houses FDA, has obtained a utility patent for the antioxidant and neuroprotective properties of plant cannabinoids. Cannabis as an antioxidant is more powerful than vitamins C and E (26). The patent explains that cannabinoids work in different ways to help reduce oxidative damage, giving the example: *"The ischemic or neurodegenerative disease may be, for example, an ischemic infarct, Alzheimer's disease, Parkinson's disease, Down's syndrome, human immunodeficiency virus (HIV), dementia, myocardial infarction, or treatment and prevention of intraoperative or preoperative hypoxic insults that can leave persistent neurological deficits following open heart surgery requiring heart/lung bypass machines, such as coronary artery bypass grafts (CABG)"* (27).

PHARMACODYNAMICS

This section will focus on the most clinically relevant cannabinoids, namely THC, CBD, and CBG, and briefly touch on CBC and CBN. Of the cannabinoids, Δ9-THC is the most well known and well researched. The actions of Δ9-THC are a result of its agonist activity on the cannabinoid receptors. The distribution of cannabinoid receptors mentioned previously should be taken into consideration to understand these effects. The interaction with CB1 receptors is primarily responsible for the analgesic effect of THC, due to their role in the transmission of nociceptive information in various tissues. CB2 receptors are highly expressed in some cells of the immune system and are believed to have a role in the immune cell function, explaining the immunomodulatory properties of THC. CB2 receptors are also considered to be involved in neuroinflammation, atherosclerosis, and bone remodeling.

CBD was discovered in 1940 and is the second most common cannabinoid in medical cannabis and the most common in hemp plants (5). CBD is a valuable nonpsychoactive compound from a pharmaceutical vantage. It has been found to possess a high antioxidant and anti-inflammatory activity, as well as neuroprotective, anxiolytic, and anticonvulsant properties (21,28). The pharmacodynamics of CBD is still an emerging science. From epilepsy studies, it has been concluded that CBD has a low affinity for endocannabinoid receptors unlike Δ9-THC (31). When Δ9-THC is active in the body, CBD is able to modulate the adverse effects of Δ9-THC by physiologically antagonizing CB1 receptors. In other words, the coadministration of Δ9-THC and CBD results in less tachycardia, anxiety, and sedation. Recently, CBD has gained popularity for being an anti-inflammatory agent. It is proposed that this anti-inflammatory action is due to an inverse agonism on the CB2 receptors subsequently blocking the migration of immune cells and therefore decreasing inflammation (29,30).

CBG was discovered in 1964 and is the precursor cannabinoid to THC, CBD, and CBC. While CBG has anti-inflammatory and analgesic activities, it is a potent antimicrobial and is superior to THC, CBD, and CBC in fighting gram-positive bacteria (31). A U.S. patent exists for CBG's potential in managing mood disorders (32). The pharmacology and therapeutic potential of CBG is an emerging field. Early studies propose that CBG has partial agonist activities at both the CB1 and CB2 receptors. CBG is nonpsychoactive, and animal data indicate that it may be helpful to increase appetite (33). The therapeutic effects of CBG are still being studied; however, it shows promise as an analgesic, anti-inflammatory, antiemetic, and anti-proliferative agent (34).

Cannabichromene (CBC) was discovered in 1966 and does not appear to interact with classical cannabinoid receptors but primarily targets TRP channels. CBC exhibits a range of effects including antibacterial and antifungal properties. Additionally, CBC may be a potential therapeutic for gastrointestinal dysfunction, as it has been found to reduce inflammation-induced hypermotility in vivo (35).

The first cannabinoid isolated was CBN in 1895, and it is the oxidized by-product of THC. CBN is one of the more common cannabinoids found in cannabis products. CBN exhibits weak psychoactivity but modulates the effect of THC. CBN is produced in minimal amounts by the cannabis plant during its growth cycle but is readily detected in older samples of dried cannabis and cannabis resin or oil. CBN is known to have anticonvulsant and anti-inflammatory properties. Because CBN has three times greater affinity for the CB2 receptor than CB1, it is believed to have a greater effect on the immune system than the CNS (31).

PHARMACOKINETICS

The tissue distribution of THC and its metabolites are governed by their physiochemical properties. Approximately 95% to 99% of THC is bound to plasma proteins, primarily lipoproteins. Metabolism of THC occurs quickly, mainly in the liver by hydroxylation, oxidation, and conjugation through the cytochrome P450 complex, specifically CYP2C9 and CYP3A (36). The majority of THC is rapidly cleared from the plasma, with 70% taken up by tissues, especially highly vascularized ones, and 30% converted by metabolism. The involvement of the cytochrome P450 complex results in considerable variance in pharmacokinetics between the oral and inhaled route (37,38). First-pass liver metabolism occurs in oral administration, and a greater proportion of 11-OH-THC, a key active metabolite, is produced compared with that which occurs in pulmonary administration. As far as complete elimination is concerned, it occurs over several days given the slow rediffusion of THC from adipose and other tissues, with adipose being the major long-term storage site of THC and its biometabolites. In the perinatal setting, cannabinoids distribute into the breastmilk of lactating mothers (where endocannabinoids are also found in appreciable quantities) (39) and diffuse across the placenta (Pregnancy Category C). Excretion of THC occurs within days and weeks, mainly as metabolites, with approximately 20% to 35% found in urine and 65% to 80% found in feces, and <5% as unchanged drug, when administered per os (40,41).

MODES OF ADMINISTRATION

There are multiple modes of administering cannabinoids, all varying in length of onset and duration. Most symptomatologies require a combination of administration routes for sustainable management.

When inhaled, cannabinoids are carried across the alveoli into the capillaries before entering the bloodstream. Cannabinoids can be inhaled through a method of combustion or vaporization and have a rapid onset of 0 to 10 minutes, with a duration of 2 to 4 hours. Patient response and metabolism is dose dependent and requires proper inhalation technique. When recommending this method, attention should be focused on the volume of inhalation and timing of breath hold. Bronchial irritation is a possible factor related to inhaling at high temperatures (42). Inhalation can be very effective in acute presentations; however, for a patient new to cannabinoids, caution is recommended when using as a first line of defense.

Cannabinoids can also be delivered orally through fluidic extractions, capsules, or infused edible products. Sublingual or buccal administration provides a rapid onset of 5 to 20 minutes with a duration of 4 to 6 hours due to absorption through the mucous membranes and sublingual venous plexus. This method may be most effective for patients seeking immediate relief from pain, nausea, and insomnia. With oral administration of cannabinoid medicines through capsules, absorption is somewhat more variable, depending on gastric contents, with a slower onset of action of 30 minutes to 2 hours, and a longer, more constant, duration of action, over 5 to 8 hours in total (40).

Cannabinoids can be compounded into a variety of products for topical application. Compounding cannabinoids into a penetrating topical cream, salve, or gel allows for localized application. Onset is typically rapid while duration varies based on concentration and anatomical placement, usually 1 to 10 minutes with a duration of 2 to 4 hours. Transdermal patches deliver cannabinoids systemically into the bloodstream through the dermis. They have a 15 to 30 minute onset with a more than 8 hour duration for patches. Conditions such as generalized pain may be treated with transdermal products.

To mitigate undesired euphoric effects, rectal administration can be an effective alternative to the modes referenced above. This form of administration allows for rapid onset due to its ability to bypass first-pass metabolism. However, the rate of rectal drug absorption is variable due to the surface area exposed and composition of the suppository. With rectal administration, the duration can be 1 to 12 hours (43).

PHARMACEUTICAL CANNABINOIDS

To date, there are three FDA-approved cannabinoid medications and one in consideration for FDA-approval. Dronabinol, nabilone, and nabiximols have been approved for cancer-related side effects while CBD is indicated for select seizure disorders. The first FDA-approved cannabinoid medicine available in the United States was dronabinol, a synthetic form of THC, also known as Marinol. Dronabinol is classified as a Schedule III drug and is indicated for chemotherapy-induced nausea and vomiting and cachexia in HIV/AIDS patients. This synthetic THC isolate is suspended in sesame oil and is available in 2.5, 5, and 10 mg strengths. Dronabinol is usually dosed orally 2 to 3 times per day and has an onset of 45 to 60 minutes. For chemotherapy-induced nausea, it is recommended that dronabinol is usually taken 1 to 3 hours before chemotherapy and then every 2 to 4 hours after for up to 4 to 6 doses in a 24-hour period (44). A 2008 systematic review showed that dronabinol had superior antiemetic activity versus neuroleptics in cancer patients (45).

Another pharmaceutical cannabinoid similar to THC is nabilone, which is sold in the United States under the brand name Cesamet. Nabilone is classified as a Schedule II drug and is indicated for chemotherapy-induced nausea and vomiting. The suggested dose for nabilone is 1 to 2 mg twice daily by mouth with a maximum dose of 6 mg. Nabilone is usually given 1 to 3 hours before chemotherapy treatments. It may also be recommended 2 or 3 times daily during chemotherapy treatment cycle, and for 48 hours after treatment ends, if needed. The effects of nabilone may last between 48 and 72 hours (46).

Nabiximols is a 1:1 CBD to THC whole plant extract. It has been approved for use in many European countries and is currently undergoing research trials in the United States as well. Nabiximols, also known as Sativex, is used to treat central neuropathic pain, cancer pain, and spasticity in multiple sclerosis. As noted by Rhan et al. 2007, recent studies suggest that cannabinoids activate the CB1 and CB2 receptors in the spinal cord lessening both visceral and somatic pain, which are often side effects of chemotherapeutic agents such as vincristine (47). Nabiximols is formulated as an oromucosal spray administered sublingually or buccally, with each spray providing 2.7-mg THC and 2.5-mg CBD. Dosing ranges between 1 and 10 sprays per day for an analgesic effect, while dosing above 10 sprays per day resulted in poor tolerability of the drug (48,49).

When considering the use of pharmaceutical cannabinoids versus phytocannabinoid medicines, it is important to review documented side effects and adverse events and to take into consideration that phytocannabinoid options, when safely available, may have a more favorable risk–benefit ratio.

CANNABINOIDS AS A POTENTIAL ANTICANCER THERAPEUTIC

It is well established that cannabinoids can be used to mitigate the adverse effects of chemotherapeutics. However, new evidence is establishing that in certain malignant tissues, the cannabinoid receptors are up-regulated. This observation suggests that cannabinoids may have a role to play as an anticancer therapeutic (50). Additionally, a 2017 review of preclinical data by Ramer and Hinz illustrated that cannabinoids also have a synergistic effect with chemotherapeutics. For example, by increasing TRPV2 activation, CBD was synergistic when used concurrently with temozolomide in glioblastoma multiforme (GBM) patient tissue samples (51). This result is encouraging for patients who are using cannabinoids for the treatment of cancer-related side effects such as nausea, appetite, and insomnia. A 2017 placebo-controlled phase II clinical trial investigated the administration of temozolomide with nabiximols versus temozolomide alone in 21 patients with GBM. Patients who were randomised to the nabiximols group had an 83% 1-year survival rate compared to 44% in the temozolomide only group (52).

More clinical data are needed to draw a conclusion on whether cannabinoids can be used as an anticancer therapeutic in addition to mitigating side effects. Patients must demonstrate caution relying on anecdotal evidence when considering cannabis use as an antiproliferative agent. Although there is promising research indicating that cannabinoids can promote apoptosis, there is also research indicating the potential for cannabinoids to have the opposite effect. Preclinical data have demonstrated that THC may increase breast cancer metastasis in hormonal and reproductive cancers (53,54). Popular protocols requiring 1,000 mg of THC per day for 60 days (known as the RSO regimen) are increasingly reported as ineffective and prohibitive due to the psychotropic side effects. However, research suggests that CBD is the most promising cannabinoid in the treatment of targeting breast cancer cell lines (55).

CONTRAINDICATIONS AND PRECAUTIONS

Although studies indicate a high safety profile, cannabinoids are contraindicated in patients who have a rare hypersensitivity to THC or allergies to any of the inert materials with which cannabinoid medicines may be formulated (56). There is some concern in the basic science literature that cannabinoid's immunomodulatory properties through CB2 activity can cause a shift from Th1 to Th2 type activity and that this might have severe consequences for a patient who is fighting an infection (such as *Legionella*) that requires Th1 immunity activity for inhibition (57,58). Cannabinoids should also be used cautiously in patients with a personal or family history of psychosis, with particular attention paid to pediatric and adolescent patient populations under psychosocial stress who may be at increased risk for developing psychosis (41).

The use of cannabinoids in a pediatric setting is a topic of controversy. Although the American Academy of Pediatrics (AAP) affirms opposition to the legalization of cannabis for both medicinal as well as recreational use, the organization updated its policy in 2015 to include "compassionate use" of medicinal cannabis for terminal or debilitating illnesses. In recent consideration, the AAP recognizes the potential therapeutic applications for adolescents with treatment resistant conditions and recommends downscheduling to facilitate this research (59). This update coincides with the process of the FDA approval of Epidiolex, a plant extract of CBD for the treatment of Lennox-Gastaut syndrome or Dravet syndrome in children 2 years or older. This medication is administered orally via spray with a starting dose of 2.5 mg/kg taken twice a day for a total of 5 mg/kg/d. After 1 week of use, dosing can be increased to a maintenance of 5 mg/kg twice a day with a total of 10 mg/kg/d (60). This approved dosing protocol has provided a guideline for dosing in palliative care for empiric treatment in pediatric populations. It is of note that development and therefore prevalence of cannabinoid receptors is age dependent. Children are known to have fewer CB1 receptors in the brain than adults and may be able to tolerate higher than expected doses of Δ8-THC, an analogue of THC. When Δ8-THC was administered as an antiemetic in a pediatric oncology population, vomiting was prevented with negligible side effects (61). Recent studies show that other analogue cannabinoids that have little to no psychotropic effect may hold more therapeutic promise than THC as an antiemetic (21).

It is always important for patients to discuss cannabinoid therapy with health care providers or pharmacists to clarify any possible pharmacological interactions with current medical regimens, before starting cannabinoid therapy.

POTENTIAL INTERACTIONS OF CANNABINOIDS WITH PHARMACEUTICALS

Despite the minimal contraindications, cannabinoids do interact with CYP450 enzymes. This interaction can potentiate the effects of pharmaceuticals and change the duration and degree to which cannabinoids and other medications are present in the patient's bloodstream (37,38,62). With the large number of individuals who have used cannabinoid botanicals concomitantly with numerous prescription medicines, no unwanted side effects of clinical relevance have been described in the literature to date. Nevertheless, cannabinoid medicines should be used with caution in patients taking the following medications: steroids, antipsychotics, antidepressants, antiepileptics, beta blockers, blood thinners, proton pump inhibitors, nonsteroidal anti-inflammatory drugs (NSAIDs), oral hypoglycemic agents, sulfonylureas, anesthetics, antibiotics, antiarrhythmics, benzodiazepines, immune modulators, HIV antivirals, prokinetics, calcium channel blockers, and HMG-CoA reductase inhibitors (41,63–65).

CLOSING THOUGHTS

The challenges faced by clinicians to palliate oncological side effects and comorbidities are increasing rapidly while the options for treatment are limited. Often inadequately treated with opioids, antidepressants, and antiemetics, patients are relying on therapies such as cannabinoids to manage their pain, nausea, vomiting, and insomnia. Current government regulatory bodies that vary from state to state determine the manner in which cannabis can be recommended, produced, and dispensed. These variations create a barrier for standardization of care for both patients and physicians. Descheduling cannabis at the U.S. federal level would allow for a more regulated market that is held to a national standard. Like many botanical medicines, cannabinoids require individualized dosing that takes into consideration the patient's constitution and current medication protocol, as well as their previous exposure to cannabinoids. Social psychologists would argue that the patient's perception of cannabinoids play a significant role in the therapeutic effect of the recommendation. Many patients come from cultural backgrounds where cannabis is stigmatized and therefore are reluctant to entertain the conversation of cannabis as a therapeutic. A successful patient interaction requires that the physician be well informed on state regulations, drug interactions, and product accessibility (66). Physicians also need to consider affordability and quality of product with awareness that the current market offers products with inconsistent cannabinoid profiles. Nevertheless, the increasing empirical evidence validates the application of cannabinoids in palliative and supportive care and sets the stage for future research.

REFERENCE

1. Amar MB. Cannabinoids in medicine: a review of their therapeutic potential. *J Ethnopharmacol.* 2006;105(1-2): 1-25. doi:10.1016/j.jep.2006.02.001.
2. Abel, E. Marihuana. The first twelve thousand years. *Ann Intern Med.* 1981;95(3):397. doi:10.7326/0003-4819-95-3-397_2.
3. Macgillivray N. Sir William Brooke O'Shaughnessy (1808–1889), MD, FRS, LRCS Ed: Chemical pathologist, pharmacologist and pioneer in electric telegraphy. *J Med Biogr.* 2015;25(3):186-196. doi:10.1177/0967772015596276.
4. Aggarwal SK. 'Tis in our nature: taking the human–cannabis relationship seriously in health science and public policy. *Front Psychiatry.* 2013;4:6. doi: 10.3389/fpsyt.2013.00006.
5. Pertwee RG. Cannabinoid pharmacology: the first 66 years. *Br J Pharmacol.* 2009;147(S1):S163-S171. doi:10.1038/sj.bjp.0706406.
6. Farag S, Kayser O. The cannabis plant: botanical aspects. In: Preedy V, ed. *Handbook of Cannabis and Related Pathologies: Biology, Pharmacology, Diagnosis, and Treatment.* London, UK: Elsevier Academic Press; 2017:3-12. doi:10.1016/b978-0-12-800756-3.00001-6.
7. Grotenhermen F. Franjo Grotenhermen. *Med Cannabis Cannabinoids.* 2018;1(1):5. doi:10.1159/000489141.
8. Marsicano G, Lafenêtre P. Roles of the endocannabinoid system in learning and memory. *Curr Top Behav Neurosci.* 2009:201-230. doi:10.1007/978-3-540-88955-7_8.
9. Pacher P, Batkai S, Kunos G. The endocannabinoid system as an emerging target of pharmacotherapy. *Pharmacol Rev.* 2006;58(3):389-462.
10. Russo E. Introduction to the endocannabinoid system. 2015. https://www.phytecs.com/wp-content/uploads/2015/02/IntroductionECS.pdf
11. Information for health care professionals: Cannabis (Marihuana, marijuana) and the cannabinoids. Canada.ca. https://www.canada.ca/en/health-canada/services/drugs-medication/cannabis/information-medical-practitioners/information-health-care-professionals-cannabis-cannabinoids.html. 2013. Accessed October 2019.
12. Herkenham M, Groen B, Lynn A, Costa BD, Richfield E. Neuronal localization of cannabinoid receptors and second messengers in mutant mouse cerebellum. *Brain Res.* 1991;552(2):301-310. doi:10.1016/0006-8993(91)90096-e.
13. Dogrul A, Gul H, Akar A, Yildiz O, Bilgin F, Guzeldemir E. Topical cannabinoid antinociception: synergy with spinal sites. *Pain.* 2003;105(1):11-16. doi:10.1016/s0304-3959(03)00068-x.
14. Zimmer A, Hohmann A, Herkenham M, Bonner T. Increased mortality, hypoactivity, and hypoalgesia in cannabinoid CB1 receptor knockout mice. *Proc Natl Acad Sci U S A.* 1999:5780-5785. doi:10.1073/pnas.96.10.5780.
15. Burns HD, Van Laere K, Sanabria-Bohorquez S, Hamil TG, Bormans G. [18F]MK-9470, a positron emission tomography (PET) tracer for in vivo human PET brain imaging of the cannabinoid-1 receptor. *Proc Natl Acad Sci U S A.* 2007;104(23):9800-9805. doi:10.1073/pnas.0703472104.
16. Brito R, Sheth S, Mukherjea D, Rybak L, Ramkumar V. TRPV1: a potential drug target for treating various diseases. *Cells.* 2014;3(2):517-545. doi:10.3390/cells3020517.
17. Grygiel-Górniak B. Peroxisome proliferator-activated receptors and their ligands: nutritional and clinical implications—a review. *Nutr J.* 2014;13(1). doi:10.1186/1475-2891-13-17.
18. Marzo VD, Melck D, Bisogno T, Petrocellis LD. Endocannabinoids: endogenous cannabinoid receptor ligands with neuromodulatory action. *Trends Neurosci.* 1998;21(12):521-528. doi:10.1016/s0166-2236(98)01283-1.
19. Marzo VD, Petrocellis LD. Why do cannabinoid receptors have more than one endogenous ligand? *Philos Trans R Soc Lond B Biol Sci.* 2012;367(1607):3216-3228. doi:10.1098/rstb.2011.0382.
20. Backes M. *Cannabis Pharmacy.* New York, NY: Black Dog & Leventhal; 2014.
21. Izzo AA, Borrelli F, Capasso R, Marzo VD, Mechoulam R. Non-psychotropic plant cannabinoids: new therapeutic opportunities from an ancient herb. *Trends Pharmacol Sci.* 2009;30(10):515-527. doi:10.1016/j.tips.2009.07.006.
22. Thomas BF, ElSohly MA. *The Analytical Chemistry of Cannabis: Quality Assessment, Assurance, and Regulation of Medicinal Marijuana and Cannabinoid Preparations.* Amsterdam, Netherlands: Elsevier/RTI International; 2016.
23. Hanuš LO, Meyer SM, Muñoz E, Taglialatela-Scafati O, Appendino G. Phytocannabinoids: a unified critical inventory. *Nat Prod Rep.* 2016;33(12):1357-1392. doi:10.1039/c6np00074f.
24. Brighenti V, Pellati F, Steinbach M, Maran D, Benvenuti S. Development of a new extraction technique and HPLC method for the analysis of non-psychoactive cannabinoids in fibre-type *Cannabis sativa L.* (hemp). *J Pharm Biomed Anal.* 2017;143:228-236. doi:10.1016/j.jpba.2017.05.049.
25. Pellati F, Brighenti V, Sperlea J, Marchetti L, Bertelli D, Benvenuti S. New methods for the comprehensive analysis of bioactive compounds in *Cannabis sativa L.* (hemp). *Molecules.* 2018;23(10):2639. doi:10.3390/molecules23102639.
26. Hampson AJ, Grimaldi M, Axelrod J, Wink D. Cannabidiol and (-) 9-tetrahydrocannabinol are neuroprotective antioxidants. *Proc Natl Acad Sci.* 1998;95(14):8268-8273. doi:10.1073/pnas.95.14.8268.
27. Hampson A, Axelrod J, Grimaldi M. Cannabinoids as antioxidants and neuroprotectants. USOO6630507B1; 2003.
28. Russo EB. Taming THC: potential cannabis synergy and phytocannabinoid-terpenoid entourage effects. *Br J Pharmacol.* 2011;163(7):1344-1364. doi:10.1111/j.1476-5381.2011.01238.x.
29. Pisanti S, Malfitano AM, Ciaglia E, et al. Cannabidiol: State of the art and new challenges for therapeutic applications. *Pharmacol Ther.* 2017;175:133-150. doi:10.1016/j.pharmthera.2017.02.041.
30. Lunn CA, Reich EP, Bober L. Targeting the CB2 receptor for immune modulation. *Expert Opin Ther Targets.* 2006;10:653-663.
31. McPartland JM, Russo EB. Cannabis and cannabis extracts. *J Cannabis Ther.* 2001;1(3-4):103-132. doi:10.1300/j175v01n03_08.
32. Musty R, Deyo R. CBG Patent. Pharmaceutical Compositions comprising cannabigerol. US8481085B2; 2007.

33. Brierley DI, Samuels J, Duncan M, Whalley BJ, Williams CM. Cannabigerol is a novel, well-tolerated appetite stimulant in pre-satiated rats. *Psychopharmacology (Berl).* 2016;233(19-20):3603-3613. doi:10.1007/s00213-016-4397-4.

34. Navarro G, Varani K, Reyes-Resina I, et al. Cannabigerol action at cannabinoid CB1 and CB2 receptors and at CB1–CB2 heteroreceptor complexes. *Front Pharmacol.* 2018;9:632. doi:10.3389/fphar.2018.00632.

35. Izzo AA, Capasso R, Aviello G, et al. Inhibitory effect of cannabichromene, a major non-psychotropic cannabinoid extracted from Cannabis sativa, on inflammation-induced hypermotility in mice. *Br J Pharmacol.* 2012;166(4):1444-1460. doi:10.1111/j.1476-5381.2012.01879.x.

36. Brenneisen R. Pharmacokinetics. In: Grotenhermen F, Russo EB, eds. *Cannabis and Cannabinoids: Pharmacology, Toxicology, and Therapeutic Potential.* Binghamton, NY: Haworth Press; 2002:67-72.

37. Abrams D, Guzman M. Cannabis in cancer care. *Clin Pharmacol Ther.* 2015;97(6):575-586. doi:10.1002/cpt.108.

38. Grotenhermen F. Pharmacokinetics and pharmacodynamics of cannabinoids. *Clin Pharmacokinet.* 2003;42(4):327-360.

39. Fride E. The endocannabinoid-CB(1) receptor system in pre and postnatal life. *Eur J Pharmacol.* 2004;500:289-297.

40. Grotenhermen F. Clinical pharmacokinetics of cannabinoids. In: Russo EB, Grotenhermen F, eds. *Handbook of Cannabis Therapeutics: From Bench to Bedside.* Binghamton, NY: Haworth Press; 2006:69-116.

41. Aggarwal S. Cannabinergic pain medicine: developing a concise clinical primer and surveying randomized-controlled trial results (S702). *J Pain Symptom Manage.* 2013;45(2):416-417. doi:10.1016/j.jpainsymman.2012.10.019.

42. Tashkin DP. Effects of Marijuana smoking on the lung. *Ann Am Thorac Soc.* 2013;10(3):239-247. doi:10.1513/annalsats.201212-127fr.

43. Bruni N, Della Pepa C, Oliaro-Bosso S, Pessione E, Gastaldi D, Dosio F. Cannabinoid delivery systems for pain and inflammation treatment. *Molecules.* 2018; 23(10):2478.

44. Calhoun V, Mcginty V, Pekar J, Watson T, Pearlson G. Investigation of marinol (THC) effects upon fMRI activation during active and passive driving using independent component analysis and SPM. *Neuroimage.* 2001;13(6):388. doi:10.1016/s1053-8119(01)91731-8.

45. Machado Rocha FC, Stéfano SC, De Cássia Haiek R, et al. Therapeutic use of Cannabis sativa on chemotherapy induced nausea and vomiting among cancer patients: systematic review and meta-analysis. *Eur J Cancer Care (Engl).* 2008;17:431-443.

46. FDA. *Cesamet™.* Costa Mesa, CA: Valeant Pharmaceuticals International; May, 2006.

47. Rahn EJ, Makriyannis A, Hohmann AG. Activation of cannabinoid CB(1) and CB(2) receptors suppresses neuropathic nociception evoked by the chemotherapeutic agent vincristine in rats. *Br J Pharmacol.* 2007;152(5):1-13.

48. Portenoy RK, Ganae-Motan ED, Allende S, et al. Nabiximols for opioid-treated cancer patients with poorly controlled chronic pain: a randomized, placebo-controlled, graded-dose trial. *J Pain.* 2012;13:438-449.

49. Johnson JR, Burnell-Nugent M, Lossignol D, et al. Multicenter, double-blind, randomized, placebo controlled, parallel-group study of the efficacy, safety, and tolerability of THC:CBD extract and THC extract in patients with intractable cancer-related pain. *J Pain Symptom Manage.* 2010;39:167-179.

50. Sanchez C, de Ceballos ML, Gomez del Pulgar T, et al. Inhibition of glioma growth in vivo by selective activation of the CB2 cannabinoid receptor. *Cancer Res.* 2001;61:5784-5789.

51. Nabissi M, Morelli MB, Amantini C, et al. Cannabidiol stimulates Aml-1a-dependent glial differentiation and inhibits glioma stem like cells proliferation by inducing autophagy in a TRPV2-dependent manner. *Int J Cancer.* 2015;137:1855-1869.

52. Schultz S, Beyer M. GW pharmaceuticals achieves positive results in phase 2 proof of concept study in glioma. 2017. http://ir.gwpharm.com/static-files/cde942fe-555c-4b2f-9cc9-f34d24c7ad27

53. McKallip RJ, Nagarkatti M, Nagarkatti PS. Δ-9-Tetrahydrocannabinol enhances breast cancer growth and metastasis by suppression of the antitumor immune response. *J Immunol.* 2005;174(6):3281-3289. doi:10.4049/jimmunol.174.6.3281.

54. McHugh D, Page J, Dunn E, Bradshaw HB. Δ9-Tetrahydrocannabinol and N-arachidonyl glycine are full agonists at GPR18 receptors and induce migration in human endometrial HEC-1B cells. *Br J Pharmacol.* 2012;165(8):2414-2424. doi:10.1111/j.1476-5381.2011.01497.x.

55. Elbaz M, Nasser MW, Ravi J, et al. Modulation of the tumor microenvironment and inhibition of EGF/EGFR pathway: Novel anti-tumor mechanisms of Cannabidiol in breast cancer. *Mol Oncol.* 2015;9(4):906-919. doi:10.1016/j.molonc.2014.12.010.

56. Sachs J, McGlade E, Yurgelun-Todd D. Safety and Toxicology of Cannabinoids. *Neurotherapeutics.* 2015;12(4):735-746. doi:10.1007/s13311-015-0380-8.

57. Klein TW, Newton C, Friedman H. Cannabinoid receptors and the cytokine network. In: Friedman H, Madden JJ, Klein TW, eds. *Drugs of Abuse, Immunomodulation, and AIDS.* New York, NY: Plenum Press; 1998:215-222.

58. Melamede R. Mechanisms in autoimmune diseases. In: Grotenhermen F, Russo EB, eds. *Cannabis and Cannabinoids: Pharmacology, Toxicology, and Therapeutic Potential.* Binghamton, NY: Haworth Press; 2002:111-119.

59. Ammerman S, Ryan S, Adelman WP. The impact of marijuana policies on youth: clinical, research, and legal update. *Pediatrics.* 2015;135(3):584-587. doi:10.1542/peds.2014-4146.

60. EPIDIOLEX® (cannabidiol) CV. EPIDIOLEX.com. https://www.epidiolex.com/. Accessed 2019.

61. Abrahamov A, Abrahamov A, Mechoulam R. An efficient new cannabinoid antiemetic in pediatric oncology. *Life Sci.* 1995;56(23-24), 2097-2102. doi:10.1016/0024-3205(95)00194-b.

62. Borgelt LM, Franson KL, Nussbaum AM, Wang GS. The pharmacologic and clinical effects of medical cannabis. *Pharmacotherapy.* 2013;33(2):195-209. doi:10.1002/phar.1187.

63. Sachse-Seeboth C, Pfeil J, Sehrt D, et al. Interindividual variation in the pharmacokinetics of Δ9-tetrahydrocannabinol as related to genetic polymorphisms in CYP2C9. *Clin Pharmacol Ther.* 2008;85(3):273-276. doi:10.1038/clpt.2008.213.

64. Lindsey WT, Stewart D, Childress D. Drug interactions between common illicit drugs and prescription therapies. *Am J Drug Alcohol Abuse.* 2012;38(4):334-343. doi:10.3109/00952990.2011.643997.

65. Grayson L, Vines B, Nichol K, Szaflarski JP. An interaction between warfarin and cannabidiol, a case report. *Epilepsy Behav Case Rep.* 2018;9:10-11. doi:10.1016/j.ebcr.2017.10.001.

66. Newhart M, Dolphin W. *The Medicalization of Marijuana: Legitimacy, Stigma, and the Patient Experience.* New York, NY: Routledge; 2019.

Special Populations

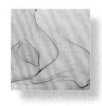 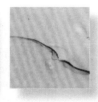 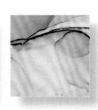 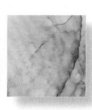 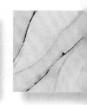

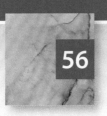

56 Geriatric Palliative Care

Jessica Israel and R. Sean Morrison

In our society, older adults make up the overwhelming majority of people living with serious medical illness. Older adults can spend years living with chronic diseases accompanied by multiple coexisting conditions, progressive dependency on others, and heavy care needs met mostly by family members. Abundant evidence suggests that the quality of life in the setting of serious illness is often poor, characterized by inadequately treated physical distress, fragmented care systems, poor to absent communication between doctors and patients and families, and enormous strains on family caregiver and support systems. In this chapter, we focus on the palliative care needs of older adults.

BIOLOGY OF AGING

Body Composition

Aging is a process that, in varying degrees over time, converts healthy adults into frail ones with diminished reserves in most physiologic systems and with an exponentially increasing vulnerability to most diseases and death (1). Aging is the most significant and common risk factor for disease in general. The body's organ system reserves and homeostatic control mechanisms steadily decline. Commonly, this slow erosion only becomes obvious in times of maximum body stress or serious illness. However, as the process continues, it takes less and less insult for the underlying physiologic weakness to become apparent. It is difficult to differentiate the effects of aging alone from those of concurrent disease or environmental factors. Eventually, a critical point is reached, when the body's systems are overwhelmed, and death ultimately results. Morbidity is often compressed into the last period of life (2).

Substantial changes occur in body composition with aging. These changes become important when related to nutritional needs, pharmacokinetics, and metabolic activity. As adults age, the proportion of bodily lipid doubles and lean body mass decreases. Bones and viscera shrink and the basal metabolic rate declines. Although specific age-associated changes occur in each organ system, changes in body composition and metabolism are highly variable from individual to individual.

Renal Function

The aging kidney loses functioning nephrons. Cross-sectional and longitudinal studies have also demonstrated a decline in creatinine clearance. There is also evidence to show decreased renal plasma flow, decreased tubular secretion and reabsorption, decreased hydrogen secretion, and decreased water absorption and excretion (3). When kidney disease complicates this aging process, the outcome can be highly deleterious.

Underlying renal function is an important issue in geriatric pharmacology. Many medications rely on the kidneys' mechanisms for excretion, and their metabolites may accumulate and lead to side effects or toxic injury in an impaired system. Commonly used medications are more likely to damage older kidneys, including nonsteroidal anti-inflammatory drugs (NSAIDs) and intravenous contrast dye (4).

Gastrointestinal and Hepatic Function

The gastrointestinal tract changes less with aging than other body systems, but there are still some deficiencies that may affect medication delivery and breakdown, as well as nutritional status and metabolism. The esophagus may show delayed transit time. The stomach may atrophy and produce less acid. Colonic transit is greatly slowed, whereas small intestinal transit appears unaffected. Pancreatic function is usually well maintained, although trypsin secretion may be decreased.

The liver usually retains adequate function, although there are variable changes seen in its metabolic pathways. The cytochrome P-450 system may decline in efficiency, and liver enzymes may be less inducible. The most significant change is the sharp decline in demethylation, the process that metabolizes medications such as benzodiazepines in the liver. This change may necessitate dosage adjustments. In addition, drugs that undergo hepatic first-pass metabolism by extraction from the blood may have altered clearance with increasing age because of decreased hepatic blood flow.

Brain and Central Nervous System Changes

The brain and central nervous system slowly atrophy with age. Neurons stop proliferating and are not replaced when they die, resulting in neuronal loss as well as loss of dendritic arborization. There are also some degrees of neurotransmitter and receptor loss. The extent of this loss is not well understood.

Age-related changes in pain perception may exist, but their clinical importance is uncertain. Although degenerative changes occur in areas of the central and autonomic nervous system that mediate pain, the relevance of these changes has yet to be determined (5). Clinical observations from elderly patients who report minimal pain and discomfort despite the presence of cardiac ischemia or intra-abdominal catastrophe suggest that pain perception may be altered in the elderly. However, experimental data suggest that significant, age-related changes in pain perception probably do not occur (6). Until further studies conclusively demonstrate that the perception of pain decreases with age, stereotyping of most elderly patients as experiencing less pain may lead to inaccurate clinical assessments and needless suffering (5).

DEMOGRAPHY OF SERIOUS ILLNESS IN THE UNITED STATES

In 2018, life expectancy from birth was 78.7 years for the total United States population (7). For perspective, in 1900, life expectancy at birth was <50 years. Those reaching 65 years can expect to live another 18 years on average and those reaching age 80 can expect to live an additional 8 years. These unprecedented increases in life expectancy (equivalent to that occurring between the Stone Age and 1900) are due primarily to decreases in maternal and infant mortality, resulting from improved sanitation, nutrition, and effective control of infectious diseases. As a result, there has been an enormous growth in the number and health of the elderly. By the year 2030, 20% of the United States' population will be over age 65, as compared with <5% at the turn of the 20th century (8).

Although death at the turn of the 20th century was largely attributable to acute infectious diseases or accidents, the leading causes of death today are chronic illness such as heart disease, cancer, stroke, and dementia. With advances in the treatment of atherosclerotic vascular disease and cancer, many patients with these diseases now survive for years. Many diseases that were rapidly fatal in the past have now become chronic illnesses.

Until recently, more than half 68% of all deaths in America occurred in hospitals or nursing homes (9). The older the patient, the higher the likelihood of death was in a nursing home or hospital, with an estimated 76% of persons over 85 years experiencing an institutional death and a similar number spending at least some time in an institution in the year prior to death (9). These statistics, however, hide the fact that most of an older person's last months and years are still spent at home in the care of family members, with hospitalization and/or nursing home placement occurring only near the very end of life. National statistics also obscure the variability in the experience of living with serious illness. For example, the need for institutionalization or paid formal caregivers in the last months of life is much higher among the poor and women. Similarly, persons suffering from cognitive impairment and dementia are much more likely to spend their last days in a nursing home compared with cognitively intact, elderly persons dying from nondementing illnesses. Interestingly, now for the first time since the early 20th century, more people in the United States are dying at home than in the hospital or the nursing home. Recent work points to about 30% in hospitals and 21% in nursing homes, a trend that is clearly in concert with patient wishes (10).

CARE SYSTEMS FOR OLDER ADULTS WITH SERIOUS ILLNESS

The needs of older adults living with serious illness are not well matched by current models of care. Specifically, multiple studies demonstrate that the personal and practical care needs of patients who are seriously ill and their families are not adequately addressed by routine office visits or hospital and nursing home stays and that this failure results in substantial burdens—medical, psychological, and financial—on patients and their caregivers (11). Neither paid personal care services at home nor nursing home costs for the functionally dependent elderly are covered by Medicare but instead are paid for approximately equally from out-of-pocket and Medicaid budgetary sources that were originally developed to provide care for the indigent. In the context of chronic progressive disease, the burden of coordinating an array of social and medical services falls on primary physicians and more often on individual families. There is much work still to do as we look at the social determinants of health and the inequities that exist when it comes to access to care.

In response to the needs of seriously ill older adults and their families, palliative care teams have become increasingly prevalent in U.S. hospitals and provide comprehensive interdisciplinary care for seriously ill patients and families in collaboration and consultation with primary physicians. Over 80% of hospitals with over 300 beds now report a palliative care team and over two third of all hospitals report a palliative care team—a steady 140% increase in prevalence since 2000 (12). Hospital palliative care teams have been shown to significantly reduce symptom burden, enhance patient and family satisfaction, and lower costs (11). Other chronic care programs, focused on reducing functional decline and delirium and improving transitions from hospitals, also show promising results (13).

In the ambulatory care setting, programs are less well developed than in hospitals. Hospice services, under the Medicare benefit, are available in most U.S. communities and provide palliative care, primarily at home, for patients with a life expectancy of 6 months or less who are willing to forgo insurance coverage for life-prolonging treatments. Overall, about 40% older adults access their hospice benefit prior to death and median length of stay on hospice is on the order of 3 weeks (14). Reasons for the low rate of utilization of the Medicare Hospice Benefit vary by community but include the inhibiting requirements that patients acknowledge that they are dying in order to access the services, that physicians certify a prognosis of 6 months or less, and that very few hours (usually 4 or less) of personal care home attendants are covered under the benefit. In addition, the fiscal structure of the Medicare Hospice Benefit lends itself well to the predictable trajectory of late-stage cancers but not so well to the unpredictable chronic course of other common causes of death in the elderly such as congestive heart failure, chronic lung disease, stroke, and dementing illnesses.

Other programs that coordinate care for patients who have complex illnesses, outside of hospice, are becoming increasingly available in many communities—primarily for younger adults or for individuals enrolled in Medicare Advantage (i.e., Medicare managed care plans). These programs typically focus on intensive telephonic case management and have been shown to improve care for those with serious illness (15). The quality, cost, and extent of the services provided are highly variable.

Finally, comprehensive multidisciplinary home care programs that serve frail older adults have been developed in several specialized settings. The Program of All-Inclusive Care for the Elderly (PACE) is a capitated Medicare and Medicaid benefit for frail older adults that offers comprehensive medical and social services at day health centers, in homes, and at inpatient facilities. Patients enrolled in PACE have higher rates of advance directive completion and lower rates of nursing home admission, hospitalization, and hospital deaths than do patients who do not use the services (11). Similar programs of team-coordinated home-based care exist within the Veterans Administration (VA) (VA home-based primary care and VA palliative care programs). All VA hospitals are required to have both a home-based primary care program for homebound veterans and a palliative care team. Furthermore, under VA regulations, all veterans are allowed access to hospice at the same time as they are receiving disease-directed or curative treatments.

In nursing homes, the site of care for many of the most seriously ill and cognitively impaired older adults, incentives promoting palliative care standard are lacking. Indeed, nursing home quality metrics focus on improvement of function and maintenance of weight and nutritional status. Evidence of the decline that accompanies the dying process is typically regarded as a measure of substandard care (16). Therefore, a death in a nursing home is often viewed as evidence particularly by state regulators of poor care rather than an expected outcome for a frail, chronically ill, older person. The financial and regulatory incentives and quality measures that currently exist in long-term care promote tube feeding over spoon feeding and transfer to hospital or emergency department in the setting of acute illness or impending death (Table 56.1). They fail to either assess or reward appropriate attention to palliative measures, including relief of symptoms, spiritual care, and promotion of continuity with concomitant avoidance of brink-of-death emergency room and hospital transfers (17). Although provision of hospice services has been shown to improve quality in nursing homes (18), penetration of hospice services into most nursing homes remains low and increasing federal scrutiny on long-lengths of stay of nursing home residents on the hospice benefit has led to concerns about enrolling this patient population.

PALLIATIVE CARE NEEDS OF OLDER ADULTS

Although death occurs far more commonly in older adults than in any other age group, remarkably little is known about the course of serious illness in the oldest old, that is, those over age 75. Most research on the experience of living with serious illness has been done in younger populations, and most studies examining pain and symptom management have focused on younger populations. Studies in older adults have focused primarily on patients' preferences for care rather than on the actual care received. Indeed, the largest study to date of the experience of living with a serious

TABLE 56.1 BENEFITS AND RISKS OF TUBE FEEDING IN OLDER ADULTS/NURSING HOME RESIDENTS

Benefits of tube feeding in older adults/nursing home patients	Risks of tube feeding in older adults/nursing home patients
Improved survival for patients in persistent vegetative state	Dementia patients more likely to be physically restrained
Improved survival for patients with extreme short bowel syndrome or proximal bowel obstruction	Increased risk of aspiration pneumonia, diarrhea, gastrointestinal discomfort, and problems associated with accidental feeding tube removal by the patient
Improved survival *AND* quality of life for patients with bulbar amyotrophic lateral sclerosis	With impaired renal function or in last days of life, patient may have choking, increased pulmonary secretions, dyspnea, pulmonary edema, and ascites
Improved survival for patients in acute phase of stroke or head injury	
Improved survival in patients receiving short-term critical care	
Improved nutritional status of patients with advanced cancer undergoing intensive radiation therapy	
No Survival Benefit in patients with dementia	

Table adapted from data summarized in Casarett D, Kapo J, Caplan A. Appropriate use of artificial nutrition and hydration—fundamental principles and recommendations. *N Engl J Med.* 2005;353:2607-2612.

illnesses in the United States (Study to Understand Prognoses and Preferences for Outcomes and Risks of Treatments [SUPPORT]) studied the hospital experience of patients with a median age of 66 (19). The median age of death in the United States is 78.6 years, and many of the oldest old die in nursing homes or at home rather than in hospital. Data from Medicare and state Medicaid registries suggest that expensive and high technology interventions are less frequently applied to the oldest patients, independent of functional status and projected life expectancy. These discrepancies may reflect patient preferences and indicate appropriate utilization of resources and patient preferences, but they may also represent a form of implicit rationing of resources based on age (20).

Aside from pain and other sources of physical distress (see section "Symptom Management: The Challenge of Pain"), the key characteristic that distinguishes the experience of serious illness in the elderly from that experienced by younger groups is the nearly universal occurrence of long periods of functional dependency and need for family caregivers in the last months to years of life. In SUPPORT, the median age of participants was 66 years and 55% of patients had persistent and serious family caregiving needs during the course of their terminal illness (21), and in another study of 988 terminally ill patients, 35% of families had substantial care needs (22). This percentage rises exponentially with increasing age. Although paid care supplements provide the sole source of care in 15% to 20% of patients (transportation, homemaker services, personal care, and more skilled nursing care),

the remaining 80% to 85% of patients receive most of their care from unpaid family members (22). Furthermore, most family caregiving is provided by women (spouses and adult daughters and daughters-in-law), placing significant strains on the physical, emotional, and socioeconomic status of the caregivers. Those ill and dependent patients without family caregivers, or those whose caregivers can no longer provide nor afford needed services, are placed in nursing homes. In the United States, this typically occurs after patients exhaust all of their financial savings in order to become eligible for Medicaid. At present, 38% of all nursing home residents are between 85 and 94 years old, about 8% are 95 years and older. These numbers are expected to continue to increase (23).

SYMPTOM MANAGEMENT: THE CHALLENGE OF PAIN

The constellation of symptoms seen in seriously ill, older, adult patients is different from that of young adults. Delirium, sensory impairment, incontinence, dizziness, cough, and constipation are more prevalent in older adults (24). The elderly, on average, have 1.5 more symptoms than younger persons in the year prior to death, and 69% of the symptoms reported for people aged 85 or more lasted more than a year as compared with 39% of those for younger adults (55 years) (24).

Studies focusing specifically on the prevalence of pain have shown consistently high levels of untreated or undertreated pain in older adults. In one study of elderly cancer patients in nursing homes, 26% of patients with daily pain received no analgesic at all and 16% received only acetaminophen, a percentage that rose with increasing age and minority status (25). A subsequent study revealed that 41% of patients who were assessed having pain on their first assessment continued to have moderate or excruciating daily pain on their second assessment 60 to 180 days later (26). Studies comparing pain management in cognitively intact versus demented elderly with acute hip fracture also found a high rate of undertreatment of pain in both groups, a phenomenon that worsened with increasing age and cognitive impairment (27,28). Similarly, a study of outpatients with cancer found that age and female sex were predictors of undertreatment, a disturbing observation given the dramatic rise in cancer prevalence with increasing age (29,30). Chronic pain due to arthritis, other bone and joint disorders, and low back pain syndrome is probably the most common cause of distress and disability in the elderly, affecting 25% to 50% of community-dwelling, older adults. It is likely that these symptoms also are consistently undertreated (31). These data suggest that the time before death among elderly persons is often characterized by significant physical distress that is neither identified nor properly treated.

Despite the high prevalence of pain and other symptoms in the elderly, most studies focusing on the assessment and treatment of pain and other symptoms have enrolled younger adults with cancer. It is unclear whether these results can be generalized to a geriatric population. Pain assessment in the elderly is often complicated by the coexistence of cognitive impairment. The assessment and management of pain in the cognitively impaired patient present special challenges to the healthcare professional. The cognitively impaired patient is often unable to express pain adequately, request analgesics, or operate patient-controlled, analgesia devices. This increases the risk of undertreatment. The fear of precipitating or exacerbating a delirious episode by employing opioids in the management of pain may also lead to inadequate pain management.

As with the cognitively intact patient, the initial step in the assessment of pain in the demented individual is to ask the patient. Although patients with severe dementia may be incapable of communicating, many patients with moderate degrees of impairment can accurately localize and grade the severity of their pain (32,33). In the noncommunicative patient, alternative means of assessment must be identified. The need for careful pain assessment in this population of patients is underscored by evidence that suggests that medical professionals undertreat pain in the presence of cognitive impairment (27,28,34) and that pain may be aggravated in the presence of cognitive deficits (32). Untreated pain can result in agitation, disruptive behavior, and may worsen or precipitate a delirious episode (35–37).

Pain assessment in the noncommunicative patient should begin with observation of both nonverbal cues, such as facial expressions (grimacing and frowning) and motor behavior (bracing, restlessness, and agitation) and verbal cues, such as groaning, screaming, or moaning. Data from cognitively intact individuals suggest that nonverbal behaviors correlate with self-reported pain in nondemented patients recovering from surgery (38,39). Pharmacologic therapy should be titrated upward in small, incremental doses until the nonverbal/verbal behavior disappears or side effects become apparent. This approach is particularly useful in the agitated patient whose behavior may well stem from untreated or undertreated pain. The risk of undertreating severe pain is generally more concerning, both medically and ethically, than the risk of worsening delirium with medications. Table 56.2 summarizes available pain assessment tools useful in care of older adults.

Pharmacologic therapy for pain must be modified in older adults. The World Health Organization's analgesic ladder approach may not be appropriate for the elderly. For example, the increased risk of side effects, including renal failure and gastrointestinal bleeding, mandates great caution in the use of NSAIDs. This caution extends to currently available parenteral NSAIDs because of the significantly increased risk of gastrointestinal bleeding, particularly with higher doses and with duration of use >5 days (40–42). The American Geriatrics Society has recommended that opioids be considered as a first-step treatment rather than NSAIDs (31). If NSAIDs are used, careful monitoring of renal function and close observation of the development of gastrointestinal bleeding must be undertaken.

Opioid therapy remains the cornerstone of pain management in palliative care, and this is also true for older adults. Some aspects of opioid therapy require special consideration in the elderly. Older adults will have a more pronounced pharmacologic effect after any weight-adjusted opioid dose than younger patients. The analgesia is more intense, and cognitive and respiratory effects, and perhaps constipation, are more severe. This enhanced effect is likely due to a lesser volume of distribution (approximately half that of younger patients), a decreased clearance, and diminished target organ reserve (central nervous system, pulmonary function, and bowel function). Age is the single most important predictor of initial opioid

TABLE 56.2 PAIN ASSESSMENT TOOLS FOR OLDER ADULTS

Brief Pain Inventory (BPI) (Charles S. Cleeland, PhD)	Originally developed for cancer pain, but validated for nonmalignant pain as well, used widely in research, widely translated into other languages, looks at pain and its impact on function
Checklist of Nonverbal Pain Indicators (CNPI) (Karen S. Feldt, PhD, RN, CS, GNP)	Designed specifically for cognitively impaired patients, looks at behavior both at rest and with movement
Faces Pain Scale (FPS) (Daivia Bieri et al.)	Designed originally as a pediatric pain assessment tool but now shown to be effective in older adults. Scale is seven faces, each depicting increasing levels of pain. This scale does not require verbal interaction so is useful in patients with expressive language problems
Functional Pain Scale (FPS) (FM Gloth III, MD, CMD, et al.)	Specifically developed for older adults, has both a subjective and objective component. Looks at a rating of "tolerable" vs. "intolerable" and the impact on function
Numeric Rating Scale (NRS) (Keela A. Herr, RN, PhD and Linda Garand, RN, PhD, CS)	This is a horizontal scale with two versions 1–20 or 0–10. Zero equals no pain, with the higher number being equal to the worst pain one can experience
Pain Assessment in Advanced Dementia Scale (PAINAD) (Victoria Warden, RN, et al.)	Specifically designed for cognitively impaired patients with advanced disease. Relies on observations of specific behaviors (breathing, facial expressions, vocalizations, consolability, and body language) to determine a level of pain
Pain Thermometer (Keela A. Herr, RN, PhD and Paula R. Mobily, RN, PhD)	Uses the visual of a vertical thermometer to rate pain. Pain increases as you move up the thermometer. Can be useful in patients with limited verbal communication and has been used in cognitively impaired patients
Verbal Descriptor Scale (VDS) (Keela A. Herr, RN, PhD and Linda Garand, RN, PhD, CS)	Uses descriptive phases to reflect differing severity of pain. Patient needs to be able to articulate symptoms, but the tool is well studied for use in older adults and even those with mild to moderate cognitive compromise
Verbal Numeric Scale (VNS) (Diane M. Young, MSN, RN, et al.)	Patients verbally rate their pain on a scale of 0–10. Again, 0 equals no pain and 10 is the worst pain imaginable. There is no visual component to this scale

Based on Compilation from the Iowa Geriatric Education Center (www.healthcare.uiowa.edu).

dose requirements for postoperative pain (43). The following formula, based on a review of records of >1,000 adults between ages 20 and 70 undergoing major surgery, provides a rough estimate of the appropriate starting dose in parenteral morphine sulfate equivalents for adult opioid-naive patients (with the exception of the oldest old): average first 24-hour morphine (mg) requirement for patients over 20 years of age = 100 minus the patient's age (43). Other factors that will influence opioid effects, but to a lesser degree than that of age, are body weight, severity of pain, abnormal renal function, nausea/vomiting, and cardiopulmonary insufficiency. After the initial dose determination, drugs should be titrated on the basis of analgesic effect.

There are no data as to appropriate starting doses for analgesia in older adults. A reasonable starting dose may be 30% to 50% of that recommended for a younger adult.

Practically speaking, however, the best advice is almost obvious. In opioid-naive older adults, one should start with the smallest dose available for the product. The key to prescribing a correct regimen is not in the first order you write, but rather, in what happens when this dose becomes effective. In an acute pain syndrome, the reassessment of the patient's level of pain at the right follow-up interval will lead to the appropriate dose titration. An intravenous medication should be effective within 6 to 15 minutes and oral medications within an hour. Reassessing effective analgesia needs to occur frequently in an acute pain crisis.

Several opioids are best avoided in older adults. Meperidine is particularly hazardous as a result of the accumulation of its toxic metabolite, normeperidine, in patients with impaired renal function. Indeed, toxic levels can accumulate in older adults with "normal kidneys" due to age-related changes in creatinine clearance. There are almost no circumstances in which meperidine should be used on older adults. Similarly, pentazocine should also be avoided in older adults because of the increased incidence of delirium and agitation associated with its use. Finally, opioids with long half-lives (e.g., methadone and levorphanol) or opioids with sustained-release preparations (e.g., sustained-release morphine, oxycodone, and hydromorphone and transdermal fentanyl) should be used with caution, rarely be used in opioid-naive geriatric patients, and should probably only be used following steady-state accumulation of shorter acting opioids.

With respect to adjuvant agents, amitriptyline and the other tricyclic antidepressants, although efficacious in some neuropathic pain syndromes, are poorly tolerated in older adults due to their anticholinergic properties. Bowel and bladder dysfunction, orthostatic hypotension resulting in falls, delirium, movement disorders, and dry mouth are very common with these medications. If tricyclics are to be used, then nortriptyline or desipramine is the agent of choice and initial dosages should be very low and dose titration should be undertaken very slowly. Safe choices in older adults may include additional adjuvants like gabapentin and pregabalin, especially for neuropathic pain. Selective serotonin reuptake inhibitors (SSRIs) serotonin–norepinephrine reuptake inhibitors (SNRIs) and steroids can also be helpful add-ons to relieve pain. Care must be given to recognize the side effect profile of these medications to be sure that they do not add to the patient's overall symptoms and are used safely. Again, starting with low doses and titrating slowly are important.

ALZHEIMER'S DISEASE AND RELATED DEMENTIAS

Irreversible dementia is a frightening and difficult diagnosis for geriatric patients and their families. A diagnosis of dementia means a certain and progressive decline in cognitive abilities over time and an eventual loss of independence. Dementia is a progressive, incurable illness, and all treatments are palliative. The average survival after a diagnosis of Alzheimer's disease ranges from 7 to 10 years. Patients with dementia require medical care that focuses on preserving dignity and quality of life. Physicians should seek to aggressively manage the symptoms that endanger these goals. This must be done in early stages of the disease, the more moderate stages, and finally the advanced stages. The needs of patients in each stage are different, but the focus is always to preserve dignity and quality of life.

In early dementia, perhaps the most important job for the physician is to recognize and diagnose the disease and then to educate patients and their families about what they can expect. At this stage, patients can still make decisions for themselves. Physicians should ask patients about their preferences for medical treatments in the later stages of their disease and facilitate these important conversations between their patients and caregivers. Specific discussions about life-prolonging treatments, such as artificial nutrition and hydration, should take place. Physicians should ask patients to designate one or more primary decision makers to speak for them in preparation for later stages of disease when they are no longer able to make decisions for themselves. Patients should be encouraged to talk with their designated caregivers and loved ones about their views about advanced medical therapies such as feeding tubes, mechanical ventilation, and cardiopulmonary resuscitation (CPR). Although it is important to explore patients' specific preferences with regard to medical technology, it is equally important to explore the patients' values and goals of medical care: What is most important in their lives? What makes their lives worth living? What religious or spiritual values may be important? There is evidence that early conversations about advance directives help to prepare families for future decision-making and may reduce the difficulty that comes with later surrogate decision-making (44).

The early stages of Alzheimer's disease may be amenable to pharmacologic therapy with cholinesterase inhibitors (donepezil, rivastigmine, or galantamine) or in combination medication that targets the glutaminergic system, specifically the NMDA receptors (memantine). Treatment with these medications may improve performance in activities of daily living, modestly improve cognitive function, or slow down the progression of the disease process. Aggressive control of vascular risk factors and the use of aspirin and cholesterol-lowering agents may slow down the progress of vascular dementia. The goals of both types of therapies are to preserve independence for as long as possible.

Many patients with early-stage disease have concurrent psychiatric issues. Depression is especially common, affecting approximately 50% of the early Alzheimer's disease population. The symptoms of depression in early disease may be atypical and include indifference, difficulties with emotional engagement, and decreased motivation. Antidepressant therapies are often indicated, and cholinesterase inhibitors may be beneficial. Support groups may also be helpful at this stage of disease, both for patients and their caregivers.

Moderate-stage dementia is the longest stage of the disease. The physician's focus should be keeping the patient's environment safe, treating psychiatric symptoms, and supporting the patient's caregivers. As patients move to this more middle stage of the disease, their need for supervision at home and help with performing activities of daily living become greater. Behavioral disturbances, agitation, and paranoia often occur in concert with increased dependence. These changes may become significant sources of caregiver stress. Palliative measures in moderate-level dementia include recognition and attention to caregiver stress, treatment of behavioral and psychiatric disturbances, and instituting environmental safety modifications. Additionally, patients with a moderate degree of cognitive impairment often exhibit impaired eating behaviors, and physicians must work with patients and their caregivers to meet nutritional demands, as well as modifying food products for easier mealtimes.

Caregiver stress is common, as relatives take on a more active and demanding role in the everyday routines of patients with progressive dementia. Many have never been in the role of primary caregiver for anyone other than their own children. Some primary caregivers may be geriatric patients themselves. Most families will face a high level of financial stress. Unless a patient has access to social services (Medicaid in the United States), out-of-pocket costs for additional help at home, pharmaceutical products, and durable medical equipment are high. Adult day programs may be hard to find, and respite programs are typically expensive. Patients with this degree of cognitive compromise may be difficult to place in nursing homes because often they do not carry other comorbid diagnoses, and the reimbursement rate for pure custodial care is low. Many caregivers leave their jobs or families behind to care for their loved ones. Some need to take on a second job to keep up with the financial burdens.

Caregivers may feel underappreciated because their loved ones fail to acknowledge how hard they are working or the sacrifices they are making. Eventually, patients fail to be able to even recognize who their caregivers are. These very real stresses need to be recognized, acknowledged, and supported. Physicians should question caregivers about fatigue, social isolation, depression, and physical symptoms. They should remind caregivers to take breaks and encourage other family members to help out. Caregiver support groups may also be helpful.

Behavioral disturbances become more frequent as dementia progresses. Although they may occur at any stage of the disease, they are associated with increasing cognitive and functional decline. Symptoms include anxiety, depression, paranoia, delusions, hallucinations, sleep disorders, agitation, and combativeness. The presence of behavioral disturbance, especially paranoia and aggression, can increase the likelihood of nursing home placement. Treatment should be aimed at improving the quality of life of the patient and caregiver and should include both pharmacologic and nonpharmacologic considerations. Careful attention should be given to alternative causes of behavioral disturbance, such as uncontrolled pain, untreated infection, or suboptimal management of concurrent

disease. Treatment of underlying medical illness may lead to sustained improvement in both cognitive status and behavior. In addition, the etiology of agitation may be based on basic human needs—hunger, thirst, or the need to change wet or soiled clothing. Identifying the root of the problem may be difficult, as patients with moderate degrees of dementia cannot tell their caregivers what exactly is bothering them. Nevertheless, the presence of a new behavioral disturbance should precipitate a medical evaluation and should not simply be considered a consequence of the underlying dementing illness.

Treating obvious etiologies as well as addressing possible modifications in the patient's care environment can be useful ways to address behavioral disturbances. For example, a careful history may demonstrate that agitated and paranoid behavior occurs at bath time. In this case, perhaps changing the water temperature or moving from a tub to a sponge bath may be less threatening for patients and lead to decreased agitation (45). Evidence suggests that involving patients actively in grooming routines may also decrease agitation. Calm environments, the use of usual routines, favorite pieces of music, and visits from children or pets may all be soothing. Attention to a patient's sleeping patterns is also important. Increasing daytime activities and decreasing daytime napping may help patients sleep better at night.

In addition to these behavioral interventions, low-dose standing as-needed major tranquilizers (common choices are haloperidol, risperidone, olanzapine, or quetiapine) may be required to successfully manage behavioral disturbances and prevent hospital admissions. It is important to consider potential cardiovascular risk when prescribing antipsychotic medications where there is an FDA black box warning of sudden cardiovascular death. However, when considering this potential toxicity, the prescriber should weigh the risk–benefit ratios. Treating a dignity and quality-of-life compromising condition at the end of life may have more gravity than the potential risk. Discussion with the patient's family about the issue is important. Bedtime dosing with major tranquilizers or with trazodone may help with sleep disturbances. Benzodiazepines may be associated with paradoxical agitation, excessive somnolence, and falls and should be avoided in most patients.

Advanced dementia is the final stage of this terminal disease. Patients with end-stage dementia are dying. Research has demonstrated a median 6-month survival rate for patients with end-stage dementia, with or without tube feeding, although the range of survival times is wide (46,47). Most patients in this stage of disease are bedbound and nonverbal. Many patients in this stage of disease are placed in a nursing home because of their increasing care demands. Although comfort care and palliation of suffering should be the paramount focus of care, patients with advanced dementia often receive nonpalliative interventions at the end of life, such as tube feedings, CPR, mechanical ventilation, and systemic antibiotics in their final days of life (27,48–51).

Surrogate decision-making in end-stage disease is inevitable. The process is made easier for all involved if, in the early stages of disease, the aforementioned critical discussions of treatment goals and end-of-life preferences have occurred. Caregivers may face multiple, difficult decisions, including emergency surgery, intubation, feeding tubes, and CPR. Even if the advance wishes were well communicated, it may still be difficult for family members to carry them out. Nonetheless, decisions should always be based on previously expressed wishes (if known) and the best interest of the patient with respect to the potential benefits or burdens of the proposed treatment. Physicians should offer caregivers continued support and offer them regular and repeated reviews of the goals of treatment and the expectations that follow interventions.

Comfort measures and the relief of suffering should be the primary palliative goals. Careful attention to potential sources of discomfort, such as pain and concurrent illness, is important. Pain is very commonly overlooked and undertreated in this population. Analgesic therapy should be empiric and preventive if an underlying source exists or the patient faces potentially uncomfortable procedures such as dressing changes or position changes. Physicians should also recognize that patients with advanced dementia may experience more discomfort from routine procedures, such as vital signs monitoring, phlebotomy, finger sticks, and bladder catheterizations, because they cannot understand what is being done to them and why. Unnecessary procedures should be discontinued. Topical anesthetic preparations may make the necessary procedures more bearable.

CONCLUSION

As a result of the unprecedented improvements in maternal and infant mortality and successes in the control, if not cure, of common chronic diseases, most people who die in the United States are old and frail. Ten thousand people in the United States turn 65 years old each day, and this is projected to continue into the 2030s. Over the next several decades, their numbers are projected to double and number over 88 million people, representing over 20% of the population by the year 2050 (arc.aarpinternational.org). The elderly die

of chronic, progressive illnesses (such as end-stage heart and lung disease, cancer, stroke, and dementia). These diseases have unpredictable clinical courses and prognoses, and current care systems are not well adapted to the trajectory of illness or the clinical needs of this group of patients. In contrast to younger adults, older adults often have unrecognized and untreated symptoms, cognitive impairment, and an extremely high prevalence of functional dependency and associated family caregiver burden. It is clear that our current systems of reimbursement are ill equipped to provide primary care with continuity, support for family caregivers, and home care and nursing home services. Because care for a frail, older adult typically includes preventive, life-prolonging rehabilitation and palliative measures in varying proportions and intensity based on the individual patient's needs and preferences, any new models of care will have to be responsive to this range of service requirements. Several "mixed management" models of care are available to address the needs of the frail elderly, including hospital palliative care teams, PACE, and new models of ambulatory care management—primarily for commercially insured or Medicare Advantage enrollees. Future research needs to be targeted at understanding the palliative care needs of older adults, developing medical interventions that address these needs, and developing models and systems of care that will meet the global needs of these patients and their families.

REFERENCES

1. Miller RA. The biology of aging and longevity. In: Hazzard WR, Blass JP, Ettinger WH, et al., eds. *Principles of Geriatric Medicine and Gerontology*. New York, NY: McGraw-Hill; 1999:1-19.
2. Fries J. Aging, natural death and the compression of morbidity. *N Engl J Med*. 1990;303:130.
3. Avorn J, Gurwitz J. Principles of pharmacology. In: Cassell C, Cohen H, Larson E, et al., eds. *Geriatric Medicine*. 3rd ed. New York, NY: Springer; 1997.
4. Perneger TV, Whelton PK, Klag MJ. Risk of kidney failure associated with the use of acetaminophen, aspirin, and nonsteroidal antiinflammatory drugs. *N Engl J Med*. 1994;331:1675-1679.
5. Ferrell B. Pain management in elderly people. *J Am Geriatr Soc*. 1991;39:64-73.
6. Harkins S. Pain perceptions in the old. *Clin Geriatr Med*. 1996;12:435-459.
7. National Center for Health Statistics. NCHS fact sheet. April 2020. https://www.cdc.gov/nchs/nvss.htm
8. Olshanksy SJ. Demography of aging. In: Cassel CK, Cohen HJ, Larson EB, et al., eds. *Geriatric Medicine*. 3rd ed. New York, NY: Springer; 1997.
9. National Vital Statistics System. *Deaths by Place of Death, Age, Race, and Sex: United States, 1999-2005*. Atlanta, GA: Center for Disease Control and Prevention. http://www.cdc.gov/nchs/nvss/mortality/gmwk309.htm. Accessed February 20, 2012.
10. Cross S, Warraich HJ. Changes in the place of death in the United States. *N Engl J Med*. 2019;381:2369-2370.

11. Morrison, RS, Meier DE. Palliative care. *N Engl J Med.* 2004;350:2582-2590.

12. Center to Advance Palliative Care/National Palliative Care Research Center. *America's Care of Serious Illness: A State-by-State Report Card on Access to Palliative Care in Our Nation's Hospitals.* New York, NY: Center to Advance Palliative Care and the National Palliative Care Research Center; 2012. http://www.capc.org/reportcard/. Accessed February 20, 2012.

13. Siu AL, Spragens LH, Inouye SK, Morrison RS, Leff B. The ironic business case for chronic care in the acute care setting. *Health Aff (Millwood).* 2009;28(1):113-125.

14. National Hospice and Palliative Care Organization. *NHPCO Facts and Figures. Hospice Care in America.* Alexandria, VA: National Hospice and Palliative Care Organization; 2012. http://www.nhpco.org/files/public/Statistics_Research/2011_Facts_Figures.pdf. Accessed February 20, 2012.

15. Spettell CM, Rawlins WS, Krakauer R, et al. A comprehensive case management program to improve palliative care. *J Palliat Med.* 2009;12:827-832.

16. Keay TJ, Fredman L, Taler GA, et al. Indicators of quality medical care for the terminally ill in nursing homes. *J Am Geriatr Soc.* 1994;42:853-860.

17. Engle VF. Care of the living, care of the dying: reconceptualizing nursing home care. *J Am Geriatr Soc.* 1998;46:1172-1174.

18. Teno JM, Gozalo PL, Lee IC, et al. Does hospice improve quality of care for persons dying from dementia? *J Am Geriatr Soc.* 2011;59:1531-1536.

19. The SUPPORT Principal Investigators. A controlled trial to improve care for seriously ill hospitalized patients. The study to understand prognoses and preferences for outcomes and risks of treatments (SUPPORT). *JAMA.* 1995;274:1591-1598.

20. Lubitz JD, Riley FF. Trends in Medicare payments in the last year of life. *N Engl J Med.* 1993;328:1092-1096.

21. Covinsky KE, Landefeld CS, Teno J, et al. Is economic hardship on the families of the seriously ill associated with patient and surrogate care preferences? SUPPORT Investigators. *Arch Intern Med.* 1996;156:1737-1741.

22. Emanuel EJ, Fairclough DL, Slutsman J, et al. Assistance from family members, friends, paid caregivers, and volunteers in the care of terminally ill patients. *N Engl J Med.* 1999;341:956-963.

23. Ferrell B. Overview of aging and pain. In: Ferrell BR, Ferrell BA, eds. *Pain in the Elderly: A Report of the Task Force on Pain in the Elderly of the International Association for the Study of Pain.* Seattle, WA: IASP Press; 1996.

24. Seale C, Cartwright A. *The Year Before Death.* Brookfield, WI: Ashgate; 1994.

25. Bernabei R, Gambassi G, Lapane K, et al. Management of pain in elderly patients with cancer. *JAMA.* 1998;279:1877-1882.

26. Teno JM, Weitzen S, Wetle T, et al. Persistent pain in nursing home residents. *JAMA.* 2001;285:2081.

27. Feldt KS, Ryden MB, Miles S. Treatment of pain in cognitively impaired compared with cognitively intact older patients with hip-fracture. *J Am Geriatr Soc.* 1998;46:1079-1085.

28. Morrison RS, Siu AL. A comparison of pain and its treatment in advanced dementia and cognitively intact patients with hip fracture. *J Pain Symptom Manage.* 2000;19:240-248.

29. Cleeland CS, Gonin R, Hatfield AK, et al. Pain and its treatment in outpatients with metastatic cancer. *N Engl J Med.* 1994;330:592-596.

30. Stein W. Cancer pain in the elderly. In: Ferrell BR, Ferrell BA, eds. *Pain in the Elderly: A Report of the Task Force on Pain in the Elderly of the International Association for the Study of Pain.* Seattle, WA: IASP Press; 1996.

31. American Geriatrics Society. The management of chronic pain in older persons: AGS panel on chronic pain in older persons. *J Am Geriatr Soc.* 1998;46:635-651.

32. Parmelee P. Pain in cognitively impaired older persons. *Clin Geriatr Med.* 1996;12:473-487.

33. Ferrell BA, Ferrell BR, Rivera LSO. Pain in cognitively impaired nursing home patients. *J Pain Symptom Manage.* 1995;10:591-598.

34. Sengstaken E, King S. The problem of pain and its detection among geriatric nursing home residents. *J Am Geriatr Soc.* 1993;41:541-544.

35. Duggleby W, Lander J. Cognitive status and postoperative pain: older adults. *J Pain Symptom Manage.* 1994;9:19-27.

36. Lynch EP, Lazor MA, Gellis JE, et al. The impact of postoperative pain on the development of postoperative delirium. *Anesth Analg.* 1998;86:781-785.

37. Morrison RS, Magaziner J, Gilbert M, et al. Relationship between pain and opioid analgesics on the development of delirium following hip fracture. *J Gerontol A Biol Sci Med Sci.* 2003;58:76-81.

38. Mateo OM, Krenzischek DA. A pilot study to assess the relationship between behavioral manifestations and self-report of pain in postanesthesia care unit patients. *J Post Anesth Nurs.* 1992;7:15-21.

39. Le Resche L, Dworkin S. Facial expressions of pain and emotions in chronic TMD patients. *Pain.* 1988;35:71-78.

40. Strom BL, Berlin JA, Kinman JL, et al. Parenteral ketorolac and risk of gastrointestinal and operative site bleeding. A postmarketing surveillance study. *JAMA.* 1996;275:376-382.

41. Camu F, Lauwers MH, Vanlersberghe C. Side effects of NSAIDs and dosing recommendations for ketorolac. *Acta Anaesthesiol Belg.* 1996;47:143-149.

42. Maliekal J, Elboim CM. Gastrointestinal complications associated with intramuscular ketorolac tromethamine therapy in the elderly. *Ann Pharmacother.* 1995;29:698-701.

43. Macintyre PE, Jarvis DA. Age is the best predictor of postoperative morphine requirements. *Pain.* 1996;64:357-364.

44. Tilden VP, Tolle SW, Nelson CA, et al. Family decision-making to withdraw life-sustaining treatments from hospitalized patients. *Nurs Res.* 2001;50:105-115.

45. Wells DL, Dawson P, Sidani S, et al. Effects of an abilities-focused program of morning care on residents who have dementia and on caregivers. *J Am Geriatr Soc.* 2000;48:442-449.

46. Meier DE, Ahronheim JC, Morris J, et al. High short-term mortality in hospitalized patients with advanced dementia: lack of benefit of tube feeding. *Arch Intern Med.* 2001;161:594-599.

47. Luchins DJ, Hanrahan P, Murphy K. Criteria for enrolling dementia patients in hospice [See comments]. *J Am Geriatr Soc.* 1997;45:1054-1059.

48. Morrison RS, Siu AL. Survival in end-stage dementia following acute illness. *JAMA.* 2000;284:47-52.

49. Mitchell SL, Kiely DK, Hamel MB, Park PS, Morris JN, Fries BE. Estimating prognosis for nursing home residents with advanced dementia. *JAMA.* 2004;291(22):2734-2740.

50. Ahronheim J, Morrison R, Morris J, et al. Palliative care in advanced dementia: a randomized controlled trial and descriptive analysis. *J Palliat Med.* 2000;3:265-273.

51. Ahronheim JC, Morrison RS, Baskin SA, et al. Treatment of the dying in the acute care hospital. Advanced dementia and metastatic cancer. *Arch Intern Med.* 1996;156:2094-2100.

Stacie Stapleton, Valerie A. Cruz Flores, Anna Sedney,
Jasmine Williams, and Laura Drach

INTRODUCTION

Epidemiology

In the previous decade, it was reported that roughly 53,000 children in the United States died each year (1–3). The Centers for Disease Control and Prevention (CDC) reported 41,881 deaths in children between the ages of 0 and 19 years in 2015 (4). The National Vital Statistics Report published in 2019 (5) showed some of the top 10 causes of death in children ages 1 through 21 included unintentional injuries, suicide, cancer, congenital malformations, and heart disease, among others. Children and families under any of these categories would benefit from early referral and intervention from a comprehensive and multidisciplinary palliative care team. However, despite palliative care medicine becoming an organized, important subspecialty, many children that might benefit from palliative care are not being reached or provided these services (2).

Palliative care is not limited to the needs of dying children. The benefit of palliative care has been established for some groups of children with chronic illnesses. For example, children with cancer in the United States are known to benefit greatly from early referral to a multidisciplinary palliative care team (6). Despite this, most of these patients are referred to palliative care only during their end-of-life period (6). A study on pediatric palliative care utilization in hospitalized children with cancer showed that only approximately 4.4% of hospitalizations for children with advanced cancer had palliative care team involvement (6). As beneficial as this is for patients and families, earlier referral would likely provide much higher benefits.

The American Academy of Pediatrics issued a policy statement including guidelines and recommendations on palliative care in August 2000 and most recently updated it in 2013. This document affirms that "pediatric palliative care and pediatric hospice care (PPC-PHC) are often essential aspects of medical care for patients who have life-threatening conditions or need end-of-life care. PPC-PHC aims to relieve suffering, improve quality of life, facilitate informed decision-making, and assist in care coordination between clinicians and across sites of care. Core commitments of PPC-PHC include being patient centered and family engaged; respecting and partnering with patients and families; pursuing care that is high quality, readily accessible, and equitable; providing care across the age spectrum and life span, integrated into the continuum of care; ensuring that all clinicians can provide basic palliative care and consult PPC-PHC specialists in a timely manner; and improving care through research and quality improvement efforts." (3) Pediatric palliative care was recognized as a medical specialty in 2006 by the American Board of Medical Specialties (7).

Development and Understanding of Death and Dying

Medical providers often lack the knowledge or still find it difficult to talk with pediatric patients about death and dying. This is the case even when guidelines and suggested language has been provided, which could assist patients to develop a clear understanding of their illness (8,9). Avoiding speaking with children about their own or a loved one's death does not protect them from their thoughts about death. Further, studies have also shown that children's capacity for understanding death is often underestimated (10–12). Some have argued that it is the child's fundamental right to discuss such matter and that doing so preserves the child's dignity (13).

In speaking with children regarding death and dying, it is essential to have an understanding of their developmental age and thoughts around death and dying and to have a working knowledge of language to use during communication of these topics with a child. Such guidance is provided in Figure 57.1 (14,15). It is important to gauge the child's level of maturity and to not rely solely on numerical age in understanding the child's concept of death and dying; Figure 57.1 provides a framework in gauging a child's understanding of death. If there are questions or concerns, addition provider support should be sought with the guidance of a pediatrician, psychologist, or other mental health professional, child life specialists, or other professional specializing in grief and bereavement.

TYPICAL QUESTIONS AND STATEMENTS ABOUT DYING	THOUGHTS THAT GUIDE BEHAVIOR	DEVELOPMENTAL UNDERSTANDING OF DEATH	STRATEGIES AND RESPONSES
MONTHS–3 YR *"Mommy, don't cry."* *"Daddy, will you still tickle me when I'm dead?"*	Limited understanding of events, future and past, and of the difference between living and nonliving	May have "sense" that something is wrong. Death is often viewed as continuous with life (analogous to being awake and being asleep).	Optimize comfort, and consistency; familiar persons, objects, routines. Use soothing songs, words, and touch. *"I will always love you."* *"I will always take care of you."* *"I will tickle you forever."*
3–5 YR *"I did something bad and so I will die."* *"Can I eat anything I want in heaven?"*	Concepts are simple and reversible. Variations between reality and fantasy.	The child may see death as temporary and reversible, and not universal. May feel responsible for illness. Death may be perceived as an external force that can get you.	Assure child that illness is not the child's fault. Provide consistent caregivers. Promote honest simple language. Use books to explain the life cycle and promote questions and answers. *"You did not do anything to cause this."* *"You are so special to us and we will always love you."* *"We know (God, Jesus, Grandma, Grandpa) are waiting to see you."*
5–10 YR *"How will I die?"* *"Will it hurt?"* *"Is dying scary?"*	The child begins to demonstrate organized, logical thought. Thinking becomes less esoteric. The child begins to problem solve concretely, reason logically, and organize thoughts coherently. However, the child has limited abstract reasoning.	The child begins to understand death as real and permanent. Death means that your heart stops, your blood does not circulate, and you do not breathe. It may be viewed as a violent event. The child may not accept death could happen to himself or herself or anyone the child knows, but starts to realize that people the child knows will die.	Be honest and provide specific details if they are requested. Help and support the child's need for control. Permit and encourage the child's participation in decision making. *"We will work together to help you feel comfortable. It is very important that you let us know how you are feeling and what you need. Will always be with you so that you do not need to be afraid."*
10–18 YR *"I'm afraid if I die my mom will Just break down."* *"I'm too young to die. I want to get married and have children."* *"Why is God letting this happen?"*	Abstract thoughts and logic possible. Body image is important. Need peer relationships for support and for validation. Altruistic values • staying alive for family • parents, siblings • donating organs/tissue Disbelief that he/she is dying.	Understand death as irreversible, inevitable and universal. Needs reassurance of continued care and love. Search for meaning and purpose of life.	Reinforce child/adolescent's self-esteem, sense of worth, and self-respect. Allow need for privacy, independence, access to friends and peers. Tolerate expression of strong emotions and permit participation in decision making. *"I can't imagine how you must be feeling. Despite it all, you are doing an incredible job. I wonder how I can help?"* *"What's most important to you now?"* *"What are your hopes...your worries?"* *"You have taught me so much, I will always remember you."*

Figure 57.1 Developmental questions, thoughts, and concepts of dying with responsive strategies.

THE INTERDISCIPLINARY PALLIATIVE CARE TEAM

Team Collaboration—Communication and Planning

Communication and planning are integral to pediatric palliative care for oncology patients. Parents face many decision points through the end-of-life process such as treatment options, withholding curative therapies, focusing on comfort and quality of life, accepting hospice or other assistance into their home, and signing documents such as do-not-resuscitate (DNR) orders. To help the parents endure the tragedy of the death of their child and support their desire to achieve their definition of being a "good parent" (16) open and consistent communication is required. Parents must trust the teams caring for their child and feel supported in their decision-making process (16).

The child, depending on the cognitive level, age and developmental stage, emotional capacity, and medical condition should be, as far as possible, involved in the decision-making process (17). Physicians may feel hesitant to discuss end of life and dying directly with the patient or the parents may not want the discussions to involve the patient due to concerns of frightening the child or feeling the child is not ready to hear such conversations. Many children, however, have a remarkable knowledge and cognizance of their own death. Therefore, it is important, often critically so, to include the patient in discussion. The child may not necessarily be ready nor may it be appropriate to burden the child with all of the information, such as specifics on the final moments of life or funeral logistics but some will have specific questions (such as asking if it will be painful or frightening) that must be addressed in open communication with the parents and child (18,19).

Effective high-quality communication is best performed by skilled professionals such as are found in an interdisciplinary pediatric palliative care team composed of professionals including an attending trained in pediatric palliative care, social worker, child life specialist, and spiritual care expert (17). Although there are some cultural differences, most studies have shown parents and patients desire to be treated as a partner and member of this team (17).

For such a partnership between caregiving team, patient, and parents to be successful, information must be communicated to the family clearly and honestly. Physicians and the clinical team, however, sometimes find it difficult to deliver bad news, and parents have been reported to feel that physicians communicate too late about the end-of-life process (20).

Providers may feel uncomfortable, angry, or sad, and they may be concerned that their patients or parents may expect that death in avoidable and blame them when it approaches. Such provider discomfort must not override the importance of the physician's presence, availability, attention, and timely effective communication (21). Barriers for physicians to communication include the following:

- Lack of time to devote as needed
- Lack of staff to devote as needed
- Does not understand prognosis
- Not aware of goals of treatment
- Conflict regarding treatment goals
- Family prefers more life-sustaining treatment than physician
- Physician prefers more life-sustaining treatment than family
- Family does not accept prognosis
- Personal or emotional discomfort
- Language barriers
- Cultural barriers
- Legal fears

The communication process takes careful and thoughtful planning. In the best cases, the primary oncologist has discussed the overall prognosis from the beginning at diagnosis. Early consultation by the palliative care team is an important part of the planning, as it takes time for the team to develop a relationship with the child and family. It is best to avoid a last minute palliative care consult at the time a DNR order is indicated or to have a team of new faces as the child is actively dying. Palliative care should ideally be part of the entire journey from diagnosis to the final outcome.

The planning continues after the initial consult to help with symptom management, social issues, school, and sibling dynamics, and to assist with intercommunication between the family and health care professionals. Each of these interactions should be thoughtful and deliberate and carried out by a skilled palliative interdisciplinary care team. The individual members of the team have a unique role, and they plan their interactions accordingly. These roles are discussed in greater detail throughout this chapter These roles are discussed in greater detail throughout this chapter but in general, each role must plan the timing of their interactions with the child and family to maximize the effect and provide the best quality care. A child with a new cancer diagnosis is typically in the midst of major medical interventions and the family is inundated with medical information, so it is crucial to plan around these processes. Many times individual meetings with the family or child with various members of the palliative care team is the best practice, while other times, a care conference is preferred to include the palliative care team and medical team, with or without the family (20,22–24). Effective communication is necessary to connect the patient, family, primary physician, other staff members, and the palliative care team and is universally the key to deliver proper and safe medical care for oncology patients—especially children—who have complex medical conditions.

Family-Centered Care

The family unit remains a vital component of any patient care experience, and focus on the family is a standard of practice in caring for children (25–27), especially those with medically complex needs, chronic illnesses, and who are nearing end of life. The family unit is the foundation, identity, and center of the life experience of the child (25).

In the psychological and social work arenas, family can be defined as having two or more people who are joined together by bond sharing and intimacy (28). It is especially important to understand that family is not limited to biological ties but encompasses adopted, step, multiple generational, blended, same-sex, and many other social arrangements (28).

It is imperative that providers understand cultural, environmental, and spiritual values and traditions possessed by each family unit in order to provide the best care and understand individual coping strategies (29,30). When a child receives life-threatening or life-limiting diagnosis, the entire family is impacted, the entire family carries the diagnosis, and the entire family could potentially be permanently altered.

Sibling(s) of a patient should also be attended to and support should be put in place for them. It is not unusual for other children to feel that they are no longer important as the sick child receives more attention or possibly feel guilty that they cannot help or save their sibling (31,32). In addition to sibling, there are "forgotten grievers" of a family (e.g., grandparents, cousins, close family friends, etc.). Grandparents often carry a unique experience as they are grieving their grandchild but also their child as well (33–35).

Families caring for children with chronic illness or a life-impacting diagnosis have reported a wide spectrum of experiences with the health care system, which can lead to increased financial burden, family role stressors, and heightened caregiver burden. A family-centered care approach is essential to help with such adaptation and coping (36–38).

It is important to recognize that all elements of family-centered care are critical (Table 57.1) (28). Relationship building is crucial for family members to be able to partner with the medical professionals to help care for the child and participate in shared decision-making to achieve the best interest of the child. In this, all providers of the team have a duty to ease concerns or feelings of abandonment (39). The interdisciplinary nature of the pediatric palliative care team allows support to be tailored to the needs of patients and their families and can help ease the fear of abandonment (40–42). Conducting family conferences can help promote ongoing relationship building, open and honest communication, and collaborative decision-making efforts (39,43). If possible, additional family members should participate and support the child's primary caregivers.

Family Structure Special Considerations

Foster Placement

Foster placement can include placement into an actual single home, a residential facility, a group home, or juvenile justice facility (44,45). Placement into a foster system can be very distressing to the child especially if multiple placements follow and/or child is not placed with sibling(s). Literature shows that increase emotional concerns and decrease medical adherence occur with children in foster care and more care from health professionals is needed (45–47). Other important matters to note with a child in foster care are that Department of Family and Children services or social services often have legal custody. This empowers them to make decisions regarding placement and medical care. Relevant state jurisdiction may impact covered services (44), and care should be taken to understand specific regulations and laws that apply to the child in foster care. The American Academy of Pediatrics continue to advocate for the establishment and support of medical homes for foster children (44). The American Academy of Pediatrics medical home model refers to high-quality primary care delivered in a planned coordinated family-centered manner that address acute and chronic care.

LGBTQ

Data have shown that children raised by gay and lesbian parents have demonstrated resilience with regard to social, psychological, and sexual health despite economic and legal disparities and social stigma (48). Studies have demonstrated that children's well-being is affected much more by their relationships with their parents, their parents' sense of security and happiness, and the presence of social and economic support for the family than by the gender or the sexual orientation of their parents (48). It should be recognized that children in these families may be from prior heterosexual relationships of one parent, adopted, or biologically related to one parent but not the other due to in vitro fertilization or surrogacy (48). Legal concerns can arise if only one parent can make medical decisions and consent for the child. Stigma still persists around these families unit, and the family may feel that they have less support. Medical provider should ensure that these families are supported and receive the equal care and respect as other families (25,48).

Single Parenting

Most single parent's voice struggles with balancing caring for an ill or medical complex child, employment obligation, childcare, and/or social support systems (36). Often the primary custodial parent or a certain parent may have more interaction with the health care team, but it is important that the health care provider understand custody issues, legal decision-making rights, and visitation policy

TABLE 57.1 COMPONENTS OF FAMILY-CENTERED CARE

- Recognizing the vital role of the family unit provided for the child
- Fostering relationships with and support immediate caregivers and immediate extended family and recognize their strengths as individuals and within the family unit
- Respecting choices the family has made regarding the child's medical care
- Ensuring and promoting normal daily patterns of living whether the child resides in the community, home, hospital, or long-term care facility
- Recognizing the importance of ongoing open communications and relationship building with families and the medical providers to endure the highest standards and quality of care

Adapted from Jones B, Gilmer MJ, Paker-Raley J, Dokken D, Freyer D, Greenberg N. Parent and sibling relationships and the family experience. In: Wolfe J, Hinds P, Sourkes B, eds. *Textbook of Interdisciplinary Pediatric Palliative Care*. Philadelphia, PA: Elsevier Saunders; 2011:135-143.

as all of these can often be shared even though one parent may be more physically present (44). Additional psychosocial concerns that can cause stress to the child include a parent getting remarried or takes on a new partner, step family relationships, or each parent having a vastly different set of home rules or parenting style (44). Provider should have a working knowledge of some of the highlighted potential concerns noted above to ensure adequate support and quality care.

Blended Families

Blended or stepfamilies occur when parents find a new partner or remarry, and the child is included in the new family units. This can sometimes create increase complexity in navigating social support and communication. Identifying decision-makers, who can receive medical and possible psychological information regarding the child, who can visit, etc., will also help to minimize any potential conflict that may arise.

Palliative Care Referrals

The goal for palliative care intervention is to help improve symptoms throughout the disease course while supporting the family psychosocially and establishing the relationship connections that will be important at the end of life to maximize the quality of life and lessen the distress of dying from cancer (49–51). Early referral to palliative care after a diagnosis of cancer is made is almost always a good idea. Whenever the referral is made, however, it is essential that the primary oncologist or referring physician discusses the upcoming consult with the family, so the family is aware that the palliative care team will be arriving. If this is not communicated clearly, it can be distressing and cause misunderstanding leading to loss of trust. This is especially true for the family who is just settling into the diagnosis of cancer. Even if the referral is later into the process, great care should be taken in making a referral. Occasionally, members of the primary oncology team may feel reluctant to consult palliative care, so a "trigger list" of conditions in which a palliative care consult is appropriate or indicated can be helpful, and it has been shown that rates of consultation increase when referral criteria are used, which helps facilitate high-quality palliative care reaching pediatric oncology patients (51). The palliative care team's purpose is to add the extra layer of an overall comprehensive medical care program to assist pediatric oncology patients. Referrals to palliative care tend to increase when a palliative medicine physician and pain specialists are already on the existing care team. The pediatric palliative care team is responsible for maintaining a high standard of care

TABLE 57.2 APPROPRIATE REFERRALS TO PEDIATRIC PALLIATIVE CARE FOR ONCOLOGY PATIENTS

New diagnosis of cancer
Relapsed cancer diagnosis
Difficult pain or symptom management
Patient or family or health care team with differing views regarding prognosis
Staff or family distress
Ethical conflicts
Frequent hospitalizations
Prolonged hospitalization
Conflicts regarding use of medical interventions in dying patient
Need for end-of-life care coordination
Need for hospice resource utilization
Imminent complex decision-making expected
Serious decline in status
High-risk medical procedures or treatments
Family with limited social support
Limited availability of family
Discharge planning regarding hospice or palliative needs

as a consultation service and ensuring all palliative care team members are trained in palliative care specific to issues of pediatric oncology patients. A list of traditional and appropriate referrals is provided in Table 57.2 (49–52).

Palliative care involvement improves quality of life and improves many symptoms including pain. In addition, it has been shown to decrease the length of stay in the hospital overall and also decrease length of stay in the PICU and decrease use of intensive care unit resources (50).

It should be noted that while some institutions have large robust pediatric palliative care teams with many members, many institutions may have limited membership, such as only a nurse practitioner and child life specialist. Even a small team, however, can provide great benefit. While, therefore, it is desirable, it is not always crucial, to have a full robust team so long as all relevant issues can be addressed. Overall, patients who have a relationship with a palliative care team have less medical interventions at the end of life, and patients without consultation from the palliative care team are more likely to die in the PICU. Pediatric patients with life-limiting illness and their families who receive care from a palliative care team may experience improved quality of life (53,54).

Goals of Care

Goals of care conversations probe the patient and family's hopes, fears, and priorities. Families usually have thoughts or fears regarding their child's illness and how it will affect their child and family both in the short term and long term. Eliciting these fears, aspirations, and goals helps the team to understand the family's values and preferences thereby allowing the medical and nursing team to provide care consistent with the beliefs and wishes of the family.

Clear and compassionate communication was associated with excellent care after children with cancer had died in a study by Mack et al. (55). When prognostic concordance between families and physicians occur, it is associated with increased quality of life and better advanced care planning. Pediatric oncologists have stated that unrealistic hopes of cure seem to be the biggest barrier in communication (56). Having goals of care conversations early and often can lead to improved communication between families and the health care team and are a technique often used by palliative care teams. Understanding a patient's and family's goals can guide medical decision-making and assist parents through their child's journey. Goals usually evolve over time for all of those involved in a child's care, so goals of care conversations should be approached as an ongoing and dynamic process rather than a "one-off" event.

When patients first present with an oncologic diagnosis, the goal is usually cure. Generally speaking, parents have been found to be more optimistic than health care teams when it comes to overall prognosis. If end-of-life planning is needed, parents will often look for continued cancer treatment. Wolfe et al. found that it took parents 3 months longer than the oncologist to recognize that there was no realistic chance at cure (22).

Continued re-assessment of goals over time is important and can be extremely helpful for children with oncologic diagnoses. It should be seen as a longitudinal discussion. Helping families reframe their goals when cure is not possible allows the health care team and family the time to achieve memory making that might not occur without advanced care planning.

Asking a patient and family what they are hoping for can provide insight to oncologic health care teams. After the family answers the first question of what they are hoping for, the follow-up question, what else are you hoping for, can provide additional insight as to what the family is thinking. What once was a goal for cure might be a switch to a goal for one last family vacation or a peaceful death at home, especially if cure is not possible. As cure becomes less likely, parental goals can differ and also change toward the end-of-life period. A family will always hope for their child to live, even in the face of death. This knowledge should not be a surprise or be seen as a sign of family denial or family misunderstanding. It should also not be seen as poor communication from the medical team. Hope will always be present; however, the meaning may change as to what the family is hoping for over time. Health care teams should not take hope away from a family when giving bad news. Rather, what is hoped for can be reframed as families will continue to be hopeful even in the face of receiving an advanced cancer diagnosis (57). Ongoing communication eliciting family goals is very important through a child's illness and life trajectory. When parents are at a crossroads with treatment decisions, a review of previous goals stated by the family can be helpful. If a family stated that they do not want their child to suffer, a discussion regarding how the family defines suffering and what choices can be made to fulfill this goal is necessary.

When parents' and providers' goals align, families are noted to be less distressed (1). Open, honest communication while eliciting patient and family goals will assist a family on their child's medical journey.

Physician Role

A hospice and palliative medicine physician has special training and certification in providing care and support to patients and their families suffering from a serious illness. Part of this training includes advanced management of pain and symptoms (nausea, vomiting, difficulty breathing, fatigue, psychological issues, end-of-life distress, and more). Communication skills are fine-tuned during this training as are skills necessary to work as a member of a palliative care team consisting of nurse practitioners, social workers, chaplains, and nurses.

Nurse Practitioner and Physician Assistants Role

Advanced practice nurses, especially those who have passed the Advanced Certified Hospice and Palliative Care Nurses (AHCPN) Exam, and physician assistants are an important component of the palliative care team. Besides having a role in symptom management, they can play many roles including educator and researcher. NPs and PAs can diagnose, treat, and prescribe medications to provide total care to a palliative care patient. They also provide specialized care to patients at end of life.

Social Work and Psychology

Social workers comprise the largest group of mental health professionals providing psychosocial services in palliative care and hospice (58). Their role is often crucial in obtaining a psychosocial assessment and ensuring a family-centered approach to care is carried out (59).

A study conducted by Jones in 2005 of the Association of Pediatric Oncology social workers

TABLE 57.3 SOCIAL WORK SKILL SET DOMAINS

Advocate/educate
- Family-centered care
- Family ability to participate in care decisions

Specialized pediatric palliative care services
- Expressive art therapy
- Play therapy
- Ongoing communications regard quality of life and transitions of care

Counselor for children
- Supportive counseling for the patient
- Supportive counseling for patient siblings

Bereavement counselor
- Bereavement support

Provider of psychosocial assessment
- Assessment of the family's needs
- Individual psychosocial assessment of the child

Confidant/companion
- Being present and providing active listening to concerns, rears, and hopes
- Supportive counseling to parents

ranked services provided and identified by social workers providing support to a palliative care patient included six principal domains shown in Table 57.3 (58,60,61).

Although not as readily found on palliative care team, the role of psychology can be very beneficial in integrating behavioral health with medical care (62) and is often obtained through consultation and referral. Psychological care aims to enable patients and/or their families to express thoughts, feelings, and concerns related to illness in addition to assessing needs for resources regarding coping and ongoing psychological support (63). Psychological care can add great value to the care of patients and families coping with life-threatening and life-limiting illnesses by assessing neurocognitive and emotional status (62,64) and treating psychopathological conditions. Social workers, psychiatrists, and psychologists thus play an integral role in a palliative care team.

Child Life

The child life specialist role began in the 1920s with the intent of helping hospitalized children have a better overall experience. Child life specialists are typically required to have an undergraduate degree in child development, then serve an internship under a certified child life specialist, and then a certification exam is offered (65) and are an integral part of a pediatric palliative care team. They support the patient, siblings, and family by providing developmentally appropriate coping and stress-reducing interventions.

Oncology patients often face frequent procedures, hospitalizations, and toxicities from their medical therapy. The child life specialist is able to work with the child to understand their thoughts, fears, and perceptions and to find ways to navigate the process with better coping strategies (65) that are developmentally appropriate. Younger children, for example, may be drawn to express their emotions in art or playtime, while an adolescent has a different concept of cancer and death, which is much more complicated (66,67) and likely to be expressed differently.

The child life specialist can be very helpful in improving communication and voicing a patient's concerns and wishes. The child life specialist can help with the informed consent process for all ages, including assenting which is the practice used with minors since they cannot legally sign a consent document but they frequently should be informed and part of the medical decision-making process. They can be helpful when research trials are discussed to ensure all involved maintain ethical principles due to the potential consequences involved in research trials (68).

The child life specialist not only works with the patient but also with the siblings, as the siblings frequently have many issue such as loneliness, neglect, behavior issues, challenges with their parents, and feeling confused about the medical condition of their brother/sister (69). The sibling's routine becomes restructured when his or her brother or sister is diagnosed with cancer and interferes with the sibling's sleep, appetite, and anxiety level. Research has shown that support of the siblings can lesson these responses. Support of the siblings through the diagnoses and end of life can improve their coping after the death of the patient (70).

Spiritual Care

Spiritual care and religious needs are an integral part of pediatric oncology and family-centered care. Addressing them helps with coping and endurance during the whole cancer journey from diagnosis through treatment and particularly at the end of life. Chaplains have specific training and board certifications in their field and can help provide valuable information and insights as part of, or consult to, the interdisciplinary team. The spiritual care professional is able to give insight into the patient's beliefs and prior spiritual and emotional experiences of the patient and family, which can help with resilience (71). It is important the chaplain have skills to work with the full spectrum of religious diversity including Jewish, Christian, Islam, Buddhist, Hindu, other traditional religions, as well as atheist and agnostic. Not all people ascribe to a religious tradition. The designation of "spiritual but not religious" is an increasingly common one in American society. These individuals and families will still have existential needs that should be addressed. Chaplains explore many areas that other professionals may not reach within the patient and family including prior losses, suffering, and grief, in addition to life-purpose, expectations, and hope (72). Tending to the spiritual needs of cancer patients has multiple positive effects such as improving overall well-being, maximizing quality of life, and minimizing emotional distress. When cancer patients are at the end of life, improving their spirituality increases their ability to cope with the terminal process. Addressing religious issues is also associated with overall lower costs of health care (73). One of the benefits of an early referral to palliative care is that spiritual care is integrated at the outset of the patient's and family's cancer journey. Spiritual needs are common and impact on end-of-life decisions and outcomes (74). Prayer is the most common expression of faith, in addition to attending worship services, reading religious materials and books, support groups, counseling, personal reflection and devotionals, music or hymns, dance or physical movements, chants, aromas and incense, partaking of certain food substances, meditation, and other forms. The age of the patient is an important consideration: young children frequently display religious expression reflective of their parents. Some may, however, choose a different form of spiritual expression. In either case, they deserve respect as an individual and the support of an understanding trained chaplain. For an adolescent who was beginning to develop their own religious thoughts separate from their parents, a cancer diagnosis may hurdle them back to their parents form or in the complete opposite direction as they question why this is happening (75,76). The spiritual care professional has the skills necessary to help with these many complex needs of the patient and is an integral part of the palliative care team.

The Learner Role

The role of the learner (from any discipline, at any level of training) in the interdisciplinary pediatric palliative care team can be challenging for a variety of reasons. For many trainees, pediatric palliative care or pediatric oncology may be their first encounter with dying children (and if it is not, reexposure to pediatric death may be personally traumatizing). Learners may not yet have developed the repertory of coping skills and resilience demonstrated by more senior members of the team. The nature of and necessity for a tightly integrated interdisciplinary team has been explored elsewhere in this chapter; however, joining a team as an outsider in a junior position is

another potential challenge. Learners and trainees are also at risk of experiencing moral distress, the "experience of cognitive–emotional dissonance that arises when one feels compelled to act contrary to one's moral requirements" (77). This can arise from their perceived or real lack of power regarding fraught clinical decisions, from a genuine moral disagreement over end-of-life care, or from a lack of knowledge or experience with the various clinical care plans, choices a patient/family may make, and potential outcomes in a given scenario that falls outside of their limited prior exposure or standard protocols. It is incumbent upon the learner to recognize and address these questions but also upon the more senior members of the team to provide a safe space for learners to explore these difficult experiences, as well as provide guidance and positive role modeling.

Exposure to palliative care can have a large positive impact on learners. Students have reported improved communication skills, ethical knowledge, teamwork abilities, holistic approach to patient care; a greater willingness to be available to patients; and reduced emotional distress after a focused palliative care teaching intervention (78,79). Longitudinal curricula have also been shown to increase residents' self-reported attitude to palliative care with specific benefits noted in breaking bad news, symptom management, goals of care, and integrative therapy—essentially the major supportive roles of palliative care (80). Satisfaction with palliative care exposure is universally high for learners, across levels of medical training, specialties, and even nations (81–84).

Given the interdisciplinary nature of palliative care, learners from any and all disciplines should be encouraged to spend time with team members from specialties outside of their own. This is especially true in pediatric palliative care, as the unique training of child life specialists has prepared them to deal with children across the developmental spectrum facing serious illness, death, and bereavement. Familiarity with age-appropriate communication tools for children and families coping with oncologic diagnoses is an invaluable skill set for anyone dealing with a pediatric population, regardless of eventual career trajectory. Learners can also benefit from well-run, high-fidelity simulation sessions to improve their communication skills without causing emotional harm to patients and families in high-stakes conversations, just as much as interventional specialists practice their procedures early in training (85,86).

Learners can also provide benefit to the interdisciplinary palliative care team. The presence of learners requires that all members of the team maintain current, evidence-based knowledge within their own disciplines. This knowledge transfer can be reciprocal as learners may also have the time and inclination to research and share the most current and up-to-date scientific literature within and across disciplines that busy clinicians may not have the wherewithal to follow. Some families and patients also enjoy the extra attention or feeling that they are able to contribute to society even at the end of their life. This is, of course, patient and learner specific (87).

SYMPTOM MANAGEMENT IN PEDIATRIC PALLIATIVE CARE

Acute and Procedural Pain

A Buddhist proverb says: "Pain is inevitable, but suffering is optional." It is easy to believe that in this day and age, and yet the literature shows that pediatric pain continues to be noted as a frustrating factor regarding patient care in both children and adults. From assessment to management of pain, many patients and family members report dissatisfaction, including in the palliative care setting. Acute and procedural pain is often ineffectively treated or even untreated (2).

The first and most critical step in pain management is assessment (88). In the pediatric population, there are several pain assessment scales available for use in the clinical setting, and their use is dependent on the patient's age and whether the patient is verbal or nonverbal. In nonverbal patients, pain assessment scales by proxy can be used. Some examples of these are the Infant FLACC (Face, Legs, Activity, Cry, and Consolability) tool, the Faces Pain Scale (or Wong-Baker FACES Pain Rating Scale) for children over 3 years of age, and the Visual Analogue Scale for older children and adolescents (89).

For acute and procedural pain management, the most commonly used guidelines are provided by the World Health Organization (WHO). The WHO guidelines recommend "Pain Ladder approach" to minimize/eliminate pain before, during, and after medical procedures or acute nonprocedural pain, including nonpharmacologic options, taking into account that emotional distress and fear can contribute to pain. The Pain Ladder approach recommends increasing from simple analgesics to weak opioids, to stronger opioids for increased pain intensity (2,90). Examples of medical procedures that can cause pain and distress in children are phlebotomy, dressing changes, and injections, to mention a few. For these procedures, preventable management of pain is important. Techniques such as distraction may be helpful for simple procedures, whereas topical analgesic agents are useful for more invasive or fearful procedures (91).

Other nonpharmacologic therapies and techniques include cuddling, general social support, acupuncture, and cognitive–behavioral techniques such as hypnosis, guided imagery, and biofeedback (90).

For moderate to severe acute pain, procedural or nonprocedural, pharmacological management is recommended and opioids are the first-line treatment. Morphine is the preferred medication for analgesia in these scenarios, as it has been thoroughly studied in the pediatric population and may be given through multiple routes of administration. Other opioid options include oxycodone, hydromorphone, fentanyl, and methadone. There are no data indicating that treatment of pain with opioids causes addition in children or that depression of respiratory drive is more common than in adults (2). Codeine and tramadol are no longer recommended for use in children due to concerns regarding their safety and efficacy (89,90).

The WHO announced a revision for their guidelines on the pharmacological treatment of persisting pain in children with medical illnesses in August 2019 (92).

Chronic Pain

Chronic pain is defined as pain that persistent in duration longer than 3 months that is often continuous but can be intermittent. The pathophysiology and other factors that contribute to pain can different between acute versus chronic pain are in Table 57.4.

It is estimated from U.S. and European studies that 15% to 25% of pediatric patients experience chronic pain (93–95). It has been estimated that roughly two-third of children and adolescents with chronic pain will become adults with chronic (96). Girls report more chronic pain than boys with a studies showing difference in coping between the sexes as well (97,98). Girls utilize more social support, positive statements, and internalizing/catastrophizing, whereas boys engage in more behavioral distraction (97). Chronic pain can be associated with increased incidence of physical disability, depression, anxiety, and decreased quality of life (99–101). Common causes of chronic pain in children and adolescents include headaches, fibromyalgia, abdominal pain, musculoskeletal pain, and complex regional pain syndrome (102–106). Due to the complex nature of chronic pain, its impact on quality of life, and other contributing psychosocial factors, a multidisciplinary approach is recommended for management (102).

Assessments should include a thorough pain history and assessment that measure day-to-day physical and psychosocial functioning (93,107). (It should be note that standard pediatric pain intensity scales or self-report should not be

TABLE 57.4 CHRONIC VERSUS ACUTE PAIN CHARACTERISTICS

	Chronic pain	Acute pain
Source/etiology	Nociceptive and/or neuropathic	Usually nociceptive
Inciting event	Can be multifactorial; source may or may not be known	Associated with an identified source or event
Duration	Greater than 3 months but resolution indeterminate	Resolution in hours, days, or weeks
Behavioral	Can display maladaptive behaviors	Adaptive behaviors
Physical symptoms	Vital signs may be normal	Tachycardia, hypertension, tachypnea may be seen
Treatment	Multidisciplinary approach with physical therapy, coping strategies, nonpharmacological intervention with minimal reliance on opioids and other pharmacological medications	Often opioids and other pharmacological medications are used

utilized in assessing chronic pain as focusing on constant intensity scoring can led to negative thoughts about pain as the underlying principle of chronic pain management is increasing functionality despite pain.) (93,108).

A multidisciplinary team consisting of a physician, physical therapist, psychologist, etc., is needed to manage chronic pain patients. Management is focus identifying the underlying etiology if possible and treatment consisting of very limited use of opioids with the goal of no opioids with use of adjuvant pain medications or modalities, physical rehabilitation, and integrative practices such as patient self-regulation practices such as biofeedback and self-hypnosis in addition to integrative practices such as acupuncture/acupressure, aromatherapy, massage, good sleep hygiene, and nutrition modifications all acting in synergy to provide the effective pediatric pain control and better long-term control (95,109–111).

Special attention should be paid to children who are nonverbal and/or neurologically impaired as recognition and treatment of pain is often lacking (112–115). Vocalizations, irritability, arching, facial expression, etc., can all be sign of pain. Common causes of chronic pain can include fractures, urinary tract infection, pancreatitis, gastroesophageal reflex disorder (GERD), constipation, feeding difficulties from delayed gut motility, positioning, spasticity, hip pain, or dental pain, etc., in this population (112–114). Therefore, it is imperative that provider recognizes potential cause of chronic pain and treat accordingly in these patients.

Neuropathic Pain

Neuropathic pain is caused by damaged, injured, or dysfunctional nerve fibers or altered excitability of the somatosensory system (116). Motor symptoms such as tremors and spasms can occur in addition to autonomic manifestations such as sweating

and erythema as well. Typical descriptions of neuropathic are an electric, tingling, burning, or crawling sensation that can also manifest as or be accompanied by itching, coldness, or numbness. Damage to the somatosensory system (e.g., effects of cancer and/or its treatment, surgery, neurodegenerative disorders, HIV/AIDS, or neuronal migration disorders) can lead to neuropathic pain. Damage to the peripheral nerves and inflammation can lead to sensitization, which can lead to amplification of pain intensity in the peripheral nerves and excitatory receptors in the spinal cord that causes increased output to the brain leading to the phenomenon of central sensitization and the output from the CNS amplifies the perception of the pain known as "wind-up" phenomenon. Neuropathic pain often presents differently in children and adolescents compared to adults (112,113,116,117). An example of this is visceral hyperalgesia.

Visceral hyperalgesia is a heightened pain response to visceral stimulation often of the gastrointestinal tract, which may manifest as retching, vomiting, flatulence, or feeding intolerance. Children with neurological impairment are at increased risk for visceral hyperalgesia (112,113). Complex regional pain syndrome is nerve damage with autonomic, sensory, and/or motor changes and symptom manifestation (112,113). Neuropathic pain is important to consider in children receiving certain chemotherapy agents and in children with neurological impairment (118,119).

There are no particular pediatric scales to grade neuropathic pain (120). Treatment often includes multimodal approach of physical, psychological, and pharmacological therapies (117,121). Most studies have been done in adults with current specific studies being undertaken in pediatrics, but gabapentin and certain selective serotonin reuptake inhibitors (SSRIs) and serotonin-noripenephrine reuptake inhibitors (SNRIs) have been shown to

TABLE 57.5 FATIGUE SYMPTOMS MANIFESTATION

Domain	Manifestation
Physical	Heaviness, weakness, lethargy, decreased endurance
Cognitive	Impaired memory, difficulty or poor concentration
Sleep	Insomnia, hypersomnia, nonrestorative sleep
Emotional	Irritability, lack of motivation

From Ullrich CK, Mayer OH. Assessment and management of fatigue and dyspnea in pediatric palliative care. *Pediatr Clin North Am.* 2007;54(5):735-756, xi.

be effective in treatment of neuropathic pain and often used as first-line treatment (121–124). Topical lidocaine has shown some effectiveness in helping managing neuropathic pain especially if a burning sequela is present (125). In addition to nonpharmacological pain adjuvants such as guided imagery, aromatherapy other modalities that have been effective include graded motor imagery exercises, visualization and mirror therapy, and laterality recognition have some benefits for neuropathic pain in pediatric cancer patients (126).

Fatigue and Somnolence

Fatigue is one of the most prevalent symptoms in patients with a life-threatening illness and/or children under cancer treatment or posttreatment (127–134). Studies have shown significant impacts on psychosocial and physical functioning affecting the child's quality of life (128,135–138). Therefore, addressing a child fatigue is very important in ensuring effective palliative care management. Fatigue symptoms may manifest in different ways as noted in Table 57.5 (127).

The National Comprehensive Cancer Network describe cancer-related fatigue as a distressing, persistent, and subjective sensation of tiredness or exhaustion that is contributed to cancer or cancer treatment that is not proportional to recent activity and interfere with usual functioning (128). Due to the subjectivity of fatigue, medical providers often rely on a parent or the child to assess it, which has led to development of self-report, observational, and performance scales that can been seen in Table 57.6.

Other studies have attempted to develop scales and measure fatigue in chronically ill patient utilizing self-report and minimally improvement quality measures and technology-based patient-centered evaluation (142–144).

Due to the effect fatigue has on a patient's quality of life, treatment and management and reassessing goals of care of fatigue symptoms are very important. Many studies have shown nonpharmacological interventions to be safe and effective at managing and/or alleviating fatigue symptoms and therefore should be considered first-line treatment (127,130–132,145–154). Interventions include physical exercise programs, music therapy, acupuncture and acupressure, healing touch, mind–body relaxation techniques, guided imagery, and good sleep hygiene (127,130–132,145–154). It is also important to consider other psychosocial and physical factors that could contribute or worsen fatigue symptoms in patients such as caffeine use, medications, anemia, infection, electrolytes disturbances, nutrition, disease progression, boredom, depression, fear, stress, anxiety, etc.

If other potential cause of fatigue have been evaluated and treated and patient does not respond well to nonpharmacological interventions, pharmacological interventions can be initiated in addition to nonpharmacological management. It is important to note that systemic pharmacological interventions should be for short-term management only (152,155–159). Short-term pharmacological treatment that could be used are corticosteroids (e.g., dexamethasone, prednisolone, prednisone) or CNS stimulants (e.g., modafinil or methylphenidate) (155–160).

Anxiety

Children and young adults with cancer face a life-threatening disease that puts them at risk for

TABLE 57.6 FATIGUE AND PERFORMANCE SCALES

Scale	Age range (in years of age)	Description
Childhood Fatigue Scale (CFS), Staff Fatigue Scale (SFS), and Parent Fatigue Scales (PFS) (139)	7–12	Utilized the child, staff, and parent evaluation of fatigue
Pediatric Quality of Life Inventory (PedsQL) (140) Multidimensional Fatigue Scale	2–18	Self-report Scale or Parent Proxy Report Scale
Modified Lansky Play Performance Scale (141)	1–16	Utilized play as a measurement of performance

comorbid anxiety. Anxiety occurs in response to a perceived or real threat and can escalate to excruciating fear (161). When anxiety affects activities of daily living and quality of life, it is considered pathologic. Cancer comes with the stress of disruption to patients' and families' lives and the ever-present fear of the unknown and possibly death. Psychological health should be addressed and managed throughout the treatment and survivorship journey.

Psychosocial support that can assist in alleviation of anxiety can be helpful to children and their families throughout the continuum of treatment and survivorship. A thorough family assessment can benefit the health care team in developing a treatment plan. In the spirit of the total pain model, spiritual, emotional, psychosocial, and physical pain should be assessed and managed appropriately, to provide patients well-rounded care (162).

Developmental staging is indicated when assisting children with their psychological health. Each stage brings its own needs. There are four stages of development to note. Infant/toddler is the period of age 0 to 3, preschool is the period of 3 to 5, school age is 6 to 12, and adolescence is 12 to 18. During each of these time periods, reactions to their illness and treatment course will change (163). Taking these factors into account may assist the health care team in providing the correct strategies for coping.

Generalized anxiety, separation anxiety, anticipatory anxiety, and anxiety regarding death are categories in which the child with cancer may be at risk for during their treatment course. Generalized anxiety is characterized by extreme worry, which can manifest as fatigue, poor concentration, and irritability.

Separation anxiety can occur in all children but is most prevalent in the infants/toddlers and school age children range. Bringing in comforting items and allowing the parents more access during procedures that may be frightening could assist the child in coping. Having articles from home may allow the child to utilize all senses to help calm them including touch, sight, and smell. Blankets, pictures, stuffed animals, familiar toys, and video games are all items that may bring comfort to a patient. Anticipatory anxiety is the most common type of anxiety that children undergoing cancer treatment face. Thinking about the hospital, taking medication, and getting their port accessed can put children into an anxious state.

Assisting children with learning cognitive–behavioral therapy (CBT), which include guided imagery, distraction, graduated exposure to anxiety provoking situations, and stress management, can mitigate the anxiety that children may be feeling. Other modalities that can be effective include music therapy, acupuncture, and hypnosis (164,165). If the anxiety continues to cause physical symptomatology such as nausea and vomiting, pharmacological treatment may be needed. Antiemetics and benzodiazepines could be useful in these situations. Children and families may also benefit from having primary nursing as continued relationships with the same team may assist with coping. Short-term pharmacological treatment may be beneficial for active symptomatology while CBT strategies are developed. If the patient is able to use the techniques taught with CBT intervention, pharmacologic treatment may no longer be necessary (166,167). In other cases, children may need both to assist them throughout their cancer treatment. If pharmacologic treatment is deemed necessary for the long term, the first line of treatment is usually an selective serotonin reuptake inhibitor (SSRI). Other therapies that may be considered are SNRIs and tricyclic antidepressants (TCAs). SNRIs and TCAs are not used as often due to cumbersome side effects. A discussion with the family regarding the FDA's black box warning and signs of suicidal ideation are warranted so that an informed decision can be made regarding use of these medications (168). Providers should be cautious when giving children the diagnosis of generalized anxiety disorder as cancer treatment is usually a short period of time. A diagnosis of adjustment disorder may be more appropriate. A collaborative team approach with psychiatrists, psychologists, mental health counselors, chaplains, and licensed clinical social workers can be very beneficial for health care teams and families when a child is living through cancer treatment.

Depression

Children are at risk for mental health conditions as they learn how to cope with their cancer diagnosis. Dysthymia, adjustment disorder, and depression should be differentiated in children suffering from a cancer diagnosis. In general, dysthymia is defined as depressed mood for most of the day, most of the time by self-report or reported by others for at least 1 year. This definition is specific to the pediatric and adolescent population. Adjustment disorder is defined as a reaction to a medical illness and is the most common mood issue in patients with cancer (161). Depression in children undergoing cancer treatment can be difficult to assess and treat due to the medical complexity of their disease. There are still not strong data to suggest that children with cancer suffer more depressive symptomatology than the general pediatric population (169). Complicating factors include issues of overlap, in that fatigue, changes in sleep and appetite, and difficulty concentrating can happen with medical illness and depression. Some of the side effects seen from cancer treatment can easily be confused with criteria used to diagnose depression.

A thorough family and patient history of current and previous psychological conditions is important when assessing the patient's mental health. Pain from cancer can affect mood, which can lead the provider to misdiagnose depression. Given this information, the medical provider should consider consulting mental health experts to assist and manage children during what could be one of the most stressful times in their life. The DSM-5 criteria for a major depressive state that five or more of the following symptoms must have been present over a 2-week period with either depressed mood or loss of interest/pleasure. In addition, the symptoms cause difficulties in activities of daily living. There should be an adequate history and physical that rules out other medical conditions (161).

a. Irritable or depressed mood almost every day by report
b. Lack of pleasure or interest in activities most of the day, almost every day
c. Weight loss/gain of more than 5% or loss of appetite every day
d. Difficulty sleeping or very sleepy every day
e. Psychomotor agitation or slowing down every day.
f. Feeling tired almost every day
g. Extreme guilt or feeling unworthy almost every day
h. Inability to concentrate or difficulty making decisions
i. Continual thoughts about death, or suicidal ideation with no specific plan/having a plan or a suicide attempt

Treatment of depression can consist of many modalities including psychosocial and medication management (170). The family and patient should assist in developing the treatment plan collaboratively with the health care team. An interdisciplinary approach utilizing psychologists, psychiatrists, social workers, or other qualified professionals in conjunction with the oncology team will bring the greatest results. CBT has been shown to be effective in depression alone, as well when in combination with SSRIs (167,171). However, it is noted that no large randomized controlled studies have been done in children with cancer and depression using SSRIs. The prescriber should educate the patient and family regarding common side effects of medications. Additionally, side effects in which they should contact the provider right away such as changes in mood, behaviors, thoughts, or feelings are important to discuss with the family. The black box warning issued in 2004 by the FDA shows concern for suicidal ideation when antidepressants are first initiated (168). An open discussion with the family regarding signs to look for with appropriate documentation is important. Currently, medication management mostly involves the use of SSRIs. Many oncologists feel very comfortable prescribing SSRIs; however, there has been difficulty in appropriate follow-up after prescribing (168). Involving mental health professionals in the treatment of patients who truly have depression will assist the patient and family in receiving the best support to prevent relapse (172).

Delirium

A high index of suspicion for delirium should be entertained in critically ill children, including those with an oncologic diagnosis, when acute mental status changes occur. Issues such as impaired consciousness, agitation, memory lapses, and poor sleep can cause a delirious state. Unfortunately, delirium is associated with poor outcomes, which is why early recognition and treatment is needed (173).

Delirium can be easily missed without proper assessment. The most common factors for delirium are infection, medications, autoimmune diseases, and malignancy. The most common medications causing delirium are opioids, anticholinergics, and benzodiazepines (174). Delirium is defined as a disturbance in attention and awareness (161). With a proper delirium assessment, the opportunity for timely treatment can occur. Without proper recognition and treatment, mortality rates can be increased (173). Unfortunately, not many studies have addressed delirium in children with cancer. In a single institution study by Traube et al., delirium affected one in five children over a 3-month time period on an oncology ward and was associated with prolonged hospital stay (175). Furthermore, consistent risk factors have been identified including use of benzodiazepines. Risk factors include young age, brain tumors, developmental delay, and malnutrition (175,176). Routine screening for delirium in the pediatric oncology population is advisable. There are five diagnostic criteria by DSM-5 to properly classify delirium (161).

A. Reduced attention and awareness.
B. Develops over a short period of time, represents a change from baseline attention and awareness, and fluctuates throughout the day.
C. An additional disruption in cognition such as memory decline or perception
D. Criteria in A and C are not better explained by another preexisting, established, or evolving

neurocognitive issue and do not occur in the setting of a coma.

E. History and physical examination or laboratory finings do not suggest another medical condition.

These are furthermore divided into subtypes: hypoactive, hyperactive, and mixed, with hypoactive being the most prevalent. Hyperactive has been described with symptoms of agitation, confusion, psychosis, loud speech, and increased motor activity. Hypoactive delirium has characteristics of slow movement, inattention, slow speech with reduced volume, and overall aloofness. It is the most common subtype found in children (175). The mixed type had characteristics of both. When assessing for delirium, the Cornell Assessment of Pediatric Delirium (CAPD) has been shown to be a reliable tool. This tool was developed from the Pediatric Anesthesia Emergence Delirium Scale. It was found to be reliable in children <2 years as well as children who were developmentally delayed (175,177). The DSM-5 criteria are considered the gold standard among psychiatrists for diagnosing pediatric delirium (178).

A more recent debate has emerged regarding the use of antipsychotics in delirium. A systematic review was completed by Nikooie et al., which does not support the routine use of Haldol or second-generation antipsychotics for use in adult patients (179). Since research is usually slower to come in the pediatric population, one can only extrapolate these data to include children.

A well-thought-out approach to preventive measures should be implemented. Interventions such as reorientation to time and place are essential. Schedules with appropriate sleep hygiene modalities can assist: routine bed time and wake up time, lights off at night, blinds open during the day, and minimal interruption by staff when patient is sleeping. All care providers have a role in minimizing noise, playing calming music, and allowing favorite activities (180). Prevention is the best modality, however, can be unavoidable in our oncology patients. Pediatric delirium is a treatable condition when recognized and managed appropriately using an interdisciplinary process.

Seizures

Seizure control can be difficult. Unfortunately, many children with cancer involving the central nervous system suffer from seizures at the end of life (181). Primary brain tumors are the second most common cause of cancer in children and the most common solid tumor. Over 4,000 children are diagnosed with brain tumors annually in the United States. Brain tumors are the leading cause of cancer death in children, and these children experience many comorbid neurologic symptoms related to their brain tumor at the end of life in addition to seizures (182). Seizures depend on area of the brain involved, occur in up to half of children with brain tumors, and can be one of the most distressful symptoms to the patient and caregivers (183). The palliative care team must establish clear and early goals of care with the patient and family as neurologic deficits can impair the patient's ability to communicate, and treating one symptom such as seizures may worsen another deficit such as weakness, fatigue, or decreased alertness, and therefore, difficult choices must be made ideally in advance. Typically, the approaches for acute seizures such as intravenous medications and intubation/ventilation are not congruous with goals of care for children at the end of life (181). Seizure surgeries are possible and rarely appropriate in the palliative setting (184). Seizure prophylaxis is not routinely recommended without clearly documented seizures as the medications can cause undesired side effects particularly fatigue or sedation; however, it is common practice to have antiseizure medication available for as needed usage for the possibility of seizures or for rare seizures (182). The route of administration of antiseizure medications is important regarding compliance, effectiveness, and quality of life, and fortunately, there are many options. If the patient has difficulty with swallowing, the sublingual or rectal route may be preferable. The various classes of drugs have certain benefits or issues. Benzodiazepines are fast acting and effective and can be given by many routes. Barbiturates are more sedating and longer lasting. Newer classes of drugs are also available and may be suggested by a neurologist. Cannabinoids have shown to be effective in Lennox-Gastaut and Dravet syndromes, with the cannabidiol component having the most evidence in seizure treatment (185).

Respiratory Symptoms

Dyspnea

Dyspnea or the sense of breathlessness is a distressing and sometimes debilitating symptom that often leads to anxiety and sense of impending doom. Although they can be subjective, dyspnea is often categorized by its symptoms, which include air hunger, chest tightness, and increased effort. Not only are the symptoms distressing to the patient but also to parents and family members who may feel the patient is suffocating (191). Patients' and their families' quality of life is often impacted when symptoms are not adequately managed (188,189,191,192). Many factors that

TABLE 57.7 POTENTIAL CONTRIBUTORS TO DYSPNEA

Causes	Examples
Physical	Pain, tumor, heart failure, cystic fibrosis, interstitial lung disease, muscle weakness, neuromuscular degenerative diseases, infections, secretions, anemia, malignancy, etc.
Psychosocial and/or spiritual	Anxiety, fear of death, fear of suffocation

From Ullrich CK, Mayer OH. Assessment and management of fatigue and dyspnea in pediatric palliative care. *Pediatr Clin North Am.* 2007;54(5):735-756, xi; Davies D. Respiratory symptoms. In: Wolfe J, Hinds P, Sourkes B, eds. *Textbook of Interdisciplinary Pediatric Palliative Care.* Philadelphia, PA: Elsevier Saunders; 2011:300-302; McGrath PJ, Pianosi PT, Unruh AM, Buckley CP. Dalhousie dyspnea scales: construct and content validity of pictorial scales for measuring dyspnea. *BMC Pediatr.* 2005;5:33; Wiseman R, Rowett D, Allcroft P, Abernethy A, Currow DC. Chronic refractory dyspnoea—evidence based management. *Aust Fam Physician.* 2013;42(3):137-140.

can contribute to dyspnea and should be investigated in addition to physiological causes as seen in Table 57.7 (127,193,194).

It is important to note that pO_2 and respiratory rate often poorly correlate with the sense of dyspnea and respiratory effort and dyspnea are not interchangeable as patient may find relief of dyspnea without a change in respiratory rate. Self-report scales of dyspnea are often used as the symptom is often subjective in nature. There are very few scales that have been created or studies that have examined dyspnea in the pediatric population. The Pediatric Dyspnea Scale (PDS) was created for and validated to measure dyspnea in pediatric asthmatic patients (195). The Dalhousie Dyspnea three construct scales were developed for self-report for dyspnea in general in pediatric patient (>8 years old). The parameters measure throat closing, effort, and chest tightness (193).

In managing dyspnea, underlying etiology and correction should be sought first. Anxiety can worsen the sensation of breathlessness providing more urgency to utilized nonpharmacological interventions such as blowing bubbles, blowing pin wheels, singing, participating in slow deep breathing, ensuring an upright comfortable position, calm environment, and companionship. Extensive studies have shown a small handheld fan to the face can help alleviate the sense of breathlessness (196–202). Although nonpharmacological interventions provide a necessary first step in managing patient with the dyspnea often, pharmacological interventions are still needed.

Opioids continue to be the standard pharmacologic management of breathlessness and when dosed appropriately have been shown to be effective in treating dyspnea by helping to suppress some respiratory awareness with some sedative effects (203–206). Starting doses for the treatment of dyspnea are typically ¼ to ½ of normal pain doses and titrated to the minimal effective dose to alleviate breathlessness (127,203–207). Benzodiazepines should not be used as first-line therapy for breathlessness but does have a role as an adjuvant to opioids if anxiety is significant (205,208). Nebulized opioids and furosemide for the treatment of dyspnea have been studied, but results examining effectiveness are mixed, and standard practices are currently to use oral or parenteral opioids for the treatment of dyspnea (203,206,209,210). Oxygen therapy can be helpful in some patients with hypoxemia; however, oxygen therapy has been shown to be ineffective in patients with dyspnea without hypoxemia and rarely effective in actively dying patients, and therefore, it is important to counsel patient and the family regarding oxygen therapy for breathlessness (194,211).

Cough

Cough is a symptom that is sometimes overlooked. However, it can lead to abdominal pain, chest pain, and/or fatigue (212). The cough reflex can be trigger by a bronchial obstruction, secretions or airway debris in the alveoli or bronchi, viral infection, postnasal drip, heart failure, environmental irritations, ciliary dyskinesia, interstitial lung disease, foreign body, aspiration, or some of irritation of the carina (213,214). Pediatric studies looking at the treatment of cough especially in cancer or palliative care patients are limited. Potential treatments include identification of underlying cause and treatment if possible. Nonpharmacological interventions could include honey, humidified air, eliminating environmental allergies, upright positioning, or chest physiotherapy. Other pharmacologic treatments such as expectorants (e.g., guaifenesin, dextromethorphan, combination products, etc.) and codeine use have been advised against by the AAP (American Academy of Pediatrics) in children <6 years old and risk versus benefits and goals of care regarding use weighed in children >6 years old. There is a concern that these medications have been associated with significant morbidity and rarely mortality related to intentional and unintentional ingestion (214–217). Honey, antihistamines, or small doses of an opioid have been shown to be effective in management of cough (216,218). Radiotherapy, surgery, or brachytherapy may be needed if obstruction or lesion occurs in the bronchi that is cause the cough (219).

Secretions

Sialorrhea can be caused by three different mechanisms: excessive production of saliva, inability to retain saliva in the mouth, or difficulty swallowing. Noisy breathing or ratting breathing both phrases used for terminal secretions is often due to secretions in the upper airway and oscillatory movements of these secretions in patients with difficulty controlling airway or unable to expectorate. Although not typically distressing or uncomfortable to the patient, it can be distressing to the parents or family members (220). Anticipatory guidance should be provided about this manifestation to parents and family members. Nonpharmacological oropharyngeal suctioning may be helpful in some cases, but deep suctioning should be avoided (220). Anticholinergic medications are often used in treatment, although some studies have shown weak evidence for effectiveness in patients with terminal secretions (221–224). Anticholinergics often used are 10% atropine eye drops administered sublingually and titrated to effect, scopolamine patch applied by the ear, or systemic use of glycopyrrolate (212). Care should be taken to monitor secretions if treatment with anticholinergics to ensure secretions does not become too thick causing the secretions to become harder to manage and potentially lead to mucous plugging, which can worsen respiratory symptoms (212).

Nausea/Vomiting

Gastrointestinal symptoms, especially nausea and vomiting, are the most distressing side effect of cancer treatment (225). Nausea not only causes immediate distress and decreased quality of life in oncology patients but also can contribute to a wide range of downstream effects such as growth failure, lack of enjoyment in previously comforting foods, inadequate nutrition, need for hospital admission, and poor wound healing or immune function. Children are more prone to chemotherapy-induced nausea and vomiting (CINV), in part because of their more toxic and emetogenic chemotherapy regimens. Fifty to fifty-seven percent of children with cancer report experiencing nausea and vomiting (226). It is important to be aware that younger children may convey nausea by behavioral changes, including food refusal.

Given the frequency and severity of these symptoms, expert palliative care practitioners approach nausea and vomiting systematically. Detailed attention should be paid to emesis pattern, associated symptoms, abdominal examination findings, and medication history. A systematic approach to identifying the underlying etiology and mechanism of action of nausea and vomiting allows targeted (or deliberately multimodal). Multiple medications targeting the same mechanism of action may increase side effects without increasing benefit, and medications that are not helpful should be discontinued.

Factors that play a role in cancer-associated nausea and vomiting include medications (chemotherapy, opioids, and antibiotics are common), mechanical and functional bowel obstruction, psychogenic effects, and impaired GI motility related to disease state. A history of motion sickness, female gender, and younger age are known predictors of worse symptoms (225,227).

The area postrema, known as the vomiting center, is in the medulla oblongata and is the final common pathway for causing emesis by triggering smooth muscle contraction in the GI tract. Neural pathways to the vomiting center originate in the cerebral cortex, the chemoreceptor trigger zone (CTZ) located on the floor of the 4th ventricle, the vestibular nuclei, and the periphery, most notably the GI tract.

The CTZ responds to medications as well as metabolic products (such as by-products of renal or hepatic failure) or toxins. Cortical stimuli can include emotional or sensory triggers, such as anticipatory nausea and vomiting or olfactory triggers, as well as increased intracranial pressure or meningeal disease. Peripheral stimuli include mechanical inputs such as obstruction, stasis, pharyngeal stimulation, as well as local GI receptors for toxins or drugs. Vestibular input can be triggered by motion or by inner ear problems.

The receptor types and neurotransmitters involved differ depending on the type of trigger for nausea and vomiting. The vestibular system is mediated by histamine type 1 and muscarinic acetylcholine receptors, and this is responsive to histamine blockers and antimuscarinics such as phenothiazines (e.g., promethazine) or anticholinergics (e.g., scopolamine).

The $5HT_3$ receptors in the GI tract respond to $5HT_3$ receptor antagonists (e.g., ondansetron, granisetron, or palonosetron). Promotility agents (e.g., metoclopramide, which antagonizes dopamine type 2 [D2] receptors in the GI tract) can be used for poor motility associated with advanced disease (228). Children are at higher risk than adults of extrapyramidal symptoms, although many experts consider this concern to be somewhat overblown (229), especially if diphenhydramine is coadministered (226). Steroids have been shown to be beneficial to reduce edema or mass effect related to bowel obstruction (230), and prevention and management of opioid-induced constipation remains obligatory.

The CTZ has D2 receptors, $5HT_3$ receptors, and neurokinin type 1 (NK1) receptors and thus is amenable to many classes of drugs, including those that also have an effect directly on the GI tract. This includes antipsychotics, both first generation such as haloperidol or atypicals such as olanzapine (which has been shown to decrease CINV by as much as 65%) (231). Aprepitant is a newer antiemetic therapy, acting on NK1 receptors, that is now considered standard of care for highly emetogenic chemotherapy regimens by the Children's Oncology Group (232) and has been shown to cut in half the risk of CINV (233). Management of cortical triggers should be based on the underlying pathology, benzodiazepines for anxiety and dexamethasone for tumor-associated elevated intracranial pressure, for example.

Nonpharmacologic management of nausea and vomiting should be considered standard and may involve simple fixes such as taking small, regular meals; remaining upright after eating; avoiding unpleasant sensory triggers, especially while eating; and addressing psychological or spiritual aspects of distress that may worsen psychogenic nausea and vomiting. Complementary therapies including aromatherapy with peppermint or ginger, guided imagery, progressive muscle relaxation, acupuncture, and acupressure wristbands have had mixed results in the pediatric literature despite more success in adults, with some studies showing benefit and others showing no change. They all have a favorable safety profile and are relatively low risk so worth attempting in interested patients (228,234–237).

Constipation and Diarrhea

Pediatric patients with chronic illnesses spent a significant amount of time in the hospital, and opioids are usually a large part of their treatment (238). Constipation is the most common side effect of treatment with opioid medications. Prevention with a safe and effective bowel regimen once opioids are instituted is essential in all patients. Commonly, one or more types of laxatives are used in combination with a motility agent (89). There are different types of laxatives, and they are osmotic laxatives (lactulose, sorbitol, magnesium citrate), stimulant laxatives (bisacodyl, Senna), bulk-forming laxatives (polyethylene glycol), and stool softeners (docusate sodium) (238). Constipation can also be a side effect of diet, dehydration, or decreased ambulation and often leads to other undesirable symptoms such as nausea or vomiting (239). Nonetheless, opioid-induced constipation is often not relieved by the use of laxatives, as these do not target the pain receptors in the gastrointestinal tract. A novel type of medications to treat opioid-induced constipation are the opioid antagonists' naloxone, naltrexone, and methylnaltrexone, all of which lack evidence-based results in the pediatric population currently but their efficacy has been suggested in pediatric case reports in the literature (238).

Diarrhea is another unwanted symptom that chronically ill patients may experience in the palliative care setting. In some cases, diarrhea may be a result of constipation, something named obstipation, where diarrhea results from overflow in a patient with constipation (226).

Hematologic/Transfusions

Despite blood product transfusions being one of the most common interventions in medical care (240), no evidence-based literature is available about their use in the pediatric palliative care setting. As a general rule, recommendations for transfusion of different blood products for the general population have undergone extensive review by international organizations, and there are specific guidelines for each of the blood components. Within these guidelines lie the need for laboratory assessment of blood counts or coagulation parameters to assess the need for blood products, something not necessarily needed during end-of-life care. However, for those palliative care patients not considered to be getting end-of-life care, laboratory evaluations are common, and the potential need for blood product transfusions may arise. It is important to note as well that the supply and availability of blood products depends on voluntary donations from healthy individuals, and more often the demand is higher. Red blood cell (RBC) units have a shelf life of up to 42 days, and platelet units have a shelf life of 5 to 7 days (241).

Anemia is a commonly encountered finding in palliative care patients, with approximately 7% of adults under palliative care requiring a transfusion (241). Generally, a RBC transfusion is recommended for hemoglobin levels between 7 and 8 g/dL. This varies depending on the clinical scenario, and patients' signs and symptoms (240,242). Symptoms and signs from significant anemia may include dyspnea, fatigue, dizziness, elevated heart rate, and low blood pressure, and the goal of a red cell transfusion is to ameliorate these. However, these symptoms can be encountered at the end of life, regardless of hemoglobin level (243).

Platelet transfusion need are also often encountered in pediatric patients undergoing palliative care, as they are used in the setting of severe thrombocytopenia to minimize the risk of bleeding or to control bleeding. For many years, the threshold to transfuse platelets to a patient, regardless of symptoms, was a platelet count of 20,000/L or below. In an attempt to decrease the number of unnecessary transfusions, multiple studies were able to prove that bleeding risk is the same between a platelet count of 10,000 and 20,000/L. Many palliative care patients have oncologic diagnoses and have received chemotherapy, which causes a hypoproliferative thrombocytopenia, prophylactic platelet transfusions are used. It was shown, however, that the risk of bleeding in patients with this specific type of thrombocytopenia is decreased when compared to other causes (240,242).

The rate of adverse reactions occurring after transfusion is similar between adult palliative and nonpalliative care patients, happening in <1% to 8% of transfusions (241). Though transfusion reactions are rare, the benefit of using blood transfusions in this population needs to be further studied. Some authors have postulated the possibility that some deaths in the palliative care population can be a result of transfusion reactions, though this would be difficult to determine (241,244). Nonetheless, the recommendations seem to lie on giving blood transfusions to those patients who are thought to have the most considerable benefit.

Dermatologic

Dermatologic complaints are common in cancer patients. Nonspecific rashes are reported by up to 85% of patients, depending on the specific therapies, and 35% report xerosis (245). Targeted therapies and monoclonal antibodies produce pruritus in up to 50% of patients (246). Alopecia associated with chemotherapy is probably the most noticeable effect of chemotherapy, but pruritus, photosensitivity, desquamation, hypersensitivity reactions, folliculitis, paronychia, xerosis, hyperpigmentation, erythema, skin thinning, and striae have all been observed from treatment or primary disease. The final common pathway of many of these conditions is breakdown in skin barrier function. Many of these effects are both cosmetically and physically distressing. High-quality, nonocclusive pigmented makeup has been shown to improve quality in life in patients with significant visible scarring (247). Permanent alopecia is a rare but reported side effect of high-dose chemotherapy, particularly for stem cell transplant conditioning, and cranial radiation (248,249).

General basic skin care is recommended with mild, nonperfumed cleansers and emollients in cream base. Cleansers should be neutral to slightly acidic. Niacinamide-containing emollients have been reported to be helpful in adults with severe xerosis. Alcohol-based cleansers are drying and should be avoided, as should most topical acne treatments that may be distressing for adolescents. Topical antimicrobials or steroids may be needed for more severe cases. Broad-spectrum sunblock should be used liberally (245).

Pruritus at the end of life can be particularly distressing as comfort becomes the goal. Dry skin as outlined above can contribute and gentle cleansing only when necessary and frequent emollient application are useful. Scratching results in temporary relief but can cause skin irritation and thickening, exacerbating itch later. There can also be a psychogenic component to pruritus. There is a role for antihistamines in some cases, and these are generally the first-line therapy. However, pruritus can also be induced by cytokines, opioids, and serotonin centrally; this is less responsive to histamine-blocking therapy. Opioid-induced pruritus occurs in 15% to 20% of patients, with incidence as high as 80% for patients receiving neuraxial opioids (250). This can be treated with opioid rotation or naltrexone. Butorphanol is frequently used but less effective. There is some debate about whether or not histamine is involved in opioid-induced pruritus (251), so antihistamines may be trialed but should not be the only therapeutic option. When they are successful, it is unclear if this is truly from histamine release blockade or the general sedating effect. Renal or hepatic failure from primary disease, medication toxicity, or terminal decline can also cause uremic or cholestatic pruritus. Cholestyramine and ursodiol may be beneficial for cholestasis. Some authors have reported using paroxetine, ondansetron, and mirtazapine to address the serotonergic component of pruritus (251–253).

Skin breakdown at the end of life can occur, especially in patients with decreased activity or mobility levels. Palliative care and even hospice do not preclude good skin care routines or wound management, as open wounds can be painful as well as psychologically distressing (254). Patients on high-dose corticosteroids, such as those with brain tumors, are at particular risk for skin breakdown and discomfort. The benefits and burdens of continuing steroid therapy should be considered on an individual basis.

INTEGRATIVE MEDICINE

Integrative medicine is often confused or used interchangeably with alternative medicine (not evidence based) or complementary medicine (use of other therapies in place of conventional medicine). Integrative medicine utilizes evidence-based complementary therapies with conventional therapies to treat the whole individual including not just the physical self but mind–body as well (255–257). Interest in integrative medicine has risen due to the prevalence of children with chronic illness, more focus on preventative health, and polypharmacy (258–260). One study showed that complementary practices were used in 31% to 84% of children with a cancer diagnosis (261). The American Academy of Pediatrics is committed to optimizing the well-being of children and therefore has recognized the increasing use of integrative therapies for children (260). It is important that providers ask patients and/or their families of integrative or complementary practices and supplements usage to provide the best care and because often families may feel providers will disapprove of usage (262,263).

The demand for integrative medicine is outpacing health providers' training (260,264,265). Although integrative medicine focuses on broad domains of the body systems to ensure complete total person care, the focus in this session will be on common dietary supplements used in children, nutrition, pain management, and mind–body practices. Some systematic reviews have shown benefits of certain therapies and shown them to be safe when used solely or in combination with conventional therapies, but there still needs to be ongoing research regarding interactions and long-term usage especially in pediatric oncology (261). There are many commonly used herbs in children such as feverfew ginkgo, lemon balm, licorice valerian, St. John's wort, etc. (266). Feverfew is used in children to help treat migraine headaches and nausea and vomiting. Abrupt discontinuation can lead to rebound headaches, and feverfew may potentiate the effects of anticoagulants (265–267). Gingko is used to improve circulation, but potential side effects include headaches, dizziness, or gastrointestinal disturbances and may also potentiate the effects of anticoagulants (265–267). Deglycyrrhizinated licorice (DGL) has been shown in many pediatric studies to help with sore throat, cough, and stomach ulcers (265–267). It is very important that DGL is used instead of glycyrrhiza-containing licorice because long-term glycyrrhiza licorice can cause mineralocorticoids effects such as potassium wasting and hypertension (265–267). St. John's wort is often used in the treatment of depression and anxiety disorders. Side effects include sedation and gastrointestinal symptoms, and it is an inducer of the metabolic enzyme CYP3A4 which means and it lower plasma concentrations of other medications metabolized by this enzyme (265–267). Herbs have relative low toxicity in short-term acute use. However, short-term nontoxicity does not equate to chronic long-term safety. Therefore, usage should follow prescribed guidelines by knowledge integrative medicine physician or practitioner. Other cautions include potential herbicides and pesticides that could cause toxicity (265).

Other commonly used supplements, botanical, and herbs in children include the following:

docosahexaenoic acid (fish oil) use for symptom improvement of neuropsychiatric disorders (such as ADHD and literature supporting use for its role in development of nervous system, brain retina, and rental cortex), melatonin in helping regulate sleep–wake cycles, probiotics to improve gut health and help restore gut microbiome after prolong antibiotic use and help with symptom control in some children with functional abdominal pain/irritable bowel syndrome (160,166–170). Magnesium and butterbur has been shown to help with migraine prevention and treatment. Echinacea is used for the prevention and treatment of viral, bacterial, and fungal infections, particularly those affecting the upper respiratory tract (260,266–270).

Nutrition

Mediterranean Diet

A balanced diet with heavy emphasis on fruits and vegetables and minimal emphasis on sugar and processed foods is very helpful in practicing good health and has shown to help prevent comorbidities such as childhood obesity, metabolic syndrome, diabetes, ADHD, headaches, celiac disease, and irritable bowel disease (271). The Mediterranean diet focuses on the incorporation of whole foods, such as nuts, fruits, vegetables, fish, and healthy fats, such as olive oil. Studies have shown that adopting a Mediterranean diet can be beneficial in children with inflammatory-based diagnoses or other inflammatory processes as it has been shown to help reduce inflammation within the body (272–274).

Ketogenic Diet

The ketogenic diet has gained popularity in helping to control seizure activity in some children with certain seizure disorders. At its core, it is one of the more extreme versions of carbohydrate restriction shifting the body to a chronic state of ketosis and deriving most of one's calories from fat. It is presumed that the ketogenic diet success in at least some cancers relies on the flexibility of normal cells (can metabolize either glucose or ketones for energy) and the inflexibility of cancer cells (reliant on glucose) that with removal of glucose normal cells easily switch to metabolizing ketones while cancerous cells cannot. Yet some cancer cells are heterogeneous in their ability to metabolize ketones, and therefore, only some cancer cells may respond to the ketogenic diet (275). Currently, most evidence for the effectiveness of the ketogenic diet is anecdotal, but more studies are currently underway regarding the utility of ketogenic diet in cancer therapy (276,277).

Medicinal Mushrooms

Certain medicinal mushrooms, widely used in Asian cultures, are thought to have some beneficial effects in as they are thought to help with immune enhancement, serve as antioxidants, and perhaps anticancer effects although anticancer effects are only anecdotal at this time as a reviews has shown no anticancer effects and limitations in some studies regarding their methodology (278–280).

Antioxidants and Oncology Treatment

There is also some debate regarding diets high antioxidants during chemotherapy or radiation treatment. Some chemotherapy (e.g., the platinum agents, alkylating agents, and antitumor antibiotics) generates free radicals; therefore, the concern is that if a patient uses antioxidant supplements during radiation or chemotherapy (with the goal of protecting normal tissues), they may in fact be inadvertently protecting the tumor or cancer cells. Although studies have been in adults, multiple studies have examined a number of antioxidants and have found that there was no evidence of diminished chemotherapy or radiation effects (281). However, at this time, expert recommendations are that patients can eat an antioxidant-rich diet during radiation or chemotherapy and use of supplemental antioxidants should be postponed until active therapy has been completed if goals of care are curative.

Medicinal Cannabis

Delta-9-tetrahydrocannabinol (THC) is the main psychoactive component of cannabis. It has been approved as dronabinol and nabilone to use in the treatment of CINV (282). Cannabis is also orexigenic (283). Research regarding cannabis and its effectiveness on pain and other symptoms has been limited due to its Schedule I classification, and effectiveness has been anecdotally driven by many patients report benefit however many studies are underway (284). Cannabis is often sought by cancer patients for pain relief in adjunct with opioids. Currently, cannabis analgesic usage is in neuropathic pain, although no supportive studies have yet been conducted in chemotherapy-induced peripheral neuropathy (283). Also to date, there are no published studies supporting calms of anticancer benefits.

Providers should also be aware that cannabis dispensaries offer patient may different selections of medical cannabis. Oral ingestion can be complicated as there is delayed peak plasma concentration, which causes even more psychoactive metabolite first pass of the THC. Also due to the prevalent use of CBD oil, highly concentrated extracts of THC and CBD could potentially interact with other medications and cancer treatment due to cytochrome P-450 interactions.

Integrative Adjuncts

Pain and other symptoms are often seen in children with chronic illness or those who are undergoing cancer treatment. Growing evidence and studies are emerging regarding the use of other modalities and therapies for symptom management. For instance, in addition to providing significant pain relief, studies have reported a reduction in the use of opioids and improve quality of life when mind–body therapies are implemented (285). Also literature shows that approximately 15% to 25% of children experience chronic pain and mind–body practices (yoga, hypnosis, guided imagery acupuncture progressive relaxation, etc.) were effective especially among female patients (286). Studies have demonstrated that acupuncture may help in alleviating pain as well (287).

A component of the overall pain treatment plan especially in children with chronic pain should include a nutrition assessment and recommendations for decreased junk food and increased whole foods including green vegetables and healthy oils. A number of dietary supplements such as vitamin D, omega-3 fatty acids, magnesium, and CoQ10 have been proposed to modulate pain; however, more studies are needed to determine efficacy (288–291). Same as with supplements, there is a paucity of evidence-based efficacy and safety data in pediatrics regarding botanicals, but a few commonly used botanicals in pediatrics that have some supporting data for their use in pain include chamomile (also helpful as an antispasmodic agent and can be used topically for mouth sores), peppermint (enteric coated can help ease pain of irritable bowel symptoms due its smooth muscle relaxation through action on calcium channels and used topically for headaches, muscle aches, and itching), pyrrolizidine alkaloids (PA)-free butterbur for headaches, and lavender for anxiety (268,289,292,293).

Integrative modalities and therapies are not just limited to pain. Cannabis in the approved form of dronabinol and nabilone is used in the treatment of CINV. Ginger root powder has been shown to reduce the effects of chemotherapy-induced nausea and vomiting in addition to conventional therapy (294). Vincristine is used in the treatment of some childhood cancer/tumors that can have some side effects of motor and sensory neuropathy. A study in the pediatric population showed that glutamine supplementation was tolerated and associated with improvement in sensory function (119).

Essential oil use has also been studied and shown effective for use in children to help has an adjunct of pain relief and other symptoms. See Table 57.8 for five common essential oils that have been studied and have been shown to be safe for use in pediatric patients (268,295,296).

TABLE 57.8 ESSENTIAL OIL USES IN CHILDREN

	Pain	Nausea	Insomnia	Anxiety	Fatigue
Lavender	X		X	X	
Lemon		X		X	
Peppermint	X	X			
Spearmint					X
Sweet orange			X	X	

From Anheyer D, Frawley J, Koch AK, et al. Herbal Medicines for Gastrointestinal Disorders in Children and Adolescents: A Systematic Review. *Pediatrics.* 2017;139(6); Kedia S. Complementary and Integrative Approaches for Pediatric Headache. *Semin Pediatr Neurol.* 2016;23(1):44-52; Weaver MS, Robinson J, Wichman C. Aromatherapy improves nausea, pain, and mood for patients receiving pediatric palliative care symptom-based consults: a pilot design trial. *Palliat Support Care.* 2020;18(2):158-163; Bikmoradi A, Khaleghverdi M, Seddighi I, Moradkhani S, Soltanian A, Cheraghi F. Effect of inhalation aromatherapy with lavender essence on pain associated with intravenous catheter insertion in preschool children: a quasi-experimental study. *Complement Ther Clin Pract.* 2017;28:85-91.

Note that true essential oils are highly concentrated and MUST be diluted in a carrier oil if topical use is indicated, although essential oils have a high safety profile for usage, applications of aromatherapy or topical application should be done by a provider trained in using these oils. Carrier oils often used in pediatrics include jojoba oil, canola oil, coconut, and safflower oil.

Mind–Body Practices

The American Academy of Pediatrics has endorsed the use of mind–body therapies (e.g., biofeedback, guided imaginary, yoga, clinical hypnosis, massage, and acupuncture in pediatrics) (260). In the 2007 to 2012 National Health Interview Survey, mind–body therapies ranked in the top 10 complementary and integrative medicine practices used by adults and children (297). Modalities often used include biofeedback, clinical hypnosis, guided imagery, meditation, and yoga (297). There have some pediatric studies analyzing specific mind–body practices (154,298,299). One randomized multicenter control trial demonstrated that acupressure could be useful to help ease symptomatology (such as nausea/vomiting/pain/fatigue) in children undergoing treatment for cancer or those undergoing stem cell transplant (150). Emerging studies are showing effective utilization of integrative therapies depending on the child age and/or developmental stage, and care should be paid to determine the most effective interventions for patients (300).

ADVANCED CARE PLANNING AND SOCIAL, ETHICAL, AND LEGAL CONSIDERATIONS AT END OF LIFE

Advanced Directives

The Patient Self-Determination Act goal was to protect a patient's autonomy at the end of life. This led more usage of advance directives such as Living Wills and Durable Powers of Attorney for health decisions (301). There are many terms that are used in advance care planning and seen below:

DNR—Do Not Resuscitate

DNAR—Do Not Attempt Resuscitate (sometimes used in place of DNR to negate the underlying assumption CPR will be successful)

AND—Allow a Natural Death (sometimes used in place of DNR to view not wanting resuscitative measures from a patient's perspective)

Power of Attorney—an individual authorized and designated to advocate on patient behalf to make medical or financial decisions

Guardianship—authority granted by the court to make decisions or advocate for the individual regarding medical, financial, or other decisions

Proxy/Surrogate Decision Maker—a designated individual who makes health care decision for a patient who is incapable (e.g., unconscious, handicap, delirious, mentally ill, or most children and adolescent since they are typically not give legal autonomy in decision-making).

Advance care planning can be difficult for any individual; however, it is something some parents never thought they would have to do for or with their child. Despite the difficulty of this topic, one study has shown that the majority of parents found advance care planning to be helpful to preserved the child's quality of life and prevent significant suffering (302). Studies have also advised that advance care planning should be a longitudinally approach to care when a life-impacting diagnosis is made or in children with chronic illness versus at a time of a crisis (303–305). It should be noted that children under state custody with diagnosis or illness where advance care planning is indicated, the child protection agency will authorize should advance care planning after multidisciplinary consultation with the medical providers (306).

Although they carry no legal weight, pediatric tools such as Five Wishes and Voicing My Choices are utilized to help make communication easier in children (who are verbal and able to comprehend) with parents and their providers. These tools seeks to address goals of care, wishes at end-of-life care, artificial nutrition and life support, etc., with the patient and family in mind at the developmental stage of the child.

Resuscitation Status

Children with progressive cancer face many decisions about treatment options, and one of the most difficult decisions is deciding on resuscitation status. As cancer is the leading cause of nonaccidental death in children in developed countries, the discussions regarding this decision is relatively frequent. The decision is complex as to the timing of implementing this status, and the options that surround it. In most states, an out-of-hospital DNR order is signed by both a licensed provider and the patient (or a parent or guardian for a minor). Inpatient DNR orders vary by institutional protocol but typically involve a physician placing an order in the electronic medical record. Regardless if in- or outpatient, the discussion with the patient and family must be clearly documented. The child should be involved in the conversation as much as they are medically, emotionally, and developmentally able. It is appropriate to have a separate conversation with only the parents and then have a conversation with the child at the developmental level. Children with cancer typically have had a long journey and understand many more medical terms than their peers, and frequently, they have only had adults as companions during long hospitalizations or confinements to home; therefore, they have had more grown-up conversations than their chronological age. On the other hand, due to lack of normal psychosocial development and lack of a peer group, they may not have the emotional capacity for processing for difficult conversations. The interdisciplinary palliative care team can help asses this situation to advise on and participate in discussions around resuscitation status (189). Not uncommonly, one parent is ready before the other parent to accept the prognosis and make advanced directive decisions or sign the DNR order for the child. It is important that both parents are aligned at the same time when signing this order, to avoid anger or guilt while the child is dying and later after the death has occurred. When there is only one parent, this scenario then frequently involves extended relatives in addition to the sole parent and pressure to make the decision sooner or later than they are willing to have conversations on resuscitation status or sign the order.

The primary oncologist should respect the decision of the family and the timing, although there could be urgency to make a decision if the child is rapidly declining from the progressive cancer. Earlier discussions and decisions about resuscitation status are associated with less suffering of the patient, better quality of life, and more preparedness of the family (307–309). The discussions for the patient and family should include specific details surrounding their wishes at the end of life. Most parents and children prefer to die at home, but sometimes, this is not possible and not all families choose this for various reasons. Cultural and religious preferences can influence their decisions as well as prior experiences with other deaths in the family. In addition to choosing a location to die, other end-of-life choices include major interventions, such as intubation, ventilations, chest compressions, and cardiac medications, and also other interventions, such as oxygen supplementation, transfusions, and palliative chemotherapy. Some therapies and treatments are withheld including antibiotics, seizure medications, and artificial nutrition, especially if any of these are causing more symptoms or discomforts than providing benefit. Pain medications and other comfort measures are standardly continued to ease suffering. The wishes of the family and patient should be honored, and the palliative care team and primary oncologist should discern the goals of care and then advise if the wishes regarding end-of-life care and specific interventions are in line with the overall goals of care.

Impact on School

Pediatric patients with chronic or life-limiting medical diagnosis must contend with how to manage with school. Treatments, hospitalizations, or symptomatology of their diagnosis may preclude them from attending school for periods of time, which can impact academic quality and prevent peer social interactions (310–312). The Rehabilitation Act of 1973 and the Disabilities Education Act (IDEA) of 2004 allows for resources to be made for continuing educational programs for young people with health concerns who are not able to attend school regularly with each state implementing the law in different ways (312). Special accommodations may be needed when the child returns to school. The parents should enquire about an Individualized Education Program (IEP) or a 504-education plan. It is also recommended that parents discuss the illness and/or ongoing medical needs and concerns with school educators and professionals to ease the burden of concerns these individuals may have when a child returns to the classroom (313,314).

If the child is unable to attend school because hospitalized or receiving home medical care, some larger pediatric hospitals provide academic teachers. Usually the patient is transferred to the hospital school for an amount of time before returning to the regular school, and usually the hospital teacher will contact the school to obtain a better understanding of the child academic history, any special needs, and coordinate curriculum, and in most cases, school credits are still usually earned, which can also provide somewhat of a sense normalcy for the child (312).

A child may be emotional ready to return to but cannot due to immunosuppression, fatigue, multiple follow-up appointments, etc. These subset of patients would possibly qualify for home-bound teaching where teacher will meet with the patient two to three times a week or online. If possible, it is very crucial that children receiving home- or hospital-based academic support maintain peer interactions and support. The social support can help with confidence regarding school reentry especially if physical changes have occurred such as weight loss, loss of hair, or utilization of medical equipment (312).

Social Media

Social media has taken the world by storm including health care, and we all are constantly immersed in it (315). What exactly is social media? The Merriam-Webster definition of social media is the form of electronic communication through which users create online communities to share information, ideas, personal messages, or other content. Some examples include Instagram, Twitter, LinkedIn, Facebook, Pinterest, YouTube, as well as wikis, blogs, and podcasts.

Patients and their parents or other family members may have developed blogs to help chronicle illness journey, found specific online support groups, and connect with other parents of children with rare disease diagnoses, participated in recruitment trials, or finding community for psychosocial support (316–319). However, social media has risk and benefits not only for patients and their families but also for health providers as certain issues such as HIPAA concerns, confidentiality, professionalism, inaccurate medical knowledge, and ethical concern have been raised (318,320,321).

Trying to promote parent's right to share his or her own story and the child's right to enter adulthood free to create his or her own digital footprint can be a hard task and is the subject of many ethical concerns (317).

Medical providers should discuss the use of social media with children and adolescents with their families. Providers can possibly help patients and parents navigate online sharing that helps protects the child's privacy, ensuring medical accuracy and mitigate any potential ethical concerns to protect the best interest of the patient while still fostering online community support (317,322).

Cultural Differences

Perspectives and opinions on medical care in general can be different depending on cultural practices, traditions, and beliefs. Culture in itself defines an individual, and it is not forgotten during illness. If anything, our cultural roots play an immense part in how we deal with illness and with end-of-life attitudes. It has been reported in the literature how services provided by palliative care are not used as often by minority groups such as African Americans, Indian Natives, or Latinos. Therefore, exceptional medical care relies on medical professionals that are sensitive and cognizant of cultural differences among patients (323), especially when providing pediatric palliative care.

Despite knowing this and despite all medical providers being taught about cultural competence, some cultural aspects tend to be significant barriers to medical care. For example, language barriers were reported to be an issue in almost 50% of end-of-life care encounters in a study about perception of barriers to palliative care in children (2). The use of a trained language interpreter, an in-person one if possible, aids in overcoming this barrier. Nonetheless, when discussing topics such as end-of-life care, many families report distrust in the medical team and feeling they are not receiving all the information they need, even when an interpreter is utilized (2).

As pediatric palliative care providers, it is imperative that we put our own cultural beliefs and expectations aside and we do our best to understand the culture of the families we are taking care of (2). Another example of how cultural differences are important in pediatric palliative care is regarding religion and spirituality, which is known to be an important aspect in decision-making for children undergoing palliative care. However, no major research examining the impact of religion and spirituality exists (1).

Other identified barriers are socioeconomic status, education level, demographics, and background history. A recently published workshop regarding multicultural pediatric palliative care was dedicated to identify specific factors that can add to conflicts within families and caretakers and attempted to create awareness of these factors in order to improve care by generating recommendations. They found that despite identifying factors such as religion and spirituality, very few physicians really explored these factors in their clinical encounters (238,324).

Transition to Adulthood

Many young adults are treated in pediatric cancer centers, and many more formerly pediatric patients will achieve legal adulthood and competency during or after their oncologic treatment. Oncology and palliative care teams should address this transition prior to the patient's 18th birthday so that the patient and the parents have a plan for how the newly legal adult may begin to control his or her own health care. Even seemingly minor issues such as scheduling appointments, signing consents and other papers, and to whom medical information may be released are potential sources of conflict for parents who have invested large amounts of time and effort in directing their child's medical care. Discussion of advance directives should be readdressed and made into legal documents; this process will be much easier if these conversations are begun early in the disease course.

Fertility Preservation

Male infertility after childhood cancer is approximately 50% in some studies and for females can range from 16% to 40% (325). While the technology does exist to allow for postpubertal patients to undergo gamete collection, for female patients especially this may delay treatment initiation. Storage is also expensive and infrequently covered by insurance. There is also significant potential for ethical dilemmas about disposition of gametes in the event of the patient's death.

Assent/Consent

Assent is the act of a child agreeing, usually verbally but sometimes in writing, to a medical treatment. The Belmont Report was a seminal work in bioethics published in 1976 by the National Commission for the Protection of Human Subjects of Biomedical and Behavioral Research that laid out the ethical framework for human subject medical research. The Commission published a subsequent report in 1977 specific to the inclusion of children as research subjects; this report recommended the age of 7 as the lower limit for obtaining assent for research. The Commission also differentiated between parental "permission" for research, instead of "consent," as consent is more directly applicable to the process by which an individual decides for themselves and is a direct outgrowth of the foundational bioethical principle of autonomy (326). It is important to respect dissent, if the child voices it (327).

Outside of research, parents or other legal guardians provide official consent for treatments and procedures. As children age and mature, their views are taken more into consideration in the event of a disagreement with the parent.

Most conflicts can be resolved with expert communication facilitation, such as from a palliative care team or ethics consultation. If the adolescent's wished are considered ethically acceptable, it is reasonable to abide by his or her choice. However, in the matter of life-saving treatment, it is generally accepted by bioethicists that teenagers do not have the right to refuse if their parents request treatment. In this case, protecting the minor's right to an open future takes precedence (328).

Some jurisdictions have mature minor statutes or case law that allow an adolescent, who independently demonstrates capacity, to make decisions. Most of the case law in the mature minor field has centered on teenage oncology patients, as their long-term experience with their disease and its treatment contributes to their presumed maturity (328). The presence of a cancer diagnosis does not exclude adolescents' right to privacy in the standard areas of contraception, pregnancy, sexually transmitted diseases, substance use, and mental health.

Clinical Trials

Treatment decisions for oncology patients are complex. When faced with progressive disease in an incurable illness, clinical trials and early-phase studies may be offered to the family as a reasonable option when there are no other medical therapies available. Up to 70% of pediatric cancer patients participate on a clinical study at some point during their treatment. As phase 1 studies are looking for toxicities and the maximum tolerated dose, patients enrolled may experience unexpected or severe side effects at any dose level and especially at the higher-dose level cohorts. In addition, there is little chance of benefit of phase 1 study drugs particularly at the lower-dose levels, and the eligibility criteria usually include the condition has no other known curative treatment options. The patients and families choose to participate with the hope of the possibility that the drug may have some effect on the cancer, such as slowing the growth and giving the patient more time. Phase 1 studies typically have very strict and frequent follow-up office visits and laboratory or other studies as part of the monitoring parameters in the protocol. The child and family are required to be present at the clinic or hospital or undergo additional testing, which may include painful procedures such as venipuncture or IV starts, which then is less time at home, more anxiety from the patient and family, and unhappy or distraught patients. These issues must all be carefully regarded to make sure this is in line with the end-of-life goals of care by the patient and family to avoid inferior quality of life, while continuing discussions on end-of-life care. The ethics of the child participating is an important consideration, as well as there can be therapeutic misconception in that the family perceives benefit (329). Sometimes parents choose to participate in a clinical study because they are not wanting to give up all treatment attempts, even though they are well informed through the extensive consent process that there is no proven benefit in most of the trials with phase 1 drugs. Families feel they need to make decisions quickly due to the pressure of very little remaining time with their child before they die. Parents are trying to meet their own internal definition of a good parent by choosing what they feel is the best option of a hope of cure despite acknowledging they understand the child has little chance of benefit. Parents also choose to participate in clinical trials to avoid any feelings of future regret of not doing enough after the child has died. In addition, the child or patient may participate for altruistic reasons in wanting to do their part in adding to research to help other children or families avoid their same outcome (330–333). Good communication is essential for these discussions, and the palliative care team is well equipped to help the primary oncologist and the family through the process of deciding to participate in a clinical trial.

Therapeutic Misconception

The therapeutic misconception occurs when a participant in research does not differentiate the purpose of the research study from his or her own clinical care (334). The risk of this is compounded in pediatric oncology, when the treating physician is frequently involved in research and when many treatment protocols are also research protocols. This is also a concern when patients enroll in phase 1 or phase 2 trials (325). However, absent intentional misleading from researchers, it is more likely that therapeutic optimism is occurring, in which a research subject hopes for therapeutic benefit from a trial, even if they understand that is not the primary purpose (334).

Disclosure

Early on, some parents do not want to tell the child about their cancer diagnosis. There may be a desire to protect the child from the negative emotional consequences of a diagnosis, a lack of knowledge about how to explain the diagnosis to their child, or an inaccurate assumption about the child's capability to understand his or her own illness. Even if they experience mood or behavior changes, overwhelmingly, children prefer to know about their diagnosis. They experience less psychological symptom burden if they are informed early about their diagnosis and are allowed open discussion.

This is increasingly true as children get older; over 80% of adolescents prefer to be involved in discussions about prognosis. Approximately half of adolescents want their parents to have a limited role in decision-making (335).

Futility

Concerns about futility are often raised when patients or families pursue aggressive medical interventions near the end of life. It is important to remember that generally (state law may vary), if a medical team truly agrees that an intervention has no chance of achieving the stated goal, they are not under any obligation to attempt such intervention. However, the much more common scenario is an intervention that has a very low chance of succeeding at the stated goal and will result in significant burdens and possible suffering. This scenario is more appropriately termed potentially inappropriate therapy and requires intensive communication and mediation to resolve (336). This process does not guarantee mutually satisfactory answers.

Pediatric Hospice and Concurrent Care

Just as with adults, children who have life-limiting terminal illness with ongoing decline with a projected lifespan of 6 months or less are eligible for hospice enrollment. The burden of choosing ongoing curative or life-prolonging treatment versus sole hospice care is often difficult for parents (337). Thus, in pediatrics, this had led to the recognition of the open access or concurrent model where hospice eligible pediatric patients can enroll in hospice and still receive life-prolonging treatment (338). Such a provision was signed into law and implemented under the passage of the Patient Protection Affordable Care Act (PPACA) in 2010 under section 2302 (Concurrent Care for Children) (338,339). Such provision requires any state Medicaid program or Child Health Insurance program to allow pediatric patients to remain eligible for hospice care while still receiving curative or life-prolong therapies if this is the goal of the family (338,339). This allows for ongoing and smoother transition of these patients and some would argue it promotes the well-being in vulnerable children and families and potentially help alleviate any inequities a child may experience at end-of-life regarding care (340).

End-of-Life Care

The death of a child is a traumatic, distressing, life-changing event for a family. Parents expect their children to grow up, living a full life. When this cycle is interrupted, it is life altering (341). How the health care team choreographs end-of-life care events can have a profound impact on how the family copes with this loss for life. Preparing for end of life can assist families to carry out their specific cultural and spiritual beliefs. Discussing end of life can be very difficult for families, children, and health care providers; however, not having these discussions can lead to poor psychological outcomes in parents and siblings (31,342).

Advance care planning conversations to facilitate decision-making should be initiated. Knowing what life-sustaining therapies the family and patient wish to have is helpful when planning for end-of-life care. Processes such as antibiotic therapy, artificial nutrition/hydration, organ donation, and respiratory support should be explored to uphold the family and patient goals (343). Physician orders for life-sustaining treatment (POLST) is available in several states, but its use varies. There are child- and adolescent-friendly resources, which are developmentally appropriate for these populations. Exploring advance directives using resources such as Voicing My Choices and My Wishes prior to the actively dying phase can be beneficial to a family and the child. Voicing My Choices is used for the adolescent and young adult population, and My Wishes is used for children. It can be implemented by all disciplines. Using these resources gives the family the opportunity to have open conversations with their children (344,345).

Preparing for where the patient and family hope for death to occur can assist clinicians in preparing for end-of-life care. Some families want their children to die at home, while others state that they feel more comfortable being in the hospital setting. If the hospital has a palliative care team, they can assist the family in navigating these choices. Not all cities have local hospices that are well prepared to care for children. There are cities that have a hospice house, which specifically care for children or hospice houses that feel quite comfortable in caring for them (346).

Having a knowledgeable palliative care social worker, case manager, or nurse coordinator may be helpful in choosing a hospice. These houses have open access to families and often times are set up like a home to make all family members feel more comfortable. Some hospitals have areas in the hospital that are set up specifically for end-of-life care. Other hospitals have carts in which supplies are kept so that a hospital room can be made more comfortable for a family needing end-of-life care. Knowing all the options so the family can make informed decisions is important.

Special attention should be paid to the family's culture, ethnicity, and religion surrounding the end of life. Some families have rituals that should be carried out. Asking the family if they have any

particular customs that they would like honored helps the family with their grief journey.

Incorporating the family's spiritual leader or the hospital chaplain can assist in fulfilling the families' customs.

The moment of death is extremely difficult for family members regardless of how long it has been expected. Even when families state that they are prepared, the clinicians should anticipate the unexpected. When the physician tells the family the time of death, the reality can be overwhelming to a family. Setting up a room for this time period is important. The family's safety should be assessed. For example, an elderly grandparent could be overcome with grief and fall to a hard floor.

Bereavement specialists can be extremely helpful to families. Getting them involved prior to the death of a child can assist in families in the future. Some local communities have bereavement programs that can assist all members of a family after a death has occurred.

The concept of a "good death" can mean many things to different people. In the palliative care world, it often means that the family had some type of preparation and that the child did not suffer. Some families would say a good death is in line with fighting until the end. Continued clinical assessment of the patient and family throughout the dying process can alert the health care team to any distress that the family may be feeling giving the team the opportunity to intervene as needed.

Managing distressing end-of-life symptoms can be difficult. Knowing what medications are available to the provider and planning for the unexpected is the key. Making sure that assurance is given to the family that everything will be done to keep their child comfortable is important. In a landmark study by Wolfe et al., it was found that the most commonly reported symptoms of children with oncologic diagnoses at end of life are pain, dyspnea, fatigue, poor appetite, nausea and vomiting, constipation, and diarrhea (347). When it comes to pain management in general, there are no ceiling doses for opioids at the end of life. Dosing is based on the patient's response to treatment. Terminal emergencies should also be planned for including hemorrhage, seizures, pneumothoraxes, airway obstruction, bowel obstruction, and delirium. Many hospitals have end-of-life care order sets, and these should be utilized when appropriate. Terminal sedation is a team decision, and all medical consultants should be included in the discussion. Terminal sedation is used when all medication management techniques are used without success, and the child must be sedated due to intractable suffering. Experts such as palliative care, anesthesia, and the hematology/oncology team or any other providers involved in the child's care should be present to be sure all therapies have been maximized. Usually terminal sedation is not needed if symptom management is aggressive. When having these discussions, it is wise to make sure families understand that this concept is different from euthanasia. If a family is asking about assisted suicide, or requesting that we hasten death, an exploration of the families suffering and wishes should be explored. If there is no resolution, an ethics consult should be considered (343,348).

Memory making and legacy building may be activities that the family and patient wish to create. Activities such as hand molds, hand prints, professional photographs, and memory boxes can provide the family with tangible memories for years to come (349). Some children wish to write letters or make decisions regarding who will receive their belongings when they die.

Staff can benefit from debriefing after the death of child. This may already be a routine event for some hospitals, and if not can be considered. This may prevent burn out of staff and increase resiliency. Often times, oncology patients have been under the care of an oncological team for a long period of time before death occurs. Sending condolence cards and attending funerals can benefit not only providers but families as well (350).

End-of-life care requires a well-thought-out plan with deliberate attention paid to physical, psychosocial, emotional, and spiritual components. If access to a palliative care team or community hospice is not available, a team of professionals well educated in end-of-life care should be consulted with for end-of-life care. A multidisciplinary approach including medical and psychosocial team members should be incorporated into the plan of care with the patient and family.

Withdrawal of Life-Sustaining Therapies

Issues such as code status and withholding or withdrawing life-sustaining therapies and/or artificial hydration and nutrition are, in principle, similar to adults. If the parents, children (if able), and treatment team are in agreement, this is not a legally or ethically challenging matter. These decisions are emotionally fraught and should be handled with compassion.

Toolkits exist for pediatric-specific end-of-life decision-making. The Conversation Project, Voicing My Choices (teenagers), and My Wishes (school-age children) are some examples of commonly used products that allow children to plan their end-of-life care and legacy.

Physician aid in dying (previously known as physician-assisted suicide) is legal in some states and the District of Columbia in the United States and some countries throughout the world; however, in the United States, this remains illegal for patients under the age of 18 (351).

Grief and Bereavement

Even though pediatric cancer cure rates continue to increase, there are children who will not be cured (352). Grief can start at the moment of diagnosis and can last through the trajectory of an illness. When one hears grief, it is usually thought of as in reference to the death of a loved one. One of the deepest sorrows known by parent report is the death of their child. It is unreasonable to ever expect that a parent will get over the death of their child. It is a lifelong process in which the parents have to learn how to cope. Grief can manifest as shock, disbelief, numbness, and denial. Studies have shown that regardless of the amount of time that has passed since the death of their child, symptoms such as depression, insomnia, and grief persist. The death of a child is an event that is seen as out of the natural order of life (341,353). How professionals assist parents through this process will determine the lifetime trajectory of coping for the family. Breaking bad news in an empathetic manner is associated with lower levels of grief in the long term. Siblings should also receive appropriate support throughout the journey. Siblings who did not receive good communication, had poor preparation for their sibling's death, or did not have a chance to say goodbye reported that they tended to have higher distress (31).

Health care professionals can play a very significant role in the healing process of families. In a study by Snaman et al., it was found that four principles were noted by families when discussing their bereavement period. They noted how important it was to have ongoing good relationships with the health care team, the importance of quality communication, the effect of negative experiences, and the importance of the hospitals role in the grief journey (354).

Writing condolence cards with fond memories, reaching out via telephone, or making home visits are all ways to communicate with families after a death (355). Health care providers have also reported that they have benefited from reaching out to families after the death of their patient.

When parents suffer the loss of a child, they also suffer the loss of the health care team that once cared for them and their child. Bereaved parents identified their health care team as an integral part of their grief journey. Bereaved parents have suggested some of the following guidelines to assist health care teams and bereaved parents: clear honest communication provided in a timely manner, incorporating goals of care and shared decision-making, involving parents in the development of skills training for health care professionals, allowing families to continue legacy building and memory making after the death of their child, and supporting ongoing relationships with provider teams (354).

Many communities offer bereavement support to families. Local hospices host programs and grief workshops for families. Bereavement support groups such as Compassionate Friends have online support and host support in their communities. They can be found at https://www.compassionate-friends.org (356).

Health care systems should strongly consider implementing bereavement programs as research is showing the long-term benefits to families (357).

Survivorship

Thanks to continued advances in cancer screening and treatment, survival of childhood cancer continues to increase. Unfortunately, we continue to deal with the late and long-term effects of a cure. Late effects occur months or years after treatment for cancer has ended. Long-term effects are effects from treatment that occur during treatment and extend beyond treatment (358). Secondary malignancies, infertility, cardiovascular disease, and endocrine issues continue to generate medical complexities for survivors for years to come. From a psychological perspective, survivors are at risk for posttraumatic stress symptoms, which are associated with depression, decreased quality of life, and overall decreased social abilities (359). Fear of relapse remains ever present for survivors of any life-threatening disease process. Preparing our survivors for what lies ahead not only from a medical perspective but also from a psychological perspective is necessary. The Institute of Medicine recommends that all patients at the end of therapy receive a treatment summary and survivorship plan. This plan should include a plan of follow-up care that is recommended as well as treatment-related effects that should be monitored (360). Childhood cancer survivors need ongoing comprehensive care to monitor and treat the late effects that may be associated with their history of disease. Many parents have also noted that they would benefit from long-term support after their child has entered into survivorship (361).

Children's Oncology Group has been collecting data on their enrolled patients for years. In 2002, COG started developing risk-based, exposure-related recommendations for late effects that occurred due to treatment for their childhood cancer. The comprehensive guidelines they developed is called *Children's Oncology Group Long Term Follow-up Guidelines for Survivors of Childhood, Adolescent and Young Adult Cancers (COG LTFU Guidelines)* (362).

It can be found at http://www.survivorship-guidelines.org/. Information on the Web site is useful for providers and survivors. It was designed to standardize follow-up care, improve survivors' quality of life, and provide guidance to health care provider teams. The role of this guideline is to assist primary care providers in assisting childhood cancer survivors with long-term medical care. As children age out of the pediatrician's care, this care plan will assist the next physician that cares for the survivor. Two-way communication between the generalist and specialist will optimize follow-up care for the survivor (363). Although it is ultimately the patient's responsibility to seek out appropriate health care for themselves after receiving cancer treatment, the oncology team and primary care physicians should partner to ensure success for the patient upon transitioning to achieve optimal long-term health.

SELF-CARE FOR PROVIDERS

"You have to take care of yourself before you take care of anyone else" is a phrase we often tell parents; however, it also rings true to the care we provide ourselves as clinicians. If we do not fill up our cup often enough, our resiliency will diminish and can lead to burnout. Burnout is described as a "syndrome characterized by emotional exhaustion, depersonalization, and low sense of accomplishment" (364). The statistics are staggering. Fifty-four percent of doctors reported at least one symptom of burnout in a recent study (365). Specifically, in pediatric oncology, 38% had high levels of burnout with 72% reporting moderate levels of burnout. The demographics are somewhat uncertain as some studies show that younger physicians are more prone to burnout, while others state that it happens in midcareer (366). Taking care of patients with life-threatening diagnoses can take an emotional toll on all those involved. Stresses such as delivering bad news, making treatment recommendations, and assisting patients with their suffering can all be very taxing. It is important that we perform self-care for ourselves and encourage our teams to do self-care as well.

Recognizing signs of burnout in ourselves, colleagues, and in our teams is important. Signs such irritability, social withdrawal, difficulty with concentration, sleep issues, physical and emotional fatigue, as well as frequent illnesses can all be individual signs of burnout. Team symptoms include low morale, high turnover, and staff conflicts (367).

Although there is no recipe that definitively prevents burnout, we know that doing things that we enjoy on a day-to-day basis can be beneficial.

Self-care is an individual process that must be cultivated by the person. Some ideas that have helped others in providing their own self-care are as follows; creating healthy lifestyles by obtaining adequate sleep, eating nutritious foods and getting regular exercise, following routine meditation practice, taking regular vacations, and maintaining healthy relationships. On a day-to-day basis, finding fulfillment outside of work can be beneficial. Activities such as volunteering, taking a class, or learning how to become mindful can be fulfilling. When at work, activities such as taking time to sit and eat lunch, getting a cup of coffee and chatting with a colleague, or pausing and taking a deep breath before going into a patient room can all be helpful. When you leave work at the end of the day, try to perform a ritual such as hanging up your stethoscope or white coat, as to emulate leaving work at work. Realizing it is easier said than done, try to leave work at work. Although more research is needed in the field, self-care has the ability to decrease the risk of burnout and promote well-being when intentionally practiced. When we practice self-care, we are not only taking care of ourselves, we are modeling behavior for the next generation of physicians (368).

QUALITY IMPROVEMENT

As the utilization of palliative care services in pediatric oncology increases, it is important to evaluate the quality of the services and implement strategies to optimize integration of the primary oncology team and the palliative care team. Palliative care attempts to reduce suffering and alleviate symptoms in many settings including the hospital, outpatient clinic, and the home, which leads to challenges in evaluating the current state and quality of services and even further challenges in engaging new practices. There are many studies that demonstrate the impact of palliative care such as decreasing hospital length of stay and improved quality of life for those who receive palliative services compared to those who do not (369). Several aspects of the palliative care services should be considered a quality perspective including:

- Full spectrum of interdisciplinary care team membership and structure
- Availability of palliative care team and response to initial consults and follow-up
- Triggers to consult palliative care
- Communication with primary oncology team
- Skill level of palliative care team including ongoing continuing education
- Appropriate information to families regarding benefits of palliative care and removing barriers of fear and resistance

The skill level of the palliative care team is particularly important when consulting on oncology patients. The ages of the children can range from neonates, to school-age children, to adolescents, to young adults, each with their own developmental level of processing their diagnosis and prognosis. Competency expectations for palliative care team members are required for a wide variety of conditions, particularly within oncology. The complexity of the patient's symptom management is challenging in the various ages due to drug dosing and formulation, and therefore, consideration must be given to avoid errors (337). Ideally, pediatric palliative care would be standardized in a way that directs core competencies of team members with practice guidelines and a system of evaluating the efficacy, safety, and quality. Practice guidelines would be across various systems such as outpatient oncology clinic, inpatient cancer ward, hospice settings, and the home at various times from cancer diagnosis to end of life (370). One of the methods of evaluating efficacy is from parent perceptions such as parents' feeling supported by the palliative care team and understanding the value of the care they receive from the team through the full journey of the disease course (371). One of the most important areas to evaluate regarding the quality of care is the quality of life of the patient. Many quality of life measures exist in the literature, and it is important to use a tool that takes into account all aspects of a child's condition that may impact the quality of life (372). The team should demonstrate benefit of services provided by evaluating and measuring performance (373). Implementation of quality improvement measures is essential for quality palliative care services for pediatric oncology patients.

REFERENCES

1. Thrane SE, Maurer SH, Cohen SM, May C, Sereika SM. Pediatric palliative care: a five-year retrospective chart review study. *J Palliat Med.* 2017;20(10):1104-1111.
2. Moody K, Siegel L, Scharbach K, Cunningham L, Cantor RM. Pediatric palliative care. *Prim Care.* 2011;38(2):327-361, ix.
3. American Academy of Pediatrics. Committee on Bioethics and Committee on Hospital Care. Palliative care for children. *Pediatrics.* 2000;106(2 Pt 1):351-357.
4. Newton K, Sebbens D. The impact of provider education on pediatric palliative care referral. *J Pediatr Health Care.* 2020;34(2):99-108.
5. Heron M. Deaths: leading causes for 2015. *Natl Vital Stat Reports.* 2017;66(5):1-76.
6. Cheng BT, Wangmo T. Palliative care utilization in hospitalized children with cancer. *Pediatr Blood Cancer.* 2020;67:e28013.
7. Section on Hospice and Palliative Medicine and Committee on Hospital Care. Pediatric palliative care and hospice care commitments, guidelines, and recommendations. *Pediatrics.* 2013;132(5):966-972.

8. Bates AT, Kearney JA. Understanding death with limited experience in life: dying children's and adolescents' understanding of their own terminal illness and death. *Curr Opin Support Palliat Care*. 2015;9(1):40-45.

9. Harrison J, Evan E, Hughes A, Yazdani S, Federman M, Harrison R. Understanding communication among health care professionals regarding death and dying in pediatrics. *Palliat Support Care*. 2014;12(5):387-392.

10. Buchwald D, Delmar C, Schantz-Laursen B. How children handle life when their mother or father is seriously ill and dying. *Scand J Caring Sci*. 2012;26(2):228-235.

11. Keeley MP, Generous MA. Advice from children and adolescents on final conversations with dying loved ones. *Death Stud*. 2014;38(1-5):308-314.

12. Nordmark-Lindberg I, Lindberg T. A child's experience of imminent death. *Acta Paediatr Scand*. 1979;68(5):645-648.

13. Cepuch G, Kruszecka-Krowka A. Child's dignity in suffering and death. *Przegl Lek*. 2017;74(1):21-24.

14. Longbottom S, Slaughter V. Sources of children's knowledge about death and dying. *Philos Trans R Soc Lond B Biol Sci*. 2018;373(1754).

15. Ullrich C, Duncan J, Joselow M, Wolfe J. Pediatric palliative care. In: Kliegman RM, St Geme JW, Blum NJ, Shah SS, Tasker RC, Wilson KM, eds. *Nelson Textbook of Pediatrics*. 20th ed. Philadelphia, PA: Elsevier; 2015:256-268.

16. Hinds PS, Oakes LL, Hicks J, et al. Parent-clinician communication intervention during end-of-life decision making for children with incurable cancer. *J Palliat Med*. 2012;15(8):916-922.

17. Ekberg S, Bradford N, Herbert A, Danby S, Yates P. Healthcare users' experiences of communicating with healthcare professionals about children who have life-limiting conditions: a qualitative systematic review protocol. *JBI Database Syst Rev Implement Rep*. 2015;13(11):33-42.

18. Beale EA, Baile WF, Aaron J. Silence is not golden: communicating with children dying from cancer. *J Clin Oncol*. 2005;23(15):3629-3631.

19. Lemus-Riscanevo P, Carreno-Moreno S, Arias-Rojas M. Conspiracy of silence in palliative care: a concept analysis. *Indian J Palliat Care*. 2019;25(1):24-29.

20. Lykke C, Ekholm O, Schmiegelow K, Olsen M, Sjogren P. End-of-life communication: a nationwide study of bereaved parents' perceptions. *BMJ Support Palliat Care*. 2019. doi: 10.1136/bmjspcare-2018-001709.

21. Meert KL, Eggly S, Pollack M, et al. Parents' perspectives on physician-parent communication near the time of a child's death in the pediatric intensive care unit. *Pediatr Crit Care Med*. 2008;9(1):2-7.

22. Wolfe J, Klar N, Grier HE, et al. Understanding of prognosis among parents of children who died of cancer: impact on treatment goals and integration of palliative care. *JAMA*. 2000;284(19):2469-2475.

23. Baker JN, Hinds PS, Spunt SL, et al. Integration of palliative care practices into the ongoing care of children with cancer: individualized care planning and coordination. *Pediatr Clin North Am*. 2008;55(1):223-250, xii.

24. Waldman ED, Levine JM. The day two talk: early integration of palliative care principles in pediatric oncology. *J Clin Oncol*. 2016;34(34):4068-4070.

25. Promoting the well-being of children whose parents are gay or lesbian. *Pediatrics*. 2013;131(4):827-830.

26. Rasmussen S, Water T, Dickinson A. Children's perspectives in family-centred hospital care. *Contemp Nurse*. 2017;53(4):445-455.

27. Smith J, Swallow V, Coyne I. Involving parents in managing their child's long-term condition-a concept synthesis of family-centered care and partnership-in-care. *J Pediatr Nurs*. 2015;30(1):143-159.

28. Jones B, Gilmer MJ, Paker-Raley J, Dokken D, Freyer D, Greenberg N. Parent and sibling relationships and the family experience. In: Wolfe J, Hinds P, Sourkes B, eds. *Textbook of Interdisciplinary Pediatric Palliative Care*. Philadelphia, PA: Elsevier Saunders; 2011: 135-143.

29. Ho K, Shaul RZ, Chapman LA, Ford-Jones EL. Standard of care in pediatrics: integrating family-centred care and social determinants of health. *Healthc Q*. 2016;19(1):55-60.

30. McKay S, Parente V. Health disparities in the hospitalized child. *Hosp Pediatr*. 2019;9(5):317-325.

31. Rosenberg AR, Postier A, Osenga K, et al. Long-term psychosocial outcomes among bereaved siblings of children with cancer. *J Pain Symptom Manage*. 2015;49(1):55-65.

32. Sood AB, Razdan A, Weller EB, Weller RA. Children's reactions to parental and sibling death. *Curr Psychiatry Rep*. 2006;8(2):115-120.

33. Charlebois S, Bouchard L. "The worst experience": the experience of grandparents who have a grandchild with cancer. *Can Oncol Nurs J* 2007;17(1):26-36.

34. Moules NJ, Laing CM, McCaffrey G, Tapp DM, Strother D. Grandparents' experiences of childhood cancer, part 1: doubled and silenced. *J Pediatr Oncol Nurs*. 2012;29(3):119-132.

35. Moules NJ, McCaffrey G, Laing CM, Tapp DM, Strother D. Grandparents' experiences of childhood cancer, part 2: the need for support. *J Pediatr Oncol Nurs*. 2012;29(3):133-140.

36. Brown RT, Wiener L, Kupst MJ, et al. Single parents of children with chronic illness: an understudied phenomenon. *J Pediatr Psychol*. 2008;33(4):408-421.

37. Crespo C, Santos S, Tavares A, Salvador A. "Care that matters": family-centered care, caregiving burden, and adaptation in parents of children with cancer. *Fam Syst Health*. 2016;34(1):31-40.

38. Nicholas DB, Beaune L, Barrera M, Blumberg J, Belletrutti M. Examining the experiences of fathers of children with a life-limiting illness. *J Soc Work End Life Palliat Care*. 2016;12(1-2):126-144.

39. Jones BL, Contro N, Koch KD. The duty of the physician to care for the family in pediatric palliative care: context, communication, and caring. *Pediatrics*. 2014;133(suppl 1):S8-S15.

40. Postier A, Catrine K, Remke S. Interdisciplinary pediatric palliative care team involvement in compassionate extubation at home: from shared decision-making to bereavement. *Children (Basel)*. 2018;5(3):37.

41. Kaye EC, Rubenstein J, Levine D, Baker JN, Dabbs D, Friebert SE. Pediatric palliative care in the community. *CA Cancer J Clin*. 2015;65(4):316-333.

42. Shafto K, Gouda S, Catrine K, Brown ML. Integrative approaches in pediatric palliative care. *Children (Basel)*. 2018;5(6):75.

43. October TW, Hinds PS, Wang J, Dizon ZB, Cheng YI, Roter DL. Parent satisfaction with communication is associated with physician's patient-centered communication patterns during family conferences. *Pediatr Crit Care Med*. 2016;17(6):490-497.

44. Wiener L, Reader S, Anne K. Special considerations in working with families. In: Wiener L, Pao M, Kazak A, Kupst MJ, Patenaude A, Arceci R, eds. *Pediatric Psycho-Oncology: A Quick Reference on the Psychosocial Dimensions of Cancer Symptom Management*. 2nd ed. New York, NY: Oxford University Press; 2015:271-278.

45. Szilagyi M. The pediatrician and the child in foster care. *Pediatr Rev*. 1998;19(2):39-50.

46. McDavid LM. Foster care and child health. *Pediatr Clin North Am*. 2015;62(5):1329-1348.

47. Wang C, Edelstein SB, Waldinger L, Lee CM, Bath E. Care of the foster child: a primer for the pediatrician. *Adv Pediatr*. 2011;58(1):87-111.

48. Perrin EC, Siegel BS. Promoting the well-being of children whose parents are gay or lesbian. *Pediatrics*. 2013;131(4):e1374-e1383.

49. Keele L, Keenan HT, Bratton SL. The effect of palliative care team design on referrals to pediatric palliative care. *J Palliat Med*. 2016;19(3):286-291.

50. Lutmer JE, Humphrey L, Kempton TM, Moore-Clingenpeel M, Ayad O. Screening criteria improve access to palliative care in the PICU. *Pediatr Crit Care Med*. 2016;17(8):e335-e342.

51. Nelson JE, Curtis JR, Mulkerin C, et al. Choosing and using screening criteria for palliative care consultation in the ICU: a report from the Improving Palliative Care in the ICU (IPAL-ICU) Advisory Board. *Crit Care Med*. 2013;41(10):2318-2327.

52. Feudtner C, Womer J, Augustin R, et al. Pediatric palliative care programs in children's hospitals: a cross-sectional national survey. *Pediatrics*. 2013;132(6):1063-1070.

53. Smith G, Bernacki R, Block SD. The role of palliative care in population management and accountable care organizations. *J Palliat Med*. 2015;18(6):486-494.

54. O'Quinn LP, Giambra BK. Evidence of improved quality of life with pediatric palliative care. *Pediatr Nurs*. 2014;40(6):284-288, 296.

55. Mack JW, Hilden JM, Watterson J, et al. Parent and physician perspectives on quality of care at the end of life in children with cancer. *J Clin Oncol*. 2005;23(36):9155-9161.

56. Rosenberg AR, Orellana L, Kang TI, et al. Differences in parent-provider concordance regarding prognosis and goals of care among children with advanced cancer. *J Clin Oncol*. 2014;32(27):3005-3011.

57. Smith TJ, Dow LA, Virago E, Khatcheressian J, Lyckholm LJ, Matsuyama R. Giving honest information to patients with advanced cancer maintains hope. *Oncology (Williston Park)*. 2010;24(6):521-525.

58. Orloff S. Pediatric hospice and palliative care: the invaluable role of the social work. In: Altilio T, Green-Otis S, eds. *Oxford Textbook of Palliative Social Work*. New York, NY: Oxford University Press; 2011:79-86.

59. Bartell AS, Kissane DW. Issues in pediatric palliative care: understanding families. *J Palliat Care*. 2005;21(3):165-172.

60. Jones BL. Pediatric palliative and end-of-life care: the role of social work in pediatric oncology. *J Soc Work End Life Palliat Care*. 2005;1(4):35-61.

61. Jones BL. Companionship, control, and compassion: a social work perspective on the needs of children with cancer and their families at the end of life. *J Palliat Med*. 2006;9(3):774-788.

62. Edlynn E, Kaur H. The role of psychology in pediatric palliative care. *J Palliat Med*. 2016;19(7):760-762.

63. Payne S, Haines R. Doing our bit to ease the pain: the potential contribution of psychology to palliative care. *Psychologist*. 2002;15(11):564-567.

64. Freyer DR, Kuperberg A, Sterken DJ, Pastyrnak SL, Hudson D, Richards T. Multidisciplinary care of the dying adolescent. *Child Adolesc Psychiatr Clin N Am*. 2006;15(3):693-715.

65. Basak RB, Momaya R, Guo J, Rathi P. Role of child life specialists in pediatric palliative care. *J Pain Symptom Manage*. 2019;58(4):735-737.

66. Pinkerton R, Donovan L, Herbert A. Palliative care in adolescents and young adults with cancer—why do adolescents need special attention? *Cancer J*. 2018;24(6):336-341.

67. Legett SM. In praise of child life. *J Palliat Med*. 2014;17(11):1284.

68. Boles J, Daniels S. Researching the experiences of children with cancer: considerations for practice. *Children (Basel)*. 2019;6(8):93.

69. Lovgren M, Kreicbergs U, Udo C. Family talk intervention in paediatric oncology: a pilot study protocol. *BMJ Paediatr Open*. 2019;3(1):e000417.

70. Newton AS, Wolgemuth A, Gallivan J, Wrightson D. Providing support to siblings of hospitalised children. *J Paediatr Child Health*. 2010;46(3):72-75.

71. Lion AH, Skiles JL, Watson BN, Young JD, Torke AM. Chaplain care in pediatric oncology: insight for interprofessional collaboration. *Pediatr Blood Cancer*. 2019;66(9):e27971.

72. Robert R, Stavinoha P, Jones BL, et al. Spiritual assessment and spiritual care offerings as a standard of care in pediatric oncology: a recommendation informed by a systematic review of the literature. *Pediatr Blood Cancer*. 2019;66(9):e27764.

73. Sinclair S, Chochinov HM. The role of chaplains within oncology interdisciplinary teams. *Curr Opin Support Palliat Care*. 2012;6(2):259-268.

74. El Nawawi NM, Balboni MJ, Balboni TA. Palliative care and spiritual care: the crucial role of spiritual care in the care of patients with advanced illness. *Curr Opin Support Palliat Care*. 2012;6(2):269-274.

75. Pravin RR, Enrica TEK, Moy TA. The portrait of a dying child. *Indian J Palliat Care* 2019;25:156-160.

76. Proserpio T, Pagani Bagliacca E, Sironi G, et al. Spirituality and sustaining hope in adolescents with cancer: the patients' view. *J Adolesc Young Adult Oncol*. 2020;9(1):36-40.

77. Berger JT. Moral distress in medical education and training. *J Gen Intern Med*. 2014;29(2):395-398.

78. Noguera A, Robledano R, Garralda E. Palliative care teaching shapes medical undergraduate students' professional development: a scoping review. *Curr Opin Support Palliat Care*. 2018;12(4):495-503.

79. Stepanyan KD, Weiss TE, Pessegueiro AM, Pietras CJ. Lessons from the development and implementation of a palliative care elective for fourth-year medical students: a pilot study. *Am J Hosp Palliat Care*. 2019;37(1):1049909119872976.

80. Weaver MS, Wichman C. Implementation of a competency-based, interdisciplinary pediatric palliative care curriculum using content and format preferred by pediatric residents. *Children (Basel)*. 2018;5(12):156.

81. Bar-Sela G, Mitnik I, Zalman D, et al. Medical students' attitudes towards participating in a palliative medicine course: a new specialty in Israel. *Palliat Support Care*. 2018;16(5):528-533.

82. Goldberg GR, Weiner J, Fornari A, Pearlman RE, Farina GA. Incorporation of an interprofessional palliative care-ethics experience into a required critical care acting internship. *MedEdPORTAL*. 2018;14:10760.

83. Mutto EM, Bunge S, Vignaroli E, Bertolino M, Villar MJ, Wenk R. Medical students' palliative care education in a Latin American university: a three-year experience at Austral University in Buenos Aires, Argentina. *J Palliat Med*. 2014;17(10):1137-1142.

84. Raoof M, O'Neill L, Neumayer L, Fain M, Krouse R. Prospective evaluation of surgical palliative care immersion training for general surgery residents. *Am J Surg*. 2017;214(2):378-383.

85. Saylor J, Vernoony S, Selekman J, Cowperthwait A. Interprofessional education using a palliative care simulation. *Nurse Educ*. 2016;41(3):125-129.

86. Sinha P, Murphy SP, Becker CM, et al. A novel inter-professional approach to end-of-life care education: a pilot study. *J Interprof Care*. 2015;29(6):643-645.

87. Gadoud A, Lu WH, Strano-Paul L, Lane S, Boland JW. A pilot study of interprofessional palliative care education of medical students in the UK and USA. *BMJ Support Palliat Care*. 2018;8(1):67-72.

88. Thomas R, Phillips M, Hamilton RJ. Pain management in the pediatric palliative care population. *J Nurs Scholarsh*. 2018;50(4):375-382.

89. Shaw TM. Pediatric palliative pain and symptom management. *Pediatr Ann*. 2012;41(8):329-334.

90. Norris S, Minkowitz S, Scharbach K. Pediatric palliative care. *Prim Care*. 2019;46(3):461-473.

91. WHO. Palliative Care. https://nam02.safelinks.protection.outlook.com/?url=https%3A%2F%2Fwww.who.int%2Fhealth-topics%2Fpalliative-care&data=04%7C01%7Cstacie.stapleton%40jhmi.edu%7Caadfb11a740f47bb345708d8915dca6a%7C9fa4f438b1e6473b803f86f8aedf0dec%7C0%7C0%7C637419179307713810%7CUnknown%7CTWFpbGZsb3d8eyJW IjoiMC4wLjAwMDAiLCJQIjoiV2luMzIiLCJBTiI6Ik1haWwiLCJXVCI6Mn0%3D%7C1000&sdata=yG3JBSdD%2FnTwu2HzAj1k2kt8ydcsRPBDEnSYUx359zQ%3D&reserved=0" https://www.who.int/health-topics/palliative-care.

92. WHO. Web statement on pain management guidance. https://www.who.int/medicines/areas/quality_safety/guide_perspainchild/en/. Accessed.

93. Saul R, Peters J, Bruce E. Assessing acute and chronic pain in children and young people. *Nurs Stand*. 2016;31(10):51-63.

94. Perquin CW, Hazebroek-Kampschreur AA, Hunfeld JA, et al. Pain in children and adolescents: a common experience. *Pain*. 2000;87(1):51-58.

95. Cooper TE, Fisher E, Gray AL, et al. Opioids for chronic non-cancer pain in children and adolescents. *Cochrane Database Syst Rev*. 2017;(7):Cd012538.

96. Pincus T, Noel M, Jordan A, Serbic D. Perceived diagnostic uncertainty in pediatric chronic pain. *Pain*. 2018;159(7):1198-1201.

97. Keogh E, Eccleston C. Sex differences in adolescent chronic pain and pain-related coping. *Pain*. 2006;123(3):275-284.

98. Boerner KE, Eccleston C, Chambers CT, et al. Sex differences in the efficacy of psychological therapies for the management of chronic and recurrent pain in children and adolescents: a systematic review and meta-analysis. *Pain*. 2017;258(4):569-582.

99. Miller MM, Meints SM, Hirsh AT. Catastrophizing, pain, and functional outcomes for children with chronic pain: a meta-analytic review. *Pain*. 2018;159(12):2442-2460.

100. Eccleston C, Clinch J. Adolescent chronic pain and disability: a review of the current evidence in assessment and treatment. *Paediatr Child Health*. 2007;12(2):117-120.

101. Logan DE, Simons LE, Kaczynski KJ. School functioning in adolescents with chronic pain: the role of depressive symptoms in school impairment. *J Pediatr Psychol*. 2009;34(8):882-892.

102. Landry BW, Fischer PR, Driscoll SW, et al. Managing chronic pain in children and adolescents: a clinical review. *PM R*. 2015;7(11 suppl):S295-S315.

103. Weiss JE, Stinson JN. Pediatric pain syndromes and noninflammatory musculoskeletal pain. *Pediatr Clin North Am*. 2018;65(4):801-826.

104. Di Lorenzo C, Colletti RB, Lehmann HP, et al. Chronic abdominal pain in children: a clinical report of the American Academy of Pediatrics and the North American Society for Pediatric Gastroenterology, Hepatology and Nutrition. *J Pediatr Gastroenterol Nutr*. 2005;40(3):245-248.

105. Di Lorenzo C, Colletti RB, Lehmann HP, et al. Chronic abdominal pain in children: a technical report of the American Academy of Pediatrics and the North American Society for Pediatric Gastroenterology, Hepatology and Nutrition. *J Pediatr Gastroenterol Nutr*. 2005;40(3):249-261.

106. Draheim N, Ebinger F, Schnobel-Muller E, Wolf B, Hauser W. [Definition, diagnostics and therapy of chronic widespread pain and the (so-called) fibromyalgia syndrome in children and adolescents: updated guidelines 2017]. *Schmerz*. 2017;31(3):296-307.

107. Manworren RC, Stinson J. Pediatric pain measurement, assessment, and evaluation. *Semin Pediatr Neurol*. 2016;23(3):189-200.

108. Birnie KA, Hundert AS, Lalloo C, Nguyen C, Stinson JN. Recommendations for selection of self-report pain intensity measures in children and adolescents: a systematic review and quality assessment of measurement properties. *Pain*. 2019;160(1):5-18.

109. Friedrichsdorf SJ. Multimodal pediatric pain management (part 2). *Pain Manage*. 2017;7(3):161-166.

110. Chen L, Michalsen A. Management of chronic pain using complementary and integrative medicine. *Br Med J*. 2017;357:j1284.

111. Fisher E, Law E, Dudeney J, Eccleston C, Palermo TM. Psychological therapies (remotely delivered) for the management of chronic and recurrent pain in children and adolescents. *Cochrane Database Syst Rev*. 2019;(4):Cd011118.

112. Hauer J. Identifying and managing sources of pain and distress in children with neurological impairment. *Pediatr Ann*. 2010;39(4):198-205; quiz 232-194.

113. Hauer J, Houtrow AJ. Pain assessment and treatment in children with significant impairment of the central nervous system. *Pediatrics*. 2017;139(6):e20171002.

114. Valkenburg AJ, de Leeuw TG, van Dijk M, Tibboel D. Pain in intellectually disabled children: towards evidence-based pharmacotherapy? *Paediatr Drugs*. 2015;17(5):339-348.

115. Ostojic K, Paget SP, Morrow AM. Management of pain in children and adolescents with cerebral palsy: a systematic review. *Dev Med Child Neurol*. 2019;61(3):315-321.

116. Howard RF, Wiener S, Walker SM. Neuropathic pain in children. *Arch Dis Child*. 2014;99(1):84-89.

117. Hyde C, Price J, Nicholl H. Neuropathic pain management in children. *Int J Palliat Nurs*. 2012;18(10):476-478,480-472.

118. Lavoie Smith EM, Li L, Hutchinson RJ, et al. Measuring vincristine-induced peripheral neuropathy in children with acute lymphoblastic leukemia. *Cancer Nurs*. 2013;36(5):E49-E60.

119. Sands S, Ladas EJ, Kelly KM, et al. Glutamine for the treatment of vincristine-induced neuropathy in children and adolescents with cancer. *Support Care Cancer*. 2017;25(3):701-708.

120. Morgan KJ, Anghelescu DL. A review of adult and pediatric neuropathic pain assessment tools. *Clin J Pain*. 2017;33(9):844-852.

121. Brown S, Johnston B, Amaria K, et al. A randomized controlled trial of amitriptyline versus gabapentin for complex regional pain syndrome type I and neuropathic pain in children. *Scand J Pain*. 2016;13:156-163.

122. Cooper TE, Heathcote LC, Clinch J, et al. Antidepressants for chronic non-cancer pain in children and adolescents. *Cochrane Database Syst Rev*. 2017;(8):Cd012535.

123. de Leeuw TG, Mangiarini L, Lundin R, et al. Gabapentin as add-on to morphine for severe neuropathic or mixed pain in children from age 3 months to 18 years—evaluation of the safety, pharmacokinetics, and efficacy of a new gabapentin liquid formulation: study protocol for a randomized controlled trial. *Trials.* 2019;20(1):49.

124. Hall GC, Carroll D, Parry D, McQuay HJ. Epidemiology and treatment of neuropathic pain: the UK primary care perspective. *Pain.* 2006;122(1-2):156-162.

125. Orellana Silva M, Yanez V, Hidalgo G, Valenzuela F, Saavedra R. 5% lidocaine medicated plaster use in children with neuropathic pain from burn sequelae. *Pain Med.* 2013;14(3):422-429.

126. Casanova-Garcia C, Lerma Lara S, Perez Ruiz M, Ruano Dominguez D, Santana Sosa E. Non-pharmacological treatment for neuropathic pain in children with cancer. *Med Hypotheses.* 2015;85(6):791-797.

127. Ullrich CK, Mayer OH. Assessment and management of fatigue and dyspnea in pediatric palliative care. *Pediatr Clin North Am.* 2007;54(5):735-756, xi.

128. Berger AM, Mooney K, Alvarez-Perez A, et al. Cancer-related fatigue, Version 2.2015. *J Natl Compr Canc Netw.* 2015;13(8):1012-1039.

129. Wolfe J, Orellana L, Ullrich C, et al. Symptoms and distress in children with advanced cancer: prospective patient-reported outcomes from the PediQUEST study. *J Clin Oncol.* 2015;33(17):1928-1935.

130. Hooke MC, Rodgers C, Taylor O, et al. Physical activity, the childhood cancer symptom cluster-leukemia, and cognitive function: a longitudinal mediation analysis. *Cancer Nurs.* 2018;41(6):434-440.

131. Lopes-Junior LC, Bomfim EO, Nascimento LC, Nunes MD, Pereira-da-Silva G, Lima RA. Non-pharmacological interventions to manage fatigue and psychological stress in children and adolescents with cancer: an integrative review. *Eur J Cancer Care (Engl).* 2016;25(6):921-935.

132. Nunes MDR, Bomfim E, Olson K, et al. Interventions minimizing fatigue in children/adolescents with cancer: an integrative review. *J Child Health Care.* 2018;22(2):186-204.

133. Ye ZJ, Zhang Z, Liang MZ, et al. Symptoms and management of children with incurable cancer in mainland China. *Eur J Oncol Nurs.* 2019;38:42-49.

134. Skeens MA, Cullen P, Stanek J, Hockenberry M. Perspectives of childhood cancer symptom-related distress: results of the state of the science survey. *J Pediatr Oncol Nurs.* 2019;36(4):287-293.

135. Antill KT. Childhood cancer-related fatigue and day-to-day quality of life. *J Pediatr Oncol Nurs.* 2019;36(2):74-85.

136. Rodgers CC, Hooke MC, Taylor OA, et al. Childhood cancer symptom cluster: leukemia and health-related quality of life. *Oncol Nurs Forum.* 2019;46(2):228-237.

137. Pan HT, Wu LM, Wen SH. Quality of life and its predictors among children and adolescents with cancer. *Cancer Nurs.* 2017;40(5):343-351.

138. Spathis A, Hatcher H, Booth S, et al. Cancer-related fatigue in adolescents and young adults after cancer treatment: persistent and poorly managed. *J Adolesc Young Adult Oncol.* 2017;6(3):489-493.

139. Hockenberry MJ, Hinds PS, Barrera P, et al. Three instruments to assess fatigue in children with cancer: the child, parent and staff perspectives. *J Pain Symptom Manage.* 2003;25(4):319-328.

140. Varni JW, Burwinkle TM, Katz ER, Meeske K, Dickinson P. The PedsQL in pediatric cancer: reliability and validity of the Pediatric Quality of Life Inventory Generic Core Scales, Multidimensional Fatigue Scale, and Cancer Module. *Cancer.* 2002;94(7):2090-2106.

141. Lansky SB, List MA, Lansky LL, Ritter-Sterr C, Miller DR. The measurement of performance in childhood cancer patients. *Cancer.* 1987;60(7):1651-1656.

142. Butt Z, Lai JS, Rao D, Heinemann AW, Bill A, Cella D. Measurement of fatigue in cancer, stroke, and HIV using the Functional Assessment of Chronic Illness Therapy—Fatigue (FACIT-F) scale. *J Psychosom Res.* 2013;74(1):64-68.

143. Lai JS, Yount S, Beaumont JL, Cella D, Toia J, Goldman S. A patient-centered symptom monitoring and reporting system for children and young adults with cancer (SyMon-SAYS). *Pediatr Blood Cancer.* 2015;62(10):1813-1818.

144. Thissen D, Liu Y, Magnus B, et al. Estimating minimally important difference (MID) in PROMIS pediatric measures using the scale-judgment method. *Qual Life Res.* 2016;25(1):13-23.

145. Bhardwaj T, Koffman J. Non-pharmacological interventions for management of fatigue among children with cancer: systematic review of existing practices and their effectiveness. *BMJ Support Palliat Care.* 2017;7(4):404-414.

146. Bogg TF, Broderick C, Shaw P, Cohn R, Naumann FL. Feasibility of an inpatient exercise intervention for children undergoing hematopoietic stem cell transplant. *Pediatr Transplant.* 2015;19(8):925-931.

147. Cheung YT, Brinkman TM, Mulrooney DA, et al. Impact of sleep, fatigue, and systemic inflammation on neurocognitive and behavioral outcomes in long-term survivors of childhood acute lymphoblastic leukemia. *Cancer.* 2017;123(17):3410-3419.

148. Duong N, Davis H, Robinson PD, et al. Mind and body practices for fatigue reduction in patients with cancer and hematopoietic stem cell transplant recipients: a systematic review and meta-analysis. *Crit Rev Oncol Hematol.* 2017;120:210-216.

149. Linder LA, Bratton H, Nguyen A, Parker K, Wawrzynski SE. Symptoms and self-management strategies identified by children with cancer using draw-and-tell interviews. *Oncol Nurs Forum.* 2018;45(3):290-300.

150. Lown EA, Banerjee A, Vittinghoff E, et al. Acupressure to reduce treatment-related symptoms for children with cancer and recipients of hematopoietic stem cell transplant: protocol for a randomized controlled trial. *Glob Adv Health Med.* 2019;8:2164956119870444.

151. Oberoi S, Robinson PD, Cataudella D, et al. Physical activity reduces fatigue in patients with cancer and hematopoietic stem cell transplant recipients: a systematic review and meta-analysis of randomized trials. *Crit Rev Oncol Hematol.* 2018;122:52-59.

152. Robinson PD, Oberoi S, Tomlinson D, et al. Management of fatigue in children and adolescents with cancer and in paediatric recipients of haemopoietic stem-cell transplants: a clinical practice guideline. *Lancet Child Adolesc Health.* 2018;2(5):371-378.

153. Shin ES, Seo KH, Lee SH, et al. Massage with or without aromatherapy for symptom relief in people with cancer. *Cochrane Database Syst Rev.* 2016;(6):Cd009873.

154. Tsai HF, Chen YR, Chung MH, et al. Effectiveness of music intervention in ameliorating cancer patients' anxiety, depression, pain, and fatigue: a meta-analysis. *Cancer Nurs.* 2014;37(6):E35-E50.

155. Tomlinson D, Robinson PD, Oberoi S, et al. Pharmacologic interventions for fatigue in cancer and transplantation: a meta-analysis. *Curr Oncol.* 2018;25(2):e152-e167.

156. Bruera E, Driver L, Barnes EA, et al. Patient-controlled methylphenidate for the management of fatigue in patients with advanced cancer: a preliminary report. *J Clin Oncol.* 2003;21(23):4439-4443.

157. Bruera E, Valero V, Driver L, et al. Patient-controlled methylphenidate for cancer fatigue: a double-blind, randomized, placebo-controlled trial. *J Clin Oncol.* 2006;24:2073-2078.

158. Kerr CW, Drake J, Milch RA, et al. Effects of methylphenidate on fatigue and depression: a randomized, double-blind, placebo-controlled trial. *J Pain Symptom Manage.* 2012;43(1):68-77.

159. Wilwerding MB, Loprinzi CL, Mailliard JA, et al. A randomized, crossover evaluation of methylphenidate in cancer patients receiving strong narcotics. *Support Care Cancer.* 2012;3:135-138.

160. Bruera E, Fainsinger R, MacEachern T, Hanson J. The use of methylphenidate in patients with incident cancer pain receiving regular opiates. A preliminary report. *Pain.* 1992;50(1):75-77.

161. Association AP. *Diagnostic and Statistical Manual of Mental Disorders: DSM5.* American Psychiatric Association; 2013. Accessed September 4, 2019. HYPERLINK "https://nam02.safelinks.protection.outlook.com/?url=https%3A%2F%2Fwww.psychiatry.org%2Fpsychiatrists%2Fpractice%2Fdsm%2520%250d373&data=04%7C01%7Cstacie.stapleton%40jhmi.edu%-7Caadfb11a740f47bb345708d8915dca6a%7C9fa4f438b1e6473b803f86f8aedf0dec%7C0%7C0%7C637419179307703816%7CUnknown%7CTWFpbGZsb3d8eyJWIjoiMC4wLjAwMDAiLCJQIjoiV2luMzIiLCJBTi6Ik1haWwiLCJXVCI6Mn0%3D%7C1000&sdata=cj9rlWcSksSRCGX6zf9yGHavfs8OkTaMp27XUyRbuAg%3D&reserved=0" https://www.psychiatry.org/psychiatrists/practice/dsm

162. Mehta A, Chan LS. Understanding of the concept of 'Total pain': a prerequisite for pain control. *J Hosp Palliat Nurs.* 2008;10(1):26-34.

163. Mavrides N, Pao M. Updates in paediatric psychooncology. *Int Rev Psychiatry.* 2014;26(1):63-73.

164. Landier W, Tse AM. Use of complementary and alternative medical interventions for the management of procedure-related pain, anxiety, and distress in pediatric oncology: an integrative review. *J Pediatr Nurs.* 2010;25(6):566-579.

165. Bradt J, Dileo C, Magill L, Teague A. Music interventions for improving psychological and physical outcomes in cancer patients. *Cochrane Database Syst Rev.* 2016;(8):Cd006911.

166. Cervin M, Storch EA, Piacentini J, et al. Symptom-specific effects of cognitive-behavioral therapy, sertraline, and their combination in a large randomized controlled trial of pediatric anxiety disorders. *J Child Psychol Psychiatry.* 2019;61(4):492-502.

167. Walkup JT, Albano AM, Piacentini J, et al. Cognitive behavioral therapy, sertraline, or a combination in childhood anxiety. *N Engl J Med.* 2008;359(26):2753-2766.

168. Kondro W. FDA urges "black box" warning on pediatric antidepressants. *CMAJ.* 2004;171:837-838.

169. Phipps S, Buckholtz KE, Fernandez L, et al. Pediatric oncologists' practices of prescribing selective serotonin reuptake inhibitors (SSRIs) for children and adolescents with cancer: a multi-site study. *Pediatr Blood Cancer.* 2012;58(2):210-215.

170. Brent DA, Kolko DJ, Birmaher B, et al. Predictors of treatment efficacy in a clinical trial of three psychosocial treatments for adolescent depression. *J Am Acad Child Adolesc Psychiatry.* 1998;37(9):906-914.

171. March J, Silva S, Petrycki S, et al. Fluoxetine, cognitive-behavioral therapy, and their combination for adolescents with depression: Treatment for Adolescents with Depression Study (TADS) randomized controlled trial. *JAMA.* 2004;292(7):807-820.

172. Kurtz BP, Abrams AN. Psychiatric aspects of pediatric cancer. *Child Adolesc Psychiatr Clin N Am.* 2010;19(2):401-421, x-xi.

173. Traube C, Silver G, Gerber LM, et al. Delirium and mortality in critically ill children: epidemiology and outcomes of pediatric delirium. *Crit Care Med.* 2017;45(5):891-898.

174. Turkel SB. Pediatric delirium: recognition, management, and outcome. *Curr Psychiatry Rep.* 2017;19(12):101.

175. Traube C, Ariagno S, Thau F, et al. Delirium in hospitalized children with cancer: incidence and associated risk factors. *J Pediatr.* 2017;191:212-217.

176. Smith HAB, Gangopadhyay M, Goben CM, et al. Delirium and benzodiazepines associated with prolonged ICU stay in critically ill infants and young children. *Crit Care Med.* 2017;45(9):1427-1435.

177. Traube C, Silver G, Kearney J, et al. Cornell Assessment of Pediatric Delirium: a valid, rapid, observational tool for screening delirium in the PICU*. *Crit Care Med.* 2014;42(3):656-663.

178. Silver G, Kearney J, Traube C, Atkinson TM, Wyka KE, Walkup J. Pediatric delirium: evaluating the gold standard. *Palliat Support Care.* 2015;13(3):513-516.

179. Nikooie R, Neufeld KJ, Oh ES, et al. Antipsychotics for treating delirium in hospitalized adults: a systematic review. *Ann Intern Med.* 2019;171(7):485-495.

180. Malas N, Brahmbhatt K, McDermott C, Smith A, Ortiz-Aguayo R, Turkel S. Pediatric delirium: evaluation, management, and special considerations. *Curr Psychiatry Rep.* 2017;19(9):65.

181. Harris N, Baba M, Mellor C, et al. Seizure management in children requiring palliative care: a review of current practice. *BMJ Support Palliat Care.* 2017;10:e22.

182. Baenziger PH, Moody K. Palliative care for children with central nervous system malignancies. *Bioengineering (Basel).* 2018;5(4):85.

183. Kuhlen M, Hoell J, Balzer S, Borkhardt A, Janssen G. Symptoms and management of pediatric patients with incurable brain tumors in palliative home care. *Eur J Paediatr Neurol.* 2016;20(2):261-269.

184. Dallas J, Englot DJ, Naftel RP. Neurosurgical approaches to pediatric epilepsy: indications, techniques, and outcomes of common surgical procedures. *Seizure* 2020;77:76-85.

185. Ali S, Scheffer IE, Sadleir LG. Efficacy of cannabinoids in paediatric epilepsy. *Dev Med Child Neurol.* 2019;61(1):13-18.

186. Bausewein C, Booth S, Gysels M, Higginson I. Non-pharmacological interventions for breathlessness in advanced stages of malignant and non-malignant diseases. *Cochrane Database Syst Rev.* 2008;(2):Cd005623.

187. Houlahan KE, Branowicki PA, Mack JW, Dinning C, McCabe M. Can end of life care for the pediatric patient suffering with escalating and intractable symptoms be improved? *J Pediatr Oncol Nurs.* 2006;23(1):45-51.

188. Rowbottom L, Chan S, Zhang L, et al. Impact of dyspnea on advanced cancer patients referred to a palliative radiotherapy clinic. *Support Care Cancer.* 2017;25(9):2691-2696.

189. Wolfe J, Hammel JF, Edwards KE, et al. Easing of suffering in children with cancer at the end of life: is care changing? *J Clin Oncol.* 2008;26(10):1717-1723.

190. Davies D. Respiratory symptoms. In: Wolfe J, Hinds P, Sourkes B, eds. *Textbook of Interdisciplinary Pediatric Palliative Care.* Philadelphia, PA: Elsevier Saunders; 2011:300-302.

191. Hechler T, Blankenburg M, Friedrichsdorf SJ, et al. Parents' perspective on symptoms, quality of life, characteristics of death and end-of-life decisions for children dying from cancer. *Klin Padiatr.* 2008;220(3):166-174.

192. Edmonds P, Higginson I, Altmann D, Sen-Gupta G, McDonnell M. Is the presence of dyspnea a risk factor for morbidity in cancer patients? *J Pain Symptom Manage*. 2000;19(1):15-22.

193. McGrath PJ, Pianosi PT, Unruh AM, Buckley CP. Dalhousie dyspnea scales: construct and content validity of pictorial scales for measuring dyspnea. *BMC Pediatr*. 2005;5:33.

194. Wiseman R, Rowett D, Allcroft P, Abernethy A, Currow DC. Chronic refractory dyspnoea—evidence based management. *Aust Fam Physician*. 2013;42(3):137-140.

195. Khan FI, Reddy RC, Baptist AP. Pediatric Dyspnea Scale for use in hospitalized patients with asthma. *J Allergy Clin Immunol*. 2009;123(3):660-664.

196. Booth S, Galbraith S, Ryan R, Parker RA, Johnson M. The importance of the feasibility study: lessons from a study of the hand-held fan used to relieve dyspnea in people who are breathless at rest. *Palliat Med*. 2016;30(5):504-509.

197. Galbraith S, Fagan P, Perkins P, Lynch A, Booth S. Does the use of a handheld fan improve chronic dyspnea? A randomized, controlled, crossover trial. *J Pain Symptom Manage*. 2010;39(5):831-838.

198. Huang SL, Lai WS, Fang SY. [Using fans to relieve dyspnea: a systematic review and clinical implications]. *Hu Li Za Zhi*. 2018;65(4):84-93.

199. Kako J, Morita T, Yamaguchi T, et al. Fan therapy is effective in relieving dyspnea in patients with terminally ill cancer: a parallel-arm, randomized controlled trial. *J Pain Symptom Manage*. 2018;56(4):493-500.

200. Luckett T, Phillips J, Johnson MJ, et al. Contributions of a hand-held fan to self-management of chronic breathlessness. *Eur Respir J*. 2017;50(2):1700262.

201. Puspawati N, Sitorus R, Herawati T. Hand-held fan airflow stimulation relieves dyspnea in lung cancer patients. *Asia Pac J Oncol Nurs*. 2017;4(2):162-167.

202. Qian Y, Wu Y, Rozman de Moraes A, et al. Fan therapy for the treatment of dyspnea in adults: a systematic review. *J Pain Symptom Manage*. 2019;58(3):481-486.

203. Currow DC, Ward AM, Abernethy AP. Advances in the pharmacological management of breathlessness. *Curr Opin Support Palliat Care*. 2009;3(2):103-106.

204. Friedrichsdorf SJ. From tramadol to methadone: opioids in the treatment of pain and dyspnea in pediatric palliative care. *Clin J Pain*. 2019;35(6):501-508.

205. Kamal AH, Maguire JM, Wheeler JL, Currow DC, Abernethy AP. Dyspnea review for the palliative care professional: treatment goals and therapeutic options. *J Palliat Med*. 2012;15(1):106-114.

206. Jennings AL, Davies AN, Higgins JP, Broadley K. Opioids for the palliation of breathlessness in terminal illness. *Cochrane Database Syst Rev*. 2001;(4):Cd002066.

207. Thomas JR, von Gunten CF. Management of dyspnea. *J Support Oncol*. 2003;1(1):23-32; discussion 32-24.

208. Navigante AH, Cerchietti LC, Castro MA, Lutteral MA, Cabalar ME. Midazolam as adjunct therapy to morphine in the alleviation of severe dyspnea perception in patients with advanced cancer. *J Pain Symptom Manage*. 2006;31(1):38-47.

209. Ferraresi V. Inhaled opioids for the treatment of dyspnea. *Am J Health Syst Pharm*. 2005;62(3):319-320.

210. Polosa R, Simidchiev A, Walters EH. Nebulised morphine for severe interstitial lung disease. *Cochrane Database Syst Rev*. 2002;(3):Cd002872.

211. Tiep B, Carter R, Zachariah F, et al. Oxygen for end-of-life lung cancer care: managing dyspnea and hypoxemia. *Expert Rev Respir Med*. 2013;7(5):479-490.

212. Davies D. Respiratory symptoms. In: Wolfe J, Hinds P, Sourkes B, eds. *Textbook of Interdisciplinary Pediatric Palliative Care*. Philadelphia, PA: Elsevier Saunders; 2011:302.

213. Ramanuja S, Kelkar PS. The approach to pediatric cough. *Ann Allergy Asthma Immunol*. 2010;105(1):3-8; quiz 9-11, 42.

214. Goldsobel AB, Chipps BE. Cough in the pediatric population. *J Pediatr*. 2010;156(3):352-358.

215. Paul IM, Yoder KE, Crowell KR, et al. Effect of dextromethorphan, diphenhydramine, and placebo on nocturnal cough and sleep quality for coughing children and their parents. *Pediatrics*. 2004;114(1):e85-e90.

216. Paul IM, Beiler J, McMonagle A, Shaffer ML, Duda L, Berlin CM, Jr. Effect of honey, dextromethorphan, and no treatment on nocturnal cough and sleep quality for coughing children and their parents. *Arch Pediatr Adolesc Med*. 2007;161(12):1140-1146.

217. Yoder KE, Shaffer ML, La Tournous SJ, Paul IM. Child assessment of dextromethorphan, diphenhydramine, and placebo for nocturnal cough due to upper respiratory infection. *Clin Pediatr (Phila)*. 2006;45(7):633-640.

218. Morice AH, Menon MS, Mulrennan SA, et al. Opiate therapy in chronic cough. *Am J Respir Crit Care Med*. 2007;175(4):312-315.

219. Klopp AH, Eapen GA, Komaki RR. Endobronchial brachytherapy: an effective option for palliation of malignant bronchial obstruction. *Clin Lung Cancer*. 2006;8(3):203-207.

220. Wee B, Hillier R. Interventions for noisy breathing in patients near to death. *Cochrane Database Syst Rev*. 2008;(1):Cd005177.

221. Bennett M, Lucas V, Brennan M, Hughes A, O'Donnell V, Wee B. Using anti-muscarinic drugs in the management of death rattle: evidence-based guidelines for palliative care. *Palliat Med*. 2002;16(5):369-374.

222. Jongerius PH, van Tiel P, van Limbeek J, Gabreels FJ, Rotteveel JJ. A systematic review for evidence of efficacy of anticholinergic drugs to treat drooling. *Arch Dis Child*. 2003;88(10):911-914.

223. Tscheng DZ. Sialorrhea—therapeutic drug options. *Ann Pharmacother*. 2002;36(11):1785-1790.

224. Van der Burg JJ, Jongerius PH, Van Hulst K, Van Limbeek J, Rotteveel JJ. Drooling in children with cerebral palsy: effect of salivary flow reduction on daily life and care. *Dev Med Child Neurol*. 2006;48(2):103-107.

225. Holdsworth MT, Raisch DW, Frost J. Acute and delayed nausea and emesis control in pediatric oncology patients. *Cancer*. 2006;106(4):931-940.

226. Santucci G, Mack JW. Common gastrointestinal symptoms in pediatric palliative care: nausea, vomiting, constipation, anorexia, cachexia. *Pediatr Clin North Am*. 2007;54(5):673-689, x.

227. Kanbayashi Y, Hosokawa T. Predictive factors for nausea or vomiting in patients with cancer who receive oral oxycodone for the first time: is prophylactic medication for prevention of opioid-induced nausea or vomiting necessary? *J Palliat Med*. 2014;17(6):683-687.

228. Wood GJ, Shega JW, Lynch B, Von Roenn JH. Management of intractable nausea and vomiting in patients at the end of life: "I was feeling nauseous all of the time ... nothing was working". *JAMA*. 2007;298(10):1196-1207.

229. Weaver M, Carter B, Keefer P, Korones D, Miller E. *Pediatric Palliative Care and Hospice*. Vol. 7. 5th ed. Chicago, IL: American Academy of Hospice and Palliative Medicine; 2017.

230. Klick JC, Hauer J. Pediatric palliative care. *Curr Probl Pediatr Adolesc Health Care*. 2010;40(6):120-151.

231. Flank J, Thackray J, Nielson D, et al. Olanzapine for treatment and prevention of acute chemotherapy-induced vomiting in children: a retrospective, multi-center review. *Pediatr Blood Cancer*. 2015;62(3):496-501.

232. Patel P, Robinson PD, Thackray J, et al. Guideline for the prevention of acute chemotherapy-induced nausea and vomiting in pediatric cancer patients: a focused update. *Pediatr Blood Cancer.* 2017;64(10).

233. Okumura LM, D'Athayde Rodrigues F, Ferreira MAP, Moreira LB. Aprepitant in pediatric patients using moderate and highly emetogenic protocols: a systematic review and meta-analyses of randomized controlled trials. *Br J Clin Pharmacol.* 2017;83(5):1108-1117.

234. Chan CW, Lam LW, Li CK, et al. Feasibility of psychoeducational interventions in managing chemotherapy-associated nausea and vomiting (CANV) in pediatric oncology patients. *Eur J Oncol Nurs.* 2015;19(2):182-190.

235. Evans A, Malvar J, Garretson C, Pedroja Kolovos E, Baron Nelson M. The use of aromatherapy to reduce chemotherapy-induced nausea in children with cancer: a randomized, double-blind, placebo-controlled trial. *J Pediatr Oncol Nurs.* 2018;35(6):392-398.

236. Suh EE. The effects of P6 acupressure and nurse-provided counseling on chemotherapy-induced nausea and vomiting in patients with breast cancer. *Oncol Nurs Forum.* 2012;39(1):E1-E9.

237. Momani TG, Berry DL. Integrative therapeutic approaches for the management and control of nausea in children undergoing cancer treatment: a systematic review of literature. *J Pediatr Oncol Nurs.* 2017;34(3):173-184.

238. Rosenberg AR, Bona K, Coker T, et al. Pediatric palliative care in the multicultural context: findings from a workshop conference. *J Pain Symptom Manage.* 2019;57(4):846-855.e842.

239. Komatz K, Carter B. Pain and symptom management in pediatric palliative care. *Pediatr Rev.* 2015;36(12):527-533; quiz 534.

240. Szczepiorkowski ZM, Dunbar NM. Transfusion guidelines: when to transfuse. *Hematology Am Soc Hematol Educ Program.* 2013;2013:638-644.

241. Raval JS. Transfusion as a palliative strategy. *Curr Oncol Rep.* 2019;21(10):92.

242. Carson JL, Guyatt G, Heddle NM, et al. Clinical practice guidelines from the AABB: red blood cell transfusion thresholds and storage. *JAMA.* 2016;316(19):2025-2035.

243. Hendricks-Ferguson V. Physical symptoms of children receiving pediatric hospice care at home during the last week of life. *Oncol Nurs Forum.* 2008;35(6):E108-E115.

244. Neoh K, Gray R, Grant-Casey J, et al. National comparative audit of red blood cell transfusion practice in hospices: recommendations for palliative care practice. *Palliat Med.* 2019;33(1):102-108.

245. Bensadoun RJ, Humbert P, Krutman J, et al. Daily baseline skin care in the prevention, treatment, and supportive care of skin toxicity in oncology patients: recommendations from a multinational expert panel. *Cancer Manag Res.* 2013;5:401-408.

246. Wu J, Lacouture ME. Pruritus associated with targeted anticancer therapies and their management. *Dermatol Clin.* 2018;36(3):315-324.

247. Wakeda T, Okamura T, Kawahara T, Heike Y. Camouflage makeup improves quality of life in cancer patients with treatment-related skin changes. *Tumori.* 2019;106(2):95-100.

248. Basilio FM, Brenner FM, Werner B, Rastelli GJ. Clinical and histological study of permanent alopecia after bone marrow transplantation. *An Bras Dermatol.* 2015;90(6):814-821.

249. Haider M, Hamadah I, Almutawa A. Radiation- and chemotherapy-induced permanent alopecia: case series. *J Cutan Med Surg.* 2013;17(1):55-61.

250. Friedman JD, Dello Buono FA. Opioid antagonists in the treatment of opioid-induced constipation and pruritus. *Ann Pharmacother.* 2001;35(1):85-91.

251. McNicol E, Horowicz-Mehler N, Fisk RA, et al. Management of opioid side effects in cancer-related and chronic noncancer pain: a systematic review. *J Pain.* 2003;4(5):231-256.

252. Dillon S, Tobias JD. Ondansetron to treat pruritus due to cholestatic jaundice. *J Pediatr Pharmacol Ther.* 2013;18(3):241-246.

253. Seccareccia D, Gebara N. Pruritus in palliative care: getting up to scratch. *Can Fam Physician.* 2011;57(9):1010-1013, e1016-e1019.

254. Langemo D. General principles and approaches to wound prevention and care at end of life: an overview. *Ostomy Wound Manage.* 2012;58(5):24-26, 28, 30 passim.

255. Becker DK. Pediatric integrative medicine. *Prim Care.* 2017;44(2):337-350.

256. Mayan M, Alvadj T, Punja S, Jou H, Wildgen S, Vohra S. Parents' experiences of an inpatient pediatric integrative medicine service for symptom management. *Explore (NY).* 2019;15(6):415-418.

257. McClafferty H. An overview of pediatric integrative medicine. *Pediatr Ann.* 2019;48(6):e216-e219.

258. Esparham A, Misra SM, Misra S, et al. Pediatric integrative medicine: vision for the future. *Children (Basel).* 2018;5(8):111.

259. McClafferty H. Integrative pediatrics: looking forward. *Children (Basel).* 2015;2:63-65.

260. McClafferty H, Vohra S, Bailey M, et al. Pediatric integrative medicine. *Pediatrics.* 2017;140(3):e20171961.

261. Ladas EJ. Integrative medicine in childhood cancer. *J Altern Complement Med.* 2018;24(9-10):910-915.

262. Steinhorn DM, Din J, Johnson A. Healing, spirituality and integrative medicine. *Ann Palliat Med.* 2017;6(3):237-247.

263. Qato DM, Alexander GC, Guadamuz JS, Lindau ST. Prevalence of dietary supplement use in us children and adolescents, 2003-2014. *JAMA Pediatr.* 2018;172:780-782.

264. Ramesh G, Gerstbacher D, Arruda J, Golianu B, Mark J, Yeh AM. Pediatric integrative medicine in academia: Stanford children's experience. *Children (Basel).* 2018;5(12):168.

265. Ziodeen KA, Misra SM. Complementary and integrative medicine attitudes and perceived knowledge in a large pediatric residency program. *Complement Ther Med.* 2018;37:133-135.

266. Gardiner P, Kemper KJ. Herbs in pediatric and adolescent medicine. *Pediatr Rev.* 2000;21(2):44-57.

267. Weydert JA, Brown ML, McClafferty H. Integrative medicine in pediatrics. *Adv Pediatr.* 2018;65(1):19-39.

268. Anheyer D, Frawley J, Koch AK, et al. Herbal medicines for gastrointestinal disorders in children and adolescents: a systematic review. *Pediatrics.* 2017;139(6):e20170062.

269. Mozurkewich EL, Klemens C. Omega-3 fatty acids and pregnancy: current implications for practice. *Curr Opin Obstet Gynecol.* 2012;24(2):72-77.

270. Crowe S, Lyons B. Herbal medicine use by children presenting for ambulatory anesthesia and surgery. *Paediatr Anaesth.* 2004;14(11):916-919.

271. Erlichman J, Hall A, Dean A, Godwin B, Mascarenhas M. Integrative nutrition for pediatrics. *Curr Probl Pediatr Adolesc Health Care.* 2016;46(6):165-171.

272. Chatzi L, Kogevinas M. Prenatal and childhood Mediterranean diet and the development of asthma and allergies in children. *Public Health Nutr.* 2009;12(9a): 1629-1634.

273. Garcia M, Bihuniak JD, Shook J, Kenny A, Kerstetter J, Huedo-Medina TB. The effect of the traditional Mediterranean-style diet on metabolic risk factors: a meta-analysis. *Nutrients.* 2016;8(3):168.

274. Velazquez-Lopez L, Santiago-Diaz G, Nava-Hernandez J, Munoz-Torres AV, Medina-Bravo P, Torres-Tamayo M. Mediterranean-style diet reduces metabolic syndrome components in obese children and adolescents with obesity. *BMC Pediatr.* 2014;14:175.

275. Chang HT, Olson LK, Schwartz KA. Ketolytic and glycolytic enzymatic expression profiles in malignant gliomas: implication for ketogenic diet therapy. *Nutr Metab (Lond).* 2013;10(1):47.

276. Martin-McGill KJ, Marson AG, Tudur Smith C, Jenkinson MD. Ketogenic diets as an adjuvant therapy in glioblastoma (the KEATING trial): study protocol for a randomised pilot study. *Pilot Feasibility Stud.* 2017;3:67.

277. Winter SF, Loebel F, Dietrich J. Role of ketogenic metabolic therapy in malignant glioma: a systematic review. *Crit Rev Oncol Hematol.* 2017;112:41-58.

278. Jin X, Ruiz Beguerie J, Sze DM, Chan GC. *Ganoderma lucidum* (Reishi mushroom) for cancer treatment. *Cochrane Database Syst Rev.* 2012;(6):CD007731.

279. Jin X, Ruiz Beguerie J, Sze DM, Chan GC. *Ganoderma lucidum* (Reishi mushroom) for cancer treatment. *Cochrane Database Syst Rev.* 2016;4:CD007731.

280. Santesso N, Wieland LS. A summary of a Cochrane review: *Ganoderma lucidum* (Reishi mushroom) for the treatment of cancer. *Eur J Integr Med.* 2016;8(5):619-620.

281. Block KI, Koch AC, Mead MN, Tothy PK, Newman RA, Gyllenhaal C. Impact of antioxidant supplementation on chemotherapeutic efficacy: a systematic review of the evidence from randomized controlled trials. *Cancer Treat Rev.* 2007;33(5):407-418.

282. Smith LA, Azariah F, Lavender VT, Stoner NS, Bettiol S. Cannabinoids for nausea and vomiting in adults with cancer receiving chemotherapy. *Cochrane Database Syst Rev.* 2015;(11):Cd009464.

283. Abrams DI, Guzman M. Cannabis in cancer care. *Clin Pharmacol Ther.* 2015;97(6):575-586.

284. Kleckner AS, Kleckner IR, Kamen CS, et al. Opportunities for cannabis in supportive care in cancer. *Ther Adv Med Oncol.* 2019;11:1758835919866362.

285. Brown ML, Rojas E, Gouda S. A mind-body approach to pediatric pain management. *Children (Basel).* 2017; 4(6):50.

286. Groenewald CB, Beals-Erickson SE, Ralston-Wilson J, Rabbitts JA, Palermo TM. Complementary and alternative medicine use by children with pain in the United States. *Acad Pediatr.* 2017;17(7):785-793.

287. Yang C, Hao Z, Zhang LL, Guo Q. Efficacy and safety of acupuncture in children: an overview of systematic reviews. *Pediatr Res.* 2015;78(2):112-119.

288. Hershey AD, Powers SW, Vockell AL, et al. Coenzyme Q10 deficiency and response to supplementation in pediatric and adolescent migraine. *Headache.* 2007;47(1):73-80.

289. Kedia S. Complementary and integrative approaches for pediatric headache. *Semin Pediatr Neurol.* 2016; 23(1):44-52.

290. Slater SK, Nelson TD, Kabbouche MA, et al. A randomized, double-blinded, placebo-controlled, crossover, add-on study of CoEnzyme Q10 in the prevention of pediatric and adolescent migraine. *Cephalalgia.* 2011;31(8):897-905.

291. Albrecht E, Kirkham KR, Liu SS, Brull R. Peri-operative intravenous administration of magnesium sulphate and postoperative pain: a meta-analysis. *Anaesthesia.* 2013;68(1):79-90.

292. Oelkers-Ax R, Leins A, Parzer P, et al. Butterbur root extract and music therapy in the prevention of childhood migraine: an explorative study. *Eur J Pain.* 2008;12(3):301-313.

293. Sadler C, Vanderjagt L, Vohra S. Complementary, holistic, and integrative medicine: butterbur. *Pediatr Rev.* 2007;28(6):235-238.

294. Pillai AK, Sharma KK, Gupta YK, Bakhshi S. Antiemetic effect of ginger powder versus placebo as an add-on therapy in children and young adults receiving high emetogenic chemotherapy. *Pediatr Blood Cancer.* 2011;56(2):234-238.

295. Weaver MS, Robinson J, Wichman C. Aromatherapy improves nausea, pain, and mood for patients receiving pediatric palliative care symptom-based consults: a pilot design trial. *Palliat Support Care.* 2020;18(2): 158-163.

296. Bikmoradi A, Khaleghverdi M, Seddighi I, Moradkhani S, Soltanian A, Cheraghi F. Effect of inhalation aromatherapy with lavender essence on pain associated with intravenous catheter insertion in preschool children: a quasi-experimental study. *Complement Ther Clin Pract.* 2017;28:85-91.

297. Mind-body therapies in children and youth. *Pediatrics.* 2016;138(3):e20161896.

298. Tsai SL, Niemtzow RC, Brown M, et al. Acupuncture and integrative medicine in pediatrics. *Med Acupunct.* 2018;30(2):61-67.

299. Kemper KJ, Wornham WL. Consultations for holistic pediatric services for inpatients and outpatient oncology patients at a children's hospital. *Arch Pediatr Adolesc Med.* 2001;155(4):449-454.

300. Yun H, Romero SAD, Record B, et al. Utilization of integrative medicine differs by age among pediatric oncology patients. *Pediatr Blood Cancer.* 2019;66(6): e27639.

301. Zinner SE. The use of pediatric advance directives: a tool for palliative care physicians. *Am J Hosp Palliat Care.* 2008;25(6):427-430.

302. Hammes BJ, Klevan J, Kempf M, Williams MS. Pediatric advance care planning. *J Palliat Med.* 2005;8(4): 766-773.

303. Jacobs HC, Truog RD, Zinner SE, et al. The Texas Advance Directives Act—is it a good model? *Semin Perinatol.* 2009;33:384-390.

304. Walsh-Kelly CM, Lang KR, Chevako J, et al. Advance directives in a pediatric emergency department. *Pediatrics.* 1999;103(4 Pt 1):826-830.

305. Lotz JD, Jox RJ, Borasio GD, Fuhrer M. Pediatric advance care planning: a systematic review. *Pediatrics.* 2013;131(3):e873-e880.

306. Savage T, Michalak DR. Finding agreement to limit life-sustaining treatment for children who are in state custody. *Pediatr Nurs.* 2001;27(6):594-597.

307. Ullrich CK, Lehmann L, London WB, et al. End-of-life care patterns associated with pediatric palliative care among children who underwent hematopoietic stem cell transplant. *Biol Blood Marrow Transplant.* 2016;22(6):1049-1055.

308. Snaman JM, Kaye EC, Lu JJ, Sykes A, Baker JN. Palliative care involvement is associated with less intensive end-of-life care in adolescent and young adult oncology patients. *J Palliat Med.* 2017;20(5):509-516.

309. Brock KE, Steineck A, Twist CJ. Trends in end-of-life care in pediatric hematology, oncology, and stem cell transplant patients. *Pediatr Blood Cancer.* 2016;63(3):516-522.

310. Cook BA, Schaller K, Krischer JP. School absence among children with chronic illness. *J Sch Health.* 1985;55(7):265-267.

311. Emerson ND, Distelberg B, Morrell HE, Williams-Reade J, Tapanes D, Montgomery S. Quality of life and school absenteeism in children with chronic illness. *J Sch Nurs.* 2016;32(4):258-266.

312. Katz E. School and academic planning. In: Wiener L, Pao M, Kazak A, Kupst MJ, Patenaude A, Arceci R, eds. *Pediatric Psycho-Oncology: A Quick Reference on the Psychosocial Dimensions of Cancer Symptom Management.* New York, NY: Oxford University Press; 2015:297-310.

313. Olson AL, Seidler AB, Goodman D, Gaelic S, Nordgren R. School professionals' perceptions about the impact of chronic illness in the classroom. *Arch Pediatr Adolesc Med.* 2004;158(1):53-58.

314. Thies KM. Identifying the educational implications of chronic illness in school children. *J Sch Health.* 1999;69(10):392-397.

315. Reid Chassiakos YL, Radesky J, Christakis D, Moreno MA, Cross C. Children and adolescents and digital media. *Pediatrics.* 2016;138(5).

316. Sedrak MS, Dizon DS, Anderson PF, et al. The emerging role of professional social media use in oncology. *Future Oncol.* 2017;13(15):1281-1285.

317. Keith BE, Steinberg S. Parental sharing on the internet: child privacy in the age of social media and the pediatrician's role. *JAMA Pediatr.* 2017;171(5):413-414.

318. McKlindon D, Jacobson JA, Nathanson P, Walter JK, Lantos JD, Feudtner C. Ethics rounds: in the eye of a social media storm. *Pediatrics.* 2016;138(3):e20161398.

319. Nagelhout ES, Linder LA, Austin T, et al. Social media use among parents and caregivers of children with cancer. *J Pediatr Oncol Nurs.* 2018;35(6):399-405.

320. Caruso Brown AE, Arthur JD, Mutrie LH, Lantos JD. Seeking a second opinion on social media. *Pediatrics.* 2020;16(3):399-400.

321. O'Keeffe GS. Social media: challenges and concerns for families. *Pediatr Clin North Am.* 2016;63(5):841-849.

322. Gage-Bouchard EA, LaValley S, Warunek M, Beaupin LK, Mollica M. Is cancer information exchanged on social media scientifically accurate? *J Cancer Educ.* 2018;33(6):1328-1332.

323. Wiener L, McConnell DG, Latella L, Ludi E. Cultural and religious considerations in pediatric palliative care. *Palliat Support Care.* 2013;11(1):47-67.

324. Derrington SF, Paquette E, Johnson KA. Cross-cultural interactions and shared decision-making. *Pediatrics.* 2018;142(suppl 3):S187-S192.

325. Sisk BA, Canavera K, Sharma A, Baker JN, Johnson LM. Ethical issues in the care of adolescent and young adult oncology patients. *Pediatr Blood Cancer.* 2019;66(5):e27608.

326. *The National Commission for the Protection of Human Subjects of Biomedical and Behavioral Research Involving Children: Report and Recommendations.* Washington, DC: NCPHSBBR; 1977. RDHEW Pub. No. (OS) 77-0004.

327. Wendler DS. Assent in paediatric research: theoretical and practical considerations. *J Med Ethics.* 2006;32(4):229-234.

328. Katz AL, Webb SA. Informed consent in decision-making in pediatric practice. *Pediatrics.* 2016;138(2):e20161485.

329. Miller VA, Feudtner C. Parent and child perceptions of the benefits of research participation. *IRB.* 2016;38(4):1-7.

330. Levine DR, Johnson LM, Mandrell BN, et al. Does phase 1 trial enrollment preclude quality end-of-life care? Phase 1 trial enrollment and end-of-life care characteristics in children with cancer. *Cancer.* 2015;121(9):1508-1512.

331. Crane S, Haase JE, Hickman SE. Parental experiences of child participation in a phase I pediatric oncology clinical trial: "We Don't Have Time to Waste". *Qual Health Res.* 2019;29(5):632-644.

332. Maurer SH, Hinds PS, Spunt SL, Furman WL, Kane JR, Baker JN. Decision making by parents of children with incurable cancer who opt for enrollment on a phase I trial compared with choosing a do not resuscitate/terminal care option. *J Clin Oncol.* 2010;28(20):3292-3298.

333. Hinds PS, Oakes LL, Hicks J, et al. "Trying to be a good parent" as defined by interviews with parents who made phase I, terminal care, and resuscitation decisions for their children. *J Clin Oncol* 2009;27(35):5979-5985.

334. Beauchamp TL, Childress JF. *Principles of Biomedical Ethics.* 7th ed. New York, NY: Oxford University Press; 2013.

335. Mack JW, Fasciano KM, Block SD. Adolescent and young adult cancer patients' experiences with treatment decision-making. *Pediatrics.* 2019;143(5):e20182800.

336. Kon AA, Shepard EK, Sederstrom NO, et al. Defining futile and potentially inappropriate interventions: a policy statement from the Society of Critical Care Medicine Ethics Committee. *Crit Care Med.* 2016;44(9):1769-1774.

337. Levine D, Lam CG, Cunningham MJ, et al. Best practices for pediatric palliative cancer care: a primer for clinical providers. *J Support Oncol.* 2013;11(3):114-125.

338. Miller EG, Laragione G, Kang TI, Feudtner C. Concurrent care for the medically complex child: lessons of implementation. *J Palliat Med.* 2012;15(11):1281-1283.

339. Keim-Malpass J, Hart TG, Miller JR. Coverage of palliative and hospice care for pediatric patients with a life-limiting illness: a policy brief. *J Pediatr Health Care.* 2013;27(6):511-516.

340. Mooney-Doyle K, Keim-Malpass J, Lindley LC. The ethics of concurrent care for children: a social justice perspective. *Nurs Ethics.* 2019;26(5):1518-1527.

341. Morris S, Fletcher K, Goldstein R. The grief of parents after the death of a young child. *J Clin Psychol Med Settings.* 2019;26(3):321-338.

342. Lichtenthal WG, Sweeney CR, Roberts KE, et al. Bereavement follow-up after the death of a child as a standard of care in pediatric oncology. *Pediatr Blood Cancer.* 2015;62(suppl 5):S834-S869.

343. Johnson LM, Snaman JM, Cupit MC, Baker JN. End-of-life care for hospitalized children. *Pediatr Clin North Am.* 2014;61(4):835-854.

344. Atherton KN. Project Five Wishes: promoting advance directives in primary care. *J Am Assoc Nurse Pract.* 2020;32(10):689-695.

345. Zadeh S, Pao M, Wiener L. Opening end-of-life discussions: how to introduce Voicing My CHOiCES, an advance care planning guide for adolescents and young adults. *Palliat Support Care.* 2015;13(3):591-599.

346. Kaye EC, Gushue CA, DeMarsh S, et al. Illness and end-of-life experiences of children with cancer who receive palliative care. *Pediatr Blood Cancer.* 2018;65(4).

347. Wolfe J, Grier HE, Klar N, et al. Symptoms and suffering at the end of life in children with cancer. *N Engl J Med.* 2000;342(5):326-333.

348. Anghelescu DL, Knapp E, Johnson LM, Baker JN. The role of the pediatric anesthesiologist in relieving suffering at the end of life: when is palliative sedation appropriate in pediatrics? *Paediatr Anaesth.* 2017;27(4):443-444.

349. Allen RS, Hilgeman MM, Ege MA, Shuster JL Jr, Burgio LD. Legacy activities as interventions approaching the end of life. *J Palliat Med.* 2008;11(7):1029-1038.

350. Macdonald ME, Liben S, Carnevale FA, et al. Parental perspectives on hospital staff members' acts of kindness and commemoration after a child's death. *Pediatrics.* 2005;116(4):884-890.

351. Brouwer M, Kaczor C, Battin MP, Maeckelberghe E, Lantos JD, Verhagen E. Should pediatric euthanasia be legalized? *Pediatrics.* 2018;141(2):7-9.

352. Kim M, Yi J, et al. A Photovoice Study on the bereavement experience of mothers after the death of a child. *Death Stud.* 2019:1-15.

353. Pohlkamp L, Kreicbergs U, Sveen J. Bereaved mothers' and fathers' prolonged grief and psychological health 1 to 5 years after loss—a nationwide study. *Psychooncology.* 2019;28(7):1530-1536.

354. Snaman JM, Kaye EC, Torres C, Gibson DV, Baker JN. Helping parents live with the hole in their heart: the role of health care providers and institutions in the bereaved parents' grief journeys. *Cancer.* 2016;122(17):2757-2765.

355. Weaver MS, Lichtenthal WG, Larson K, Wiener L. How I approach expressing condolences and longitudinal remembering to a family after the death of a child. *Pediatr Blood Cancer.* 2019;66(2):e27489.

356. The Compassionate Friends. https://www.compassionatefriends.org/. Accessed October 28, 2019.

357. van der Geest IM, Darlington AS, Streng IC, Michiels EM, Pieters R, van den Heuvel-Eibrink MM. Parents' experiences of pediatric palliative care and the impact on long-term parental grief. *J Pain Symptom Manage.* 2014;47(6):1043-1053.

358. Shapiro CL. Cancer survivorship. *N Engl J Med.* 2018;379(25):2438-2450.

359. Ross WL, Mitchell HR, Iyer NS, Santacroce SJ, Kadan-Lottick NS. Impact of survivorship care on young adult survivors of childhood cancer with post-traumatic stress symptoms. *Oncol Nurs Forum.* 2019;46(1):33-43.

360. Beaupin LK, Uwazurike OC, Hydeman JA. A roadmap to survivorship: optimizing survivorship care plans for adolescent and young adult cancer survivors. *J Adolesc Young Adult Oncol.* 2018;7(6):660-665.

361. Christen S, Mader L, Baenziger J, et al. "I wish someone had once asked me how I'm doing": disadvantages and support needs faced by parents of long-term childhood cancer survivors. *Pediatr Blood Cancer.* 2019;66(8):e27767.

362. Group CsO. *Long-Term Follow-Up Guidelines for Survivors of Childhood, Adolescent and Young Adult Cancers. Version 5.0.* Monrovia, CA: Group CsO; 2018.

363. Long-term follow-up care for pediatric cancer survivors. *Pediatrics.* 2009;123(3):906-915.

364. Shanafelt TD, Boone S, Tan L, et al. Burnout and satisfaction with work-life balance among US physicians relative to the general US population. *Arch Intern Med.* 2012;172(18):1377-1385.

365. Shanafelt TD, West CP, Sinsky C, et al. Changes in burnout and satisfaction with work-life Integration in physicians and the general US working population between 2011 and 2017. *Mayo Clin Proc.* 2019;94(9):1681-1694.

366. Whitford B, Nadel AL, Fish JD. Burnout in pediatric hematology/oncology-time to address the elephant by name. *Pediatr Blood Cancer.* 2018;65(10): e27244.

367. Kearney MK, Weininger RB, Vachon ML, Harrison RL, Mount BM. Self-care of physicians caring for patients at the end of life: "Being connected… a key to my survival". *JAMA.* 2009;301(11):1155-1164, e1151.

368. Sanchez-Reilly S, Morrison LJ, Carey E, et al. Caring for oneself to care for others: physicians and their self-care. *J Support Oncol.* 2013;11(2):75-81.

369. Spruit JL, Prince-Paul M. Palliative care services in pediatric oncology. *Ann Palliat Med.* 2019;8(suppl 1): S49-S57.

370. Jagt-van Kampen CT, Kars MC, Colenbrander DA, et al. A prospective study on the characteristics and subjects of pediatric palliative care case management provided by a hospital based palliative care team. *BMC Palliat Care.* 2017;16(1):1.

371. Verberne LM, Schouten-van Meeteren AY, Bosman DK, et al. Parental experiences with a paediatric palliative care team: a qualitative study. *Palliat Med.* 2017;31(10):956-963.

372. Avoine-Blondin J, Parent V, Fasse L, et al. How do professionals assess the quality of life of children with advanced cancer receiving palliative care, and what are their recommendations for improvement? *BMC Palliat Care.* 2018;17(1):71.

373. Jones E, Thienprayoon R, Hidalgo M, Stapleton S. *Patient Safety and Quality in Pediatric Hematology/Oncology and Stem Cell Transplantation.* New York, NY: Springer; 2017.

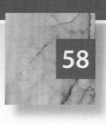

58 Hematopoietic Cell Transplantation and Supportive Care

Nina L. Bray and Ann M. Berger

INTRODUCTION

Over 50,000 people undergo hematopoietic cell transplantation (HCT) annually throughout the world, a number that continually increases with advances in technology and access to care (1). We have reached a mark of over 1 million HCTs reported worldwide in the last six decades (2). HCT refers to the administration of hematopoietic progenitor cells from any source (e.g., bone marrow, peripheral blood, umbilical cord blood) or donor (e.g., allogeneic, autologous) to reconstitute the bone marrow in efforts to treat disorders such as malignancies, genetic disorders, and bone marrow failure due to other causes.

HCT is a lengthy process endured by patients and their families with many substantial side effects and complications (Table 58.1). It dramatically changes the lives of these patients and families in many dimensions, and improved transplantation strategies have contributed to survival increments of 10% per decade (2). Patients who survive for 2 years after allogeneic HCT now have survival rates of 80% to 92% at 10 years (3,4), and survival rates approach 70% at 10 years following autologous HCT (5). However, these patients still must contend with numerous short- and long-term complications; thus, it is important to increase the emphasis of their care on additional supportive techniques that will bolster them through the process of survival. Our goal is to address the challenges of this process and how the medical community can address them. Some of the obstacles these patients face have overlap with the topics that are covered in other chapters in this text; thus, this chapter will focus on the specific concerns pertaining to overall quality of life (QOL) to enhance in the holistic supportive care of the HCT patient.

QUALITY OF LIFE

As we discuss some of the complications and the proposed interventions, it is important to note that patients do not experience these complications in discrete units, but in symptom clusters of varying magnitude and scope (6,7). There are models of these symptom clusters; however, it is of critical importance to recognize these not just as symptoms or clusters of symptoms but to realize that these clusters occur in the wider context of their lives. This realization is critical because it helps the clinician recognize that while each symptom is of great concern at the time of presentation, these symptoms are just a portion of the overall effect on the patient. Specifically, as patients consider the process of HCT, they question not only what these individual complications will be but also what their QOL will be following transplant. Generally, QOL is difficult to measure as inherently it is a multidimensional, dynamic, and subjective concept that encompasses every dimension of a person's life including good health, adequate housing, employment, personal and family safety, good relationships, education, and enjoyment of leisurely pursuits. As the numbers of survivors increase, it is more and more important to further evaluate and improve QOL, especially as issues related to QOL are routinely cited by cancer survivors as among their greatest concerns (8). However, there is evidence that suggest that transplant physicians consider QOL as secondary to the curative potential of HCT, underestimate patient's symptoms, and overestimate QOL (9,10). Patients often describe significantly more distress from their symptoms then are even recognized by their medical providers (11).

Bury (12) describes illness as a "biographical disruption" in which a person's life story is disrupted in the light of their illness, the treatment demands and the many changes that occur. In this chapter, we hope to emphasize that supportive care of the HCT patient centers on the patient's life story, relating both to their QOL and their need for holistic supportive care. In covering some of the complications of the process of HCT, we hope to highlight some of the main factors that affect QOL and propose interventions that can help improve QOL in these patients. In addition, we also hope to help the clinician to better listen and more fully appreciate the stories of our patients so we can truly help all.

TABLE 58.1 COMPLICATIONS OF HEMATOPOIETIC CELL TRANSPLANT

Constitutional
- Pain—physical, psychosocial, spiritual
- Fatigue
- Cachexia
- GVHD (multisystem)
- Infections
- Engraftment syndrome
- Impaired growth

Dermatological
- Rash/skin changes
- Alopecia

Gastrointestinal
- Mucositis
- Nausea
- Vomiting
- Anorexia
- Diarrhea
- Constipation
- Esophageal stricture
- Veno-occlusive disease
- Hepatitis
- Liver failure

Ophthalmologic
- Cataracts
- Keratoconjunctivitis sicca
- Retinopathy

Pulmonary
- Interstitial pneumonitis
- Bronchiolitis obliterans
- BOOP
- COPD

Renal
- Renal failure/nephropathy
- Bladder dysfunction
- Hemorrhagic cystitis

Musculoskeletal
- Myopathies
- Osteopenia
- Avascular necrosis

Endocrine/reproductive
- Hypothyroidism
- Infertility
- Sexuality

Vascular/cardiovascular
- Thrombotic microangiopathy
- Arrhythmias
- Cardiomyopathy
- Cardiac tamponade

Hematologic
- Neutropenia
- Anemia
- Thrombocytopenia
- Eosinophilia
- Bleeding/hemorrhage

Neurologic
- Delirium
- Peripheral neuropathies
- Cognitive decline
- Learning deficits
- Impaired memory

Rheumatologic
- Autoimmune diseases

Psychological
- Depression
- Anxiety
- PTSD
- Adjustment disorder

General health/psychosocial/other
- QOL
- Sleep disorders
- Dental caries
- Family stress
- Secondary malignancies
- Graft failure
- Financial burden
- Employment discrimination
- Spiritual needs/concerns

HEALTH CARE TEAM/MULTIDIMENSIONAL MODEL OF CARE

Evaluation of HCT transplantation is a complex process, it has wide variability across transplant centers, and there are no formal guidelines to conduct pre-HCT evaluation (12). There is also wide variation in supportive care practices in HCT (13). From the time patients contemplate the process through the time years later when they are looking back on it, likely forever changed, they experience the effects in all dimensions of their lives—physical, psychological, social, and spiritual (Fig. 58.1). The effects extend beyond these groupings, but the model is a useful starting place from which health care team can better address and support the patients through the many HCT complications. This not only requires physicians from nearly every specialty but also nurses from a wide variety of backgrounds, social workers, mental health specialists, pastoral care, nutritionists, and many others. As a team, we can better encompass treatment aimed at helping patients in all aspects of their care.

PHYSICAL

Graft versus Host Disease

Graft versus host disease (GVHD) is one of the most common complications after allogeneic HCT. Historically, acute GVHD is defined as disease that occurs in the first 100 days after transplant and chronic GVHD is defined as disease after 100 days (13).

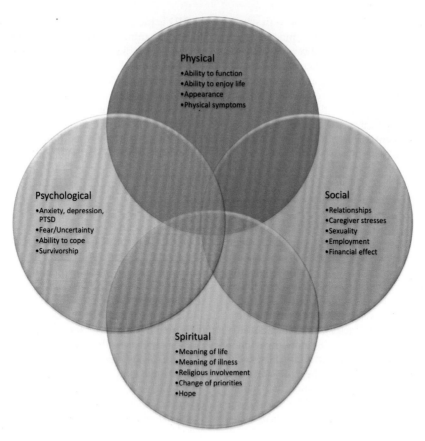

Figure 58.1 Multidimensional model of care summarizing the components of quality of life.

It is recognized that a temporal distinction is rather arbitrary and that disease manifestations would be a more appropriate means to make the distinction between acute and chronic GVHD as they appear to involve different immune cell subsets, different cytokine profiles, somewhat different host targets, and respond differently to treatment. Accordingly, in 2014 the NIH Consensus Conference has suggested a more complex categorization of acute and chronic GVHD (14,15). In either case, acute and chronic GVHD have a significant impact on short- and long-term morbidity as well as mortality in patients undergoing HCT. As a result of the physical and emotional aspects of the transplant process and development of GVHD, QOL in transplant survivors can be adversely affected. The strongest association between reduced QOL and impaired functional status following HCT is the presence of chronic GVHD (16). Even mild chronic GVHD symptoms are associated with impaired physical and general QOL (17). For patients with acute GVHD, they had measurable declines in their QOL over the first 6 months after HCT compared to those with no acute GVHD; however, this effect did not persist at 12 months after HCT unless the patient developed chronic GVHD (18).

Acute GVHD

Occurring at rates 10% to 80% depending on the study, underlying disease, prophylaxis regimens, and other factors, acute GVHD is the most frequent cause of mortality following allogeneic HCT due to its clinical toxicity, requirement for intensive immunosuppressive management, and associated infections (19–21). It generally develops within 2 to 8 weeks after transplantation. The most common manifestation of acute GVHD is dermatologic (21,22), which in most cases accompanies other manifestations in the liver or gastrointestinal tract, but each can occur independently.

The rash of acute GVHD is most commonly maculopapular, but can also be morbilliform, or sometimes a confluent erythematous exanthema. It may be pruritic or painful, and it may often involve the palms and soles, which can help distinguish it from drug eruptions that are usually not in this location (23,24). It can be mild and affect <25% of the body but also can be severe, leading to whole body erythema, desquamation, bullae formation, and sloughing of the skin (25). Patients with severe skin GVHD have similar features and the need for similar treatments as those of severely burned patients. Hepatic GVHD is difficult to diagnose due to a lack of definitive testing and these patients have many other reasons to present with hepatic dysfunction (drug toxicity, TPN, infection, cholelithiasis, veno-occlusive disease, etc.). Gastrointestinal involvement can lead to nausea, anorexia, pain, watery secretory diarrhea, and/or abnormal liver function tests. In more severe cases, it may lead to mucosal denudation causing bloody diarrhea, hemorrhage, protein-losing enteropathy, or ileus (26).

There have been many advances in the prevention of acute GVHD but currently older immunosuppressive drugs such as methotrexate, cyclosporine, and calcineurin inhibitors are the mainstay in the prevention of GVHD (27). Initial treatment is with corticosteroids, with about 40% to 50% of patients responding (28). Alternative therapies for steroid refractory cases include antithymocyte globulin, cyclosporine alone, mycophenolate mofetil, anti-iL-2 receptor, anti-cD5-specific immunotoxin, and numerous others. These agents can be used alone or in combination, but unfortunately there aren't sufficient studies comparing these regimens (27). Many of these agents produce a response to the acute GVHD; however, the risk of infectious mortality remains high as the treatment of acute GVHD leads to further immunosuppression and thus infectious susceptibility.

As these patients can quickly become critically ill, it is important to provide immediate disease-based treatment as outlined above. In addition, organ-specific supportive measures are critically important. Specific therapies for the skin include the use of topical emollient therapy and meticulous wound care, with considerations for care in a burn unit when appropriate and possible. For gastrointestinal tract complications, bowel rest, hyperalimentation, and antimotility agents may be required. In cases of bloody diarrhea, transfusion support may be necessary. Octreotide may help control the secretory component of gastrointestinal GVHD (29). As the majority of patients with steroid-refractory GVHD have a high mortality due to infection (30), systematic monitoring and judicious use of antibiotics for prophylaxis against infectious pathogens are essential.

Chronic GVHD

Chronic GVHD affects 27% to 60% of patients receiving allogeneic transplants from sibling donors and 42% to 72% from those receiving transplants from unrelated donors (31,32). There is some recent evidence that the incidence of chronic GVHD is increasing due to the adverse impact of protracted immunological derangements associated with chronic GVHD (33). The median onset of chronic GVHD is 4 to 6 months after HCT (34). The major risk factors for chronic GVHD are human leukocyte antigen disparity, increasing age, and preceding acute GVHD (35,36). Treatment of chronic GVHD is usually less aggressive than that of acute GVHD; however, most of the chronic GVHD patients require prolonged treatment lasting many months to years (20). In addition, combined with the stress of the existing diagnosis, the added stressor of developing chronic GVHD represents the most important cause of nonrelapse mortality beyond 2 to 3 months after transplantation. This is usually due to its significant immune dysfunction and the resultant increased infectious susceptibility (21). Detailed grading systems have been developed by the 2005 and 2014 NIH Consensus Conference to standardize the terminology and classify the severity of chronic GVHD, which help predict long-term survival (14,15,37). Generally, risk factors for worse prognosis are extensive skin involvement, progressive onset of chronic GVHD following acute GVHD, thrombocytopenia at diagnosis, and direct progression from acute GVHD (38).

First-line treatment for patients with moderate to severe chronic GVHD is steroids with or without a calcineurin inhibitor. Just as in acute GVHD, approximately 50% of patients are steroid-refractory patients, which is associated with a worse prognosis. There is no standard agreed-upon second-line therapy as there is a lot of new research being done. Extracorporeal photopheresis, rituximab, IL-2, mTOR inhibitors, mycophenolate mofetil, and numerous others are currently being studied (39). Assessment of effectiveness of treatment is at 8 to 12 weeks (37); however, the treatment in most cases continues for many years, leading to risks of continued progression, issues with side effects from medications, and many other complications.

With all these complications and the resultant prolongation of illness, it is not surprising that the strongest association between reduced QOL and impaired functional status following HCT is the presence of chronic GVHD (16). These patients continue to battle with the process and effects of HCT. The individual symptoms discussed below lead to numerous physical and emotional disturbances that effect QOL, and thus it is critical to aggressively support each patient through each symptom using innovative and creative solutions. Supportive care should include education, prevention of flares, infectious disease prophylaxis, physical and occupational therapy, nutrition, alleviation of chronic manifestations and effects of treatments, and promotion of coping mechanisms or resources to help patients deal with the psychosocial, sexual, and financial consequences of the disease (40). Below, we will address the skin, oral, ocular, and gynecological manifestations as these are key places where supportive care can aid in the overall care for the chronic GVHD patient.

Skin. The cutaneous manifestations of chronic GVHD are broad but can be classified into three groups: lichen planus–like lesions, sclerotic skin manifestations, and poikilodermatous changes. Lichenoid chronic GVHD presents as an erythematous papular rash that resembles lichen planus; sclerodermatous GVHD may involve the dermis or muscle fascia leading to dermal fibrosis and fasciitis, while poikilodermatous skin changes appear as patches of mottled pigmentation and telangiectasias (23,25,31). All these changes can lead to fragile skin with increased risk of erosions and ulceration or the skin can become thickened and tight with resultant detriment to the range of motion and poor wound-healing capacity. Any of these changes can lead to intense pruritus or pain. Hair loss and destruction of sweat glands are common; blistering may occur in severe cases. These symptoms are compounded by the patients' perception of their further worsening appearance, especially if widespread.

Oral and topical steroids serve as the primary treatment for cutaneous chronic GVHD (31,34,41). Petrolatum-based emollients are helpful for those patients with xerotic skin. In addition, topical calcineurin inhibitors (tacrolimus and pimecrolimus), phototherapy, and extracorporeal photophoresis can be helpful. Oral antipruritic agents such as antihistamines and tricyclic antidepressants such as doxepin should be used with caution as they can worsen oral and ocular sicca symptoms. Topical hydrocortisone, pramoxine, menthol-based creams/lotions, doxepin cream, or colloidal oatmeal powder bathtub soaks can also be used for short-term relief of intractable pruritus. For patients with thickened/tight skin and decreased range of motion, deep muscle/fascial massage is recommended, as well as daily stretching and referral to physical and/or occupational therapy. Surgical release can be considered in extreme cases. For patients with erosions and ulcerations, topical or oral antimicrobials, wound dressings, and debridement should all be considered. It is also important to instruct patients to take preventive measures such as avoidance of sun exposure, use of sunscreens (SPF > 20 with broad-spectrum UVA and UVB protections), and the use of protective clothing as there is an increased risk of skin cancer in patients with chronic GVHD (41–45).

Oral. Almost 80% of patients diagnosed with chronic GVHD demonstrate some degree of oral involvement, making this one of the most common clinical manifestations of chronic GVHD. The clinical findings can include erythema, leukoplakia, lichenoid lesions, ulcers, mucosal atrophy, cicatricial changes, and xerostomia (44,45). These can range from very mild changes to severe ones that can be functionally debilitating and lead to a decreased QOL due to significant pain, weight loss, malnutrition, and the loss of the ability to enjoy food and the process of eating. There are also many reports of oral squamous cell cancer in patients with chronic GVHD; thus, patients should be closely monitored for oral malignancies (46).

Like the treatment of skin chronic GVHD, topical high-potency corticosteroids are often used for the treatment of oral chronic GVHD (47). Additionally, supportive interventions for patients with oral chronic GVHD include encouraging good oral hygiene and utilizing of topical anesthetic agents, such as viscous lidocaine, to reduce pain and facilitate oral intake. Patients with xerostomia may benefit from salivary stimulants (sugarless gum or candy), oral lubricants or saliva substitutes, and frequent water sipping. Cholinergic agonists to stimulate saliva production (e.g., pilocarpine and cevimeline) may be useful in patients in whom the use of these agents is not contraindicated. Xerostomia can increase the risk of tooth decay, so it is also important to encourage the use of topical fluorides (48). Advise patients to avoid mint-flavored toothpastes and whitening products, as these can further aggravate the oral mucosa.

Ocular. Keratoconjunctivitis sicca is the most frequent presentation of chronic GVHD of the eye (41,49). Other eye chronic GVHD consequences are acute conjunctival inflammation and pseudomembranous and cicatricial conjunctivitis. These can lead to ocular irritation, dry eye syndrome, pain, or visual changes. Topical cyclosporine eye drops are the mainstay of treatment and are recommended by some prior to transplant to reduce the severity of ocular chronic GVHD (50). Other topical treatments include artificial tear liquids, ointments, slow dissolving hydroxypropyl methylcellulose, serum eye drops, and judicious use of topical steroid drops. Oral medications include cevimeline, pilocarpine, flaxseed oil, and doxycycline. Occlusive eye wear, warm compresses, humidified environments, or specialized contact lenses can also be used. Surgical interventions can also be considered in refractory cases (41,49,51).

Vulvar/Vaginal. Gynecological presentations of chronic GVHD are not as frequently studied as the other complications of chronic GVHD, and currently only case reports and retrospective reviews have been done to study these complications and their treatment (52,53). However, the effects of chronic GVHD on the female reproductive tract can be difficult for women, and thus it is important to ask about these issues, assess them, and treat them aggressively or refer to a physician that can do so. Symptoms can include dysuria, dryness, tenderness to touch, and dyspareunia. On examination, there may be erosions and fissures, introital stenosis, resorption of the labia minora, vaginal synechiae, or vaginal narrowing. Treatment includes the avoidance of mechanical and chemical irritants, the use of emollients such as lanolin cream applied to external genitalia, and water-based lubricants internally for the vagina. Short-term use of ultrahigh potency corticosteroid or topical calcineurin ointments can also be tried. In addition, topical and systemic estrogen or hormone treatment can be tried for patients who do not have contraindications. Dilators can be helpful in vaginal GVHD that leads to fibrotic vaginal scarring, and only in extreme cases, surgical interventions should be performed (41,43,52–55). Though they are limited in number, gynecologists with familiarity of GVHD are the best physicians to treat these patients; nevertheless, it is of most importance to ask about these symptoms and refer to a gynecologist in a timely manner.

PSYCHOLOGICAL

Psychological Effects

An important survey of 600 HCT survivors was conducted in 2006 by the Bone Marrow Transplant Information Network, which found that 73% of respondents endorsed emotional/psychological health as the most significant issue facing them following transplantation (56). Studies also have shown that biopsychosocial models will better predict cancer treatment–related pain and distress than a strictly biomedical model (57). The transplant process can be psychologically devastating, which consequently can be destructive in a patient's personal and family life. Patients who undergo this process have many sources of stress as they are faced with many questions about the process and how they will fare in comparison to the statistics they are given. There undoubtedly will be fear: fear that the transplant will not cure, fear that it might kill, fear of pain, fear of the complications, fear that they will never be the same, fear for their family, etc. Even if they are cured of the disease they had, studies show that HCT patients have a sense of feeling different from "normal people" despite having physical recovery (58).

These patients have been forever changed by their experience of illness and all the psychosocial changes a prolonged illness can bring. Unfortunately, in 2008, The Institute of Medicine report identified that meeting psychosocial needs of patients and family is the exception rather than the common occurrence in the current health care climate (59). As of 2019, there has been further research about specific guidelines for evaluation and treatment strategies to help HCT patients specifically; however, there still is a lot of research to be done to help these patients (60,61). This is not an unsurprising finding as the psychological and social issues can be more challenging for the health care team than the medical issues (62). We hope that this improves in the future, but this will require an increased awareness of these issues as well as a dedicated approach to identifying, recognizing, and treating the reality of the psychosocial distress that endangers these patients. Attention to psychosocial factors in cancer patients before transplantation is important because social support, optimism, and self-efficacy measured prior to HCT predicted health-related QOL 1-year posttransplantation (63). Not surprisingly, patients with previous psychiatric morbidity such as those patients with anxiety or depression are at risk for poorer health outcomes, longer length of hospital stay, and higher mortality (64–68).

During HCT, between 37% and 53% of patients experience mental disorders that meet the diagnostic criteria for psychiatric illness (69,70). Mood disturbances occur more frequently in patients undergoing HCT than in other types of cancer patients (71,72). The most common diagnosis is mixed anxiety and depressive reaction (69). In long-term survivors, defined as those who have survived >1-year posttransplant, 20% to 43% reported clinically significant global psychological distress (73,74). Of HCT survivors, only a minority consider themselves to have "returned to normal" following HCT. Discordance between pre-HCT expectations for returning to normal and current functional status was associated with greater current psychological distress; however, it is important to note that the rates of anxiety, depression, and posttraumatic stress disorder do decline with time after transplant (75,76). Some studies show that treatment-related distress decreases to baseline 5 years posttransplant, but there is a wide variability on the trajectory of recovery following HCT that depends on numerous factors such as physical limitations, social support, and coping styles (74,76–78). There is a large European study that shows HCT survivors had a higher incidence of suicidal and accidental death than the general population occurring between 1 year and >15 years posttransplant (79).

Unfortunately, only about 50% of distressed HCT survivors receive mental health services due to time limitations, lack of awareness of services available, embarrassment or discomfort associated with the need for mental health services, and physical limitations (80). It is important for clinicians to be aware of these barriers and address them. In addition to medications for psychiatric disturbances, clinicians should encourage patients to use mental health services and complementary services such as guided imagery, life review, relaxation breathing, and healing touch and increase physical activity or even simply go outside and experience sunshine. There is new data that show that using technology such as wearable sensor information to determine circadian rhythm, which can then help predict recovery of QOL after HCT (81). Clinicians can also further support the patient during regular visits by thorough empathic listening, providing information about both feelings and procedures, reframing negative statements, improving coping strategies, distraction, humor, giving opportunities to discuss fears and losses, arranging meetings with others who have had an HCT or suggesting an appropriate support group, and including family in all interventions, as appropriate. Reducing fears with these interventions has helped patients maintain hope (82).

Psychological effects of HCT are not only negative. HCT patients also report positive sequelae in conjunction with negative sequelae. The concept of posttraumatic growth has been evolving in the past decade and increasing numbers of studies are being done to evaluate the benefits that come from stressful ordeals such as HCT (83). Some of these benefits are having a new philosophy of life, having a greater appreciation of life, making changes in personal characteristics or attributes, finding support within the family, improving relationships within the family, and finding help and support from friends. The poorer the patient's prognosis and the more risk associated with the process predicted more positive sequelae. However, just as negative sequelae, positive sequelae diminished with time (80). Predictors of posttraumatic growth are good social support, the ability to approach rather than avoid, young age, less education, greater use of positive reinterpretation or cognitive appraisal sense of mastery, self-efficacy, problem solving, seeking alternative rewards, more stressful appraisal of the experience, and more negatively biased recall of pretransplant levels of psychological distress (71,83,84).

As the concept of posttraumatic growth becomes real, so does the concept of survival and survivorship. Mullan, a physician, faced with his own battle with cancer grappled with his own concept of survivorship and broke it into three phases:

- Acute survival—Surviving the initial diagnosis and treatment
- Extended survival—The time after treatment ceases and when the patient is most concerned about the disease returning or the treatment not working
- Permanent survival—When it appears the disease has been permanently eradicated or "cured" and the patient recommences his or her life but knowing that things have changed (85)

Survivorship is in part a psychological understanding that shows that the process of cancer and its treatment has psychological effects. They can be devastating, or they can lead to growth, but regardless, it is important to understand and appreciate that the psyche is forever changed in the process.

SOCIAL

Caregiver Effects

Caregivers are the unsung heroes of the HCT process. They give invaluable emotional and physical support during the patients' long hospital stays. Their presence alone protects the patients from loneliness and complete isolation. They are also an invaluable, though very ill-defined, part of the health care team. Without the caregiver, the health care team would be less able to understand the patient's specific and occasionally unspoken needs and, in addition, would not have the help in coaching, guiding, and motivating the patient throughout the long and volatile recovery period.

The presence of a caregiver has been associated with improved survival at 1 year after transplantation versus patients without a dedicated caregiver (86). HCT caregivers are females in 51% to 72% of cases, the patient's spouse 71% to 90% of the time, with a mean age of 43 to 50 years (37). Predictors of strain in family caregivers are younger age of persons with cancer, younger age of the caregiver, being a female caregiver, and being a spouse rather than a nonspouse. The strain is also most apparent in those of lower socioeconomic status (36). These caregivers are tasked with the responsibility of taking on unfamiliar roles without adequate support, which can lead to the potential for the development of interpersonal conflict within the family because of high levels of stress and the duty of managing multiple roles.

One of the earliest papers about HCT effects on the family was that of Lesko (88) published in 1994. Factors that were reported to affect better outcomes for caregivers and patients were awareness of the transplant process, preparation, and understanding of probable side effects and toxicities including those that would affect body image and patients' coping abilities. Around this time, the concept of primary caregiver as psychologically a "second-order patient" began to be more widely acknowledged (89). Further studies described five factors that affect caregiver vulnerability during the acute phase of HCT:

- Preexisting stress related to the initial cancer diagnosis
- The high level of uncertainty associated with the transplant process, especially if treatment is not curative
- The struggle to maintain one's sense of personal control over the situation
- The major disruption in the caregiver's personal life
- The financial burden and/or strain on family resources (90,91)

Multiple complications requiring repeated hospitalizations caused worse outcomes on all fronts. With all these vulnerabilities, it is not incredibly surprising that despite not having to go through the physical process of HCT, the effects of the patient's illness on the caregiver can cause emotional and functional distress at levels equal to or even greater than that of the patients themselves. They frequently feel that they must "be strong" and be the support and strength to their loved one. They end up suppressing their own emotional responses and are less likely to obtain mental health intervention than the patient (92).

In a 5-year longitudinal study comparing marital satisfaction after HCT, female spouses that were the caregivers of HCT recipients reported decreased martial satisfaction from 6 months through 5 years after transplant (93). In another study of QOL in spouse/partner caregivers and HCT recipients, caregivers and healthy controls reported better physical health than did HCT recipients; however, both partners and recipients reported more depressive symptoms and sleep and sexual problems than did controls. Moreover, caregivers reported less social support, decreased dyadic satisfaction and spiritual well-being, as well as more loneliness than both recipients and health controls. Furthermore, caregivers also reported less posttraumatic growth than did HCT recipients (92).

HCT caregivers in multiple studies have consistently identified early, in-depth education and physical and emotional aspects of care as most important to their well-being (87,94). Importance of open and early communication regarding the peritransplant process, expectations for discharge, long-term goals, and overall prognosis has been shown to decrease tension and foster a trusting relationship with the health care team (89). Psychoeducational interventions combine the use of written, group, and individual instruction to provide a thorough understanding of the type of care that is expected in terms of medications, adverse effects, symptoms, psychological support, and procedures to be performed—these interventions aid in satisfying the caregiver's educational needs and feelings of mastery with the transplant process (94–96). This is a beginning, but more studies need to be done as the process of HCT transitions from inpatient to outpatient. Will these changes increase or decrease strain on the caregiver? These are important questions, as caregiver presence is vitally important to patient outcomes and the changing trends in medical practice will continue to affect the caregiver.

Sexual Dysfunction/Infertility

Since the 1970s, sexual function has been identified as an important aspect of patient care (97). It may be difficult to discuss due to the sensitive and private nature of the subject, but, when asked, patients acknowledge that this is a significant concern (59). All aspects of the human sexual response can be affected by the transplantation process, and this is an important part of many patients' return to normalcy.

There are numerous factors that can lead to sexual dysfunction, such as a changed physique, reduced self-esteem, increased fear/uncertainty, fatigue, impotence, decreased libido, incontinence, infertility, premature ovarian failure/menopause, vaginal dryness, dyspareunia, depression, anxiety, and loss of meaning (98). Sexual dysfunction is a common complaint after transplantation but tends to be more common in women. One study by Syrjala et al. showed that 3 years after transplant, 80% of women reported at least one sexual problem as against 29% of men. Variables that predicted lower sexual satisfaction in men were older age, poorer psychological function, not being married, and lower sexual satisfaction prior to transplant. In contrast, there were no pretransplant predictors for women's posttransplant satisfaction (99). Another study by Syrjala et al. showed that both sexes declined in sexual activity at 6 months after HCT, but 77% of men recovered by 1 year while only 55% of women did in the same time period (100). This conclusion highlights the importance of posttransplant screening of sexual dysfunction, which is even more important in females. Adult women posttransplant should be evaluated by a gynecologist, and it is likely that many will need hormone replacement therapy, if not contraindicated, to maintain libido, sexual function, and bone density.

The PLISSIT model has been widely available for addressing sexual concerns since 1976 (101). It addresses the best way for clinicians to approach the subject and help both male and female patients with this very private matter. It consists of four major considerations:

- P—Permission: Create a comfortable climate that gives permission for patient to discuss sexual concerns, validating sexuality as a legitimate health issue.
- LI—Limited Information: Address specific sexual concerns and attempt to correct misinformation.
- SS—Specific Suggestions: Offer practical advice on how to deal with specific sexual problems.
- IT—Intensive Therapy: Refer to a specialist such as sex therapist, gynecologist, urologist, and psychiatrist if problem is not resolving.

In addition to addressing and supporting patients through their sexual concerns posttransplant, it is extremely important to also address their fertility concerns as loss of fertility can have a significant influence on QOL and is frequently reported as a "loss" by female HCT recipients (102–104). Some survivors, male and female, have reported that dealing with their loss of fertility was as painful as confronting cancer itself (105). For males, sperm banking is the cornerstone of fertility preservation; however, in one study only 91% of oncologists agreed that sperm banking should be offered to all eligible men. Yet in practice, only 48% offered it at all and those who did so did it <25% of the time, citing the difficulty in finding sperm banks, financial implications, and insufficient time (106). Another study showed that when offered, patients do elect for gamete/embryo preservation. After transplant, the collected material is used frequently and pregnancies in partners of male patients were often successful despite prolonged storage times (107). The frequency of pregnancy complications (caesarean section, preterm delivery, and low birth weight) was much higher in female allograft recipients compared with the normal population. This was more pronounced for females that received total body irradiation as part of their conditioning regimens. However, partners of male HCT recipients had uncomplicated pregnancies (108). Another study reported that HCT survivors of both genders had a lower prevalence of conception compared with their siblings but if pregnancy did occur, the outcome was likely to be favorable. Increased risk of infertility was reported when the HCT recipient was female, age at HCT was >30 years, and with use of total body irradiation in conditioning (109). Numerous studies show no increase in congenital abnormalities in patients that have undergone HCT (110).

Oncofertility is a new and rapidly growing field and one that should not be ignored as patients approach the perilous process of HCT (111). There are various options to preserve fertility, and they should be fully reviewed with patients before proceeding with the treatment.

Financial Burden

HCT is a highly technical process that involves many disciplines of care, and thus, it is very expensive and important to determine financial coverage early in the transplant process. Hematological cancers are significantly more expensive to treat than other common types of cancers (breast, colon, lung, and prostate) (112). There is a wide variation in estimates of cost of the transplant, from approximately $150,000 to approximately $600,000 depending on the type of transplant, adult or pediatric patient, source of stem cells, and whether it can be performed as an outpatient or inpatient basis (113). Costs include physician charges, medication cost, blood product and transfusion costs, graft procurement, hospitalization, and laboratory and radiologic investigations. In addition, there are many complications that can occur, and thus these complications can further increase the overall cost of the procedure. These complications (graft failure, dialysis, mechanical ventilation, and prolonged inpatient stay) are the main source of an increase in the total direct costs of HCT (114). There are numerous indirect costs associated with HCT such as lost wages and travel costs, as some patients need to travel and stay a significant distance from home. In addition, caregivers separately incur costs of care through money spent directly as well as time lost from work (115). There has been a trend to transition from inpatient to outpatient monitoring posttransplant that is helpful to reduce the cost of HCT but that will undoubtedly put more stress on caregivers.

In an ideal health care system, this is where insurance coverage would help. Unfortunately, limits on benefits and various types of cost-sharing in insurance plans may quickly lead to high out-of-pocket costs once cancer treatment begins. Some patients report more than $100,000 in medical bills, despite having an insurance policy throughout their treatment (116). In addition, people who depend on their employer for health insurance may not be protected from catastrophically high health care costs if they become too sick to work. While cancer patients who are unable to work can usually continue their employer-sponsored insurance coverage for up to 18 months by paying the full premium, that additional cost can be a substantial burden since these patients are typically living on a reduced income. In addition, the HCT process can last much longer than this especially if there are numerous posttransplant complications. Patients who survive for years after HCT may have trouble finding affordable insurance and others that try to apply for government programs such as Medicare or Medicaid face long waiting periods and strict eligibility guidelines. Medical costs are increasingly becoming the sole reason for bankruptcy, with a conservative estimate of two-thirds of all bankruptcies having a medical cause despite the fact that >75% of these people do have medical insurance (117). The National Donor Marrow Program (NDMP) provides a booklet titled "Mapping the Maze: A Personal Financial Guide to Blood Stem Cell Transplant," which helps patients through the financial, insurance, and legal obstacles of HCT and which at this time is also available for free download through the NDMP web site (118). Resources such as this are invaluable and of critical importance to helping the patient and caretaker navigate the financial burdens of care and find help in learning about grants and fundraising options.

Undoubtedly, these financial stressors can be significant in the patient's and caregiver's psychosocial distress. Unfortunately, there is a paucity of studies that have assessed the role of the health care team in addressing these financial burdens. As patients face the overwhelming process of HCT, it is important to provide resources for addressing their insurance coverage and limitations of their coverage, and possibly guiding them to other resources that can aid in paying their medical bills. Having a health care team member who is familiar with the patient's history, the transplant process, the insurance terminology, and other resources to help raise funds is a very important asset to the patient with yet another overwhelming task associated with the disease. This is especially important as sometimes insurance and cost issues can delay the transplant procedure, which then has the possibility of negatively affecting the process itself.

SPIRITUAL

From the beginning of the planning stages through the entire journey of HCT, this process will bring changes at many levels to the patient and the family. Any life-threatening illness can become a crisis time for the patient and family, which can bring up questions of mortality, the meaning of life, and the meaning of illness and test the bonds of relationships (119). These changes and questions can be even more pronounced in patients undergoing the long arduous process of HCT. Medicine has a long history of attempting to cure and relieve

suffering; however, from diagnosis through treatment and ideally into survivorship, the existential questions can be disconcerting and uncomfortable, thereby adding another dimension of suffering that medicine is not always equipped to address. The search for meaning is ongoing, is multifaceted, and may be lived out in a variety of ways. Living with illness and the harsh but powerful treatment it demands brings many changes, some of which lead to a sense of loss of control. The health care team, while often supportive, sometimes fails to see these needs of those they cared for, specifically these deeper spiritual ones (120).

In a small study in 1996 by Steeves, patients were interviewed within the first 100 days of HCT about the meaning of their lives during and following the transplant. In finding meaning, patients renegotiated their social position in their new situation and tried to reach an understanding of their experiences as a whole (121). The conclusion of the study was a focus on the concept of holism and the importance of listening to the patient perspective. Another study looked at global meaning (the belief that life has a purpose and coherence) and showed that having global meaning was associated with less psychological distress (122). Chronic GVHD patients typically have lower QOL scores; however, a higher level of spiritual well-being was a significant independent predictor of contentment with QOL in these patients (123). Disappointingly, about 50% of cancer patients report that their spiritual needs are not being supported by a religious community and about 70% report that their spiritual needs are not being supported by the medical system. Spiritual support by religious communities or the medical system is associated with improvements in patient's QOL (124). If this was any other medical outcome, it would be considered a treatment failure and rapidly addressed. While there is increasing research in this area, it is imperative that this support be addressed more aggressively and more seriously in this fragile population.

As we know that addressing spiritual matters improves patient's QOL, we as clinicians should encourage these behaviors or, at the very least, have someone on the team that can do so. Often patients and families turn to the health care team to help directly or indirectly answer these spiritual concerns. Clinicians can easily miss the importance of how that which is not present gives depth, perspective, and clues to the real meaning of social action in clinical encounters (125). People with a religious faith may find it helpful talking to a priest, pastor, imam, rabbi, or other religious leader, while others may find it important to have quiet time to reflect, read, walk in nature, be artistic, spend time with loved ones, or do other things that bring meaning to their lives. We cannot continue

TABLE 58.2 SUPPORTING SPIRITUAL DISTRESS

- Being present for the patient without the need of "doing" something
- Allowing time, space, and privacy to explore issues
- Asking questions directly and indirectly about meaning
- Watching and listening for cues of spiritual distress
- Being aware of own spirituality
- Caring for self
- Showing humility
- Being aware of the patient's culture and religious spiritual needs
- Involving pastoral support/prayer
- Offering use of labyrinths
- Art therapy/Mandalas
- Healing touch/Reiki
- Meditation apps

to miss the opportunities to further explore these profound concerns (Table 58.2).

The clinician who dares to ask about spirituality imparts a vital message to the patients that they are being cared for by someone who has not forgotten that a broken patient remains a whole person and that healing transcends survival (126). As one approaches this topic, it is central to realize that supportive care is not always about fixing the situation. It is about awareness of the patient's inner life and remembering it does not want to be fixed, but often it wants simply to be seen and heard. In the text, *Sharing the Darkness,* by Cassidy, she describes moments that occur when a doctor or nurse is confronted with a painful situation and there seems to be nothing that can be done. However, she implores that if the doctor or nurse can simply stay with that person during the uncomfortable and difficult time, then they will have shared a moment of that person's darkness, which thereby

gives support (127). Quinn goes so far as to state that the clinical team member will find it difficult to recognize or support the patient/family in this search if that team member is unaware of his or her own search to find meaning and own need for support (120). There are many proponents for further medical education on spirituality needs of self and patient (128,129). In addition, specific courses have been developed for clinicians to explore and support spiritual and religious issues confronting critically ill patients and their families (130).

Moving from the numinous to the tangible, there are many discrete treatment plans and modalities that have been shown to be effective in positively affecting the patient's spiritual needs. Art therapy is shown to help patients who have difficult family relationships prior to admission and those who wish to explore existential/spiritual issues (131). The meaning-making intervention is a novel psychological intervention that consists of discrete tasks that address the normative distress associated with the search for meaning within the context of cancers of many types (132). Negative spiritual coping is associated with worse outcomes in HCT patients (133). More studies need to be done, but it would make sense that candidly helping patients explore their existential issues can possibly help them improve their coping skills and hopefully lead to improved outcomes and QOL.

CONCLUSION

Support for the HCT patient and family is greatly needed as the effects of transplantation are far-reaching and profound. In this chapter, we have highlighted only a few of the many physical, psychological, social, and spiritual effects and interventions of HCT (Table 58.3). It is our hope that

TABLE 58.3 SUPPORTIVE CARE INTERVENTIONS

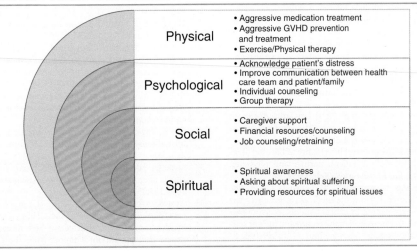

Physical	• Aggressive medication treatment • Aggressive GVHD prevention and treatment • Exercise/Physical therapy
Psychological	• Acknowledge patient's distress • Improve communication between health care team and patient/family • Individual counseling • Group therapy
Social	• Caregiver support • Financial resources/counseling • Job counseling/retraining
Spiritual	• Spiritual awareness • Asking about spiritual suffering • Providing resources for spiritual issues

in compiling this information in one location, the body of the present research as well as its shortcomings can be viewed, and a more unified holistic approach could be developed. This is just the beginning of understanding and supporting patients as they try to maintain their QOL throughout the process of HCT. The diverse effects and highly individual patient responses often require a team approach that is large and flexible. There are an increasing number of proposals to incorporate palliative care teams in the management of all patients preparing to endure the process of HCT (134,135). Palliative care team expertise in symptom management and holistic care with an interdisciplinary team approach would benefit patients and the HCT team as they help address the comprehensive care of the HCT patient. Just as the biomedical cornerstones of care must be addressed to treat the diseases leading to HCT, early and continuous interventions in supportive physical, psychological, social, and spiritual care must become the standard of care in order to effectively treat the patient.

REFERENCES

1. Gratwohl A, Baldomero H, Aljurf M, et al. Hematopoietic stem cell transplantation a global perspective. *JAMA*. 2010;303:1617-1624.
2. Gratwohl A, Pasquini MC, Aljurf MD, et al. Global hematopoietic stem cell transplantation (HSCT) at one million: an achievement of pioneers and foreseeable challenges for the next decade. A report from the Worldwide Network For Blood and Marrow Transplantation (WBMT). *Blood*. 2013;122(21):213.
3. Wingard JR, Majhail NS, Brazauskas R, et al. Long-term survival and late deaths after allogeneic hematopoietic cell transplantation. *J Clin Oncol*. 2011;29(16):2230-2239.
4. Pidala J, Anasetti C, Jim H. Quality of life after allogenic hematopoietic cell transplantation. *Blood*. 2009;114:7-19.
5. Kopp M, Schweigkofler H, Holzner B, et al. EORTC QLQ-C30 and FACT-BMT for the measurement of quality of life in bone marrow transplant recipients: a comparison. *Eur J Haematol*. 2000;65:97-103.
6. Bevans MF, Mitchell SA, Marden S. The symptom experience in the first 100 days following allogeneic hematopoietic stem cell transplantation. *Support Care Cancer*. 2008;16:1243-1254.
7. Kirkova J, Walsh D, Aktas A, Davis MP. Cancer symptom clusters: old concept but new data. *Am J Hosp Palliat Care*. 2010;27:282-288.
8. Baker, F, Denniston M, Smith T, West MM. Adult cancer survivors: how are they faring? *Cancer*. 2005;104: 2565-2576.
9. Lee SJ, Joffe S, Kim HT, et al. Physicians' attitudes about quality-of-life issues in hematopoietic stem cell transplantation. *Blood*. 2004;104:2194-2200.
10. Hendrinks MG, Schouten HC. Quality of life after stem cell transplantation: a patient, partner and physician perspective. *Eur J Intern Med*. 2002;13:52-56.
11. Strömgren AS, Groenvold M, Pedersen L, Olsen AK, Spile M, Sjøgren P. Does the medical record cover the symptoms experienced by cancer patients receiving palliative care? A comparison of the record and patient self-rating. *J Pain Symptom Manage*. 2001;21(3):189-196.
12. Bury M. Chronic illness as a biographical disruption. *Social Health Illn*. 1982;4:167-182.
13. Schaffer JV. The changing face of graft-versus-host disease. *Semin Cutan Med Surg*. 2006;25:190-200.
14. Filipovich AH, Weisdorf D, Pavletic S, et al. National Institutes of Health consensus development project on criteria for clinical trials in chronic graft-versus-host disease: I. Diagnosis and staging working group report. *Biol Blood Marrow Transplant*. 2005;11:945-956.
15. Pavletic SZ, Vogelsang GB, Lee SJ. 2014 National Institutes of Health Consensus Development project on criteria for clinical trials in chronic graft-versus-host disease: preface to the series. *Biol Blood Marrow Transplant*. 2015;21(3):387-388.
16. Baker KS, Fraser CJ. Quality of life and recovery after graft-versus-host disease. *Best Pract Res Clin Haematol*. 2008;21:333-341.
17. Kurosawa S, et al. Quality of life after allogeneic hematopoietic cell transplantation according to affected organ and severity of chronic graft-versus-host disease. *Biol Blood Marrow Transplant*. 2017;23(10):1749-1758.
18. Lee SJ, Kim HT, Ho VT, et al. Quality of life associated with acute and chronic graft-vs-host disease. *Bone Marrow Transplant*. 2006;38:305-310.
19. Joachim Deeg H, Flowers ME. Acute graft-versus-host disease. In: Treleaven J, Barrett AJ, eds. *Hematopoietic Stem Cell Transplantation in Clinical Practice*. Elsevier Limited; 2009:387-400.
20. Weisdorf D. GVHD the nuts and bolts. *Hematology Am Soc Hematol Educ Program*. 2007:62-67.
21. Jacobsohn DA, Vogelsang GB. Acute graft versus host disease. *Orphanet J Rare Dis*. 2007;2:35.
22. Ferrara JL, Levine JE, Reddy P, Holler E. Graft-versus-host disease. *Lancet*. 2009;373:1550-1561.
23. Saurat JH. Cutaneous manifestations of graft versus-host disease. *Int J Dermatol*. 1981;20:249-256.
24. Cutler C, Antin JH. Manifestations and treatment of acute graft-versus-host disease. In: Appelbaum FR, Forman SJ, Negrin RS, Blume KG, eds. *Thomas' Hematopoietic Cell Transplantation: Stem Cell Transplantation*. Wiley-Blackwell; 2009:1287-1303.
25. Chavan R, el-Azhary R. Cutaneous graft-versus-host disease: rationales and treatment options. *Dermatol Ther*. 2011;24:219-228.
26. Ross WA. Treatment of gastrointestinal acute graft-versus-host disease. *Curr Treat Options Gastroenterol*. 2005;8:249-258.
27. Nassereddine S, Rafei H, Elbahesh E, Tabbara IA. Acute graft versus host disease: a comprehensive review. *Anticancer Res*. 2017;37(4):1547-1555.
28. Saliba RM, de Lima M, Giralt S, et al. Hyperacute GVHD: risk factors, outcomes, and clinical implications. *Blood*. 2007;109:2751-2758.
29. Ippoliti C, Champlin R, Bugazia N, et al. Use of octreotide in the symptomatic management of diarrhea induced by graft-versus-host disease in patients with hematologic malignancies. *J Clin Oncol*. 1997;15:3350-3354.
30. Bolaños-Meade J, Vogelsang GB. Novel strategies for steroid-refractory acute graft-versus-host disease. *Curr Opin Hematol*. 2005;12:40-44.
31. Lee SJ, Vogelsang G, Flowers ME. Chronic graft-versus-host disease. *Biol Blood Marrow Transplant*. 2003;9: 215-233.
32. Socié G, Salooja N, Cohen A, et al. Nonmalignant late effects after allogeneic stem cell transplantation. *Blood*. 2003;101:3373-3385.
33. Arai S, Arora M, Wang T, et al.; Graft-vs-Host Disease Working Committee of the CIBMTR. Increasing incidence of chronic graft-versus-host disease in allogeneic transplantation: a report from the Center for

International Blood and Marrow Transplant Research. *Biol Blood Marrow Transplant*. 2015;21(2):266–274.

34. Lee, SJ Have we made progress in the management of chronic graft-v-host disease? *Best Pract Res Clin Haematol*. 2010;23:529-535.

35. Wagner JL, Seidel K, Boeckh M, et al. De novo chronic graft-versus-host disease in marrow graft recipients given methotrexate and cyclosporine: risk factors and survival. *Biol Blood Marrow Transplant*. 2000;6:633-639.

36. Remberger M, Kumlien G, Aschan J, et al. Risk factors for moderate-to-severe chronic graft-versus-host disease after allogeneic hematopoietic stem cell transplantation. *Biol Blood Marrow Transplant*. 2002;8:674-682.

37. Wolff D, Schleuning M, von Harsdorf S, et al. Consensus conference on clinical practice in chronic GVHD: second-line treatment of chronic graft-versus-host disease. *Biol Blood Marrow Transplant*. 2011;17:1-17.

38. Akpek G, Zahurak ML, Piantadosi S, et al. Development of a prognostic model for grading chronic graft-versus-host disease. *Blood*. 2001;97:1219-1226.

39. Flowers ME, Martin PJ. How we treat chronic graft-versus-host disease. *Blood*. 2015;125(4):606-615.

40. Shlomchik WD, Lee SJ, Couriel D, Pavletic SZ. Transplantation's greatest challenges: advances in chronic graft-versus-host disease. *Biol Blood Marrow Transplant*. 2007;13:2-10.

41. Couriel DR. Ancillary and supportive care in chronic GVHD. *Best Pract Res Clin Haematol*. 2008;21:291-307.

42. Wingard JR, Vogelsang GB, Deeg HJ. Stem cell transplantation: supportive care and long-term complications. *Hematol Am Soc Hematol Educ Program*. 2002;2002:422-444.

43. Couriel D, Carpenter PA, Cutler C, et al. Ancillary therapy and supportive care of chronic graft-versus-host disease: national institutes of health consensus development project on criteria for clinical trials in chronic graft-versus-host disease: V. Ancillary Therapy and Supportive Care Working Group Report. *Biol Blood Marrow Transplant*. 2006;12:375-396.

44. Ratanatharathorn V, Ayash L, Lazarus HM, Fu J, Uberti JP. Chronic graft-versus-host disease: clinical manifestation and therapy. *Bone Marrow Transplant*. 2001;28:121-129.

45. Cowen EW, Hymes SR. Cutaneous manifestations of chronic graft versus host disease. In: Vogelsang GB, Pavletic SZ, eds. *Chronic Graft Versus Host Disease: Interdisciplinary Management*. Cambridge University Press; 2009:169-181.

46. Demarosi F, Lodi G, Carrassi A, Soligo D, Sardella A. Oral malignancies following HSCT: graft versus host disease and other risk factors. *Oral Oncol*. 2005;41:865-877.

47. Imanguli MM, Alevizos I, Brown R, Pavletic SZ, Atkinson JC. Oral graft-versus-host disease. *Oral Dis*. 2008;14:396-412.

48. Schubert MM, Sullivan KM. Recognition, incidence, and management of oral graft-versus-host disease. *NCI Monogr*. 1990;9:135-143.

49. Livesey SJ, Holmes JA, Whittaker JA. Ocular complications of bone marrow transplantation. *Eye*. 1989;3:271-276.

50. Malta JB, Soong HK, Shtein RM, et al. Treatment of ocular graft-versus-host disease with topical cyclosporine 0.05% *Cornea*. 2010;29(12):1392-1396.

51. Kim SK, Smith JA, Dunn JP. Chronic ocular graft versus host disease. In: Vogelsang GB, Pavletic SZ, eds. *Chronic Graft Versus Host Disease: Interdisciplinary Management*. Cambridge University Press; 2009:199-206.

52. Turner ML, Stratton P. Gynecological manifestations of chronic graft versus host disease. In: Vogelsang GB, Pavletic SZ, eds. *Chronic Graft versus Host Disease: Interdisciplinary Management*. Cambridge University Press; 2009:207-215.

53. Chung CP, Sargent RE, Chung NT, et al. Graft-versus-host disease associated vulvovaginal symptoms after bone marrow transplantation. *Biol Blood Marrow Transplant*. 2016;22(2):378-379.

54. Spiryda LB, Laufer MR, Soiffer RJ, et al. Graft-versus-host disease of the vulva and/or vagina: diagnosis and treatment. *Biol Blood Marrow Transplant*. 2003;9:760-765.

55. Anderson M, Kutzner S, Kaufman RH. Treatment of vulvovaginal lichen planus with vaginal hydrocortisone suppositories. *Obstet Gynecol*. 2002;100:359-362.

56. McQuellon RP, Andrykowski M. Psychosocial issues in hematopoietic cell transplantation. In: Appelbaum FR, Forman SJ, Negrin RS, eds. *Thomas' Hematopoietic Cell Transplantation: Stem Cell Transplantation*. 4th ed. Oxford, UK: Wiley-Blackwell; 2009:488-501.

57. Schulz-Kindermann F, Hennings U, Ramm G, Zander AR, Hasenbring M. The role of biomedical and psychosocial factors for the prediction of pain and distress in patients undergoing high-dose therapy and BMT/PBSCT. *Bone Marrow Transplant*. 2002;29:341-351.

58. Sherman RS, Cooke E, Grant M. Dialogue among survivors of hematopoietic cell transplantation support-group themes. *J Psychosoc Oncol*. 2005;23:1-24.

59. Adler NE, Page AEK, eds. *Cancer Care for the Whole Patient: Meeting Psychosocial Health Needs*. Washington, DC: Institute of Medicine. The National Academies Press; 2008.

60. Nakamura ZM, Nash RP, Quillen LJ, et al. Psychiatric care in hematopoietic stem cell transplantation. *Psychosomatics*. 2019;60:227-237.

61. Amonoo HL, Massey CN, Freedman ME, et al. Psychological considerations in hematopoietic stem cell transplantation. *Psychosomatics*. 2019;60(4):331-342.

62. Eldredge DH, Nail LM, Maziarz RT, Hansen LK, Ewing D, Archbold PG. Explaining family caregiver role strain following autologous blood and marrow transplantation. *J Psychosoc Oncol*. 2006;24:53-74.

63. Hochhausen N, Altmaier EM, McQuellon R, et al. Social support, optimism, and self-efficacy predict physical and emotional well-being after bone marrow transplantation. *J Psychosoc Oncol*. 2007;25:87-101.

64. Prieto JM, Blanch J, Atala J, et al. Stem cell transplantation: risk factors for psychiatric morbidity. *Eur J Cancer*. 2006;42:514-520.

65. Garcia C Jr, Botega NJ, De Souza CA. A psychosocial assessment interview of candidates for hematopoietic stem cell transplantation. *Haematologica*. 2005;90:570-572.

66. Prieto JM, Blanch J, Atala J, et al. Psychiatric morbidity and impact on hospital length of stay among hematologic cancer patients receiving stem-cell transplantation. *J Clin Oncol*. 2002;20:1907-1917.

67. Goetzmann L, Klaghofer R, Wagner-Huber R, et al. Psychosocial need for counseling before and after a lung, liver or allogenic bone marrow transplant—results of a prospective study. *Z Psychosom Med Psychother*. 2006;52:230-242.

68. Goetzmann L, Klaghofer R, Wagner-Huber R, et al. Quality of life and psychosocial situation before and after a lung, liver or an allogeneic bone marrow transplant. *Swiss Med Wkly*. 2006;136:281-290.

69. Khan AG, Irfan M, Shamsi TS, Hussain M. Psychiatric disorders in bone marrow transplant patients. *J Coll Physicians Surg Pak*. 2007;17:98-100.

70. Fritzsche K, Struss Y, Stein B, Spahn C. Psychosomatic liaison service in hematological oncology: need for psychotherapeutic interventions and their realization. *Hematol Oncol.* 2003;21:83-89.

71. Cooke L, Gemmill R, Kravits K, Grant M. Psychological issues of stem cell transplantation. *Semin Oncol Nurs.* 2009;25:139-150.

72. Andrykowski MA, Henslee PJ, Barnett RL. Longitudinal assessment of psychosocial functioning of adult survivors of allogeneic bone marrow transplantation. *Bone Marrow Transplant.* 1989;4:505-509.

73. Rusiewicz A, DuHamel KN, Burkhalter J, et al. Psychological distress in long-term survivors of hematopoietic stem cell transplantation. *Psychooncology.* 2008;17:329-337.

74. McQuellon RP, Russell GB, Rambo TD, et al. Quality of life and psychological distress of bone marrow transplant recipients: the 'time trajectory' to recovery over the first year. *Bone Marrow Transplant.* 1998;21:477-486.

75. Andrykowski MA, Brady MJ, Greiner CB, et al. 'Returning to normal' following bone marrow transplantation: outcomes, expectations and informed consent. *Bone Marrow Transplant.* 1995;15:573-581.

76. Sun CL, Francisco L, Baker KS, Weisdorf DJ, Forman SJ, Bhatia S. Adverse psychological outcomes in long-term survivors of hematopoietic cell transplantation: a report from the Bone Marrow Transplant Survivor Study. *Blood.* 2011;118(17):4723-4731.

77. Syrjala KL, Langer SL, Abrams JR, et al. Recovery and long-term function after hematopoietic cell transplantation for leukemia or lymphoma. *J Am Med Assoc.* 2004;291:2335-2343.

78. Fromm K, Andrykowski MA, Hunt J. Positive and negative psychosocial sequelae of bone marrow transplantation: implications for quality of life assessment. *J Behav Med.* 1996;19:221-240.

79. Tichelli A, Labopin M, Rovo A. Increase of suicide and accidental death after hematopoietic stem cell transplantation: a cohort study on behalf of the Late Effects Working Party of the European Group for Blood and Marrow Transplantation (EBMT). *Cancer.* 2013;119:2012-2021.

80. Mosher CE, DuHamel KN, Rini CM, et al. Barriers to mental health service use among hematopoietic SCT survivors. *Bone Marrow Transplant.* 2010;45:570-579.

81. Hoogland AI, Bulls HW, Gonzalez BD, et al. Circadian rhythmicity as a predictor of quality of life in allogeneic hematopoietic cell transplant patients. *J Pain Symptom Manage.* 2019;57(5):952-960.

82. Cohen MZ, Ley CD. Bone marrow transplantation: the battle for hope in the face of fear. *Oncol Nurs Forum.* 2000;27:473-480.

83. Widows MR, Jacobsen PB, Booth-Jones M, Fields KK. Predictors of posttraumatic growth following bone marrow transplantation for cancer. *Health Psychol.* 2005;24:266-273.

84. Jacobsen PB, Sadler IJ, Booth-Jones M, et al. Predictors of posttraumatic stress disorder symptomatology following bone marrow transplantation for cancer. *J Consult Clin Psychol.* 2002;70:235-240.

85. Mullan F. Seasons of survival: reflections of a physician with cancer. *N Engl J Med.* 1985;313:270-273.

86. Bolwell BJ, Foster L, McLellan L, et al. The presence of a caregiver is a powerful prognostic variable of survival following allogeneic bone marrow transplantation. *Proc Am Soc Hematol.* 2001;98:202A (abstract 845).

87. Chow K, Coyle N. Providing palliative care to family caregivers throughout the bone marrow transplantation trajectory: research and practice: partners in care. *J Hosp Palliat Nurs.* 2011;13:7-13.

88. Lesko LM. Bone marrow transplantation: support of the patient and his/her family. *Support Care Cancer.* 1994;2:35-49.

89. Lederberg MS. The family of the cancer patient. In: Holland JC, ed. *Psycho-Oncology.* 1st ed. New York, NY: Oxford University Press; 1998:981.

90. Fife BL, Monahan PO, Abonour R, Wood LL, Stump TE. Adaptation of family caregivers during the acute phase of adult BMT. *Bone Marrow Transplant.* 2009;43:959-966.

91. Simon RW. The meanings individuals attach to role identities and their implications for mental health. *J Health Soc Behav.* 1997;38:256-274.

92. Bishop MM, Beaumont JL, Hahn EA, et al. Late effects of cancer and hematopoietic stem-cell transplantation on spouses or partners compared with survivors and survivor-matched controls. *J Clin Oncol.* 2007;25:1403-1411.

93. Langer SL, Yi JC, Storer BE, Syrjala KL. Marital adjustment, satisfaction and dissolution among hematopoietic stem cell transplant patients and spouses: a prospective, five-year longitudinal investigation. *Psychooncology.* 2010;19:190-200.

94. Cooke L, Grant M, Eldredge DH, Maziarz RT, Nail LM. Informal caregiving in hematopoietic blood and marrow transplant patients. *Eur J Oncol Nurs.* 2011;15:500-507.

95. Honea NJ, Brintnall R, Given B, et al. Putting evidence into practice: nursing assessment and interventions to reduce family caregiver strain and burden. *Clin J Oncol Nurs.* 2008;12:507-516.

96. Grimm PM, Zawacki KL, Mock V, Krumm S, Frink BB. Caregiver responses and needs: an ambulatory bone marrow transplant model. *Cancer Pract.* 2000;8:120-128.

97. Hughes MK. Alterations of sexual function in women with cancer. *Semin Oncol Nurs.* 2008;24:91-101.

98. Quinn B. Psychologic and supportive care issues in the transplant setting. In: Treleaven J, Barrett AJ, eds. *Hematopoietic Stem Cell Transplantation in Clinical Practice.* Elsevier Limited; 2009:369-377.

99. Syrjala KL, Roth-Roemer SL, Abrams JR, et al. Prevalence and predictors of sexual dysfunction in long-term survivors of marrow transplantation. *J Clin Oncol.* 1998;16:3148-3157.

100. Syrjala KL, Kurland BF, Abrams JR, et al. Sexual function changes during the 5 years after high-dose treatment and hematopoietic cell transplantation for malignancy with case-matched controls at 5 years. *Blood.* 2008;111:989-996.

101. Annon, JS. *Behavioral Treatment of Sexual Problems: Brief Therapy.* New York, NY: Harper & Row; 1976.

102. Hammond C, Abrams JR, Syrjala KL. Fertility and risk factors for elevated infertility concern in 10-year hematopoietic cell transplant survivors and case-matched controls. *J Clin Oncol.* 2007;25:3511-3517.

103. Watson M, Wheatley K, Harrison GA, et al. Severe adverse impact on sexual functioning and fertility of bone marrow transplantation, either allogeneic or autologous, compared with consolidation chemotherapy alone: analysis of the MRC AML 10 trial. *Cancer.* 1999;86:1231-1239.

104. Curbow B, Legro MW, Baker F, Wingard JR, Somerfield MR. Loss and recovery themes of long-term survivors of bone marrow transplants. *J Psychosoc Oncol.* 1993;10:1-20.

105. Schover LR. Motivation for parenthood after cancer: a review. *J Natl Cancer Inst Monogr.* 2005;34:2-5.

106. Schover LR, Brey K, Lichtin A, Lipshultz LI, Jeha S. Oncologists' attitudes and practices regarding banking sperm before cancer treatment. *J Clin Oncol.* 2002;20:1890-1897.

107. Babb A, Farah N, Lyons C, et al. Uptake and outcome of assisted reproductive techniques in long-term survivors of SCT. *Bone Marrow Transplant.* 2011;47(4):568-573. http://www.nature.com/bmt/journal/vaop/ncurrent/full/bmt2011134a.html

108. Salooja N, Szydlo RM, Socie G, et al. Pregnancy outcomes after peripheral blood or bone marrow transplantation: a retrospective survey. *Lancet.* 2001;358:271-276.

109. Carter A, Robison LL, Francisco L, et al. Prevalence of conception and pregnancy outcomes after hematopoietic cell transplantation: report from the Bone Marrow Transplant Survivor Study. *Bone Marrow Transplant.* 2006;37:1023-1029.

110. Loren AW, Chow E, Jacobsohn DA, et al. Pregnancy after hematopoietic cell transplantation: a report from the late effects working committee of the Center for International Blood and Marrow Transplant Research. *Biol Blood Marrow Transplant.* 2011;17:157-166.

111. Woodruff TK. The emergence of a new interdiscipline: oncofertility. *Cancer Treat Res.* 2007;138:3-11.

112. Greenberg D, Earle C, Fang CH, Eldar-Lissai A, Neumann PJ. When is cancer care cost-effective? A systematic overview of cost-utility analyses in oncology. *J Natl Cancer Inst.* 2010;20;102:82-88.

113. Broder MS, Quock TP, Chang E, et al. The cost of hematopoietic stem-cell transplantation in the United States. *Am Health Drug Benefits.* 2017;10(7):366-374.

114. Majhail NS, Mothukuri JM, Brunstein CG, Weisdorf DJ. Costs of hematopoietic cell transplantation: comparison of umbilical cord blood and matched related donor transplantation and the impact of posttransplant complications. *Biol Blood Marrow Transplant.* 2009;15:564-573.

115. Meehan KR, Fitzmaurice T, Root L, Kimtis E, Patchett L, Hill J. The financial requirements and time commitments of caregivers for autologous stem cell transplant recipients. *J Support Oncol.* 2006;4(4):187-190.

116. Schwartz K, Claxton G, Martin K, Schmidt C. *Spending to Survive: Cancer Patients Confront Holes in the Health Insurance System.* Kaiser Family Foundation & American Cancer Society; February 2009. http://www.kff.org/insurance/upload/7851.pdf

117. Himmelstein DU, Thorne D, Warren E, Woolhandler S. Medical bankruptcy in the United States, 2007: results of a national study. *Am J Med.* 2009;122:741-746.

118. Jolley P, Storey J, Richetts J. *Mapping the Maze, National Marrow Donor Program*; October 2015. https://bethematch.org/uploadedfiles/bethematch-content/patients_and_families/before_transplant/planning_how_things_will_get_done/612%20mm%20financial%20planning%20before%20transplant.pdf. Accessed September 10, 2019.

119. Bolen JS. *Close to the Bone: Life-Threatening Illness and the Search for Meaning.* New York, NY: Touchstone; 1996.

120. Quinn B. Cancer and the treatment: does it make sense to patients? *Hematology.* 2005;10(suppl 1):325-328.

121. Steeves RH. Patients who have undergone bone marrow transplantation: their quest for meaning. *Oncol Nurs Forum.* 1992;19:899-905.

122. Vehling S, Lehmann C, Oechsle K, et al. Global meaning and meaning-related life attitudes: exploring their role in predicting depression, anxiety, and demoralization in cancer patients, *Support Care Cancer.* 2011;19:513-520.

123. Harris BA, Berger AM, Mitchell SA, et al. Spiritual well-being in long-term survivors with chronic graft-versus-host disease after hematopoietic stem cell transplantation. *J Support Oncol.* 2010;8:119-125.

124. Balboni TA, Vanderwerker LC, Block SD, et al. Religiousness and spiritual support among advanced cancer patients and associations with end-of-life treatment preferences and quality of life. *J Clin Oncol.* 2007;25:555-560.

125. Buetow SA. Something in nothing: negative space in the clinician-patient relationship. *Ann Fam Med.* 2009;7:80-83.

126. Ferrell B. Meeting spiritual needs: what is an oncologist to do? *J Clin Oncol.* 2007;25:467-468.

127. Cassidy S. *Sharing in the Darkness.* London, UK: Darton, Longman and Todd; 1988.

128. Graves DL, Shue CK, Arnold L. The role of spirituality in patient care: incorporating spirituality training into medical school curriculum. *Acad Med.* 2002;77:1167.

129. Barnett KG, Fortin AH VI. Spirituality and medicine. A workshop for medical students and residents. *J Gen Intern Med.* 2006;21:481-485.

130. Todres ID, Catlin EA, Thiel MM. The intensivist in a spiritual care training program adapted for clinicians. *Crit Care Med.* 2005;33:2733-2736.

131. Gabriel B, Bromberg E, Vandenbovenkamp J, Walka P, Kornblith AB, Luzzato P. Art therapy with adult bone marrow transplant patients in isolation: a pilot study. *Pyscho-oncology.* 2001;10:114-123.

132. Lee V. The existential plight of cancer: meaning making as a concrete approach to the intangible search for meaning. *Support Care Cancer.* 2008;16:779-785.

133. Sherman AC, Plante TG, Simonton S, Latif U, Anaissie EJ. Prospective study of religious coping among patients undergoing autologous stem cell transplantation. *J Behav Med.* 2009;32:118-128.

134. Chung HM, Lyckholm LJ, Smith TJ. Palliative care in BMT. *Bone Marrow Transplant.* 2009;43:265-273.

135. Mitchell SA, Palliative care during and following allogeneic hematopoietic stem cell transplantation. *Curr Opin Support Palliat Care.* 2018;12(1):58-64.

59 Survivorship Issues in Pediatrics

Rebecca Berger and Lynda Kwon Beaupin

INTRODUCTION

Currently, there are over 15 million survivors of cancer in the United States—over 400,000 of whom are survivors of pediatric cancers (1,2). Due to continued advancements in cancer treatment, the overall survival of children with cancer is >80% after 5 years from diagnosis (3). Cancer treatment is, however, often associated with long-term and late effects that increase risk of adverse health and decreased quality life compared to healthy peers (4). These include increased chronic health conditions (5), hospitalizations (6), physical limitations (7), psychological distress (8), and neurocognitive dysfunction (9). In 2005, a seminal report from the Institute of Medicine (IOM), "From Cancer Patient to Cancer Survivor: Lost in Transition," highlighted the need to recognize survivorship as a distinct phase in cancer care and the need to address the concerns of survivors (10). "Cancer survivorship" encompasses the myriad of issues faced by those who have completed cancer treatment. In pediatric oncology, "survivorship" typically refers to the time after a patient is approximately 2 or more years from completion of treatment.

Although long-term health outcomes among pediatric cancer survivors have been studied since the 1970s, advances in treatment of pediatric cancers, and in medicine's knowledge of late effects of therapy, make ongoing research in survivorship imperative. Findings help guide clinical care for patients and assist in developing effective screening guidelines to reduce long-term morbidity. In this chapter, we review some of the more common medical and psychosocial conditions for which childhood cancer survivors are at risk, discuss models of care and the need for risk-based monitoring for the said health conditions, and provide information on resources available to health care providers following childhood cancer survivors. We also address some of the unique issues faced by patients who are diagnosed with cancer during their adolescent and young adult (AYA) years.

LATE-TERM COMORBIDITIES

The survival rate of pediatric cancer has increased to >80% in the past several decades (11). However, the same treatments that cure cancer put survivors at risk for a host of late-term complications including cardiovascular, pulmonary, endocrine, and central nervous system (CNS) changes. These, in turn, have significant impact on morbidity and mortality. Greater than 80% of survivors will develop serious, life-threatening health conditions by age 45 (12). (See Table 59.1 for list of late-term health complications of childhood cancer survivors.) Survivors of pediatric and young adult cancer tend to pursue lifestyles, which may further increase their risk and exacerbate long-term complications: they tend to have suboptimal diets, are more sedentary than their siblings, and are at increased risk of substance abuse. Providers must focus on the lifestyle of young survivors to mitigate the risk of late-term effects (14).

Cardiovascular

Cardiovascular complications of childhood cancer survivors are among the most serious, causing significant morbidity and mortality. Highest risk is with survivors treated with anthracyclines, with 65% of survivors treated with anthracyclines, including doxorubicin, daunorubicin, and mitoxantrone, experiencing late cardiovascular toxicities (11). Antineoplastic agents work by destroying rapidly dividing malignant cells and in the process destroy healthy cells with high division rates including cardiomyocytes. Cardiomyocytes have limited ability to repair themselves unlike the bone marrow, gastrointestinal cells, and other healthy cells that are damaged during treatment, leading to long-term damage. Anthracyclines lead to cardiotoxicity through a variety of mechanisms, but the most acknowledged is the "oxidative stress hypothesis." When anthracyclines enter cells and form complexes with iron, they form free radicals leading to cell death and damage (15). Around 50% of childhood cancer survivors will be exposed to anthracyclines during treatment (15). Besides anthracycline exposure, several other treatments involved in childhood cancer cause cardiac damage including chest radiation, cyclophosphamide, cranial irradiation, ifosfamide, paclitaxel, 5-fluorouracil, cisplatin, and tyrosine kinase inhibitors (11,15). Risk factors for chemotherapy-induced

TABLE 59.1 LATE-TERM COMORBIDITIES IN CHILDHOOD CANCER SURVIVORS

System impacted	Late effect	Exposures	Other risk factors
Cardiovascular	Cardiomyopathy Subclinical left ventricular dysfunction Congestive heart failure Arrhythmia	Radiation therapy Anthracyclines Platinums	Hypertension, lipid abnormalities, diabetes, obesity, smoking, illicit drug use, alcohol
Pulmonary	Pulmonary fibrosis Interstitial pneumonitis	Radiation therapy Bleomycin Alkylating agents	Aging, smoking, illicit drug use
Endocrine	Growth hormone deficiency Precocious puberty Hyperprolactinemia Central hypothyroidism Gonadotropin deficiency Thyroid nodules Obesity Diabetes/insulin resistance	Radiation therapy Alkylating agents	Smoking, alcohol, carbonated beverages, lack of exercise, younger age at treatment
Nervous system	Peripheral sensory or motor neuropathy Cognitive dysfunction Learning disabilities Clinical leukoencephalopathy Cerebrovascular complications	Radiation therapy Heavy metals High-dose IV cytarabine Methotrexate—IO, IT, high-dose IV Vincristine/vinblastine	Age younger than 3 at time of treatment, preexisting learning disability or family history, sickle cell higher rates of stroke
Renal/urological	Hemorrhagic cystitis Hydronephrosis Vesicoureteral reflux Bladder malignancy Glomerular toxicity Renal insufficiency Hypertension Tubular injury	Radiation therapy Platinums Ifosfamide/cyclophosphamide	Alcohol, illicit drug use, diabetes, hypertension, nephrectomy
Secondary malignancies	Solid tumors AML/myelodysplasia	Radiation therapy Alkylating agents Epipodophyllotoxins Heavy metals Anthracyclines	Cancer genetic predisposition syndromes
Psychosocial	Mental health disorders Posttraumatic stress Employment and educational problems Insurance discrimination Risky behaviors	Cancer	Preexisting mental health disorders
Auditory	Ototoxicity	Carboplatin Cisplatin Radiation	
Visual	Cataracts Ocular toxicity	Busulfan Corticosteroids Radiation	
Dental	Dental abnormalities	Cancer	Preexisting poor oral hygiene

From Nass SJ, Beaupin LK, Demark-Wahnefried W, et al. Identifying and addressing the needs of adolescents and young adults with cancer: summary of an Institute of Medicine workshop. *Oncologist*. 2015;20(2):186-195; Children's Oncology Group. Long-Term Follow-Up Guidelines for Survivors of Childhood, Adolescent, and Young Adult Cancers. 2018. http://www.survivorshipguidelines.org. Accessed January 10, 2020; Berger A, Hinds P, Puchalski C, eds. *Handbook of Supportive Oncology and Palliative Care*. Demos Medical; 2018. Ref. (13).

cardiotoxicity include young age during treatment, female sex, black race, trisomy 21, higher cumulative anthracycline dose, higher anthracycline dose rates, longer time since treatment, and presence of preexisting cardiovascular disease (11,15). Risk of

cardiotoxicity is significantly higher in children who receive cumulative anthracycline dose >300 mg/m^2; however, there are subclinical cardiac abnormalities at lower dosages at well, suggesting that any dose of anthracycline increases the risk of cardiac toxicity (11,15). Studies have shown that the presence of traditional cardiovascular risk factors, such as elevated insulin levels, elevated cholesterol, and elevated blood pressure, are higher among survivors of childhood cancer, especially as time passes since treatment, compared to healthy siblings, which further heightens their risk for cardiac toxicity (11). Recent studies have looked at genetic causes of cardiac toxicity, to further delineate patients who are high of risk and help prevent such toxicity, especially given that the course of toxicity varies in each patient and even patients with low doses of anthracyclines can have significant cardiac toxicity (11,15).

Anthracycline cardiotoxicity can be acute or chronic, with chronic toxicity divided into early-onset and late-onset. Acute toxicity occurs during treatment and is rare, occurring in <1% of patients. It manifests as arrhythmias, electrocardiographic abnormalities, or occasionally heart failure (HF) and usually resolves when treatment is stopped, although may recur in follow-up. Early-onset cardiotoxicity includes left ventricular (LV) dysfunction, electrocardiographic changes, and HF. Late-onset toxicity shows changes such as reduced LV dimensions, reduced LV wall thickness, reduced LV shortening fraction, and reduced LV contractility similar to patients with restrictive cardiomyopathy (15).

Of utmost importance is the prevention of cardiac toxicity in children treated for cancer. The only medication approved for cardio prevention is dexrazoxane. Dexrazoxane was initially studied in beagles in the 1980s (15). Dexrazoxane is an iron chelator that binds to iron complexes, thus preventing the formation of anthracycline–iron complexes. It also hinders the action of topoisomerase 2, the enzyme which regulates DNA formulation. The use of dexrazoxane has been limited in women with metastatic breast cancer who are being treated with >300 mg/m² of anthracyclines. However, recently there have been several studies looking at the use of dexrazoxane in children treated with anthracyclines with different tumor types, which has shown decreased risk of cardiac injury. There have been fears of the cardioprotective impact of dexrazoxane extending to malignant cells, leading to secondary malignancies and decreased efficacy of the chemotherapy; however, several studies have failed to support this (11,15). Studies have been performed looking at enalapril for cardioprotection in survivors who receive anthracyclines; however, the benefits are transient (11). Studies have looked at continuous dosing of doxorubicin versus bolus dosing for improved cardioprotective measures; however, several studies fail to show statistically significant benefits to continuous dosing. With

that in mind, many pediatric cancer centers do incorporate continuous infusion anthracyclines for cardioprotection (11). There are limited studies in pediatrics looking at the use of liposomal anthracyclines and anthracycline analogs to prevent cardiotoxicity (15).

Screening such as echocardiograms, radionuclide ventriculography, and cardiac magnetic resonance imaging (MRI) detects changes to the heart after damage has occurred, making it difficult to screen for cardiotoxicity before irreversible damage has occurred. Cardiac biomarkers including cTnT, which is an indicator of myocardial damage, and n-terminal pro–brain natriuretic peptide (NT-proBNP) have been studied in survivors of childhood cancer and may become useful early screening biomarkers as more is known about their relationship with long-term cardiotoxicity (11,15). Children's Oncology Group (COG) recommends echocardiograms every 2 to 5 years for survivors who have anthracycline exposure (15,16). It is important to remember that screening must continue for life, as the risk of cardiotoxicity is lifelong after anthracycline exposure. There is no established standard of care in treating chemotherapy-induced cardiac disease. Medications that have been used include angiotensin-converting enzyme inhibitors (ACEI), beta-blockers, and growth hormone replacement therapy. However, these have been found to delay LV dysfunction and HF, but not prevent progression of disease, which highlights the need for new strategies aimed at treating anthracycline-related cardiotoxicity (15).

Pulmonary

The lungs are particularly sensitive to damage from chemotherapy, radiation, and the effects of hematopoietic stem cell transplant. The risk of pulmonary complications increases with time, and 5-year childhood cancer survivors have an 8.8-fold excess risk of pulmonary complications compared to peers without cancer (12,17). Pulmonary toxicities primarily manifest as pulmonary fibrosis, but patients who receive radiation therapy or bleomycin are also at risk of interstitial pneumonitis (17). Pulmonary toxicities can range from subclinical to life-threatening. They can occur early following treatment or develop years following treatment (12). Risk factors for pulmonary toxicity include young age at treatment, combined chemotherapy and chest radiation, combined chemotherapy and total body irradiation (TBI), combined chest radiation and TBI, multiple combined pulmonary toxic chemotherapy agents, active chronic graft versus host disease (GVHD), inhaled illicit drug use, and smoking (17). Highest prevalence is among survivors treated with chest radiation, followed by those treated with bleomycin, followed by those who underwent thoracotomy (12).

The biggest risk factor for pulmonary toxicity is radiation. Acute toxicity while receiving radiation therapy is rare in modern times; however, pulmonary fibrosis may occur for an extended time following radiation exposure. Survivors who receive radiation are also at risk of chronic cough, exercise-associated dyspnea, chronic pneumonia, and abnormal chest wall (17). Dose of radiation $\geq$15 Gy or TBI $\geq$ 6 Gy in a single fraction or $\geq$12 Gy fractionated puts survivors at highest risk of long-term pulmonary toxicities (17).

The chemotherapy agent with the highest risk of pulmonary toxicity is bleomycin, especially in older adolescents and adults. Risk of toxicity is worsened with doses >400 units/m^2 and when given with chest radiation. Bleomycin is at risk of causing both interstitial pneumonitis and pulmonary fibrosis (17). Other chemotherapy agents that increase risk of pulmonary toxicity are alkylating agents including carmustine (BCNU) and lomustine (CCNU). Risk of pulmonary fibrosis with BCNU is seen at doses in the nontransplant setting of 700 to 1,800 mg/m^2 and in the transplant setting at doses of 500 to 600 mg/m^2. Busulfan, melphalan, and cyclophosphamide also increase risk of pulmonary toxicity. Busulfan is at risk of causing interstitial fibrosis and bronchopulmonary dysplasia, especially in doses >500 mg (17).

Pulmonary toxicity is especially high in survivors of hematopoietic transplantation and is in fact one of the greatest causes of posttransplant morbidity and mortality. Manifestations include delayed interstitial pneumonitis, restrictive lung disease, obstructive lung disease, bronchiolitis obliterans, and bronchiolitis obliterans with organizing pneumonia. Survivors who receive unfractionated TBI as part of their conditioning have higher risk of pulmonary toxicity than those who receive fractionated TBI. Patients with chronic GVHD are at high risk of obstructive lung disease, which can persist for years after transplant. Bronchiolitis obliterans can occur months to years following transplantation and is often hard to detect on imaging studies and hard to treat (17).

Unfortunately, there is nothing currently available to prevent pulmonary toxicities associated with childhood cancer treatment. Due to the high morbidity and mortality, long-term follow-up (LTFU) for life is required for any patient at high risk. COG does provide guidelines based on specific exposures of each survivor. As pulmonary toxicities can present subclinically, often survivors will not be aware they are experiencing toxicity, which highlights the need for continued follow-up (12). Follow-up should include yearly pulmonary examination and detailed history focusing on symptoms such as chronic cough shortness of breath, wheezing, and dyspnea on exertion. Pulmonary function tests should be performed at entry into LTFU and repeated as clinically indicated, including before general anesthesia if abnormal. All survivors should be counseled routinely on the dangers of illicit drug use and smoking, as this further increases the risk of pulmonary toxicity (17). Aging itself causes pulmonary deterioration including pulmonary inflammation and lung structure changes, which suggests need for increased surveillance as survivors age (12).

Endocrine

Endocrine complications of childhood cancer treatment are a result of chemotherapy, radiation, and surgical interventions. The most common endocrine complications occur in the thyroid gland, including hypothyroidism, hyperthyroidism, and thyroid tumors, which were previously discussed with secondary malignancies. Risk factors for thyroid disease include female sex, radiation to the cranium, head, neck mantle, TBI with increasing doses, and young age at treatment (17). White race confers a higher risk for hypothyroidism (18). Newer agents, including tyrosine kinase inhibitors and checkpoint inhibitors, may also cause long-term damage to the thyroid (18). Up to 20% of adult survivors of childhood cancer experience thyroid dysfunction. Survivors of Hodgkin's lymphoma, brain tumors, and malignant extracranial solid tumors who undergo head and/or neck radiation or I-MIBG in neuroblastoma are at particularly high risk (17,18). Up to 50% of survivors of hematopoietic transplant experience hypothyroidism with TBI being an independent risk factor (18). Screening should include yearly history with particular attention to thyroid signs and symptoms; yearly physical examination with attention to height, weight, eyes, hair, skin, and thyroid; and yearly checks of thyroid-stimulating hormone and free T4 level (17). Survivors who are considering pregnancy or are pregnant should have increased monitoring as thyroid dysfunction may be unmasked during pregnancy. Treatment is per standard recommendations for thyroid dysfunction (18).

There is research to support that survivors of childhood cancer are at risk of metabolic syndrome, including obesity, insulin resistance, dyslipidemia, hypertension, hyperglycemia, and proinflammatory state (17). Survivors who receive doses of cranial radiation $\geq$20 Gy are at particularly high risk of developing obesity, as are those who receive TBI and abdominal radiation (17,18). Females and those who are treated at younger ages are at higher risk as well, as are those survivors who have prolonged glucocorticosteroid use, familial dyslipidemia, growth hormone deficiency, hypothyroidism, hypogonadism, and surgery in suprasellar region (17). Survivors at highest risk are those with sellar and suprasellar tumors and those with direct damage to the hypothalamus either through the tumor itself or surgery. These survivors are at high risk of developing hypothalamic obesity, which has been most studied in survivors of craniopharyngioma, but also occurs in survivors of other CNS tumors. The other main group of survivors at high risk of developing obesity are those with acute lymphoblastic leukemia (ALL), particularly those who were young females when treated (18). Survivors at high risk of weight-related complications should be screened annually focusing on height, weight, body mass index (BMI), and blood pressure. Survivors who underwent cranial radiation should also be screened for comorbid conditions and should be counseled on the risk of obesity (17).

Cranial radiation at doses ≥24 Gy and TBI used for conditioning in hematopoietic transplant have significant risk of causing growth hormone deficiency and causing significant growth retardation. This is primarily seen in survivors of brain tumors and ALL, although the rate of cranial radiation is decreasing with advances to current childhood treatment modalities. Younger age at treatment confers a higher risk. For those at risk, detailed history and physical focusing on nutritional status, height, weight, and BMI should be performed every month until linear growth is complete, then annually, and Tanner staging every 6 months until sexual maturity. Consider endocrine consultation for poor growth or decline in growth velocity for high-risk survivors to assess need for growth hormone replacement. Thyroid function should also be checked in all survivors who experience poor growth (17).

Cancer treatment can lead to deficiency in hormones produced by the hypothalamus and the pituitary. Chemotherapy may play some part in this; however, radiation therapy is the biggest risk factor. Over half of childhood cancer survivors have at least one deficiency of the hypothalamic pituitary (HP) axis by 25 years following treatment. Patients with CNS tumors and those who undergo irradiation to surrounding areas including spinal radiation and head and neck radiation are at high risk of HP dysfunction. Symptoms can vary from mild to life-threatening depending on the specific hormone deficiency. Workup and treatment is the same in survivors of childhood cancers as any patient with HP axis hormone deficiencies (18).

Auditory

Radiation and chemotherapy, specifically platinum-based regimens, are at risk of causing damage to the cochlea, causing ototoxicity. Supportive care medications including aminoglycoside antibiotics and loop diuretics further increase this risk. Cisplatin confers a higher risk of irreversible sensorineural hearing loss than carboplatin, which only causes hearing loss at myeloablative doses. Risk factors include younger age, brain tumor history, doses of cisplatin >400 mg/m^2, and doses of radiation >30 Gy. The advent of proton beam radiation has minimized the risk of ototoxicity (17). Refer to COG guidelines for specific screenings; however, in general, survivors with high-risk chemotherapy exposure should have auditory screening at entry into survivorship program, and survivors with radiation doses ≥30 Gy to cranial region should be completed yearly after completion of therapy until age 10 or for 5 years off treatment, if older than 10, then every 5 years. Survivors with hearing loss should be referred to audiology and speech and language therapy and should have guidance navigating special accommodations at school (17).

Secondary Primary Malignancies

Secondary malignant neoplasms (SMNs) remain the second leading cause of mortality in survivors of childhood cancer behind recurrence of the original cancer (19,20). In a large study at Kaiser Permanente Southern California of AYA survivors of cancer, survivors with a SMN were at 7-fold greater risk of dying than survivors who did not have a diagnosis of SMN (19). SMNs are any histologically distinct neoplasm occurring at least 2 months after completion of treatment of primary malignancy (21). There is a cumulative incidence of SMNs of 3% within 15 years of diagnosis, which increases to 10% to 20% by 30 years from diagnosis, which is a 6-fold increased risk from the general public (19,21,22). Recent changes in therapy including minimizing radiation have led to decreased risk of SMNs, but the risk is not eliminated (19). Survivors tend to be diagnosed with SMNs at a younger age than other adults are diagnosed with similar malignancies (28.04 vs. 47.55 years) (19). Survivors are most at risk of solid tumors including breast cancer, nonmelanoma skin cancer, thyroid cancer, benign CNS tumors, bone cancer, soft tissue sarcomas, and hematologic malignancies (19,21,23). Nonmelanoma skin cancers are the most common SMN in survivors, comprising 41% of all SMNs (24). The time from primary malignancy to SMN varies based on specific type of malignancy. Hematologic malignancies tend to have a shorter latency period of 2 to

3 years if due to exposure from etoposide and 5 to 7 years if due to exposure from alkylating agents, while meningioma and other solid tumors have a latency of 10 to 15 years, and even up to 30 years (21,25). The main risk factors for developing SMNs include exposure to chemotherapy, exposure to radiation therapy, and hematopoietic stem cell transplantation (21). Alkylating agents, including cyclophosphamide, ifosfamide, melphalan, busulfan, dacarbazine, nitrosoureas, and cisplatin increase the risk of therapy-related acute myeloid leukemia (t-AML) often associated with preceding myelodysplastic syndrome (21). T-AML due to alkylating agents has a latency period of 5 to 7 years and has distinct cytogenetic features including monosomy or partial deletions of chromosomes 5 (−5/del[5q]) and 7 (−7/del[7q]) (21,25). Alkylating agents are used in protocols for both Ewing sarcoma and Hodgkin's lymphoma, both of which have known significant increases in risk of t-AML (21). Topoisomerase II inhibitors, including anthracyclines, anthracenediones such as mitoxantrone, and epipodophyllotoxins such as etoposide and teniposide increase the risk of t-AML as well, usually with a latency period of 2 to 3 years (21). Specific cytogenetic changes of t-AML associated with epipodophyllotoxins include MLL-gene 11q23, t(8;21)(q22;q22), and fusion AML1-ETO (21,25). Prolonged low-dose exposure to etoposide may decrease the risk of t-AML compared to intermittent treatment schedules (21). In a large-scale Dutch study of >6,000 survivors of childhood cancer, chemotherapy, especially doxorubicin and cyclophosphamide, increased the risk of subsequent solid tumors independent of radiation exposure. Doxorubicin had a dose-dependent increased risk of female breast cancer, and cyclophosphamide had a dose-dependent increase risk of sarcoma (23).

Radiation therapy is the strongest independent risk factor for development of SMN and is used for many childhood cancers including solid tumors, CNS tumors, Hodgkin's lymphoma, and part of conditioning for stem cell transplant. The latency period of SMN development is 10 to 15 years. The SMN often corresponds to the area of the body that was exposed to radiation therapy. For example, survivors of Hodgkin's lymphoma have known increased risk of breast cancer and thyroid cancer due to the use of mantle radiation. Common SMNs seen following radiation therapy include meningiomas, nonmelanoma skin cancer, breast cancer, thyroid cancer, and bone tumors. Doses >30 Gy to the mediastinum increase the risk of breast and thyroid cancer, while any radiation exposure increases the risk of subsequent sarcomas (21). The greatest risk of SMNs is in survivors who received TBI compared to other types of radiation (23). In recent years, less craniospinal irradiation is used in protocols for ALL except in certain high-risk populations due to the higher risk of SMNs especially meningiomas and other impacts on cognitive development, which should decrease the rate of SMNs in this population (21). Additionally, with the recent advances of proton radiation therapy, which has been shown to lower cancer risk by a factor of 2 to 10, fewer childhood cancer survivors should develop radiation-related SMNs in the future (21).

Survivors of hematopoietic stem cell transplantation are at particularly high risk of developing SMNs, 8-fold higher incidence compared to the general population (21). Risk factors in survivors of stem cell transplants include chemotherapy exposures and TBI used during conditioning. Additionally, a unique risk factor is that of chronic GVHD. Survivors with GVHD are at high risk of squamous cell carcinoma of the skin and oropharynx, especially when GVHD is severe and when on chronic immunosuppression (21).

Several studies have been conducted to look at survival patterns of SMNs with primary malignant neoplasms (PMNs) of the same origin in patients who have not previously had cancer. In one study looking at 1,409 SMNs from the NCIs SEER database compared to 1,332,203 similar PMNs in those without previous cancer history, those with a SMN had lower overall survival (19). Even when controlling for other factors, history of childhood cancer was significantly associated with worse overall survival (19). In a large study in the Dutch Childhood Cancer Oncology Group-Long-Term Effects After Childhood Cancer (DCOG-LATER), survivors with subsequent sarcomas, breast cancers, and melanomas were compared to patients with similar cancers who did not have a history of previous cancer (26). Survivors with subsequent sarcomas had significantly decreased survival compared to those without previous cancer history, while those with breast cancer and melanoma SMNs did not have poorer overall survival (26). However, those with breast cancer SMNs were more likely to have mastectomies without chemotherapy or radiation therapy than those with primary breast cancers (26). The lower overall survival and differences of treatment options of childhood cancer survivors with SMNs compared to patients with similar PMNs may in part be since treatment during childhood limits treatment options for SMNs due to cumulative exposures of radiation therapy and anthracyclines (19,26). Also, treatment exposures during childhood may result in SMNs with specific genetic mutational profiles impacting therapy response (19).

It is reported that survivors are not concerned about their risk of SMNs or other long-term health complications, which may limit how often they get appropriate screening. In a large study using the Childhood Cancer Survivor Study (CCSS), 30.7% of survivors reported lack of concern of future health and 39.9% reported lack of concern of developing subsequent malignancy (22). Survivors more likely to report concern were female, had already been diagnosed with cancer or grade 3 or 4 chronic condition, had clinical anxiety, and were older (22). It is possible that survivors may not fully understand their increased risk of subsequent cancer and other late effects. In the CCSS, fewer than half of high-risk survivors are compliant to cancer screening guidelines; however, only 70% can recall location of their radiation therapy if given and fewer than half of survivors knew if they received anthracycline therapy (22). It is the responsibility of the pediatric oncologist and the providers who continue to follow survivors long term to educate about exposures and subsequent cancer risks, to ensure they are getting appropriate screening.

Prevention, when possible, and early detection of SMNs is vital for the survival of childhood cancer survivors due to their morbidity and mortality (20,21). Refer to COG and United States Preventive Services Task Force (USPSTF) for screening guidelines based on specific cancer risk (17,21,27). All survivors exposed to radiation should conduct monthly self-exams of the skin and have annual exams of the skin done by a qualified provider (20). The American Academy of Dermatology and the USPSTF fail to give specific recommendations regarding skin evaluations, and currently only 30.9% of survivors have ever had a clinical skin examination (23). Survivors with a family history of breast cancer and/or a history of mantle radiation should have yearly mammography at age 25 or 8 years after radiation, whichever occurs later, and should have clinical breast examinations yearly to every 6 months starting at age 25. Breast MRI can be used yearly as adjunct to mammography as well (16,20). All survivors should have education regarding risk reduction, including smoking cessation/avoidance, exercise, healthy diet, and sun protection (16,20).

NEUROCOGNITIVE EFFECTS

"Chemo brain" commonly refers to cancer-associated cognitive impairment. Symptoms include trouble with executive function, short-term memory issues, concentration and attention difficulties, and reduced information processing speeds (28). Research on the neurocognitive effects of cancer treatment among children showed that those who receive directed therapy to the brain have the greatest risk to its structure and function (29). In pediatric oncology, CNS tumors and ALL are the most common diseases with CNS-directed therapy with survivors of CNS tumors at greatest risk for neurocognitive impairment (9). A review of adult survivors of pediatric cancer found the most salient issues to be impaired intelligence, processing speed, and executive function, and the greatest risk factors were younger age, higher cranial irradiation dose, larger brain volume irradiated, and longer time since treatment exposure (30). Hydrocephalus with shunt placement and revisions were also associated risk factors (31). Similarly, among children who received cranial radiation therapy (CRT) for ALL, similar neurocognitive impairments were found with severity dependent on dose of CRT, younger age at diagnosis, female sex, and longer time since diagnosis (32). Interestingly, though CRT is largely avoidable in contemporary ALL therapy, we have learned that chemotherapy alone, either via intrathecal and or systemic administration, correlates with impairment in intelligence, attention, memory, processing speed, and executive function (33).

Due to neurocognitive issues, affected pediatric cancer survivors have social development issues such as attaining educational achievement, establishing reliable employment, developing meaningful friendships and intimate relationships, and being able to live independently (34–36). As social goals are negatively impacted, quality of life is also affected. Indeed, long-term survivors of CNS tumors report the poorest health-related quality of life among all childhood cancers (37).

The current survivorship guidelines set forth by COG recommend neurocognitive evaluation for survivors who received neurotoxic or CNS-directed therapy. This should be evaluated after completion of cancer treatment as a baseline assessment, followed by period testing at different timepoints of educational transition (16). The goal is for early recognition of potential neurocognitive dysfunction and delivering effective strategies to succeed in school and attaining educational goals.

REPRODUCTIVE HEALTH AND GU EFFECTS

Gonadotoxicity is a significant issue many pediatric cancer patients face while undergoing cancer treatment. Any surgery, radiation, or chemotherapy that negatively affects any component of the hypothalamic–pituitary–gonadal axis may pose a risk to fertility in childhood cancer survivors (38). There are various ways cancer treatment can affect one's ability to have biological offspring. For both boys and girls, surgery involving reproductive organs (orchiectomy, oophorectomy) affects fertility potential directly. Radiotherapy and chemotherapy also affect reproductive potential and depends on age at the time of exposure and the cumulative exposure dose (Table 59.2).

Radiotherapy involving the pelvic area or the spine, including whole body irradiation, can cause gonadal damage. Cranial irradiation impairs fertility by disruption to the hypothalamic–pituitary–gonadal axis. In pediatric and adolescent males, testicular damage occurs when there is direct irradiation of the testes. Most commonly for children, radiation is used in the management of testicular disease in ALL. In such cases, 24 Gy is used, resulting in permanent azoospermia (39). In females, whole body irradiation and radiation to the abdomen and pelvis can impact gonadal function. It has been shown that the risk of premature ovarian failure increased with lower dose of radiation when age of exposure is later with sterilizing doses of radiation: 20.3 Gy at birth, 18.4 Gy at 10 years, 16.5 Gy at 20 years, and 14.3 Gy at 30 years (40). In addition, pelvic irradiation has been associated with low birth weight and preterm delivery (41,42).

Various chemotherapy agents pose a risk to fertility. Anthracyclines, such as doxorubicin, and platinum agents, cisplatin and carboplatin, impart a risk of gonadotoxicity, although usually less than that of alkylating agents. And the cumulative effect in multidrug regimens has not been well studied. The risk of infertility depends on the medication exposure, cumulative dose, age of exposure, and sex of the patient. Previous studies on long-term

male pediatric cancer survivors showed that cumulative cyclophosphamide equivalent doses (CED) of <4,000 mg/m^2 poses a small risk of spermatogenesis (43), whereas a CED of >7,500 mg/m^2 is expected to cause gonadal failure (44). For females, ovarian reserve is expected to be greater in prepubertal and adolescent girls as they have a greater complement of primordial follicles than adult females (45). Overall, the risk of infertility may be significant when treatment includes combined modality therapy with alkylating agent chemotherapy and abdominal/pelvic radiation or dose-intensive alkylating agents for myeloablative conditioning before hematopoietic cell transplantation (46,47). And due to the high risk of infertility following childhood cancer treatment, fertility preservation efforts have evolved with ongoing efforts to reduce cumulative doses of radiation and chemotherapy in treatment protocols (48).

Fortunately, when fertility is preserved, studies on pregnancy outcomes have shown that offspring of childhood cancer survivors do not have an excess of birth defects or adverse health outcomes (48,49). The most significant risk is associated with high doses of abdominopelvic radiation for females, which can lead to uterine vascular insufficiency, spontaneous abortion, neonatal death, low–birth-weight infants, fetal malposition, and premature labor (48,50).

PHYSICAL DISFIGUREMENT

Little attention is given to long-term outcomes of childhood cancer treatment such as scarring, permanent hair loss, and disfigurement that impact quality of life and psychosocial functioning. In the Western world, dissatisfaction with physical appearance and a desire to have a perfect appearance are common. For survivors of childhood cancer, who have outward disfigurement, this desire and subsequent feelings of unattractiveness are magnified (51). Persistent alopecia is reported in survivors of cranial radiation and certain chemotherapies including busulfan and high-dose cyclophosphamide. Permanent disfigurement occurs from amputation of limb, radical surgeries to resect tumors, weight loss or gain, and head and neck radiation therapy, which can lead to spinal deformities. Scarring results from tissue biopsies, placement of central lines, surgeries, and secondary nonmelanoma skin cancers, which occur in survivors treated with radiation therapy (52).

One study showed 33% of adult survivors of childhood cancer reported treatment-related scarring, compared to 1.5% to 4.5% of the general population (52). In a study using survivors from the CCSS compared to siblings, survivors were more

TABLE 59.2 CANCER TREATMENT AFFECTING REPRODUCTIVE POTENTIAL

Chemotherapy	• Alkylating agents (most
• Class of chemotherapy	detrimental): busulfan, carmustine, lomustine,
• Cumulative dose received	cyclophosphamide, ifosfamide,
• Age at time of treatment; higher risk with increasing age	mechlorethamine (nitrogen mustard), melphalan, procarbazine, thiotepa
	• Platinum-based: carboplatin, cisplatin
Radiotherapy	• Pelvis/testicles
• Site of radiation therapy	• Lower spine
• Total dose of radiation therapy	• Total body irradiation
	• Cranial irradiation ≥30 Gy (3,000 cGy/rads)

From Children's Oncology Group. Long-Term Follow-Up Guidelines for Survivors of Childhood, Adolescent, and Young Adult Cancers. 2018. http://www.survivorshipguidelines.org. Accessed January 10, 2020.

likely to have scarring, persistent hair loss, and disfigurement in all sites including the head, neck, arms, legs, chest, and abdomen. Survivors with scarring and disfigurement, especially of the head and neck, report increased depressive symptoms. Those with persistent hair loss report increased anxiety. Health-related quality of life scored using the Medical Outcomes Short Form to self-report general health in the past 4 weeks was adversely affected by scarring, hair loss, and disfigurement as well. Past research has shown that melanoma patients with visible scarring report increased distress (52).

Additionally, studies of young adult survivors report on the impact of losing a breast, impact of masculinity among testicular cancer survivors, and difficulties with head and neck scarring (51). It appears that outward physical appearance, with visible scars and hair loss, cause the most distress and impact on quality of life. Adolescents and young adults with scarring and disfigurement report feelings of unattractiveness and a decrease in participation in social activities due to these feelings (51). Providers often do not think about disfigurement as they are thinking more about treatment and curing the patient. Although it may not be possible to avoid all scarring and disfigurement with current modalities of treatment for childhood cancer patients, providers should be aware of the impact it has on them, well into adulthood.

PAIN

Many pediatric patients experience pain during their cancer treatment. The pain may be due to the disease itself or from the side effects of treatment. Pain may also be acute, episodic, or chronic. Though pain typically resolves over time, especially after treatment has ended, pain may become a chronic issue for many survivors. Studies have shown that up to 58.7% of survivors report pain and are four times more likely to experience pain compared with their siblings (53,54). Up to one-half of pediatric cancer survivors report experiencing at least mild pain-related impairment, and pain has been associated with elevated suicidal ideation and distress (54,55). A recent literature review on pain among pediatric cancer survivors reported that pain does not appear to be more prevalent in survivors of childhood cancer than in the general population, except for specific subgroups of patients (56). Pediatric cancer survivors with cancer-related pain tend to be those who were diagnosed at a younger age, female sex, greater time since diagnosis, and certain diagnoses (CNS tumors, bone tumors, and sarcomas). Fatigue and persistent emotional distress were also associated

with cancer-related pain. Migraines, headaches, and back pain were the most common types of pain. The CCSS report on pain among adult survivors of pediatric cancer also identified minority status, unemployment, and being single as associated risks for reporting pain conditions (53).

Psychological distress likely plays a factor in chronic pain. Though not well studied, pain can cause distress by suggesting there may be an underlying concern for disease recurrence of treatment effect, or distress can exacerbate a painful experience. Future research is needed to better understand psychosocial distress and its relationship with pain and how to identify and address these issues.

FATIGUE

Cancer-related fatigue (CRF) is one of the most common and disruptive symptoms among cancer survivors (57) though not well understood in the pediatric population. As a result, CRF is often unrecognized and untreated though it may contribute to diminished social functioning, reduced quality of life, and socioeconomic consequences (58).

Among pediatric cancer survivors, two different studies examining fatigue among long-term pediatric cancer survivors did not show that they have increased fatigue compared to their peers (59,60). When compared to their siblings, pediatric cancer survivors have increased fatigue, sleep disturbance, and daytime sleepiness (61), though predictors of fatigue, disturbed sleep, and daytime sleepiness were similar among both survivors and siblings. Furthermore, there was a significant association between fatigue, disordered sleep, and daytime sleepiness with overall health-related quality of life identified in both groups.

The limited data among pediatric cancer survivors highlight the need for further research on this issue, especially as fatigue correlates with psychosocial factors including quality of life.

NUTRITION

The effects of childhood cancer on the nutritional and physical status of pediatric cancer survivors varies for each individual. With the risk of acquiring a chronic medical condition due to long-term and late effects from cancer treatment, the role of nutrition may play an important role in the etiology or severity of comorbid issues.

In pediatric oncology, obesity has been identified as a late effect seen particularly in survivors of ALL and CNS tumors, likely from the use of glucocorticoids and cranial radiotherapy (62,63). However, more recent studies have shown that pediatric cancer survivors' overweight characteristics do not differ from that in the general population, suggesting that environmental factors could be associated with the development of obesity (64,65).

While we understand that nutrition and lifestyle modifications may have an impact on health outcomes of pediatric cancer survivors, interventional studies examining diet and exercise are limited. The current survivorship guidelines from COG recommends adhering to a healthy, balanced diet and incorporating regular physical activity (16).

VOCATIONAL

Education

A diagnosis of cancer often puts a hold on a child's education while undergoing treatment. Education is important for children's social development and for socioeconomic progress.

Around 35% of survivors of childhood cancer have neurocognitive decline that have the potential to impact schooling. Additionally, while undergoing treatment and even into survivorship, patients miss school, which affects their future education (66). Neurocognitive declines can present themselves up to 5 years following treatments and can be a result of the treatment or cancer itself. Neurocognitive declines are especially common in survivors of CNS tumors. Deficits are common in math, reading, spelling, fine motor, and perpetual motor skills, which all impact academic performance. Additionally, survivors may suffer from chronic pain and fatigue, which further impact academic performance (67).

In one systemic review of education following treatment for childhood cancer, survivors of CNS tumors had lower educational attainment than peers without cancers, while the data was inconclusive for survivors of other cancers (66). In a small Italian study looking at educational and employment of childhood cancer survivors, survivors were less likely to complete secondary education and postsecondary education than peers. Survivors of CNS tumors had the highest risk of not obtaining educational qualifications. Other risks for not obtaining educational qualifications include female gender, younger age at diagnosis, and cranial radiation. Unfortunately, survivors with lower educational attainment and therefore lower employment opportunities have higher rates of poverty, unhealthy lifestyles including drug use and alcohol, and social marginalization (68). In a large meta-analysis of 28,434 survivors, survivors were less likely to progress to secondary education or to complete postsecondary education. Again, survivors with CNS tumors were at the greatest

risk; however, decreased educational attainment was seen for survivors of all cancers (69).

There are several laws that protect students with disabilities that providers of childhood cancer survivors should be aware of. Public schools that receive federal funds must adhere to these laws, while private schools are not mandated but oftentimes do. The Individuals with Disabilities Education Act 2004 (IDEA) provides a written Individual Education Program (IEP) for students with learning disabilities, speech and language impairments, vision and hearing impairments, and other health impairments. Section 504 of the Rehabilitation Act of 1973 protects individuals from discrimination based on their disability. A 504 Plan provides students with disabilities accommodations while in school such as extra time to complete tests and access to elevators (67).

Employment

Employment is important for the survivor not only for financial stability and obtaining health insurance but also for fulfilling a purpose, elevating self-esteem, and providing a sense of normalcy (70). Unfortunately, due to the long-term chronic health conditions, which survivors of childhood cancer face that last for decades, adult survivors of childhood cancer have a greater risk of unemployment, employment in low-income jobs, and need for assistance from the government than their siblings and peers. This is particularly true of survivors of CNS tumors due to long-term neurocognitive dysfunction and survivors treated at <4 years of age (71). In a large British meta-analysis, overall survivors of childhood cancer were 5 times more likely, survivors of CNS malignancies were 8 times more likely, and survivors of CNS malignancies who received cranial radiation were 15 times more likely to be unemployed than their peers. Survivors of CNS malignancies and survivors of leukemia who received CNS-directed radiation were more likely to not work in managerial/professional positions; however, survivors of other tumor types had no difference compared to peers (72).

In addition to cognitive difficulties following cancer treatment, there are social and physical reasons that survivors do not return to work or change career paths following treatment. Survivors have chronic pain that may affect their ability to sit or stand for long periods, therefore affecting career choices. Survivors may also have frequent medical appointments and may get sick more often than healthy peers, influencing their work performance. Unfortunately, survivors do take more time off than peers due to health concerns. Socially, survivors report changing their goals posttreatment in regard to careers. Some survivors are not able to plan long term due to the uncertainty regarding their health, while others change career paths to one in health care following their own cancer experience (73).

Adult survivors of childhood cancer have a higher rate of "job lock" than peers, in which they feel they are unable to leave their job due to fear of loss of health insurance. This is more common among females, survivors who have problems paying their medical bills, and survivors with chronic, life-threatening, and disabling conditions. Survivors may feel stuck in their current job and be unable to have upward mobility or work in small businesses due to fear of losing insurance coverage and how this will impact their health (74).

The American with Disabilities Act (ADA) of 1990 was designed to protect individuals with physical illness, including cancer, in the workplace. Individuals with disabilities are not to be excluded if they can perform the job with reasonable accommodations. Unfortunately, despite these protections, survivors report job discrimination. They are less likely to obtain jobs at all, and when they do, they are viewed as less capable candidates for professional advancement. Discrimination in the workplace, even when subtle, does influence an employee's job performance and satisfaction. Unfortunately, cancer survivors report more job discrimination than those with any other disability (70).

Providers should be aware of the challenges that survivors face in both school and employment and offer support and guidance. This support should start from the beginning of treatment and continue through survivorship, as the survivor matures and reaches adulthood seeking a career path. Survivors should be aware of the laws that protect them at school and in the workplace.

FINANCIAL STRESSORS

Childhood cancer survivors are at risk of economic burden as they mature into adulthood. Cancer survivors face more economic hardship than those without cancer history. Financial burden can worsen physical and psychological health, due to inability to obtain adequate health care and stress it may impose on the individual; however, in the reverse, physical and psychological late effects that survivors face can lead to financial hardship (75). In a large population study, survivors of CNS cancers had lower incomes than peers, likely due to the long-term neurocognitive sequela they experience. Older females were also an economically vulnerable population, earning significantly less than peers (76).

In a study looking at adult survivors of childhood cancer, annual productivity losses per capita was $8,169 compared with $3,083 among individuals without cancer history. The majority of this productivity loss was from employment disability where people are not able to work due to physical or mental health, followed by missed days of work. The survivors in this study were more likely to have public insurance than those without cancer history. They were also more likely to be in fair or poor health, need help with routine care, and be limited in the work they can perform due to their health compared to those without cancer history (77).

Survivors may have more limited access to employer-sponsored insurance than those without cancer history. Fortunately, the Affordable Care Act (ACA) has provisions such as prohibiting coverage exclusions for preexisting conditions and elimination of the annual coverage limits, which does make insurance more widely available to survivors through the Health Insurance Marketplace or expanded Medicaid eligibility (75,77). However, even with these provisions, survivors are oftentimes left with high deductible plans. In one large study of adult survivors of childhood cancer, females, those who were hospitalized in the past year, those with lower household incomes, those unemployed, and those with severe to life-threatening medical conditions were all more likely to pay >10% of their income on out-of-pocket medical costs. Due to the chronic, debilitating, life-threatening conditions that survivors face, continued risk-based screening and health care throughout adulthood remains important. Survivors with no insurance or with costly, restrictive insurance with higher out of pocket medical expenses report less survivor-focused care than those with adequate health insurance. These survivors often report thoughts of filing bankruptcy, frequent worries of affording health care, and taking smaller doses of medications than prescribed due to costs (78). Providers need to be aware of the insurance challenges survivors face, as they may be less likely to seek continued care if they do not have adequate health coverage. Providers should routinely screen survivors for financial hardship and refer to appropriate resources when applicable.

SURVIVORSHIP AND MENTAL HEALTH DISORDERS

As discussed throughout this chapter, the late- and long-term effects of cancer treatment on children are vast and dependent upon details of the treatment received such as cumulative dose, age of exposure, site of radiation, or type of chemotherapy. Our knowledge in understanding the impact of treatment on different organ systems has improved, and we are able to better predict or determine which patients may be more at risk of cognitive issues or cardiac dysfunction. And yet the long-term psychosocial effects of cancer treatment is more challenging to characterize. Though many pediatric cancer survivors thrive after completing treatment, some survivors face significant psychosocial challenges that may be debilitating. Pediatric cancer survivors are at risk for disrupted psychosocial development secondary to their primary diagnosis, treatment, and physical late effects. Additionally, the missed educational opportunities and socialization with peers during the time of active cancer treatment may impact achieving social developmental milestones. The emergence of any medical late effects may further affect psychosocial health. Indeed, studies have shown that certain long-term treatment-related issues increase the risk of emotional distress, such as cancer-related pain and disfigurement, neurocognitive challenges (79), and fears related to fertility, mortality, and overall well-being (80). Additional factors associated with adverse psychological symptoms include female sex, low income, lower education, disability status, and unmarried status (81). However, it is difficult to discern whether these are contributing risk factors or are consequences of adverse psychosocial health. We have learned that compared to their siblings, pediatric cancer survivors are significantly more likely to have anxiety and depression, inattention, antisocial behavior, and impaired social competence (82) along with more comorbid distress (83).

A major contributing factor to psychosocial outcomes is their success in social relationships. Studies among long-term pediatric survivors have shown that they were more likely to be never married compared to their siblings and patients with CNS tumors were at greatest risk (84,85). A small study also illustrated the struggle pediatric cancer survivors may have with romantic relationships whereby they have fewer reported relationships and greater distress when a relationship ends (86).

Anxiety and Depression

Symptoms of anxiety and depression have been reported among pediatric cancer survivors many years after they have completed therapy (81). Among long-term pediatric CNS survivors, those who self-reported their physical health status as poor also reported significantly more symptoms of depression and anxiety (8). Similarly, when compared to siblings, pediatric cancer survivors with a history of a chronic medical conditions correlated with increased symptoms of depression (81). Screening for anxiety and depression among pediatric cancer survivors is an important aspect in LTFU.

Posttraumatic Stress

Posttraumatic stress symptoms (PTSS) include rearousal, or reexperiencing an unwanted memory or event; avoidance of reminders of the experience, such as hospitals and doctors; or increased response to sudden noise or heightened awareness of surrounding risk and potential dangers. Studies have shown that while pediatric cancer survivors exhibit significant PTSS, actual diagnostic criteria for posttraumatic stress disorder (PTSD) is found in a minority with as few as 3% in survivors 8 to 20 years of age (87) to 20% in older pediatric cancer survivors (88,89). The increased prevalence among older survivors may affect their educational goals and achievement of other social developmental milestones. And among adult survivors of childhood cancer, only 14.5% identified cancer as a traumatic event, and PTSD evaluation scores were comparative to normal controls. It may be important to recognize that long-term survivors may have distress that is not directly related to their cancer experience.

Risky Behaviors

Despite having increased risk factors that may negatively impact psychosocial factors, pediatric cancer survivors have similar or lower rates of risk-taking compared to their siblings or peers (90,91). A broad review of health behaviors among pediatric cancer survivors reported that tobacco use varies but in general is less among survivors than the general population or not different than their siblings though rates differed by cancer diagnosis (92). Alcohol use varied widely with some studies demonstrating decreased intake compared to siblings or either no difference or increased consumption compared to controls. And for illicit drugs, pediatric cancer survivors were less likely to drug use than the general population or no difference with their siblings.

Overall, the psychosocial aspect of pediatric cancer survivorship is vast and warrants ongoing research. While pediatric cancer survivors have many risk factors that may impact their mental health, we have learned that the majority of them experience few psychosocial problems in long-term survivorship (93). But in the subset that may have issues, they may be significant and debilitating. Further studies on screening and intervention may improve identifying survivors at risk at different timepoints throughout survivorship.

CANCER AFTER CARE

Around 80% of survivors of childhood cancer will develop serious, disabling, or life-threatening chronic health conditions by the age of 45 (12). Oftentimes, survivors in their twenties and thirties have the endurance and muscle strength of healthy peers 60 to 70 years of age (12). LTFU and surveillance must be continued for life for survivors of childhood cancer, and due to increasing morbidity the further survivors are from active treatment, there is increased need for surveillance as survivors age (12). The IOM has identified four components of survivorship care, including prevention and surveillance of new cancers and late effects, interventions for long-term medical and psychological consequences of cancer, and long-term coordination of care between specialists and primary care provider. The report recommends that every survivor of cancer be given a survivorship care plan (SCP) to ensure adequate communication between the oncology team, the patient, and the primary care provider (PCP) (94).

COG has published Long-Term Follow-Up Guidelines for Survivors of Childhood, Adolescent, and Young Adult Cancers (16), which is periodically updated, to provide evidence-based guidelines for screening survivors of childhood cancer who are at least 2 years from the completion of their cancer therapy. These are risk-based, exposure-related guidelines for screening and management of late-term toxicities commonly seen in pediatric malignancies, which are for use by oncologists, oncology nurse practitioners and physician assistants, PCPs, and other specialists who take care of survivors of childhood cancer. The COG guidelines provide a framework for documenting each patient's individual treatment course and then tailoring follow-up based on the individual treatment received. These guidelines exist to attempt to standardize the follow-up that survivors of childhood cancer undergo throughout their lifespan and to allow for early detection and intervention of any complications.

Upon completion of cancer therapy, each patient should be provided with a SCP or a cancer treatment summary, which includes demographic information, cancer diagnosis including stage, date of diagnosis, and date therapy was completed, names of all chemotherapy agents received, cumulative mg/m² dosing of all anthracyclines received, whether any dose of carboplatin was myeloablative, route of administration of cytarabine and methotrexate and information regarding whether IV doses were "high dose" ($\geq 1,000$ mg/m²) versus "standard dose," names of all radiation fields and total dose including boost dose in Gy, whether patient underwent hematopoietic cell transplant and whether autologous versus allogeneic, whether

patient has history of or currently active chronic GVHD, list of all surgical procedures, whether patient received radioiodine therapy or systemic MIBG, and name of treating provider (16). The guidelines provide potential late effects and evaluations applicable to all childhood cancer survivors including adverse psychosocial, mental health disorders, fatigue, sleep disorders, and risky behaviors. It also provides screenings applicable to survivors treated at certain timepoints including those diagnosed prior to 1972 due to risk of chronic hepatitis B, those diagnosed prior to 1993 due to risk of chronic hepatitis C, and those diagnosed between 1977 and 1985 due to the risk of HIV infection. For each therapeutic exposure, the guidelines provide potential late effects with periodic evaluations including history, physical examination, and any screening examinations with timelines of frequency and health counseling and further considerations for the provider (16,95).

Also important in the discussion of survivorship care is the transition of young adult childhood cancer survivors from pediatric care to adult focused care. As previously stated, lifelong health screening of survivors of childhood cancer is vital, even as they age out of pediatric practices (96). Many late effects, such as secondary malignancies and risk of sudden onset cardiac arrhythmia, can occur 20 years or longer following diagnosis (97). Several barriers exist to transitioning young adult survivors to adult care, from both the survivor and the provider point of view. Young adult survivors and their parents oftentimes desire continued pediatric-centered care, after years of trust with their pediatric team. Survivors are oftentimes not psychologically ready to seek adult-centered care (96). Additionally, young adult survivors frequently miss follow-up appointments, regardless of the setting. In one study, nearly three-quarters of adult survivors of childhood cancer had not had a cancer-related health visit in the past 2 years, and only 41% reported that they planned to do so in the next 2 years (97). Many survivors of childhood cancer have little knowledge of their treatment and its risks, likely because they were young when treated and not part of the upfront conversations with their care team. Those with moderate or severe life-threatening health complications are twice as likely as those with no complications to follow-up with cancer-related visits (97). Young adult survivors often have multiple times of transition, such as when moving to a new geographic location, which further challenges LTFU (12). There are often barriers due to the young adult survivor's insurance coverage of where they can be seen, which also may cause frequent transitions in care

(12,96). Barriers to transition from the provider standpoint include lack of adult providers, both PCPs and subspecialists, to partner with and lack of knowledge of the needs of survivors among adult providers. Also, pediatric survivorship providers are oftentimes unwilling to let go of their adult survivors following years of care (96). Due to the challenges many AYAs face as patients and survivors, many resources have been developed for this population. Table 59.3 lists relevant resources that may be helpful for AYAs.

Several models of LTFU have been identified, based on survivor risk. In the most current models, survivors with the highest risk for serious late effects continue to follow with multidisciplinary survivor clinics. Those with moderate risk follow with a shared model of both PCP and cancer center care. Those with low risk for late effects continue LTFU with their PCPs and should be provided with a SCP and guidelines for continued surveillance (12,97). Important in LTFU, whether survivors follow in a multidisciplinary oncology setting or with a PCP, is education about the treatment they received, possible late effects, and surveillance. Every survivor should be given a personalized SCP and should have access to portable electronic personal health records (12). Often, at diagnosis, although patients and families are given information about long-term effects of cancer and its treatment, they are in survival mode, not survivor mode. Following the completion of therapy, it is vital to ensure that survivors and their parents are aware of the potential long-term effect of their treatment, the need for continued surveillance, and the importance of maintaining a healthy lifestyle and available psychosocial support (97).

TABLE 59.3 RESOURCES FOR ADOLESCENT AND YOUNG ADULT ONCOLOGY PATIENTS AND SURVIVORS

Organization	Web site
LIVESTRONG	https://www.livestrong.org/we-can-help/young-adults
Teen Cancer America	https://teencanceramerica.org/
Stupid Cancer	https://stupidcancer.org
13Thirty Cancer Connect	13thirty.org
Ulman Cancer Fund for Young Adults	https://ulmanfoundation.org/
First Descents	https://firstdescents.org/
Young Survival Coalition	https://www.youngsurvival.org/

CONCLUSION

Significant improvements in the outcomes of pediatric cancers has resulted in more children living well into adulthood as long-term survivors. These survivors are at risk of long- and late-term physical and psychological complications and benefit from the medical care provided at a survivorship focused clinic. The goal of long-term survivorship care is to help survivors attain a high quality of life through screening, recognizing, and addressing long- and late-term effects.

Clinical Bullets

- The number of pediatric cancer survivors continues to rise due to improvements in treatment outcomes.
- Pediatric cancer survivors are at risk for long- and late-term physical and psychosocial effects due to their cancer and its treatment.
- All survivors should be provided a comprehensive treatment summary detailing the treatment received.
- Treatment summary details help develop a personalized SCP for survivors to use as they transition into adulthood.
- More salient issues for pediatric cancer survivors are fertility risk, long-term organ damage, and disrupted social development that may impact education and career goals and intimate relationships.

REFERENCES

1. Howlader N, Noone AM, Krapcho M, et al. *SEER Cancer Statistics Review, 1975-2016.* Bethesda, MD: National Cancer Institute; 2019. https://seer.cancer.gov/csr/1975_2016/. Accessed January 8, 2020.
2. National Cancer Institute Cancer Control and Population Sciences. Estimated US Cancer Prevalence. 2010. http://cancercontrol.cancer.gov/ocs/prevalence/prevalence.html. Accessed.
3. Phillips SM, Padgett LS, Leisenring WM, et al. Survivors of childhood cancer in the United States: prevalence and burden of morbidity. *Cancer Epidemiol Biomarkers Prev.* 2015;24(4):653-663.
4. Robison LL, Hudson MM. Survivors of childhood and adolescent cancer: life-long risks and responsibilities. *Nat Rev Cancer.* 2014;14(1):61-70.
5. Oeffinger KC, Mertens AC, Sklar CA, et al. Chronic health conditions in adult survivors of childhood cancer. *N Engl J Med.* 2006;355(15):1572-1582.
6. Sieswerda E, Font-Gonzalez A, Reitsma JB, et al. High hospitalization rates in survivors of childhood cancer: a longitudinal follow-up study using medical record linkage. *PLoS One.* 2016;11(7):e0159518.
7. Hoffman MC, Mulrooney DA, Steinberger J, Lee J, Baker KS, Ness KK. Deficits in physical function among young childhood cancer survivors. *J Clin Oncol.* 2013;31(22):2799-2805.
8. Zebrack BJ, Zevon MA, Turk N, et al. Psychological distress in long-term survivors of solid tumors diagnosed

in childhood: a report from the childhood cancer survivor study. *Pediatr Blood Cancer.* 2007;49(1):47-51.

9. Krull KR, Hardy KK, Kahalley LS, Schuitema I, Kesler SR. Neurocognitive outcomes and interventions in long-term survivors of childhood cancer. *J Clin Oncol.* 2018;36(21):2181-2189.

10. National Academies of Sciences, Engineering, and Medicine; Health and Medicine Division; Board on Health Care Services; National Cancer Policy Forum. *Long-Term Survivorship Care after Cancer Treatment: Proceedings of a Workshop.* Washington, DC: National Academies Press (US); 2018.

11. Franco VI, Lipshultz SE. Cardiac complications in childhood cancer survivors treated with anthracyclines. *Cardiol Young.* 2015;25(suppl 2):107-116.

12. Record EO, Meacham LR. Survivor care for pediatric cancer survivors: a continuously evolving discipline. *Curr Opin Oncol.* 2015;27(4):291-296.

13. Berger A, Hinds P, Puchalski C, eds. *Handbook of Supportive Oncology and Palliative Care.* Demos Medical; 2018.

14. Nass SJ, Beaupin LK, Demark-Wahnefried W, et al. Identifying and addressing the needs of adolescents and young adults with cancer: summary of an Institute of Medicine workshop. *Oncologist.* 2015;20(2):186-195.

15. Bansal N, Amdani S, Lipshultz ER, Lipshultz SE. Chemotherapy-induced cardiotoxicity in children. *Expert Opin Drug Metab Toxicol.* 2017;13(8):817-832.

16. Children's Oncology Group. Long-Term Follow-Up Guidelines for Survivors of Childhood, Adolescent, and Young Adult Cancers. 2018. http://www.survivorshipguidelines.org. Accessed January 10, 2020.

17. Galligan A. Childhood cancer survivorship and long-term outcomes. *Adv Pediatr.* 2017;64(1):133-169. doi:10.1016/j.yapd.2017.03.014.

18. Gebauer J, Higham C, Langer T, Denzer C, Brabant G. Long-term endocrine and metabolic consequences of cancer treatment: a systematic review. *Endocr Rev.* 2019;40(3):711-767.

19. Brown AL, Arroyo VM, Agrusa JE, Scheurer ME, Gramatges MM, Lupo PJ. Survival disparities for second primary malignancies diagnosed among childhood cancer survivors: a population-based assessment. *Cancer.* 2019;125(20):3623-3630.

20. Chao C, Bhatia S, Xu L, et al. Incidence, risk factors, and mortality associated with second malignant neoplasms among survivors of adolescent and young adult cancer. *JAMA Netw Open.* 2019;2(6):e195536.

21. Choi DK, Helenowski I, Hijiya N. Secondary malignancies in pediatric cancer survivors: perspectives and review of the literature. *Int J Cancer.* 2014;135(8):1764-1773.

22. Gibson TM, Li C, Armstrong GT, et al. Perceptions of future health and cancer risk in adult survivors of childhood cancer: a report from the Childhood Cancer Survivor Study. *Cancer.* 2018;124(16):3436-3444.

23. Teepen JC, van Leeuwen FE, Tissing WJ, et al. Long-term risk of subsequent malignant neoplasms after treatment of childhood cancer in the DCOG LATER Study Cohort: role of chemotherapy. *J Clin Oncol.* 2017;35(20):2288-2298.

24. Sharma D, Lee T, Friedman AJ, Redbord KP. Need for improved skin cancer surveillance in pediatric cancer survivors. *Am J Clin Dermatol.* 2017;18(2):165-168.

25. Ueda T, Migita M, Itabashi T, et al. Therapy-related secondary malignancy after treatment of childhood malignancy: cases from a single center. *J Nippon Med Sch.* 2019;86(4):207-214.

26. Teepen JC, Kremer LC, van der Heiden-van der Loo M, et al. Clinical characteristics and survival patterns of subsequent sarcoma, breast cancer, and melanoma after childhood cancer in the DCOG-LATER cohort. *Cancer Causes Control.* 2019;30(9):909-922.

27. Published Recommendations. 2019. https://www.uspreventiveservicestaskforce.org/BrowseRec/Index/browse-recommendations

28. Chatalian L. Managing Chemo Brain in Pediatric Survivors of Childhood Cancer. 2018. https://www.oncologynurseadvisor.com/home/departments/from-cancercare/managing-chemo-brain-in-pediatric-survivors-of-childhood-cancer/. Accessed January 8, 2020.

29. Moore BD. Neurocognitive outcomes in survivors of childhood cancer. *J Pediatr Psychol.* 2005;30(1):51-63.

30. Brinkman TM, Krasin MJ, Liu W, et al. Long-term neurocognitive functioning and social attainment in adult survivors of pediatric CNS tumors: results from the St Jude Lifetime Cohort Study. *J Clin Oncol.* 2016;34(12):1358-1367.

31. Pietilä S, Korpela R, Lenko HL, et al. Neurological outcome of childhood brain tumor survivors. *J Neurooncol.* 2012;108(1):153-161.

32. Edelstein K, D'agostino N, Bernstein LJ, et al. Long-term neurocognitive outcomes in young adult survivors of childhood acute lymphoblastic leukemia. *J Pediatr Hematol Oncol.* 2011;33(6):450-458.

33. Cheung YT, Krull KR. Neurocognitive outcomes in long-term survivors of childhood acute lymphoblastic leukemia treated on contemporary treatment protocols: a systematic review. *Neurosci Biobehav Rev.* 2015;53:108-120.

34. Barrera M, Shaw AK, Speechley KN, Maunsell E, Pogany L. Educational and social late effects of childhood cancer and related clinical, personal, and familial characteristics. *Cancer.* 2005;104(8):1751-1760.

35. de Boer AG, Verbeek JH, van Dijk FJ. Adult survivors of childhood cancer and unemployment: a metaanalysis. *Cancer.* 2006;107(1):1-11.

36. Gurney JG, Krull KR, Kadan-Lottick N, et al. Social outcomes in the Childhood Cancer Survivor Study Cohort. *J Clin Oncol.* 2009;27(14):2390-2395.

37. Schreiber JE, Gurney JG, Palmer SL, et al. Examination of risk factors for intellectual and academic outcomes following treatment for pediatric medulloblastoma. *Neuro Oncol.* 2014;16(8):1129-1136.

38. Hudson MM. Survivors of childhood cancer: coming of age. *Hematol Oncol Clin North Am.* 2008;22(2):211-231, v-vi.

39. Castillo LA, Craft AW, Kernahan J, Evans RG, Aynsley-Green A. Gonadal function after 12-Gy testicular irradiation in childhood acute lymphoblastic leukaemia. *Med Pediatr Oncol.* 1990;18(3):185-189.

40. Wallace WH, Thomson AB, Saran F, Kelsey TW. Predicting age of ovarian failure after radiation to a field that includes the ovaries. *Int J Radiat Oncol Biol Phys.* 2005;62(3):738-744.

41. Green DM, Whitton JA, Stovall M, et al. Pregnancy outcome of female survivors of childhood cancer: a report from the Childhood Cancer Survivor Study. *Am J Obstet Gynecol.* 2002;187(4):1070-1080.

42. van de Loo LEXM, van den Berg MH, Overbeek A, et al. Uterine function, pregnancy complications, and pregnancy outcomes among female childhood cancer survivors. *Fertil Steril.* 2019;111(2):372-380.

43. Green DM, Liu W, Kutteh WH, et al. Cumulative alkylating agent exposure and semen parameters in adult survivors of childhood cancer: a report from the St Jude

Lifetime Cohort Study. *Lancet Oncol.* 2014;15(11):1215-1223.

44. Kenney LB, Laufer MR, Grant FD, Grier H, Diller L. High risk of infertility and long term gonadal damage in males treated with high dose cyclophosphamide for sarcoma during childhood. *Cancer.* 2001;91(3):613-621.

45. Levine J. Gonadotoxicity of cancer therapies in pediatric and reproductive-age females. In: Gracia C, Woodruff T, eds. *Oncofertility Medical Practice: Clinical Issues and Implementation.* New York, NY: Springer Science + Business Media; 2012:3-14.

46. Müller J. Impact of cancer therapy on the reproductive axis. *Horm Res.* 2003;59(suppl 1):12-20.

47. Green DM, Sklar CA, Boice JD, et al. Ovarian failure and reproductive outcomes after childhood cancer treatment: results from the Childhood Cancer Survivor Study. *J Clin Oncol.* 2009;27(14):2374-2381.

48. Hudson MM. Reproductive outcomes for survivors of childhood cancer. *Obstet Gynecol.* 2010;116(5):1171-1183.

49. Green DM, Whitton JA, Stovall M, et al. Pregnancy outcome of partners of male survivors of childhood cancer: a report from the Childhood Cancer Survivor Study. *J Clin Oncol.* 2003;21(4):716-721.

50. Signorello LB, Mulvihill JJ, Green DM, et al. Congenital anomalies in the children of cancer survivors: a report from the childhood cancer survivor study. *J Clin Oncol.* 2012;30(3):239-245.

51. Olsson M, Enskar K, Steineck G, Wilderang U, Jarfelt M. Self-perceived physical attractiveness in relation to scars among adolescent and young adult cancer survivors: a population-based study. *J Adolesc Young Adult Oncol.* 2018;7(3):358-366.

52. Kinahan KE, Sharp LK, Seidel K, et al. Scarring, disfigurement, and quality of life in long-term survivors of childhood cancer: a report from the childhood cancer survivor study. *J Clin Oncol.* 2012;30(20):2466-2474.

53. Lu Q, Krull KR, Leisenring W, et al. Pain in long-term adult survivors of childhood cancers and their siblings: a report from the childhood cancer survivor study. *Pain.* 2011;152(11):2616-2624.

54. Alessi D, Dama E, Barr R, et al. Health-related quality of life of long-term childhood cancer survivors: a population-based study from the Childhood Cancer Registry of Piedmont, Italy. *Eur J Cancer.* 2007;43(17):2545-2552.

55. Recklitis CJ, Diller LR, Li X, Najita J, Robison LL, Zeltzer L. Suicide ideation in adult survivors of childhood cancer: a report from the childhood cancer survivor study. *J Clin Oncol.* 2010;28(4):655-661.

56. Reinfjell T, Zeltzer L. A systematic review of self-reported pain in childhood cancer survivors. *Acta Paediatr.* 2020;109(1):56-70.

57. Servaes P, Verhagen C, Bleijenberg G. Fatigue in cancer patients during and after treatment: prevalence, correlates and interventions. *Eur J Cancer.* 2002;38(1):27-43.

58. Minton O, Berger A, Barsevick A, et al. Cancer-related fatigue and its impact on functioning. *Cancer.* 2013;119(suppl 11):2124-2130.

59. Mulrooney DA, Mertens AC, Neglia JP, Green DM, Zeltzer L, Robison LL. Fatigue and sleep in survivors of childhood cancer: a report from the Childhood Cancer Survivor Study (CCSS). *J Clin Oncol.* 2004;22(14 suppl):8129.

60. Langeveld NE, Grootenhuis MA, Voûte PA, de Haan RJ, van den Bos C. No excess fatigue in young adult survivors of childhood cancer. *Eur J Cancer.* 2003;39(2):204-214.

61. Mulrooney DA, Ness KK, Neglia JP, et al. Fatigue and sleep disturbance in adult survivors of childhood cancer: a report from the childhood cancer survivor study (CCSS). *Sleep.* 2008;31(2):271-281.

62. Zhang FF, Kelly MJ, Saltzman E, Must A, Roberts SB, Parsons SK. Obesity in pediatric ALL survivors: a meta-analysis. *Pediatrics.* 2014;133(3):e704-e715.

63. Pietilä S, Mäkipernaa A, Sievänen H, Koivisto AM, Wigren T, Lenko HL. Obesity and metabolic changes are common in young childhood brain tumor survivors. *Pediatr Blood Cancer.* 2009;52(7):853-859.

64. Lindemulder SJ, Stork LC, Bostrom B, et al. Survivors of standard risk acute lymphoblastic leukemia do not have increased risk for overweight and obesity compared to non-cancer peers: a report from the Children's Oncology Group. *Pediatr Blood Cancer.* 2015;62(6):1035-1041.

65. Warner EL, Fluchel M, Wright J, et al. A population-based study of childhood cancer survivors' body mass index. *J Cancer Epidemiol.* 2014;2014:531958.

66. Molcho M, D'Eath M, Thomas AA, Sharp L. Educational attainment of childhood cancer survivors: a systematic review. *Cancer Med.* 2019;8(6):3182-3195. doi:10.1002/cam4.2154.

67. Hauff M, Abel R, Hersh J, et al. Adolescent survivors' information needs for transitions to postsecondary education and employment. *Pediatr Blood Cancer.* 2019;66(4):e27547.

68. Maule M, Zugna D, Migliore E, et al. Surviving a childhood cancer: impact on education and employment. *Eur J Cancer Prev.* 2017;26(4):351-356.

69. Saatci D, Thomas A, Botting B, Sutcliffe AG. Educational attainment in childhood cancer survivors: a meta-analysis. *Arch Dis Child.* 2019;105(4):339-346.

70. Crom DB, Ness KK, Martinez LR, et al. Workplace experiences and turnover intention among adult survivors of childhood cancer. *J Cancer Surviv.* 2018;12(4):469-478.

71. Gunnes MW, Lie RT, Bjorge T, et al. Economic independence in survivors of cancer diagnosed at a young age: a Norwegian National Cohort Study. *Cancer.* 2016;122(24):3873-3882.

72. Frobisher C, Lancashire ER, Jenkinson H, et al. Employment status and occupational level of adult survivors of childhood cancer in Great Britain: The British childhood cancer survivor study. *Int J Cancer.* 2017;140(12):2678-2692.

73. Vetsch J, Wakefield CE, McGill BC, et al. Educational and vocational goal disruption in adolescent and young adult cancer survivors. *Psychooncology.* 2018;27(2):532-538.

74. Kirchhoff AC, Nipp R, Warner EL, et al. "Job Lock" among long-term survivors of childhood cancer: a report from the childhood cancer survivor study. *JAMA Oncol.* 2018;4(5):707-711.

75. Nathan PC, Henderson TO, Kirchhoff AC, Park ER, Yabroff KR. Financial hardship and the economic effect of childhood cancer survivorship. *J Clin Oncol.* 2018;36(21):2198-2205.

76. Teckle P, Peacock S, McBride ML, Bentley C, Goddard K, Rogers P. Long-term effects of cancer on earnings of childhood, adolescent and young adult cancer survivors—a population-based study from British Columbia, Canada. *BMC Health Serv Res.* 2018;18(1):826.

77. Guy GP Jr, Berkowitz Z, Ekwueme DU, Rim SH, Yabroff KR. Annual economic burden of productivity losses among adult survivors of childhood cancers. *Pediatrics.* 2016;138(suppl 1):S15-S21.

78. Nipp RD, Kirchhoff AC, Fair D, et al. Financial burden in survivors of childhood cancer: a report from the childhood cancer survivor study. *J Clin Oncol.* 2017;35(30):3474-3481.

79. Oancea SC, Brinkman TM, Ness KK, et al. Emotional distress among adult survivors of childhood cancer. *J Cancer Surviv.* 2014;8(2):293-303.

80. Lehmann V, Grönqvist H, Engvall G, et al. Negative and positive consequences of adolescent cancer 10 years after diagnosis: an interview-based longitudinal study in Sweden. *Psychooncology.* 2014;23(11):1229-1235.

81. Zeltzer LK, Recklitis C, Buchbinder D, et al. Psychological status in childhood cancer survivors: a report from the childhood cancer survivor study. *J Clin Oncol.* 2009;27(14):2396-2404.

82. Brinkman TM, Li C, Vannatta K, et al. Behavioral, social, and emotional symptom comorbidities and profiles in adolescent survivors of childhood cancer: a report from the childhood cancer survivor study. *J Clin Oncol.* 2016;34(28):3417-3425.

83. D'Agostino NM, Edelstein K, Zhang N, et al. Comorbid symptoms of emotional distress in adult survivors of childhood cancer. *Cancer.* 2016;122(20):3215-3224.

84. Janson C, Leisenring W, Cox C, et al. Predictors of marriage and divorce in adult survivors of childhood cancers: a report from the childhood cancer survivor study. *Cancer Epidemiol Biomarkers Prev.* 2009;18(10):2626-2635.

85. Rauck AM, Green DM, Yasui Y, Mertens A, Robison LL. Marriage in the survivors of childhood cancer: a preliminary description from the childhood cancer survivor study. *Med Pediatr Oncol.* 1999;33(1):60-63.

86. Thompson AL, Marsland AL, Marshal MP, Tersak JM. Romantic relationships of emerging adult survivors of childhood cancer. *Psychooncology.* 2009;18(7):767-774.

87. Kazak AE, Barakat LP, Meeske K, et al. Posttraumatic stress, family functioning, and social support in survivors of childhood leukemia and their mothers and fathers. *J Consult Clin Psychol.* 1997;65(1):120-129.

88. Stuber ML, Kazak AE, Meeske K, et al. Predictors of posttraumatic stress symptoms in childhood cancer survivors. *Pediatrics.* 1997;100(6):958-964.

89. Hobbie WL, Stuber M, Meeske K, et al. Symptoms of posttraumatic stress in young adult survivors of childhood cancer. *J Clin Oncol.* 2000;18(24):4060-4066.

90. Marjerrison S, Hendershot E, Empringham B, Nathan PC. Smoking, binge drinking, and drug use among childhood cancer survivors: a meta-analysis. *Pediatr Blood Cancer.* 2016;63(7):1254-1263.

91. Cantrell MA, Posner MA. Engagement in high-risk behaviors among young adult survivors of childhood cancer compared to healthy same-age peers surveyed in the national longitudinal study of adolescent health. *J Adolesc Young Adult Oncol.* 2016;5(2):146-151.

92. Ford JS, Barnett M, Werk R. Health behaviors of childhood cancer survivors. *Children (Basel).* 2014;1(3):355-373.

93. Bitsko MJ, Cohen D, Dillon R, Harvey J, Krull K, Klosky JL. Psychosocial late effects in pediatric cancer survivors: a report from the Children's Oncology Group. *Pediatr Blood Cancer.* 2016;63(2):337-343.

94. Mayer DK, Nekhlyudov L, Snyder CF, Merrill JK, Wollins DS, Shulman LN. American Society of Clinical Oncology clinical expert statement on cancer survivorship care planning. *J Oncol Pract.* 2014;10(6):345-351.

95. Berger A, Shuster J, Von Roenn J, eds. *Principles and Practice of Palliative Care and Supportive Oncology.* 4th ed. Philadelphia, PA: Lippincott Williams & Wilkins; 2013.

96. Sadak KT, Szalda D, Lindgren BR, et al. Transitional care practices, services, and delivery in childhood cancer survivor programs: a survey study of U.S. survivorship providers. *Pediatr Blood Cancer.* 2019;66(8):e27793.

97. Schwartz CL. Creating a bridge for transition: from pediatric cancer survival to life-long, risk-based health care of the adult cancer survivor. *Cancer.* 2020;126(3):473-476.

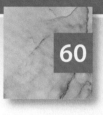

60 Survivorship Issues in Adults

Rachel Ombres, M. Jennifer Cheng, and Schuyler C. Cunningham

BACKGROUND AND SIGNIFICANCE

With continued advances in strategies to detect cancer early and treat it effectively along with the aging of the population, the number of individuals living years beyond a cancer diagnosis can be expected to continue to increase. It is estimated that as of 2019, there are 16.9 million cancer survivors in the United States, which will increase by 29.1% to 21.7 million by 2029 (1). According to the National Cancer Institutes' widely accepted definition, "an individual is considered a cancer survivor from the time of diagnosis, through the balance of his or her life. Family members, friends, and caregivers are also affected by the survivorship experience and are therefore included in their definition."

Fitzhugh Mullan, a physician diagnosed with and treated for cancer himself, first described the concept of cancer survivorship (2). Mullan described the survivorship experience as similar to the seasons of the year. Mullan recognized three seasons or phases of survival: acute (extending from diagnosis to the completion of initial treatment, encompassing issues dominated by treatment and its side effects); extended (beginning with the completion of initial treatment of the primary disease, remission of disease, or both, dominated by watchful waiting, regular follow-up examinations, and, perhaps, intermittent therapy); and permanent survival (not a single moment; evolves from extended disease-free survival when the likelihood of recurrence is sufficiently low). An understanding of these phases of survival is important for facilitating an optimal transition into and management of survivorship. This chapter will primarily focus on extended and permanent phases of cancer survivorship.

Although beneficial and often lifesaving against the diagnosed malignancy, most therapeutic modalities for cancer are associated with long-term health sequelae and a spectrum of late effects ranging from minor and treatable to serious or, occasionally, potentially lethal (3–7). *Late effects* refer specifically to unrecognized toxicities that are absent or subclinical at the end of therapy and become manifest later with the unmasking of hitherto unseen injury caused by any of the following factors: developmental processes, the failure of compensatory mechanisms with the passage of time, and/or organ senescence. *Long-term effects* refer to any side effects or complications of treatment for which a patient with cancer must compensate; also known as persistent effects, they begin during treatment and continue beyond the end of treatment (8–11). Late effects, in contrast, appear months to years after the completion of treatment (12–17).

Questions of particular importance to cancer survivors include surveillance for late- and long-term effects of treatment; the development of new (second) cancers; and recurrence of their original cancer. In recent years, health promotion and preventative care, psychological care, and care coordination among a multidisciplinary team (including transition back to primary care physicians [PCP]) are recognized as additional crucial components of survivorship care (18). There is today a greater recognition of the physical–psychosocial challenges facing cancer survivors after the completion of treatment and that arise years after primary therapy (6,19,20). The study of late effects, originally within the realm of pediatric cancer, is now germane to cancer survivors at all ages because concerns may continue to surface throughout the life cycle (21). These concerns underscore the need to routinely follow up and screen survivors of cancer for these complications and to develop and provide effective interventions.

This chapter focuses on survivorship issues in adults; examines late effects of cancer treatment; discusses long-term physical symptoms and psychosocial challenges among survivors of adult cancer; and reviews current standards for survivorship care, including assessment during survivorship visits.

REVIEW OF LATE- AND LONG-TERM EFFECTS: ORGAN SYSTEM SEQUELAE AND SYNDROMES (TABLE 60.1)

Cardiac Sequelae

Therapeutic irradiation and chemotherapeutic agents are both potential culprits of long-term

TABLE 60.1 POSSIBLE LATE EFFECTS OF RADIOTHERAPY AND CHEMOTHERAPY

Organ system	Late effects/ sequelae of radiotherapy	Late effects/ sequelae of chemotherapy	Chemotherapeutic drugs responsible	Other
Bone and soft tissues	Short stature, atrophy, fibrosis, osteonecrosis	Avascular necrosis	Steroids	Exercise resistance training improves muscle strength, maintenance/ improvement in bone density (22) Most allogeneic hematopoietic cell transplant (HCT) survivors have accelerated bone loss (23)
Cardiovascular	Pericardial effusion, pericarditis, coronary arterial disease	Cardiomyopathy (CM), congestive cardiac failure	Anthracyclines Cyclophosphamide	Early heart failure intervention results in better long-term cardiac function (24) HER2-targeted agents, angiogenesis inhibitors, and immunotherapies may cause CM or other myopathies (25,26)
Pulmonary	Pulmonary fibrosis, decreased lung volumes	Pulmonary fibrosis Interstitial pneumonitis	Bleomycin, BCNU Methotrexate, adriamycin	Bronchiolitis obliterans syndrome is the most frequent and potentially lethal post-HCT complication (27)
Central nervous system	Neuropsychological deficits, structural changes, hemorrhage	Neuropsychological deficits, structural changes Hemiplegia, seizure	Methotrexate	There is suggestion that cancer itself, chemotherapy, hormone therapy, and radiation can induce cognitive disorders (28)
Peripheral nervous system		Peripheral neuropathy, hearing loss	Cisplatin, vinca alkaloids	NCCN guidelines for survivorship have recommendations for seven categories of pain: neuropathic, chronic pain syndromes, myalgias/ arthralgias, skeletal, myofascial, GI/pelvic, postradiation (29)
Hematologic	Cytopenia, myelodysplasia	Myelodysplastic syndromes	Alkylating agents	Acute myeloid leukemia/ myelodysplastic syndrome as secondary malignant neoplasm from exposure to alkylators
Renal	Decreased creatinine clearance Hypertension	Decreased creatinine clearance Increased creatinine, renal filtration Delayed renal filtration	Cisplatin Methotrexate Nitrosoureas	Three clinical syndromes of kidney disease post-HCT thrombotic microangiopathy, nephrotic syndrome, and idiopathic or graft vs. host disease–related CKD (30)

TABLE 60.1 POSSIBLE LATE EFFECTS OF RADIOTHERAPY AND CHEMOTHERAPY *(Continued)*

Organ system	Late effects/ sequelae of radiotherapy	Late effects/ sequelae of chemotherapy	Chemotherapeutic drugs responsible	Other
Genitourinary	Bladder fibrosis, contractures	Bladder fibrosis, hemorrhagic cystitis	Cyclophosphamide	
Gastrointestinal	Malabsorption, stricture, abnormal LFT	Abnormal LFT, hepatic fibrosis, cirrhosis	Methotrexate, BCNU	Late effect after HCT includes chronic graft vs. host disease of the upper and lower GI tracts. GVHD should be distinguished from reactivation of herpesvirus (HSV, CMV, VZV)
Pituitary	Growth hormone deficiency, pituitary deficiency			
Thyroid	Hypothyroidism, nodules			
Reproductive/ sexual health	Men: direct exposure or scatter when other nearby organs are targeted	Men: impact on spermatogenesis through direct damage to spermatogonia	Alkylating and platinum-based agents	Certain surgical procedures can impair sexual function, such as radical pelvic surgery, removal of prostate, and seminal vesicles from prostate and bladder surgery; retroperitoneal lymph node dissection can interrupt sympathetic nerves and orchiectomy (31)
	Women: ovarian failure, early menopause. The severity of depletion depends on the proximity of ovaries to the irradiated field, the dose of radiation	Women: sterility, premature menopause	Alkylating and platinum-based agents Procarbazine	
Dental/oral health	Poor enamel and root formation, dry mouth			Oral complications of cGVHD affect almost 50% of adult patients post-HCT
Ophthalmologic	Cataracts, retinopathy	Cataracts	Steroids	Late effects after HCT include ocular cGVHD. Therapeutic goals are to reduce symptom, control disease activity, and prevent tissue damage. Severe cases may require gas-permeable scleral lens (32)

BCNU, carmustine; LFT, liver function test.

and late cardiac sequelae faced by survivors. Several types of damage have been reported including pericardial, myocardial, and vascular. Cardiac damage is most pronounced after treatment with the anthracycline drugs doxorubicin and daunorubicin, used widely in the treatment of most childhood cancers and as adjuvant chemotherapy for breast and many other adult cancers. An additive effect has also been reported when anthracyclines are used in conjunction with cyclophosphamide and radiation therapy. The incidence of anthracycline-induced cardiomyopathy, which is dose dependent, may exceed 30% among patients receiving cumulative doses in excess of 600 mg/m^2. Anthracyclines cause myocardial cell death, leading to a diminished number of myocytes and compensatory hypertrophy of residual myocytes (33). Major clinical manifestations include reduced cardiac function, arrhythmias, heart failure, and blunted hemodynamic responses to exercise. Chronic cardiotoxicity usually manifests as cardiomyopathy, pericarditis, and congestive heart failure and may also include significant valvular and conduction defects (34).

Cardiac injury that becomes clinically manifest during or shortly after completion of chemotherapy may progress, stabilize, or improve after the first year of treatment. This improvement may either be transient or last for a considerable length of time. There is also evidence of a continuum of injury that will manifest itself throughout the lives of these patients (34). From a risk factor perspective, patients who exhibit reduced cardiac function within 6 months of completing chemotherapy are at increased risk for the development of late cardiac failure (35). However, a significant incidence of late cardiac decompensation manifested by cardiac failure or lethal arrhythmia occurring 10 to 20 years after the administration of these drugs has also been reported (36).

Effects of radiation on the heart may be profound and include valvular damage, pericardial thickening, and ischemic heart disease. Adult patients with radiation-related cardiac damage have a markedly increased relative risk (RR) of both angina and myocardial infarction (RR 2.56) years after mediastinal radiation (37).

Chronic cardiotoxicity associated with radiation alone most commonly involves pericardial effusion or constrictive pericarditis, sometimes in association with pancarditis. Symptomatic pericarditis, which usually develops 10 to 30 years after irradiation, is found in 2% to 10% of patients (38). Coronary artery disease has been reported after radiation to the mediastinum, although mortality rates have not been significantly higher in patients who receive mediastinal radiation than in the general population (37).

Given the known acute and long-term cardiac complications of therapy, prevention of cardiotoxicity is a focus of active investigation.

Pulmonary Sequelae

Similar to cardiac toxicities, the pulmonary sequelae faced by cancer survivors may be due to either chemotherapy, radiation, or both. Stem-cell transplantation may also lead to late pulmonary complications such as idiopathic pneumonia syndrome and bronchiolitis obliterans (39). Newer cancer therapies, including immunotherapy agents such as erlotinib, cetuximab, panitumumab, and rituximab, have been associated with pulmonary fibrosis, although more studies are necessary (40).

Among the well-studied chemotherapeutic agents, bleomycin is most widely implicated in the development of long-term toxicity, although drugs such as alkylating agents, methotrexate, and nitrosoureas may also lead to pulmonary fibrosis especially when combined with radiation therapy (41). In adults, bleomycin is used to treat Hodgkin's disease and germ cell tumors. In these patients, the most common manifestation of bleomycin-related pulmonary toxicity is pneumonitis and has an incidence up to 46% (42). Older patients who smoke or have renal dysfunction are at increased risk, as are those who receive higher cumulative bleomycin doses and/or mediastinal radiation (42). A majority of people who develop bleomycin-induced pneumonitis (BIP) will recover, but a small number will progress to pulmonary fibrosis and have persistent symptoms such as dyspnea on exertion and nonproductive cough (43). Respiratory failure and cor pulmonale are late and often fatal complications of pulmonary fibrosis.

Mediastinal radiation, usually used to treat lung cancer, HD, and breast cancer, can cause long-term radiation pneumonitis. Similar to BIP, radiation-induced pneumonitis is usually self-limited, with a minority of patients progressing to pulmonary fibrosis (44). Other nonspecific ventilatory defects attributed to mediastinal radiation can occur as late as 10 to 20 years after treatment and include reduced lung volumes and restrictive lung disease with symptoms of dyspnea in 20% of patients (45).

The long-term outcome of pulmonary toxicity is determined by factors such as the severity of the acute injury, the degree of tissue repair, and the level of compensation possible. Pulmonary dysfunction is usually subclinical and may be manifested by subconscious avoidance of exercise owing to symptoms. Premature respiratory insufficiency, especially with exertion, may also become evident with aging.

Endocrinologic Sequelae

Thyroid

Radiation exposure to the head and neck is a known risk factor for subsequent abnormalities of the thyroid. Among survivors of HD and, to a lesser extent, survivors of leukemia, abnormalities of the thyroid gland, including hypothyroidism, hyperthyroidism, and thyroid neoplasms, have been reported to occur at rates significantly higher than those found in the general population (46–49). Hypothyroidism is the most common nonmalignant late effect involving the thyroid gland. Following radiation doses above 15 Gy, laboratory evidence of primary hypothyroidism is evident in 40% to 90% of patients with a history of HD, NHL, or head and neck malignancies (48–51). Most of the adult cases occur in the first 5 years, but the risk is lifelong and should be monitored regularly.

Bone Health

Osteoporosis and osteopenia are prevalent conditions in the general population, especially among women, and is a prevalent health problem among cancer survivors (52–55). Data of Twiss et al. indicate that 80% of older breast cancer patients have T-scores <−1, clinically confirmed osteopenia. Other cancer populations, such as premenopausal breast and prostate cancer patients, may possess good skeletal integrity at the onset of their disease, but are at risk for developing osteopenia that may ensue with treatment-induced ovarian suppression or androgen ablation.

Metabolic Syndrome–Associated Diseases: Obesity, Diabetes, and Cardiovascular Disease

Obesity is a well-established risk factor for cancers of the breast (postmenopausal), colon, kidney (renal cell), esophagus (adenocarcinoma), and endometrium; therefore, a large proportion of patients with cancer are overweight or obese at the time of diagnosis (56,57). Additional weight gain can also occur during or after active cancer treatment, an occurrence that has been frequently documented among individuals with breast cancer, but has been reported among patients with testicular and gastrointestinal cancers as well (43,58). Given data that obesity is associated with cancer recurrence in both breast and prostate cancers as well as reduced quality of life among survivors, there is compelling evidence to support weight control efforts in this population (59–61). Also, gradual weight loss has proven benefits in controlling hypertension, hyperinsulinemia, pain, and dyslipidemia and in improving levels of physical functioning, conditions that are significant problems in the survivor population (59,62,63). Accordingly,

the American Cancer Society's Recommendations for Cancer Survivors lists the "achievement of a healthy weight" as a primary goal (59).

Obesity represents one of several metabolic disorders that are frequently present among cancer survivors; disorders that are grouped under the umbrella of "the metabolic syndrome" include diabetes and cardiovascular disease (CVD). Insulin resistance is the underlying event associated with metabolic syndrome, and insulin resistance and diabetes have been reported as health concerns among cancer survivors (64–66). As Brown et al. (67) observed, diabetes may play a significant role in the increased number of non–cancer-related deaths among survivors; however, its role in progressive cancer is still speculative.

Although there is one study that suggests that older breast cancer patients derive a cardioprotective benefit from their diagnosis and/or associated treatments (tamoxifen) (68), most reports indicate that CVD is a major health issue among survivors, evidenced by mortality data that demonstrate half of the non–cancer-related deaths are attributed to CVD (69). Risk is especially high among men with prostate cancer who receive hormone ablation therapy, as well as with patients who receive adriamycin and radiation treatment to fields surrounding the heart (70). Although more research is needed to explore the potential benefits of lifestyle interventions specifically within survivor populations, the promotion of a healthy weight through a low saturated fat diet with ample amounts of fruits and vegetables and moderate levels of physical activity is recommended (59).

Gonadal and Sexual Dysfunction

Treatment-related gonadal dysfunction has been well documented in both men and women following childhood malignancies (71). Manifested as amenorrhea or azoospermia, treatment-related gonadal dysfunction can lead to infertility in both male and female survivors of cancer and may have its onset during therapy (72). Infertility can be transient, especially in men, and may eventually recover after therapy. Reversibility is dependent on the dose of gonadal radiation or alkylating agents. Ovarian function is unlikely to recover long after the immediate treatment period because long-term amenorrhea commonly results from loss of ova. Cryopreservation of sperm before treatment is an option for men (73), but limited means are available to preserve ova or protect against treatment-related ovarian failure for women (74–76). Among survivors of adult cancer, the risk of premature onset of menopause in women treated with chemotherapeutic agents such as alkylating agents and procarbazine, or with abdominal radiation therapy, is age-related, with women older than age 30 at the time of treatment having the greatest risk of treatment-induced amenorrhea and menopause (77). While ovarian suppression is becoming a more common adjuvant treatment for hormone receptor–positive (HRP) breast cancer, in premenopausal patients with HRP tumors, ovarian ablation is rarely recommended as primary treatment. Its use as adjuvant therapy in high-risk or relapsed premenopausal women is mixed when risks and benefits are considered (78,79). Regardless of menopausal status in breast cancer survivors, sexual dysfunction is most common among patients treated with aromatase inhibitors compared to those treated with tamoxifen, chemotherapy, and/or radiation (78). Cytoreductive surgery, a mainstay treatment for ovarian cancer, causes premature menopause in premenopausal patients.

Sexual health and function can be impacted at any time during or after cancer treatment and have lasting consequences for survivors and their partners. Prevalence estimates range from 40% to 100% and include a variety of manifestations, such as dysfunctional sexual response (i.e., erectile and/or ejaculatory dysfunction, inability to reach orgasm, vaginal dryness), low libido, loss of sensation, and pain (80,81). Some of these symptoms may be related to the onset of premature menopause in women cancer survivors, yet the safety of hormone replacement therapy in survivors of gynecologic malignancies remains controversial (81). In addition to physical symptoms, body image concerns, especially following cancer-related surgery, are likely underreported and may contribute to diminished sexual desire and responsiveness. Despite its prevalence and potential to profoundly impact quality of life, surveyed providers report discomfort about communicating with their cancer survivor patients about sexual health and often avoid the issue entirely (82,83). Nonetheless, this is a domain of social functioning that is important to proactively discuss with patients.

Survivors of genitourinary tract and gastrointestinal malignancies, including prostate, testicular, bladder, and colorectal cancer, also face increased rates of sexual dysfunction. Erectile and ejaculatory dysfunction, diminished sexual desire, and body image disturbances are especially prevalent in these populations (84–87).

GENITOURINARY TRACT SEQUELAE

Several drugs such as cisplatin, methotrexate, and nitrosoureas have been associated with both acute and chronic toxicities such as glomerular and tubular injury (88). Glomerular injury may recover over time, whereas tubular injury generally persists. Hemodialysis to counteract the effects of chronic renal toxicity may be warranted for some patients. Ifosfamide may cause Fanconi syndrome with glycosuria, phosphaturia, and aminoaciduria and may affect glomerular filtration. Hypophosphatemia may result in slow growth in children, with possible bone deformity if untreated.

Radiation therapy may cause tubular damage and hypertension as a result of renal artery stenosis, especially in doses >20 Gy, particularly among children (89). Radiation and chemotherapy may act synergistically, the dysfunction occurring with only 10 to 15 Gy.

The bladder is particularly susceptible to certain cytotoxic agents. Acrolein, a metabolic by-product of cyclophosphamide and ifosfamide, may cause hemorrhagic cystitis, fibrosis, and occasionally diminished bladder volume. An increased risk of developing bladder cancer also exists. Radiation may lead to bladder fibrosis, diminished capacity, and decreased contractility, the severity of which is proportional to dose and area irradiated. The resultant scarring may diminish urethral and ureteric function.

GASTROINTESTINAL/HEPATIC SEQUELAE

Chronic gastrointestinal toxicity is often a result of radiotherapy. The syndrome known as "pelvic radiation disease" (PRD) can occur following radiation to the pelvic area and includes a wide range of gastrointestinal symptoms including abdominal bloating and flatulence, chronic diarrhea or constipation, nausea and vomiting, pain, loss of anal sensation, and chronic gastrointestinal bleeding. In varying severity, it is estimated that up to 80% of patients experience symptoms of PRD (90,91). Chronic fecal incontinence, one element of PRD, affects up to 44% of anal cancer survivors who received radiotherapy, and of these, up to 10.9% require a colostomy for symptom control (92). Other potential treatments to manage fecal incontinence include the use of topical phenylephrine, sacral nerve stimulation, biofeedback, and constipating agents, although evidence supporting these modalities is limited (92–94).

Notably, while chronic toxicity from immune checkpoint inhibitors is still an area of active investigation, diarrhea is a well-described side effect that may itself persist as a long-term effect following treatment (95,96).

There are few studies describing long-term hepatic effects faced by survivors, either due to underdetection or due to a longer latency period than for other organs. Hepatic sequelae may result from the deleterious effects of many chemotherapeutic agents and radiotherapy, and transfusions received during cancer treatment may increase the risk of viral hepatitis.

IMMUNE SYSTEM SEQUELAE

Hematologic and immunologic impairments can occur after either chemotherapy or radiation and are usually acute in nature. They are temporally related to the cancer treatment. Occasionally, cytopenias may persist after pelvic radiation or in patients who have received extensive therapy with alkylating agents. Alkylating agents may cause myelodysplastic syndrome or leukemia as a late sequela. Immunologic impairment is seen as a long-term problem in HD, relating to both the underlying disease and the treatments used. HD patients are also at risk for serious bacterial infections if they have undergone splenectomy.

NEUROCOGNITIVE SEQUELAE

Fatigue

Fatigue has been reported as a prevalent and persistent side effect of cancer and its treatment in many studies (97–101). Treatment-related fatigue may be associated with various factors and comorbidities, such as anemia, infection, changes in hormone levels, lack of physical activity, and sleep disorders (58). Other psychosocial stressors may also impact fatigue and impair daily functioning, such as depression, anxiety, chronic pain, and existential distress. Given its extensive prevalence and potential to impair quality of life, screening for fatigue in cancer survivors is essential. Nevertheless, data suggest that fatigue is often underreported by patients and insufficiently addressed by health care providers (102).

To adequately address and treat fatigue, a thorough history and examination are necessary in order to rule out reversible physiological causes, optimize contributing comorbidities, and distinguish fatigue from other psychological illnesses. In addition to treating and optimizing contributing comorbid conditions and factors, cancer-related fatigue (CRF) may be treated using a multimodal and multidisciplinary approach. Exercise has the most evidence in terms of the nonpharmacologic approaches and is recommended for cancer survivors as a method to treat fatigue in addition to other common cancer-related quality-of-life parameters, such as physical functioning, anxiety, and depression (103,104). Cognitive behavioral therapy (CBT) also has data supporting its use for CRF and has been shown to improve not only fatigue but also related parameters such as health-related well-being, likely by its potential to promote self-care

management through relaxation strategies, emotional expression, and encouragement to seek support from others (105,106). Pharmacotherapy for fatigue in cancer survivors is more controversial due to its potential for harm with long-term use. Psychostimulants and steroids, not uncommonly prescribed for cancer-related fatigue during active cancer treatment or in end-stage disease, have long-term side effects that limit their chronic use in survivors. More studies are needed to further elucidate appropriate pharmacotherapy for CRF in the survivor population (107).

Cognitive Impairment

Cancer-related cognitive impairment (CRCI) is increasingly recognized as a potential lasting consequence of cancer and its treatment. A syndrome of dysfunction in multiple neurocognitive domains including memory, processing speed, executive functioning, concentration, and attention, it can persist for months to years following treatment and can have significant effects on quality of life for cancer survivors (108). The literature suggests variability between the prevalence of subjective, patient-reported cognitive concerns and objectively identified cognitive impairment based on neuropsychologic testing, with the former being more common, although this may highlight the failure of current tools to adequately test and detect this unique syndrome. Over 50% of breast cancer patients report cognitive deficits following chemotherapy, even though the current testing methods detect decline in only 15% to 20% of these patients (109).

Risk factors for the development of CRCI include patient-related and treatment-related variables. Implicated genes are apolipoprotein E and brain-derived neurotrophic factor, both of which regulate neural repair and are also thought to be involved in the pathogenesis of Alzheimer's disease (110). Older patients are also at greater risk for developing CRCI than younger patients. Possible treatment-related mechanisms include a combination of chemotherapy-induced cytotoxicity and cytokine dysregulation leading to neurotoxicity and oxidative stress, triggering cell death, DNA damage, and shortening of telomeres (110). Most research has focused on the prevalence of CRCI in breast cancer survivors, although similar data are emerging in survivors of lymphoma and colorectal and ovarian cancer (109,111).

Chemotherapy is not the only culprit treatment implicated in the development of CRCI. While still limited, there is growing evidence that endocrine therapies for breast and prostate cancer, as well as targeted immunotherapies, can affect cognition following treatment (112–114). Intracranial radiotherapy, both for primary intracranial malignancies and for metastatic lesions, may lead to lasting cognitive deficits, although some studies have shown that stereotactic radiosurgery leads to less cognitive decline compared to whole-brain radiation (115). Due to the prevalence of cognitive dysfunction in the setting of brain radiation and the improved long-term survival of patients, numerous studies have attempted to identify strategies to mitigate cognitive dysfunction in an effort to improve the quality of life in survivors. Now, a common component of treatment for patients undergoing intracranial radiotherapy is memantine, a NMDA receptor antagonist often used in the treatment of Alzheimer's disease. Patients treated with memantine while undergoing intracranial radiation show better cognitive function, including better outcomes in the domains of memory, executive function, and processing speed (116).

Unlike cognitive dysfunction related to intracranial radiation, CRCI related to chemotherapy does not have well-established preventative or treatment modalities. Nonpharmacologic therapies, such as CBT and other forms of cognitive rehabilitation, are being studied, as are certain pharmaceuticals, such as acetylcholinesterase inhibitors and stimulants (111,117). Preliminary data are mixed and more studies are needed in order to confidentially support the use of these therapies.

AGING CANCER SURVIVORS

The U.S. Census Bureau predicts that between 2016 and 2060, the population of adults aged 65 and older will nearly double (118). By then, for the first time in history, older adults will outnumber the population of children in the United States. The demographics of cancer survivors will also reflect this population shift, with nearly 75% of survivors belonging to the geriatric age group by 2050 (1). Caring for older adults often must balance the management of acute and chronic diseases with the preservation of function, all of which may be more complex in cancer survivors. Compared to age-matched individuals, older adult cancer survivors have more deficits with activities of daily living (ADLs), such as maintaining personal hygiene, dressing, and eating, as well as with instrumental activities of daily living (IADLs), including managing finances and medications (119,120). This relationship becomes even more pronounced in those cancer survivors with other medical comorbidities and is directly related to increased mortality, with cancer survivors who have functional deficits at highest risk for mortality compared to matched noncancer adults (119). Anticipating this trend,

addressing functional status in older adult cancer survivor should be a mainstay of their primary care, including aggressive interventions aimed at maintaining function and independence.

Older adult cancer survivors may also face different concerns regarding lasting disease and treatment-related side effects compared to younger survivors. More research is emerging regarding chemotherapy-related cognitive impairment. While this can affect all ages, it poses particular implications for older adults whose age alone increases their baseline risk for neurocognitive deficits. For example, in studies of breast cancer patients, older women were more susceptible to developing cognitive deficits following chemotherapy than younger women (121). It is postulated that posttreatment cognitive performance may also vary depending on cognitive reserve prior to treatment. Using these data, physicians can better inform patients and families especially when making treatment decisions and also help to manage expectations regarding outcomes in older adults.

PAIN

Cancer-related pain can occur at the onset of a diagnosis and persist through treatment. Once a survivor has ended cancer treatment, up to 40% may be faced with a new, chronic pain syndrome often related to the treatment that enabled their cure (122). Beyond feeling uncomfortable, chronic pain affects global function and quality of life. Cancer survivors with chronic pain have higher rates of depression and unemployment and more functional limitations compared to cancer survivors without chronic pain (123). Managing chronic pain in a cancer survivor differs from managing chronic pain unrelated to prior malignancy. Firstly, there is often identifiable tissue damage, which can often help guide therapy. Secondly, a cancer survivor is at higher risk for recurrent disease and secondary malignancies, mandating careful evaluation of new pain complaints (124). Lastly, many cancer survivors with chronic pain will have already been receiving opioids for cancer-related pain during active treatment, necessitating a thoughtful transition to the management of opioids in the chronic setting.

In addition to providing an overview of chronic cancer pain and its management in survivors, the following section will address in more detail two common chronic pain syndromes that occur secondary to cancer treatment: chemotherapy-induced peripheral neuropathy and secondary lymphedema. See Table 60.2 for additional chronic pain syndromes prevalent in cancer survivors.

TABLE 60.2 CHRONIC CANCER-RELATED PAIN SYNDROMES

Surgery	Postmastectomy pain Breast reconstruction Postthoracotomy pain Post–neck dissection pain Phantom limb pain Lymphedema	**Hematopoietic Stem-Cell Transplant**	Esophageal strictures Painful fibrosis Osteonecrosis Peripheral neuropathy
Radiation Therapy	Osteoradionecrosis Nerve entrapment GI adhesions Mucositis Painful fibrosis	**Chemotherapy**	Peripheral neuropathy

Chronic Chemotherapy-Induced Peripheral Neuropathy

Chronic chemotherapy-induced peripheral neuropathy (CIPN) affects up to 40% of individuals treated with neurotoxic chemotherapies (125). The condition is due to damage of the dorsal root ganglion neurons or their axons and leads to pain and sensory loss usually in the hands and/or feet. The pain can include allodynia, hyperalgesia, and dysesthesia, in addition to chronic burning and tingling sensations. Some people also have motor involvement or sensory ataxia, which contributes to the CIPN-related functional deficits that survivors may face. Certain tasks, such as dressing, writing, preparing meals, and walking, become challenging. Due to diminished proprioception in the feet, driving may become dangerous. For these reasons in addition to the associated chronic pain, CIPN has been associated with poor quality of life in survivors (126). Higher survivor-reported severity of CIPN correlates with higher frequencies of insomnia, falls, and lower quality of life (126,127).

Research elucidating predictors of chronic CIPN and preventative measures is limited, although growing. Undoubtedly, the type of chemotherapy is critical to the development of CIPN, and the major culprits include the taxanes, platinum compounds, vinca alkaloids, and proteasome inhibitors. Some research suggests that more severe acute CIPN during chemotherapy may be a predictor for the development of chronic symptoms. Lower income, a higher number of comorbidities, diabetes mellitus, and alcohol consumption continue to demonstrate inconclusive findings (125).

Treatment for chronic CIPN includes pharmacologic and complementary therapies. Pharmacologically, the only medication currently recommended by the American Society of Clinical Oncology (ASCO) to treat established, painful CIPN is duloxetine (125). Clinically, other serotonin–norepinephrine reuptake inhibitors, gabapentinoids, tricyclic antidepressants, and antiepileptics are employed.

Opioids may be effective, but they should not be first-line therapy for chronic pain syndromes due to their side effect profile. Complementary therapies including acupuncture, electrocutaneous nerve stimulation (scrambler therapy), and exercise have limited and mixed data, but may be discussed with survivors as part of a comprehensive approach to managing this chronic pain syndrome (125).

Lymphedema

Lymphedema can occur following treatment for cancer, including surgery and radiation therapy, due to damage to the lymphatic system. The risk for lymphedema is lifelong, and its onset may be delayed for several decades following cancer treatment (128). Upper extremity lymphedema is reported most commonly after breast cancer treatment with incidence rates between 6% and 48% (129). It is often a chronic and incurable condition that manifests with physical symptoms, functional impairment, and diminished quality of life (130). Physical symptoms include pain, limb swelling, sensory alterations, limited range of motion, and fatigue. These symptoms can lead to decreased physical activity and difficulty completing certain ADL. As salient as its physical manifestations are chronic lymphedema's effects on quality of life. In several studies including a recent qualitative study by Anbari et al. in 2019, depression, irritability, and loss of body confidence were identified as common themes among breast cancer survivors with chronic lymphedema (130).

Timely intervention to treat lymphedema is crucial in order to limit its progression and prevent its complications. As the condition progresses untreated, tissue fibrosis can make treatment attempts less successful, and the resulting stagnation of lymphatic fluid puts the limb at risk for soft tissue infection (129). The mainstay treatment for lymphedema is multimodal and long-term, including skin care, massage, bandaging for compression, and exercise.

Opioids in the Chronic Pain Management of Cancer Survivors

Recent guidelines stipulating limitations on opioid prescriptions for pain management often include a caveat that the recommendation applies to "noncancer pain" (131). These policies do not adequately address the estimated 40% of cancer survivors who have chronic cancer–related pain and may have preexisting opioid prescriptions, leaving prescribing physicians to navigate this potentially complicated domain without standardized guidance or consensus (122). Opioids are often not the most effective or the safest choice for long-term treatment. Nevertheless, opioid prescribing rates in cancer survivors are higher than matched controls without cancer, including 10 years or more past a cancer diagnosis (132).

In the climate of today's opioid addiction crisis, prescribing oncologists and palliative care providers face novel challenges. Acknowledging the growing population of survivors, even in the active cancer treatment phase, prescribers must weigh potential long-term risks from opioid therapy. Survivors may have preexisting substance abuse problems, and those who do not may still be at risk of developing them during their cancer treatment. Nevertheless, data on the incidence of opioid misuse in cancer patients are sparse, with wide estimates between 0% and 43% in studies with small patient numbers and variable assessment tools (133). A small trial of opioid-naïve stage I and II cervical cancer survivors showed that 25% were still using opioids following their cancer treatment and that persistent use was associated with history of substance abuse, depression, and anxiety (134).

Despite the known prevalence of chronic pain in cancer survivors, guidelines addressing its management remain limited. Using an expert review panel and an extensive literature search, the ASCO published a special report in 2016 to begin to address this need. Considerations from these guidelines include (135):

- Management of chronic cancer pain should balance pharmacologic and nonpharmacologic techniques, often necessitating the involvement of a multidisciplinary team.
- Goals of treatment should focus on improving function and limiting long-term adverse effects of pain and its treatment. This is in contrast to the common goal of treating acute cancer pain, which is to provide comfort.
- All providers who interact with cancer survivors should be trained to implement best practices in the management of chronic pain.

For more detailed recommendations on the assessment of pain and pain management in the cancer survivor, see Table 60.3.

MENTAL HEALTH DIAGNOSING IN THE SETTING OF SURVIVORSHIP

Diagnosing mental health conditions in the setting of cancer or survivorship can be complicated. In large part, this is due to the overlapping symptoms and side effect profiles with physiological conditions. Moreover, often a mental health assessment is in the context of knowing no baseline pretreatment unless the patient is able to reliably report their mental health history. Nonetheless, mental health conditions negatively impact survivors and can also have a negative impact on the clinical care team.

To further illustrate the intricacies of mental health in survivorship, consider the following:

Ms. Smith recently finished treatment for lymphoma. She returns for her 3-month checkup and reports symptoms similar to those she had during treatment. She reports a constellation of the following: fatigue, panic attacks, shallowing breathing, loss of interest in regular activities, loss of appetite, prolonged periods of being in bed, decreased optimism or ability to be future focused, significant weight loss, insomnia or hypersomnia, decreased memory or ability to concentrate, and/or suicidal thinking.

During treatment, it is likely that all of these symptoms would be seen in the context of side effects of chemotherapy, especially, if Ms. Smith did not report a previous mental health diagnosis. While these symptoms can be side effects of treatment, they are also very well aligned with a depressive disorder, anxiety, or even posttraumatic stress disorder (PTSD). For this reason, it is important to refer to a mental health professional to establish a mental health diagnosis whenever possible:

- 95% reported at least one emotional concern, and only 45% received care for their reported emotional concern (136).
- 80% reported fears of recurrence.
- 60% reported issues with grief or identity or emotional distress.
- 50% reported concerns about body image or risk of cancer for family members.

DEPRESSION

The prevalence of depression in the United States among adults is 7% (137). Depression rates in survivorship can be as high as 17% (138). In a pooled sample of 51,381 cancer survivors, the prevalence

TABLE 60.3 ASSESSMENT AND TREATMENT OF PAIN IN CANCER SURVIVORS

Assessment	Content of clinical visit

	• Conduct an initial comprehensive pain assessment:
	  • Explore the nature of pain and its functional, psychological, social, and spiritual impact
	  • Characterize pain and clarify its cause
	  • This should be accompanied by a physical exam and any appropriate diagnostic testing
	
	• Screen for pain at every subsequent encounter:
	  • Always consider the possibility of cancer reoccurrence, secondary malignancy, or late-onset treatment effects when a new pain report arises in a cancer survivor
	
	• Assess for and treat comorbid conditions known to impact pain intensity in chronic pain sufferers (135), such as:
	  • Depression
	  • Anxiety
	  • Personality disorders
	  • Posttraumatic stress disorder

Treatment	• Aims
	  • Improve quality of life by decreasing pain, improving function, and limiting adverse effects
	  • Patient and caregivers should be active participants in care plan
	
	• Nonpharmacologic interventions:
	  • Include appropriate nonpharmacologic interventions as part of a comprehensive care plan
	  • Physical therapy, occupational therapy, recreational therapy, and orthotics
	  • Complementary medicine, such as massage therapy and acupuncture
	  • Interventional pain management, for example, nerve blocks, neuraxial infusions, and neurostimulatory therapies
	  • Psychological health providers and spiritual counseling
	
	• Pharmacologic interventions:
	  • Pharmacologic interventions should resemble those for chronic, non–cancer-related pain
	  • Evidence-based consensus is to prioritize trials with systemic, nonopioid analgesics in order to relieve chronic pain, improve function, and minimize harm:
	    • NSAIDs
	    • Acetaminophen
	    • Adjuvant analgesics
	    • Topical analgesics, such as commercially available NSAIDs, local anesthetics, or compounded agents that include baclofen, amitriptyline, and ketamine

Treatment—use of opioids	• Use of opioids
	  • In carefully screened cancer survivors who continue to have chronic pain despite the use of the nonpharmacologic and nonopioid interventions described above, a time-limited trial of opioids may be appropriate. In these patients:
	    • Assess risk for opioid misuse using standardized risk tool, such as the Opioid Risk Tool (ORT)
	    • Only prescribe opioids if the potential for opioid-related harm is deemed less than the potential for benefit
	    • Engage multidisciplinary care providers, such as social workers and addiction medicine specialists, in patients who fall into moderate- or high-risk category
	    • Formulate patient-specific safe prescribing plan for moderate- to high-risk patients, including provisions such as frequent urine drug screens, frequent clinic follow-up appointments, and providing short supply of medications at one time
	    • Educate patients and their families/caregivers on risks and benefits of long-term opioid therapy, safe storage, and safe disposal, regardless of patient's ORT score
	    • Ensure short follow-up intervals to assess efficacy. If opioids fail to provide pain relief and/or improve function, consider taper and discontinuation
	  • Provide ongoing assessment for adverse short-term and long-term effects. Short-term/persistent effects:
	    • Constipation
	    • Cognitive impairment
	    • Nausea
	    • Fatigue
	    • Myoclonus
	    • Opioid-induced hyperalgesia
	    • Long-term effects
	    • Osteoporosis/osteopenia
	    • Infertility

Adapted from Paice JA, Portenoy R, Lacchetti C, et al. Management of chronic pain in survivors of adult cancers: American Society of Clinical Oncology Clinical Practice guideline. *J Clin Oncol*. 2016;34(27):3325-3345.

of depression was 12% (139). This indicates a much higher than normal proclivity toward depressive symptoms and clinical depression in the survivor population.

For adult survivors of childhood cancer, up to 11% reported persistent depressive symptoms, and up to 12% reported anxiety symptoms after treatment. Among long-term survivors of adult cancer, up to 20% report anxiety symptoms (139). Risk factors include being female, shorter time since diagnosis, younger age of diagnosis, living alone, and a diagnosis of lung cancer or melanoma.

In many instances, physical symptoms can be related to depressive symptoms (140). These may present differently in different diagnostic groups. For example, Badr and colleagues reported that oral cancer survivors who reported dental health, problems with smelling, and issues with range of motion were associated with both depressive and anxiety symptoms (141). The literature reports that survivors of prostate cancer who also had higher levels of urinary and androgen deprivation therapy had higher levels of depressive symptoms and in head and neck cancer survivors, reduced sexual function was associated with depressive symptoms (142,143). Also of note, not receiving follow-up care instructions significantly increased the odds of symptoms of current depression in survivors within the first 5 years post treatment (144). A survivorship care plan is required by the American College of Surgeons (145).

Identifying depression in this population can be as simple as a basic screening and referral for a mental health assessment. Given the physiological complexities of survivorship, a thorough medical workup is often warranted in survivors who present with symptoms reflective of depression. That is not to say that their mental health symptoms are less impactful than other symptoms. Instead, it is to ensure a thorough medical and mental health workup.

Basic screenings include the Patient Health Questionnaire-9 (PHQ-9), the Beck's Depression Inventory (BDI), the Edinburgh Depression Scale (EDS), or the Hospital Anxiety and Depression Scale (HADS). These include questions about self-harm and self-injury. If a survivor answers positively to a self-harm or self-injury question, he or she should be immediately assessed.

For information regarding medication for depression in the setting of cancer survivorship, please refer to the chapter in this book on depression.

SUICIDE RISK

Suicide risk among cancer survivors is another important aspect of the survivorship continuum.

Compared to the general population, cancer suicide rate among patients is nearly double (146). This gives serious concern for the identification and treatment of self-harm and self-injury among this population.

Overall, out of approximately 8.5 million survivors studied, only 13,311 (0.15%) committed suicide (147). Overall men and people with metastatic disease at diagnosis had the highest death rates from suicide at 13% (147).

Osazuwa-Peters et al. presented a poster at the 2018 ASCO and reported results of suicide rates among survivors. They reported that the rate of male cancer survivor suicide was 2.5 times higher in men over 70 years old than in men between 20 and 39 years old. They reported the opposite phenomenon in women. Women between 20 and 39 years old were twice as likely to die of suicide than women over 70 years old. Men represented approximately 84% of the suicides (148).

Screening for suicide risk is quite simple. Clinics can utilize robust screening instruments or ultra-short measures depending on the risk level in a specific population as well as other logistical considerations. One method is to include a self-harm–related question on a distress screening tool, like the National Comprehensive Cancer Network's (NCCN) ubiquitous distress thermometer. Another option is to use the free Ask Suicide-Screening Questions Toolkit. This tool was created by the National Institute of Mental Health and consists of four yes/no questions that takes about 20 seconds to administer (149). Once a screening process is in place, it is also vital to have a process by which survivors get assessed by a mental health provider (e.g., medical social workers) if they screen positive. For this reason, doing phone screenings can be challenging as it is harder to ensure an immediate follow-up assessment.

ANXIETY

Anxiety is common among survivors. Anxiety is an emotion characterized by feelings of tension, worried thoughts, and physical changes like increased blood pressure (150). It can present with other physiological symptoms including, but not limited to, excessive sweating, shortness of breath, fluttery sensation in the stomach, narrow vision, difficulty concentrating, and panic attacks. Identifying and treating anxiety can improve the quality of life in the survivorship population as in any other population.

In terms of prevalence, in a pooled sample of 48,964 cancer survivors, the prevalence of anxiety was 18% (139), whereas the prevalence of generalized anxiety disorder (GAD) among those over 18 years old in the United States is 3% (151). While symptoms of anxiety and a diagnosis of GAD differ, the symptoms of anxiety experienced by those in survivorship must be understood to negatively impact their quality of life.

Risk factors for developing anxiety are important guides when considering survivors' experience. The literature suggests that females were twice as likely to experience anxiety in survivorship than males (152). Other risk factors for anxiety include shorter time since diagnosis, higher number of comorbid conditions, younger age, living alone, and a diagnosis of lung cancer or melanoma (153,154). Risk factor profiles are important as a shorthand guide to use in screening so that survivors with anxiety can be quickly identified and referred to the appropriate clinician for intervention.

Fear of recurrence (FOR) is another factor that survivors cope with and is quite similar to anxiety. Survivors considered FOR as one of the greatest concerns and the most frequently endorsed unmet need (155). Almost 80% of respondents to a national survey of cancer survivors reported some level of FOR as a concern. It was as high as 38% in survivors of colorectal cancer (136,156). Somewhat counterintuitively, risk factor for FOR included living with someone. This could be due to a newfound difficulty managing the relationship post cancer, changes in ability related to sexual intimacy, and/or the function of intimacy in the relationship. It could also be a sense of guilt for the negative impacts of treatment on their partner's physical and/or mental health. Additional risk factors include being female, 60 years old or younger, as soon as 5 years postdiagnosis, social isolation, and <10 years of education (157).

ONCOLOGY-RELATED PSYCHOSOCIAL DISTRESS

The theoretical foundation that oncology-related distress rests on is often guided by the transactional model of stress and coping, also called the stress model theory (SMT), developed by Lazarus and Folkman and expanded over the past three decades (158). SMT was originally developed from systems theory and uses cognitive, motivational, and relational theories to understand and explain how emotions are generated based on a stressful event, the outcome of an appraisal of the event, and how coping mediates between the appraisal and the outcome or reaction to the event (159).

One of the major expansions of SMT was the inclusion of preevent factors that influence how one reacts to a stressor or event were added to the theory (160,161). The preevent factors include person factors and situation factors. The person factors include commitments and beliefs, gender, and culture, while situation factors include previous experience with the event, the timing of the event, ambiguity, and timing within the life cycle of the individual and the family (159,161,162).

The outcome of the stressful event in an oncology setting manifests as psychosocial distress and traumatic stress symptomatology, or the emotional reaction. Experiences in a patient's history, in addition to an oncology diagnosis and treatment, known to cause traumatic stress are an aspect of preevent experiences, both personal and situational, which includes a cancer diagnosis. A patient's demographic profile is predisposing, as these are aspects of the individual that are preexisting. Illness-related data combine both information that might influence situational factors and the actual stressful event. Figure 60.1 illustrates how all these factors feed into the emotional reaction.

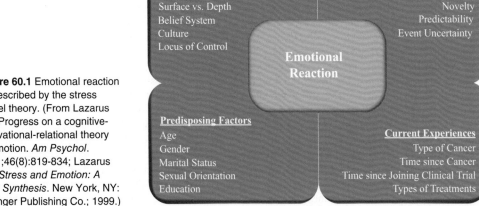

Figure 60.1 Emotional reaction as described by the stress model theory. (From Lazarus RS. Progress on a cognitive-motivational-relational theory of emotion. *Am Psychol.* 1991;46(8):819-834; Lazarus RS. *Stress and Emotion: A New Synthesis.* New York, NY: Springer Publishing Co.; 1999.)

Person Factors
Vulnerability
Surface vs. Depth
Belief System
Culture
Locus of Control

Situational Factors
Temporal Factors
Novelty
Predictability
Event Uncertainty

Emotional Reaction

Predisposing Factors
Age
Gender
Marital Status
Sexual Orientation
Education

Current Experiences
Type of Cancer
Time since Cancer
Time since Joining Clinical Trial
Types of Treatments

In 2015, the American College of Surgeons Commission on Cancer required all accredited cancer hospitals to begin screening oncology patients for psychosocial distress (145). Distress is an unpleasant experience of an emotional, psychological, social, or spiritual nature that interferes with the ability to cope with cancer treatment. It extends along a continuum, from common normal feelings of vulnerability, sadness, and fears, to problems that are disabling, such as depression, anxiety, panic, and feeling isolated or in a spiritual crisis (163).

Psychosocial distress in people with cancer can be debilitating (164). Distress can impact an individual's ability to cope with a cancer diagnosis and participate in treatment (165,166). Increased levels of psychosocial distress have been associated with decreased treatment adherence (167,168), surveillance screening (169), adoption of prevention behaviors (170), and communication between patient and provider (171). It has also been found that distressed individuals with cancer have longer inpatient stays (172) and increased health care costs (173). Distress may also negatively influence quality of life (174,175). The literature shows that preexisting psychosocial factors such as social support, past history of substance abuse, medical illness, health, employment, finances, self-appraisal, and education also play a role in a person's adjustment and ability to cope with oncology-related distress (176).

Zabora et al. (177) performed a seminal study on the prevalence and level of distress by cancer type, replicating earlier studies but substantially increasing the sample size to approximately 4,500 subjects. The results of their study showed the mean level of psychosocial distress for all cases was 35%. The distress level was highest at 45.5% for individuals with lung cancer, 37.8% for Hodgkin's lymphoma, 36% for non-Hodgkin's lymphoma, 32.7% for leukemia, and 30.5% for prostate cancer (178).

Accurate and early recognition of psychosocial distress often results in a timely intervention and improvement in outcome of co-occurring physical illness (179,180). Although patient distress levels and need for services are positively related, many clinics are unable to provide a full psychosocial assessment as resources are limited and there is a high demand for services (180,181). Nonetheless, if distress is not screened for the compounding effects, it could make survivorship more difficult.

In 2014, the Association for Oncology Social Work (AOSW) established the *Project to Assure Quality Cancer Care* (*APAQCC*), which consists of a group of oncology social workers who represented 65 Commission on Cancer-accredited cancer programs throughout the United States and two in Canada. The APAQCC examines the capacity of cancer programs to provide quality psychosocial

support and to evaluate the implementation of distress screening. Overall adherence rate to distress screening protocol was 63% (182). The highest rates of adherence to the screening guidelines were 76% in community cancer programs, whereas the lowest rates were National Cancer Institute–designated cancer programs at 43% (182).

Self-reported screening tools for distress are easily cost-effective for use in high-volume medical settings (179,183). If implemented in the clinical setting, distress screening can reliably identify emotionally distressed survivors, thereby ensuring better mental health care (184,185). Evidence indicates that the use of psychosocial screening instruments among cancer patients results in reductions in emotional distress, increased quality of life, and improved patient–provider communication (181,184,186,187). The NCCN offers the distress thermometer, which is free to use and free to adapt to a specific setting (188).

ONCOLOGY-RELATED TRAUMATIC STRESS

While it is well established that a cancer diagnosis and treatment may cause distress, there is evidence in the literature to suggest that distress related to cancer can also lead to traumatic stress symptoms and even fully diagnosed acute stress disorder (ASD) or PTSD. It has been shown that a cancer diagnosis represents a threat to life and bodily integrity and can create a sense of loss of social and occupational roles, causing one's adaptive capacity to become overwhelmed (189–192). Becoming overwhelmed due to a stressor that threatens one's life and bodily integrity and a loss of social roles is the definition of traumatic stress (193). A sense of feeling overwhelmed when a stressful trigger is not present is further evidence that a cancer diagnosis and treatment are producing traumatic stress (194).

The incidence of fully diagnosed PTSD in individuals recently diagnosed with early-stage cancer was 3% to 4% (195). The incidence rose to 35% following the completion of cancer treatment (196). Gurevich et al. (194) reviewed 39 studies between 1992 and 2001, looking at the prevalence of posttraumatic stress of individuals with a variety of types of cancer. They compared the site of disease, design of the study, sample, PTSD measure, PTSD predictors, and major significant results reported by the researcher of each study. They found that known risk and protective factors in other trauma contexts are relevant to cancer as well as empirical support for the use of a trauma-informed psychosocial support model of care in cancer (194).

Evidence supports the existence of substantial traumatic stress in the oncology population, whether or not the individual meets the full criteria for a diagnosis of PTSD. Cella et al. (197) found that 20% of patients diagnosed with early-stage cancer exhibited traumatic stress symptoms, even if they did not meet full criteria for PTSD. That rose to 80% among those with recent recurrences. Patients that had traumatic stress symptoms reported significantly reduced quality of life compared to patients without these symptoms (195). Poor health behaviors and decreased adherence to medical treatment have also been documented in this patient population (198).

People experiencing traumatic stress symptoms may present with intrusive or avoidant thoughts or memories, nightmares, flashbacks, amnesia, and reactivity. They may have negative thoughts or beliefs or feel a distorted sense of blame. They may exhibit reduced interest in activities or feel detached or isolated from the world and people around them. They may also experience difficulty concentrating and exhibit sleep disturbances. Some may even exhibit increased arousal, hypervigilance, or irritability (151). The specific nature of these symptoms warrants evidenced-based trauma-informed interventions (194).

Predictors of traumatic stress symptoms in people with cancer include prior negative life stressors, psychological problems, and elevated distress after diagnosis, being female, young age at diagnosis, lower social economic status, limited education, avoidant coping style, limited social support, and reduced physical functioning. Several studies have shown that cancer recurrence and more advanced disease may be associated with increased variety and severity of traumatic stress symptoms in comparison to the initial diagnosis (194,199,200).

The three most stressful experiences reported were receiving the diagnosis, waiting for the results of diagnostic testing, and waiting for surgery. As noted before, the outcome of these events can lead to overwhelming feelings and trigger active trauma symptoms. These can then be recalled or triggered again at a later date by diagnostic and treatment procedures, witnessing adverse outcomes of other individuals with cancer, psychoeducational interventions, and routine follow-up care (194).

The American College of Surgeons issued a strong stance by requiring accredited oncology clinics and hospitals to screen for psychosocial distress. The literature supports the need for further investigation into traumatic stress symptoms in people with cancer by providing data regarding the prevalence, rates, and the negative impact of traumatic stress in the oncology population, regardless of whether full criteria for PTSD have been met. There is work being done by Cunningham and colleagues to develop and put forward an oncology trauma syndrome (201).

Cancer-related traumatic stress is becoming more articulated in the literature. From clinical observation, many oncology providers—doctors, nurses, social workers, and other allied health care professionals—informally acknowledge the severity of traumatic stress symptoms in patients during and after treatment.

Here is a case example

A 30-year-old single female was receiving CBT from an oncology social worker. She was having trouble integrating back into life after successfully completing a bone marrow transplant. Prior to bone marrow transplant for lymphoma, she had survived pediatric lymphoma. Her mental health symptoms reflected what the provider believed to be classic depressive and anxious symptoms. After a number of months in treatment, this provider discussed the case with a social worker experienced in trauma-informed mental health care, and it was decided that the patient needed to be assessed for PTSD. She was assessed and found to have PTSD as a result of her oncology treatment. She began a course of trauma-informed therapy, using eye movement desensitization and reprocessing (EMDR), and about 3 months later, her trauma symptoms were significantly decreased in intensity, frequency, and duration. This ended up being a durable response in the significant reduction of her PTSD symptoms for years post EMDR treatment.

What was striking about this case is that during the CBT treatment, the patient felt as if her symptoms were getting worse. She expressed this to the provider and also shared that she felt as if she was going crazy as she was doing everything that the provider recommended and working hard during therapy sessions. She also reported that she felt as if she was to blame for her symptoms getting worse as she was doing what the therapist said but not improving. This was a clear indication that she required trauma-informed mental health care post oncology treatment. It also points to the possibility that normal talk therapy, including traditional CBT, can exacerbate mental health symptoms if a patient requires trauma-informed mental health care as opposed to more general mental health care.

SCREENING FOR DISTRESS AND PTSD

Self-report screening tools can be cost-effective for use in busy general medical settings (179,183). Implementation of distress screening in a clinical setting can help to reliably identify emotionally distressed patients and enhance provision of access to mental health services (184,185). This can improve patient outcomes and maximize the use of limited treatment resources. Identification of patient needs results in early referrals and allows for the optimum outcome in the shortest possible duration of hospitalization (202).

Numerous studies have addressed improved patient outcomes resulting from distress screening in oncology settings (183,184,203). Evidence indicates that the use of psychosocial screening instruments among cancer patients results in reductions in emotional distress, increased quality of life, and improved patient–provider communication (181,184,186,187).

In high-volume settings with limited resources, there is a need to effectively identify and support patients with unmet psychosocial needs and enhance the integration of psychosocial care in patient care (187).

Research of distress screening indicates the need for measures that incorporate a score above a particular cutoff point that identifies patients in need of available services that they are currently not receiving (187,204).

Various reliable and valid patient self-report screening tools are well documented in the literature, including the PHQ-9, Center for Epidemiologic Studies Depression Scale (CES-D), BDI, Beck Anxiety Inventory (BAI), HADS, Brief Symptom Inventory-18 (BSI-18), and Brief Symptom Inventory-53 (BSI-53). The Brief Symptom Inventory-18 (BSI-18) will be used to assess psychosocial distress, one of the independent variables (205). It is an 18-item self-report instrument that measures psychological distress and produces one global symptoms index (GSI) and three subscales scores including anxiety, depression, and somatization (205). The BSI-18 has been normed and validated on oncology patients and survivors over age 18.

The most ubiquitous instrument for distress screening is the NCCN Distress Thermometer (DT) with associated problem list. This is an ultra-short measure that could be paired with population-specific demographic questions to target a broader set of psychosocial factors. The NCCN DT has a picture of a thermometer on the left side of the instrument for patients to indicate their level of distress from 0 to 10. On the right side of the instrument is a problem list that includes seven domains with check boxes for patients to indicate yes or no to a specific question.

For screening traumatic stress, the PTSD Checklist for DSM-5 (PCL-5) is an instrument developed by the U.S. Department of Veterans Affairs and is free to obtain and use (206). It is a 20-item self-report measure that assesses for DSM-5 symptoms of PTSD and takes 5 to 10 minutes to complete. It can be scored for total symptom severity and can identify PTSD symptom cluster severity per the DSM-5 diagnostic criteria for PTSD. The Life Events Checklist for DSM-5 (LEC-5) can be used to assess potentially traumatic events in a survivor's lifetime (207). This is an instrument developed by the U.S. Department of Veterans Affairs and is free to obtain and use.

MENTAL HEALTH CARE

For depression, anxiety, and traumatic stress, the standard of care is medication and talk therapy. There are a number of different evidenced-based forms of talk therapy. The Substance Abuse and Mental Health Services Administration (SAMHSA) maintains the Evidenced-Based Practices Resource Center to provide information about evidenced-based interventions for more information.

CBT has been widely used in the oncology population to treat mental health conditions in survivorship. While much of the research is conducted on breast cancer survivors, the overall outcomes are very promising. However, some believe that CBT is beginning to lose up to half of its efficacy in clinical trials, especially for treating depressive symptoms (208).

Nonetheless, the literature still supports the use of CBT with survivors and has been shown to be effective in reducing mood symptoms in cancer survivors as well as improving survivors' sleep and reducing fatigue among a host of other benefits (209–213). In one study with almost 1,500 survivors, the authors investigated the effectiveness of CBT versus patient education to reduce symptoms of anxiety and depression and quality of life. They found that CBT intervention was effective for reducing anxiety and depression as well as improving quality of life as compared to patient education, where there was no improvement in outcomes (214).

In addition to CBT, mindfulness-based approaches have been gaining in use and validity among the survivorship population. Mindfulness-based approaches include present moment focus, decentering, and an approach to orientation (215). While it is too difficult to distill mindfulness-based approaches to a few key words, it should be understood as supporting survivors to make a profound shift in the way they experience thoughts, feelings, and physical sensations and ultimately relate to their experiences (215). This is what is referred to as decentering. Overall, mindfulness also has demonstrated efficacy in reducing anxiety and depressive symptoms in survivors (216–221).

Psychosocial trauma is different than non–trauma-related stress. The key difference was articulated by Bessel van der Kolk in his seminal article published in 1994. van der Kolk's findings define the difference thusly:

> Trauma is stored in somatic memory and expressed as changes in the biological stress response. Intense emotions at the time of the trauma initiate the

long-term conditional responses to reminders of the events, which are associated both with chronic alterations in the physiological stress response and with the amnesias and hypermnesias characteristic of posttraumatic stress disorder (PTSD). Continued physiological hyperarousal and altered stress hormone secretion affect the ongoing evaluation of sensory stimuli as well. Although memory is ordinarily an active and constructive process, in PTSD failure of declarative memory may lead to organization of the trauma on a somatosensory level (as visual images or physical sensations) that is relatively impervious to change. The inability of people with PTSD to integrate traumatic experiences and their tendency, instead, to continuously relive the past are mirrored physiologically and hormonally in the misinterpretation of innocuous stimuli as potential threats (222).

For shorthand, providers often say "the issues are in the tissues," which in this case is not only an ironic double entendre but a way to describe how traumatic stress is primarily a psychological experience instead of simply behavioral, characterological, or cognitive. That is the primary reason that trauma-informed mental health care is distinct from typical mental health counseling.

A review of 39 studies conducted between 1992 and 2001 reported empirical support for the use of trauma-informed psychosocial support model of care in cancer (194). The SAMHSA published *SAMHSA's Concept of Trauma and Guidance for a Trauma-Informed Approach* in July 2014 (223). In it, they lay out their concept of trauma to include "individual trauma results from an event, series of **events**, or set of circumstances that is **experienced** by an individual as physically or emotionally harmful of life threatening and that has lasting adverse **effects** on the individual's functioning and mental, physical, social, and emotional, or spiritual well-being." They provide further guidance on trauma-informed care by stating "a program, organization, or system that is trauma-informed **realizes** the widespread impact of trauma and understands potential paths for recovery; **recognizes** the signs and symptoms of trauma in clients, families, staff, and others involved with the system; and **responds** by fully integrating knowledge about trauma into policies, procedures, and practices, and seeks to actively **resist retraumatization**." Lastly, they provide their six principles of a trauma-informed approach including safety; trustworthiness and transparency; peer support; collaboration and mutuality; empowerment, voice, and choice; and cultural, historical, and gender issues.

Known trauma-informed mental health care interventions include trauma-focused cognitive behavioral therapy (TF-CBT), EMDR, somatic experiencing, neurofeedback, and other exposure-based mental health treatments. Trauma-informed care is exposure based with the idea that the survivor will remember but not experience their stressor(s) in an effort to desensitize the intensity of the symptoms associated with the event(s) and this is primarily done by having the survivor. Often, survivors experiencing traumatic stress symptoms require medication. This can help reduce the pathological symptoms and provide a stronger foundation to better leverage trauma-informed talk therapy.

Other forms of treatment are also available to survivors. In a small study, hypnosis has reduced anxiety symptoms in breast cancer survivors (212). Telehealth approaches may improve access to mental health resources especially for those with limited online access or lack of online skill (211,224,225). Reiki is a form of biofield energy, consists of moving energy to induce a reduction in unwanted symptoms. Many oncology clinics offer reiki and other complementary and alternative treatments to survivors.

PUTTING IT TOGETHER: SURVIVORSHIP CARE AND CARE PLAN

Optimal follow-up of survivors includes both ongoing monitoring and assessment of persistent and late effects of cancer treatment and the successful introduction of appropriate interventions to ameliorate these sequelae. The prevention of late effects, second cancers, and recurrences of the primary disease requires watchful follow-up and optimal utilization of early detection screening techniques. Physical symptom management is as important in survivorship as it is during treatment, and effective symptom management during treatment may prevent or lessen lasting effects. There is also growing awareness of the psychological, social, and financial difficulties cancer survivors face as they undergo cancer treatment and as they reintegrate into posttreatment life.

Regular monitoring of health status after cancer treatment is recommended, because this should:

1. Permit the timely diagnosis and treatment of long-term complications of cancer treatment
2. Permit the detection of functional, physical, or psychological difficulties
3. Provide the opportunity to institute preventive strategies such as diet modification, tobacco cessation, and other lifestyle changes
4. Facilitate screening for, and early detection of, a second cancer
5. Ensure timely diagnosis and treatment of recurrent cancer

The ASCO expert panels identified and developed recommendations for practice for posttreatment follow-up of specific cancer sites (www.asco.org). In addition, the ASCO and NCCN have also created an expert panel tasked with the development of follow-up care guidelines geared toward the prevention or early detection of late effects among survivors diagnosed and treated as adults.

There are several models of survivorship care, including survivorship clinics within cancer centers, community survivorship clinics run by primary care clinicians, and survivorship care in primary care settings. With the expected increase in cancer survivors over the next decades, the need for survivorship follow-up care is expected to grow, with primary care clinicians taking on an increasing role. While a randomized clinical trial comparing family physician versus specialist care found no difference in disease-related outcomes (226,227), PCP often are not familiar with specific needs of cancer survivors and often support a shared care model with oncologists (228,229). Surveys of survivors also suggest a preference for oncologist-driven follow-up care over PCP follow-up care, and PCP should provide care under a shared care model (230).

Although evidence for use of survivorship care plan is lacking, the NCCN Survivorship Panel currently recommends the use of survivorship care plans to enhance communication and information sharing between oncology and primary teams (7). A survivorship care plan can also be informative for palliative care clinicians in addressing symptoms and quality-of-life concerns.

A survivorship care plan should include summary of treatment received, information on follow-up care and surveillance recommendations, information on posttreatment needs (treatment-related effects and health risks), oncologist and PCP role delineation and timing of transfer of care if appropriate, and healthy living recommendations (29) (Tables 60.4 and 60.5).

TABLE 60.4 SURVIVORSHIP CARE PLAN

Follow-up visit	Content of clinic visit	Suggested evaluative procedures and ancillary actions
Summary of treatment received	1. Cancer type/location/histology subtype 2. Surgical procedure/location/findings 3. Radiation 4. Systemic therapy (chemotherapy, hormonal therapy, immunotherapy)	• Provide patient with a copy of the survivorship care plan • Familial cancer risk assessment if indicated, including hereditary risk factor(s) or predisposing conditions. Genetic counseling if appropriate
Information regarding follow-up care and surveillance recommendations	1. Need for ongoing (adjuvant) treatment for cancer 2. Schedule of clinic visits (when and how often) and coordinating providers 3. Cancer surveillance and related tests (what/when/how often) 4. All general health care recommendations, including cancer screening tests 5. Symptoms that should be brought to attention of a provider: new or persistent symptoms and indications that cancer may have recurred	See Table 60.5
Information on treatment-related effects and health risks	1. Persistent symptoms or side effects at completion of treatment 2. Possible late- and long-term effects that someone with this type of cancer and treatment may experience (Table 60.1) 3. Review with patient any areas of concerns	Areas of concern: • Emotional and mental health • Physical functioning • Memory or concentration loss • Fatigue • Pain (Table 60.3) • Weight changes • Insurance • Financial advice or assistance • School/work • Fertility • Sexual functioning
Healthy behavior recommendations	1. Lifestyles/behaviors that can affect ongoing health: smoking cessation, diet, alcohol use, sunscreen use, weight management (loss/gain), physical activity 2. Survivorship resources	https://www.cancer.net/survivorship (ASCO cancer.net survivorship section)

Adapted from ASCO. ASCO Cancer Treatment and Survivorship Care Plans. https://www.cancer.net/survivorship/follow-care-after-cancer-treatment/asco-cancer-treatment-and-survivorship-care-plans. Accessed October 22, 2019. Ref. (231).

TABLE 60.5 FOLLOW-UP CARE AND SURVEILLANCE FOR LATE EFFECTS

Follow-up visit	Content of clinic visit	Suggested evaluative procedures and ancillary actions
Chemotherapy/treatment cessation visit	1. Review complete treatment history 2. Calculate cumulative dosages of drugs 3. Document regimen(s) administered 4. Radiation ports, dosage, machine 5. Document patient age at diagnosis/treatment 6. Side effects during treatment 7. Identify likely late effects 8. Baseline "grading" of late effects (Garre or Swiss Pediatric Oncology Group [SPOG])	Develop late effect risk profile Summarize all information in the previous column Provide copy to patient (or parent if minor child) Instruct that this summary should be provided to primary care or other health care providers Keep a copy of summary in patient chart
General measures at every visit	1. Detailed history 2. Complete physical examination 3. Review systems 4. Medication, maintenance, prophylactic antibiotics 5. Education: grade point average, school performance 6. Employment history 7. Menstrual status/cycle 8. Libido, sexual activity 9. Pregnancy and outcome	Evaluate symptomatology, patient reports of issues Review any intercurrent illnesses Evaluate for disease recurrence, second neoplasms Systematic evaluation of long-term (persistent) and late effects (see specific measures) Grade long-term and late effects: Garre or SPOG criteria Complete blood cell, urinalysis; other tests depending on exposure history and late effect risk profile
Specific measures to evaluate late effects Relevance differs by: 1. Age at diagnosis/ treatment	Growth: includes issues such as short stature, scoliosis, hypoplasia	Monitor growth (growth curve), sitting height, parental heights, nutritional status/diet; evaluate scoliosis, bone age, growth hormone assays, thyroid function; endocrinologist consult; orthopedic consult
2. Specific drugs, regimens 3. Combinations of treatment modalities 4. Dosages administered	Cardiac	Electrocardiogram, echo, afterload reduction, cardiologist consult Counsel against isometric exercises if high risk, advice ob/gyn risk of cardiac failure in pregnancy
5. Expected toxicities (based on mechanics of action of cytotoxic drugs; cell cycle–dependent; proliferation kinetics)	Neurocognitive	History and examination Communicate: school, family, special education Compensatory remediation techniques
6. Exceptions occur to the theoretical assumption that least susceptible organs/tissues are those that replicate slowly or not at all (vinca, methotrexate, adriamycin)		Neuropsychology consult; computed tomography or magnetic resonance imaging; cerebrospinal fluid; basic myelin protein Written instructions, appointment cards
7. Combinations of radiation/ chemotherapy more often associated with late effects	Neuropathy	History/examination: neurologic examination, sensory changes hands/ feet, paresthesias, bladder, gait, vision, muscle strength Neurologist consult

(Continued)

TABLE 60.5 FOLLOW-UP CARE AND SURVEILLANCE FOR LATE EFFECTS *(Continued)*

Follow-up visit	Content of clinic visit	Suggested evaluative procedures and ancillary actions
	Gonadal toxicity	History for primary vs. secondary dysfunction, gonadal function (menstrual cycle, pubertal development/delay, libido); hormone therapy; interventions (bromocriptine) Premature menopause: hormone replacement unless contraindicated; dual-energy X-ray absorptiometry scans for osteoporosis; calcium Endocrinologist consult Reproductive technologies
	Pulmonary	Chest X-ray; pulmonary function tests; pulmonologist consultation
	Urinary	Urinalysis; blood urea nitrogen/creatinine; urologist if hematuria
	Thyroid	Annual thyroid-stimulating hormone; thyroid hormone replacement; endocrinologist
	Weight history	Evaluate dietary intake (food diary)/physical activity Nutritionist and/or endocrinologist consult
	Lymphedema	History/examination: swelling, sensations of heaviness/fullness
	Fatigue	Rule out hypothyroidism, anemia, cardiac/pulmonary sequelae; evaluate sleep habits Evaluate physical fitness and activity levels Regular physical activity unless contraindicated
	Surgical toxicity	Antibiotic prophylaxis (splenectomy)
	Gastrointestinal/hepatic	Liver function, hepatitis screen, gastroenterologist consult
Screening for second malignant neoplasms	Screening guidelines differ by age	Follow guidelines for age-appropriate cancer screening (mammogram, Pap smear, fecal occult blood test/flexible sigmoidoscopy)
	Oncologist consult	Mammogram at age 30 if history of mantle radiation for Hodgkin's disease Screen for associated cancers in hereditary nonpolyposis colorectal cancer family syndrome Screen for ovarian cancer if history of breast cancer and BRCA I and II
Assess/manage comorbidities	Osteoporosis, heart disease, arthritis, etc.	History/examination; be cognizant of risk; appropriate consult

Evaluations are suggestions only. Relevance will differ by treatment history and late effect risk profile.

REVIEW AND CONCLUSIONS

In recent years, there is increased emphasis on whole-person approach to survivorship care, including physical, psychosocial, and existential explorations and support. In a 2019 National Coalition for Cancer survivorship online survey of adult cancer patients, key areas of survivorship needs identified by cancer patients include the following:

1. Depression and anxiety are common and not well addressed by health care providers.
2. While most patients have spoken with health care providers about posttreatment care, few

discuss financial services/support, survivorship plans, or emotional support.

3. There is generally a strong interest among cancer patients in access to resources/programs for insurance coverage, financial support, long-term symptom management, and emotional health.

4. Immunotherapy patients tend to be more satisfied with their posttreatment experiences (feeling more prepared and informed) while sharing similar concerns around financial and emotional issues.

Each person with cancer has unique needs based on the extent of the disease, effects of treatment, prior health, functional level, coping skills, support systems, and many other influences. This complexity requires an interdisciplinary approach that is organized, systematic, and geared toward the provision of high-quality care. Additional studies will help guide how to best integrate psychosocial needs into survivorship care.

REFERENCES

1. Bluethmann SM, Mariotto AB, Rowland JH. Anticipating the "silver tsunami": prevalence trajectories and comorbidity burden among older cancer survivors in the United States. *Cancer Epidemiol Biomarkers Prev.* 2016;25(7):1029-1036.

2. Mullan F. Seasons of survival: reflections of a physician with cancer. *N Engl J Med.* 1985;313(4):270-273.

3. Head KJ, Iannarino NT. "It changed our outlook on how we want to live": cancer as a transformative health experience for young adult survivors and their family members. *Qual Health Res.* 2019;29(3):404-417.

4. Robison LL, Green DM, Hudson M, et al. Long-term outcomes of adult survivors of childhood cancer. *Cancer.* 2005;104(11 suppl):2557-2564.

5. Sklar CA. Overview of the effects of cancer therapies: the nature, scale and breadth of the problem. *Acta Paediatr Suppl.* 1999;88(433):1-4.

6. Friend AJ, Feltbower RG, Hughes EJ, Dye KP, Glaser AW. Mental health of long-term survivors of childhood and young adult cancer: a systematic review. *Int J Cancer.* 2018;143(6):1279-1286.

7. NCCN guidelines for supportive care. 275 Commerce Drive, Suite 300, Fort Washington, PA 19034, National Comprehensive Cancer Network. https://www.nccn.org/professionals/physician_gls/default.aspx#supportive

8. Lovelace DL, McDaniel LR, Golden D. Long-term effects of breast cancer surgery, treatment, and survivor care. *J Midwifery Womens Health.* 2019;64:713-724.

9. Davis KM, Kelly SP, Luta G, Tomko C, Miller AB, Taylor KL. The association of long-term treatment-related side effects with cancer-specific and general quality of life among prostate cancer survivors. *Urology.* 2014;84(2):300-306.

10. Paoli D, Gallo M, Rizzo F, et al. Testicular cancer and sperm DNA damage: short- and long-term effects of antineoplastic treatment. *Andrology.* 2015;3(1):122-128.

11. Haugnes HS, Bosl GJ, Boer H, et al. Long-term and late effects of germ cell testicular cancer treatment and implications for follow-up. *J Clin Oncol.* 2012;30(30):3752-3763.

12. Loescher LJ, Welch-McCaffrey D, Leigh SA, Hoffman B, Meyskens FL Jr. Surviving adult cancers. Part 1: physiologic effects. *Ann Intern Med.* 1989;111(5):411-432.

13. Welch-McCaffrey D, Hoffman B, Leigh SA, Loescher LJ, Meyskens FL Jr. Surviving adult cancers. Part 2: psychosocial implications. *Ann Intern Med.* 1989;111(6):517-524.

14. Harris C, Sander CR. Late respiratory effects of cancer treatment. *Curr Opin Support Palliat Care.* 2017;11(3):197-204.

15. Skitch A, Mital S, Mertens L, et al. Novel approaches to the prediction, diagnosis and treatment of cardiac late effects in survivors of childhood cancer: a multi-centre observational study. *BMC Cancer.* 2017;17(1):519.

16. Pillai US, Kayal S, Cyriac S, et al. Late effects of breast cancer treatment and outcome after corrective interventions. *Asian Pac J Cancer Prev.* 2019;20(9):2673-2679.

17. Livinalli A, Silva MT, Lopes LC. Late adverse effects related to treatment in a cohort of survivors of childhood and adolescent cancer. *Medicine (Baltimore).* 2019;98(12):e14921.

18. Haines LS, Charles L. Cancer survivorship. In: Oh WK, Chari A, eds. *Mount Sinai Expert Guides.* Hoboken, NJ: John Wiley & Sons Ltd 2019:535-542.

19. Gurney JG, Krull KR, Kadan-Lottick N, et al. Social outcomes in the childhood cancer survivor study cohort. *J Clin Oncol.* 2009;27(14):2390-2395.

20. Brandenbarg D, Maass S, Geerse OP, et al. A systematic review on the prevalence of symptoms of depression, anxiety and distress in long-term cancer survivors: implications for primary care. *Eur J Cancer Care (Engl).* 2019;28(3):e13086.

21. Aziz NM, Rowland JH. Trends and advances in cancer survivorship research: challenge and opportunity. *Semin Radiat Oncol.* 2003;13(3):248-266.

22. Strasser B, Steindorf K, Wiskemann J, Ulrich CM. Impact of resistance training in cancer survivors: a meta-analysis. *Med Sci Sports Exerc.* 2013;45(11):2080-2090.

23. Pundole X, Cheema HI, Petitto GS, Lopez-Olivo MA, Suarez-Almazor ME, Lu H. Prevention and treatment of bone loss and fractures in patients undergoing a hematopoietic stem cell transplant: a systematic review and meta-analysis. *Bone Marrow Transplant.* 2017;52(5):663-670.

24. Thakur A, Witteles RM. Cancer therapy-induced left ventricular dysfunction: interventions and prognosis. *J Card Fail.* 2014;20(3):155-158.

25. Ky B, Vejpongsa P, Yeh ET, Force T, Moslehi JJ. Emerging paradigms in cardiomyopathies associated with cancer therapies. *Circ Res.* 2013;113(6):754-764.

26. Bonaca MP, Olenchock BA, Salem JE, et al. Myocarditis in the setting of cancer therapeutics: proposed case definitions for emerging clinical syndromes in cardio-oncology. *Circulation.* 2019;140(2):80-91.

27. Hakim A, Cooke KR, Pavletic SZ, Khalid M, Williams KM, Hashmi SK. Diagnosis and treatment of bronchiolitis obliterans syndrome accessible universally. *Bone Marrow Transplant.* 2019;54(3):383-392.

28. Lange M, Joly F. How to identify and manage cognitive dysfunction after breast cancer treatment. *J Oncol Pract.* 2017;13(12):784-790.

29. Sanft T, Denlinger CS, Armenian S, et al. NCCN guidelines insights: survivorship, version 2.2019. *J Natl Compr Canc Netw.* 2019;17(7):784-794.

30. Hingorani S. Chronic kidney disease in long-term survivors of hematopoietic cell transplantation: epidemiology, pathogenesis, and treatment. *J Am Soc Nephrol.* 2006;17(7):1995-2005.

31. Kort JD, Eisenberg ML, Millheiser LS, Westphal LM. Fertility issues in cancer survivorship. *CA Cancer J Clin.* 2014;64(2):118-134.

32. Inamoto Y, Valdes-Sanz N, Ogawa Y, et al. Ocular graft-versus-host disease after hematopoietic cell

transplantation: expert review from the Late Effects and Quality of Life Working Committee of the CIBMTR and Transplant Complications Working Party of the EBMT. *Bone Marrow Transplant.* 2019;54(5):662-673.

33. Lipshultz SE, Colan SD, Gelber RD, Perez-Atayde AR, Sallan SE, Sanders SP. Late cardiac effects of doxorubicin therapy for acute lymphoblastic leukemia in childhood. *N Engl J Med.* 1991;324(12):808-815.

34. Bu'Lock FA, Mott MG, Oakhill A, Martin RP. Left ventricular diastolic function after anthracycline chemotherapy in childhood: relation with systolic function, symptoms, and pathophysiology. *Br Heart J.* 1995;73(4): 340-350.

35. Goorin AM, Borow KM, Goldman A, et al. Congestive heart failure due to adriamycin cardiotoxicity: its natural history in children. *Cancer.* 1981;47(12):2810-2816.

36. Steinherz LJ, Steinherz PG, Tan C. Cardiac failure and dysrhythmias 6–19 years after anthracycline therapy: a series of 15 patients. *Med Pediatr Oncol.* 1995;24(6):352-361.

37. Hancock SL, Donaldson SS, Hoppe RT. Cardiac disease following treatment of Hodgkin's disease in children and adolescents. *J Clin Oncol.* 1993;11(7):1208-1215.

38. Ruckdeschel JC, Chang P, Martin RG, et al. Radiation-related pericardial effusions in patients with Hodgkin's disease. *Medicine (Baltimore).* 1975;54(3):245-259.

39. Carver JR, Shapiro CL, Ng A, et al. American Society of Clinical Oncology clinical evidence review on the ongoing care of adult cancer survivors: cardiac and pulmonary late effects. *J Clin Oncol.* 2007;25(25):3991-4008.

40. Barber NA, Ganti AK. Pulmonary toxicities from targeted therapies: a review. *Target Oncol.* 2011;6(4): 235-243.

41. Horning SJ, Adhikari A, Rizk N, Hoppe RT, Olshen RA. Effect of treatment for Hodgkin's disease on pulmonary function: results of a prospective study. *J Clin Oncol.* 1994;12(2):297-305.

42. Sleijfer S. Bleomycin-induced pneumonitis. *Chest.* 2001; 120(2):617-624.

43. Nuver J, Smit AJ, Postma A, Sleijfer DT, Gietema JA. The metabolic syndrome in long-term cancer survivors, an important target for secondary preventive measures. *Cancer Treat Rev.* 2002;28(4):195-214.

44. McDonald S, Rubin P, Phillips TL, Marks LB. Injury to the lung from cancer therapy: clinical syndromes, measurable endpoints, and potential scoring systems. *Int J Radiat Oncol Biol Phys.* 1995;31(5):1187-1203.

45. Gustavsson A, Eskilsson J, Landberg T, et al. Long-term effects on pulmonary function of mantle radiotherapy in patients with Hodgkin's disease. *Ann Oncol.* 1992;3(6):455-461.

46. Shalet SM, Beardwell CG, Twomey JA, Jones PH, Pearson D. Endocrine function following the treatment of acute leukemia in childhood. *J Pediatr.* 1977;90(6): 920-923.

47. Robison LL, Nesbit ME Jr, Sather HN, Meadows AT, Ortega JA, Hammond GD. Height of children successfully treated for acute lymphoblastic leukemia: a report from the Late Effects Study Committee of Childrens Cancer Study Group. *Med Pediatr Oncol.* 1985;13(1):14-21.

48. Hancock SL, Cox RS, McDougall IR. Thyroid diseases after treatment of Hodgkin's disease. *N Engl J Med.* 1991;325(9):599-605.

49. Sklar C, Whitton J, Mertens A, et al. Abnormalities of the thyroid in survivors of Hodgkin's disease: data from the Childhood Cancer Survivor Study. *J Clin Endocrinol Metab.* 2000;85(9):3227-3232.

50. Glatstein E, McHardy-Young S, Brast N, Eltringham JR, Kriss JP. Alterations in serum thyrotropin (TSH) and thyroid function following radiotherapy in patients with malignant lymphoma. *J Clin Endocrinol Metab.* 1971;32(6):833-841.

51. Rosenthal MB, Goldfine ID. Primary and secondary hypothyroidism in nasopharyngeal carcinoma. *JAMA.* 1976;236(14):1591-1593.

52. Schultz PN, Beck ML, Stava C, Vassilopoulou-Sellin R. Health profiles in 5836 long-term cancer survivors. *Int J Cancer.* 2003;104(4):488-495.

53. Twiss JJ, Waltman N, Ott CD, Gross GJ, Lindsey AM, Moore TE. Bone mineral density in postmenopausal breast cancer survivors. *J Am Acad Nurse Pract.* 2001;13(6):276-284.

54. Ramaswamy B, Shapiro CL. Osteopenia and osteoporosis in women with breast cancer. *Semin Oncol.* 2003;30(6):763-775.

55. Diamond TH, Higano CS, Smith MR, Guise TA, Singer FR. Osteoporosis in men with prostate carcinoma receiving androgen-deprivation therapy: recommendations for diagnosis and therapies. *Cancer.* 2004;100(5):892-899.

56. Bergstrom A, Pisani P, Tenet V, Wolk A, Adami HO. Overweight as an avoidable cause of cancer in Europe. *Int J Cancer.* 2001;91(3):421-430.

57. World Health Organization. *IARC Handbook of Cancer Prevention.* Vol. 6. Geneva: World Health Organization; 2002.

58. Mock V, Atkinson A, Barsevick A, et al. NCCN practice guidelines for cancer-related fatigue. *Oncology (Williston Park).* 2000;14(11A):151-161.

59. Schwartz CL. Long-term survivors of childhood cancer: the late effects of therapy. *Oncologist.* 1999;4(1):45-54.

60. Freedland SJ, Aronson WJ, Kane CJ, et al. Impact of obesity on biochemical control after radical prostatectomy for clinically localized prostate cancer: a report by the Shared Equal Access Regional Cancer Hospital database study group. *J Clin Oncol.* 2004;22(3):446-453.

61. Chlebowski RT, Aiello E, McTiernan A. Weight loss in breast cancer patient management. *J Clin Oncol.* 2002;20(4):1128-1143.

62. Marina N. Long-term survivors of childhood cancer. The medical consequences of cure. *Pediatr Clin North Am.* 1997;44(4):1021-1042.

63. Argiles JM, Lopez-Soriano FJ. Insulin and cancer (Review). *Int J Oncol.* 2001;18(4):683-687.

64. Bines J, Gradishar WJ. Primary care issues for the breast cancer survivor. *Compr Ther.* 1997;23(9):605-611.

65. Yoshikawa T, Noguchi Y, Doi C, Makino T, Nomura K. Insulin resistance in patients with cancer: relationships with tumor site, tumor stage, body-weight loss, acute-phase response, and energy expenditure. *Nutrition.* 2001;17(7-8):590-593.

66. Balkau B, Kahn HS, Courbon D, Eschwege E, Ducimetiere P; Paris Prospective Study. Hyperinsulinemia predicts fatal liver cancer but is inversely associated with fatal cancer at some other sites: the Paris Prospective Study. *Diabetes Care.* 2001;24(5):843-849.

67. Brown BW, Brauner C, Minnotte MC. Noncancer deaths in white adult cancer patients. *J Natl Cancer Inst.* 1993; 85(12):979-987.

68. Lamont EB, Christakis NA, Lauderdale DS. Favorable cardiac risk among elderly breast carcinoma survivors. *Cancer.* 2003;98(1):2-10.

69. Shusterman S, Meadows AT. Long term survivors of childhood leukemia. *Curr Opin Hematol.* 2000;7(4): 217-222.

70. Hull MC, Morris CG, Pepine CJ, Mendenhall NP. Valvular dysfunction and carotid, subclavian, and coronary artery disease in survivors of hodgkin lymphoma treated with radiation therapy. *JAMA.* 2003;290(21): 2831-2837.

71. Thomson AB, Critchley HO, Wallace WH. Fertility and progeny. *Eur J Cancer.* 2002;38(12):1634-1644; discussion 1645-1636.

72. Lamb MA. Effects of cancer on the sexuality and fertility of women. *Semin Oncol Nurs.* 1995;11(2):120-127.

73. Brougham MF, Kelnar CJ, Sharpe RM, Wallace WH. Male fertility following childhood cancer: current concepts and future therapies. *Asian J Androl.* 2003;5(4): 325-337.

74. Wallace WH, Anderson R, Baird D. Preservation of fertility in young women treated for cancer. *Lancet Oncol.* 2004;5(5):269-270.

75. Opsahl MS, Fugger EF, Sherins RJ, Schulman JD. Preservation of reproductive function before therapy for cancer: new options involving sperm and ovary cryopreservation. *Cancer J Sci Am.* 1997;3(4):189-191.

76. Oktay K, Newton H, Aubard Y, Salha O, Gosden RG. Cryopreservation of immature human oocytes and ovarian tissue: an emerging technology? *Fertil Steril.* 1998;69(1):1-7.

77. Goodwin PJ, Ennis M, Pritchard KI, Trudeau M, Hood N. Risk of menopause during the first year after breast cancer diagnosis. *J Clin Oncol.* 1999;17(8):2365-2370.

78. Kuehn R, Casaubon J, Raker C, Edmonson D, Stuckey A, Gass J. Sexual dysfunction in survivorship; the impact of menopause and endocrine therapy. *Ann Surg Oncol.* 2019;26(10):3159-3165.

79. Nourmoussavi M, Pansegrau G, Popesku J, Hammond GL, Kwon JS, Carey MS. Ovarian ablation for premenopausal breast cancer: a review of treatment considerations and the impact of premature menopause. *Cancer Treat Rev.* 2017;55:26-35.

80. Zhou ES, Nekhlyudov L, Bober SL. The primary health care physician and the cancer patient: tips and strategies for managing sexual health. *Transl Androl Urol.* 2015;4(2):218-231.

81. Whicker M, Black J, Altwerger G, Menderes G, Feinberg J, Ratner E. Management of sexuality, intimacy, and menopause symptoms in patients with ovarian cancer. *Am J Obstet Gynecol.* 2017;217(4):395-403.

82. Wiggins DL, Wood R, Granai CO, Dizon DS. Sex, intimacy, and the gynecologic oncologists: survey results of the New England Association of Gynecologic Oncologists (NEAGO). *J Psychosoc Oncol.* 2007;25(4):61-70.

83. Park ER, Bober SL, Campbell EG, Recklitis CJ, Kutner JS, Diller L. General internist communication about sexual function with cancer survivors. *J Gen Intern Med.* 2009;24(suppl 2):S407-S411.

84. Donovan JL, Hamdy FC, Lane JA, et al. Patient-reported outcomes after monitoring, surgery, or radiotherapy for prostate cancer. *N Engl J Med.* 2016;375(15):1425-1437.

85. La Vignera S, Cannarella R, Duca Y, et al. Hypogonadism and sexual dysfunction in testicular tumor survivors: a systematic review. *Front Endocrinol (Lausanne).* 2019;10:264.

86. Matsuda T, Aptel I, Exbrayat C, Grosclaude P. Determinants of quality of life of bladder cancer survivors five years after treatment in France. *Int J Urol.* 2003;10(8):423-429.

87. Thyo A, Elfeki H, Laurberg S, Emmertsen KJ. Female sexual problems after treatment for colorectal cancer—a population-based study. *Colorectal Dis.* 2019;21(10): 1130-1139.

88. Vogelzang NJ. Nephrotoxicity from chemotherapy: prevention and management. *Oncology (Williston Park).* 1991;5(10):97-102, 105; discussion 105, 109-111.

89. Dewit L, Anninga JK, Hoefnagel CA, Nooijen WJ. Radiation injury in the human kidney: a prospective analysis using specific scintigraphic and biochemical endpoints. *Int J Radiat Oncol Biol Phys.* 1990;19(4):977-983.

90. Theis VS, Sripadam R, Ramani V, Lal S. Chronic radiation enteritis. *Clin Oncol (R Coll Radiol).* 2010;22(1): 70-83.

91. Teo MT, Sebag-Montefiore D, Donnellan CF. Prevention and management of radiation-induced late gastrointestinal toxicity. *Clin Oncol (R Coll Radiol).* 2015;27(11):656-667.

92. Pan YB, Maeda Y, Wilson A, Glynne-Jones R, Vaizey CJ. Late gastrointestinal toxicity after radiotherapy for anal cancer: a systematic literature review. *Acta Oncol.* 2018;57(11):1427-1437.

93. Badvie S, Andreyev HJ. Topical phenylephrine in the treatment of radiation-induced faecal incontinence. *Clin Oncol (R Coll Radiol).* 2005;17(2):122-126.

94. Maeda Y, Hoyer M, Lundby L, Buntzen S, Laurberg S. Temporary sacral nerve stimulation for faecal incontinence following pelvic radiotherapy. *Radiother Oncol.* 2010;97(1):108-112.

95. Cramer P, Bresalier RS. Gastrointestinal and hepatic complications of immune checkpoint inhibitors. *Curr Gastroenterol Rep.* 2017;19(1):3.

96. Johnson DB, Friedman DL, Berry E, et al. Survivorship in immune therapy: assessing chronic immune toxicities, health outcomes, and functional status among long-term ipilimumab survivors at a single referral center. *Cancer Immunol Res.* 2015;3(5):464-469.

97. Loge JH, Abrahamsen AF, Ekeberg O, Kaasa S. Hodgkin's disease survivors more fatigued than the general population. *J Clin Oncol.* 1999;17(1):253-261.

98. Andrykowski MA, Curran SL, Lightner R. Off-treatment fatigue in breast cancer survivors: a controlled comparison. *J Behav Med.* 1998;21(1):1-18.

99. Broeckel JA, Jacobsen PB, Horton J, Balducci L, Lyman GH. Characteristics and correlates of fatigue after adjuvant chemotherapy for breast cancer. *J Clin Oncol.* 1998;16(5):1689-1696.

100. Greenberg DB, Kornblith AB, Herndon JE, et al. Quality of life for adult leukemia survivors treated on clinical trials of Cancer and Leukemia Group B during the period 1971–1988: predictors for later psychologic distress. *Cancer.* 1997;80(10):1936-1944.

101. Bower JE, Ganz PA, Desmond KA, et al. Fatigue in long-term breast carcinoma survivors: a longitudinal investigation. *Cancer.* 2006;106(4):751-758.

102. Berger AM, Gerber LH, Mayer DK. Cancer-related fatigue: implications for breast cancer survivors. *Cancer.* 2012;118(8 suppl):2261-2269.

103. Cramp F, Byron-Daniel J. Exercise for the management of cancer-related fatigue in adults. *Cochrane Database Syst Rev.* 2012;11:CD006145.

104. Campbell KL, Winters-Stone KM, Wiskemann J, et al. Exercise guidelines for cancer survivors: consensus statement from international multidisciplinary roundtable. *Med Sci Sports Exerc.* 2019;51(11):2375-2390.

105. Ebede CC, Jang Y, Escalante CP. Cancer-related fatigue in cancer survivorship. *Med Clin North Am.* 2017; 101(6):1085-1097.

106. van der Lee ML, Garssen B. Mindfulness-based cognitive therapy reduces chronic cancer-related fatigue: a treatment study. *Psychooncology.* 2012;21(3):264-272.

107. Yennurajalingam S, Bruera E. Review of clinical trials of pharmacologic interventions for cancer-related fatigue: focus on psychostimulants and steroids. *Cancer J.* 2014;20(5):319-324.

108. Ahles TA, Saykin AJ, Furstenberg CT, et al. Neuropsychologic impact of standard-dose systemic chemotherapy in long-term survivors of breast cancer and lymphoma. *J Clin Oncol.* 2002;20(2):485-493.

109. Lange M, Joly F, Vardy J, et al. Cancer-related cognitive impairment: an update on state of the art, detection,

and management strategies in cancer survivors. *Ann Oncol.* 2019;30:1925-1940.

110. Ahles TA, Saykin AJ. Candidate mechanisms for chemotherapy-induced cognitive changes. *Nat Rev Cancer.* 2007;7(3):192-201.

111. Vega JN, Dumas J, Newhouse PA. Cognitive effects of chemotherapy and cancer-related treatments in older adults. *Am J Geriatr Psychiatry.* 2017;25(12):1415-1426.

112. Mulder SF, Bertens D, Desar IM, et al. Impairment of cognitive functioning during Sunitinib or Sorafenib treatment in cancer patients: a cross sectional study. *BMC Cancer.* 2014;14:219.

113. Nead KT, Gaskin G, Chester C, Swisher-McClure S, Leeper NJ, Shah NH. Association between androgen deprivation therapy and risk of dementia. *JAMA Oncol.* 2017;3(1):49-55.

114. Schilder CM, Seynaeve C, Beex LV, et al. Effects of tamoxifen and exemestane on cognitive functioning of postmenopausal patients with breast cancer: results from the neuropsychological side study of the tamoxifen and exemestane adjuvant multinational trial. *J Clin Oncol.* 2010;28(8):1294-1300.

115. Brown PD, Jaeckle K, Ballman KV, et al. Effect of radiosurgery alone vs radiosurgery with whole brain radiation therapy on cognitive function in patients with 1 to 3 brain metastases: a randomized clinical trial. *JAMA.* 2016;316(4):401-409.

116. Brown PD, Pugh S, Laack NN, et al. Memantine for the prevention of cognitive dysfunction in patients receiving whole-brain radiotherapy: a randomized, double-blind, placebo-controlled trial. *Neuro Oncol.* 2013;15(10):1429-1437.

117. Chung NC, Walker AK, Dhillon HM, Vardy JL. Mechanisms and treatment for cancer- and chemotherapy-related cognitive impairment in survivors of non-CNS malignancies. *Oncology (Williston Park).* 2018;32(12):591-598.

118. United States Census Bureau. 2017 National Population Projections Tables. https://www.census.gov/data/tables/2017/demo/popproj/2017-summary-tables.html. Accessed October 22, 2019.

119. Blair CK, Jacobs DR Jr, Demark-Wahnefried W, et al. Effects of cancer history on functional age and mortality. *Cancer.* 2019;125:4303-4309.

120. Grov EK, Fossa SD, Dahl AA. Activity of daily living problems in older cancer survivors: a population-based controlled study. *Health Soc Care Community.* 2010;18(4):396-406.

121. Ahles TA, Saykin AJ, McDonald BC, et al. Longitudinal assessment of cognitive changes associated with adjuvant treatment for breast cancer: impact of age and cognitive reserve. *J Clin Oncol.* 2010;28(29):4434-4440.

122. van den Beuken-van Everdingen MH, Hochstenbach LM, Joosten EA, Tjan-Heijnen VC, Janssen DJ. Update on prevalence of pain in patients with cancer: systematic review and meta-analysis. *J Pain Symptom Manage.* 2016;51(6):1070-1090.e1079.

123. Sanford NN, Sher DJ, Butler SS, et al. Prevalence of chronic pain among cancer survivors in the United States, 2010–2017. *Cancer.* 2019;125:4310-4318.

124. Glare PA, Davies PS, Finlay E, et al. Pain in cancer survivors. *J Clin Oncol.* 2014;32(16):1739-1747.

125. Kanzawa-Lee GA, Knoerl R, Donohoe C, Bridges CM, Smith EML. Mechanisms, predictors, and challenges in assessing and managing painful chemotherapy-induced peripheral neuropathy. *Semin Oncol Nurs.* 2019;35(3):253-260.

126. Mols F, Beijers T, Vreugdenhil G, van de Poll-Franse L. Chemotherapy-induced peripheral neuropathy and its association with quality of life: a systematic review. *Support Care Cancer.* 2014;22(8):2261-2269.

127. Bao T, Basal C, Seluzicki C, Li SQ, Seidman AD, Mao JJ. Long-term chemotherapy-induced peripheral neuropathy among breast cancer survivors: prevalence, risk factors, and fall risk. *Breast Cancer Res Treat.* 2016;159(2):327-333.

128. Brennan MJ, Weitz J. Lymphedema 30 years after radical mastectomy. *Am J Phys Med Rehabil.* 1992;71(1):12-14.

129. Lawenda BD, Mondry TE, Johnstone PA. Lymphedema: a primer on the identification and management of a chronic condition in oncologic treatment. *CA Cancer J Clin.* 2009;59(1):8-24.

130. Anbari AB, Wanchai A, Armer JM. Breast cancer-related lymphedema and quality of life: a qualitative analysis over years of survivorship. *Chronic Illn.* 2019. doi:10.1177/1742395319872796.

131. Dowell D, Haegerich TM, Chou R. CDC guideline for prescribing opioids for chronic pain-United States, 2016. *JAMA.* 2016;315:1624-1645.

132. Sutradhar R, Lokku A, Barbera L. Cancer survivorship and opioid prescribing rates: a population-based matched cohort study among individuals with and without a history of cancer. *Cancer.* 2017;123(21):4286-4293.

133. Hojsted J, Sjogren P. Addiction to opioids in chronic pain patients: a literature review. *Eur J Pain.* 2007;11(5):490-518.

134. Ward K, Ramzan A, Sheeder J, Fischer S, Lefkowits C. Persistent opioid use after radiation therapy in opioid-naive cervical cancer survivors. *Int J Gynecol Cancer.* 2019;29(7):1105-1109.

135. Paice JA, Portenoy R, Lacchetti C, et al. Management of chronic pain in survivors of adult cancers: American Society of Clinical Oncology Clinical Practice guideline. *J Clin Oncol.* 2016;34(27):3325-3345.

136. Beckjord EB, Reynolds KA, van Londen GJ, et al. Population-level trends in posttreatment cancer survivors' concerns and associated receipt of care: results from the 2006 and 2010 LIVESTRONG surveys. *J Psychosoc Oncol.* 2014;32(2):125-151.

137. American Psychiatric Association. *Diagnostic and Statistical Manual of Mental Disorders.* 5th ed. Arlington, VA: American Psychiatric Publishing; 2013.

138. Stanton AL, Wiley JF, Krull JL, et al. Depressive episodes, symptoms, and trajectories in women recently diagnosed with breast cancer. *Breast Cancer Res Treat.* 2015;154(1):105-115.

139. Mitchell AJ, Ferguson DW, Gill J, Paul J, Symonds P. Depression and anxiety in long-term cancer survivors compared with spouses and healthy controls: a systematic review and meta-analysis. *Lancet Oncol.* 2013;14(8):721-732.

140. Vehling S, Mehnert A, Hartmann M, Oing C, Bokemeyer C, Oechsle K. Anxiety and depression in long-term testicular germ cell tumor survivors. *Gen Hosp Psychiatry.* 2016;38:21-25.

141. Badr H, Lipnick D, Gupta V, Miles B. Survivorship challenges and information needs after radiotherapy for oral cancer. *J Cancer Educ.* 2017;32(4):799-807.

142. Sharp L, O'Leary E, Kinnear H, Gavin A, Drummond FJ. Cancer-related symptoms predict psychological wellbeing among prostate cancer survivors: results from the PiCTure study. *Psychooncology.* 2016;25(3):282-291.

143. Suzuki M, Deno M, Myers M, et al. Anxiety and depression in patients after surgery for head and neck cancer in Japan. *Palliat Support Care.* 2016;14(3):269-277.

144. Oancea SC, Cheruvu VK. Psychological distress among adult cancer survivors: importance of survivorship care plan. *Support Care Cancer.* 2016;24(11):4523-4531.

145. American College of Surgeons. Cancer Program Standards: Ensuring Patient-Centered Care. 2016. https://www.facs.org/quality-programs/cancer/coc/standards. Accessed October 19, 2019.

146. Misono S, Weiss NS, Fann JR, Redman M, Yueh B. Incidence of suicide in persons with cancer. *J Clin Oncol.* 2008;26(29):4731-4738.

147. Zaorsky NG, Zhang Y, Tuanquin L, Bluethmann SM, Park HS, Chinchilli VM. Suicide among cancer patients. *Nat Commun.* 2019;10(1):207.

148. Osazuwa-Peters N, Boakye EA, Simpson MC, et al. Gender differences and trends in suicide risk among cancer survivors. *J Clin Oncol.* 2018;36(15_suppl):10087.

149. National Institute of Mental Health. Ask Suicide-Screening Questions (ASQ) Toolkit. https://www.nimh.nih.gov/research/research-conducted-at-nimh/asq-toolkit-materials/index.shtml. Accessed October 19, 2019.

150. Kazdin AE. *Encyclopedia of Psychology.* 6th ed. Washington, DC: American Psychological Association; 2000.

151. American Psychiatric Association. *Diagnostic and Statistical Manual of Mental Disorders.* 5th ed. Washington, DC: American Psychiatric Association Press; 2013.

152. Yi JC, Syrjala KL. Anxiety and depression in cancer survivors. *Med Clin North Am.* 2017;101(6):1099-1113.

153. Braamse AM, van Turenhout ST, Terhaar Sive Droste JS, et al. Factors associated with anxiety and depressive symptoms in colorectal cancer survivors. *Eur J Gastroenterol Hepatol.* 2016;28(7):831-835.

154. Boyes AW, Girgis A, D'Este C, Zucca AC. Flourishing or floundering? Prevalence and correlates of anxiety and depression among a population-based sample of adult cancer survivors 6 months after diagnosis. *J Affect Disord.* 2011;135(1-3):184-192.

155. Simard S, Thewes B, Humphris G, et al. Fear of cancer recurrence in adult cancer survivors: a systematic review of quantitative studies. *J Cancer Surviv.* 2013;7(3):300-322.

156. Custers JAE, Gielissen MFM, Janssen SHV, de Wilt JHW, Prins JB. Fear of cancer recurrence in colorectal cancer survivors. *Support Care Cancer.* 2016;24(2):555-562.

157. Koch-Gallenkamp L, Bertram H, Eberle A, et al. Fear of recurrence in long-term cancer survivors-Do cancer type, sex, time since diagnosis, and social support matter? *Health Psychol.* 2016;35(12):1329-1333.

158. Lazarus RS, Folkman S. *Stress, Appraisal, and Coping.* 6th ed. New York, NY: Springer Publishing Co.; 1984.

159. Lazarus RS. Progress on a cognitive-motivational-relational theory of emotion. *Am Psychol.* 1991;46(8):819-834.

160. Lazarus RS. *Stress and Emotion: A New Synthesis.* New York, NY: Springer Publishing Co.; 1999.

161. Nilsson D. Adapting coping theory to explain the concept of adjustment. *Soc Work Health Care.* 2007;45(2):1-20.

162. Helgeson VS. *Gender, Stress, and Coping.* New York, NY: Oxford Press; 2011.

163. NCCN practice guidelines for the management of psychosocial distress. National Comprehensive Cancer Network. *Oncology (Williston Park).* 1999;13(5A):113-147.

164. Mosher CE, Duhamel KN. An examination of distress, sleep, and fatigue in metastatic breast cancer patients. *Psychooncology.* 2012;21(1):100-107.

165. American Cancer Society. Distress in People with Cancer. http://www.cancer.org/treatment/treatments-and-side-effects/emotional-side-effects/distress.html. Accessed October 20, 2019.

166. Allen JO, Zebrack B, Wittman D, Hammelef K, Morris AM. Expanding the NCCN guidelines for distress management: a model of barriers to the use of coping resources. *J Community Support Oncol.* 2014;12(8):271-277.

167. DiMatteo MR, Lepper HS, Croghan TW. Depression is a risk factor for noncompliance with medical treatment: meta-analysis of the effects of anxiety and depression on patient adherence. *Arch Intern Med.* 2000;160(14):2101-2107.

168. Stoudemire A, Thompson TL II. Medication noncompliance: systematic approaches to evaluation and intervention. *Gen Hosp Psychiatry.* 1983;5(4):233-239.

169. Katz ML, Donohue KA, Alfano CM, Day JM, Herndon JE II, Paskett ED. Cancer surveillance behaviors and psychosocial factors among long-term survivors of breast cancer. Cancer and Leukemia Group B 79804. *Cancer.* 2009;115(3):480-488.

170. Carmack CL, Basen-Engquist K, Gritz ER. Survivors at higher risk for adverse late outcomes due to psychosocial and behavioral risk factors. *Cancer Epidemiol Biomarkers Prev.* 2011;20(10):2068-2077.

171. Lerman C, Daly M, Walsh WP, et al. Communication between patients with breast cancer and health care providers. Determinants and implications. *Cancer.* 1993;72(9):2612-2620.

172. Torer N, Nursal TZ, Caliskan K, et al. The effect of the psychological status of breast cancer patients on the short-term clinical outcome after mastectomy. *Acta Chir Belg.* 2010;110(4):467-470.

173. Simpson JS, Carlson LE, Trew ME. Effect of group therapy for breast cancer on healthcare utilization. *Cancer Pract.* 2001;9(1):19-26.

174. Shim EJ, Mehnert A, Koyama A, et al. Health-related quality of life in breast cancer: a cross-cultural survey of German, Japanese, and South Korean patients. *Breast Cancer Res Treat.* 2006;99(3):341-350.

175. Skarstein J, Aass N, Fossa SD, Skovlund E, Dahl AA. Anxiety and depression in cancer patients: relation between the Hospital Anxiety and Depression Scale and the European Organization for Research and Treatment of Cancer Core Quality of Life Questionnaire. *J Psychosom Res.* 2000;49(1):27-34.

176. Weisman AD. *Psychosocial Screening and Intervention with Cancer Patients: Research Report.* Project Omega, Department of Psychiatry, Harvard Medical School, Massachusetts General Hospital; 1980.

177. Zabora J, BrintzenhofeSzoc K, Curbow B, Hooker C, Piantadosi S. The prevalence of psychological distress by cancer site. *Psychooncology.* 2001;10(1):19-28.

178. Kazak AE, Barakat LP, Meeske K, et al. Posttraumatic stress, family functioning, and social support in survivors of childhood leukemia and their mothers and fathers. *J Consult Clin Psychol.* 1997;65(1):120-129.

179. Young QR, Ignaszewski A, Fofonoff D, Kaan A. Brief screen to identify 5 of the most common forms of psychosocial distress in cardiac patients: validation of the screening tool for psychological distress. *J Cardiovasc Nurs.* 2007;22(6):525-534.

180. Keefler J, Duder S, Lechman C. Predicting length of stay in an acute care hospital: the role of psychosocial problems. *Soc Work Health Care.* 2001;33(2):1-16.

181. Vodermaier A, Linden W, Siu C. Screening for emotional distress in cancer patients: a systematic review of assessment instruments. *J Natl Cancer Inst.* 2009;101(21):1464-1488.

182. Zebrack B, Kayser K, Bybee D, et al. A practice-based evaluation of distress screening protocol adherence and medical service utilization. *J Natl Compr Canc Netw.* 2017;15(7):903-912.

183. Katon W, Lin EH, Kroenke K. The association of depression and anxiety with medical symptom burden in patients with chronic medical illness. *Gen Hosp Psychiatry.* 2007;29(2):147-155.

184. Gentilello LM, Ebel BE, Wickizer TM, Salkever DS, Rivara FP. Alcohol interventions for trauma patients treated in emergency departments and hospitals: a cost benefit analysis. *Ann Surg.* 2005;241(4):541-550.

185. Katz MR, Kopek N, Waldron J, Devins GM, Tomlinson G. Screening for depression in head and neck cancer. *Psychooncology.* 2004;13(4):269-280.

186. Mystakidou K, Tsilika E, Parpa E, Smyrniotis V, Galanos A, Vlahos L. Beck depression inventory: exploring its psychometric properties in a palliative care population of advanced cancer patients. *Eur J Cancer Care (Engl).* 2007;16(3):244-250.

187. van Scheppingen C, Schroevers MJ, Smink A, et al. Does screening for distress efficiently uncover meetable unmet needs in cancer patients? *Psychooncology.* 2011;20(6):655-663.

188. National Comprehensive Cancer Network. NCCN distress thermometer and problem list for patients. https://www.nccn.org/patients/resources/life_with_cancer/pdf/nccn_distress_thermometer.pdf. Accessed October 22, 2019.

189. Barakat LP, Kazak AE, Meadows AT, Casey R, Meeske K, Stuber ML. Families surviving childhood cancer: a comparison of posttraumatic stress symptoms with families of healthy children. *J Pediatr Psychol.* 1997;22(6):843-859.

190. Holland JC, Rowland JH, eds. *Handbook of Psychooncology: Psychological Care of the Patient with Cancer.* New York, NY: Oxford University Press; 1989.

191. Irvine D, Brown B, Crooks D, Roberts J, Browne G. Psychosocial adjustment in women with breast cancer. *Cancer.* 1991;67(4):1097-1117.

192. Baum A, Posluszny DM. *Psychosocial Interventions for Cancer.* Washington, DC: American Psychological Association; 2001.

193. International Society for Traumatic Stress Studies. What is traumatic stress? http://www.istss.org/public-resources/what-is-traumatic-stress.aspx. Accessed October 20, 2019.

194. Gurevich M, Devins GM, Rodin GM. Stress response syndromes and cancer: conceptual and assessment issues. *Psychosomatics.* 2002;43(4):259-281.

195. Einsle F, Kraft D, Kollner V. Post-traumatic stress disorder (PTSD) in cardiology and oncology—which diagnostic tools should be used? *J Psychosom Res.* 2012;72(6):434-438.

196. Mundy EA, Blanchard EB, Cirenza E, Gargiulo J, Maloy B, Blanchard CG. Posttraumatic stress disorder in breast cancer patients following autologous bone marrow transplantation or conventional cancer treatments. *Behav Res Ther.* 2000;38(10):1015-1027.

197. Cella DF, Mahon SM, Donovan MI. Cancer recurrence as a traumatic event. *Behav Med.* 1990;16(1):15-22.

198. Rustad JK, David D, Currier MB. Cancer and posttraumatic stress disorder: diagnosis, pathogenesis and treatment considerations. *Palliat Support Care.* 2012;10(3):213-223.

199. Kangas M, Henry JL, Bryant RA. Predictors of posttraumatic stress disorder following cancer. *Health Psychol.* 2005;24(6):579-585.

200. Butler LD, Koopman C, Classen C, Spiegel D. Traumatic stress, life events, and emotional support in women with metastatic breast cancer: cancer-related traumatic stress symptoms associated with past and current stressors. *Health Psychol.* 1999;18(6):555-560.

201. Exploring the Influence of Psychosocial Distress and Lifetime Trauma Exposure on Traumatic Stress Among Oncology Patients on Clinical Trials. https://clinicalstudies.info.nih.gov/ProtocolDetails.aspx?B_2017-CC-0010.html. Accessed November 7, 2019.

202. Sollner W, DeVries A, Steixner E, et al. How successful are oncologists in identifying patient distress, perceived social support, and need for psychosocial counselling? *Br J Cancer.* 2001;84(2):179-185.

203. Garcia SF, Cella D, Clauser SB, et al. Standardizing patient-reported outcomes assessment in cancer clinical trials: a patient-reported outcomes measurement information system initiative. *J Clin Oncol.* 2007;25(32):5106-5112.

204. Ma X, Zhang J, Zhong W, et al. The diagnostic role of a short screening tool—the distress thermometer: a meta-analysis. *Support Care Cancer.* 2014;22(7):1741-1755.

205. Derogatis, L.R.(1993). BSI Brief Symptom Inventory: Administration, Scoring, and Procedure Manual (4th Ed.). Minneapolis, MN: National Computer Systems.

206. Weathers FW, Litz BT, Keane TM, Palmieri PA, Marx BP, Schnurr PP. PTSD Checklist for DSM-5 (PCL-5). 2013. https://www.ptsd.va.gov/professional/assessment/adult-sr/ptsd-checklist.asp. Accessed October 20, 2019.

207. Weathers, F.W., Blake, D.D., Schnurr, P.P., Kaloupek, D.G., Marx, B.P., & Keane, T.M. (2013). The Life Events Checklist for DSM-5 (LEC-5). Instrument available from the National Center for PTSD at HYPERLINK "http://www.ptsd.va.gov"www.ptsd.va.gov

208. Johnsen TJ, Friborg O. The effects of cognitive behavioral therapy as an anti-depressive treatment is falling: a meta-analysis. *Psychol Bull.* 2015;141(4):747-768.

209. Brothers BM, Yang HC, Strunk DR, Andersen BL. Cancer patients with major depressive disorder: testing a biobehavioral/cognitive behavior intervention. *J Consult Clin Psychol.* 2011;79(2):253-260.

210. Jassim GA, Whitford DL, Hickey A, Carter B. Psychological interventions for women with non-metastatic breast cancer. *Cochrane Database Syst Rev.* 2015;(5):CD008729.

211. DuHamel KN, Mosher CE, Winkel G, et al. Randomized clinical trial of telephone-administered cognitive-behavioral therapy to reduce post-traumatic stress disorder and distress symptoms after hematopoietic stem-cell transplantation. *J Clin Oncol.* 2010;28(23):3754-3761.

212. Johnson JA, Rash JA, Campbell TS, et al. A systematic review and meta-analysis of randomized controlled trials of cognitive behavior therapy for insomnia (CBT-I) in cancer survivors. *Sleep Med Rev.* 2016;27:20-28.

213. Gielissen MF, Verhagen CA, Bleijenberg G. Cognitive behaviour therapy for fatigued cancer survivors: long-term follow-up. *Br J Cancer.* 2007;97(5):612-618.

214. Osborn RL, Demoncada AC, Feuerstein M. Psychosocial interventions for depression, anxiety, and quality of life in cancer survivors: meta-analyses. *Int J Psychiatry Med.* 2006;36(1):13-34.

215. Crane RS, Brewer J, Feldman C, et al. What defines mindfulness-based programs? The warp and the weft. *Psychol Med.* 2017;47(6):990-999.

216. Carlson LE, Tamagawa R, Stephen J, Drysdale E, Zhong L, Speca M. Randomized-controlled trial of mindfulness-based cancer recovery versus supportive expressive group therapy among distressed breast cancer survivors (MINDSET): long-term follow-up results. *Psychooncology.* 2016;25(7):750-759.

217. Dawson G, Madsen LT, Dains JE. Interventions to manage uncertainty and fear of recurrence in female breast cancer survivors: a review of the literature. *Clin J Oncol Nurs.* 2016;20(6):E155-E161.

218. Johns SA, Brown LF, Beck-Coon K, et al. Randomized controlled pilot trial of mindfulness-based stress reduction compared to psychoeducational support for persistently fatigued breast and colorectal cancer survivors. *Support Care Cancer.* 2016;24(10):4085-4096.

219. Lengacher CA, Reich RR, Paterson CL, et al. Examination of broad symptom improvement resulting from mindfulness-based stress reduction in breast cancer survivors: a randomized controlled trial. *J Clin Oncol.* 2016;34(24):2827-2834.

220. Reich RR, Lengacher CA, Alinat CB, et al. Mindfulness-based stress reduction in post-treatment breast cancer patients: immediate and sustained effects across multiple symptom clusters. *J Pain Symptom Manage.* 2017;53(1):85-95.

221. Piet J, Wurtzen H, Zachariae R. The effect of mindfulness-based therapy on symptoms of anxiety and depression in adult cancer patients and survivors: a systematic review and meta-analysis. *J Consult Clin Psychol.* 2012;80(6):1007-1020.

222. van der Kolk BA. The body keeps the score: memory and the evolving psychobiology of posttraumatic stress. *Harv Rev Psychiatry.* 1994;1(5):253-265.

223. SAMHSA's Trauma and Justice Strategic Initiative. SAMHSA's concept of trauma and guidance for a trauma-informed approach. 2014. http://www.trau-mainformedcareproject.org/resources/SAMHSA%20 TIC.pdf. Accessed October 20, 2019.

224. Okuyama S, Jones W, Ricklefs C, Tran ZV. Psychosocial telephone interventions for patients with cancer and survivors: a systematic review. *Psychooncology.* 2015;24(8):857-870.

225. Wenzel L, Osann K, Hsieh S, Tucker JA, Monk BJ, Nelson EL. Psychosocial telephone counseling for survivors of cervical cancer: results of a randomized biobehavioral trial. *J Clin Oncol.* 2015;33(10):1171-1179.

226. Grunfeld E, Levine MN, Julian JA, et al. Randomized trial of long-term follow-up for early-stage breast cancer: a comparison of family physician versus specialist care. *J Clin Oncol.* 2006;24(6):848-855.

227. Wattchow DA, Weller DP, Esterman A, et al. General practice vs surgical-based follow-up for patients with colon cancer: randomised controlled trial. *Br J Cancer.* 2006;94(8):1116-1121.

228. Cheung WY, Aziz N, Noone AM, et al. Physician preferences and attitudes regarding different models of cancer survivorship care: a comparison of primary care providers and oncologists. *J Cancer Surviv.* 2013;7(3):343-354.

229. Lawrence RA, McLoone JK, Wakefield CE, Cohn RJ. Primary care physicians' perspectives of their role in cancer care: a systematic review. *J Gen Intern Med.* 2016;31(10):1222-1236.

230. Hudson SV, Miller SM, Hemler J, et al. Adult cancer survivors discuss follow-up in primary care: 'not what i want, but maybe what i need'. *Ann Fam Med.* 2012;10:418-427.

231. ASCO. ASCO Cancer Treatment and Survivorship Care Plans. https://www.cancer.net/survivorship/follow-care-after-cancer-treatment/asco-cancer-treatment-and-survivorship-care-plans. Accessed October 22, 2019.

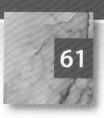

61 Cancer Genetics and Palliative Care

Xiao P. Peng, Ruthann M. Giusti, and Joann N. Bodurtha

INTRODUCTION

Genetics, the study of how characteristics of living organisms are transmitted from one generation to the next via DNA, and genomics, the study of the entirety of an organism's genes, the genome, using high throughput data collection and analysis, have been essential for developing strategies to prevent and treat cancer and furthering our understanding of the family experience of cancer in the 21st century (1). The availability of direct-to-consumer testing and increasing array of genetic testing options place all health care providers (HCPs) in a position to be asked about family history risk and testing (2). Palliative care (PC) providers are no exception and, in fact, may play a particularly important role when a cancer is diagnosed with genetic implications at the end of life.

Next-generation sequencing (NGS) has enabled the identification of countless somatic DNA changes in tumor tissues, as well as germline mutations in approximately 5% to 10% of all adult and 8% of all pediatric cancers (3). The paradigm is emerging that atypical cancers or presentations of common cancers may involve genetically encoded cancer risk even in the absence of a clear family history. This has, in turn, shaped evolving guidelines for cancer genetics evaluation, testing, and management. For example, the National Comprehensive Cancer Network (NCCN) guidelines now recommend genetic counseling and testing for all new patients with pancreatic cancer and all men with very high risk, high risk, metastatic, or regional prostate cancer (4). In 2019, the US Preventive Services Task Force (USPSTF) recommended that primary care providers use a family history screening tool to guide referral for genetic counseling and testing in breast cancer patients (USPSTF) (5). Other key oncology organizations such as the American Society of Clinical Oncology (ASCO) and American Association for Cancer Research (AACR) have likewise been evolving consensus guidelines for timely evaluation and management of adult and pediatric patients at potential genetic risk for cancer (6–8).

Although family-centeredness is a core tenet of the PC ethos, integrating cancer genetics into palliative medicine has been challenging (9). However, many oncology patients in PC have concerns about genetic predisposition to cancer that it is imperative to address (10). While PC providers are increasingly recognizing that the end-of-life (EOL) setting may provide greatest opportunity for facilitating such much-needed discussions about cancer genetics assessment, genetics is still far from being a core element of PC practice (11,12). Provider-reported barriers to the introduction of genetics discussion in PC include uncertainty about how to broach the topic and concern about incurring distress, difficulties surrounding obtaining an accurate family history, lack of confidence and knowledge about genetics, and low awareness of genetic services and how to access them (11–15).

One problem is the assumption that the need for cancer genetics evaluation and testing has already been addressed prior to a cancer patient's entry into PC (18). However, the PC setting may often be the first and last opportunity to obtain vital genetic material and family history that could prove life-saving for surviving family members. Approximately one-third of cancer patients have a family history of cancer, with significant impact on relatives' perceptions and emotions surrounding the possibility of inherited cancer risk (16,17).

Rapid communication of information (whether accurate or not) through our current forms of media have impacted patient awareness and expectations regarding genetic testing, surveillance, and treatment options (18,19). Dying patients frequently voice concern for the health of surviving family members and find a sense of beneficence in preserving their DNA for future testing (11). Current genetic testing is most high yield when initiated with a known affected patient and then expanded to other family members after a pathogenic change has been identified. Once a patient dies, however, their DNA becomes unavailable for future analysis unless it has been properly preserved by DNA banking—a practice that is unfamiliar to most HCPs (11,15). As always, decisions about genetic testing and DNA banking should involve partnered and iterative discussions with families, given their potentially profound psychosocial and economic impact (20).

This chapter addresses some fundamental issues in contemporary cancer genetics, including the personal, psychosocial, and cultural considerations relevant to families with potentially heritable cancers, with associated resources to help clinicians identify and refer families to specialized genetic services, including genetic counseling and DNA banking.

CANCER GENETICS: OVERVIEW

Though the vast majority of cancers occur sporadically from random somatic mutations or carcinogenic exposures, approximately 30% of cancers are familial, meaning that the proportion of cancers observed in a family exceeds general population risk levels (21). Currently, an estimated 5% to 10% of the heritable fraction of cancer can still be attributed to highly penetrant, monogenic, dominantly inherited syndromes (21). The advent of high-throughout, NGS-based technologies has significantly accelerated the discovery of new germline cancer mutations.

Traditionally, the clinical identification of such hereditary cancer syndromes (HCS) involved clinical recognition of a syndrome, followed by identification of the implicated gene and pathogenic variant. When optimally used, genetic testing can help to identify the underlying etiology for cancers observed in a family, help clarify a patient's future cancer risks, bring relatives to attention for evaluation and testing, and inform preventive strategies and treatment options tailored to an individual's genetic makeup and personal values.

Cancer genetics is evolving rapidly as it adapts to the ever-expanding repertoire of available genetic tests (18). This makes it more imperative than ever for HCPs, including PC clinicians, to partner with genetics providers whenever possible for the optimal delivery of genetically informed care. HCPs involved in the care of patients with cancer and their families should gain a level of comfort with and awareness of the basic elements and process of cancer genetics risk assessment, counseling, testing, and follow-up including when to seek and where to find additional resources.

Evolution of Genetic Testing for Hereditary Cancer

Historically, cancer genetic testing (CGT) involved step-wise, single-gene testing for mutations in highly penetrant genes based on differential diagnoses informed by clinical features (23–25). This single-gene testing strategy is still useful in select circumstances, but NGS now allows for the simultaneous interrogation of many genes at marginally higher cost. Current clinical platforms, for example, can enable the sequencing and analysis of a patient's whole genome within several days.

Most cancer gene panels continue to assess for mutations in a handful of highly penetrant genes (associated with 18- to 20-fold increased cancer risk) (26). However, after the 2013 US Supreme Court decision invalidating patents on specific genes, the number of commercially available laboratory tests blossomed. Now, there is a rapidly expanding cohort of less well-studied, moderately penetrant genes (associated with 2- to 5-fold increased cancer risk) increasingly included in multigene panel tests (MGPTs) (23–25). Currently, over 100 Clinical Laboratory Improvement Amendments (CLIA)-certified tests are available in the United States for diagnosing BRCA1/2-associated hereditary breast and ovarian cancer (HBOC) alone (23).

Important factors guiding the use of these tests include institutional availability, the number of genes included in the test, depth and coverage of genes of interest, detection rates, inclusion of large rearrangements, and finally testing costs and insurance coverage.

Evaluation of Suspected Hereditary Cancer

Palliative and supportive oncology care is an interdisciplinary undertaking. When a hereditary etiology of cancer is suspected, genetics expertise must be recruited into the care of the patient and family (see below). According to the NIH, comprehensive cancer risk assessment and counseling includes clinical assessment, genetic testing when appropriate, and risk management recommendations delivered in the context of one or more genetic counseling sessions (27).

Although providers of all backgrounds and roles have the potential to deal with genetics issues, the rapid evolution of genetic medicine mandates that an interdisciplinary cancer care team find ways to maintain currency in the field and provide the most up-to-date information to the patient and family. Familiarity by all HCPs with the basic process below leads to greater recognition and initiation of cancer risk assessment where needed:

1. Information gathering—including a cancer-focused family history
2. Interpretation—determining whether a concern for hereditary cancer susceptibility exists
3. Communication—conveying concerns from risk assessment to patients and families
4. Follow-up—coordinating necessary referrals for or providing pre-/posttest counseling and testing

Role of Cancer Genetics Providers

If a patient's personal and/or family history is suggestive of HCS, referral to a Cancer Genetics Clinic and/or Cancer Genetic Counselor (CGC) is warranted, either to conduct the initial risk assessment or to follow up on the findings of a referring HCP who has identified a patient or family at risk for HCS.

CGCs and cancer geneticists are board-certified professionals specially trained to perform personalized risk assessments based on a combination of both personal factors and family history, as well as the use of mathematical risk assessment tools where appropriate (23). Specific services provided by cancer genetics professionals:

- Pre- and posttest counseling on medical, legal, and financial ramifications of testing
- Assessment for and management of patient-specific barriers or concerns
- Proper informed consent and managing logistics of genetic testing
- Results interpretation in the context of a patient's medical and family history
- Resources for family members dealing with the psychosocial impact of results
- Facilitating communication among and testing for additional family members
- Helping to develop individualized management plans for risk reduction and treatment
- Coordinating EOL genetics discussions and DNA banking
- Helping other HCPs provide ongoing education and identify high-risk patients

Pre- and posttest genetic counseling is now recommended by the ASCO as part of the CGT process and many major insurance companies now require documentation of counseling to cover the cost of genetic testing. Cancer genetic professionals are uniquely equipped to understand the process of genomic sequencing analysis and variant classification, which is essential for helping patients and other clinicians interpret test results. Finally, one of the most valuable and under-appreciated aspects of their job involves the provision of longitudinal follow-up for families with HCS to ensure that the concerns of each generation are appropriately managed and addressed.

PRINCIPLES OF HEREDITARY CANCER RISK ASSESSMENT (22–27)

HCS risk assessment can occur in a variety of different settings and may be conducted to various extents by any HCP. In cancer genetics clinics, these sessions have traditionally taken place during face-to-face visits, but many clinics now perform the initial risk assessment via telephone, video conference, or in group sessions and provide results by telephone. Whatever the modality, these basic steps are necessary for completeness of information on the clinician's part and voluntary, informed decision-making on the patient's part:

- Obtain a detailed personal medical history
- Obtain a detailed family cancer history (at least three generation pedigree)
- Provide education on the implications of testing for patient and family members
- Obtain informed consent
- Psychosocial assessment

In practice, the first two steps can be performed by any HCP, but they can refer a patient/family for formal counseling and genetic testing at any stage of concern. See **Resources** section for additional Web sites, guides, and tools to aid in cancer risk assessment.

Taking a Personal History (27)

Eliciting a full health history is one of the most important skills for HCPs to have. A comprehensive personal history includes direct questioning about medical, surgical, family, social, and reproductive factors, as well as risk factors known to contribute to cancer (Table 61.1). Understanding patterns of sporadic (nonhereditary) cancer can also help identify suspicious histories outside the norm.

Obtaining a Cancer Family History (27)

Accuracy of family history taking is crucial to cancer risk assessment (Table 61.2). An NIH consensus statement defines the critical elements of a cancer risk pedigree as:

- First-degree (children, siblings, and parents) relatives
- Second-degree (grandparents, aunts, uncles, and half-siblings) relatives
- Their types and ages at diagnosis of cancer
- Lineage relationships (maternal or paternal)

Third-degree relatives can also impact testing criteria or eligibility, but information for them may not always be available. Studies have found that patient reporting is usually most accurate for first-degree relatives and common cancers, such as breast, while others, particularly gynecologic cancers, are more often misreported. Additional considerations when taking a family history:

- Pedigrees should be expanded and updated over time
- Limited family structure may affect pedigree-based assessment, that is, small family size, early ages at death in family members, few female relatives
- Ancestry may affect risk, that is BRCA1/2 in the Ashkenazi Jewish population
- Note adoption, consanguinity, nonpaternity, or use of donor sperm or egg

TABLE 61.1 COMMON CANCER RISK FACTORS[27]

Risk factor	Cancer type
Age	Advancing age is a risk factor for most cancers
Alcohol (>1 drink/day)	Oral, throat, esophagus, larynx, liver, breast, colorectal cancers
Precancerous lesions	Lobular carcinoma in situ (LCIS), atypical ductal hyperplasia (ADH), and atypical lobular hyperplasia (ALH) are risk markers for future breast cancer
	Cervical dysplasia and cervical cancer
	Colon polyps and colon cancer
Hormones	Exposure to DES (diethylstilbestrol) in utero and vaginal cancer
	Postmenopausal hormone replacement therapy and breast cancer
	Estrogen replacement without progesterone in a woman with a uterus and endometrial cancer
Immune suppression	Those on immunosuppressants because of transplant at risk for non-Hodgkin's lymphoma, leukemia, lung, kidney, liver, and cervical cancer
	Those with HIV immunosuppression at risk for Kaposi's sarcoma, liver, cervical, and other cancers
Infectious agents	Epstein-Barr virus and lymphoma, cancers of the nose and throat
	Human papillomavirus (HPV) and cervical, penile, vulvar, vaginal, and oral cancers
	Hepatitis C virus, hepatitis B virus, and liver cancer
	H. pylori and gastric cancer
Inflammatory bowel disease	Colon cancer
Obesity	Postmenopausal breast cancer, endometrial, colorectal, esophagus, kidney, pancreas, and gallbladder
Radiation	Women with a history of Hodgkin's lymphoma who received mantle radiation before age 30 are at high risk for breast cancer
Reproductive risk factors	Prolonged exposure to endogenous hormones leading to higher risk for breast cancer (nulliparity, early menarche, late menopause, no breast-feeding)
Smoking	Lung, oral cancers, esophagus, bladder, kidney, liver, stomach, pancreas, colorectal, acute myeloid leukemia, and cervical cancers
	Smokeless tobacco and mouth/oral cancers, esophagus, and pancreas
UV radiation	Skin cancers because of sun or tanning bed exposures

Adapted from Forman A, Schwartz S. Guidelines-based cancer risk assessment. *Semin Oncol Nurs.* 2019;35(1):34-46.

- History of birth defects or multiple miscarriages (suggestive of possible chromosomal anomalies)

A thorough family history also includes ethnographic and psychosocial details to help providers understand family dynamics and health beliefs, assess communication patterns, create rapport with patients, and support communication among family members regardless of the type of CGT being offered.

Identifying Patients to Refer for Genetic Testing

Specific testing criteria vary among HCS, but some broadly applicable red flags that warrant additional investigation or referral include:

- Patients with a personal or close family history of earlier-than-expected onset of cancer (i.e.,

colon cancer at <50 years of age, premenopausal breast cancer)
- Multiple primary cancers in a single individual (i.e., colorectal and endometrial cancer)
- Bilateral cancer in paired organs or multifocal disease (i.e., bilateral breast cancer, multifocal renal cancer)
- Multiple family members with the same or related cancers within the same lineage, particularly if clustered over successive generations (i.e., mother, daughter, and sisters with breast cancer)
- High-risk or unusually aggressive cancers (i.e., triple negative breast cancer, Gleason 7+ prostate cancer)
- Uncommon presentation (i.e., male breast cancer)
- Uncommon tumor histology (i.e., medullary thyroid carcinoma)

TABLE 61.2 ELEMENTS OF A FAMILY HISTORY[27]

Key elements for minimum adequate cancer risk pedigree:
- First- and second-degree relatives
- Ethnicity
- Assessment of both maternal and paternal lineage
- Age at diagnosis and type of primary cancer for each affected family member
- Results of prior genetic testing in family members

Expanded elements:
- Third-degree relatives
- Histology and treatment details for relatives' cancer history
- Exposure history, for example, smoking, mantle radiation
- Current ages and or ages at death for all family members
- Cause of death for all family members
- History of benign tumors or other features suggestive of hereditary cancer risk, for example, adenomatous polyps
- History of preventive surgeries, for example, prophylactic oophorectomy

Adapted from Forman A, Schwartz S. Guidelines-based cancer risk assessment. *Semin Oncol Nurs.* 2019;35(1):34-46.

- Rare cancer types (i.e., retinoblastoma, adrenocortical carcinoma, sebaceous carcinoma, ocular melanoma; serous ovarian or granulosa cell tumor of the ovary; fallopian tube, ureteral, diffuse gastric, or primary peritoneal cancer)
- Rare cancers associated with birth defects (i.e., Wilms' tumor and genitourinary abnormalities)
- Geographic or ethnic populations at high risk of hereditary cancers, especially if a known founder effect is present (i.e., Ashkenazi Jewish heritage and BRCA1/2)

Cancer Predisposition in Children (28)

Large gene sequencing panels, chromosomal microarrays, and whole exome sequencing are being used with increased frequency in pediatric care. In combination with routine tumor genomic profiling, a greater number of pediatric patients with HCS are being identified. Germline variants play a role in approximately 8.5% to 10% of all pediatric cancer diagnoses, a rate mirroring that seen for adult cancers, with TP53, APC, BRCA2, NF1, PMS2, RB1, and RUNX1 highlighted as the most commonly identified germline mutations in their cohort (29). A number of pediatric tumors are highly suggestive of hereditary cancer risk and warrant additional genetic evaluation.

Established protocols exist for many known HCS with childhood onset, including:

- Von Hippel-Lindau syndrome (VHL)
- Multiple endocrine neoplasia type I and type II (MEN1, MEN2A, MEN2B)

- PTEN hamartoma tumor syndrome
- Familial paraganglioma/pheochromocytoma syndrome
- Peutz-Jeghers syndrome (PJS)
- Beckwith Wiedemann syndrome (BWS)
- Li-Fraumeni syndrome (LFS)

Although there can be many morbidity and mortality benefits when at-risk children are appropriately tested for HCS, genetic testing for pediatric cancer syndromes is rarely straightforward. Many issues need to be considered before testing is offered, including:

- Optimal timing of testing for at-risk pediatric patients
- Interpretation of results and explanation to patients and families
- Utility of testing and availability of follow-up management recommendations
- Emotional ramifications and available support for patients and families
- Informed consent and assent for minors undergoing CGT
- Disclosure of genetic test results after a child has died from cancer

Before genetic testing is offered, it is also essential to consider the emotional impact of CTG results for each child and the family as a whole. Testing can be associated with:

- A complexity of emotions (i.e., guilt, anxiety, denial) and, especially in adolescence, feelings of guilt and self-blame for disease
- Significant impact on family dynamics, including disruption of parent–child or sibling–sibling relationships
- Concerns that children with a known HCS may be treated differently than those without the syndrome in a manner that may impact growth and development, including potential loss of autonomy for the child

It is important to recognize and address these and other psychosocial issues when helping families navigate the CTG process. As a general rule, genetic testing in pediatric patients is only recommended when the HCS being tested for is associated with childhood onset of disease AND there are effective and safe screening tools and/or intervention options. When genetic testing is performed appropriately for children, those that test positive for an HCS may be candidates for additional cancer screening. Screening may result in early detection, which may translate into better treatment options and improved survival. However, it also harbors potential disadvantages:

- Ability to cause significant anxiety on the part of patient and family

- The potential for additional, possibly invasive, work-up
- Time taken away from school or work and possible long-distance travel for hospital visits
- Unclear clinical benefit or actionability of screening
- Negative impact of false positive results on families and their relationships with providers

Given the vulnerability of this patient population, developmentally appropriate counseling for the patient and awareness of the social/environmental context of the family is even more paramount.

Emerging Genetic Testing Concerns

CGCs have been rapidly adapting their clinical practices to accommodate the ever-expanding panoply of reported germline cancer mutations and available genetic tests. However, they are faced with increasingly difficult decisions, as most recently developed tests, including most MGPTs, have little to no associated validity or outcomes data. Moreover, little to no evidence exists to guide recommendations regarding follow-up management of patients with variants of uncertain significance (VUS) or more recently identified variants for which the genotype–phenotype correlations remain unclear.

Additionally, pathology-based population screening for adult cancers, such as colorectal and endometrial, may soon become common practice. This would occur without informed consent or prior genetic counseling involvement. The abrupt need to consider further HCS testing shortly after a cancer diagnosis is likely to create additional stress for patients. Thus, dissemination of additional educational support and preparative information in nongenetics facilities such as oncology clinics may be warranted to help prepare patients emotionally for this additional diagnostic hurdle.

Cultural and Individual Context (30–35)

While we live in an era of increasingly personalized medicine, it is important to remain aware of the historical experiences of ethnic minority groups that harbor potentially significant impact on attitudes toward health care and genetics. For example, the ambivalent relationship that many African-Americans have with HCPs may be influenced by our country's unfortunate legacy of often institutionalized racism and exploitation, of which the Tuskegee Syphilis Study has been only one notable example. Levels of gender-specific comfort discussing cancer with members of the opposite sex and levels of cancer fatalism, which may be positively or negatively motivating, are also commonly reported themes by minorities (30). Finally, some ethnic groups, such as South Asians, hold differing concepts of the meaning of "close family members" from Westerners and this has the potential to impact family history reporting and thus risk assessment (30). For more specific information about themes and beliefs influencing cancer-associated decision-making among minority populations, see Licqurish et al. (32).

Ethnocultural concepts of illness, suffering, and dying greatly inform PC, shaping communication and decision-making about EOL care for patients, families, and HCPs. One systematic review identified significant differences in the processes, preferences, and beliefs of ethnic minority cancer patients surrounding EOL care (33). When providers fail to appreciate, overlook, or inadequately address such differences, PC patients are at risk of receiving inferior care, which may involve inequality in utilization of and access to services and EOL planning. For more specific information about how to approach urgent EOL cancer genetics evaluation and testing, including EOL adaptations to informed consent, see Roeland et al. (34).

INTEGRATING GENETICS INTO PALLIATIVE AND SUPPORTIVE ONCOLOGY CARE (9–17)

Care of the individual patient in the context of the family is central to the ethos of PC revolves around two themes: First, what is the role of the PC provider in identifying individuals and families at high genetic risk of cancer and referring these for genetic testing and/or DNA banking? Second, how does understanding the psychosocial impact of genetic cancer risk on a family help the PC provider to better support the unique communication and decision-making needs of each member?

All the literature to date suggest that there is substantially more room for cancer genetics to play a role in the PC setting, whether to optimize EOL care and planning for the affected patient, or to address cancer risk and prevention for surviving family members. One study found that 25% of PC patients had no prior documentation of family history, while 32% of all pedigrees warranted referral to genetic services, comparable to the 21% reported in a prior study (10,15). These studies identified suboptimal genetic assessment practices surrounding palliative oncology patients and their providers. Their findings are echoed in other studies that identified the following major provider barriers to the initiation of genetic discussions in a PC setting (9,17):

1. *Assumption that genetics was addressed earlier in the disease trajectory*—Suboptimal genetic referral rates within the oncology setting are well documented, with genetic issues often overlooked at the time of initial diagnosis. Patients with particularly aggressive cancers may not present until the advanced stages of their disease, and concerns about the family history may only surface as the affected individual becomes

increasingly unwell. For these patients, the option of genetic testing or DNA storage may only become available in the PC setting.

2. *Concerns that initiating a discussion about genetics would cause patient distress*—Distress from genetic testing for cancer susceptibility has been measured primarily in the setting of predictive genetic testing for a known mutation. One study exploring patient experiences of genetics in the PC setting found that patients with a family history are often already concerned about an HCS and fearful about cancer risk for subsequent generations. Thus, genetic evaluation may not only alleviate distress but PC patients may also perceive the provision of a DNA sample as a positive, comforting and altruistic experience, given the potential benefits for their family.

3. *Lack of knowledge and poor confidence addressing genetic issues*—Given the complexity of genetic information, most HCPs felt that it was beyond the scope of their practice and required specialist referral, unrealistic when the window of opportunity is limited. One study examining DNA banking for dying cancer patients found that only 10% of physicians were aware of the availability of DNA banking and few reported confidence with discussing or facilitating the process (15). Genetics services also need to be proactive about ensuring that PC providers have the skills, knowledge, and confidence to discuss and assess cancer risk and refer when needed. Nurses in one study reported routinely obtained a family history, but for the purposes of gauging family support rather than identifying genetic risk. Expanding their scope of questioning to familial cancer occurrences may help identify patients who may benefit from genetic assessment.

Given the current demand on genetic services, efforts have been made to facilitate the translation of genetics to mainstream clinical environments to ensure equitable access to genetic testing (9). This often involves the provision of pretest information and counseling by a nongenetics provider. Such mainstreaming within the oncology setting has shown good preliminary results in the United Kingdom and provides a model by which cancer genetics can be integrated within the PC setting.

A genetics framework applicable to any cancer patient in the PC setting includes the following (15):

1. Do not assume patients have had genetics assessment.
2. Record family history for all patients.
3. Offer DNA banking and genetics consult if appropriate (see section on **Principles of Hereditary Cancer Risk Assessment** for details).
4. Know how to access genetics resources and DNA banking as an option at the end of life.

DNA Banking (11,15)

In the PC setting, DNA banking may be the most practical approach to genetic testing in patients with cancer. However, most patients, even those at high risk for hereditary cancer, know little about DNA banking. Even family members who consider the PC period an inopportune time for discussing familial cancer risk may be open to DNA banking, especially at the patient's request. DNA banking involves drawing blood for long-term storage at a DNA banking facility. Not typically covered by insurance, costs vary from one to a few hundred dollars. Facilities offering DNA banking vary in their informed consent requirements and documentation for sample ownership (e.g., who is authorized to submit a sample to a laboratory for genetic testing). Banking can be particularly helpful in view of the long turn-around time for genetic testing and possibility of more informative analysis options in the future. In addition, given the complex and emotional decision-making that can be involved in genetic testing, banking gives family members time to seek counseling and to carefully consider such decisions without feeling pressure to pursue testing before a loved one dies.

DNA banking in the PC setting is also associated with a host of ethical, social, and legal issues only just beginning to be systematically examined. Who will have access to the banked DNA after the donor has died? This can be specified on DNA banking consent forms, establishing a line of access. However, family decisions about testing and disclosure are often not unanimous and may change over time. How can it be assured that potentially important genetic information is disseminated among family members? Despite these challenges, the potential benefits to surviving family members are real.

See **Resources** for additional information.

THE EXPERIENCE OF FAMILIES AFFECTED BY HCS

Families with heritable cancer risk live with a heavy burden of repetitive loss and uncertainty. However, it has been challenging to systematically understand the psychosocial impact of familial cancer and its unique impact on individual families.

Much of available literature is derived from studies assessing the psychosocial impact of genetic testing rather cancer genetic risk per se, though it is likely that some key concepts can be extrapolated. A family's experience is likely to be influenced by characteristics of the specific genetic condition, such as its penetrance and expressivity (i.e., the likelihood that an individual with the gene will get cancer and what type(s) of cancer(s), age of onset, lethality, etc.) and options available for diagnosis and management. Moreover, different individuals with the same genetic risk from the same family may have different psychosocial responses, a concept called "multifinality." One individual may become distressed; another might use adaptive coping strategies. In addition, stress associated with familial cancer may be one among many stressors contributing to the same psychosocial outcome, a concept called "equifinality." For example, a cancer patient's depression may stem from living in a high-risk family, recent job loss, disease morbidity, child-care worries, or some combination thereof (35).

Finally, the illness and death of a loved one may prove the seminal event that fosters communication about cancer risk among family members, providing an opportunity to be referred for potential genetic counseling, evaluation, and management for surviving family members (17).

Vignettes for Discussion (36–40)

We use the following case studies to illustrate some of the feelings and concerns that have been voiced by families of pediatric and adult patients affected by HCS:

Case 1: Mark and Judy

Mark is a previously healthy, active 15-year-old boy with an unremarkable past medical history. He presents with 6 months of increasing left lower extremity leg pain with a now palpable mass on exam. Imaging is concerning for osteosarcoma. He is referred to a pediatric oncologist for further workup and staging. During the initial oncology visit, his stepmother Anne also mentions that his biological mother Judy is currently in hospice care for a brain tumor. After reading criteria developed by the Cancer Predisposition Working Group of the Society for Pediatric Oncology and Hematology (the "Jongmans Criteria"), his oncologist discusses referring Mark and his family to a cancer geneticist.

Mark, Anne, and his dad Jim meet with Dr. Lee, a Cancer Genetics provider and Kristen Wall, a genetic counselor. Judy and her designated health care proxy join them over the phone as she is no longer able to travel. Prior to the meeting, Kristen reviewed Mark and Judy's oncology records from their outside providers. During the meeting, she takes a detailed history, including a 3-generation pedigree from both Mark and Judy families. Judy was adopted, so she knows very little about her family history. She does recall being told that at least one of her parents passed away at a young age. In addition, a maternal cousin she found later in life had survived an unspecified blood cancer. Dr. Lee conducts a full physical exam on Mark and notes no findings concerning for dysmorphology, skeletal dysplasia, or skin or nervous system involvement. After reviewing Mark's presumptive diagnosis of osteosarcoma and Judy's two primary diagnoses of choroidal plexus carcinoma and glioblastoma multiforme, the Cancer Genetics team then recommends beginning with focused testing for Li-Fraumeni syndrome by TP53 sequencing in Judy, with the understanding that if Judy is found to be positive, they will then test Mark for her variant. Judy is indeed found to have a pathogenic variant in TP53 and Mark is subsequently found to carry the same variant.

Theme 1: Referral Uptake by Cancer Patients.

Judy: This is actually my second cancer—I had radiation earlier in life for another and my doctors thought that maybe I had this brain tumor because of that. They had wanted me to get a gene test at the time, but I wasn't interested. Later on, was interested in learning more about my genetic heritage, hoping I would learn more about my birth family. I figured if there was anything unusual in my genes, it would show up. I never heard that there was a problem.

Anne: My stepchildren know that their mother has been sick for a while but we don't know all the details of her diagnoses. I am concerned about them and about the risk for the children Jim and I have together and may have in the future. If there is a cancer gene responsible for Mark's tumor, maybe it comes from Jim's side of the family.

Jim: If that's what needs to be done, let's do the testing. Now that both my ex-wife and my son have cancer, it doesn't sound random. I'd like an answer.

Theme 2: Perceived Benefits of Testing.

Judy: Knowing for me is still really important, even though I've already made peace with my own situation. I need to know for Mark and for his older sister, Julie, so that they can be prepared and know what they need to do to beat cancer. If there's any chance I could help out other family members, I want to at least be able to do that.

Mark: I just would really not have to deal with this. But more with the cancer diagnosis in general. I think just knowing why and being able to have some control over it would be good. So that I won't end up like my mom, not knowing what was going on until it was too late.

Jim: I really learned a lot from the counseling and testing process. Having Dr. Lee and Kristen explain what was going on was definitely a lot more helpful than my looking up stuff online, which was too overwhelming. With all those genes out there, I was a bit taken aback when they said they only wanted to test for one gene, but it made sense after they explained why. I was worried about what they would do if Judy's testing came back negative but it sounded like they had a reasonable back-up plan, banking DNA for future testing when more info might be available.

Theme 3: Involving Children in Conversations About Genetic Cancer Risk.

Jim: Mark's always been a smart kid, but he's getting to an age now where he's starting to understand things a lot better. He was always very curious and asking a lot of questions when he was younger and his mother was sick, but I was feeling too overwhelmed back then to do much explaining. The geneticists have been great about helping me figure out how to talk with him about these things and connecting me to other parents who have had to go through similar situations.

Judy: I like that the Genetics team dealt with Mark directly, asked his opinion and treated him as an individual. Their respect for him has been very positive. I really appreciate their helping us communicate with Julie as well about what's been going on. I know it's tough for her right now, being on the other coast and just starting grad school.

Case 2: Cindy

Cindy is a 41-year-old African-American woman, a nurse and single mother of two, with a strong family history of gastric cancer. She was found to carry a *CDH1* mutation and has been referred to your institution for a prophylactic gastrectomy. Pain and Palliative Care has been consulted in advance of surgery to plan for postoperative pain management. You begin your consult by interviewing Cindy to obtain information concerning her family history and to better understand her family relationships and dynamics.

Theme 1: The Evolving Nature of Genetic Information.

You: What is your current understanding of your diagnosis?

Cindy: I first learned that I had the CDH1 mutation about 15 years ago. My doctor referred me for genetic testing because we have a lot of cancer in my family. My mom and her sister both had breast cancer in their forties. My aunt was tested and they told her she had a suspicious change in the CDH1 gene, but they didn't know exactly what it meant because CDH1 was not a gene that they had seen in families with breast cancer. Now, of course, I'm told that they know for sure the CDH1 gene causes both stomach and breast cancers.

Theme 2: Motivation for Testing.

You: What ultimately helped you decide to go through with the tough step of getting tested?

Cindy: My mother did not want anything to do with testing. She thought it was tempting fate. I have always been proactive about my health and I wanted to know if I had the mutation. I figured if I had the gene I would be more regular with mammograms. I wanted to know since would also impact the lives of my children. I went for testing and they found the CDH1 gene change in me too.

Theme 3: Posttesting Responses.

You: What was your immediate reaction? How has the genetic testing result affected your life since then?

Cindy: When I first heard about the risk of gastric cancer, my heart sank. I had gotten used to the idea of breast cancer and there seemed to be ways to manage the risk. I was already getting yearly mammograms and MRIs. When I was 13, my grandmother—who was my age at the time—went into the hospital and died within a few days. It was sudden and very unexpected. She may have had stomach cancer, but it happened so fast and I'm not sure they ever figured it out. I decided to go through with the gastrectomy because I want to be there for my kids. I'm thinking about getting mastectomies too.

Theme 4: The Importance of an Updated Family History.

You: Do you know if any other members of your family may potentially be affected? Have you had a chance to connect with them about the diagnosis?

Cindy: About a year ago, I got a call from Tom, my mother's uncle's son. I was surprised to hear from him because his parents don't usually have much contact with the rest of the family. Tom told me that his father and his brother had both been diagnosed with stomach cancer and that they found the CDH1 mutation in them as well. Tom said his father had already died and his brother wasn't doing well. That was the first I knew that the mutation could be related to something besides breast cancer. Tom said his family were all going in for testing—four had already been found to carry the gene and two had already opted for gastrectomy to prevent stomach cancer.

Theme 5: Involving Children.

You: What have you been able to share about your diagnosis with your children? How have they responded?

Cindy: I have two daughters—Emily is 21 and Ella is 12. I took them with me to the genetic counseling session because this affects them too and they have a right to know about it. Emily decided to be tested. I was really proud of her for making the decision for herself. I was so relieved to find out that she was not a carrier. Ella is only 12 so she is a bit farther from the age when she could get breast or gastric cancer; we decided that she should wait until she is older and then make the decision about testing for herself.

Theme 6: Impact on Family Relationships.

You: How has the diagnosis affected your relationship with your family? Who have you been able to share your diagnosis with? What have been some of their own thoughts on testing?

Cindy: Coming here has been difficult. I feel pretty much alone in dealing with all of this. I haven't gotten much support from my family. Talking to my cousin, Tom, was helpful. It's tough for me that my mother and older brother Anthony refuse testing, even though Anthony knows this could affect his two kids. We've had some big arguments over it. My mom is very religious and feels that we should accept life as God gives it to us. But I wonder if she is also just afraid of having to deal with the idea that she might have passed down the gene to her kids. At least my other brother Gabe is still thinking about it—I think his wife would like him to be tested. They haven't had kids yet and if Gabe found out he has the gene, he might think about adoption.

Case 3: Oscar and his Family

Oscar is a 78-year-old gentleman admitted to home hospice care after he progressed on standard therapy for a glioblastoma diagnosed 6 months ago. His seizures are now controlled; he appears comfortable and is alert and oriented but unable to move his left side. You are visiting him for the first time. He is at home with his wife, his two surviving children and their spouses, and Oscar's son-in-law Edward. His older son, Jason, holds medical power of attorney.

You learn from Edward that his wife Elena, Oscar's youngest child, died 4 years ago at age 40 during treatment for metastatic colon cancer: "We're all still reeling from losing her. I feel like we're all suffering from posttraumatic stress. Here we are again, so soon after Elena passed. And Oscar's brother, Javier died of a brain tumor 2 years ago. Just so much loss. All this death in our family really scares me, especially thinking about what it means for my daughter, Alison, who just turned 16."

Theme 1: Introducing the Concept of DNA Banking.

You ask Edward whether anyone had discussed genetic counseling and testing with the family, but he does not recall that this has been mentioned. He is concerned about raising the issue with his in-laws while Oscar is dying, though the family has talked among themselves about whether their family is "cursed" with cancer.

You meet Oscar surrounded by his family. Cuddled up next to him is his 5-year-old granddaughter who runs off to play. After talking to him for some time, you mention having learnt of the recent bereavements the family has suffered. "I have always tried to take good care of my family," Oscar says, "but with all these deaths, I am worried about them. At this point, if there's a way to know what is going on, I'm prepared to try it—for them."

Theme 2: Discussing the Logistics of DNA Banking.

After your discussion with Oscar, he gives you permission to broach the subject of banking his DNA for genetic testing with his entire family

present. You introduce this as the best way to help them understand their family's cancer risk. Oscar's wife and sons only want to focus on taking care of Oscar right now. You continue, "If we obtain a sample of genetic material from Oscar, usually blood or some cheek cells from inside the mouth, we can always store this sample for future testing, when you decide you would like to know if there is a specific gene potentially causing your family's increased risk for cancer."

When asked for details, you explain that saving the sample usually costs several hundred dollars a year, that insurance may not cover this cost, and that having a sample from someone in the family affected by cancer usually makes it more certain that if there is a "cancer gene" in the family that it can be identified. "In addition," you say, "sometimes identifying whether individual family members have a cancer predisposing gene can lead to preventive measures such as more regular screening, which may help detect cancers earlier on when they can more easily be treated."

Theme 3: Step-wise Decisions and Planning for Follow-up.

You also explain the need for clear agreement in the family about who decides when and under what circumstances the sample is tested. Oscar is thoughtful. "I think it is important for me to do this for my family." He looks at Jason. "You will need to be the one to decide about this," he says. You make a plan with the family to send them additional resources on DNA banking and CGT, as well as arrange for a follow-up phone call to touch base with them after they've gone through the materials.

Theme 4: Referral to Genetic Counseling and DNA Banking Services.

Back at your office, you look on the National Society of Genetic Counselors (NSGC) Web site and find the contact number for a genetics counselor at your local institution who would be happy to work with the family if they are interested. You also identify a local laboratory that provides DNA storage and banking services and e-mail their consent form and some additional information to the family and to the other members of Oscar's palliative care team.

During the follow-up call, it becomes clear that the family has a lot more questions, some of which you feel are beyond your scope of expertise. The family sounds overall more positive about the cancer genetics evaluation process, especially given Oscar's interest. You arrange for a follow-up meeting with you and the genetic counselor to address the families' questions and concerns and potentially begin the evaluation process (Tables 61.3 to 61.5).

TABLE 61.3 PREDOMINANTLY SOLID OR MIXED TUMOR SYNDROMES[4-7,23-25,28,53-67]

Syndrome	Gene(s) (inheritance)	Tumors and other clinical findings	Risk assessment and management guidelines
Peutz-Jeghers syndrome (PJS)	*STK11/LKB1* (AD)	*Cancers:* • GU (Ovarian and fallopian tube mucinous carcinomas, ovarian Sertoli-Leydig cell, ovarian sex cord tumors with annular tubules, cervical adenoma malignum, endometrial/uterine carcinoma, testicular, other) • GI (colorectal, gastric, pancreatic) • Breast • Lung *Other:* • Melanocytic macules • Hamartomatous benign polyps (GI tract, ureters, bladder, lungs, bronchi, gallbladder) • Intussusception risk	• National Comprehensive Cancer Network (NCCN): www.nccn.org/professionals/physician_gls/default.aspx • American Society of Clinical Oncology (ASCO): www.ncbi.nlm.nih.gov/pmc/articles/PMC5321096/ • American College of Medical Genetics and Genomics (ACMG) and National Society of Genetic Counselors (NSGC): www.acmg.net/docs/ACMG_Practice_Guideline_Referral_Indications_for_cancer_predisposition.pdf • American College of Gastroenterology (ACG): www.ncbi.nlm.nih.gov/pmc/articles/PMC4695986/
Juvenile polyposis syndromes (JPS)	*SMAD4, BMPR1A* (AD)	*Cancers:* • GI (esophagus, gastric, pancreatic, small bowel, colorectal) *Other:* • GI polyps • Hereditary hemorrhagic telangiectasia (if SMAD4 carrier)	• American College of Obstetricians and Gynecologists (ACOG): www.acog.org/Clinical-Guidance-and-Publications/Committee-Opinions/Committee-on-Genetics/Hereditary-Cancer-Syndromes-and-Risk-Assessment • Canadian Partnership Against Cancer Guidelines Database: www.partnershipagainstcancer.ca/tools/cancer-guidelines-database/ • European Society for Pediatric Gastroenterology Hepatology and Nutrition (ESPGHAN): www.espghan.org/fileadmin/user_upload/Society_Papers/Management_of_Juvenile_Polyposis_Syndrome_in_Children.pdf; www.espghan.org/fileadmin/user_upload/Society_Papers/Management_of_Familial_Adenomatous_Polyposis.pdf • International Society for Gastrointestinal Hereditary Tumours (InSiGHT): www.insight-group.org/syndromes/ • GeneReviews • National Organization for Rare Disorders (NORD)
Familial adenomatous polyposis (FAP) spectrum Gardner's syndrome (colorectal polyposis + osteomas and soft tissue tumors) Attenuated FAP (increased CRC risk, fewer polyps, later age of onset)	*APC* (AD)	*Cancers:* • GI (gastric, pancreatic, hepatobiliary, colorectal) • CNS • Thyroid *Other:* • Adenomatous GI polyps • Extra-GI polyps (spleen, cerebellum) • Osteomas • Dental anomalies • Congenital hypertrophy of the retinal pigment epithelium (CHRPE) • Benign skin/soft tissue tumors (epidermoid cysts, fibromas, desmoid tumors)	

Syndrome	Gene	Manifestations
MUTYH-associated polyposis	*MUTYH* (AR)	*Cancers:* • GI (colorectal, pancreatic) • Skin • GU (ovary, endometrial, bladder) • Breast • Sebaceous neoplasms • Thyroid *Other:* • GI polyps • Benign skin/soft tissue tumors (fibrous histiocytoma, capillary hemangioma, pilar cyst, dermatofibroma, follicle cyst) • Thyroid anomalies • Dental anomalies • CHRPE
Turcot syndrome (colorectal polyposis + CNS tumors)	Type II: *APC (2/3)* (AD) Type I: *MMR genes (1/3)* (AR)	*Cancers:* • Medulloblastoma (type II) • Glioblastoma or astrocytoma (type I) • GI (colorectal, other intra-abdominal) • Thyroid • Adrenal • Skin (BCC) *Other:* • Café-au-lait spots • Lipomas
Lynch syndrome (LS)/ hereditary nonpolyposis colorectal cancer (HNPCC) Muir–Torre (sebaceous neoplasm + visceral malignancy)[41]	Mismatch repair (MMR) genes (AD): *MLH1, MSH2/ EPCAM, MSH6, PMS2*	*Cancers:* • GU (ovarian mucinous or endometrial/uterine carcinoma, testicular) • CNS (glioblastoma) • GI (gastric, small bowel, colorectal, hepatobiliary, pancreatic) • Pheochromocytoma • Adrenocortical carcinoma • Melanoma • Sebaceous carcinomas • Sarcomas (fibrous histiocytomas, rhabdomyosarcomas, leiomyosarcoma, liposarcoma) *Other:* • Benign skin/soft tissue tumors (sebaceous adenomas, sebaceous epitheliomas, keratocanthomas)

(Continued)

TABLE 61.3 PREDOMINANTLY SOLID OR MIXED TUMOR SYNDROMES (Continued)

Syndrome	Gene(s) (inheritance)	Tumors and other clinical findings	Risk assessment and management guidelines
PTEN hamartoma tumor syndrome (PHTS)	PTEN (AD)	*Cancers:* • GU (endometrial/uterine carcinoma, leiomyoma) • Breast • GI (colorectal, gastric) • CNS • Melanoma • Thyroid • Vascular *Other:* • Lipomas (breast, GI tract) • Acral keratosis (extremities) • Papillomatous skin papules • Mucosal papillomas (nose, mouth) • Trichilemmomas (hair follicles) • Fibromas • GI polyps • Benign breast, thyroid, and uterine lesions • Arteriovenous malformations • Macrocephaly • Autism spectrum • Intellectual disability • Developmental delay	• NCCN • ACOG • GeneReviews • NORD • Mutation risk calculator: http://www.lerner.ccf.org/gmi/ccscore/
Li-Fraumeni syndrome (LFS)/ sarcoma, breast, leukemia and adrenal gland (SBLA)	TP53, CHEK2 (AD)	*Cancers:* • Osteosarcoma, soft tissue sarcoma • Breast • CNS • Adrenocortical • Melanoma • GI (stomach, colon, pancreas, esophagus) • Lung • Thyroid • Renal, Wilms' tumor • Gonadal germ cell • Hematologic (leukemia, lymphoma)	• GeneReviews • NORD • ASCO • ACOG • Expert Review (AACR): clincancerres.aacrjournals.org/content/23/11/e38

Syndrome	Gene	Cancers/Other	Resources
Hereditary breast and ovarian cancer syndrome (HBOC)	*BRCA1/2* (AD)	*Cancers:* • GU (ovarian, fallopian tube and peritoneal serous carcinomas, ovarian endometrioid and clear cell carcinomas, prostate) • GI (colorectal, gastric, pancreatic) • Breast (male and female) • Melanoma • Hematologic (leukemia, lymphoma)	• NCCN (2019) • ACMG and NSGC (2014) • U.S. Preventive Services Task Force (USPSTF) (2013, being updated): www.uspreventiveservicestaskforce.org/Page/Document/UpdateSummaryFinal/brca-related-cancer-risk-assessment-genetic-counseling-and-genetic-testing • ACOG (2015, 2017): Practice Bulletin No. 182, Committee Opinion No. 634 • ASCO (2010)
Familial atypical multiple mole melanoma (FAMMM)	*CDKN2A* (AD; 40%); *CDK4* (rare)	*Cancers:* • Pancreatic adenocarcinoma • Melanoma • Oropharyngeal or pancreatic SCC *Other:* • Dysplastic nevi	• Cancer Syndromes (Book): www.ncbi.nlm.nih.gov/books/NBK7030/ • American Association of Family Physicians (AAFP): www.aafp.org/afp/2015/0115/p125.html • Skin Cancer Foundation • American Academy of Dermatology (AAD): www.ncbi.nlm.nih.gov/pmc/articles/PMC4761105/; www.jaad.org/article/S0190-9622(15)02108-8/abstract
Neurofibromatosis type 1 (NF1)	*NF1* (AD)	*Cancers:* • MPNST • Neurofibromas • Optic gliomas • Juvenile xanthogranuloma • Hematologic (myeloid leukemias) • Pheochromocytomas • Paragangliomas (rare) *Other:* • Café-au-lait spots • Axillary/inguinal freckling • Lisch nodules • Bony dysplasia (i.e., scoliosis, pseudoarthrosis, sphenoid dysplasia) • Osteopenia/osteoporosis • Hypertension • Precocious puberty • ADHD	• NCCN • GeneReviews • NORD • American Association of Pediatrics (AAP): pediatrics.aappublications.org/content/121/3/633 • Children's Tumor Foundation: www.ctf.org/news/updated-guidelines-published-about-nf1-diagnosis-and-management-in-children • American Academy of Dermatology (AAD): www.jaad.org/article/S0190-9622(97)70182-8/fulltext

(Continued)

TABLE 61.3 PREDOMINANTLY SOLID OR MIXED TUMOR SYNDROMES *(Continued)*

Syndrome	Gene(s) (inheritance)	Tumors and other clinical findings	Risk assessment and management guidelines
Multiple endocrine neoplasia type 1	*MEN1* (AD)	*Cancers:* • Pituitary adenoma • Duodenopancreatic NETs • Bronchial, thymic, or gastric carcinoid • Thyroid adenoma • Meningioma • Spinal ependymoma • Esophageal, lung, uterine leiomyoma • Facial angiofibroma • Collagenoma • Lipoma • Adrenal cortical adenoma, diffuse or nodular hyperplasia, carcinoma *Other:* • Primary hyperparathyroidism • Parathyroid hyperplasia > adenoma	• NORD • GeneReviews • Endocrine Society (International guidelines): MEN I: academic.oup. com/jcem/article/97/9/2990/2536740/; MEN I and II: academic.oup.com/jcem/article/86/12/5658/2849111/
Multiple endocrine neoplasia type 2	*RET* (AD)	*Cancers:* • Medullary thyroid carcinoma • Pheochromocytoma • Paraganglioma (rare) • Mucocutaneous neuroma *Other:* • Parathyroid adenoma/hyperplasia • Hyperparathyroidism • MEN2B: • Distinctive facies • Polycythemia • Marfanoid body habitus • Joint laxity • Skeletal malformations	• NORD • GeneReviews • Endocrine Society (International guidelines): MEN I and II: academic.oup.com/jcem/article/86/12/5658/2849111/
Von Hippel-Lindau	*VHL* (AD)	*Cancers:* • CNS hemangioblastomas (brain, spinal cord, retina) • Renal clear cell carcinomas • Pheochromocytomas • Paragangliomas (infrequent) • Pancreatic NETs *Other:* • Renal cysts (often multiple and bilateral) • Endolymphatic sac tumors • Epididymal and broad ligament cystadenomas	• NORD • GeneReviews • Expert Review (AACR): clincancerres. aacrjournals.org/content/23/12/e68.long • Von Hippel Lindau Alliance: www.vhl.org/wp-content/uploads/2017/07/Active-Surveillance-Guidelines.pdf

Syndrome	Gene	Tumors/Features	Resources
Familial pleuropulmonary blastoma tumor predisposition[a]	DICER1 (AD; 60%–70%)	*Cancers:* • Pleuropulmonary blastoma • GU (ovarian gynadroblastoma, juvenile type granulosa cell, Sertoli-Leydig cell tumors, cervical botryoid-type embryonal rhabdomyosarcoma) • Ocular (intraocular medulloepithelioma) • CNS (supratentorial primitive neuroectodermal tumor) • Wilms' tumor (rare) • GU (cystic nephroma) *Other:* • Thyroid (multinodular goiter)	• NORD • GeneReviews • Expert Review (AACR): clincancerres.aacrjournals.org/content/24/10/2251.long
Hereditary leiomyomatosis and renal cell carcinoma (HLRCC)	FH (Fumarate hydratase) (AD)	*Cancers:* • GU (endometrial/uterine leiomyoma, leiomyosarcoma, testicular Leydig-cell tumors of the testes, ovarian cystadenomas, bladder) • Pheochromocytoma • Renal (type II papillary clear cell carcinoma, tubulo-papillary and renal collecting duct carcinomas) • Breast • Gastrointestinal stromal tumors *Other:* • Adrenal incidentaloma • Cutaneous leiomyomata	• NORD • GeneReviews • ESMO (European Society for Medical Oncology) Guidelines: academic.oup.com/annonc/article/27/suppl_5/v58/1741525 • Expert Review: www.ncbi.nlm.nih.gov/pmc/articles/PMC4574691/
Rhabdoid tumor predisposition (RTPS)[a]	SMARCA4, SMARCB1/INI1 (AD)	*Cancers:* • Atypical teratoid/rhabdoid tumor • Rhabdoid tumor of the kidney • Other extracranial malignant rhabdoid tumors (soft tissue, ovary, lung, liver) • MPNST • Ovarian small cell carcinoma of the hypercalcemic type *Other:* • Multiple benign schwannomas	• NORD • GeneReviews • NCI: www.cancer.gov/types/brain/hp/child-cns-atrt-treatment-pdq • Expert Review (AACR): clincancerres.aacrjournals.org/content/23/12/e62

(Continued)

TABLE 61.3 PREDOMINANTLY SOLID OR MIXED TUMOR SYNDROMES (Continued)

Syndrome	Gene(s) (inheritance)	Tumors and other clinical findings	Risk assessment and management guidelines
Noonan and Noonan spectrum (including Leopard, cardio-facio-cutaneous syndrome (CFC), Costello)[a]	PTPN11, KRAS, RAF1, NRAS, BRAF, MAP2K1, SOS1, RIT1, CBL (AD); LZTR1 (AD or AR)	*Cancers:* • CNS • Hematologic (JMML, ALL) • Neuroblastoma *Other:* • Myeloproliferative disorders resembling JMML • Short stature • Congenital heart defects • Dysmorphic facies • Developmental delay (variable) • Broad or webbed neck • Pectus • Widely set nipples • Cryptorchidism in males • Coagulation defects • Lymphatic dysplasias	• NORD • GeneReviews • Expert Review: www.ncbi.nlm.nih.gov/pmc/articles/PMC4099190/
Hereditary paragangliomas and pheochromocytoma syndromes (HPPS)[a]	MAX, SDHB, SDHD, SDHC, SDHA, SDHAF2, TMEM127 (AD)	*Cancers:* • Adrenal • Pheochromocytoma • Thyroid, renal, or GI stromal tumors • Parasympathetic paragangliomas (head and neck) • Sympathetic paragangliomas (thoracic, abdominal, pelvic)	• NORD • GeneReviews • Expert Reviews: www.ncbi.nlm.nih.gov/pmc/articles/PMC5508015/; www.ncbi.nlm.nih.gov/pubmed/30536464
Hereditary pancreatitis (HP)	PRSS1 (AD), SPINK1 (AR), CFTR (AR), others (i.e., CTRC, CASR, CPA1, GGT1, CLDN2, CL, UBR1, SBDS)	*Cancers:* • Pancreatic *Other:* • Recurrent and/or chronic pancreatitis • Abdominal pain, nausea, vomiting • Exocrine/endocrine pancreatic insufficiency	• Genereviews • Pancreapedia: www.pancreapedia.org/reviews/hereditary-pancreatitis • National Pancreas Foundation

[a]Predominantly pediatric cancers.

AD, autosomal dominant; AR, autosomal recessive; XR, X-linked recessive; GI, gastrointestinal; GU, genitourinary; CNS, central nervous system; BCC, basal cell carcinoma; SCC, squamous cell carcinoma; MPNST, malignant peripheral nerve sheath tumors; JMML, juvenile myelomonocytic leukemia; NET, neuroendocrine tumors.

TABLE 61.4 GENOME INSTABILITY SYNDROMES WITH INCREASED SOLID AND LIQUID CANCER RISK[a51,53-55]

Syndrome	Gene(s) (inheritance)	Cancers	Other clinical features
Fanconi anemia	*FANCA, FANCC, FANCD1/BRCA2, FANCD2, FANCE, FANCF, FANCG/XRCC9, FANCI, FANCJ/BRIP1, FANCL/ PHF9, FANCM, FANCN/ PALB2, FANCO/RAD51C, FANCP/SLX4, FANCQ/ ERCC4, FANCT/UBE2T, FANCU/XRCC2, FANCV/ MAD2L2* (AR); *FANCB* (XR); *FANCR/RAD51* (AD)	• Leukemia (MDS/AML) • Lymphoma • Breast • Ovarian • Prostate • GI (gastric, pancreatic, liver) • Wilms' tumor • Medulloblastoma • Neuroblastoma • SCC (oral, esophageal, vulvar)	• Microcephaly • Short stature/growth retardation • Congenital anomalies (radial limb, GU) • Hip dysplasia • Café-au-lait spots
Ataxia-telangiectasia	*ATM* (AR)	• Lymphoma (B cell) • Leukemia (T cell) • Ovarian • Breast • GI (gastric, pancreatic) • Melanoma • Leiomyoma • Sarcoma	• Neurological changes: Ataxia, apraxia, choreoathetosis, slurred speech • Telangiectasias • Radiation sensitivity • Immunodeficiency • Insulin-resistant diabetes • Premature aging
Bloom	*BLM/RECQL3* (AR)	• Leukemia • Lymphoma • Oropharyngeal • GI (esophageal, gastric, colorectal) • GU • Breast • Skin • Renal, Wilms' tumor • Lung	• Microcephaly • Short stature/growth retardation • Dysmorphic facial features • Immunodeficiency • Bone marrow failure • Hypogonadism, infertility (men), early menopause (women) • Radiation sensitivity • Insulin resistance • COPD
Werner[48-49]	*WRN* (AR)	• Sarcomas (osteosarcoma, leiomyosarcoma, rhabdomyosarcoma) • Leukemia (MDS/AML) • Meningioma • Thyroid • Lung • Skin (melanoma, BCC) • Head/neck and skin SCC • GI (hepatobiliary, gastric, pancreatic) • MPNST • Breast • Female GU	• Bilateral cataracts • Premature aging • Scleroderma-like skin changes • Short stature/growth retardation • Type 2 diabetes • Osteoporosis, osteosclerosis • Soft tissue calcification • Premature atherosclerosis • Dysmorphic facial features • Hypogonadism
Nijmegen breakage[47]	*NBN* (AR)	• Lymphoma (B and T cell) • Medulloblastoma • Rhabdomyosarcoma • Glioma • Breast • Prostate • Melanoma • *Heterozygous carriers may have increased cancer risk*	• Microcephaly • Dysmorphic facial features • Short stature/growth retardation • Radiation sensitivity • Intellectual disability • Immunodeficiency • Impaired fertility

(Continued)

TABLE 61.4 GENOME INSTABILITY SYNDROMES WITH INCREASED SOLID AND LIQUID CANCER RISK[a] (Continued)

Syndrome	Gene(s) (inheritance)	Cancers	Other clinical features
Rothmund-Thomson	*RECQL4* (AR)	• Osteosarcoma • Skin (BCC, SCC, melanoma) • Leukemia • Lymphoma	• Characteristic evolving rash progressing to poikiloderma +/– hyperkeratotic lesions • Small size • Sparse hair, eyelashes, and/or eyebrows • Skeletal anomalies: Distal upper limb, absent or hypoplastic patella • Dental abnormalities • Cataracts • Impaired fertility • Osteopenia • Cytopenias
Xeroderma pigmentosum[50]	*DDB2, ERCC1, ERCC2, ERCC3, ERCC4, ERCC5, POLH, XPA, XPC* (AR)	• Skin cancer within 1st decade of life (BCC, SCC, melanoma) • CNS (glioma, glioblastoma) • Lung • GI (gastric, pancreatic) • GU (uterine, testicular) • Breast • Renal • Leukemia	• Skin: Acute sun sensitivity, early-onset lentigos • Ocular involvement: Photophobia, conjunctival injection, severe keratitis, atrophy of eyelids and eyelashes • CNS: Diminished or absent DTRs, peripheral neuropathy, acquired microcephaly, progressive SNHL, progressive cognitive impairment
Short telomere syndromes (dyskeratosis congenita spectrum)	*TERC, TINF2* (AD); *DKC1* (XR); *CTC1, NHP2, NOP10, PARN, WRAP53* (AR); *TERT, ACD, RTEL1* (AD or AR)	• Leukemia (MDS/AML) • Head/neck and skin SCC • Anogenital adenocarcinoma	• Nail dystrophy • Livedo reticularis • Oral leukoplakia • Pulmonary fibrosis • Liver cirrhosis • Cytopenias
Constitutional mismatch repair deficiency (CMMRD)	MMR genes: *MLH1, MSH2/EPCAM, MSH6, PMS2* (AR)	• Lymphoma • CNS • GI (colorectal, gastric) • Skin/soft tissue	• Skin: Cafe-au-lait spots, axillary freckling, hyperpigmented spots • CNS (in some patients): Agenesis of the corpus callosum, gray matter heterotopia, intracerebral cysts • Immunodeficiency
Diamond-Blackfan anemia[46]	More common: *RPL5, RPL11, RPL35A, RPS10, RPS17, RPS19, RPS24, RPS26* (AD) Less common: *GATA1, TSR2* (XR); *RPL15, RPL18, RPL26, RPL27, RPL35* (AD); *RPS7, RPS15A, RPS27, RPS28, RPS29* (AD)	• Leukemia (MDS/AML) • Osteogenic sarcoma • Colorectal • Female GU	• Pallor, weakness • Failure to thrive • Growth retardation (30%) • Congenital malformations (~30%–50%): Craniofacial, upper limb, heart, GU
Immunodeficiency with centromeric instability and facial anomalies (ICF1-4)[45]	*DNMT3B, ZBTB24, CDCA7, HELLS* (AR)	• Lymphoma • Leukemia • Adrenocortical adenoma • Angiosarcoma	• Dysmorphic facial features • Developmental delay • Macroglossia • Malabsorption • Cytopenias • Immunodeficiency

[a]For Management, see Expert Review on DNA Repair Disorders (AACR): clincancerres.aacrjournals.org/content/23/11/e23
AD, autosomal dominant; AR, autosomal recessive; XR, X-linked recessive; GI, gastrointestinal; GU, genitourinary; CNS, central nervous system; BCC, basal cell carcinoma; SCC, squamous cell carcinoma; MPNST, malignant peripheral nerve sheath tumors; AML, acute myeloid leukemia; MDS, myelodysplastic syndrome; DTR, deep tendon reflex; COPD, chronic obstructive pulmonary diseases.

Lymphoma and Adaptive Immune Dysregulation (Inheritance)

Familial hemophagocytic lymphohistiocytosis
PRF1 (AR)
FHL1 (AR)
STXBP2 (AR)
UNC13D (AR)

Autoimmune lymphoproliferative syndromes (ALPS) and ALPS-like
TNFRSF6/FAS (AD)
TNFSF6/FASLG (AD)
PRKCD (AR)
LRBA (AR)
STAT3 GOF (AD)
CTLA4 (AD)[a]

X-linked lymphoproliferative syndromes
SH2D1A/SAP (XR)
XIAP (XR)

Activated phosphoinositide 3-kinase delta syndromes (APDS)
PIK3CD (AD)
PIK3R1 (AR, AD)

EBV-associated lymphoproliferative disorders
ITK (AR)
TNFRSF7/CD27 (AR)
TNFSF7/CD70 (AR)
IL10RA, IL10RB (AR)
MAGT1 (XR)
CTPS1 (AR)
MST1/STK4 (AR)
RLTPR/CARMIL2 (AR)
IFNGR1 (AR)
RASGRP1 (AR)[a]
ADA (AR)

Hyper-IgM syndromes
UNG (AR)
TNFSF5/CD40LG (XR)[a]

Other immune dysregulation syndromes
TNFAIP3 (AD)
CXCR4 (AD)
TNFRSF13C/BAFFR (AR)
TNFRSF13B/TACI (AD, AR)
CARD11 (AD)
RHOH (AR)[a]

Syndromes with developmental defects
SMARCAL1 (AR)
RMRP (AR)[a]
TP63 (AD)

Leukemia/MDS and Bone Marrow Failure (Inheritance)

Severe congenital neutropenia and other phagocyte disorders
HAX1 (AR)
ELA2/ELANE (AD)
GFI1 (AD)
GATA2 (AD)
SBDS (AR)[a]

Familial thrombocytopenia
RUNX1 (AD)
ANKRD26 (AD)
ETV6 (AD)
DDX41 (AD)

Neuro/endocrine syndromes
SAMD9 (AD)
SAMD9L (AD)

Other
CEBPA (AD)

(Continued)

TABLE 61.5 GERMLINE MUTATIONS ASSOCIATED WITH INCREASED HEMATOLOGIC MALIGNANCY RISK *(Continued)*

Leukemia and Lymphoma

Hyper-IgE syndromes
STAT3 (AD)
TYK2 (AR)
DOCK8 (AR)a

Other
LIG4 (AD)
WAS (XR)
IKZF1 (AD)

aSolid tumors have also been described.
AD, Autosomal dominant; AR, Autosomal recessive; XR, X-linked recessive; MDS, myelodysplastic syndrome.

RESOURCES[27]

Resource	Organization	Web site	How they can help
Education	Cancer.Net	http://www.cancer.net/navigating-cancer-care/cancer-basics/genetics	Patient-oriented information on cancer care from the American Society of Clinical Oncology and the Conquer Cancer Foundation
	American Society of Clinical Oncology (ASCO)	www.asco.org/practice-guidelines/cancer-care-initiatives/genetics-toolkit	Tools and resources to integrate hereditary cancer risk into practice
	Cancer Genetics Risk Assessment and Counseling (PDQ)	www.cancer.gov/about-cancer/causes-prevention/genetics/risk-assessment-pdq#section/_1004	Evidence-based review on topics related to cancer risk assessment, including links to tools for helping identify candidates for cancer genetics referrals
	City of Hope	https://www.cityofhope.org/education/health-professional-education/cancer-genetics-education-program/intensive-course-in-cancer-risk-assessment-overview	Intensive course on genetics; great for those practicing in genetics and those without internal resources
	National Institutes of Health	www.genome.gov/17517037/health-professional-education	Multiple sources of education regarding genetics/genomics
	Jackson Laboratories	www.jax.org/education-and-learning/clinical-and-continuing-education/family-history	Family history resources for health care providers
	Global Alliance for Genomics and Health: Genomic Data Toolkit	http://www.ga4gh.org/	Family History Tools Inventory offers in-depth pedigree tools and additional tools for genetic analysis
HCS information	National Comprehensive Cancer Network (NCCN)	www.nccn.org/professionals/physician_gls/#detectionUSPSTF.gov	Testing criteria and medical management guidelines for hereditary cancer syndromes
	US Preventative Services Task Force: BRCA-related cancer: risk assessment, genetic counseling, and genetic testing	www.uspreventiveservicestaskforce.org/Page/Document/RecommendationStatementFinal/brca-related-cancer-risk-assessment-genetic-counseling-and-genetic-testing	Guidelines for testing of the BRCA1/2 genes
	American College of Medical Genetics and Genomics and the National Society of Genetic Counselors	https://www.nature.com/articles/gim2014147#recommendations	Consensus practice guidelines and referral indications for cancer predisposition assessment (Hampel et al. Genet Med 2015)

RESOURCES[27] (*Continued*)

Resource	Organization	Web site	How they can help
	GeneReviews	www.ncbi.nlm.nih.gov/books/NBK1116/advanced	Thorough clinical summaries of hereditary cancer syndromes
	OMIM (Online Mendelian Inheritance in Man)	https://www.ncbi.nlm.nih.gov/omim	Comprehensive, authoritative compendium of human genes and genetic phenotypes that is freely available and updated daily
	GTR (Genetic Testing Registry) **Also for DNA Banking**	https://www.ncbi.nlm.nih.gov/gtr/	Voluntary registry of genetic tests and laboratories, with detailed information and context-specific links to practice guidelines, published literature, and genetic data/information. Includes single gene tests, arrays, panels, pharmacogenetic tests and facilities offering **DNA banking**.
Cancer genetics providers	National Society of Genetic Counselors (NSGC)	www.findageneticcounselor.com (http://www.nsgc.org or by phoning the NCI information service at 1-800-4-CANCER)	Find a local or telegenetics genetic counselor for patient referral or clinical support
	NCI cancer genetics services directory	www.cancer.gov/about-cancer/causes-prevention/genetics/directory	Providers for adult genetic issues or high-risk cancer clinics
	InformedDNA	http://informeddna.com/	Offers individualized genetic counseling by telephone for patients and physicians in rural areas
Nursing-specific resources	International Society of Nurses in Genetics	https://www.isong.org	Organization that provides leadership and education for nurses integrating genetics and genomics across nursing education, research and care
	Oncology Nursing Society	www.ons.org/education/courses-activities?combine=genomics	Free and on-demand CNE offerings
Subspecialty providers	American Society of Breast Surgeons	www.breastsurgeons.org/new_layout/membership/membersearch/index.php	May manage high-risk breast cancer screening
	National accreditation program for breast centers (NAPBC)	www.facs.org/search/find-a-surgeon	May organize and interpret MRI screening for breast cancer
	American Academy of Dermatology	www.aad.org/find-a-derm	Skin screening
	American Gastroenterological Association	https://mygi.health/find-a-specialist	Colon cancer screening/colonoscopy
	Society for Gynecologic Oncologists (SGO)	www.sgo.org/seek-a-specialist	For preventative surgery (BSO) or have high-risk GYN cancers (abnormal paps, etc.)
	American Society of Clinical Oncology (ASCO)	www.cancer.net/find-cancer-doctor	Find medical oncologists for discussion of management and chemoprevention
DNA Banking			**See above (Genetic Testing Registry)**

Modified from Forman A, Schwartz S. Guidelines-based cancer risk assessment. *Semin Oncol Nurs.* 2019;35(1):34-46.

REFERENCES

1. Manolio TA, Rowley R, Williams MS, et al. Opportunities, resources, and techniques for implementing genomics in clinical care. *Lancet.* 2019;394(10197): 511-520.

2. Jacobs C, White S, Phillips J. Genetics in palliative care: too much to ask? *Int J Paliatl Nurs.* 2019;25(5):212-213.

3. Kindler O, Quehenberger F, Benesch M, Seidel MG. The Iceberg Map of germline mutations in childhood cancer: focus on primary immunodeficiencies. *Curr Opin Pediatr.* 2018;30(6):855-863.

4. National Comprehensive Cancer Network (NCCN). *NCCN Guidelines' & Clinical Resources.* 2020. www.nccn.org/professionals/physician_gls. Last accessed January 4, 2020.

5. U.S. Preventive Services Task Force (USPSTF). *Recommendations for Primary Care Practice.* 2017. www.uspreventiveservicestaskforce.org/Page/Name/recommendations. Last accessed January 4, 2020.

6. American Society of Clinical Oncology (ASCO). *Guidelines, Tools & Resources.* 2020. www.asco.org/research-guidelines/quality-guidelines/guidelines. Last accessed January 4, 2020.

7. American Association for Cancer Research (AACR). *Pediatric Cancer Predisposition and Surveillance.* 2020. www.aacr.org/MEMBERSHIP/PAGES/SCIENTIFIC%20WORKING%20GROUPS/PEDIATRIC-CANCER-PRE-DISPOSITION-AND-SURVEILLANCE.ASPX. Last accessed January 4, 2020.

8. Druker H, Zelley K, McGee RB, et al. Genetic counselor recommendations for cancer predisposition evaluation and surveillance in the pediatric oncology patient. *Clin Cancer Res.* 2017;23(13):e91-e97.

9. Morrow A, Jacobs C, Best M, et al. Genetics in palliative oncology: a missing agenda? A review of the literature and future directions. *Support Care Canc.* 2018;26: 721-730.

10. Lillie AD, Clifford C, Metcalfe A. Caring for families with a family history of cancer: why concerns about genetic predisposition are missing from the palliative agenda. *Palliat Med.* 2011;25(2):117-124.

11. Quillin JM, Emidio O, Ma B, et al. High-risk palliative care patients' knowledge and attitudes about hereditary cancer testing and DNA banking. *J Genet Couns.* 2018;27(4):834-843.

12. Dearing A, Taverner N. Mainstreaming genetics in palliative care: barriers and suggestions for clinical genetic services. *J Community Genet.* 2018;9:243-256.

13. Metcalfe A, Pumphrey R, Clifford C. Hospice nurses and genetics: implications for end-of-life care. *J Clin Nurs.* 2010;19(1–2):192-207.

14. Abusamaan MS, Quillin JM, Owodunni E, et al. The role of palliative medicine in assessing hereditary cancer risk. *Am J Hosp Palliat Care.* 2018;35(12):1490-1497.

15. Quillin J, Bodurtha J, Siminoff L, et al. Physicians' current practices and opportunities for DNA banking of dying patients with cancer. *J Oncol Pract.* 2011;7(3): 183-187.

16. Rodríguez VM, Corona R, Bodurtha JN, Quillin JM. Family ties: the role of family context in family health history communication about cancer. *J Health Commun.* 2016;21(3):346-355.

17. Gonthier C, Pelletier S, Gagnon P, et al. Issues related to family history of cancer at the end of life: a palliative care providers' survey. *Fam Cancer.* 2018;17(2): 303-307.

18. Hooker GW, Clemens KR, Quillin J, et al. Cancer genetic counseling and testing in an era of rapid change. *J Genet Couns.* 2017;26(6):1244-1253.

19. Ghandourh WA. Palliative care in cancer: managing patients' expectations. *J Med Radiat Sci.* 2016;63: 242-257.

20. Johnson LM, Sykes AD, Lu Z, et al. Speaking genomics to parents offered germline testing for cancer predisposition: use of a 2-visit consent model. *Cancer.* 2019;125:2455-2464.

21. Lahiri Batra S. Management of gynecologic cancers in relation to genetic predisposition. *Semin Oncol Nurs.* 2019;35(2):182-191.

22. Hampel H, Bennett RL, Buchanan A, et al. A practice guideline from the American College of Medical Genetics and Genomics and the National Society of Genetic Counselors: referral indications for cancer predisposition assessment. *Genet Med.* 2015;17(1):70-87.

23. Samadder NJ, Giridhar KV, Baffy N, Riegert-Johnson D, Couch FJ. Hereditary cancer syndromes-a primer on diagnosis and management: part 1: breast-ovarian cancer syndromes. *Mayo Clin Proc.* 2019;94(6):1084-1098.

24. Samadder NJ, Baffy N, Giridhar KV, Couch FJ, Riegert-Johnson D. Hereditary cancer syndromes-a primer on diagnosis and management, part 2: gastrointestinal cancer syndromes. *Mayo Clin Proc.* 2019;94(6):1099-1116.

25. Kanth P, Grimmett J, Champine M, Burt R, Samadder NJ. Hereditary colorectal polyposis and cancer syndromes: a primer on diagnosis and management. *Am J Gastroenterol.* 2017;112(10):1509-1525.

26. Esteban I, Lopez-Fernandez A, Balmaña J. A narrative overview of the patients' outcomes after multigene cancer panel testing, and a thorough evaluation of its implications for genetic counselling. *Eur J Med Genet.* 2019;62(5):342-349.

27. Forman A, Schwartz S. Guidelines-based cancer risk assessment. *Semin Oncol Nurs.* 2019;35(1):34-46.

28. Mitchell SG, Pencheva B, Porter CC. Germline genetics and childhood cancer: emerging cancer predisposition syndromes and psychosocial impacts. *Curr Oncol Rep.* 2019;21(10):85.

29. Zhang MY, Keel SB, Walsh T, et al. Genomic analysis of bone marrow failure and myelodysplastic syndromes reveals phenotypic and diagnostic complexity. *Haematologica.* 2015;100(1):42-48.

30. Etchegary H, Potter B, Perrier C, Wilson B. Cultural differences in family communication about inherited cancer: implications for cancer genetics research. *J Cult Divers.* 2013;20(4):195-201.

31. Hann KEJ, Freeman M, Fraser L, et al.; PROMISE study team. Awareness, knowledge, perceptions, and attitudes towards genetic testing for cancer risk among ethnic minority groups: a systematic review. *BMC Public Health.* 2017;17(1):503.

32. Licqurish S, Phillipson L, Chiang P, Walker J, Walter F, Emery J. Cancer beliefs in ethnic minority populations: a review and meta-synthesis of qualitative studies. *Eur J Cancer Care (Engl).* 2017;26(1).

33. LoPresti MA, Dement F, Gold HT. End-of-life care for people with cancer from ethnic minority groups: a systematic review. *Am J Hosp Palliat Care.* 2016;33(3):291-305.

34. Roeland EJ, Dullea AD, Hagmann CH, Madlensky L. Addressing hereditary cancer risk at the end of life. *J Oncol Pract.* 2017;13(10):e851-e856.

35. Wade CH. What is the psychosocial impact of providing genetic and genomic health information to individuals? an overview of systematic reviews. *Hastings Cent Rep.* 2019;49(suppl 1):S88-S96.

36. Vetsch J, Wakefield CE, Warby M, et al. Cancer-related genetic testing and personalized medicine for adolescents: a narrative review of impact and understanding. *J Adolesc Young Adult Oncol.* 2018;7(3):259-262.

37. Bleiker EM, Esplen MJ, Meiser B, Petersen HV, Patenaude AF. 100 years Lynch syndrome: what have we learned about psychosocial issues? *Fam Cancer.* 2013;12(2):325-339.

38. Bleiker EM, Hahn DE, Aaronson NK. Psychosocial issues in cancer genetics—current status and future directions. *Acta Oncol.* 2003;42(4):276-286.

39. French DP, Howell A, Evans DG. Psychosocial issues of a population approach to high genetic risk identification: behavioural, emotional and informed choice issues. *Breast.* 2018;37:148-153.

40. Jacobs C, Patch C, Michie S. Communication about genetic testing with breast and ovarian cancer patients: a scoping review. *Eur J Hum Genet.* 2019;27(4):511-524.

41. Biller LH, Syngal S, Yurgelun MB. Recent advances in Lynch syndrome. *Fam Cancer.* 2019;18(2):211-219.

42. Leeksma OC, de Miranda NF, Veelken H. Germline mutations predisposing to diffuse large B-cell lymphoma. *Blood Cancer J.* 2017;7(2):e532. doi:10.1038/bcj.2017.15. Review. Erratum in: Blood Cancer J. 2017 Mar 10;7(3):e541.

43. de Miranda NF, Peng R, Georgiou K, et al. DNA repair genes are selectively mutated in diffuse large B cell lymphomas. *J Exp Med.* 2013;210(9):1729-1742.

44. Riaz IB, Faridi W, Patnaik MM, Abraham RS. A systematic review on predisposition to lymphoid (B and T cell) neoplasias in patients with primary immunodeficiencies and immune dysregulatory disorders (inborn errors of immunity). *Front Immunol.* 2019;10:777.

45. van den Brand M, Flucke UE, Bult P, Weemaes CM, van Deuren M. Angiosarcoma in a patient with immunodeficiency, centromeric region instability, facial anomalies (ICF) syndrome. *Am J Med Genet A.* 2011;155A(3):622-625.

46. Vlachos A, Rosenberg PS, Atsidaftos E, Alter BP, Lipton JM. Incidence of neoplasia in Diamond Blackfan anemia: a report from the Diamond Blackfan anemia registry. *Blood.* 2012;119(16):3815-3819.

47. Ciara E, Piekutowska-Abramczuk D, Popowska E, et al. Heterozygous germ-line mutations in the NBN gene predispose to medulloblastoma in pediatric patients. *Acta Neuropathol.* 2010;119(3):325-334.

48. Wang Z, Xu Y, Tang J, et al. A polymorphism in Werner syndrome gene is associated with breast cancer susceptibility in Chinese women. *Breast Cancer Res Treat.* 2009;118(1):169-175.

49. Lauper JM, Krause A, Vaughan TL, Monnat RJ Jr. Spectrum and risk of neoplasia in Werner syndrome: a systematic review. *PLoS One.* 2013;8(4):e59709.

50. Bradford PT, Goldstein AM, Tamura D, et al. Cancer and neurologic degeneration in xeroderma pigmentosum: long term follow-up characterises the role of DNA repair. *J Med Genet.* 2011;48(3):168-176.

51. Walsh MF, Chang VY, Kohlmann WK, et al. Recommendations for childhood cancer screening and surveillance in DNA repair disorders. *Clin Cancer Res.* 2017;23(11):e23-e31.

52. Tangye SG, Al-Herz W, Bousfiha A, et al. Human inborn errors of immunity: 2019 update on the classification from the International Union of Immunological Societies Expert Committee [published online ahead of print, 2020 Jan 17]. *J Clin Immunol.* 2020;40:24-64. doi:10.1007/s10875-019-00737-x.

53. Riegert-Johnson DL, Boardman LA, Hefferon T, et al., eds. *Cancer Syndromes* [Internet]. Bethesda, MD: National Center for Biotechnology Information (US); 2009. https://www.ncbi.nlm.nih.gov/books/NBK1825/

54. Adam MP, Ardinger HH, Pagon RA, et al., eds. *GeneReviews*® [Internet]. Seattle, WA: University of Washington, Seattle; 1993–2019. GeneReviews® Copyright Notice and Usage Disclaimer. 2013 Jun 3 [Updated 2016 Jul 29]. https://www.ncbi.nlm.nih.gov/books/NBK138602/

55. National Organization for Rare Disorders (NORD). *Rare Disease Resources.* 2019. www.rarediseases.org/for-clinicians-and-researchers/resources/rare-disease-information/. Last accessed January 1, 2020.

56. National Cancer Institute (NCI). *The Genetics of Cancer.* 2017. www.cancer.gov/about-cancer/causes-prevention/genetics. Last accessed November 30, 2019.

57. American College of Medical Genetics and Genomics (ACMG). *Practice Guidelines.* 2019. www.acmg.net/ACMG/Medical-Genetics-Practice-Resources/Practice-Guidelines.aspx. Last accessed January 4, 2020.

58. National Society of Genetic Counselors (NSGC). *NSGC Practice Guidelines.* 2020. www.nsgc.org/page/practice-guidelines. Last accessed January 4, 2020.

59. American College of Gastroenterology (ACG). *Guidelines.* 2019. gi.org/guidelines. Last accessed January 4, 2020.

60. American College of Obstetricians and Gynecologists (ACOG). *Clinical Guidance and Publications.* 2019. www.acog.org/Clinical-Guidance-and-Publications/Search-Clinical-Guidance?IsMobileSet=false. Last accessed January 4, 2020.

61. Canadian Partnership Against Cancer. *Cancer Guidelines Database.* 2019. www.partnershipagainstcancer.ca/tools/cancer-guidelines-database. Last accessed January 4, 2020.

62. European Society for Medical Oncology. *ESMO Clinical Practice Guidelines.* 2020. www.esmo.org/Guidelines. Last accessed January 4, 2020.

63. American Academy of Dermatology (AAD). *Clinical Guidelines.* 2020. www.aad.org/member/clinical-quality/guidelines. Last accessed January 4, 2020.

64. International Society for Gastrointestinal Hereditary Tumours (InSiGHT). *Syndromes.* 2020. www.insight-group.org/syndromes. Last accessed January 4, 2020.

65. European Society for Pediatric Gastroenterology Hepatology and Nutrition (ESPGHAN). *Gastroenterology Guidelines.* 2020. www.espghan.org/guidelines/gastroenterology. Last accessed January 4, 2020.

66. Endocrine Society. *Clinical Practice Guidelines.* 2020. www.endocrine.org/clinical-practice-guidelines. Last accessed January 4, 2020.

67. American Association of Family Physicians (AAFP). *Clinical Practice Guidelines.* 2020. www.aafp.org/patient-care/browse/type.tag-clinical-practice-guidelines.html. Last accessed January 4, 2020.

Palliative and Supportive Care: The Global Context

Joseph O'Neill and Stephen Connor

INTRODUCTION

This chapter provides a global overview of palliative and supportive care with an emphasis on cancer in lower income and middle-income regions and countries as defined by the World Bank (1). This is done in recognition of long-standing local and indigenous traditions of caring for those who suffer and with awareness of how formal palliative care as defined by the World Health Organization (2) (Table 62.1) has augmented, and has the potential to further enhance, these efforts. The intent of this chapter is to place supportive and palliative cancer care in a global context so that the many challenges cancer patients and providers face outside high-income regions can be better understood and supported.

Recent decades have witnessed a growing comprehension of the interconnectedness of, and disparities between, members of the global community. The maldistribution of the burden of disease across the globe has been especially compelling to public, academic, policy, and other sectors of the health care community. Academic health institutions in the United States have, for example, dramatically ramped up their engagement in global health at all levels (3).

One meaningful measure of health disparities is healthy life expectancy at birth (Fig. 62.1). Other measures tracked by the World Health Organization are equally compelling (Table 62.2). Simply put, some people on the globe live longer and healthier lives than do others, not because of inherent genetic predisposition to illness but because of socioeconomic determinants of health.

Not surprisingly, local government expenditures on health care vary widely (6) as do availability of trained nurses, midwives (7), and doctors (8).

The dramatic treatment advances in oncology, infectious diseases (especially HIV/AIDS and TB) and other fields of medicine that have been achieved in recent years, when viewed against this backdrop, heighten demand for, and urgency of, creative and fulsome responses from wealthier public and private health care sectors. The need is especially compelling in cancer care.

CANCER

There were about 9.6 million cancer related (excluding non–melanoma-related skin cancer) deaths globally in 2018. Fifty-six percent of these deaths were in males and 44% in females (9). Cancer remains the second leading cause of death (after cardiovascular disease) worldwide with deaths from cancer projected by the World Health Organization to surpass 13 million in 2030, with a disproportionate 10 to 11 million of these cases in low- and middle-income countries. Of the 9.6 million cancer deaths in 2018, the most common were lung (2.09 million), breast (2.09 million), colorectal (1.8 million), prostate (1.28), skin (1.04 million), and stomach (1.03 million) (10).

Common issues contributing to poor cancer outcomes in low-income countries include late-stage presentation, inadequate diagnosis, and poor access to cancer treatment. For example, only about one quarter of low-income countries reported that they had pathology services available in the public sector in 2017 and only 30% had treatment available (10). A 2016 analysis of global access to radiotherapy services (11) found that the majority of low-income countries had no radiotherapy services available at all. A Lancet Commission on Global Surgery estimated that 5.3 billion people globally do not have access to safe, timely surgical care and anesthesia care when needed. This translates into an estimate that, in low- and middle-income countries, 94% of the population lacks access to such care (compared to 14.9% of the population in high-income countries) (12). A follow-on report focusing specifically on oncology surgery is in the offing (13).

The American Society of Clinical Oncology (ASCO)'s Global Oncology Leadership Task Force has identified professional development and training, quality of care and need for research as being key issues in low- and middle-income countries (14). Recommendations were then stratified between low- and middle-income countries (while recognizing that in many middle-income countries there are geographic regions that closely resemble low-income conditions). Key elements of these

TABLE 62.1 WORLD HEALTH ORGANIZATION DEFINITIONS OF PALLIATIVE CARE FOR ADULTS AND CHILDREN

Palliative care is an approach that improves the quality of life of patients and their families facing the problem associated with life-threatening illness, through the prevention and relief of suffering by means of early identification and impeccable assessment and treatment of pain and other problems, physical, psychosocial, and spiritual.

Palliative care:
- provides relief from pain and other distressing symptoms;
- affirms life and regards dying as a normal process;
- intends neither to hasten or postpone death;
- integrates the psychological and spiritual aspects of patient care;
- offers a support system to help patients live as actively as possible until death;
- offers a support system to help the family cope during the patient's illness and in their own bereavement;
- uses a team approach to address the needs of patients and their families, including bereavement counseling, if indicated;
- will enhance quality of life, and may also positively influence the course of illness;
- is applicable early in the course of illness, in conjunction with other therapies that are intended to prolong life, such as chemotherapy or radiation therapy, and includes those investigations needed to better understand and manage distressing clinical complications.

WHO definition of palliative care for children

Palliative care for children represents a special, albeit closely related field to adult palliative care. WHO's definition of palliative care appropriate for children and their families is as follows; the principles apply to other pediatric chronic disorders:

- Palliative care for children is the active total care of the child's body, mind, and spirit, and also involves giving support to the family.
- It begins when illness is diagnosed, and continues regardless of whether or not a child receives treatment directed at the disease.
- Health providers must evaluate and alleviate a child's physical, psychological, and social distress.
- Effective palliative care requires a broad multidisciplinary approach that includes the family and makes use of available community resources; it can be successfully implemented even if resources are limited.
- It can be provided in tertiary care facilities, in community health centers, and even in children's homes.

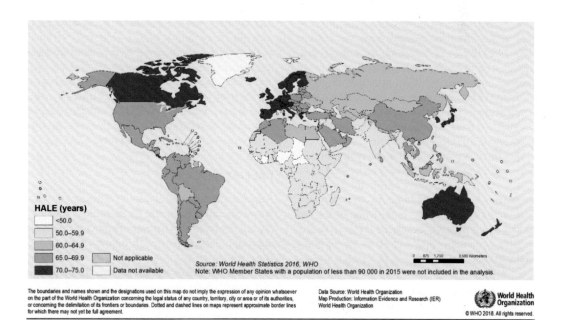

HALE (years)
- <50.0
- 50.0–59.9
- 60.0–64.9
- 65.0–69.9
- 70.0–75.0
- Not applicable
- Data not available

Source: World Health Statistics 2016, WHO
Note: WHO Member States with a population of less than 90 000 in 2015 were not included in the analysis.

The boundaries and names shown and the designations used on this map do not imply the expression of any opinion whatsoever on the part of the World Health Organization concerning the legal status of any country, territory, city or area or of its authorities, or concerning the delimitation of its frontiers or boundaries. Dotted and dashed lines on maps represent approximate border lines for which there may not yet be full agreement.

Data Source: World Health Organization
Map Production: Information Evidence and Research (IER)
World Health Organization

World Health Organization
© WHO 2018. All rights reserved.

Figure 62.1 WHO Member States Healthy Life expectancy (HALE) at birth, both sexes, 2016. (From http://gamapserver.who.int/mapLibrary/Files/Maps/Global_HALE_2016.png. Ref. (4).)

TABLE 62.2 GLOBAL HEALTH DISPARITIES

- Today, there is a 36-year gap in life expectancy between countries. A child born in Malawi can expect to live for only 47 years while a child born in Japan could live for as long as 83 years. In Chad, every fifth child dies before reaching the age of 5, while in the WHO European Region, the under-5 mortality rate is 13 out of 1,000. There is no biological or genetic reason for these alarming differences in health and life opportunity.
- In Afghanistan, Somalia, and Chad, the maternal mortality ratio is over 1,000 (out of 100,000 live births) while the same average figure for the WHO European Region is 21. Developing countries account for 99% of annual maternal deaths in the world, with the decline being the slowest in WHO's Eastern Mediterranean and African Regions.
- Worldwide, about 150 million people a year face catastrophic health care costs because of direct payments such as user fees, while 100 million are driven below the poverty line. Even if they could pay, access to doctors would be a challenge. Low-income countries have 10 times fewer physicians than do high-income countries. Nigeria and Myanmar have about 4 physicians per 10,000, while Norway and Switzerland have 40 per 10,000.
- According to the latest estimates, the number of people living in hunger in the world is over a billion, the highest on record. Half of the world's workers—nearly 1.53 billion people—are in vulnerable employment. These workers do not tend to have formal work arrangements or receive social security and health benefits.

From https://www.who.int/sdhconference/background/news/facts/en. Accessed October 2019. Ref. (5).

recommendations included the need to strengthen health systems and the importance of deepening relationships between high-income health institutions, professional schools, and other stakeholders.

Although palliative care was not specifically addressed in these recommendations, the overall picture painted of the status of oncology care in underresourced regions of the world provides an important framework for any discussion of the potential need for palliative and supportive oncology care.

It is relevant to note that one-third of all cancer deaths could be avoided by modifying or avoiding key risk factors (15). Many cancers common in low-income and middle-income countries could be prevented by smoking cessation, adoption of more active lifestyles, weight loss, vaccination (HPV and HBV), and screening for cancers that, if detected early, can be easily treated (e.g., cervical cancer). Given these realities, provision of public health prevention measures will, especially in low-income regions, likely be viewed as relatively more cost-effective than expenditures on oncology care for advanced disease for some time to come.

These factors underscore that the symptom mitigation and supportive care that can be offered by palliative care are extremely important for oncology patients in low- and middle-income countries. Because, moreover, these underlying issues are unlikely to significantly change in the near future, the value of palliative and supportive care is likely to remain crucial.

DEMAND FOR PALLIATIVE CARE AND EPIDEMIOLOGY OF HEALTH-RELATED SUFFERING

The estimated global need for palliative care for adults at the end of life is over 19 million (78%

living in low- and middle-income countries) and for children almost 1.2 million (89% living in low- and middle-income countries) (16). Because, however, not all health-related suffering ends in death, estimates based solely on mortality statistics significantly underestimate the need for palliative and supportive care. To account for those needing palliative care before the end of life, the number was doubled to a total of 40 million, a likely minimum estimate. Only 34% of this need was for cancer patients. Globally, it was estimated in 2014 that <10% of the need for palliative care is being met.

A Lancet Commission (17) developed an index to estimate serious health-related suffering (SHS) that defined "health related" as being associated with illness or injury of any kind and "serious" as that which cannot be relieved without medical intervention and encompasses physical, emotional, and social functioning. Estimates were based upon numbers of patients with one of 20 specific common diseases and days associated with that disease that could be relieved with palliative care. Results of this analysis are compelling (Table 62.3).

PALLIATIVE CARE

Any discussion of the status of contemporary palliative care must recognize that countless individuals and organizations have, throughout history and across the globe, organized themselves, and devoted their resources to mitigating human suffering as best they can. The contemporary world of palliative care stands on the shoulders of these efforts.

Despite many obstacles, considerable progress has been made in advancing palliative care in global health policy as well as in many regional and local communities. Exactly how the elements of palliative care are brought online and sequenced,

TABLE 62.3 LANCET COMMISSION ESTIMATES OF ACCESS TO PALLIATIVE CARE AND PAIN RELIEF 2015

- More than 61 million people experienced serious health-related suffering (SHS), 25.5 million of whom died
- 45% of global deaths were accompanied by SHS
- 1/3 of children who died experienced SHS
- Patients with SHS accrued at least 6 billion days of suffering
  - 80% of those days were accumulated in low- and middle-income countries (LMICs)
- In low- and middle-income countries, over 20 million deaths were associated with SHS
- More than 95% of all patients in need of palliative care and pain relief associated with HIV, premature birth, birth trauma, TB, and malnutrition live in LMIC
- More than 98% of children aged 15 years or younger who die with SHS live in low- and middle-income countries

From Knaul FM, Farmer PE, Krakauer EL, et al. Alleviating the access abyss in palliative care and pain relief—an imperative of universal health coverage: the Lancet Commission report. *Lancet.* 2018;391(10128):1391-1454. doi:10.1016/S0140-6736(17)32513-8. https://www.thelancet.com/journals/langlo/article/PIIS2214-109X(18)30082-2/fulltext

what form they take, and how they are delivered vary across geography, levels of economic development, and culture. The earliest modern hospices in Europe and North America, for example, date back to the 1960s and 1970s and largely focused on cancer and noncommunicable diseases. These spawned a global expansion of the hospice movement (18). This stands in contrast to the development of hospice and palliative care on the African continent where response to communicable diseases has predominated and inspired dissemination of models of care.

The HIV/AIDS pandemics have heightened awareness of the need for palliative care in high-income regions prior to availability of effective treatment and in lower income regions currently because of poor access to health care and lifesaving HAART therapy. It is not surprising therefore that, although the World Health Organization began advocating for pain control and access to opioids in the early 1980s, it wasn't until 2002 that their Program on Cancer Control collaborated with the WHO's Department of Care for HIV/AIDS, to initiate a project entitled "Community Health Approach to Palliative Care for HIV and Cancer Patients in Africa" (19). A number of other public sector global HIV/AIDS initiatives, including the US Government's PEPFAR (President's Emergency Plan for AIDS Relief) (20) and the United Kingdom's Department for International Development (21) have encouraged and supported palliative and hospice care as part of their HIV/AIDS undertakings.

Private sector global health initiatives have also made significant contributions to the development of palliative care in low- and middle-income countries. These have included the American Cancer Society's Treat the Pain (22) initiative, the National Hospice and Palliative Care Organization's Foundation for Hospices in Sub-Saharan Africa, now Global Partners in Care (23), the Open Society Foundations (24), and the Diana, Princess of Wales Memorial Fund (25).

Increasingly access to health care, specifically including access to palliative care, is being viewed as a human right (26). The Worldwide Hospice Palliative Care Alliance and other proponents of this view secured an enormous advance for it on May 24, 2014, when the World Health Organization adopted resolution WHA67.19 on Strengthening of Palliative Care as a Component of Comprehensive Care Throughout the Life Course (27) at the 67th World Health Assembly (WHA), the governing body of the World Health Organization (WHO).

WHA resolutions carry the weight of policy and significantly influence individual country health polices and international donor organizations. The resolution's urging of Member States to include palliative care in national health plans as part of the continuum of care at all levels, including education of health care providers, has made local advocacy for palliative care much easier and more impactful.

Further advances in policy have been made recently including the inclusion of palliative care in the UN Sustainable Development continuum of Universal Health Coverage under SDG 3.4 (28). The continuum is now described as promotion, prevention, treatment, rehabilitation, and palliative health services. Therefore, we can now say that health care coverage is not universal without palliative care.

STATUS OF PALLIATIVE CARE DEVELOPMENT AROUND THE GLOBE

The Worldwide Hospice Palliative Care Alliance (WHPCA) describes itself as "a global action network focusing exclusively on hospice and palliative care development worldwide. Its members are national and regional hospice and palliative care organizations and affiliate organizations supporting hospice and palliative care" (29). Together with the WHO, WHPCA published a Global Atlas of Palliative Care at the End of Life (29,30). Based upon information compiled from a variety of sources, including opinion leaders, published literature, informal literature, hospice directories, and more, the Atlas assigned each country a category

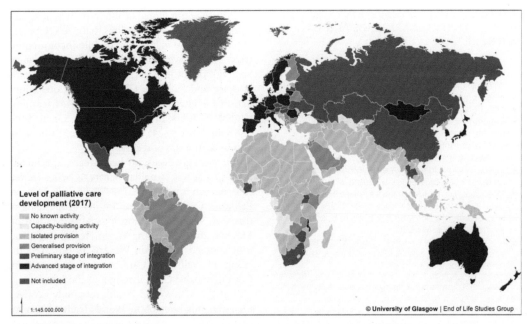

Figure 62.2 Status of development of palliative care. (From file:///Users/josephoneill/Downloads/Global_Atlas_ of_Palliative_Care%20(4).pdf)

of palliative care development based upon presence of specific factors, including presence of models of palliative care delivery, access to opioids and other pain-relieving drugs, level of awareness and activism in policy arenas, presence of relevant professional associations, and presence of educational centers.

Analysis in 2011 yielded compelling results: No palliative care activity was found in 75 (32%) countries; some activity was detected in 136 (58%), and advanced integration of palliative care into health care systems was found in 45 (19%) of countries. In the follow-up study in 2017, the situation had improved considerably with fewer countries in the no palliative care activity category (22%) and more countries in the advanced integration group (25%).

These 2017 findings for general palliative care and pediatric palliative care are graphically displayed (31) (Figs. 62.2 and 62.3).

BARRIERS

The Lancet Commission on Palliative Care and Pain Relief (17) identified several key barriers to expansion of palliative care: (a) focus of existing health outcome measures that emphasize extending life and productivity but neglect needs for dignity and relief of suffering; (b) fear and avoidance of opioids; (c) diversion of opioids; (d) focus of contemporary medicine on cure and extending life; (e) limited patient advocacy for palliative care; and (f) global neglect of noncommunicable diseases.

Access to opioids is an especially thorny issue. The United States and other developed countries focus on an "opioid crisis" related to unwise and illegal-use opioids that have been diverted from their intended use to relieve pain associated with disease to recreational and addictive behavior.

In other regions another type of "opioid crisis" exists—lack of access to essential pain medicines by those who need them. Opioids have been included in the World Health Organization's list of essential medicines since 1977 (32), yet as late as 2011, an estimated 80% of the world's population could not access them (33) (Fig. 62.4).

In addressing the problem of access to opioids, it must be kept in mind that illicit production, diversion, and abuse of opioids is a significant health issue in its own right. According to the United Nations Office on Drugs and Crime's World Drug Report 2018 (34), 76% of the approximately 450,000 drug related deaths globally in 2015 were due to opioids. This is not meant to imply that efforts to provide access to morphine for those needing palliative care should not be increased. It does mean that greater efforts to control misuse of opioids are warranted as is better cooperation and understanding between health and law enforcement interests at all levels.

While clearly necessary, access to opiates alone is not sufficient to provide comprehensive palliative care. The Lancet Commission recommended a suite of essential human resources, medicines, and equipment to be part of universal health care coverage, the cost of which was estimated to be about $2 to $16 per capita per year (35) (Fig. 62.5).

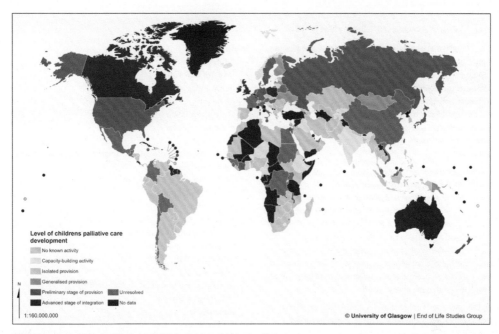

Clelland D, van Steijn D, Macdonald ME et al. Global development of children's palliative care: the picture in 2017 [version 1]. Wellcome Open Res 2020, 5:99 (doi: 10.12688/wellcomeopenres.15815.1)

Wellcome Open Research

Figure 62.3 Status of development of pediatric palliative care. (From file:///Users/josephoneill/Downloads/Global_Atlas_of_Palliative_Care%20(4).pdf)

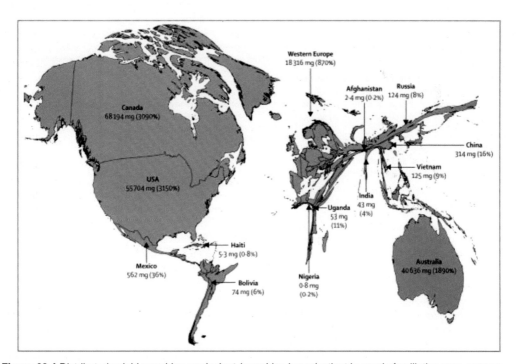

Figure 62.4 Distributed opioid morphine-equivalent (morphine in mg/patient in need of palliative care, average 2010–2013), and estimated percentage of need that is met for the health conditions most associated with serious health-related suffering. (From Knaul FM, Farmer PE, Krakauer EL, et al. Alleviating the access abyss in palliative care and pain relief—an imperative of universal health coverage: the Lancet Commission report. *Lancet*. 2018;391(10128):1391-1454. doi:10.1016/S0140-6736(17)32513-8. https://www.thelancet.com/journals/langlo/article/PIIS2214-109X(18)30082-2/fulltext)

Panel 2: An Essential Package Of Palliative Care And Pain Relief Health Services

The Essential Package contains the inputs for safe and effective provision of essential palliative care and pain relief interventions to alleviate physical and psychological symptoms, including the medicines and equipment that can be safely prescribed or administered in a primary care setting. The list of essential medicines in the Essential Package is based on WHO's list of essential medicines, and considers the medicines, doses, and administration routes for palliative care for both adults and children.

The Essential Package is designed to be lowest cost by including only off-patent formulations, frugal innovation for needed equipment, and a staffing model based on competencies rather than professions. Tasks often undertaken by specialised medical personnel in high-income countries can be performed by other specialised and general practitioners and nurses or by community health workers empowered with the necessary training and medical supervision to participate effectively in the delivery of palliative care and pain treatment at all levels of care, from the hospital to the home.

With the key exception of morphine, the medicines in the Essential Package are available in most countries even if supply is limited. For morphine, an essential palliative care medicine, assuring safety and accessibility is complex. Ensuring a balance between appropriate medical access to controlled medicines and the prevention of their diversion and nonmedical use is crucial, and the Commission not only designed appropriate human resource models but also the strategies to provide the complementary policy and stewardship to expand access to an Essential Package that includes morphine.

The health services of the Essential Package must be complemented by interventions for the relief of social and spiritual suffering to preserve the dignity of patients, facilitate access to health interventions, and prevent financial hardship and impoverishment. Yet, these social supports are neither part of the remit of health ministries nor should they be financed from a health budget.

Antipoverty and social development policies, publicly funded safety nets, programmes, and ministries must give special attention to ensure that families do not sacrifice their basic needs in desperate attempts to care for loved ones. These persons with life-limiting or life-threatening health conditions and their families should be mainstreamed into existing social support and social welfare programmes, yet they are often ignored, excluded, or marginalised, preventing them from being effectively integrated into these programmes.

Medicines
- Amitriptyline
- Bisacodyl (Senna)
- Dexamethasone
- Diazepam
- Diphenhydramine (chlorpheniramine, cyclizine, or dimenhydrinate)
- Fluconazole
- Fluoxetine or other selective serotonin-reuptake inhibitors (sertraline and citalopram)
- Furosemide
- Hyoscine butylbromide
- Haloperidol
- Ibuprofen (naproxen, diclofenac, or meloxicam)
- Lactulose (sorbitol or polyethylene glycol)
- Loperamide
- Metoclopramide
- Metronidazole
- Morphine (oral immediate-release and injectable)
- Naloxone parenteral
- Omeprazole
- Ondansetron
- Paracetamol
- Petroleum jelly

Medical equipment
- Pressure-reducing mattress
- Nasogastric drainage or feeding tube
- Urinary catheters
- Opioid lock box
- Flashlight with rechargeable battery (if no access to electricity)
- Adult diapers (or cotton and plastic, if in extreme poverty)
- Oxygen

Human resources (varies by referral, provincial or district hospital, community health center, or home)
- Doctors (specialty and general, depending on level of care)
- Nurses (specialty and general)
- Social workers and counsellors
- Psychiatrist, psychologist, or counsellor (depending on level of care)
- Physical therapist
- Pharmacist
- Community health workers
- Clinical support staff (diagnostic imaging, laboratory technician, nutritionist)
- Non-clinical support staff (administration, cleaning)

Additional detail is provided in the additional online material.

Figure 62.5 Essential package of palliative care and pain services. (From Gomez-Batiste X, Connor S, eds. *Building Integrated Palliative Care Programs & Services*. Vic, Spain: Eumo Editorial, University of Vic; 2017. https://www.thewhpca.org/resources/building-integrated-palliative-care-programs-and-services. Ref. (36).)

Even when medicines and materials are accessible and available to providers, professional and lay, they must be trained to use them and, especially when to use them. There should be a general level of understanding of principles of palliative care with competency-based training in pain and symptom management mainstreamed into all levels of health education for professional health workers and lay health workers who act as nurse and physician extenders to suffering patients.

Additional training must also be provided sufficient to produce a cadre of palliative care specialists able to care for those suffering with complex and difficult to manage suffering.

Academic institutions, professional organizations, and public sector health entities are producing, reviewing, and disseminating clinical guidelines and training materials, but more efforts along these lines are needed. Advanced training in palliative care for physicians and nurses is available in only a few academic intuitions outside high-income regions. Given the rapid expansion of online capacity, however, there are an expanding number of opportunities for training collaboration between academic institutions that can be developed.

Palliative care needs better integration into formal national health care systems including in primary care (37), rather than being siloed as a specialization. The unmet need for palliative care, especially in low- and middle-income countries, will never be met without serious efforts to ensure that this care is included in Universal Health Coverage plans at national levels. The need for palliative care, based on expected increases in mortality and health-related suffering, is expected nearly to double by 2060 (38).

CONCLUSION

The unmet need for supportive and palliative care for adult and pediatric cancer is expanding in middle- and low-income regions of the world. The policy framework to address this need is in place at the international level and to varying degrees at national levels and in some private sector institutions.

Even though the expense of bridging this gap is relatively modest, sufficient resources remain elusive. It is critical that those who understand the contribution that supportive oncology and palliative care can make for those suffering from cancer advocate for it.

REFERENCES

1. Lower income GNI/Capita < $996; middle income $996–3,895; upper-middle income $3,896–$12,055; high income >$12,055. https://blogs.worldbank.org/opendata/new-country-classifications-income-level-2018-2019. Accessed November 2019.
2. https://www.who.int/cancer/palliative/definition/en/. Accessed October 2019.
3. Adams LV, Wagner CM, Nutt CT, Binagwaho A. The future of global health education: training for equity in global health. *BMC Med Educ.* 2016;16(1):296. doi:10.1186/s12909-016-0820-0. PMID: 27871276.
4. http://gamapserver.who.int/mapLibrary/Files/Maps/Global_HALE_2016.png
5. https://www.who.int/sdhconference/background/news/facts/en. Accessed October 2019.
6. https://data.worldbank.org/indicator/SH.XPD.GHED.PP.CD

7. https://data.worldbank.org/indicator/SH.MED.NUMW.P3?view=map&year=2010
8. https://data.worldbank.org/indicator/SH.MED.PHYS.ZS?view=map&year=2010
9. Cancer Research UK. https://www.cancerresearchuk.org/health-professional/cancer-statistics/worldwide-cancer/mortality#heading-Zero. Accessed October 2019.
10. https://www.who.int/news-room/fact-sheets/detail/cancer
11. Yap ML, Zubizarreta E, Bray F, Ferlay J, Barton M. Global access to radiotherapy services: have we made progress during the past decade? *J Glob Oncol.* 2016;2(4):207-215. doi:10.1200/JGO.2015.001545. Published online on jgo.ascopubs.org on March 16, 2016. Accessed October 2019.
12. Global distribution of surgeons, anaesthesiologists, and obstetricians. *Lancet Glob Health.* 2015;3(suppl 2):S9-S11.
13. https://www.uicc.org/sites/main/files/atoms/files/Lancet%20Oncology%20Commission%20on%20Global%20Cancer%20Surgery.pdf. Accessed October 2019.
14. Hortobagyi GN, Pyle D, Cazap EL, et al. American Society of Clinical Oncology's Global Oncology Leadership Task Force: findings and actions. *J Glob Oncol.* 2018;4:1-8. doi:10.1200/JGO.17.00060.
15. https://www.who.int/cancer/resources/keyfacts/en/. Accessed October 2019.
16. https://www.who.int/nmh/Global_Atlas_of_Palliative_Care.pdf
17. Knaul FM, Farmer PE, Krakauer EL, et al. Alleviating the access abyss in palliative care and pain relief—an imperative of universal health coverage: the Lancet Commission report. *Lancet.* 2018;391(10128):1391-1454. doi:10.1016/S0140-6736(17)32513-8. https://www.thelancet.com/journals/langlo/article/PIIS2214-109X(18)30082-2/fulltext
18. https://www.thelancet.com/journals/lanonc/article/PIIS1470-2045(07)70138-9/fulltext
19. Sepulveda C, Marlin A, Yoshida T, Ulrich A. Palliative care: the World Health Organization's global perspective. *J Pain Symptom Manage.* 2002;24(2):91-96.
20. https://www.congress.gov/bill/108th-congress/house-bill/1298/text Section 104 (d) (2) (B)
21. https://www.gov.uk/government/speeches/hiv-care-and-support
22. http://www.treatthepain.org/
23. https://globalpartnersincare.org/
24. https://www.opensocietyfoundations.org/voices/topics/palliative-care
25. https://www.nhpco.org/hospice-care-overview/history-of-hospice/
26. Radbruch L, Payne S, de Lima L, Lohmann D. The Lisbon Challenge: acknowledging palliative care as a human right. *J Palliat Med.* 2013;16(3):301-304.
27. http://apps.who.int/gb/ebwha/pdf_files/WHA67/A67_R19-en.pdf. Accessed October 2019.
28. https://www.who.int/health_financing/universal_coverage_definition/en/
29. Connor SR, ed. *Global Atlas of Palliative Care.* 2nd ed. London, United Kingdom: Worldwide Hospice Palliative Care Alliance; 2020. http://www.thewhpca.org/resources/global-atlas-on-end-of-life-care
30. https://www.researchgate.net/publication/231223923_Mapping_Levels_of_Palliative_Care_Development_A_Global_Update
31. https://www.researchgate.net/publication/337442942_Mapping_Levels_of_Palliative_Care_Development_in_198_Countries_The_Situation_in_2017
32. The selection of essential drugs: report of a WHO expert committee. *World Health Organ Tech Rep Ser.* 1977;615:1-36.

33. Milani B, Scholten W. *The World Medicines Situation 2011. Access to Controlled Medicines*. Geneva, Switzerland: World Health Organization; 2011.

34. https://www.unodc.org/unodc/en/frontpage/2018/June/world-drug-report-2018_-opioid-crisis--prescription-drug-abuse-expands-cocaine-and-opium-hit-record-highs.html. Accessed October 2019.

35. https://www.thelancet.com/action/showPdf?pii=S0140-6736%2817%2932513-8

36. Gomez-Batiste X, Connor S, eds. *Building Integrated Palliative Care Programs & Services*. Vic, Spain: Eumo Editorial, University of Vic; 2017. https://www. thewhpca.org/resources/building-integrated-palliative-care-programs-and-services

37. Gomez-Batiste X, Connor S, eds. *Building Integrated Palliative Care Programs & Services*. Vic, Spain: Eumo Editorial, University of Vic; 2017. https://www.thewhpca.org/resources/building-integrated-palliative-care-programs-and-services

38. Sleeman KE, de Brito M, Etkind S, et al. The escalating global burden of serious health-related suffering: projections to 2060 by world regions, age groups, and health conditions. *Lancet Glob Health*. 2019;7: e883-e892.

Research Issues in Supportive Palliative Care

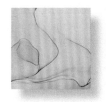 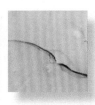 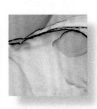 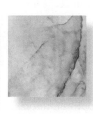 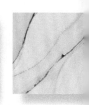

Accountability has been called the *third revolution* in medical care (1). Health care providers are now often faced with new questions. For example, what are the outcomes of palliative care that justify its continued institutional support? Or, what is the evidence for the use of a certain medical intervention for a specific patient? Fundamental to answering these questions are defining quality of care for seriously ill persons and determining how care is measured.

Quality care at the end of life is different than during any other period of time. Dying persons, their families, and health care providers are often faced with decisions that involve tradeoffs between length of life and quality of life. Reasonable persons may differ in such decisions. Therefore, preferences and values are important to shaping treatment decisions in ways unlike other time periods. Outcomes assessment for the dying must take this into consideration. In this chapter, a practical approach to examining outcomes, whether it is part of an audit prior to quality improvement efforts or for the ongoing assessment of institutional quality of care, will be discussed.

WHY EXAMINE OUTCOMES?

The first response of staff to auditing the quality of care is, "Why?" A typical response is that their work cannot be measured. Yet, audits and ongoing quality monitoring through examining administrative data, reviewing medical records, and/or speaking with dying persons and families lead to important opportunities to improve the quality of care. Simply stated, "If you don't measure it, you won't improve it" (2).

The results of assessing the outcomes of palliative medicine can help create the needed attention to the issue of improving the quality of care. Such tension can create the awareness among health care providers of opportunities to improve and enhance their current practices. Examining the outcomes can be critical to detecting early problems with new medications or other unintended consequences from medical interventions. Examining outcomes can guide organizational efforts to improve the quality of care. For example, knowing

that one in four persons now die in a nursing home provides important information for the planning of new programs to meet the needs of the dying (3).

WHAT OUTCOMES TO MEASURE?

Reflecting on the thirtieth anniversary of St. Christopher's Hospice, Dame Cicely Saunders said, "We have never lost sight of the values that were so important to David: commitment to openness, openness to challenge, and the absolute priority of patients' own views on what they need" (4). Fundamental to palliative care is meeting the needs and expectations of patients and families. Quality in a 42-year-old with an acute myocardial infarction can be measured by whether interventions have been done that minimize infarct size, such as the use of aspirin or percutaneous transluminal angioplasty. The vast majority of persons would want efforts to focus on restoring function under these circumstances. On the other hand, the circumstances of a 92-year-old dying of stage IV lung cancer are quite different. Technological interventions require weighting of their impact on both quality and quantity of life—decisions that require the input of an informed patient.

The importance of preferences is reflected in the Institute of Medicine's (IOM) definition of quality of care: the "degree to which health services for individuals and populations increased the likelihood of desired health outcomes and are consistent with professional knowledge" (5). This definition implies that conceptual models for quality care (as well as instruments measuring quality) must be based on both professional knowledge *and* informed patient preferences. To date, most conceptual models have been built either around expert opinion *or* qualitative data from patients, families, or health care providers.

Fortunately, both experts and consumers agree in many ways about what is important for the end-of-life care—physical comfort, emotional support, and autonomy. However, they have significant areas of disagreement as well, for example, unmet needs (Table 63.1). Family members want more information on what to expect and how they can

TABLE 63.1 COMPARISON OF DOMAINS OF EXPERT, PATIENTS, FAMILY MEMBERS, HEALTH CARE PROVIDERS, AND PROPOSED COMBINED MODEL IN MEASURING QUALITY OF CARE AT THE END OF LIFE

Expert opinion				Consumer opinion	Bereaved family members	Combined model
Emanuel and Emanuel (6)	Institute of Medicine approaching death: improving care at the end of life (7)	NHO pathway (8)	Patients with human immunodeficiency virus, renal failure on dialysis, and nursing home residents (9)	Patients, families, and health care providers		Person-centered, family-centered medical care (10)
Physical symptoms	Overall quality of life	Safe and comfortable dying	Receiving adequate pain and symptom management	Pain and symptom management	Providing desired physical comfort	Providing desired level of physical comfort and emotional support
Psychological and cognitive symptoms	Physical well-being and functioning	Self-determined life closure	Avoiding inappropriate prolongation of the dying	Clear decision-making	Achieving control over health care decisions and everyday decisions	Promote shared decision-making
Social relationships and support	Psychosocial well-being and functioning	Effective grieving	Achieving sense of control	Preparation for death	Burden of advocating for quality medical care	Focus on the individual that includes closure, respect, and dignity of the patient
Economic demands and caregiving demands	Family well-being and perceptions		Relieving burden	Completion	Educating on what to expect and increasing confidence in providing care	Attend to the needs of the family for information, increasing their confidence in helping with patient care and providing emotional support prior to and after the patient's death
Hopes and expectations			Strengthening relationship	Contributing to others	Emotional support prior to and after the patient's death	Coordination and continuity of care
Spiritual and existential beliefs				Affirmation of the whole person		Informing and educating

From Nelson EC, Splaine ME, Batalden PB, et al. Building measurement and data collection into medical practice. *Ann Intern Med.* 1998;128:460-466.

help their dying loved ones. Patients and families emphasize the importance of closure at the end of life, including issues of personal relationships. Families often speak of frustration with a lack of coordination of medical care. It is often not clear who is in charge; different health care providers provide conflicting information, and transitions can be fraught with confusion (10).

One conceptual model, patient-focused, family-centered medical care (Table 63.1), is based on a review of existing professional guidelines *and* results from focus groups conducted with bereaved family members (10,11). According to this model, institutions and care providers striving to achieve person-centered, family-centered medical care for the seriously ill patient should:

- provide the desired level of physical comfort and emotional support;
- promote shared decision-making, including care planning in advance;
- focus on the individual patient by facilitating situations in which patients achieve their desired levels of control, staff members treat patients with respect and dignity, and patients are aided in achieving their desired levels of closure;
- attend to the needs of caregivers for information and skills in providing care for the patient and provide emotional support to the family before and after the patient's death; and
- coordinate patients across disease trajectory, health care providers, and settings of care.

On the basis of this model, a survey intended to be used as part of an initial quality audit of the quality of end-of-life care has been developed and validated. Two surveys have been created including the Consumer Assessment and Reports of End of life Care (CARE) that was used in national mortality followback survey (12) and Brown University Family Evaluation of Hospice Care (13). In part, this research and the Clinical Practice Guidelines for Quality Palliative Care (14) informed the development of the CAHPS Hospice Survey that is used for the purpose of accountability and publicly reported for US Hospice Programs (15).

WHEN ARE OUTCOMES MEASURED?

The question of when outcomes are measured is an extremely important consideration. Dying is unlike any other period of time. Often, the dying person and the health care providers are balancing the hope for longevity versus the need to make appropriate preparation. Although many outcome measures are not clearly linked to disease trajectory and patient readiness, several outcomes are linked to either. For example, issues around

closure are clearly linked to the dying person and family readiness to discuss that the patient is dying. Therefore, the wording of questions and timing of administration of survey must be done in a sensitive manner to reflect where the dying person is in their readiness to discuss existential issues. Other process measures, such as counseling on advance directives or discussion of hospice, should reflect the recommendation of professional guidelines with measures of quality of care to include counterbalancing measures about whether such discussions were done in a sensitive and compassionate manner.

HOW ARE OUTCOMES MEASURED?

Assessment of outcomes refers to measuring the "end results"—the impact or effect of medical care on the dying person and/or the family. Measuring outcomes allows you to judge the effectiveness of medical interventions, innovative programs, and new medications. In addition to examining outcomes, process measures provide important information for quality improvement and examination of the effect of new programs. A *process measure* examines what a service or intervention does for patients and their families. For example, a process measure focuses on whether there is a regular assessment of pain noted in the medical record, while an *outcome measure* examines whether patients report that they received their desired amount of pain relief. Both are important and critical to measure. Ultimately, the quality of medical care is judged by changes in outcome indicators. Yet, an organization will not achieve those outcomes if it does not implement key processes of care that are known to benefit medical care.

Key to choosing an outcome or process measure is the intended use of the quality measures. Table 63.2 notes the four potential uses of measurement tools.

The areas of emphasis and desired characteristics vary for measurement tools intended for different purposes (Table 63.3). For example, the intended audience for quality improvement measures is the institutional and quality improvement team, whereas the intended audience for public accountability is the health care purchaser and consumer.

Measurement tools used for public accountability need further evidence that justifies their use. For example, given the intended audiences and implications of the use of measurement tools for public accountability, more stringent psychometric properties must be used for these measures. In addition, there must be either normative or

TABLE 63.2 PURPOSES OF QUALITY MEASURES

1. Quality improvement—measures to provide information for health care institutions to reform or shape how care is provided
2. Clinical assessment—measures to guide individual patient management
3. Research—measures that assess the phenomenon of interest
4. Accountability—measures that allow comparison of quality of care for the purposes of quality assurance or for consumer choice between health care institutions or practitioners

From Teno JM, Byock I, Field MJ. Research agenda for developing measures to examine quality of care and quality of life of patients diagnosed with life-limiting illness. White paper from the conference on Excellent Care at the End of Life through Fast-Tracking Audit, Standards, and Teamwork (EXCELFAST), September 28–30, 1997. *J Pain Symptom Manage*. 1999;17:75-82.

empirical research that substantiates a claim that the construct being measured for public accountability is under the control of that health care institution.

Typically, measurement tools can review the electronic medical record, examine administrative data (such as death certificate or billing data), or conduct interviews with a patient or a proxy such as a family member. Each potential source of data has strengths and limitations that should be considered when selecting a measurement tool or strategy.

Medical records are legal documents that should reflect the medical care that patients receive. Yet, medical records reflect staff perceptions, and their contents are subject to reporting bias. For example, a nurse may document that a patient understands how to take his/her medications on hospital discharge; this documentation reflects the nurse's perception. Yet, patients and families often report that they did *not* understand that explanation when interviewed after hospital discharge (16). Furthermore, not all discussions are documented in the medical record. Discussions about resuscitation preferences are usually only documented when the patient or family consents to a "do not resuscitate" order. Therefore, a physician and patient may have talked about resuscitation preferences and decided *not* to forgo cardiopulmonary resuscitation, but there is nothing documented in the medical record because cardiopulmonary resuscitation is the default in most of the US hospitals.

Administrative data, such as death certificate data, billing data, and the Minimum Data Set, are readily assessable information that can provide invaluable information. Examining death certificate data that are published on the Internet (see www.cdc.gov) and available in public use files can provide hospice and palliative programs with information about their "market share," that is, what proportion of persons for whom they provide medical care in a certain geographic area. This information can highlight areas that are underserved

TABLE 63.3 AREAS OF EMPHASIS BASED ON THE PURPOSE OF QUALITY MEASURE

	Purpose of measure			
	Clinical assessment	Research	Improvement	Accountability
Audience	Clinical staff	Science community	Quality improvement team and clinical staff	Payers, public
Focus of measurement	Status of patient	Knowledge	Understand care process	Comparison
Confidentiality	Very high	Very high	Very high	Purpose is to compare groups
Evidence base to justify use of the measure	Important and the measure should have face validity from a clinical standpoint	Builds off existing evidence to generate new knowledge	Important	Extremely important in that proposed domain ought to be under control of that institution
Importance of psychometric properties	Important to the individual provider	Extremely important to that research effort	Important within that setting	Valid and responsive across multiple settings

This table was adapted from an article by Solberg LI, Mosser G, McDonald S. The three faces of performance measurement: improvement, accountability, and research. *Jt Comm J Qual Improv*. 1997;23:135-147. On the Three Faces of Performance Measurement: Improvement, Accountability, and Research and reproduced from an article by Teno JM, Byock I, Field MJ. Research agenda for developing measures to examine quality of care and quality of life of patients diagnosed with life-limiting illness. White paper from the conference on Excellent Care at the End of Life through Fast-Tracking Audit, Standards, and Teamwork (EXCELFAST), September 28–30, 1997. *J Pain Symptom Manage*. 1999;17:75-82.

and opportunities for program expansion. Users of administrative data need to be aware that it can be inaccurate because of coding problems, key punch errors, or economic incentives to upgrade a patient's condition to get more reimbursement. For example, one prospective cohort study of nursing home residents with advance dementia found that 37% did not have dementia mentioned on their death certificate (17).

The Minimum Data Set is used in US nursing homes to systematically collect information on more than 300 items on a quarterly basis. This instrument can provide institution-specific and national estimates of outcomes, such as pain management (18). Yet, these data reflect staff perceptions of patients' levels of pain. Therefore, ascertainment bias is an important concern in the use of these data.

Surveys, either self- or telephone administered, provide information directly from the patient and family perspective about the quality of care. Typically, satisfaction measures which ask a person to rate the quality of care with response categories that vary from "poor" to "excellent" have not yielded discriminating information about the quality of care. The respondents' task with these rating questions includes several steps: first, determine whether that event occurred; second, formulate their expectations regarding that aspect of care; and third, choose a category from the response categories. Often, persons have lowered expectations regarding their medical care, which, at least in part, explains the finding of high satisfaction in the face of indicators of poor quality of care, for example, severe pain (18,19).

Newer methods have begun using either "patient-centered reports" or "preference-based questions" (i.e., unmet needs) to capture the consumer perspective (Fig. 63.1) (20). These methodologies, unlike typical satisfaction questions that rely on rating questions, provide information that guide improvement of the quality of care. For example, knowing that 85% of patients believe a health care provider is "very good" does not tell that provider in what ways and specific processes of care that he/she can improve. On the other hand, knowing that 20% of patients did not understand a provider's directions for taking pain medications does provide a tangible target for improving and enhancing the quality of care. Moreover, patient-centered reports and preference-based questions have strong face validity with health care providers. In the future, surveys need to rely on all three methodologies—ratings, patient-centered reports, and preference-based questions—to capture the consumer perspective on the quality of care at the end of life.

WHICH TOOL SHOULD BE USED?

Selecting a measurement tool should be guided by its intended use and the characteristics of the particular tool. The goals of measurement should be clear. As noted in Table 63.3, different psychometric properties (i.e., reliability, validity, and responsiveness of the tool) are needed for different intended uses. In addition, the intended audience is different for each of the four key purposes of measurement listed in Table 63.3. Measurement tools used for accountability, for example, have an intended audience of health insurers, the government, and other such institutions that pay for health care services. The focus of measurement is to compare health care institutions or plans. Given this purpose, it is very important that there is evidence that what is being measured is under the control of that health care institution and that the chosen instrument is reliable, valid, and responsive across the settings.

Reliability is necessary but not sufficient evidence of validity of an instrument or measurement tool. Reliability examines the degree to which the measurement tool is capable of reproducing the same results over time. Therefore, a person should give the same response to a question if asked within a short period of time.

A measurement tool is valid if there is evidence that it measures what it purports to measure. In essence, one is asking whether the measurement tool is reporting the truth. Often, the intent of the measurement tool is to identify a perception or attitude of the respondent. In this case, there is no "gold standard" by which to judge whether the measurement tool is accurately representing the construct that is being measured.

Content validity asks whether the measurement tool examines the correct concepts at face value. Were experts involved as advisors in the creation of the tool? Was the selection of concepts based on a theoretical model? *Construct validity* examines the degree to which the results from that measurement tool are associated with preestablished and known relationships. For example, a measure of overall satisfaction should be associated with consumer choice of health care plans.

Responsiveness examines the degree to which a measurement tool changes as a result of interventions or historical events. Often, responsiveness is not reported in the initial validation of a measurement tool. Rather, responsiveness is reported at a later date after the measurement tool has been utilized in intervention studies or research that tracks quality over time.

Over the past several decades, an increasing number of measurement tools have been developed

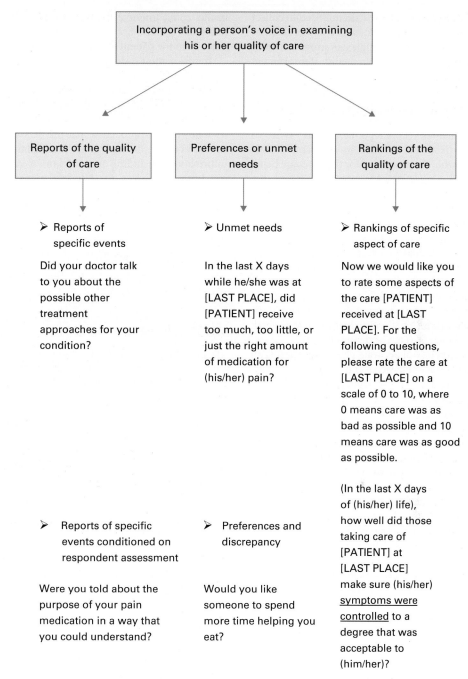

Figure 63.1 Proposed classification scheme for measuring a patient and family voice about the quality of medical care. (Adapted from Teno JM. Putting the patient and family voice back into measuring the quality of care for the dying. *Hosp J*. 1999;14(3–4):167-176.)

for examining the quality of end-of-life care. There are web-based resources from organizations such as the Palliative Care Research Cooperative Group that identifies instruments to measure the quality of palliative care (21).

For a seriously ill and dying population, the time burden on respondents and staff is an important

consideration for selecting an instrument. Limiting the scope of domains covered and the number of individual cases for which data are collected can reduce time burden. For an interview respondent—especially a seriously ill patient—it is particularly important to limit the scope of domains that are covered in the interview. For the purpose of quality improvement, you do not need to collect a large number of cases. A small number of cases collected by a random sample can provide invaluable information to guide a quality improvement effort.

HOW IS THE SAMPLE SELECTED?

A fundamental, yet often perplexing, step is deciding who is to be included in the sample. This relates to the "denominator" for the outcome being measured. Simply stated, a rate is composed of a numerator and a denominator. Determining who is in the denominator can be difficult in palliative medicine. For example, three decades ago, most persons would have considered patients with leukemia in childhood to be among those patients with a terminal illness. However, this no longer is the case due to the tremendous strides made in treating cancers in childhood. Researchers and quality improvement teams, then, must make decisions about which patients to include in the overall group of interest (i.e., the denominator).

The difficulty of accurate prognostication is an additional issue. Physicians are often overly optimistic in their prognoses, resulting in uncertainty about patients' actual time before death. Even the best statistical models are inaccurate because they are applying historical information from a previous cohort of similar patients to predict the future. There is a certain error in those estimates. Moreover, new treatments can invalidate even the best estimates by prediction models.

Although the timing of the interview is not as critical for certain domains, such as pain assessment, other domains are very sensitive to the time from death at which the interview takes place. Communication about prognosis, current medical treatment, and advance care planning are complex social interactions for which the timing of discussions should be based on the patient and family readiness and preferences to undertake these conversations. Thus, the timing of prospective surveys can't assume that all persons would be ready or want to have a conversation about their impending mortality (22). Additionally, it is possible that institutions will interview persons at different time periods prior to death. This situation may result in differences in observed quality measures that reflect timing of the interview more than differences in the quality of care provided.

Given these prognostication issues, retrospective interviews with bereaved family members may be more suited to collect information on whether care was consistent with patient goals of care. Doing a prospective patient data collection has important advantages. First and foremost, the results could improve the quality of care of that individual patient. Second, the information originates from the patient and not a surrogate.

If information is desired about the last week of life, often a family member is the only person that is able to provide a consumer perspective on the quality of end-of-life care delivered to the deceased and his/her family. The advantage of this "mortality followback" approach is that the denominator can be precisely defined, given that demographic information (including next of kin) is reported on death certificates to state-level departments of vital registries. Therefore, data collection can occur quickly without the costs of case finding for the prospective sample of patients. Because of this, mortality followback surveys have been used by both the United Kingdom (23,24) and the United States to collect (25–27) information on the last year of life of decedents, quality of decision-making, and the benefits of hospice services.

WHAT ARE THE NEXT STEPS?

The first step in improving the quality of end-of-life care is taking stock—identifying and understanding the opportunities to improve. Simply stated, if you do not measure it, you will not improve it (2). Measuring or conducting an audit is the first step (Fig. 63.2). A metaphor for the audit is the physician review of system. A review of system only provides with a symptom. The next step is to ask further questions and consider ordering diagnostic tests to understand the diagnosis or in the case of audit—the root cause or high leverage process of care where an intervention would improve the quality of care. The second step is to engage stakeholders and define the goal. Engaging stakeholders means to present the results of the audit in a way that does not assign blame, but rather looks for shared opportunities to improve and enhance the quality of care. Key to the success of this second step is raising awareness and developing a shared goal.

The third step is actually improving the quality of end-of-life care through interventions and measuring whether these interventions succeed in creating change. Often, persons believe that education which provides knowledge and impacts attitudes will achieve change. Many times, even knowledge is not sufficient to change behavior. Instead, changes must be made in the processes of care that provide the cues and default pathways that ensure persons will choose the right behavior. Often, this change can be achieved through a model of rapid improvement that utilizes multiple plan, do, check, and act (PDCA) cycles (28). PDCA cycles allow testing of interventions first on

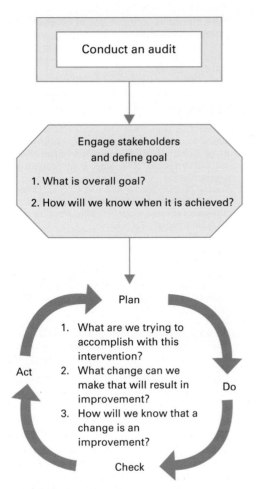

Figure 63.2 Quality improvement model.

a small scale (sometimes as small as only one nurse with one patient). From the information learned, the intervention can be refined or a different one can be tested.

Three key questions help to frame the work of the PDCA cycle. First, what is one trying to accomplish with this intervention? Just as an overall goal was identified in step 2 of the quality improvement model, a goal must be stated for each PDCA cycle. Second, what changes can one make that will result in improvement? This may involve brainstorming with a team of colleagues about what interventions can achieve the goal of the cycle. An effort should be made to be creative, yet one should not be afraid to copy the success of others. Third, how will one know that change is an improvement? It is important to choose either a process or outcome variable that examines whether the goal of that cycle is being met and that data are tracked for the goal of that cycle, as well as the overall goal for the improvement effort. Often, a quality improvement team must test multiple interventions and conduct

multiple PDCA cycles to achieve the overall goal. Two recent studies suggest that application of rapid cycle quality improvement can result in substantial gains of the quality of pain management in the nursing homes or feeding tube decision-making (29,30).

CONCLUSIONS

Outcomes assessment is key to improving the quality of end-of-life care. At this early stage of development of supportive and palliative care, we urgently need both research and quality improvement efforts that will contribute to the scientific evidence base. Care at the end of life is quite different than care at other time periods. Patients' informed preferences play an even more central role in decision-making and outcomes. Not all persons with stage IV lung cancer, for example, will want experimental chemotherapy, and quality indicators must take into account that reasonable persons have different treatment preferences. Hence, measuring the quality of end-of-life care often requires interviews to examine the consumer perspective.

Even at this early stage, there are several promising measurement tools for quality improvement audits, for research, and for accountability. Selection of these measurement tools must be guided by the intended use of the data. The use of measurement tools for accountability carries two key requirements: an evidence base that suggests that the domain of interest is under the control of health care providers and demonstration of satisfactory psychometric properties of the tool across settings of care.

With an increased focus on accountability, health care providers will need to become familiar with methods to improve the quality of medical care. Measurement plays an important role in quality improvement efforts—from the initial audit that raises awareness of an opportunity to improve to ongoing assessments of whether interventions are achieving their goals. The ideal quality monitoring system for palliative care should strongly link guidelines such as the current 4th edition of the Clinical Practice Guidelines for Quality Palliative Care and proposed quality indicators (14). Guidelines should be based on both normative and empirical research. Quality indicators can measure information about the structure of a health care institution (e.g., availability of certain services and existence of policies) about processes of care (i.e., the interactions of health care providers, patients, and family members), and about outcomes of care (i.e., the effectiveness of treatment).

Currently, most quality indicators measure either structure or processes of care. Outcome measures are intuitively more attractive, but they are more difficult to apply because of our limited ability to adjust for differences in patient characteristics and the relatively small numbers of people with a particular condition treated at institutions each year. One argument in favor of collecting process data is that they are a more sensitive measure of quality because adverse outcomes do not occur every time there is an error in the provision of medical care. Furthermore, important outcomes—both positive and negative—often appear months or even years after care has been given. Quality indicators based on measures of structure or process, however, are only as good as their ability to predict outcomes of importance.

ACKNOWLEDGMENTS

This chapter in part is based on a background paper prepared for the National Cancer Policy Board of the IOM. The author acknowledges the helpful comments by Ms. Helen Gelband.

REFERENCES

1. Relman AS. Assessment and accountability: the third revolution in medical care [editorial]. *N Engl J Med.* 1988;319(18):1220-1222.
2. Nelson EC, Splaine ME, Batalden PB, Plume SK. Building measurement and data collection into medical practice. *Ann Intern Med.* 1998;128(6):460-466.
3. Teno JM. Facts on dying: brown Atlas site of death 1989–1997. http://www.chcr.brown.edu/dying/factson-dying.htm. Accessed February 26, 2004.
4. Saunders C, ed. *Monograph in Commemoration of the 30th Anniversary of St. Christopher's Hospice.* London: St. Christopher's Hospice; 2001.
5. Institute of Medicine, ed. *Medicare: A Strategy for Quality Assurance.* Washington, DC: National Academy Press; 1990.
6. Emanuel EJ, Emanuel LL. The promise of a good death. *Lancet.* 1998;351(suppl 2):SII21-SII29.
7. Institute of Medicine, Committee on Care at the End of Life, eds. *Approaching Death: Improving Care at the End of Life.* Washington, DC: National Academy Press; 1997.
8. National Hospice Organization, ed. *A Pathway for Patients and Families Facing Terminal Illness: Self-Determined Life Closure, Safe Comfortable Dying and Effective Grieving.* Alexandria, VA: National Hospice Organization; 1997.
9. Singer PA, Martin DK, Kelner M. Quality end-of-life care: patients' perspectives. *JAMA.* 1999;281(2):163-168.
10. Teno JM, Casey VA, Welch L, Edgman-Levitan S. Patient-focused, family-centered end-of-life medical care: views of the guidelines and bereaved family members. *J Pain Symptom Manage.* Special Section on Measuring Quality of Care at Life's End II. 2001;22(3):738-751.
11. Teno JM, Connor SR. Referring a patient and family to high-quality palliative care at the close of life: "we met

12. Teno JM, Clarridge BR, Casey V, et al. Family perspectives on end-of-life care at the last place of care. *JAMA.* 2004;291(1):88-93.
13. Connor SR, Teno J, Spence C, Smith N. Family evaluation of hospice care: results from voluntary submission of data via website. *J Pain Symptom Manage.* 2005;30(1):9-17.
14. National Consensus Project for Quality Palliative Care. *Clinical Practice Guidelines for Quality Palliative Care.* 4th ed. Richmond, VA: National Coalition for Hospice and Palliative Care; 2018. https://www.nationalcoalitionhpc.org/ncp
15. Anhang-Price R, Stucky B, Parast L, et al. Development of valid and reliable measure of patient and family experiences of hospice care for public reporting. *J Palliat Med.* 2018;21(7):924-932.
16. Cleary PD, Edgman-Levitan S, Roberts M, et al. Patients evaluate their hospital care: a national survey. *Health Aff (Millwood).* 1991;10(4):254-267.
17. Wachterman M, Keily DK, Mitchell SL. Reporting dementia on the death certificate of nursing home residents dying with end-stage dementia. *JAMA.* 2008;300(22):2608-2610.
18. Teno JM, Weitzen S, Wetle T, Mor V. Persistent pain in nursing home residents. *JAMA.* 2001;285(16):2081.
19. Desbiens NA, Wu AW, Broste SK, et al. Pain and satisfaction with pain control in seriously ill hospitalized adults: findings from the SUPPORT research investigations. For the SUPPORT Investigators. Study to understand prognoses and preferences for outcomes and risks of treatment. *Crit Care Med.* 1996;24(12):1953-1961.
20. Quality improvement guidelines for the treatment of acute pain and cancer pain. American Pain Society Quality of Care Committee. *JAMA.* 1995;274(23):1874-1880.
21. PCRC Instrument Library. https://palliativecareresearch.org/corescenters/measurement-core/pcrc-instrument-library
22. Teno JM, Price RA, Makaroun LK. Challenges of measuring quality of community-based programs for seriously ill individuals and their families. *Health Aff (Millwood).* 2017;36(7):1227-1233.
23. Teno JM. Putting the patient and family voice back into measuring the quality of care for the dying. *Hosp J.* 1999;14(3–4):167-176.
24. Cartwright A. Changes in life and care in the year before death 1969–1987. *J Public Health Med.* 1991;13(2):81-87.
25. Addington Hall J, McCarthy M. Regional study of care for the dying: methods and sample characteristics. *Palliat Med.* 1995;9(1):27-35.
26. NCHS. *The National Mortality Followback Survey—Provisional Data, 1993.* Public User Data File Documentation. Hyattsville, MD: Centers for Disease Control and Prevention; 1998.
27. Teno JM, Gozalo PL, Lee IC, et al. Does hospice improve quality of care for persons dying from dementia? *J Am Geriatr Soc.* 2011;59(8):1531-1536.
28. Teno JM, Mitchell SL, Kuo SK, et al. Decision-making and outcomes of feeding tube insertion: a five-state study. *J Am Geriatr Soc.* 2011;59(5):881-886.
29. Langley G, Nolan K, Nolan T, Norman C, Provost L, eds. *The Improvement Guide: A Practical Approach to Enhancing Organizational Performance.* San Francisco, CA: Jossey-Bass Publishers; 1996.
30. Baier RR, Gifford DR, Patry G, et al. Ameliorating pain in nursing homes: a collaborative quality-improvement project. *J Am Geriatr Soc.* 2004;52(12):1988-1995.

a new personality. with this level of compassion and empathy". *JAMA.* 2009;301(6):651-659.

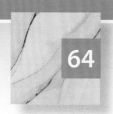

64 Research Issues: Ethics and Study Design

Ryan D. Stephenson, Biren Saraiya, and Eric A. Singer

INTRODUCTION

The goal of good palliative care is to relieve suffering and to improve quality of life. However, it is apparent that access to palliative care is inconsistent and standards to guide palliative care have not been established clearly. These deficiencies exist, at least in part, because of a lack of solid evidence on which to base clinical decisions (1,2). Therefore, there is an urgent need for research that can provide evidence to define the standard of care and to increase access to quality care.

Recent years have seen a dramatic increase in palliative care research, defined broadly as activities that are designed to contribute to generalizable knowledge (3) about symptom management and end-of-life care. This growth has created a heterogeneous field that encompasses both qualitative and quantitative techniques, and descriptive as well as interventional study designs (4). Although the past 10 years have seen impressive growth in all of these areas, this rate of growth appears to be particularly rapid for interventional research, including controlled trials of pain medications (5,6), interventional procedures for pain (7), and other nonpharmacologic interventions to improve a variety of aspects of end-of-life care (8–12). In 2005, clinical trials represented only 7.22% of the published palliative care literature (13).

Despite the valuable knowledge that has been produced by this research, and the promise of important advances in the future, progress has been slowed by a persistent uncertainty about the ethics of these studies (14). Indeed, there have been concerns raised from several quarters about whether patients near the end of life should ever be asked to participate in any form of research (15,16). Others have objected to this extreme position (1,17). Nevertheless, many providers, Institutional Review Boards (IRBs), ethics committees, study sections, and even investigators remain uncertain about the ethical limits of research involving dying patients.

These concerns have considerable intuitive appeal and must be taken seriously. Indeed, it would be unfortunate if the progress of palliative care research was slowed by the sorts of ethical scandals that have threatened other fields of research that involve vulnerable populations, such as those with mental illness (18). However, strict overseeing and tight limits on palliative care research have the potential to do equal damage to the growing field (19). Therefore, in order to avoid potential scandals, without excessive regulation and overseeing, it will be important that palliative care investigators and clinicians consider these concerns in a fair and balanced way.

Emanuel et al. proposed a general framework elucidating seven requirements to make clinical research ethical, which are summarized in Table 64.1 (20). Palliative care ethics must satisfy these requirements but may require special attention in certain areas, particularly protecting voluntariness and minimizing the burdens of follow-up near the end of life. This chapter will discuss the seven domains of ethical research noted in Table 64.1 as they specifically relate to the intricacies of palliative care research design and conduct.

SOCIAL OR SCIENTIFIC VALUE

Palliative care research is designed to produce knowledge that will advance understanding of symptom management and end-of-life care. Implicit in this goal is the expectation that this knowledge will eventually improve care for future patients. Therefore, the first ethical aspect of palliative care research that deserves consideration is its potential benefits for future patients.

Broadly, value can be defined as the likelihood that a study's results will improve the health and well-being of future patients (21). Value is an essential aspect of a study's ethical design because a central goal of research is to produce knowledge that will ultimately be "important," (3,22) "fruitful," (23) or "valuable" (24). In fact, one reason that subjects participate in clinical research is to produce knowledge that will benefit others (25,26). Because subjects are willing to accept risks and burdens of research at least in part in order to benefit others, investigators have accepted an ethical responsibility to maximize the probability that a study will be able to do so. Therefore, in addition to widely accepted scientific arguments for valuable research, there are compelling ethical arguments as well.

TABLE 64.1 SEVEN REQUIREMENTS FOR DETERMINING WHETHER A RESEARCH TRIAL IS ETHICAL

Requirement	Explanation	Justifying ethical values	Expertise for evaluation
Social or scientific value	Evaluation of a treatment, intervention, or theory that will improve health and well-being or increase knowledge	Scarce resources and nonexploitation	Scientific knowledge; citizen's understanding of social priorities
Scientific validity	Use of accepted scientific principles and methods, including statistical techniques, to produce reliable and valid data	Scarce resources and nonexploitation	Scientific and statistical knowledge; knowledge of condition and population to assess feasibility
Fair subject selection	Selection of subjects so that stigmatized and vulnerable individuals are not targeted for risky research and the rich and socially powerful not favored for potentially beneficial research	Justice	Scientific knowledge; ethical and legal knowledge
Favorable risk–benefit ratio	Minimization of risks; enhancement of potential benefits; risks to the subject are proportionate to the benefits to the subject and society	Nonmaleficence, beneficence, and nonexploitation	Scientific knowledge; citizen's understanding of social values
Independent review	Review of the design of the research trial, its proposed subject population, and risk–benefit ratio by individuals unaffiliated with the research	Public accountability; minimizing influence of potential conflicts of interest	Intellectual, financial, and otherwise independent researchers; scientific and ethical knowledge
Informed consent	Provision of information to subjects about purpose of the research, its procedures, potential risks, benefits, and alternatives, so that the individual understands this information and can make a voluntary decision whether to enroll and continue to participate	Respect for subject autonomy	Scientific knowledge; ethical and legal knowledge
Respect for potential and enrolled subjects	Respect for subjects by 1. Permitting withdrawal from the research 2. Protecting privacy through confidentiality 3. Informing subjects of newly discovered risks or benefits 4. Informing subjects of results of clinical research 5. Maintaining welfare of subjects	Respect for subject autonomy and welfare	Scientific knowledge; ethical and legal knowledge; knowledge of particular subject population

Reproduced with permission from Emanuel EJ, Wendler D, Grady C. What makes clinical research ethical? *JAMA*. 2000;283(20):2701-2711.

Scientific Validity

Research must be conducted in a manner to produce valid results. That is, it must incorporate techniques of design and data analysis that peer reviewers can agree as appropriate. In addition, all studies must be designed to produce knowledge that is generalizable (3,27). These requirements collectively describe a study's validity (28). Validity is a threshold requirement for all research, because it is unethical to expose human subjects to risks in studies that peer reviewers agree cannot adequately answer a research question (29). Therefore, at a minimum, investigators must routinely consider a study's validity.

First, a study's sample size should be adequate to answer the research question that is posed. Problems of underpowered studies, and particularly clinical trials, are both widespread and well described (30). But issues of power and sample size are particularly relevant to pain and symptom research, in which random variation can be quite large (31). To minimize these problems, the establishment of consortia or collaborative groups can facilitate the conduct of multicenter studies. Such arrangements have been highly effective in promoting research on rare disorders and may be applicable to palliative care research as well, in which investigators are limited and available patients are often sparse. To that end, the Palliative Care Research Cooperative Group was founded in 2010 with the principal aim "to facilitate conduct of collaborative, rigorous, multi-site end-of-life and palliative care research," which presently includes over 550 members at over 180 locations in the United States (32).

Second, palliative care investigators can enhance the ethical quality of a study by taking reasonable steps to increase the generalizability of its results. These steps might include sample size calculations that permit subgroup analysis of groups of patients that have typically not been the focus of investigation, such as patients with noncancer diagnoses, or special populations such as elderly patients or postoperative patients, or patients with addiction. The generalizability of a study's results might also be enhanced by recruiting subjects outside academic medical settings, because preliminary evidence suggests that these patients, and their needs for care, may be different than those who receive care in academic settings (33).

In addition, palliative care investigators can enhance the generalizability, and therefore the value, of their research by making reasonable efforts to include patients who are receiving care at home and particularly those who are enrolled in a home hospice program. Substantial barriers may make it difficult to include these patients in research. Nevertheless, few data exist to guide the management of home care patients near the end of life, and palliative care investigators can enhance the value of their research by including this population whenever possible (34).

Of course, all of these improvements in generalizability come at a substantial cost. For instance, studies that recruit subjects from several different settings require more elaborate designs for recruitment and follow-up. In addition, investigators who include plans for subgroup analysis in their sample size calculations face rapidly escalating sample size requirements and costs. Nevertheless, steps such as these offer an important way to enhance the value of a palliative care study and therefore its ethical quality. Therefore, it will also be important that funding agencies understand the ethical importance of generalizability and that generalizability comes with a financial cost.

Fair Subject Selection

For knowledge gained from research to be truly generalizable, as required by value and validity, the selection of study participants must be fair (26,27). Studies should be designed to include the patients about whom the question is being raised. History is replete with examples of unethical research in which "easier" groups were studied, only to have the benefits of research used by those who did not accept the burdens of risk (35). Further, for the study intervention to be valid, it should be tested on those closest to the study patient as possible.

In palliative care research, the target population frequently includes patients in the final months, weeks, and days of their life. It is a particularly vulnerable moment in life; but it would be unethical to exclude such patients due to the nature of the vulnerability. Including such patients in study recruitment respects the ethical principal of autonomy (36). Studies should specifically recruit such patients and include methodologies that collect data while minimizing burdens.

Favorable Risk–benefit Ratio

Investigators can also enhance a study's ethical soundness by taking steps to minimize a study's risks and burdens. Although the distinction between risks and burdens is not always clear, a rough heuristic is useful. In general, a *risk* can be considered as the probability of an adverse medical event or undesirable outcome. Risks might include side effects of a medication or increased pain during a study. The term *burden* can be used to describe those unpleasant features of participation in a study that are more certain and which are better thought of as inconveniences. Additional visits to the clinic, time spent filling out questionnaires, or time spent waiting in the clinic might be described as burdens.

Attention to the ethical design of pain research, and to the minimization of research risks and burdens, requires a clear agreement about how they should be defined. The criteria by which study risks and burdens are identified and evaluated use the concept of incremental or "demarcated" risks imposed by participation in a study (37). The application of this standard to interventional pain research would mean that investigators designing a trial to compare the effectiveness of two opioids (38), for moderate to severe pain, need not go to great lengths to justify the risks of the opioids being evaluated, if subjects in the trial would have received similar medications, with similar risks, as standard of care. Of course, the risks of any medication in a clinical trial should be disclosed in the informed consent process (3). Nevertheless, investigators are not under the obligation to minimize or justify these risks as they would be if, for instance, the same medications were being given to patients with mild pain, who would not receive them as part of standard care.

Perhaps, one of the most contentious and emotional questions in palliative care research (39,40), and indeed in research generally (41–43), is whether a placebo or sham control arm is ethically appropriate. Some have advocated for a "middle ground" balancing the competing demands of the scientific validity of placebo controls with minimizing risks of active controls (44). Broadly, placebos can be defined as interventions that are "ineffective or not specifically effective" for the symptom or disorder in question (45). Increased attention to the ethical issue of placebo controls in recent years has produced a growing consensus that all subjects in a clinical trial should have access to the best available standard of care, including supportive care and palliation (46). Therefore in infectious disease research, for instance, all subjects with meningitis would have access to an antimicrobial agent that has proved effective. However, this requirement may be difficult to apply to studies of treatment for pain, other symptoms, or depression, in which the placebo response can be quite substantial. These difficulties are compounded when the symptom being studied is transient, such as incident pain (6).

For these reasons, it may not be practical to prohibit placebos in palliative care research, and a placebo control may be ethically acceptable in several situations. First, placebos are acceptable if subjects receive a placebo in addition to the standard care. For example, subjects might be randomly assigned to receive either an opioid or an opioid plus an adjuvant agent. Second, a placebo arm is justified if the symptom under study has no effective treatment. For example, the transient nature of incident pain often defies adequate treatment on an as-needed basis, and a placebo control might be justified in a randomized controlled trial of a novel agent for the treatment of incident pain. Third, a placebo control is justified if subjects have adequate access to breakthrough or "rescue" treatment. This may in turn alter a trial's end points. For instance, the free use of breakthrough dosing in a trial suggests the possible inclusion of these doses as a study end point either directly (47,48) or as part of a composite end point (5,49). If placebo control is used, thorough informed consent must address that subjects assigned to placebo will not receive effective therapy and must explore the risks of forgoing such treatment (44).

Concrete recommendations about sham procedures are somewhat more elusive, in part because sham procedures themselves are difficult to define. In general, although sham procedures in palliative care research involve the use of a control procedure such as a nerve block, which is administered in a way that makes it ineffective (7), these procedures create ethical concerns because some subjects, or all subjects, depending on the study's design, are exposed to the risks of the procedure without hope of its benefits (41). Like placebo controls, shams also have a role in research, because the nonspecific therapeutic effects of surgery may be substantial. For instance, Leonard Cobb's research in the 1950s effectively debunked a widely used cardiac procedure that, if it had been widely disseminated, would eventually have put thousands of patients at risk.

Investigators have an opportunity to reduce these concerns substantially in the design of a sham-controlled study. For instance, investigators might conduct these studies in a setting in which the procedure itself (whether sham or real) poses few if any additional or "incremental" risks above and beyond the usual care. Investigators might insert a sham epidural catheter that would then be used for postoperative analgesia (50). When this is not possible, investigators can choose a crossover design, in which subjects are assigned to receive either the sham or the real procedure, followed by the other. This design does not decrease the incremental risks of the sham procedure. However, it does ensure that all subjects who bear the risks of the sham procedure also have access to the real procedures' potential benefits. This crossover sham design has been used in other settings (51) and might be appropriate for pain research when the risks or discomforts of the sham procedure are substantial.

For the most part, opportunities to minimize burdens are readily apparent. For instance, it seems reasonable wherever possible to minimize surveys, interviews, and additional study visits (52). These are all burdens that investigators routinely consider carefully in designing studies. However, there may be other needs and concerns that may be unique to, or more common in, patients near the end of life.

Although it is intuitively obvious that all research subjects would like to avoid the added time commitment and inconvenience of travel to and from additional appointments, this concern may be especially important to patients near the end of life, for whom long periods of time spent sitting in a car can exacerbate discomfort. Similarly, patients may view surveys and questionnaires not only as time-consuming but also as a drain on their energy. Therefore, investigators who conduct palliative care research may have an added reason to minimize the burdens of extra visits and data collection procedures and to rely on telephone data collection (or use of technology such as online surveys accessible via web portal) strategies whenever possible.

Palliative care investigators may also need to consider the burdens that a study creates for friends and family members who often take on substantial burdens as caregivers (53–56). Although most of the burdens of research participation are borne by the subject, the requirements of time, travel, and perhaps time off from work create burdens for others. Patients may be very sensitive to these burdens, and, for some patients with chronic pain, burdens to others can be influential in the decision whether or not to enroll in a study (25). By building flexibility into a study design (e.g., use of brief telephone interviews and multiple options for timing of clinic visits), investigators may be able to reduce the burdens of research participation on others.

Independent Review

Independent review is essential to the ethical conduct of clinical trials. Clinical researchers are faced with conflicting priorities of developing important clinical questions into rigorous trials in a timely and cost-effective manner that promotes patient well-being. Independent review takes multiple forms from grant review committees, scientific review boards, data and safety monitoring boards, and local IRBs. Guidance for independent review has its origins in the Declaration of Helsinki (22) and Belmont report (27) and in the United States is codified in the Federal Register by the Common Rule (3). The Common Rule was first enacted in 1991 to bring human subjects regulations across 15 federal agencies into harmony. It was updated slightly in 2009 and most recently underwent substantive revisions in 2018 known as the "Revised Common Rule" with far-reaching implications on the conduct of clinical research (3,57).

Several provisions have already taken effect, including revised informed consent document requirements intended to provide a more concise and focused delineation of the reasons why patients may or may not want to participate in research (3). It reduced administrative burdens by removing the requirement for annual review of low-risk research and centralizing the IRB of multicenter studies to a single IRB review at the institution of the principal investigator. Such changes aim to streamline the review process and eliminate redundancy (57).

The mandate of IRBs remains to ensure that clinical research conforms to the ethical standards of beneficence, respect, and autonomy by ensuring that clinical research does not place participants at undue risk and that participants give free and uncoerced consent. To that end, the revised Common Rule has updated the definition of vulnerable populations, substituting "impaired decision-making capacity, or economically or educationally disadvantaged" for the previously designated "handicapped or mentally disabled persons" (57). By the nature of cognitive changes at the end of life and potential for loss of decision-making capacity, many palliative care research participants may fall into this protected category. Conducting research at the end of life (and thus palliative care) has been challenging among IRB panelists due to ethical uncertainties (17). IRBs have expressed concerns regarding the impact of cognitive or functional impairment on the ability of participants to provide informed consent, identification of an appropriate surrogate to make study discontinuation decisions if a patient loses decisional capacity, whether a patient's proxy also needs to be consented, and burdens surrounding data collection (19).

It is too often the case that IRBs may lack members with expertise in caring for patients near the end of life (19). There has been a call for increased education of IRB members in the special needs of palliative care patients (57), as there have previously been calls for inclusion of other vulnerable populations such as homeless persons involved in pharmaceutical research (58) or minority children with mental health research (59). In addition to increased education of IRB members, it has been recommended to involve palliative care practitioners and family members among IRB membership, in accordance with Common Rule regulations calling for IRB membership associated with the intended population (19,36). By the nature of cognitive changes at the end of life and potential for loss of decision-making capacity, many palliative care research participants may fall into this protected category.

INFORMED CONSENT

Patients who consent to participate in research should have adequate decision-making capacity, which refers to the subjects' ability to understand relevant information, to appreciate the significance of that information, and to reason through to a conclusion that makes sense for them (60). These concerns are parallel to concerns in research involving patients with dementia (61), psychiatric illness, and patients in the intensive care setting (62). However, deficits in decision-making capacity may create several additional challenges for palliative care investigators.

First, concern about capacity is reasonable given the prevalence of cognitive impairment at the end of life (63,64). Cognitive impairment occurs in 10% to 40% of patients in the final months and in up to 85% of patients in the last days of life (63,64). Cognitive impairment may be difficult to identify in palliative care research because decision-making capacity varies over time (64) and because impairment may result from the experimental or therapeutic medications themselves, such as opioids, benzodiazepines, and corticosteroids (65–67). Investigators who conduct trials of medications will encounter these challenges even more frequently if trials are designed to evaluate treatments for delirium, for which impairment is an inclusion criterion (68).

Second, the effects of cognitive impairment on comprehension may be complicated by clinical depression, which occurs in 5% to 25% of patients near the end of life (69–72). Clinically significant adjustment disorders may be even more common (69). It is possible that these disorders may impair either comprehension or decision-making, or both (73), but studies have not yet supported this conclusion.

Third, even in the absence of overt cognitive impairment or depression, it is possible that severe symptoms or affective disorders may impair subjects' ability to understand the risks and benefits of research participation. For some studies, particularly clinical trials, the presence of one or more of these intractable symptoms is an inclusion criterion (74–76). It is possible that severe symptoms may impair comprehension if patients are unable to concentrate on the information offered in the informed consent process (77).

Finally, these challenges may be compounded in prospective studies that require participation over days or weeks. In these studies, even if patients have the capacity to consent at the time of enrollment, they may not retain that capacity throughout the study. Therefore, days or weeks after patients give consent to participate, they may be unable to understand changes in their condition clearly enough to withdraw. The result can be a "Ulysses contract" of sorts, in which research subjects find it easier to enroll than they do to withdraw (78).

None of these challenges is easily remedied. Indeed, it is the obstacles such as these that lead some authors to argue that patients near the end of life should not be allowed to enroll in research (15,16). Nevertheless, palliative care investigators have several concrete opportunities to enhance the ethical quality of palliative care research when decision-making capacity is uncertain.

First, at a minimum, investigators whose research involves patients near the end of life who are likely to lack decision-making capacity might institute brief assessments of understanding.

Although this strategy cannot assess decision-making capacity, a few simple questions in either open-ended or multiple-choice format provide a brief assessment of understanding (78–80). In some situations, investigators may wish to assess decision-making capacity more formally using validated instruments (81). Incorporation of a capacity assessment team, such as that used by the National Institutes of Health's Human Subjects Protection Unit, provides another strategy to protect vulnerable patients (57). The team consists of clinical research advocates who are independent from the study and clinical team who serve as impartial observers (82,83). They are study participant advocates that observe study personnel during the informed consent process and intervene when they observe impaired decision-making capacity. They may also perform formal capacity assessments when indicated and maintain oversight for the duration of a participant's involvement with a research trial.

These sorts of safeguards need not be employed in all studies. Instead, their use should be guided by the prevalence of cognitive impairment in a study population and by the balance of risks and benefits that a study offers (34). For instance, when palliative care research involves only interviews or behavioral interventions that pose minimal risks, informal capacity assessments are generally sufficient. "Minimal risks" are defined as those risks that are encountered during a patient's usual care or in everyday life (3). When research poses greater than minimal risks but offers potential benefits, some assessment of understanding may be appropriate. This research includes studies that involve a placebo (6) or invasive interventions such as nerve blocks (84) or epidural catheters (85). When a study that poses greater than minimal risks does not offer potential benefits or is conducted in a population in which the prevalence of cognitive impairment is high (e.g., an inpatient hospice unit), a formal evaluation of capacity should be considered. This research includes studies that involve a placebo when an effective agent is available (5) and some pharmacokinetic/pharmacodynamic studies that required blood samples and prolonged observation, without potential benefits (86). In such a situation, the MacArthur Competence Assessment Tool (MacCAT-CR) should be used to formally assess decision-making capacity as it has been studied in a variety of settings and modified specifically for clinical research (60,87–91).

If a patient does not have the capacity to give consent, a legally authorized representative may be able to give consent for research. This follows from federal guidelines governing research involving children (3) and is justified by the argument that surrogate decision-makers should be allowed to consent to research, just as they are allowed to consent to medical therapy. Advanced directives provide an opportunity for patients to provide guidance on whether they would agree to participate in research should they lose capacity to make informed decisions. However, as with other research that involves patients without capacity to consent, investigators should be aware of applicable state laws that may restrict or even prohibit surrogate consent for research.

If a patient does not have the capacity to consent but is still able to participate in decisions, investigators should obtain assent from the patient and informed consent from the patient's surrogate (92,93). This "dual consent" ensures that patients are as involved in the decision as possible yet provides the additional protection of a surrogate's consent.

If a patient has decision-making capacity intermittently or is expected to lose capacity, investigators may obtain advance consent (14). This approach has been used in a study of treatment for delirium, in which informed consent was obtained from patients while they had decision-making capacity (68). Advance consent should be obtained only for specific studies and should be obtained close to the planned start of research, for instance, at the time of hospitalization or enrollment in a hospice or palliative care program. Another strategy involves identification of a surrogate decision-maker who can make decisions on the patient's behalf if the patient loses decision-making capacity (36). In studies where it is likely that patients will lose decision-making capacity, dual consent of both the patient and the surrogate decision-maker is obtained at the time of study entry, which ensures that both the patient and surrogate understand the risks and benefits of the study, while assuring that the surrogate is ready to assume the responsibility of decision-making in the event the patient loses capacity (92).

Respect for Potential and Enrolled Subjects

Respect extends far beyond ensuring the informed consent of enrolled subjects. Respect must be extended to all persons, whether enrolled or not, who may be touched by the clinical research in question. This includes not only the enrolled study participant but also their caretakers, those who are approached for participation but declined or are excluded, and those who refuse participation after being enrolled. Emanuel et al. noted five domains of demonstrating respect, noted in Table 64.1 (20). Privacy and confidentiality of the subject is essential. Enrolled subjects must be free to withdraw

their consent for participation at any time without coercion. Subjects must be provided with new information as it becomes available and reconsented as informed consent documents are revised. All subjects must promptly and appropriately be treated for any adverse effects and if required be removed from the study. Given their crucial role in producing data, subjects should be entitled to learn of the outcomes from their research.

Investigators can also enhance the ethics of a study's design by ensuring that subjects are able to withdraw at any time. Although a subject's ability to withdraw should be a fundamental aspect of any ethical research (3), there may be unique barriers to withdrawal from palliative care research. For instance, subjects who withdraw from clinical pain research that involves one or more medications will usually need access to a different medication upon withdrawal. This problem may be straightforward in many cases but can be very challenging if in an interventional study, the investigational medication is an opioid, which requires the subject to get a new prescription and get it filled. Most states have created considerable barriers to opioid prescribing, including triplicate prescriptions, which may make it very difficult for a subject to obtain a new prescription and get it filled in a timely manner. If a subject has his or her medication available, the process may be easier. Nevertheless, considerable challenges of calculating an equianalgesic dose remain. For both of these reasons, investigators can enhance the ethical design of pain research by developing mechanisms to ensure that subjects who drop out continue to receive adequate pain treatment with as little interruption as possible.

CONCLUSION

The field of palliative care, and the standard of care that it represents, depends upon rigorous research to provide data that will guide clinical care. Although this research raises substantial ethical questions, these questions need not curtail what promises to be a valuable and highly productive area of inquiry. Of course, the concerns discussed in the preceding text should be taken seriously. To do otherwise is to risk the sorts of ethical missteps that have produced scandals in other fields. Nevertheless, these ethical questions can be addressed through careful planning, and with attention to the adequacy of a study's design, and to the informed consent process.

ACKNOWLEDGMENT

The authors would like to acknowledge David Casarett who authored the previous version of this chapter.

REFERENCES

1. Mount BM, Cohen R, MacDonald N, Bruera E, Dudgeon DJ. Ethical issues in palliative care research revisited. *Palliat Med.* 1995;9(2):165-166.
2. Krouse RS, Easson AM, Angelos P. Ethical considerations and barriers to research in surgical palliative care. *J Am Coll Surg.* 2003;196(3):469-474.
3. Department of Health and Human Services. Protection of Human Subjects. Title 45 Part 46. Code of Federal Regulations. 2018.
4. Corner J. Is there a research paradigm for palliative care? *Palliat Med.* 1996;10(3):201-208.
5. Dhaliwal HS, Sloan P, Arkinstall WW, et al. Randomized evaluation of controlled-release codeine and placebo in chronic cancer pain. *J Pain Symptom Manage.* 1995;10(8):612-623.
6. Farrar JT, Cleary J, Rauck R, Busch M, Nordbrock E. Oral transmucosal fentanyl citrate: randomized, double-blinded, placebo-controlled trial for treatment of breakthrough pain in cancer patients. *J Natl Cancer Inst.* 1998;90(8):611-616.
7. Polati E, Finco G, Gottin L, Bassi C, Pederzoli P, Ischia S. Prospective randomized double-blind trial of neurolytic coeliac plexus block in patients with pancreatic cancer. *Br J Surg.* 1998;85(2):199-201.
8. Elliott TE, Murray DM, Oken MM, et al. Improving cancer pain management in communities: main results from a randomized controlled trial. *J Pain Symptom Manage.* 1997;13(4):191-203.
9. de Wit R, van Dam F, Zandbelt L, et al. A pain education program for chronic cancer pain patients: follow-up results from a randomized controlled trial. *Pain.* 1997;73(1):55-69.
10. Kravitz RL, Delafield JP, Hays RD, Drazin R, Conolly M. Bedside charting of pain levels in hospitalized patients with cancer: a randomized controlled trial. *J Pain Symptom Manage.* 1996;11(2):81-87.
11. Teno J, Lynn J, Connors AF Jr, et al. The illusion of end-of-life resource savings with advance directives. SUPPORT Investigators. Study to Understand Prognoses and Preferences for Outcomes and Risks of Treatment. *J Am Geriatr Soc.* 1997;45(4):513-518.
12. Bredin M, Corner J, Krishnasamy M, Plant H, Bailey C, A'Hern R. Multicentre randomised controlled trial of nursing intervention for breathlessness in patients with lung cancer. *BMJ.* 1999;318(7188):901-904.
13. Tieman J, Sladek R, Currow D. Changes in the quantity and level of evidence of palliative and hospice care literature: the last century. *J Clin Oncol.* 2008;26(35):5679-5683.
14. Casarett DJ, Knebel A, Helmers K. Ethical challenges of palliative care research. *J Pain Symptom Manage.* 2003;25(4):S3-S5.
15. de Raeve L. Ethical issues in palliative care research. *Palliat Med.* 1994;8(4):298-305.
16. Annas G. *Some Choice: Law, Medicine, and the Market.* New York, NY: Oxford University Press; 1998.
17. Casarett DJ, Karlawish JH. Are special ethical guidelines needed for palliative care research? *J Pain Symptom Manage.* 2000;20(2):130-139.
18. Hilts P. VA Hospital is told to halt all research. *New York Times.* March 25, 1999.
19. Abernethy AP, Capell WH, Aziz NM, et al. Ethical conduct of palliative care research: enhancing communication between investigators and institutional review boards. *J Pain Symptom Manage.* 2014;48(6):1211-1221.
20. Emanuel EJ, Wendler D, Grady C. What makes clinical research ethical? *JAMA.* 2000;283(20):2701-2711.
21. Casarett DJ, Karlawish JH, Moreno JD. A taxonomy of value in clinical research. *IRB.* 2002;24(6):1-6.
22. World Medical Association. World Medical Association Declaration of Helsinki: ethical principles for medical research involving human subjects. *JAMA.* 2013;310(20):2191-2194.
23. The Nuremberg Code. Reprinted. In: Brody B, ed. *The Ethics of Biomedical Research. An International Perspective.* New York, NY: Oxford University Press; 1947:213.
24. Freedman B. Placebo-controlled trials and the logic of clinical purpose. *IRB.* 1990;12(6):1-6.
25. Casarett D, Karlawish J, Sankar P, Hirschman KB, Asch DA. Obtaining informed consent for clinical pain research: patients' concerns and information needs. *Pain.* 2001;92(1-2):71-79.
26. *Advisory Committee on Human Radiation Experiments.* Final Report. Vol 061 00000848–9. Washington, DC: Government Printing Office; 1995.
27. The Belmont Report. Ethical principles and guidelines for the protection of human subjects of research. *J Am Coll Dent.* 2014;81(3):4-13.
28. Freedman B. Scientific value and validity as ethical requirements for research: a proposed explication. *IRB.* 1987;9(6):7-10.
29. Rutstein D. The ethical design of human experiments. In: Freund P, ed. *Experimentation with Human Subjects.* New York, NY: George Braziller; 1970:383-401.
30. Meinert C. *Clinical Trials. Design, Conduct, and Analysis.* Oxford: Oxford University Press; 1986.
31. Moore RA, Gavaghan D, Tramer MR, Collins SL, McQuay HJ. Size is everything—large amounts of information are needed to overcome random effects in estimating direction and magnitude of treatment effects. *Pain.* 1998;78(3):209-216.
32. Palliative Care Research Cooperative Group. Palliative care research cooperative group. Updated September 9, 2019. https://palliativecareresearch.org/about-us. Accessed February 27, 2020.
33. Casarett DJ. Differences between patients referred to hospice from academic vs. non-academic settings. *J Pain Symptom Manage.* 2001;21(3):197-203.
34. Casarett D, Ferrell B, Kirschling J, et al. NHPCO task force statement on the ethics of hospice participation in research. *J Palliat Med.* 2001;4(4):441-449.
35. Millum J. Sharing the benefits of research fairly: two approaches. *J Med Ethics.* 2012;38(4):219-223.
36. Laneader A, Angelos P, Ferrell BR, et al. Ethical issues in research to improve the management of malignant bowel obstruction: challenges and recommendations. *J Pain Symptom Manage.* 2007;34(1 suppl):S20-S27.
37. Freedman B, Fuks A, Weijer C. Demarcating research and treatment: a systematic approach for the analysis of the ethics of clinical research. *Clin Res.* 1992;40(4):653-660.
38. Ahmedzai S, Brooks D. Transdermal fentanyl versus sustained-release oral morphine in cancer pain: preference, efficacy, and quality of life. The TTS-Fentanyl Comparative Trial Group. *J Pain Symptom Manage.* 1997;13(5):254-261.
39. Kirkham SR, Abel J. Placebo-controlled trials in palliative care: the argument against. *Palliat Med.* 1997;11(6):489-492.
40. Hardy JR. Placebo-controlled trials in palliative care: the argument for. *Palliat Med.* 1997;11(5):415-418.
41. Macklin R. The ethical problems with sham surgery in clinical research. *N Engl J Med.* 1999;341(13):992-996.
42. Rothman KJ, Michels KB. The continuing unethical use of placebo controls. *N Engl J Med.* 1994;331(6):394-398.

43. Temple R, Ellenberg SS. Placebo-controlled trials and active-control trials in the evaluation of new treatments. Part 1: ethical and scientific issues. *Ann Intern Med.* 2000;133(6):455-463.

44. Emanuel EJ, Miller FG. The ethics of placebo-controlled trials—a middle ground. *N Engl J Med.* 2001;345(12):915-919.

45. Shapiro AK, Shapiro ES. The placebo: is it much ado about nothing? In: Harrington A, ed. *The Placebo Effect.* Cambridge, MA: Harvard University Press; 1998.

46. World Medical Association International Code of Medical Ethics; amended by the 57th World Medical Assembly, Pilansberg, South Africa October 2006.

47. Broomhead A, Kerr R, Tester W, et al. Comparison of a once-a-day sustained-release morphine formulation with standard oral morphine treatment for cancer pain. *J Pain Symptom Manage.* 1997;14(2):63-73.

48. Maxon HR III, Thomas SR, Hertzberg VS, et al. Rhenium-186 hydroxyethylidene diphosphonate for the treatment of painful osseous metastases. *Semin Nucl Med.* 1992;22(1):33-40.

49. Silverman DG, O'Connor TZ, Brull SJ. Integrated assessment of pain scores and rescue morphine use during studies of analgesic efficacy. *Anesth Analg.* 1993;77(1):168-170.

50. Haak van der Lely F, Burm AG, van Kleef JW, et al. The effect of epidural administration of alfentanil on intraoperative intravenous alfentanil requirements during nitrous oxide-oxygen-alfentanil anaesthesia for lower abdominal surgery. *Anaesthesia.* 1994;49(12):1034-1038.

51. Hahn AF, Bolton CF, Pillay N, et al. Plasma-exchange therapy in chronic inflammatory demyelinating polyneuropathy. A double-blind, sham-controlled, crossover study. *Brain.* 1996;119(Pt 4):1055-1066.

52. Bruera E. Ethical issues in palliative care research. *J Palliat Care.* 1994;10(3):7-9.

53. Steele RG, Fitch MI. Needs of family caregivers of patients receiving home hospice care for cancer. *Oncol Nurs Forum.* 1996;23(5):823-828.

54. Emanuel EJ, Fairclough DL, Slutsman J, Alpert H, Baldwin D, Emanuel LL. Assistance from family members, friends, paid care givers, and volunteers in the care of terminally ill patients. *N Engl J Med.* 1999;341(13):956-963.

55. Takesaka J, Crowley R, Casarett D. What is the risk of distress in palliative care survey research? *J Pain Symptom Manage.* 2004;28(6):593-598.

56. *Family Caregiving: Agenda for Action, Improving Services and Support for America's Family Caregivers.* Washington, DC: National Health Council; 1999.

57. DeRenzo EG, Moss J, Singer EA. Implications of the revised common rule for human participant research. *Chest.* 2019;155(2):272-278.

58. Beauchamp TL, Jennings B, Kinney ED, Levine RJ. Pharmaceutical research involving the homeless. *J Med Philos.* 2002;27(5):547-564.

59. Fisher CB, Hoagwood K, Boyce C, et al. Research ethics for mental health science involving ethnic minority children and youths. *Am Psychol.* 2002;57(12):1024-1040.

60. Grisso T, Appelbaum PS. *Assessing Competence to Consent to Treatment.* New York, NY: Oxford University Press; 1998.

61. Marson DC, Schmitt FA, Ingram KK, Harrell LE. Determining the competency of Alzheimer patients to consent to treatment and research. *Alzheimer Dis Assoc Disord.* 1994;8(suppl 4):5-18.

62. Lemaire F, Blanch L, Cohen SL, Sprung C. Informed consent for research purposes in intensive care patients in Europe—part II. An official statement of the European Society of Intensive Care Medicine. Working Group on Ethics. *Intensive Care Med.* 1997;23(4):435-439.

63. Breitbart W, Bruera E, Chochinov H, Lynch M. Neuropsychiatric syndromes and psychological symptoms in patients with advanced cancer. *J Pain Symptom Manage.* 1995;10(2):131-141.

64. Pereira J, Hanson J, Bruera E. The frequency and clinical course of cognitive impairment in patients with terminal cancer. *Cancer.* 1997;79(4):835-842.

65. Bruera E, Franco JJ, Maltoni M, Watanabe S, Suarez-Almazor M. Changing pattern of agitated impaired mental status in patients with advanced cancer: association with cognitive monitoring, hydration, and opioid rotation. *J Pain Symptom Manage.* 1995;10(4):287-291.

66. Bruera E, Macmillan K, Hanson J, MacDonald RN. The cognitive effects of the administration of narcotic analgesics in patients with cancer pain. *Pain.* 1989;39(1):13-16.

67. Stiefel FC, Breitbart WS, Holland JC. Corticosteroids in cancer: neuropsychiatric complications. *Cancer Invest.* 1989;7(5):479-491.

68. Breitbart W, Marotta R, Platt MM, et al. A double-blind trial of haloperidol, chlorpromazine, and lorazepam in the treatment of delirium in hospitalized AIDS patients. *Am J Psychiatry.* 1996;153(2):231-237.

69. Derogatis LR, Morrow GR, Fetting J, et al. The prevalence of psychiatric disorders among cancer patients. *JAMA.* 1983;249(6):751-757.

70. Kathol RG, Mutgi A, Williams J, Clamon G, Noyes R Jr. Diagnosis of major depression in cancer patients according to four sets of criteria. *Am J Psychiatry.* 1990;147(8):1021-1024.

71. Brown JH, Henteleff P, Barakat S, Rowe CJ. Is it normal for terminally ill patients to desire death? *Am J Psychiatry.* 1986;143(2):208-211.

72. Massie MJ, Holland JC. Depression and the cancer patient. *J Clin Psychiatry.* 1990;51(suppl):12-17; discussion 18-19.

73. Elliott C. Caring about risks. Are severely depressed patients competent to consent to research? *Arch Gen Psychiatry.* 1997;54(2):113-116.

74. Eisenach JC, DuPen S, Dubois M, Miguel R, Allin D. Epidural clonidine analgesia for intractable cancer pain. The Epidural Clonidine Study Group. *Pain.* 1995;61(3):391-399.

75. Pappas GD, Lazorthes Y, Bes JC, Tafani M, Winnie AP. Relief of intractable cancer pain by human chromaffin cell transplants: experience at two medical centers. *Neurol Res.* 1997;19(1):71-77.

76. Plancarte R, de Leon-Casasola OA, El-Helaly M, Allende S, Lema MJ. Neurolytic superior hypogastric plexus block for chronic pelvic pain associated with cancer. *Reg Anesth.* 1997;22(6):562-568.

77. Kristjanson LJ, Hanson EJ, Balneaves L. Research in palliative care populations: ethical issues. *J Palliat Care.* 1994;10(3):10-15.

78. Dresser R. Bound to treatment: the Ulysses contract. *Hastings Cent Rep.* 1984;14(3):13-16.

79. Miller CK, O'Donnell DC, Searight HR, Barbarash RA. The deaconess informed consent comprehension test: an assessment tool for clinical research subjects. *Pharmacotherapy.* 1996;16(5):872-878.

80. Penman DT, Holland JC, Bahna GF, et al. Informed consent for investigational chemotherapy: patients' and

physicians' perceptions. *J Clin Oncol*. 1984;2(7):849-855.

81. Grisso T, Appelbaum PS. The MacArthur Treatment Competence Study. III: abilities of patients to consent to psychiatric and medical treatments. *Law Hum Behav*. 1995;19(2):149-174.

82. Nugent AC, Miller FG, Henter ID, Zarate CA Jr. The ethics of clinical trials research in severe mood disorders. *Bioethics*. 2017;31(6):443-453.

83. National Institute of Mental Health. Human subjects protection unit (HSPU). Published 2020. https://www.nimh.nih.gov/research/research-conducted-at-nimh/scientific-director/office-of-clinical-director/administrative-research-support/human-subjects-protection-unit-hspu.shtml. Accessed February 27, 2020.

84. Mercadante S. Celiac plexus block versus analgesics in pancreatic cancer pain. *Pain*. 1993;52(2):187-192.

85. Boswell G, Bekersky I, Mekki Q, Eisenach J. Plasma concentrations and disposition of clonidine following a constant 14-day epidural infusion in cancer patients. *Clin Ther*. 1997;19(5):1024-1030.

86. Hoffman M, Xu JC, Smith C, et al. A pharmacodynamic study of morphine and its glucuronide metabolites after single morphine dosing in cancer patients with pain. *Cancer Invest*. 1997;15(6):542-547.

87. Grisso T, Appelbaum PS, Hill-Fotouhi C. The MacCAT-T: a clinical tool to assess patients' capacities to make treatment decisions. *Psychiatr Serv*. 1997;48(11):1415-1419.

88. Appelbaum PS, Grisso T, Frank E, O'Donnell S, Kupfer DJ. Competence of depressed patients for consent to research. *Am J Psychiatry*. 1999;156(9):1380-1384.

89. Kim SY, Caine ED, Currier GW, Leibovici A, Ryan JM. Assessing the competence of persons with Alzheimer's disease in providing informed consent for participation in research. *Am J Psychiatry*. 2001;158(5):712-717.

90. Carpenter WT Jr, Gold JM, Lahti AC, et al. Decisional capacity for informed consent in schizophrenia research. *Arch Gen Psychiatry*. 2000;57(6):533-538.

91. Casarett DJ. Assessing decision-making capacity in the setting of palliative care research. *J Pain Symptom Manage*. 2003;25(4):S6-S13.

92. High DM, Whitehouse PJ, Post SG, Berg L. Guidelines for addressing ethical and legal issues in Alzheimer disease research: a position paper. *Alzheimer Dis Assoc Disord*. 1994;8(suppl 4):66-74.

93. High DM. Advancing research with Alzheimer disease subjects: investigators' perceptions and ethical issues. *Alzheimer Dis Assoc Disord*. 1993;7(3):165-178.

INDEX

Note: The letters '*f*' and '*t*' following the locators refer to figures and tables respectively.

CCS0321